The Lumbar Spine

THE INTERNATIONAL SOCIETY FOR THE STUDY OF THE LUMBAR SPINE

The Lumbar Spine

EDITORIAL COMMITTEE

JAMES N. WEINSTEIN
Director, Spine Diagnostic and Treatment Center
Department of Orthopaedic Surgery
The University of Iowa Hospitals and Clinics
Iowa City, Iowa

SAM W. WIESEL
Professor and Chairman
Department of Orthopaedic Surgery
Georgetown University Medical Center
Washington, D.C.

W.B. SAUNDERS COMPANY
Harcourt Brace Jovanovich, Inc.
Philadelphia London Toronto Montreal Sydney Tokyo

W. B. SAUNDERS COMPANY
Harcourt Brace Jovanovich, Inc.

The Curtis Center
Independence Square West
Philadelphia, PA 19106

Library of Congress Cataloging-in-Publication Data

The Lumbar spine / editorial committee, James N. Weinstein, Sam W. Wiesel; the International Society for Study of the Lumbar Spine.

p. cm.

1. Backache. 2. Vertebrae, Lumbar—Diseases.
I. Weinstein, James N. II. Wiesel, Sam W.
III. International Society for Study of the Lumbar Spine.
[DNLM: 1. Lumbar Vertebrae. 2. Spinal Diseases.
WE 750 L95665]

RD771.B217L86 1990 617.5′6—dc20 90–8115

ISBN 0–7216–9337–7

Editor: Edward H. Wickland, Jr.
Developmental Editor: Kathleen McCullough
Designer: W. B. Saunders Staff
Production Manager: Bill Preston
Manuscript Editor: Leslie Fenton
Illustration Coordinator: Walt Verbitski
Indexer: Roger Wall

The Lumbar Spine: The International Society for the Study of the Lumbar Spine ISBN 0–7216–9337–7

Printed in the United States of America.

Last digit is the print number: 9 8 7 6 5 4 3 2

Contributors

Gunnar B. J. Andersson, M.D., Ph.D.
Professor and Associate Chairman, Rush Medical College, Senior Attending and Associate Chairman, Department of Orthopedic Surgery, Rush-Presbyterian-St. Luke's Medical Center, Chicago, Illinois.
Chapter 4. Biomechanics: Occupational Biomechanics; Chapter 17. Low Back Pain in Pregnancy

Michele Crites Battié, P.T., Ph.D.
Research Associate, Department of Orthopaedics, School of Medicine, University of Washington, Seattle, Washington. Associate Director, Spine Resource Clinic, University of Washington, Seattle, Washington.
Chapter 18. Industrial Low Back Pain: Risk Factors

Gordon R. Bell, M.D.
Orthopaedic Surgeon, Section of Spinal Surgery, Department of Orthopaedic Surgery, Cleveland Clinic Foundation, Cleveland, Ohio.
Chapter 2. Anatomy of Low Back Pain: Anatomy of the Lumbar Spine: Developmental to Normal Adult

Michel Benoist, M.D.
University of Paris VII. Consultant Rheumatologist of Paris Hospitals, Paris, France.
Chapter 11. Inflammatory Disorders: Inflammatory Spondyloarthropathies

Stanley J. Bigos, M.D.
Associate Professor, Department of Orthopaedics, School of Medicine, University of Washington, Seattle, Washington. Director, Spine Resource Clinic, University of Washington, Seattle, Washington.
Chapter 18. Industrial Low Back Pain: Risk Factors

David S. Bradford, M.D.
Professor of Orthopaedic Surgery and Director of Spine Service and Twin Cities Scoliosis Center, Department of Orthopaedic Surgery, University of Minnesota. Professor of Orthopedic Surgery, University of Minnesota Hospital and Clinic. Attending Physician/Surgeon, Abbott Northwestern Hospital and Minneapolis Children's Hospital, Minneapolis, Minnesota.
Chapter 8. Lumbar and Lumbosacral Spondylolisthesis: Operative Treatment: Adults

Paul Brinckmann, Prof. Dr. rer. nat.
Professor, Institut für Experimentelle Biomechanik, Universität Münster, Münster, West Germany.
Chapter 4. Biomechanics: Effects of Repeated Loads and Vibration

Mark D. Brown, M.D., Ph.D.
Professor and Chairman, Department of Orthopaedics and Rehabilitation, University of Miami School of Medicine. Chief of Service, Jackson Memorial Hospital and The Veterans Administration Hospital, Miami, Florida.
Chapter 7. Clinical Entities: Chemonucleolysis

Charles V. Burton, M.D.

Medical Director, Institute for Low Back Care, Minneapolis, Minnesota.
Chapter 23. Fusion: Where It's Been and Where It's Going

Bradford L. Currier, M.D.

Fellow in Spine Surgery, Department of Orthopaedics and Rehabilitation, University of Miami School of Medicine, Miami, Florida.
Chapter 7. Clinical Entities: Chemonucleolysis

Frank J. Eismont, M.D., F.A.C.S.

Professor of Orthopedic Surgery, Department of Orthopedic Surgery and Rehabilitation, University of Miami School of Medicine. Co-Director of Spinal Cord Injury Service, Jackson Memorial Hospital, Miami, Florida.
Chapter 12. Trauma of the Lumbar Spine: Classification and Treatment

Jeremy C.T. Fairbank, M.D., F.R.C.S.

Consultant, Orthopaedic Surgery, Woodlands Northfield Royal Orthopaedic Hospital, Woodlands, Northfield, Birmingham, England.
Chapter 3. Diagnosis and Neuromechanisms: History Taking and Physical Examination: Identification of Syndromes of Back Pain

Henry L. Feffer, M.D.

Professor of Orthopaedic Surgery, The George Washington University Medical Center. Director of Medical Research, Health Care Excellence, Inc., Washington, District of Columbia.
Chapter 7. Clinical Entities: A Lumbar Spine Algorithm

Yizhar Floman, M.D.

Professor of Orthopaedic Surgery, Hebrew University—Hadassah Medical School, Jerusalem, Israel. Professor of Orthopaedic Surgery, Department of Orthopaedics, Hadassah University Hospital, Jerusalem, Israel.
Chapter 16. Rehabilitation: Psychologic Approaches to the Management and Treatment of Chronic Low Back Pain

Robert D. Fraser, M.B., B.S., M.D. (Adel.), F.R.A.C.S.

Senior Lecturer, University of Adelaide, Adelaide, Australia. Senior Visiting Orthopaedic Surgeon and Head of the Spinal Unit, Royal Adelaide Hospital, Adelaide, Australia.
Chapter 13. Spinal Infections: Iatrogenic Discitis

Bruce E. Fredrickson, M.D.

Associate Professor of Orthopaedic Surgery and Attending Physician, SUNY Health Science Center, Syracuse, New York. Active Staff, Crouse-Irving Memorial Hospital, Syracuse, New York.
Chapter 21. Spinal Instrumentation: Internal Fixation

John W. Frymoyer, M.D.

Professor, Department of Orthopaedics and Rehabilitation, University of Vermont; Director, McClure Musculoskeletal Research Center. Attending in Orthopaedics, Medical Center, Hospital of Vermont, Burlington, Vermont.
Chapter 1. Epidemiology: Magnitude of the Problem; Chapter 10. Segmental Instability

Steven R. Garfin, M.D.
Associate Professor of Surgery, Division of Orthopaedics and Rehabilitation, University of California, San Diego Medical Center, San Diego, California.
Chapter 7. Clinical Entities: The Intervertebral Disc: Disc Disease—Does It Exist?

Harry K. Genant, M.D.
Professor of Radiology, Medicine, and Orthopaedic Surgery, Department of Radiology, University of California, San Francisco, California.
Chapter 6. Radiology: Magnetic Resonance Imaging of the Lumbar Spine

Stanley D. Gertzbein, M.D., F.R.C.S.(C.)
Associate Professor of Surgery, University of Toronto. Director, Spinal Clinic, Sunnybrook Medical Centre, Toronto, Ontario, Canada.
Chapter 12. Trauma of the Lumbar Spine: Classification and Treatment

John Getty, M.S., F.R.C.S.
Honorary Lecturer in Orthopaedics, University of Sheffield. Consultant Orthopaedic Surgeon and Director, Sheffield Problem Back Unit, Northern General Hospital, Sheffield, England.
Chapter 22. Surgical Approaches: Laminectomies

Vijay K. Goel, Ph.D.
Associate Professor and Director, Biomechanics Laboratory II, Department of Biomedical Engineering, University of Iowa, Iowa City, Iowa.
Chapter 4. Biomechanics: Biomechanics of Spine Stabilization

David P. Guy, R.P.T., M.S.
Senior Associate, Department of Orthopaedics and Rehabilitation, Vanderbilt University School of Medicine, Nashville, Tennessee. Director of Programs, Ability Assessment Center, Vanderbilt University Hospital, Nashville, Tennessee.
Chapter 18. Industrial Low Back Pain: Industrial Low Back Pain: A Practical Approach

Scott Haldeman, M.D., Ph.D.
Assistant Clinical Professor, Department of Neurology, University of California, Irvine, California.
Chapter 3. Diagnosis and Neuromechanisms: Clinical Neurophysiology and Electrodiagnostic Testing in Low Back Pain

Hamilton Hall, M.D.
Orthopaedic Surgeon, Toronto, Ontario, Canada.
Chapter 3. Diagnosis and Neuromechanisms: History Taking and Physical Examination: Identification of Syndromes of Back Pain

Edward N. Hanley, Jr., M.D.
Associate Professor and Director of Spine Surgery, Department of Orthopaedic Surgery, University of Pittsburgh. Active Staff, Presbyterian University Hospital and Children's Hospital of Pittsburgh, Pittsburgh, Pennsylvania.
Chapter 8. Lumbar and Lumbosacral Spondylolisthesis: Operative Treatment: Children and Adolescents

Kenneth B. Heithoff, M.D.
Medical Director, Center for Diagnostic Imaging, Minneapolis, Minnesota.
Chapter 6. Radiology: Computed Tomography and Plain Film Diagnosis of the Lumbar Spine

Harry N. Herkowitz, M.D.

Co-Director, Ability Assessment Center, Department of Orthopaedics and Rehabilitation, Vanderbilt University Medical Center, Nashville, Tennessee.
Chapter 7. Clinical Entities: The Intervertebral Disc: Disc Disease—Does It Exist?

Sten H. Holm, Ph.D.

Associate Professor, University of Gothenburg, Gothenburg, Sweden. Director, Laboratory of Experimental Surgery, Sahlgren Hospital, Gothenburg, Sweden.
Chapter 5. Biochemistry: Nutrition of the Intervertebral Disc

Shun-ichi Inoue, M.D.

Late Professor, Department of Orthopedic Surgery, School of Medicine, Chibu University, Chibu City, Chibu, Japan.
Chapter 7. Clinical Entities: Surgical Indications and Techniques

Roger P. Jackson, M.D.

Assistant Clinical Professor, Department of Surgery, Section of Orthopaedics, University of Kansas School of Medicine, Kansas City, Kansas, and Co-Director, Rae R. Jacobs Memorial Spine Fellowship at Kansas City. Staff Surgeon, North Kansas City Hospital, North Kansas City, Missouri.
Chapter 6. Radiology: Computed Tomography—Discography

Rae R. Jacobs, M.D.

Late Professor, Department of Surgery, Section of Orthopaedics, University of Kansas School of Medicine, Kansas City, Kansas.
Chapter 6. Radiology: Computed Tomography—Discography

Malcolm I. V. Jayson, M.D.

Professor of Rheumatology, University of Manchester, Manchester, England. Professor of Rheumatology, Rheumatic Diseases Centre, Hope Hospital, Salford, England.
Chapter 11. Inflammatory Disorders: Fibrosis, Chronic Inflammation, and Vascular Damage in Back Pain Syndromes

Neil Kahanovitz, M.D.

Specialist in Spinal Surgery and Rehabilitation, Anderson Clinic, Inc., Arlington, Virginia.
Chapter 15. Osteoporosis

Kiyoshi Kaneda, M.D.

Professor and Chairman, Department of Orthopedic Surgery, Hokkaido University School of Medicine, Sapporo, Japan.
Chapter 22. Surgical Approaches: Anterior Surgical Approach to the Thoracolumbar, Lumbar, and Lumbosacral Spine

Young E. Kim, Ph.D.

Assistant Professor, Department of Mechanical Engineering, College of Engineering, Dankook University, Dong, Yongsan-Ku, Seoul, Korea.
Chapter 4. Biomechanics: Biomechanics of Spine Stabilization

William H. Kirkaldy-Willis, M.D.

Emeritus Professor, Department of Orthopaedic Surgery, University Hospital, Saskatoon, Saskatchewan, Canada.
Chapter 2. Anatomy of Low Back Pain: The Three-Joint Complex

John P. Kostuik, M.D., F.R.C.S.C.
Professor of Orthopedics, University of Toronto. Head of Orthopedics, Toronto General Hospital and Mount Sinai Hospital; Director, Spinal Unit, Toronto General Hospital; Director, Biomechanics Laboratory, Toronto General Hospital, Toronto, Ontario, Canada.
Chapter 20. Adult Scoliosis

Martin H. Krag, M.D.
Associate Professor, Department of Orthopaedics and Rehabilitation, University of Vermont. Staff, Orthopaedics and Rehabilitation Service, Medical Center, Hospital of Vermont, Burlington, Vermont.
Chapter 21. Spinal Instrumentation: Biomechanics of Transpedicle Spinal Fixation

Henry La Rocca, M.D.
Clinical Professor of Orthopaedic Surgery, Tulane University, New Orleans, Louisiana. Editor-in-Chief of Spine. Active Staff, Elmwood Medical Center, Jefferson, Louisiana.
Chapter 19. Failed Lumbar Surgery: Principles of Management

Casey K. Lee, M.D.
Orthopaedic Surgeon, Department of Orthopaedics, New Jersey Medical School, College of Medicine, Newark, New Jersey.
Chapter 4. Biomechanics: Lumbar Orthosis (Brace)

John C.Y. Leong, M.B.B.S.(H.K.), F.R.C.S., F.R.C.S.E., F.R.A.C.S.
Professor and Head, Department of Orthopaedic Surgery. Dean, Faculty of Medicine, University of Hong Kong. Chief of Orthopaedic Surgery, Queen Mary Hospital and Duchess of Kent Children's Hospital, Hong Kong.
Chapter 13. Spinal Infections: Pyogenic and Tuberculous Infections

Stephen J. Lipson, M.D.
Assistant Professor of Orthopedic Surgery, Harvard Medical School. Orthopedic Surgeon, Brigham and Women's Hospital, Boston, Massachusetts.
Chapter 5. Biochemistry: Aging Versus Degeneration of the Intervertebral Disc

Y. King Liu, Ph.D.
Professor and Director, Center for Materials Research, Department of Biomedical Engineering, University of Iowa, Iowa City, Iowa.
Chapter 4. Biomechanics: Biomechanics of Spine Stabilization

Tom G. Mayer, M.D.
Clinical Professor, Department of Orthopedic Surgery, University of Texas Southwestern Medical School, Dallas, Texas.
Chapter 16. Rehabilitation: Functional Restoration for the Patient with Chronic Low Back Pain

John A. McCulloch, M.D., F.R.C.S.(C.)
Professor of Orthopedics, Northeastern Ohio Universities College of Medicine, Rootstown, Ohio. Crystal Clinic, Akron, Ohio.
Chapter 7. Clinical Entities: Surgical Indications and Techniques

Robin McKenzie, F.N.Z.S.P., D.I.P. M.T.
International Director, McKenzie Institute, Wellington, New Zealand.
Chapter 16. Rehabilitation: Mechanical Diagnosis and Therapy for Low Back Pain: Toward a Better Understanding

Thomas W. McNeill, M.D.

Associate Professor, Rush Medical College, Chicago, Illinois. Senior Attending Surgeon, Rush-Presbyterian-St. Luke's Medical Center, Chicago, Illinois.
Chapter 7. Clinical Entities: Pelvic Visceral Dysfunction—Cauda Equina Syndrome

Kazimiera Milanowska, M.D.

Professor, Faculty of Medicine, University of Poznan, Poznan, Poland. Head of Rehabilitation Department, Institute of Orthopaedics and Rehabilitation, Poznan, Poland.
Chapter 8. Lumbar and Lumbosacral Spondylolisthesis: Conservative Treatment

Vert Mooney, M.D.

Professor, Division of Orthopaedic Surgery, Department of Surgery, Irvine Medical Center, University of California, Irvine, California.
Chapter 7. Clinical Entities: Facet Syndrome

Hideshige Moriya, M.D.

Orthopaedic Surgeon, Department of Orthopaedic Surgery, School of Medicine, Chibu University, Chibu City, Chibu, Japan.
Chapter 7. Clinical Entities: Surgical Indications and Techniques

Alf Nachemson, M.D.

Professor, Department of Orthopaedic Surgery, Sahlgren Hospital, Gothenburg, Sweden.
Chapter 1. Epidemiology: The Future of Low Back Pain

Noboru Nakano, M.D., Ph.D.

Instructor, Sapporo Medical College, Sapporo, Japan. Director, Nakano Orthopaedic Hospital, Sapporo, Japan.
Chapter 22. Surgical Approaches: Anterior Extraperitoneal Lumbar Discectomy Without Fusion

Tohru Nakano, M.D.

Vice Director, Nakano Orthopaedic Hospital, Sapporo, Japan.
Chapter 22. Surgical Approaches: Anterior Extraperitoneal Lumbar Discectomy Without Fusion

Arthur Naylor, Ch.M., M.Sc., M.B., F.R.C.S.(Ed.), F.R.C.S.(Eng.)

Formerly Honorary Lecturer, Department of Fibre Science, Bradford University, Leeds, England. Honorary Consultant in Orthopaedic Surgery, Bradford Hospitals and Woodlands Orthopaedic Hospital, Leeds, England.
Chapter 1. Epidemiology: Historical Perspective

Margareta Nordin, Ph.D.

Adjunct Associate Professor, New York University, New York, New York. Director, Occupational Industrial Orthopaedic Center, Hospital for Joint Diseases, Orthopaedic Institute, New York, New York.
Chapter 18. Industrial Low Back Pain: Trunk Strength and Endurance: Measurement Techniques

T. Okuma, M.D.

Orthopedic Surgeon, Department of Orthopedic Surgery, School of Medicine, Keio University, Tokyo, Japan.
Chapter 4. Biomechanics: Biomechanics of Spine Stabilization

Manohar M. Panjabi, Ph.D., Dr. Tech.

Professor, Department of Orthopaedics and Rehabilitation and Department of Mechanical Engineering, Yale University, New Haven, Connecticut.
Chapter 4. Biomechanics: Degeneration, Injury, and Spinal Instability

Stanley V. Paris, Ph.D., P.T.
President, Institute of Graduate Health Sciences, Atlanta, Georgia. Co-Director, Flagler Physical Therapy, Flagler Hospital, St. Augustine, Florida.
Chapter 16. Rehabilitation: Manipulation of the Lumbar Spine

Malcolm H. Pope, Ph.D.
McClure Professor of Orthopaedic Surgery and Professor of Mechanical Engineering; Co-Director of Rehabilitation Engineering, Medical Center, Hospital of Vermont, Burlington, Vermont.
Chapter 4. Biomechanics: Effects of Repeated Loads and Vibration; Chapter 10. Segmental Instability

Richard Porter, M.D., F.R.C.S., F.R.C.S.E.
Fellow, University of Hull, Hull, England. Consultant Orthopaedic Surgeon, Doncaster Royal Infirmary, Doncaster, Yorkshire, England.
Chapter 9. Lumbar Spinal Stenosis: Development of the Vertebral Canal

Franco Postacchini, M.D.
Associate Professor of Orthopaedic Surgery, University "La Sapienza" of Rome, Italy.
Chapter 9. Lumbar Spinal Stenosis: Classification and Treatment

Wolfgang Rauschning, M.D., Ph.D.
Assistant Teaching Professor, Department of Orthopaedic Surgery, University Hospital, Uppsala, Sweden.
Chapter 6. Radiology: Imaging Anatomy of the Lumbar Spine

Richard H. Rothman, M.D., Ph.D.
Professor and Chairman, Department of Orthopaedic Surgery, Thomas Jefferson University, Philadelphia, Pennsylvania.
Chapter 7. Clinical Entities: A Lumbar Spine Algorithm

Stephen L.G. Rothman, M.D.
Medical Director, Multiplanar Diagnostic Imaging, Inc., Torrance, California. Active Medical Staff, Rancho Los Amigos Hospital, Downey, California.
Chapter 8. Lumbar and Lumbosacral Spondylolisthesis: Classification, Diagnosis, and Natural History

Björn L. Rydevik, M.D., Ph.D.
Associate Professor of Orthopaedic Surgery, University of Gothenburg, Gothenburg, Sweden. Associate Professor, Department of Orthopaedics, Sahlgren Hospital, Gothenburg, Sweden.
Chapter 3. Diagnosis and Neuromechanisms: Etiology of Sciatica

Albert B. Schultz, Ph.D.
Vennema Professor of Mechanical Engineering and Applied Mechanics, The University of Michigan, Ann Arbor, Michigan.
Chapter 4. Biomechanics: Biomechanical Analyses of Loads on the Lumbar Spine

David K. Selby, M.D.
Orthopaedic Surgeon, Dallas, Texas.
Chapter 7. Clinical Entities: Posterior Spinal Fusion

David L. Spencer, M.D.

Associate Professor of Orthopaedics, University of Illinois, Lutheran General Hospital, Park Ridge, Illinois.
Chapter 3. Diagnosis and Neuromechanisms: The Biomechanical Mechanisms of Nerve Root Compression Due to a Herniated Disc

Dan M. Spengler, M.D.

Professor and Chairman, Department of Orthopaedics and Rehabilitation, Vanderbilt University School of Medicine, Nashville, Tennessee. Professor and Chairman, Department of Orthopaedics and Rehabilitation, Vanderbilt University Medical Center, Nashville, Tennessee.
Chapter 18. Industrial Low Back Pain: Industrial Low Back Pain: A Practical Approach

Daniel Stein, M.D.

Head, Department of Adolescent Psychiatry, Abrabanel Mental Health Center, Bat-Yam, Israel.
Chapter 16. Rehabilitation: Psychologic Approaches to the Management and Treatment of Chronic Low Back Pain

Ian A.F. Stokes, Ph.D.

Research Associate Professor, University of Vermont, Burlington, Vermont.
Chapter 6. Radiology: Reliability of Radiographic Studies

David W. Stoller, M.D.

Director, California Institute for Musculoskeletal Imaging. Assistant Clinical Professor of Radiology, University of San Francisco, San Francisco, California.
Chapter 6. Radiology: Magnetic Resonance Imaging of the Lumbar Spine

Kazuhisa Takahashi, M.D.

Orthopaedic Surgeon, Department of Orthopaedic Surgery, School of Medicine, Chibu University, Chibu City, Chibu, Japan.
Chapter 7. Clinical Entities: Surgical Indications and Techniques

Keiichi Takata, M.D.

Orthopaedic Surgeon, Department of Orthopaedic Surgery, School of Medicine, Chibu University, Chibu City, Chibu, Japan.
Chapter 7. Clinical Entities: Surgical Indications and Techniques

Jill Urban, Ph.D.

Research Fellow, Physiology Laboratory, University of Oxford, Oxford, England.
Chapter 5. Biochemistry: Disc Biochemistry in Relation to Function

Pieter F. van Akkerveeken, M.D., Ph.D.

Orthopedic Surgeon, Dr. A. Mathysen Hospital, Utrecht, The Netherlands. Chairman, Verbiest Institute Foundation, Utrecht, The Netherlands.
Chapter 3. Diagnosis and Neuromechanisms: Pain Patterns and Diagnostic Blocks

Henk Verbiest, M.D., Ph.D., Hon. F.R.C.S.

Emeritus Professor of Neurosurgery, Utrecht University, Utrecht, The Netherlands. Private Practice, Utrecht, The Netherlands.
Chapter 9. Lumbar Spinal Stenosis: Morphology, Classification, and Long-Term Results

Gordon Waddell, B.Sc., M.D., F.R.C.S.
Director, West of Scotland Back Pain Research Unit, University of Glasgow. Consultant Orthopaedic Surgeon, Western Infirmary, Glasgow, Scotland.
Chapter 1. Epidemiology: A New Clinical Model for the Treatment of Low Back Pain

Henrik Weber, M.D.
Consultant, Ullevaal Hospital, Oslo, Norway.
Chapter 7. Clinical Entities: Natural History of the Herniated Disc

James N. Weinstein, D.O.
Director, Spine Diagnostic and Treatment Center. Associate Professor, Department of Orthopedics and Biomedical Engineering, University of Iowa College of Medicine, Iowa City, Iowa. Orthopaedic Surgeon, The University of Iowa Hospitals and Clinics, Iowa City, Iowa.
Chapter 4. Biomechanics: Biomechanics of Spine Stabilization; Chapter 14. Spinal Tumors

Arthur H. White, M.D.
Orthopaedic Spine Surgery Consultant to San Francisco Combined Orthopaedic Residency Training Program. Medical Director, Spinecare Medical Group, Daly City, California. Staff, Seton Medical Center, Daly City, California.
Chapter 16. Rehabilitation: Back School: State of the Art

Sam W. Wiesel, M.D.
Professor and Chairman, Department of Orthopaedic Surgery, Georgetown University Medical Center, Washington, District of Columbia.
Chapter 7. Clinical Entities: A Lumbar Spine Algorithm

David G. Wilder, Ph.D., P.E.
Research Assistant Professor, Department of Orthopaedics and Rehabilitation, University of Vermont School of Medicine, Burlington, Vermont.
Chapter 10. Segmental Instability

Leon L. Wiltse, M.D.
Clinical Professor of Orthopaedic Surgery, University of California at Irvine, Irvine, California. Active Medical Staff, Memorial Medical Center of Long Beach, California.
Chapter 8. Lumbar and Lumbosacral Spondylolisthesis: Classification, Diagnosis, and Natural History

Ken Yong-Hing, M.D.
Associate Professor and Head, University Hospital, University of Saskatchewan, Saskatoon, Saskatchewan, Canada.
Chapter 2. Anatomy of Low Back Pain: The Three-Joint Complex

Hansen A. Yuan, M.D.
Professor, Attending Staff, and Chairman of Orthopaedic Surgery, SUNY Health Science Center, Syracuse, New York. Active Staff, Crouse-Irving Memorial Hospital, Syracuse, New York.
Chapter 21. Spinal Instrumentation: Internal Fixation

Preface

It is important to emphasize that the first edition of *The Lumbar Spine* focuses on the broad range of lumbar spine care. Emphasis is placed on the newer techniques and advances, such as magnetic resonance imaging, new spinal instrumentation, perfected pharmacologic agents, and conservative treatment programs. It also reflects on the art of physical examination and diagnosis and on the treatment of difficult spinal problems, including tumors, trauma, and infections. In many cases, model systems using animal and human subjects are discussed in terms of the author's past research achievements and future research directions.

It is hoped that this first edition will stimulate further research involving the care of patients with lumbar spine problems. The International Society for the Study of the Lumbar Spine brings together many medical and nonmedical disciplines in an attempt to provide a forum for sharing new directions and ideas of spinal research. Through the forum of the International Society for the Study of the Lumbar Spine we present a multidisciplinary book for the multidimensional problem.

It is impossible to acknowledge all those who helped in the preparation of this book. I would, however, like to thank a few special people, including my wife, Mimi; my two daughters, Brieanna, and Shelsey; my secretary, Margie; and my friends in the International Society for the Study of the Lumbar Spine. Thank you for your help and for your encouragement.

JAMES N. WEINSTEIN

Contents

1
Epidemiology 1

- HISTORICAL PERSPECTIVE 1
  Arthur Naylor
- MAGNITUDE OF THE PROBLEM 32
  John W. Frymoyer
- A NEW CLINICAL MODEL FOR THE TREATMENT OF LOW BACK PAIN 38
  Gordon Waddell
- THE FUTURE OF LOW BACK PAIN 56
  Alf Nachemson

2
Anatomy of Low Back Pain 71

- ANATOMY OF THE LUMBAR SPINE: DEVELOPMENTAL TO NORMAL ADULT 71
  Gordon R. Bell
- THE THREE-JOINT COMPLEX 80
  Ken Yong-Hing and William H. Kirkaldy-Willis

3
Diagnosis and Neuromechanisms 88

- HISTORY TAKING AND PHYSICAL EXAMINATION: IDENTIFICATION OF SYNDROMES OF BACK PAIN 88
  Jeremy C.T. Fairbank and Hamilton Hall
- PAIN PATTERNS AND DIAGNOSTIC BLOCKS 107
  Pieter F. van Akkerveeken
- ETIOLOGY OF SCIATICA 132
  Björn L. Rydevik
- MECHANISMS OF NERVE ROOT COMPRESSION DUE TO A HERNIATED DISC 141
  David L. Spencer
- CLINICAL NEUROPHYSIOLOGY AND ELECTRODIAGNOSTIC TESTING IN LOW BACK PAIN 146
  Scott Haldeman

4
Biomechanics 160

■ BIOMECHANICAL ANALYSES OF LOADS ON THE LUMBAR SPINE 160
Albert B. Schultz

■ EFFECTS OF REPEATED LOADS AND VIBRATION 171
Paul Brinckmann and Malcolm H. Pope

■ DEGENERATION, INJURY, AND SPINAL INSTABILITY 188
Manohar M. Panjabi

■ BIOMECHANICS OF SPINE STABILIZATION 195
Vijay K. Goel, James N. Weinstein, Y. King Liu, Young E. Kim, and T. Okuma

■ OCCUPATIONAL BIOMECHANICS 212
Gunnar B.J. Andersson

■ LUMBAR ORTHOSIS (BRACE) 224
Casey K. Lee

5
Biochemistry 231

■ DISC BIOCHEMISTRY IN RELATION TO FUNCTION 231
Jill Urban

■ NUTRITION OF THE INTERVERTEBRAL DISC 244
Sten H. Holm

■ AGING VERSUS DEGENERATION OF THE INTERVERTEBRAL DISC 261
Stephen J. Lipson

6
Radiology 266

■ IMAGING ANATOMY OF THE LUMBAR SPINE 266
Wolfgang Rauschning

■ COMPUTED TOMOGRAPHY AND PLAIN FILM DIAGNOSIS OF THE LUMBAR SPINE 283
Kenneth B. Heithoff

■ MAGNETIC RESONANCE IMAGING OF THE LUMBAR SPINE 320
David W. Stoller and Harry K. Genant

■ RELIABILITY OF RADIOGRAPHIC STUDIES 337
Ian A.F. Stokes

■ COMPUTED TOMOGRAPHY—DISCOGRAPHY 346
Roger P. Jackson and Rae R. Jacobs

7
Clinical Entities 358

■ A LUMBAR SPINE ALGORITHM 358
Sam W. Wiesel, Henry L. Feffer, and Richard H. Rothman

■ THE INTERVERTEBRAL DISC: DISC DISEASE—DOES IT EXIST? 369
Steven R. Garfin and Harry N. Herkowitz

■ NATURAL HISTORY OF THE HERNIATED DISC 381
Henrik Weber

■ SURGICAL INDICATIONS AND TECHNIQUES 393
John A. McCulloch, Shun-ichi Inoue, Hideshige Moriya, Kazuhisa Takahashi, and Keiichi Takata

■ FACET SYNDROME 422
Vert Mooney

■ CHEMONUCLEOLYSIS 441
Mark D. Brown and Bradford L. Currier

■ PELVIC VISCERAL DYSFUNCTION—CAUDA EQUINA SYNDROME 449
Thomas W. McNeill

■ POSTERIOR SPINAL FUSION 456
David K. Selby

8
Lumbar and Lumbosacral Spondylolisthesis 471

■ CLASSIFICATION, DIAGNOSIS, AND NATURAL HISTORY 471
Leon L. Wiltse and Stephen L.G. Rothman

■ CONSERVATIVE TREATMENT 500
Kazimiera Milanowska

■ OPERATIVE TREATMENT: CHILDREN AND ADOLESCENTS 515
Edward N. Hanley, Jr.

■ OPERATIVE TREATMENT: ADULTS 528
David S. Bradford

9
Lumbar Spinal Stenosis 546

■ MORPHOLOGY, CLASSIFICATION, AND LONG-TERM RESULTS 546
Henk Verbiest

■ DEVELOPMENT OF THE VERTEBRAL CANAL 589
Richard Porter

■ CLASSIFICATION AND TREATMENT 594
Franco Postacchini

10
Segmental Instability 612
John W. Frymoyer, Malcolm H. Pope, and David G. Wilder

11
Inflammatory Disorders 637

■ INFLAMMATORY SPONDYLOARTHROPATHIES 637
Michel Benoist

■ FIBROSIS, CHRONIC INFLAMMATION, AND VASCULAR DAMAGE IN BACK PAIN SYNDROMES 649
Malcolm I.V. Jayson

12
Trauma of the Lumbar Spine: Classification and Treatment 662
Stanley D. Gertzbein and Frank J. Eismont

13
Spinal Infections 699

■ PYOGENIC AND TUBERCULOUS INFECTIONS 699
John C.Y. Leong

■ IATROGENIC DISCITIS 723
Robert D. Fraser

14
Spinal Tumors 741
James N. Weinstein

15
Osteoporosis 760
Neil Kahanovitz

16
Rehabilitation 770

■ BACK SCHOOL: STATE OF THE ART 770
Arthur H. White

■ MECHANICAL DIAGNOSIS AND THERAPY FOR LOW BACK PAIN: TOWARD A BETTER UNDERSTANDING 792
Robin McKenzie

■ MANIPULATION OF THE LUMBAR SPINE 805
Stanley V. Paris

■ PSYCHOLOGIC APPROACHES TO THE MANAGEMENT AND TREATMENT OF CHRONIC LOW BACK PAIN 811
Daniel Stein and Yizhar Floman

■ FUNCTIONAL RESTORATION FOR THE PATIENT WITH CHRONIC LOW BACK PAIN 827
Tom G. Mayer

17
Low Back Pain in Pregnancy 840
Gunnar B.J. Andersson

18
Industrial Low Back Pain 846

■ RISK FACTORS 846
Stanley J. Bigos and Michele Crites Battié

■ TRUNK STRENGTH AND ENDURANCE: MEASUREMENT TECHNIQUES 859
Margareta Nordin

■ INDUSTRIAL LOW BACK PAIN: A PRACTICAL APPROACH 869
Dan M. Spengler and David P. Guy

19
Failed Lumbar Surgery: Principles of Management 872
Henry La Rocca

20
Adult Scoliosis 882
John P. Kostuik

21
Spinal Instrumentation 916

■ BIOMECHANICS OF TRANSPEDICLE SPINAL FIXATION 916
Martin H. Krag

■ INTERNAL FIXATION 941
Bruce E. Fredrickson and Hansen A. Yuan

22
Surgical Approaches 956

■ LAMINECTOMIES 956
John Getty

■ ANTERIOR SURGICAL APPROACH TO THE THORACOLUMBAR, LUMBAR, AND LUMBOSACRAL SPINE 975
Kiyoshi Kaneda

1 □ Epidemiology

Arthur Naylor
John W. Frymoyer
Gordon Waddell
Alf Nachemson

HISTORICAL PERSPECTIVE

Arthur Naylor

Felix qui potuit verum cognoscere causas.

Lumbosacral pain, alone or in association with leg pain, has been a recognized human affliction for a long time. Jacob, in chapter 32 of Genesis, was the first person reported to suffer from sciatica. Hippocrates described the treatment of lumbosacral pain with tractions and manipulations that sometimes involved the medical attendant jumping on and walking over the patient's back, a therapeutic measure that still endures. The incidence of the syndrome of lumbosacral and related leg pain over the past 40 years has increased, attracting the attention of the legal and medical professions, industrialists, and governments, not only with regard to the possible causes, but also concerning means of prevention. In Great Britain, 4% of the patients on a general medical practitioner's list see consultants each year because of back pain.[127] Between 1971 and 1981 in the United States, the number of persons disabled with low back pain increased to 14 times that of the growth population.[95]

When the writer was a medical student in the mid-1930s, low back pain and sciatica, other than that due to infective or malignant conditions, received scant attention, and those who suffered from what is now called mechanical backache never—or very rarely—attended outpatient clinics, and few orthopedic departments existed. The reasons for the increase are difficult to elucidate but must partly be attributed to the increases in population, patients' knowledge, and treatments available in medicine and surgery.

The development of orthopedic surgery and neurosurgery as specialties separate from general surgery as well as the fact that we have a more prosperous and more compensation-minded population, are some factors explaining the increase; however, these cannot be the sole explanation. Despite the increase, the cause of back symptoms is never diagnosed for many people, and 86% return to work within 1 month. Of those referred to a hospital, some 40% have recovered before being seen. Much of present day treatment is still empirical. The relatively benign, short-term nature of low back pain and its tendency to resolve spontaneously are factors restricting specific statistical evaluation of many treatments, both orthodox and unorthodox. Such a startling increase in incidence has required an equal expansion of investigations of the etiology, epidemiology, diagnosis, and treatment of low back pain. In many patients, the cause and site of origin of their pain cannot be accurately located; identifying these is essential to successful treatment.

The various factors responsible for the development of low back pain were long poorly understood. Theories of the roles played by these various factors and spinal structures have come and gone in a manner reminiscent of the fickleness of fashion trends and are often based on ill-defined and unproven concepts.

The first investigations were naked-eye descriptions of the normal and degenerate spine found in the writings of Vesalius in 1555[297] and Cotugno in 1765[54] explaining the symptom of sciatica as the result of a change in the cerebrospinal fluid, a view that is not unusual when considered in the light of the present-day knowledge of the role of endorphins in the cerebrospinal fluid. Forst[90] believed that sciatica resulted from a neuritis that evolved following chronic neuralgia. Lasègue[90] described this sign, which is related to sciatic pain, in 1880.

Low back pain, leg pain, or neck and arm pain were thought to be associated with that idiopathic speculative clinical morass of imprecisely defined disorders known as "muscular rheumatism," "neuritis," "sciatic and brachial neuritis," and "fibrositis," which were usually accompanied by fruitless searches for supposedly causal focal sepsis. A high proportion of the population had their good normal teeth sacrificed on this altar. It was evident that progress in the diagnosis and treatment of low back and leg pain required the removal of preconceived nonscientific ideas. Hypotheses have to be made, concepts must be constantly reviewed, and the Hunterian method of "putting it to the experiment" is essential.

It became increasingly evident that we in our profession needed to harness the vast expanse of knowledge and expertise gained over the last 40 years in the basic sciences, particularly in biochemistry, bioengineering, biophysics, and cell biology. During that time we have passed from naked-eye examination and light microscopy to the study of the ultrastructure of the intervertebral disc by biophysical techniques such as x-ray crystallography and electron microscopy, along with the study of the constituents of the spine with the help of our biochemical, biophysical, bioengineering colleagues and others in the basic sciences fields. Despite current studies of cell biology, mechanisms of cell membranes, lysosomes, and immune responses, as well as the enormous advances made in our knowledge of the various constituents of the lumbar spine, its structure, metabolism, and function, in many instances we remain ignorant about the source of chronic low back pain.

Virchow[299] first described what is now known as a lumbar disc prolapse in 1857, but its significance and relationship to back and leg pain were not recognized at the time.

Intensive naked-eye and histologic studies were made by the Dresden School of Morbid Anatomy, seeking gross cellular defects as possible sources of back disorders, notably by Schmorl,[259] Andrae,[9] Beadle,[16] and Böhmig.[29] Middleton and Teacher[192] first described lumbar disc herniation at postmortem examination. The latter studies called attention to nuclear herniation through the bony end plate into the cancellous vertebral body and posteriorly through the annulus fibrosus, often at multiple levels in the same subject and notably in some who had no history of back problems. These studies did not produce any definite information as to the source of low back pain, possibly excepting findings of arthrosis of the facet joints. Histologic changes described were initially thought to be simple age changes, but the knowledge that similar changes appear in some subjects at much earlier decades in life led to the progression of histologic studies reported by Keyes and Compere,[162] Coventry and associates,[56] Key,[161] and Ross Smith.[248] However, no distinction could be shown between the discs of patients who had suffered from back pain and those of patients who had not. At that time, mechanical concepts of lumbosacral and sacroiliac strains as causes of low back pain were propounded by Goldthwaite and Osgood in 1905.[108] These terms were applied to suspected sites of origin for pain for which there was no proof. Treatment was directed to eliminating these strains by bed rest, immobilization in plaster jackets and corsets, in particular by the specially designed Goldthwaite belt and in many cases by manipulation. Failed conservative treatment was often followed by arthrodesis of the lumbosacral or sacroiliac joints, a popular surgical procedure in the orthopedist's armamentarium from that time until the early 1930s, although this was more common in North America than in Europe. Its lack of popularity in Great Britain was evident in discussions about fusion for unspecified back pain in a small series of cases from four orthopedic centers presented at the British Orthopaedic Association Meeting in 1942 and 1943. At that meeting it was revealed that such procedures carried a 4% mortality in the immediate postoperative period and that the incidence of improvement in symptoms was not encouraging.

The first clinical description of a lumbar disc prolapse was offered by Goldthwaite[109] in describing the result of manipulating the lower back of a patient who was thought to be suffering from a sacroiliac subluxation that had occurred while the individual was getting out of a bath. The patient had previously had a number of a similar attacks that were successfully treated by manipulation, but following the last incident, the maneuver consisted simply of hyperextending the spine to apply a plaster jacket. The patient developed cauda equina compression with sphincter paralysis. Recovery within 2 hours was followed by recurrences of the problem. The patient was turned in bed, and the next day he had virtually complete paraplegia with a sensory deficiency. Harvey Cushing performed a laminectomy, but findings at the operation showed nothing more than a "narrowing of the spinal canal at the lumbosacral junction," no doubt the first description of what we now know to be lumbar spinal stenosis. A slow recovery ensued. I am indebted to the late Sir Harry Platt, resident at the Massachusetts General Hospital at the time, for information about the operative findings. Goldthwaite attributed the pathologic process to the instability resulting from facet unlocking with the rotation and forward displacement of the lumbosacral joint (i.e., a dynamic spondylolisthesis with nerve root compression). In describing another case, Goldthwaite postulated a rupture of the annulus fibrosus of the L5-S1 disc with posterior protrusion as a cause of back and leg pain. Unfortunately, he never applied these ideas to his treatment. These experiences led Goldthwaite to investigate the significance of anatomic variations of the lumbosacral junction, which were already well known to anatomists. He thought unilateral facet asymmetry was a potent source of instability of the lumbosacral joint that could lead to nerve root compression. His views gained little attention until Mixter and Barr described lumbar disc prolapse as a cause of leg pain.[193] In 1916 the neurosurgeon Elsberg[73] described the appearance and operative removal of "enchondromas" that were causing nerve root disorders. It was not evident that the latter were really disc herniations until the material removed by Mixter and Barr at operation was subjected to pathologic study and compared with the tissue then known as enchondroma.

At the time of these studies, considerable attention was directed to the possibility that lumbosacral anatomic segmental anomalies were factors in the production of low back and leg pain.[244, 301, 320]

The problems found were very similar to those encountered today: The patients are those with previous attacks of minimal back pain and industrial injury who have a subsequent increase in symptoms, but often negative radiologic and clinical findings, other than a segmental anomaly. The reported symptoms were frequently attributable to lumbosacral strains due to segmental anomalies, asymmetric facets, and nonfusion of spinous processes. This attribution was largely based on radiologic appearances and the supposition that these anomalies are the cause of such symptoms. Knowledge of the biomechanical effects of these anomalies has only been elucidated in the past 15 to 16 years, particularly by the work of Farfan,[82, 83] Adams and Hutton,[2] and Cyron and Hutton,[61] who demonstrated the abnormal stresses these anomalies placed on the spinal segments above.

More recently, interest has been revived in the possibilities of low back and leg pain arising from mechanical defects of the sacroiliac joint. Some manipulative procedures have also been restored for pain presumed to arise from stresses, strains, and "subluxations" of the sacroiliac joint; these treatments have long been valued by orthodox, but more so by unorthodox, practitioners. Despite the descriptions of signs and symptoms thought to be produced by mechanical defects of the sacroiliac joint, these studies are characterized by poor diagnostic accuracy. They are also marked by an inability to demonstrate incontrovertibly by modern radiologic techniques and biomechanical studies that the sacroiliac joint is actually moving alone (rather than in combination with the lumbosacral joint) and that the symptoms actually arise therefrom. Treatment outcome has never been reliably proved and certainly not for a long follow-up period. There have been no randomized double-blind trials in patients with proven sacroiliac joint subluxation, as opposed to those with diseases of the sacroiliac joints and those with nonspecific low back pain. Most of the studies have been anatomic.

Weissl,[312–314] in a comprehensive study of cadaveric specimens and clinical and radiologic methods in human subjects, showed that the largest and most consistent movement of the sacral promontory occurred when the individual moved from a recumbent to a standing position. In most, the conjugate diameter of the pelvis was reduced by 5 to 6 mm with trunk extension; the sacrum moved dorsally only on standing. Changes were more marked when hip flexion was added to trunk flexion, and Weissl found the axis of rotation to be 10 cm below the promontory in normal subjects, during both recumbency and standing. The axis moved more than 5 cm following changes in posture. The difference in range of movements was not correlated with height, weight, sacral curve index, or sex. The sacroiliac joint was found to be divided, by two transverse planes, into the cranial caudocondyloid joint and an intermediate saddle joint. The sacroiliac joints were conjoined into a pelvic ring, and dorsoventral movement could only occur with slight movements of the sacrum. Extreme sacroiliac joint movement was restricted by the very strong sacroiliac joint ligaments, and the movement of one sacroiliac joint must affect movement at the symphysis pubis and the contralateral sacroiliac joint. No well-defined evidence of independent, one-joint movement has been clinically demonstrated. Early clinical tests said to affect sacroiliac joints must have also affected the lumbosacral regions and to some extent the hip joints. It is very difficult to distinguish completely, or to isolate, the force on one sacroiliac joint.

Bowen and Cassidy[30] identified an atypical synovial joint; the iliac side of the joint is covered with fibrocartilage, whereas the sacral component is covered with hyaline cartilage. The difference in cartilages persists throughout life. They thought that mechanical derangements produced pain that was referred to the buttock and posterior thigh, but this has not been proved by subjecting the patient to nerve block. Relief by manipulation does not prove that the joint is the origin of the pain, nor is there any biomechanical proof that the joint alone is being manipulated.

Gunterberg[111] performed biomechanical testing of fresh autopsy specimens of the pelvis, including the sacrum, and compared the load-bearing capacities demonstrated under various conditions. The studies showed that sacroiliac joint articulations remain intact when the specimens are loaded vertically with loads twice the estimated normal physiologic load. Solonen[273] then suggested that irregularities of the articular surface and the thick sacroiliac joint ligaments inhibit movement.

Wilder and colleagues,[316] using the implantation of wires into the posterior superior iliac crests, could not show any rotation movement. They showed that motion during rotation cannot occur exclusively on the axis of rotation that was previously proposed. Any rotation has to involve some measure of translation, and it is minimal because the motion is resisted by bony opposition and tightening of the ligaments. All agree that the rotation alone cannot occur without a significant separation of the joint surfaces.[52]

Positive technetium scintigraphy of the joint has some value in elucidating sacroiliac joint disease. Chisin and colleagues,[49] using this method to assess the effects of stressful physical activity, showed some abnormal uptake that resolved with rest in 4 of 181 tested military recruits. As yet, no conclusive scientific evidence shows that a purely mechanical disturbance of the sacroiliac joints alone is a cause of low back and leg pain.

Theories about nerve root entrapment developed in the 1930s. Williams[318] postulated that a nerve root could be compressed as it emerged from the neural canal when marked narrowing of the L5-S1 disc space was evident. He suggested that fusion was the appropriate treatment, but many years elapsed before Crock[58, 59] elucidated the pathologic process and the clinical treatment by nerve root decompression.

The report of Mixter and Barr was followed by a great increase in the use of surgical enucleation of intervertebral discs for treating low back pain alone (as opposed to low back and leg pain). Overenthusiasm led to a large number of patients being unnecessarily operated upon in this manner. This problem became clear when the natural history of lumbar disc herniation, and its marked tendency to resolve spontaneously became evident. A tendency existed to regard all low back pain problems as resulting from disc herniation, and treatment was based on this view. Simultaneously, the views concerning the role of sacroiliac and lumbosacral stress and strain faded. We had entered what Ian McNab has called the period of the "disc dynasty." However, not all were convinced that disc herniation was the sole cause of the problem. Some held the view that the osteoarthritic facet joint was a cause of nerve root irritation that produced lumbosacral and leg pain.[63] Sicard[268] postulated that sciatica might be due to irritation of the spinal nerve roots at the intervertebral foramen; this idea was elaborated by Putti,[242] who postulated that arthritic changes in the lower lumbar articular facet joints might be subject to acute exacerbations, producing sciatic scoliosis and back and leg pain. The treatment consisted of heat, rest, and plaster immobilization. For more persistent cases, a total facetectomy was performed to decompress the nerve root. Similar views were held by Blundell-Bankart in Great Britain[26] and by Delchef in Belgium,[65] who discounted the ideas of Mixter and Barr. Subsequently, however, problems of instability due to total facetectomy were evident in many cases. Enthusiasm for disc enucleation for back and leg pain continued unabatedly, until controlled clinical studies of the long-term results of disc enucleation and more scientific investigations of the many factors involved in low back and leg pain came under critical scrutiny. The slipped-disc concept needed to be removed, and the role of possible mechanical factors, then considered the main cause of disc herniation, needed reconsideration.

Marked advances in basic and applied scientific disciplines needed to be applied to understanding the etiology of low back pain. The cooperation of medical and basic scientists and biochemists, biophysicists, and bioengineers became a reality in the last 30 years. During that time, the members of the International Society for the Study of the Lumbar Spine (ISSLS), with contributions of the interdisciplinary international sabbatical interchange and with the development of multicenter cooperation on particular projects, produced considerable advances in our knowledge of the function and disorders of the lumbar spine.

The questions raised are as follows:

1. Is it possible to define the structural changes in the various constituents of the lumbar spine that disturb function sufficiently to produce pain?
2. What structural changes occur with aging or as a result of injury?
3. What forces cause injury to various elements of the spine?
4. When disc degeneration occurs, are the stability of the intervertebral disc and the segments of the spine, as a whole, reduced? How does this cause pain?
5. Which comes first: injury that causes structural change and thus disordered function, or disturbances of stress or varied mechanical forces that cause structural changes?

The damaging effect of mechanical forces had always been considered the main factor in producing disturbed lumbar spinal function and was thus presumed to render the spine painful. Naked-eye and histologic changes were the only evidence of disturbed structure, but these did not indicate what produced pain. Attempts to answer the above questions led to a steady increase in scientific investigations of the structure, function, and innervation of the various spinal structures in which pain might be produced. This was investigated little before the early 1950s. The major advances in the basic sciences provided those in medicine with the expertise necessary to solve these problems.

BIOMECHANICAL STUDIES

The biomechanical and biochemical behavior of the motion segment is interdependent and indivisible. A major step toward determining the effects of mechanical forces on the components of the lumbar spine came when the concept of the motion segment was developed by Junghanns[153] and Schmorl.[259, 260] They suggested that the intervertebral disc was part of a compound three-point joint at each single vertebral level. The segment consisted of the intervertebral disc; the two facet joints and their controlling ligaments, muscles, and segmental contents of the intervertebral canal and foramen as one functional anatomic unit. It is preferable to include the adjacent halves of the vertebrae above and below these structures. Some physical properties of the intervertebral disc were first examined by Püschel.[241] He demonstrated the high fluid content of the nucleus pulposus at birth (i.e., 88% by weight); this decreases to 80% by 18 years of age, and to 69% by 77 years. However, the annulus fibrosus, which was 78% at birth, showed a reduction to 70% by the age of 30 years. Fick[87] made the first observation of the marked swelling properties of the disc nucleus pulposus. These observations suggested that the intervertebral disc was prone to viscoelastic properties. Göcke[107] examined the variations produced in the swelling of the disc tissue when it was immersed in acid, alkaline, and saline media. He observed that nuclear tissue immersed in saline absorbed the equivalent of 50% to 60% of its weight, but in aged subjects the tissue absorbed only 25%.

Charnley[48] and Naylor and Smare[205, 206] studied the possibility that a swelling nucleus may produce back pain by exerting internal pressure, affecting the annulus fibrosus and posterior longitudinal ligaments, and thus stimulating nociceptors in the spinal structures. Hirsch[132] had already shown that an increase in intradiscal pressure could produce back pain. Intranuclear injection of saline was found to produce low back pain that could be abolished by a subsequent injection of local anesthetic agent into the posterior longitudinal ligament or into the disc itself. Using a plethysmograph, Charnley measured the force produced by the swelling of isolated nuclear tissue when it was immersed in isotonic and hypertonic saline solutions. He demonstrated the high expansile force so produced, and suggested that this was an imbibition phenomenon. Bush and associates[42] and Naylor and Smare[205, 206] measured internal disc pressures generated by the immersion of disc and adjacent bony end plates in saline and water. They noted the high intradisc pressures so generated, except in discs showing advanced degeneration, and they demonstrated the production of disc herniation resulting from annular or end plate ruptures produced by the high pressures. This led to their hypothesis concerning the sequence of changes leading to lumbar pain and disc prolapse. They proposed that these changes resulted from the breakdown of the glycosoaminoglycans (GaGs) in the nucleus pulposus, in turn leading to an increase in the power of the nucleus to absorb water. Fluid, they hypothesized, enters the disc by diffusion through the end plate, thus increasing intradisc pressure; this changes the responses of the disc to mechanical forces and stimulates the nociceptors in the posterior part of the annulus and posterior longitudinal ligaments. Although imbibition was thought to be one factor in producing the fluid change, these authors thought that the breakdown of GaG increased the osmotic pressure within the disc. Hendry[125] noted that a degenerate disc retains less fluid than does a normal one and suggested that the aforementioned observations indicated that the discs were less fully hydrated prior to immersion; he maintained that imbibition pressure—not osmotic pressure—was the important force in maintaining the hydration of the nucleus. More recent extensive biochemical investigations by Urban and colleagues[292] have shown that ionic concentration, rather than molecular size, affects osmotic pressure and that partial degradation of GaG does not increase the magnitude of the osmotic pressure within the disc.

Sylven[279] and Hirsch and coworkers[132–134] made histochemical and electron microscope investigations of the intervertebral disc and showed the nucleus to have a loose three-dimensional lattice collagen structure with a gel matrix containing undetermined GaG. Nachemson[197, 198] and Nachemson and Morris[202, 203] then carried out epoch-making studies on intradisc pressure, both in vitro and in vivo and demonstrated the effects of compression loading of the discs and the variations of intradiscal pressure resulting from this loading, as well as from age and varying posture. They demonstrated the function of the intervertebral disc in redistributing the axial load radially to the inner layer of the annulus fibrosus, in addition to vertical compression to the end plates, thus converting a compressive load to tension within the annulus. The mechanism of redistributing such a compressive force was elucidated by the research of Happey and associates,[121] Naylor and associates,[211] Horton,[142] and Naylor[207, 209] on the ultrastructure of lumbar intervertebral discs using x-ray crystallographic and polarizing microscopic techniques. These demonstrated the annulus fibrosus to consist of collagen sheets arranged in alternate layers set at angles to one another. The fibers passed obliquely around the wall of the annulus, and the angle varied in different portions of the annulus. Such an arrangement of the fibers conveyed an elastic function on the disc. The obliquity of the fibers indicated that the tension on them was maximal with rotational forces. In older specimens the fibers showed increased crystallinity, fibrillation, and thickening. The oblique fibrous structure of the annulus allowed large compressive forces to be redistributed by the movement of the alternate sheaths on one another, producing very little disturbance in the annular wall. In the nucleus, the collagen was seen to be randomly arranged, and the fibrils were coarser and thicker with increasing age. Similar examination of prolapse nuclei showed the prolapsed tissue to have more collagen, and this was associated with an increased quantity of DNA in the nucleus.[59] Electron microscopic studies[120] showed the nucleus to have few chondrocyte cells, but the cells in the annulus were of the fibroblast type. The nuclear collagen was Type II.

Hickey and Hukins[128–131] and Klein and Hukins[164] et al examined, by x-ray crystallography, the effect of loading in the disc, noting the changes in orientation of the annular fibers with offset loading and tilting. They showed that flexion forces caused stretching of the posterior collagen fibers of the annulus, which provided reinforcement, but slackening of the anterior fibers. In torsion, the outer lamellae moved further than the inner lamellae of the annulus (i.e., the annulus is subject to shear stress). Excess force caused concentric fissures to develop in the inner lamellae, reducing resistance to nuclear pressure. The fiber orientation does not change with age, contrary to the thinking of previous workers.[119]

Inoue[147] and Inoue and Takeda[148] re-examined the three-dimensional collagen framework in the disc and noted no difference between prolapsed intervertebral disc tissue and the changes seen in normal aging.

Postacchini and colleagues[237] studied the differences between normal and recurrent disc herniations using light and elecron microscopy. Their findings suggest that newly formed disc tissue found in early recurrent prolapses resulted mainly from remnants of the original herniation. However, in late recurrent prolapsed tissue there was newly formed material from the annulus fibrosus with granulation invading the disc space after previous discectomy. Previous workers had not been able to detect elastic tissue in the intervertebral disc, but Sylvest and colleagues,[280] using modern techniques and methods of preparation, noted the presence of elastic fibers at the annular-nuclear junction, although the fibers were few in number.

Epidemiologic studies have shown that, among the diverse factors that affect the onset of low back pain and disc herniation, abnormal stresses and strains placed on the spine are very evident.[47, 159, 160] Numerous studies have been made on postmortem specimens of the whole motion segment or isolated structures, noting the effects of axial compression, axial compression with offset loading, and rotational forces on the various parts of the motion segment, whereas mathematic modeling has been used to estimate the stresses in the human spine in vivo.

Virgin,[300] demonstrating the hysteretic properties of the intervertebral disc, showed that purely axial loading could not produce disc herniation, even when the posterolateral aspects of the annulus were divided. This work was subsequently substantiated by extensive biomechanical studies by Farfan,[82] Farfan and coworkers,[84, 85] Markol and Morris,[189] Hirsch,[132, 135, 136] Horst and Brinckman,[141] Brinckman and colleagues,[33, 34] and Jayson and colleagues.[151] They have shown that the first structure to fail in axial compression is the vertebral end plate, in which the nucleus herniates into the vertebral body. This occurs in discographically normal and abnormal nuclei. Brinckman and associates[33] and Horst and Brinckman[141] noted bulging of the end plates toward the vertebral body before breaking, when axial loads were applied to isolated specimens. Again, they noted that the division of the annular fibers did not allow nuclear herniation to occur, despite the marked axial forces applied.

It had been assumed that herniation and degeneration adversely affected the biomechanical properties of the disc, but the above investigations showed that there was no consistent relationship between disc degeneration and mechanical behavior, although Kazarian[155] showed the viscoelastic behavior of the disc was significantly altered in degeneration (i.e., such discs demonstrate less creep than formal discs).

Farfan[82] and Farfan and colleagues[84, 85] used stress analysis techniques to demonstrate effectively that, contrary to belief at that time, the degenerate disc was stronger than the normal when subjected to compression; in addition to circumferential lateral bulging, the annulus bulged into the nucleus. Anterior bulging of the annulus was seen on flexion, and posterolateral bulging was found on extension. Lateral bulging,

Muir,[79, 80] Herbert and associates,[126] and Jayson and associates,[151] located some Type I collagen in the nucleus in the layers adjacent to the nuclear-annular junction. The annulus was found to contain 30% Type II and 70% Type I collagen, the proportions of these two types varying with the levels examined. Meanwhile, the synthesis of new collagen, predominantly Type I in both annulus and nucleus was noted in discs above the level of any degeneration. The degenerative process was unevenly distributed throughout the tissue of a particular disc. Some evidence suggests that other collagens, particularly Types V and VI, exist in normal discs, whereas Type III collagen has been shown to be a component of a degenerate disc.[208]

Once the chemical structures and their relationship to the fluid content of the intervertebral disc were established, the possible pathways of fluid to and from the general path of circulation to the relatively avascular disc needed investigation. Impedance of such flow would affect disc homeostasis and function and thus could be a factor in development of low back pain. It had been assumed that the flow between the disc and the general circulation was via the vertebral end plate, passing from the avascular nucleus to the vascular network in the intervertebral body adjacent to the end plate. Such a pathway of nutrition was demonstrated by Brodin[35] using fluorescent techniques, and by investigators of iodine diffusion using radiography.[207] Holm and colleagues,[139] Nachemson and associates,[201] and Urban and colleagues[289, 290] demonstrated a lesser pathway of diffusion from the nucleus through the annulus fibrosus to the blood vessels at the periphery of the annulus. They also confirmed that the central portion of the end plate of healthy discs was permeable to solutes, but there was a significant degree of impermeability in the presence of macroscopic disc degeneration. The central portion of the end plate was more permeable than the peripheral parts. Diffusion depended on the proportion of the blood vessel content at each situation and the type of solute (i.e., its charge and size), glucose, and oxygen entering the discs through the end plates. The rates of metabolism of various elements, their rates of diffusion, and the oxygenation of various areas of the intervertebral disc were demonstrated. Metabolism in the center of the nucleus was shown to be virtually anaerobic. Fluid flow in normal discs, although small, depends on the charges of the various solutes. The fluid flows via molecular diffusion carrying the fluid with the particular solutes; however, the flow is also controlled by the pumping action of the varying loads on the intervertebral disc. The latter has been extensively investigated by Krämer[166, 167] and Krämer and associates,[168] who showed the mass effects generated by loading and unloading the discs through varying postures and spinal movement to be important in solute transport. Intradiscal pressures greater than 80 kilopounds inhibited diffusion of ^{14}C glucose and ^{35}S into the disc, suggesting the operation of a pumping mechanism to aid the flow of nutrients into the disc coincidentally with outflow of metabolites. They showed an influx of fluid into the disc in the supine position, whereas fluid was extruded from the disc on standing, sitting, and walking. Using color diffusion tests, they showed that only molecules with molecular weights of 400 or less could pass freely to and from the disc, although large plasma proteins with larger molecular weights have been demonstrated in the annulus fibrosus of the disc. A significant decrease in fluid flow and disc permeability with increasing age has been noted.

The importance of movement in maintaining normal disc nutrition has been shown by the progression of investigations into the nutrition of the disc, the movements of solutes from the bloodstream into the intervertebral disc, the oxygenation of the disc, and variations of nutrition induced by motion. Thus, the significance of exercise for the normal maintenance of disc homeostasis and the harmful effects of lack of movement interfering with disc nutrition is scientifically well supported.[137, 138, 289, 290] The possibility of such factors being involved in development of low back pain has become evident. Holm and Nachemson[138] demonstrated the adverse effects of localized fusion on the nutritional efficiency in the discs above and below the level of fusion induced by the lack of movement the fusion produces.

Studies of the sites and rates of synthesis of the GaG and collagen became necessary. Hansen and Ullberg[116] and Soutar and Taylor,[274] using microautoradiographic techniques, showed that the maximum synthesis of the GaG occurs at the nuclear-annular junction, while synthesis and degradation of both GaG and collagen were studied in experimental models of intervertebral disc degeneration by Lipson and Muir.[173] Considerable variations in the metabolisms of GaG in immature and mature pathologic tissues have been noted, but the effects of this on dysfunction have yet to be fully demonstrated.

Evidence of the enzymic activity within the intervertebral disc necessary for the development of degradative and synthetic processes within the disc was shown initially by Naylor,[208] who demonstrated the presence of lysosomal enzymes capable of breaking down GaG in the intervertebral disc nucleus. This led him to reiterate the concept of autoimmune activity as a possible initiator of disc degeneration.[207] Disturbances of normal enzyme regulation within the disc appear to result from one of the following:

1. Alternative one—faulty genetic programming seen in the chondrodystrophoid degeneration in dogs, which is associated with increased incidence of disc prolapse in those breeds.
2. Alternative two—defective synthesis of the normal enzymes regulating the metabolism of the disc.
3. Alternative three—decreased synthesis or accumulation of enzyme inhibitors normally present in the intervertebral disc matrix.

Subsequent to this discovery of GaG degradative enzymes, research has been particularly directed toward investigation of the collagenolytic enzymes and protease inhibitors. The effects of these and GaG degradative enzymes and other specific granules of phagocytes producing collagenase, either in latent form or in combination with inhibitors or proenzymes, have been investigated.[14, 195] Plasmin occurs in almost all tissues as its precursor plasminogen. Its activity is controlled by the balance of tissue activators and inhibitors in the serum. Ghosch and colleagues,[101, 102] Gibson and colleagues,[104] and Knight and associates[165] have demonstrated these effects in cartilage and intervertebral disc tissue. Sedowofia and coworkers[265] established the presence of neutral proteolytic enzymes within the human intervertebral disc, which were capable of degrading the matrix. They isolated collagenase, gelatinase, and the elastolytic proteases in both the annulus and the nucleus. Collectively, these studies reveal that the human intervertebral disc contains a system of degradative enzymes active at neutral pH, capable of metabolizing the major components of the disc matrix. Failure, decline, or reduced activity of the enzymic activities with aging could be an important factor in producing intervertebral disc degeneration. Protease inhibitors produced by the chondrocytes inhibit the action of the serum protease and collagenase; that is, they have a protective function against enzymic destruction of collagen and GaG, but an imbalance produced by damage to the end plate of the annulus could change the balance in favor of degradation leading to the development of degenerative change. Autoimmune responses could lead to a similar enzyme imbalance, producing similar degenerative changes and failure of the disc with disordered motion segment function.

Avascularity of the intervertebral disc, and thus its relative isolation from immune systems, predisposes it to intense reactions when sequestration occurs. The possibility of such reactions being responsible for the development of degenerative processes and disc herniation led to the hypothesis that such reactions[207] might alter cartilage end plate permeability and possibly the production of plasminogen, thus altering enzymic balance and activity with a degradative effect on the disc tissues. Fissuring of the annulus or end plate fracture, which has been seen to result from chronic repetitive rotation stresses[84] followed by the ingrowth of granulation tissue, is the probable route of vascularization; this may lead to the development of autoimmune processes. Such a pathologic condition was demonstrated by Smith and Walmsley.[271] In their study, the experimental division of animal disc annulus was seen to heal in the outer layers only, and the nucleus invaded the deeper, divided layers of the annulus. Such granulation tissue invading peripheral annular tears is seen in advanced degeneration.

Cell-mediated immunity by the intervertebral disc nucleus was effected by Bobechko and Hirsch,[27] while Keiser and Sandson[156] demonstrated the presence of antigenic determinants in cartilage proteoglycans. Support for the autoimmune hypothesis was provided by the evidence of increased γ-globulins in patients with prolapsed intervertebral discs, produced by Naylor[210] and Naylor and colleagues.[212] Leukocyte migration inhibition tests in patients with intervertebral disc disorders also produced some confirmatory evidence.[97, 98, 123, 174] The latter demonstrated the presence of a cellular immune response in patients whose intervertebral discs were found to be sequestered at the time of surgery for disc prolapse, but no humeral antibody had been detected in disc or serum.

Tait and Devlin,[282] using lymphocyte transformation techniques for cell-mediated immunity, examined patients with disc disease and obtained positive reactions in those with sequestered disc material. They showed that the proteoglycans extracted from the nucleus of cadaveric discs had antigenic properties, confirming the observations of Pankowich and Korngold.[226] Little further investigation of this aspect of the problem has been made, despite the promise of the earlier research. Although the evidence to support this thesis is considerable, it has been impossible to find antibodies in patient serum. Further immunologic investigations appear to be necessary.

The possible effect of the degradative agents from intervertebral disc prolapse leaking and causing irritation of the nerve root has not been substantiated. Further studies using immunologic processes combined with MRI and CT monitoring of degenerative processes may prove to be useful means of investigation.

The involvement of genetic factors in disc degeneration has been questioned, although the subject has received scant attention. Hansen[115] drew attention to the chondrodystrophoid degeneration of intervertebral discs in certain breeds of dogs known to be susceptible to neurologic defects associated with disc degeneration and herniation, pointing out that these changes were often at multiple and adjacent levels. Naylor and Horton[213] suggested the possibilities of a basic systemic factor being responsible for degeneration that appears at many levels, even in patients with single-level prolapse. This has received some confirmation by the recent MRI studies by Gibson and colleagues showing the degenerative changes at many levels in the lumbar spine in children suffering from single level disc herniation.[105, 106] Berry[22] produced some evidence of a genetic influence when he showed that a pin-tail mutation in mice is associated with intervertebral disc anomalies in the tail and lumbar regions. The tail was reduced in size with a lower GaG content, showing advanced age changes. Additional genetic studies may be rewarding. The prospect of endocrine control of chondroitin sulfate synthesis, or of the GaG synthesis degradation balance being disturbed by such influences, was raised by Scott,[263] who showed the effects of increased adrenocortical activity on the volume of the nucleus pulposus; supporting evidence was provided in a study of the treatment of lumbar disc herniation with adrenocorticotropic hormone (ACTH).[215]

Despite the extensive research into the biochemistry of intervertebral discs, the vast knowledge accumulated during the past 30 years, and the consequent biomechanical changes, we still need to understand how biochemical factors could be responsible for low back pain. We need the quantification of the various enzymes at different ages and various stages of degeneration and prolapse. We need more information on the role of noncollagenous proteins, which are seen to be changed in quantity and character in disc prolapse.

Recent biochemical studies with important therapeutic implications include those of McNicol,[184] who reported that small proteins (catabolins) produced by joint synovium appear to play important parts in the degradation of the connective tissue matrix. Cellular messenger proteins appear to be involved in the balance between matrix degradation and synthesis, although little is known about these control mechanisms. Both steroids and nonsteroidal anti-inflammatory drugs appear to influence the synthetic activity of synovial cells and chondrocytes. Specific receptors for sulfated polysaccharides present on lymphocytes and macrophages may play an important role in the matrix homeostasis. McNicol's work demonstrated, for the first time, the presence of receptors for sulfated polysaccharides in cells of normal joint fluid and synovial membrane. The breakdown products of matrix degradation, including sulfated polysaccharides released from the proteoglycans of the matrix, may conceivably be involved in the control mechanisms. These receptors in the synovial cells were activated by matrix degradation products, and produced through a process of cell messengers an inhibition of release of factors that degrade the matrix.

It is likely that polysulfated glycosoaminoglycans (Arteparon), a polysulfated polysaccharide, could have such an inhibitory effect. The use of polysulfated glycosoaminoglycans in modifying disc degeneration was attempted by Australian workers Cole and colleagues.[53] Using animal studies, they produced the first report that a systemically administered drug could influence the turnover of disc proteoglycans and suggested that polysulfated glycosoaminoglycans may therefore be valuable in the management of disc disease. These ideas were further developed by Gill and colleagues,[105] who used rabbit models to produce herniation of the nucleus in the lumbar spine. They then studied the effects of this herniation as well as the effects of immobilization and polysulfated glycosoaminoglycans injection on the subsequent regeneration of the components of intervertebral disc and speculated on possible degenerative changes that might develop. They compared the effects of immobility, activity, and polysulfated glycosoaminoglycans in reducing the progression of degenerative disease, examining the spines radiographically and histologically. Disc space narrowing and osteophyte formation were noted. The animals treated with polysulfated glycosoaminoglycans showed less osteophyte formation, less narrowing of disc space, and better repair than the untreated groups. This result showed that experimental disc degeneration was prevented, at least in part, by intramuscular injections of the polysulfated glycosoaminoglycans. These biochemical studies confirm the importance of disc biochemistry and metabolism in the development of low back pain and have important therapeutic implications. Earlier it was thought that the "disc dynasty" had perished. Perhaps we are about to witness its "phoenix."

NEUROLOGIC INVESTIGATIONS AND THEIR IMPLICATIONS

It is increasingly evident that low back pain is not only a problem of the back, but also part of the more general problem of pain mechanism and control. During the past 20 years, considerable basic research into both aspects has been generated. Research on pain mechanisms and control is largely linked to the great achievements in neurobiology.

Despite frequent searches, no nerve endings had been noted in the intervertebral disc nucleus, but some were noted in the posterior aspect of the annulus.[247] Pedersen and colleagues[230] demonstrated the distribution of the posterior rami of the spinal nerves to the posterior aspects of the annulus and associated ligamentous structures. They showed a segmental distribution of single nerve roots throughout the lumbar spine. Paris[227] has confirmed this, also showing the multilevel segmental innervation of single facet joints. More recent examination of fresh intervertebral disc tissue removed at operation has revealed the presence of fine nerve fibers in the annulus fibrosus of the posterior third of the disc, but no nerve receptors were demonstrated in the nucleus.[329] Evidence for the presence of nociceptor nerve endings that are sensitive to mechanical and chemical tissue dysfunction had been elicited following extensive researches in the anatomic and neurochemical field, whereas restriction of the nociceptor system to the anterior aspects of the spinal dura and dural nerve root sheaths had already been observed by Edgar and colleagues[70, 71] and Hovelacque.[143] In normal circumstances, this nociceptor receptor system is largely inactive. It becomes active, however, when its constituent unmyelinated nerves are depolarized by mechanical forces applied to the tissue containing them, which sufficiently stress, deform or damage the tissue. This may happen, for example, by pressure distraction, distention, or laceration or by exposure to a concentration of tissue fluid containing irritating substances such as lactic acid, potassium ions, polypeptide, kianins, 5-hydroxytryptamine, prostaglandins, and histamine that are released from affected or metabolically abnormal tissues, especially when exposed to factors producing ischemia.[144, 145, 324–326]

The differentiation of pain referred from spinal structures, as opposed to nerve root pain, heralded the end of the "disc dynasty." At that time it became evident that pain in the back, alone or combined with leg pain resembling that associated with disc herniation, could arise from the sclerotogenous components of the motion segment. The distribution of the spinal nerves had been well demonstrated by Foerster.[89] Kellgren,[157, 158] in the late 1930s, revealed the value of clinical scientific investigations in the differentiation of the two types of pain affecting the back and leg. He demonstrated the distribution of pain arising from the deep somatic structures when they were stimulated by injections of normal and hypertonic saline. The finding was subsequently confirmed by Inman and Saunders[146] and Sinclaire and colleagues.[269] This work indicated that disc enucleation had no place in the relief of pain arising from such structures, and this idea coincided with clinical analyses of the causes of failure of lumbar surgery.

Reference to the possibility of pain arising from facet joint disease has already been made.[26, 243, 268] Ghormley[99] used the term *facet syndrome* in reference to the role of facet joints in causing nerve root compression. The use of this term was different from its current meaning. It is now used to describe pain referred from the articular structure and surrounding tissues of the facet joint (i.e., referred pain, rather than root pain).

Facet joint nerve block as a means of differentiating sites of pain origin in the low back was first used by Steindler and Luck,[277] who injected a local anesthetic in the region of facet joints and obtained substantial relief of back pain in some cases. Meanwhile, Badgeley,[13] in his series of patients with low back and leg pain, noted fewer than 20% showing any nerve root irritation or neurologic defect. No further developments in this field were made until Rees,[245] in Australia, described a method of surgical denervation of facet joint by using a percutaneous procedure.[188] Whether the facet joints were actually denervated by these procedures is open to question, but the method did show that back pain and referred leg pain could arise from the tissues on the posterior aspects of the facet joint. Shealy[266] modified this procedure using a radiofrequency method of destroying tissues in the vicinity of the facet joint. Whether the injection is made into the pericapsular or interarticular tissues is not related to the result.[81, 180] These and other clinical studies using radiologically controlled facet joint periarticular injections[194, 224] showed that coincidental injections of a long-acting anesthetic agent with steroids can produce persistent and often prolonged relief of low back and leg pain for variable periods. However, relief is temporary as it is unlikely to cure degenerative disease. This is a useful diagnostic tool in eliminating possible sources of pain and does allow pain relief, which can then be augmented by rehabilitation measures. The results suggest that simple muscle stripping, laterally, in the process of laminectomy and partial facetectomy may inadvertently relieve discomfort as a result of partial joint denervation.

Epidural injections have been used for many years to relieve sciatic pain radiation. Initially these consisted of injections of some 30 to 40 ml of normal saline, but the method became unfashionable in the late 1930s with the advent and increasing use of discectomy. Its limited use has been revived during the past 20 years with increased empirical use in many pathologic conditions. Epidural injection now involves the use of a long-acting local anesthetic agent combined with steroids and is used largely in the conservative treatment of disc prolapse with root pain. Success rates of 20% to 30% relief have been obtained. Although relief is often temporary, the treatment allows other supportive rehabilitation measures to be employed.

Anatomic, clinical scientific, and basic scientific investigations of the spinal nerves and their functions reveal the roots in the lumbosacral region to be structurally, vascularly, and metabolically unique. Smyth and Wright[272] observed the hypersensitivity of the nerve root when it was subjected to compression by the disc prolapse, as compared with the minimal effect of traction on a nerve root in which no prolapse is present. Parke and Wattenabe[228] showed that spinal nerves may respond to mechanical stresses and inflammatory conditions in a manner different from peripheral nerves. This is because the spinal nerve has no epineurium to resist mechanical stress, being encased in a thin pial sheath. Rydevik and colleagues[251] demonstrated the diffusion of endorphins in the CSF into the spinal nerve root sheath. Thus, the blockage of the sheath by nerve root compression in disc herniation or spinal stenosis—or by adhesion formation and arachnoiditis—is liable to be followed by inadequate nerve root perfusion by the CSF, so eliminating the modulating effects of the endorphins it contains and allowing pain to persist. The significance of endorphin levels in the CSF may affect the modulation of pain. Diminished levels of endorphins in the CSF in patients with chronic back pain have been demonstrated by Puig and colleagues,[240] Terenius and Tamsen,[284] and Dahlin and colleagues.[62]

Newer ideas on nerve root conduction and on the modulating effect of applying additional nociceptors and other stimuli followed from the works of Melzack and Wall.[190, 191] They have shown that a polypeptide, substance P, can modify nociception by lumbar nerve roots when they are stimulated mechanically, although the mechanism stimulating the synthesis and the transport and release of peptides from the dorsal root ganglion is not yet understood. Recently, Weinstein[311] and Badalamente and colleagues[12] showed the neurotransmitter substance P emerging from the dorsal root ganglion. They demonstrated the way in which this can be caused by vibration and that mechanical factors can produce chemical changes affecting pain.

Advances in neuropharmacology and neurobiology have led to the development of methods of relieving chronic pain.[276, 327] Of particular interest has been the discovery of prostaglandin PGE_2, estimated by radioimmune assay techniques,[182] in a greater concentration in discs enucleated for disc prolapse than in those from patients operated on for paralytic spinal deformities. Whether the prostaglandin has a central or peripheral role is uncertain.

The increasing knowledge of the modulating effects of mood and other central nervous system mechanisms on pain has had a considerable effect on the management of chronic pain, and on back pain in particular, with an increasing trend toward the use of nonsurgical methods of pain control and relief. Newer concepts of neural transmission have changed the surgical approach to pain control, diminishing the use of ablative methods such as neurectomy, rhizotomy, and tractotomy. Operative central stimulation of periaqueductal and periventricular gray matter for relief of pain increases the secretion of endorphins into the CSF and has produced gratifying results, despite the risks attached to the method. It has the advantage of using the body's own natural mediator for pain alleviation. The continuous epidural perfusion of morphine, by means of silastic percutaneously introduced catheters, has reduced pain by activating opiate receptors in the spinal cord, selectively inhibiting the release of substance P and suppressing nociceptor input to the substantia gelatinosa in the spinal cord. It has the advantage of not depressing the central nervous system. Its effect can be reversed by naloxone, but tolerance develops rapidly.

Neurobiologic research has led to some explanation of the effect of placebos. They appear to act on β-endorphin release in the third ventricle. Newer studies of axoplasmic transport of macromolecules within the axons of the nervous system have led to the revision of ideas about neuronal function and about the production and relief of pain. This may provide some clues to the mechanism of low back pain where no specific localized cause can be detected. The contribution of exercise therapy to pain relief has given support to the treatment of chronic low back pain using "back school" methods. Exercise increases the levels of endorphins in the CSF and so reduces pain sensitivity, thereby contributing to the trend of the last 10 years toward using nonsurgical methods in the treatment of chronic low back pain.[91, 264, 330]

It is increasingly apparent that a patient's psyche has an important effect on the outcome of a physical treatment; this idea is particularly applicable to the treatment of low back and leg pain. Psychosomatic reactions are closely related to an individual's capacity to deal with stress, and considerable research has been done to assess the possible effects of stress—particularly psychologic stress—in the production and modification of low back pain. A surgeon has to consider the degree of integration of the intellectual and emotional aspects of a patient's personality as well as the possible presence of any psychologic disorders. The importance of these assessments in selecting patients for specific procedures has led to the use of many methods of psychologic assessment. The Minnesota Multiphasic Personality Inventory (MMPI) is a sophisticated tool for the assessment of the patient's index of hypochondriasis and hysteria. High hypochondriasis and hysterical scores are considered to be inversely related to the successful outcome of any surgical intervention for disc disorders and low back pain, but subsequent surgical reviews correlating predictions by the MMPI with the surgical findings and the ultimate outcome have not always proved the prediction to be accurate. The results of the surgery are often better than was anticipated. Other methods of assessment include the modified somatic perception questionnaire (MSPQ).[186, 332] There is an apparent need for separate predictive indices for patients who have prominent physical signs and those having only marginal findings. Testing is time consuming, and the help of a clinical psychologist is not always available. A simple and rapid clinical assessment is given by the use of pain diagrams.[244] Various predictive signs pointing to good or poor outcomes assist in improved selection of patients.[304, 305]

A new view of the development and treatment of low back pain, combining clinical and psychologic factors, has been developed by Waddell and colleagues.[302, 306a, 306b] The various psychologic factors associated with disability include increased bodily awareness related to anxiety and symptoms of depression. The majority of patients with backache are not personality deficient, neurotic, hypochondriacal, hysterical, or insane; they are simply distressed by their physical problems. Waddell prefers to consider these as illness behavior, rather than as separate psychologic entities, and emphasizes the value of assessing inappropriate descriptions of symptoms and inappropriate responses. He notes that the philosophy of rest for reducing pain should be replaced by more active restoration of function. He further points out that the lasting value of rest, which is commonly prescribed, is doubtful and that prolonged bed rest may be harmful. Conversely, there is no evidence that activity is harmful, and it does not necessarily make the pain worse. Controlled exercise can restore function, reduce stress and illness behavior, and thus expedite a return to work. Such a regimen does reduce pain, and clinical studies have confirmed the value of active rehabilitation.

Chronic pain resulting in multiple absences or a prolonged absence from work and repeated hospitalization leads to psychologic upset. Pain persisting for more than 3 months will cause additional psychologic problems. In the treatment of these disorders, programs involving the elimination of addictive pain medication and relief of psychologic factors need to be combined with "back school" methods of physical re-education, which will certainly produce results better than those of repetitive surgery.

ADVANCES RESULTING FROM CLINICAL RESEARCH

Advances have been made by retrospective and prospective clinical scientific studies, in which the value of both conservative and surgical measures used to treat back pain have been researched.

To assess these treatments, it has been necessary to define the various back pain syndromes. Unfortunately, many studies of clinical treatments—particularly of conservative measures—have tended to assess large groups with unspecified diagnoses. The failure to identify, as separate groups, those with nonspecific back pain, root pain, stenotic symptoms, and referred back pain reduced the value of many studies. Simple separation into (1) acute short-term backache, (2) backache with marked leg pain, and (3) chronic back pain has been necessary. Treatment by conservative methods has shown that most patients with acute short-term cases are relieved by, or in spite of, whatever method of treatment is used. There is some evidence that short-term relief can be afforded by manipulative techniques, but in the longer term the outcome is little affected by the method of treatment. Of those with acute short-term back pain, 90% are not absent for more than 1 week. In cases of back pain with leg pain, manipulation may ease some of the back symptoms, but the relief of sciatic symptoms appears to be no greater than that obtained with a placebo treatment.[113] The results of rotatory manipulation show that such activity had no effect on the size of a disc herniation predicted by myelography.[50] Treatment by traction, anti-inflammatory drugs, muscle relaxants, and ultrasound therapy had no significant effect on the length of the absence from work. Studies of the natural history of lumbar disc herniation have shown the natural tendency toward resolution in a high proportion of cases, thus making it difficult to assess the value of various therapies.

Epidemiologic studies reveal that chronic back pain appears to diminish considerably in severity within 4 years of onset, sufficiently to allow return to work. Schmorl's (see above) studies showed the incidence of herniations of the nucleus pulposus in patients who never had back and leg symptoms. Weber,[310] in a prospective randomized study, showed that patients with myelographically proven herniated discs obtained relief of pain and return of function, regardless of surgical intervention. The benefit of surgery was to speed recovery, particularly to bring about the rapid relief of pain. The outcome of surgical treatments was better than that of conservative treatments after 1 year, but the difference between the two groups progressively narrowed after 4 years. The natural progress of patients with radiculopathy associated with disc disease was more rapid than had been expected, and patients became much better adjusted to factors of daily living, in spite of their back disease, as the years passed. The 10-year results emphasized the value of back school for teaching the patient about his or her disability and how to adjust to it. Spinal fusion was scarcely necessary as part of the initial operation of disc enucleation, but studies showed that surgery, when indicated, should preferably be performed within 3 months of the onset of leg pain to obtain optimal results. Spangfort,[275] in a computer analysis of 2,504 patients treated by surgery for lumbar disc herniation, compared these with a series of patients who did not undergo surgery. He had previously shown the results at the end of 10 years to be indistinguishable. Of the patients who were operated on, 20% to 45% had persistent backache, despite simultaneous fusion.

Currently, there is a trend to avoid using combined disc enucleation and fusion. In the past, the combined procedure was recommended in patients who had many previous attacks of low back pain that suggested instability, and in whom it was believed that considerable instability would follow the disc enucleation in view of the associated advanced degeneration. Young and colleagues[331] found the combined procedure to yield long-term results that were marginally superior. However, Frymoyer and coworkers,[94] in a 10-year follow-up of 312 patients, found residual backache, nerve root symptoms, and functional impairment to be as common in those with simultaneous fusion as in those with simple enucleation (i.e., in 30%). Seven percent of patients with fusion had symptoms from the donor site for the bone grafts. In Great Britain, the practice has invariably been not to do simultaneous enucleation and fusion, but to reserve fusion for a later time, as a possible second procedure, if indicated. This would be required by few. The results of Troup and coworkers[287, 288] show increasing evidence that both back and leg pain in most patients last for a certain period of time only, approximately 3 to 4 years. No late recurrences are expected, indicating no haste for fusion.

Along with the reduced incidence of surgical intervention, there has been a trend toward using both minimal surgical exposure and microsurgical techniques.[46, 319] This has the advantage of reducing the patient's hospitalization and returning him or her more rapidly to work, but it has the disadvantage of not revealing all pathologic conditions, especially lateral stenosis and intraligamentous herniation. In view of its economic advantages, the procedure is gaining popularity.

Many studies of the surgical results of intervention for failed surgery have shown the inefficacy of multiple surgical assaults on the lumbar spine.[88, 231, 249, 303]

A significant new concept concerning the mechanism leading to back and leg pain in certain patients is that the size of the spinal canal is incompatible with the size of its contents. Congenital narrowing of the spinal canal was first reported by Sarpyener,[255, 256] but its possible relationship to clinical symptoms was unrecognized until descriptions of the clinical aspects of spinal stenosis were published by Verbiest[295, 296] and Brain.[32] Verbiest noted the constriction of the dural sheath by bony compression in a narrowed spinal canal. This constriction was often mistakenly believed to be responsible for the symptoms of intermittent claudication due to peripheral vascular disease and those commonly presumed to result from psychologic disturbance, not from any physical defect or disease. He demonstrated the value of wide decompressive laminectomy to relieve these symptoms. Further descriptions and classifications of the results of treatment for this condition, which we had previously ignored and patients had maligned, followed.[7, 11, 72, 76, 257, 321, 322] The importance of stenosis in the chondrodystrophies, particularly achondroplasia, was noted by Nelson,[216] whereas Kirkaldy-Willis and Farfan[163] and Naylor[210] emphasized the role of chronic rotational stresses in increasing the compromise of the contents of the spinal canal by

preliminary skin testing and premedication with H and H_2 blockers and steroids. As the diagnosis of disc prolapse has become more accurate, by clinical means and by myelography and CT scanning, and as a more purified chymopapain has been developed, the treatment has become more popular over the past five years. However, we still do not have long-term follow-up studies of outcome (i.e., beyond 10 or more years). Fraser,[92, 93] in a well-controlled prospective double-blind trial, compared the effects of normal saline injection with chymopapain treatment after the failure of a 3-week conservative treatment. Seventy-five per cent of patients tested with chymopapain were relieved within 6 weeks, whereas 37% of those treated with saline were relieved in the same period; but is 3 weeks of conservative treatment a period sufficient to determine failure? The successful relief of pain can be consistent with persistence of the prolapse seen on radiculography. A 70% to 75% success rate appears to be the standard for all forms of treatment, including placebos, but a lower rate holds for intradiscal hydrocortisone and saline. One "successful chymotherapy trial" uses intradiscal alcohol prior to the use of the enzyme; the results appear to be the same as for those without the alcohol—yet, it has been definitely shown that alcohol application to chymopapain will destroy its enzyme activity.[214] The preliminary instillation of radiopaque dyes prior to discography has been shown not to have any adverse effect on the chymopapain action.[214] The question arises: Why does saline produce such a reasonable amount of relief or any relief at all? Failures of chymopapain are seen to occur, as happens with other methods of intradiscal therapy, if there is an extruded degenerate nucleus; surgery is required in such cases.

Double-blind prospective trials[278] have compared the results of chymopapain treatment with surgery. Chymopapain yields good results in the short term and when the herniation is small and the clinical pattern indicates slight or moderate nerve compression. For all large herniations and medium-sized ones causing severe root signs, surgery is preferable, because it provides a significantly higher short- and long-term success rate. Animal studies[31, 307] have demonstrated a loss of proteoglycans from the normal canine disc annulus, nucleus, and end plate after the intradisc injection of chymopapain, but regeneration follows and is complete within 6 months. Biomechanical properties adversely affected initially by the injection are reversed to normal within 3 months. These operations were made on normal discs. Whether prolapsed and degenerate discs respond and reconstitute to the same degree is questionable, but investigations of the long-term effects by magnetic resonance imaging (MRI)[281] have shown scarring and fibrous tissue within the nucleus following chymopapain injection; these changes appear to be irreversible and analogous to gross disc degeneration.

Aprotonin (Transxylol) has been used with varying degrees of success, although the success rate is not as high as with chymopapain.[169] Aprotonin suppresses inflammatory responses and inhibits proteases. This action is shown in patients with rheumatoid arthritis, in whom intra-articular injection is equally as effective as corticosteroids. It is thought the aprotonin acts by inhibiting the activation of plasmin and lysosomal cathepsins, notably cathepsin D, neutralizing 10% of the charges on the acidic groups of chondroitin sulfate. It has an affinity for the chondroitin sulfate and forms complexes that do not pass out of the disc because of their high molecular weight. Its advantage is that it does not appear to produce serious complications.

Intradiscal instillation of collagenase was first utilized by Bromley and associates,[36, 37] who reported successful relief in 78% of patients with disc herniation symptoms without any systemic local toxic effects. As was found with the use of chymopapain, failures appear to be associated with disc sequestration and extrusion. The effect of epidural and intrathecal injection of collagenase in animals was tested by Olmarker and coworkers[220] and Rydevik and colleagues.[253] Clinical comparisons of chymopapain and collagenase have primarily produced approximately similar success rates.[39, 124] Although collagenase effectively relieves pain, it attacks the collagen of the disc—of both the annulus and the nucleus—particularly its supporting structure; therefore, it is likely to damage both parts of the disc and affect its subsequent mechanical properties, in view of the very slow regeneration of collagen. The possible deleterious long-term effects have yet to be assessed.

The similar success rates of intradiscal medication suggest that the net effects of the biochemical degradation must have some common effect, which is probably biomechanical (i.e., the reduction of intradiscal pressure).[214] It has been shown that the breakdown products do not produce any ill effects on the nerve root; nor do they produce pain. Further investigation as to the mode of relief by assessing the biochemical effects of the various medicaments is needed.

Analyses of the failure of surgery to relieve lumbar disc prolapse show that the most frequent causes are misdiagnosis and enucleation of the disc in the absence of prolapse. Other causes are nonrecognition of spinal stenosis, recurrent herniation, and arachnoiditis and perineural fibrosis. Studies have been made to prevent arachnoiditis and perineural adhesions. Some have attempted to insert plastic sheets to separate the theca from surrounding muscles; fat grafts and grafts from the deepest layer of the dermis have been used to this end. Free fat grafts, which are apt to shrink and become replaced by fibrous tissue, have been superseded by pedicle fat grafts taken from surrounding subcutaneous tissues. They have been shown to remain viable and considerably minimize perineural adhesion formation.[106, 149, 170]

A nonsurgical approach to the problem of postoperative adhesion and arachnoiditis has been initiated by Jayson and coworkers.[150, 152] Clinical recognition of arachnoiditis and nerve root sheath fibrosis requires further radiculography, CT, and MRI; repetitive surgery for such conditions has produced an unsatisfactory outcome. Jayson showed that many patients with such adhesion formation and arachnoiditis have a defect in fibrinolytic activity. The defect leads to the failure to clear fibrin and to persistent chronic inflammation, resulting in scar tissue formation. He proposed that this is a possible factor in the development of chronicity of low back pain and suggested that fibrinolytic enhancement may offer a new approach to the management of this condition. He hypothesized that venous obstruction is probably a factor in the development of extraneural and perineural fibrosis.

Major contributions to the diagnosis of low back problems have been made by advances in the fields of radiology and electrophysiology. Before 1970, myelography was undertaken with oil-based media, which were associated with a high incidence of complications, particularly arachnoiditis. The development of water-based radiopaque media during the past 15 years was a significant advance, bringing together a lower complication rate and greater accuracy in defining nerve root sleeve obstruction. CT scanning developed by Hounsfield in England in the 1970s promised equally good delineation of such pathologic changes without the risk associated with an invasive procedure. Both myelography and CT scanning reveal the presence and extent of any spinal stenosis. CT is of considerable value in evaluating spinal trauma, especially if it is complemented by metrizamide enhancement. These techniques provide information not afforded by conventional radiography, demonstrating soft tissue abnormalities within the spinal canal, especially if these methods are combined with multiplanar reconstruction. Rothman and colleagues[250] compared the relative values of CT scanning and disc myelography in 122 patients with the surgically confirmed disorders of either prolapsed intervertebral disc or spinal stenosis, or both. They found myelography to be more accurate than CT in the diagnosis of disc prolapse. In the diagnosis of spinal stenosis, myelography was slightly more accurate, but CT offers no side effects, less radiation, and clearer visualization of lateral pathologic conditions, and it avoids hospitalization. They found that 55% of asymptomatic subjects had abnormal CT scans. The study received considerable criticism because it did not discuss gradations of disc disease from internal derangement with anular bulging, frank herniation, or recurrent herniation and did not distinguish central stenosis from lateral foraminal and extraforaminal defects. When CT alone is used to assess defects of the lumbosacral canal, disorders of the conus and cauda equina may be overlooked, if the separation of the sections is too great; a degenerative process may be diagnosed as disc prolapse when root symptoms are present.

An important advance in radio diagnosis came with the development of MRI. Mansfield and Grannell[188] of Nottingham first reported the use of MRI in the Journal of Physics in 1973. This concept of MRI was simultaneously considered by Lauterbaur in

Poland.[170a] The first images were produced in the Department of Physics at the University of Nottingham in 1976, and the first whole body image was demonstrated there in 1978. In the same department, Moore initiated a related system that was subsequently developed into the present-day commercial MRI imaging method. Moore's group developed the first head image in 1979, and this appears to be the first true published image. Mansfield's system is still being developed and promises to produce body images more rapidly than does the present-day system. It is possible that a second generation of nuclear magnetic resonance (NMR) machines will adopt this system, as it has the advantage of producing images far more rapidly. These would possibly be capable of producing dynamic pictures of the intervertebral disc and spinal function.

MRI is a noninvasive procedure that does not require hospitalization and shows anomalies of the cord, such as pathologic cavitation in the cervical region and Arnold-Chiari defects and tumors. The recorded signals indicate the degree of hydration of discs, and the absence of extradural fat can be demonstrated in stenotic lesions. The demonstration of extraneous compression of the cord by spondylitic disc disease, skeletal and neoplastic disease with cord compression (e.g., neurofibromata and spinal metastases) is liable to render myelography or CT redundant. At present, CT scan is superior to MRI for evaluating various spondylitic root encroachment syndromes, but, when disc extrusion is present, CT and MRI are equally effective. The reduction of water content in the prolapsed intervertebral disc is evident. Gibson and colleagues[103, 104] showed the value of MRI in diagnosing disc degeneration in the absence of evidence on plain radiographs. In protrusion, degeneration is seen as a diminished signal that indicates reduced water content and is present at multiple levels in three quarters of patients with a single-level prolapse. This supports the hypothesis of Naylor and coworkers.[213] Demonstrating disc degeneration at various levels in the lumbar spine is a valuable means of assessing the suitability of patients for whom spinal fusion is to be considered, when the effects of the fusion on other levels that may be degenerate can be assessed.

Discography was described by Lindblom[172] and Hirsch[132] in 1948 as a means of localizing the sites of origin of discogenic leg pain. Adoption was slow.[77] In 1952, Cloward and Buzaid[51] described the use of discography as an indicator in the evaluation of the normal and abnormal intervertebral discs prior to surgical intervention. They described the appearance and size of normal and abnormal discs. Its further use over the past 30 years, with attempts to reproduce patients' symptoms by injecting the annulus and then the nucleus with a radiopaque dye to show the exact placement and localization, has led to disappointment regarding its efficacy. The degree of pain produced by an injection of saline into the disc varies with the degree of degeneration and the speed and amount of injection; moreover, in its simple form it did not accurately locate the source of the patient's pain, although it did reveal the extent of the disc degeneration. Adams and colleagues[1] have described the standard discograms showing the four stages of degeneration, which can be clearly defined. More valuable information is now available if discography is combined with CT scanning. This is a much more accurate investigative tool, especially if enhancement with metrizamide and computer integration with lateral and axial views are employed. Discography has experimentally been shown to have no adverse effect on the intervertebral disc.[154] Vaharanter and colleagues[294] and Videman and coworkers[254, 298] have developed a sophisticated method of classifying CT discography. Four stages, from normal through progressive degeneration to disruption, are shown. Disruption is noted to be most likely to be the source of exact pain reproduction.[294] The use of such CT axial and lateral views should now allow a much more accurate indication of the level and the site of discogenic pain.

The additional information afforded by electromyography that is conducted by a skilled clinical physiologist is invaluable in the assessment of nerve root involvement, in the exclusion of other neurologic disorders, and in the prognosis of nerve root involvement in disc disease. Meanwhile, nerve root infiltration at the point of emergence of the nerve from the canal is a useful method of demonstrating the level of pain production.[113, 183, 308]

The increased incidence of low back pain disorders during the last 30 years has led to a swell of research, both in the basic scientific and clinical fields. Our understanding of the spine—of its basic structure and ultrastructure, its chemical constitution, and its biochemical function—has been considerably advanced as a result of the cooperation of many medical specialties, together with the wider basic scientific fields of biochemistry, biomechanics and neurobiology. It has become more evident that acute short-term back pain resolves spontaneously, irrespective of methods of treatment. It has also become evident that surgery should not be employed in the absence of specific proof of a causal factor with proven anatomic source. Ample evidence is now available to show that multiple surgical interventions are liable to be followed by failure to give relief; thus, surgery or intradiscal therapy, with specific exceptions, should be used only after strict and thoroughly controlled conservative treatments have failed. Activity, and, in most cases, return to work are likely to be more beneficial for the patient.

Clinical research has shown that the integrity of the disc annulus should be maintained, except where it has been breached by a proven herniation (i.e., enucleation should be reserved for definite nuclear extrusion; the best results are obtained when sequestrated tissue is removed). Bulging degenerate discs should be left intact, as enucleation does not improve their function.

As an unstable condition usually stabilizes naturally, any surgical fusion must be believed to offer rapid and certain relief and to offer more benefits than conservative back school therapy. Although fusion has a definite place for spondylolisthesis, it must usually be combined with decompression when degenerative spondylolisthesis is present. Lateral, posterolateral, anterior, and posterior interbody fusions have ardent proponents, as do the improved internal fixation devices. However, evidence suggests that a careful assessment of the possible advantages of surgery over a nonsurgical method is imperative and is more important than the technical methods employed. The use of surgery and other invasive methods in treating low back pain has become far more restricted, selective, and carefully defined and has been aided by advances in diagnostic methods; this trend suggests that the low back surgeon might be "doomed to become a physician." The continued cooperation of basic and clinical scientific researchers is essential to achieve the goal of minimizing the use of invasive and surgical methods to treat those who suffer from low back pain.

References

1. Adams, M.A., Dolan, P., and Hutton, W.C.: The states of disc degeneration are revealed by discograms. J. Bone Joint Surg. 68B:36, 1986.
2. Adams, M.A., and Hutton, W.C.: The role of the apophyseal joints in resisting intervertebral compressive force. J. Bone Joint Surgery, 62B:358–363, 1980.
3. Adams, M.A., and Hutton, W.C.: The mechanical function of the lumbar apophyseal joints. Spine 8:327–330, 1983.
4. Adams, M.A., and Hutton, W.C.: The relevance of torsion to the mechanical derangements of the lumbar spine. Spine 6:241–248, 1981.
5. Adams, M.A., and Hutton, W.C.: Prolapsed intervertebral disc. A hyperflexion injury. Spine 7:184–191, 1982.
6. Adams, P., and Muir, H.: Qualitative changes with age of proteoglycans of human intervertebral discs. Ann. Rheum. Dis. 35:289–296, 1976.
7. Ake, W.E.: Results of decompression for lumbar spinal stenosis. Clin. Orthop. Rel. Res. 115:96–113, 1976.
8. Andersson, G.B.J., and Schultz, A.B.: Effects of fluid injection on the mechanical properties of intervertebral discs. J. Biomech. 12:453–458, 1979.
9. Andrae, B.: Über Knorpelknotchen in hinteren Ende des Wirbelbandscheiben im Bereich des Spinal Kanals. Beitragen Pathol. Anat. 82:464, 1929.
10. Antonopoulos, C.A.: Glycosaminoglycans of human nucleus pulposus: Identification and variation in their concentration with age. Acta Universitatis Lund 11:3–7, 1965.
11. Arnaldi, C.L., Brodsky, A.E., Cauchoix, J., et. al.: Lumbar spinal stenosis and nerve root entrapment. Clin. Orthop. Rel. Res. 115:4–5, 1976.
12. Badalamente, M.A., Dee, R., Ghillani, R., Chien-Putan, and Daniels, K.: Mechanical stimulation of dorsal root ganglion induces increased production of substance P. A mechanism for pain following nerve root compromise? Spine 12:552–555, 1987.
13. Badgeley, C.E.: The articular facets and relationship to low back pain and sciatic radiation. J. Bone Joint Surg. 23A:481–496, 1941.
14. Barrett, A.J.: The possible roles of neutral proteases in damage to articular cartilage. Agents Actions 8:11–18, 1978.
15. Bartelink, D.L.: The role of abdominal pressure in relieving the pressure on the lumbar intervertebral disc. J. Bone Joint Surg. 39B:718–725, 1957.
16. Beadle, A.O.: Special Report. Series Medical Research Council London, p. 161, 1931.
17. Beard, H.K., and Stevens, R.L.: Biochemical changes in intervertebral discs. *In* Jayson, M.I.V. (ed.): Lumbar Spine & Back Pain, 2nd Ed. London, Pitman, pp. 407–436, 1980.
18. Beard, H.K., Ryvar R., Brown R., and Muir H.: Immunochemical localisation of collagen types and proteoglycans in pig intervertebral discs. Immunology 41:491–507, 1980.

19. Beard, H.K., Roberts, S., and O'Brien, J.P.: Immunofluorescent staining for collagens and proteoglycans in normal and scoliotic intervertebral discs. J. Bone Joint Surg. 633:529–534, 1981.
20. Belytschko, T., Andriacchi, T., Schultz, A., and Galante, J.: Analog studies of forces in human spine. Computational techniques. J. Biochem. 6:361, 1973.
21. Bernadi, G., Happey, F., and Naylor, A.: Mucopolysaccharides from cartilage and nucleus pulposus. Nature 180:1341, 1957.
22. Berry, R.J.: Genetically controlled degeneration of the nucleus pulposus in the mouse. J. Bone Joint Surg. 43B:387, 1961.
23. Bisla, R.S., Marchisello, P.J., Lockshin, M.D., et al.: Auto-immune basis of disc degeneration. Clin. Orthop. Rel. Res. 121:205–211, 1976.
24. Blakey, P.R., Happey, F., Naylor A., and Turner, R.L.: Protein in the nucleus pulposus of the intervertebral disc. Nature 195:73, 1962.
25. Blau, J.N., Rushworth, G.: Observations of blood vessels of the spinal cord and their responses to motor activity. Brain 81:354–363, 1958.
25a. Blau, J.N., and Logue, V.: Intermittent claudication of the cauda equina. An unusual syndrome resulting from central protrusion of an intervertebral disc. Lancet 1:1081–1086, 1961.
26. Blundell-Bankart, A.S., and Newman, P.: Personal communication.
27. Bobechko, P., and Hirsch, C.: Auto-immune response of the nucleus pulposus in the rabbit. J. Bone Joint Surg. 47B:574, 1965.
28. Bogduk, N., and McIntosh, J.: The applied anatomy of the thoraco-lumbar fascia. Spine 9:164–170, 1984.
29. Böhmig, R.: Die Degenerationen der Wirbelbandscheiben und ihre Bedeutung fur die Klinik. München Mediziniche Wochenschrift 76:1318, 1929.
30. Bowen, V., and Cassidy, J.D.: Macroscopic and microscopic anatomy of the sacroiliac joint from embryonic life until the eighth decade. Spine 6:620–628, 1981.
31. Bradford, D.S., Cooper, K., and Oegema, T.R. Jr.: Chymopapain chemonucleolysis and nucleus pulposus degeneration and regeneration. A biochemical and biomechanical study (Volvo Prize). Spine 9:135–147 and J. Bone Joint Surg. 65A:1215, 1984.
32. Brain, R.: Cerebral spondylosis—the known and the unknown. Lancet 1:687–693, 1954.
33. Brinckman, P., Philbin, W., Hierholzer, E., and Horst, M.: Deformation of the vertebral endplate under axial loading of the spine. Spine 8:851–856, 1983.
34. Brinckman, P., and Horst, M.: The influence of vertebral body fracture, intradiscal injection and partial discectomy on radial bulge and height on human lumbar discs. Spine 10:138–145, 1985.
35. Brodin, H.: Paths of nutrition in articular cartilage. Acta Orthop. Scand. 24:177–183, 1955.
36. Bromley, J.W.: Results of intradiscal injection of collagenase in intervertebral disc prolapse. (Communication to the International Society for the Study of the Lumbar Spine. Paris Meeting, May, 1981.) Spine 8:322, 1983.
37. Bromley, J.W., Varma, A., Santoro, A., et al.: Double blind evaluation of collagenase injections for herniated lumbar discs. Spine 9:486–488, 1984.
38. Brown, M.: Pathophysiology of disc disease. Orthop. Clin. North Am. 2:359–370, 1971.
39. Brown, M.D., and Tompkins, J.S.: Chemoneucleolysis (Discolyses) with collagenase. Spine 11:123–130, 1986.
40. Brown, M., and Tsaltas, T.T.: Studies on the permeability of intervertebral discs during skeletal maturation. Spine 1:240, 1976.
41. Brown, T., Hanson, R., and Yarra, A.: Some mechanical tests on the lumbar spine with particular reference to the intervertebral disc. J. Bone Joint Surg. 39A:1135, 1957.
42. Bush, H.D., Horton, W.G., Smare, D.L., and Naylor, A.: Fluid content of the nucleus pulposus as a factor in the disc syndrome. Br. Med. J. 2:81, 1956.
43. Bushell, G.R., Ghosch, P., Taylor, T.K.F., and Alkeson, W.H.: Proteoglycans chemistry of intervertebral discs. Clin. Orthop. Rel. Res. 129:115–121, 1977.
44. Buttle, D.J.: Biochemical basis for the use of chymopapain in the treatment of sciatica. Ph.D. Thesis. London, British Library, 1985.
45. Buttle, D.J., Abrahamson, M., and Barrett, A.J.: Biochemistry of the action of chymopapain in relief of sciatica. Spine 11:688–694, 1986.
46. Caspar, W., and Iwa, H.: A microsurgery operation for lumbar disc herniation. Neurol. Surg. 6:657, 1979.
47. Chaffin, D.B.: Human strength capability and low back pain. J. Occup. Med. 16:248, 1974.
48. Charnley, J.: Imbibition of fluid as a cause of herniation of the nucleus pulposus. International Congress of Orthopaedic Surgery 5, Stockholm. Lancet 1:124, 1952.
49. Chisin, R., Milgrom, C., Margonlier J., et al.: Unilateral sacro-iliac overuse syndrome in military recruits. Br. Med. J. 289:590–591, 1984.
50. Chrisman, O.D., Mittracht, A., and Snook, G.A., A study of the results following rotatory manipulation in lumbar intervertebral disc syndrome. J. Bone Joint Surg. 46A:517–524, 1964.
51. Cloward, R.B., and Buzaid, L.L.: Discography, technique indications, evaluation of normal and abnormal intervertebral discs. A.J.R. 68:552, 1952.
52. Colachis, S.C., Warden, R.E., Becktol, C.O., and Strohm, B.R.: Movement of the sacro-iliac joint in the adult male. Preliminary report. Arch. Phys. Med. Rehab. 44:490–498, 1963.
53. Cole, T.C., Ghosch, P., Taylor, T.K.F.: Arteparon modifies proteoglycans turnover in the intervertebral disc. 46th Scientific Meeting, Australian Orthopaedic Association, Sydney, September 1986. J. Bone Joint Surg. 70B:164, 166, 1988.
54. Contugno, D.F.A.: Quoted by Ehni, G., Presidential Address, International Society for the Study of the Lumbar Spine. May, 1980.
55. Copeman, W.S.C. (ed.): Textbook of Rheumatic Diseases, 3rd Ed. Edinburgh, Livingstone, 1984.
56. Coventry, M.B., Ghormley, R.K., and Kernohan, J.W.: The intervertebral disc. Its microscopic anatomy and pathology. Part I. Anatomy and development and physiology. J. Bone Joint Surg. 27:105–112, 1945; Part II. Changes in the intervertebral disc concomitant with age. J. Bone Joint Surg. 27:233–242, 1945; Part III. Pathological changes in the intervertebral disc. J. Bone Joint Surg. 27:460–474, 1945.
57. Crawshaw, C., Fraser, A.M., Merriam, W.F., et al.: A comparison of surgery and chemonucleolysis

in the treatment of sciatica. Prospective randomised trials. Spine 9:194–198, 1984.
58. Crock, H.V.: A reappraisal of intervertebral disc lesions. Med. J. Aust. 1:983, 1970.
59. Crock, H.V.: Isolated disc resorption as a cause of nerve root canal stenosis. Clin. Orthop. Rel. Res. 115:109, 1976.
60. Crock, H.V., and Ishiwara, H.: The blood supply of the vertebral column and spinal cord in man. New York, Springer-Verlag, 1977.
61. Cryon, B.M., and Hutton, W.: Articular tropism and stability of the lumbar spine. Spine 6:168–172, 1980.
62. Dahlin, L.B., Rydevik, B., and Lundborg, G.: Pathophysiology of nerve entrapments and nerve compression injuries. *In* Hargens, A.R. (ed.): Tissue Nutrition and Viability. New York, Springer-Verlag, 1987.
63. Danforth, M.W., and Wilson, P.D.: Anatomy of the lumbosacral region in relief of sciatic pain. J. Bone Joint Surg. 7:109, 1925.
64. Davidson, E.A., and Woodall, B.: Biochemical alterations in herniated intervertebral discs. Biochem. J. 11:251; J. Biol. Chem. 234:2951–2954, 1959.
65. Delchef, J.: [The advantages and disadvantages of ischio-femoral arthrodesis; A curious myographic image.] Acta Orthop. Belg. 27:476–485, 515–518, 1961.
66. De Puky, P.: The physiological oscillation of the length of the body. Acta Orthop. Scand. 6:338, 1935.
67. Diamant, B., Karlson, J., and Nachemson, A.: Correlation between lactate levels and pH in discs of patients with lumbar rhizopathies. Experentia (Basel) 24:1195–1196, 1968.
68. Domisse, G.F.: Arteries and veins of the lumbar nerve roots and cauda equina. Clin. Orthop. Rel. Res. 115:22–29, 1976.
69. Douglas, D.L., Duckworth, T., Cannis, J.A., et al.: Spinal cord dysfunction in Paget's disease of bone. Has medical treatment a vascular basis? J. Bone Joint Surg. 63B:495–503, 1981.
70. Edgar, M.A., and Nundy, S.: Innervation of spinal dura mater. J. Neurol. Neurosurg. Psychiatr. 29:530–534, 1966.
71. Edgar, M.A., and Park, W.M.: Induced pain patterns in passive straight leg raising lower disc protrusion. J. Bone Joint Surg. 56B:658, 1974.
72. Ehni, G.: A significance of the small lumbar spinal canal cauda equina syndrome due to spondylosis. Part I. Introduction. J. Neurosurg. 31:490, 1969; Part IV. Acute compression artificially induced during operation. J. Neurosurg. 31:507, 1969.
73. Elsberg, C.A.: Diagnosis and treatment of surgical diseases of the spinal cord and its membranes. Philadelphia, W.B. Saunders, 1916.
74. Elwes, M.W., Bucknill, T., and Sullivan, M.: In vitro inhibition of leucocyte migration in patients with intervertebral disc lesions. Orthop. Clin. North Am. 6:59–65, 1975.
75. Emes, J.H., and Pearce, R.H.: Proteoglycans of the human intervertebral disc. Biochem. J. 145:545–556, 1975.
76. Epstein, J.A., Epstein, B.S., and Lavine, L.: Nerve root compression with narrowing of the lumbar spinal canal. J. Neurol. Neurosurg. Psychiatr. 25:165, 1962.
77. Erlacher, P.R.: Nucleography. J. Bone Joint Surg. 34B:204–210, 1952.
78. Eyre, D.R.: Biochemistry of intervertebral disc. Internat. Rev. Conn. Tiss. Res. 8:227–291, 1979.
79. Eyre, D.R., and Muir, H.: Types I and II collagens in intervertebral disc. Interchanging radial distribution in annulus fibrosus. Biochim. Biophys. Acta 492:29–42, 1976.
80. Eyre, D.R., and Muir, H.: Quantitative analysis of types I and II collagens in human intervertebral discs at various ages. Biochim. Biophys. Acta 492:29–42, 1977.
81. Fairbank, J.C.T., Park, W.M., McCall, I.W., and O'Brien, J.P.: Apophyseal injection of local anaesthetic as a diagnostic aid in primary low back syndromes. Spine 6:598–605, 1981.
82. Farfan, H.: Mechanical Disorders of the Low Back. Philadelphia, Lea & Febiger, 1973.
83. Farfan, H.: Muscular mechanism of the lumbar spine and the position of power and efficiency. Orthop. Clin. North Am. 6:135–144, 1975.
84. Farfan, H., Cossett, J.W., Robertson, G.H., et al.: Effect of torsion on the lumbar intervertebral joints. The role of torsion in the production of disc degeneration. J. Bone Joint Surg. 52A:468, 1970.
85. Farfan, H., Hubidor, R.M., Dubow, H.I.: Lumbar intervertebral disc degeneration. J. Bone Joint Surg. 54A:492, 1972.
86. Feffer, H.: Treatment of low back pain and sciatica by injection of hydrocortisone into degenerated discs. J. Bone Joint Surg. 38A:585, 1956.
87. Fick, R.: Handbuch der Anatomie und Mechanik der Glenke. Jena, Gustav Fischer Verlag, 1904.
88. Finnegan, W.J., Fenlan, J.M., Marvel, J.P., et al.: Results of surgical intervention in the symptomatic multiple operated back patient. J. Bone Joint Surg. 61A:10, 70, 1979.
89. Foerster, O.: The dermatomes in man. Brain 56:1–39, 1933.
90. Forst, J.J.: Quoted by Cauchoix, J., Presidential Address, International Society for the Study of the Lumbar Spine, June, 1978.
91. Frailoli, F., Moretti, C., Paolucci, D., et al.: Physical exercise stimulates marked concomitant release of beta endorphin and adrenocorticotrophic hormone (ACTH) in peripheral blood in man. Experiencia 36:987, 1980.
92. Fraser, R.D.: Chymopapain for the treatment of intervertebral disc prolapse. A double blind study. Spine 7:608, 1982.
93. Fraser, R.D.: Chymopapain for the treatment of intervertebral disc prolapse. A double blind study. Spine 9:815–818, 1984.
94. Frymoyer, J.W., Harley, E., Howe, J., et al.: Disc excision and spine fusion in the management of disc disease. Spine 3:1, 7, 1978.
95. Frymoyer, J.W., and Mooney, V.: Current Concepts Review. Occupational Orthopaedics. J. Bone Joint Surg. 68A:468–473, 1986.
96. Gardell, S., Rastgeldie, S.: The mucopolysaccharides of nucleus pulposus. Acta Chem. Scand. 8:362, 1954.
97. Gerztbein, S., Tile, M., Gross, A., and Falk, R.: Autoimmunity in degenerative disc disease of lumbar spine. Orthop. Clin. North Am. 6:67, 1975.
98. Gertzbein, S., Tait, J.H., and Devlin, S.R.: Stimulation of lymphocytes by nucleus pulposus in

patients with degenerative disc disease of lumbar spine. Clin. Orthop. Rel. Res. 123:149, 1977.
99. Ghormley, R.K.: Low back pain with special reference to the articular facets, with presentation of an operative procedure. J. Am. Med. Assoc. 1:1773, 1933.
100. Ghosch, P., Knight, J., Stevens, R.W., et al.: Comparative study of the proteoglycanase inhibitors in intervertebral discs of various mammalian species. Proc. Aust. Biochem. Soc. 12:27, 1979.
101. Ghosch, P., Taylor, T.K.F., Bushell, J.R., and Stevens, R.W.: Neutral protease inhibitors from human intervertebral discs and femoral head cartilage. Trans. Orthop. Res. Soc. 4:47, 1971.
102. Ghosch, P., Taylor, T.K.F., and Horsborough, B.A.: The composition and protein metabolism in immature rabbit intervertebral disc. Cell Tiss. Res. 163:223–238, 1975.
103. Gibson, M.J., Buckley, J.M., Worthington, B.S., and Mulholland, R.C.: Magnetic resonance imaging of the intervertebral disc. Read at Manchester meeting of the British Back Pain Research Society. *In* Hukins, D.W.L., and Mulholland, R.C. (eds.): Back Pain. Methods for Clinical Investigation and Assessment. Manchester, University Press, 1986.
104. Gibson, M.J., Szypryt, E.P., Buckley, J.M., et al.: Magnetic resonance imaging of adolescent disc herniations. J. Bone Joint Surg. 69B:699–703, 1987.
105. Gill, K., Videman, T., Shimizu, T., and Mooney, V.: Effect of Arteparon in rabbit degenerative disc model. Read at International Society for the Study of the Lumbar Spine Meeting, Rome, May, 1987.
106. Gill, C.G., Sacowicz, L., and Thompson, E.: Pedicle fat grafts for prevention of scar formation after laminectomy. An experimental study in dogs. Spine 4:176, 1979.
107. Göcke, C.: Uber die quellung des Wirbelsbandscheiben. Das Verhalten des Bandscheiben bei Wirbelverletzungen. Arch. Orthop. Unfall-Chirurg. 31:43.
108. Goldthwaite, J.E., and Osgood, R.B.: Boston Med. Surg. J. 21:22, 1905.
109. Goldthwaite, J.E.: The lumbosacral articulation. An explanation of many cases of "lumbago," sciatica and paraplegia. Boston Med. Surg. J. 164:365–372, 1911.
110. Gracovetsky, S., and Farfan, H.: The abdominal mechanism. Spine 10:317–324, 1985.
111. Gunterberg, B.: Effects of major resection of the sacrum. Clinical studies on urogenital and rectal fusion and a biochemical study on pelvic strength (thesis). Goteborg, Uno. Lungren Tryckeri, A.B., 1975.
112. Haldemann, S.: Spinal manipulative therapy—a status report. Clin. Orthop. Rel. Res. 179:62–70, 1983.
113. Haldemann, S.: The electrodiagnostic evaluation of nerve root function. Spine 9:42, 1984.
114. Hannai, K.: Dynamic measurements of interosseous pressures in lumbar spinal vertebrae with special reference to spinal canal stenosis. Spine 5:568–574, 1980.
115. Hansen, H.J.: A pathologic-anatomical interpretation of disc degeneration in dogs. Acta Orthopaedica Scandinavica 20–208. Acta Orthop. Scand. supplement II (1952).
116. Hansen, H.J., and Ullberg, S.: Uptake of S^{35} after injection of S^{35} sulphate. An auto-radiographic study. J. Bone Joint Surg. 52B:371, 1960.
117. Hansson, T., and Roos, B.: The relationship between bone mineral content, experimental fracture and disc degeneration. Spine 6:147, 1981.
118. Hansson, T., Roos, B., Sandström, J., et al.: The bone mineral content of the lumbar spine in patients with chronic low back pain. Spine 10:158, 1985.
119. Happey, F.: Studies in the structure of the human intervertebral disc in relation to its function and aging processes. *In* Solcoloff, L. (ed.): The Joints and Synovial Fluid. 2: 95–137. New York, Acad. Press, 1980.
120. Happey, F., Johnson, A.G., Naylor, A., and Turner, R.L.: Preliminary observations concerning the fine structure of the intervertebral disc. J. Bone Joint Surg. 46B:563, 1964.
121. Happey, F., Naylor, A., and MacRae, T.: Collagenous changes in the intervertebral disc. Symposium on Collagen. London, Faraday Society, 1953.
122. Happey, F., Wiseman, A., and Naylor, A.: Polysaccharide content of the prolapsed nucleus pulposus of the human intervertebral disc. Nature 192:868, 1961.
123. Hayes, M.A., Howard, T.C., Grewal, C.R., and Copter, J.A.: Roentgenographic evaluation of lower spine flexion and extension in normal individuals (abstr.). New Orleans, Federation Spinal Association, Feb., 1986.
124. Hedtmann, A., Steffan, R., and Krämer, J.: Prospective comparative study of intradiscal high-dose and low-dose collagenase versus chymopapain. Spine 12:388–392, 1987.
125. Hendry, N.G.C.: Hydration of the nucleus pulposus and its relation to intervertebral disc derangement. J. Bone Joint Surg. 40B:132, 1958.
126. Herbert, C.M., Lindberg, K.A., Jayson, M.I.V., and Bailey, A.J.: Changes in collagen of human intervertebral discs during aging and degenerative disc disease. J. Mol. Med. 1:79–91, 1975.
127. Her Majesty's Stationery Office Publications, No. 36: Morbidity statistics from general practice (1971–1972). London, Her Majesty's Stationery Office, 1979.
128. Hickey, D.S., and Hukins, D.W.O.: The relationship between structure of the annulus fibrosus on function and failure of the intervertebral disc. Spine 5:106–116, 1980.
129. Hickey, D.S., and Hukins, D.W.O.: Aging changes in the macromolecular organization of the intervertebral disc: An X-ray diffraction and electron microscopic study. Spine 7:234–242, 1982.
130. Hickey, D.S., and Hukins, D.W.O.: Collagen fibril diameters and elastic fibres of human foetal intervertebral discs. J. Anat. 133:351–357, 1987.
131. Hickey, D.S., and Hukins, D.W.O.: X-ray diffraction studies of the arrangement of collagenous fibres in human foetal intervertebral disc. J. Anat. 131:81–90, 1980.
132. Hirsch, C.: An attempt to diagnose the level of a disc lesion clinically by disc puncture. Acta Orthop. Scand. 18:132, 1948.
133. Hirsch, C., Paulsson, S., Sylven, B., and Snellman, O.: Biophysical and physiological investigations on cartilage and other mesenchymal tissues. II. The ultrastructure of bovine and human nuclei pulposi. J. Bone Joint Surg. 33A:333, 1951.

134. Hirsch, C., Paulsson S., Sylven, B., and Snellman, O.: Biophysical and physiological investigations on cartilage and other mesenchymal tissue. IV. Characteristics of human nuclei pulposi during aging. Acta Orthop. Scand. 22:175, 1952.
135. Hirsch, C.: Studies on the mechanism of low back pain. Acta Orthop. Scand. (Suppl. 20):261, 1951.
136. Hirsch, C.: The reaction of the intervertebral disc to compression forces. J. Bone Joint Surg. 37A:1188, 1955.
137. Holm, S., and Nachemson, A.: Variations in the nutrition of the canine intervertebral disc induced by motion. Spine 8:866–873, 1983.
138. Holm, S., and Nachemson, A.: Nutritional changes in canine intervertebral discs after spinal fusion. Clin. Orthop. Rel. Res. 169:243–258, 1982.
139. Holm S., Maroudas, A., Urban, J.P.G., et al.: Nutrition of the intervertebral disc. Solute transport and metabolism. Connect. Tissue Res. 8:101–119, 1987.
140. Holm, S., and Selstam, G.: In vivo measurements of relationship between arterial intradiscal oxygen tension. Uppsala J. Med. 87:163–174, 1982.
141. Horst, P., and Brinckman, P.: Measurements of the distribution of axial stress on the end plate of the vertebral body. Spine 6:217–232, 1981.
142. Horton, W.G.: Further observations on the elastic mechanism of the intervertebral disc. J. Bone Joint Surg. 40B:552, 1958.
143. Hovelacque, A.: Le nerf sinu vertebral. Ann. Anat. Pathol. Med. J. 2:435, 1925.
144. Iggo, A.: Non-myelinated visceral muscular and cutaneous afferent fibres and pain. *In* Keele, C.A., and Smith, R. (eds.): U.F.A.W. Symposium, Assessments of Pain in Man and Animals. London, Livingstone, 1962, p. 74.
145. Iggo, A.: The case for pain receptors. *In* Jansen, R., Keidel, W.D., Hirst, A., and Steichele, C. (eds.): Pain. Basic Principles. Pharmacology and Therapy. Stuttgart, Thieme, 1974, p. 60.
146. Inman, V.T., and Saunders, J.B.: Referred pain from skeletal structures. J. Nerv. Ment. Dis. 99:660–667, 1944.
147. Inoue, H.: Three dimensional collagen framework of collagen intervertebral discs in rats, dogs and humans. Arch Histolog. Jpn. 36:39–56, 1973.
148. Inoue, H., and Takeda, T.: Three dimensional observations of collagen framework of intervertebral discs. Acta Orthop. Scand. 46:949–956, 1975.
149. Jacobs, R.R., and McLaine, F.J.: Control of post laminectomy scar formation. Spine 5:223, 1980.
150. Jayson, M.I.V.: Chronic inflammation and fibrosis in back pain syndromes. *In* Jayson, M.I.V. (ed): Lumbar Spine and Back Pain, 3rd Ed. London, Pitman, 1987.
151. Jayson, M.I.V., Herbert, C.M., and Barks, J.S.: Intervertebral disc morphology and bursting pressures. Ann. Rheum. Dis. 32:308–315, 1973.
152. Jayson, M.I.V., Keegan, A., Million, R., and Tomlinson, I.: A fibrinolytic defect in chronic back pain syndrome. Lancet 2:1186–1187, 1984.
153. Junghanns, H.: Der Lumbosacralwinkel. Deutsch Zeitschrift Chirurgic 213:322, 1929.
154. Kahanowicz, N., Arnoczky, S.P., Sisson, H.A., et al.: The effects of discography on the canine intervertebral disc. Spine 11:26–27, 1986.
155. Kazarian, L.E.: Pre-characteristics of the human spinal column. Orthop. Clin. North Am. 6:3, 1975.
156. Keiser, P., and Sandson, J.: Immunology of cartilage proteoglycans. Federat. Proc. 32:1474–1477, 1973.
157. Kellgren, J.H.: Observations of referred pain arising from muscle. Clin. Sci. Mol. Med. 175:190, 1938.
158. Kellgren, J.H.: On the distribution of pain rising from deep somatic structures with charts of segmental pain areas. Clin. Sci. Mol. Med. 4:35–46, 1939.
159. Kelsey, J.L., Githens, P.B., White, A.A., et al.: An epidemiological study of lifting and twisting on the job and risk for acute prolapsed intervertebral disc. J. Orthop. Res. 2:61–68, 1984.
160. Kelsey, J.L., and Hardy, R.J.: Driving of motor vehicles as a risk factor in acute herniated lumbar intervertebral disc. Am. J. Epidemiol. 102:63–75, 1975.
161. Key, J.A.: Intervertebral disk lesions are most common cause of low back pain with or without sciatica. Ann. Surg. 121:534, 1945.
162. Keyes, D.C., and Compere, D.L.: The normal and pathological physiology of the nucleus pulposus of the intervertebral disc. An anatomical and clinical and experimental study. J. Bone Joint Surg. 14:897, 1932.
163. Kirkaldy Willis, W.H., and Farfan, H.F.: Instability of the lumbar spine. Clin. Orthop. 165:110–123, 1982.
164. Klein, J.A., and Hukins, D.W.O.: Collagen fibre orientation in the annulus fibrosus of intervertebral disc during bending and torsion measured by X-ray diffraction. Biochim. Biophys. Acta 719:98–101, 1982.
165. Knight, J., Stevens, R.W., Bushell, J.R., et al.: Neutral proteins inhibitors from human intervertebral discs and femoral cartilage. Biochim. Biophys. Acta 584:304–310, 1979.
166. Krämer, J.: Biopolymer and Biomechanic von Bindegewebs system. New York, Springer-Verlag, 1974.
167. Krämer, J.: Pressure dependent fluid shifts in the intervertebral disc. Orthop. Clin. North Am. 8:211, 1972.
168. Krämer, J., Kolditz, D., and Gowin, R.: Water and electrolyte content of human intervertebral disc under variable load. Spine 10:69–71, 1985.
169. Krämer, J., and Laternous, H.: Lumbar intradiscal instillation with aprotinin (Transxylol). Spine 7:73, 1982.
170. LaRocha, H., and McNab, I.: The laminectomy membrane. Studies of evolution, characteristics and effects of prophylaxis in dogs. J. Bone Joint Surg. 56B:545–550, 1974.
170a. Lauterbaur, P.C.: Image formation by induced local inter-reactions. Examples employed in NMR. Nature 242:190–191, 1973.
171. Lidstrom, A. and Zachrisson, M.: Physical therapy in low back pain and sciatica. An attempt in evaluation. Scand. J. Rehab. Med. 2:37, 1970.
172. Lindblom, K.: Diagnostic puncture of intervertebral disc in sciatica. Acta Orthop. Scand. 17:231, 1948.
173. Lipson, S.J., and Muir, H.: Experimental intervertebral disc degeneration. Arth. Rheum. 24:12–21, 1981.
174. Liu, K.Y., Ray, G., and Hirsch, C.: Resistance of the lumbar spine to direct shear. Orthop. Clin. North Am. 6:33, 1975.

175. Lorenz, M., Patwardham, A., and Vanderby, R., Jr.: Load bearing characteristics of lumbar facets in normal and surgically altered spinal segments. Spine 8:122, 1983.
176. Lyman Smith, Garvin, P.J., and Gesler, R.M.: Enzyme dissolution of the nucleus pulposus. Nature 4887:1311–1312, 1963.
177. Lyman Smith: Enzyme dissolution of the nucleus pulposus in humans. J. Am. Med. Assoc. 187:137–140, 1964.
178. Lyman Smith, and Brown, J.E.: Treatment of lumbar intervertebral disc lesions by direct injections of chymopapain. J. Bone Joint Surg. 49B:502–519, 1967.
179. Lyons, H., Jones, E., Quinn, F., and Sprunt, D.: Changes in protein polysaccharide fractions of nucleus pulposus from human intervertebral discs with age and herniation. J. Lab. Clin. Med. 68:930, 1966.
180. McCall, I.W., Park, W.M., and O'Brien, J.P.: Induced pain referral from posterior lumbar elements in normal subjects. Spine 4:441–446, 1979.
181. McCullough, J.A.: Chemonucleolysis. J. Bone Joint Surg. 57B:45, 1977.
182. McEwan, S.J., Sherlock, D., Kinross, R., et al.: Prostaglandins in disc nuclei. Read at British Back Pain Research Society Meeting, Manchester, March, 1986.
183. McNab, I.: Backache. Baltimore, Williams & Wilkins, 1977.
184. McNicol, D.: Cell receptors to sulphated polysaccharides in normal synovial joint. 46th Scientific Meeting, Australian Orthopaedic Association, Sydney, Sept., 1986. J. Bone Joint Surg. 70B:164, 1988.
185. Magnaes, B.: Clinical recording of pressure on the spinal cord and cauda equina. J. Neurosurg. 57:63, 1982.
186. Main, C.J.: The modified somatic perception questionnaire (M.S.P.Q.). J. Psychosom. Res. 27:503–514, 1983.
187. Malmgren, H., and Sylven, B.: Biophysical and physiological investigations on cartilage and other mesenchymal tissues. 5. Identification of the polysaccharide of bovine nuclei pulposi. Biochim. Biophys. Acta (Amst.) 9:706, 1952.
188. Mansfield, P., and Grannell, P.K.: Spacial structure in solids. NMR "diffraction" in solids? (letter to editor). J. Phys. C. Solid State Physics. 6:422–425, 1973.
189. Markol, K., and Morris, J.M.: The structural components of the intervertebral disc. A study of their contributions to the ability of the disc to withstand compressive forces. J. Bone Joint Surg. 56a:675–687, 1974.
190. Melzack, R., and Wall, P.D.: Pain mechanisms. A new theory. Science 150:971, 1965.
191. Melzack, R., and Wall, P.D.: Gate control theory of pain. *In* Soulairac, A., Cahn, N.J., and Sharpantia, J. (eds.): Pain. New York, Academic Press, 1968.
192. Middleton, G.S., and Teacher, J.H.: Injury of the spinal cord due to rupture of an intervertebral disk during muscular effort. Glasgow Med. J. 76:1, 1911.
193. Mixter, W.J., and Barr, J.S.: Rupture of the intervertebral disc with involvement of the spinal canal. N. Engl. J. Med. 211:210, 1934.
194. Mooney, V., and Robertson, J.: The facet syndrome. Clin. Orthop. Rel. Res. 115:149–156, 1976.
195. Morrison, R.I.G., Barrett, A.J., Dingle, J.T., and Prior, D.: Cathepsins B and D action on human cartilage proteoglycans. Biochim. Biophys. Acta 302:411–419, 1973.
196. Muir, H.: Biochemistry of articular cartilage. *In* Freeman, M.A.R. (ed): Adult Cartilage, 2nd Ed. London, Pitman, 1979.
197. Nachemson, A.: Measurement of intradiscal pressure. Acta Orthop. Scand. 28:269, 1959.
198. Nachemson, A.: Lumbar intradiscal pressure. Experimental studies on post mortem material. Acta Orthop. Scand. (Suppl. XLIII):7–104, 1960.
199. Nachemson, A.: Intradiscal measurements of pH in patients with lumbar rhizopathies. Acta Orthop. Scand. 40:23, 1969.
200. Nachemson, A., and Evans, J.H.: Some mechanical properties of the third lumbar interlaminar ligament (ligamentum flavum). J. Biomech. 1:211–220, 1968.
201. Nachemson, A., Lewin, T., Maroudas, A., and Freeman, M.A.R.: In vitro diffusion of dye through the endplates of the annulus fibrosus of human intervertebral discs. Acta Orthop. Scand. 41:589–607, 1970.
202. Nachemson, A., and Morris, J.M.: Lumbar discometry—measurements in vivo. Lancet 1:1140, 1963.
203. Nachemson, A., and Morris, J.M.: In vivo measurement of intradiscal pressure. Discometry—a method for the determination of pressure in the lower intervertebral discs. J. Bone Joint Surg. 46A:7–92, 1964.
204. Nade, S., Pell, E., and Wyke, B.D.: Articular neurology of the feline lumbar spine. Proc. Austr. N. Z. Orthop. Assoc. Oct. 1977, p. 6.
205. Naylor, A.: Fluid content of nucleus pulposus as a factor in the disc syndrome. Communication to British Orthopaedic Association. Sheffield, Oct., 1952.
206. Naylor, A., and Smare, D.L.: Fluid content of the nucleus pulposus as a factor in the disc syndrome. Br. Med. J. 2:1975, 1953.
207. Naylor, A.: The biophysical and biochemical aspects of intervertebral disc herniation and degeneration. Ann. R. Coll. Surg. Engl. 9:31–73, 1962.
208. Naylor, A.: Biochemical changes in the human intervertebral disc in degeneration and nuclear prolapse. Orthop. Clin. North Am. 2:343–359, 1971.
209. Naylor, A.: Intervertebral disc prolapse and degeneration. A biochemical and biophysical approach. Spine 1:108–114, 1976.
210. Naylor, A.: Factors in the development of the spinal stenosis syndrome. J. Bone Joint Surg. 61B:306–309, 1979.
211. Naylor, A., Happey, F., and MacRae, T.: The collagenous changes in the intervertebral disc with age—a biophysical study. An X-ray crystallographic study. Br. Med. J. 2:570, 1954.
212. Naylor, A., Happey, F., Turner, R.L., et al.: Enzymic and immunological activity in the intervertebral disc. Orthop. Clin. North Am. 6:51–73, 1975.
213. Naylor, A., and Horton, W.G.: The hydrophilic properties of the intervertebral disc. Rheumatism 11:32–35, 1955.
214. Naylor, A., Earland, C., and Robinson, J.: The

effect of diagnostic radio-opaque fluids used in discography on the chymopapain activity. Read to International Society for the Study of the Lumbar Spine, Toronto, June, 1982. Spine 8:875, 1983.
215. Naylor, A., and Turner, R.L.: ACTH in treatment of lumbar disc prolapse. Proc. R. Soc. Med., 54:282–284, 1961.
216. Nelson, M.A.: Orthopaedic aspects of the chondrodystrophies. (Robert Jones Prize Essay, British Orthopaedic Association.) Ann. R. Coll. Surg. Engl. 47:185–210, 1970.
217. Newman, P.H.: Sprung back. J. Bone Joint Surg. 34B:30–37, 1952.
218. Nordby, E.J., and Lucas, J.L.: Comparative analysis of lumbar disc disease treated by laminectomy or chemonucleolysis. J. Bone Joint Surg.
219. O'Brien, J.: Anterior spinal tenderness in low back pain syndromes. Spine 4:279, 1979.
220. Olmarker, K., Rydevik, B., Dahlin, L.B., et. al.: Effects of epidural and intrathecal application of collagenase in the lumbar spine. An experimental study in rabbits. Spine 12:477–482, 1987.
221. Onofrio, B.: Injecting chymopapain into intervertebral discs. J. Neurosurg. 42:384, 1975.
222. Ooi, Y., Mita, F., and Satoh, Y.: Pathophysiological study of intermittent claudication in the lumbar spinal stenosis. Read at International Society for Study of the Lumbar Spine Meeting, Dallas, May 31, 1986.
223. Orpen, L.A., Singer, F.R.: Paget's Disease. Reversal of severe paraparesis with calcitonin. Spine 4:213–219, 1979.
224. Oudenhoven, R.C.: The results of facet denervation. Presented at International Society for Study of the Lumbar Spine Meeting, Paris, 1981.
225. Panjabi, M.M., and Brand, R.A.: Three dimensional flexibility and stiffness properties of the human thoracic spine. J. Biomech. 9:185–192, 1976.
226. Pankovich, A. M., and Korngold, L.: A comparison with antigenic properties of nucleus pulposus and cartilage protein polysaccharides. J. Immunol. 99:431, 1967.
227. Paris, S.B.: Functional anatomy of the lumbar spine. Ph.D. Thesis, University of Atlanta, 1983.
228. Parke, W.W., and Wattenabe, R.: The intrinsic vacculature of the lumbosacral spinal nerve roots. Spine 10:510, 1985.
229. Pearcey, M.J., and Tilsewal, S.B.: Axial rotation and lateral bending in normal lumbar spine measured by 3-dimensional radiography. Spine 6:582, 1984.
230. Pedersen, H.S., Blunck, C.J.F., and Gardener, E.D.: Anatomy of the lumbosacral posterior rami and meningeal branches of spinal nerves (sinovertebral nerves) with an experimental study of their function. J. Bone Joint Surg. 38A-377, 1956.
231. Pheasant, H.C., and Dyck, P.: Failed lumbar disc surgery. Cause, assessment, treatment. Clin. Orthop. Rel. Res. 164:93, 1982.
232. Pope, M.H., Wilder, D.G., Mattireri, R.E., and Frymoyer, J.W.: Experimental measures of vertebral motion under load. Orthop. Clin. North Am. 8:155, 1977.
233. Porter, R.W., Wicks, M., and Ottewell, D.: Measurement of the spinal canal by diagnostic ultrasound. J. Bone Joint Surg. 60B:481–487, 1978.
234. Porter, R.W., and Hibbert, C.: Calcitonin treatment for neurogenic claudication. Spine 8:585–592, 1983.
235. Porter, R.W., Hibbert, C., and Wilman, P.: Backache and the lumbar spinal canal. Spine 5:99–105, 1980.
236. Posner, J., White, A.A., Edwards, W.T., and Hayes, M.A.: Biomechanical analysis of clinical stability of lumbar and lumbo-sacral spines. Spine 7:374, 1982.
237. Postacchini, F., Bolotchi, M., Ricciardi-Pollini, P.T., and Modesti, A.: Ultrastructural study of recurrent disc herniations. A preliminary report. Spine 7:492–497, 1982.
238. Postacchini, F., Lami, R., and Massobrio, M.: Chemonucleolysis versus surgery in lumbar disc herniations—correlation of results of pre-operative clinical pattern and size of herniation. Spine 12:87–96, 1987.
239. Potts, E., Hutchinson, G., Stern, J., and Clark, K.: A comparison of intervertebral disc disease treatment by chymopapain injection and open surgery. J. Neurosurg. 42:397, 1975.
240. Puig, M.M., Laordin, M.L., Miralles, F.S., and Olassa, M.H.: Endorphin levels in cerebrospinal fluid in patients with post-operative chronic pain. Anaesthesiology 57:1, 1982.
241. Püschel, J.: Der Wassergehalt normaler und degenereiter zwischen Wirbelscheiben. Beitrazen Pathol. Anat. Allgemeine Pathol. 84:123, 1930.
242. Putti, V.: New concepts in the pathogenesis of sciatic pain, Lancet 2:53–60, 1927.
243. Pyle, E.: Congenital abnormalities of the lumbosacral region as causes of persistent low back pain. N. Engl. J. Med. 204:1083–1088.
244. Ransford, A.O., Cairns, D., and Mooney, V.: The pain diagram as an aid to the psychological evaluation of patients with low back pain. Spine 1:127, 1976.
245. Rees, W.S.: Multiple bilateral subcutaneous rhizolysis of segmental nerves in the treatment of intervertebral disc syndrome. Ann. Gen. Pract. 26:126–127, 1971.
246. Reichert, F.L., Rytand, D.A., and Brook, D.L.: Arteriosclerosis of the lumbar segmental arteries producing ischaemia of the spinal cord and consequent claudication of the thighs. Am. J. Med. Sci. 187:794–806, 1935.
247. Roofe, P.G.: Innervation of annulus fibrosus and posterior longitudinal ligament. Arch. Neurol. Psychiatr. 44:100, 1940.
248. Ross-Smith, N.R.: Br. J. Surg. 18:358, 1931.
249. Rothman, R.H., and Booth, R.: Failures of spine fusion. Orthop. Clin. North Am. 6:299, 1975.
250. Rothman, R.H., Booth, R., Cuckler, J.M., et al.: A study of computer assisted tomography. Comparison of metrizamide myelography and CAT in diagnosis of herniated lumbar disc and spinal stenosis. Spine 9:552–556, 1984.
251. Rydevik, D., Holm, S., Brown, M.D., and Lundborg, H.: Nutrition of spinal nerve roots. The role of diffusion from the cerebrospinal fluid. Transactions of the 30th Orthopaedic Research Society Meeting. 9:276, 1984.
252. Rydevik, B., Branemark, P.I., Nordberg, C., et al.: Effects of chymopapain on nerve tissue. Spine 1:137, 1976.
253. Rydevik, B., Brown, M.D., Thira, T., and Nordberg, C.: Effects of collagenase on nerve tissue. An

experimental study on acute and long term effects in rabbit. Spine 10:562–566, 1985.
254. Sachs, B.L., Vaharanter, H., Spivery, M.A., et al.: The Dallas discogram: A new classification of CT discography in low back disorders. Spine 2:287–293, 1987.
255. Sarpyener, M.A.: Congenital stricture of the spinal canal. J. Bone Joint Surg. 27:70, 1945.
256. Sarpyener, M.A.: Spina bifida apperta. The congenital structure of the spinal canal. J. Bone Joint Surg. 29:817, 1947.
257. Schatzker, J., and Pennel, G.F.: Spinal stenosis. A cause of cauda equina compression. J. Bone Joint Surg. 50B:606, 1968.
258. Schmorl, G.: Über die an den Wirbelsbandscheiben vorkommenden Ausdehnungs und Zerreissungsvorgange und die dadurch an irhen und der Wirbels spongiosa hervorgerufenen Veranderungen. Verh. Dtsch. Orthop. Ges.21:3, 1927; Arch. fur Klin. Chir. 153:35, 150, 420, 1928; Klin. Wochenschr. 8:43, 1929.
258a. Schmorl, G.: Über Knorpelknocken an den Wirbelbandscheiben. Fortsch. Gebiet Roent. 41:359, 1930.
259. Schmorl, G., and Junghanns, H.: Die Gesunde und kranke Wirbelsaule im Roentgenbild. Pathologische Anatomische untersuchungen. Fortschrift am dem Gebiet des Roentgenstrahlen. Leipzig, G. Thieme, 1932.
260. Schmorl, G., and Junghanns, H.: Human spine in health and disease. New York, Grune & Stratton, 1959.
261. Schultz, A., Andersson, G.B.J., Ortengren, R., et al.: Analysis and quantitative myoelectric measurements of loads on the lumbar spine with holding weights in standing postures. Spine 7:390–397, 1982.
262. Schultz, A., Andersson, G.B.J., Ortengren, R., et. al.: Loads on the lumbar spine. J. Bone Joint Surg. 63A:713–720, 1982.
263. Scott, J.C.: Stress factor in disc syndrome. J. Bone Joint Surg. 37B:107, 1955.
264. Scott, V., and Gijsbers, K.: Pain reception in competitive swimmers. Br. Med. J. 283:91, 1984.
265. Sedowofia, K.A., Tomlinson, I.W., Weiss, J.B., et al.: Collagenous enzyme systems in human intervertebral disc. Spine 7:213–222, 1982.
266. Shealy, C.N.: Percutaneous radiofrequency denervation of spinal facets. Treatment for chronic back pain and sciatica. J. Neurosurg. 43:448–451, 1975.
267. Shiraz, A.M., Shirvasta, S.C., and Ahmed, A.M.: Stress analysis of the lumbar disc-body unit in compression. Spine 9:120–134, 1984.
267a. Shiraz, A.M., Shirvasta, S.C., and Ahmed, A.M.: Mathematical models: Finite-element technique. *In* Jayson, M.I.V. (ed.): Lumbar Spine and Back Pain, 3rd Ed. 1984, p. 183.
268. Sicard, R.: Personal communication.
269. Sinclaire, D.C., Feindle, W.H., Waddell, G., and Falconer, M.A.: The intervertebral ligaments as a source of segmental pain. J. Bone Joint Surg. 30B:515–521, 1948.
270. Smit, A.M.: Department of Health and Education letter to Dr. R.S. Knighton, July 17, 1975. Distributed by American Association of Neurological Surgeons.
271. Smith, J.W., and Walmsley, R.: Experimental incision of the intervertebral disc. J. Bone Joint Surg. 33B:612–625, 1957.
272. Smyth, M.J., and Wright, V.: Sciatica. The intervertebral disc—an experimental study. J. Bone Joint Surg. 40A:1401, 1958.
273. Solonen, K.A.: Sacro-iliac joint in the light of anatomical and roentgenological and clinical studies. Acta Orthop. Scand. (Suppl. 27), 1957.
274. Soutar, W.A., and Taylor, T.K.F.: Sulphated acid mucopolysaccharide metabolism in rabbit intervertebral disc. J. Bone Joint Surg. 52B:371, 1970.
275. Spangfort, E.V.: The lumbar disc herniation—a computer-aided analysis of 2504 operations. Acta Orthop. Scand. (Suppl. 142), 1972.
276. Stein, J.: Transcutaneous nerve stimulation technique. Central stimulation of periaqueduct and periventricular grey matter for relief of pain. Spine 10:100–101, 1985.
277. Steindler, A., and Luck, J.V.: Differential diagnosis of pain in the low back. Allocation of the source of pain by procaine hydrochloride method. J. Am. Med. Assoc. 1:106–113, 1938.
278. Sussman, B.: Inadequacies and hazards of chymopapain injections as treatment for intervertebral disc disease. J. Neurosurg. 42:389, 1974.
279. Sylven, B.: On the biology of the nucleus pulposus. Acta Orthop. Scand. 20:275, 1950.
280. Sylvest, J., Hentzer, B., and Takosi, K.: Ultrastructure of the intervertebral disc. Acta Orthop. Scand. 48:32–40, 1977.
281. Szypryt, E.P., Gibson, M.J., Mulholland, R.C., and Worthington, B.S.: The long term effect of chemonucleolysis on the intervertebral disc as assessed by magnetic resonance imaging. Spine 12:707–711, 1987.
282. Tait, J.H., and Devlin, S.R.: Stimulation of lymphocytes by nucleus pulposus in patients with degenerative disc disease of lumbar spine. Clin. Orthop. Rel. Res. 123:149, 1977.
283. Taylor, T.K.F.: The scientific basis of treatment of intervertebral disc disorders. *In* Owen, R., Goodfellow, J., and Bullough, P. (eds.): Scientific Foundations of Orthopaedics and Traumatology. London, Heinemann, 1980, 387–406.
284. Terenius, L., and Tamsen, A.: Endorphins and the modulation of acute pain. Acta Anaesthesiol. Scand. 74(Suppl.):21, 1982.
285. Thoczuen, H.: Tensile properties of spinal ligaments. Acta Orthop. Scand. (Suppl. 115), 1968.
286. Thomas, L.: Reversible collapse of rabbits' ears after intravenous repair, and prevention of recovery by cortisone. J. Exp. Med. 104:245, 1958.
287. Troup, J.D.G.: Recurrent back pain and its prediction. J. Soc. Occup. Med. 33:66–74, 1983.
288. Troup, J.D.G., Martin, J.W., and Lloyd, D.C.F.: Back pain in industry. A prospective survey. Spine 6:61, 1981.
289. Urban, J.P.G., Holm, S., Maroudas, A., and Nachemson, A.: Nutrition of intervertebral disc. An in vivo study of the solute transport. J. Clin. Orthop. 170:296–302, 1977.
290. Urban, J.P.G., Holm, S., Maroudas, A., and Nachemson, A.: Nutrition of intervertebral disc. Effect of fluid flow in solute transport. J. Clin. Orthop. 170:296–302, 1982.
291. Urban, J., and Maroudas, A.: The chemistry of the intervertebral disc in relation to its physiological function and requirements. Clin. Rheum. Dis. 6:51–76, 1980.
292. Urban, J.P.G., Maroudas, A., Bayliss, M.T., and Dillon, J.: Swelling pressures of proteoglycans at

the concentrations found in cartilagenous tissues. Biorheology. 16:447–464, 1979.
293. Urtsberg, L., and Bailey, C.: Spinal cord syndrome due to non-compressible Paget's disease of bone. A spinal artery steal phenomenon reversible with calcitonin. Lancet 2:13–15, 1980.
294. Vaharanter, H., Sachs, B.L., Spidery, M.A., et al.: The relationship of pain provocation to lumbar disc deterioration as seen by CT/discography. Spine 12:295–298, 1987.
295. Verbiest, H.: Surtain formes rares de compression de la kueue de cheval. Homage à Chloris. Paris, Vincent, 1949.
296. Verbiest, H.: A radicular syndrome with developmental narrowing of the lumbar vertebral canal. J. Bone Joint Surg. 36B:230, 1954.
297. Vesalius, A.: De Humani Corporis Fabrica. Libri Septum, 1555. Quoted in Bradford, F.K., and Spurling, R.G.: Intervertebral Disc. Springfield, Charles C Thomas.
298. Videman, T., Malmivarra, A., and Mooney, V.: The value of axial views in assessing discograms. An experimental study with cadavers. Spine 12:299–307, 1987.
299. Virchow, R.: Untersuchung uber die Entwickelung des Schadelgrund. Berlin, G. Reimer, 1857.
300. Virgin, W.J.: Experimental investigations into the physical properties of the intervertebral disc. J. Bone Joint Surg. 33B:607, 1951.
301. Von Lackum, H.L.: The lumbosacral region. An anatomical study and some clinical observations. J.A.M.A. 82:1109–1114, 1924.
302. Waddell, G.: Understanding the patient with back pain. *In* Jayson, M.I.V. (ed.): Lumbar Spine and Back Pain, 3rd Ed. London, Churchill Livingstone, 1987, pp. 417–434.
303. Waddell, G., Cummell, E.G., and McCullough, J.A.: Failed lumbar disc surgery. Repeat surgery following industrial injury. J. Bone Joint Surg. 61A:201, 1979.
304. Waddell, G., and Main, C.: Assessment of severity in low back disorders. Spine 9:204, 1984.
305. Waddell, G., McCullough, J.A., Cummell, E., and Venner, R.M.: Non-organic physical signs in low back pain. Spine 5:117, 1979.
306a. Waddell, G., Main, C., Morris, E.W., et al.: Chronic low back pain. Psychological stress and illness behaviour. Spine 9:208, 1984.
306b. Waddell, G., Birchner, M., Finlayson, D., and Main, C.J.: Symptoms and signs. Physical disease or illness behaviour. Br. Med. J. 289:739–741, 1984.
307. Wakano, K., Kasman, R., Cheo, E.Y., et al.: Biochemical analysis of canine intervertebral discs after chymopapain injection. Spine 8:59–68, 1983.
308. Waluch, H.V.: MRI in lumbar disc disease. Clinical potential limitations. Paper read at International Society for Study of the Lumbar Spine Meeting, Dallas, May, 1987.
309. Waters, R.L., and Morris, J.M.: An in vitro study of normal and scoliotic interspinous ligaments. J. Biomech. 1:211–220, 1973.
310. Weber, H.: Lumbar disc herniation. A controlled prospective study with ten-year observation. Spine 8:131–140, 1983.
311. Weinstein, J.: Mechanism of spinal pain. The dorsal root ganglion and its role as a mediator of low back pain. Spine 11:999–1001, 1986.
312. Weissl, H.L.: The articular surfaces of the sacro-iliac joint and their relation to the movements of the sacrum. Acta Anat. 22:1–14, 1954.
313. Weissl, H.L.: The ligaments of the sacro-iliac joint examined with particular reference to their function. Acta Anat. 20:201–213, 1954.
314. Weissl, H.L.: Movements of the sacro-iliac joint. Acta Anat. 23:80, 81, 1955.
315. White, A.A., and Panjabi, M.: Clinical Biomechanics of Spine. Philadelphia, J.B. Lippincott, 1978.
316. Wilder, D.G., Selickson, D., Frymoyer, J.W., and Pope, M.H.: Objective measurement of L4–5 instability. Spine 5:56, 1980.
317. Wilder, D.G., Pope M.H., and Frymoyer, J.: The functional topography of the sacro-iliac joint. Spine 5:575–579, 1980.
318. Williams, P.C.: The reduced lumbo-sacral joint space. J.A.M.A. 19:1677, 1932.
319. Williams, R.W.: A conservative surgical approach to virgin herniated disc. Spine 3:175, 1978.
320. Willis, T.A.: An analysis of vertebral anomalies. Am. J. Surg. N.S. 6:162–168, 1939.
321. Wilson, C.B., Ehni, G., and Gray J.: Neurogenic intermittent claudication. Clin. Neurosurg. 18:62–85, 1971.
322. Wiltse, L., Kircaldy Willis, W.H., and MacIvor, G.W.D.: Treatment of spinal stenosis. Clin. Orthop. Rel. Res. 115:83–91, 1976.
323. Wiltse, L., Widdell, E.H., and Howson, A.L.: Chymopapain chemonucleolysis in lumbar disc disease. J.A.M.A. 231:1754, 1975.
324. Wyke, B.D.: Lumbar spine and back pain. *In* Jayson, M.I.V., and Wyke, B.D. (eds): Neurological Aspects of Low Back Pain, 1st Ed. 1976. London, Pitman, p. 189–256.
325. Wyke, B.D.: Neurological mechanisms of spinal pain. *In* Hernandez, S., and Connesa, J. (eds.): Pathology of the vertebral column. Murcia, Ferrer International, 1977, p. 45.
326. Wyke, B.D.: Neurological aspects of low back pain. *In* Jayson, M.I.V. (ed): Lumbar Spine and Back Pain, 3rd Ed. London, Pitman Medical, 1987, pp. 56–59.
327. Wyke, B.D., Keele, C.A., and Armstrong, D.: Mediators of pain. *In* Lyme, R.K.S., Armstrong, D., and Pardoe, E.G. (eds.): Pharmacology of Pain. Oxford, Pergamon Press, 1968, p. 3.
328. Yong, K.H., and King, A.I.: Mechanisms of facet load transmission as a hypothesis for low back pain. Spine 9:557, 1984.
329. Yoshizawa, H., O'Brien, J.P., Smith, W.T., et al.: The neuropathology of intervertebral discs removed for low back pain. J. Pathol. 132:95–104, 1980.
330. Young, R.J.: The effect of regular exercise on cognitive functioning and personality. Br. J. Sports Med. 3:110, 1979.
331. Young, H.H., Love, J.G., and Svien, H.J.: Low back pain and sciatic pain—long term results after removal of protruded intervertebral disc with or without pain. Clin. Orthop. Rel. Res. 5:128, 1975.
332. Zung, W.W.K.: A self rating depression scale. Arch. J. Psychiatr. 12:70, 1965.

MAGNITUDE OF THE PROBLEM

John W. Frymoyer

The magnitude of low back problems in our society can be measured in many different ways, such as by the incidence and prevalence of symptoms, the impact of the problem on the utilization of health care services, the resultant impairments or disability, or its cost to society. Depending on the approach used, the apparent magnitude of the problem may appear inflated or deflated.

Many approaches have been used in the epidemiologic research of low back pain, including retrospective analyses of populations, cross-sectional surveys, case control studies, and prospective studies of selected cohorts. Each of these methods provides a somewhat different perspective to the problem and its magnitude. Because of major differences in the socioeconomic systems among countries, the discussion here focuses primarily on the United States.

MAGNITUDE OF THE PROBLEM: LOW BACK PAIN SYMPTOMS

Hult,[17] Horal,[16] and Kellgren and Lawrence[19] are credited with conducting the first epidemiologic studies of the prevalence of low back symptoms among Swedish and English populations. In these and later studies, the percentage of the population who have experienced low back pain at any time in their lives (lifetime prevalence) has ranged from 51.4% to 70%. However, a lower lifetime prevalence of 40% was reported in less industrialized societies. Fahrni and Trueman suggest that increased lumbar lordosis in primitive populations is protective.[8] These figures demonstrate that low back pain is a very common symptom and they are often cited as evidence that low back pain is a major health problem. However, it is well known that low back complaints are usually self-limiting, and the majority of patients get well within 1 month. Only 5% to 10% continue to have symptoms after 3 months, as Nachemson discusses elsewhere in this chapter.

In an attempt to refine this information, other analyses have been performed to measure the severity and duration of symptoms. The National Center for Health Statistics asked the question "Have you ever had low back pain which lasted more than 1 month?" In a cohort that was representative of the United States population, ages 25 to 74, only 16% of the subjects responded affirmatively. This figure closely approximates the 18% positive response rate in the survey population studied by Nagi and colleagues,[27] when they asked, "Are you often bothered by pain in the back?" We utilized a similar approach by asking respondents to quantify their low back symptoms on a modified Likert scale of severity. Although 70% of the male respondents, ages 18 to 55, reported low back pain sometime during their life, only 22% classified the complaint as "severe."

The prevalence of low back pain is also modified by age and by sex, as shown in Figure 1. Note the increase up to age 50 in males, and the subsequent decrease. However, in women beyond the age of 50, low back complaints continue to increase, an

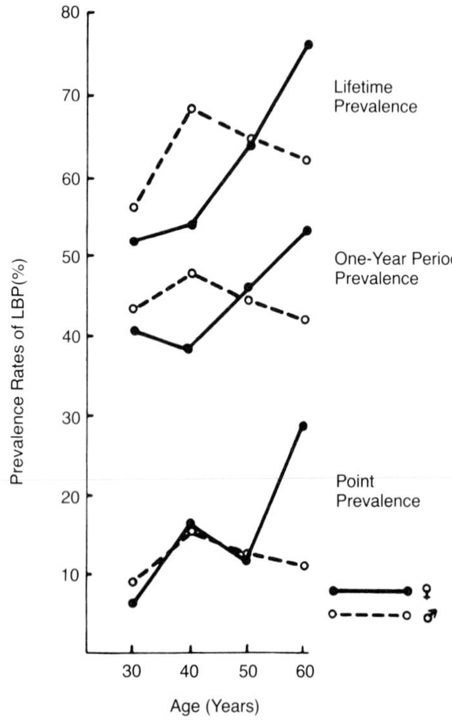

Figure 1 □ The lifetime prevalence and incidence of low back pain with 1-year period and point-prevalence data. (From Biering-Sorenson, F.: Low back trouble in a general population of 30-, 40-, 50-, and 60-year-old men and women. Study design, representativeness and basic results. Dan. Med. Bull. 29:289–99, 1982.)

observation also made by Valkenburg and Haanen.[37]

The incidence of low back complaints offers yet another different perspective to the problem. Overall, 5% of the population have a low back complaint in any given year, but the incidence ranges from 1% to 20% if different industrial populations are surveyed. At any given time (point prevalence) 12.2%[25] to 52%[38] report they are symptomatic with back pain.

As another measure of the severity of low back symptoms, one can analyze recurrence rates, which range from 85% in the study of Valkenburg and Haanen[37] to 60% in the industrial survey of Troup and colleagues.[36]

MAGNITUDE OF THE PROBLEM: SCIATICA AND CLAUDICATION

The lifetime prevalence of sciatica is 40%, based on cross-sectional studies.[2] The complaint of leg pain has been highly associated with a history of numbness and/or weakness, and is also far more common in patients with severe low back pain, suggesting that these patients may have a discogenic basis for their complaints. However, only 2.5% of the American population report they have ever had a ruptured disc.

The annual incidence of sciatica is much lower and has been reported to be 1%.

The prevalence and incidence of claudication is unknown, but is anecdotally reported to be increasing in the aging population. Radiographic evidence of degenerative spondylolisthesis is identified in 5.8% of males and 9.1% of females, but many are asymptomatic.

MAGNITUDE OF THE PROBLEM: EFFECTS OF LOW BACK PAIN ON SOCIETY

Utilization of Health Services

The National Center for Health Statistics reports that 14.3% of new-patient visits to physicians are for low back complaints. Annually, 12,900,000 visits are made for chronic low back pain, and 4,114,000 visits are for back symptoms. Orthopedists see about 15% of these patients (2,758,000). By comparison, it has been estimated that of the 100,000,000 patient visits made to chiropractors each year, one half are for back complaints.[26] An additional 5,259,000 office visits are made for physiotherapy services per year.[29] Symptoms severe enough to require hospitalization account for 2.8% of all hospital discharges in the United States. The utilization of these services again varies as a function of the patient's perception of the severity of the symptoms (Table 1). Note that in this population the utilization of health services was twice as great for those who reported having severe low back pain, compared with those who reported moderate low back pain. Also note the relatively low utilization of chiropractors, which emphasizes the wide regional variations in what services are available and used. For comparison, the health services used in the United Kingdom are described in Table 2.

Table 1 □ Type of Health-Care Services and Treatment Utilized by Men with Low Back Pain

	PERCENT MODERATE (n = 565)	PERCENT SEVERE (n = 288)
Health care practitioner		
Family physician	30.5	66.7
Orthopedic surgeon	8.8	32.3
Neurosurgeon	2.7	9.5
Osteopath	7.0	23.8
Chiropractor	12.7	27.5
Physiotherapist	3.8	16.1
Other	5.0	12.1
Treatment		
Bed rest	35.1	72.8
Muscle relaxant	17.1	52.6
Prescription pain medication	21.1	58.0
Physiotherapy	9.5	23.9
Back support	11.3	37.4
Other nonsurgical treatment	12.6	27.4
Lumbar spine surgery	2.0	10.5

From Frymoyer, J. W., Pope, M. H., Clements, J. C., et al.: Risk factors in low-back pain. An epidemiological survey. J. Bone Joint Surg. 65A:213–18, 1983.

Table 2 □ The Back Patient's Need for Medical and Social Services (Expressed as Rates per 1,000 Persons, Both Sexes, at Risk Per Year)

	Number Subjects per 1,000 per year	
Handicapped/pension	2.0	
General practitioner	20.0	(58 visits)
Referrals	9.0	
Admissions	1.0	
Operations	0.1	
Spinal braces/corsets	7.0	

Modified from Benn, R. T., and Wood, P. H. N.: Pain in the back: An attempt to estimate the size of the problem. Rheumatol. Rehab. 14:121–28, 1975.

LOW BACK PAIN: MAGNITUDE OF THE SURGICAL PROBLEM

Only a small percentage of the population require surgical intervention for low back pain, sciatica, and claudication. The lifetime prevalence of lumbar spinal surgery has been reported as 4% by Nagi and colleagues,[27] 3% by Frymoyer[9] in the United States cohorts, 1% by Andersson[2] in Sweden, and 1% in a Danish population.[5] The annual incidence of lumbar spinal surgery is surprisingly low. Table 3 shows the 4-year trend for the United States as reported by Rutkow.[31] However, wide regional variations appear to exist in the utilization of surgical treatment. Kane has reported that the incidence of surgery is four times higher in the western, in comparison with the central, United States.[18] Additionally, the risk of disc herniation requiring surgery is higher in smokers, truck drivers, commuters, and those whose occupations require more twisting.

As a subset of the surgical problem, the magnitude of failed low back surgery is far greater in complexity than it is in magnitude. A gross estimate of the magnitude can be derived based on a calculation of a 15% surgical failure rate requiring further surgical intervention. On this basis it is estimated that 30,000 to 70,000 people will enter the failed surgical group each year.

LOW BACK PAIN: SOCIOECONOMIC CONSEQUENCES

Impairment and Disability

It is estimated that 9,200,000 Americans are currently impaired and 2,400,000 are currently disabled by low back pain, one

Table 3 □ Orthopedic Surgery: The 20 Most Frequent Operations

PROCEDURE*	1983 TOTAL	PERCENTAGE OF ALL ORTHOPEDIC OPERATIONS PERFORMED IN 1983	1981 TOTAL	1979 TOTAL
Open reduction of a fracture and internal fixation [79.3]	331,000	9.3	293,000	274,000
Arthroscopy [80.2]	260,000	7.3	228,000	130,000
Excision or destruction of an intervertebral disc [80.5]	188,000	5.3	129,000	132,000
Closed reduction of a fracture without internal fixation [79.0]	183,000	5.2	193,000	238,000
Excision of a bunion or bunionette [77.5]	182,000	5.1	139,000	112,000
Placement or removal of an internal fixation device without reduction of a fracture [78.5 and 78.6]	173,000	4.9	202,000	160,000
Arthroplasty of the knee or ankle [81.4]	161,000	4.5	148,000	123,000
Total hip replacement or arthroplasty of the hip [81.5 and 81.6]	159,000	4.5	155,000	130,000
Excision of semilunar cartilage of the knee [80.6]	147,000	4.1	155,000	155,000
Local excision of a lesion or tissue of bone [77.6]	136,000	3.8	120,000	95,000
Amputation of the lower limb [84.1]	118,000	3.3	90,000	80,000
Toe	35,000			
Foot	11,000			
Below the knee	37,000			
Above the knee	35,000			
Division of bone [77.3]	116,000	3.3	85,000	56,000
Arthroplasty of the foot or toe [81.3]	103,000	2.9	71,000	43,000
Partial ostectomy [77.8]	95,000	2.7	78,000	84,000
Spinal fusion [81.0]	70,000	2.0	59,000	52,000
Division of joint capsule, ligament, or cartilage [80.4]	68,000	1.9	56,000	40,000
Division of muscle, tendon, and fascia [83.1]	61,000	1.7	45,000	48,000
Arthrodesis of the foot or ankle [81.1]	58,000	1.6	33,000	28,000
Arthroplasty of the upper extremity, except the hand [81.8]	57,000	1.6	41,000	34,000
Local excision or destruction of a lesion of the knee joint [80.86]	48,000	1.4	21,000	16,000

*The numbers in brackets are the codes in the International Classification of Disease, 9th Revision, Clinical Modification. From Rutkow, I. M.: Orthopaedic operations in the United States, 1979 through 1983. J. Bone Joint Surg. 68A:716–19, 1986.

half of whom (1,200,000) are chronically disabled. In the United Kingdom, the figure is lower, with 0.158% of the population disabled versus 0.4% in the United States. In the United States the rate of disabling low back pain is increasing at a rate estimated to be four times the growth of the population. Low back pain represents 10% of all chronic health conditions[21] and is the most common source of activity limitation in the population under the age of 64. Kelsey and White estimated that an average of 28.6 days per 100 workers are lost each year.[22] The corresponding figures are 36 days in Sweden and 32.6 days in the United Kingdom. However, the figures can be much higher when specific industrial populations are analyzed. For example, Anderson[1] reported that in British postal workers, 70 weeks per 100 employees were lost each year. However, these figures demonstrate only one facet of the problem. Another consequence of low back pain is change in employment and job classification, with one out of every 25 English workers changing jobs annually because of low back pain. In the Netherlands, 8% of men and 4% of women have changed jobs because of back symptoms.

Table 4 □ Annual Costs of Musculoskeletal Conditions: Back Pain

Direct Costs	
Hospital inpatient services	$4,462,770,000
Outpatient and emergency room institutional services	259,690,000
Outpatient diagnostic and therapeutic services	1,010,590,000
Physician inpatient services	1,075,750,000
Physician office, outpatient and emergency room services	1,048,120,000
Other practitioner services	233,630,000
Drugs	121,340,000
Nursing home services	2,933,520,000
Prepayments and administration	501,530,000
Non–health sector goods and services	1,275,800,000
Total Direct Costs	$12,922,740,000
Indirect Costs	
Lost earnings—wage earners	2,524,370,000
Lost earnings—homemakers	425,650,000
Total Indirect Costs	$2,950,020,000
Total Costs	$15,872,760,000

From Holbrook, T. L., Grazier, K., Kelsey, J. L., and Stauffer, R. N.: The Socioeconomic Impact of Selected Musculoskeletal Disorders. Chicago, American Academy of Orthopaedic Surgeons, 1984.

Economic Consequences

The economic consequences of low back pain in the United States have been reported to range from $16 billion to over $50 billion each year. The lower figure was calculated from an analysis of National Health Data statistics, and a breakdown of those costs is provided in Table 4. In an earlier publication, I argued the cost figure of $16 billion appeared to be low, based on the reported data for component costs of medical diagnosis and treatment, compensation, and the indirect costs associated with time lost from work.

The cost of diagnostic tests for low back disease is uncertain. In 1978, Scavone and coworkers[32] calculated the cost of plain radiographs alone to be $600 million, and based on inflation alone, this figure must now exceed $1 billion. Additional estimates are not available for the cost of computed tomographic (CT) scans, myelography, magnetic resonance imaging (MRI), electrodiagnostic procedures, and thermography.

The treatment costs are also incompletely understood. In the analysis in which estimated overall costs were $16 billion, 14% were for outpatient treatment, 36% for hospital care, and 19% for nursing home care. Other components of treatment costs were not calculated; these include physical therapy, rehabilitation programs, pain clinics, drugs, braces, and transcutaneous electrical nerve stimulation (TENS) units, to name a few.

The costs of surgery, likewise, are not certain, although they can be estimated. Based on an annual surgical rate of 258,000,[31] and a cost per case of $10,000,[26] a reasonable estimate is $2.58 billion/year. However, there appears to be a very costly subset of patients, namely, patients with a compensable cause of their symptoms. Norton[30] has calculated the costs for a successful outcome for chemonucleolysis or laminectomy to be $128,000 for chymopapain, and $48,000 for surgery. Of course, some of that cost is related to compensation payment.

The costs of compensation in low back disease have been analyzed in depth. It is known that these disorders are the single greatest cause of compensable injury in the working age population, and the second most common cause of work loss time. Snook[33, 34] has analyzed compensation costs and estimated an annual expense of $4.6

Table 5 □ Cost per Case of Compensable Back Pain

YEAR	SOURCE	MEAN COST	MEDIAN COST
1967	Leavitt, Johnston, and Beyer (1971)	$2911	$404
1976	Snook (1984)	4500	566
1978	Antonakes (1981)	6600	—
1979	Klein, Jensen, and Sanderson (1983)	5081	—
1979	National Council on Compensation Insurance (1983)	5500	—

From Snook, S. H., and Jensen, R. C.: Cost. *In* Pope, M. H., Frymoyer, J. W., and Andersson, G. (eds.): Occupational Low Back Pain. New York, Praeger, 1984.

billion. In a survey of nine states, back injuries constituted 21% of all compensable work injuries but accounted for 33% of the cost. Snook[34] also calculated the cost per case, based on a review of the literature. These figures are given in Table 5. A further breakdown of cost per case showed that one third was for medical care, and two thirds for disability payment. He made a very important additional observation that 90% of the total compensation costs in the United States were produced by 25% of those suffering low back injuries.

Lastly, the work loss time component of low back pain costs has only been estimated. In our analysis of a male population, ages 18 to 55, we estimated the cost to be $11 billion annually. As did Snook, we found that a small percentage of the cases produced the highest cost; 1.7% of the population surveyed produced 75% ($8 billion) of the total cost. This finding also conforms to that of Leavitt and colleagues,[24] who reported that high-cost cases were those with prolonged lag times from injury to treatment, delays in hospitalization and diagnosis, and surgery that was mentioned as a treatment alternative but not performed.

Based on our analysis of the component costs for low back pain, the data support a significantly higher economic impact than $16 billion.

REAPPRAISAL OF THE MAGNITUDE OF THE PROBLEM

Although low back pain is a prevalent, costly health problem, its impact is overestimated if one critically examines the available information. For the population as a whole, low back disease is a common occurrence, but it is self-limiting, requires little treatment, and should have a low cost. As a surgical problem, relatively few members of the population are affected, and the socioeconomic consequences should ideally be minimal. It is clear that the magnitude of low back disease is magnified by a relatively small percentage of the population who have chronic or recurrent disabling low back symptoms, who seek multiple health practitioners and treatments, and whose surgery, if performed, is often not successful. This population has been analyzed in detail and its members are characterized by psychosocial problems such as job dissatisfaction, psychologic distress, and high-cost work-

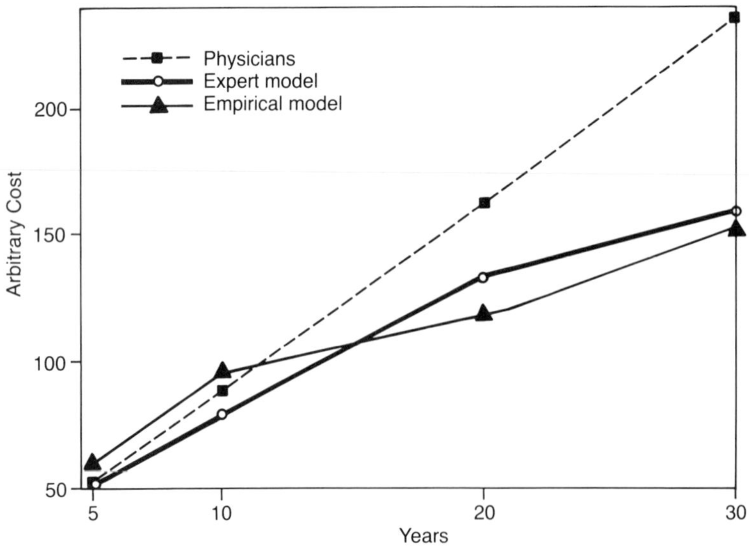

Figure 2 □ Graph shows projected costs for low back pain.

men's compensation claims. This group is also the one that is increasing at a rate four times that of the growth of the population. We have mathematically modeled the costs for low back pain in the future based on available data, using the changes that are occurring in disability and impairment. Figure 2 illustrates these projections, and it is clear that if these trends continue, the magnitude of the low back problem will indeed be enormous.

References

1. Anderson, J.A.D.: Back pain and occupation. *In* Jayson, M.I.V. (ed.): The Lumbar Spine and Back Pain, 2nd Ed. Pitman, London Medical, pp. 57–82, 1980.
2. Andersson, G.B.J., Pope, M.H., and Frymoyer, J.W.: Epidemiology. *In* Pope, M.H., Frymoyer, J.W., and Andersson, G. (eds.): Occupational Low Back Pain. New York, Praeger, 1984.
3. Beals, R.K., and Hickman, N.W.: Industrial injuries of the back and extremities. Comprehensive evaluation—an aid in prognosis and management: A study of one hundred and eighty patients. J. Bone Joint Surg. 54A:1593–1611, 1972.
4. Benn, R.T., and Wood, P.H.N.: Pain in the back: An attempt to estimate the size of the problem. Rheumatol. Rehab. 14:121–28, 1975.
5. Biering-Sorensen, F.: Low back trouble in a general population of 30-, 40-, 50-, and 60-year old men and women. Study design, representativeness and basic results. Dan. Med. Bull. 29:289–99, 1982.
6. Bremner, J.M., Lawence, J.S., and Miall, W.E.: Degenerative joint disease in a Jamaican rural population. Ann. Rheum. Dis. 27:326–32, 1968.
7. Brunarski, D.J.: Clinical trials of spinal manipulation: A critical appraisal and review of the literature. J. Manip. Physiol. Ther. 7:243–49, 1984.
8. Fahrni, W.H., and Trueman, G.E.: Comparative radiological study of the spines of a primitive population with North Americans and Northern Europeans. J. Bone Joint Surg. 47B:552–55, 1965.
9. Frymoyer, J.W.: The role of spine fusion. Question 3. Spine 6:284–90, 1981.
10. Frymoyer, J.W., Pope, M.H., Clements, J.C., et al.: Risk factors in low-back pain. An epidemiological survey. J. Bone Joint Surg. 65A:213–18, 1983.
11. Frymoyer, J.W., Rosen, J.C., Clements, J., and Pope, M.H.: Psychologic factors in low-back-pain disability. Clin. Orthop. Rel. Res. 195:178–84, 1985.
12. Frymoyer, J.W., and Cats-Baril, W.: Predictors of low back pain disability. Clin. Orthop. Rel. Res. 221:89–98, 1987.
13. Frymoyer, J.W.: Epidemiologic aspects of back pain. *In* Danchik, K.M., Drury, T.S., and Ganz, A. (eds.): National Center for Health Statistics: An Evaluation of Adequacy, Epidemiologic Uses and National Data Needs. Vital and Health Statistics, Series 4. Public Health Service (in preparation).
14. Haber, L.D.: Disabling effects of chronic disease and impairment. J. Chron. Disabil. 24:469–87, 1971.
15. Holbrook, T.L., Grazier, K., Kelsey, J.L., and Stauffer, R.N.: The socioeconomic impact of selected musculoskeletal disorders. Chicago, Am. Acad. Orthop. Surgeons, 1984.
16. Horal, J.: The clinical appearance of low back disorders in the city of Gothenburg Sweden. Acta Orthop. Scand. (Suppl.) 118:1–109, 1969.
17. Hult, L.: Cervical, dorsal and lumbar spinal syndromes. Acta Orthop. Scand. 24:174–75, 1954.
18. Kane, W.: The incidence rate of laminectomy in the United States. Presented at the International Society for Study of the Lumbar Spine, New Orleans, 1980.
19. Kellgren, J.H., and Lawrence, J.S.: Osteo-arthrosis and disk degeneration in an urban population. Ann. Rheum. Dis. 17:388–97, 1958.
20. Kelsey, J.L., Pastides, H., and Bisbee, G.E., Jr.: Musculo-skeletal disorders: Their frequency of occurrence and their impact on the population of the United States. Prodist, New York, 1978.
21. Kelsey, J.L., and White, A.A., III: Epidemiology and impact on low back pain. Spine 5:133–42, 1980.
22. Kelsey, J.L., Githens, P.B., White, A.A., et. al.: An epidemiologic study of lifting and twisting on the job and risk for acute prolapsed lumbar intervertebral disc. J. Orthop. Res. 2:61–66, 1984.
23. Kelsey, J., Githens, P.B., O'Connor, T., et. al.: Acute prolapsed lumbar intervertebral disc: An epidemiologic study with special reference to driving automobiles and cigarette smoking. Spine 9:608–13, 1984.
24. Leavitt, S.S., Johnston, T.L., and Beyer, R.D.: The process of recovery: Patterns in industrial back injury. Part I: Costs and other quantitative measures of effort. Indust. Med. Surg. 40:7–14, 1971.
25. Magora, A., and Taustein, I.: An investigation of the problem of sick-leave in the patient suffering from low back pain. Indust. Med. Surg. 38:398–408, 1969.
26. McCulloch, J.: Costs: Surgery vs. chemonucleolysis. Alt. Spinal Surg. 2:3–4, 1985.
27. Nagi, S.Z., Riley, L.E., and Newby, L.G.: A social epidemiology of back pain in a general population. J. Chron. Disabil. 26:769–79, 1973.
28. National Center for Health Statistics. Prevalence of Selected Impairment, United States—1977. D.H.H.S. Publication (P.H.S.), Hyattsville, Maryland, series 10, no. 134, 1981.
29. National Center for Health Statistics: Physiotherapy office visits: National Ambulatory Medical Care Survey: United States 1980–81. Advance Data from Vital and Health Statistics, no. 120, D.H.H.S. publication # (PHS) 86-1250. Public Health Service, Hyattsville, MD, July 11, 1986.
30. Norton, W.L.: Chemonucleolysis versus surgical discectomy: Comparison of costs and results in workers' compensation claimants. Spine 11:440–43, 1986.
31. Rutkow, I.M.: Orthopaedic operations in the United States, 1979 through 1983. J. Bone Joint Surg. 68A:716–19, 1986.
32. Scavone, J.G., Latshaw, R.F., and Rohrer, G.V.: Use of lumbar spine films: Statistical evaluation at a university teaching school. J.A.M.A. 246:1105–08, 1981.
33. Snook, S.H.: Low back pain in industry. *In* White, A.A., and Gordon, S.L., (eds.): American Academy of Orthopaedic Surgeons Symposium on Idiopathic Low Back Pain. St. Louis, C.V. Mosby Company, 1982.

34. Snook, S.H., and Jensen, R.C.: Cost. *In* Pope, M.H., Frymoyer, J.W., and Andersson, G., (eds.): Occupational Low Back Pain. New York, Praeger, 1984.
35. Svensson, H.O., and Andersson, G.B.J.: Low back pain in 40- to 47-year-old men: Work history and work environment factors. Spine 8:272–76, 1983.
36. Troup, J.D.G., Martin, J.W., and Lloyd, D.C.E.F.: Back pain in industry: A prospective survey. Spine 6:61–9, 1981.
37. Valkenburg, H.A., and Haanen, H.C.M.: The epidemiology of low back pain. *In* White, A.A., and Gordon, S.L., (eds.): American Academy of Orthopaedic Surgeons Symposium on Idiopathic Low Back Pain. St. Louis, C.V. Mosby Company, 1982.
38. Vallfors, B.: Acute, subacute and chronic low back pain. Clinical symptoms, absenteeism and working environment. Scand. J. Rehab. Med. (Suppl. 11):1985.
39. Westrin, C.G.: Sicklisting Because of Low Back Pain. A Nosologic and Medical Insurance Investigation. Göteborg (doctoral dissertation, in Swedish), 1970.
40. Westrin, C.G.: Low back sicklisting. A nosological and medical insurance investigation. Scand. J. Soc. Med. 7(Suppl.):1–116, 1973.

A NEW CLINICAL MODEL FOR THE TREATMENT OF LOW BACK PAIN

Gordon Waddell

There is growing concern about our present epidemic of low back disability.[25, 121, 131, 148, 151, 158] Ever-increasing medical and health care resources are being consumed, but they fail to alleviate the problem.[174] There is a constant demand from all directions for more research, both in basic sciences and in clinical treatment. Equally and more fundamentally important is the need to question our entire approach to back pain. These questions have been raised many times over the past 100 years, but only in the last few years has any real attempt been made to face them.[100, 101, 123, 148, 186] This review will try to analyze the theoretic and philosophic framework on which any real breakthrough in treatment depends.

OBSERVATIONS ON THE NATURAL HISTORY OF LOW BACK PAIN AND DISABILITY

The following observations have been made in regard to the natural history of this disorder:

1. Of all people, 80% experience low back pain at some time in their lives. Each year, 2% to 5% of adults will attend a doctor or lose time from work because of low back pain.[11, 25, 71, 73, 78, 131] Up to 60% of normal people will have experienced some degree of low back pain in the past year, although they will not necessarily have visited a doctor or lost time from work.[27, 28, 38, 129, 179]

2. Of all patients who have attacks of low back pain, 90% recover within about 6 weeks, irrespective of the type of treatment or, indeed, regardless of whether they receive treatment (Fig. 1).[11, 24, 71–73, 143, 187]

3. Newly introduced orthopedic services in rapidly developing countries such as Oman are flooded with patients seeking treatment for low back pain. As we would expect from the above studies of Western populations, low back pain seems to be almost universal. In Oman, the striking observation is that there is very little actual disability here, where western medicine has not been introduced. Patients in Oman are crippled by polio, tuberculosis, or spinal fractures, but no one goes to bed, no one stops daily life, and no one is permanently disabled by simple backache.[165]

4. There has been a dramatic increase in low back disability in all Western countries (Table 1 and Figs. 2 to 4). In view of Observations 1 and 5, this does not necessarily mean that there has been such an increase in low back pain or even in low back injuries. More specifically, there are increases in work loss, sick certification, compensation, and long-term disability because of low back pain. Use of the diagnosis of disc prolapse may also have increased.[80] However, there is

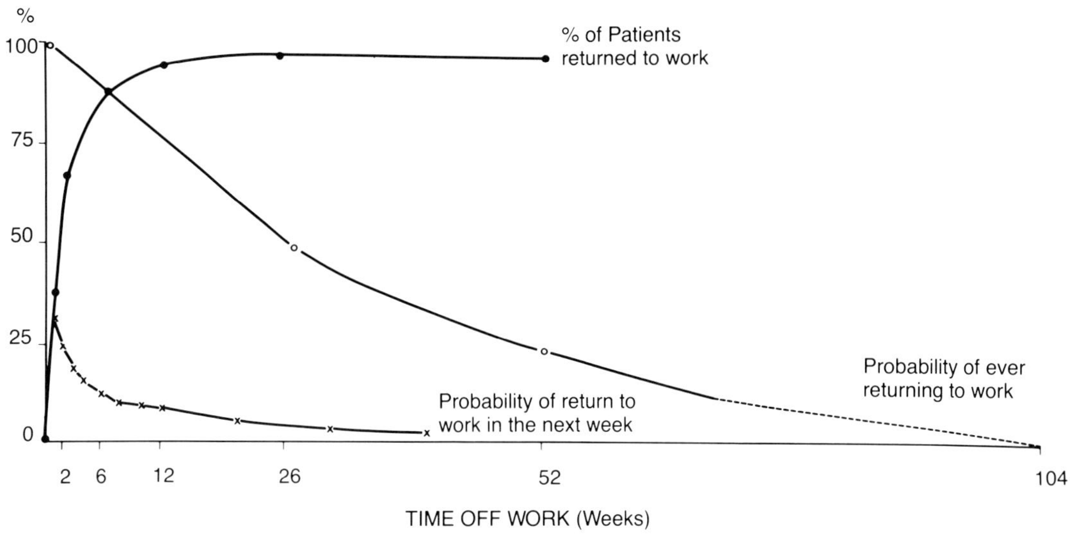

Figure 1 □ Return to work as a function of time off from work as a consequence of low back pain. The graph shows the proportion of patients returning to work with time[11, 24, 71, 73, 143] and the diminishing probability of returning to work in the short term[72, 187] or ever.[92] (Based on data from Hrudey[72] and the Workmen's Compensation Board of British Columbia.[187])

Table 1 □ United Kingdom Sick Certification*

	ALL INCAPACITIES				BACK INCAPACITIES			
	Spells/1,000		Days/1,000 at Risk		Spells/1,000		Days/1,000 at Risk	
YEAR	MALE	FEMALE	MALE	FEMALE	MALE	FEMALE	MALE	FEMALE
1953–4	404	406	—	—	21.7	8.0	—	—
'54–5	432	444	14,140	17,095	22.3	8.8	506	329
'55–6	439	444	14,107	16,807	23.8	9.5	538	352
'56–7	410	423	13,462	16,102	25.3	9.9	545	331
'57–8	536	574	13,736	17,596	25.3	10.2	560	365
'58–9	479	489	14,549	16,927	27.4	11.2	595	400
'59–60	444	459	14,005	16,177	29.1	11.9	638	438
'60–1	488	507	14,423	16,449	29.2	12.2	630	422
'61–2	491	526	—	—	30.5	12.9	—	—
'62–3	494	501	15,049	15,944	31.9	13.9	720	447
'63–4	484	497	14,999	15,919	34.9	14.5	724	530
'64–5	505	518	15,418	16,135	37.3	15.3	761	451
'65–6	562	565	16,562	16,487	39.1	14.9	791	423
'66–7	512	529	16,169	15,861	41.1	16.4	863	479
'67–8	576	600	17,704	17,237	43.8	17.3	941	491
'68–9	582	599	17,951	16,919	43.3	18.7	976	521
'69–70	627	631	18,780	17,365	44.1	19.0	1,051	512
'70–1	509	542	16,976	16,152	42.5	19.7	1,054	547
'71–2	504	561	17,002	16,144	41.3	20.8	1,032	565
'72–3	554	619	17,727	16,780	45.1	21.9	1,097	612
'73–4	553	621	17,895	16,630	47.3	24.1	1,133	634
'74–5	534	605	17,339	16,151	47.9	24.8	1,150	642
'76–7	535	616	18,126	15,182	51.0	29.5	1,254	763
'77–8	571	688	19,262	17,975	55.9	34.3	1,432	954
'78–9	589	752	20,210	18,307	56.9	41.3	1,455	1,035
'79–80	503	705	19,337	17,966	56.1	44.6	1,720	1,330
'80–1	505	690	19,314	17,433	58.2	44.7	1,852	1,457
'81–2	468	655	19,859	18,171	54.6	47.7	1,882	1,622

*For all forms of sickness and for back incapacities including Sickness and Invalidity Benefit and Injury Benefit, expressed as the annual number of spells or episodes of incapacity and as total days of sick certification per 1,000 persons at risk. No comparable figures are available from 1982, owing to changes in the recording system. Back incapacities include all spinal disorders and diagnoses.
Calculated from statistics supplied by the DHSS.[145]

7. The majority of people with low back pain cope with it themselves without medical treatment.[131] People do not go to the doctor simply because they experience pain or even because of the severity of pain. There is surprisingly little difference between patients with low back pain who see a doctor and those who cope with it alone (Table 3).[27, 28, 129] Many everyday bodily symptoms are interpreted as minor nociceptive stimuli that generate little anxiety. Some people deal with the symptoms by ignoring or resting the affected part in expectation of a natural resolution, which results in little interference with normal life.[1, 2] The decision to seek health care appears to depend on the person's perception and interpretation of the significance of the symptoms. It also depends on the availability and expectations of treatment and on learned and cultural patterns of illness behavior.[1, 2, 6, 70, 103–105, 134, 175, 176] The decision to go to the doctor is more likely to be made if the person is suffering from anxiety and emotional distress,[104, 107, 159] or as a result of life events and stress.[105–109, 116]

8. Once a patient reaches the doctor, medical assessment and treatment are influenced by the patient's distress and illness behavior more than by the actual physical disorder.[104, 167] Medical treatment may, in theory, be prescribed on logical physical indications. In practice, however, both conservative[167] and surgical[118, 172] treatments for a poorly understood condition such as low back pain are determined—to a much greater extent than most doctors realize or like to admit—by the patient's distress and illness behavior (Table 4).

Table 3 □ Amount and Severity of Back Pain in People Who Have Attended a Doctor and Those Who Have Received No Medical Attention in the Past 12 Months

	MEDICAL ATTENTION IN THE PAST 12 MONTHS	
	Own Doctor	**None**
Duration of Back Pain in the Past 12 Months		
None	12	211
Part of the year	132	310
All or most of the year	126	79
Severity of Back Pain in the Past 12 Months on a Scale of 0–10		
0–4	48	190
4–7	111	141
7–10	99	59

Calculated from data from the Consumer's Association Back Pain Survey.[27]

Table 4 □ Analysis of Elements of Illness Influencing How Much Conservative Treatment Patients Received for Low Back Pain*

MAIN ELEMENTS OF ILLNESS	EXTENT TO WHICH THESE ACCOUNT FOR THE AMOUNT OF TREATMENT RECEIVED
Duration of symptoms	14%
Physical severity	11%
Psychologic distress	9%
Abnormal illness behavior	15%
Total identified†	50%

*Waddell, G., Bircher, M., Finalyson, D., and Main, C. J.: Symptoms and signs: Physical disease or illness behaviour? Br. Med. J., 289:739–741, 1984.
†See footnote for Table 1.

9. Many claims have been made by individual practitioners about the symptomatic success of various treatments for low back pain; but every controlled trial has shown remarkably few differences among all conceivable treatments.[25, 32, 62, 122, 144, 174] Very few effects have reached statistical significance, and even these are usually so small as to be of no practical clinical significance. It is also important to distinguish between temporary or symptomatic relief and an actual change in the underlying disease or natural history. It is the duty of every doctor to help patients in pain. It is entirely ethical to achieve this by unscientific means, even by using placebos.[10] However, this pragmatic relief of symptoms must be recognized for what it is and must not be confused with the strict scientific proof of the effect of treatment. Viewing the situation in this light, one can see that there is no real evidence that any of our treatments for low back pain is much better than a combination of natural history (Observation 2) and placebo effect.[174]

10. Chronic pain is a clinical syndrome completely different from acute pain.[43, 90, 153, 154, 160] Acute and chronic pain are not only different in time scale;[125] they are fundamentally different in kind. Acute and experimental pains usually bear a straightforward relationship to peripheral stimulus, nociception, and tissue damage.[75] There may be some understandable anxiety about the meaning and consequences of the pain.[153, 154] However, acute pain, acute disability, and acute illness behavior are generally proportionate to the physical findings. Appropriate treatment directed to the underlying physical disorder is usually highly effective in

Table 5 □ Cause of Pain in Patients Admitted to the Johns Hopkins Pain Clinic*

Total admissions	1,541
Spinal pain	1,032
Low back pain with multiple surgery	826
Low back pain with no previous surgery	52

*From Workmen's Compensation Board Symposium: Low Back Pain: A Multi-Disciplinary Approach. Vancouver, 1986.

relieving acute pain. Chronic pain, chronic disability, and chronic illness behavior, in contrast, become increasingly dissociated from the physical problem.[90, 137, 185, 190] There may indeed be very little objective evidence of any remaining nociceptive stimulus.[57, 90, 123] Instead, chronic pain and disability become increasingly associated with emotional distress, depression, disease conviction, and adaptation to chronic invalidity.[18, 43, 128, 157, 171] Chronic pain progressively becomes a self-sustaining condition that is resistant to traditional medical management. Physical treatment directed to a hypothetic but unidentified and possibly nonexistent nociceptive source not only is unsuccessful but may cause additional physical damage. Failed treatment may then reinforce and aggravate pain, distress, disability, and illness behavior.[53, 54, 155, 168, 172, 182] Pain clinics are now full of patients who have undergone failed back surgery (Table 5).

11. Time off work and return to work after treatment are poorly explained by physical severity. They appear to be more dependent on socioeconomic and job-related influences (Table 6).[8, 115, 172, 176] Prolonged time off work *in itself* makes recovery and return to work less likely (see Fig. 1).[39, 156] In all Western countries, however, regardless of the social or medical system, work loss of more than a brief duration depends on sickness certification. The medical profession, therefore, bears the responsibility for not only sanctioning but often advising patients with low back pain to continue to take time off from work.

Preliminary Conclusions

1. Low back pain, based on its natural history, should be a benign self-limiting condition.
2. Low back disability, as opposed to low back pain, appears to be a relatively recent Western epidemic that is not explained by any demonstrable change in the physical disorder.
3. Traditional medical treatment for low back pain has failed, and the role of medicine in the present epidemic of low back disability must be critically examined.

DISEASE MODEL OF ILLNESS

Modern medicine traces its roots to the European Renaissance of the sixteenth and seventeenth centuries. The work of Francis Bacon (1561–1616), Galileo Galilei (1564–1642), and Isaac Newton (1642–1717) epitomized the scientific method. Careful observation, systematic collection of information, and logical reasoning enabled the unlocking of nature's secrets without the influence of religious revelation. Paracelsus (1493–1541), Andreas Vesalius (1514–1564), and William Harvey (1578–1657) successfully challenged the authority of Galen and applied the scientific method to the practice of medicine. Studies of human anatomy and physiology provided the basis for careful clinical observation and understanding of illness. René Descartes (1596–1650), the foremost philosopher of the Renaissance, divided human existence into "mind" and "body." According to this dichotomy pain was characterized as a simple reflex re-

Table 6 □ Comparison of Elements of Illness Influencing Assessment of Outcome of Surgery, Subjective Disability, and Return to Work After Surgery, Based on Separate Regression Analyses of Each Measure

PATIENT'S AND SURGEON'S ASSESSMENT OF OUTCOME OF SURGERY[172]		DISABILITY[171]		RETURN TO WORK AFTER SURGERY[172]	
Postoperative physical impairment	55%	Physical impairment	40%	Postoperative disability	28%
Postoperative pain	20%	Psychologic distress / Abnormal illness behavior	31%	Few identified social factors*	22%
Total identified	75%	Total identified	71%	Total identified	50%

*Very limited social information was available, and this is likely to be an underestimate.

sponse to a physical stimulus.[31] Practical interpretation of pain could then be used to elucidate disease.

> A pain, an ache, a discomfort—these are the common complaints of those who seek the doctor's help. Pain issues a warning with kindly intent. She calls to action and, pointing the way, brooks no delay. And thus the ancient [sic] cycle is served, from pain to cause, to treatment to cure.[135]

Sydenham (1624–1689) is the father of modern clinical medicine. He distinguished illness from underlying disease and developed our present concept of individual diseases with characteristic symptoms and signs. However, it was only two centuries later, when Louis Pasteur (1822–1895) discovered that infectious disease was caused by microbes[134] and Rudolf Virchow (1821–1902) proposed the concept of cellular pathology,[163] that this philosophic approach to medicine could be turned into daily practice. Since that time, modern medicine has been based on the following disease model of illness:

- Recognize patterns of illness behavior (symptoms and signs)
- Infer underlying pathologic condition (diagnosis)
- Conduct physical therapy for underlying pathologic condition (treatment)
- Expect illness behavior to improve (cure)

The industrial revolution, increasing material resources, and the explosion of technology after World War II have given us powerful new investigative and therapeutic tools. We can now treat disease in a way that previous ages would have regarded as miraculous, although twentieth century Western society takes it for granted. This physical approach to medicine reached its peak when the mystery of life itself was unraveled in the DNA molecule.[26] It became possible to replace hip joints[23] and even to transplant hearts.[142] In this mood of medical achievement and euphoria it was possible to assert confidently that the primary role of the doctor was the control and, ideally, the relief of all pain.[43, 188]

This physical approach to disease depends on being able to identify the physical disorder. Symptoms and disability must be directly related to this. Any psychologic elements must be relatively unimportant. Clinical diagnosis of the underlying pathologic condition then provides the basis of rational physical treatment of the illness. Unfortunately, in low back pain none of these assumptions is true, so it is not surprising that conventional medical treatment for low back pain has been unsuccessful.

BIOPSYCHOSOCIAL CONCEPT OF ILLNESS

Medicine has a much more ancient and much richer lineage than science. Since before the time of Plato the relationship between mind and body has been held to be of fundamental importance to human existence and to medicine. Aristotle recognized that human beings are social animals who live and act—and fall ill—in a social relationship with other humans. Hippocrates emphasized the already well-established tradition that the doctor's practical role as healer cannot be separated from the social role of helping humans to cope with illness and suffering.[69]

There is no logical reason why scientific treatment of disease should not be combined with human care of the patient.[4] It is only because of the limitations of human nature that increased time, training, and concentration on the physical aspects of disease have led doctors to neglect the psychologic and social aspects of illness.[48] All doctors agree in principle with the need to treat each patient as a human being, but in a busy practice we too quickly proceed with the practicalities of treating perceived disease. Yet, from the time of Claude Bernard[14] to the present day there has been a recurring note of concern and criticism from eminent members of the profession[141] and independent observers.[79] A too-mechanistic approach may cure many serious diseases but addresses only one half—and not necessarily the more important half—of the role of medicine in society.

Practical application of these humanitarian principles to the daily practice of medicine has fallen behind the physical therapy of disease. Nearly a century ago, Sigmund Freud (1856–1939) reaffirmed the importance of psychologic factors in medicine. He showed that psychoneurotic symptoms could be assessed clinically to provide insight into emotional processes.[58] Adolf Meyer (1866–1950) originally developed the concept of *multicausality* in psychiatry.

However, he recognized that psychosocial factors influenced the course and outcome of every illness and that each patient must be seen and assessed as a person.[114] Such a holistic view of medicine has been the hallmark, inspiration, and source of the preeminence of American psychiatry.[87] It has rightly been claimed that an understanding of the psychosocial aspects of illness is one of the most important contributions that the behavioral sciences can make to medicine.[86] Because mental illness has never comfortably fit the disease model, psychiatrists have raised fundamental questions about illness. They have proposed an alternative biopsychosocial model, which includes physical, psychologic, and social elements.[44–47, 86–88] This is very much a model of human illness, rather than disease, and applies equally well to physical illness (Fig. 6).

The gate control theory of pain[112] provided the physiologic basis of the biopsychosocial model. Pain can no longer be regarded as merely a physical sensation of noxious stimulus and disease. Conscious experience of pain may be modulated by mental, emotional, and sensory mechanisms. It includes both sensory and emotional components.[75, 105, 111, 161] The major conceptual contribution of the gate control theory is that it replaces the Cartesian mind—body dichotomy and allows for the complexity of clinical pain phenomena. It explains how psychologic and social influences may indeed modulate individual perception and response to disease. The gate control theory has stimulated and contributed greatly to the new clinical approach to illness. However, we should avoid overemphasizing pain as the single most important element of human illness and even as the sole focus of medical treatment.[43, 173] The gate control theory should not be clinically misapplied, merely perpetuating the errors of the disease model in a new direction. The physical treatment of pain should not be completely divorced from our ability to diagnose disease or carried out without due consideration of nonphysical factors. The gate mechanism should not be invoked simply to move failed physical treatment to a higher level in the neural pathway. The true clinical application of the gate control theory lies in a fuller understanding of human pain and illness.

Several elements of the biopsychosocial model have been developed further in the behavioral sciences. Early hopes that personality tests would predict individual responses to illness have not been realized,[64, 99] although they have led to a number of simple psychologic questionnaires used to measure distress.[9, 97, 192] Medical sociology,[106, 108, 109] behavioral psychology,[51, 54, 161] and psychiatry[138, 139] have combined to develop the concept of illness behavior. This can be assessed clinically as "observable and potentially measurable actions and conduct which express and communicate the individual's own perception of disturbed health."[167] Sociologists have considered illness to be a social phenomenon or sick role.[102–109, 133]

The whole biopsychosocial concept emphasizes human illness, rather than disease. This idea must now be applied to clinical practice.[83, 95]

ANALYSIS OF SUCCESS AND FAILURE IN LOW BACK DISORDERS

We can now treat and even prevent many serious spinal diseases, such as polio, tuberculosis, spinal deformities, and paralysis. Since the identification of the disc prolapse,[117] surgical relief has become routine for nerve compression that fails to resolve naturally. Disc surgery has survived the test

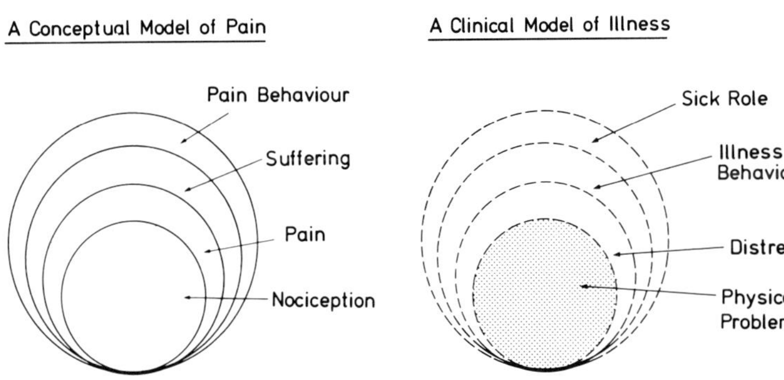

Figure 6. □ The biopsychosocial concept of illness[44]: Loeser's conceptual model of pain[80, 89] and the Glasgow Illness Model[167, 171]—an operational model for clinical practice.

of time; at least 70% to 80% of carefully selected patients experience relief.[149] Such dramatic surgical successes, unfortunately, apply to only some 1% of patients with low back disorders.[131] Our failure is in the remaining 99% of patients with simple backache, for whom, despite new investigations and all our treatments, the problem has become progressively worse (see Figs. 2 to 4).

Medical diagnosis may be one of two fundamentally different kinds: substantive or nominal.[191] Substantive diagnoses have objective clinical features, and investigations confirm a definite pathologic process. This permits rational and successful treatment. In most patients with simple backache, however, we cannot identify any definite pathologic condition or even the exact anatomic source of pain.[121] Because human beings dislike uncertainty and fear the unknown, we search for the meaning of strange events as the first stage to regaining control.[104] The preference of doctors and patients for even a nominal diagnosis is clearly demonstrated by the vogue of the diagnosis of the disc prolapse (see Fig. 3). Mixter's and Barr's original insistence on the need for definite clinical and radiologic proof before making the diagnosis[117] was soon forgotten. Indeed, by 1945 Key[80] could dogmatically state that 99% of all low back pain, apart from tumor and infection, was a result of lesions of the intervertebral disc. Of patients coming to our clinic, 60% believe or have been told that they have a disc prolapse, although only 11% show any evidence of nerve root involvement.[164] Radiologically observed changes of degeneration are an equally irresistible causal explanation of symptoms, if one ignores their normal, age-related occurrence (Observation 6).

Patients and doctors alike are much more comfortable and happier with even nominal diagnosis. Unfortunately, once such a diagnosis has been made, we easily forget that it was only a convenient label and begin to treat it as if it were substantive. Not unexpectedly, the success rate of treatment based on such a nominal diagnosis is low.[149] Unjustified pseudopathologic diagnoses must be avoided and replaced by clear unambiguous terms such as *simple backache* or *simple back strain*.[42] Physical treatment, particularly potentially harmful treatment such as surgery, should be directed to the objective pathologic conditions that they are likely to help. A study of the indications for spinal surgery suggests that, in practice, decisions to operate are frequently based on the duration and severity of the patient's pain and disability, the patient's distress and illness behavior, and the failure of conservative treatment. However, the outcome of surgery depends on the accuracy of diagnosis of a surgically treatable lesion.[172] The patient's demand and the doctor's desire to help must not confuse logical, rational decisions about physical treatment based on substantive diagnosis.

When the number of operations escalated after World War II, it was soon realized that the failures of spinal surgery were catastrophic.[29, 59, 66, 77, 168, 172] Every study for the past 30 years has stressed the association of surgical failure with psychologic disturbance.[65, 168, 172, 182] In 1975 Wiltse and Rocchio first demonstrated that preoperative psychologic tests could actually predict how patients would respond to treatment.[182] A number of prospective studies have since shown that psychologic factors influence how patients respond to any form of physical treatment, regardless of whether it is physiotherapy,[12, 23] rehabilitation,[8, 49] chemonucleolysis,[91, 182] surgical decompression,[41, 132, 136] fusion,[183] repeat spinal surgery,[40] or pain tract surgery.[17] The most important psychologic disturbances associated with low back pain are anxiety, increased bodily awareness, and depressive symptoms, which are best interpreted clinically as psychologic distress.[104, 153, 171, 172] This distress is largely secondary to the physical disorder and becomes better or worse, depending on the success or failure of treatment.[155, 172] Furthermore, distress arising from unrelated causes may aggravate and perpetuate physical pain.

Clinical observation should distinguish the symptoms and signs of physical disease from those of distress and illness behavior.[140, 169, 171] This is most simply illustrated by the pain drawing.[140] The *way* that patients draw their pain is influenced by distress. So the patient's apparently straightforward description of pain provides both physical information about the pain and psychologic information about the response to the pain (Fig. 7). Similarly, the adjectives that patients use to describe pain fall into two distinct patterns. Some describe the sensory qualities of pain, whereas others are mainly about the emotional qualities of the pain

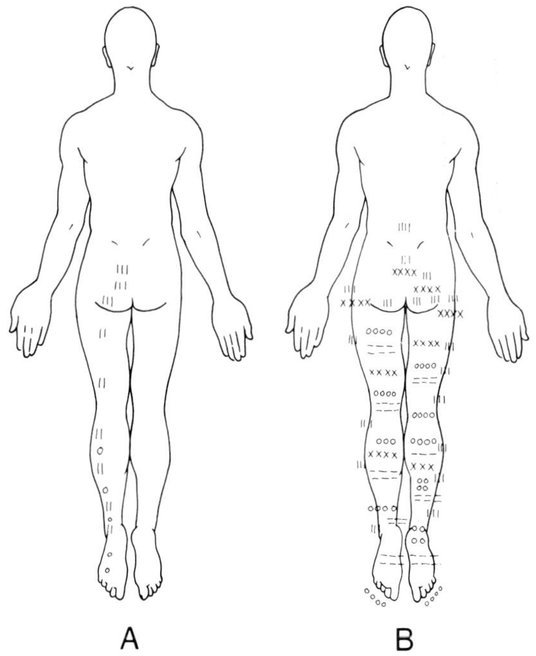

Figure 7 □ The pain drawing provides clinical information about the physical and emotional characteristics of the patient's pain.[140] Patient A describes the anatomic pattern of S1 pain and paraesthesia from a disc prolapse. Patient B with simple low-back pain does not have cauda equina involvement but is communicating distress. Many patients' symptoms communicate a combination of both physical information and distress to various degrees. (00 = pain; 0 = pins and needles; x = ache; = = = numbness). (From Waddell, G., Bircher, M., Finalyson, D., and Main, C. J.: Symptoms and signs: Physical disease or illness behaviour? Br. Med. J., 289:739–741, 1984.)

experience.[82, 110] Behavioral symptoms and signs have also been described in low back pain and provide a clinical measure of distress and illness behavior (Table 7).[169, 171]

We have tested the biopsychosocial model in clinical practice by analyzing the mathematic relationship among the elements of illness in chronic low back pain. We measured the relationship between pain and disability and physical impairment (see Fig. 4).[166] The psychologic disturbance, we found, is simply distress about the continuing pain.[171] We were able to distinguish the symptoms and signs of illness behavior and

Table 7 □ Comparison of the Symptoms and Signs of Physical Disease and Abnormal Illness Behavior in Chronic Low Back Pain

	PHYSICAL DISEASE, NORMAL ILLNESS BEHAVIOR	INAPPROPRIATE OR BEHAVIORAL SYMPTOMS AND SIGNS
Pain Drawing[140]	Localized Neuroanatomic Proportionate	Nonanatomic Regional Magnified
Pain Adjectives[110]	Sensory	Emotional
Symptoms[171]		
Pain	Localized	Whole leg pain Tailbone pain
Numbness	Dermatomal	Whole leg numbness
Weakness	Myotomal	Whole leg giving way
Time pattern	Varies with time	Never free of pain
Response to treatment	Variable benefit	Intolerance of treatments Emergency admissions to hospital
Signs[169]		
Tenderness	Localized	Superficial Widespread nonanatomic
Axial loading	No lumbar pain	Lumbar pain
Simulated rotation	No lumbar pain	Lumbar pain
Straight-leg raising	Limited on distraction	Improves with distraction
Sensory	Dermatomal	Regional
Motor	Myotomal	Regional, jerky, giving way
General response	Appropriate pain	Over-reaction

those of physical disease (see Table 7).[171] Distress and illness behavior were found to be secondary to the physical disorder and improve or deteriorate with successful or failed treatment[172]. We showed how physical disorder, distress, and illness behavior combine to produce disability (see Table 2).[171] Medical decisions about conservative[167] and surgical[172] treatment are influenced, we found, by distress and illness behavior more than by physical indications (see Table 3). Our studies showed how physical and psychologic factors interact to determine the outcome of treatment.[172] Finally, we found that work loss and return to work are determined more by social factors than by the physical disorder (see Table 6).[172] All of our studies confirm that the biopsychosocial concept of illness can be used as an operational clinical model (see Fig. 6*B*), which explains many of the observations on the natural history of low back pain and disability.

REST OR RECOVERY?

Rest, restriction of activity, and bed rest is now standard treatment for backache. Rest is the treatment most commonly prescribed by doctors, apart from symptomatic analgesics (Table 8*A*). Bed rest is unanimously taught as the first line of treatment for "acute attacks." Yet bed rest became the accepted "conservative" treatment only in recent times. One of the patients in Mixter's and Barr's original description of disc prolapse[117] had "several months in absolute recumbency on a Bradford frame without relief" (sic) before surgery. By as early as 1923, a standard orthopedic text suggested that immediate recumbency was required for the most severe cases of back strains. It also cautioned against excessive bed rest and advised that "as soon as possible, movement must be encouraged and bed forbidden." Personal experience,[7] however, suggests that this was very much the exception and was employed only in rare cases before World War II. Even by as late as 1966, family doctors could write that "little discussion (of acute backache or its treatment) is given in the standard textbooks of orthopaedics."[35] It appears that bed rest has been widely prescribed only within the last generation.

The rationale of rest, and particularly bed rest, is not nearly as obvious as might be imagined. It appears to be based on the clinical observation that lying down may relieve pain, although this applies to only one person in two (Table 8*B*). The pathophysiologic argument[32, 61] seems to be a combination of a nominal diagnosis of disc prolapse[117] and the biomechanical finding that intradiscal pressure is lowest in the lying position.[119, 120, 127] However, this argument contains a number of completely illogical steps. Symptomatic relief of pain is not necessarily associated with alteration of the natural history or cure of the pain: compare parts *B* and *C* of Table 8. Disc prolapse accounts for only a small percentage of those with back pain, and treatment for disc prolapse cannot be extrapolated to that for all low back pain. Because of the difference between acute and chronic pain, treatment directed to the noxious stimulus of acute pain may be quite inappropriate for chronic pain.

Remarkably little scientific or clinical evidence is available to support the advisability of bed rest for low back pain or sciatica. There are only four controlled studies of bed rest.[33, 62, 84, 180] Only the trial by Weisel and colleagues[180] showed an advantage to bed rest, but this study suffered major methodologic defects.[61, 94] It was carried out on army recruits and compared admissions to sick bay with continued, albeit modified, army duties. No allowance was made for the pa-

Table 8 □ Treatment for Low Back Pain

A. INCIDENCE REPORTED BY 500 PATIENTS ATTENDING ORTHOPEDIC CLINICS[36]

Treatment	1 Course	>1 Course
Analgesics	18%	69%
Bed rest	21%	27%
Corset	14%	17%
Physiotherapy	10%	14%
Manipulation	5%	5%

B. EFFECT OF ACTIVITY ON LOW BACK PAIN[27, 28]

	Relieves Pain	No Difference	Makes Pain Worse
Lying down	58%	30%	10%
Walking	16%	45%	36%

C. MOST EFFECTIVE TREATMENT/CURE FOR LOW BACK PAIN[27, 28]

Analgesics	35%
Local heat/Applications/Massage	30%
Exercise/Physiotherapy/Manipulation	20%
Rest/Lying down	14%

tients' attitudes to the treatment or to training. In the particular military context, there was considerable observer bias in assessing the results. Yet this is the only clinical trial suggesting that bed rest is better than continued ambulation. In complete contrast, Gilbert and colleagues[62] found no statistically significant differences between bed rest, exercise, and no treatment, although the results tended to favor early mobilization. Lidstrom and Zachrisson[84] found little difference between exercise and rest, except that exercise improved muscle strength. Deyo and colleagues[33, 34] showed that 2 days of bed rest were more beneficial than 7 days. However, their results could also be interpreted to show that 7 days of bed rest were proportionately more harmful than 2 days! No studies compare bed rest in the hospital with bed rest at home. Consequently, it is difficult to justify the admission of 40,000 to 50,000 patients to the hospital each year in Britain for bed rest for low back pain. Yet 2,000 hospital beds are permanently occupied in this way while other patients are kept waiting up to 3 years for the proven procedure of hip replacement for osteoarthritis.[130, 131]

There is little doubt about the harmful effects of bed rest, particularly if it is prolonged.[18, 100, 101] This is part of basic medical and nursing teachings. Protracted rest leads to a catabolic state with general malaise.[18] There is demineralization of bone[146] and 3% loss of muscle strength per day.[150] Cardiovascular fitness decreases.[100, 101] Rest and inactivity actually inhibit healing.[18] More generally, prolonged rest causes increased psychologic distress and depression. There are loss of the work habit, increasing difficulty in starting rehabilitation, progressive loss of job opportunity, and decreasing probability of ever returning to work (Fig. 1).[72, 156] Perhaps the final test is to observe how doctors treat themselves. At a recent meeting,[186] 60% of 230 doctors reported personal experience of backache. Only two had stayed in bed for as long as 2 weeks, and none for longer periods. Yet doctors continue to treat their patients with prolonged bed rest, a way in which they would never treat themselves. Some patients with simple backache are actually treated as if they were more seriously ill than patients with myocardial infarction who now routinely receive early ambulation.[74]

Conversely, there is no evidence that activity is harmful. Contrary to medical belief, it does not necessarily even aggravate the pain (Table 8*B*). With increasing biomechanical understanding, it is possible to avoid specific activities that increase the load on the spine.[12, 115, 116, 189] Several studies have shown that patients with backache or sciatica can perform selected activities almost normally without increasing their pain.[13, 93, 126] Indeed, there is evidence that increased activity may promote bone and muscle strength.[18, 84, 146] It improves disc and cartilage nutrition,[123] and it increases systemic endorphin levels, perhaps actually reducing pain.[123] No evidence suggests that early return to work increases the likelihood of future recurrences. On the contrary, physically fit people have fewer and shorter attacks of low back pain and are more tolerant of pain.[16, 20, 123]

Fordyce and other behavioral psychologists have investigated the relationship between chronic pain and physical activity.[57, 85] They suggest that pain behaviors are influenced and modified by their consequences.[54, 56] Exercise to the limit of pain tolerance is strongly influenced by conscious feedback about the amount of exercise that has been done. In the absence of such feedback, patients with chronic pain perform the same amount of exercise as normal pain-free people.[52] The exercise tolerance of chronic pain patients is also markedly improved by verbal praise and encouragement from a physiotherapist.[21] Patients with chronic backache almost universally report lower levels of activity, but careful observation shows that subjective reports of pain are largely unrelated to activity levels.[57, 85] Observed pain behavior is, in fact, inversely proportional to the amount of exercise performed.[57] In an elegant experiment,[53] Fordyce and colleagues compared traditional medical treatment with a behavioral approach to acute low back pain. Traditional treatment was rest, analgesics, and activity on a PRN basis; the patient was advised to "let pain be your guide." This was compared with a fixed regimen of incremental activity based on tissue healing times. At 1 year follow-up, patients treated on the traditional basis reported that disability had actually increased. Patients treated on the rehabilitation regime had returned to preonset levels of activity. Dolce and coworkers[37] independently confirmed the value of a fixed exercise quota. They showed increased exercise tolerance, an increased self-estimate of exercise capability, and decreased anxiety about the effects of exercise. Berntzen and Gotestam[15] confirmed that regular analgesics provided greater relief than PRN medication and also reduced drug dependency.

An improved understanding of the relationship between pain and physical activity has already been tested in clinical practice. Industrial physicians and occupational therapists have always emphasized the physical, psychologic, and social value of an early return to work,[30, 63, 178] although this has never been scientifically confirmed.[22, 94] Improved spinal ergonomics combined with physiotherapy has produced the back school approach to patient education. Improved understanding reduces fear and improves the ability of patients to cope with their back problems.[67, 177, 189] The goal of most pain management program is rehabilitative rather than symptomatic and tries to improve functional capacity and reduce illness behavior. Patients have to take a more active role, in which they accept responsibility and begin to manage the problems themselves.[50, 98, 104] Mayer and colleagues[100, 101] have combined these principles into a sports medicine approach to the clinical rehabilitation of patients with chronic backache. They used objective functional capacity measurements to guide patients on an active exercise program with the emphasis on improving function rather than solely on pain. Psychologic support and education were also provided. Some temporary increase in pain occurred, but over the long term, patients improved their objective functional capacity, and this was associated with less pain, less distress, less health care utilization, and an 86% return to work. An active approach to illness can indeed be used in clinical practice to treat the whole person.

The evidence is clear. There is a fundamental antithesis between the passive and active strategies of rest or activity. There is no evidence that rest has any beneficial effect on the natural history of backache. On the contrary, there is strongly suggestive evidence that rest, particularly prolonged bedrest, may be the most harmful treatment ever devised for backache and a potent cause of iatrogenic disability (Table 9). There is clear evidence that, despite medical belief, activity is not harmful for backache and active rehabilitation can not only restore function but actually reduce pain. It remains to be proven whether a policy of active mobilization and early return to work can be put into widespread clinical practice.[94] However, the questions can no longer be avoided: rest or rehabilitation? rest or restoration of function? rest or recovery?

Table 9 □ Chronic Backache—A Disuse Syndrome

Loss of 3% muscle bulk per day on bedrest
Loss of muscle strength and endurance
Loss of cardiovascular fitness
Demineralization of bone
Tissue healing inhibited
General debility and malaise
Anxiety, distress, and depression
Anger
Disease conviction
Illness behavior
Restriction of social activities
Economic loss
Job loss
Loss of interest and motivation
Slowing mental processes
Physically and mentally progressively more difficult to start rehabilitation
Adopt chronic invalid role
Avoid iatrogenic disability—bedrest is bad for backs.

CONCLUSIONS

Backache affects most human beings at some time in their lives and is recorded throughout human history. Chronic disability due to simple backache is a relatively recent Western epidemic. Modern medicine can successfully treat many serious spinal diseases but has completely failed to cure the vast majority of patients with simple backache. Much worse, our concentration on physical therapy may be contributing to the problem. We place too much emphasis on pain to the exclusion of other aspects of illness. We overdiagnose disc lesions. We overprescribe rest. We have actually prescribed low back disability!

Much remains to be learned about backache. It is necessary that we relate improved biomechanical understanding to clinical observation in the individual patient. We must develop methods of localizing the exact source of the pain, and we must differentiate low back syndromes. Furthermore, we must conduct proper, controlled trials to determine which treatments are most effective for which types of backache. Only in this way can we develop a rational basis for choosing the most effective treatment for each patient.

But equally and more fundamentally important, we must change our entire approach to backache. In principle, we all agree about the need to treat people rather than spines. To make this a practical reality we must consider low back disability as an illness, rather than low back pain as a disease. We all recognize, in theory, the need to consider the physical, psychologic, and social aspects of illness. To put this into practice we must distinguish pain from disability, distinguish the symptoms and signs of distress and illness behavior from those of physical disease, and direct treatment to restoration of function as well as the relief from pain.

This leads to a fundamental shift in our strategy for managing backache (Table 10). Backache is only a symptom; it is not a serious disease unless we make it so. We must provide whatever relief from pain we can, but our aim must be to help patients to lead a life that is as normal as possible. They should either stay at work or return to work as rapidly as possible. Whatever the modalities of treatment we use, they must be directed toward helping the patient. We must confess honestly that we do not have a magic cure for backache, and the doctor's role as healer must be accompanied by the more ancient role as counselor helping patients to cope with their problems. Correspondingly, the patient's role must change from that of a passive recipient of treatment to a more active sharing of responsibility for one's own progress. Above all, we must stop causing iatrogenic disability. Our basic strategy of management must change from rest to rehabilitation and active restoration of function.

This requires a change in medicine, in patients, and in society. Some change must occur at political and managerial levels. Nevertheless, doctors cannot escape the primary responsibility, both as the final providers of health care and for providing society with a new understanding and model of illness, which alone makes real change possible.

Table 10 □ Management Strategy for Backache

Aim to keep the patient as active as possible.
Aim to return the patient to work as soon as possible.
Make sure that there is no serious pathologic condition.
Reassure the patient that this is simple backache. Use words such as strain, muscle pain, or rheumatics. Avoid words such as rupture, degeneration or arthritis.
Reassure the patient that he or she will get better, usually quite quickly, provided that he or she gets going.
Most patients can simply modify their activities in the acute stage. Only the most acute patients need bed rest, and then usually for only 1 to 2 days.
Patients do need adequate pain relief in the acute stage.
Encourage early mobilization, usually within a few days, and always by 2 weeks at the very latest—even if it hurts a bit at first (hurt and harm are not the same). Reassure patients that they will not do any damage by moving; they will incur more harm by staying in bed. Use a sports medicine analogy.
Use whatever treatment modalities you find successful, provided that they help the patient to get back to normal activities.
Work is good for people with backache. Get the patient back to work as soon as possible, usually within 1 to 2 weeks, and almost always by 6 weeks. Consider the possibility of modified work, at first. Advising someone to give up his or her livelihood because of simple backache is rarely justified.
Avoid iatrogenic disability.

Acknowledgments

This chapter was adapted from and reproduced with permission from Spine 12:632–644, 1987. The studies on which it is based were supported by the Medical Research Council, the Back Pain Association, and the MacTaggart Trust. I would particularly like to thank David Allan, Bill Fordyce, David Hamblen, Bill Hrudey, John Loeser, Chris Main, Alf Nachemson, Henrik Weber, and Philip Wood for their ideas, information, and assistance. Further data and detailed analyses were supplied by the Consumer's Association, London, the Department of Health and Social Security Headquarters Division SR8B, Newcastle upon Tyne, and the Workmen's Compensation Board of British Columbia. The interpretation and views expressed, however, are entirely my own responsibility.

References

1. Alonzo, A.A.: Acute illness behaviour: A conceptual exploration and specification. Soc. Sci. Med. 14A:515–526, 1980.
2. Alonzo, A.A.: An illness behaviour paradigm: A conceptual exploration of a situational-adaptation perspective. Soc. Sci. Med. 19:499–510, 1984.
3. American Academy of Orthopaedic Surgeons: Manual for Orthopaedic Surgeons in Evaluating Permanent Physical Impairment. Chicago (undated), pp. 1–30.
4. American Board of Internal Medicine: Clinical competence in internal medicine. Ann. Intern. Med. 90:402–411, 1979.
5. American Medical Association: A guide to the evaluation of permanent impairment of the extremities and back. J.A.M.A. 166(Suppl.):1–122, 1958.

6. Balint, M.: The Doctor, His Patient and the Illness, 2nd Ed. London, Pitman, 1968.
7. Barnes, R.: Unpublished data, University of Glasgow.
8. Beals, R.K., and Hickman, N.W.: Industrial injuries of the back and extremities. J. Bone Joint Surg. 54A:1593–1611, 1972.
9. Beck, A.T., Ward, C.H., Mendelson, M.M., et al.: An inventory for measuring depression. Arch. Gen. Psychiatr. 4:561–571, 1961.
10. Beecher, H.K.: Measurement of subjective responses: Quantitative effect of drugs. New York, Oxford University Press, 1959.
11. Benn, R.T., and Wood, P.H.N.: Pain in the back: An attempt to estimate the size of the problem. Rheumatol. Rehab. 14:121–128, 1975.
12. Bergquist-Ullman, M., and Larsson, U.: Acute low back pain in industry. Acta Orthop. Scand. 170(Suppl.):1–117, 1977.
13. Berkson, M., Schultz, A., Nachemson, A., and Andersson, G.B.J.: Voluntary strengths of male adults with acute low back pain. Clin. Orthop. 129:84–95, 1977.
14. Bernard, C.: Leçons sur les Phénomènes de la Vie Commune aux Animaux et aux Végétaux. Paris, Baillière, 1878.
15. Berntzen, D., Gotestam, K.G.: Effects of on-demand or fixed interval schedules in the treatment of chronic pain with analgesia compounds: An experimental study (in press, J. Consult. Clin. Psychol.).
16. Biering-Sorensen, P.: Physical measurements as risk indicators for low back trouble over a one year period. Spine 9:106–119, 1984.
17. Blumetti, A.E., and Modesti, L.M.: Psychological Predictors of Success or Failure of Surgical Intervention for Intractable Back Pain, *In* Bonica, J.J., Albe-Fessard, D. (eds.): Advances in Pain. Research and Therapy. Vol 1. New York, Raven Press, 1976.
18. Bortz, W.M.: The disuse syndrome. West. J. Med. 141:691–694, 1984.
19. Brown, T., Barr, J.S., Nemiah, J.C., and Barry, H.: Psychological factors in low back pain. N. Engl. J. Med. 251:123–128, 1954.
20. Cady, L., Bischoff, D., and O'Connel, E.: Strength and fitness and subsequent back injuries in firefighters. J. Occup. Med. 21:269–272, 1979.
21. Cairns, D., and Pasino, J.: Comparison of verbal reinforcement and feedback in the operant treatment of disability due to chronic low back pain. Behav. Ther. 8:621–630, 1977.
22. Catchlove, R., and Cohen, K.: Effects of a directive return to work approach in the treatment of workmen's compensation patients with chronic pain. Pain 14:181–191, 1982.
23. Charnley, J.: Arthroplasty of the hip: A new operation. Lancet 1:1129–1132, 1961.
24. Choler, U., Larsson, R., Nachemson, A., and Paterson, L.-E.: Ont y ryggen—farsok med vardsprogram for patienter med lumbala smattillstrand. Stockholm, S.P.R.I. Report 188/85, 1985.
25. Cochrane Report: Working Group on Back Pain. London, H.M.S.O., 1979.
26. Cochrane, W., and Crick, F.H.C.: Evidence of the Pauling-Covey α-helix in synthetic polypeptides. Nature 169:234–235, 1952.
27. Consumer's Association: Back Pain Survey. London, 1986.
28. Consumer's Association: Back pain: The which report—Which? Feb.: 58–63, 1986.
29. De Palma, A.F., and Rothman, R.H.: The Intervertebral Disc. Philadelphia, W.B. Saunders, 1970.
30. Derebery, W.J., and Tullis, W.H.: Delayed recovery in the patient with a work compensable injury. J. Occup. Med. 25:829–835, 1983.
31. Descartes, R.: L'Homme (translated by M. Foster). New York, Cambridge University Press, 1644.
32. Deyo, R.A.: Conservative therapy for low back pain: Distinguishing useful from useless therapy. J.A.M.A. 250:1057–1062, 1983.
33. Deyo, R.A., Diehl, A.K., and Rosenthal, M.: How much bed rest for backache? A randomised clinical trial. Clin. Res. 33:248A, 1985.
34. Deyo, R.A., Diehl, A.K., and Rosenthal, M.: How many days of bed rest for acute low back pain? N. Engl. J. Med. 315:1064–1070, 1986.
35. Dillane, J.B., Fry, J., and Kalton, G.: Acute back syndrome—a study from general practice. Br. Med. J. 2:82–84, 1966.
36. Di-Paola, M., Waddell, G.: Unpublished data, University of Glasgow.
37. Dolce, J.J., Crocker, M.F., Moletteire, C., and Doleys, D.M.: Exercise quotas, anticipatory concern and self-efficacy expectancies in chronic pain: A preliminary report. Pain 24:365–372, 1986.
38. Dunnell, K., and Cartwright, A.: Medicine Takers, Prescribers and Hoarders. London, Routledge & Kegan Paul, 1972.
39. Dworkin, R.H., Handlin, D.S., Richlin, D.M., et al.: Unravelling the effects of compensation, litigation and employment on treatment response in chronic pain. Pain 23:49–59, 1985.
40. Dzioba, R.B., and Doxey, N.C.: Predictors of outcome of repeat back surgery following industrial injuries. Presented at the annual meeting of the American Academy of Orthopaedic Surgeons, 1984.
41. Dzioba, R.B., and Doxey, N.C.: A prospective investigation into the orthopaedic and psychologic predictors of outcome of first lumbar surgery following industrial injury. Spine 9:614–623, 1984.
42. Editorial: Back pain—what can we offer? Br. Med. J. 1:706, 1979.
43. Engel, G.L.: Psychogenic pain and the pain prone patient. Am. J. Med. 26:899–918, 1959.
44. Engel, G.L.: The need for a new medical model: A challenge for biomedicine. Science 196:129–136, 1977.
45. Engel, G.L.: The biopsychosocial model and medical education. N. Engl. J. Med. 306:802–805, 1982.
46. Fabrega, H.: The position of psychiatry in the understanding of human disease. Arch. Gen. Psychiatr. 32:1500–1512, 1972.
47. Fabrega, H.: The need for an ethnomedical science. Science 189:969–975, 1975.
48. Flexner, A.: Medical Education in the United States and Canada. New York, Carnegie Foundation, 1910.
49. Flynn, R.J., Salomone, P.R.: Performance of the MMPI in predicting rehabilitation outcome: A discriminant analysis, double-cross validation assessment. Rehab. Lit. 38:12–15, 1977.

50. Follick, M.J., Smith, T.W., and Ahern, D.K.: Sickness impact profile: A global measure of disability in chronic low back pain. Pain 21:67–76, 1985.
51. Fordyce, W.E.: Behavioural Methods for Chronic Pain and Illness. St. Louis, C.V. Mosby, 1976.
52. Fordyce, W.E.: A behavioural perspective on chronic pain. Br. J. Clin. Psychol. 21:313–320, 1982.
53. Fordyce, W.E., Brockway, J.A., Bergman, J.A., and Spengler, D.: Acute back pain: A control group comparison of behavioural vs. traditional management methods. J. Behav. Med. 9:127–140, 1986.
54. Fordyce, W.E., Fowler, R.S., Lehmann, J.F., and DeLateur, B.J.: Some implications of learning in problems of chronic pain. J. Chron. Dis. 21:179–190, 1968.
55. Fordyce, W.E., Roberts, A.H., and Sternbach, R.A.: The behavioural management of chronic pain: A response to critics. Pain 22:113–125, 1985.
56. Fordyce, W.E., Shelton, J.L., and Dundore, D.E.: The modification of avoidance learning pain behaviours. J. Behav. Med. 5:405–414, 1982.
57. Fordyce, W.E., McMahon, R., Rainwater, G., et al: Pain complaint-exercise performance relationship in chronic pain. Pain 10:311–321, 1981.
58. Freud, S.: Collected Papers. New York, Basic Books, 1959.
59. Frymoyer, J.W., and Donaghy, R.M.P.: The ruptured intervertebral disc: Follow-up report on the first case fifty years after recognition of the syndrome and its surgical significance. J. Bone Joint Surg. 67A:1113–1116, 1985.
60. Fullenlove, T.M., and Williams, A.J.: Comparative roentgen findings in symptomatic and asymptomatic backs. J.A.M.A. 168:572–574, 1957.
61. Gilbert, J.R.: Management of low back pain in family practice: A critical review. Can. Fam. Phys. 32:1855–1861, 1986.
62. Gilbert, J.R., Taylor, D.W., and Hildebrand, A.: Clinical trial of common treatments for low back pain in family practice. Br. Med. J. 291:791–794, 1985.
63. Goldberg, R.T.: The social and vocational rehabilitation of persons with chronic pain. Rehab. Lit. 43:274–283, 1982.
64. Graham, J.R.: The MMPI: A practical guide. New York, Oxford University Press, 1977.
65. Gray, I.C.M., Main, C.J., and Waddell, G.: Illness behaviour and the role of psychological assessment in general orthopaedic practice. Clin. Orthop. 184:258–263, 1984.
66. Greenwood, J., McGuire, T.H., and Kimbell, F.: A study of causes of failure in the herniated vertebral disc operation. J. Neurosurg. 9:15–20, 1952.
67. Hall, H.H., and Iceton, J.A.: Back School: An overview with specific reference to the Canadian Back Education Units. Clin. Orthop. 179:10–17, 1983.
68. Harris, R.I., and Macnab, I.: Structural changes in the intervertebral discs. J. Bone Joint Surg. 36B:304–323, 1954.
69. Hippocrates: Translated by W.H.S. Jones. Cambridge, Harvard University Press, 1923.
70. Hirschfield, A., and Behan, R.C.: The accident process. J.A.M.A. 186:84–90, 193–199, 1963; 197:125–129, 1966.
71. Horal, J.: The clinical appearance of low back pain disorders in the city of Gothenburg, Sweden. Acta Orthop. Scand. 118(Suppl.):1–109, 1969.
72. Hrudey, W.P. Unpublished data, Workmen's Compensation Board of British Columbia.
73. Hult, L.: The Munkfors investigation. Acta Orthop. Scand. 16(Suppl.), 1954.
74. Hurst, J.W.: Ambulation after myocardial infarction (editorial). N. Engl. J. Med. 292:746–748, 1975.
75. International Association for the Study of Pain: Pain terms: A list with definitions and notes on usage. Pain 6:249–252, 1979.
76. Jones, R., and Lovett, R.W.: Orthopaedic Surgery. London, Hodder & Stoughton, 1923.
77. Kelly, J.N., Voris, D.C., Swien, H.J., and Ghormley, R.K.: Multiple operations for protruded lumbar vertebral discs. Proc. Staff Meet. Mayo Clin. 29:546–550, 1954.
78. Kelsey, J., and White, A.A.: Epidemiology and impact of low back pain. Spine 6:133–142, 1980.
79. Kennedy, I.: The unmasking of medicine. London, Allen & Unwin, 1981.
80. Key, J.A.: Intervertebral disc lesions are the most common cause of low back pain with or without sciatica. Ann. Surg. 121:534–544, 1945.
81. La Rocca, H., Macnab, I.: Value of pre-employment radiographic assessment of the lumbar spine. Can. Med. Assoc. J. 101:383–388, 1969.
82. Leavitt, F., Garron, D.C., Whistler, W.W., and Sheinkop, M.B.: Affective and sensory dimensions in back pain. Pain 4:273–281, 1978.
83. Leigh, H., and Reiser, M.F.: The patient: Biological, psychological and social dimensions of medical practice. New York, Plenum Press, 1980.
84. Lidstrom, A., and Zachrisson, M.: Physical therapy on low back pain and sciatica: An attempt at evaluation. Scand. J. Rehab. Med. 2:37–42, 1970.
85. Linton, S.J.: The relationship between activity and chronic pain. Pain 21:289–294, 1985.
86. Lipowski, Z.J.: Psychosocial aspect of disease. Ann. Intern. Med. 71:1197–1206, 1969.
87. Lipowski, Z.J.: Holistic-medical foundations of American psychiatry: A bicentennial. Am. J. Psychiatr. 138:888–895, 1981.
88. Lipowski, Z.J.: Psychosocial reactions to physical illness. Can. Med. Assoc. J. 128:1069–1072, 1983.
89. Loeser, J.D.: Concepts of Pain: Chronic Low Back Pain. New York, Raven Press, 1982.
90. Loeser, J.D., and Fordyce, W.E.: Chronic Pain. Behavioural Science in the Practice of Medicine. Carr, J.E., and Dengerink, H.A. (eds.): New York, Elsevier, 1983.
91. McCulloch, J.A.: Chemonucleolysis. J. Bone Joint Surg. 59B:45–52, 1977.
92. McGill, C.M.: Industrial back programmes: A control program. J. Occup. Med. 10:174–178, 1968.
93. McNeill, T., Warwick, D., Andersson, G.B.J., and Schultz, A.: Trunk strength in attempted flexion, extension and lateral bending in healthy subjects and patients with low back disorders. Spine 5:529, 1980.
94. McVeigh, E.L.: Occupational Back Pain and Modified Work: A Randomised Control Trial. MSc Thesis, McMaster University, 1986.
95. McWhinney, I.R.: Beyond diagnosis: An approach to the integration of behavioural science and clinical medicine. N. Engl. J. Med. 287:384–387, 1972.
96. Magora, A., Schwartz, A.: Relation between the low back pain syndrome and X-ray findings. Scand. J. Rehab. Med. 8:115–125, 1976.

97. Main, C.J.: The modified somatic perception questionnaire. J. Psychosom. Res. 27:503–514, 1983.
98. Main, C.J.: Psychological approaches to management and treatment. *In* Jayson, M.I.V. (ed.): The Lumbar Spine and Back Pain. Tunbridge Wells, Pitman, 1987.
99. Main, C.J., Waddell, G.: Personality assessment in the management of low back pain. Clin. Rehab. 1:139–142, 1987.
100. Mayer, T.G., Gatchell, R.J., Kitchino, N., et al.: Objective assessment of lumbar function following industrial injury. Spine 10:482–493, 1985.
101. Mayer, T.G., Gatchel, R.J., Kishino, N., et al.: A prospective short-term study of chronic low back pain patients utilising novel objective functional measurement. Pain 25:53–68, 1986.
102. Mayou, R.: Sick role, illness behaviour and coping. Br. J. Psychiatr. 144:320–322, 1984.
103. Mechanic, D.: Medical Sociology. New York, Free Press, 1968.
104. Mechanic, D.: Illness behaviour, social adaptation and the management of illness. J. Nerv. Ment. Dis. 165:79–87, 1977.
105. Mechanic, D.: The experience and reporting of common physical complaints. J. Health Soc. Behav. 21:146–155, 1980.
106. Mechanic, D.: The concept of illness behaviour: culture, situation and personal predisposition (Editorial). Psychol. Med. 16:1–7, 1986.
107. Mechanic, D., Cleary, P.D., and Greenely, J.R.: Distress syndrome, illness behaviour, access to care and medical utilisation in a defined population. Med. Care 20:361–372, 1982.
108. Mechanic, D., and Volkart, E.H.: Illness behaviour and medical diagnosis. J. Health Hum. Behav. 1:86–96, 1960.
109. Mechanic, D., and Volkart, E.H.: Stress, illness behaviour and the sick role. Am. Sociol. Rev. 26:51–58, 1961.
110. Melzack, R.: The McGill pain questionnaire: Major properties and scoring methods. Pain 1:277–299, 1975.
111. Melzack, R., and Casey, K.L.: Sensory, motivational and central control determinants of pain. *In* Kenshalo, D.R. (ed.): The Skin Senses. Springfield, Illinois, Charles C Thomas, 1968.
112. Melzack, R., and Wall, P.D.: Pain mechanisms: A new theory. Science 150:971–979, 1965.
113. Mensor, M.C., and Duvall, G.: Absence of motion at the fourth and fifth lumbar interspaces. J. Bone Joint Surg. 41A:1047–1054, 1959.
114. Meyer, A.: Progress in teaching psychiatry. J.A.M.A. 69:861–863, 1917.
115. Miller, J.H.: Preliminary report on disability insurance. To the Committee on Ways & Means of the U.S. House of Representatives. Washington, D.C., U.S. Government Printing Office, 1976.
116. Miller, P.M.C., Ingham, J.G., and Davidson, S.: Life events, symptoms and social support. J. Psychosom. Res. 20:515–522, 1976.
117. Mixter, W.J., and Barr, J.S.: Rupture of the intervertebral disc with involvement of the spinal canal. N. Engl. J. Med. 211:210–215, 1934.
118. Morris, E.W., DiPaola, M., Vallance, R., and Waddell, G.: Diagnosis and decision making in lumbar disc prolapse and nerve entrapment. Spine 11:436–439, 1986.
119. Nachemson, A.: The load on lumbar discs in different positions of the body. Clin. Orthop. 45:107–122, 1966.
120. Nachemson, A.: Towards a better understanding of low back pain: A review of the mechanics of the lumbar disc. Rheumatol. Rehab. 14:129–143, 1975.
121. Nachemson, A.: The lumbar spine: An orthopaedic challenge. Spine 1:9–21, 1976.
122. Nachemson, A.: A critical look at conservative treatment for low back pain. *In* Jayson, M. (ed.): The Lumbar Spine and Low Back Pain. London, Pitman, 1976.
123. Nachemson, A.: Work for all, for those with low back pain as well. Clin. Orthop. 179:77–85, 1983.
124. Nachemson, A.: Advances in low back pain. Clin. Orthop. 200:266–278, 1985.
125. Nachemson, A., and Andersson, G.B.J.: Classification of low back pain. Scand. J. Work Environ. Health 8:134, 1982.
126. Nachemson, A., and Lindh, M.: Measurement of abdominal and back muscle strength with or without low back pain. Scand. J. Rehab. Med. 1:60, 1965.
127. Nachemson, A., and Morris, J.M.: In vivo measurement of intradiscal pressure. J. Bone Joint Surg. 46A:1077–1092, 1964.
128. Naliboff, B.D., Cohen, M.J., Swanson, G.A., et al.: Comprehensive assessment of chronic low back pain patients and controls: Physical abilities, level of activities, psychological adjustment and pain perception. Pain 23:121–134, 1985.
129. The Nuprin Pain Report: New York, Louis Harris and Associates, 1985.
130. Office of Health Economics: Hip Replacement and the NHS. London, 1982.
131. Office of Health Economics: Back Pain. London, 1985.
132. Oostdam, E.M., Duidenwoorden, H.J., and Pondaag, N.: Predictive value of some psychological tests on the outcome of surgical intervention in low back pain patients. J. Psychosom. Res. 25:227–235, 1981.
133. Parsons, T.: The Social System. New York, Free Press, 1951.
134. Pasteur, M.L.: Mémoire sur la fermentation appellée lactique. Comptes Rendus Acad. Sci. 45:913–916, 1857.
135. Penfield, W.: Foreword. Pain and the Neurosurgeon. Springfield, Illinois, Charles C Thomas, 1969.
136. Pheasant, H., Gilbert, D., Goldfar, J., and Heron, L.: The MMPI as a predictor of outcome in low back surgery. Spine 4:78–84, 1979.
137. Philips, H.C., and Jahanshahi, M.: The components of pain behaviour report. Behav. Res. Ther. 24:117–125, 1986.
138. Pilowsky, I.: Abnormal illness behaviour. Br. J. Med. Psychol. 42:347–351, 1969.
139. Pilowsky, I.: A general classification of abnormal illness behaviours. Br. J. Med. Psychol. 51:131–137, 1978.
140. Ransford, A.O., Cairns, D., and Mooney, V.: The pain drawing as an aid to the psychological evaluation of patients with low back pain. Spine 1:127–134, 1976.
141. Reiser, S.J.: Medicine and the reign of technology. Cambridge, Cambridge University Press, 1978.
142. Rider, A.W., et al.: The status of cardiac transplantation. Circulation 52:531, 1975.
143. Rowe, M.L.: Low back pain in industry. J. Occup. Med. 11:161–169, 1969.
144. Sackett, D.L.: How to read clinical journals: V. To

distinguish useful from useless or even harmful therapies. Can. Med. Assoc. J. 124:1156–1162, 1981.
145. Sample sickness and/or invalidity benefit 1967–1985: D.H.S.S. Headquarters Division SR 8B, Newcastle-upon-Tyne. Unpublished data.
146. Sandstrom, J., Hansson, T., Jonson, R., et al.: The bone mineral content of the lumbar spine in patients with chronic low back pain. Spine 10:158–160, 1985.
147. Social Security Bulletin: Annual Statistical Supplement. Washington, D.C., U.S. Government Printing Office, 1984–1985.
148. Social Security Commission on the Evaluation of Pain: Report to U.S. Congress. Washington, D.C., U.S. Government Printing Office, 1986.
149. Spangfort, E.V.: The lumbar disc herniation: A computer aided analysis of 2504 operations. Acta Orthop. Scand. 142(Suppl.):1–95, 1972.
150. Spengler, D.: Unpublished data, University of Washington.
151. Spitzer, W.O.: Rapport du groupe de travail Québecois sur les aspects cliniques des affections vertebrales chez les travailleurs. Institût du recherche en santé et en sécurité du travail de Québec, 1986.
152. Splithoff, C.A.: Lumbosacral junction: Roentgenographic comparison of patients with and without backache. J.A.M.A. 152:1610–1613, 1953.
153. Sternbach, R.A.: Pain Patients: Traits and Treatment. New York, Academic Press, 1974.
154. Sternbach, R.A.: Psychological aspects of chronic pain. Clin. Orthop. 129:150–155, 1977.
155. Sternbach, R.A., and Timmermans, G.: Personality changes associated with reduction of pain. Pain 1:177–181, 1975.
156. Strang, J.P.: The chronic disability syndrome. Evaluation and Treatment of Chronic Pain. *In* Aronoff, G.M. (ed.): Baltimore, Urban & Schwarzenberg, 1985.
157. Szasz, T.S.: The painful person. J. Lancet 88:18–22, 1968.
158. Task Force on Backs: Ontario Council of Safety Associations. Toronto, 1984.
159. Tessler, R., Mechanic, D. and Dimond, M.: The effect of psychological distress on physician utilisation: A prospective study. J. Health Soc. Behav. 17:353–364, 1976.
160. Torgeson, W.R., and Dotler, W.E.: Comparative roentgenographic study of the asymptomatic and symptomatic lumbar spine. J. Bone Joint Surg. 58A:850–853, 1976.
161. Turk, D.C., Meichenbaum, D., and Genest, M.: Pain and behavioural medicine. New York, Guildford Press, 1983.
162. Urban, J., and Maroudas, A.: The chemistry of the intervertebral disc in relation to its physiological functions and requirements. Clin. Rheum. Dis. 6:51–76, 1980.
163. Virchow, R.: Die Cellular pathologie in Ihrer Begrundurg auf physiologische und pathologische. Berlin. A. Hirschwald, 1858.
164. Waddell, G.: An approach to backache. Br. J. Hosp. Med. 28:187–219, 1982.
165. Waddell, G.: Provision of Orthopaedic Services for Backache in Oman. Report to the Minister of Health. Muscat, Sultanate of Oman, 1986.
166. Waddell, G.: Clinical assessment of lumbar impairment. Clin. Orthop. 221:110–120, 1987.
167. Waddell, G., Bircher, M., Finlayson, D., and Main, C.J.: Symptoms and signs: Physical disease or illness behaviour? Br. Med. J. 289:739–741, 1984.
168. Waddell, G., Kummel, E.G., Lotto, W.N., et al.: Failed lumbar disc surgery and repeat surgery following industrial injury. J. Bone Joint Surg. 61A:201–207, 1979.
169. Waddell, G., McCulloch, J.A., Kummel, E.G., and Venner, R.M.: Non-organic physical signs in low back pain. Spine 5:117–125, 1980.
170. Waddell, G., and Main, C.J.: Assessment of severity in low back disorders. Spine 9:204–208, 1984.
171. Waddell, G., Main, C.J., Morris, E.W., DiPaola, M., and Gray, I.C.M.: Chronic low back pain, psychological distress and illness behaviour. Spine 9:209–213, 1984.
172. Waddell, G., Morris, E.W., DiPaola, M., et al.: A concept of illness tested as an improved basis for surgical decisions in low back disorders. Spine 11:712–719, 1986.
173. Wall, P.D.: Causes of intractable pain. Hosp. Update 12:969–974, 1986.
174. Weber, H.: Conservative management of back pain: Critical evaluation of conservative treatment programmes. Presented at the First European Congress on Back Pain Current Concepts and Recent Advances. Helsinki, 1986.
175. Weinstein, M.R.: The illness process. J.A.M.A. 204:117–121, 1968.
176. Weinstein, M.R.: The concept of the disability process. Psychosomatics 19:94–97, 1978.
177. White, A.: AAOS Instructional Course Lectures. Back School. St. Louis, C.V. Mosby, 1979.
178. White, A.W.M.: Low back pain in men receiving workmen's compensation. Can. Med. Assoc. J. 95:50–56, 1966.
179. White, K.L., Williams, F., and Greenberg, B.: The ecology of medical care. N. Engl. J. Med. 265:885–892, 1961.
180. Wiesel, S.W., Cuckler, J.M., Deluca, F., et al.: Acute low back pain: An objective analysis of conservative therapy. Spine 5:324–330, 1980.
181. Wiltse, L.L.: The effect of the common anomalies of the lumbar spine upon disc degeneration and low back pain. Orthop. Clin. North Am. 2:569–582, 1971.
182. Wiltse, L.L., and Rocchio, P.D.: Pre-operative psychological tests as predictions of success of chemonucleolysis in the treatment of the low back syndrome. J. Bone Joint Surg. 57A:478–483, 1975.
183. Wing, P.C., Wilfling, F.J., and Kokan, P.J.: Psychological, demographic and orthopaedic factors associated with prediction of outcome of spinal fusion. Clin. Orthop. 90:153–160, 1973.
184. Wolff, B.B., and Langley, S.: Cultural factors and the response to pain. Am. Anthropol. 70:494–501, 1968.
185. Wood, P.L.R., and Main, C.J.: The changing influence of physical and psychological factors on subjective disability in low back pain. Presented to the First International Congress of the International Back Pain Society, Vienna, 1985.
186. Workmen's Compensation Board Symposium: Low Back Pain: A Multi-Disciplinary Approach. Vancouver, 1986.
187. Workmen's Compensation Board of British Columbia: Vancouver, Canada. Unpublished data, 1986.

syndrome can be demonstrated to be modulated by psychologic factors, by the physician as well as by regulatory agencies.

The current availability of various types of isodynamic and isokinetic muscle testing machines[65, 74, 75] for use among patients with low back pain calls for more research into the physiology of muscle training. Sports medicine experts already have obtained some useful basic knowledge in this area after years of studying the quadriceps muscle.[99]

In the lower back, we know that endurance training, especially for the extensor group of muscles, is of some clinical importance.[9, 65, 75] The manner by which these as well as the intersegmental muscles should be trained must be subjected to further study. The availability of portable fine-wire electromyogram (EMG) equipment, MRI, and muscle testing machines already brings such research within reach today. It is the responsibility of the manufacturer to demonstrate whether very expensive machines are necessary to muscle training. At present, the only area of proven efficacy is in the demonstration of intrapatient strength gain.

Discs

Certain genetic traits among patients with disc disorders should be investigated, specifically in regard to cells in the nucleus.[23] The search to find eternal youth—or to avoid disc aging—will probably continue. Instead, the discs should be studied to elucidate the means by which they stay nondegenerated for such considerable lengths of time without a direct blood supply and only with nutrition from diffusion.[24, 45, 46, 73, 118, 119] We already know how to increase nutrition by motion.[22, 58] The negative influences of immobilization,[57, 114] smoking,[59] and vibration can be seen in animal models, and these findings are supported by observations from epidemiologic studies.[84]

The mechanical competence of the discs depends on both collagen and proteoglycans. Preliminary studies using MRI,[33] which is still in its infancy as a scientific methodology, and using MR spectroscopy point to some possibilities for further research.

I do not believe that it will ever be possible to differentiate between aging and degeneration, nor do I believe in a specific "degenerative disc" disease.[28] Rather, normal or genetically produced premature age change renders the disc mechanically incompetent, abnormal motion patterns occur and then subject the ligaments, joints, and muscles to undue stress that might cause pain. Also the dorsal root ganglion might be sensitized in that manner.[122]

Discs do not carry pain fibers. However, the surrounding structures carry them as do, perhaps, the subchondral bony end plates. All of these could be reached by chemical breakdown products resulting from disc aging.[31, 84] We know that only some disc hernias cause sciatica.[7, 14, 56] In 20% to 30% of healthy volunteers no sciatica is produced, despite the clear demonstration of herniation by computed tomography (CT)[7, 22, 60] or myelogram.[56] Maybe mechanical irritation is not enough. Perhaps sciatica requires additional chemical irritation resulting from breakdown products in the aging disc. The hydrogen ion, for example, can cause nociception, and a low pH has been measured in some patients.[31]

Again, MR spectroscopy should eventually clarify this question. Some of these breakdown products can probably be detected in the bloodstream by means of new sensitive immunoessay methods.[137]

Motion Segment Mechanics

Most of the efforts of basic science during the last decade have been directed toward motion segment mechanics. The reason is obvious, because low back pain is such a mechanical problem. Biomechanical studies of various types, both in vivo and in vitro, and increasingly sophisticated mathematic models and ingenious testing equipment have yielded useful basic information. Some of the findings fit our epidemiologic data and clinical observations; others do not.[42, 84] More is to be gained now from a combination of biomechanics and biochemistry, an observation already made during the search for pathomechanics of osteoarthritis.[66, 73]

Several investigators have proposed further study of "instability" as a cause of low back pain to determine what chemical changes of collagen and proteoglycans are behind it[84, 89] and to what extent muscles can stabilize.

It must be clear, however, that our attempts to measure instability from ordinary x-ray films correlated with clinical findings has failed dismally.[41, 43] The ordinary x-ray methods, even the biplanar ones, seem too crude. They can detect only gross abnormal translations of 5 mm or more or 15 to 20 degrees of excess angulation. However, such large abnormal motions rarely occur, except in patients with spondylolisthesis and in some older patients following surgical destabilization.[63]

The Selvik method is already available.[88, 89, 108] Can we allow patients' lumbar spines to be "raped" by surgeons for undefined instability syndromes? We must allow the insertion of small tantalum ball bearings around the motion segment to detect normal or abnormal motions and the correlation of these with clinical syndromes. By means of this method measurements as exact as 0.3 degrees and 0.1 mm can be made.[108] An unpublished study using this method for the SI joints clearly demonstrated that no abnormal motion can be detected by any external palpation technique. No difference existed between symptomatic SI patients and normals. It was previously demonstrated[93] that our clinical tests for determination of such mobility of hypermobility are unreliable.

Systematic examination of the facet joints by CT, ordinary x-ray studies, or injection studies in normal and patient populations have failed to pinpoint a facet syndrome.[4, 44, 60, 61, 71, 78, 79] This was recently underscored by Jackson and coworkers.[61] On the other hand, facet arthritis does exist, and certainly rheumatoid arthritis and severe osteoarthritic changes can cause specific but rare syndromes.[84] However, these are detectable by serologic tests and CT measurements of central canal stenosis. On the other hand, root canal stenosis remains an unproven entity that needs scientific evaluation by a combined approach from those studying nerve root anatomy, nutrition, and biomechanics, together with those carrying out various radiologic investigations using three-dimensional CT and MRI. For central stenosis we are approaching the goal,[107] whereas for root canal stenosis, questions remain about the means of properly diagnosing it and correlating it with symptoms.[92] Again, clinicians should make efforts using somatosensory evoked potential (SEP) recordings, three-dimensional CT and MRI, and clinical trials.[98, 103] The diagnosis itself is used much too often for operating, in the absence of any proper studies supporting the benefits of such surgery.[92]

Diagnosis

As stated earlier, a number of conditions can be diagnosed as causes of low back pain and sciatica. Some methods used to diagnose such conditions have shown sensitivity, specificity, and adequate predictive value.[13, 86] They include CT, myelography, MRI, and CT discography for sciatica due to disc hernia, instability of more than 4 mm of excessive motion in the young with spondylolisthesis; x-ray studies and laboratory tests for tumors, infections, and rheumatic diseases; and CT measurements of dural sac area for spinal stenosis. Discography is used in many places to diagnose discogenic back pain, but specificity, sensitivity, and predictive value have not been proven.[90, 121, 122] For the diagnosis of disc herniation, it has proven less useful than both myelography and CT, with a specificity of only 35%.[60] No study in the literature demonstrates the clinical usefulness of discography. Therapy, including lumbar fusion based on the discographic picture and/or the pain response at injection has also been poorly evaluated; few—if any—studies have validated outcome measures[13, 85] or adequate follow-up by unbiased observers.[32, 101]

Various types of scientific studies have failed to prove the existence of a clinical facet syndrome, SI joint syndrome, lumbar compartment syndrome, fibrositis, or spasm. Likewise, the importance of the abdominal pressure mechanism for the relief of low back load has seriously been questioned and remains unproven.

For the majority of those who have low back pain without sciatica, we still are uncertain. This deplorable state of missing knowledge was clearly demonstrated in a recent effort[86] by a 22-member task force, who worked for nearly 3 years scrutinizing about 800 articles out of 7,000 titles written up to 1985 in the scientific literature. This uncertainty of diagnosis is certainly mirrored by the multiplicity of treatment methods used for the many unproven and sometimes already disproven diagnostic labels that exist. The Quebec task force simplified diagnosis into 11 categories (Table 1) and tabulated, for these various diagnostic entities, the scientific evidence provided by various types of examinations.

Table 1. SCIENTIFIC GRADING FOR DIAGNOSTIC PROCEDURES — SPINAL DISORDERS

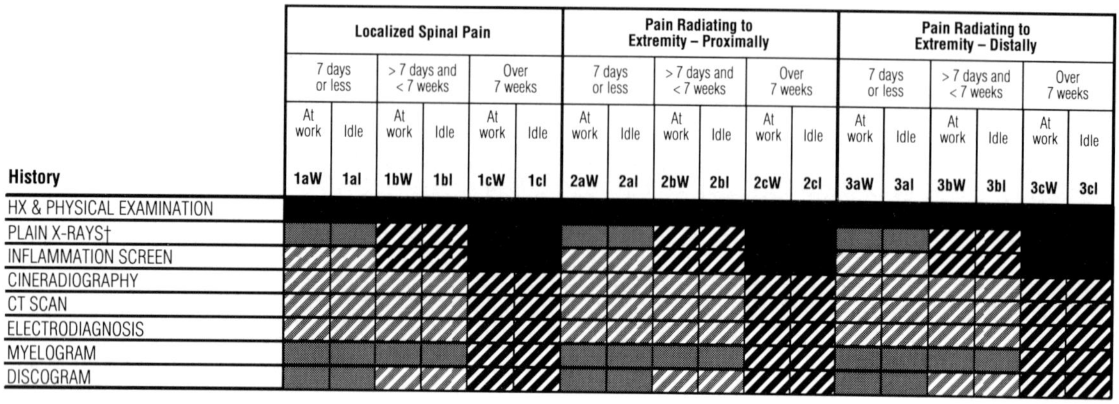

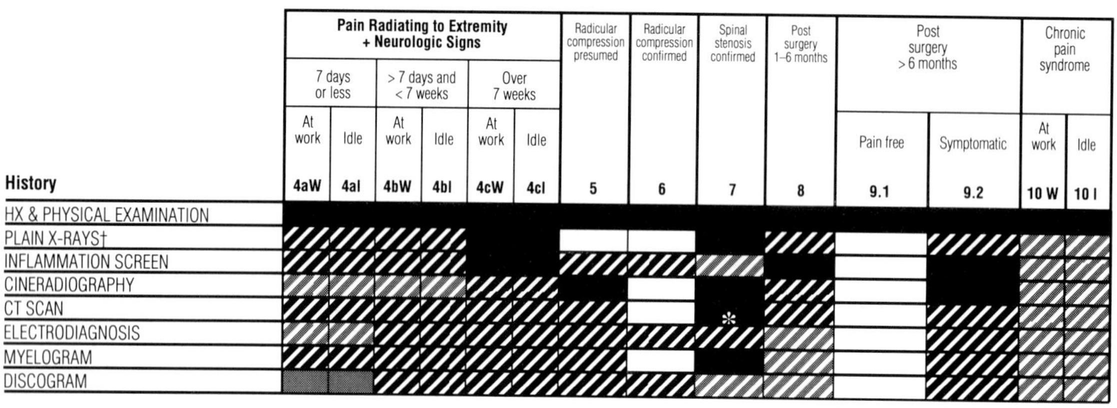

- (Black with ✻) Usefulness **demonstrated** by randomized controlled trial.
- (Black) Usefulness **demonstrated** by nonrandomized controlled trial.
- (Gray) **Contraindicated** on basis of scientific evidence.
- (Heavy hatching) Common practice but **no** scientific evidence.
- (Light hatching) **Not** in common practice and **no** scientific evidence.
- (White) Not applicable.

†Contraindicated as shown, given the *absence* of specific orienting elements: age below 20 or above 50, history or sign of trauma, neoplasm, fever, neurologic deficit, or recurrent nature of the spinal disorder.

(From Nachemson, A., Spitzer, W.O., et al.: Scientific approach to the assessment and management of activity-related spinal disorders. A monograph for clinicians. Report of the Quebec Task Force on Spinal Disorders. Spine 12 (suppl.):S1–S59, 1987.)

Treatment of Low Back Pain and Sciatica

Most of the various treatment methods commonly used have specific goals, and in the Quebec study[86] these were listed as follows: promote rest, diminish spasm, diminish inflammation, reduce pain, increase strength, increase range of motion, increase endurance, alter joint tissue, alter nerve tissue, increase function, modify work environment, modify social environment, and modify psychologic states (Table 2). In that study we applied the presumed effect of a given treatment method to the simplified diagnostic grid. The scientific literature was reviewed against such a system and categorized for scientific validity. Only 50 articles were found on high-quality, well-controlled prospective randomized trials, published through 1985.[80, 103] Since then, 10 to 15 others have appeared, demonstrating clinical efficacy for only a limited number of methods used for the clinically strictly definable diagnostic categories (Table 2).

It must be pointed out, however, that the fact that no proof exists for a certain method applied to a certain condition does not rule out a potential effect. It means only that scientific studies are lacking. If such studies exist and show negative results, the method is actually contraindicated.

This same state of affairs certainly also applies to the surgical treatment of some of the rarer syndromes. I have already mentioned the fact that lumbar discectomy and fusion for "instability" is performed very often in the United States, 10 times more frequently than in Europe,[83, 125] and that the value of operating for not clearly defined root canal stenosis is doubtful. Even though there are established diagnostic criteria for lumbar disc herniation, these obviously are not always fulfilled, judging from various reports in the United States,[69, 72, 102] where surgery is performed five to eight times more often for presumed disc prolapse than it is in Europe. Surgery based on scientifically unproven or misdiagnosed criteria also leads to a great increase in the number of reoperations;[130] this is certainly a North American problem.[77, 139] Because the failed surgery syndrome is one of the most devastating problems for the individual and for society, it is of the utmost importance to encourage satisfactory randomized studies for all operations performed for ill-defined syndromes, in order to determine which patient (meeting certain criteria) would benefit. Given the excellent state of knowledge in epidemiology and clinical statistics,[13, 98, 103] such prospective center or surgeon randomized studies[120] can and must be performed, and they certainly have been proposed recently in all the leading orthopedic journals.[13, 85, 86, 98, 103]

Psychology and Idiopathic Low Back Pain

Today there is clear evidence from several sources that psychosocial factors play a role in the reporting of an acute low back "injury."[11] Some evidence suggests that these factors cause overmorbidity,[18, 134] and the prominence of such factors in the chronic low back pain syndrome is particularly well known and established.[36, 37, 40, 97, 112, 113, 134] In the study by Bigos and Battié,[11] reporting a prospective study of more than 3,000 workers who during a 4-year follow-up period suffered attacks of low back pain, these psychosocial factors—particularly those at work—were more important than the workload. Also in the Andersson and Svensson and Vällfors studies of population samples from Gothenburg, Sweden,[106, 112, 134] the same trends were noted.[132, 133] It seems that the psychologic characteristics of the worker and his or her environment play a role equal to or perhaps even more prominent than the biomechanical factors,[106, 129, 131, 134] in regard to the industrial back pain problem. It is imperative to continue the study of psychologic factors and to evaluate the biochemical changes that may influence, for example, muscle fatigue and/or nociceptive pain.[96]

Several authors[39, 96, 110] have studied the effects of exercise and fitness on the production of enkephalins and other pain-reducing substances. The interrelationship of psychologic states and the production of endorphins, as well as the effects of depression and anxiety on endorphins, is well known.[3] Perhaps less well known is the fact that psychologic factors must also be considered in developing treatment programs for patients with low back pain. Using behavioral models,[38, 70] some psychologists have proved that treatment programs aimed at reducing disability by activation have beneficial ef-

Table 2. SCIENTIFIC GRADING FOR THERAPEUTIC MODALITIES — LUMBAR SPINAL DISORDERS

	Low Back Pain						LBP Radiating to Posterior Thigh					
	7 days or less		> 7 days and < 7 weeks		Over 7 weeks		7 days or less		> 7 days and < 7 weeks		Over 7 weeks	
	At work	Idle	At work	Idle	At work	Idle	At work	Idle	At work	Idle	At work	Idle
	1aW	1aI	1bW	1bI	1cW	1cI	2aW	2aI	2bW	2bI	2cW	2cI
1. Promote Rest												
1.1.1 Bed rest for < 2 days		*		*				*		*		
1.1.2 Bed rest for > 2 days												
1.2.1 Orthosis												
1.2.2 Support												
1.3 Work cessation												
2. Diminish Spasm												
2.1 Systemic medication												
2.2 Thermotherapy (heat)												
2.3 Cryotherapy (cold)												
2.4 Biofeedback (EMG)												
2.5 Mobilization/manipulation												
2.6 Massage												
3. Diminish Inflammation												
3.1.1 Systemic medication												
3.1.2 Local medication												
3.2 Cryotherapy (cold)												
4. Reduce Pain												
4.1.1 Systemic medication												
4.1.2 Local medication												
4.2 Electroanalgesia												
4.3 Pain clinic												
4.4 Acupuncture												
4.5 Cryotherapy (cold)												
4.6 Thermotherapy (heat)												
4.7.1 Bed rest for < 2 days		*		*				*		*		
4.7.2 Bed rest for > 2 days												
5. Increase Strength												
5.1 Strengthening exercises												
6. Increase Range of Motion												
6.1 Stretching exercises												
6.2 Mobilization/manipulation												
6.3 Traction												
7. Increase Endurance												
7.1 Home exercises												
7.2 Exer. in special. centre												
8. Alter Joint Tissue												
8.1 Surgery												
8.2 Chemonucleolysis												
9. Alter Nerve Tissue												
9.1 Denervation												
10. Increase Function												
10.1 Postural information												
10.2 Functional training												
10.3 Back to school		*		*				*		*		
10.4 Return to work												
11. Modify Work Environment												
11.1 Ergonomic intervention												
12. Modify Social Environment												
12.1 Social services												
13. Modify the Psyche												
13.1 Psychological support												
13.2 Psychopharmacology												
13.3 Psychotherapy												
13.4 Combined therapy												

* Usefulness **demonstrated** by randomized controlled trial.

Usefulness **demonstrated** by nonrandomized controlled trial.

Contraindicated on basis of scientific evidence.

Common practice but **no** scientific evidence.

Not in common practice and **no** scientific evidence.

Not applicable.

Table 2. SCIENTIFIC GRADING FOR THERAPEUTIC MODALITIES — LUMBAR SPINAL DISORDERS *Continued.*

LBP Radiating to Calf ± Foot						LBP Radiating to Leg + Neurologic Signs						Radicular compression presumed	Radicular compression confirmed	Spinal stenosis confirmed	Post surgery 1–6 months	Post surgery > 6 months		Chronic pain syndrome	
7 days or less		>7 days and <7 weeks		over 7 weeks		7 days or less		>7 days and <7 weeks		over 7 weeks									
At work	Idle	At work	Idle	At work	Idle	At work	Idle	At work	Idle	At work	Idle					Pain free	Sympto-matic	At work	Idle
3aW	3aI	3bW	3bI	3cW	3cI	4aW	4aI	4bW	4bI	4cW	4cI	5	6	7	8	9.1	9.2	10 W	10 I

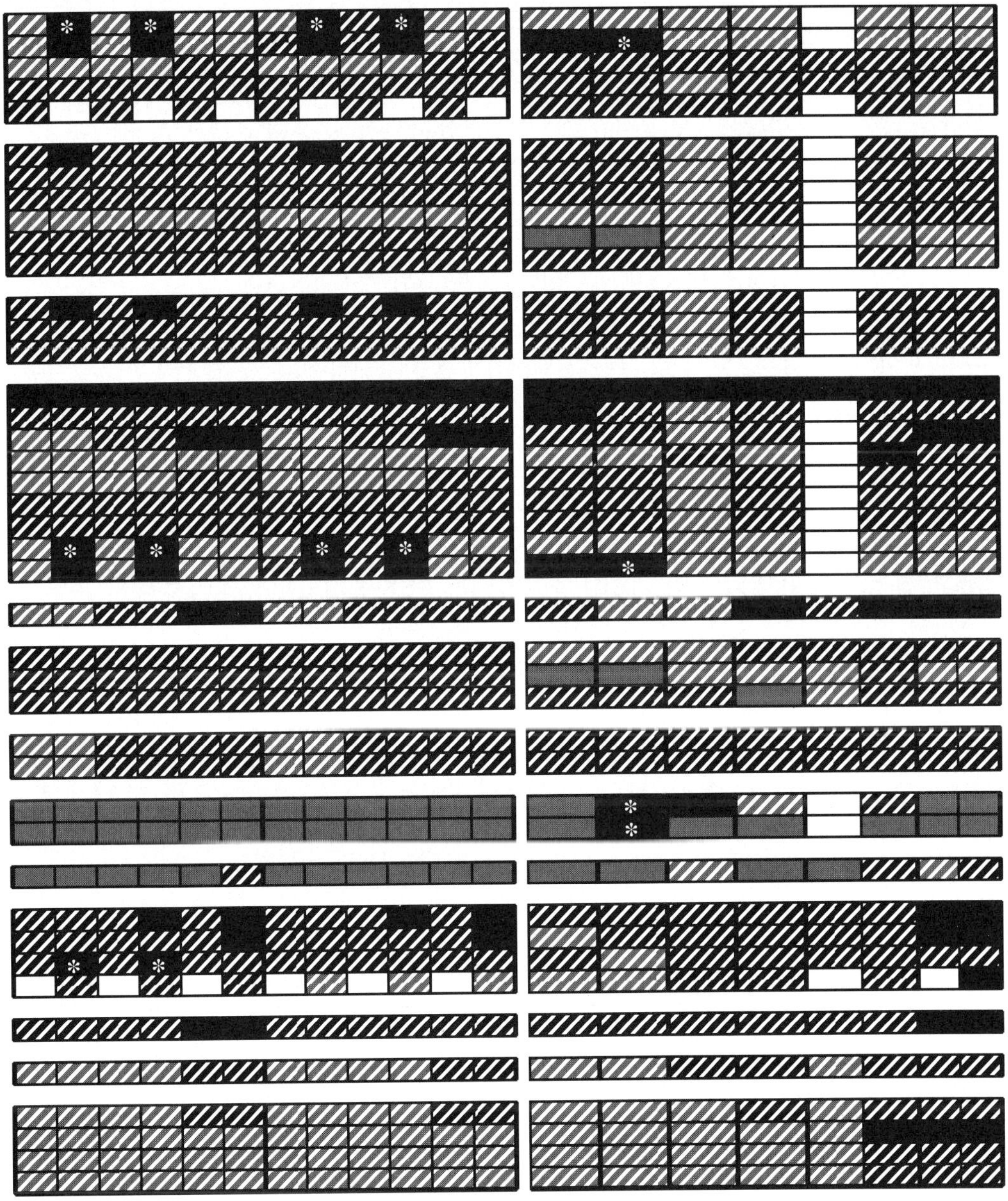

fects. Other authors[133, 139] have demonstrated that reducing depression clearly benefits these patients.

Exercise, Fitness, and Back Pain

Basic scientific knowledge supports the idea that motion benefits the tissues that may cause low back pain; there is some proof that they become mechanically stronger when exercised, and there is evidence that the lack of both exercise and fitness, (i.e., the result of immobilization) is detrimental.[17, 30, 51, 52, 117, 124, 128] These effects also apply to the intervertebral disc.[58]

The minimum amount of motion necessary to maintain or enhance the strength of healing of the various tissues involved in low back pain is not known.[137] Some guidelines can be inferred, however, from animal studies and clinical observations of the relationship between physical fitness and the occurrence of low back pain.

For disc and cartilage, the animal models suggest that about 30 minutes of running each day is beneficial.[1, 68] More violent or longer periods of motion did not result in any improvement. Kiviranta,[66] in an unpublished study, demonstrated that extensive running of rabbits resulted in a negative effect on the proteoglycans of their joints.

It seems reasonable that for the disc, which has no direct blood supply, exercises improving the general circulation are more beneficial than very strong muscles. In our prospective study of 3,000 workers,[5] those with strong muscles did not demonstrate fewer back pain attacks. Epidemiologic studies have generally shown a weak correlation among lack of physical fitness, reduced activity at work and during leisure time, and an increase in the incidence and prevalence of back pain, as well as an increase in absence from work as a result of this pain. However, in our search for a means of *preventing* low back pain, this relationship becomes less clear. In the much-quoted studies by Cady and coworkers,[19, 20] a clear relation between fitness and reported low back injury was established over a 10 year period in a select population of fire fighters in Los Angeles. The least fit group reported 10 times more low back pain accidents than did the most fit group. In a recent report, Deyo and colleagues[29, 30] demonstrated that the three combined factors of body weight, smoking and decreased physical activity, were highly significant in regard to the occurrence of low back pain. Weaker associations have been found by Frymoyer[42] and coworkers, Svensson[112] and colleagues, and others.[6, 134]

In one prospective study, cardiovascular fitness[105] was investigated as a risk factor for industrial back pain. We could not verify its significance for acute injury in the 2,400 subjects who underwent a treadmill test.[5] The study suggested that higher cardiovascular fitness alone does not reduce the risk of an incident of low back pain for workers who perform a wide variety of tasks. On the other hand, that study demonstrated that patients who eventually develop *chronic* disabling back pain have a significantly lower cardiovascular fitness level to begin with, as compared with age- and sex-matched controls.

Absolute evidence that fitness prevents low back pain is not at hand. However, several studies have demonstrated the benefits of increased body awareness through programs that promote general health and fitness, as well as exercises of large muscles groups in various cohorts. Followed for various lengths of time, these programs reduce absenteeism in general, and absenteeism from low back pain in particular.[8, 10, 12, 25, 26] Nevertheless, the converse seems to be more convincing, that is, the limited endurance of large muscle groups, in particular the back extensors, seems to put one at a greater risk of experiencing long-standing back pain within the next year.

A summary of the reports from a recent NIH symposium on the injury and repair of the musculoskeletal soft tissues are listed in Tables 1, 2, and 3.[137]

Treatment Aspect

In treating the patient with acute (<7 days) low back pain, there is little evidence that general fitness and exercise play a major role. However, as the duration of an attack of low back pain increases, there is evidence that some types of activation programs aimed at increasing endurance have a beneficial effect. Immobilization by bed rest for more than 1 or 2 days also seems to be contraindicated.[29]

The benefits of motion and activation can occur at several levels. At the tissue level, discs have been demonstrated to improve

Table 3 □ Summary of Reports from an NIH Symposium

LOAD DEPRIVATION—BED REST, OUTER SPACE	
Muscles	− − −
Bone	− − −
Ligaments	− −
Cartilage	− − −
Discs	− −
MODERATE LOADING—ACTIVITY GENERAL FITNESS EXERCISE 30 MINUTES, 3× WEEKLY	
Muscles	+ +
Bone	+
Ligaments	+
Cartilage	+ +
Discs	+
EXTREME LOADING—ACTIVITY SEVERAL HOURS HARD TRAINING, EXTREME POSITION	
Muscles	−
Bone	+ +
Ligaments	+
Cartilage	− ?
Discs	?

−: Negative influences.
+: Positive influences.

their nutritional status by motion. The general oxygenation process probably plays a part, as does the pumping effect at the disc level.

The pain level governed by endorphins and substance P, both of which are reduced in low back pain patients, is influenced by exercising large muscle groups, and the perception of pain can be diminished by exercise.[96]

A study[8] performed at the Volvo plant in Gothenburg in the 1970s demonstrated that a 4-hour back school program aimed at activation and return to work resulted in patient returning to work 1 week sooner than the group that received mostly passive physical therapy, including manipulative treatment. Both patient groups recovered from the pain as quickly as and significantly more rapidly than the third randomized group, who received "detuned" short-wave diathermia only. Most of the patients in the back school group returned to work with some pain but also with knowledge of how to move more "biomechanically" correctly at the work place. Perhaps the most interesting finding at the 1 year follow-up was the lack of a significant difference in the rate of recurrence in these three groups. There was a tendency for the back school group, who returned 1 week earlier than the two other groups, to exhibit fewer and less severe recurrences during the follow-up year. This tendency was even more pronounced in the community-based study,[21] in which we asked the health officers to refer patients who did not recover within 3 weeks. Overall, in the community the recurrence rate was again approximately 50%. In the group exposed to information and activation, the recurrence rate was only one third of that. Numerous reports are available on the benefit of information and activation programs for patients with acute and subacute low back pain.[10, 123]

In another randomized study at the Volvo plant in Gothenburg, recently concluded but yet not published, we have been able to demonstrate a highly significant reduction in low back disability; 50 subjects suffering from idiopathic low back pain of 9 week duration were activated to perform an increasing number of exercises per quota established by Fordyce.[36] They were compared with a control group of equal size who did not receive any particular treatment but were allowed to continue with their general practitioner or industrial health officer after our first thorough investigation and randomization. The screening, performed by an orthopedic surgeon, served to eliminate those patients from the study who exhibited signs of disorders, which included not only back-related diseases but also a few patients with obvious medical diseases like obstructive emphysema, recent myocardiac infarction, and substance abuse.

In acute and subacute patients Fordyce and colleagues,[38] have demonstrated that a behavioral approach to activation provides good results and reduces recurrence over the next years.

Even in the most "deconditioned" patients who have demonstrable deficits in strength, endurance, and fitness, goal-oriented activation using group and behavioral psychologic methods has demonstrated an astonishingly rapid improvement of these parameters as well as a high percentage of patients returning to work.[53, 75] Actually, the recovery was far more rapid than was thought possible based on other studies of injured individuals. Muscle strength was tripled by this 3-week program. This clearly points to the psychologic part in the deconditioning of the chronic low back pain patient.

Biomechanically, we know what limits to set for the exercise program for patients with low back pain.[81] In the beginning, any vigorous muscular activities combined with large motions of the spine should be avoided, particularly in the upright positions. Isometric training and probably limited eccentric muscle training should be used for leg, back, and abdominal muscles. The principal aim should be to increase the endurance of the large and small back muscles.

The physician dictates this increase—not the patient, who should be assured that even if he or she experiences some pain, the exercise is not dangerous. Such advice necessitates a thorough clinical examination to exclude any contraindication.

Continuous positive reinforcement is of paramount importance, and pain behavior should be ignored. The success of such activation programs in randomized studies for acute, subacute, and chronic patients clearly confirm that exercise and fitness are among the more important factors in the overall treatment of patients with idiopathic low back pain. In studies in which endurance, strength, and fitness were measured, their increases mirror the recovery from low back disability.

DISCUSSION

Our present knowledge seems to suggest that, although physical fitness alone does not prevent low back pain, a general healthy lifestyle, including moderate motion and exercise of the lumbar spine and abstinence from smoking, may have some preventive effects. However, it is also clear that so-called "wellness programs" must include organizational changes at the work place, in order to reduce monotony and increase worker satisfaction by other means (some still unknown), in order to significantly reduce the epidemiologically increasing incidence of absenteeism resulting from low back pain.

For patients struck by an acute attack of low back pain, studies have also shown that minimal immobilization is beneficial. Basic experiments also underline this clinical observation (Table 3). Little proof exists of beneficial effects for most of the many other treatment modalities that exist for these patients (Table 2). The studies presented above indicate that patients suffering from back pain of longer duration also can benefit from activity.

For patients with sciatica due to a disc herniation[135, 136] or central spinal stenosis and for a few other proven diseases, treatment programs exist that are proven by well-designed studies, either randomized[8, 29, 38] or case series judged by independent observers.[34, 101] Fitness and exercise programs alone are not a global solution to the low back problem. A cohesive effort by basic scientists, biostatisticians, physicians, politicians, and employers is necessary to solve the most expensive medical problem of today's industrialized societies.

SUMMARY

The last decade has brought new understanding to some important aspects of the low back problem. First, the importance of moderate loading and moderate activity for the maintenance of the wellness of all the structures in the back has been demonstrated, as has the negative effect of load deprivation. In the study of the pain, further knowledge of opioids and their regulation will probably clarify how psychologic factors modulate the levels of these important pain-reducing substances. For the majority of patients with "idiopathic" low back pain, treatment programs seem to exist that can significantly reduce back morbidity. However, further studies are necessary to elucidate whether improvement can be gained with a combination of other types of treatment. Treatment methods and modalities that have not been proven, especially those that unnecessarily label the patient, seem to be contraindicated.

Some 8% to 10% of sufferers of chronic back pain (i.e., those who do not recover within 3 months) are found to have rheumatoid disease; some may even have a fibrinolytic defect.

Instability needs to be further clarified, and the means to accomplish this in the clinical setting already exist. This research should have a high priority, as should randomized studies to determine which patients will benefit from surgery, not only for instability syndromes but also for root canal stenosis and "degenerative disc disease."

Clinical practice of the future depends on the experimental findings of today. In regard to the detrimental effect of immobilization, the evidence is clear—in general and in particular for the lumbar spine and the various types of tissue that exist in the low back. Experimental and clinical evidence clearly suggests that graded activity is beneficial. Behavioral psychologic approaches to exercise and activation programs for back patients also have demonstrable positive effects.

References

1. Akeson, W. H., Amiel, D., Abel, M. F., et al.: Effects of immobilization on joints. Clin. Orthop. 219:28–37, 1987.
2. Almay, B. G. L., Johansson, F., Von Knorring, L., et al.: Substance P in CSF of patients with chronic pain syndromes. Pain 33:3–9, 1988.
3. Andersson, S. A., Carlsson, C. A., and Eriksson, M.: Akupunktur. Från tro till vetenskap. Malmö, Liber Förlag, 1984.
4. Badgley, C. E.: The articular facets in relation to low back pain and sciatic radiation. J. Bone Joint Surg. 23:481–491, 1941.
5. Battié, M. C., Bigos, S. J., Fisher, L. D., et al.: A prospective study of the role of cardiovascular risk factors and fitness in industrial back pain complaints. Spine 14:141–147, 1989.
6. Beals, R. K., and Hickman, N. W.: Industrial injuries of the back and extremities. J. Bone Joint Surg. 51A:1593–1611, 1972.
7. Bell, G., Rothman, R., Booth, R. E., et al.: A study of computor assisted tomography. II. Comparison of metrizamide of herniated lumbar disc and spinal stenosis. Spine 9:552–556, 1984.
8. Bergquist-Ullman, M., and Larsson, U.: Acute low back pain in industry. A controlled prospective study with special reference to therapy and confounding factors. Acta Orthop. Scand. Suppl. 170:1–115, 1977.
9. Biering-Sörensen, F.: Physical measurements as risk indicators for low-back trouble over a one-year period. Spine 9:106–119, 1984.
10. Bigos, S. J., Battié, M. C.: Acute care to prevent back disability. Ten years of progress. Clin. Orthop. 221:121–130, 1987.
11. Bigos, S. J., Battié, M. C., Fisher, et al: The prospective study of risk factors for the report of industrial back problems: A univariate analysis. ISSLS Meeting, Miami, Fla., April 13–17, 1988.
12. Blair, S. N., Oiserchia, P. V., Wilbur, C. S., and Crowder, J. H.: A public health intervention model for work-site health promotion. Impact on exercise and physical fitness in a health promotion plan after 24 months. J.A.M.A. 255:921–926, 1986.
13. Bloch R: Methodology in back pain trials. Spine 12:430–432, 1987.
14. Boden, S. D., Davis, D. O., Dina, T. S., et al: The incidence of abnormal lumbar spine MRI-scans in asymptomatic patients. Spine. Unpublished data, 1989.
15. Bogduk, N., Tynan, W., and Wilson, A. S.: The nerve supply to the human lumbar intervertebral discs. J. Anat. 132:39–56, 1981.
16. Booth, F. W.: Physiologic and biochemical effects of immobilization on muscle. Clin. Orthop. 219:15–20, 1987.
17. Bortz, W. M.: The disuse syndrome. West. J. Med. 141:691–694, 1984.
18. Brennan, G. P., Ruhling, R. O., Hood, R. S., et al.: Physical characteristics of patients with herniated lumbar discs. Spine 12:699–702, 1987.
19. Cady, L. D., Bischoff, D. P., O'Connell, E. R., et al.: Strength and fitness and subsequent back injuries in firefighters. J. Occup. Med. 4:269–272, 1979.
20. Cady, L. D., Thomas, P. C., and Karvaski, R. J.: Program for increasing health and physical fitness of fire-fighters. J. Occup. Med. 2:111–114, 1985.
21. Chöler, U., Larsson, R., Nachemson, A., and Peterson, L. E.: Ont i ryggen. Sprirapport 188, Stockholm, 1985.
22. Cole, T.-C., Burkhardt, P., Ghosh, P., et al: Effects of spinal fusion on the proteoglycans of the canine intervertebral disc. J. Orthop. Res. 3:277–291, 1985.
23. Cole, T.-C., Ghosh, P., Hannan, N. J., et al: The response of the canine intervertebral disc to immobilization produced by spinal arthrodesis is dependent on constitutional factors. J. Orthop. Res. 5:337–347, 1987.
24. Cole, T.-C., Ghosh, P., Taylor, T.: Variations of the proteoglycans of the canine intervertebral disc with aging. Biochim. Biophys. Acta 880:209–219, 1986.
25. Cox, M., Shephard, R. J., and Corey, P.: Influence of an employee fitness programme upon fitness, productivity, and absenteeism. Ergonomics 24:795–806, 1981.
26. Cox, M., Shephard, R. J., and Corey, P.: Absenteeism, fitness and worker satisfaction (abstr.). Can. J. Appl. Sports Sci. 8:227, 1983.
27. Crawford, W. C., Yang, J. C., and Janal, M. N.: Altered pain and visual sensitivity in humans: The effects of acute and chronic stress. Ann. N. Y. Acad. Sci. 467:116–129, 1986.
28. Crock, H. V.: Internal disc disruption. A challenge to disc prolapse fifty years on. The Presidential Address: I. S. S. L. S. Spine 11:650–653, 1986.
29. Deyo, R. A., Diehl, A. K., Rosenthal, M.: How many days bed rest for acute low back pain? A randomized clinical trial. N. Engl. J. Med. 315:1064–70, 1986.
30. Deyo, R. A., and Bass, J. E.: Lifestyle and low back pain: The influence of smoking, exercise and obesity. Clin. Res. 35:577A, 1987.
31. Diamant, B., Karlsson, J., and Nachemson, A.: Correlation between lactate levels and pH in discs of patients with lumbar rhizopathies. Experientia 24:1195–1196, 1968.
32. Ejeskär, A., Nachemson, A., Herberts, P., et al.: Surgery versus chymonucleolysis for herniated lumbar discs. A prospective standard random study with random assignment. Clin. Orthop. 174:236–242, 1983.
33. Evans, W., Jobe, W., Seiberg, C.: A cross-sectional prevalence study of lumbar disc degeneration in a working population. Spine 14:60–64, 1989.
34. Flynn, J. C., and Hoque, M. P. A.: Anterior fusion of the lumbar spine. End result study with long-term follow-up. J. Bone Joint Surg. 61A:1077–1080, 1979.
35. Fordyce, W. E.: Behavioral conditioning concepts in chronic pain. Pain 1(Suppl):163, 1981.

36. Fordyce, W. E.: Behavioral/cognitive methods for treating tissue injury pain. *In* Foley K. M., and Payne, R.: Current Therapy for Pain. Philadelphia, B. C. Decker, 1987.
37. Fordyce, W. E., Brena, S. F., Halcomb, R. J., et al.: Relationship of patient semantic pain description to physician diagnostic judgements, activity level measures, and MMPI. Pain 5:293–303, 1978.
38. Fordyce, W. E., Brockway, J. A., Bergman, J. A., and Spengler, D.: Acute back pain; A control-group comparison of behavioral vs. traditional management methods. J. Behav. Med. 9:127–140, 1985.
39. Fordyce, W. E., McMahon, R., Rainwater, G., et al.: Pain complaint—exercise performance relationship in chronic pain. Pain 10:311–321, 1981.
40. Fordyce, W. E., Roberts, A. H., and Sternbach, R. A.: The behavioral management of chronic pain: A response to critics. Pain 22:113–125, 1985.
41. Friberg, O.: Lumbar instability: a dynamic approach by traction-compression radiography. Spine 110:119–129, 1987.
42. Frymoyer, J. W., Cats-Baril, W.: Predictors of low back pain disability. Clin. Orthop. 221:89–98, 1987.
43. Frymoyer, J. W., Hanley, E., Howe, J., et al.: A comparison of radiographic findings in fusion and nonfusion patients. Ten or more years following lumbar disc surgery. Spine 4:435–440, 1979.
44. Ghormley, R. K.: 1933. Low back pain with special reference to the articular facets with presentation of an operative procedure. J.A.M.A. 101:1773–1777, 1933.
45. Ghosh, P., Taylor, T. K. F., and Braund, K. G.: Variation of the glycosaminoglycans of the canine intervertebral disc with aging. I. Chondrodystrophoid breed. Gerontology 23:87–98, 1977.
46. Ghosh, P., Taylor, T. K. F., and Braund, K. G.: Variation of the glycosaminoglycans of the intervertebral disc with ageing. II. Non-chondrodystrophoid breed. Gerontology 23:99–109, 1977.
47. Gibson, M. J., Buckley, J., Mawhinney, R., et al.: Magnetic resonance imaging and discography in the diagnosis of disc degeneration. A comparative study of 50 discs. J. Bone Joint Surg. 68B:369–373, 1986.
48. Gray, I. C. M., Main, C. J., and Waddell, G.: Psychologic assessment in general orthopaedic practice. Clin. Orthop. 194:258–264, 1985.
49. Hadler, N. M.: A critical reappraisal of the fibrositis concept. A. J. M. 81(Suppl. 3A):26–30, 1986.
50. Hadler, N. M.: Regional musculoskeletal diseases of the low back cumulative trauma versus single incident. Clin. Orthop. 221:33–41, 1987.
51. Hansson, T., Roos, B., and Nachemson, A.: Development of osteopenia in the fourth lumbar vertebra during prolonged bed rest after operation for scoliosis. Acta Orthop. Scand. 46:621–630, 1975.
52. Hansson, T., Sandström, J., Roos, B., et al.: The bone mineral content of the lumbar spine in patients with chronic low back pain. Spine 2:158–160, 1985.
53. Hazard, R. G., Fenwick, J., Kalish, S., et al.: Functional restoration with behavioral support: A one year prospective study of chronic low back pain patients. I.S.S.L.S. Meeting, Miami, Fla., April 13–17, 1988.
54. Hirsch, C., Ingelmark, B. E., and Miller, M.: The anatomical basis for low back pain. Acta Orthop. Scand. 33:1–17, 1963.
55. Hitchcock, T. F., Light, T. R., Bunch, W. H., et al.: The effect of immediate controlled mobilization on the strength of flexor tendon repairs. *In* Proc. 32nd Ann. O.R.S., New Orleans, Feb. 17–20, 1986.
56. Hitselberger, W. E., and Witten, R. M.: Abnormal myelograms in asymptomatic patients. J. Neurosurg. 28:204–206, 1968.
57. Holm, S., and Nachemson, A.: Nutritional changes in the canine intervertebral disc after spinal fusion. Clin. Orthop. 169:243–258, 1982.
58. Holm, S., and Nachemson, A.: Variations in the nutrition of the canine intervertebral disc induced by motion. Spine 8:866–874, 1983.
59. Holm, S., and Nachemson, A.: Nutrition of the intervertebral disc: Acute effects of cigarette smoking. Ups. J. Med. Sci. 93:91–99, 1988.
60. Jackson, R. P., Becker, G. J., Jacobs, R. R., and Mortesano, P. X.: The neuroradiographic diagnosis of lumbar herniated nucleus pulposus. Spine (in press).
61. Jackson, R. P., Jacobs, R. R., and Montesano, P. X.: Facet joint injections in low back pain: A prospective statistical study. Spine 13:966–971, 1988.
62. Jayson, M. I. V., Keegan, A. L., Million, R., and Tomlinson, I.: A fibrinolytic defect in chronic back pain syndromes. Lancet 24:1186–1187, 1984.
63. Johnsson, K.-E., Willner, S., and Johnsson, K.: Postoperative instability after decompression for lumbar spinal stenosis. Spine 11:107–110, 1986.
64. Järvinen, M. J., and Lehto, M. U. K.: Biological background of the treatment of muscle injuries. A review with special reference to the effects of early mobilization or immobilization on the healing process. Acta Orthop. Scand. (in press).
65. Kahanovitz, N., Nordin, M., Verderame, R., et al. Normal trunk muscle strength and endurance in women and the effect of exercises and electrical stimulation and exercises to increase trunk muscle strength and endurance. Spine 12:112–118, 1987.
66. Kiviranta, I.: Joint loading influences on the articular cartilage of young dogs. Thesis. Kuopio University Printing Office, Kuopio, Finland, 1987.
67. Komi, P. V.: Neuromuscular biomechanics: Selective correlates between structure and function. *In* Maehlum, S., Nilsson, S., and Renström, P. (eds.): An Update on Sports Medicine. Proceedings from the Second Scandinavian Conference in Sports Medicine, Oslo, March 9–15, 1986. Syntex, Norway AS, Oslo, 1987, pp. 60–78.
68. Langenskiold, A., Michelsson, J.-E., and Videman, T.: Osteoarthritis of the knee in the rabbit produced by immobilization. Attempts to achieve a reproducible model for studies on pathogenesis and therapy. Acta Orthop. Scand. 50:1–14, 1979.
69. Lehmann, T. R., Spratt, K. F., Tozzi, J. E., et al.: Long-term follow-up of lower lumbar fusion patients. Spine. 12:97–104, 1987.
70. Linton, S. J.: The relationship between activity and chronic pain. Pain 21:289–294, 1985.
71. Lippitt, A. B.: The facet joint and its role in spine pain. Management with facet joint injections. Spine 7:746–750, 1984.
72. Long, D. M., Filtzer, D. L., Ben Debba, M., and Hendler, N. H.: Clinical features of the failed-back syndrome. J. Neurosurg. 69:61–71, 1988.
73. Maroudas, A., Stockwell, R. A., Nachemson, A.,

and Urban, J.: Factors involved in the nutrition of the human lumbar intervertebral disc; cellularity and diffusion of glucose in-vitro. J. Anat. 120:113–130, 1975.
74. Mayer, T. G.: Assessment of lumbar function. Clin. Orthop. 221:99–109, 1987.
75. Mayer, G., Gatchel, R. J., Kishino, N., et al.: Objective assessment of spine function following industrial injury. A prospective study with comparison group and one-year follow-up. Spine 10:482–493, 1985.
76. Mooney, V.: The syndromes of low back disease. Orthop. Clin. North Am. 14:505–515, 1983.
77. Mooney, V.: The failed back: An orthopaedic view. Int. Disabil. Stud. 10:32–36, 1988.
78. Mooney, V., and Robertson, J.: The facet syndrome. Clin. Orthop. 115:149–156, 1976.
79. Moran, R., O'Connell, D., and Walsh, M. G.: The diagnostic value of facet joint injections. Spine 13:1407–1410, 1988.
80. Morris, R. W.: A statistical study of papers in the Journal of Bone and Joint Surgery [Br.], 1984. J. Bone Joint Surg. 70B:242–296, 1988.
81. Nachemson, A.: Work for all. For those with low back pain as well. Clin. Orthop. 179:77–85, 1983.
82. Nachemson, A.: Advances in low-back pain. Clin. Orthop. 200:266–278, 1985.
83. Nachemson, A.: Editorial letter. Acta Orthop. Scand. 56:285–286, 1985.
84. Nachemson, A., and Bigos, S.: The low back. *In* Cruess, R. L. and Rennie, W. R. J. (eds.): Adult Orthopaedics, Vol. II. New York, Churchill Livingstone, 1984, pp. 843–935.
85. Nachemson, A., LaRocca, H.: Editorial letter. Spine 12:427–429, 1987.
86. Nachemson, A., Spitzer, W. O., et al.: Scientific approach to the assessment and management of activity-related spinal disorders. A monograph for clinicians. Report of the Quebec Task Force on Spinal Disorders. Spine 12 (suppl. 1):S1–S59, 1987.
87. Nettelbladt, E.: Antalet reumatikerinvalider i Sverigo undor on 30-årsperiod. O. P. M. E. A. R. 30:54–56, 1985.
88. Olsson, T. H., Selvik, G., and Willner, S.: Kinematic analysis of spinal fusions. Invest. Radiol. 11:202–209, 1976.
89. Olsson, T. H., Selvik, G., and Willner, S.: Mobility in the lumbosacral spine after fusion studied with the aid of roentgen stereophotogrammetry. Clin. Orthop. 129:181–190, 1977.
90. Park, W. M.: Radiological investigation of the intervertebral disc. *In* Jayson, M. I. V.: The Lumbar Spine and Back Pain, 2nd Ed. Bath, Pitman Medical Publishing, 1980, pp. 185–230.
91. Parke, W. W., and Watanabe, R.: The intrinsic vasculature of the lumbosacral spinal nerve roots. Spine 10:508–515, 1985.
92. Porter, R. W., Hibbert, C., and Evans, C.: The natural history of root entrapment syndrome. Spine 9:418–421, 1984.
93. Potter, N. A., Rothstein, J. M.: Intertester reliability for selected clinical tests of the sacroiliac joint. Phys. Ther. 65:1671–1675, 1985.
94. Pountain, G. D., Keegan, A. L., and Jayson, M. I. V.: Impaired fibrinolytic activity in defined chronic back pain syndromes. Spine 12:83–86, 1987.
95. Powell, M. C., Wilson, M., Szypryt, P., and Symonds, E. M.: Prevalence of lumbar disc degeneration observed by magnetic resonance in symptomless women. Lancet, 13:1366–1367, 1986.
96. Puig, M. M., Laorden, M. L., Miralles, F. S., et al.: Endorphin levels in cerebrospinal fluid of patients with postoperative and chronic pain. Anesthesiology 57:1, 1982.
97. Ransford, A. O., Cairns, D., and Mooney, V.: The pain drawing as an aid to the psychologic evaluation of patients with low-back pain. Spine 1:127–134, 1976.
98. Raskob, G. E., Lofthouse, R. N. and Hull, R. D.: Current concepts review. Methodological guidelines for clinical trials evaluating new therapeutic approaches in bone and joint surgery. J. Bone Joint Surg. 67A:1294–1297, 1985.
99. Renström, P., and Johnsson, R. J.: Overuse injuries — a great problem in sports. *In* An Update on Sports Medicine. Maehlum, S., Nilsson, S., and Renström, P. (eds.): Proceedings from the Second Scandinavian Conference in Sports Medicine, Oslo. March 9–15, 1986. Syntex, Norway AS, Oslo, 1987, pp. 169–190.
100. Report of the Commission on the Evaluation of Pain. Soc. Sec. Bul. vol. 50, 1987.
101. Roberts, N., Smith, R., Bennett, S., et al.: Health beliefs and rehabilitation after lumbar disc surgery. J. Psychosom. Res. 28:139–149, 1984.
102. Rothman, R. H. and Booth, R.: Failures of spinal fusion. Orthop. Clin. North Am. 6:299–304, 1975.
103. Rudicel, S., and Esdaile, J.: The randomized clinical trial in Orthopaedics: Obligation or option? J. Bone Joint Surg. 67A:1284–1293, 1985.
104. Rydevik, B., Brown, M., and Lundborg, G.: Pathoanatomy and pathophysiology of nerve root compression. Spine 9:7–15, 1984.
105. Sahltin, B.: The physiological and biochemical basis of aerobic and anaerobic capacities in man: Effect of training and range of adaption. *In* An update on sports medicine. Maehlum, S., Nilsson, S., and Renström, P. (eds.): Proceedings from the Second Scandinavian Conference in Sports Medicine, Oslo. March 9–15, 1986. Syntex, Norway AS, Oslo, 1987, pp. 16–60.
106. Saraste, H., and Hultman, G.: Life conditions of persons without low-back pain. Scand. J. Rehab. Med. 19:109–115, 1986.
107. Schönström, N.: The narrow lumbar spinal canal and the size of the cauda equina in man. Thesis. Gothenburg University, Göteborg, 1988.
108. Selvik, G.: A roentgen stereophotogrammetric method for the study of the kinematics of the skeletal system. Thesis. The University of Lund, Lund, 1974.
109. Shapiro, R.: Lumbar discography: An outdated procedure. J. Neurosurg. 64:686–691, 1986.
110. Shuy, B. C., Andersson, S. A., and Thorén, P.: Endorphin-mediated increase in pain threshold induced by long-lasting exercise in rats. Life Sci. 30:833–840, 1982.
111. Sturesson, B., Selvik, G., and Udén, A.: Movements of the sacroiliac joint. A roentgenstereophotogrammetric analysis. Spine (in press).
112. Svensson, H.-O.: Low back pain in forty to forty-seven-year-old men: A retrospective cross-sectional study. Thesis. Gothenburg University, Göteborg, 1982.

113. Svensson, O. H., Vedin, A., Wilhelmsson, C., and Andersson, G. B. J.: Low-back pain in relation to other diseases and cardiovascular risk factors. Spine 8:277–285, 1983.
114. Taylor, T. K. F., Ghosh, P., Braund, K. G., et al.: The effect of spinal fusion on intervertebral disc composition: An experimental study. J. Surg. Res. 21:91–104, 1976.
115. Terenius, L.: Endorphins and pain. Front Horm. Res. 8:162–167, 1981.
116. Tidball, J. G.: Myotendinous junction: Morphological changes and mechanical failure associated with muscle cell atrophy. Exp. Mol. Pathol. 40:1–12, 1984.
117. Tipton, C. M., Vailas, A. C., and Matthes, R. D.: Experimental studies on the influences of physical activity on ligaments, tendons and joints: A brief review. Acta Med. Scand. 711(Suppl.):157–168, 1985.
118. Urban, J. P. G., Holm, S., Maroudas, A., and Nachemson, A.: Nutrition of the intervertebral disk—an in-vivo study of solute transport. Clin. Orthop. 129:101–114, 1977.
119. Urban, J. P. G., Holm, S. Maroudas, A., and Nachemson, A.: Nutrition of the intervertebral disc. Effect of fluid flow on solute transport. Clin. Orthop. 170:296–302, 1982.
120. Van der Linden, W.: On the generalisation of surgical trial results. Acta Chir. Scand. 146:229–294, 1980.
121. Vanharanta, H., Sachs, B. L., Spivey, M. A., et al.: Dallas discogram description: A new classification of CT/discography in low back disorders. Spine 13:321–324, 1988.
122. Weinstein, J., Claverie, W., and Gibson, S.: The pain of discography. Spine 13:1344–1351, 1988.
123. Versloot, J. M., Schilstra, A. J., Tolen, F. J. and van Akkerveeken, P. F.: Backschool in industry. A prospective longitudinal controlled study (3 years). I.S.S.L.S. Meeting, Miami, Fla., April 13–17, 1988.
124. Videman, T.: Connective tissue and immobilization. Key factors in musculoskeletal degeneration? Clin. Orthop. 221:26–32, 1987.
125. Volinn, E., Lai, D., McKinney, S., and Loeser, D.: When back pain becomes disabling: A regional analysis. Pain 33:33–39, 1988.
126. Von Knorring, L., Almay, B. G. L., Johansson, F., and Terenius, L.: Pain perception and endorphin levels in cerebrospinal fluid. Pain 5:359–365, 1978.
127. Von Knorring, L., Almay, B. G. L., and Johansson, P.: Personality traits in patients with idiopathic pain disorders. Acta Psychiatr. Scand. 76:490–498, 1987.
128. Vuorinen, J., and Rokkanen, P.: The effect of immobilization of the spine of rats. Acta Orthop. Scand. 58:458, 1987.
129. Waddell, G.: A new clinical model for the treatment of low back pain. Spine 12:632–644, 1987.
130. Waddell, G., Kummel, E. G., Lotton, W. N., et al.: Failed lumbar disc surgery and repeat surgery following industrial injuries. J. Bone Joint Surg. 61A:201–207, 1979.
131. Waddell, G., and Main, C.: Assessment of severity of low-back pain disorders. Spine 9:204–208, 1984.
132. Waddell, G., Main, C. J., Morris, E. W., et al.: Normality and reliability in the clinical assessment of backache. Br. Med. J. 284:1519–1523, 1982.
133. Waddell, G., Main, C., Morris, E. W., et al.: Chronic low back pain, psychologic distress and illness behaviour. Spine 9:209–213, 1984.
134. Vällfors, B.: Acute, subacute and chronic low back pain. Clinical symptoms, absenteeism and working environment. Scand. J. Rehabil. Med. 11(Suppl.):1–98, 1985.
135. Weber, H.: Lumbar disc herniation. Part I. J. Oslo City Hosp. 28:33–40, 1978.
136. Weber, H.: Lumbar disc herniation. Part II. J. Oslo City Hosp. 28:89–95, 1978.
137. Woo S. L.-Y., Buckwalter, J. A.: Injury and repair of the musculoskeletal soft tissues. American Academy of Orthopaedic Surgeons Symposium. Park Ridge, American Academy of Orthopaedic Surgeons, 1988.
138. Wyke, B.: The neurology of low back pain. *In* Jayson, M. I. V., (ed.): The Lumbar Spine and Back Pain, 3rd Ed. London, Churchill Livingstone, 1987, pp. 56–99.
139. Young, A., and Wynn Parry, C. B.: The assessment and management of the failed back. Part I. Int. Disabil. Stud. 10:21–43, 1988.

2 □ Anatomy of Low Back Pain

Gordon R. Bell
Ken Yong-Hing
William H. Kirkaldy-Willis

■ ANATOMY OF THE LUMBAR SPINE: DEVELOPMENTAL TO NORMAL ADULT

Gordon R. Bell

EMBRYOLOGY

The nervous system, with its associated structural support system, is clearly the most complicated anatomic system of the human body. Its 100 billion neurons and 1 trillion glial cells form a complex network of connections that constitute the structural framework of nature's most complicated piece of biologic architecture: the human body. Metamerism, whereby an organism is formed by the serial repetition of similar anatomic segments (metameres), is retained in vertebrate embryology from its higher invertebrate evolutionary origin. In addition, Stromer's law defines the economy of function that is characteristic of higher life forms. According to this principle, many similar anatomic segments decrease in number by their deletion or fusion with other segments, and the remaining segments diversify their function and become more specialized.

Fetal development may be conceptually divided into three stages: pre-embryonic, embryonic, and fetal. The *pre-embryonic period* begins at fertilization and lasts for approximately 3 weeks. The three primary germ layers (ectoderm, mesoderm, and endoderm) develop during this period. The second stage, the *embryonic period*, is the most active period and the one in which the organ systems form. It lasts from approximately the third to eighth week of development. The *fetal period* is the final stage of development and lasts from approximately eight weeks to birth. The organ systems formed during the embryonic period undergo further growth and development during this stage.

At approximately 16 days, the embryo is transformed from a two-layered structure, consisting of a dorsally situated ectoderm and amniotic cavity and a ventrally situated endoderm and yolk sac, to a trilaminar structure. At this stage, a proliferation of midline ectodermal cells becomes the primitive streak. Just cranial to this area, the ectoderm begins to invaginate to form the primitive pit. The ectodermal cells adjacent to this opening are known as the primitive knot, and their cranial proliferation produces Hensen's node (Fig. 1*A*). This tubular notochordal process is destined to become the notochord. The hollow cavity and ventral surface of the notochordal process disappear so that the dorsal surface of the process comes to lie in direct contact with the underlying endoderm and yolk sac, forming a flat notochordal plate. Further, in a craniocaudal direction, the lateral edges of the notochor-

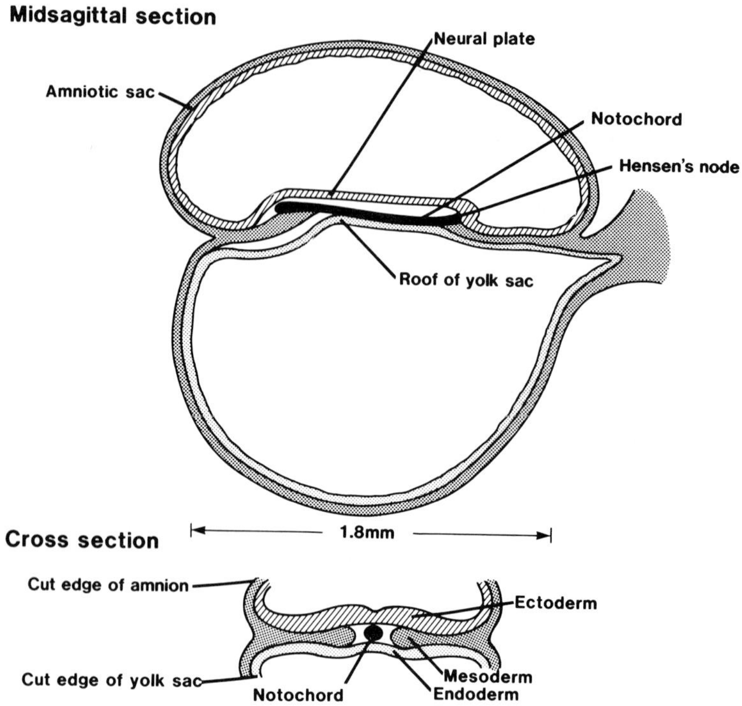

Figure 1 □ Human embryo at approximately 16 days. *A,* Sagittal view shows relationship of developing neural structures to amniotic sac and yolk sac. *B,* Cross section through notochord shows relationship of notochord to the layers of the trilaminar embryo.

dal plate curl under, uniting the edges of the endoderm and producing the true notochord, which thus comes to lie between the underlying endoderm and overlying ectoderm (Fig. 1*B*).

During the third week of fetal development, a the ectoderm overlying the notochord thickens, producing the neural plate. The lateral edges of this plate proliferate dorsally and eventually curl over the neural plate to create a tubular structure known as the neural tube (Fig. 2*A,B*).

By the end of the third week, the third layer of the trilaminar embryonic structure forms. This layer, known as the mesoderm, is situated between the dorsal ectoderm and the ventral endoderm and lies lateral to the notochord. By approximately the 19th day, the mesoderm has divided into three distinct areas by virtue of its complex differentiation in both a mediolateral and a craniocaudal direction. The most cellular portion of this mesodermal structure lies immediately lateral to the notochord and is known as the *paraxial mesoderm.* From this paired structure, two additional areas form on each side by its further lateral proliferation. These are the *intermediate mesoderm columns* and a more laterally situated *lateral mesodermal plate.* The intermediate mesoderm ultimately differentiates into the urogenital system, while the lateral mesoderm divides into the somatic mesoderm, which forms the ventrolateral body wall musculature, and the splanchnic mesoderm, which forms the muscular layer of the gut.

The paraxial mesoderm gives rise to the somites, 42 to 44 paired segments that will give rise to the major skeletal, muscular, and integumentary systems of the body. The central portion of the somite comprises a cavity known as the myocoele. The cells situated dorsolaterally to the myocoele become the *dermomyotome,* while the more ventromedially located cells become the *sclerotome* (Fig. 2*B,C*). The dermomyotome further divides into a lateral *dermatome,* which becomes the integument, and a medial *myotome,* which is destined to become the posterolateral body wall musculature. The sclerotome undergoes further migration and differentiation to become the skeletal structures (Fig. 2*C,D*).

The sclerotome is not homogeneous, but is divided into a cranial and caudal portion by the sclerotomic fissure of von Ebner. A resegmentation of the sclerotome occurs in which the caudal portion of one sclerotome unites with the cranial portion of the next caudal sclerotome to form the primordium of the future vertebral body, or *centrum* (Fig. 3). Thus, a centrum receives equal contributions from adjacent sclerotomes. The segmental vessels, which originally lay between somites, ultimately come to lie over the center of the centrum. Conversely, the segmental nerve, which originally lay in the center of the sclerotome, comes to lie between adjacent centra opposite the intervertebral disc (Fig. 3*D*).

As the sclerotome surrounds the notochord, the notochordal cells within the centrum degenerate such that, by adulthood, notochordal remnants within the vertebral body are usually absent. Occasionally, however, such notochordal rests may persist and thus have the potential for the development of a malignant chordoma. Between centra, the notochord undergoes mucoid degeneration resulting in a gelatinous mass of cells that become the intervertebral disc (Fig. 3*D*).

Additional migration of other sclerotome cells results in the formation of the remainder of the embryonic vertebrae. Dorsally migrating cells become the *neural arch*, while ventrolateral sclerotomal cell migration results in *costal process* formation (Fig. 3*D*). In the thoracic vertebrae, the costal process becomes a rib, and, in the cervical vertebrae, it forms the anterior portion of the transverse foramen. In the lumbar vertebrae, the costal process forms the transverse process (Fig. 4). Thus, although only the thoracic vertebrae typically bear ribs, all vertebrae, except the coccyx, have a costal process and are therefore capable of bearing ribs. This can clinically be seen when a rudimentary cervical rib may give rise to brachial plexus compression.

The first 6 weeks of fetal development as described above result in a mesenchymal anlage of the vertebral column. During the sixth week, this mesenchymal structure undergoes chondrification. A typical vertebra chondrifies via six chondrification centers. Two centers appear in the vertebral centrum, one on each side of the notochord. These fuse around the notochord to form the center for the centrum. Two additional centers form and fuse dorsally to become the neural arch. The final two centers appear lateral to the junction of the neural arch and centrum to provide the chondrification center for each transverse process.

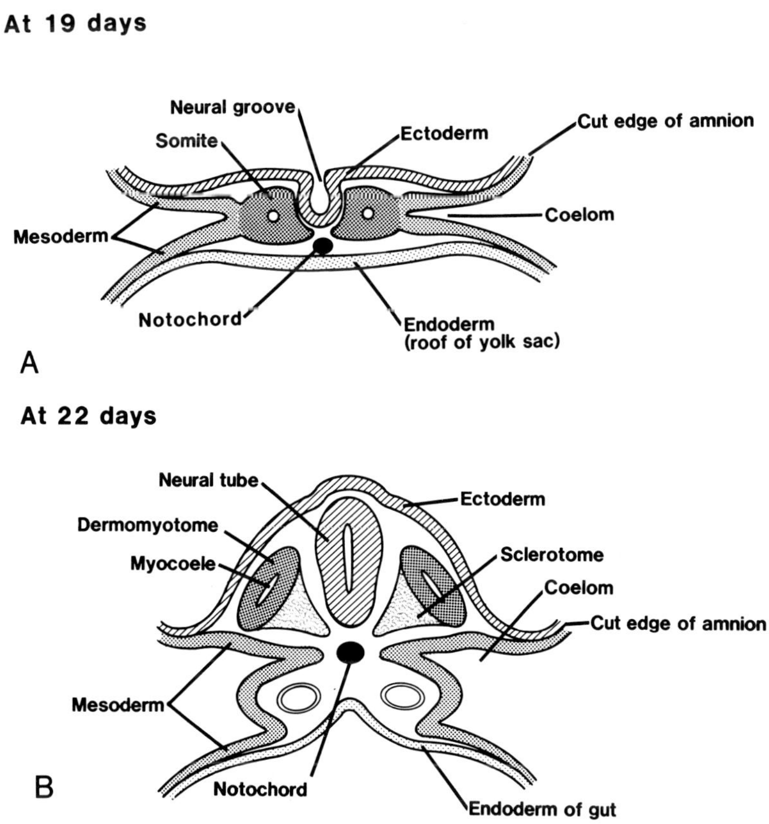

Figure 2 □ Cross section of human embryo showing formation and differentiation of somite. *A, B,* The dermomyotome and sclerotome form from somite.

Illustration continued on following page

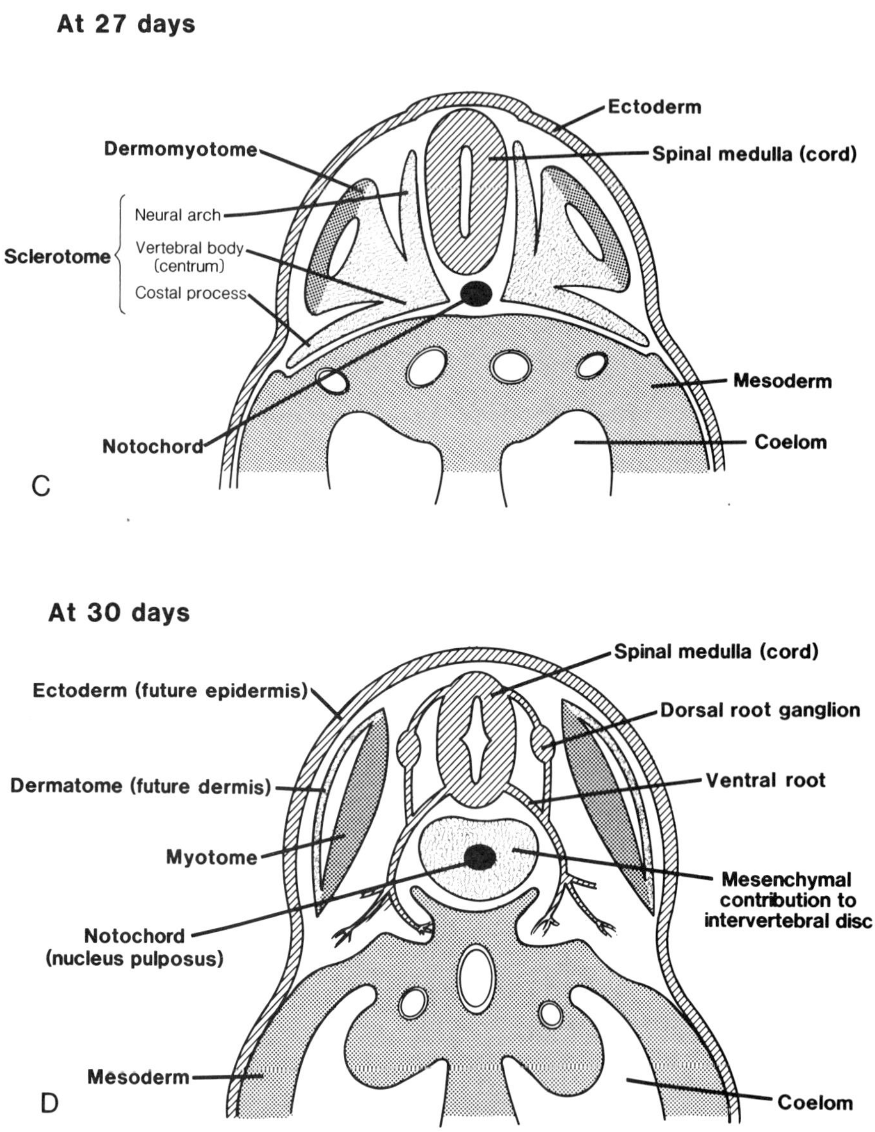

Figure 2 *Continued C, D,* Sclerotome further differentiates and migrates to form portions of vertebra.

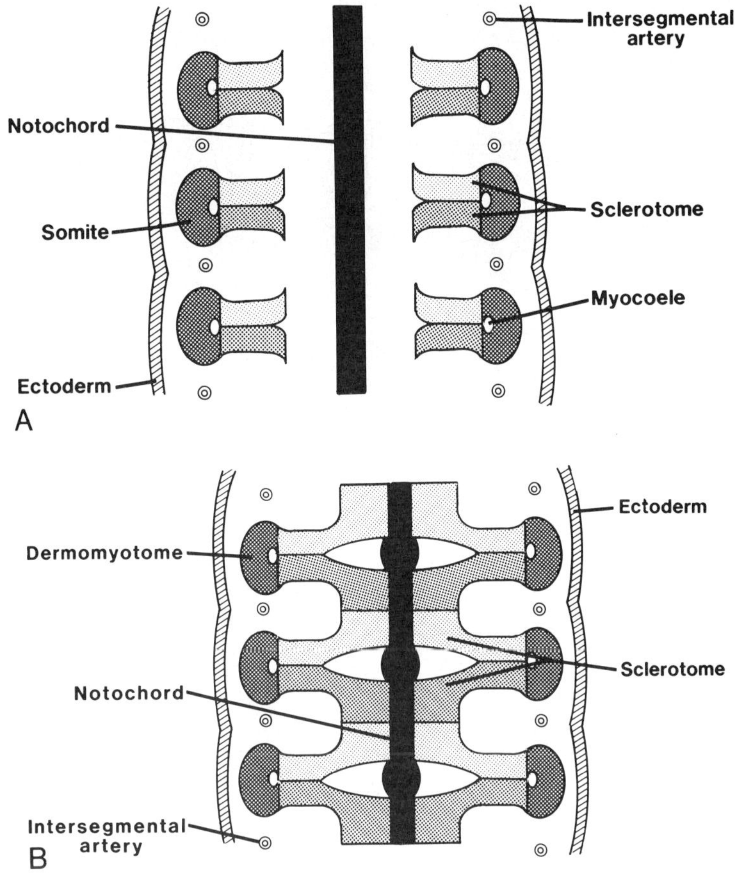

Figure 3 □ Formation of vertebral column and related neuromuscular structures. *A–C,* Note that centrum is formed from equal contributions of two adjacent sclerotomes.
Illustration continued on following page

Ossification of the cartilaginous model just described begins by approximately 9 weeks with the invasion by perichondral blood vessels. Three primary and three secondary ossification centers exist for each typical vertebra. Ossification of the centrum occurs from a single center, while the neural arch ossifies from two centers. Ossification of the vertebral arch center begins by about the eighth week, beginning in the cervical areas first and proceeding caudally. Ossification of the centrum begins later, commencing by about the 16th week. Centra ossification centers appear initially at the thoracolumbar junction, and caudal development is more rapid than cranial development. The ossified centrum and neural arch are joined by a cartilaginous connection known as the *neurocentral synchondrosis.* This junction is situated anterior to the pedicles far enough that the true vertebral body is formed not only by the centrum but also by an adjacent portion of the neural arch (Fig. 4). The centrum fuses to the neural arch late during fetal growth, beginning in the upper lumbar area. Fusion then continues cranially and caudally.

Three secondary ossification centers develop during adolescence. One appears for each transverse process tip and one for the tip of the spinous process by approximately 15 or 16 years of age. By the third decade, these centers fuse with the remaining portion of the vertebrae. Occasionally, these centers may remain as distinct entities and may be confused with a fracture of the involved process.

APPLIED ANATOMY

Osteology and Arthrology

The human spinal column is an articulated segmental structure that serves the dual purposes of protection and motion. Thirty-three vertebrae, segmentally connected with one another, form a protective housing for the spinal cord and nerves. The spine contains each of the three major types of joints: synarthroses, diarthroses, and am-

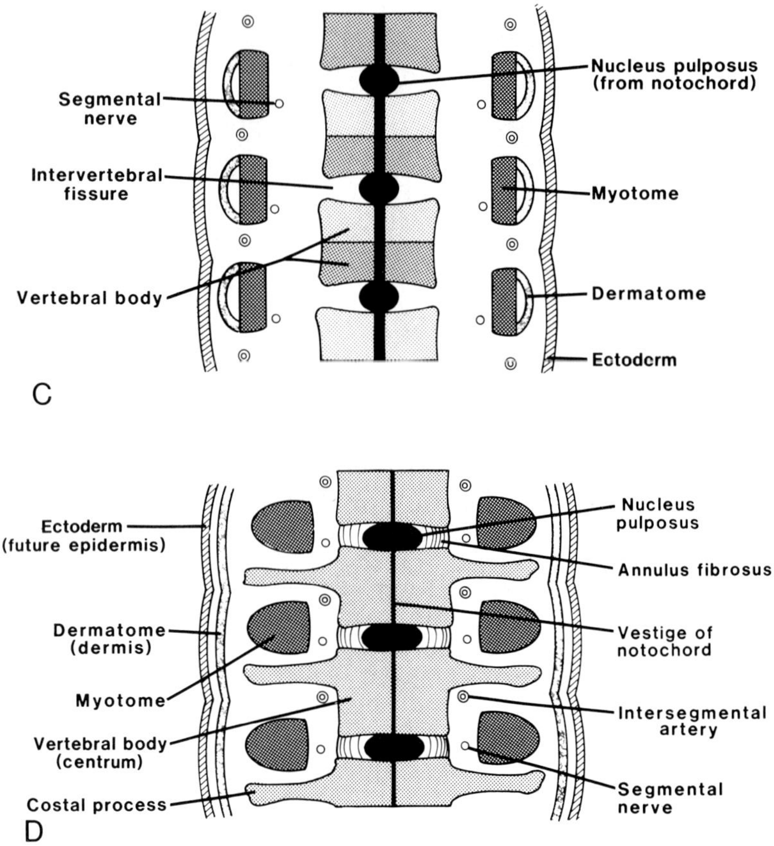

Figure 3 *Continued C, D,* The segmental artery, originally lying between sclerotomes, comes to lie opposite the centrum. *D,* The spinal nerve comes to lie opposite the intervertebral disc. Note that the intervertebral disc develops from notochordal tissue between centra, whereas notochordal tissue enclosed by the centrum ultimately degenerates (*D*).

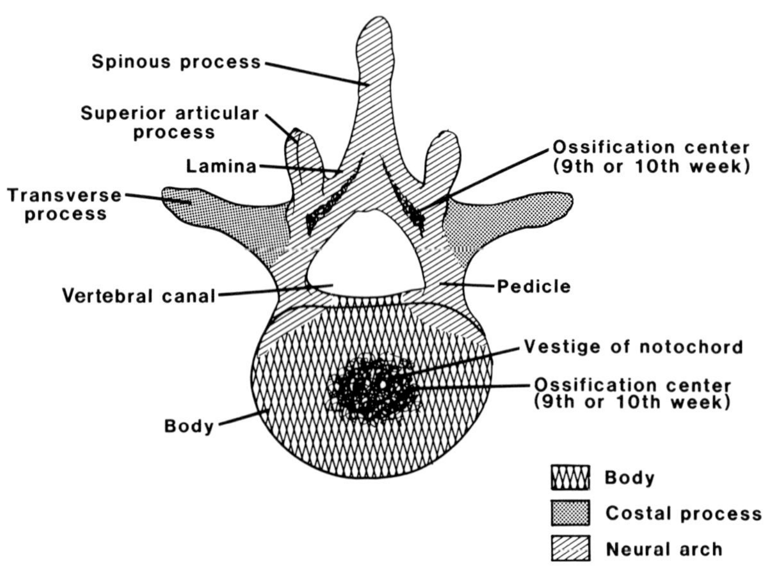

Figure 4 □ Formation of typical lumbar vertebra. Note that the vertebral body is formed by centrum and a portion of the neural arch.

phiarthroses. Together they allow various intersegmental motions, which differ in each region of the spine. A *synarthrosis*, such as the neurocentral synchondrosis, is an immobile joint in which two bones are joined by a thin cartilaginous plate. *Diarthroses* are synovial joints of the gliding variety (arthrodial), such as the lumbar facet joints. The *amphiarthroses*, slightly moveable nonsynovial joints, are of two types: *symphysis* and *syndesmosis*. The fibrocartilage of the intervertebral disc is typical of a symphysis type of amphiarthrosis. Ligamentous connections between the vertebrae constitute the syndesmotic type of amphiarthrosis.

A typical vertebra is composed of an outer cancellous vertebral body and a posterior vertebral arch, which is connected to the body by two pedicles (Fig. 5). The lumbar vertebrae are the largest vertebrae of the spine. The bodies are often (although not necessarily) wedge shaped, being wider anteriorly than posteriorly. The body is kidney shaped in cross section, as opposed to that of a typical thoracic vertebra, which is heart shaped. The posterior surface is flatter than that of a typical thoracic vertebra. The discs between the lumbar vertebrae are wedge shaped, and these are primarily responsible for the normal lordosis that is characteristic of the lumbar spine.

The pedicles are attached to the superior aspect of the vertebral body and form the upper boundary of the neural foramen. The vertebral body, pedicles, and vertebral arch enclose a triangular vertebral foramen. As described previously, the vertebral body is composed of the centrum, the ossified adjacent neurocentral synchondrosis, and a portion of the vertebral arch. The transverse processes from the upper four lumbar vertebrae are more posteriorly located than those of the L5 vertebra, sitting well back on the pedicle. The fourth transverse process is usually the longest and frequently angles slightly superiorly, as well as projecting laterally. The fifth lumbar transverse processes are shorter, thicker, and more anteriorly situated, projecting from the anterior aspect of the pedicle and the lateral aspect of the vertebral body. Embryologically, the transverse process is formed from the costal process, which develops from the ventrolateral migration of sclerotomal cells. The true transverse element of the lumbar vertebra, corresponding to the rudimentary transverse process of a thoracic vertebra, consists of the mamillary process and the accessory tubercle. The mamillary process is a small elevation that projects posteriorly from the superior articular process behind the articular facet. The accessory tubercle lies below the mamillary process at the base of the transverse process. These two projections serve as muscle attachments for the erector muscle of the spine.

Adjacent vertebral arches are joined together by a superior and inferior articular process to form the facet joint, which allows a gliding type of motion. The capsules of these diarthroses are attached to the articular margins. The plane of motion of these joints is determined by the orientation of the articular processes themselves and not by the ligamentous anatomy. The uppermost lumbar articular processes face the middle. As we proceed in a caudal direction, the plane of the facets becomes posteriorly oriented as well, such that at the L4–L5 and L5–S1 levels the orientation is approximately midway between sagittal and coronal.

A syndesmotic type of amphiarthrosis between the vertebral arches is formed by strong ligamentous connections. Such ligaments include the flaval ligaments, the intertransverse ligaments, the interspinous ligaments, and the supraspinous ligament. The flaval ligaments form a shingle-like arrangement between the laminae, attaching to the superior aspect of the inferior laminae and the ventral (deep) aspect of the superior laminae. This arrangement is readily visible once the loose areolar tissue overlying the flaval ligaments is removed. This unique aspect of the superior attachment of the flaval ligaments is of particular clinical significance during the performance of a laminectomy. The flaval ligaments meet in the midline where a raphe-like slit exists for passage of small blood vessels.

The vertebral bodies are also interconnected by a syndesmotic type of amphiarthrosis (anterior longitudinal ligament and posterior longitudinal ligament as well as by a symphysis type of amphiarthrosis (intervertebral disc). The anterior longitudinal ligament in the lumbar spine is firmly attached to the vertebral body periosteum but lies freely over the intervertebral disc. Its deepest fibers span one segment only, whereas its intermediate and superficial layers extend over several vertebrae.

Figure 5 □ Anatomic specimen of lumbar spine. *A* shows the posterior view of lumbar spine. *B* shows a close-up posterior view of L4 and L5. *C* illustrates the lateral aspect of the lumbar spine. *D* shows an anterior-oblique projection. (1 = body, 2 = pedicle, 3 = lamina, 4 = transverse process, 5 = spinous process, 6 = facet joint, 7 = mamillary process, 8 = accessory tubercle, 9 = pars interarticularis, 10 = superior articular process, 11 = inferior articular process.)

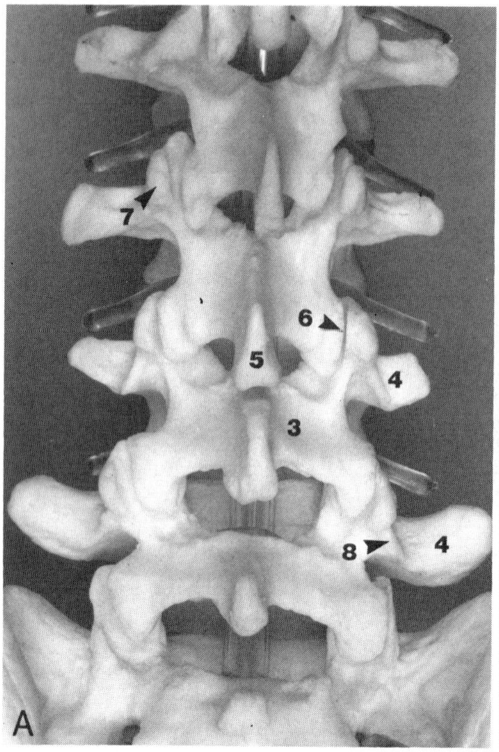

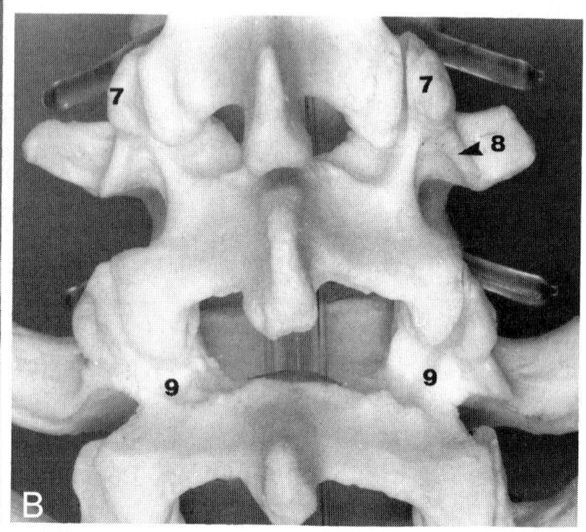

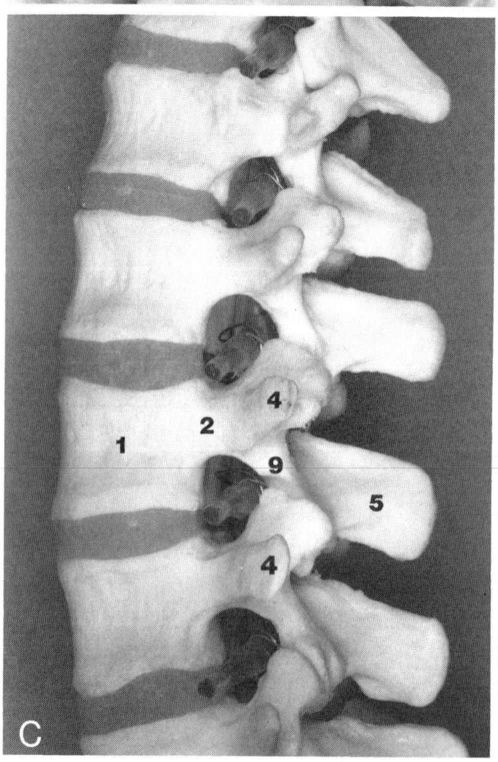

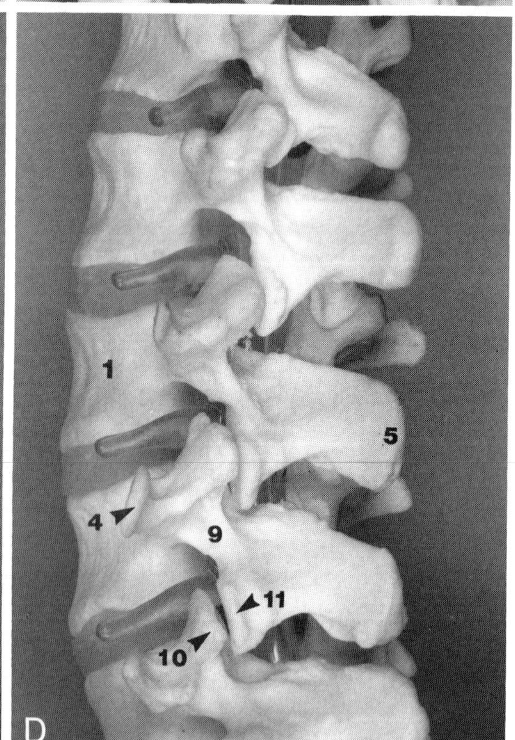

The posterior longitudinal ligament, on the other hand, is firmly attached to the intervertebral disc, particularly laterally, and is not attached to the posterior surface of the vertebral body. It is strung across the posterior vertebral concavity from which it is separated by the basivertebral veins. The deep layer of the posterior longitudinal ligament spans two vertebral levels. It has firm lateral attachments along the dorsum of the disc extending through the neural foramen, but it is weaker in its more central portions. The stronger superficial layer bridges several bodies and is particularly strong at the center. This arrangement explains the more usual lateral location of disc herniations, because the stronger superficial layer of the posterior longitudinal ligament prevents direct midline herniations, whereas the firm lateral attachments of the deep layer of the posterior longitudinal ligament usually prevent lateral extrusion into the intervertebral foramen. The weakest portion of the posterior longitudinal ligament, therefore, is in its deep portion and is slightly lateral to the midline.

The intertransverse ligaments pass between the transverse processes and are anatomically most distinct in the lumbar spine. The interspinous ligaments are attached from the base of the superior spinous process to the superior aspect of the immediately subjacent inferior spinous process. The supraspinous ligament is an unpaired ligament extending from the C7 spinous process to the end of the sacrum.

A symphysis type of amphiarthrosis is typified by the intervertebral disc. This structure forms a fibrocartilaginous articulation between the vertebral bodies and is composed of the nucleus pulposus and the annulus fibrosus. The nucleus pulposus is composed of a gelatinous mass of cells that embryologically result from mucoid degeneration of the notochordal tissue located between the vertebral centra. The nucleus pulposus responds as a viscid fluid under pressure, being able to resist and redistribute compressive forces. Although centrally located within the embryonic annulus fibrosus, it comes to lie eccentrically in the adult such that it sits closer to the posterior margin of the disc.

The annulus fibrosus consists of a series of fibrous lamellae, each having a different orientation to the others and to the vertebral body itself. Its architecture and lamellar orientation have been compared to the alternating layers of a radial tire. This unique arrangement allows the annulus to resist tensile forces. Because of the posterior location of the nucleus pulposus within the adult disc, the posterior lamellae of the annulus fibrosus are thinner than the anterior lamellae. This arrangement partially explains the predisposition to posterior disc herniations.

The annulus is primarily attached to a peripheral ring of compact bone on the margin of the vertebral body. The outermost lamellae of the annulus penetrate this ring as Sharpey fibers. Radiographically, this attachment is sometimes visible as a *traction spur*, which MacNab[5] states is a radiographic sign of segmental instability. This spur is typically located approximately 2 mm from the edge of the vertebral body and corresponds to the attachment of the annulus fibrosus. The outer margins of the annulus have additional more diffuse attachments to the vertebral body periosteum and to the longitudinal ligaments.

Neurology and Myology

The spinal nerve, containing a mixture of sensory and motor fibers, divides into an anterior and a posterior primary ramus immediately upon exiting the intervertebral foramen. The *posterior ramus* supplies the extensor muscles of the spine (spinal erector muscle of the spine) and much of the overlying skin. It also supplies sensory innervation to the facet joints, interspinous ligaments, and flaval ligaments. The *anterior ramus* supplies all three layers of body wall musculature, exclusive of the spinal erector muscle of the spine.

The *sinuvertebral* nerve is a recurrent branch of the spinal nerve, which originates just distal to the dorsal root ganglion and reenters the neural foramen. It divides into superior and inferior branches, which arborize to supply the periosteum, the posterior longitudinal ligament, the dura, the outermost layers of the annulus fibrosus, and the epidural vessels of several adjacent segments. This diffuse anastomotic arrangement, whereby a single sinuvertebral nerve provides sensation to several levels, helps to explain why many clinicians doubt the reliability of discography to accurately predict the source of discogenic low back pain. It should be emphasized that the nucleus pulposus and the inner layers of the annulus fibrosus have no known nerve supply.

The musculature of the body wall has been conveniently divided into three layers, which are described by their relationship to the ribs: an inner layer passing inside the ribs, an external layer passing outside the ribs, and an intermediate layer reinforced by the ribs. All three layers, except the spinal erector muscle portion of the external muscle layer, are supplied by anterior primary rami. The erector muscle of the spine, as mentioned previously, is supplied by posterior primary rami.

The innermost layer of the lumbar region is represented by flexor muscles such as the psoas. The intermediate layer is confined to the rib layer and contains the external and internal intercostal muscles. The quadratus lumborum is included in this layer. In the lumbar region, the external layer is composed of the erector muscle of the spine. This muscle runs along the entire length of the spine, from skull to sacrum. It consists of three layers, each containing three muscles. The deepest layer consists of the interspinal muscles (passing between spinous processes), the intertransverse muscles (running between adjacent transverse processes), and the rotator muscles (passing from the base of a transverse process to the spinous process above). The rotator muscles are found in the thoracic spine only.

The intermediate layer of the erector muscle of the spine is well developed and consists of the multifidus spinal muscles, the semispinal muscles, and the levator muscles of the ribs. The multifidus extends from the lamina and mamillary process to the spinous process of the vertebra two or three levels above. The semispinal muscles and levator muscles of the ribs are not represented in the lumbar spine.

The superficial layer of the erector muscle of the spine is powerful and consists of three parts. From lateral to medial they are the sacrospinal muscle, the longissimus muscle of the thorax, and the spinalis muscle. The sacrospinal muscle is the most powerful of the three parts, extending from the sacrum and inner aspect of the iliac crest to the transverse processes of the lower four cervical vertebrae.

References

1. Crelin, E. S.: Development of the nervous system: A logical approach to neuroanatomy. Clin. Symp. 28:1, 1976.
2. Crelin, E. S.: Development of the musculoskeletal system. Clin. Symp. 33:1, 1981.
3. Last, R. J.: Anatomy: Regional and Applied. London, J. & A. Churchill, 1970.
4. Lonstein, J. E.: 1. Spine embryology. *In* Winter, W. B. (ed.): Congenital Deformities of the Spine. New York, Thieme-Stratton, 1983.
5. MacNab, I.: Backache. Baltimore, Williams & Wilkins, 1977.
6. Parke, W. W.: 1. Development of the spine. 2. Applied anatomy of the spine. *In* Rothman, R. H., and Simeone, F. A. (eds.): The Spine. Philadelphia, W. B. Saunders, 1982.

■ THE THREE-JOINT COMPLEX

Ken Yong-Hing
William H. Kirkaldy-Willis

The three-joint complex is part of the motion segment. Schmorl and Junghanns first introduced the concept of the motor segment, which was later referred to as the motion segment or functional spinal unit.[6] The motion segment is the smallest segment of the spine that contains all the components of the rest of the spine and demonstrates the characteristics of the entire spine. A motion segment can be studied in the laboratory, and the findings related to it may be assumed to reflect the behavior of the rest of the spine.[8]

The motion segment consists of two vertebrae, three joints (two posterior joints and one intervertebral disc), and the soft tissue structures, including joint capsules, ligaments, and muscles. The ligaments are the interspinous, supraspinous, intertransverse, yellow, anterior longitudinal, and posterior longitudinal ligaments. The intrinsic muscles of the spine, which, unlike the extrinsic ones, do not span more than one motion segment, are the splenius, erector spinae, transversospinalis and segmental muscles.[4] The functions of all these structures interact so that they determine the strength and movement of the motion segment. Many aspects of the motion segment have been studied: stiffness, loading to failure, response to surgical fusion, partial ablation, and chemonucleolysis.[8]

Notwithstanding its usefulness as a model for the study of the spine, the motion segment concept has obvious limitations that must qualify the extrapolation of data from a motion segment to the entire spine. For example, one cannot ignore the effect exerted on the behavior of a motion segment by the extrinsic muscles of the spine, such as the latissimus dorsi, transverse and oblique abdominis, quadratus lumborum, and psoas, which span more than one motion segment.[3] In life, the abdominal viscera lend support to the spine. Furthermore, at different levels the size and shape of the transverse processes, muscles, vertebral bodies, joints, and other components of the motion segment vary tremendously. Congenital variations, including transitional vertebrae and spina bifida, add to the limitations. Finally, aging, even in the absence of disease, probably influences each component of the individual motion segments in a different manner to affect their strength and behavior.

TYPES OF DEGENERATION

The three-joint complex consists of an intervertebral disc and two facet joints. It forms the intervertebral articulation between the two vertebrae of the motion segment. The disc forms a joint between the vertebral bodies, and the two facet or posterior joints are articulations between the posterior articular processes. All three joints are affected by the intrinsic and extrinsic muscles, which act across the two vertebrae of the motion segment. The three joints of a motion segment function together so that there are twelve freedoms of movement.[8]

A list of diseases of the spine is also a list of the diseases that affect a motion segment. Aging and degenerative changes of the motion segment are described in the following sections by first describing the changes in the facet joints, then the changes in the disc, and lastly the changes in the three-joint complex (Fig. 1). They are described in this manner for convenience; in fact, however, malfunctioning of one component affects the functioning of the other two components of the three-joint complex (Fig. 2). Abnormal movement, immobility, disease, major trauma, and possibly repetitive microtrauma that affect one of the three joints inevitably affect the other two. When one component becomes structurally abnormal, the other two become progressively more abnormal. When there is a disc herniation, for example, there is nearly always degeneration in the posterior joints; and when the posterior joints degenerate, so does the disc.

Posterior Joint Degeneration

Degeneration of the posterior joints is similar to the degeneration that occurs in other diarthrodial joints. A nonspecific synovial reaction to an initiating factor, such as a major traumatic injury or repetitive minor trauma, is the first detectable disorder. The hyaline cartilage that covers the facets becomes fibrillated and loses its thickness. It is likely that effusions in the joints distend the capsules, which become stretched. Capsular laxity is the result of the stretching of the capsules and thinning of the cartilage on the articular surfaces; because the supporting properties of the capsules are compromised, the laxity permits subluxation of the joints. The articular surfaces of the facets produce osteophytes, which cause the facets to enlarge, sometimes massively. The inferior facets enlarge in a medial direction to encroach on the central canal, while the superior facets enlarge in an anterior direction to narrow the lateral recesses.

Disc Degeneration

The disc starts to degenerate in the second decade of life. At first, no evidence of this is obvious on plain x-ray films or computed tomographic (CT) scans, but abnormalities can be demonstrated by magnetic resonance imaging (MRI). In places, especially at the posterolateral corners of the annulus, the lamellae of the annulus fibrosus separate to form circumferential tears. Radial tears form when several circumferential tears coalesce.

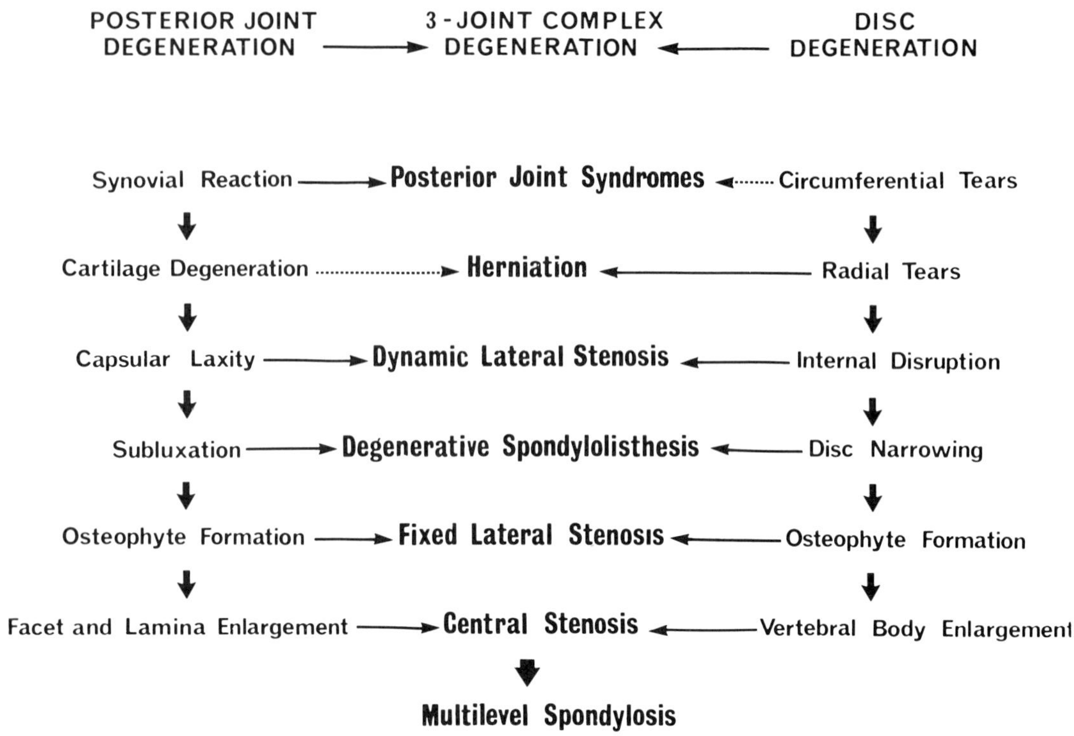

Figure 1 □ Scheme shows the pathologic changes in the posterior joints (left column) and in the disc (right column) that lead to the changes in the three-joint complex (center column).

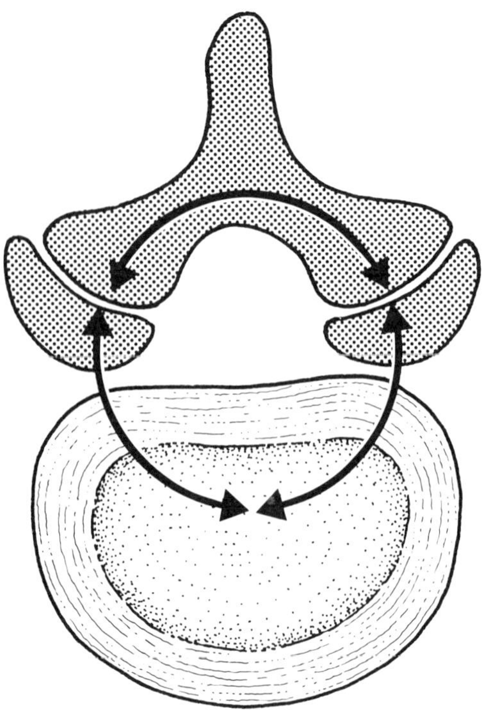

Figure 2 □ The three-joint complex. Changes in any one joint affect the other two, and vice versa.

Tears also extend into the fibrous nucleus so that a continuous cavity extends in the disc, from front to back and from side to side. The disc bulges circumferentially and loses height and mechanical stability. In reaction to the instability, osteophytes form around the periphery of the vertebral bodies at the attachments of the annulus. In this manner, the vertebral bodies enlarge centrifugally, including backward into the spinal canal.

Combined Three-Joint Complex Degeneration

The degenerative changes in the two posterior joints and the anterior joint (disc) occur together to produce the changes in the three joints of the motion segment.

The posterior joint syndrome is probably due to some manner of malfunction or dysfunction of the posterior joints and the disc. Migration of nuclear material through radial tears, which is a disc herniation, usually occurs at a stage when the loss of both disc height and posterior joint cartilage is not severe.

Lateral stenosis is a narrowness of the lateral parts of the spinal canal. Instability in the disc resulting from disc disruption and instability in the posterior joints because of capsular laxity permit subluxation of the facets, which narrows the lateral canal (Fig. 3). Early on, the subluxation is intermittent and is altered by movement of the spine; this causes intermittent narrowing of the lateral recesses or dynamic lateral stenosis. Later, osteophytes form around the facets and vertebral bodies and cause a permanent or fixed lateral stenosis that does not change with alterations in position (Figs. 4, 6).

Degenerative spondylolisthesis is produced when the degeneration occurs unequally in the posterior joints and disc. Anterior spondylolisthesis follows when the narrowing is found predominantly in the posterior joints, and posterior spondylolisthesis follows when the narrowing is found primarily in the disc. It is unknown why one or the other pattern of degeneration occurs (Fig. 5).

Central spinal stenosis is circumferential narrowing of the central spinal canal by the enlarged vertebral body and posterior joints (Fig. 6).

Whether the first pathologic changes begin in the disc, in the facet joints, in the disc and facet joints simultaneously, or, for that matter, in the muscles or ligaments is not known. In many patients with back pain the muscles of the spine are tender, in spasm, or atrophic. Do these changes in the muscles *lead to* or *result from* the three-joint changes?[5] The ligament and muscle insertions are two other possible sources of pain and possible sites of the initial insult. Is a spinal equivalent of the tennis elbow or lateral epicondylitis displayed at the spinal muscle insertions? Enthesitis or inflammation of ligament insertions occurs in the seronegative spondyloarthritides. Does a similar process occur in the ligaments of the spine without the other features of a classic spondyloarthritis?

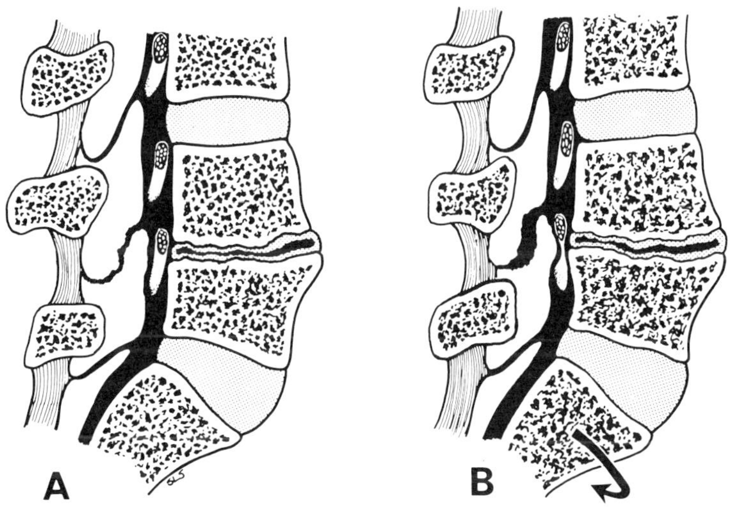

Figure 3 □ Drawing of a spine cut in the midsagittal plane and viewed from the middle. It shows dynamic lateral stenosis at the unstable L4-L5 three-joint complex. In the unstressed state there is no narrowing (*A*), but with rotation there is narrowing of the lateral recess and pinching of the fifth spinal nerve (*B*).

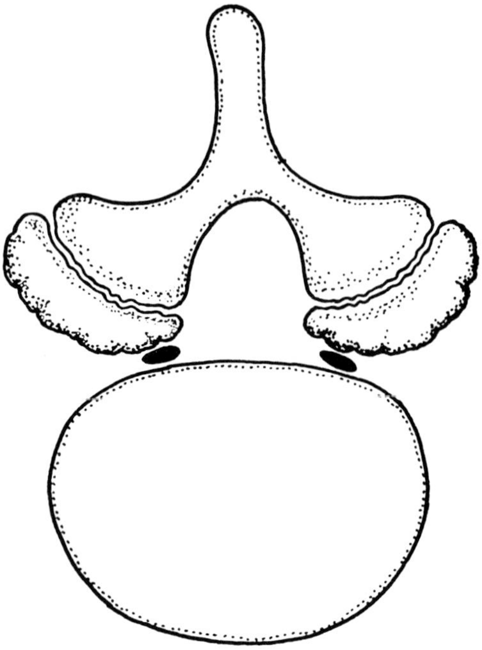

Figure 4 □ Fixed lateral stenosis results from osteophytic enlargement of the superior facets, and the nerve compression does not change with alterations of position.

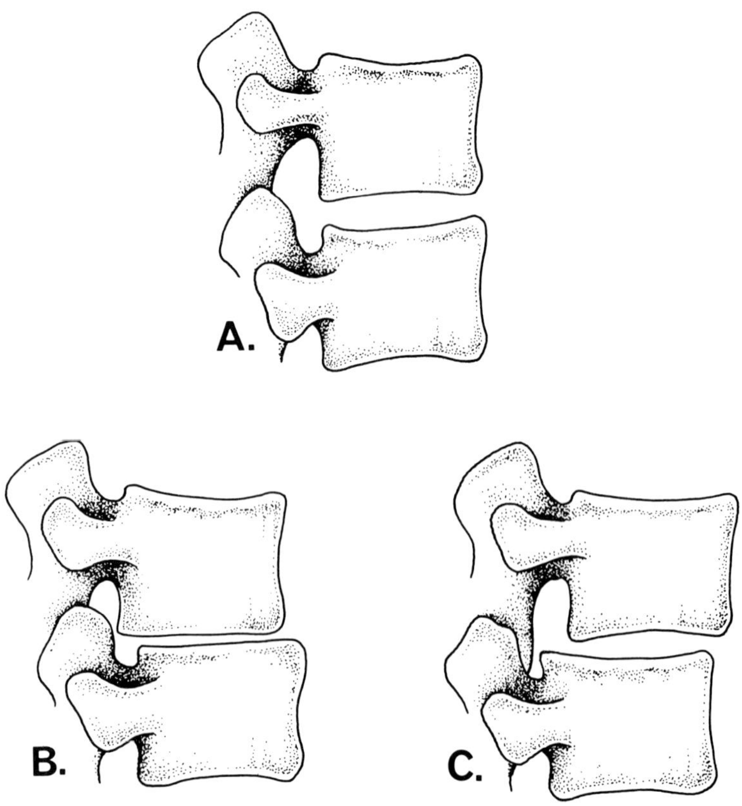

Figure 5 □ Degenerative spondylolisthesis is the result of unequal degeneration of the three joints. *A,* The normal three-joint complex is shown. *B,* Retrolisthesis occurs when disc narrowing is greater than posterior joint degeneration. *C,* Anterolisthesis occurs when the posterior joints are more degenerated than the disc.

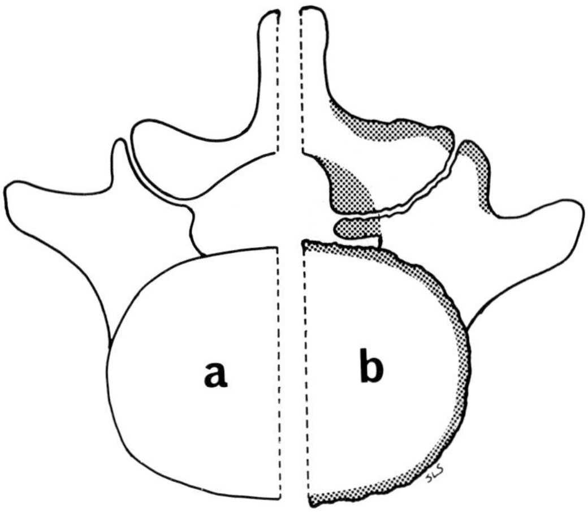

Figure 6 □ Lateral and central stenosis result from enlargement (illustrated by shaded areas in b) of the vertebral body and facets. Enlargement of the superior facet encroaches on the lateral recess, and enlargement of the inferior facet encroaches on the central canal.

The theory that the disc is the site of the initial injury is advocated by some, while others believe that the posterior joint is the site of the initial injury.[2, 3]

Furthermore, it is unknown whether these changes first occur in one motion segment and then are propagated to adjacent motion segments or whether they affect several segments simultaneously, in the manner of a generalized diathesis. To support the first theory, we can adduce the accelerated degeneration that affects the motion segment immediately adjacent to a surgical or congenital spinal fusion.[5] Presumably, stress is concentrated at the junction between the fused and mobile parts, and this abnormal stress causes the degeneration (Fig. 7). The second theory, that two or more levels are affected simultaneously, gains support from a recent study of adolescent patients by MRI. Fifteen of twenty symptomatic subjects with a disc herniation had more than one degenerated disc. The suggestion is that the etiologic factor in the degeneration, regardless of its nature, simultaneously affected the discs of two or more motion segments.[2]

Perhaps the MRI changes resulting from degeneration at two adjacent three-joint complexes are evidence of subtle interference with the function of joints at one level by the joints at the adjacent level, rather than evidence of a generalized diathesis. For example, could a disc herniation at L5–S1 cause a posterior joint syndrome at L4–5? Could spondylolisthesis at L5–S1 cause instability at L4–L5?

PHASES OF DEGENERATION

Degeneration of the spine was described above. The pathologic changes of degeneration lead to alterations in the behavior of the affected three-joint complex over time. The behavior falls into three stages, or phases, which blend into each other (Fig. 8).

Dysfunction Phase

In this phase, the plain x-ray and CT findings may be normal. MRI studies often show

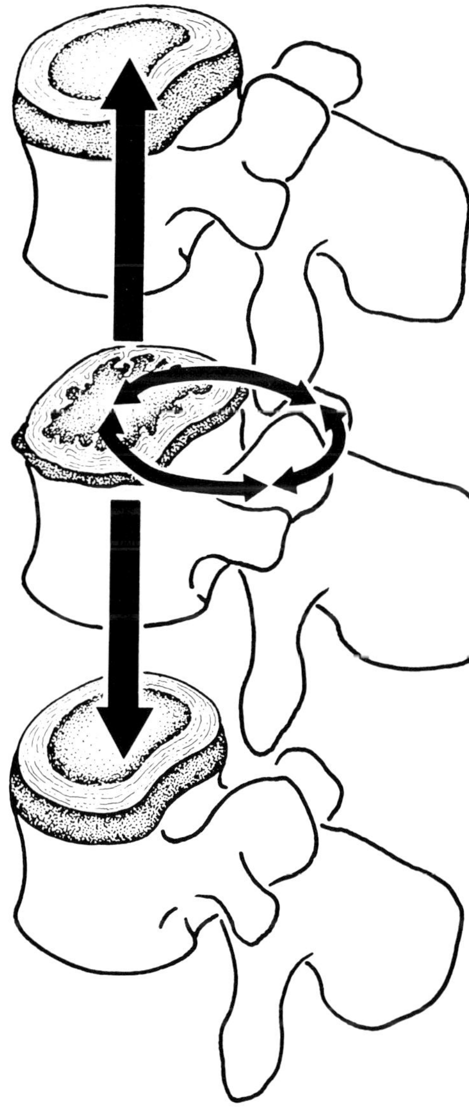

Figure 7 □ The degenerative changes at one three-joint complex may affect the adjacent levels.

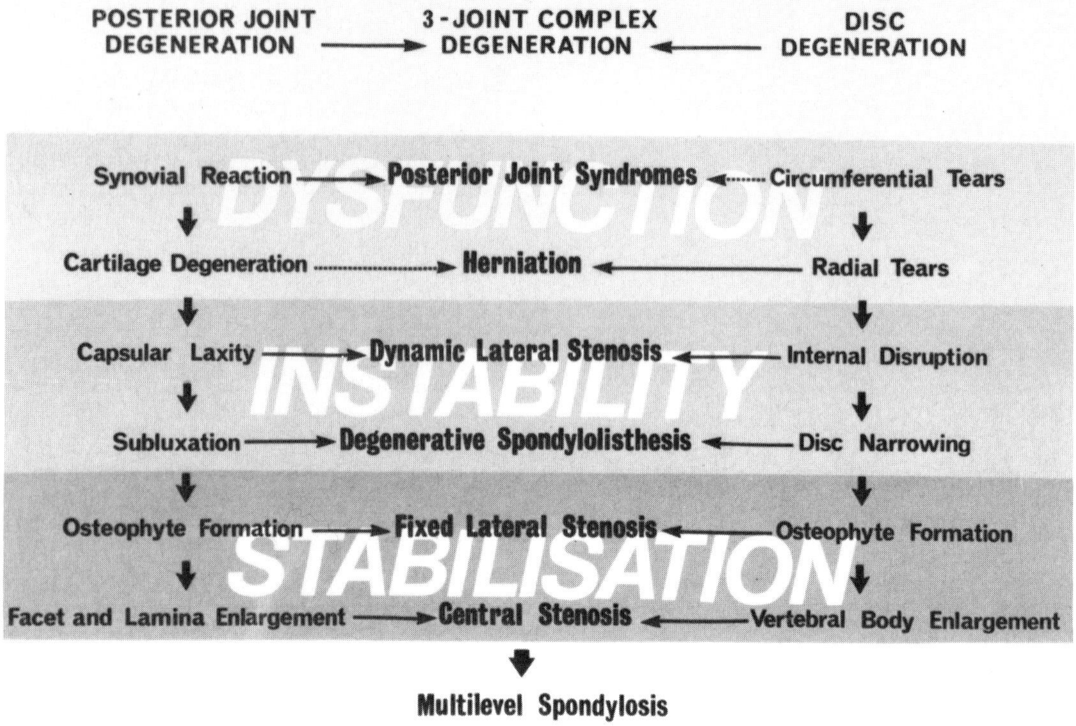

Figure 8 □ The degeneration of the three-joint complex passes through three phases.

degenerated discs when the plain x-ray studies are normal. This clearly demonstrates that our current routine methods of investigation are much too crude to detect early degeneration. The physical signs are subtle. The movement of the motion segment is normal. When treatment is necessary, conservative measures such as injections, manipulations, exercise, or drugs are sufficient.

Instability Phase

The motion segment moves abnormally because the three-joint complex is unstable. Treatment is logically directed at regaining stability by bracing, exercises, or surgical fusion. In this phase, radiologic changes of degeneration are obvious in all three joints.

Stabilization Phase

The abnormal movement of the earlier phase gives way to decreased movement. Teleologically, it seems that the motion segment produces osteophytes on the facets to stabilize the posterior joints and on the vertebral bodies to increase the area of bone in contact across the disc in order to stabilize the anterior joint. The three-joint complex becomes stiff or even fixed, and, when nerves become entrapped, surgical decompression may be needed.

Matching the clinical symptoms and signs to the pathologic findings in a particular patient remains an unsolved problem. Why can a patient be in excruciating pain at one time and then later completely free of pain, in the absence of any degenerative changes on repeated x-ray or CT studies. Perhaps a mismatch in the phases of degeneration of the three joints of the three-joint complex is a cause of pain. When the phase of the slowest joint "catches up" to the other joints, the pain is reduced although the x-ray findings do not change. This theory is attractive but purely speculative.

Additionally, degenerative changes like those described above are common in asymptomatic individuals. Why do the same radiologic changes seem to cause pain in one patient but not in another? Individual differences in pain perception may be an explanation. In some individuals, developmental narrowing of the spinal canal or abnormally large conjoined nerve roots may compromise the tolerance of the spine for degenerative changes acquired later in life.[2, 7]

Why do forms of treatment as widely different as manipulation, surgery, anti-inflammatory drugs, exercises, and posterior joint injections all seem to help patients who have the same type of back pain? The usual assumption is that they all occupy the physician and patient while a self-limiting condition takes its natural course. However, other explanations are possible. Could the pain-free state of a three-joint complex result from some sort of "balance" that may be achieved, equally effectively, by Treatment A, B, C, or D, each of which alters any one of several undefined determinants in either the disc or posterior joints to regain this balance?

What is the explanation for the pain relief that many derive from local anesthetic injections into either the disc or posterior joints? Might this mean simply that in a painful three-joint complex pain is often produced in the disc as well as in the posterior joints? Alternatively, perhaps the elimination of the pain impulses from the disc alone, or from the posterior joints alone, may reduce the number of pain impulses to a critical level below which the three-joint complex and patient are pain free. That pain may arise from the posterior joint, as well as from the disc, in the patient with a disc herniation may provide an explanation of the persistence of pain in some patients following a straightforward discectomy. The residual pain is presumably produced by the unresolved pre-existing posterior joint dysfunction or instability, and it may need treatment after discectomy by manipulation, exercise, drugs, injection, or even fusion.

SUMMARY

We have deliberately set out to be controversial in order to provoke thought. Plato wrote "education is not so much teaching new things as bringing to mind things already known." We all know about the three-joint complex but often forget the meaning of this simple concept. When a three-joint complex is demonstrably abnormal we need to consider, rule out, or treat dysfunction, instability, lateral stenosis, and central stenosis at either the same or the adjacent three-joint complex.

References

1. Arnoldi, A. E., et al.: Lumbar spinal stenosis and nerve root entrapment syndromes. Clin. Orthop. 115:4, 1976.
2. Gibson, M. J., Szypryt, E. P., Buckley, J. H., et al.: Magnetic resonance imaging of adolescent disc herniation. J. Bone Joint Surg. 69B:699, 1987.
3. Gracovetsky, S., Farfan, H. F., and Hellerer, C.: The abdominal mechanism. Spine 11:317, 1985.
4. Hollinshead, W. H.: Anatomy for Surgeons, Vol. 3, 2nd Ed. New York, Harper & Row, 1969.
5. Kirkaldy-Willis, W. H.: Managing Low Back Pain, 2nd Ed. New York, Churchill Livingstone, 1988.
6. Schmorl, G. and Junghanns, H.: The Human Spine in Health and Disease, 2nd Ed. New York, Grune & Stratton, 1977.
7. Verbiest, H.: A radicular syndrome from developmental narrowing of the lumbar vertebral canal. J. Bone Joint Surg. 36B:230, 1954.
8. White, A. A. and Panjabi, M. M.: Clinical Biomechanics of the Spine. Philadelphia, J. B. Lippincott, 1978.

3 □ Diagnosis and Neuromechanisms

Jeremy C. T. Fairbank
Hamilton Hall
Pieter F. van Akkerveeken
Björn L. Rydevik
David L. Spencer
Scott Haldeman

HISTORY TAKING AND PHYSICAL EXAMINATION: IDENTIFICATION OF SYNDROMES OF BACK PAIN

Jeremy C.T. Fairbank
Hamilton Hall

Conventional Western medical therapy is practiced on the basis of a diagnosis that is made from a synthesis of information acquired from the patient's history, physical examination, and special investigations. Back pain is a common presenting symptom, and its diagnosis should be approached in the same manner as that of any other complaint. The clinician needs a framework on which to base a diagnosis. This framework and its application to the history and physical examination are the subjects of this chapter. Ideally, a set of symptoms and signs (a "syndrome") should be identified, which can be related to a particular anatomic structure (a "pain source")[86] that is undergoing an identified pathologic process; a diagnosis should then be established, on which subsequent management is based.[120] We are far from reaching such an ideal in back pain, but it is helpful to clarify the areas of our knowledge and ignorance. In contrast, abdominal pain is an example of a symptom whose syndromes have been established much more clearly, partly because of the availability of the laparotomy.[29]

One example of the problems of correlating a back pain symptom with its pain source and pathologic condition is the symptom of claudication; when the patient walks a distance, he or she has to stop and wait to relieve increasing leg pain before carrying on. Various features of the clinical picture help the clinician to classify this symptom as part of either a vascular or a neurogenic claudication syndrome. The diagnosis is usually based on the patient's history but may be modified based on the presence or absence of peripheral pulses and neurologic signs. Other physical signs may support or refute the working hypothesis developed from the patient's history. Essentially, the skilled clinician makes a working diagnosis simply by listening to the patient. Subsequently, this diagnosis may be confirmed by a special investigation such as CT scanning, Doppler studies, or arteriography. The severity of symptoms, the age and activity of the patient, the presence of other diseases, social factors, and the expectations of the patient will help to dictate whether reassurance, further investigation, conservative therapy, or surgery is indicated.

The symptom of claudication can also be used to illustrate the problems of relating symptoms to disease. Doctors have been aware of this symptom since Charcot described it in 1858.[19] Dejeurine first described intermittent claudication involving the cauda equina in 1911.[30] Verbiest drew attention to the pathology of spinal stenosis,[153] but not until the 1960s did the syndrome of neurogenic claudication start to be distinguished clinically from vascular claudication.[12, 41, 80] The 1970s saw an increased understanding of lateral canal stenosis.[40] In the 1980s, we are able to subdivide syndromes of neurogenic claudication.[79, 90] However, it still is not always possible to distinguish on clinical grounds the precise level or pathologic lesion that is causing the symptoms and signs. For example, neurogenic claudication may be caused by a spinal tumor.[1, 87] Even with the sophisticated imaging techniques available, we are not always able to correlate the degree of claudication with the pathologic process. We do not know why one patient with a degenerative spondylolisthesis may have so much more pain than another. This reflects our lack of knowledge about the actual mechanism of the pain, which is presumed to be of vascular origin and which may occur at the arteriolar, capillary, or venous level. Evidence is accumulating that local venous obstruction[76] and possibly the flow of cerebrospinal fluid among the axons of the nerve roots[159] are important factors. In spite of this ignorance, neurogenic claudication is a condition in which there is a reasonably good correlation between symptoms and lesions and for which a rational treatment that has a good chance of success may be offered. Most other back pain syndromes are much less clearly established.

HISTORICAL ASPECTS OF THE DIAGNOSIS OF BACK PAIN

Back pain has always been with us. Gerard, who published the first herbal in English in 1597, had a diagnostic index that included the terms lumbago and sciatica, indicating which herbs were appropriate for treatment.[56] These terms were familiar to Shakespeare and presumably to his public. Cotunnius wrote the first major treatise on sciatica in 1775,[23] but the skills of neurologic examination were developed in the nineteenth century. Lasègue was credited with the description of the straight leg raise test by one of his pupils, J. J. Forst,[53] although Lasègue's famous paper on sciatica does not mention it,[93] and its clinical significance may not have been clear to its author. Other variants on this test were reported by Lazarevic,[96] who in 1884 described the exacerbation of the leg pain by dorsiflexion of the ipsilateral foot; Fajerszdahn,[46] who in 1901 described the "well-leg raising test," when the unaffected limb is raised, inducing pain in the opposite and symptomatic limb; Gower,[63] who in 1902 noted that pressure in the popliteal fossa intensified the leg pain (redescribed by Cram in 1953);[25] and Deutsch,[31] who in 1924 described the internal rotation of the affected hip during straight-leg raising, which exacerbated leg pain (redescribed by Breig and Troup in 1979).[14] Henry Head's description of the dermatomes through detailed observation of patients with herpes zoster infections was an important advance.[73] Other descriptions of the dermatomes were made by Foerster,[52] who used accumulated clinical observations of patients with isolated nerve root lesions, and by others who observed patients with intervertebral disc prolapses.[47, 81, 82]

Research of the nineteenth and twentieth centuries has yielded the detailed description of the anatomy and pathology of most of the potential sources of back pain, including the intervertebral discs, the sacroiliac joints, the facet joints, and the spinal ligaments.[102, 146] In Boston, at the turn of the century, the interest (which persisted into the 1920s) in the medical literature was focused on the sacroiliac joint as a source of back pain.[6, 62] This joint has subsequently remained important to physiotherapists, chiropractors, and osteopaths, but less so to physicians.[28, 157] The pathology of the intervertebral disc was studied in Germany by Schmorl,[9, 146] and the clinicopathologic descriptions of Middleton and Teacher,[110] Goldthwait,[61] Dandy,[27] and Compere and Keyes[22] culminated in the description of intervertebral disc prolapse by Mixter and Barr in 1934,[112] heralding what Macnab christened the "dynasty of the disc." Certainly this paper blinded many clinicians to other possible sources of pain, and even to other mechanisms of root compression, for many years.[15] Whether or not the intervertebral disc is a pain source in its own right has been argued for over 50 years,[3, 24, 118, 125, 126, 148] although strong support for its pain-producing properties has come from the identification of unmyelinated nerve fibers in the outer half of the annulus fibrosus.[160]

The apophyseal joints have been of interest since Vittorio Putti first drew attention to them in 1927.[134] Ghormley[4, 5] associated joint pathologic conditions with clinical symptoms in 1933,[57] coining the term *facet syndrome*. Descriptions of apophyseal pathologic conditions were made by Putti and Logroscino,[135] Lewin,[97] and Eisenstein.[37, 39] Subluxation,[67, 69] inflammation,[127] foraminal encroachment,[68] the effect of orientation,[48, 50, 58, 59] fracture,[143] and the innervation of the synovium[59] have all been studied. The concept of a facet syndrome was revived by Mooney and Robertson in 1976.[117] McCall and colleagues[105] and Fairbank and coworkers[43] have used injection techniques to try to establish the clinical features of facet joint pain. A recent study by Jackson and colleagues[78] has not been able to distinguish clinically between responders and nonresponders, among those given facet joint injections.

In the 1930s, the work of Kellgren, with Sir Thomas Lewis, showed that pain could be referred by mechanisms other than direct nerve root irritation.[83, 98] This process was called sclerodermal pain by Inman and Saunders.[77] Feindel and colleagues[51] and Sinclair and coworkers[147] attempted to refute the phenomenon, but Kellgren's findings were confirmed by the work of Whitty and Willison,[158] Hockaday and Whitty,[74] and McCall and associates.[105] Sclerodermal pain referral is still poorly understood, and is one of the most common reasons for clinical confusion over back pain syndromes.[91, 99] It is likely that pain arising in the ligaments,[66] dura,[26, 35] facet joints,[105] and discs[86] may be referred in this manner.[148]

The distribution of dermatomes and, to a lesser extent, motor innervation tends to be viewed as a static anatomic fact by many clinicians, but in fact it is quite variable. Some of this variation may be explained by prefixation and postfixation of the spinal cord. Another explanation may be that the axial musculature is innervated by motor neurons whose cell bodies have dendrites crossing the midline, whereas the limb musculature motor dendrites do not cross the midline. This may influence the distribution of muscle spasm and, hence, the location of pain. Further confusion is probably attributable to physiologic adaptation of the nervous system and to pathologic fiber interaction.[64] The problem in the assessment of referred pain has been compounded by the observation of Kibler and Nathan[89] that local anesthetic injected into a peripheral nerve, say the median nerve, could block referred pain from a central source, such as a tumor in the cervical spinal cord. This observation means that the results of diagnostic nerve root blocks must always be treated with caution.

There have been considerable advances in the understanding of pain mechanisms over the last 30 years, much of this prompted by the publication of the Gate Control Theory by Melzack and Wall in 1955.[108] For example, interest has been increasing in the concept of inflammation as a factor in the genesis of root irritation.[104] Most basic research has concentrated on the mechanisms involved in the perception of acute pain following injury. It is clear that various processes are involved in chronic pain, which may even manifest itself as reflex sympathetic dystrophy.[10] This work has revealed the complex involvement of the spinal cord in the genesis of pain influenced by a number of different polypeptides, including the endorphin system.

The present knowledge of the mechanism of back pain, and hence specific diagnoses, consists of a thorough understanding of the clinical features manifested when nerve root compression exists, but increasing uncertainty in identifying the causes of leg pain when nerve root compression cannot be demonstrated. The clinical features, pathology, and natural history of intervertebral disc protrusion are well known when the pathologic condition can be demonstrated. Similarly, the syndrome of neurogenic claudication can be fairly easily recognized and distinguished from vascular claudication; the pathologic conditions related to this syndrome can usually be demonstrated. At the other end of the spectrum, we have a range of more or less defined clinical syndromes, which we try to correlate with pathologic entities, such as facet joint and intervertebral disc degeneration, and other structures, such as the sacroiliac joint and the various muscles and ligaments[122, 140, 141] of the lumbar spine.

HISTORY

A detailed history obtained from the patient is essential for making a diagnosis, assessing disability, and dictating management. Time spent listening to the patient will not be wasted. Back pain has a wide variety of causes, and many of these can be revealed during history taking. Although most experienced clinicians glean an accurate history by listening and using astute questioning, it is easier for some, particularly in the research setting, to use a structured questionnaire to ensure that all the relevant questions are answered. Others have found that a preliminary interview with a computer-based questionnaire is an effective method of gathering data from a patient in a standardized format.[55, 136] Questionnaires with specific applications are available, such as those designed to assess disability (the Oswestry Disability Questionnaire;[42] the St. Thomas' Questionnaire[142]) or psychologic status (the Minnesota Multiphasic Personality Inventory; the Zung Questionnaire[161]).

Some work has been done on the reliability of history taking.[11, 121] Most investigators have found a low degree of reliability, often because of the patient's difficulties recalling the precise nature and onset of symptoms, but also because of so-called illness behavior, that is, a patient exaggerating symptoms to try to obtain secondary gain, such as greater sympathy from the doctor. A recent study in one of our institutions found that an analysis of 40 different aspects of a standard clinical history taken by a consultant had a major error rate of 0.9%, with a 3.75% minor error rate. This was compared with a major error rate of 3.4% and a minor error rate of 1.9%, when the same history was taken by a computer-based interview.[150]

Various aspects of the history are of particular importance. An accurate history depends on the patience and skill of the doctor. Some patients have difficulty in recall, are easily distracted from answering a question, or may not understand. Because the accuracy of the diagnosis depends so greatly on the history, the skilled clinician must be able to assess the reliability of the patient's answers. The history forms pieces of a puzzle, which can be most misleading if taken out of context. Illness behavior is a particular problem in the patient with chronic back pain, and Waddell and colleagues have published a number of papers in this field.[155, 156] Some doubt has been cast on the isolated value of these symptoms and signs by further work on Canadian Workers' Compensation patients.[13] The skilled clinician relies heavily on the consistency of the patient's history in making an assessment and arriving at a provisional diagnosis.

Age

Age can be a good indicator of the nature of likely pathology; for example, discitis in the absence of an invasive procedure is normally seen only in children and in adults over the age of 60. The behavior of the pain is different between these age groups. In older patients, this condition is probably caused by bacterial contamination,[54] although this has not been established in the young. Of course, discitis may occur at any age following violation of the disc for discograms or chemonucleolysis, inadvertently during lumbar puncture, or after disc surgery. Disc prolapse is unusual under the age of 20 years and over the age of 60. Neurogenic claudication is unusual below the age of 40. Posterior annular tears tend to occur in the age group of up to 40 years.[128] Spondylolysis and spondylolisthesis may manifest themselves at any age, but they tend to cause back pain under the age of 40 years and neurogenic symptoms in older patients.[131, 145]

Sex

Although the overall incidences of back pain in the two sexes are similar,[45] as are the prevalences of disc degeneration and disc prolapse, lytic spondylolysis and spondylolisthesis are more common in males. Degenerative spondylolisthesis may be more common in females.[146]

Occupation

It has proved difficult to link the incidence of back pain to occupation. This is largely attributable to the problems of assigning diagnoses in epidemiologic surveys.[2] An "injury" to the back is essential in most workers' compensation schemes, and therefore tends to be over-reported. Rowe[144] suggests that only about 4% of back pain episodes in industry can be clearly related to a single injury. In general terms, the incidence of back pain does not vary greatly among occupations, although the presence of low back discomfort is clearly more disabling in specific work situations. Prolonged sitting or standing in one position, particularly if repetitive lifting is involved as well, appears to be a factor in increasing the incidence of back pain. The nature of the occupation may have a profound effect on whether or not a patient with back pain will return to work. The longer an individual has been absent from work, the less likely he or she is to return to it.[2] Litigation and compensation are recognized factors in prolonging the time off from work of patients with back pain complaints, and they may affect the results of treatment.

Porter has produced evidence that coal miners are less likely to have an intervertebral disc prolapse but are more likely to develop disc degeneration at an earlier age than a control population of manual workers.[133] Pope[129] has shown an accelerated rate of disc degeneration in the operators of vibrating equipment.

Onset of Symptoms

Most patients and their doctors are anxious to find a precipitating cause of back pain. It is important to examine the original onset of symptoms, although some patients have difficulty in recalling this episode.[150] Back pain may start suddenly or insidiously; sudden onset is usually accurately recalled, but insidious onset may occur over hours, days, or even weeks and is hard to define. Sometimes a patient may recall an episode that he or she believes initiated the back pain, although the pain itself did not start for some time afterward. If this period is more than 2 weeks, we find it impossible to accept a causal relationship between the episode and the pain. In some cases, a patient describes an incident when lifting or bending when something is felt to "go" in the back. This may not be immediately painful but may be followed in a few hours by slowly increasing pain that often radiates into one or both legs. It is useful to inquire about the details of the position and movement of the individual in these circumstances. Farfan[49] has argued that a rotational injury is more likely to involve the L4–L5 disc, whereas axial or flexion strains are more likely to affect the lumbosacral level.

In a few patients there is a clear episode of trauma such as a fall, violent twisting injury, or traffic accident. There is usually considerable energy involved in these types of injuries which may precipitate an annular tear.[128] The largest proportion of patients do not have an episode of trauma to explain their symptoms. In a study at the Canadian Back Institute, 70% of 6,000 noncompensation responders were unable to identify a specific injury to account for the onset of their symptoms (unpublished data). Pain may start suddenly, such as during rising from a chair, getting out of a car, or bending down, or it may begin gradually over hours or days with no precipitating event. Some patients describe repeated episodes of back pain, starting abruptly or slowly, then resolving over variable periods. We believe it is important to determine the nature of the onset. As a result of careful questioning, many patients can provide a clear account. In a detailed analysis of patients suffering their first attack of back pain, it was found that a facet joint block could eliminate the symptoms of back pain in those whose pain started suddenly, but not in those whose pain started insidiously.[43]

Periodicity of Pain

Most back pain is variable in the intensity, duration, and frequency of attacks. Pain arising in connection with fractures, infections, and tumors may be continuous and unremitting. Many patients with chronic back pain, particularly those in whom the pain itself has become a problem, complain of continuous symptoms and sleep disruption. Most, on direct questioning, admit sleeping several hours every day and concede there are times when pain is not felt. In general, the pattern of periodicity is not of much help in diagnosing back pain syndromes, although it is of value in assessing disability.

Exacerbating and Relieving Factors

The most common factors that are analyzed are the effects of the following: lying down, including the most and least favorable positions; sitting, including the act of getting out of a chair; and walking, including the effect of slopes and stairs. Changes in the weather, or, more specifically, changes in barometric pressure often influence back pain. It is now widely accepted that coughing frequently exacerbates mechanical back pain with muscle spasm, as well as the more commonly recognized increase with dural and nerve root pain.

Neurogenic symptoms are usually made worse by walking. Neurogenic claudication may be distinguished from vascular claudication by the duration of recovery. Vascular claudicants usually can carry on walking after 1 to 3 minutes, whereas cauda equina claudication requires 5 to 20 minutes for recovery.[79] Neurogenic claudicants frequently report the relief of symptoms by lying, sitting, bending, or squatting. Some patients have fewer symptoms if they walk uphill, in contrast to vascular claudicants, who have more pain walking uphill.[33]

Discogenic pain is often severe, regardless of the position adopted, although lying prone may reduce the pain. Some authors find that disc pain is most exacerbated by flexion. Extension-induced pain is classically associated with facet pain. In a diagnostic facet joint injection study, we found responding patients' symptoms tended to be exacerbated by sitting or standing still, and relieved by walking.[43]

Diurnal Pattern

Night pain is classically related to benign spinal tumors. This observation, however, was not found helpful in the diagnosis of a series of patients with spinal tumors described by Ker and Jones.[88] Night pain was found in 70% of patients with spinal tumors reviewed by Kaneda. In our experience, some patients with intervertebral disc prolapse suffer with severe night pain. Some physiotherapists distinguish patients whose symptoms are most severe in the morning from those whose symptoms become worse through the day. Morning stiffness is a classic symptom of ankylosing spondylitis, as it is in other types of arthropathy. The Birmingham computer interview has revealed to us that this symptom is present in 70% of our back pain sufferers. This may reflect an initial pain on movement in osteoarthritic motion segments after night-time immobility. We use a linear analog scale, and ask for the duration of morning stiffness in an attempt to distinguish those with severe morning stiffness of greater than 30 minutes, typical of ankylosing spondylitis.[17, 18]

Pain Pattern

The pattern of pain is of considerable importance in distinguishing syndromes of back pain. Monoradicular symptoms are usually felt in a dermatomal distribution. L4 root involvement usually causes pain in the front of the thigh, whereas L5 root pain usually radiates to the dorsomedial aspect of the foot. S1 root pain spreads to the lateral side and sole of the foot. There are frequent variations of pattern in clinical practice. For instance, S1 root pain may involve only the posterior thigh, perhaps an example of referred pain, rather than radicular pain.

Kellgren showed that referred pain could radiate to the limbs, and that this is usually, although not always, confined to the thigh.[85] Referred pain tends to radiate farther down the leg when it is more severe. The term sciatica may be misleading, as it has come to be used indiscriminately to describe both referred and radicular pain. If this term is used, it should be confined to radicular pain syndromes. Barker,[7] in a family practice study, used pain patterns to distinguish groups of back patients. Those with greater radiation to the legs tended to take longer to recover. In the Consumers Association survey,[45] pain in the leg was rated as more disabling than pain in the back, with more absence due to sickness, greater personal costs, and more medical help being sought. Lawrence has used pain patterns in epidemiologic surveys to classify his patients according to Kellgren's ideas of referred pain.[94, 95] The Quebec group has also used pain patterns to classify patients with back pain.[137]

Myofascial pain syndromes[149, 151] have characteristic pain patterns that may be small and localized. One such syndrome has trigger points over the posterior iliac crest and an associated pain pattern. In the absence of an associated pain source within the spine, this condition is unusual, representing perhaps 1% to 2% of new patients referred with back pain (unpublished data). It usually responds to local anesthetic injection, and is, therefore, satisfying to diagnose.[44] This syndrome has also been called the "multifidus triangle syndrome."[8] Maigne has suggested that this pain may be due to a localized posterior nerve entrapment at the iliac crest.

If a pain drawing is used to identify pain patterns, patients with excessive illness behavior may be identified by the extent of their pain pattern and the graffiti that they add to the drawing.[138]

Pain arising in the hip joint is usually felt in the groin. It frequently radiates into the anterior thigh or knee. This pain is usually exacerbated by walking, although in the early stages of osteoarthritis of the hip, continued exercise can relieve pain after the initial painful movement. These symptoms can be fully evaluated by examining the hip. Gauvain's test, in which the extended leg is gently rolled by the examiner while the patient is lying and relaxed, produces either pain or involuntary ipsilateral abdominal contracture. It is a useful maneuver to elucidate hip symptoms. Internal rotation of the flexed hip may also reproduce pain. The physical examination is an important supplement to accurate history taking.

Pain Type

The words used to describe back pain are often culturally determined. This has caused many doctors to discount the importance of the descriptive phrases. Although the Magill pain questionnaire uses precise descriptive terms to estimate the severity of pain,[107] in our own practices we have not found this technique helpful in assessing our patients. Some descriptive terms such as "burning," "pins and needles," or "numbness," may be associated with radicular pain, whereas "cramp" or "ache" tends to relate to vascular or referred pain. These terms may have some value in eliciting the source of pain in the individual, but they have resisted useful analysis.[101]

General Medical Questions

Some systemic conditions may, on occasion, present with back pain. Tuberculosis and other infections, metastases, lymphomas, pancreatitis, or a leaking aortic aneurysm can all cause pain in the back. Pain arising from metastases and from infection is frequently unremitting and may be worse at night. The patient should be asked about weight loss, eating habits, disturbances of digestion, bowel and bladder function, night sweats, drugs, and allergies. Diabetes mellitus, hypothyroidism, osteoporosis, osteomalacia and other metabolic bone diseases, psoriasis, and pregnancy may all be factors in the development of back pain.

Family History

Back pain is so common that a family history of back pain may be of little value, although some work suggests that spinal stenosis[123] and intervertebral disc prolapse may run in families.[133]

Psychologic Factors

The most effective way of assessing the psychologic component of a patient's history is to spend enough time listening to the patient. Inconsistencies in the patient's history will become apparent to the experienced clinician. Although the inappropriate symptoms described by Waddell have merit in deciding treatment strategies, they are of little value in arriving at a diagnosis. The patient who gives a history full of psychogenic features may still have organic disease. It is important to obtain the social and economic details related to a patient with back pain, particularly when the symptoms have become chronic. As long as we do not fully understand the causes of back pain, a few patients, exploiting this ignorance, may seek financial support, increased attention, or avoidance of work because of their symptoms. Emotional magnification becomes increasingly important when major surgery is contemplated for back symptoms.

Disability

It is of critical importance to assess the patient's disability. An effective diagnosis depends on issues broader than merely identifying the pain source and the pathologic process. It depends on the psychologic status and assessment of disability, or severity of symptoms as perceived by the patient.[154] Disability, the degree of physical impairment, can usually be assessed by the astute clinician who has spent time listening to and observing the patient. Quantifying this opinion is difficult, however, and may vary markedly from one clinician to another, or indeed, from one culture to another. There have been numerous attempts to quantify disability, usually involving questionnaires of varying complexity. A recent editorial[119] has recommended the use of one or more of the following for patients who have back pain: Oswestry Disability Questionnaire;[42] Million Questionnaire;[111] St. Thomas' Questionnaire;[142] Waddell Questionnaire; MMPI; Magill Pain Questionnaire.[107]

PHYSICAL EXAMINATION

Objective evidence obtained on physical examination should enhance and support the diagnostic hypotheses arising from the patient's history. In orthopedic practice, the physical examination for back pain is often confined to a musculoskeletal assessment of the back and lower limbs, and appropriate tests of neurologic function. Clearly, however, a full physical examination should be part of the work-up, whether performed by the referring physician or by the specialist. Specific areas of emphasis in the general examination will often be determined by information obtained in the general medical history. In this chapter, however, we have chosen to focus on those aspects of the physical examination pertaining to disease within the spine and the adjacent musculoskeletal structures.

Because the back examination relies heavily on patient cooperation, and since many of the required movements are painful, it is important to examine quickly and efficiently without duplication. For example, eliciting an ankle reflex in one position is sufficient. Demonstrating the same reflex at various other times during the examination adds no new information but wastes time and the patient's endurance.

To conduct a complete physical assessment in a minimum of time and with the least amount of discomfort, the patient should be examined in a fixed sequence of positions. We employ nine positions starting with the patient erect and finishing with the patient lying prone. Each position allows optimum examination of the musculoskeletal system, the nervous system, and the common sites of referred back pain. Examination of these three areas is combined in each position, because examining sequentially would necessitate considerable repetition. The examination requires the use of a chair as well as an examining table. The examining room should contain adequate space to allow the patient free movement.

Position 1: Standing

Musculoskeletal

With the patient erect and facing away from the examiner, the back is exposed and inspected for curvatures and other visible postural deformities. The patient is asked to bend forward at the waist while keeping the knees straight. Both the range of movement and the apparent production of pain were observed. Repetitive forward bending can be instructive. Pain that increases with repetition suggests discogenic pain or a problem in the anterior column of the spine. Forward bending in patients with discogenic back pain is often associated with a list to one side. It produces an effect as if the patient were attempting to bend forward and around an obstacle directly in front of him or her.

The range of movement is recorded in relation to some easy reference point such as the distance of the fingertips from the floor, or the relation of the hands to the knees. Precise measurement is unnecessary since minor variations in range are of no diagnostic significance. The range of forward bending is most useful when compared with repeat examinations.

The rhythm of spinal movement and the pattern of pain production are more than mere measures of range. The patient is instructed to straighten slowly from the forward bent position. Normally, extension begins in the low back and proceeds smoothly up the spine, with most movement occurring in the lumbar region. Patients with mechanical back pain often fix the lower back, flex the knees, and then straighten through the hips. This "hitch" reduces spinal movement and minimizes irritation in a painful motion segment. Abnormal spinal rhythm is often a feature in the clinical diagnosis of "segmental instability."

During spinal extension, one should ensure that the patient's hips and knees remain locked. Particular attention should be paid to movement in the lumbar area, and this should be distinguished from hip extension. Increasing pain with repetitive extension suggests a pain source in the posterior elements of the spine.

In place of lateral bending, the patient should be examined with a side shift.[106] The pelvis is gently pushed in one direction while the thorax is moved in the opposite direction. This maneuver allows assessment of lateral movement without the rib cage impinging on the pelvis, the usual limiting factor in side bending.

Spinal rotation is performed while the examiner holds the pelvis to prevent movement. A modification of rotation testing is an excellent means of uncovering functional magnification. With arms at the sides, the patient's hands are held firmly against the greater trochanters while the examiner rotates the patient's torso by rotating the pelvis. With the arms held down, the patient's shoulders and hips maintain a fixed relationship to each other, and no movement occurs within the spine. The first 30 degrees of rotation occur through the hip joints, and back pain produced by this maneuver indicates a psychogenic pain response.

Neurologic

The power of plantar flexion is tested by having the patient perform 10 toe raises standing on both feet and then 10 more standing on each foot separately. Repeated activity causes fatigue of the calf and uncovers minimal differences in the strength of muscles innervated predominantly by the first sacral root. This method is more accurate than the conventional technique in which the supine patient plantar flexes against resistance from the examiner's hand. As long as the remaining strength in the patient's calf muscles is greater than the strength in the examiner's arm, a slight decrease in power cannot be detected. Although the patient may be aware of greater effort on the affected side, no objective measure is possible.

Hip abductor power, predominantly a fifth lumbar root function, is assessed in the standing position with the Trendelenburg test. The examiner's thumbs are placed on the patient's posterior superior iliac spines to gauge the obliquity of the pelvis. Weakness of hip abduction allows the opposite side of the pelvis to sag when the patient stands on the affected leg.

An increase in radicular leg pain may be produced in patients with acute nerve root compression by jugular venous compression. The mechanism is presumably a distention of the inflamed dural sac resulting from an increase in cerebrospinal fluid pressure.

Related Conditions

While the patient remains standing, it is convenient to measure the range of chest excursion. Less than a 4.5 cm difference between full inspiration and full expiration demonstrates the retardation of movement that is suggestive of ankylosing spondylitis.

Position 2: Kneeling on a Chair

Nervous System

A kneeling position accentuates the ankle reflex. To provide further reinforcement for this predominantly S1 function, have the patient squeeze the back of the chair with both hands at the moment of hammer strike. The reflex may be rendered more obvious by having the patient sustain plantar flexion of the ankle against light resistance from the examiner's hand.

Position 3: Sitting on a Chair with the Feet on the Floor

Nervous System

Keeping the heel on the floor, the seated patient maintains elevation of the forefoot against strong downward pressure by the examiner. The mechanical advantage achieved by positioning the examiner's upper body above the patient's foot, allowing the use of both arm strength and gravity, is sufficient to overcome even normal dorsiflexor power. Only with the ability to judge the full range of normal power is it possible for the examiner to document objectively minor degrees of weakness.

In measuring dorsiflexor power, a predominantly L5 function, it is necessary to differentiate between a voluntary release and legitimate power loss. When genuinely overpowered, the patient's muscles give way smoothly, and the examiner has a sensation of uniform resistance as the forefoot descends. Voluntary release will occur in one of two ways. Some patients will successfully resist the examiner's downward pressure for a few moments and then suddenly let go. Others will attempt to simulate the gradual release of true weakness. Deliberate relaxation, however, always produces a series of small "cogwheel" steps. With practice, the patient can minimize this effect but cannot eliminate it completely.

Although it is important to establish the patient's honesty during the examination, the presence of a voluntary release does not necessarily exclude organic pathologic conditions. Patients may demonstrate excessive weakness to ensure that the examiner will not miss a minor degree of real power loss. Unfortunately, the opposite often occurs; convinced that the patient is malingering, the doctor may ignore genuine and valid objective findings.

Position 4: Bending Forward over the Examining Table

Musculoskeletal

The patient bends forward, supporting the weight of the upper body with arms on the table. First the spine is inspected for obvious asymmetry, abnormal bony landmarks, or scars from previous surgery. Palpate down the length of the spine for local tenderness, muscle spasm, soft tissue masses, or bony defects.

Palpation of the bony structures can identify only the spinous processes. The laminae and apophyseal joints cannot be felt through the layers of muscle and fascia. Because of this and because of the wide variation in the patterns of pain referral, the precise localization of trigger points, palpable fibrocytic nodules, or areas of muscle spasm, is of little diagnostic importance.

Position 5: Sitting on the Examining Table with the Legs Hanging Free

Nervous System

The knee reflex subtends a predominantly L4 function. To be best seen, the reflex is elicited with the patient sitting so that the edge of the examining table is at the proximal edge of the popliteal fossa. The reflex can be reinforced by having the patient lock the fingers of both hands together, then suddenly trying to pull the hands apart at the moment of hammer strike.

Minor asymmetry in the reflex pattern is usually the result of the patient's failure to completely relax the hamstrings or quadriceps. A marked asymmetry should be considered valid only when it is present on repeat testing.

Pathologic conditions in the low back below the level of L2 can produce only a lower motor neuron impairment. Findings of upper motor neuron involvement place a lesion at or above the conus. For this reason, a screen for long tract signs should be part of every low back assessment. With the patient seated, test the plantar response by stroking the sole of the patient's foot along its lateral border. To perform this test, it is convenient to lift each leg, in turn, to a horizontal position. This produces a straight-leg raise comparable to the formal test to be carried out with the patient supine, and the maneuver should therefore elicit the same pain response. The patient should remain sitting upright. In cases of active nerve root irritation, the patient may lean backward as the leg is lifted to limit the amount of leg elevation.

Hip flexor strength is assessed by having the patient attempt to lift the thigh off the table against strong downward pressure from the examiner. The same mechanical advantage discussed in the examination of ankle dorsiflexion can be applied here.

Position 6: Lying Supine

Musculoskeletal

Differentiation between pain arising in the low back and the hip joint can be difficult. Typical pain produced on hip flexion and internal rotation suggests an intra-articular source and requires a more complete hip examination. Hip pain tends to radiate into the anterior groin and down the anteromedial thigh to the top of the knee. Back pain spreads typically through the buttock and posterior thigh. While back pain referred to the groin is not unusual, pain from the hip joint rarely reaches the back of the leg.

The sacroiliac joint can be stressed by applying pressure to the medial aspect of the ipsilateral knee with the hip flexed and abducted, and the knee bent so that the heel of the foot rests on the anterior aspect of the opposite thigh. An alternate method of exerting stress on both sacroiliac joints is to apply pressure simultaneously on the inner aspects of the anterior superior iliac spines. The examiner is positioned directly above the patient's pelvis and applies force with the arms crossed to push laterally. In both instances, a positive test is pain occurring posteriorly in the region of the affected joint. Anterior groin pain is not significant.

Patients suffering acute discogenic back pain will be unable to perform an unassisted bent knee sit-up with the feet free because the attempt will greatly increase the pain. In the pain-free patient, a sit-up is a convenient way to assess abdominal strength and muscle tone.

Nervous System

The classic test of sciatic nerve irritation is passive straight-leg raising.[152] In order to obtain a valid comparison to the straight-leg lift performed while testing the plantar response with the patient sitting, the patient must now lie with the contralateral hip and knee flexed and the sole of the foot flat on the table. This position mimics the seated posture of the pelvis and low back. Straight-leg lifting in this position is normally 10 degrees to 20 degrees better than with the contralateral leg extended.

With the knee straight, the leg is lifted at the heel. An unequivocally positive result produces pain radiating down the back of the thigh below the buttock while the leg is elevated 60 degrees or less at the hip. Symptoms produced at elevations above 60 degrees may represent irritation of the nerve root but frequently reflect referred mechanical back pain or hamstring tightness.

If unilateral root irritation is present, the examiner can usually raise both the patient's legs together, without producing radiating pain, to an elevation greater than is possible when lifting the affected leg alone. To heighten the sensitivity of this variation of passive straight-leg raising, the single leg lift should be performed with the contralateral leg extended. The greater elevation obtained with both legs together is due to the additional movement gained by flexing the lumbar spine and the lack of tethering in the contralateral nerve roots. Where psychogenic magnification exists, double straight-leg raising is routinely more painful at a lower elevation than the passive single-leg lift. These patients anticipate that if lifting one leg hurts, lifting both legs should hurt even more.

It is important to differentiate between well-leg lifting and cross-over pain.[36, 75] In both cases, lifting the affected limb produces the anticipated posterior thigh pain. Well-leg lifting denotes pain on the affected side when the normal leg is tested. This demonstrates an extreme irritability of the affected nerve root but denotes a unilateral problem. Cross-over pain describes a situation in which pain is also produced in the normally asymptomatic limb when the affected leg is lifted. Cross-over pain is indicative of a central disc herniation with compromise of the neural elements across the midline.

Other tests of sciatic nerve root irritation include digital pressure by the examiner in the midline of the popliteal fossa and variation of straight-leg raising in which the foot is dorsiflexed while the straight leg is held just below the elevation producing a positive response. In both cases, a positive test results in pain radiating into the posterior thigh or calf.

Tests of root irritation can localize the site of a lesion only to one of the segments supplying a major nerve. Tests of nerve function are more specific. In the supine position, quadricep and hamstring power are tested, and a sensory examination is performed from the L3 to the S1 dermatomes.

Related Causes

In addition to the hip and sacroiliac joints, the other common sources of referred pain to be assessed in the supine patient are intra-abdominal, retroperitoneal, and vascular. Palpation of the abdomen, costovertebral angles, and the peripheral pulses complete this phase of the examination.

Positions 7 and 8: Lying on the Left and Right Sides

Musculoskeletal

With the patient lying on the side and the lower knee drawn up, forceful downward and anterior pressure applied at the side of the pelvis exerts stress on the uppermost sacroiliac joint. A positive test produces localized pain in the region of the uppermost posterior superior iliac spine.

Nervous System

The power of hip abduction is most efficiently tested when the examiner can gain a substantial mechanical advantage. With the knee extended, the patient elevates the upper leg against downward pressure from the examiner that is applied below the knee. The patient must avoid flexing or extending the hip to ensure that only the abductor muscles, principally innervated by the fifth lumbar nerve root, are used. The combination of gravity and the leverage obtained by pressing on the lower leg enable the examiner to overcome the normal hip abductors, ensuring that minor degrees of weakness on one side will be objectively demonstrated.

Position 9: Lying Prone

Musculoskeletal

Lying prone produces extension in the low back. This position may reduce discogenic back pain or cause a shift in the pain pattern from the leg into the lumbar region. Back pain arising in the posterior elements of the spine is generally intensified. Any effect produced by the prone posture can be further accentuated by having the patient use the arms to raise the upper body.

Pain produced by passive rotation of the lumbar spine is believed by Farfan to represent one type of disc disruption.[49] Standing beside the table, the examiner reaches across the patient and grips the front of the pelvis at the anterior superior iliac spine. Stabilizing the rib cage with the other hand, the examiner rotates the pelvis and lumbar spine backwards. The test is repeated with the examiner standing on the opposite side of the table. To be significant, pain should be produced in only one direction of rotation.

Nervous System

The femoral stretch test demonstrates nerve root irritation at the L2, L3 and L4 levels. The test is comparable to passive straight-leg raising, which identifies irritation in the roots of the sciatic nerve. With the patient prone and the knee straight, the examiner lifts the patient's leg, extending the hip and tightening the femoral nerve across the front of the pelvis. Pain radiating into the anterior thigh constitutes a positive test.

The femoral stretch is performed with the knee extended to avoid increasing tension within the quadriceps and rectus femoris. Flexing the knee while extending the hip may produce anterior thigh pain on the basis of muscle tension only. The femoral stretch also increases lumbar lordosis and, in cases of posterior element involvement, may increase the patient's low back pain. A failure to determine the correct source and location of the pain can lead to the erroneous diagnosis of femoral nerve root irritation.

Gluteus maximus is the major hip extensor and is supplied primarily by the first sacral component of the sciatic nerve. Occasionally, a major nerve deficit can be recognized by easily visible wasting of one buttock. Testing power in the gluteus maximus by having the patient actively extend the hip against resistance is awkward and, because of a lack of mechanical advantage, insensitive. Since muscle tone is an equally valid reflection of normal muscle function, a better quantitative assessment of the gluteus maximus can be obtained by palpating the buttocks as the patient attempts to clench them tightly together. Gross weakness is easily detected on palpating a flaccid muscle. Minor degrees of weakness will become apparent through early fatigue with repetitive tightening.

Because it is difficult to tighten only one buttock voluntarily, and since the patient has no knowledge of what constitutes a positive test, this examination is also a valid indication of the patient's cooperation.

The hamstring reflex is the only reflex most conveniently elicited with the patient prone. The tendons of semitendinosus and semimembranosus are struck at the medial side of the popliteal fossa. Because the hamstring muscles are supplied by both the L5 and S1 nerve roots, this reflex may be lost with a conduction deficit at either level. Its diagnostic value requires comparison with the other positive physical findings. For example, loss of the hamstring reflex with preservation of the ankle reflex on the same side suggests a fifth lumbar root lesion.

The examiner can test sensation in the dermatomes supplied by the first through fifth sacral nerve roots. Because of the serious implications of a sensory loss in the area between the upper buttocks supplied by the third, fourth, and fifth sacral roots, sensory testing in this area should be part of every low back examination. Together with cross-over leg pain, and a reduction in anal sphincter tone and loss of the anal reflex, saddle anesthesia is a feature of central disc herniation causing midline pressure on the cauda equina.

Additional Observations

A comprehensive low back assessment often includes a rectal examination. Palpable intrapelvic masses may indicate the cause of the back pain. If the diagnosis of central disc herniation is being seriously considered, a rectal examination is mandatory to gauge sphincter tone and to elicit the anal reflex, a sudden contraction of the sphincter with a light touch of the examining finger. Both tone and reflex, functions of the lower sacral roots, can be affected by pressure on the dural sac within the spinal canal, but may also be diminished with multiple pregnancies or repeated anal intercourse.

Separating functional from organic findings is difficult and, although clinical judgment improves with practice, even the experienced examiner usually relies on several specific tests. Acetabular rotation, voluntary muscle release, and alteration in straight-leg raising between the seated and formal test position are helpful. Although paresthesia involving the entire leg may be present in the acute stage of root irritation, the persistence of a nondermatome sensory abnormality suggests nonorganic problems. A slow painful gait with heavy reliance upon a cane is more indicative of a psychogenic abnormality than a mechanical back disorder. Sudden lurching, starts or jumps caused by the examiner's light touch on the patient's spine are not the reactions found in a painful mechanical condition. Observing the patient in an unguarded moment, talking to a receptionist, or leaving the examining room, may add valuable information to the clinical picture. It is the consistency of the physical examination, both intrinsically and in relation to the patient's history, that supports the diagnosis of organic disease.

SYNDROME CLASSIFICATION

The concept of defining syndromes of back pain is an attractive one. The clear definitions are probably essential to making progress in understanding of the pathologic processes involved in the genesis of back pain and in improving its treatment. However, specific syndromes have proved extremely elusive to the many clinicians who have attempted a classification. There is, on one hand, the strong clinical impression that some patients describe symptoms in a pattern that has been seen many times before, but on the other hand, that most patients present with such a mixture of symptoms that it defies organization. It is tempting to explain these symptoms in terms of a particular pathologic process or dysfunction of a particular structure, but in our view, this temptation should be indulged with care.

In writing this chapter, we found that we have very considerable agreement in defining our principal diagnostic categories. These categories are presented in combination with a system of levels of diagnostic precision, suggested to us by Dr. Paul Pynsent, which provides a framework for the analysis of a patient's history and physical examination. In our view, a classification should be of practical value to the working clinician and should be capable of expansion and adaptation as more becomes known of the pathologic processes.

Recently, a number of syndrome classifications of the common types of back pain have been published.[55, 92, 116, 120, 124, 137] None of these symptoms entirely satisfies the current need. Most appreciate the difficulty in obtaining reproducible information from the patient, particularly when different cultures and medical practitioners are involved. To add to the available literature, we present our own classification.

Hall-Fairbank-Pynsent Classification

There are a large number of pathologic processes that may produce back pain. To include these within a diagnostic format, one may look at the process of diagnosing back pain as the penetration of a number of levels, providing a hierarchy of diagnostic precision. This approach, which is helpful in clarifying the extensive and generally anecdotal material on this subject, may satisfy both the "splitters" and "lumpers" of back pain syndromes.

The hierarchy of syndromes is shown in Table 1 and consists of a series of levels, from Level 0 to Level N. At the top, Level 0, there is the presenting complaint of back pain, and at the bottom, Level N, there is a long list of all the pathologic processes which are thought to cause back pain with a number of intervening levels of increasing complexity between.

We have avoided the conventional algorithm structure, as it would entail identifying a large number of junction points, which would produce an intimidating diagram and force a rigidity that probably does not exist. At Level 1, a distinction is made between pain of spinal and extraspinal origin. The latter group is the subject of conventional medical inquiry into inflammatory, gastrointestinal, genitourinary, metabolic, and cardiovascular symptoms beyond the scope of this chapter. This group also includes psychogenic pain. At Level 2, a distinction is made between back and leg pain. Back pain includes pain in the buttock, while leg pain denotes pain radiating to the thigh, lower leg, and foot. At Level 3, a distinction is made between leg pain, which is referred (sclerodermal), and radicular (neurogenic)

Table 1 □ Hall-Fairbank-Pynsent Diagnostic Scheme

Level 0	Back pain
Level 1	Spinal pain Extraspinal pain (genitourinary, gastrointestinal, cardiovascular, psychologic)
Level 2	Back pain Thigh pain Leg/foot pain
Level 3	Back pain Referred pain Radicular Pain
Level 4	Back pain (Type 1)—facet pain Back pain (Type 2)—disc pain Back pain (Type 3)—radicular pain Back pain (Type 4)—neurogenic claudication Back pain (Type 5)—unclassifiable
Level 5	Examples: Discitis (Type 2) Instability syndrome (Type 1, Type 2) Posterior annular tear (Type 2) Central stenosis (Type 4) Lateral stenosis (Type 3, Type 4) Spondylolysis/spondylolisthesis (Type 1, Type 2, Type 3, Type 4)
Level N	**Congenital** Spondylolisthesis Spondylolysis Spina bifida Diastematomyelia Achondroplasia
	Acquired (spinal) Infection—*M. tuberculosis, Brucella, Staphylococcus,* others Neoplasia—Tumors, benign, malignant Inflammatory—Rheumatoid, osteoarthritis, Reiter syndrome, ankylosing spondylitis
	Others Degenerative—Disc, facet, arthrosis, spondylolisthesis Metabolic—Paget disease, osteoporosis Iatrogenic—Stenosis, spondylolisthesis, postlaminectomy syndrome Traumatic—Fracture, posterior annular tear, stress fracture, crush fracture
	Acquired (extraspinal causes) Infection—Guillain-Barré, other viral illness Neoplasia—Direct invasion, testicular tumors, lymphomas, etc. Inflammatory—Rheumatoid, osteoarthritis, Reiter syndrome, ankylosing spondylitis Cardiovascular system—Aortic aneurysms, ischemia Digestive system—Pancreatitis, gallbladder disease, etc. Genitourinary system—Renal pain, uterine pain, etc. Central nervous system—Psychologic, central pain syndromes

pain. At Level 4, we classify back pain of spinal origin into five main groups: Type 1 through Type 5.

We see all these groups as consisting of a spectrum of symptoms and signs, some of which overlap. These labels do not imply that a particular lesion is causing each type, but focus instead on the principal location of pain. Thus, we postulate that the posterior joint complex is the site of pain for most Type 1 patients and that Type 2 pain is usually discogenic in origin. Type 3 is nerve root pain caused by direct and acute root irritation, typically the result of intervertebral disc prolapse, whereas Type 4 pain denotes neurogenic claudication, which, although often caused by spinal stenosis, may have a number of causes. Type 5 includes those syndromes of back pain not already defined. In practice, it is not always possible to assign a patient to a particular group, and some patients may have features of more than one syndrome. But this system provides a valuable clinical classification and framework that will encompass most patients with back pain.

It is clear to us that there are a number of subsets of these main diagnostic groups; for instance, Type 3 pain may arise at different anatomic levels, and although it is usually caused by a disc prolapse, it may on occasion be caused by a spinal tumor or infection. Type 4 pain may result from central spinal stenosis, lateral recess entrapment, or chronic lumbar disc protrusion. Some patients' symptoms are unclassifiable at this level, and the diagnosis will remain as a classification of leg pain at Level 3. Spondylolisthesis in its various forms may cause any of the first four types of pain, emphasizing our attention to the source of pain, rather than to the pathologic process. To make a diagnosis in Level 5 and beyond, it will be necessary to use special investigations.

This concept of a hierarchy of levels can be continued until Level N is reached, when all the sources of back pain can be listed. We recognize that there are numerous blank spots in our knowledge between Level 5 and Level N, but we are comfortable in assigning most of our patients to the categories in Level 4. An outline of the different pain types is given in Table 2.

Critics of Level N will point out that many of these pathologic processes occur in combination, and therefore it is impossible and unrealistic to attempt to distinguish one from another. This is true enough but the criticism can be responded to by taking the description back one stage to Level N-1, where it is possible to amalgamate combi-

Table 2 □ Types of Back Pain

Type 1

This patient describes onset of back pain spontaneously or following a minor incident. The pain is mainly felt in the back or buttock with some radiation into the posterior thigh or groin. The pain is aggravated on extension or straightening from a forward bent position. It is most noticeable after prolonged sitting or standing, and may be temporarily relieved by walking or swimming. Discrete attacks last from a few days to a few weeks.

The physical examination reveals pain aggravated on extension. Straight-leg raising is normal, or produces only back pain. There are no neurologic abnormalities.

Type 2

Usually this patient can recall something "giving" in the back. This is usually painful but may cause only minor irritation followed by the gradual onset of increasing low back and buttock pain. Episodes may be precipitated by an unexpected lift, sudden twist of the trunk, or a slip without falling. Pain is increased on prolonged sitting or standing, particularly in a forward flexed position. Individual episodes last from a few weeks to several months before gradually subsiding.

The physical examination reveals pain on forward flexion and often some relief of pain on extension. Straight-leg raising is full or produces back pain only, and the neurologic examination is normal.

Type 3

The principal feature is the dominance of leg pain. In some cases, no back pain may be present. In others, the back pain may increase gradually following an initial painful episode, usually related to flexion or rotation. Over time, the patient commonly complains of pain radiating below the knee.

The physical examination is marked by positive root irritation signs with or without evidence of a conduction deficit.

Type 4

The patient is usually older and often has a history of chronic back discomfort. The predominant symptom is leg pain produced by walking and relieved by several minutes of rest. Occasionally, the patient notes a more rapid relief of symptoms after assuming a particular position.

The physical examination is often normal or demonstrates back pain only. Positive neurologic findings in the lower limbs may appear with provocation. The peripheral circulation is normal.

Type 5

Patients in this group may exhibit a variety of nonorganic findings or present with a history that is incompatible with the physical examination. Patients who present with aspects of several of the other types may be categorized here, although, where possible, the dominant features of the clinical picture are used to select a more specific syndrome.

nations of one or more features of Level N and to associate them with particular clinical features descending from the higher levels. This system is clearly a simplification of the truth, but it provides a line on which to hang our knowledge and, seeing it on display, we hope to advance our understanding.

References

1. Allen, I.M.: Tumours involving the cauda equina: A review of their clinical features and differential diagnosis. J. Neurol. Psychopath. 11:111–143, 1930.
2. Anderson, J.A.D.: Back pain and occupation. *In* Jayson, M.I.V. (ed.): The Lumbar Spine and Back Pain, 3rd ed. Edinburgh, Churchill Livingstone, 1987, pp. 16–37.
3. Armstrong, J.R.: Lumbar Disc Lesions, 2nd Ed. Edinburgh, E&S Livingstone, 1958.
4. Ayers, C.E.: Further case studies of lumbosacral pathology with consideration of the involvement of the intervertebral discs and the articular facets. N. Engl. J. Med. 213:716–721, 1935.
5. Badgley, C.E.: The articular facets in relation to low back pain and sciatic radiation. J. Bone Joint Surg. 23:481–496, 1941.
6. Baer, W.S.: Sacro-iliac strain. Bull. Johns Hopkins Hosp. 28:159–163, 1917.
7. Barker, M.E.: Pain in the back and leg: A general practice survey. Rheumatol. Rehab. 16:37–45, 1977.
8. Bauwens, P., and Coyer, A.B.: The "multifidus triangle" syndrome as a cause of recurrent low back pain. Br. Med. J. 2:1306–1307, 1955.
9. Beadle, O.A.: The intervertebral discs. Medical Research Council Special Report Series No. 161. London, His Majesty's Stationery Office, 1931.
10. Bernini, P.M., and Simeone, F.A.: Reflex sympathetic dystrophy associated with low lumbar disc herniation. Spine 6:180–184, 1981.
11. Biering-Sorenson, F., and Hilden, J.: Reproducibility of the history of low-back trouble. Spine 9:280–286, 1984.
12. Blau, J.N., and Logue, V.: Claudication of the cauda equina. An unusual syndrome resulting from central protrusion of a lumbar intervertebral disc. Lancet 1:1081–1086, 1961.
13. Bradish, C.F., Lloyd, G.L., Aldam, G.H., Albert, J., Dyson, P., Doxey, N.C.S., and Mitson, G. L.: Do not organic signs help to predict the return to activity of patients with low-back pain? Spine 13:557–560, 1988.
14. Breig, A., and Troup, J.D.G.: Biomechanical considerations in the straight leg raising test. Cadaveric and clinical studies of the effect of medial hip rotation. Spine 4:242–250, 1979.
15. Brown, H.A.: Enlargement of the ligamentum flavum: A cause of low-back pain with sciatic radiation. J. Bone Joint Surg. 20:325–338, 1938.
16. Burton, A.K.: Regional lumbar sagittal mobility related to back pain: A pilot study. *In* Hukins, D.W.L., and Mulholland, R.C. (eds.): Back pain: Methods for Clinical Investigation and Assessment. Manchester, Manchester University Press, 1986, pp. 16–22.
17. Calin, A., Porta, J., Fries, J.F., and Schurman, D.J.: Clinical history as a screening test for ankylosing spondylitis. J. Am. Med. Assoc. 237:2613–2614, 1977.
18. Cats, A., van der Linden, S.J., Goei The, H.S., and Khan, M.A.: Proposals for diagnostic criteria of ankylosing spondylitis and allied disorders. Clin. Exp. Rheumatol. 5:167–171, 1987.
19. Charcot J.M.: Cited by Gilfillan, R.S., Jones, O.W., Roland, W.I., and Wylie, E.J. *In* Arterial occlusions simulating neurological disorders in lower limbs. J. Am. Med. Assoc. 154:1149, 1954.
20. Clague, G.E., and Macmillan, R.R.: Backache and the Guillain-Barré syndrome: A diagnostic problem. Br. Med. J. 293:325–326, 1986.
21. Cole, R.P.: Low back pain and testicular cancer. Br. Med. J. 295:840–841, 1987.
22. Compere, E.L., and Keyes, D.C.: Roentgenological studies of the intervertebral disc: A discussion of the embryology, anatomy, physiology, clinical and experimental pathology. Am. J. Radiol. 29:774–797, 1933.
23. Cotunnius, D.: A treatise on the nervous sciatica or nervous hip gout. London, translated by Henry Crantz, 1775.
24. Coventry, M.B., Ghormley, R.K., and Kernohan, J.W.: The intervertebral disc: Its microscopic anatomy and pathology. Part I: Anatomy, development, and physiology. Part II: Changes in the intervertebral disc concomitant with age. Part III: Pathological changes in the intervertebral disc. J. Bone Joint Surg. 27:105–112, 233–247, 460–474, 1945.
25. Cram, R.H.: A sign of sciatic nerve root pressure. J. Bone Joint Surg. (Br.) 35–B:192–195, 1953.
26. Cyriax, J.: Dural pain. Lancet 1:919–921, 1978.
27. Dandy, W.E.: Loose cartilage from intervertebral disc simulating tumour of the spinal cord. Arch. Surg. 19:660–672, 1929.
28. Davis, P., and Lentle, B.C.: Evidence for sacro-iliac disease as a common cause of low back ache in women. Lancet 2:496–497, 1978.
29. de Dombal, F.T.: Computer aided diagnosis of acute abdominal pain—the British experience. Rev. Epedemiol. Sante Publique 32:50–56, 1984.
30. Dejeurine, J.: La claudication intermittente de la molle epiniere. Press Med., Paris 9:981, 1911.
31. Deutsch, F.: Cited by Alexander, W. *In* Neuralgie und Neuritis; Specielle Pathologie und Therapie. Berlin, Wein, Urban and Swarzenburg, Band 1: Nervenkrankheiten, 341–608, 1924.
32. Dillane, J.B., Fry, J., and Kalton, E.: Acute back syndrome—a study from general practice. Br. Med. J. 2:82–84, 1966.
33. Dong, D., and Porter, R.W.: Walking and Cycling in Neurogenic and Intermittent Claudication. Paper read to I.S.S.L.S., Miami, 1988.
34. Edgar, M.A., and Ghadially, J.A.: Innervation of the lumbar spine. Clin. Orthop. 115:35–41, 1976.
35. Edgar, M.A., and Nundy, S.: Innervation of the spinal dura mater. J. Neurol. Neurosurg. Psychiatr. 29:530–534, 1966.
36. Edgar, M.A., and Park, W.M.: Induced pain patterns on passive straight-leg raising in lower lumbar disc protrusions. J. Bone Joint Surg. (Br.) 56B:658–667, 1974.

37. Eisenstein, S.: The morphometry and pathological anatomy of the lumbar spine in South African negroes and caucasoids with specific reference to spinal stenosis. J. Bone Joint Surg. (Br.) 59B:173–180, 1977.
38. Eisenstein, S.: Spondylolysis: A skeletal investigation of two population groups. J. Bone Joint Surg. (Br.) 60B:488–499, 1978.
39. Eisenstein, S., and Parry, C.R.: The lumbar facet arthrosis syndrome: Clinical presentation and articular surface changes. J. Bone Joint Surg. (Br.) 69B:3–7, 1987.
40. Epstein, J.A., Epstein, B.S., and Rosenthal, A.D.: Sciatica caused by nerve root entrapment in the lateral recess: The superior facet syndrome. J. Neurosurg. 36:584–589, 1972.
41. Evans, J.G.: Neurogenic intermittent claudication. Br. Med. J. 2:985–987, 1964.
42. Fairbank, J.C.T., Davies, J., Couper, J., and O'Brien, J.P.: Oswestry disability questionnaire. Physiotherapy 66:271–273, 1980.
43. Fairbank, J.C.T., Park, W.M., McCall, I.M., and O'Brien, J.P.: Apophyseal injection of local anaesthetic as a diagnostic aid in primary low-back syndromes. Spine 6:598–605, 1981.
44. Fairbank, J.C.T., and O'Brien, J.P.: Iliac crest syndrome: A treatable cause of back pain. Spine 8:220–224, 1983.
45. Fairbank, J.C.T.: The incidence of back pain in Britain. *In* Hukins, D.W.L., and Mulholland, R.C. (eds.): Back pain: Methods for Clinical Investigation and Assessment. Manchester, Manchester University Press, 1986, pp. 1–12.
46. Fajerszdahn, J.: Uber dasgekreutze Iscias Phaenomen. Wein Klin. Wchnschr. 14:41–47, 1901.
47. Falconer, M.A., Glasgow, G.L., and Cole, D.S.: Sensory disturbances occurring in sciatica due to intervertebral disc protrusions: Some observations on the fifth lumbar and first sacral dermatomes. J. Neurol. Neurosurg. Psychiatr. 10:72–84, 1974.
48. Farfan, H.F.: Effects of torsion on the intervertebral joints. Can. J. Surg. 12:336–341, 1969.
49. Farfan, H.F.: Mechanical Disorders of the Low Back. Philadelphia, Lea & Febiger, 1973.
50. Farfan, H.F., and Sullivan, J.D.: The relation of facet orientation to intervertebral disc failure. Can. J. Surg. 10:179–185, 1967.
51. Feindel, W.H., Weddell, G., and Sinclair, D.C.: Pain sensibility in deep somatic structures. J. Neurol. Neurosurg. Psychiatr. 11:113–117, 1948.
52. Foerster, O.: Dermatomes in man. Brain 56:1–39, 1933.
53. Forst, J.J.: Contibution a l'étude clinique sur la sciatique. Paris, Thesis No. 33, 1881.
54. Fraser, R.D., Osti, O.L., and Vernon-Roberts, B.: Discitis after discography. J. Bone Joint Surg. (Br.) 69B:26–35, 1987.
55. Gardner, A.D.H., Pursell, L.M., Murty, K., and Smith, D.G.: The management of the clinical problem of spinal pain with the assistance of a microcomputer. *In* Hukins, D.W.L., and Mulholland, R.C. (eds.): Back Pain: Methods for Clinical Investigation and Assessment. Manchester, Manchester University Press. 1986, pp. 23–41.
56. Gerard, J.: The Herbal or General Historie of Plants. London, 1597.
57. Ghormley, R.K.: Low back pain with special reference to the articular facets, with presentation of an operative procedure. J. Am. Med. Assoc. 101:1773–1777, 1933.
58. Giles, L.G.F.: Lumbo-sacral zygapophyseal joint tropism and its effect on hyaline cartilage. Clin. Biomech. 2:2–6, 1987.
59. Giles, L.G.F., and Taylor, J.R.: Human zygapophyseal joint capsule and synovial fold innervation. Br. J. Rheumatol. 26:93–98, 1987.
60. Glover, J.R.: Back pain and hyperaesthesia. Lancet 1:1165–1169, 1960.
61. Goldthwait, J.E.: The lumbo-sacral articulation: An explanation of many cases of "lumbago," "sciatica" and paraplegia. Boston Med. Surg. J. 164:365–372, 1911.
62. Goldthwait, J.E., and Osgood, R.B.: A consideration of the pelvic articulations from an anatomical, pathological and clinical standpoint. Boston Med. Surg. J. 152:593–601, 643–648, 1905.
63. Gower, Sir W.R.: Diseases of the Nervous System, Vol. 1. Philadelphia, Blakiston, 1901, p. 127.
64. Granit, G., Leksell, L., and Skoglund C.R.: Fibre interaction in injured or compressed region of nerve. Brain 67:125–140, 1944.
65. Gunn, C.C., and Milbrandt, W.E.: Tenderness at motor points. J. Bone Joint Surg. (Am.) 58A:815–825, 1976.
66. Hackett, G.S.: Referred pain from low back ligament disability. Am. Med. Assoc. Arch. Surg. 73:878–883, 1956.
67. Hadley, L.A.: Subluxation of the apophyseal articulations with bony impingement as a cause of back pain. Am. J. Radiol. 33:209–213, 1935.
68. Hadley, L.A.: Intervertebral foramen studies: Foramen encroachment associated with disc herniation. J. Neurosurg. 7:347–351, 1950.
69. Hadley, L.A.: Anatomico-roentgenographic studies of the posterior spinal articulations. Am. J. Radiol. 86:270–276, 1961.
70. Hall, H.: Examination of the patient with low back pain. Bull. Rheum. Dis., Vol. 33, No. 4, 1983.
71. Hall, H.: The Back Doctor. New York, Berkley Books, 1982.
72. Hall, H.: More Advice from the Back Doctor. Toronto, McClelland and Stewart, 1987.
73. Head, H.: On disturbances of sensation with special reference to the pain of visceral disease. Brain 16:1–133, 1893.
74. Hockaday, J.M., and Whitty, C.W.M.: Patterns of referred pain in the normal subject. Brain 90:481–496, 1967.
75. Hoppenfield, S.: Physical Examination of the Spine and Extremities. New York, Appleton-Century-Crofts, 1976, pp. 257–258.
76. Hoyland, J.A., Freemont, A.J., and Jayson, M.I.V.: Intervertebral foramen venous obstruction: A cause of periradicular fibrosis? Spine 14, 558–568, 1989.
77. Inman, V.T., and Saunders, J.B. de C.M.: Referred pain from skeletal structures. J. Nerv. Ment. Dis. 99:660–664, 1944.
78. Jackson, R.P., Jacobs, R.A., and Montesano, P.X.: Facet joint injection in low-back pain. A prospective statistical study. Spine 13, 966–971, 1988.
79. Johansson, J.E., Barrington, T.W., and Ameli, M.: Combined vascular and neurogenic claudication. Spine 7:150–158, 1982.
80. Jones, R.A.C., and Thomson, J.L.G.: The narrow lumbar canal: A clinical and radiological review. J. Bone Joint Surg. (Br.) 50B:595–605, 1968.

81. Keegan, J.J.: Dermatome hypalgesia associated with herniation of the intervertebral disc. Arch. Neurol. Psychiatr. 50:67–83, 1943.
82. Keegan, J.J., and Garrett, F.D.: The segmental distribution of the cutaneous nerves in the limbs of man. Anat. Rec. 102:409–437, 1948.
83. Kellgren, J.H.: Observations on referred pain arising from muscle. Clin. Sci. 3:175–190, 1938.
84. Kellgren, J.H.: On the distribution of pain arising from deep somatic structures with charges of segmental pain areas. Clin. Sci. 4:35–46, 1939.
85. Kellgren, J.H.: Sciatica. Lancet 1:561–564, 1941.
86. Kellgren, J.H.: The anatomical source of back pain. Rheumatol. Rehab. 16:3–12, 1977.
87. Kelly, M.: Is pain due to pressure on nerves? Spinal tumours and the intervertebral disc. Neurology 6:32–36, 1956.
88. Ker, N.B., and Jones, C.B.: Tumours of the cauda equina: The problem of differential diagnosis. J. Bone Joint Surg. 67B:358–362, 1985.
89. Kibler, R.F., and Nathan, P.W.: Relief of pain and paraesthesiae by nerve block distal to a lesion. J. Neurol. Neurosurg. Psychiatr. 23:91–98, 1960.
90. Kikuchi, S.: Classification of syndromes of neurogenic claudication. Personal communication, 1985.
91. King, J.S., and Lagger, R.: Sciatica viewed as a referred pain syndrome. Surg. Neurol. 5:46–50, 1976.
92. Kirkaldy-Willis, W.H., and Hill, R.J.: A more precise diagnosis for low-back pain. Spine 4:102–108, 1979.
93. Lasègue, E.C.: Consideration sur la sciatique. Archive Generale de Médecine 6:558–580, 1864.
94. Lawrence, J.S.: Disc degeneration: Its frequency and relationship to symptoms. Ann. Rheum. Dis. 28:121–138, 1969.
95. Lawrence, J.S.: The epidemiology of low back pain. Curr. Orthop. 1:361–365, 1987.
96. Lazarevic, L.: Ischias postica Cotunnii-Ein Beitrag zu deren Differential-diagnose. Med. Allgem. Wein Med. Ztg. 29:425–426, 1884.
97. Lewin, T.: Osteoarthritis in lumbar synovial joints: A morphological study. Acta Orthop. Scand. 73 (Suppl.):1–112, 1964.
98. Lewis, T., and Kellgren, J.H.: Observations relating to referred pain, viscero-motor reflexes, and other associated phenomena. Clin. Sci. 1:47–71, 1939.
99. Lewit, K.: The needle effect in the relief of myofascial pain. Pain 6:83–90, 1979.
100. Lindahl, O.: Hyperalgesia of the lumbar nerve roots in sciatica. Acta Orthop. Scand. 37:367–374, 1966.
101. Ljunggren, A.E.: Descriptions of pain and other sensory modalities in patients with lumbago-sciatica and herniated intervertebral discs. Interview administration of an adapted McGill pain questionaire. Pain 16:267–276, 1983.
102. Luschka, H.: Die Nerven des menschlichen Wirbelkanals. Tubingen, 1850.
103. Luschka, H.: Die Halbgelenke des menschlichen Korpers. G. Reiner, Berlin, 1858.
104. Marshall, L.L., Trethewie, E.R., and Curtain, C.C.: Chemical radiculitis: A clinical, physiological and immunological study. Clin. Orthop. Rel. Res. 129:61–67, 1977.
105. McCall, I.W., Park, W.M., and O'Brien, J.P.: Induced pain referral from posterior lumbar elements in normal subjects. Spine 4:441–446, 1979.
106. McKenzie, R.A.: The Lumbar Spine, Mechanical Diagnosis and Therapy. Waikanae, New Zealand, Spinal Publications, 1981.
107. Melzack, R.: The McGill pain questionaire: Major properties and scoring methods. Pain 1:277–299, 1975.
108. Melzack, R., and Wall, P.D.: Pain mechanisms: A new theory. Science 150:971–975, 1965.
109. Meyer, T.G., Tencer, A.F., Kristoferson, S., and Mooney, V.: Use of noninvasive techniques for quantification of spinal range-of-motion in normal subjects and chronic low-back dysfunction patients. Spine 9:588–594, 1984.
110. Middleton, G.S., and Teacher, J.H.: Injury of spinal cord due to rupture of the intervertebral disc during muscular effort. Glasgow Med. J. 76:1–6, 1911.
111. Million, R., Nilson, K.H., Baker, R.D., and Jayson, M.I.V.: Assessment of progress of the back pain patient. Spine 7:204–212, 1982.
112. Mixter, W.J., and Barr, J.S.: Rupture of the intervertebral disc with involvement of the spinal canal. N. Engl. J. Med. 211:210–215, 1934.
113. Moll, J.M.H., Liyanage, S.P., and Wright, V.: An objective clinical method to measure spinal extension. Rheumatol. Phys. Med. 11:293, 1972.
114. Moll, J.M.H., and Wright, V.: Normal range of spinal mobility: An objective clinical study. Ann. Rheum. Dis. 30:381–386, 1971.
115. Moll, J.M.H., and Wright, V.: An objective clinical method to measure lateral flexion. Rheumatol. Phys. Med. 11:225, 1972.
116. Mooney, V.: The syndromes of low back disease. Orthop. Clin. North Am. 14:505, 1983.
117. Mooney, V., and Robertson, J.: The facet syndrome. Clin. Orthop. 115:149–156, 1976.
118. Morgan, F.P., and King, T.: Primary instability of lumbar vertebrae as a common cause of low back pain. J. Bone Joint Surg. (Br.) 39B:6–22, 1957.
119. Nachemson, A.L., and LaRocca, H.: Editorial: Spine 1987. Spine 12:427–429, 1987.
120. Nelson, M.: The identification of back pain syndromes. *In* Hukins, D.W.L., and Mulholland, R.C. (eds.): Back Pain: Methods for Clinical Investigation and Assessment. Manchester, Manchester University Press, 1986, pp. 13–15.
121. Nelson, M.A., Allen, P., Clamp, S.E., and de Dombal, F.T.: Reliability and reproducibility of clinical findings in low back pain. Spine 4:97–101, 1979.
122. Newman, P.H.: Sprung back. J. Bone Joint Surg. (Br.) 34B:30–35, 1952.
123. Nightingale, S.: Personal communication.
124. O'Brien, J.P.: Mechanisms of spinal pain. *In* Wall, P.D., and Melzack, R. (eds.): Textbook of Pain. Edinburgh, Churchill Livingstone, 1984, pp. 240–251.
125. O'Connell, J.E.A.: Sciatica and the mechanism of the production of the clinical syndrome in protrusions of the lumbar intervertebral discs. Br. J. Surg. 30:315–327, 1943.
126. O'Connell, J.E.A.: Protrusion of the lumbar intervertebral discs: A clinical review based on five hundred cases treated by excision of the protrusion. J. Bone Joint Surg.(Br.) 33B:8–30, 1951.
127. Oppenheimer, A.: Development, clinical manifestations and treatment of rheumatoid arthritis of the apophyseal intervertebral joints. Am. J. Radiol. 49:49–76, 1943.
128. Park, W.M., McCall, I.W., O'Brien, J.P., and Webb,

J.K.: Fissuring of the posterior annulus fibrosus in the lumbar spine. Br. J. Radiol. 52:382–387, 1979.
129. Pope, M.H., Wilder, D.G., and Frymoyer, J.W.: Vibration as an aetiologic factor in low back pain. Proc. Conf. Engineer. Aspects Spine, meeting Br. Orthop. Assoc. Inst. Engl., U.K., 1980.
130. Porter, R.W., Hibbert, C.S., and Wellman, P.: Backache and the lumbar spinal canal. Spine 5:99–105, 1980.
131. Porter, R.W., and Hibbert, C.S.: Symptoms associated with lysis of the pars interarticularis. Spine 9:755–758, 1984.
132. Porter, R.W., Hibbert, C.S., Wicks, M.: The spinal canal in symptomatic lumbar disc lesions. J. Bone Joint Surg. (Br.) 60B:485–487, 1978.
133. Porter, R.W., and Oakshott, G.H.L.: Familial aspects of disc protrusion. Personal communication, 1988.
134. Putti, V.: New conceptions in the pathogenesis of sciatic pain. Lancet 2:53–60, 1927.
135. Putti, V., and Logroscino, D.: Anatomia dell' artritismo vertebrale apofisario. Bologna-Licinio cappelli editore. XVI, 1938.
136. Pynsent, P.B., and Fairbank, J.C.T.: A computer interview system for patients with back pain. J. Biomed. Engineer. 11:25–29, 1989.
137. Quebec Task Force on Spinal Disorders. Scientific approach to the assessment and management of activity-related spinal disorders. Spine 12(7S): S16–S21, 1987.
138. Ransford, A.O., Cairns, D., and Mooney, V.: The pain drawing as an aid to the psychological evaluation of patients with low back pain. Spine 1:127–134, 1976.
139. Reynolds, P.M.G.: Measurement of spinal mobility: A comparison of three methods. Rheumatol. Rehab. 14:180–185, 1975.
140. Rissanen, P.M.: The surgical anatomy and pathology of the supraspinous and interspinous ligaments of the lumbar spine, with special reference to ligament ruptures. Acta Orthop. Scand. Suppl. 44:1–100, 1960.
141. Rissanen, P.M.: Comparison of pathologic changes in intervertebral discs and interspinous ligaments of the lower part of the lumbar spine in the light of autopsy findings. Acta Orthop. Scand. 34:54–65, 1964.
142. Roland, M., and Morris, R.: A study of the natural history of low back pain. Part 1: Development of a reliable and sensitive measure of disability in low-back pain. Spine 8:141–144, 1983.
143. Rothman, S.L.G., Glen, W.V., and Kerber, C.W.: Postoperative fractures of lumbar articular facets: Occult cause of radiculopathy. Am. J. Radiol. 145:779–784, 1985.
144. Rowe, M.L.: Low back pain disability in industry: Updated position. J. Occup. Med. 13:476–478, 1971.
145. Saraste, H.: Long-term clinical and radiological follow-up of spondylolysis and spondylolisthesis. J. Pediatr. Orthop. 7:631–638, 1987.
146. Schmorl, E., and Junghans, M.: The human spine in health and disease. New York, Grune & Stratton, 1959.
147. Sinclair, D.C., Feindel, W.H., Weddell, G., and Falconer, M.A.: The intervertebral ligaments as a source of segmental pain. J. Bone Joint Surg. (Br.) 30B:515–521, 1948.
148. Smyth, M.J., and Wright, V.: Sciatica and the intervertebral disc. J. Bone Joint Surg. (Am.) 40A:1401–1418, 1958.
149. Sola, A.E., and Williams, R.L.: Myofascial pain syndromes. Neurology 6:91–95, 1956.
150. Thomas, A.M.C., Fairbank, J.C.T., Pynsent, P.B., and Baker, D.: A computer interview system for patients with back pain: A validation study. Spine, 1989. (In press.)
151. Travell, J., and Rinzler, S.H.: Myofascial genesis of pain. Postgrad. Med. 11:425–434, 1952.
152. Troup, J.D.G.: Straight leg raising (SLR) and the qualifying tests for increased root tension. Spine 6:526–527, 1981.
153. Verbiest, H.: A radicular syndrome from developmental narrowing of the lumbar vertebral canal. J. Bone Joint Surg. (Br.) 36B:230–237, 1954.
154. Waddell, G., and Main, C.J.: Assessment of severity in low-back disorders. Spine 9:204–213, 1984.
155. Waddell, G., Main, C.J., and Morris, E.W.: Normality and reliability in the clinical assessment of backache. Br. Med. J. 284:1519–1523, 1982.
156. Waddell, G., McCulloch, J.A., and Kummel, E.: Nonorganic physical signs in low back pain. Spine 5:117–125, 1980.
157. Waisbrod, H., Krainick, J.U., Gerbershagen, H.U.: Sacroiliac joint arthrodesis for chronic lower back pain. Arch. Orthop. Traumat. Surg. 106:238–240, 1987.
158. Whitty, C.W.M., and Willison, R.G.: Some aspects of referred pain. Lancet 2:226–231, 1958.
159. Yoshizawa, H.: Papers read to I.S.S.L.S. Miami, 1988, Kyoto, 1989.
160. Yoshizawa, H., O'Brien, J.P., Smith, W.T., and Trumper, M.: The neuropathy of intervertebral discs removed for low-back pain. J. Pathol. 132:95–104, 1980.
161. Zung, W.W.K.: A self-rated depression scale. Arch. Gen. Psychiatr. 32:63, 1965.

PAIN PATTERNS AND DIAGNOSTIC BLOCKS

Pieter F. van Akkerveeken

As defined by Merskey, pain is an unpleasant sensory and emotional experience associated with actual or potential tissue damage or described in terms of such damage.[28] According to this definition, pain is not related to the stimulus. It is always a psychologic state and not merely activity in nociceptive pathways.[39] Indeed, the amount of pain reported by the patient is not dependent on the amount or severity of tissue damage but on a number of psychologic factors, such as anxiety, insecurity, and loss of perspective.[34] Therefore, if a patient has incapacitating low back pain that needs to be evaluated to provide a rationale for treatment, psychologic variables as well as physical factors have to be assessed. Low back pain is a multicausal phenomenon. This chapter describes the patterns of pain radiation in the leg that are caused by lesions of structures in the low back, specifically, radicular pain resulting from the lesion of a nerve root and nonradicular pain caused by lesions of other tissues. The patterns of these two types and the two diagnostic tests that differentiate between them are described. These tests are also necessary to differentiate between *asymptomatic* and *symptomatic* lesions.

The incidence of radiologically observed degenerative changes of the lumbar spine steadily increases with age; however, the incidence of low back symptoms is at its maximum in the fourth decade and decreases gradually after the fifth decade. Hence, many older people have degenerative changes of the lumbar spine without manifesting any symptoms at all. Similarly, people can have radiologic signs of root entrapment, that is, morphologic changes indicating restricted space for the neural contents, without any symptom or sign of root entrapment. This has been shown with myelography[16] and with computed tomography (CT).[41]

RADICULAR VERSUS NONRADICULAR PAIN

Definitions

Radicular pain is usually defined as pain caused by a lesion of a spinal nerve root, radiating from the back into the dermatome of that root along the femoral or sciatic nerve trunk.[40] It may be a lesion outside the nerve root leading to entrapment or to abnormal tension of the root, such as a disc protrusion, a lateral recess stenosis caused by degeneration of a facet joint, or metastases in the pedicle narrowing the root canal. The root itself may be damaged, as occurs in radiculitis and a "battered" nerve root.

In a patient with radicular pain, positive signs of nerve root irritation, such as found during the straight-leg raising test, may be observed. However, if these signs are negative the only evidence of the presence or absence of radicular pain is the pattern of pain. According to the above definition, the

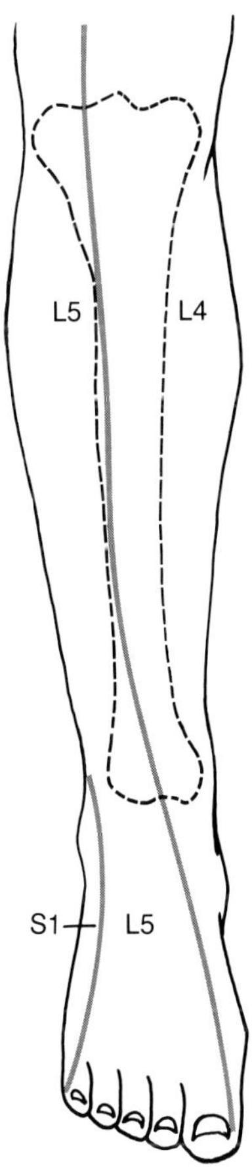

Figure 1 □ Dermatomes as defined by Keegan are illustrated.

radicular pain pattern of an L5 nerve root problem has to extend into the dorsum of the foot and the big toe. In the case of an S1 root problem, the pain radiates into the lateral aspect of the foot (Fig. 1).

Nonradicular pain is defined as pain caused by a lesion of a spinal motion segment, located in the back and radiating into the buttock and the leg in a nondermatomal pattern. Pain can be located in the area of the sacroiliac joint, the origin of the medial gluteal muscle, the area of the posterior iliac crest, the anterosuperior iliac spine, the greater trochanter, the area along the posterolateral or anterolateral aspect of the thigh, and even sometimes in the calf muscle (Fig. 2). This type of pain can be caused by a sprain of the paraspinal muscle or the spinal ligaments and by pathologic changes in the disc, the facet joint, or other structures of the motion segment.

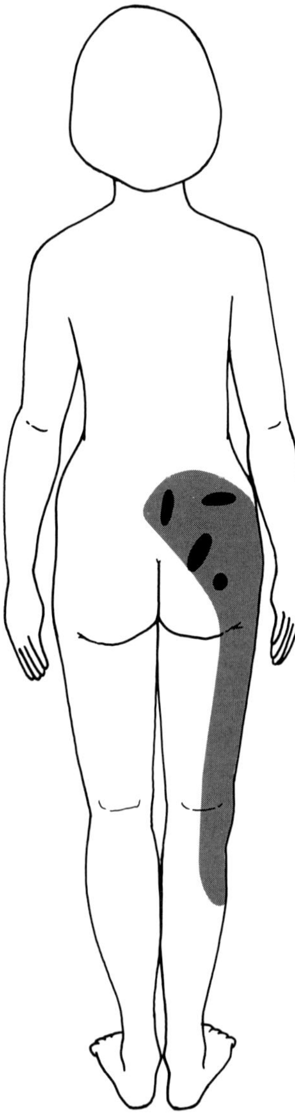

Figure 2 □ Nonradicular pain pattern. Pain can be experienced by the patient in the low back, the buttock, the outer aspect of the thigh, and the lateral aspect of the calf. Tenderness can be found at the posterior iliac crest, the sacroiliac joint, the anterosuperior iliac spine, the greater trochanter, and the lateral aspect of the thigh.

Table 1 □ Synonyms of Radicular and Nonradicular Pain

RADICULAR PAIN	NONRADICULAR PAIN
Root pain	Referred pain
Ischialgia	Pseudoradicular pain
Sciatica	Vertebrogenic pain
Neuropathic pain	Facet pain
Neuritic pain	Discogenic pain

These definitions are clear and straightforward. However, to differentiate between radicular and nonradicular pain in daily clinical practice is not so easy. This may be illustrated by the numerous synonyms for nonradicular pain (Table 1) and by the following three case histories. The inconsistency of radicular pain patterns has also been demonstrated[36] by describing in detail the pain patterns of patients with a surgically verified disc protrusion syndrome.

■ ***CASE 1:*** This case was described by Lasègue in 1864.[22] A sturdy 27-year-old employee of the department of bridges and roads of the city of Paris suddenly felt a lancinating pain in his left thigh during his regular walk. The pain steadily increased and he had to leave his job because of sickness, which he had not done in the last 10 years. He went to bed, but the pain increased, and during the night he did not sleep well. The next morning the pain was gone. However, 1 day later he got out of bed, and the lancinating stabbing pain returned. He was admitted to the hospital.

At examination, Dr. Lasègue observed normal extension, flexion, and abduction in the left hip without causing pain. He wrote "la flection brusque ou graduelle et sous l'angle le plus aigu de la cuisse sur le tronc ne reveille pas la moindre souffrance et n'exagere pas d'avantage celle qui existe." In other words, the straight-leg raising sign, the "Lasègue sign," was negative. He continued to note that, although the passive movements were painless, as soon as the patient actively flexed his hip joint, he experienced pain locally in his back, Lasègue believed that the pain syndrome in this man was "plus musculair que sciatic." The patient improved rapidly, and Lasègue saw no threat of deterioration in this patient.

□ *COMMENT:* In the detailed and clear style of the great French pioneers of medicine of the nineteenth century, Lasègue described a patient with a severe acute back pain syndrome and pain radiation into his leg without the characteristics typical of a radicular syndrome. He demonstrated the pattern of nonradicular pain, the high morbidity resulting in hospital admission, and the spontaneous regression.

■ ***CASE 2:*** This case was described by H. Verbiest in 1962.[37] A 24-year-old woman, 4 years after a laminectomy for a disc-protrusion syndrome, still had the same pain syndrome as she had before the operation. At operation no disc protrusion or other lesions causing root irritation were observed. Over the years, the pain had gradually increased. It was in the low back, radiating into both buttocks at the posterior aspect of both legs and into the ankle joint.

Bending forward was restricted and painful and was carried out with a fixed lordosis of the lumbar spine. Tenderness at the spinous process of L4 and L5 was observed.

The straight-leg raising sign was positive for both legs at about 45 degrees. Pain was indicated during this maneuver at the posterior aspect of the entire leg. The test of Bragard caused pain in the hollow of the knee. The sign of Naffziger was negative. No signs of neurologic deficit were found.

Radiologically, a normal state was observed after laminectomy. After the patient was placed in a prone position, Verbiest injected procaine 1% in the area of the interspinal ligaments between L4 and L5 and between L5 and S1.

After this injection, the woman was able to bend forward with a normal pattern of motion of the lumbar spine without any restriction; she could touch the ground with her fingers. The maneuver could be accomplished without any pain. At examination, the Lasègue test was negative for both legs at an angle of 90 degrees. About half a day later, all symptoms and signs returned, and the injection was repeated with the same result.

□ *COMMENT:* Verbiest described a patient with a radicular syndrome, demonstrating a typical pain pattern and positive signs of root tension. By injecting nonradicular structures with an anesthetic, the syndrome disappeared completely. In the original publication, the cause of the pain syndrome was not described.

■ ***CASE 3:*** A 23-year-old private soldier presented to the author with severe pain in his left buttock only, which developed gradually after a shooting exercise. No accident had occurred. The pain in his left buttock increased with coughing and sneezing. He had no complaints about pins and needles or weakness in his leg.

During the examination, I observed diminished lumbar lordosis fixed in flexion with a list to the right side. The patient was not able to move his back. All signs indicating nerve root irritation were positive at the left side. A slight loss of strength was noticed in the musculus extensor hallucis at the left side.

The clinical diagnosis, L5 root compression syndrome, was confirmed by subsequent myelography (Fig. 3*A,B*). At operation, protrusion of the L4–L5 disc at the left side was found in combination with a sequestered piece of disc in the root canal. At follow-up, no signs of root irritation were found, and the pain in the left buttock had disappeared completely.

□ *COMMENT:* The pain pattern, in itself, is typically nonradicular, whereas the signs at physical examination indicate a lumbar root compression. A similar nonradicular pain pattern may also be caused by compression of the dura. After removal of the sequestered and protruded part of the disc, the pain completely disappeared.

In the first case, Lasègue described a patient with a severe pain syndrome, which he recognized to be of nonradicular origin. Because of the severity of the syndrome, the patient was admitted and treated in the hospital conservatively. The second patient, presented by Verbiest, showed a typical ra-

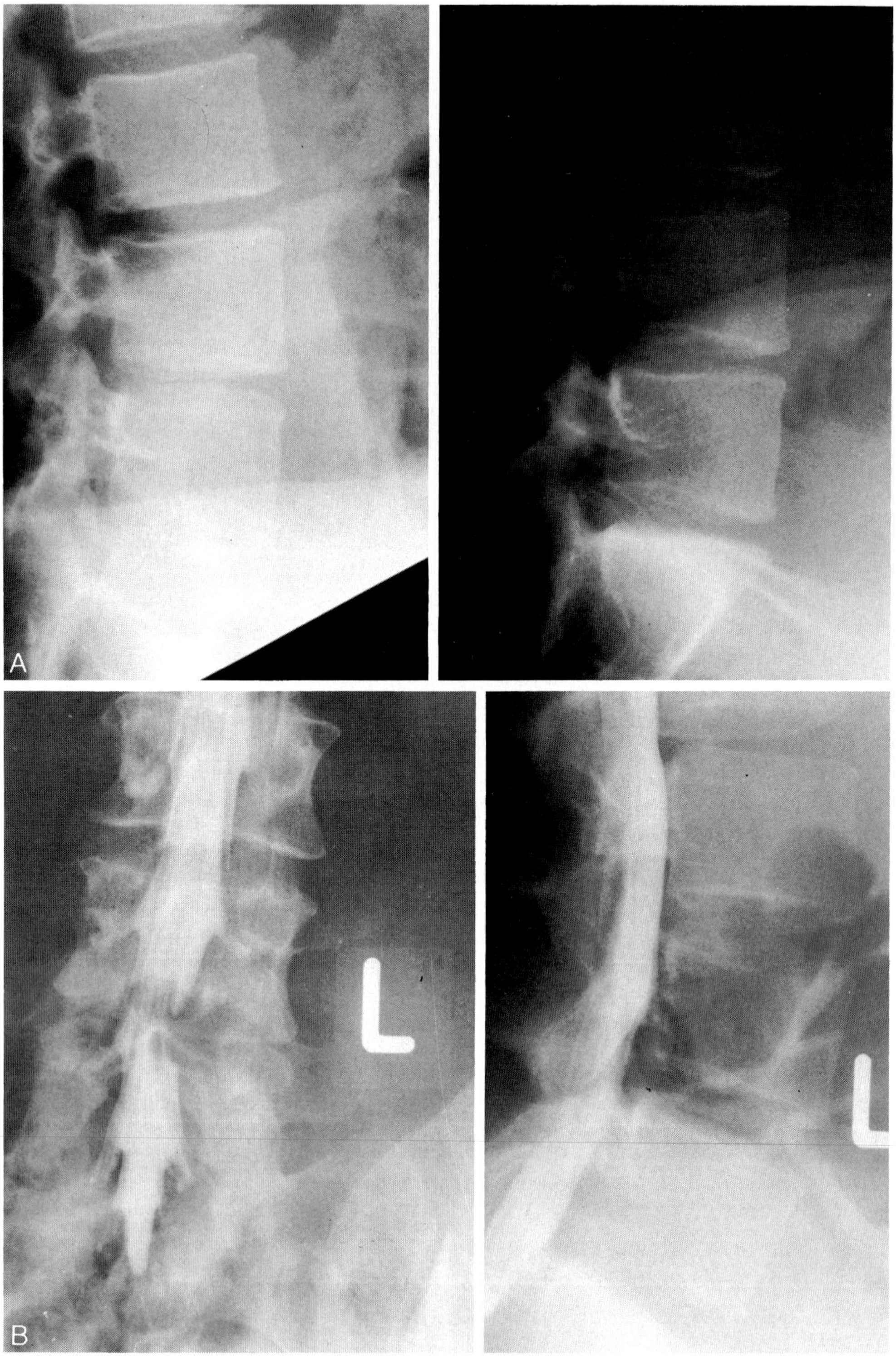

Figure 3 □ *A,* Lateral views of the lumbar spine of Case 3 in extension and in flexion. Note the absence of segmental motion at L4–L5. *B,* On the myelogram, lack of filling of the left L5 root is observed. The column of dye is pushed to the right. The lateral view shows an asymmetric protrusion of the L4–L5 disc.

dicular syndrome regarding the pain pattern and signs. However, by injecting the interspinal ligaments, structures distant from the nerve root, with procaine, the "radicular" pain was completely relieved. The third patient presented with a typical nonradicular pain pattern in combination with positive signs of root irritation. During an operation, a protruded disc stretching and compressing the nerve root was found.

These examples demonstrate the inconsistencies in distinguishing radicular and nonradicular pain patterns. As Farfan[11] pointed out, a disc protrusion is a "nonradicular" lesion and can be the cause of a nonradicular pain pattern. However, the same disc protrusion also causes nerve root irritation, thereby causing radicular pain. Because in the last patient the pain pattern was nonradicular, it may be concluded that the root irritation caused diminished root function but no root pain. As stated earlier this pain syndrome can also be explained on the basis of compression of the dura, which is, strictly speaking, nonradicular.

Dermatomes and Sclerotomes

The area of skin innervated by a spinal nerve is called a dermatome. Dermatomes have been defined by a number of researchers: by Bolk,[4] using anatomic dissections (Fig. 4); by Head,[14] observing cutaneous lesions in patients with herpes zoster; by Foerster,[12] observing the remaining sensibility after sectioning the neighboring nerve roots; and by Keegan and Garret[18] (among others), by observing hypalgesia from a proven lesion of a single nerve root. One has to realize that no area of skin is exclusively innervated by one nerve root for the following reasons:

1. A sharp boundary between dermatomes is lacking; on the contrary, series of overlapping areas innervated by different nerve roots are observed.[20]

2. A lesion of one nerve root disturbs the neurons in the cord, causing a spread of impulses exciting neighboring cord segments, which subsequently may cause pain in a wider distribution than caused by the original lesion.[8]

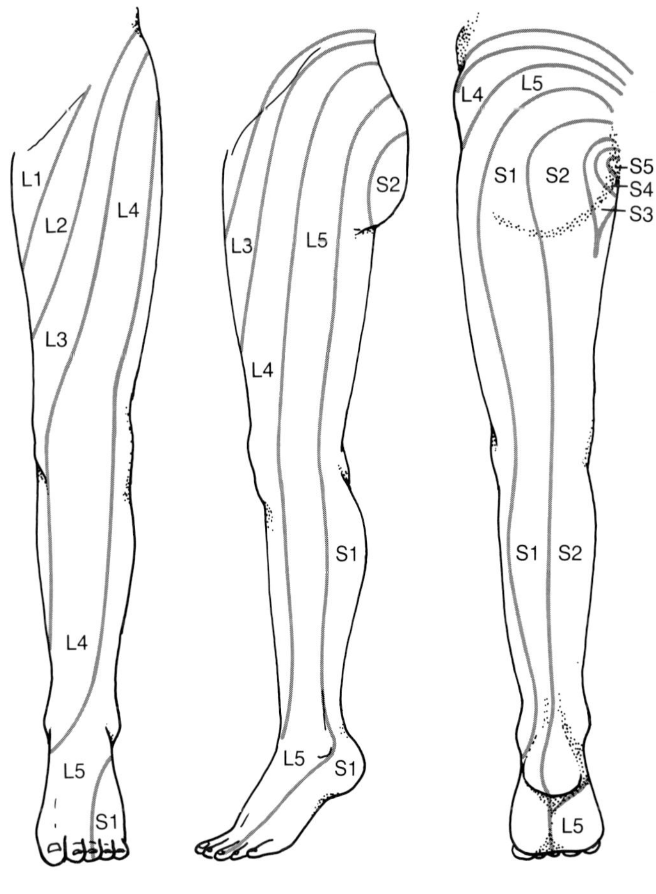

Figure 4 □ Dermatomes as defined by Bolk, a Dutch anatomist, around the turn of the century. He used painstaking effort to dissect the bundles of nerve fibers.

3. In the central part of the dermatome the innervation is more dense than in its margins, where the overlap of nerves is presumed to be present.[21] In regard to this overlap, opinions are not unanimous. The method used to assess dermatomes seems to be a cause of the differences.

By injecting structures in the back with hypertonic saline, Kellgren provoked pain radiating into one leg.[19] He called the pain in the leg *referred pain*, and the area of the pain located by the patient *sclerotome*. He tried systematically to outline these areas in order to create an atlas of sclerotomes to be used in clinical practice. However, he and later McCall[26] proved the inconsistency of the phenomenon of referred pain. That is, pain provoked by injecting high lumbar facet joints can be noted in different locations in different patients, in the groin and the anterior part of the thigh as well as along the posterolateral aspect of the thigh into the knee (Fig. 5). Similar patterns were observed for the provocation of the lower lumbar facet joints. Therefore, the systematic use of sclerotomal pain as a localizing symptom is not feasible. However, the concept of nonradicular pain is useful in clinical practice. The variability of these referred pain patterns between patients, and in the same patient over time, is tremendous.

FACET ARTHROGRAPHY

In 1927, before the golden age of the disc, in which the disc was considered the source of nerve root entrapment, Putti[32] described a syndrome of neuralgia in one leg caused by hypertrophy of a facet joint resulting from degeneration. However, the role of the facet joint as a direct source of pain was first described by Badgley,[2] who in 1941 postulated that irritation of the capsule of the lumbar intervertebral joint is able to cause pain by firing nociceptive stimuli from the facet joint capsule through the posterior primary ramus into the sensory dorsal root ganglion. Although a number of experimental studies were carried out since the original ones by Kellgren[19] in the early 1930s, not until the 1970s did the facet joint draw the attention of the medical profession at large as a primary source of back pain. In particular, the original work of Mooney and Robertson[29] inspired many clinicians in their research and resulted in numerous publications about the therapeutic effects of facet arthrography[5, 9, 17, 23, 33] and a number of well-performed anatomic studies.[1, 3, 13, 15, 31]

Facet arthrography is often used in combination with a corticosteroid drug as a therapeutic modality. When the technique is successful, in some centers it is followed by destruction of the primary posterior ramus to denervate the facet joint.

In the mid-1970s, Park and McCall started to use lumbar facet arthrography systematically in the evaluation of patients with incapacitating chronic back pain, most of them having had a laminectomy. Facet arthrography was part of the assessment to define the so-called symptomatic level. Subsequently many of these patients were treated by lumbar fusion. This section is restricted to facet arthrography as a diagnostic procedure and does not discuss its therapeutic value.

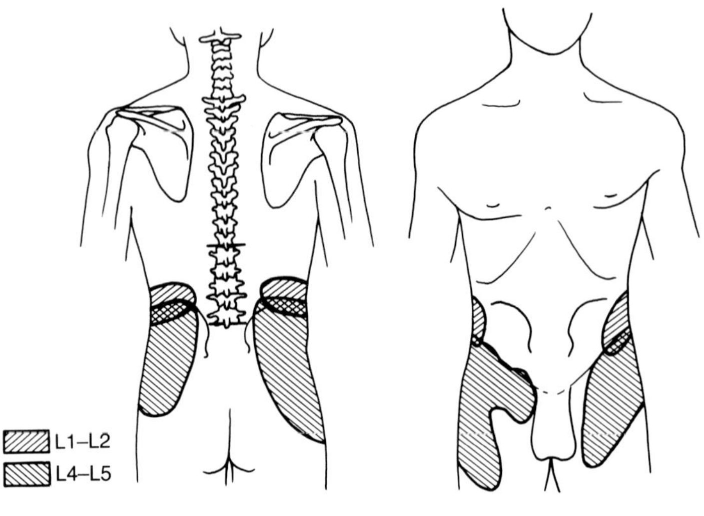

Figure 5 □ Pain referral in "normals" after intracapsular facet-joint injections of 6% saline, according to McCall and colleagues. (From McCall, I. W., Park, W. M., and O'Brien, J. P.: Induced pain referral from posterior lumbar elements in normal subjects. Spine 4:441–446, 1979.) Note the overlap around the iliac crest.

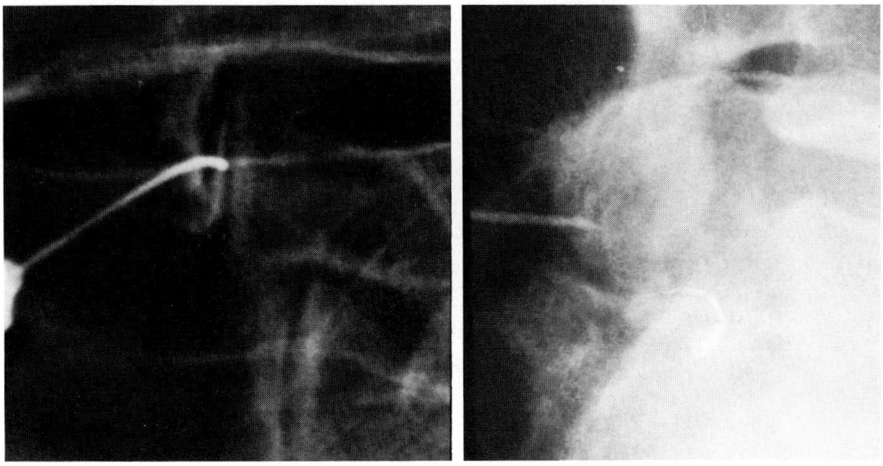

Figure 6 □ An oblique and lateral view of a L4–L5 facet joint with a needle inserted intra-articularly. The radiograph is made after injection of a very small amount of contrast medium.

Technique

The test is performed as an outpatient procedure with premedication of 10 mg of diazepam, if indicated. Radiologic monitoring in the anteroposterior and lateral views is mandatory. The patient is placed in the prone position. The radiography table is slowly rotated around a longitudinal axis until the articular surfaces are projected in the anteroposterior view as parallel lines. The more distally the facet joints are located, the more transverse they are aligned; hence, a greater degree of rotation has to be applied. A 23-gauge 10-cm disposable spinal needle is introduced through the skin perpendicularly into the joint under direct radiologic control (Fig. 6). In most patients, the easiest entrance to the joint is at the lower margin of the parallel projections of the joint surfaces. In some patients it is easier to approach the joint in the proximal area. The capsule is rather tough and when the needle has passed the capsule a sensation of giving way may be observed.

To check the correct position of the needle tip, a very small amount of water-soluble contrast medium is injected (0.1 to 0.2 ml) (Fig. 6). If the correct position is confirmed, slow injection of anesthetic (lidocaine 1% or bupivacaine hydrochloride [Marcaine] 0.5%) follows. Because quantities of 2 to 3 ml of contrast medium will rupture the capsule, only about 0.4 to 0.6 ml is used.[25] Some patients may have large recesses originating from the capsule into which up to 2 ml of contrast material may escape (Fig. 7). Therefore, a slow injection is recommended, and the injection should be stopped when the pressure is increasing.

Symptoms occurring at injection of the contrast material are noted; the patient is followed up for at least 4 hours and asked to report symptoms at regular intervals. If all symptoms are relieved by the injection, the test is considered positive. If only the back pain or leg pain is relieved, the test is considered to be a partial success and the

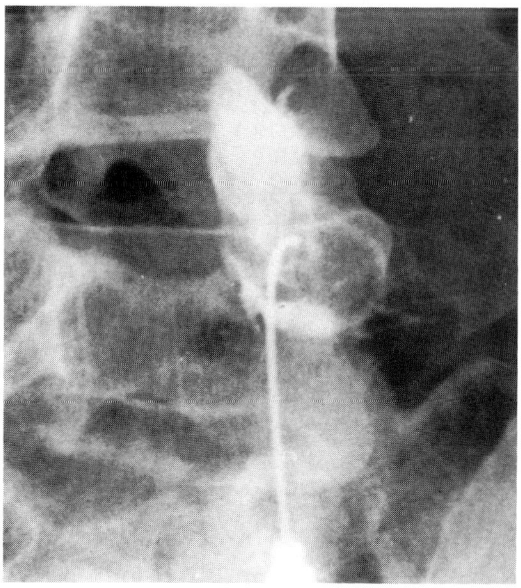

Figure 7 □ Facet arthrography of an L4–L5 joint demonstrates a large recess seen superiorly, containing 1.6 ml of contrast medium. No symptoms were provoked at injection.

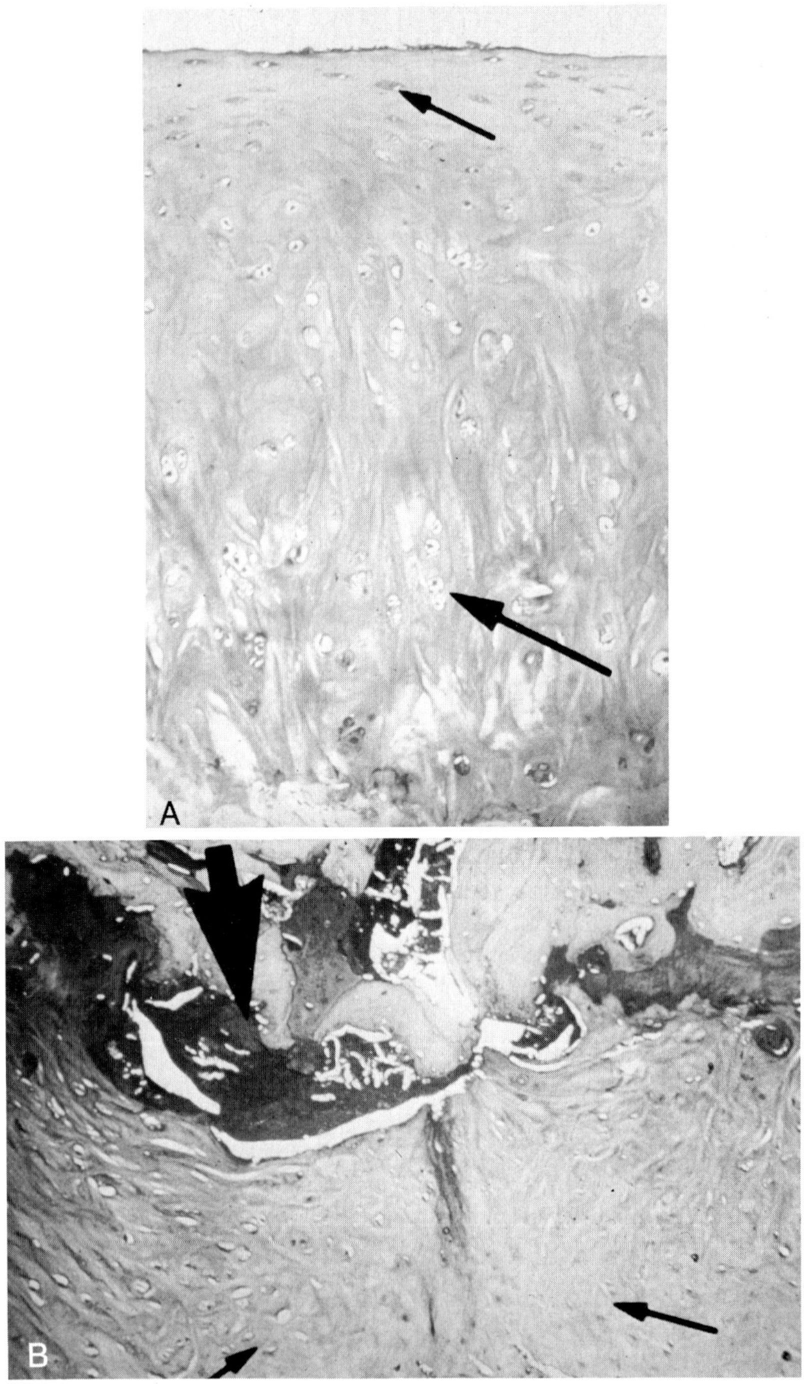

Figure 8 □ *A* shows the normal articular cartilage of a 48-year-old male. The arrow at the top demonstrates the normal horizontal orientation of the chondrocytes near the surface. The lower arrow points to the perpendicular orientation of the collagen fibrils. *B* is a high-power magnification view of the cartilage-bone interface of the L4–L5 facet joint of Case 4. Between the small arrows an area of necrosis is seen. The large arrow indicates a separation between bone and cartilage filled with exudate.

outcome is classified as doubtful. If no relief of symptoms occurs, the test result is classified as negative.

Diagnostic Value

In most reports about facet arthrography,[2, 5, 9, 10, 17, 23, 29, 33] the therapeutic value is described. Many authors have been using large quantities of anesthetic, and in many cases more than one facet joint in the same patient has been blocked. As McCall stated, the specificity of facet arthrography as a diagnostic test partly depends on "the quantity of fluid injected into the joint."[25] Because the capacity of the facet joint is limited and because large quantities of anesthetic will penetrate the surrounding sensitive tissues, such as the dura and nerve root sheath, the dorsal root ganglion, the ligamentum flavum, and the periosteum, structures other than the facet joint are blocked. More recently, an attempt was made to define the diagnostic value.[25] However, clear answers on the questions of indications and significance have not yet been provided.

Indications

As a diagnostic procedure, facet arthrography has two indications.

Indication 1

In the first instance, facet arthrography is used in the assessment of patients suffering from severe incapacitating back and nonradicular leg pain to differentiate between an asymptomatic and a symptomatic facet joint. Eisenstein has demonstrated pathologic changes of facet joint cartilage in patients treated surgically (Fig. 8).[10]

■ *CASE 4:** A 24-year-old female suffered from low back pain from the age of 15. The pain increased over the years. Occasionally the pain radiated into her left lower leg down to the calf. The leg pain was felt only when low back pain was particularly severe. Her pain generally decreased by gentle motion and was aggravated by rest. All standard modes of conservative treatment were given; mobilization of the back was most helpful, while lumbosacral spinal support immediately aggravated her symptoms (Fig. 9). By the time she consulted the department for spinal disorders at Oswestry, she had already undergone myelography, intravenous pyelography (IVP), scintigraphy, and CT (Fig. 10). No abnormal

*Courtesy of Mr. S. Eisenstein, F.R.C.S., Ph.D., Oswestry, United Kingdom.

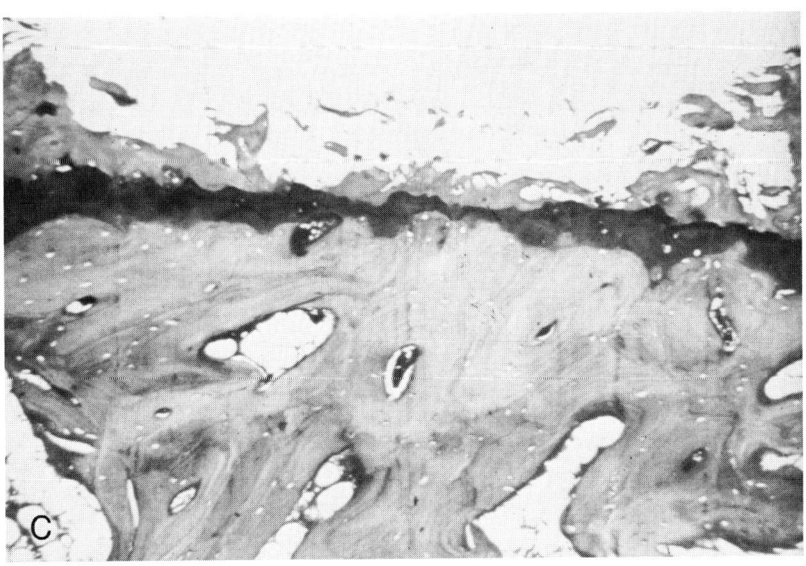

Figure 8 *Continued* C shows the cartilage-bone interface of a facet joint from a 38-year-old female who presented with a syndrome similar to that of Case 4. A large area of cartilage necrosis is seen to produce a crater that penetrates to the bone. This stage of degeneration follows that seen in Case 4. (By courtesy of Mr. S. Eisenstein).

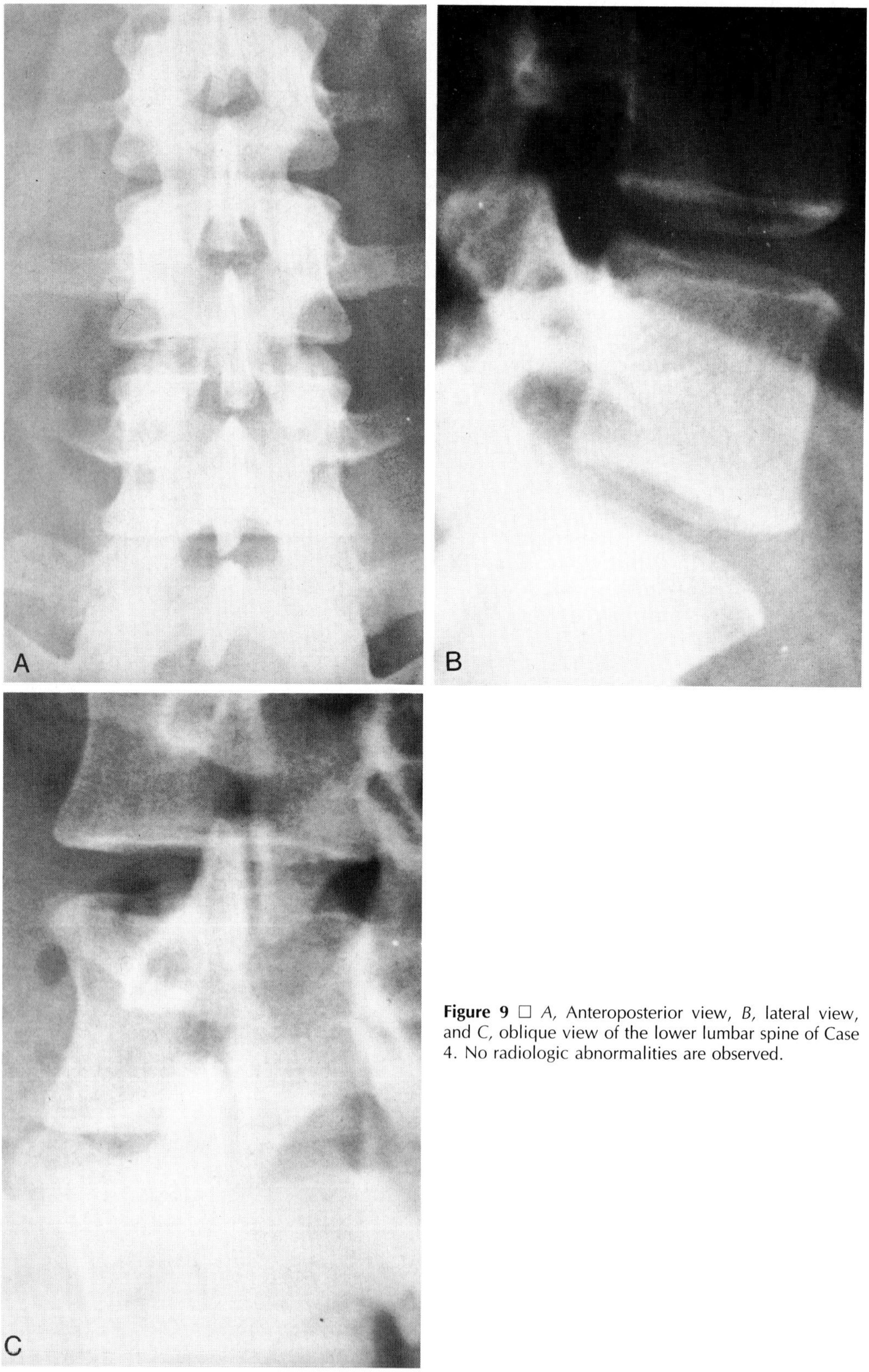

Figure 9 □ *A,* Anteroposterior view, *B,* lateral view, and C, oblique view of the lower lumbar spine of Case 4. No radiologic abnormalities are observed.

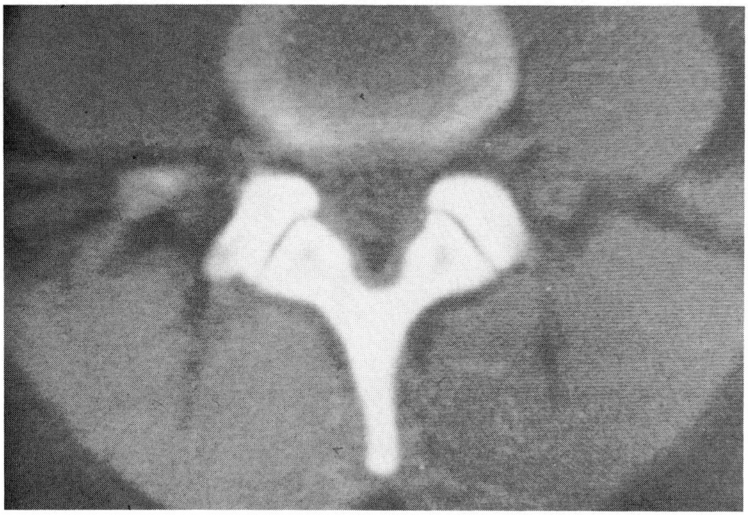

Figure 10 □ A computed tomographic (CT) image of the L4–L5 disc and facet joints of Case 4. Normal periradicular and epidural fats are observed. The disc and facet joints also have normal appearances.

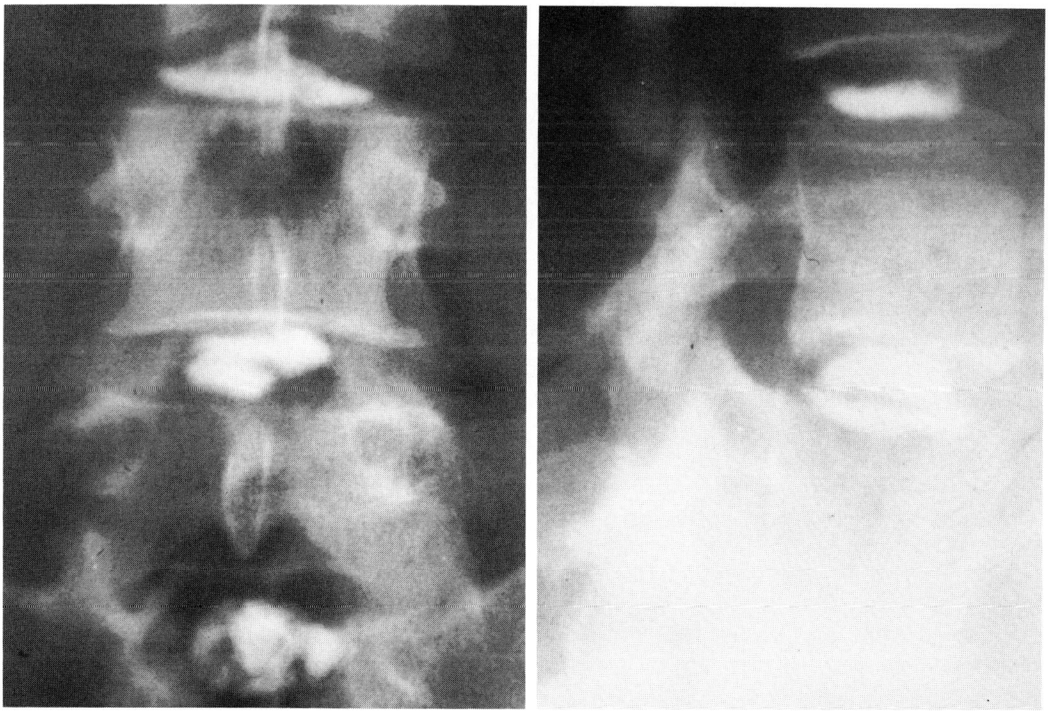

Figure 11 □ Anteroposterior and lateral views of the lumbar spine of Case 4 after discography at L3–L4, L4–L5, and L5–S1. Morphology is normal; at injection of contrast medium no symptoms were elicited.

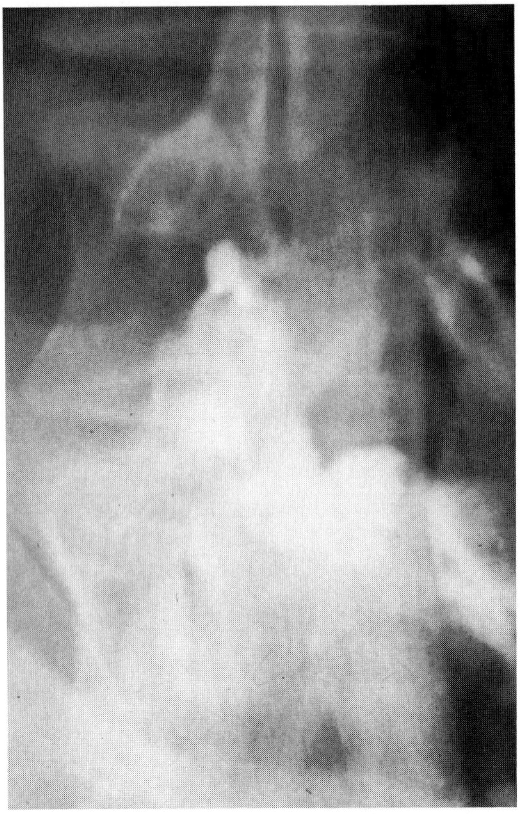

Figure 12 □ An oblique view of the left L4–L5 facet joint of Case 4 after facet arthrography. Note the rupture of the capsule and subsequent leaking of contrast medium at the lower aspect of the joint. At the moment of leakage, the "typical" symptoms were provoked. After injection of lidocaine, the patient's symptoms were relieved.

findings were demonstrated. Her disability was considered to be significant because she was unable to do her daily work as a secretary. Consequently, ancillary investigations were carried out. At discography, morphologic findings were normal at the lower three levels (Fig. 11). Facet arthrography, however, exactly reproduced her symptoms upon injection of contrast material in the L4–L5 facet joint at the left side (Fig. 12). After lidocaine infiltration in the joint, she had several hours of relief.

Subsequently, the patient underwent posterolateral fusion at L4–L5–S1 without instrumentation, and at follow-up 2 years later she had an excellent result. She was able to lead a full life, professionally and socially and had no need for analgesics or treatment. Occasionally she had vague pain.

Indication 2

The second indication is to assess the symptomatic segment in patients with severe incapacitating back and leg pain following an operation on the lumbar spine. In patients who have symptoms after a lumbar decompression or after an interbody fusion, facet arthrography must be part of the assessment protocol.

■ ***CASE 5:*** A 65-year-old woman presented with low back pain and nonradicular pain radiating in the left leg. The pain began about a year before and gradually increased. It was experienced in the buttock, the groin, and the anteromedial aspect of the thigh.

Five years previously, an interlaminar decompression of the L5 root at the left side by a partial medial undermining facetectomy at L4–L5 was performed. At that time, a diagnosis was made by water-soluble myelography and nerve root sheath infiltration with bupivacaine hydrochloride. The neurogenic intermittent claudication syndrome was completely relieved after this procedure. The current pain was described by the patient as completely different from the previous pain syndrome.

Plain radiographs (Fig. 13*A*) demonstrate the partial medial facetectomy and laminotomy at the left side. The lateral view shows the degenerative spondylolisthesis L4–L5, Grade 1. Discography (Fig. 14) resulted in no symptoms at injection. Facet arthrography of the L4–L5 joint at the left side provoked the symptoms, which, after a bupivacaine hydrochloride injection, disappeared completely (Fig. 15).

The diagnosis of degenerative spondylolisthesis with symptomatic facet joint degeneration was made, and the patient was subsequently treated by intertransverse fusion at L4–L5 (Fig. 13*B*). At follow-up 1 year and 7 months after the operation, the patient is virtually pain free and is leading a normal life. Walking, biking and swimming are part of her daily routine. An examination revealed a 67-year-old woman in good physical condition, with a normal and pain-free range of movement of the back. Radiologically, she had a solid fusion of L4–L5 as shown by extension and flexion views.

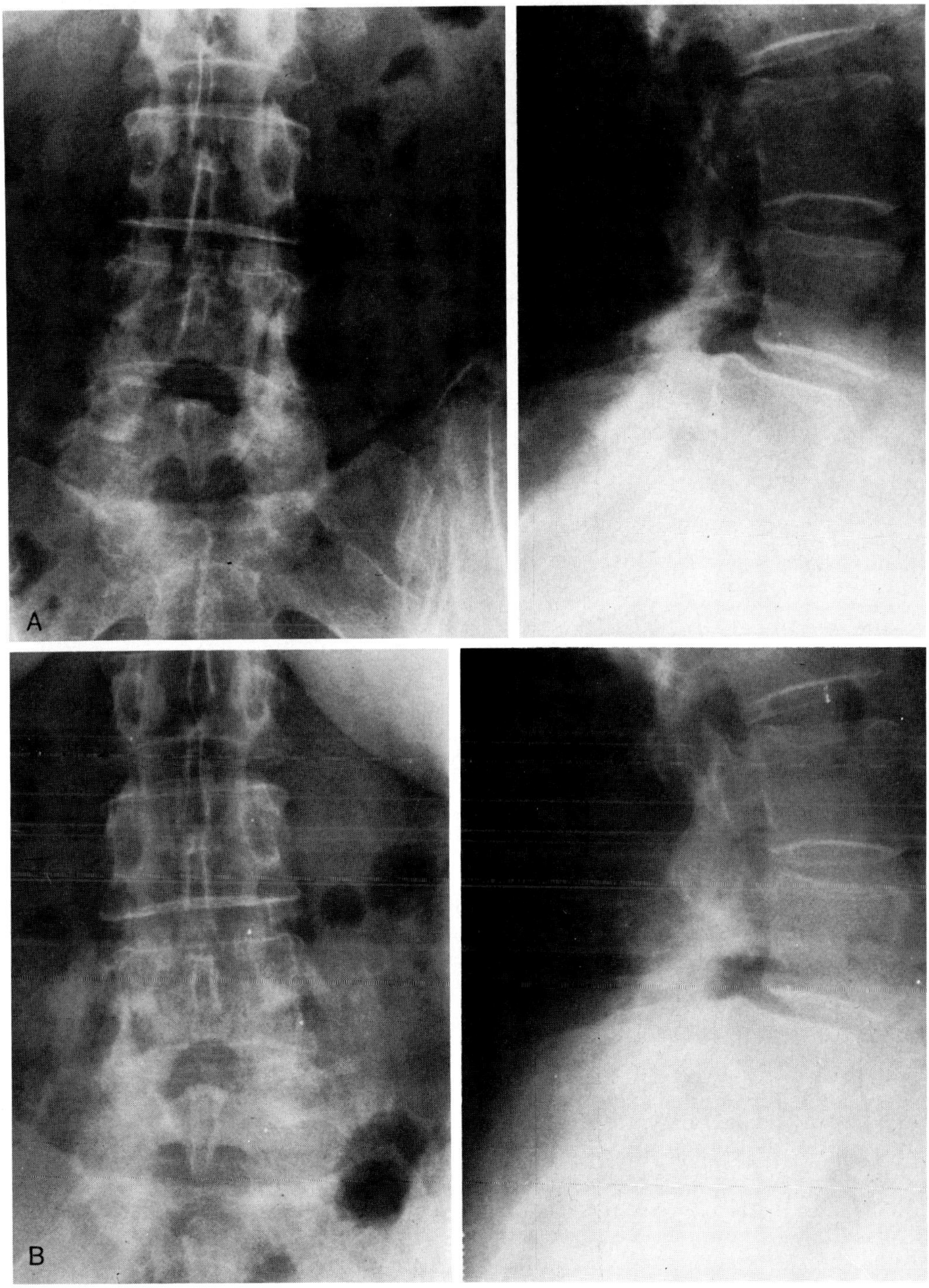

Figure 13 □ *A*, Anteroposterior and lateral radiographs of Case 5. Note the degenerative L4–L5 facet joint at the left side and the partial laminotomy at the upper margin of the lamina of L5. *B*, The situation is shown 1 year after intertransverse fusion: solid bony fusion can be observed between the transverse processes and between articular facets.

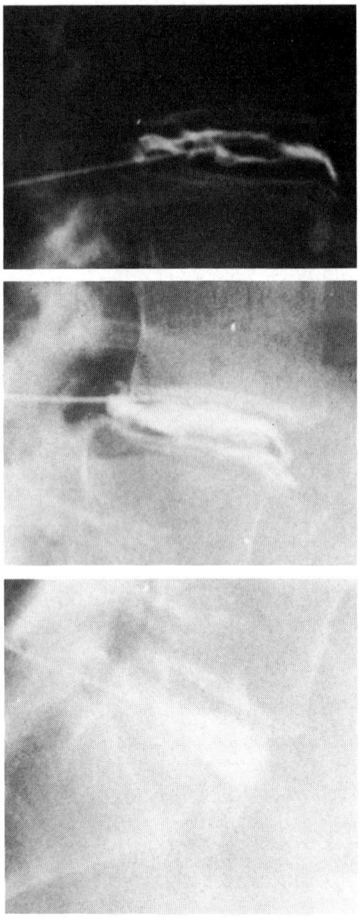

Figure 14. □ Discography of L3–L4, L4–L5, and L5–S1 of Case 5. Degenerative morphologic findings are observed at L3–L4 and L4–L5. The injection at L5–S1 is annular, and therefore inconclusive. At injection of contrast medium, no symptoms were reproduced at any level (asymptomatic degeneration).

Recommendations and Studies Needed

Since Putti addressed the Royal College of Surgeons in 1928,[32] numerous papers on the facet joint as a source of low back pain have been written. In most papers the therapeutic value of facet arthrography is retrospectively described. Systematic assessment is lacking; a set of variables that permit discrimination regarding the outcome of treatment is not known.

To ascertain which type of patient will benefit from this invasive procedure, controlled multifactorial studies have to be carried out.

Regarding the diagnostic value, the situation is even worse. Until now, no attempt

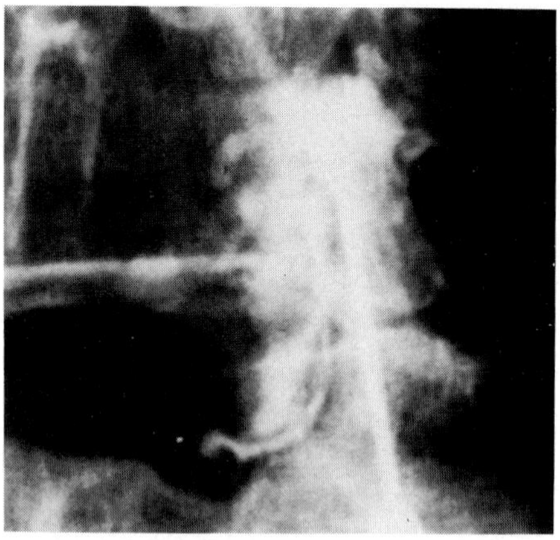

Figure 15 □ Facet arthrography of the L4–L5 joint at the left side. Following the injection of contrast medium, the symptoms of the patient were provoked, at the moment of dye escaping from the superior recess of the joint capsule. After an intra-articular injection of bupivacaine hydrochloride (Marcaine) all symptoms were relieved.

has been made to define the replicability and validity of facet arthrography. Finally, animal experiments must be performed, for example, to assess the spread of the fluid used, in order to define the anatomic selectivity of the procedure.

LUMBAR NERVE ROOT SHEATH INFILTRATION

The neurogenic claudication syndrome has been defined by Verbiest[38] as "a syndrome in which the patient will feel pain, tension, and weakness in one or both legs upon walking, progressively increasing until walking becomes impossible, and disappearance of the symptoms after a period of rest." The syndrome can be caused by a narrowing of the vertebral canal, leading to cauda equina dysfunction, or by entrapment of a nerve root in a narrow lateral recess or root canal. In the latter, the diagnosis may be difficult for the following reasons:

1. Radiologic signs of root entrapment have been observed in asymptomatic people.[16, 41]

2. Patients can have radiologic signs of root entrapment at more than one level.

3. Patients may have an atypical claudication syndrome, without root tension signs, such as pain in a nonradicular pattern in one leg that is constantly present and increases during standing and walking.

To differentiate between asymptomatic and symptomatic lesions, in other words, to identify the root that causes the symptoms, nerve root sheath infiltration with an anesthetic is indicated.

As a diagnostic aid in patients who may have root problems after a lumbar decompression operation, this procedure was described in 1971 by Macnab.[24] Later, the diagnostic value of this procedure was systematically evaluated by van Akkerveeken.[6, 36]

Lumbar nerve root sheath infiltration may also be helpful in patients with a so-called failed-back surgery syndrome, in particular, if morphologic changes indicating a possible root entrapment are shown by myelography, CT, and/or MRI. However, the interpretation of the test in these patients is less straightforward; a nerve root may be situated within a dense postoperative fibrosis without entrapment but may be damaged, a so-called battered root. In such a case the result of the nerve root sheath infiltration will be positive, although an operation aimed at decompression of that nerve root will not yield any success.

Technique

The test is performed as an outpatient procedure. When it is indicated, patients are premedicated with 10 mg diazepam. The procedure is explained to the patient, not only its aims and technical details, but also what the patient may expect in terms of pain and pain relief. It is important that the patient is optimally relaxed when the procedure starts. A terrified patient will distract the observer who has to concentrate on a technically demanding procedure.

An image intensifier working in two directions is used. If a lumbar root sheath at the right side has to be infiltrated, the patient is lying prone with a pillow under his or her right side in order to make possible a vertical approach to the nerve root.

A 21- or 23-gauge, 6-inch-long discography needle is used. The needle is introduced vertically, in a manner resembling the lateral approach in discography (Fig. 16).[27] The advancement of the needle is checked radiologically in the anteroposterior and lateral views. The needle is not aimed at the disc but, rather, at the lower border of the pedicle just proximal to the nerve root. The nerve root is passing immediately under the pedicle and is proceeding forward, downward, and laterally (Fig. 17*A*).

When the needle hits the pedicle, the needle is drawn backward about one inch and then brought forward again, aiming at a point just under the pedicle.

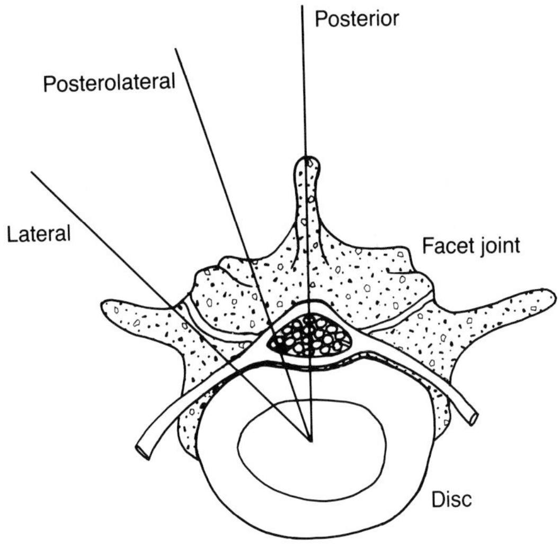

Figure 16 □ Diagram showing a transverse section through a lumbar disc, which illustrates the three approaches to the disc. The lateral approach is also used in lumbar root sheath infiltrations.

If the needle point is at the line between the centers of the two adjacent pedicles, as seen on the anteroposterior view, it must hit the nerve root sheath (Fig. 17*B*). On the lateral view, the needle point has to be located about 2 mm below the lower margin of the pedicle, in the middle of the intervertebral foramen (Fig. 18).

When the nerve root sheath is hit, the patient will experience a sharp pain with an electric sensation in the leg, usually into the dermatome of the nerve. Most patients will also experience paresthesia. If the observer is convinced that the needle is at the right place, he or she injects 0.2 ml of radiopaque dye. A radiograph is obtained in the anteroposterior and lateral views (Fig. 19). Subsequently, 0.2 to 0.5 ml bupivacaine hydrochloride 0.5% or lidocaine 1% is injected slowly.

The reaction of the patient and the effect of the anesthetic on the pain pattern are noted. The patient is asked to walk and, again, the pain pattern is documented. A number of patients will also experience motor weakness for a couple of hours, such as a drop-foot in the case of the L5 root. However, not all patients with provoked pain, paresthesia, and a positive reaction on the root block will experience motor weakness.

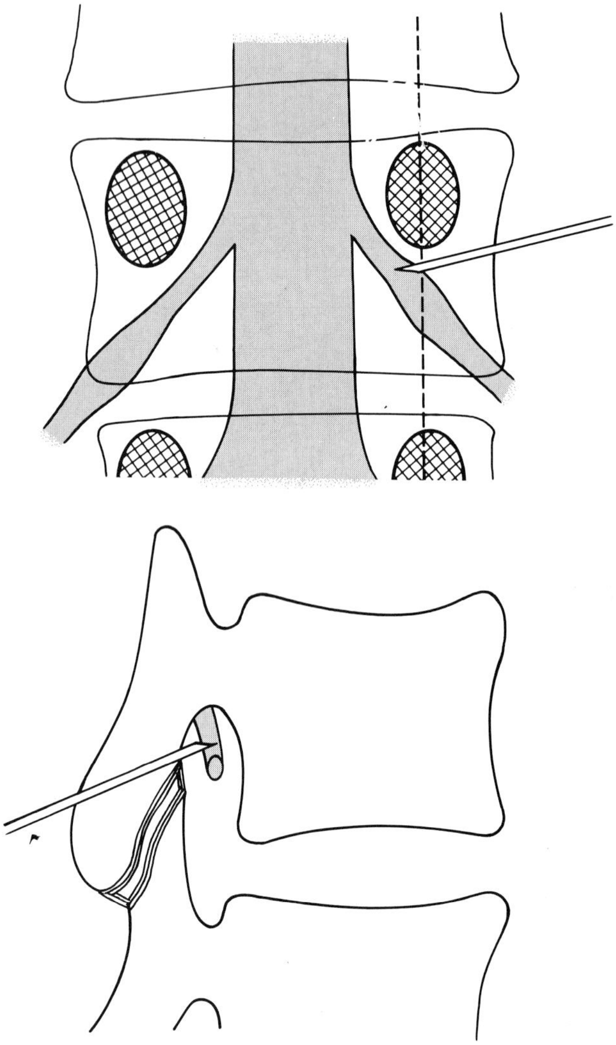

Figure 17 □ Diagram demonstrates, with a needle, the relationship of a lumbar nerve root to the surrounding bony landmarks in *A*, anteroposterior, and *B*, lateral, projections (see text).

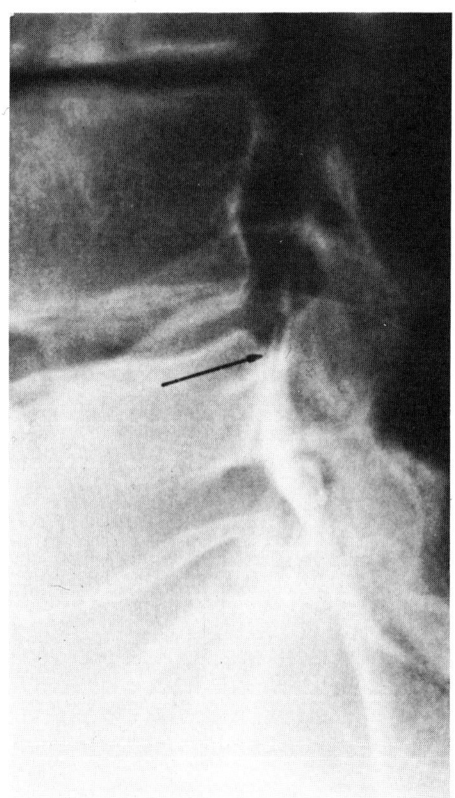

Figure 18 □ A lateral radiograph made after infiltration with contrast medium of the root sheath of L4 in the L4–L5 intervertebral foramen (Case 6). The arrow points to contrast outlining the nerve root. Symptoms of the patient were not affected by the injection of bupivacaine hydrochloride (see also Figs. 22–24).

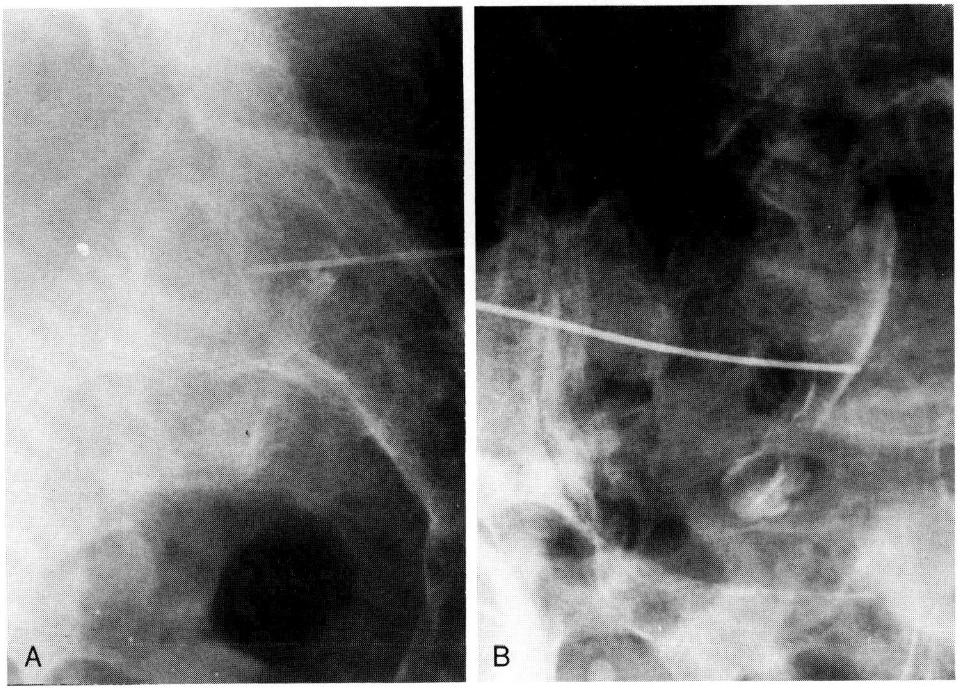

Figure 19 □ *A,* Anteroposterior view, and *B,* lateral view, after S1 root sheath infiltration. Note the location of the needle tip in relation to bony landmarks and the anteroposterior diameter of the sacrum.

To be as selective as possible, that is, to anesthetize the nerve root sheath only and not the facet joint capsule and the primary posterior ramus, care is taken to inject a minimal quantity of the anesthetic agent.

If the observer is convinced that the procedure was technically correct, the test result is defined as positive when the patient is able to walk and stand for 1 hour or more without pain in his or her leg. A negative result is observed when the pain in the leg of the patient is not influenced at all. Finally, the result can be dubious when the patient hesitates and indicates that the pain may be less or that some components of the pain are relieved but others are not.

If the S1 root sheath has to be infiltrated, the approach is slightly different. The patient is lying prone and the needle is introduced in the first sacral foramen from a posterior point under radiologic control and in an anteroposterior direction. About halfway into the sacral root canal, the root will be met. On the lateral view the needle point should not cross the anterior border of the sacrum (Fig. 19).

The unexperienced observer has to be aware of the following pitfalls that may cause an incorrect interpretation of the test results.

1. *Finding the correct root.* The L5 nerve root must be approached in the L5–S1 intervertebral foramen. The L4–L5 intervertebral foramen is the location of the L4 nerve root (Fig. 20). Being used to a disc protrusion syndrome in which the L4–L5 disc causes an entrapment of the L5 root, the inexperienced observer may be inclined to approach the L5 root in the L4–L5 foramen. To avoid this pitfall, it is necessary to describe to the radiologist, in detail, the nerve root that has

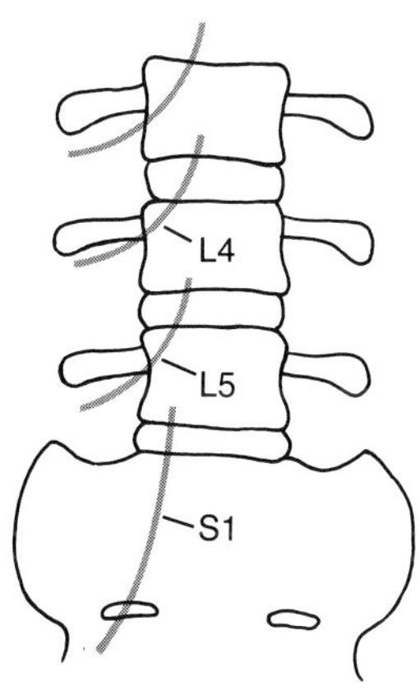

Figure 20 □ Diagram demonstrating the L4 root passing the L4–L5 intervertebral foramen, and the L5 root similarly passing the L5–S1 foramen.

to be blocked: for example, the right L5 root in the L5–S1 foramen. As a second check, one has to insist on obtaining anteroposterior and lateral radiographs with the needle in situ, so as to document the exact location of the needle (see Fig. 19).

2. *Finding the correct site of the entrapment of the root.* For example, the L5 root can be entrapped in the lateral recess at the L4–L5 level; this is also called a subarticular entrapment (Fig. 21). This entrapment is caused by a hypertrophic superior articular process of L5 and the posterior aspect of the vertebral body and/or disc.

The L5 nerve root can also be entrapped more laterally and distally in the root canal between the superior articular facet of S1 and the lower aspect of the lamina and pedicle of L5 (Fig. 21). In both cases, a nerve root sheath infiltration of L5 will be positive. However, the surgical approach will be different in each case.

3. If a lesion is more distally located, in the lumbar plexus or the sciatic nerve, the root sheath block will be positive. Obviously, a lumbar decompression will not solve this problem.

4. As stated earlier, the interpretation of a positive test result in patients who have had a lumbar decompression can be erroneous: a battered nerve root is not an indication for a redecompression.

Diagnostic Value

The diagnostic value of a procedure is usually described in terms of replicability and validity.[7]

Replicability

Replicability is a measure of precision and defines the variance in the results of a test when the test is repeatedly performed on the same patient. Replicability is subdivided into reproducibility and repeatability.

If the test is repeated in the same patient by different observers, the reproducibility is defined. As far as I know, no study has been done to define the reproducibility. However, in our experience of more than 400 root sheath injections, the procedure was performed on the same root in 27 patients two times or more by different observers; in four cases a negative test result was noted, whereas the test result of the other procedure

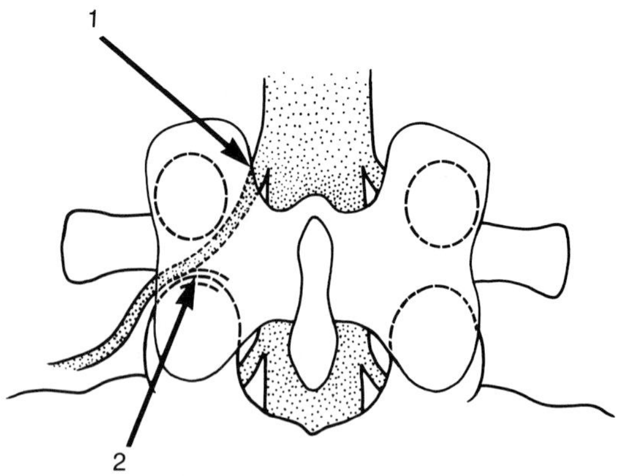

Figure 21 □ Posterior schematic view of an L5–S1 segment. At site *1*, the L5 root can be trapped in the lateral recess between the superior articular facet of L5 and the posterior aspect of the vertebral body, a so-called front-back entrapment. At site *2*, the L5 nerve root can be trapped between the superior articular facet of S1 and the lower aspect of the pedicle of L5, a so-called up-down entrapment.

was positive. Because these four patients did give different responses following an injection of contrast medium and also following an injection of anesthetic agent and because the location of the needle point was radiologically not correct, these tests were considered technically incorrect. In the other 23 patients the same test result was obtained by different observers on different occasions.

If the diagnostic test is repeated in a patient by the same observer the repeatability is defined. Again, no quantitative data are available. However, in 11 of our patients the test was repeated at least once by the same observer. In all 11 patients the same test result was obtained. In 9 patients, the root sheath infiltration was performed for chronic pain, on the basis that metastases in the pedicle and root canal caused root entrapment. In these patients, a series of root injections were performed as a mode of palliative treatment.

Even if the diagnostic test is proved to be highly replicable, it may not be measuring what it should measure. A good test has to be reliable, and the reliability of root sheath infiltration as a diagnostic test, again, is not established. If the injection has to block the nerve root only, very small quantities of anesthetic agent have to be used.

Validity

To define the validity of a diagnostic test, its performance is measured in terms of sensitivity and specificity.

Sensitivity

Sensitivity measures the percentage of patients with a positive test having the disease. If the number of false-negative test results is high the sensitivity will be low.

The sensitivity of lumbar nerve root sheath infiltration was defined in a group of patients with a lumbar nerve root compression syndrome caused by a disc protrusion.[6] The clinical and radiologic signs were confirmed by surgical findings. In 24 consecutive patients the nerve root sheath infiltration was positive. Hence, no false negatives were observed. Therefore, the sensitivity is 100% with a 95% confidence interval of 88% to 100%.

Specificity

Specificity measures the percentage of people not suffering from the disease with a negative test. It is obvious that this invasive procedure is not performed on people without a radicular syndrome. Therefore studies to define specificity are lacking. However, in a number of patients with symptomatic degeneration of a lumbar motion segment proved by provocative discography and facet block, a root sheath infiltration was also performed in seven patients. In all seven patients the test result of the root sheath infiltration was negative; the nonradicular pain in the leg was not affected by the root block. To define the specificity a larger group of patients with nonradicular pain in one leg has to be subjected to lumbar root sheath infiltration. In this way the number of true negatives and false positives can be counted. On ethical grounds such a study appears unacceptable.

Predictive Value

Another important measure of test performance is predictive value; it measures the percentage of patients with a positive test result who in fact have the disease. This is also called the predictive value positive. In a similar way, the predictive value negative is defined.

The predictive value positive of lumbar nerve root sheath infiltration was defined by prospectively studying a group of patients with degenerative lateral stenosis causing root entrapment. Included in the study were 30 patients: the predictive value positive in 18 surgically treated patients was 95% with a 95% confidence interval of 77% to 100%.[36] If the positive test results of the eight patients not operated upon are considered as false positives, the predictive value was 70%.

Indications

Atypical Neurogenic Claudication Syndrome □ Neurogenic claudication syndrome is characterized by pain, tension, and weakness in one or both legs upon walking, progressively increasing until walking becomes impossible; the symptoms disappear after a period of rest.[38] If the radiologic observations on CT or myelogram are clear, the diagnosis is made.

However, if radiologic signs of lumbar root entrapment on more than one level are found, or if the history of the pain is not typical and neurologic signs are lacking, the diagnosis is uncertain. These patients may have pain in one leg that is aggravated by standing and walking, although they are able to continue walking. The pain may present in a vague pattern and may even be limited to the buttock and the posterior part of the thigh. Classically, bending forward relieves the pain in the leg, as do sitting and biking. However, in a number of patients this phenomenon is not observed.

In other patients, pain is localized in a dermatome. For example, in some patients, pain in the lateral aspect of the foot is not increased by walking and standing and there are no signs of root irritation. Such a pain syndrome may result from root entrapment. Again, the diagnosis is uncertain.

To determine the value of root sheath infiltration in predicting the outcome of treatment for patients with an atypical neurogenic claudication syndrome, a prospective longitudinal study was performed.[36] Patients with signs of a neurologic deficit or root tension were excluded. All patients had definite radiologic signs of root entrapment. After root sheath infiltration, all patients were operated on. During a 6-year period, 62 patients qualified for this study.

A positive test result did not significantly improve the diagnostic capability of myelography and CT. However, a negative test result allowed a more reliable prediction of a negative outcome following decompression of the tested root, and a positive test result of an adjacent root predicted a positive outcome following decompression.[36]

■ *CASE 6:* A 52-year-old woman with a long history of back pain had complained for 2 years about increasing pain in her left leg that was aggravated by standing and walking. The pain was radiating into her buttock and the posterolateral aspect of her thigh, and into her calf muscle. Sitting on a chair or riding a bicycle relieved her leg pain. The pain in the back and in the left buttock also bothered her while she was sitting and made her change her posture at short intervals.

At physical examination, no signs of root entrapment were found. The straight-leg raising test, for example, was bilaterally negative at 90 degrees. Radiologically degenerative changes at multiple levels were observed (Fig. 22). A myelogram showed a diminished filling of the root sleeve of L5 at the left side and displacement of the dural sac to the median line by a degenerate facet joint of L4–L5 (Fig. 23). On the oblique view, the L4 root at the L3–L4 facet joint seems to be entrapped. The lateral view shows a large diffuse bulging of the L3–L4 disc, leading to a relative narrowness of the vertebral canal. To define precisely the source of pain and to determine the extent to which a decompression operation should be performed, root sheath infiltration was done (see Figs. 18 and 21). After injection of the L5 root sheath with bupivacaine hydrochloride, the patient was relieved of the pain in her left leg and could walk with a normal gait pattern (Fig. 24). However, her back pain was barely diminished. Infiltration of the L4 root was negative (see Fig. 18).

Subsequently, a minor operation was performed: an interlaminar partial medial facetectomy at L4–L5, at the left side only, to decompress the L5 nerve root.

Four years and 4 months postoperatively the patient was progressing well, could walk normally, and had no pain in her legs, although she still had backache similar to the one she had before the operation.

Hip-Spine Dilemma □ Most patients with symptomatic degeneration of a hip joint

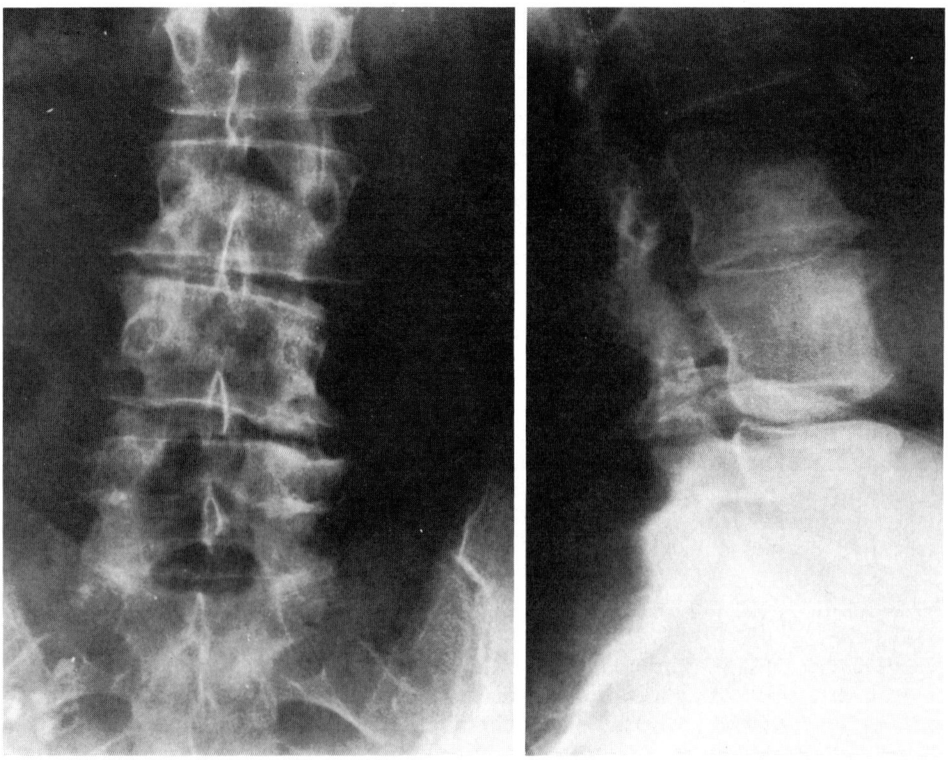

Figure 22 □ Anteroposterior and lateral view of the lumbar spine of Case 6. Note the degenerative changes on multiple levels.

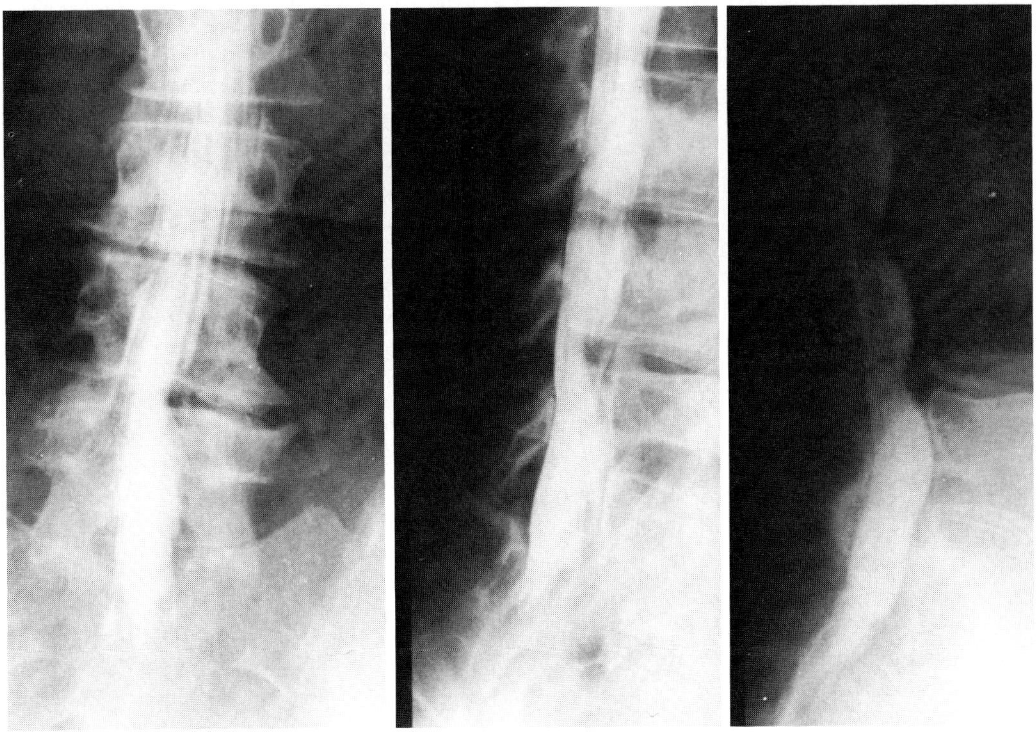

Figure 23 □ Lumbar myelogram of Case 6. Definitive radiologic signs of entrapment of L5 at the left side by degenerated facet joint. Dubious sign of L4 entrapment at the L3–L4 facet joint, as seen on the oblique view.

Figure 24 □ Anteroposterior view of L5 root sheath infiltration at the left side of Case 6. The symptoms of the patient were relieved and she was able to walk normally. The infiltration with bupivacaine hydrochloride of the L4 root did not affect the symptoms (see Fig. 18).

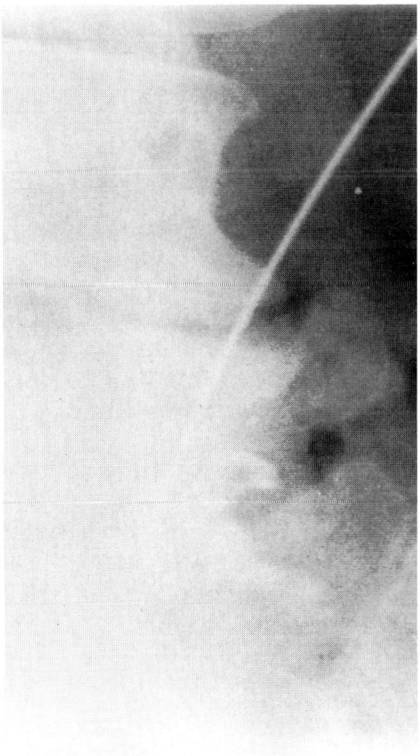

have a typical pain pattern, which is pain in the groin radiating down the medial aspect of the thigh to the knee. Often the pain is aggravated by walking and is relieved by sitting. Some patients, however, have an atypical pain pattern, characterized by pain in the buttock radiating down the posterolateral aspect of the thigh.

A minority of patients have both pain patterns. In those patients it may be difficult to differentiate between the hip joint and the degenerative back as the main source of pain. Degenerative stenosis of L3–L4 with entrapment of L3 or L4 may, in part, mimic the pain pattern of a degenerative hip joint, which consists of pain in the groin radiating down the anterior aspect of the thigh.[30]

On the other hand, lateral stenosis of the lower lumbar segments with entrapment of L5 and/or S1, causing pain in the buttock, along the posterior and posterolateral aspect of the thigh, and into the calf muscle, may be mimicked by an atypical pain pattern of a degenerative hip joint.

To evaluate these patients, hip arthrography with bupivacaine hydrochloride injection, myelography, CT, and nerve root sheath infiltration is used. In a 6-year period, about 850 total hip arthroplasties were performed in our department. In the same period, only 32 patients were subjected to this protocol of evaluation.

■ *CASE 7:* A 73-year-old woman had pain in her right leg. The pain was located in the buttock, the groin, the posterolateral aspect of the thigh, and the calf, and it was aggravated by walking. During walking, she hit small irregularities of the walking surface with her right foot. Furthermore, she tended to bend her back forward during walking. The pain in her groin also was slowly aggravated.

Since undergoing a total hip arthroplasty at the left side 8 years before, her left leg had been completely pain free. At clinical examination, a small but significant reduction in the range of motion in the right hip was observed. Signs of root compression were negative.

Radiologically degenerative changes of the lower lumbar segments and of the right hip joint (Fig. 25) were observed. At myelography (Fig. 26) the S1 root sleeve at the right side showed a filling defect and dislocation of the dural sac to the median line. After S1 root sheath injection (Fig. 27), some of her symptoms were relieved, specifically pain in the right buttock and the posterolateral aspect of the thigh. After injection of bupivacaine hydrochloride in the hip joint, the pain in the groin was relieved (Fig. 27). On the basis of this evaluation, the patient was operated on in two stages. The first was a total hip arthroplasty, and the second was an interlaminar partial medial facetectomy at L5–S1 (also at the right side).

More than 3 years later, the patient presented to the emergency department with a fracture of the left calcaneus. She reported being without pain in her right leg since the operative procedures. She was able to walk normal distances, for her age, without discomfort and without a tendency to bend forward.

Patients with Failed Back Surgery □ Patients who have pain below the knee in one or both legs, not necessarily in a dermatome, and who have undergone a lumbar decompression are considered to have radicular pain until proved otherwise. If these patients are severely restricted in their daily life, suffering from serious disability and not able to work, they are extensively evaluated. If the leg pain predominates, the patient is subjected to myelography, CT, and nerve root sheath infiltration, followed by psychologic evaluation. In a number of patients, neurophysiologic studies, including somatosensory evoked potentials, are done. If back pain is predominant and a nonradicular type of pain pattern is presented, provocative discography and facet arthrography are added. If fusions have been undertaken in the past, conventional tomography and bone scintigraphy are also indicated.

Patients in this group may have had a period without symptoms or with no relief at all after an operative procedure. Many patients show pain behavior with or without symptomatic lumbar lesions. In some of these patients, surgery is indicated but nearly all need psychotherapy and behavioral modification.

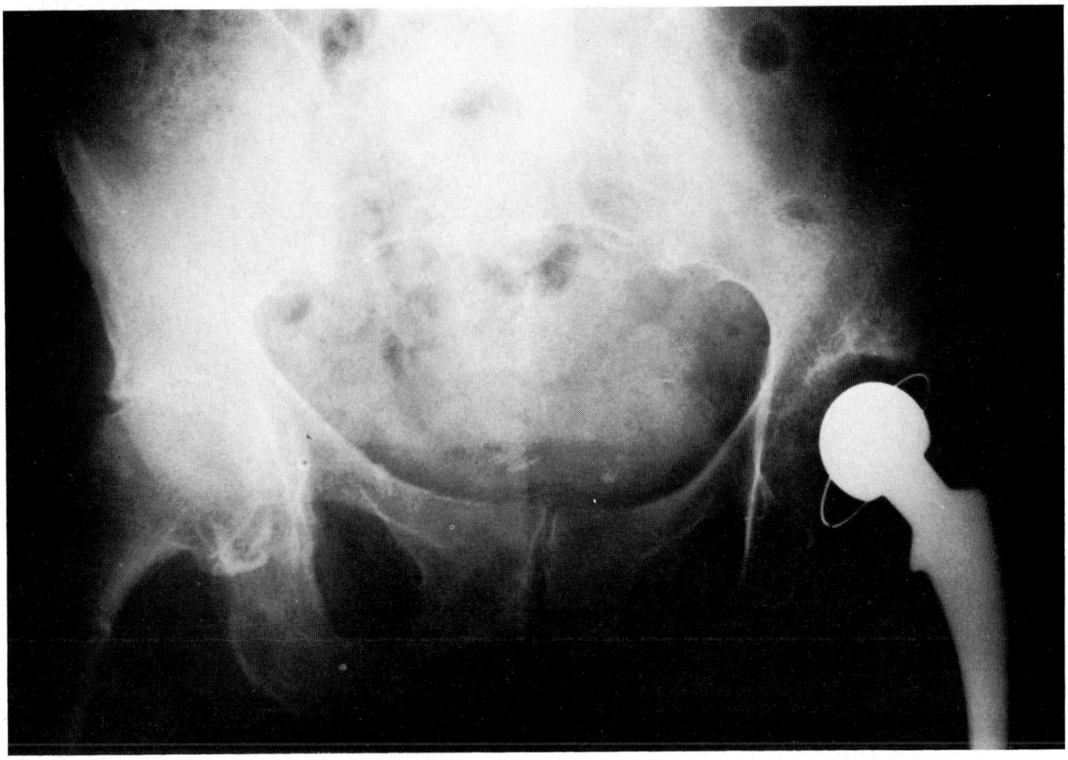

Figure 25 □ Anteroposterior view of the pelvis of Case 7. Degenerative changes of the right hip joint are obvious.

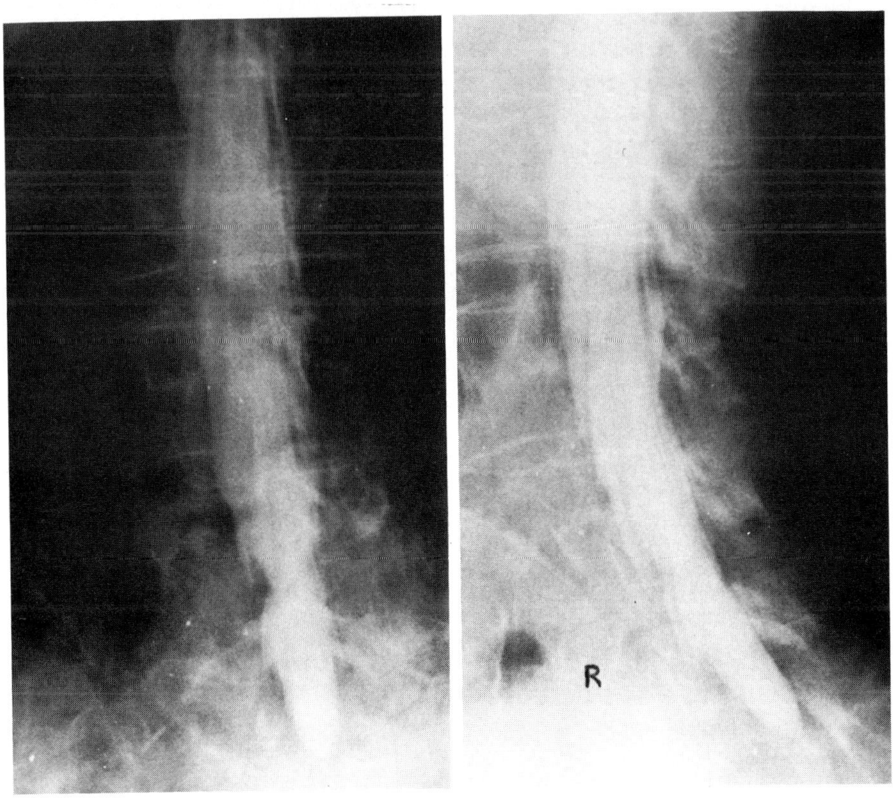

Figure 26 □ Lumbar myelogram of Case 7 shows diminished filling of the root sleeve of S1 and displacement of the column of dye to the median line by a degenerate L5–S1 facet joint.

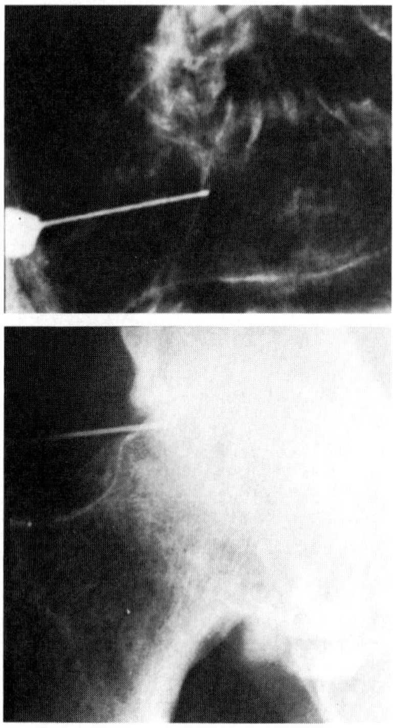

Figure 27 □ The top radiograph shows the outline of the S1 root at the right side by contrast medium in Case 7. The symptoms of the patient were partially relieved after injection of bupivacaine hydrochloride. The bottom radiograph shows the needle positioned intra-articularly in the hip joint. After injection of contrast medium, the symptoms were partially provoked; subsequently, they were partially relieved by bupivacaine hydrochloride.

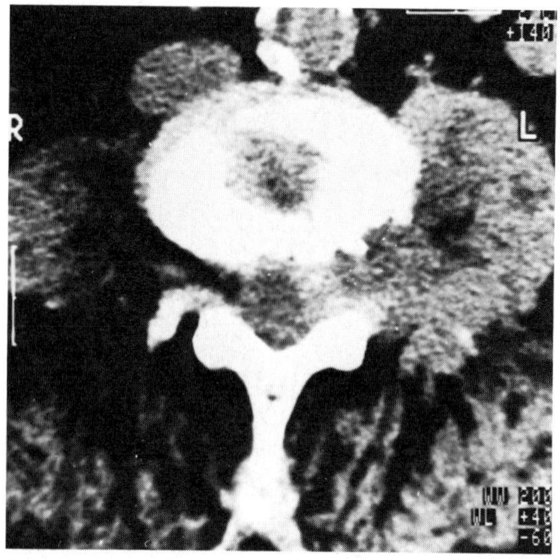

Figure 28 □ CT scan of the lower border of L3 of a 67-year-old woman. Eight years previously, her left eye had been removed because of malignant melanoma. She presented with a typical intermittent neurogenic claudication syndrome at the left leg. Tumor tissue is invading the left L3–L4 root canal, the pedicle, and the adjoining vertebral bodies, as was proved by needle biopsy.

Recommendations and Studies Needed

Nerve root sheath infiltration as a diagnostic test has been used by the author since 1981. In the last 2 years the procedure has also been made part of a therapeutic program for patients suffering from malignancies that cause lumbar nerve root entrapment (Fig. 28). It has also been used for patients having severe pain in one leg as a result of nerve root tension caused by an acute disc protrusion, in order to overcome the time they have to wait for surgery.

The author relies heavily upon this test in the evaluation of patients with dubious chronic radicular pain.

In patients with a so-called deep-seated L5 vertebra (Fig. 29), it can be technically impossible to approach the L5 root in the intervertebral foramen. If such a patient has clear-cut radiologic signs of root entrapment of L5 and negative root sheath infiltration of the adjoining roots, the L5 root entrapment is considered to be symptomatic and treatment is installed on this basis.

Although at other levels the procedure is relatively simple, still it is a difficult one demanding concentration and precision. Furthermore, the observer must empathize with the patient, for whom the procedure is sometimes very uncomfortable, although in most patients the test does not cause much pain.

Along with the increasing number of root sheath infiltrations, an increase in the frequency of dubious results of the test was observed, as well as an increase in the number of "technically impossible" procedures. If the department of radiology is very busy,

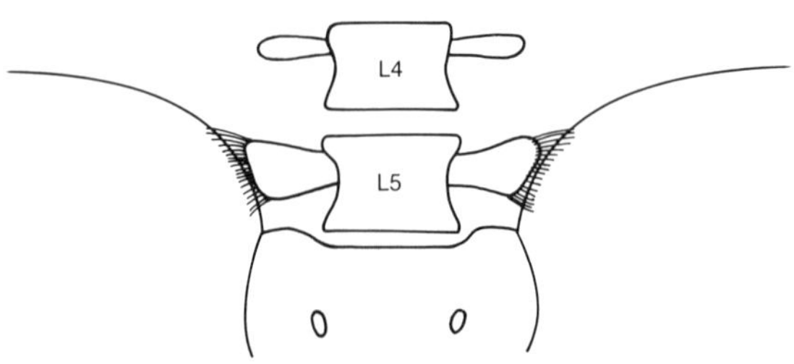

Figure 29 □ Diagram of a so-called deep-seated L5 vertebra, characterized by large transverse processes, nearly forming a joint with the iliac crest. The disc L5–S1 is narrow because of hypoplasia, not as a result of degeneration.

the time spent by the radiologist with one patient decreases, resulting in poorer test quality. One has to take time to explain the procedure to the patient, to make the patient feel comfortable, and to perform the procedure slowly with care for details.

Another mistake, made even by experienced people and usually on a very busy day, is the infiltration of the wrong root, one segment too high. In itself, this is not a serious complication, if recognized, and is followed by an infiltration of the correct root on another day. To facilitate recognition of the lumbar level for the referring clinician, it is mandatory to make radiographs in anteroposterior and lateral views with the needle in situ.

We have begun to define the diagnostic value and indications of lumbar root sheath infiltration.[36] However, larger series of patients who suffer from typical or atypical neurogenic claudication syndrome and have radiologic signs of multiple level root involvement must be studied in relation to this diagnostic procedure.

Acknowledgment

The knowledge and experience of Iain W. McCall, F.R.C.R., Oswestry, United Kingdom, was invaluable in writing the section Facet Arthrography.

References

1. Auteroche, P.: Innervation of the zygapophyseal joints of the lumbar spine. Anat. Clin. 5:17–28, 1983.
2. Badgley, C. E.: The articular facets in relation to low back pain and sciatic radiation. J. Bone Joint Surg. 23:481–496, 1941.
3. Bogduk, H.: The innervation of the lumbar spine. Spine 8:162–167, 1983.
4. Bolk, L.: De segmentale innervatie van romp en ledematen bij de mens. Haarlem, Bohn, 1910.
5. Carrera, G. F.: Lumbar facet joint injection in low back pain and sciatica. Radiology 137:665–667, 1980.
6. Castro, W. H. M., and van Akkerveeken, P. F.: Selective Lumbar Nerve Root Infiltration, a Diagnostic Procedure. Paper read at the Annual Meeting of the I.S.S.L.S. Sidney, April 14–19, 1985.
7. Committee for Evaluation Medical Technologies in Clinical Use, Institute of Medicine: Assessing Medical Technologies. Washington, National Academy Press, 1985.
8. Denny-Brown, D., et al.: The tract of Lissauer in relation to sensory transmission in the dorsal horn of spinal cord in the macaque monkey. J. Comp. Neurol. 151:175, 1973.
9. Destouet, J., et al.: Lumbar facet joint injection: Indication, technique, clinical correlation and preliminary results. Radiology 145:321–325, 1982.
10. Eisenstein, S. M., and Parry, C. R.: The lumbar facet arthrosis syndrome. J. Bone Joint Surg. 69B:3–7, 1987.
11. Farfan, H.: Personal communication, 1986.
12. Foerster, O.: The dermatomes in man. Brain 56:1–39, 1933.
13. Giles, L. G. F., and Taylor, J. R.: Innervation of lumbar zygapophyseal joint synovial folds. Acta Orthop. Scand. 58:43–46, 1987.
14. Head, C. A. W.: The pathology of herpes zoster and its bearing on sensory localization. Brain 23:323–353, 1900.
15. Hirsch, C., Ingelmark, V. E., and Miller, N.: The anatomic basis for low back pain studies on the presence of sensory endings in ligamentous capsular and intervertebral structures in the human lumbar spine. Acta Orthop. Scand. 33:1–17, 1963.
16. Hitselberger, W. E., and Written, R. M.: Abnormal myelograms in asymptomatic patients. J. Neurosurg. 28:204–206, 1968.
17. Jackson, R. P., and Craven, S. D.: Facet joint injections in mechanical low back pain. A prospective study. Orthop. Trans. 8:428, 1984.
18. Keegan, J. J., and Garret, F. D.: The segmental distribution of the cutaneous nerves in the limbs of man. Anat. Rec. 102:409–437, 1948.
19. Kellgren, J. H.: Observations on referred pain arising from deep somatic structures with charts of segmental pain areas. Clin. Sci. Mol. Med. 4:35–46, 1939.
20. Kirk, E. J., and Denny-Brown, D.: Functional variation in dermatomes in the macaque monkey following dorsal root lesions. J. Comp. Neurol. 151:175, 1973.
21. Kuhn, R. A.: Organisation of tactile dermatomes in cat and monkey. J. Neurophysiol. 16:169, 1953.
22. Lasègue, C. H.: Consideration sur la sciatique. Arch. Gen. Med. 6:558–580, 1864.
23. Lippit, A. B.: The facet joint and its role in spine pain. Spine 9:746–750, 1984.
24. Macnab, I.: Negative disc exploration. J. Bone Joint Surg. 53A:891–903, 1971.
25. McCall, I. W.: Facet arthrography (in press).
26. McCall, I. W., Park, W. M., and O'Brien, J. P.: Induced pain referral from posterior lumbar elements in normal subjects. Spine 4:441–446, 1979.
27. McCulloch, J. A., Waddell, G.: Lateral lumbar discography. Br. J. Radiol. 51:498, 1978.
28. Merskey, H.: Pain terms: A list with definitions and notes on usage. Pain 6:249–252, 1979.
29. Mooney, V., Robertson, J.: The facet syndrome. Clin. Orthop. 115:149–156, 1976.
30. Offierski, C. M., and Macnab, I.: Hip-spine syndrome. Spine 8:316–321, 1983.
31. Paris, S. V.: Anatomy as related to function and pain. Orthop. Clin. North Am. 14:475–489, 1983.
32. Putti, V.: Lady Jones Lecture. On new conceptions in the pathogenesis of sciatic pain. Lancet 2:53–60, 1927.
33. Schroeder, W. F.: Facet arthrography: Diagnosis and treatment. Orthop. Trans. 8:439–440, 1984.
34. Smith, G., and Covino, B. (eds.): Acute Pain. London, Butterworths, 1985.
35. Sunderland, S.: Nerve and Nerve Injuries, 2nd Ed. New York, Churchill Livingstone, 1978.

36. van Akkerveeken, P. F.: Lateral stenosis of the lumbar spine. Thesis at the University of Utrecht, 1989 (in press).
37. Verbiest, H.: Echte en schijnbare lumbo-sacrale pijn. Ned. Tijdschr. Geneesk. 106:2561–2569, 1962.
38. Verbiest, H.: Neurogenic Intermittent Claudication. Amsterdam, North-Holland Elsevier, 1976.
39. Wall, P. D., and Melzack, R. (eds.): Textbook of Pain. Edinburgh, Churchill Livingstone, 1984.
40. Watkins, R. G., Collis, J. S. Jr.: Lumbar Discectomy and Laminectomy. Rockville, Maryland, Aspen Publications, 1987, p. 37.
41. Wiesel, S. W., et al.: The incidence of positive CAT-scans in an asymptomatic group of patients. Spine 9:549–552, 1984.

■ ETIOLOGY OF SCIATICA*

Björn L. Rydevik

The nerve roots in the lumbar spine are often involved in disease processes and injuries, such as disc herniation, spinal stenosis, and vertebral fractures. Under such conditions, the nerve roots can be mechanically deformed by the surrounding tissue components, often resulting in various degrees of neurologic deficit and/or pain. The mechanical compression may lead to a series of intraneural tissue reactions, including edema formation, demyelination, and fibrosis. However, the correlation between such tissue changes and functional disorders remains incompletely understood. In the following text, some problems related to the etiology of sciatica will be discussed.

STRUCTURE AND FUNCTION OF NERVE ROOTS

The spinal nerve roots constitute the anatomic and physiologic connection between the central and peripheral nervous systems (Fig. 1). The nerve roots within the spinal column are not homogeneous structures like the peripheral nerves. A given nerve root has certain structural characteristics when it is located in the cauda equina and other anatomic features at its location in the lateral nerve root canal (Fig. 2*A*,*B*). At this latter location, each nerve root is surrounded by the dural sleeve, within which is a motor root, a sensory root, and a dorsal root ganglion (Fig. 2*B*,*C*). Thus, pathologic processes impinging upon nerve roots in disorders such as central spinal stenosis and disc herniation involve anatomically different components of neural tissue.

Nerve Fibers

The nerve roots, spinal nerves, and peripheral nerves contain various parts of the long cellular extensions from the nerve cell bodies, which are located in the anterior horn of the spinal cord (motor neurons) or in the dorsal root ganglia (sensory neurons) (Fig. 1). These cellular extensions, the axons, may be more than 100 cm long. This is a remarkable length, considering the size of the nerve cell body, which usually is about 100 μm. Changing to a larger scale more dramatically demonstrates this relative length; a nerve cell body 100 cm in diameter would have an axon about 10 cm in diameter and an axonal length in the range of 10 km. The function of the axons is not only to conduct impulses, but also to serve as transport medium for proteins and other essential substances, which are synthesized in the nerve cell bodies. This transferal of material is maintained by the axonal transport systems. These systems carry proteins and organelles from the centrally located place of synthesis to the periphery (anterograde axonal transport) and also in the opposite direction (retrograde axonal transport). Two main phases of anterograde axonal transport have been identified: slow and fast axonal transport.

Slow anterograde axonal transport takes place at a velocity of 1 to 6 mm/day. By means of this component, mainly cytoskeletal elements, such as microtubuli and microfilaments, are transported. Fast anterograde axonal transport takes place at speeds of up to about 400 mm/day and involves

*This review is in part based on work supported by the Swedish Medical Research Council (No. 8685) and the Swedish Medical Society.

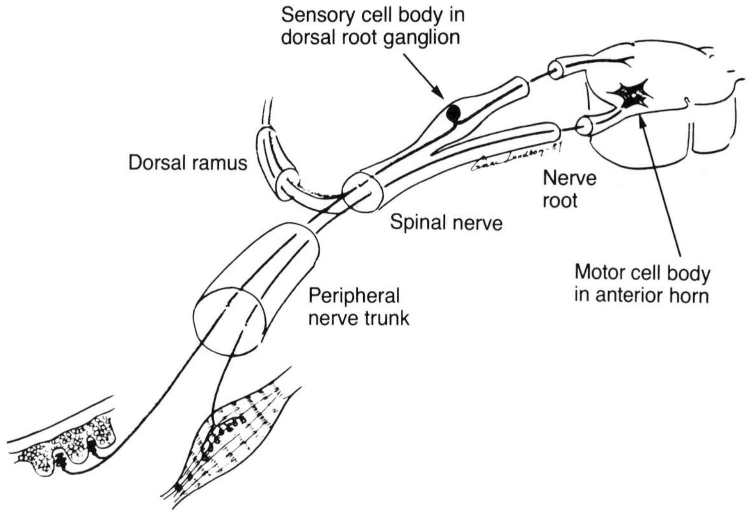

Figure 1 □ Schematic drawing shows the anatomic arrangement of nerve roots, spinal nerve, and peripheral nerve, including target organs for innervation by sensory and motor neurons. From Rydevik, B., Brown, M.D., and Lundborg, G.: Pathoanatomy and pathophysiology of nerve root compression. Spine 9:7–15, 1984.

glycoproteins, lipids, and transmitter substance vesicles as well as various enzymes.[4, 5, 13, 19, 23, 50] Interference with axonal transport as a result of, for example, nerve root compression may deplete the distal parts of the axons of proteins and other essential components.[34]

Connective Tissue

In peripheral nerves, the nerve fibers are located in the endoneurium (endoneurial space), inside the perineurium that surrounds each nerve fascicle (Fig. 3*A*). This sheath has considerable mechanical

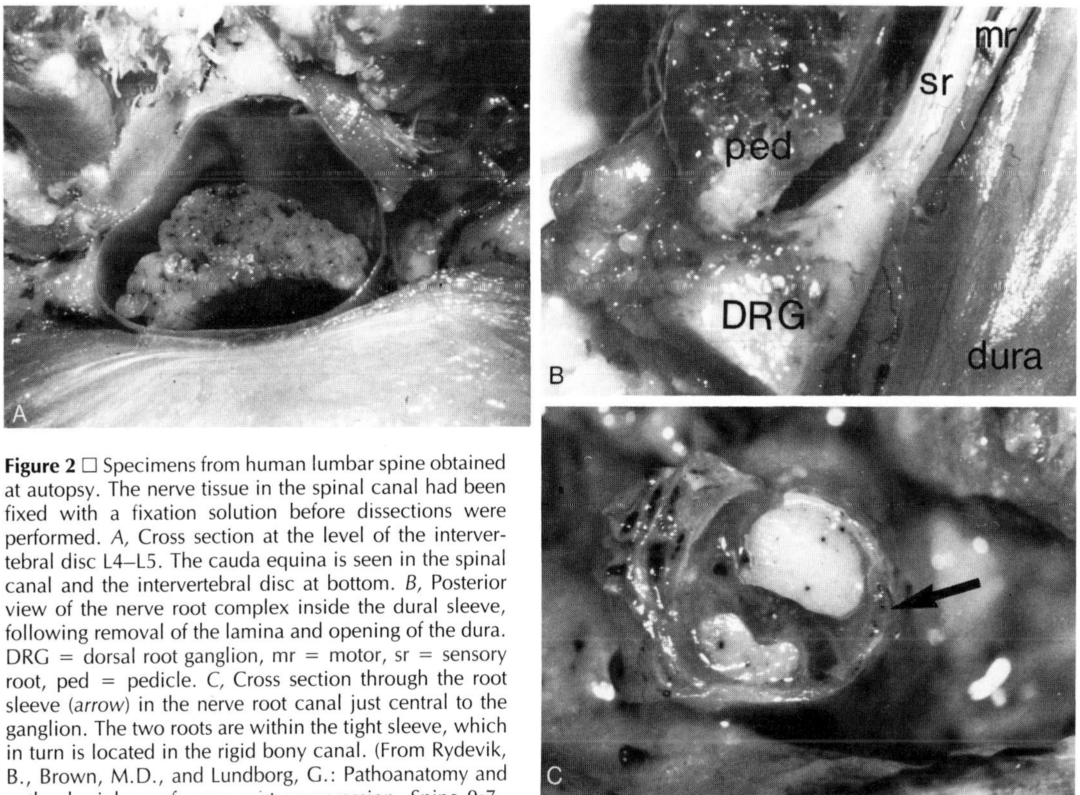

Figure 2 □ Specimens from human lumbar spine obtained at autopsy. The nerve tissue in the spinal canal had been fixed with a fixation solution before dissections were performed. *A,* Cross section at the level of the intervertebral disc L4–L5. The cauda equina is seen in the spinal canal and the intervertebral disc at bottom. *B,* Posterior view of the nerve root complex inside the dural sleeve, following removal of the lamina and opening of the dura. DRG = dorsal root ganglion, mr = motor, sr = sensory root, ped = pedicle. *C,* Cross section through the root sleeve (*arrow*) in the nerve root canal just central to the ganglion. The two roots are within the tight sleeve, which in turn is located in the rigid bony canal. (From Rydevik, B., Brown, M.D., and Lundborg, G.: Pathoanatomy and pathophysiology of nerve root compression. Spine 9:7–15, 1984.

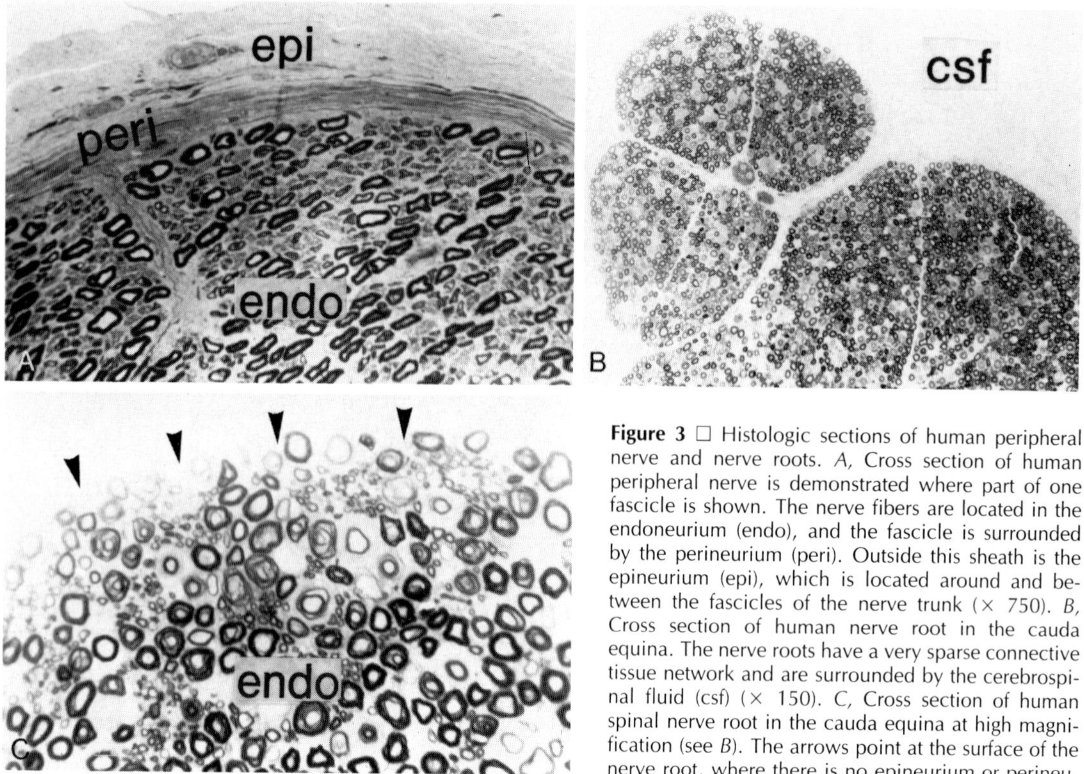

Figure 3 □ Histologic sections of human peripheral nerve and nerve roots. *A,* Cross section of human peripheral nerve is demonstrated where part of one fascicle is shown. The nerve fibers are located in the endoneurium (endo), and the fascicle is surrounded by the perineurium (peri). Outside this sheath is the epineurium (epi), which is located around and between the fascicles of the nerve trunk (× 750). *B,* Cross section of human nerve root in the cauda equina. The nerve roots have a very sparse connective tissue network and are surrounded by the cerebrospinal fluid (csf) (× 150). *C,* Cross section of human spinal nerve root in the cauda equina at high magnification (see *B*). The arrows point at the surface of the nerve root, where there is no epineurium or perineurium. The irregularities seen in the myelin sheaths of some nerve fibers are probably attributable to postmortem changes (× 750). (From Rydevik, B., Brown, M.D., and Lundborg, G.: Pathoanatomy and pathophysiology of nerve root compression. Spine 9:7–15, 1984).

strength, and it also possesses certain diffusion barrier properties.[14, 27, 33, 39] The nerve roots in the cauda equina are devoid of perineurium (Fig. 3*B*) and have a very loose, thin "epineurial" layer, which corresponds to the pia layer of the spinal cord. However, the nerve roots are surrounded by the cerebrospinal fluid, the arachnoid membrane, and the dura (Fig. 3C). These structures act together with the bony components of the spinal column to mechanically protect the nerve roots from external trauma. Furthermore, the cerebrospinal fluid seems to play a role in nutrition for the nerve roots in the cauda equina (see below).

Because of the lack of perineurium and significant epineurium, the nerve roots in the cauda equina would probably be more functionally susceptible to deterioration under certain degrees of mechanical deformation than would the peripheral nerves. Within the lateral nerve root canals, the sensory and motor roots for each level are adjacent to each other; the sensory root is dorsal to the motor root. Here the roots are surrounded by the root sleeve and other connective tissue components. The dura of the root sleeve is continuous with the epineurium in the peripheral nerves.[46, 47]

Blood Supply

The nerve roots, dorsal root ganglia, and spinal nerves receive their blood supply from segmental arteries entering the spinal nerve lateral to the foramen and from central arteries coursing caudally from the spinal cord.[29, 30] These vessels in the nerve roots form an intraneural microvascular system with some anatomic characteristics. Parke and coworkers[29, 30] have shown that, in a region of relative hypovascularity in the nerve roots in the cauda equina, these two vascular supply systems approach each other. Furthermore, it has been shown that the number of microvessels per unit cross-sectional area of the lumbar nerve roots is lower than the number of microvessels in human peripheral nerves.[30] Studies of the nutritional mechanisms of spinal nerve roots indicate that the cerebrospinal fluid may serve as a nutritional transport medium for the nerve root tissue.[9, 35] Thus, the intrathecal parts of the nerve roots seem to have dual nutritional pathways, which are as follows: (1) via the intraneural microvessels and (2) via diffusion from the cerebrospinal fluid.

The blood supply to the dorsal root ganglia is different from that to other parts of the nerve roots in that the ganglia have a very rich microvascular network.[1] Moreover, the blood vessels in the ganglia are more permeable to proteins, for example, than are the intraneural blood vessels at other levels of the nerve roots and peripheral nerves.[1, 28] The rich vascular supply and higher vascular permeability of the microvessels in the ganglia may reflect the greater metabolic demand at this level; here are sensory nerve cell bodies that synthesize, for example, proteins that supply the entire neuron.

BIOMECHANICAL ASPECTS OF NERVE ROOT DEFORMATION

Mechanical deformation of nerve roots in association with disc herniation, for example, can result in a variety of clinical symptoms. Deformation characteristics, as well as critical limits for compression and tension, are not well defined. This is partly attributed to the fact that the mechanical properties of the nerve roots and their various components are incompletely known and defined. Also, the mechanical strength of the attachment of nerve roots to the surrounding tissues is incompletely known. Some of the data available in the literature regarding these issues is summarized here.

Mechanical Properties of Nerve Roots

The length of the nerve roots from the spinal cord to the intervertebral foramina varies from about 60 mm (L1) to about 170 mm (S1).[45] As stated above, the nerve roots in the central spinal canal lack epineurium, but with tensile loading they show both elasticity and tensile strength properties.[44] The values for ultimate load at failure for human anterior spinal nerve roots from the central spinal canal are between 2 and 22 newtons (N) and, for posterior nerve roots from the central spinal canal, between 5 and 33 N.[44, 46] The mechanical properties of human spinal nerve roots have recently been shown to be different for L5 and S1 nerve roots when they are located in the central spinal canal and when the same nerve root is located in the lateral nerve root canals. The ultimate load for the intrathecal portion of the S1 nerve root was found to be about 13 N and, for the foraminal portion of the same root, about 73 N. For human L5 nerve roots the corresponding values were found to be 16 N and 71 N, respectively.[11]

Thus, the foraminal segments of the nerve roots showed values for the ultimate load approximately five times higher than those for the intrathecal portion of the same nerve root under tensile loading. However, the cross-sectional area of the nerve root in the intervertebral foramen is significantly larger than that of the same nerve root in the thecal sac, and thereby the values for ultimate tensile stress were of more comparable magnitude for the two nerve root locations.

Motion of Spinal Nerve Roots

The nerve roots in the spine are not static structures; they move relative to the surrounding tissues with every spinal movement. In order to allow for such motion, there must be a gliding capacity of the nerve roots in the nerve root canals. The normal range of movements of nerve roots in the human lumbar spine has been measured in cadaver experiments.[8] It was found that with straight-leg raising, the nerve roots at the level of the nerve root canals move approximately 2 to 5 mm.

Chronic tissue irritation with fibrosis around the nerve roots, in association with a disorder such as disc herniation and/or lateral canal stenosis might result in impaired gliding capacity of the nerve roots with repeated "microstretching" injuries of the nerve roots, even during normal spinal movement. Thus, a vicious circle of continued tissue irritation in the nerve root components may be initiated.

Nerve Root Deformation Due to Disc Herniation

When a nerve root is deformed by a protruding portion of an intervertebral disc, there is a unilateral compression of nerve root tissue. Thus, the situation is different from nerve entrapments such as the carpal tunnel syndrome, in which the pressure is presumably applied in a more circumferential manner to the nerve tissue. In patients with nerve root compression by disc herniation, the deformation characteristics may be divided into two components: (1) local compression at area of contact and (2) intraneural tension in the nerve root segments extending above and below the area of contact.

The local compression is likely to mechanically deform all the tissue components (i.e., nerve fibers, connective tissue, and intraneural blood vessels). In cases of local compression, the nerve fibers are displaced from the center of the compressed area toward the noncompressed areas. This longitudinal displacement is maximal at the edges of the compressed segment[22, 33, 38] and may be called "the edge effect" (Fig. 4). At the edges, where the mechanical deformation is maximal, the damage to both nerve fibers and intraneural microvessels is most pronounced. Tissue damage does not occur where the hydrostatic pressure in the nerve tissue is the highest (i.e., in the center).

Unilateral compression of a nerve root in patients with disc herniation may induce intraneural tension, because the nerve roots are normally adherent to the surrounding tissues above and below each intervertebral disc.[36, 42, 43] Experimentally, it has been noted that this tension, as well as the contact force between the disc herniation and the nerve root, is lowered if the disc height is reduced.[43] These observations might explain some of the sciatic pain relief that has followed chemonucleolysis and possibly the "spontaneous" relief of sciatic pain over time as disc herniation progresses and disc height decreases.[43]

Nerve root deformation in association with disc herniation is a complex phenomenon for which only sparse data are available and for which the correlation between the mechanical nerve root deformation and physiologic changes including pain production are incompletely known.

BIOLOGIC EFFECTS OF NERVE ROOT COMPRESSION

Mechanical deformation of the nerve root tissue can induce a series of intraneural tissue reactions, which may, in turn, induce neurologic deficit and/or pain. A rather limited amount of information has been available in the literature regarding the effects of local compression on spinal nerve roots in

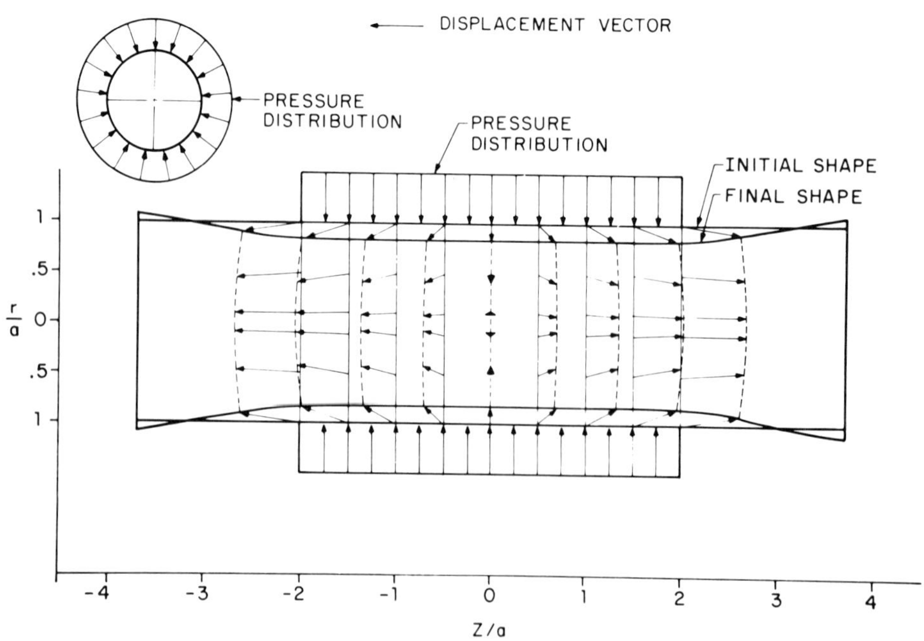

Figure 4 □ Theoretic displacement field under a pressure cuff applied to a model cylindric nerve with the radius A. Displacement in radial (r) and longitudinal (z) directions are computed on the basis of isotropic material properties and elastic series, so the deformation is proportional to the pressure. Note that the displacement is maximal at the edges of the compressed segment. (From Rydevik, B.L., Lundborg, G., and Skalak, R.: Biomechanics of peripheral nerves. *In*: Frankel, V.H., Nordin, M. [eds]: Basic Biomechanics of the Musculo-Skeletal System, 2nd Ed. Philadelphia, Lea & Febiger, 1988 [in press].)

vivo. Previous neurophysiologic studies[6, 40] indicate that nerve roots may be more susceptible to compression than are peripheral nerves. However, no critical pressure limits for various changes in nerve roots during compression were identified as they have been for peripheral nerves. Neurophysiologic effects of mechanical deformation on chronically injured nerve roots have been analyzed.[10]

Certain data regarding the biologic effects of nerve root compression have been obtained in a porcine model, in which the nerve roots in the cauda equina were subjected to graded compression in vivo.[25, 31, 38] Using this model, the effects of various pressure levels on nerve root blood flow, solute transport to the nerve root tissue, and impulse conduction and structural properties have been analyzed. It has been found that even a slight compression of the nerve roots (about 5 to 10 mmHg) can induce pronounced changes of venous congestion in the intraneural microcirculation.[25] Total ischemia in the compressed nerve root segments is induced at about 130 mmHg compression in this model, a pressure level that correlates well with the mean arterial blood pressure of the experimental animal. Analysis of the transport of H3 labeled methylglucose to the nerve root tissue during graded compression showed that there was about 45% reduction of the solute transport to the nerve roots at 10 mmHg compression.[24] Intraneural edema, as seen in the fluorescence microscope by extravasation of Evans-blue–labeled albumin, was induced after compression at 50 mmHg for only 2 minutes.[26] However, if the pressure on the nerve roots was applied slowly, the intraneural edema formation was not as pronounced. Electrophysiologic analyses in this model showed that compression at 50 mmHg as well as sham application of the compression device for 2 hours induced no significant changes in motor or sensory nerve root conduction. On the other hand, compression at 100 mmHg during 2 hours induced a more pronounced impairment of impulse conduction in sensory nerve roots (75% reduction of the recorded compound nerve action potential amplitude) than it did in motor nerve roots (45% reduction of the recorded electromyogram [EMG] amplitude).[31] The analyses also indicate that the impulse conduction in motor nerve roots recovered faster and more completely than in the sensory roots, following pressure release.

The observations indicate that local compression of the cauda equina induces a more pronounced deterioration of sensory nerve root function than of motor nerve root function. Furthermore, the impairment of the nutritional supply to the nerve root tissue in the cauda equina, in regard to reduced solute transport to the roots and impaired intraneural blood flow, can be acutely affected at low levels of pressure (i.e., 10 to 20 mmHg). Long-standing compression of nerve roots at these or greater pressure levels may, therefore, lead to a reduction of the nutritional supply to the nerve fibers and possibly an accumulation of waste products within the nerve root tissue. These factors may cause various kinds and degrees of functional changes, including pain.

PAIN MECHANISMS

Back and nerve root pain in connection with disc herniation and nerve root compression have an unclear pathophysiologic basis. Acute compression of a normal peripheral nerve does not cause pain, but rather numbness, paresthesia, motor weakness, and related signs and symptoms. This is seen in common situations such as when the peroneal nerve is compressed during sitting with crossed legs. Experimental investigations on compression of the human medial nerve in the carpal canal in vivo indicate that the induced numbness results from ischemia, not from mechanical nerve fiber deformation of the compressed nerve segment.[15] Mechanical deformation of normal spinal nerve roots seems to induce similar sensory and motor symptoms without associated pain.[16, 41] The observations regarding the reaction of human spinal nerve roots to compression were obtained by placing sutures or inflatable balloons close to nerve roots at the time of laminectomy. Postoperatively, mechanical deformation of normal nerve roots primarily induced numbness and paresthesia, but if the nerve roots had been compressed by a herniated disc before this test was performed (i.e., if the root was irritated), even minimal mechanical deformation resulted in reproduction of the sciatic pain.[16, 41] Brown and coworkers[3] have reported that compressed nerve roots in patients undergoing laminectomy and disc excision under epidural anesthesia are very sensitive to mechanical manipulation. These authors described that, although all tissues in the lumbar spine were well anesthetized, even careful retraction of an inflamed nerve root caused radiating leg pain. Such observations of humans correlate well with data from experimental investigations on the neurophysiologic response of normal versus inflamed nerves and nerve roots.[10] It seems, therefore, that inflammation of the nerve root tissue is a significant factor that has to be present in order for mechanical nerve root deformation to induce radiating pain.

Several questions arise regarding possible causes of intraneural and extraneural inflammation as well as the histologic and biochemical characteristics of such inflammation. Furthermore, can such inflammation be treated? Obviously, mechanical factors such as compression and/or traction and irritation of the nerve roots can induce the sequence of tissue reactions in the nerve roots, which leads to intraneural inflammation. The exact nature of the inflammation is not known. It is likely to be characterized by edema, inflammatory cell reaction, and probably segmental demyelination of the nerve fibers.

It has been proposed that certain biochemical mechanisms, as well as mechanical factors, may be involved in the production of nerve root inflammation. Breakdown products from degenerating nucleus pulposus tissue might leak into the epidural space and induce a "chemical radiculitis" along the nerve root.[17, 18] Intraoperative measurements of pH in the nucleus pulposus at the level of disc herniation have demonstrated low pH values, particularly in patients who had extensive adhesion formations around the nearby nerve root.[20, 21] These observations indicate a possible chemical interaction between the degenerating intervertebral disc and the nerve root that courses over it. Such "radiculitis" may be initiated by directly irritating effects of proteoglycans from the disc[17] and/or by an autoimmune reaction from exposure to disc tissues.[2, 7] However, no conclusive experimental or clinical studies are available to demonstrate that these mechanisms actually exist at the tissue level. On the other hand, current knowledge does not exclude the possibility that chemical irritation of nerve roots by disc degeneration may be significant in the pathophysiology of nerve root pain.[34] If such chemical mechanisms are found to be important in the pathogenesis of nerve root pain, a better understanding of their development and prevention might lead to the development of new and improved treatment modalities. Perhaps certain pharmacologic substances that would interfere with the chemical nerve root irritation could be obtained.

Dorsal Root Ganglion

Dorsolateral disc herniations in the lumbar spine often impinge upon the dorsal root ganglion (DRG) of the nerve roots.[12] These observations are interesting in relation to more recent experimental studies, which show that compression of normal DRG may produce a neurophysiologic response, corresponding to the neural activity induced when an irritated nerve or nerve root is compressed.[10] Thus, there are reasons to believe that the compression of a normal DRG, as distinct from the compression of a normal spinal nerve more proximally, may induce radiating pain. Recent investigations by Weinstein and coworkers[48, 49] have indicated a possible role of neuropeptides, such as substance P and vasoactive intestinal peptides (VIP) in the DRG, in the production of low back pain.

CONCLUDING REMARKS

The tissue reactions that occur in nerve roots in association with mechanical compression, such as disc herniation, have a complex basis that involves mechanical and possibly certain biomechanical factors. The functional changes in the nerve roots may be of two different modalities: (1) loss of nerve function, which is seen as sensory deficit and/or muscle weakness and (2) hypersensitivity of the nerve tissue (Fig. 5). The latter phenomenon implies that the nerve root tissue is easily excited to generate impulses by further mechanical stimulus and the nerve roots thus become the site of ectopic impulse generation,[32] which may be related to pain.[10] The two kinds of functional changes (loss of nerve function and hyperexcitability) can be present simultaneously; that is, the involved nerve roots demonstrate impaired electrophysiologic parameters in regard to blocked impulse transmission in nerve fibers and/or decreased conduction velocity at the site of injury, although they

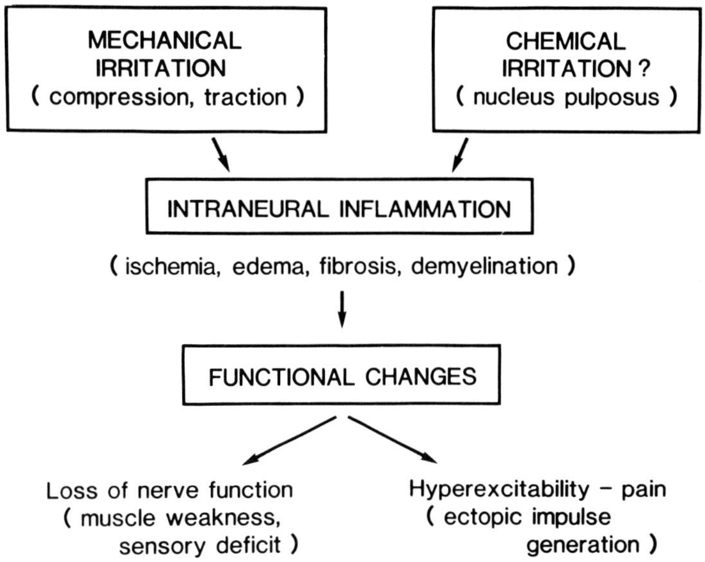

Figure 5 □ Proposed sequence of events leading to nerve root involvement in connection with disc herniation (i.e., sciatica). Mechanical, and possibly chemical, irritation may lead to intraneural inflammation, which in turn may induce various functional changes. Note that loss of nerve function is distinct from hyperexcitability. (From Rydevik, B., and Garfin, S.: Spinal nerve root compression. *In* Szabo, R.M. (ed.): Nerve Compression Syndromes—Diagnosis and Treatment. Thorofare, NJ, Charles B. Slack, Inc., 1989.)

remain hypersensitive to further mechanical stimulus at the injured segments. Clinically, the loss of nerve function can be assessed by analyzing EMG abnormalities and impaired sensory nerve conduction. However, these neurophysiologic phenomena may not necessarily correlate with the degree of nerve root pain experienced by the patient. The neurophysiologic evaluation merely supplies information about whether a nerve root is "affected" and allows only certain degrees of quantification of such involvement. Moreover, there are no experimental data regarding the possible correlation between a loss of nerve conduction, and hyperexcitability in association with nerve root injury induced by a disorder such as disc herniation.

References

1. Arvidson, B.: Distribution of intravenously injected protein tracers in peripheral ganglia of adult mice. Exp. Neurol. 63:388–410, 1979.
2. Bobechko, W. P., and Hirsch, C.: Auto-immune response to nucleus pulposus in the rabbit. J. Bone Joint Surg. 47B:574–580, 1965.
3. Brown, M. D., Gepstein, R., and Pallares, V.: Somatosensory evoked potentials during epidural anaesthesia. 32nd Annual Meeting Orthopaedic Research Society (Trans.), New Orleans, Feb., 1986.
4. Dahlström, A.: Axoplasmic transport (with particular respect to adrenergic neurons). Philos. Trans. R. Soc. Lond. (Biol.) 261:325–358, 1971.
5. Droz, B.: Synthetic machinery and axoplasmic transport: Maintenance of neuronal connectivity. *In* Tower DB (ed.): The Nervous System, Vol. 1. The Basic Neurosciences. New York, Raven Press, 1975, pp. 111–127.
6. Gelfan, S., and Tarlov, J. M.: Physiology of spinal cord, nerve root, and peripheral nerve compression. Am. J. Physiol. 185:217–229, 1956.
7. Gertzbein, S. D., Tile, M., Gross, A., and Falk, R.: Auto-immunity in degenerative disc disease of the lumbar spine. Orthop. Clin. North Am. 6:67–73, 1975.
8. Goddard, M. D., and Reid, J. D.: Movements induced by straight leg raising in the lumbo-sacral roots, nerves and plexus, and in the intrapelvic section of the sciatic nerve. J. Neurol. Psychiatr. 28:12–18, 1965.
9. Holm, S., and Rydevik, B. L.: Nutrition of spinal nerve roots—quantification of the contribution from intraneural microvessels and cerebrospinal fluid (to be published 1989).
10. Howe, J. F., Loeser, J. D., and Calvin, W. H.: Mechanosensitivity of dorsal root ganglia and chronically injured axons: A physiological basis for the radicular pain of nerve root compression. Pain 3:25–41, 1977.
11. Kwan, M., Rydevik, B., Brown, R., et al.: Selected biomechanical properties of lumbosacral nerve roots. Proc. Internat. Soc. Lumbar Spine, Miami, Apr., 1988.
12. Lindblom, K., and Rexed, B.: Spinal nerve injury in dorso-lateral protrusions of lumbar discs. J. Neurosurg. 5:413–432, 1948.
13. Lubinska, L.: Axoplasmic streaming in regenerating and in normal nerve fibres. Prog. Brain Res. 13:1–71, 1964.
14. Lundborg, G., Nordborg, G., Rydevik, B. L., and Olsson, Y.: The effect of ischemia on the permeability of the perineurium to protein tracers in rabbit tibial nerve. Acta Neurol. Scand. 49:287–294, 1973.
15. Lundborg, G., Gelbermann, R., Minteer-Convery, M., et al.: Median nerve compression in the carpal tunnel: The functional response to experimentally induced controlled pressure. J. Hand Surg. 7:252–259, 1982.
16. Macnab, I.: The mechanism of spondylogenic pain. *In* Hirsch, C., and Zotterman, Y. (eds.): Cervical Pain. New York, Pergamon Press, 1972, pp. 89–95.

17. Marshall, L. L., and Trethewie, E. R.: Chemical irritation of nerve root in disc prolapse. Lancet 2:320, 1973.
18. Marshall, L. L., Trethewie, E. R., and Curtain, C. C.: Chemical radiculitis—A clinical, physiological and immunological study. Clin. Orthop. Rel. Res. 129:61–67, 1977.
19. McLean, W. G., McKay, A. L., and Sjöstrand, J.: Electrophoretic analysis of axonally transported proteins in rabbit vagus nerve. J. Neurobiol. 14:227–236, 1983.
20. Nachemson, A.: Intradiscal measurements of pH in patients with lumbar rhizopathies. Acta Orthop. Scand. 40:23–42, 1969.
21. Nachemson, A.: The lumbar spine—an orthopaedic challenge. Spine 1:59–71, 1976.
22. Ochoa, J., Fowler, T. J., and Gilliatt, R. W.: Anatomical changes in peripheral nerves compressed by a pneumatic tourniquet. J. Anat. 113:433–455, 1972.
23. Ochs, S.: Axoplasmic transport. *In* Tower, D. (ed.): The Nervous System, Vol. 1. The Basic Neurosciences. New York, Raven Press, 1975, pp. 137–146.
24. Olmarker, K., Holm, S., Hansson, T., and Rydevik, B.: Experimental graded compression of the cauda equina: Effects on nerve root nutrition. Proc. Internat. Soc. Lumbar Spine, Dallas, May, 1986.
25. Olmarker, K., Rydevik, B. L., Holm, S., et al: Graded compression of the porcine cauda equina modifies nerve root nutrition, blood flow and impulse conduction. 33rd Annual Meeting, Orthopaedic Research Society (Trans.), San Francisco, 1987.
26. Olmarker, K., Rydevik, B. L., Holm, S.: Intraneural edema formation in spinal nerve roots of the porcine cauda equina induced by experimental, graded compression. 34th Annual Meeting, Orthopaedic Research Society (Trans.), Atlanta, 1988.
27. Olsson, Y., Kristensson, K., and Klatzo, I.: Permeability of connective tissue sheaths in the peripheral nervous system to exogenous proteins. Acta Neuropath. (Berl.) 5(Suppl.):61–69, 1971.
28. Olsson, Y.: Vascular permeability in the peripheral nervous system. *In* Dyck, P. J., Thomas, P. K., Lambert, E. H., and Bunge, R. P. (eds.): Peripheral Neuropathy, Vol. 1. Philadelphia, W. B. Saunders, 1984, pp. 579–598.
29. Parke, W. W., Gamell, K., and Rothman, R. H.: Arterial vascularization of the cauda equina. J. Bone Joint Surg. 63A:53–62, 1981.
30. Parke, W. W., and Watanabe, R.: The intrinsic vasculature of the lumbosacral spinal nerve roots. Spine 10:508–515, 1985.
31. Pedowitz, R. A., Rydevik, B. L., Hargens, A. R., et al.: Motor and sensory nerve root conduction deficit induced by acute graded compression of the pig cauda equina. 34th Annual Meeting, Orthopaedic Research Society (Trans.), Atlanta, 1988.
32. Rasminsky, M.: Ectopic generation of impulses in pathological nerve fibers. *In* Jewett, D. L., and McCarroll, H. R. (eds.): Nerve Repair and Regeneration—Its Clinical and Experimental Basis. St. Louis, CV Mosby, 1980, pp. 178–185.
33. Rydevik, B., and Lundborg, G.: Permeability of intraneural microvessels and perineurium following acute, graded experimental nerve compression. Scand. J. Plast. Reconstr. Surg. 11:179–187, 1977.
34. Rydevik, B. L., Brown, M. D., Ehira, T., et al.: Effects of graded compression and nucleus pulposus on nerve tissue—an experimental study in rabbits. Acta Orthop. Scand. 54:670–671, 1983.
35. Rydevik, B. L., Holm, S., Brown, M. D., and Lundborg, G.: Nutrition of spinal nerve roots. 30th Annual Meeting, Orthopaedic Research Society, Atlanta, Feb., 1984.
36. Rydevik, B. L., Brown, M. D., and Lundborg, G.: Pathoanatomy and pathophysiology of nerve root compression. Spine 9:7–15, 1984.
37. Rydevik, B., Pedowitz, R. A., Garfin, S. R., et al.: Effects of graded compression on function and structure of sensory and motor nerve roots. An experimental study on the porcine cauda equina (to be published, 1989).
38. Rydevik, B. L., Lundborg, G., and Skalak, R.: Biomechanics of peripheral nerves. *In* Nordin, M., and Frankel, V. (eds.): Basic Biomechanics of the Musculoskeletal System, 2nd Ed. Philadelphia, Lea & Febiger, 1989.
39. Shanta, T. R., and Bourne, G. Gh.: The peripheral epithelium—a new concept. *In* Bourne, G. H. (ed.): Structure and Function of Nervous Tissue, Vol. 1. Structure. London, Academic Press, 1969, pp. 379–459.
40. Sharpless, S. K.: Susceptibility of spinal nerve roots to compression block. *In* Goldstein, M. (ed.): The Research Status of Spinal Manipulative Therapy. N.I.H. Workshop, Feb. 2–4, N.I.N.C.D.S. Monograph No. 15, 1975, pp. 155–161.
41. Smyth, M. J., and Wright, V.: Sciatica and the intervertebral disc. An experimental study. J. Bone Joint Surg. 40A:1401–1418, 1958.
42. Spencer, D. L., Irwin, G. S., and Miller, J. A. A.: Anatomy and significance of fixation of the lumbosacral nerve roots in sciatica. Spine 8:672–679, 1983.
43. Spencer, D. L., Miller, J. A. A., and Bertolini, J. E.: The effects of intervertebral disc space narrowing on the contact force between the nerve root and a simulated disc protrusion. Spine 9:422–426, 1984.
44. Sunderland, S., and Bradley, K. C.: Stress-strain phenomena in human spinal nerve roots. Brain 84:120–124, 1961.
45. Sunderland, S.: Avulsion of nerve roots. *In* Vinken, P. J., and Bruyn, G. W. (eds.): Handbook of Clinical Neurology, Vol. 25. Injuries of the Spine and Spinal Cord. New York, American Elsevier, 1975, pp. 393–435.
46. Sunderland, S.: Nerves and Nerve Injuries, 2nd ed. New York, Churchill Livingstone, 1978.
47. Thomas, P. K., and Olsson, Y.: Microscopic anatomy and function of the connective tissue components of peripheral nerve. *In* Dyck, P. J., Thomas, P. K., Lambert, E. H., and Bunge, R. P. (eds.): Peripheral Neuropathy. Philadelphia, W. B. Saunders, 1984, pp. 97–120.
48. Weinstein, J. N.: Mechanisms of spinal pain: The dorsal root ganglion and its role as a mediator of low back pain. Spine 11:999–1001, 1986.
49. Weinstein, J., Pope, M., Schmidt, R., and Serrousi, R.: Effects of low frequency on the dorsal root ganglion. Neuro-Orthopaedics 4:24–30, 1987.
50. Weiss, D. G.: General properties of axoplasmic transport. *In* Weiss, D. G. (ed.): Axoplasmic Transport. Berlin, Springer-Verlag, 1982, pp. 1–14.

MECHANISMS OF NERVE ROOT COMPRESSION DUE TO A HERNIATED DISC

David L. Spencer

Sciatica due to a herniated lumbar intervertebral disc is one of the commonly recognized and diagnosed afflictions of the lumbar spine. Because it is such a common disorder, a large body of clinical experience has accumulated, focusing primarily on the natural history and the clinical course of the condition resulting from various treatment modalities. Surprisingly, little research has been done on the biomechanics of nerve root compression due to a disc herniation. Many of the well-recognized clinical characteristics of the disorder are perplexing; for example, spontaneous resolution of sciatic pain commonly occurs, even though there is no apparent diminution in the size of the disc herniation.[1] Recent interest in innovative nonsurgical treatment of sciatica due to a herniated disc (chemonucleolysis and percutaneous nuclectomy) has led to basic research into the mechanisms of nerve root compression due to a disc herniation that increases our understanding of the syndrome.

Experimental simulation of a disc herniation using an instrumented probe in fresh cadaver specimens has demonstrated that pressure can be applied to the extrathecal intraspinal nerve root* without compression against the posterior wall of the neural canal. Furthermore, experimental widening of the disc space at the level of the herniation increases the pressure, while narrowing the space decreases the pressure on the nerve root.[11] This means that when a disc herniation protrudes into the neural canal, displacing everything in its path as it must, the extrathecal intraspinal nerve root resists displacement. As a result, there is pressure on the nerve at the point of contact between the nerve root and the disc herniation, even though it is not compressed against the posterior wall of the neural canal. This implies that the extrathecal interspinal nerve root is fixed in its location in the neural canal. Specifically because of this fixation, the nerve root resists being displaced by a disc protrusion and becomes stretched over or around the disc herniation, producing compression of the nerve against the herniation by virtue of the tension in the nerve root without any impingement against the posterior wall of the neural canal. The nerve rootlets of the cauda equina inside the thecal sac cannot be stretched over or around a disc herniation and compressed against the disc herniation, unless direct impingement against the posterior wall of the neural canal occurs, because they lie loosely inside the thecal sac and can easily be displaced.

The extrathecal intraspinal nerve root is attached distally at its foraminal exit by radially directed fibers that suspend the nerve root from the walls of the foraminal exit. This suspension fixation has been likened to a membrane perforated in the center by the nerve root.[12] This fixation arrangement allows a finite amount of longitudinal translational movement of the nerve root in either direction, with a definite end point. Thus, traction on the lumbosacral plexus, for example, as during the straight-leg raising maneuver, can result in longitudinal translation of the nerve root inside the neural canal proximal to the foraminal attachments, as has been experimentally observed.[4]

The dural root sleeve of the extrathecal interspinal nerve root is proximally continuous with the main dural sac, which is attached proximally at the foramen magnum and distally at the filum terminale. The significance of this proximal fixation is demonstrated when flexion of the head and neck applies traction to the dural sac at its foramen magnum attachment. Traction is transmitted all the way down the inelastic dura caudally to the nerve root stretched over the disc herniation, increasing the tension in the

*The extrathecal intraspinal lumbar nerve root is defined as that portion of the nerve root and dural sleeve between the main dural sac and the foraminal exit.[3]

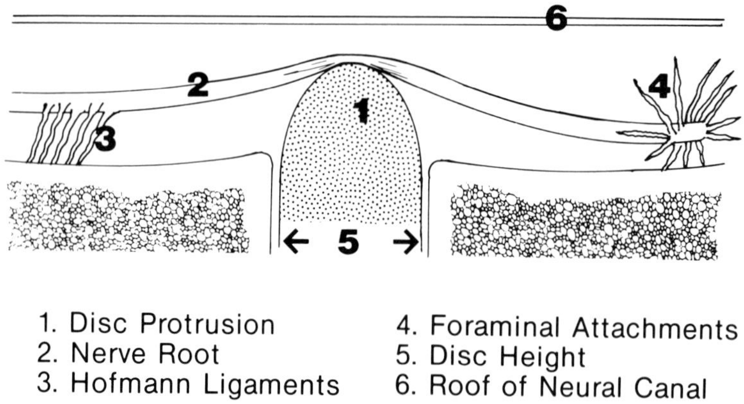

Figure 1 □ The nerve root is stretched over the disc herniation, not compressed against the posterior wall of the neural canal.

nerve root resulting in increased pressure on the nerve root and increased sciatic pain.

The extrathecal intraspinal nerve root is also attached ventrally to the neural canal by the Hofmann ligaments.[2] These ligaments are filamentous bands and are sometimes mesentery-like sheets that attach the dura of the nerve root and the main thecal sac to the posterior longitudinal ligament and posterior vertebral periosteum. There is considerable individual variability in the tenacity of these filamentous bands.[9] These ligaments are situated to resist dorsal displacement of the dura and the extrathecal interspinal nerve root within the neural canal.

In summary, the nerve rootlets of the cauda equina within the main dural sac are free to move about within the dural sac in the neural canal. On the other hand, the extrathecal interspinal nerve root is relatively fixed in its location in the neural canal. This means that when a disc herniation protrudes into the neural canal the extrathecal interspinal nerve root, because of its attachment, resists displacement. The nerve root is stretched over the prominence of the protrusion, resulting in pressure on the nerve without impingement against the posterior wall of the neural canal. The nerve rootlets of the cauda equina inside the main thecal sac are not subjected to pressure from the disc herniation protruding into the neural canal, unless the herniation is large enough or the canal small enough to compress the rootlets against the posterior wall of the neural canal. This compression of the nerve root against the disc herniation because of the tension of the nerve root is termed the TENSION mechanism of nerve root compression (Fig. 1). The second mechanism of nerve root compression by a disc herniation is, of course, direct impingement against the posterior wall of the neural canal. This obviously is the COMPRESSION mechanism (Fig. 2).

The nerve rootlets of the cauda equina, as has been pointed out, can be subjected to pressure from a disc herniation only by the COMPRESSION mechanism. The extrathecal interspinal nerve root, because of its fixation in the neural canal, can be subjected

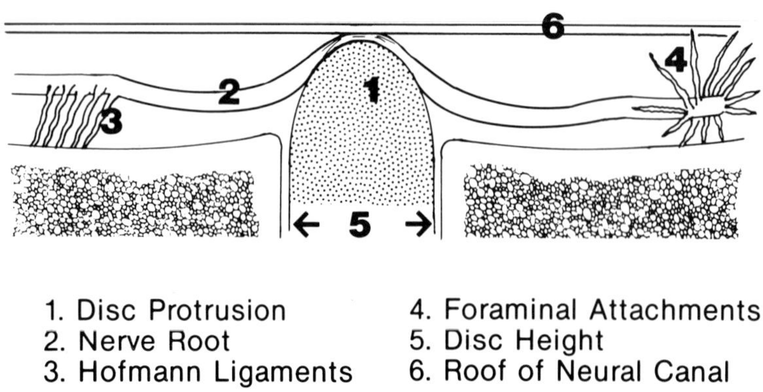

Figure 2 □ The nerve root is compressed against the posterior wall of the neural canal, not stretched over the disc herniation.

to pressure from a disc herniation by either the TENSION or the COMPRESSION mechanism, or both. In a neural canal of normal dimensions in a young individual who has no advanced degenerative disc disease, the nerve root is stretched over or around the disc herniation in a pure TENSION mechanism that applies pressure to the nerve root. In a neural canal of markedly diminished size, either congenital or due to advanced degenerative changes, the nerve root may be compressed against the posterior wall of the neural canal by the disc herniation with absolutely no tension in the nerve root—a pure COMPRESSION mechanism. Between these two extremes, depending on local anatomy, a combination of both mechanisms may apply.

Well-documented studies confirm that the clinical picture of sciatica due to a disc herniation varies depending upon the age of the patient.[8] In fact, it has been suggested that the syndrome is actually composed of two relatively distinct clinical subgroups: the young and the old.[5] The fundamental clinical finding that separates the two groups is the straight-leg raising (SLR) or tension test. In the young subgroup, the SLR test is characteristically markedly positive, whereas in the older group it may be negative. On closer scrutiny, other, more subtle, differences are found. The young subgroup frequently reports that the sciatic pain is most severe during sitting, less painful during recumbency, and least painful during standing or walking. The old subgroup frequently reports just the opposite, that is, relief during recumbency, minimal discomfort during sitting, and more severe pain during standing and walking.

Standard x-ray films of the lumbar spine characteristically show significantly more degeneration at the involved motion segment in the older subgroup, compared with the young. The CT scan in the young subgroup usually demonstrates a focal disc herniation without any associated spinal stenosis (Fig. 3). In the older group, the CT picture is more often less distinct with evidence of degenerative spinal stenosis and disc herniation (Fig. 4). The myelogram in both groups demonstrates a filling defect commensurate with the size of the disc herniation and the size of the neural canal at the level of the disc herniation. In a small or stenotic neural canal, a larger filling defect on myelogram is produced by an equivalent-sized disc herniation than in a larger canal.

Combining the young and the old clinical subgroups with the two mechanisms of

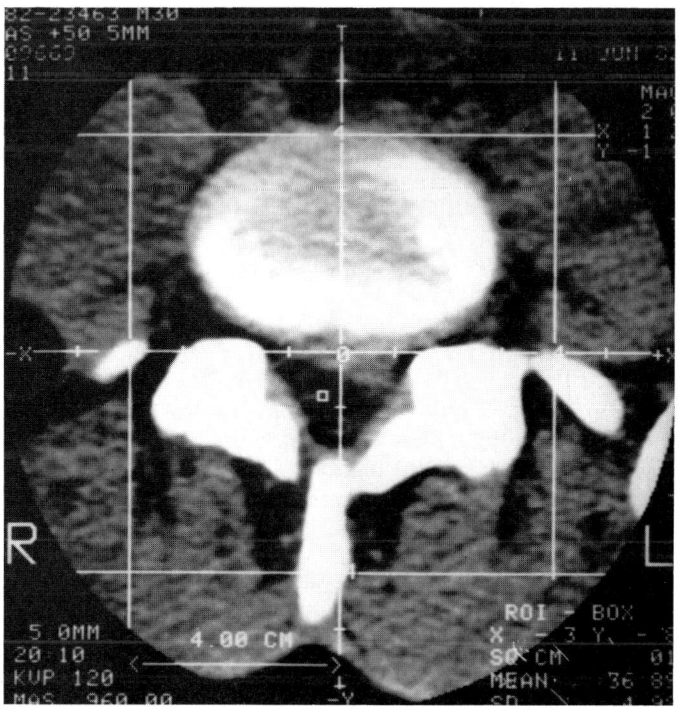

Figure 3 □ The nerve root is stretched over the disc herniation, not compressed against the posterior wall of the neural canal.

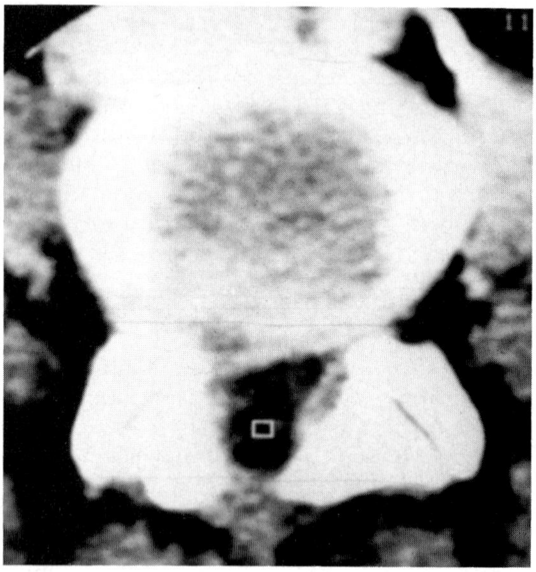

Figure 4 □ The nerve root is compressed against the posterior wall of the neural canal, not stretched over the disc herniation.

nerve root compression due to a disc herniation results in a consistent and logical conceptualization of the pathomechanics of nerve root compression due to disc herniation. The two distinct clinical subgroups of sciatica—the old subgroup with negative straight-leg raising and the young subgroup with prominently positive straight-leg raising—represent the two different mechanisms by which pressure can be exerted on the nerve by a disc herniation. The nerve can be directly compressed against the posterior wall of the neural canal by the disc herniation, which is COMPRESSION (the old subgroup). It can be stretched over or around the disc herniation without compression against the posterior wall of the neural canal, which is TENSION (the young subgroup). Obviously, the clinical picture of sciatica and the underlying pathomechanics is a continuum, extending from pure TENSION in the young to pure COMPRESSION in the old, and including a large number of combinations of both forms of pressure.

The typical patient in the young subgroup has sciatic pain, and a prominently positive SLR test, made worse by the lumbar flexion of sitting because the nerve root is stretched over or around the disc herniation and not compressed against the posterior wall of the neural canal.

The typical patient in the old subgroup has negative SLR and has no pain during sitting, but does have pain during standing and walking, because the nerve is compressed against the posterior wall of the stenotic neural canal by the disc herniation, with no nerve root tension.

Viscoelasticity is a fundamental property of biologic tissue, in general, and of collagen, in particular.[13] One could predict that spontaneous resolution of pressure on the nerve root, and thus resolution of sciatic pain due to disc herniation, would occur in the young subgroup more predictably than in the old subgroup, without any change in size of disc herniation, owing to the stress relaxation in the nerve root and its attachments. Clinical experience confirms this prediction.[8] In the old subgroup, in whom the nerve root is compressed against the posterior wall of the neural canal rather than stretched over the disc herniation, stress relaxation of the nerve root and its attachments does not occur, and, therefore, spontaneous reduction of the pressure on the nerve root and resolution of sciatic pain occurs less predictably than in the young subgroup.

In the young subgroup, any procedure or manipulation that reduces the tension in the nerve root stretched over the disc herniation results in a decrease in pressure on the nerve root and should result in a decrease in sciatic pain, even though the size of the disc herniation does not change. The converse is, of course, also true. Increased tension (the SLR test) results in greater pressure and more pain.

Since the axis of flexion and extension of the motion segment lies anterior to the disc herniation and nerve root,[13] flexion (sitting) should increase the pressure and pain, whereas extension (standing) should decrease the pressure and pain in the young subgroup.

Disc-space narrowing at the site of a disc herniation reduces the tension in the nerve root by reducing the distance traversed by the nerve root.[11] Chemonucleolysis has repeatedly been shown to decrease sciatic pain with no diminution in size of the disc herniation.[6] Clinical follow-up studies and serial lateral x-ray studies have shown that the sciatic pain gradually resolves and the SLR test returns toward normal over the same 6-week postchemonucleolysis interval during which the disc space narrowing occurs.[10] Obviously, if the nerve root is compressed against the posterior wall of the neural canal, as in the old subgroup, disc space narrowing would be of no benefit in resolving sciatic pain. Therefore, chemonucleolysis could be predicted to be less effective in the old subgroup, just as clinical experience has demonstrated.[7]

To the extent that any procedure produces disc-space narrowing (percutaneous nuclectomy) at the site of the disc herniation that is producing sciatic pain by virtue of tension in the nerve root and not compression against the posterior wall of the neural canal, it can be expected to reduce the pressure on the nerve root and reduce the sciatic pain without any change in the size of the disc herniation. On the other hand, in the old subgroup with compression of the nerve root against the posterior wall of the neural canal, disc-space narrowing cannot be expected to diminish the pressure on the nerve root and reduce sciatic pain.

Partial spontaneous resolution of sciatic pain may, in some patients, represent resolution of the TENSION component, owing to stress relaxation of the nerve root and its attachments, but persistence of the COMPRESSION component, which is unaffected by reduction in nerve root tension. Similarly, one would predict that the indirect techniques of reduction in nerve root pressure (chemonucleolysis and percutaneous nuclectomy) would produce a spectrum of results ranging from complete resolution of sciatic pain to no relief, depending on the underlying mechanism of nerve root compression.

In conclusion, there are two distinct and separate mechanisms whereby a disc herniation can apply pressure to the extrathecal interspinal nerve root: TENSION and COMPRESSION. Because of the fixation of the extrathecal interspinal nerve root, which resists nerve root displacement by the disc herniation, pressure can be applied to the nerve root by the herniation without compression against the posterior wall of the neural canal. These two mechanisms of nerve root compression explain many of the previously perplexing clinical observations, including the following: (1) spontaneous resolution of sciatic pain without a change in disc herniation size, (2) asymptomatic disc herniation, (3) resolution of sciatic pain by indirect methods that narrow the disc space but do not reduce disc herniation size, and (4) most importantly, the clinical observation that the syndrome of sciatica due to a disc herniation is a continuum of two separate subgroups (old and young) representing the two mechanisms of nerve root compression by a disc herniation.

References

1. Falconer, M. A., McGeorge, M., and Bogg, A. C.: Observations on the cause and mechanism of symptom-production in sciatica and low back pain. J. Neurol. Neurosurg. Psychiatr. 11:13–26, 1948.
2. Hofmann, M.: Die befestigung der dura Mater im Wirbelcanal. Arch. F. Anat. Physiol. (Anat. Abstract) 403, 1898.
3. Hollinshead, W. H.: Anatomy for Surgeons, Vol. 3. The Back and Limbs. New York, Harper & Row, 1969.
4. Inman, V. T., and Saunders, J. B. deC. M.: The Clinico-anatomical aspects of the lumbo-sacral region. Radiology 38:669, 1942.
5. Lipson, S. J., and Dassow-Warburg, R. G.: A Review of Clincal Signs in Low Back Pain with Sciatica Caused by Herniated Discs: Are There Two Groups Dependent Upon Age? Presented at the Annual Meeting of the International Society for the Study of the Lumbar Spine, Dallas, May, 1986.
6. Macnab, I.: Chemonucleolysis. Can. Med. Assoc. J. 14:280–289, 1971.
7. McCulloch, J. A., and Macnab, I.: Sciatica and Chymopapain. Baltimore, Williams and Wilkins, 1983.
8. Rothman, R., and Simeone, F.: The Spine, 2nd Ed., Philadelphia, W. B. Saunders, 1982.
9. Spencer, D. L., Irwin, G. S., and Miller, J. A. A.: Anatomy and significance of fixation of the lumbosacral nerve roots in sciatica. Spine 8:672–679, 1983.
10. Spencer, D. L., Watt, D., and Miller, J. A. A.: Chymopapain Chemonucleolysis: A Clinical Study of Results and Correlations with Size of Disc Protrusion and Post-Injection Disc Space Narrowing. Presented at the 51st Annual Meeting of the American Academy of Orthopaedic Surgeons, Atlanta, February, 1984.
11. Spencer, D. L., Miller, J. A. A., and Bertolini, J. E.: The effect of intervertebral disc space narrowing on the contact force between the nerve root and a simulated disc protrusion. Spine 9:422–426, 1984.
12. Testut, L., and Latarjet, A.: Traite d'anatomic humaine, Vol. 3. Paris, G. Doin et Cie, 1959.
13. White, A. A., and Paojabi, M.: Clinical Biomechanics of the Spine. Philadelphia, J. B. Lippincott, 1978.

■ CLINICAL NEUROPHYSIOLOGY AND ELECTRODIAGNOSTIC TESTING IN LOW BACK PAIN

Scott Haldeman

As in other fields of spine research, there has been a rapid expansion in the field formerly represented simply by electromyography. In the field of radiology, the reading of radiographs has been supplemented by the advanced techniques of myelography, computerized tomography (CT), magnetic resonance imaging (MRI), and various contrast studies to form the field of clinical imaging with its own subspecialization and skilled technical and interpretative requirements. In the same way, electromyography has been supplemented by a wide variety of electrodiagnostic tests such as evoked responses and reflex and nerve conduction studies. In addition, other techniques have been developed to measure neurologic function. Many of these techniques no longer use electric measurement and often look indirectly at the function of the nervous system through the measurement of end organ function. Thus, cystometry, colonometry, penile tumescence, thermography, galvanic skin response, and so forth, have been included in the potential armamentarium of the spine diagnostician. This has led to the evolution of electromyography and electrodiagnosis into the more complex and interesting field of "clinical neurophysiology."

The 1980s have seen the coming of age of the field of clinical neurophysiology. It is no longer adequate for a clinician to order an electromyographic examination and assume that he or she is fully cognizant of neurologic function of the lumbar spine any more than it would be sufficient to order a standard x-ray study and feel that he or she was fully cognizant of all the structural relationships and disorders in the spine. Table 1 lists the potential tests available to document neuronal deficits in the lumbar spine. Such tests have the capacity not only to document abnormal nerve function but also to localize the source, nature, chronicity, and severity of such deficits. Each of these tests has specific indications, advantages, and disadvantages.

The test most commonly ordered in patients with low back pain is electromyography in the search for radiculopathy or sciatica.[10, 18, 19, 29, 31, 40, 64] Such a request has often resulted in a simple yes-or-no answer. This can be very confusing to clinicians if, for

Table 1 □ List of Clinical Neurophysiologic Tests and Their Utilization

Test	Utilization
ELECTROMYOGRAPHY	Acute denervation Chronic denervation Myopathies
MOTOR NERVE CONDUCTION	Peripheral neuropathies Entrapment neuropathies
SENSORY NERVE CONDUCTION	Peripheral neuropathies Entrapment neuropathies Postganglionic nerve injuries
H REFLEXES	S1 radiculopathies Cauda equina lesions Sciatic neuropathies Peripheral neuropathies
F RESPONSES	Motor radiculopathies Sciatic neuropathies Peripheral neuropathies
MIXED NERVE SOMATOSENSORY EVOKED RESPONSES	Peripheral and sciatic neuropathies, myelopathies Brainstem and cortical lesions
SMALL SENSORY NERVE EVOKED POTENTIALS	Sensory radiculopathies Sensory peripheral neuropathies Myelopathies
DERMATOMAL SOMATOSENSORY EVOKED RESPONSES	Root-specific sensory radiculopathies Sensory peripheral neuropathies Myelopathies
BULBOCAVERNOSUS REFLEXES	Cauda equina lesions Pudendal nerve lesions Impotence, bladder dysfunction
CYSTOMETRY	CNS lesions affecting bladder PNS lesions affecting bladder
NOCTURNAL PENILE TUMESCENCE AND RIGIDITY	Impotence
COLONOMETRY AND COLON MOTILITY	Neurogenic constipation, bowel incontinence
THERMOGRAPHY	Reflex sympathetic dystrophy

Table 2 □ Questions That Can Be Answered by Clinical Neurophysiologic Testing in Patients With Low Back Pain

Does a neurologic deficit exist and can it be documented?
What is the severity of the deficit?
Is the neurologic deficit progressive?
Is the deficit acute or chronic?
Where is the deficit localized?
What is the level of the radiculopathy?
Is there a peripheral neuropathy?
Is there an entrapment neuropathy?
Is there a sacral or cauda equina lesion?
Is there a spinal cord lesion?
Is there any change in spinal cord or nerve root function during surgery?
Is bowel, bladder, or sexual dysfunction present and neurologic in origin?
Is there evidence for reflex sympathetic dystrophy?

some reason, the answer does not fit their conceptualization of the clinical picture.[55] The answer one receives is likely to depend on the question that is asked and the clinical setting in which the test is performed. If the clinician fails to ask the correct question, the test will frequently give conflicting, frustrating and often irrelevant information. If, however, the question is accurately posed and one completely understands the sensitivity and weaknesses of each of the electrodiagnostic tests, then they can greatly enhance the clinician's ability to understand the neurologic deficits of a particular patient. The remainder of this chapter outlines the questions that are most commonly addressed to clinical neurophysiologists (Table 2) and describes the tests that lead to answers to these questions.

DOCUMENTATION OF NEUROLOGIC DEFICIT

The first question that inevitably arises in any clinical investigation is: Does a neurologic deficit exist? Many clinical decisions are made on the basis of the answer to that question. The major indication for lumbar surgery is documented radiculopathy.[48, 50] Performing surgery on an emergency basis for a patient with bladder incontinence depends on the determination that such incontinence results from neurologic cauda equina compression, rather than stress incontinence or some other form of local bladder disturbance.[50] At the same time, many forms of conservative care, such as spinal manipulation, have been demonstrated to be more effective in patients without neurologic deficits.[37, 49]

It is becoming evident that a large disc herniation or other structural abnormality, such as spondylosis, spondylolisthesis, or spinal stenosis as seen on imaging studies, can exist without causing nerve compression. Many prominent structural abnormalities can exist in individuals who are asymptomatic.[1, 9, 39, 46, 63] Similarly, in chronic patients it has been demonstrated that there is a breakdown in the relationship between the degree of disc herniation or spinal stenosis and many clinical findings such as neurologic deficit and straight-leg raising.[26] It is possible to have very large disc herniations with negative straight-leg raising and no neurologic deficits, whereas in other situations a relatively small disc protrusion may result in neurologic deficits and radiating pain in the leg and foot. Clinical findings and documented neurologic deficits make the abnormalities seen on imaging studies relevant. The increasing sophistication of imaging studies has, therefore, led to a greater need for sophisticated functional tests to look for neurologic deficits.

In the diagnosis of lower extremity neurologic deficits, a natural progression of tests adds information to the clinical examination (Fig. 1). The clinical examination is often capable of accurately determining the presence and defining the nature of a neurologic deficit. If motor, sensory, and reflex function all follow well-defined, consistent patterns then the presence of a particular neurologic deficit can be assumed with a high degree of confidence. Unfortunately, in many patients with low back pain, especially chronic pain, such findings become blurred on clinical examination. Leg pain and paresthesia, which the patient may describe as numbness, have been noted on stimulation of muscles and ligaments of the spine and do not necessarily indicate nerve root dysfunction.[12, 31] Muscle testing can be influenced by pain as well as by the effort and cooperation by the patient, and a nonanatomic weakness may camouflage true weakness.[26] In these situations, electrodiagnostic studies are crucial in determining whether clinical signs are the result of neurologic deficits.

Each of the electrodiagnostic and clinical neurophysiologic tests listed in Table 1 documents a certain type of neurologic deficit.

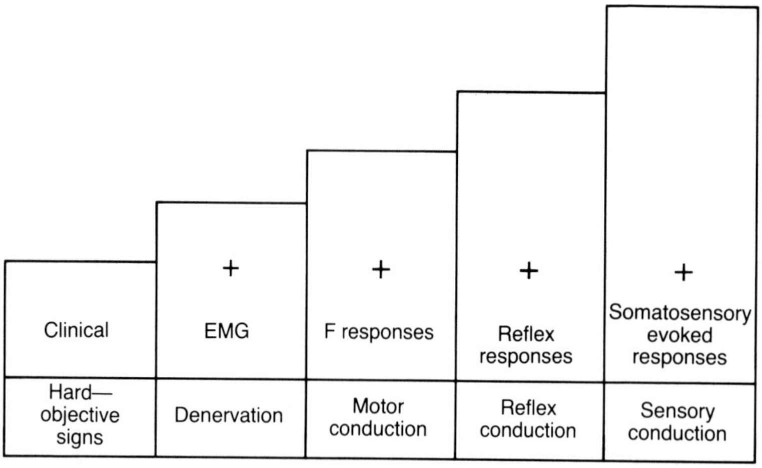

Figure 1 □ This illustration shows the manner in which each electrodiagnostic family of tests adds information to the clinical examination. (From Haldeman, S.: The electrodiagnostic evaluation of nerve root function. Spine 9:42–48, 1984.)

Unfortunately, no single test has been developed to document all types of neurologic deficit. Electromyography, in particular, can be difficult to interpret.[55] Although it is a very sensitive test for radiculopathy and neuronal deficits,[2, 30, 38, 40, 54, 64] it requires a very high level of technical experience.[58] In addition, this test does not become positive until 3 to 4 weeks after the onset of a deficit.[10, 31] Electromyography measures denervation and reinnervation, and these are slow ongoing processes. It takes approximately 3 to 4 weeks for the membrane of the muscle to react to denervation by becoming hypersensitive and spontaneously generate its own electric activity in the form of fibrillation potentials and positive sharp waves. These potentials can be picked up by the electromyographic needle. In the case of radiculopathy, there is a progression from proximal to distal muscles over time, the proximal muscles showing denervation changes before the more distal muscles in the leg. It is, therefore, common practice to wait 4 weeks before ordering electromyographic evaluation of the lower extremities, unless one is looking for a baseline electromyographic evaluation at the time of onset of the symptoms.[10, 19, 35]

Direct nerve conduction tests do not pose the problem that is presented by electromyography. The reflex tests and somatosensory evoked responses become abnormal immediately following onset of a neuronal injury.[5, 8, 60] However, other weaknesses in these tests exist, and a normal evoked response or F response test result, by itself, may not exclude the presence of a neuropathic process.

F responses, for example, exclusively measure motor nerve pathways between the point of stimulation in the leg and the anterior horn.[13, 14, 47] This test, which is performed by stimulating a motor nerve in the leg, results in an impulse traveling up the motor nerve to the anterior horn, where it makes a loop connection through a Renshaw-type cell. This results in an orthodromic response in the same motor nerve, which in turn can be recorded in the muscle to which that nerve travels. This test has been reported to be abnormal in a high percentage of patients with myelographically confirmed disc herniations.[11] This response, however, is independent of the sensory nerve root and will therefore remain normal in the presence of a purely sensory radiculopathy or neuropathy. In addition, many of the F responses are not represented in single nerve roots, and a single-level radiculopathy may not be detected by an F response recording.[13, 14] Examples of normal bilateral F responses can be seen in Figure 3, and a unilateral abnormal response is seen in Figure 2.

The H reflex does not pose the same problems presented by the F response. The H reflex consists of a sensorimotor monosynaptic reflex arc, which is measured as a response recorded over the soleus/gastrocnemius muscle group on stimulation of the posterior tibial nerve in the popliteal fossa.[5, 6, 8, 45] This response has been shown to have a 90% correlation with the Achilles reflex and measures the presence or absence of an S1 radiculopathy with a high degree of accuracy.[2, 53] Unfortunately, H reflexes are obtainable on a routine basis in the soleus/

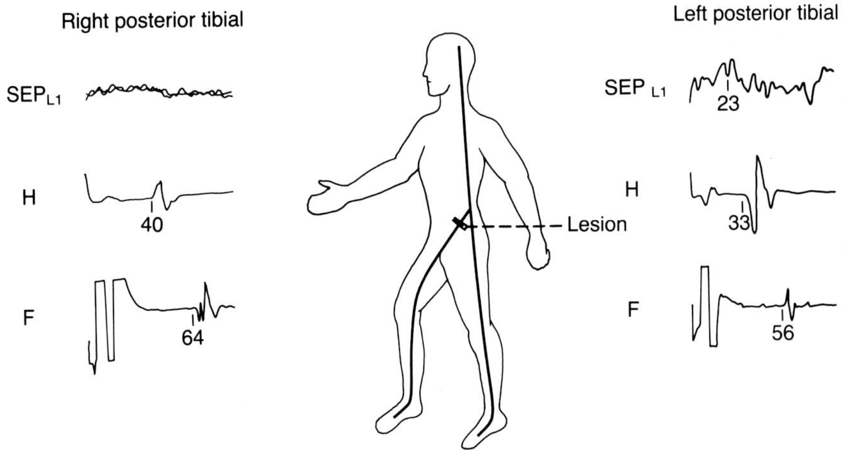

Figure 2 □ This illustrates the diagnosis of a sciatic nerve lesion by three different tests (somatosensory evoked potentials [SEP], H reflexes, and F responses).

gastrocnemius muscle group only and can only assess the S1 nerve root. Similar H reflexes have not been obtained, except under very special experimental conditions, in other lower-extremity nerves and therefore cannot be used to determine the presence or absence of radiculopathy at other levels. Examples of normal and abnormal responses can be seen in Figures 2 and 3.

Somatosensory evoked responses can be used to complement the F response in looking for the sensory component of a radiculopathy. However, multiple and often confusing methods exist by which a somatosensory evoked response can be elicited. The easiest and most common means of eliciting these responses is by stimulation of large mixed nerves, such as the peroneal

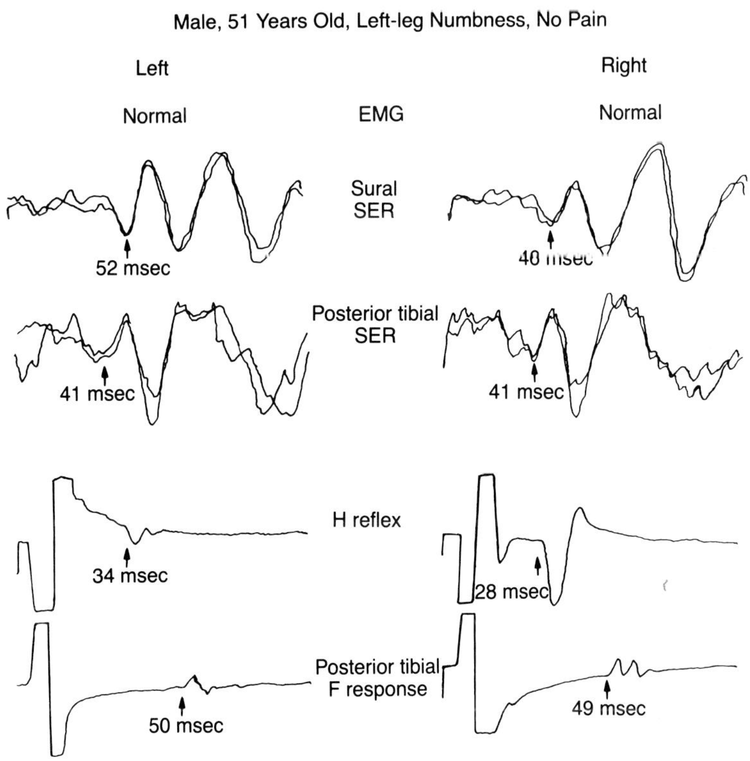

Figure 3 □ An example of a diagnostic battery of tests in a 51-year-old man with a purely sensory S1 radiculopathy. This illustrates how certain tests (F responses and posterior tibial somatosensory evoked response [SER]) can be normal, while other tests (H reflexes, sural SER) can confirm the diagnosis. (From Haldeman, S.: The electrodiagnostic evaluation of nerve root function. Spine 5:42–48, 1984.)

posterior tibial nerve at the ankle or knee.[7, 32] On stimulation of these nerves and by computerized averaging of the responses, it is possible to obtain a well-defined and reproducible response over both the spinal cord and the scalp. By measuring the latency of these responses and relating them to normal values for individuals of the same height and leg length,[24] it is possible to document disturbances in the primary sensory pathways from the point of stimulation to the scalp. Unfortunately, the stimulation of large mixed nerve fibers results in impulses traveling along multiple nerve roots. Thus, a single-level radiculopathy often does not significantly alter somatosensory evoked responses on stimulation of these large mixed nerves. Posterior tibial and peroneal somatosensory evoked responses have, therefore, been of very little value in documenting radiculopathy, although these tests are still used to measure spinal cord function.

In order to more accurately localize the nerve root that is stimulated, two alternative techniques have been developed. The first is the stimulation of small sensory nerves that fairly accurately represent a single nerve root.[10] Thus, the stimulation of the sural nerve represents S1 fibers, the stimulation of the superficial peroneal nerve represents L5 fibers, and the stimulation of the saphenous nerve represents L4 fibers. Figure 3 illustrates how a mixed major nerve evoked response (posterior tibial) may miss a radiculopathy, which is then diagnosed by a small sensory nerve (sural) evoked response. The second technique is to stimulate the skin area that represents a specific dermatome.[19, 52] By placing electrodes over the skin representing the S1, L5, and L4 dermatomes and by repeatedly stimulating and computer averaging 500 or more responses recorded over the scalp, it is possible to obtain a reproducible response that depends on the intactness of the sensory pathways in those specific dermatomes. Both small sensory nerve evoked responses and dermatomal evoked responses have been shown to have a high correlation with radiculopathy.[10, 52] It is not yet evident which of these tests is the more accurate or easier to perform. Each of these tests requires a reasonable degree of technical skill in order to achieve an accurate result. Figure 4 illustrates how a single parameter such as stimulation intensity can influence a response. Changing this and other simple technical parameters, such as skin temperature, recording electrode placement, or resistance, can lead to abnormal results. For this reason, evoked responses should be performed in experienced laboratories only.

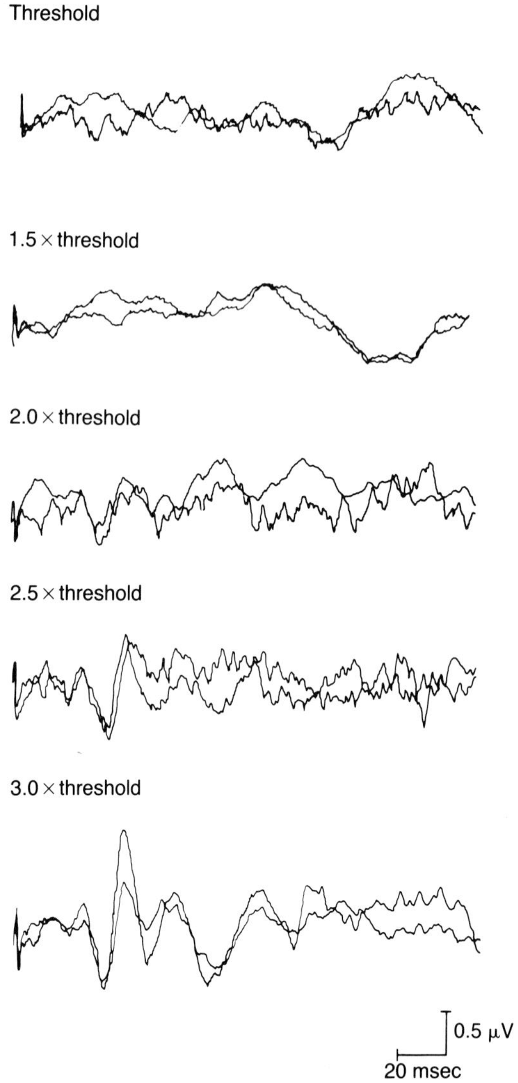

Figure 4 □ This shows the effect of stimulus intensity on the form and amplitude of a small nerve-evoked response.

For the reasons listed, it is evident that no single test is sufficient to rule out all forms of neuronal deficit. Those that are ordered and performed have to fit with the clinical picture and take into account chronicity, expected location of the lesion, and whether a primarily motor or sensory abnormality is anticipated.

SEVERITY OF THE DEFICIT

In many patients, a deficit is known to exist, but the severity of the deficit is not clear from the clinical examination. This is particularly true in severe neurologic deficits in which minimal, if any, motor activity is palpable on clinical examination. Under these circumstances, it is important to know whether a nerve has been severed and is therefore totally inactive, or whether the nerve remains intact. Again, this may influence a clinical decision about the nature and timing of surgical intervention or other treatment protocols, as well as determine whether exercise and other rehabilitation techniques are worth attempting in order to build muscle strength.

The most sensitive test for determining whether a nerve is intact is needle electromyography.[35] Activity in single motor units can be picked up by needle electromyography on voluntary contraction of the muscle. Often these single motor units are not sufficient to cause any appreciable resistance to clinical examination, but nonetheless they generate electric activity in the muscle that can be recorded electromyographically. To a lesser extent, needle electromyography can be used to determine the degree of severity of a denervation process by measuring recruitment and interference patterns.[10, 31, 35] Recruitment is the process whereby an increasing number of motor units are activated as the muscle contracts. The interference pattern is a crude evaluation of the total amount of electric activity generated by a muscle on maximum contraction. By measuring recruitment and interference patterns, the degree of denervation can be roughly estimated.

F responses are of minimal value in determining the severity of a lesion.[13, 14] Admittedly, the 10-msec delay of a response would suggest a degree of neuronal compromise greater than the delayed response of 3 or 4 msec. It has not, however, been determined how this translates into quantification. The H reflex, similarly, is very crude in its ability to quantify neuronal loss. The amplitude of the H reflex does diminish, but there can be a fair amount of variation from side to side and in a normal population. As a general rule, a 50% diminution in amplitude of the H reflex and a 2-msec delay on one side compared with the other is believed to be significant.[10] One assumes that greater degrees of amplitude diminution or conduction delay would reflect increasing degrees of deficit, but this has not been quantified in the literature.

Many clinical neurophysiologists attempt to estimate the degree of neuronal deficit on a four- or six-point scale, as follows: I—normal, II—minimal loss presumably without clinical evidence of deficit, III—slight loss with some degree of clinical deficit, IV—moderate loss with very obvious clinical deficit, V—severe loss that would reflect only minimal residual neuronal function, and VI—profound or total loss of neurologic function in a particular nerve.

LOCALIZATION OF THE DEFICIT

One of the major advantages of electrodiagnostic and clinical neurophysiologic techniques is their ability to accurately localize where a neurologic lesion exists and to differentiate among neurologic lesions with similar clinical patterns. This is particularly important in the case of contemplated surgery. Surgery is only as valuable as its ability to remove a compressive lesion and depends on accurate localization of such a lesion prior to surgical intervention. It is not unusual for patients with lumbar lesions to have spinal stenosis or disc herniations at multiple levels, with or without peripheral entrapment or other neuropathies. Under these circumstances, an electrodiagnostic evaluation should help to accurately define the location of the nerve entrapment and direct the surgeon to that area.

Radiculopathy

By far, the greatest number of electrodiagnostic studies will be performed in an attempt to localize the level of a suspected radiculopathy. The highest level of surgical success can be expected when a structural lesion accurately coincides with the level of radicular deficit.

Localization to a particular level is not as easy as it may seem. Needle electromyography as a primary tool is only as accurate as the innervation of the muscles that are tested.[18, 31, 35] Most muscles in the lower extremities are innervated by two or more nerve root levels. Therefore, it is necessary to sample multiple muscles in each nerve root distribution in order to provide the necessary overlap to accurately document the level of a lesion. Deep paraspinal muscles show a reasonable segmental innervation pattern, but superficial paraspinal muscles show considerable segmental overlap and cannot be used for localization of a radiculopathy.[10] H reflexes are probably the most accurate in documenting the level of a lesion. Their correlation with an S1 radiculopathy is extremely high, about 90%.[5, 6, 8, 53] The combination of electromyography, H reflexes, and F responses has been proposed as the most accurate method of documenting the level of a radiculopathy.[60] Dermatomal somatosensory evoked responses and small sensory nerve evoked responses have also shown a high correlation with the level of radiculopathy and are very specific to each level.[52] However, accurate technical placement of the electrodes is necessary because the dermatomes can vary among individuals. Direct stimulation of nerve roots has been proposed[44] as another method of accurately investigating root and plexus lesions, but because of the invasive nature of this testing it has not been widely investigated.

Peripheral Neuropathy

The differentiation between peripheral neuropathy as a cause of motor, sensory, and reflex changes in the lower extremities and radiculopathy is often clear-cut after the clinical examination is completed. It is, however, sometimes difficult to differentiate between the two when the history of back pain and leg pain is more diffuse, and when the clinical findings are not clear.

The primary tools for documenting peripheral neuropathy are motor and sensory nerve conduction studies. Motor nerve conduction can be studied in either the posterior tibial or peroneal nerves, whereas sensory nerve conduction can be studied in the sural or saphenous nerves.[35] As a routine procedure, posterior tibial motor nerve conduction and sural sensory nerve conduction seem to be more widely used. Somatosensory evoked responses, reflex studies, and cystometry also show abnormalities in the presence of peripheral neuropathies.[21] Sensory responses appear to be affected before motor responses in many of the common forms of peripheral neuropathy, but sensory responses in the lower extremities often require computer averaging, in order to obtain well-formed responses from which nerve conduction velocity and amplitude can be measured. In severe peripheral neuropathies, needle electromyography may also show denervation in the small muscles of the foot, but this occurs only later in the neuropathic process.

Entrapment Neuropathies

One of the major errors in the diagnosis of lower extremity neurologic deficits is the failure to differentiate between a peripheral entrapment neuropathy and a radiculopathy.[24, 51] Entrapment of the peroneal nerve at the fibular head fairly often occurs concomitantly with blows to the leg, tight stockings, or sleeping under the influence of alcohol or a sedative, which results in pressure over the fibular head. This can lead to a drop foot and sensory changes in the dorsum of the foot, very similar to those noted in an L5 radiculopathy. Similarly, tarsal tunnel entrapment of the posterior tibial nerve at the ankle can result in weakness of the intrinsic muscles of the foot; this may be confused with an S1 radiculopathy. Injury or entrapment of branches of the sciatic nerve in various locations is also a potential cause of neurologic deficit in the lower extremities.[44]

Saal and colleagues[51] have demonstrated that a significant proportion of patients sent to an electrodiagnostic laboratory for the documentation of radiculopathy have peripheral entrapment syndromes that were clinically misdiagnosed. The primary method of documenting these peripheral entrapment neuropathies is by nerve conduction studies and, to a lesser extent, needle electromyography. The nerve conduction studies require direct stimulation of the nerve being tested, above and below the level of suspected entrapment.[35] Thus, the diagnosis of a peroneal nerve entrapment at the fibular head is accomplished by recording over the extensor digitorum brevis muscle while stimulating the peroneal nerve at the ankle, below the fibular head and above the fibular head. If the nerve conduction velocity shows slowing across the fibular head, an entrapment of the peroneal nerve at that level has occurred. Motor and sensory nerves can be followed either by percutaneous stimulation and recording, when they are close to the surface, or by the insertion of needles close to the nerves when they are deeper in the leg.

Sacral Nerve and Cauda Equina Entrapment

Needle electromyography, H reflexes and F responses, and dermatomal somatosensory evoked responses often miss sacral nerve and cauda equina lesions. Such lesions are often of major significance, as they can affect bowel, bladder, and sexual function. The recent development of electrodiagnostic tests has allowed direct investigation of the sacral and pudendal nerves.[20, 22, 23] Because it is a potential surgical emergency, the documentation of a cauda equina lesion may be very important. The neuronal pathways that innervate the pelvic organs are illustrated in Figure 5. The primary pathways are via the pudendal nerve.

The electrodiagnostic tools for evaluating the sacral nerve roots are the pudendal somatosensory evoked response and the bulbocavernosus reflex response.[20, 22, 57] The pudendal somatosensory evoked response is obtained by stimulating the dorsal nerve of the penis or of the clitoris and measuring the computer-averaged response over the scalp. The stimuli can be applied bilaterally or unilaterally. This test measures the sensory pathways within the pudendal and sacral nerves from S2 through S4. The bulbocavernosus reflex has the advantage of recording both motor and sensory pathways within the pudendal nerve. The response is obtained by stimulating the dorsal nerve of the penis or clitoris and recording over the bulbocavernosus or some other pelvic floor muscle.

Spinal Cord

The documentation and localization of spinal cord lesions have become feasible with the development of somatosensory evoked responses. It is possible to measure somatosensory evoked responses at each level along the spinal cord simply by placing electrodes over the spinous processes at multiple levels and over the scalp.[24] The scalp response demonstrates the integrity of the entire neuraxis.[7] By recording responses at multiple levels along the spine on stimulation of the nerves of both upper and lower extremities, it is possible to determine the level within the spinal cord at which a suspected lesion is interfering with the primary sensory pathways. The weakness of this test is that somatosensory evoked responses record transmission only in the dorsal columns of the spinal cord.[32] Spinal cord lesions affecting other portions of the cord may be missed by this test. Figures 6 and 7 illustrate two different patients with spinal cord injuries. Figure 6 illustrates a complete spinal cord injury and shows intact spinal evoked responses but absent cortical evoked responses during the stimulation of both the pudendal and posterior tibial nerves. The integrity of the distal spinal cord and peripheral nervous system is confirmed by a bulbocavernosus reflex and sural sensory nerve conduction test. Figure 7 illustrates a partial spinal cord injury with an absent posterior tibial evoked response but a definite, although abnormal, pudendal evoked response. There is some suggestion that pu-

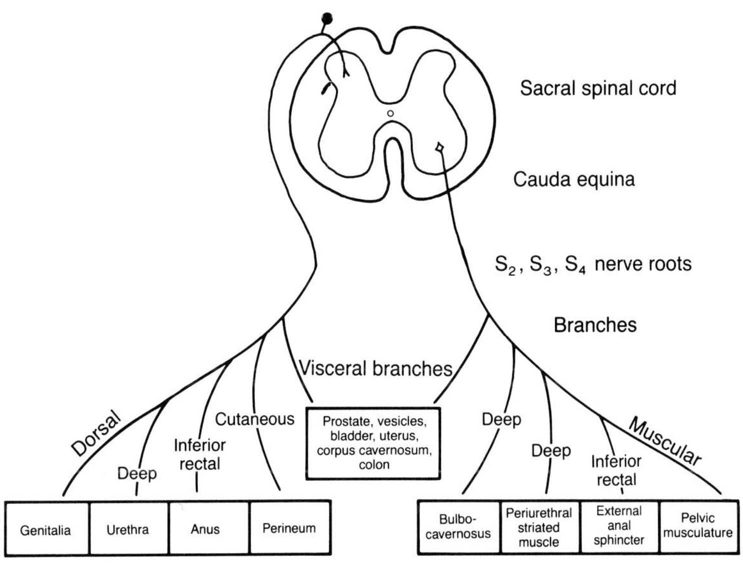

Figure 5 □ Illustrated are the primary neurologic pathways to the bowel, bladder, and sexual organs, which can be influenced by cauda equina and pudendal nerve lesions. (From Haldeman, S., Bradley, W.E., and Bhatia, N.N.: Evoked responses in clinical neuro-urology. Bull. Los Angeles Neurol. Soc. 47:76–90, 1982.)

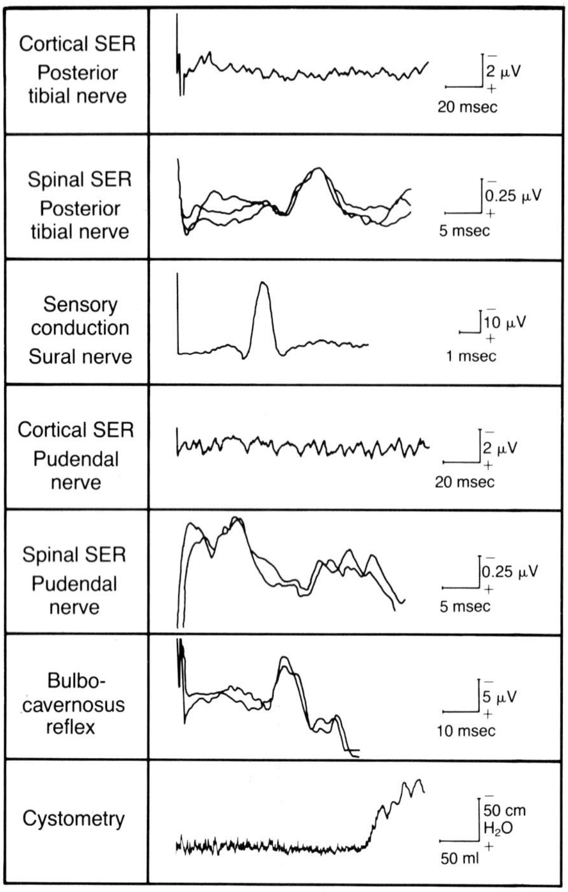

Figure 6 □ This demonstrates the effect of a complete spinal cord lesion on somatosensory evoked responses, bulbocavernosus reflex response, sacral sensory conduction, and cystometry. (From Haldeman, S., Bradley, W.E., and Bhatia, N.N.: Evoked responses in clinical neuro-urology. Bull. Los Angeles Neurol. Soc. 47:76–90, 1982.)

dendal evoked responses may follow different routes in the spinal cord, but these routes have not yet been defined.

More recent efforts have been made to access the autonomic nervous system directly by stimulation or by recording from deeper structures in the urethra and bladder.[25] Figure 8 illustrates an example of the response obtained from the anal sphincter on stimulation of the proximal urethra. The latter structure is thought to be innervated by the pelvic nerve. This urethral-to-anal-sphincter reflex has the potential of further increasing the sensitivity of electrodiagnostic testing of the cauda equina and sural nerve roots innervating the bowel, bladder, and sexual organs.

Attempts to measure spinal cord function by directly stimulating the brain and recording descending motor responses may prove beneficial in the future. These responses, which have recently been documented in animals[56] and humans,[42, 43] have not yet been studied in depth, although they hold great promise.

SURGICAL MONITORING

The evolution of equipment and experience for recording somatosensory evoked responses has allowed these electrodiagnostic procedures to enter the operating room.[41, 59, 65] It has become common practice to monitor the somatosensory evoked responses from the upper and lower extremities during spinal surgery for scoliosis and fractures. Periodic monitoring of these responses can alert the surgeon to excessive stretching or ischemia of the cord, and it has successfully reduced complications from spinal surgery. Somatosensory evoked responses, however, do not guarantee that postoperative radicular changes will be prevented.[27] Furthermore, they may not be as valuable in monitoring patients undergoing surgery who have incomplete spinal cord lesions.[36]

The monitoring of dermatomal somatosensory evoked responses during intervertebral disc surgery has been proposed in an attempt to determine when adequate decompression of a nerve root has taken place.[28] Although

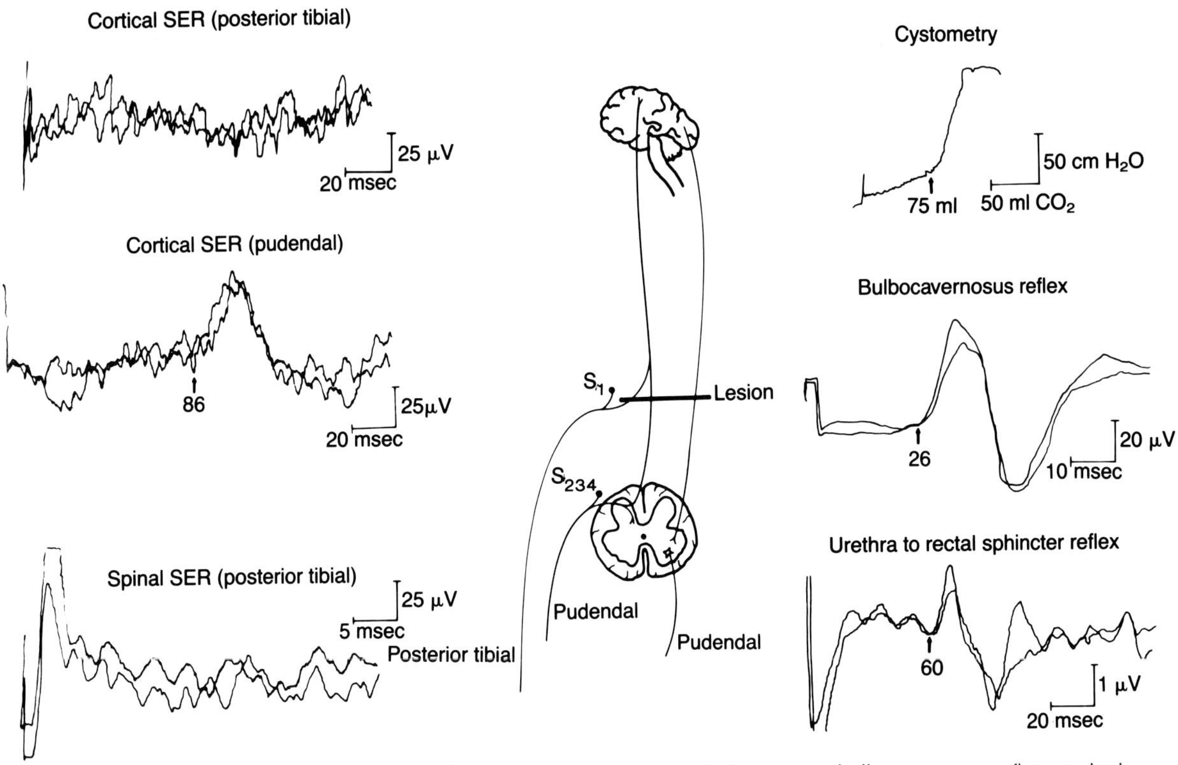

Figure 7 □ The effect of a partial spinal cord lesion on somatosensory evoked responses, bulbocavernosus reflex, urethral-to-rectal sphincter reflex responses, and cystometry. Note the difference in cortical responses on stimulation of the posterior tibial and pudendal nerves.

Figure 8 □ The reflex response of the anal sphincter to stimulation of the urethra is shown. (From Haldeman, S., Bradley, W.E., and Bhatia, N.N.: Evoked responses in clinical neuro-urology. Bull. Los Angeles Neurol. Soc. 47:76–90, 1982.)

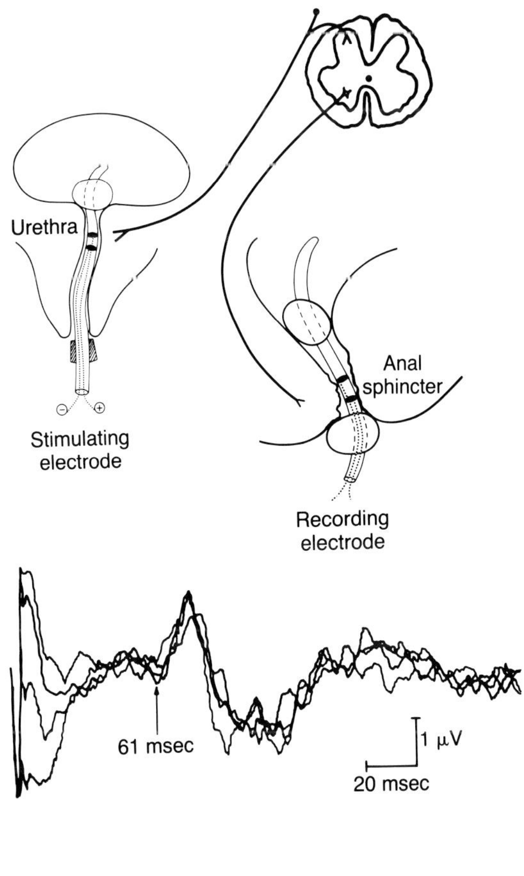

these techniques are promising, it remains to be proved that they will increase the success rate of lumbar disc surgery. Attempts to monitor somatosensory evoked responses before and after surgery to document successful decompression have also been proposed; however, they are not yet established as a method of determining the success of surgical decompression.

The Diagnosis of Bowel, Bladder, and Sexual Dysfunction

Clinical neurophysiologic techniques have expanded beyond the use of electrophysiologic techniques, and end organ monitoring is being explored. This promises to be useful in monitoring visceral organ functions. The primary organs innervated by lumbar and sacral nerves are in the pelvis. They include the bowel, the bladder, and the sexual organs. As mentioned above, it is possible to measure function in the pudendal nerve directly by means of bulbocavernosus reflex and pudendal somatosensory evoked response studies; however, they do not measure autonomic nervous system control of these organs. Because impotence and other visceral nerve dysfunctions can occur as part of a lumbar intervertebral disc herniation, or even after lumbar surgery, direct monitoring of these organs is increasingly important.

Classically, urodynamic studies, including cystometry, have been the tools of choice in measuring bladder function. Cystometry is performed by inserting a catheter into the bladder, gradually filling the bladder with water or carbon dioxide, and measuring the pressure in the bladder. In this way, the reflex contraction in the bladder and the ability of the patient to suppress that reflex contraction can be measured.[21] Figure 9 illustrates a normal cystometrogram, whereas Figures 6 and 7 show examples of abnormal cystometry in patients with upper motor neuron lesions. Recent simultaneous measures of bladder and urethral pressure and 24-hour monitoring of these pressures have led to greater sensitivity in monitoring the neurogenic reflexes associated with voiding and the retention of urine.[3, 4]

The measurement of impotence has also become increasingly more sophisticated.[33, 61] Initially, nocturnal penile tumescence studies required hospitalization of the patient and expensive and intricate measurement using simultaneous electroencephalography. Instruments have been developed that measure both tumescence and penile rigidity and that can be taken home and used on an outpatient basis. These tests have greatly

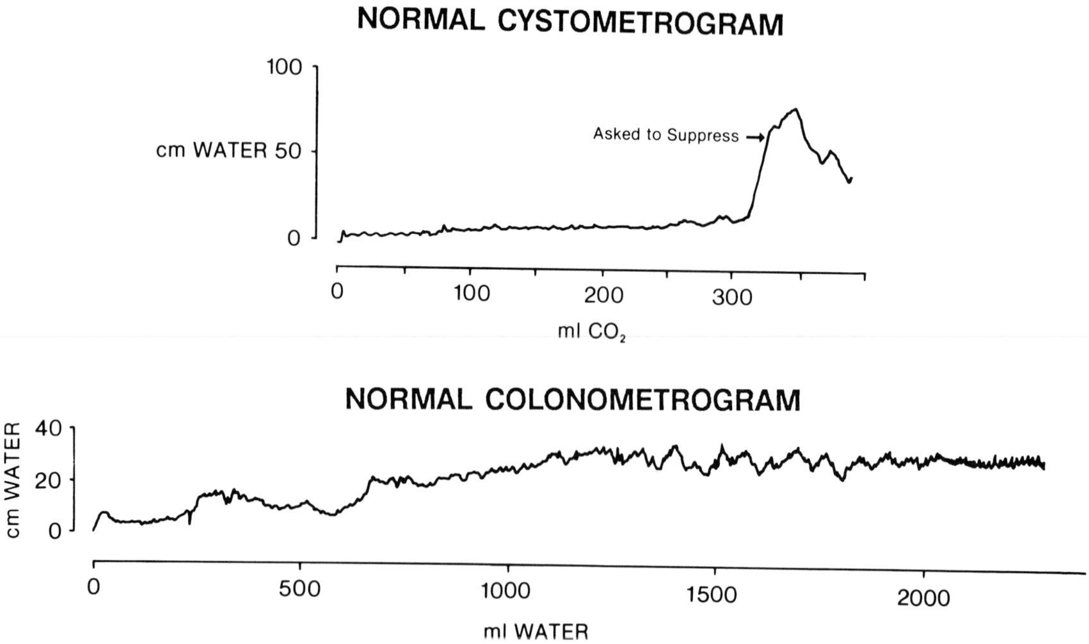

Figure 9 □ Normal cystometrogram (upper figure) and normal colonometrogram or colonic compliance tests (lower figure) are illustrated.

increased the number of impotent patients identified and, together with the evoked response studies, can differentiate neurogenic from non-neurogenic organic impotence.

The evaluation of neurogenic bowel disturbances is in an early stage of development.[16, 17] It is possible to measure colon compliance, or colonometry, by inserting a catheter into the bowel and filling the bowel with water. Reflex contraction of the bowel musculature is measured as well as the compliance of the bowel, as illustrated in Figure 9. By means of this technique it is possible to differentiate lesions of lower motor neurons from those of upper motor neurons affecting the bowel. Additional tests have allowed for direct measurement of bowel motility and myoelectric activity in normal and spinal-cord-injured patients. These tests help to explain the effect of spinal cord lesions on the bowel but have not yet been applied to patients with cauda equina lesions and isolated radiculopathies.

REFLEX SYMPATHETIC DYSTROPHY

One of the most controversial clinical neurophysiologic techniques has been thermography. Thermography has been proposed for the diagnosis of virtually every pain-related syndrome in the spine, but most authorities remain very skeptical about its use. Recent papers have suggested that its clinical value in spinal stenosis is less than that of other conventional testing procedures.[15]

Despite the skepticism concerning thermography in spinal pain syndromes, it appears to have some value in the diagnosis of reflex sympathetic dystrophy. Uematsu and associates[62] have demonstrated a high correlation between reflex sympathetic dystrophy associated with nerve injuries and thermographic changes. Thermography can also be used in monitoring the changes following sympathetic block and is probably one of the more accurate methods of determining the success of a sympathetic block or sympathectomy in patients with reflex sympathetic dystrophy.

PAIN

No discussion of electrodiagnostic and clinical neurophysiologic techniques is complete without considering the relationship of these tests to pain. One of the common reasons for referring patients for testing is the presence of radiating pain in the lower extremities. Unfortunately, none of the electrodiagnostic or clinical neurophysiologic tests has been demonstrated either to determine the presence or absence of pain or to measure its degree. It is possible for a patient to have major neurologic deficits, including disturbances from bowel or bladder dysfunction, total paralysis, and total loss of sensation, in the absence of pain. It is also possible for one to have extreme pain in the absence of neurologic deficit. Clinical neurophysiologic tests are valuable only when the pain is associated with an actual neurologic deficit. The same is true for other spinal diagnostic tests; clinical imaging studies of disc herniations, spinal stenosis, and severe degenerative changes do not relate directly to pain.

At this time, the diagnosis of spinal pain remains elusive. Fortunately, in many patients with pain, there are close correlations among the pain, a lesion seen on imaging, and neurologic deficits. The clinician should not be disillusioned, however, if the clinical neurophysiologist is unable to document the presence of a painful lesion. Pain remains a subjective response of a patient influenced by a wide variety of pathologic, psychologic, and social factors, which remain poorly understood and unproven. However, the clinical neurophysiologist can, with increasing sophistication, answer questions about the nature, localization, and extent of a suspected neurologic deficit. When these correlate with the patient's symptoms and a lesion seen on imaging, then these tests will facilitate a more accurate diagnosis and, one hopes, more effective treatment.

References

1. Barton, P. N.: The significance of anatomical defects of lower spine. Indust. Med. 17:37–40, 1948.
2. Baylan, S. P., Yu, J., and Grant, A. E.: H reflex latency in relation to ankle jerk electromyographic, myleographic, and surgical findings in back pain patients. Electromyogr. Clin. Neurophysiol. 21:201–206, 1981.
3. Bhatia, N. N., Bradley, W. E., Haldeman, S., and Johnson, B. K.: Continuous ambulatory urodynamic monitoring. Br. J. Urol. 54:357–359, 1982.
4. Bhatia, N. N., Bradley, W. E., Haldeman, S., and Johnson, B. K.: Continuous monitoring of bladder and urethral pressures: A new technique. Urology 18:207–210, 1981.
5. Braddon, R. L., and Johnson, E. W.: Standardization

of H reflex and diagnostic use in S1 radiculopathy. Arch. Phys. Med. Rehab. 55:161–166, 1974.
6. Braddon, R. L., and Johnson, E. W.: H reflex: Review and classification with suggested clinical uses. Arch. Phys. Med. Rehab. 55:412–417, 1974.
7. Cracco, R. O.: Spinal evoked response: Peripheral nerve stimulation in man. Electroencephalogr. Clin. Neurophysiol. 35:379–386, 1973.
8. Deschuytere, J., and Rosselle, N.: Diagnostic use of monosynaptic reflexes in L5 and S1 root compression. *In* Desmedt, J. E. (ed.): New Developments in Electromyography and Clinical Neurophysiology, Vol. 3. Basel, Karger, 1973, pp. 360–366.
9. Dively, R. L., and Oglevie, R. R.: Pre-employment examinations of the low back. J. Am. Med. Assoc. 160:856–858, 1956.
10. Eisen, A., and Hoirch, M.: The electrodiagnostic evaluation of spinal root lesion. Spine 8:98–106, 1983.
11. Eisen, A., Schamer, D., and Melmed, C.: An electrophysiological method for examining lumbosacral root compression. Can. J. Neurol. Sci. 2:117–122, 1977.
12. Feinstein, B.: Referred pain from paravertebral structure. *In* Buerger, A. A., and Tobis, J. S. (eds.): Approaches to the Validation of Manipulation Therapy. Springfield, Charles C Thomas, 1977, pp. 139–174.
13. Fisher, M. A., Shivde, A. J., Teixera, C., and Grainer, L. S.: Clinical and electrophysiological appraisal of the significance of radicular injury in back pain. J. Neurol. Neurosurg. Psychiatr. 41:303–306, 1978.
14. Fisher, M. A., Shivde, A. J., Teixera, C., and Grainer, L. S.: The F response—a clinically useful physiological parameter for the evaluation of radicular injury. Electromyogr. Clin. Neurophysiol. 19:65–75, 1979.
15. Getty, C. J. M.: Bony sciatica—the value of thermography, electromyography and water soluble myelography. Clin. Sports Med. 5:327–342, 1986.
16. Glick, M. E., Meshkinpour, H., Haldeman, S., et al.: Colonic dysfunction in multiple sclerosis. Gastroenterology 83:1002–1007, 1982.
17. Glick, M. E., Meshkinpour, H., Haldeman, S., et al.: Colonic dysfunction in patients with thoracic spinal cord injury. Gastroenterology 86:287–294, 1984.
18. Gough, J. G., and Koepke, G. H.: Electromyographic determination of motor root levels in erector spinae muscles. Arch. Phys. Med. Rehab. 47:9–11, 1966.
19. Haldeman, S.: The electrodiagnostic evaluation of nerve root function. Spine 9:42–48, 1984.
20. Haldeman, S., Bradley, W. E., and Bhatia, N.: Evoked responses from the pudendal nerve. J. Urol. 128:974–980, 1982.
21. Haldeman, S., Bradley, W. E., Bhatia, N. N., et al.: Neurologic evaluation of bladder, bowel, and sexual disturbances in diabetic men. *In* Goto, Y., Horiuchi, A., and Kogure, K. (eds.): Diabetic Neuropathy: Proceedings of the International Symposium on Diabetic Neuropathy and Its Treatment. Tokyo, Sept. 1981. Excerpta Med. (Amsterdam) 298–301, 1982.
22. Haldeman, S., Bradley, W., Bhatia, N., et al.: Pudendal evoked responses in neurologic disease. Neurology 32:A67, 1982.
23. Haldeman, S., Bradley, W. E., Bhatia, N. N., and Johnson, B. K.: Pudendal evoked responses. Arch. Neurol. 39:280–283, 1982.
24. Haldeman, S.: Spinal clinical neurophysiology. *In* Cauthen, J. C. (ed.): Lumbar Spine Surgery, 2nd Ed. Baltimore, Williams & Wilkins, 1988, pp. 128–143.
25. Haldeman, S., Bradley, W. E., and Bhatia, N. N.: Evoked responses in clinical neuro-urology. Bull. Los Angeles Neurol. Soc. 47:76–90, 1982.
26. Haldeman, S., Shouka, M., and Robboy, S.: Computed tomography, electrodiagnostic and clinical findings in chronic Workers' Compensation patients with back and leg pain. Spine (accepted for publication).
27. Harper, C. M., Jr., Daube, J. R., Litchy, W. J., and Klassen, R. A.: Lumbar radiculopathy after spinal fusion for scoliosis. Muscle Nerve 11:386–391, 1988.
28. Herron, L. D., and Trippi, A. C.: Intraoperative use of dermatomal somatosensory evoked potentials in lumbar spinal surgery. Proc. North Am. Spine Soc. Annu. Meet., Bolton Landing, New York, July 20–23, 1986.
29. Hoover, B. B., Caldwell, J. W., Krusen, E. M., and Muckelroy, R. N.: Value of polyphasic potentials in diagnosis of lumbar root lesions. Arch. Phys. Med. 51:546, 1970.
30. Jacobson, R. E.: Lumbar stenosis. An electromyographic evaluation. Clin. Orthop. 115:68–71, 1976.
31. Johnson, E. W., and Melvin, J. L.: Value of electromyography in lumbar radiculopathy. Arch. Phys. Med. Rehab. 52:239–243, 1971.
32. Jones, S. J., and Small, D. G.: Spinal and sub-cortical evoked potentials following stimulation of the posterior tibial nerve in man. Electroencephalogr. Clin. Neurophysiol. 44:299–306, 1978.
33. Karacan, I., Solis, P. J., and Williams, R. L.: The role of the sleep laboratory in the diagnosis and treatment of impotence. *In* Williams, R. L., Karacan, I., and Frazier, S. H. (eds.): Sleep Disorders: Diagnosis and Treatment. New York, John Wiley & Sons, 1978.
34. Kellgren, J. H., and Lewis, T.: Observations related to referred pain, visceromotor reflexes and other associated phenomena. Clin. Sci. 4:47, 1939.
35. Kimura, J.: Electrodiagnosis in diseases of nerve and muscle: Principles and practice. Philadelphia, F. A. Davis, 1983.
36. King, D. C., Dall, B. E.: Cortical somatosensory evoked potentials: Its efficacy in patients with incomplete neurological lesions (Abstr.). Meeting of International Society for the Study of the Lumbar Spine, Miami, Apr. 13–17, 1988.
37. Kirkaldy-Willis, W. H., and Cassidy, J. D.: Spinal manipulation in the treatment of low back pain. Can. Fam. Phys. 31:535–540, 1985.
38. Knuttson, B.: Comparative value of electromyographic, myelographic, and clinical-neurological examination in diagnosis of lumbar root compression syndrome. Acta Orthoped. Scand. 49(Suppl.): 1–135, 1961.
39. La Rocca, H., Macnab, I.: Value of pre-employment radiographic assessment of the lumbar spine. Can. Med. Assoc. J. 101:383–388, 1969.
40. Lane, M. D., Tamhankar, M. N., and Demopoulos, J. T.: Discogenic radiculopathy. Use of electromyography in multidisciplinary management. New York State J. Med. 32–36, 1978.

41. Leuders, H., Gurd, A., Hahn, J., et al.: A new technique for intraoperative monitoring of spinal cord function: Multichannel recording of spinal cord and subcortical evoked potentials. Spine 7:110–115, 1982.
42. Levy, W. J., York, D. H., McCaffrey, M., and Tanzer, F.: Motor evoked potentials from transcranial stimulation of the motor cortex in humans. Neurosurgery 15:287–302, 1984.
43. Levy, W. J., and York, D. H.: Evoked potentials from the motor tracts in humans. Neurosurgery 12:422–429, 1983.
44. MacLean, I. C.: Nerve root stimulation to evaluate conduction across the brachial and lumbosacral plexuses. Third Annual Continuing Education Course, American Association of Electromyography and Electrodiagnosis, Philadelphia, Sept. 25, 1980.
45. Malcolm, D. S.: A method of measuring reflex times applied in sciatica and other conditions due to nerve root compression. J. Neurol. Neurosurg. Psychiatr. 14:15–24, 1951.
46. McCrae, D. L.: Asymptomatic intervertebral disc protrusions. Acta Radiol. 46:9–27, 1956.
47. McLeod, J. G., and Wary, S. H.: An experimental study of the F wave in the baboon. J. Neurol. Neurosurg. Psychiatr. 29:196–200, 1966.
48. Nachemson, A. L.: An orthopedic challenge. Spine 1:59–71, 1976.
49. Potter, G. E.: A study of 744 cases of neck and back pain treated with spinal manipulation. J. Can. Chiropract. Assoc. 21:154–156, 1977.
50. Rothman, R. H., and Simeone, F. A.: Lumbar disc disease. *In* Rothman, R. H., and Simeone, F. A. (eds.): The Spine, Vol. 2. Philadelphia, W. B. Saunders, 1975, pp. 443–468.
51. Saal, J. A., Dillingham, M. F., Gamburd, R. G., and Fanton, G. S.: The pseudoradicular syndrome: Lower extremity peripheral entrapment masquerading as lumbar radiculopathy. A report of thirty-one cases. Proc. North Am. Spine Soc. Annu. Meet. Banff, Canada, June 25–28, 1987.
52. Scarff, T. B., Ballmann, D. E., and Toleikis, J. R.: Dermatomal somatosensory evoked potentials in the diagnosis of lumbar root entrapment. Surg. Forum 32:489–491, 1981.
53. Schuchmann, J. A.: H reflex latency in radiculopathy. Arch. Phys. Med. Rehab. 59:185–187, 1978.
54. Seppalainen, A. M., Alaranta, H., and Saini, J.: Electromyography in the diagnosis of lumbar spinal stenosis. Electromyogr. Clin. Neurophysiol. 21:55–66, 1981.
55. Shapiro, D., Hanley, E., and Wright, K.: Limited usefulness of electromyography in lumbar radiculopathy (Abstr.). Meeting of International Society for the Study of the Lumbar Spine, Miami, Apr. 13–17, 1988.
56. Simpson, R. K., Jr., and Baskin, D. S.: An animal model for studying spinal cord injury using corticomotor evoked potentials. Neuro-Orthopedics 5:10–24, 1988.
57. Siroky, M. B., Sax, D. S., and Krane, R. S.: Sacral signal tracing: The electrophysiology of the bulbocavernosus reflex. J. Urol. 122:661–664, 1979.
58. Skaggs, H.: Guidelines in EMG. Professional Standards Committee, American Association of Electromyography and Electrodiagnosis, 1979.
59. Spielholz, N. I., Benjamin, M. V., Engler, G. L., and Ransohoff, J.: Somatosensory evoked potentials during decompression and stabilization of the spine: Methods and findings. Spine 4:500–505, 1979.
60. Tonzola, R. F., Ackil, A. A., Shahani, B. T., and Young, R. R.: Usefulness of electrophysiological studies in the diagnosis of lumbosacral root disease. Ann. Neurol. 9:305–308, 1981.
61. Torrens, M. J.: Neurologic and Neurosurgical disorder associated with impotence. *In* Krane, R. J., Siroky, M. B., and Goldstein, I. (eds.): Male Sexual Dysfunction. Boston, Little, Brown & Company, 1983.
62. Uematsu, S., Hendler, N., Hungerford, D., et al: Thermography and electromyography in the differential diagnosis of chronic pain syndromes and reflex sympathetic dystrophy. Electromyogr. Clin. Neurophysiol. 21:165, 1982.
63. Wiesel, S. W., Tsourman, N., Feffer, H. L., et al: A study of computer-assisted tomography. 1. The incidence of positive CAT scans in an asymptomatic group of patients. Spine 9:549–551, 1984.
64. Wise, C. S., and Ardizzone, I.: Electromyography in intervertebral disc protrusions. Arch. Phys. Med. Rehab. 35:442–446, 1954.
65. York, D. H., Chabot, R. J., and Gaines, R. W.: Response variability of somatosensory evoked potentials during scoliosis surgery. Spine 12:864–876, 1987.

4 □ Biomechanics

Albert B. Schultz
Paul Brinckmann
Malcolm Pope
Manohar M. Panjabi
Vijay K. Goel
James N. Weinstein
Y. King Liu
Young E. Kim
T. Okuma
Gunnar B. J. Andersson
Casey K. Lee

BIOMECHANICAL ANALYSES OF LOADS ON THE LUMBAR SPINE

Albert B. Schultz

The chief reason to study the way in which physical activity loads the structures of the lumbar trunk is the evidence that heavy trunk loads and low back pain are related. This association has been documented in both classical[8, 11] and more recent studies[10] showing that workers with physically stressful jobs are more likely to develop low back pain or lumbar disc herniations. The evidence is not conclusive, for a recent study of over 30,000 aircraft workers[6] showed that the incidence of back-related disabilities was not associated significantly with any of 32 job classifications. On the other hand, that same study showed that lifting or materials handling was the reason most often cited for the onset of back pain. Perhaps the most compelling evidence that low back pain and loads on the spine are related is the everyday observation of individuals with low back pain who are unwilling to move as fast or push as hard as they would in the absence of pain.

It is impractical to measure directly the loads internal to the lumbar trunk that are imposed by the performance of a physical task. Although they can be estimated from experimental measurements, those usually require a laboratory setting, skilled personnel, and expensive equipment. Biomechanical model calculations of internal loads are safe, quick, and inexpensive. Because of this, most current knowledge about lumbar trunk internal loads has been derived from biomechanical model calculations.

Morris and colleagues[14] reported one of the earliest biomechanical model analyses of loads on the lumbar spine. Over the past 10 years many other studies have been reported. Several recent reviews of them are available.[2, 22, 23] This chapter summarizes what has been learned about loads on the lumbar spine from biomechanical model calculations and laboratory measurements. It also illustrates the use of new features in biomechanical models that may enable realistic predictions of lumbar trunk loads to be made in a wider variety of circumstances.

NET REACTIONS ON THE LUMBAR SPINE

The main determinant of the loads on any musculoskeletal joint is the set of contraction forces in the muscles that cross that joint. That set of forces is determined largely by the net reaction across the joint. In the case of the lumbar spine, imagine a transverse plane passed through the trunk at the level of the L3–L4 intervertebral disc. All the body segments superior to that plane are in equilibrium when a task is performed slowly. The weights of the body segments superior to that plane and the moments of

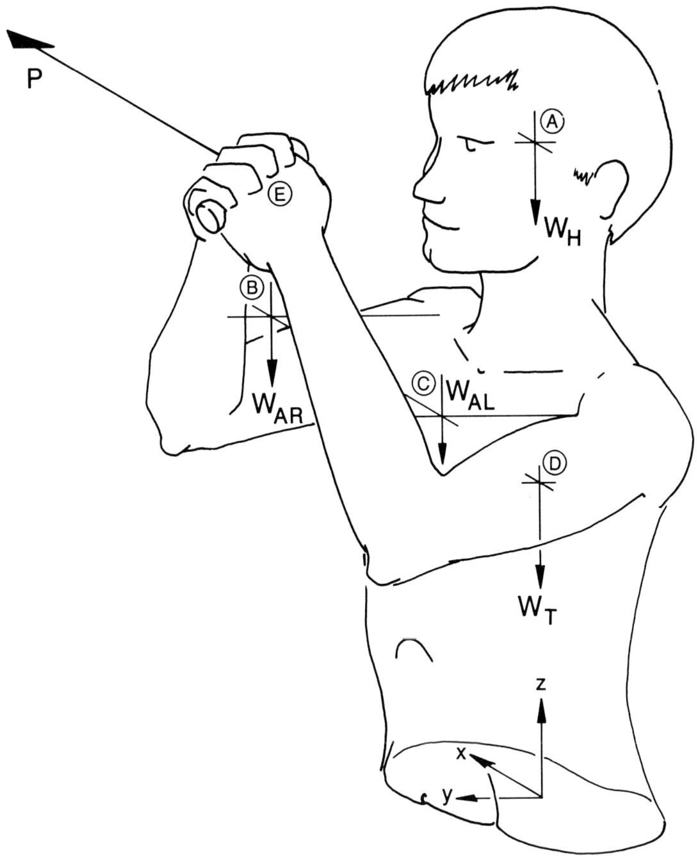

Figure 1 □ Schematic diagram shows variables involved in the calculation of the net reaction needed across the L3 transverse cross section to equilibrate the body segments superior to that plane.

those weights, and any forces and moments externally applied superior to that plane, need to be equilibrated. The net reaction consists of three components of the force and three components of the moment that must be supplied by the inferior body segments across the imaginary cutting plane to maintain equilibrium (or, in a rapidly performed task, to maintain force and moment balance). Figure 1 and Table 1 illustrate a sample calculation of net reaction components.

TRUNK MUSCLE CONTRACTION FORCES

Once the net reactions that need to be supplied for performance of a task have been

Table 1 □ Sample Calculation of a Net Reaction[1]

	NET REACTION FORCES (N)			FORCE LOCATION COORDINATES (cm)			NET REACTION MOMENTS (Nm)		
BODY SEGMENT WEIGHTS	F_x	F_y	F_z	Ant	Right	Sup	M_x	M_y	M_z
A Head (0.050*BW)	0	0	34	−0.9	0		−0.3	0.0	0.0
B Left Arm (0.045*BW)	0	0	31	20.9	−12.5		6.5	0.0	0.0
C Right Arm (0.045*BW)	0	0	31	20.9	12.5		6.5	0.0	0.0
D Trunk (0.361*BW)	0	0	248	−1.1	0		−2.7	0.0	0.0
Applied Load									
E	74	0	0	61.0	0.0	40.8	0.0	44.8	−30.0
Total Net Reaction	74	0	344				10.0	44.8	−30.0

BW = Body weight. The letters correspond to the points shown and the locations of force application points as expressed in the coordinate system shown in Figure 1.

[1]The calculation is for the task illustrated in Figure 1. A pull to the right of 73.5 N is applied to the hands, which are held symmetrically in front of the face. Body weight is assumed to be 686 N.

calculated from considerations of either equilibrium or dynamics, a set of muscle contraction forces that can supply that net reaction can be calculated. If enough simplifying assumptions are made, so that only a few unknown muscle contraction forces need to be calculated, this is easily accomplished. If more realistic assumptions are used, this calculation is more complicated. The complexity occurs because the number of unknown muscle contraction forces exceeds six, while there are no more than six requirements for achieving force and moment balance. In other words, calculations of trunk internal loads are usually statically indeterminate.

Optimization techniques are used to make statically indeterminate calculations. An objective function is chosen and a set of internal loads is found that minimizes that function. For example, in some models internal loads have been calculated using an objective of minimum compression force on the spine. Table 2 summarizes the results of trunk internal load calculations from a number of earlier studies. In the first two summarized studies the calculations were rendered statically determinate, either by modeling only a few muscles or by assuming, a priori, how loads were to be shared among synergistic muscles. In the last four summarized studies, optimization techniques were used. In the third study listed, spine compression was minimized, whereas in the remaining studies two objective functions were minimized. The first objective was to minimize the maximum contraction intensity required from any muscle to equilibrate the net reaction moment components (this is referred to subsequently as the min/max contraction intensity). The second objective function was to minimize spine compression within the bounds of the min/max contraction intensity.

EXPERIMENTAL METHODS TO TEST MODEL VALIDITY

Although it is not practical to measure trunk internal loads directly, they can be gauged from laboratory measurements. The main use of such measurements has been to validate biomechanical model analyses. Chiefly, two techniques have been used to make those estimates. The first is quantitative electromyography.[16] If the magnitudes of myoelectric signals are measured at a muscle site while a series of quasistatic tasks are performed, the relative signal strengths relate monotonically (often linearly) to the muscle contraction forces. This enables those forces to be estimated. Electromyographic measurements are particularly useful when obtained within a population of individuals performing those tasks, for the inherent noisiness of myoelectric signals can be averaged over the population. The validity of a biomechanical model can be tested by observing how well the set of model-predicted muscle contraction forces correlates with the set of measured myoelectric activities.

The second load-gauging technique is to measure intradiscal pressures. These have often been shown[15] to relate directly to spine compression. However, such measurements are difficult, and only one comprehensive study reporting correlations of intradiscal pressure measurements with model-predicted spine compressions has so far been reported. That is the third study summarized in Table 2.

VALIDITY OF EARLIER MODELS

Table 2 also provides a summary regarding the validity of the model predictions made in the listed representative studies. Validation was by myoelectric signal measurement, except in the one study in which intradiscal pressure measurements were made as well. The first studies listed examined only situations that were simple to analyze mechanically. The correlation data summarized in Table 2 suggest that the models predicted the trunk loads adequately in those situations. The later studies examined situations that were mechanically more complex and so more difficult to analyze with a biomechanical model because of the multiplicity of feasible solutions. In these situations the models seemed to predict some of the internal loads very well, but in others not as well as desired. This is discussed in detail in the following section.

TYPICAL VALUES OF PREDICTED LUMBAR TRUNK LOADS

Typical values of lumbar trunk loads predicted by the models used to date are given in the Table 2 summary. The moments that

Table 2 □ Summary of Selected Model Calculations/Laboratory Studies of Lumbar Spine Loads

	SUBJECT, TASK NUMBERS	LARGEST MOMENTS (N•m)				MAXIMUM PREDICTED MUSCULAR FORCE PER SIDE (N)				MAXIMUM PREDICTED COMPRESSION (N)	MIN/MAX INTENSITY (kPa)	APPROXIMATE CORRELATION COEFFICIENT[1]	
		Flexion	Extension	Lateral	Twist								
Andersson et al (1980)	10, 30	33	0	43	0	ES	500	OM	290	720		ES	0.98
Schultz et al (1982a)	10, 42	105	0	0	0	ES RA	2270 370	OM	900	2660		ES	0.98
Schultz et al (1982b)[2]	4, 25	98	24	43	28	ES RA	890 130	XOM IOM	260 160	2350		ES RA OM	0.90 0.55 .20–.57
Schultz et al (1983)	10, 25	53	47	45	60	ESM ESL ESI RA	99 199 199 92	XOM IOM XOL IOL	133 145 145 158	1647	300	ES RA OM	0.90 0.90 .61-.90
Schultz et al (1987)	10, 45	191	204	180	91	ESM ESL ESI RA	337 674 674 315	XOM IOM XOL IOL	388 441 329 441	5049	740	ES[3] RA OM OL	0.90 0.90 0.90 0.74
Zetterberg et al (1987)	10, 8	153	186	142	0	ESM ESL ESI RA	325 325 650 258	XOM IOM XOL IOL	318 361 270 359	4886	660	ES[4] RA OM	0.90 0.90 .43-.88

Data given are mean values over the subject populations.
ES = erector spinae, RA = rectus abdominis, IO = internal oblique, XO = external oblique. For the ES, M = multifidus, L = longissimus, I = iliocostalis. For the obliques, M = medial, L = lateral.
[1]For linear regressions of predicted contraction forces on measured myoelectric signal levels.
[2]Also measured intradiscal pressures to 1620 kPa, intra-abdominal pressures to 6.1 kPa. Compression values derived from disc pressures approximately 30% lower than predicted values.
[3]The coefficients quoted are for less strenuous tasks. Correlations for strenuous tasks were weaker. Use of "antagonistic" contractions in abdominal muscles clearly seen.
[4]"Antagonistic" contractions in abdominal muscles are 38% to 68% of maximum voluntary contraction values observed.

can be developed in a slowly performed, maximum voluntary strength test by a healthy young male standing upright have mean values of approximately 200 N•m in attempted trunk extension, 150 N•m in either attempted trunk flexion or lateral bending, and 100 N•m in attempted axial twist. The levels of effort called for in the tabulated studies can be seen by comparing the tabulated moments with these maximum voluntary strength moments.

In the summarized study results, predicted spine compressions ranged from approximately 400 N, the weight of the body segments above the L3 level of the spine, to in excess of 5,000 N. Muscle contraction intensities exceeded 700 kPa in the heaviest exertions.

In the study in which they were measured, intradiscal pressures ranged to approximately 1,600 kPa, and abdominal cavity pressures to approximately 6 kPa. Predicted peak muscle contraction forces per side ranged in those studies to approximately 1,600 N in the erector spinae groups, 300 N in the rectus abdominis, 900 N in the internal abdominal oblique groups, and 700 N in the external abdominal oblique groups.

If the data summarized in Table 2 are studied in detail from the original papers, it can clearly be seen that predicted trunk internal load magnitudes are strongly dependent on net reaction moment magnitudes. The net reaction moments range widely, from just a few N•m during quiet standing to well over 100 N•m during heavy exertions. The predicted internal loads, correspondingly, also range widely. Their magnitudes are much more sensitive to the net reaction moment magnitudes than they are to any of the details of the models used to predict them. However, it will subsequently be seen that the predicted values just quoted for internal loads in the last two summarized studies, both of which involved heavy exertions, may be too high.

SHORTCOMINGS OF EARLIER MODELS

The above discussion points out that the biomechanical models used to date are able to predict the loads on the lumbar spine well in many situations. That is, the models yield sets of predicted muscle contraction forces and spine loads that correlate well with measurements of myoelectric activities and intradiscal pressures, as shown by the first sets of entries in Table 2. Recent work has subjected these models to more critical tests of their validity. The last sets of Table 2 entries show that there are situations in which these models do not predict results as well as would be desired.

At least four issues seem to be involved. First, consider the study in which intradiscal pressure measurements were obtained. Analyses subsequent to the reporting of that study show that, although the relative changes from task to task in predicted spine compressions are in keeping with the changes in the measured disc pressures, their absolute values seem high by approximately 30%. Model improvements are needed to bring predicted spine compressions into better agreement with the compression values derived from the intradiscal pressure measurements. Second, although the earlier models are capable of accounting for the effects of abdominal cavity pressurization if supplied with experimentally measured values of that pressure, they do not predict a priori the use of cavity pressurization. Model improvements are needed to capture this phenomenon.

Third, in studies that have examined equilibration of axial twisting moments, the agreement between predictions and measurements in the tasks involving twist moments has been considerably weaker than in other tasks. The ability of the models to more correctly predict twist responses needs improvement.

Fourth, in studies that have examined heavy exertions, substantial contraction forces in the abdominal wall muscles have been observed during, for example, flexion-resist or attempted extension tasks. Lumbar trunk models used to date have not incorporated any features that would predict the occurrence of these forces. Mechanically, this phenomenon must be linked to the need to produce the abdominal wall tensions required to equilibrate the abdominal cavity when it is pressurized. These tensions can be produced passively, merely by stretching the ligamentous tissues of the wall. Calculations suggest that moderate stretches are all that are required to produce the needed tensions. So, the longitudinal tensions could readily be produced by extending the trunk a few degrees only. Although the transverse tensions needed for equilibrium could be developed by allowing the abdominal wall to expand, subjects in laboratory tests have often been observed to draw the wall inward upon exertion. This suggests that equilibrium is achieved circumferentially, often by active contractions of the external oblique, internal oblique or transverse abdominal wall muscles.

MODELING CONSIDERATIONS

Although the vertebral level of most interest for studies of low back impairment is the L5 level, it is more reasonable to construct a biomechanical model based on a cross section at the L3 level. The reason for this is that an L3 section does not cut any bony structures other than the spine, whereas an L5 section cuts major pelvic bones. Load transmission paths through bony structures can be complex, and an L3 section avoids most of this complexity. Loads at the levels of L3 and L5 probably differ little, and the amount of the difference can be estimated.

Most trunk cross-section models assume that the spine motion segment can passively develop significant resistances to compression and shear forces, but negligible resistance to bending moments. This assumption is based on the mechanical properties of lumbar spine motion segments.[5, 24] Substantial resistances to compression and shear forces are developed by only small relative translations of the vertebrae, but the stiffnesses in bending at small rotations are, at most, about 5 N•m/degree. In many of the positions of the trunk of interest, relative rotations between the L3 and L4 vertebrae are less than a degree. The 5-N•m or smaller moment that these produce can often be neglected, compared with the 100- or 200-N•m external moments that are sometimes present.

On the other hand, this assumption is not always valid. Miller and colleagues[13] found that when large relative rotations of adjacent vertebrae are allowed, bending resistances of up to 65 N•m can be developed. Panjabi and associates[17] found that, when motion segments are placed under substantial compressive loads, their stiffnesses in torsion increase significantly. Thus, it would be useful to have a model that does not require the assumption that the motion segments have negligible resistances to moments.

The role of abdominal cavity pressurization in relieving loads on the lumbar spine was recognized as early as 1900.[9] Bartelink[3] discussed the issue, and Morris and colleagues[14] analyzed the amount of relief that cavity pressurization might provide. A number of studies[7] have shown that maximum cavity pressures developed in ordinary circumstances are on the order of 100 mmHg (13.3 kPa). The abdominal cavity has a cross section of about 300 cm^2. The centroid of this cavity lies approximately 5 cm anterior to the L3 disc center. Thus, at a 100-mmHg pressure, the extension moment about that center provided by cavity pressurization would be approximately 20 N•m. In comparison with the approximately 200-N•m maximum voluntary extension moments that the back muscles can develop, this value is relatively small. However, abdominal cavity pressurization may indirectly exert more profound effects on trunk loads.

A factor that is sometimes important in the determination of trunk internal loads is the objective function chosen to enable solution of the statically indeterminate calculation problem. In mechanically simple situations, many different objective functions produce nearly the same set of internal load predictions. For example, if tasks calling for only the development of trunk extension moments are considered, the muscle contraction force sets will be almost independent of the choice of objective function. This occurs because the back muscles are the chief producers of trunk extension moments. They produce those moments without involving any substantial lateral bending or twisting moments. Any reasonable objective function entails the back muscles contracting just enough to produce the required moment. In this situation, the constraint of having to produce the needed extension moment, rather than the objective function, dominates muscle recruitment.

In mechanically more complicated situations, different objective functions lead to significantly different predicted sets of muscle contraction forces. Tasks that call for use of the oblique abdominal muscles, for example, are mechanically more complicated, because their contractions simultaneously develop moments in flexion, lateral bending, and twisting, and all three of these moments must be equilibrated. The extent to which the oblique abdominals are contracted in model simulations is then influenced substantially by objective function choice.

Care must be taken in designing laboratory experiments aimed at testing the validity of a given objective function in biomechanical model calculations of spine loads. A laboratory study primarily involving tasks that require use of the back muscles only would show almost any physiologically reasonable objective function to be valid.

The earliest biomechanical models for predicting spine loads used an objective function that minimized spine compression. The chief rationale for this objective was to avoid recruitment of antagonistic muscles. Its use amounted to the assumption that an experienced subject would perform a task by means of the least effort consistent with achieving equilibrium. Although a minimum compression objective does minimize antagonistic contractions, it results in the sole recruitment of the muscles with the largest moment arms up to the contraction level required to produce the required net reaction moment, unless an upper bound is placed on the contraction intensity in that muscle. Myoelectric data show that recruitment schemes such as this are not used in vivo.

Later models used two objective functions, the first of which minimized the maximum value of the contraction intensity needed in any muscle to achieve equilibrium, as already noted. When this objective is used, all muscles that can contribute to equilibrating a moment are called on to do so, generally with the calculated min/max value of contraction intensity. This recruits muscles with small as well as large moment arms, and so loads the spine heavily in compression. While myoelectric data show that this scheme more accurately predicts actual muscle recruitment patterns than does minimum compression alone, they also show that actual recruitment patterns can be best predicted by using assumptions that lie somewhere between these two extremes. In other words, more realistic muscle force predictions can be obtained if the min/max contraction intensity is first calculated and then spine compression is minimized, subject to a constraint that the allowable contraction intensity is some factor larger than 1.0 times the min/max intensity. This tends to minimize antagonistic contractions and recruit all muscles that can contribute to moment equilibration, but those with larger moment arms contract more intensely than those with smaller moment arms.

A MORE COMPREHENSIVE MODEL FOR SPINE LOADS CALCULATION

The model now to be described incorporates new features to rectify some of the shortcomings of earlier spine loads models described in the foregoing sections. These new features are as follows: (1) allowance for muscle contraction intensities larger than the initially calculated min/max required value; (2) allowance for abdominal cavity pressurization, without having to prescribe what pressure is to be used; (3) inclusion of the transverse abdominal muscles and constraints requiring that the abdominal wall tensions possibly needed to equilibrate the abdominal pressures can be developed; and (4) development of motion segment passive resistances to moments, as well as to forces.

The cross-sectional geometry currently employed for this model is described in Table 3 and illustrated in Figure 2. It is similar to the geometry used in earlier models, but a few numbers have been altered to reflect the availability of better cross-sectional data. Moreover, medial and lateral sections of the transverse abdominal muscles have been incorporated bilaterally, bringing the total number of muscles in the model to 26.

The scheme for calculating internal forces is the same as that provided by Bean and colleagues.[4] The net reaction moment components to be equilibrated (M_i) are supplied. The subscript i takes on values 1, 2, and 3, corresponding to flexion/extension, lateral bending, and axial twist directions. The first calculation minimizes the min/max contraction intensity (I_{mmx}) subject to 40 constraints. The first 26 of these ensure that no muscle contraction intensity exceeds this min/max value.

$$I_m - I_{mmx} \leq 0 \qquad m = 1, .. 26$$

where I_m is the contraction intensity in muscle, m.

The next three constraints ensure that the net reaction moments are equilibrated. The transverse abdominal muscles do not participate in this equilibration. The effective

Table 3 □ Data Incorporated into the 26 Single Equivalent Muscle L3 Cross-Sectional Model

MUSCLE	LINE OF ACTION[a]	AREA RATIO PER SIDE[b]	LOCATION OF CENTROID	
			AP Ratio[c]	Lateral Ratio[d]
Erector spinae				
Multifidus		0.0078	0.060	0.230
Longissimus		0.0156	0.140	0.210
Iliocostalis		0.0156	0.220	0.190
Latissimus dorsi	In frontal plane, 45 degrees to longitudinal	0.0074	0.210	0.280
Quadratus lumborum		0.0057	0.170	0.120
Psoas		0.0130	0.113	0.030
Rectus abdominis		0.0125	0.120	0.615
Oblique abdominals	All inclined 45 degrees to longitudinal			
Internal, medial	In plane 30 degrees to sagittal plane	0.0084	0.413	0.335
External, medial		0.0074	0.413	0.335
Internal, lateral	In sagittal plane	0.0084	0.462	0.081
External, lateral		0.0074	0.462	0.081
Abdominal cavity		0.4650	0.000	0.240

The vertebral body center is located in the midsagittal plane at 0.66 times the trunk depth from the anteriormost edge of the cross section.

[a]If not specified, it is longitudinal.

[b]In ratio to trunk width times trunk depth.

[c]From vertebral body center, in ratio to trunk depth.

[d]From vertebral body center, in ratio to trunk width.

In addition to the 22 muscles listed above, there are a pair of medial and a pair of lateral transverse abdominal muscles incorporated. These are called upon only to equilibrate circumferential wall tensions, so only their thicknesses need be specified. The thicknesses of each of the oblique and the transverse abdominals is assumed to be 0.50 cm.[26]

Abdominal wall circumferential tensions per unit longitudinal length must be large enough to allow radii of curvature to be no more than 14 cm medially and 7 cm laterally.

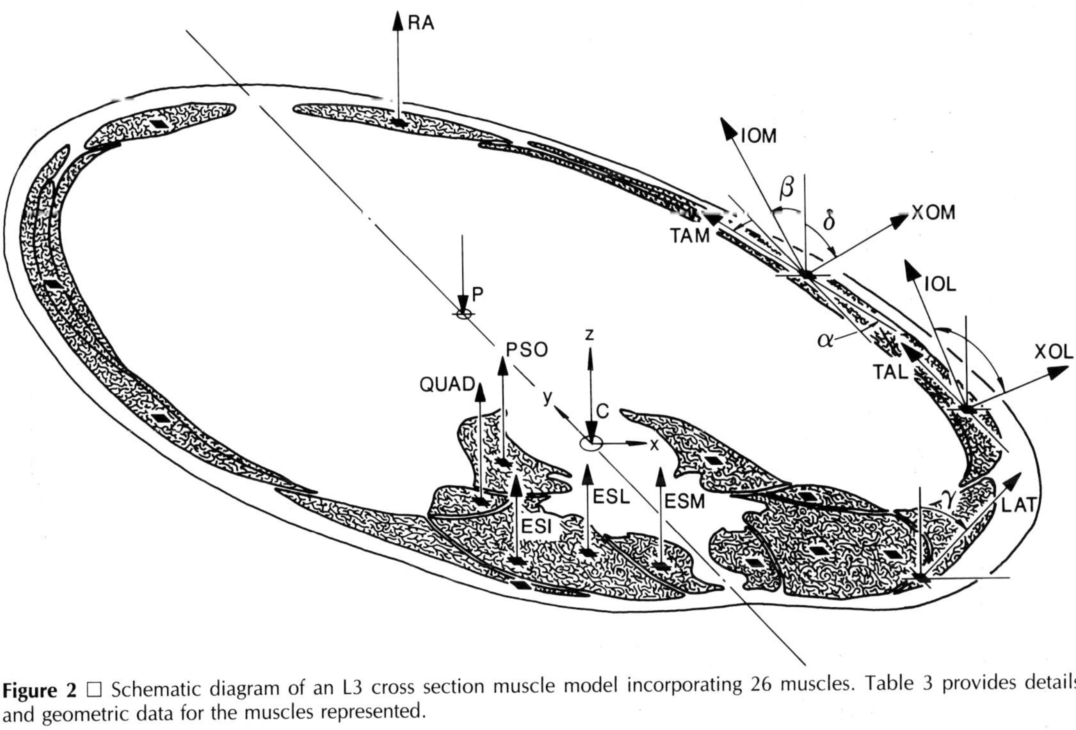

Figure 2 □ Schematic diagram of an L3 cross section muscle model incorporating 26 muscles. Table 3 provides details and geometric data for the muscles represented.

moment arms for muscle m is a_{im}, P is abdominal cavity pressure, A_m the muscle cross-sectional area, subscript *a* refers to the abdominal cavity, and R_i^+ and R_i^- are positive and negative components of the motion segment passive moment resistances. The linear programming technique requires that these two components both be unknowns. One of them will always be found to be zero.

$$\sum_{m=1}^{22} (a_{im}A_mI_m) - a_{ia}A_aP + R_i^+ - R_i^- = M_i \qquad i = 1,2,3$$

The next six constraints insure that the motion segment passive bending resistances do not exceed α_i times the motion segment compression, either for the positive or negative component of these resistances. The β_m multipliers are to account for muscle lines of action that may not be longitudinal.

$$\alpha_i\left(\sum_{m=1}^{22} \beta_mA_mI_m - A_aP\right) - R_i^+ \geq 0 \qquad i = 1,2,3$$

$$\alpha_i\left(\sum_{m=1}^{22} \beta_mA_mI_m - A_aP\right) - R_i^- \geq 0 \qquad i = 1,2,3$$

The next four constraints ensure that transverse tensions per unit longitudinal length sufficient to equilibrate the abdominal cavity pressure are actively developed by combinations of external and internal oblique and transverse abdominal muscle contractions. The first of these, for the left medial muscle groups, is

$$I_{xo}T_{xo} \cos\delta \sin\delta + I_{io}T_{io} \cos\beta \sin\beta + I_tT_t - Pr \geq 0$$

where the subscripts xo = external oblique, io = internal oblique, and t = transverse abdominal.

The T are muscle thicknesses, δ and β are inclination angles for the force vectors (Fig. 2), and r is the maximum abdominal wall circumferential radius of curvature at that location. The I values are muscle contraction intensities, and P is abdominal cavity pressure. Similar equations govern pressure equilibration for the left lateral and for the right medial and right lateral muscle groups.

The last constraint equation ensures that the abdominal pressure, P, developed does not exceed a given upper bound, P_{allow}.

$$P \leq P_{allow}$$

Thus, this first linear program is one in 34 unknowns (26 muscle contraction intensities, the min/max intensity, the abdominal cavity pressure, and the six components of the motion segment passive resistances) subject to the 40 constraints just outlined.

The second linear program minimizes the compression on the motion segment.

$$\sum_{m=1}^{22} (\beta_mA_mI_m) - A_aP$$

The above is subject to the same 40 constraints, except that the first 26 of these now take the following form:

$$I_m \leq I_{allow} \qquad m = 1, \ldots 26$$

These 26 constraints ensure that no muscle contraction intensity exceeds the allowable contraction intensity, I_{allow}, which is larger by a specified factor than the previously calculated min/max intensity. Thus, this program involves 33 unknowns subject to 40 constraints.

SAMPLE RESULTS FROM THE COMPREHENSIVE MODEL

Table 4 presents selected results obtained using the model just outlined, for five sets of input parameters. In each case, spine loads have been calculated when the trunk is upright and subject to net reaction moments that approximate maximum voluntary strengths in healthy young males; 200 N•m in attempted extension, 150 N•m in each of attempted flexion and attempted lateral bending, and 100 N•m in attempted twist. The approximately 400 N of upper body segment weights has not been added into the quoted spine compression values.

The first of the five parameter sets shows the internal loads that result when none of the new features is incorporated. That is, no abdominal cavity pressurization or motion segment passive moment resistances are al-

Table 4 □ Summary of Predictions Made with the 26 Muscle Model

INPUT PARAMETERS	MAXIMUM PREDICTED COMPRESSION (N) Ex,	Fl,	LB,	Tw	MAXIMUM ACP USED (kPa) Ex,	Fl,	LB,	Tw	MIN/MAX INTENSITY (kPa) Ex,	Fl,	LB,	Tw	MAXIMUM TRANSVERSE ABDOMINAL INTENSITY (kPa) (Medial,	Lateral)	MAXIMUM MUSCULAR FORCES (N), PER SIDE			
Set 1																		
IR = 1.0	5922	2111	2323	1216	0	0	0	0	788	507	410	488	0	0	ESM	309	RA	380
ACP = 0															ESI	738	IOM	256
TWP = 0															ESL	738	XOM	225
																	IOL	256
																	XOL	219
Set 2																		
IR = 1.13	4553	1413	1678	1053	0	0	0	0	788	507	410	488	0	0	ESM	479	RA	494
ACP = 0															ESI	959	IOM	269
TWP = 0															ESL	517	XOM	292
																	IOL	320
																	XOL	282
Set 3																		
IR = 1.15	3849	1450	1581	2079	13.3	7.4	13.3	0	718	507	399	248	374	187	ESM	386	RA	437
ACP = 13.3 kPa															ESI	772	IOM	294
TWP = 0.02 m															ESL	693	XOM	259
																	IOL	231
																	XOL	204
Set 4																		
IR = 1.30	3775	1307	1351	407	13.3	13.3	13.3	13.3	718	507	404	488	374	187	ESM	437	RA	494
ACP = 13.3 kPa															ESI	873	IOM	265
TWP = 0															ESL	492	XOM	292
																	IOL	320
																	XOL	282
Set 5																		
IR = 1.30	3775	1307	1351	1698	13.3	13.3	13.3	2.3	718	507	399	248	374	187	ESM	437	RA	494
ACP = 13.3 kPa															ESI	873	IOM	332
TWP = 0.02 m															ESL	485	XOM	230
																	IOL	261
																	XOL	230

IR = $I_{allow}/I_{min}/_{max}$. ACP = Abdominal cavity pressure (input value is maximum allowed). TWP = Motion segment passive resistance multiplier in twist. Those in flexion/extension and lateral bending are zero. ES = erector spinae, M = multifidus, I = iliocostalis, L = longissimus. RA = rectus abdominis. IO = internal oblique, XO = external oblique; M = medial, L = lateral.

Ex = extension. FL = flexion. LB = lateral bending. Tw = twist.

*Predictions are for applied moments of 200 Nm in attempted extension, 150 Nm in each of flexion and lateral bending, and 100 Nm in twisting.

lowed to be developed, and no contraction intensity can exceed the initially calculated min/max value. The other four sets show the results of relaxing those bounds, so that the effects of various combinations of abdominal cavity pressures up to 13.3 kPa (100 mmHg), passive resistances in twist up to 0.02 m times spine compression (e.g., up to 20 Nm for a compression of 1000 N), and contraction intensities up to 30% in excess of the min/max value can be seen.

The Table 4 results show that the incorporation of the new features has the potential to rectify at least some of the shortcomings of the models used earlier. Any one of the new features lowers the predicted spine compressions, sometimes quite substantially. The provision for abdominal pressurization, even under the constraint that appropriate abdominal wall transverse tensions are required for this pressurization, leads to use of this load-relieving mechanism, often to the full extent allowed. The use of abdominal pressurization is qualitatively in keeping with experimental observations; quantitatively, however, in the relevant study reviewed, pressures of up to only 6 kPa were measured, compared with the 13 kPa allowed in the model load calculations. The recruitment of the transverse abdominal muscles to provide abdominal wall tensions in attempted extension tasks, for which no other anterior wall muscles are recruited, may explain the experimental detection of myoelectric activities by abdominal wall surface electrodes during such task performances.

An inspection of the results in Table 4 shows that the different parameter sets lead to internal load predictions that vary over a possible twofold range. This uncertainty as to the exact values of internal loads probably reflects conditions in vivo. The central nervous system likely has many choices as to how a given set of external loads is to be equilibrated. It may be unrealistic to expect the set of internal loads that a task performance imposes in vivo to be unique.

Nevertheless, at least the order of magnitude of those internal loads would seem to be correctly predicted. Despite the wide range of model parameter values used in the five sets of load predictions, the internal loads do not vary greatly. Experience with modeling has shown that limited cross-sectional geometry differences affect the loads predicted only slightly. Similarly, although reasonable sets of changes in model parameters do produce differences in the loads predicted, those differences are not major. The major determinant of internal loadings across any body joint is the net reaction moments that must be equilibrated. In vivo, these moments vary widely. Different models may predict different sets of internal loads, but their variation is relatively small, compared with the variation resulting from different net reaction moments. Thus, at least an approximate picture of the internal loads is provided by any one of the model parameter sets. The Table 4 data give a picture of the orders of magnitude of the internal loads on the lumbar trunk structures when tasks that call for near maximum voluntary trunk strengths are performed.

CLOSURE

The past 10 years has produced the intensive development of biomechanical models to predict what loads internal to the lumbar trunk are imposed by the performance of physical tasks. Although the models have become more sophisticated, a general conclusion reached in the early days of model development remains valid: To keep the loads on the lumbar trunk structures small, keep the net reaction moments that need to be equilibrated small. In other words, avoid positions involving substantial trunk flexion or lateral bending, and keep any loads lifted as close to the spine as is possible.

References

1. Andersson, G., Ortengren, R., and Schultz, A.: Analysis and measurement of the loads on the lumbar spine during work at a table. J. Biomech. 13:513–520, 1980.
2. Ashton-Miller, J.A., and Schultz, A.B.: Biomechanics of the human spine and trunk. *In* Pandolf, K.B., (ed.): Exercise and Sport Science Reviews. New York, Macmillan, 1988, pp. 169–204.
3. Bartelink, D.: The role of abdominal pressure in relieving the pressure on the lumbar intervertebral discs. J. Bone Joint Surg. 39B:718–725, 1957.
4. Bean, J.C., Chaffin, D.B., and Schultz, A.B.: Biomechanical model calculation of muscle contraction forces: A double linear programming method. J. Biomech. 21:59–66, 1988.
5. Berkson, M.H., Nachemson, A., and Schultz, A.B.: Mechanical properties of human lumbar spine motion segments—Part II: Responses in compression and shear; influence of gross morphology. J. Biomech. Engineer. 101:53–57, 1979.

6. Bigos, S.J., Spengler, D.M., Martin, N.A., et al.: Back injuries in industry: A retrospective study. II. Injury factors. Spine 11:246–251, 1986.
7. Eie, N., and Wehn, P.: Measurements of the intra-abdominal pressure in relation to weight bearing of the lumbosacral spine. J. Oslo City Hosp. 12:205–217, 1962.
8. Hult, L.: The Monkfors Investigation. Acta Orthop. Scand. 16 (Suppl.):1–76, 1954.
9. Keith, A.: Man's posture: Its evolution and disorders. Br. Med. J. 1:587–590, 1923.
10. Kelsey, J.L., Githens, P.B., Walter, S.D., et al.: An epidemiological study of acute prolapsed cervical intervertebral disc. J. Bone Joint Surg. 66A:907–914, 1984.
11. Magora, A.: Investigation of the relation between low-back pain and occupation. Indust. Med. 39:504–510, 1970.
12. Miller, J.A.A., Schultz, A.B., and Andersson, G.B.J.: Load displacement behavior of sacroiliac joints. J. Orthop. Res. 5:92–100, 1987.
13. Miller, J.A.A., Schultz, A.B., Warwick, D.N., and Spencer, D.L.: Mechanical properties of lumbar spine motion segments under large loads. J. Biomech. 19:79–84, 1986.
14. Morris, J.M., Lucas, D.B., and Bresler, R.: Role of the trunk in stability of the spine. J. Bone Joint Surg. 43A:327–351, 1961.
15. Nachemson, A.L.: Disc pressure measurements. Spine 6:93–97, 1981.
16. Ortengren, R., and Andersson, G.B.J. Electromyographic studies of trunk muscles, with special reference to the lumbar spine. Spine 2:44–52, 1977.
17. Panjabi, M., Krag, M., White, A., and Southwick, W.: Effects of preload on load displacement curves of the lumbar spine. Orthop. Clin. North Am. 8:181–193, 1977.
18. Schultz, A., Andersson, G., Ortengren, R., et al.: Analysis and quantitative myoelectric measurements of loads on the lumbar spine when holding weights in standing postures. Spine 7:390–397, 1982a.
19. Schultz, A., Andersson, G., Ortengren, R., et al.: Loads on the lumbar spine. J. Bone Joint Surg. 64A:713–720, 1982b.
20. Schultz, A., Cromwell, R., Warwick, D., and Andersson, G.: Lumbar trunk muscle use in standing isometric heavy exertions. J. Orthop. Res. 5:320–329, 1987.
21. Schultz, A.: Loads on the lumbar spine. *In* Jayson, M.I.V. (ed.): The Lumbar Spine and Back Pain. New York, Churchill Livingstone, 1987, pp. 204–214.
22. Schultz, A., and Miller, J.A.A.: Biomechanics of the Human Spine. *In* Mow, V.C., and Hayes, W.C. (eds.): Basic Orthopaedic Mechanics. New York, Raven Press, 1988.
23. Schultz, A.B.: Biomechanics of the human spine and trunk. *In* Skalak, R., and Chien, S. (eds.): Handbook of Bioengineering. New York, McGraw-Hill, 1987, pp. 41.1–41.20.
24. Schultz, A., Warwick, D., Berkson, M., and Nachemson, A.: Mechanical properties of human lumbar spine motion segments—part I: Responses in flexion, extension, lateral bending, and torsion. J. Biomech. Engineer. 101:46–52, 1979.
25. Schultz, A., Haderspeck, K., Warwick, D., and Portillo, D.: Use of lumbar trunk muscles in isometric performance of mechanically complex standing tasks. J. Orthop. Res. 1:77–91, 1983.
26. Strohl, K.P., Mead, J., Banzett, R.B., et al.: Regional differences in abdominal muscle activity during various maneuvers in humans. Am. Physiol. Soc., 1981, pp. 1471–1476.
27. Zetterberg, C., Andersson, G.B.J., and Schultz, A.B.: The activity of individual trunk muscles during heavy physical loading. Spine 12:1035–1040, 1987.

EFFECTS OF REPEATED LOADS AND VIBRATION

Paul Brinckmann
Malcolm H. Pope

Epidemiologic studies point to repeated loading of the spine as one possible cause of low back problems. Repeated loading of the lumbar spine occurs in handling tasks in industrial work, in athletic exercises, and in environments that expose the body to vibration. The prevalence of low back problems, which are believed to be caused by repeated loading of the spine, increases with increasing load magnitude and with increasing exposure time (i.e., with increasing numbers of load cycles). It seems that small loads applied over a large number of cycles may have noxious effects similar to those caused by larger loads applied only a few times.

In this review, a distinction is made between loads that derive from anticipated, voluntary actions of the individuals and loads that are caused by an exposure of the body to vibration. The frequency range of anticipated, repetitive tasks and of vibration is well discriminated. With few exceptions—jogging or running, for example—repetitive, voluntary tasks have frequencies of less than 1 Hz; spinal loading caused by lifting may be of interest even at a frequency of one lift per hour. The domain of vibration frequencies in the present context is 1 to 50 Hz. A similar difference holds for the total number of load cycles sustained, say, per workday. In addition, the epidemiologic, clinical, and experimental methods used to explore both fields are different. It seems appropriate, therefore, to review separately the effects of voluntary repetitive tasks and vibration.

BIOMECHANICAL TERMS AND DEFINITIONS

The fracture behavior of a material is characterized by the stress at the yield limit. Depending on the loading mode of a probe, a fracture may be initiated when the limit of the maximum compressive, tensile, or shear stress is reached. Stress is expressed in units of newtons per square meter (N/m^2).

The ultimate strength, compressive or tensile, of a structure is determined by the amount of force necessary to cause the structure to begin to fail. The ultimate strength (or shorter: strength) of a structure depends on the properties of the materials employed, on the geometry and architecture of the structural elements, and on the specific loading mode. Strength is expressed in newtons (N).

Like all solid materials, bone and soft tissue are subject to mechanical fatigue; under repetitive loading, the yield stress of these materials and the strength of structures built from these materials is reduced with respect to the stress or strength observed under a single load cycle. Fractures induced by repetitive loading are called fatigue fractures. In order to explain the phenomenon of mechanical fatigue, it is assumed that under cyclic loading microdamage is initiated and gradually enhanced until gross, macroscopic failure occurs. In a given loading situation, the probability of observing a fatigue fracture increases with increasing load cycle numbers and decreases with decreasing load magnitude.

When applying this concept to living tissues, it has to be kept in mind that in vivo repair processes will always compete with the generation of microdamage by minor traumatic events. In the medical literature, fatigue fractures are sometimes termed "stress fractures"; this is misleading and should be avoided because stress is always the cause of fracture, regardless of whether it occurs under a single load or after a certain number of load cycles.

Several terms are important in our understanding of vibrational phenomena. The natural frequency is the frequency at which resonance occurs (the oscillation of the body is much greater than the input). Frequency is measured in units of hertz (Hz). For the seated human subject, resonance is at 5 to 6 Hz. Another term encountered is mechanical impedance, which is defined as the force transmitted from the seat to the body divided by the vibration velocity. The impedance reaches a peak at resonance.

REPETITIVE TASKS AND LOW BACK PROBLEMS

Mechanical failure of structural elements of the lumbar spine, bone, and ligaments is frequently seen as result of single traumatic events. In many cases of patients with low back problems, however, patient history shows evidence of repeated loading of the lumbar spine, rather than evidence of major traumatic events. This led to the hypothesis that repeated loadings may cause certain structural elements of the lumbar spine to yield by mechanical fatigue. Thus, accumulated microtrauma could have noxious effects similar to the effects of single traumatic events.

Epidemiologic information about the effects of repetitive tasks stems largely from three fields: industrial work, military exercises, and athletic training. These studies are reviewed below; additional references to related topics are contained in the review papers by Andersson,[6] Sandover,[115] and Troup and Edwards[130] or in the monograph by Junghanns.[70]

A specific lesion of the lumbar spine, fracture of the pars interarticularis and subsequent spondylolisthesis, can be readily identified on roentgenograms. However, this lesion causes clinical problems in only a fraction of the persons involved. Several authors consider repetitive loading of the spine a possible cause of spondylolysis. This hypothesis has not been confirmed explicitly by epidemiologic studies; rather it has been corroborated by the examination of small groups in specialized occupations and by case reports, specifically from persons engaged in athletic training.

Risk Factors Identified in Industrial Labor Environments

Partridge and associates[103] investigated rheumatic complaints in workers in iron foundries. The highest prevalence of lumbar disc disease among the various occupational groups investigated was seen in iron molders (floor molders). This occupational group performed work much of the time in a stooped position; work included shoveling and heavy lifting (50 to 100 kg), as well.

Magora[92] studied 3316 individuals in eight preselected occupations. A high incidence of low back pain was found in persons sitting for prolonged periods of time or in those unable to sit at all during the working day. Weight lifting (5 kg or more for an average of at least 10 times per hour of the working day) was found to be important for low back pain when related to a poor technique in lifting.

Chaffin[19] reported an evaluation of 103 jobs having various amounts of required two-handed load lifting; the 411 people populating these jobs were also evaluated. For a 1-year period, any low back problems in the group were noted. The field study showed that high loads on the lumbar spine, depending on both the location and magnitude of the load lifted, correlate with the incidence of low back pain. It followed that lifting, if a certain load limit in the lumbar spine is exceeded, has to be considered potentially hazardous.

Undeutsch and associates[131] found a high prevalence of back pain in airport transport workers who were engaged in physical heavy work in unfavorable body positions. The prevalence of back pain correlated positively with the past duration of exposure to transport work.

Frymoyer and colleagues[42] analyzed records of 3,920 patients, approximately 10% of whom had reported an episode of low back pain in a certain 3-year interval. The complaint of medically reported low back pain was significantly related to occupational factors such as truck driving, lifting, carrying, pulling, pushing, and twisting as well as to vibrational exposure. In a subsequent survey on 1,221 men between 18 and 55 years of age, Frymoyer and associates[41] identified repetitive heavy lifting, the use of jackhammers or machine tools, and the operation of motor vehicles as risk factors for severe low back pain.

Svensson and Andersson[127] studied the relationship of low back pain to work history and work environment factors in a randomized sample of 940 men from 40 to 47 years of age. Among the variables investigated, only three had a direct association with low back pain: less overtime work, monotonous work, and a high degree of lifting.

Luttmann and colleagues[87, 89, 90] compared the incidence of spine problems of 249 persons engaged in heavy handling and packing work with an age-matched control group of 267 persons. The authors showed the incidence of disease in the lumbar spine to be significantly increased in the heavy manual handling group. In contrast, degenerative disease and postural or morphologic anomalies were uniformly distributed among both groups. In the manual handling group, spine problems tended to occur at a younger age and after a shorter work history than in the control group.

Risk Factors Identified in Athletic Training

Jaros and Cech[69] investigated 20 top-performance weight lifters with an average past training of 7 years. During a training unit, two to three times per week, between 6,000 and 10,000 kg were lifted. All athletes in the group could lift more than 120 kg. Every third athlete reported back pain, but this was only in the initial stage of training; thereafter the symptoms ceased. As compared with wrestlers, weight lifters showed less symptoms involving the spine. Two persons of the group had a spina bifida occulta; they reported no clinical symptoms.

Groher[49] examined a group of top-performance high divers. The athletes had between 5 and 15 years of past training of 16 hours per week, on the average. All complained of back pain, and frequently of neck and shoulder pain. The author postulates that the clinical symptoms result from the high forces on the shoulder and the spine when a diver hits the water surface perpendicularly. In those jumps in which the water surface is hit at an oblique angle, very rapid flexion or extension movements of the lumbar spine can be observed in the submersion

determined maximum acceptable lifting workloads by the use of psychophysical methods. These studies employed realistic simulations of work environments. Snook[122] determined maximum acceptable weights as a function of lifting frequency. For example, a lift of 18 kg from floor to knuckle height at a frequency of one per minute (equivalent to about 400 per day) was acceptable for a male worker. Legg and Myles[81] determined a mass of 17.5 kg lifted 900 times per day to be an acceptable workload for young male military personnel. Mital and Okolie[82] determined one lift per minute of a 25-kg container filled with liquid to be an acceptable workload.

Conclusions

The epidemiologic investigations reviewed above agree in one respect: repetitive lifting, pushing or carrying heavy objects, or performing work in the flexed or hyperextended posture represent risk factors for low back problems. Biomechanical model analyses or direct electromyogram (EMG) or disc pressure measurements have shown that such tasks effect large tensile forces in muscles and ligaments and large compressive forces on bones and cartilaginous joint surfaces. It is therefore inferred that the risk connected to the tasks mentioned above is attributable to injury by mechanical overload of the tissues. However, it must be stressed that the epidemiologic studies provide no information with respect to specific injury responsible for the observed low back problems: mechanically induced damage could occur on the vertebral body, in the disc, in the posterior elements, or in the ligaments.

Minor back problems seem to occur frequently in the initial period of a "risky" task; a subsequent decrease of the risk is interpreted as being a training or a selection effect. More severe problems tend to occur after a certain time of exposure to a repetitive task, rather than after a single maneuver. These findings have prompted many authors to consider mechanical fatigue failure of structural elements of the lumbar spine to be responsible for the low back problems encountered. However, at present there appears to be no substantial evidence to prove this conjecture.

Mechanical damage of a structure (i.e., fracture of a vertebra) may result from a single overload or from mechanical fatigue after a certain number of load cycles. In practice, it is usually difficult to decide on either cause, because it is impossible to closely monitor persons during the time span of an epidemiologic investigation. The interpretation difficulties arise because, during the course of a repetitive task, the occurrence of single, traumatic events that overload the lumbar spine can never be ruled out. Examples are stumbling while lifting or carrying a heavy container or a hard landing from a jump during an athletic exercise or a ballet rehearsal. The probability of the occurrence of such events rises with the increasing physical demand of the work or exercise performed; it also rises in proportion to the time of exposure to such tasks. Thus, the probability of such events depends on load magnitude and exposure time, as does the occurrence of true fatigue fractures. In addition, clinical symptoms need not develop immediately after an accidental overloading episode; consequently, the episode may not be included in the patient's history.

Present knowledge on the effects of athletic exercises on the lumbar spine is still fragmentary. With respect to athletic exercises, there is conflicting evidence in regard to risk factors. Some disciplines that carry high spinal loads and high repetition rates or that require a frequent adoption of unfavorable body positions, such as hyperextension, seem to have a high risk of injury. According to Alexander[5] these disciplines are gymnastics, weightlifting, and football; the most common types of lower back injuries found in athletes are muscle strains, ligament sprains, lumbar vertebral fractures, disc injuries, and neural arch fractures.

Some high-performance athletes seem to be at a risk of back problems that is lower than for the general population. At present, it is difficult to determine whether the low rate of back problems in these athletes is because of an unexpectedly low risk of trauma or the result of favorable training effects. Alternatively, a low rate of back problems in some groups of athletes may result from a selection of the individuals who engage in intense training. The high percentage of persons who discontinue athletic training in the first year of training and in subsequent stages supports this latter inference.

There is evidence that the bone mineral

content (and, hence, strength) of lumbar vertebrae can be increased by physical exercises. Granhed and colleagues[47] compared the bone mineral content of the L3 in a group of top-performance power lifters with that of a matched group of "normal" individuals. The bone mineral content of the athletes was significantly higher than that of the normal group. Within the group of athletes, the mineral content correlated closely with the estimated annual weight lifted. This finding is in accord with the increase of the mineral content in the distal femur of athletes, as compared with normal persons, as shown by Nilsson and Westlin.[100] In addition, physical exercise has been shown to bring about an increase of the vertebral bone mineral content in persons with a subnormal mineral content.[77]

The comparison of athletic exercises with respect to industrial labor is complicated by the fact that in the athletic field one deals with young, healthy subjects, that there is a selection of individuals for the specific tasks, and that the specific task is always accompanied by remedial exercises. In industrial labor, one is dealing with the average population. There is almost no selection of the individuals, and there are many monotonous tasks that are not interrupted by remedial exercises.[52]

In the past, much attention has been given to spondylolysis: this lesion can be readily identified on radiographs and by means of bone scans. Spondylolysis is often observed in athletes whose profession requires them to frequently adopt a hyperextended and rotated posture of the lumbar spine. For this reason, many authors postulate that spondylolysis is caused by mechanical fatigue of the bone of the pars interarticularis. However, there is no hard evidence to prove this hypothesis; fracture of the pars may also occur in a single overload episode. In addition, the observed fractures in the pars differ from fatigue fractures elsewhere in the body, in that the pars interarticularis lesions do not show new periosteal bone formation; there is a high potential for fibrous union.[22]

Future work performed to elucidate the chain of events leading to low back problems after repeated loading of the spine will have to rely on a very close monitoring of the persons under investigation. A detailed biomechanical analysis of the stresses and forces created in the lumbar spine as well as strength and endurance data of the tissues will then allow identification of the primary cause of the low back problems, at least in a certain proportion of cases.

IN VITRO INVESTIGATIONS OF THE MECHANICAL EFFECTS OF REPETITIVE LOADING OF COMPONENTS OF THE LUMBAR SPINE

Repetitive Loading of Lumbar Vertebrae

Hardy and associates[57] reported the first experiment on fatigue fracture of lumbar vertebrae. Cyclic compressive loads were applied to five specimens (one fresh, four embalmed), each consisting of five lumbar vertebrae. Loading was performed at 2 Hz; the load magnitudes ranged from 0.5 to 4.5 kN. Compression fractures of the vertebral bodies occurred after 200 to 1,200,000 cycles.

Liu and colleagues tested 11 specimens of human lumbar spine motion segments consisting of two vertebral bodies and the intervening disc. A cyclic axial load was applied, between 37% and 80% of the ultimate compressive strength of vertebral bodies, as determined from the mean values of failure strength compiled by White and Panjabi.[137] The temporal course of the load corresponded to a sine wave at a frequency of 0.5 Hz. The authors noted an abrupt increase in the maximum compressive displacement at load cycle numbers below 2,000 in five specimens loaded at between 60% and 80% of the mean ultimate compressive strength. This increase in compressive displacement, equivalent to an irreversible height loss of the specimens, was interpreted as sign of a compression fracture. Post-test radiographic investigations of transverse end plate slices showed crack propagation from the periphery of the subchondral bone inward. A removal of the organic matrix from the fractured specimens resulted in their physical disintegration into small particles.

Hansson and coworkers[56] tested 17 lumbar motion segments from eight spines under a cyclic axial compressive load. The load magnitude was expressed as a percentage of the ultimate compressive load, the latter predicted from the bone mineral content of lumbar vertebrae determined by dual-photon absorptiometry. The applied load (expressed as a percentage of the ultimate compressive strength) varied between 60% and 100%. Failure occurred between 1 and 950 cycles; one specimen sustained 1,000 load cycles, the maximum number of cycles applied in this experiment. The fractures observed were all in the end-plate region; no lesions were observed in the outer fibers of the annulus fibrosus. According to the authors' analysis, cycles to failure relate to the relative stress (stress range divided by yield stress) by a power of approximately −14. This is in general agreement with published data on the fatigue of cortical bone, by Lafferty and colleagues.[80]

Brinckmann and associates[13, 14] tested 70 lumbar motion segments from 35 spine specimens under an axial cyclic compressive load at 0.25 Hz. The load magnitude varied between 20% and 70% of the ultimate compressive strength of the vertebrae. In this experiment, the ultimate compressive strength of a motion segment to be tested was predicted from the experimentally measured compressive strength of a neighboring segment from the same spine specimen. The probability of a motion segment being fractured after 10, 100, 500, 1,000 or 5,000 load cycles is shown in Figure 1. This probability increases as the relative load and number of load cycles are increased. At loads above 70%, specimens sustained only a few number of cycles; at loads below 30%, almost all specimens sustained 5,000 load cycles (the maximum number applied in this experiment) without fracture. Under axial compression, fractures occurred invariably in the end-plates; the annuli were not damaged. The results of this experiment are in general agreement with the data of Hansson and coworkers,[56] although the latter tended to show slightly more cycles to fracture.

Repetitive Torsion of Lumbar Motion Segments

Farfan and colleagues[35] measured torsional strength of human lumbar intervertebral joints. They showed that disc injury can be produced by slowly applied rotation in amounts within the range of normal lumbar movement. Because the articular processes stabilize the intervertebral joint against torsion, they suggest that impairment of the function of the posterior elements may result in a higher risk of disc degeneration.

Adams and Hutton[3] simultaneously loaded specimens of intervertebral joints in compression and torsion. It was shown that torsion of the lumbar spine is resisted by the apophyseal joint that is in compression; the compression facet is the first structure to yield at the limit of torsion (i.e., 1 to 2 degrees of rotation) in joints with nondegenerated discs. The authors conclude that torsion seems unimportant in the etiology of disc degeneration and prolapse, since much

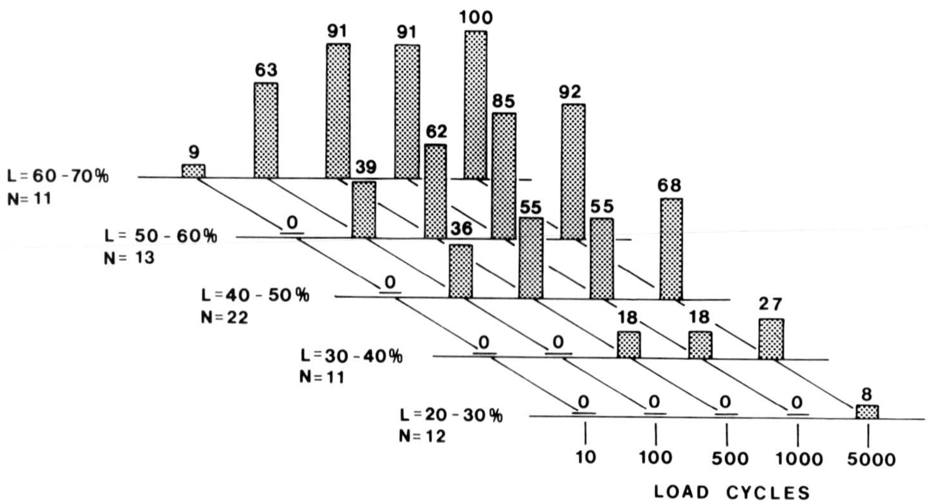

Figure 1 □ Probability of human lumbar vertebrae to fracture as a function of load magnitude and load cycle numbers. The load magnitude is expressed in percent of the ultimate compressive strength of the vertebrae. N is the number of specimens tested in each load range. (From Brinckmann, P., Johannleweling, N., Hilweg, D., and Biggemann, M.: Fatigue fracture of human lumbar vertebrae. Clinical Biomechanics 1987, 2:94–96 by permission of the publishers, Butterworth & Co (Publishers) Ltd ©.)

greater angles are required to damage the intervertebral disc.

Liu and colleagues[85] investigated the effect of cyclic torsional loads on the behavior of intact lumbar intervertebral joints. Angular displacement, rather than torque, was proven to be the determinant in the production of fatigue fractures: specimens that exceeded a motion range of more than ±1.5 degree failed in fatigue. Cycles to fracture varied between 50 and 10,000. Failure occurred in the end plates, facets, laminae and capsular ligaments. All cartilagenous surfaces exhibited fibrillation upon post-test inspection, regardless of whether the intervertebral joint failed in fatigue.

Repetitive Flexion and Extension Tests

The effect of repetitive loading on lumbar intervertebral discs was investigated by Adams.[2] The intervertebral joints were loaded in the flexed position. The cyclic load varied between 1.5 and 6.0 kN; the total number of load cycles amounted to 9,600. This loading was devised to simulate a day of work involving moderate to heavy lifting. Macroscopic inspection of the bisected discs showed distortions of the lamellae and in a few cases complete radial fissures in the posterior region. Distortions and fissures were interpreted as representing the initial stages of disc protrusions.

Adams and colleagues[4] subjected lumbar motion segments to fatigue loading in axial compression and bending. The load, applied at 0.67 Hz, ranged between 800 and 6,000 N. The bending angle varied between 7 and 16 degrees. The number of load cycles varied between approximately 2,000 and 20,000. The failure mode most commonly observed was an end-plate fracture; some specimens showed a gradual disc prolapse. Discs most commonly affected were from the lower lumbar spine of young cadavers.

Repetitive Loading of the Neural Arch

Hutton and coworkers[61] and Cyron and Hutton[30] investigated the fatigue strength of the neural arch. A cyclic compressive force was applied at the inferior articular processes of human lumbar vertebrae. The force direction was selected to simulate the physiologic shear force in the L5–S1 joint. The force magnitude was 570 ±190 N; a force of this magnitude had been calculated to act during every step of walking with a 50-kg pack on the back. The frequency was set to 100 cycles per minute, simulating walking with 100 steps per minute. Seventy-four vertebrae were tested. The cycles to fracture ranged between 17 and 440,000; in the young and old age groups, fractures always occurred in less than 55,000 cycles. Most of the specimens fractured across the partes interarticulares, some across the pedicles and some across the pedicle on one side and the pars on the other. The authors concluded that strenuous activity such as walking with a heavy pack or working for long periods in the flexed position can cause mechanical fatigue of the neural arch.

Lafferty and colleagues[80] determined the fatigue strength of vertebral posterior elements by applying a repetitive force to the inferior joints of human and rhesus monkey vertebrae. The force acted in the plane of the disc, perpendicular to the direction of the long axis of the spine. In approximately half of the 17 specimens tested, fracture occurred in the pars interarticularis and the remaining half in the pedicles. On the basis of the experimentally derived dependence of the cycles to failure on the relative stress (maximum stress divided by cyclic stress), the authors estimate that in vivo forces are of sufficient magnitude to induce fatigue fractures.

Suezawa and Jacob[126] and Jacob and Suezawa[65] presented a critical review of previous attempts to provoke fractures in the pars interarticularis. The authors argued that former experiments were inconclusive with respect to the etiology of such fractures, since the neural arch of the specimens tested had been constrained in such a way that possible fractures were forced to occur in the pars. It was proposed, instead, that such fractures may occur during hyperextension of the spine when the caudal rim of the inferior facets of one vertebra comes into contact with the lamina of the inferior vertebra. Experimentally, fractures of the pars interarticularis could be produced in hyperextension under loads of between 3 and 12 kN. For specimens in which contact of the facets with the lamina was hindered in pure extension, contact (although usually one-sided) could be achieved after applying a minute amount of rotation. The authors concluded that the identical mechanism could easily cause fatigue fractures of the pars, since submaximal spinal loads, in addition to hyperextension and axial rotation, occur frequently during manual handling and athletic exercises.

Conclusions

In vitro experiments are performed to elucidate the chain of events that lead to mechanical failure of the lumbar spine. In addition, by varying the loading modes, magnitudes, and load frequencies, identifying the components of the structure that are most susceptible to injury is attempted. Until now, interest has been primarily on the vertebral body, the bones of the neural arch and the apophyseal joints, the hyaline cartilage, and the intervertebral disc. Most experiments determined the strength of the structures under a single load cycle; the review given above shows that only a few experiments quantify the mechanical behavior under cyclic loading. The situation is further complicated by the fact that effects of cyclic loading (fatigue fractures) in bone are easier to detect and to quantify than in discs or ligaments. This accounts for our fragmentary insight into the mechanical behavior of these important structures under everyday loading conditions or during specialized repetitive tasks. At the same time, it leaves ample room for hypotheses about the cause of low back problems.

In vitro experiments employing cyclic loading indicate that the safety margin between the fatigue strength of vertebral bodies under axial load and that under in vivo loading is small. The same seems to apply (although this is not as well documented) to the strength of the neural arch loaded by shear forces or placed in the hyperextended posture. In general, the disc seems to be less susceptible to injury under cyclic loads: in axial compression, as well as in torsion, the bone yields first. At lower load magnitudes, at which the bone is not damaged, the information on disc properties under cyclic loading is limited by the short time interval that is available before a tested disc specimen deteriorates. At present, the important issue of mechanical contributions to the etiology of disc protrusions has not been resolved.

In mechanical engineering, the identification of fatigue fractures is simplified by the fact that the loading regime is usually well known; additional information about the mechanism of a fracture can be obtained from an inspection of the fracture surfaces. In vivo, the latter is impossible, however, fatigue fractures seem to be characterized as less catastrophic than fractures due to single traumatic events.[97] Displacement of the fragments is less because the energy absorbed per load cycle is smaller. To identify existing fractures as resulting from mechanical fatigue, it is necessary to estimate the fracture probability on the basis of the load history and the experimental data on the bone material properties. At present, such an estimate is possible for vertebral compression fractures only. There is histologic evidence regarding fractures of trabeculae in vertebral bodies,[75, 133] which hypothetically could result from mechanical fatigue. The important question—are such fractures "physiologic" (i.e., desirable and beneficial for bone remodeling) or do they indicate spinal overloading leading to disease?—is controversial and unresolved.

VIBRATION AND LOW BACK PROBLEMS

Rosegger and Rosegger[113] and Bremner and associates[12] were among the first to suggest that the interface of modern man with machinery may be associated with the low back problem. Frymoyer and coworkers,[42] Heliovaara,[58] Kelsey,[71, 72] Kelsey and Hardy,[73] Kelsey and White,[74] Rosegger,[112] and Radke[110] subsequently reported the apparent relationships between various kinds of machinery and low back pain. Seidel and Heide[117] reviewed 185 articles and concluded that people who sit in a vibrating environment that exceeds the ISO exposure limit[63a] place their musculoskeletal systems at risk. Their review covers 43,000 workers exposed to whole-body vibration and 24,000 controls. These data suggest an increased health risk to the spine after intense, long-term whole-body vibration. They concluded that certain vibration exposures are a health risk for the back and the ISO exposure limit (1978) should be set at a more conservative level. In addition, Christ[21] presented strong suspicions of vibration-induced injury in the spine, as seen on x-ray films and by orthopedic examination.

Many studies have revealed that shipyard workers, sheet metal workers, miners, and those using vibrational hand tools have demonstrable abnormal changes in the musculoskeletal, cardiovascular and gastrointestinal systems.[17, 20, 24, 27, 40, 43, 50, 53, 91, 114, 128, 135, 136]

Automobiles and Other Vehicles

Frymoyer and coworkers[42] determined that low back pain was more common in individuals driving trucks and tractors and operating heavy construction equipment. Evaluation of field vibration data also showed that the vibration environment in subjects utilizing common construction vehicles ranges in frequency from 3.5 to 8.9 Hz with vertical accelerations of up to 2.6 g. Both Heliovaara[58] and Kelsey[71, 72] found an increased incidence of herniated discs with long-term exposure to automobiles and trucks. Kelsey and colleagues[73] determined the odds of sustaining a prolapsed disc for each additional 5 hours of driving each week. The use of Swedish or Japanese cars was associated with a lower-than-average risk. Newer cars were less risky than older ones.

Clayberg[23] discussed the strong association he observed between severe low back pain in officers riding in jeeps and other unsprung vehicles. Fishbein and Salter[40] surveyed 1,474 orthopedists and found an association between truck and tractor driving and disorders of the spine and supporting structures. In his retrospective, epidemiologic study of whole-body vibration and interstate truck drivers, Gruber[50] compared truck drivers with air traffic controllers. Vibration was found to be a factor in vertebrogenic pain and deformities of the spine occurring at an earlier age than controls. Snook[121] reported that truck drivers are at high risk of low back pain.*

Rosegger and Rosegger[113] found that x-ray examinations of the spines of 371 tractor operators revealed degenerative changes in the spine occurring earlier and in proportion to the length of service as a tractor driver. Rosegger[112] believed so strongly that early degenerative changes in the spines of tractor drivers were attributable to vibration that he suggested the medical-social welfare system should cater more closely to them. Barbaso[8] also suggested that changes should be made to reduce the high incidence of spine lesions in workers (43% of 213 studied) employed for transport services.

Backman[7] found that spine trouble was common in a health survey of 633 male professional drivers. The drivers studied were as follows: 165 local bus drivers, 122 long distance bus drivers, 154 stock delivery drivers, 159 truck drivers, and 33 tank truck drivers. The health inquiry revealed that 40% of the drivers often had back trouble, and bus drivers reported the most trouble. Increasing age was associated with an increasing prevalence of back pain. Low back pain was the second most common reason for early retirement (18 individuals). Among all the drivers, shoulder and neck pain and back trouble were the most common complaints.

Burton and Sandover[16] reported that the reduction of stiffness of Grand Prix race car suspensions resulted in a significant decrease in the incidence and severity of back pain in the drivers. This suggests that shock and vibration are significant factors in the production of low back pain related to driving and can be reduced by redesigning the cars.

Troup[129] indicated the need for a good, case-controlled study of the effects of vibration on the back. The closest to date has been conducted by Heliovaara.[58] In his attempt to identify risk groups and generate causal hypotheses, Heliovaara[58] found that motor vehicle drivers were at a high risk of being hospitalized for herniated lumbar intervertebral disc or sciatica. His is an important study because it controlled for age, sex, and place of residence. Of 57,000 people who participated in the baseline examinations, 592 were later discharged from hospital (during an 11-year follow-up), having had herniated lumbar intervertebral disc or sciatica. When compared with 2,140 controls (from the same group), motor vehicle drivers were found to be at a greater risk of herniated disc or sciatica. This finding was also suggested by others.[18, 129]

Aircraft

The exposure to aircraft vibration has also been related to low back pain. In a survey of 200 professional pilots, 300 flight attendants, and 200 sedentary, nonflying controls, Buratti[15] found, on x-ray examination, the

*From reports of the California Department of Industrial Relations and the Wisconsin Department of Industry, Labor and Human Relations.

following rates of disc disease and arthrosis: 32% in each of the flight attendant and sedentary control groups, in contrast to 45.5% in the pilot group. Beck,[11] Gearhart,[45] and Fischer and coworkers[39] found that helicopter vibration can cause changes in the musculoskeletal system. In contrast, Shanahan and Reading[118] found no difference between the subjective reports of pain in 11 pilots in either vibrating or nonvibrating UH-1H helicopter seating simulations. However, the simulations used a 10.8-Hz vibration similar to that found during cruise flight. This vibration differs from the natural frequency of 4.5 to 5.5 Hz to which sitting individuals are known to be sensitive.[139, 143] Hence, these findings implicate posture as the more serious problem in this situation.

Earth-Moving Equipment

Kunz and Meyer[78] evaluated drivers of heavy construction machinery; 33% were found to have complaints of disabling low back pain. Even half of these with no low back pain had clinically detectable changes to the musculoskeletal system. Cremona found that 70% of those in the iron industry and those in the mining industry have low back pain. Kohne and Zerlett[76] studied drivers of heavy earth-moving equipment, compared with miners not exposed to vibration. Many more of the vibrated group complained of low back pain and spinal disorders.

Conclusions

The studies described above show an unusual relationship between vibration exposure and low back pain and other musculoskeletal changes. The prevalence of low back pain is as high as 70% in certain occupations, but it appears to be at an unacceptable level for many workers.

HUMAN RESPONSE TO VIBRATION

Mechanical studies have been performed by numerous investigators to evaluate the effect of vibrating the human in either seated, standing, or supine postures, and in single or multiple directions. Most mechanical studies of vibration of the human have utilized the following outcome measures: resonant frequency, transmissibility, impedance, spinal muscle activity, or subjective assessment of discomfort. Mechanical studies are, in general, an improvement on psychophysical studies, as they have the potential of demonstrating the behavior of mechanical elements in the body. When a structure fails as a result of resonant vibration, the failure occurs because the structure oscillates at its maximum possible excursion, thus creating the greatest possible strains in its components. As a result, the structure is at its greatest point of susceptibility to fatigue failure.

Natural Frequency (Resonance)

The natural frequency of a structure of a single degree of freedom can be determined by two means: acceleration transmissibility and driving point impedance. Using the acceleration transmissibility method (transmissibility being defined as the ratio of output acceleration to input acceleration), a comparison is made between the output acceleration in the simple structure resulting from the input, or driving, acceleration. At resonance, this ratio becomes much greater than one. In studies of mechanical driving point impedance, resonance occurs when both the driving force and resultant velocity are in phase, and the curve in the impedance versus frequency plot reaches a maximum.[105]

Mechanical studies to determine the resonant frequency of the seated human operator subjected to vertical vibration have been reported by Bastek and coworkers,[9] Coermann,[25, 26] Dieckmann,[32] Dupuis,[33] Edwards and Lange,[34] Ferraioli and Nightingale,[38] Goldman and von Gierke,[46] Guignard and Irving,[51] Hagena and coworkers,[54] Loach,[86] Müller,[99] Panjabi and coworkers,[102] Pope and colleagues,[105] Radke,[108–110] Seidel and coworkers,[116] Stayner,[124] Stayner and coworkers,[125] Varterasian and Thompson,[132] Vogt,[134] White and coworkers,[138] and Wilder and associates.[139, 140, 142] Some of the above-mentioned studies also reported resonant frequencies of standing and supine subjects, and resonant frequencies of seated subjects as affected by side-to-side or fore–aft vibrations.[59] The natural frequency has been found to be about 5 to 6 Hz, and many vehicles excite that frequency.[105]

Transmissibility

The degree to which the operator moves in a vibration environment is demonstrated by the magnitude of the acceleration transmissibility at the frequency of interest.

At the resonant frequency, the acceleration transmissibility (hence the motion) will be greatest. Work reported by Bastek and associates,[9] Dieckmann,[32] Dupuis,[33] Ferraioli and Nightingale,[38] Goldman and von Gierke,[46] Griffin,[48] Guignard and Irving,[51] Hagena and colleagues,[54] Hornick and coworkers,[59] Matthews,[94] Mertens,[96] Müller,[99] Panjabi and colleagues,[102] Pope and colleagues,[105] Radke,[108–110] Seidel and coworkers,[116] Simons,[119] Sjoflot and Suggs,[120] and Wilder and associates[139, 140, 142] showed transmissibilities greater than 1.0 for the first resonant frequency of the seated operator.

Dieckmann[32] established that, in the standing posture, the first vertical natural frequency is about 5 Hz and the second is 12 Hz. Under horizontal excitation, 1 to 3 Hz is found to be particularly severe. These data are important, because some occupations impart vibration to individuals in the standing posture (e.g., fishermen).

Studies Specific to the Lumbar Spine

Most of the above studies determined transmissibilities by comparing the output acceleration at the head with the input acceleration at the seat. Although this indicates that the resultant motion of the head exceeds the input motion at the seat, these data provide no indication of the relative motion in the lumbar region. Using accelerometers and pins implanted in the lumbar region, the work by Panjabi and coworkers and Dupuis[33] showed that the resonant frequency in the human lumbar region of the vertically vibrated seated operator was 4.5 Hz. By vibrating primates in seated postures, Quandieu and Pellieux,[146] and Slonim[147] showed relative motion between lumbar levels and the upper and lower spine, respectively, via accelerometry. In addition, Coermann[26] found relative motion between the pelvis and the neck in humans by using mercury strain gauges between aluminum shells surrounding and tightly fitting the pelvic and chest regions. Zagorski and associates,[145] using accelerometers taped to the backs of human subjects, found greater acceleration at L3 than at the sacrum in the frequency range of 2 to 5 Hz. Wilder and colleagues[139] found relative motion on the surface of the lumbar region by means of filming seated subjects vibrating at their natural frequency as a moiré fringe pattern was projected on to their backs. Finally, Pope[104] found low levels of relative motion at the seated human's first natural frequency by using a computerized video digitizer (Selspot) system and accelerometers on pins placed into the sacrum and L3. He also reported on artifacts that resulted from skin movement if the accelerators were not rigidly mounted to the spine. Using pins with accelerometers mounted to them, Panjabi and colleagues[102] found little or no relative motion between L1 and L3. This was performed, with similar methodology, by Pope and colleagues.[106]

Electromyographic Studies

Dupuis[33] first reported that under cyclic loading the dorsal muscles also respond cyclically with bursts of activity synchronous with the cyclic excitation. Similar activity levels were reported in the dorsal neck musculature by Cursiter and Harding.[29] In a simulation of helicopter vibration, Pope and coworkers[107] found evidence of muscle fatigue using a medium frequency shift.

Pope and associates[106] found that by vibrating seated individuals near their natural frequency without any foot support, spinal muscle activity was significantly greater. It was assumed that pelvic rocking was an important factor in the production of the first natural frequency of the seated individual.

These studies indicate that maximum strain occurs in the seated operator's lumbar region at the first natural frequency. In addition, Seidel and Heide[117] have monitored the timing of the back muscle response with respect to the vibration stimulus. They found that the muscles were not able to protect the spine from adverse loads. At many frequencies, the muscle responses are so far out of phase that their forces are effectively added to those of the stimulus.

Conclusions

The human spine is susceptible to large oscillations and, thus, potential damage at its natural frequencies. In the seated individual these occur at 5 Hz and 10 Hz, and in the standing individual at 5 Hz and 12 Hz. Many vehicles excite these frequencies. The main reasons for the first resonance appear to be pelvic rocking, and little increased transmissibility occurs in the lumbar spine itself. Vibration causes muscle contracture that can increase the effective spinal load. Such exposure, if prolonged, can lead to muscular fatigue.

References

1. Abel, M.S.: Jogger's fracture and other stress fractures of the lumbar spine. Skeletal Radiol. 13:221–227, 1985.
2. Adams, M.H.: The effect of fatigue on the lumbar intervertebral disc. J. Bone Joint Surg. 65B:199–203, 1983.
3. Adams, M.A., and Hutton, W.C.: The relevance of torsion to the mechanical derangement of the lumbar spine. Spine 6:241–248, 1981.
4. Adams, M.A., and Hutton, W.C.: Gradual disc prolapse. Spine 10:524–531, 1985.
5. Alexander, M.J.L.: Biomechanical aspects of lumbar spine injuries in athletes: A review. Can. J. Appl. Sport Sci. 10:1–20, 1985.
6. Andersson, G.: Epidemiologic aspects of low back pain in industry. Spine 6:53–60, 1981.
7. Backman, A.L.: Health survey of professional drivers. Scand. J. Work Environ. Health 9:30–35, 1983.
8. Barbaso, E.: Sull'incidenza delle alterazioni della colonna vertebrale nel personale viaggante di una azienda auto-tramviaria. [Incidence of changes of the vertebral column in travelling personnel of a bus-streetcar company.] Med. Lav. 49:60–634, 1958.
9. Bastek, R., Buchholz, Ch., Denisov, E.I., et al.: Comparison of the effects of sinusoidal and stochastic octave-band-wide vibrations—a multi-disciplinary study. Part I: Experimental arrangement and physical aspects. Part II: Physiological aspects, Part III: Psychological investigations, Internat. Arch. Occup. Environ. Health 39:143–179, 1977.
10. Beals, R.K., and Hickman, N.W.: Industrial injuries of the back and extremities. Comprehensive evaluation—an aid in prognosis and management. A study of one hundred and eighty patients. J. Bone Joint Surg. 54A:1593–1611, 1972.
11. Beck, A., Radiologische Beurteilung de Wirbelsaule aus fliegerarztlicher Sicht. Wehrmed. Monatsschr. 267–276, 1973.
12. Bremner, J.M., Lawrence, J.S., and Miall, W.E.: Degenerative joint disease in a Jamaican rural population. Ann. Rheum. Dis. 27:326–332, 1968.
13. Brinckmann, P., Johannleweling, N., Hilweg, D., and Biggemann, M.: Fatigue fracture of human lumbar vertebrae. Clin. Biomech. 2:94–96, 1987.
14. Brinckmann, P., Biggemann, M., and Hilweg, D.: Fatigue fracture of human lumbar vertebrae. Clin. Biomech. Suppl. 1 (in press).
15. Buratti, L., Ruggieri, G., and Spuri, L.: Spinal degeneration found in pilots greater than in flight attendants. Rheumatology News 5, 1978.
16. Burton, A.K., and Sandover, J.: Back pain in Grand Prix drivers: A "found" experiment. Appl. Ergon. 18:3–8, 1987.
17. Casciu, G., Cossu, F., and Spinazzola, A.: Sulla incidenza della alterazioni radiologiche dell'apparato osteoarticolare negli operai dell'industria estrattiva sarda con particolare riguardo ai perforatori. [The frequency of radiological changes in the osteoarticular apparatus in Sardinian miners, especially in workers using pneumatic hammers.] I: Lo scheletro delle mani e dei polsi. II: L'articolazione del gomito. Folia Medica (Napoli) 51:370–395, 1968.
18. Cecchitti, E.: Lumbar pains in a group of professional drivers. Difera Sociale 24:82–94, 1963.
19. Chaffin, D.B., and Park, K.S.: A longitudinal study of low back pain as associated with occupational weight lifting factors. Am. Indust. Hygiene Assoc. J. 34:513–524, 1973.
20. Chierchi, P., et al.: Study of the vibrations produced by pneumatic hammers. Securitas 53:65–90, 1968.
21. Christ, V.W.: Belastung durch mechanische Schwingungen und moegliche Gesundheitsschaedigungen im Bereich der Wirbelsaeule. 2. Moeglichkeit von Gesundheitsschaedigungen. [Stress through mechanical vibrations and possible damage to health in the area of the spine.] Fortschritte der Medizin. 92:705–708, 1974.
22. Ciullo, J.V., and Jackson, D.W.: Pars interarticularis stress reaction, spondylolysis and spondylolisthesis in gymnasts. Clin. Sports Med. 4:95–110, 1985.
23. Clayberg, H.D.: Pathologic physiology of truck and car driving. Military Surgeon. 105:299–311, 1949.
24. Coermann, R.R.: Mechanical vibrations. Proceedings of a Symposium of Ergonomics and Physical Environmental Factors, Sept. 16–21, 1968, Geneva, Switzerland. The International Labour Office.
25. Coermann, R.R., Ziegenrucker, G.H., Wittwer, A.L. and von Gierke, H.E.: The passive dynamic mechanical properties of the human thorax-abdomen system and of the whole body system. Aerospace Med. 31:443–455, 1960.
26. Coermann, R.R.: The mechanical impedance of the human body in sitting and standing position at low frequencies. Acoustic Systems Division Technical Report #61–492, Aerospace Medical Research Labs, Wright Patterson Air Force Base. Sept., 1961.
27. Coermann, R.R.: Physiological problems of vibration in motor vehicles. Zentralblatt fur Verkehrs-Medizin 11:150–166, 1965.
28. Cremona, E.: Die Wirbelsaule bei den Schwerarbeitern der Eisen—und Stahlindustrie sowie des Bergbaus. Kommiss. Europ. Gen. Generaldir. Soz. Angelegenheiten Dok. Nr. 1911/72, 1972.
29. Cursiter, M.C., and Harding, R.H.: Electromyographic recordings of shoulder and neck muscles of seated subjects exposed to vertical vibrations. Proc. Physiol. Soc. I Physiol. 239:117–118, 1974.
30. Cyron, B.M., and Hutton, W.C.: The fatigue strength of the lumbar neural arch in spondylolysis. J. Bone Joint Surg. 60B:234–238, 1978.
31. Damkot, D.K., Pope, M.H., Lord, J., and Frymoyer, J.W.: The relationship between work history, work environment and low back pain in males. Spine 9:395–399, 1984.
32. Dieckmann, D.: A study of the influence of vibration on man. 1:347–355, Ergonomics, 1958.
33. Dupuis, H.: Belastung durch mechanische Schwingungen und moegliche Gesundheitsschaedigungen im Bereich der Wirbelsaeule. [Impact through mechanical vibrations and possible dam-

age to health in the area of the spine.] Fortschritte der Medizin. 92:618–620, 1974.
34. Edwards, R.G., and Lange, K.O.: A mechanical impedance investigation of human response to vibration. A.M.R.L.-T.R.-64-91, Final Report. A.D.-609-006, 1964.
35. Farfan, H.F., Cossette, J.W., Robertson, G.H., et al.: The effects of torsion on the lumbar intervertebral joints: The role of torsion in the production of disc degeneration. J. Bone Joint Surg. 52A:468–497, 1970.
36. Farfan, H.F., Osteria, V., and Lamy, C.: The mechanical etiology of spondylolysis and spondylolisthesis. Clin. Orthop. Rel. Res. 117:40–55, 1976.
37. Ferguson, R.J.: Low back pain in college football linemen. J. Bone Joint Surg. 56A:1, 300, 1974.
38. Ferraioli, A., and Nightingale, J.M.: A design of a vibrating platform and transmission of low frequency vertical vibrations of the seated man. Technic. Ital. 44:213–219, 1979.
39. Fischer, V., et al.: Vibrationsbedingte Wirbelsaulenschaden bei Hubschrauberpiloten. Arb. Med. Soz. Med. Prav. Med. 7:161–163, 1980.
40. Fishbein, W.I., and Salter, L.C.: The relationship between truck and tractor driving and disorders of the spine and supporting structures. Indust. Med. Surg. 19:444–445, 1950.
41. Frymoyer, J.W., Pope, M.H., Clements, J.H., et al.: Risk factors in low-back pain. J. Bone Joint Surg. 65A:213–218, 1983.
42. Frymoyer, J.W., Pope, M.H., Costanza, M.C., et al.: Epidemiologic studies of low back pain. Spine 5:419–423, 1980.
43. Fusco, M., Paggi, E., Rossi, A., and Sessa, G.: L'azione delle vibrazioni sull'apparato circulatorio periferico e sulla colonn vertebrale. [Effect of vibration on the peripheral vascular system and on the vertebral column]. Folia Medica (Napoli) 46:361–372, 1963.
44. Gaynor, B.J., Hagen, R.J., and Allen, W.C.: Biomechanics of the spine in the polevaulter as related to spondylolysis. Am. J. Sports Med. 11:53–57, 1983.
45. Gearhart, J.R.: Response of the skeletal system to helicopter-unique vibration. Aviat. Space Environ. Med. 49:253–256, 1978.
46. Goldman, D.E., von Gierke, H.E.: The effects of shock and vibration on man. Lecture and Review Series, No. 60-3, Naval Medical Research Institute, Bethesda, Jan. 8, 1960. American National Standards Institute #S3-W-39.
47. Granhed, H., Jonson, R., and Hansson, T.: The loads on the lumbar spine during extreme weight lifting. Spine 12:146–149, 1987.
48. Griffin, M.J.: Vertical vibration of seated subjects: Effects of posture, vibration level, and frequency. Aviat. Space Environ. Med. 46:269–276, 1975.
49. Groher, W.: Kreuzschmerzen und Wirbelsaulenveranderungen bei Kunst—und Turmspringern. Sport. Sportmed. 11:444–450, 1969.
50. Gruber, G.J.: Relationships between whole-body vibration and morbidity patterns among interstate truck drivers. D.H.E.W. (N.I.O.S.H.) Publication No. 77–167. U.S. Department of Health, Education and Welfare, National Institute of Occupational Safety and Health, Cincinnati, 1976.
51. Guignard, J.C., and Irving, A.: Effects of low frequency vibration on man. Engineering (London) 190:364–367, 1960.
52. Häublein, H.G.: Berufsbelastung und Bewegungsapparat. Berlin, V.E.B. Verlag Volk und Gesundheit, 1979.
53. Haack, M.: Human tolerance to vibrations in farm machines. Agric. Engineer. 4:253–257, 1956.
54. Hagena, F.W., Wirth, C.J., Piehler, J., et al.: *In-vivo* experiments on the response of the human spine to sinusoidal G_z vibration. A.G.A.R.D. Conf. Proceedings No. 378 N.T.I.S. Springfield, Virginia, U.S.A.; Paris, E.S.A./Information Retrieval Service; British Lending Library Division, West Yorkshire, U.K., 1985.
55. Hall, S.J.: Mechanical contribution to lumbar stress injuries in female athletes. Med. Sci. Sports Exerc. 18:599–602, 1986.
56. Hansson, T.H., Keller, T.S., and Spengler, D.M.: Mechanical behavior of the human lumbar spine. II. Fatigue strength during dynamic compressive loading. J. Orthop. Res. 5:479–487, 1987.
57. Hardy, W.G., Lissner, H.R., Webster, J.E., and Gurdjian, E.S.: Repeated loading tests of the lumbar spine. Surg. Forum 9:690–695, 1958.
58. Heliovaara, M.: Occupation and risk of herniated lumbar intervertebral disc or sciatica leading to hospitalization. J. Chron. Dis. 40:259–264, 1987.
59. Hornick, R.J., Boettcher, C.A., and Simons, A.K.: The effect of low frequency high amplitude, whole body, longitudinal and transverse vibration upon human performance. Final report, contract No. DA-11-022-509-ORD-3300, Ordnance Project No. TEI-1000, Bostrom Research Labs, Milwaukee, 1961.
60. Hoshina, H.: Spondylolysis in athletes. Physician Sportsmed. 8:75–79, 1980.
61. Hutton, W.C., Stott, J.R.R., and Cyron, B.M.: Is spondylolysis a fatigue fracture? Spine 2:202–209, 1977.
62. Ichikawa, N., Ohara, Y., Morishita, T., et al.: An aetiological study on spondylolysis from a biomechanical aspect. Br. J. Sports Med. 16:135–141, 1982.
63. Ireland, M.L., Michell, L.M.: Bilateral stress fracture of the lumbar pedicles in a ballet dancer. J. Bone Joint Surg. 69A:140–142, 1987.
63a. I.S.O.: Guide for the evaluation of human exposure to whole body vibration. Internat. Organ. Standard. Ref. No. I.S.O. 2631-1978 (E).
64. Jackson, D.W., Wiltse, L.L., and Cirincione, R.J.: Spondylosis in the female gymnast. Clin. Orthop. Rel. Res. 117:68–73, 1976.
65. Jacob, H.A.C., and Suezawa, Y.: Zur Aetiologie der Spondylolyse infolge mechanischer Einwirkung. *In* Hackenbroch, M.H., Refior, H.J., Jager, M., (eds.): Biomechanik der Wirbelsaule. Thieme, Stuttgart, 1983.
66. Jäger, M., and Luttmann, A.: Biomechanische Analyse ausgewahlter Tatigkeiten im Baugewerbe. *In* Laurig, W., Gerhard, L., Luttmann, A., Jäger, M., and Nau, H.E.: Untersuchungen zum Gesundheitsrisiko beim Heben und Umsetzen schwerer Lasten. Schriftenreihe der Bundesanstalt fur Arbeitsschutz Fb Nr. 409, Dortmund, 1985.
67. Jäger, M.: Biomechanisches Modell des Menschen zur Analyse und Beurteilung der Belastung der Wirbelsaule bei der Handhabung von Lasten. Fortschritt-Berichte Reihe 17: Biotechnik Nr. 33, V.D.I. Verlag, Dusseldorf, 1987.
68. Jäger, M., and Luttmann, A.: Biomechanical model calculations of spinal stress for different working

137. White, A.A., and Panjabi, M.M.: Clinical biomechanics of the spine. Philadelphia, J.B. Lippincott, 1978.
138. White, G.H., Lange, K.O., and Coermann, R.R.: The effects of simulated buffeting on the internal pressure of man. Hum. Fact. 4:275–290, 1962.
139. Wilder, D.G., Frymoyer, J.W., and Pope, M.H.: The effect of vibration on the spine of the seated individual. Automedica 6:5–35, 1985.
140. Wilder, D.G., Pope, M.H., and Frymoyer, J.W.: Cyclic loading of the intervertebral motion segment. *In* Hansen, E.W. (ed.): Proceedings of Tenth Northeast Bioengineering Conference, March 15–16, 1982, Dartmouth College, Hanover, pp. 9–11. Institute of Electrical and Electronic Engineers, Inc., Catalog #82CH1747–5, New York, 1982.
141. Wilder, D.G., Seroussi, R.E., Dimnet, J., and Pope, M.H.: How the lumbar motion segment responds to sustained sitting. *In* American Society of Mechanical Engineers: Advances in Bioengineering, American Society of Mechanical Engineers, New York, 1986.
142. Wilder, D.G., Woodworth, B.B., Frymoyer, J.W., and Pope, M.H.: Energy Absorption in the Human Spine. *In* Paul, I. (ed.): Proceedings of Eighth Northeast (New England) 1980 Bioengineering Conference, March 27–28, 1980, M.I.T., Cambridge, pp. 442–445, 1980.
143. Wilder, D.G., Woodworth, B.B., Frymoyer, J.W., and Pope, M.H.: Vibration and the human spine. Spine 7:243–254, 1982.
144. Wiltse, L.L., Widell, E.H., and Jackson, D.W.: Fatigue fracture: The basic lesion in isthmic spondylolisthesis. J. Bone Joint Surg. 57A:17–22, 1975.
145. Zagorski, J., Jakubowski, R., Solecki, L., et al.: Studies on the transmissions of vibrations in human organism exposed to low-frequency whole-body vibration. Acta Physiol. Polonica 27:347–354, 1976.
146. Quandieu, P. and Pellieux, L. (1982) Study in situ et in vivo of the acceleration of lumbar vertebrae of a primate exposed to vibration in the z-axis. J. Biomed. 15, 985–1002.
147. Slonim, A.R. (1983) Some vibration data on a primate implanted with accelerometers on the upper and lower spine: methodology and results in Rhesus monkeys. AMRL-TR-81-153.

DEGENERATION, INJURY, AND SPINAL INSTABILITY

Manohar M. Panjabi

Although the cause of most cases of low back pain (LBP) is unknown,[35] spinal instability is considered to be one of the most common[17] and the most important causes.[18] It is hypothesized that mechanical derangement by degeneration, injury, or muscle dysfunction is the cause of spinal instability that results in pain and/or dysfunction. It is assumed that an underlying intervertebral motion abnormality exists, which is magnitude- and direction-dependent. It is further hypothesized that the spinal stability is provided by two inter-related systems: the spinal column and the muscular control system. One may think of the former as the passive system and the latter as the active system. Instability results when a single or multiple components fail or malfunction in any of the two systems. Except as otherwise noted, this discussion pertains to the spinal column and its components, as little is known about the muscular control of stability. Although the phrase "spinal instability" is commonly used in a clinical setting, there is no single accepted definition.[37]

Like any other disease, spinal instability may be described by its causes, diagnostic methods, and treatments. Presently the causes are thought to be injury, degeneration, and muscle dysfunction or insufficiency—or a combination of all three. Diagnostic methods generally include static or functional roentgenograms. Treatment methods include exercises and surgery. Past research concerned with these aspects of spinal instability is described. Also presented are future directions for research.

This work was supported in part by NIH grants AR 34699 and AR 30361.

CAUSES OF SPINAL INSTABILITY

Injury

Microtrauma occurring for long periods of time may lead to accelerated degeneration and spinal instability.[5] A major overload may fracture facets and end plates, produce annular tears of the disc, and/or rupture ligaments, which may also lead to spinal instability. Surgical procedures (e.g., total facetectomies) may also cause instability.

What roles do the ligaments, facets, and disc components play in providing stability? Conversely, how much and what kind of stability is lost because of injury to any one or more of these passive spinal components? Farfan and associates[4] experimentally determined the contribution of the facet joints to be nearly 50% in resisting torsional loads. However, the axis of rotation was fixed in the experiments, and that has been shown to enhance the role of the facet joints.[31] A more detailed study of the role of the various spinal components in providing spinal stability was conducted by Posner and coworkers.[29] Fresh cadaveric functional spinal units were subjected to either flexion or extension loads, whereas the various spinal components were transected from either a posterior-to-anterior direction or vice versa. Vertebral movements were monitored in the sagittal plane. Results of this study formed the basis of the guidelines for determining the thresholds of clinical instability in the lumbar spine.[36] This was, however, a sagittal plane study. More recently, using pure moment loads and measuring three-dimensional 6 degrees-of-freedom motions, the effects of posterior ligamentous injury and of partial and total facetectomies were recorded.[1] Using physiologic loads of 8 N•m, the average ranges of motion (and neutral zones) for the intact lumbar spine were found to be as follows: flexion = 8.2 (0.93) degrees; extension = 4.0 (0.93) degrees; lateral bending = 6.2 (0.97) degrees; and axial rotation = 3.5 (1.1) degrees (Fig. 1). (The concept of neutral zone is indicated in Fig. 3 and is explained later.) Cutting of supraspinous and interspinous ligaments produced a 2-degree increase in flexion, but no change in other motions. Unilateral facetectomies produced significant increases of 4.2 degrees in flexion and 1.8 degrees in rotation, but no marked changes in other motions. Bilateral total facetectomy, compared with the intact spine, produced increases of 63% in flexion, 78% in extension, 15% in lateral bending and 126% in axial rotation. Thus, facets do play a significant mechanical role, especially in rotatory stability. They concluded that the partial facetectomy of one or both facets at a single level does not cause spinal instability, whereas the loss of a complete facet joint on one or both sides makes the spine acutely unstable. These in vitro experimental results should be carefully interpreted for clinical use.

Does the injury to the disc repair itself? Is this possible? It is known from pathologic studies that the disc does not have the healing potential of most other structures in the body because it lacks a blood supply.[10] The concept of a self-sealing phenomenon of a mechanical nature that would seal off the defect (e.g., microfractures in the end plate or tears in the annulus) was advocated[15] but was later shown to be a fallacy, especially for multidirectional instabilities.[8, 24]

The process of repair and restabilization after injury, if it occurs, cannot be studied by in vitro biomechanical studies. Neither can the clinical studies provide any useful information concerning the natural time course of an injury, as all significant injuries in the humans are most often surgically or otherwise stabilized. Thus the natural history of most spinal injuries is presently unknown. In a recent set of in vivo experiments using two different animals, three graded spinal injuries (interspinous and supraspinous ligament transections, laminectomy, and facetectomy) at the C4–C5 level were studied by functional flexion–extension stereoradiographs for up to 24 weeks.[25, 34]

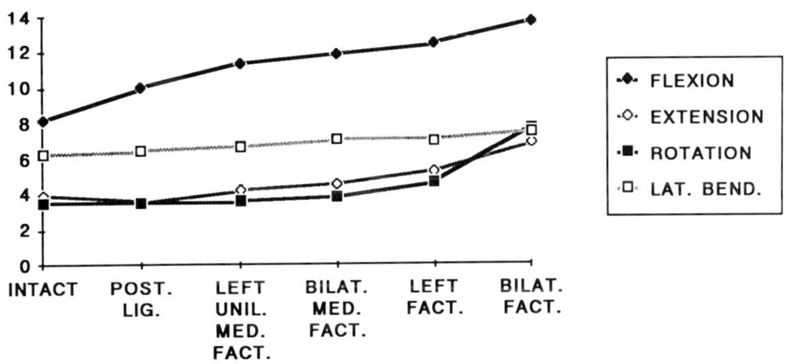

Figure 1 □ Average intervertebral ranges of motion of fresh cadaveric lumbar spine specimens as functions of injury. The motions are as follows: flexion, extension, lateral bending, and axial rotation; the injuries are sequential transactions from posterior ligaments to bilateral facetectomy. (Based upon data from Abumi and colleagues.[1])

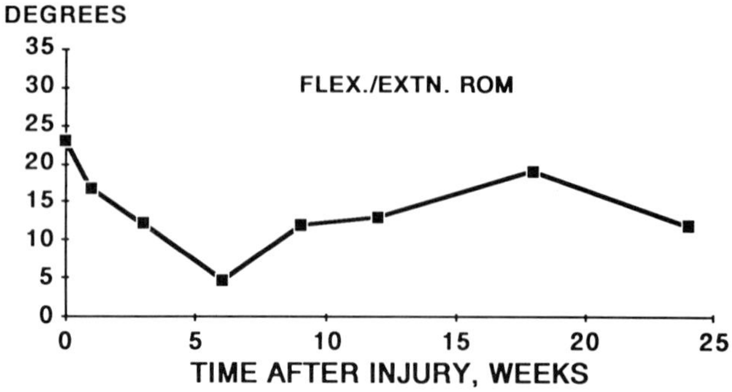

Figure 2 □ Motion at injury site as function of healing time. The injury was bilateral facetectomy at C4–C5 in a canine model. The injury was unprotected during the entire healing phase, and the motion measurements were made using functional flexion-extension radiographs. (Based upon data from Panjabi and colleagues.[25])

Contrary to expectations, the spine at the injury site became more stable (even compared with the intact spine) as measured by standardized flexion–extension x-rays during the healing period (Fig. 2). Although the facetectomy resulted in the largest increase in motion acutely, it also had the largest decrease in motion in vivo. At 6 weeks after the injury, the range of motion decreased from 23 degrees preoperatively to 5 degrees postoperatively. These findings are supported by studies of Whitehill and coworkers.[38] Although no such experimental studies have been conducted in the lumbar region, one may expect similar responses.

Degeneration

With age the human spine degenerates, as do most other structures in the body. This normal process results in altered mechanical characteristics. It may also lead to low back problems. Kirkaldy-Willis[12] has provided a classification of degeneration of the spine based on three stages. *Dysfunction* (1st stage) includes LBP with a nonspecific syndrome. The facet capsule may be lax and disc degeneration is of Grade 1 to 2 on a scale of 1 to 4. *Instability* (2nd stage) has increased facet laxity and a disc degeneration of Grade 2 to 3. A clinical syndrome can be identified and the instability may be measured by functional x-rays. *Restabilization* (3rd stage) is reached with fibrosis in posterior joints and osteophytic formations leading to decreased overall motion. Disc degeneration has reached the final stage (Grades 3 to 4).

In the second degeneration stage, the spine may become more mobile and, thus, unstable. This effect on the mechanical properties of the spine is quite specific and direction dependent. From load-displacement curves of a lumbar spine specimen, several parameters may be obtained to quantify the mechanical properties. These are as follows: the neutral zone, representing "looseness of the specimen"; the elastic zone, which may be equated with elastic deformation; and the range of motion (Fig. 3). For example, in an in vitro study using fresh cadaveric lumbar spine specimens, results showed that as the spine degenerated, the range of motion in flexion decreased; in axial rotation the range increased, and it remained constant in lateral bending.[23] In the same study, the neutral zone was affected differently. As the spine degenerated, the neutral zone increased both in flexion (especially the coupled anteroposterior translation) and in axial rotation, but in lateral bending it was unaffected. Creep, representing more of the viscous properties, has also been found to be significantly altered with degeneration.[11] Although some of the mechanical properties change with degeneration, and the degeneration increases with age, there does not seem to be a direct relationship between the mechanical property changes and age.[19]

In a recent study by Wilder and coworkers,[39] another phenomenon has been observed in the biomechanical behavior of the spinal column, which may explain the clinical observation of spine suddenly "giving way." In this in vitro study, when axial compression was applied to a fresh cadaveric two-vertebra functional spinal unit, the authors observed a sudden increase in flexion and/or lateral bending. They characterized this buckling phenomenon as a possible mechanism of spinal instability.

The above knowledge has been obtained mostly from in vitro experiments. The general degeneration of the spine, seen on x-rays as decreased disc height, deformed end plates, and osteophyte formations, has not been found to be a reliable predictor of LBP.

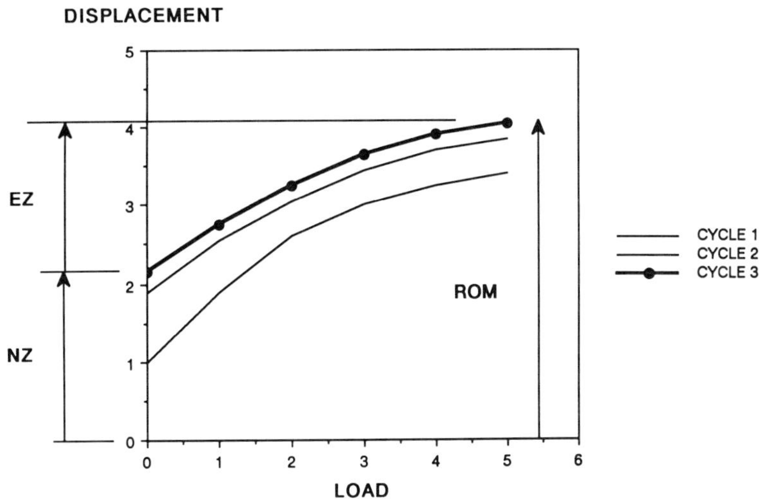

Figure 3 □ Load displacement curves of a spine specimen obtained by three load-unload cycles. The lower two curves represent preconditioning. From the final curve parameters of neutral zone (NZ), the elastic zone (EZ), and range of motion (ROM) are obtained.

On the other hand, there is evidence to suggest that increased disc degeneration carries a significantly higher risk of LBP problems.[33] During discography 23% of patients with nondegenerated discs reported pain, and 77% felt either pressure only or no pain at all. On the other hand, among the patients with a severely degenerated annulus, 90% reported pain during discography, whereas only 10% felt no pain or only some pressure. Thus, a significant relationship seems to exist between disc degeneration and low back pain, even though it may not be a one-to-one correspondence. This and similar in vivo studies provide a link between the in vitro biomechanical studies, by which the mechanical characteristics of the spine and the clinical symptoms of LBP may be precisely quantified.

Muscle Dysfunction

A spinal column that is devoid of musculature is an extremely unstable structure, with a load carrying capacity of less than 25 N.[14] However, with properly coordinated muscle action, the spine can sustain very large loads, which is exemplified by the action of weightlifters. Electromyographic (EMG) signals of the paraspinal and abdominal muscles have been studied both in normal subjects and in patients with LBP. The results have been rather unclear, showing both the difficulty of the subject matter and the inherent variability of the EMG signals. In one of the recent studies using EMG measurements, the only conclusion reached was that the EMG patterns showed some abnormalities in low back pain patients compared with the normal group. This was true during flexion but not during rotation and lateral bending.[20] It is believed that interabdominal pressure plays an important role in stabilizing the spine, although its significance in relieving the load on the spine is minimal.[9]

In spite of these facts, the role of the muscles in providing a major part of spinal stability is not well understood. Muscle dysfunction may result from muscle weakness, in the form of decreased strength or endurance, and possibly from a disturbance in the neuromuscular control system. There are few, if any, studies dealing with this specific aspect of muscle function.

DIAGNOSTIC METHODS

Besides the grades of disc degeneration, which are related to a greater risk of LBP, there are other motion and posture parameters that may be obtained from radiographs or computed tomographic (CT) scans. Functional radiographs (i.e., a pair of radiographs taken, generally, at the extremes of a motion in a certain plane) form the basis of most clinical studies of motion. Knutsson was probably the first to indicate a relationship between excessive anteroposterior translation seen on flexion-extension radiographs and low back problems. These observations have been confirmed in recent studies.[7, 13] In another study, patients with LBP were followed in lateral bending, and centers of rotation were calculated for various positions of the lumbar spine. The area occupied by the locus of the centers of rotation at a particular level was found to be directly related to the LBP associated with that level.[3] In other words, the greater the spread in the locations of the centers of rotation at a particular level, as the spine bends from left to right, the greater is the risk of LBP associated with that level. More recently, similar results were found by Seligman and colleagues[30] in an in vitro study of the parameter of the length of the path of the center of rotation in flexion–extension. However, this promising biomechanical tool of the centers of rotation was found to be a poor predictor in an in vivo study of LBP patients conducted by the same research team, Gertzbein and associates,[7] primarily because of significant errors associated with the technique of determining the centers of rotation.

More than the increased quantity of motion, the quality of motion may be affected by instability and, therefore, may be its best indicator. The spinal movements of LBP patients suspected of having instability may not always be greater in magnitude. In fact, it is known clinically, and has been quantified using three-dimensional X-ray analysis that the patients with LBP have restricted flexion–extension intervertebral motion. The total flexion (L1–S1) of about 50 degrees in the normals decreased to less than 20 degrees in LBP patients with nerve root tension signs.[26] Associated with the restricted flexion–extension spinal motion were increased coupled motions (i.e., lateral bends and axial rotations). Both observations may be explained by the fact that the spinal instability resulted in activation of the muscular system. Increased muscle forces restricted the overall motion of the spine and at the same time, owing to muscle imbalance, resulted in asymmetric spinal movements (i.e., out-of-sagittal-plane coupled motions during flexion–extension).

Stokes and Frymoyer[32] used a stereoradiographic technique to analyze flexion–extension motion in LBP patients suspected of segmental spinal instability on clinical grounds. The average angular range of motion in patients at the unaffected level (9.67 degrees) was not found to be significantly different from that at the affected levels (8.45 degrees). The same was true for the anteroposterior shear values, which were 1.54 versus 0.92 mm, respectively. But the ratio, that is, coupled shear translation divided by the flexion angle, was significantly different (+0.18 versus −0.13 mm/degrees, respectively) at the unaffected and affected levels at a p-value of less than 0.001. The retrodisplacement (anterior-to-posterior translation during flexion from extended position) was associated with the restricted motion, especially for sagittal plane rotations of less than 5 degrees, but was not correlated with the specific clinically unstable levels.

In a recent innovative study using functional x-ray, the two extremes of motion were obtained (1) by spinal traction (suspending the individual from his or her hands) and (2) by compression (using weighted backpack during standing).[6] Anteroposterior translation measurements were taken from lateral x-rays of patients who had spondylolisthetic or retro-olisthetic displacement. Depending on the severity of symptoms, the patients were divided into the following groups: (1) asymptomatic patients; (2) those with moderate symptoms; (3) and severe symptoms. The degree of primary anterior slip was almost equal in all three groups, but the translatory movement differed significantly among them, as follows: 0.7 mm, 5.2 mm, and 7.5 mm, respectively.

Other Measures of Instability

It has been suggested that stability in purely mechanical terms may be equated to stiffness.[28] The stiffness is defined as the applied load divided by the produced motion. Because it is difficult, if not impossible, to measure the loads in the spine in vivo, it is equally difficult or impossible to measure the in vivo stiffness of the spine. Accurate measurement of spinal motion in vivo, on the other hand, is relatively less difficult. For this reason the range of motion has often been used as an indicator of instability. Unfortunately, the range of motion is not related to clinical instability, as exemplified by a young gymnast who may have a hyper-range of motion but no clinical symptoms of instability. Further, the measurement of the range of motion is affected by (1) voluntary effort the subject applies at the time of examination, and (2) motion limitation because of pain. Thus, investigating other parameters of motion as possible indicators of instability has merit. One such parameter is the coupled motion coefficient. This is defined as the ratio of an associated motion to the main motion, for example, lateral bending or axial rotation with flexion. For every spinal motion, there may be two to five coupled motion coefficients. Another parameter is the neutral zone, which represents "looseness" of the spinal column around the neutral position. Support for the coupled motions is provided by Pearcy and colleagues,[26] who documented the presence of these motions in patients with suspected clinical instability. The neutral zone has been studied only in vitro. The increase of the neutral zone was found to be associated with disc degeneration, and its decrease with simulated muscle force application.[22, 23] No direct clinical evidence is yet available. As both parameters are generally smaller in magnitude compared with the range of motion, new and more accurate diagnostic methods are needed.

TREATMENTS

Spinal instability is treated clinically by diverse methods, some of which seem to be paradoxical. Both the flexion exercises, which strengthen abdominal muscles, and the extension exercises, which strengthen back muscles, have been found to be effective.[10, 40] Rotational exercises have been effective in patients who did not respond to other treatments.[27] The concept of exercise-treatment is supported by other observations that exercises in general reduce the risk of low back pain.[2] In contrast to the motion-producing exercises, complete rest has also been found to be beneficial and has been used as an absolute indicator of spinal instability.[21]

FUTURE RESEARCH DIRECTIONS

Seen from the biomechanical viewpoint, several aspects of spinal instability need to be investigated. A short list is provided.

1. Investigate the role of muscles, intersegmental (deep) as well as multisegmental (superficial), in providing spinal stability by means of in vitro simulations, using human cadaveric material, and mathematic model simulations.
2. Study the role of healing and adaptation after injury in altering spinal stability, using in vivo animal models.
3. Develop new and more accurate diagnostic methods of determining abnormalities of coupled motions, neutral zones, and other motion parameters, which may help provide more sensitive and specific measurements of spinal instability than are presently available.
4. Conduct clinical studies (prospective, double-blind, and controlled), that correlate carefully measured instability parameters of intervertebral motions (representing spinal column) and muscle function (representing neuromuscular control) to the clinical symptoms. These studies may help bridge the gap between instability indicators and clinical symptoms.
5. Conduct clinical studies (prospective, double-blind, and controlled) to evaluate the effect of sagittal and out-of-sagittal plane exercises on the instability parameters and clinical symptoms.

References

1. Abumi, K., Panjabi, M.M., Duranceau, J. and Kramer, K.: Lumbar Spinal Instability Due to Graded Facetectomies. Annual Meeting International Society for Lumbar Spine, Miami, 1988.
2. Cady, L.D., Bischoff, D.P., O'Connell, E.R., et al.: Strength, fitness and subsequent back injuries in firefighters. J. Occup. Med. 21:269–272, 1979.
3. Dimnet, J., Fischer, L.P., Gonon, G., and Carr, J.P.: Radiographic studies of lateral flexion in the lumbar spine. J. Biomech. 11:143–150, 1978.
4. Farfan, H.F., Cosette, J.W., Robertson, G.H., et al.: The effects of torsion on the lumbar intervertebral joints: The role of torsion in the production of disc degeneration. J. Bone Joint Surg. 52A:368, 1970.
5. Farfan, H.F.: Mechanical Disorders of the Low Back. Philadelphia, Lea & Febiger, 1973.
6. Friberg, O.: Lumbar Instability: A dynamic approach by traction-compression radiograph. Spine 12:119–129, 1987.
7. Gertzbein, S.D., Wolfson, N., and King, G.: The diagnosis of segmental instability in vivo by centroide length. Trans. Int. Soc. Study Lumbar Spine, Vol. 7, 1988.
8. Goel, C.K., Nishiyama, K., Weinstein, J.N., and Liu, Y.K.: Mechanical properties of lumbar spinal motion segments as affected by partial disc removal. Spine 11:1008–1012, 1986.
9. Gracovetsky, S., Farfan, H., and Helleur, C.: The abdominal mechanism. Spine 10:317–324, 1985.
10. Hirsch, C.: The mechanical response in normal and degenerated lumbar discs. J. Bone Joint Surg. 38A:242, 1956.
11. Kazarian, L.E.: Creep characteristics of the human spinal column. Orthop. Clin. North Am. 6:3, 1975.

12. Kirkaldy-Willis, W.H.: Managing Low Back Pain. New York, Churchill Livingstone, 1983.
13. Lehman, T., and Brand, R.: Instability of the Lower Lumbar Spine. Int. Soc. Study Lumbar Spine. Toronto, Canada, 1982.
14. Lucas, D., and Bresler, B.: Stability of ligamentous spine. Biomech. Lab. Report 40. University of California, San Francisco, 1961.
15. Markolf, K.L., and Morris, J.M.: The structural components of the intervertebral disc. J. Bone Joint Surg. 56A:675, 1974.
16. McKenzie, R.A.: The Lumbar Spine. Lower Hutt, New Zealand, Spinal Publications, 1981.
17. Moran, F.P., and King, T.: Primary instability of lumbar vertebrae as a common cause of low back pain. J. Bone Joint Surg. 39B:6–22, 1957.
18. Nachemson, A.: Lumbar spine instability: A critical update and symposium summary. Spine 10:290–291, 1985.
19. Nachemson, A., Schultz, A., and Berkson, M.: Mechanical properties of human lumbar spine motion segments: Influence of age, sex, disc level and degeneration. Spine 4:1–8, 1979.
20. Nouwen, A., van Akkerveeken, P.F., and Versloot, J.M.: Patterns of muscular activity during movement in patients with chronic low-back pain. Spine 12:777–782, 1987.
21. Olerud, S., Sjostrom, L., Karlstrom, G., and Hamberg, M.: Spontaneous effect of increased stability of the lower spine in cases of severe chronic back pain—the answer of an external transpeduncular fixation test. Clin. Orthop. 203:67–74, 1986.
22. Panjabi, M.M., Abumi, K., and Duranceau, J.: Spinal stability and intersegmental muscle forces. Trans. Int. Soc. Study Lumbar Spine, Vol. 14, 1988.
23. Panjabi, M.M., Goel, V., and Summers, D.: Relationship between Chronic Instability and Disc Degeneration. International Society for Study of the Lumbar Spine. Toronto, 1982.
24. Panjabi, M.M., Krag, M.H., and Chung, T.Q.: Effects of disc injury on mechanical behavior of the human spine. Spine 9:707–713, 1984.
25. Panjabi, M.M., Pelker, R.R., Crisco, J.J., and Thibodeau, L.L.: Biomechanics of Healing of Posterior Spinal Injuries in a Canine Model. Fifteenth Annual Cervical Spine Research Society Meeting, Washington, D.C., 1987.
26. Pearcy, M., Portek, I., and Shepherd, J.: The effect of low-back pain on lumbar spinal movements measured by three-dimensional x-ray analysis. Spine 10:150–153, 1985.
27. Polermo, F., and Panjabi, M.M.: Role of trunk rotation endurance exercise in failed back treatment. Arch. Phys. Med. Rehab. 67:620, 1986.
28. Pope, M., and Panjabi, M.: Biomechanical definition of spinal instability. Spine 10:255–256, 1985.
29. Posner, I., White, A.A., Edwards, W.T., et al.: A biomechanical analysis of the clinical stability of the lumbar and lumbosacral spine. Spine 7:374–388, 1982.
30. Seligman, J.V., Gertzbein, S.D., Tile, M., and Kapasouri, A.: Computer analysis of spinal segment motion in degenerative disc disease with and without axial bending. Spine 9:566–573, 1984.
31. Shiraziadl, A., Ahmed, A.M., and Shrivastava, S.C.: Mechanical response of a lumbar motion segment in axial torque alone and combined with compression. Spine 11:914–927, 1986.
32. Stokes, I.A.F., and Frymoyer, J.W.: Segmental motion and instability. Spine 12:688–691, 1987.
33. Vanharanta, H., Sachs, B.L., Spivey, M.A., Guyer, R.D., et al.: The relationship of pain provocation to lumbar disc deterioration as seen by CT/Discography. Spine 12:295–298, 1987.
34. Wetzel, F.T., Panjabi, M.M., Pelker, R.R., and Summers, D.J.: Temporal biomechanics of healing of posterior cervical spine injuries. Trans. 31st Annu. Orthop. Res. Soc. 10:306, 1985.
35. White, A., and Gordon, S.: Synopsis: Workshop on idiopathic low-back pain. Spine 7:141–149, 1982.
36. White, A.A., Panjabi, M.M., Posner, I., et al.: Spinal Stability: Evaluation and Treatment. Am. Acad. Orthop. Surg. Instructional Course Lectures, Vol. 30. St. Louis, C.V. Mosby, 1981, pp. 457–484.
37. White, A.A., and Panjabi, M.M.: The Clinical Biomechanics of the Spine. Philadelphia, J.B. Lippincott, 1978.
38. Whitehill, R., Stowers, S.F., Fechner, R.E., et al.: Posterior cervical fusions using cerclage wires, methylmethacrylate cement and autogenous bone graft. An experimental study of a canine model. Spine 12:12–22, 1987.
39. Wilder, D.G., Pope, M.H., Seroussi, R.E., and Dimnet, J.: Buckling or "Giving Way" in the Lumbar Spine Following Exposure to Sitting. 34th Annual Meeting, Orthopaedic Research Society, Atlanta, 1988.
40. Williams, P.C.: Examination and conservation treatment for disc lesions of lower spine. Clin. Orthop. 5:28–35, 1955.
41. Knutsson, F.: The instability associated with disc degeneration in the lumbar spine. Acta Radiol. 25:593–609, 1944.

BIOMECHANICS OF SPINE STABILIZATION

Vijay K. Goel
James N. Weinstein
Y. King Liu
Young E. Kim
T. Okuma

The activation of nociceptors (nerve endings) may trigger pain stimuli to the brain. Nociceptors, located within almost all spinal elements,[1] may be activated in the following situations: compression fractures, disc bulge (herniation), spinal stenosis, excessive strains, and sprains leading to inflammation and ligamentous trauma. Frequently, the removal of these mechanical forces may relieve pain. In some cases, pain can be resolved with bed rest, bracing, appropriate low back exercises, and medication.[45] However, patients who do not respond to conservative treatment may require surgical intervention when indicated.

The basic principle underlying surgery, from a biomechanical viewpoint, is either to dissect or to remove the structures impinging on the nociceptors. However, these procedures, depending on the amount and location of structures removed, may lead to spinal instability.

The natural history of lumbar fusion is unclear, yet it continues to be a procedure frequently employed in the surgical treatment of low back pain. Fusion of the lumbar spine segments (single level and multilevel) for instability following extensive decompression or degenerative spondylolisthesis and/or excessive retrodisplacement is undertaken using bone chips (mass) with or without spinal instrumentation. Internal fixation through instrumentation is accomplished primarily to augment spinal stability and enhance postoperative mobilization of the patient. A number of devices—Harrington rods, Weiss springs, Knodt rods, Synthese locking hook devices, Luque rods and loops, screw plates, the C-D system, and anterior devices like the Kaneda device—are available to the surgeon. Selection of a proper internal fixation system for a given clinical situation depends on the type of injury or disease, the capabilities of the fixation system, and the preference of the surgeon. Despite a plethora of literature comparing the results of discectomy alone with the results of discectomy and lumbar fusion, meaningful information about the long-term effects of lumbar arthrodesis is relatively scarce.[12, 33] In other words, lumbar and lumbosacral spinal fusion for relief of low back pain is a highly disputed and controversial subject.[10, 31, 32, 41, 46, 50]

The rationale for using spinal fusion procedures as treatments for low back pain is predicated on the idea that painful symptoms can be relieved by eliminating the pressure exerted on inflamed nerve tissue as a result of degenerated and/or unstable spinal motion segment. A few of the clinical studies supporting this viewpoint are described below.

Callahan and colleagues[3] suggested fusion following laminectomy in order to prevent progressive deformity as well as to eliminate motion and its pathologic consequences. Mooney[40] stated that painful hypermobility above the fusion site is seldom a source of disability, although complaints were found to increase with continuing age and with the duration of the fusion. Deorio and Bianco[8] discovered that children and adolescents were much better off after a discectomy with fusion than after a discectomy alone. In a follow-up study of 2,690 patients operated on for lumbar disc herniation between 1950 and 1981, Eie and coworkers[9] concluded that posterior spinal fusion postdiscectomy provided more effective protection against recurrent low back pain than did simple removal of the herniated disc material. Inoue and colleagues[22] found a 94.3% success rate in a follow-up evaluation of 350 patients in whom lumbar disc herniation was treated by anterior discectomy and interbody fusion. Tile[51] suggested spinal fusion following laminectomy to prevent intractable back pain for patients with segmental instability, degenerative spondylolisthesis, or significant prior back pain. A recent in vivo study by Kornblatt and Jacobs[29] demonstrated that the use of rigid internal fixation produced a significantly more rapid fusion rate. Hutter[21] suggested that fusion should accompany the first excision of degenerated or protruding disc material, since the majority of his patients developed foraminal or scar stenosis following decompression procedures. This suggestion is important because the success of fusion decreased as the number of decompressive procedures increased. Feffer and coworkers[10] reviewed two groups of surgically treated patients with degenerative spondylolisthesis and concluded that those who had decompression accompanied by fusion had more favorable outcomes than those treated with decompression alone. Schneck[47] suggests that re-establishing the disc space was the ideal corrective surgery to prevent secondary spondylotic changes. Cloward[5] strongly asserted his belief, based on clinical experience over the past 45 years, in the necessity of eliminating (1) the simple discectomy, which cures the sciatica but not the back pain; (2) the "decompressive laminectomy," which leaves the patient with painful instability and nerve root scarring; and (3) chemonucleolysis, which does not provide permanent relief of either low back or leg pain. According to Cloward, the answer to the treatment of lumbar disc disease (with or without sciatica) is posterior lumbar interbody fusion (PLIF).

On the other hand, some authors believe that spinal fusion procedures should not be encouraged, as the adverse iatrogenic effects outweigh the positive results. For example, an early study by Harris and Wiley[19] cautioned that spondylolysis may result from the stress concentrations at the vertebral levels adjacent to a fusion. Hirabayashi and associates[20] noted an increase in spinal stenosis both above and below the anterior fusion level, which they believed was caused by excessive stress on the adjacent intervertebral discs. They also cautioned that one must consider the possible adverse effects on the adjacent discs when deciding the level at which to perform vertebral body fusion. This view was supported by Leong and coworkers,[34] who found radiologic evidence of disc degeneration adjacent to the fused segment in 52.5% of the patients who had anterior spinal fusion for intervertebral disc prolapse. Lipson[35] found lumbar spinal stenosis above the fusion level. Louis[37] noted herniated discs above the fusion site in a follow-up study of screw-plate fusions performed between 1972 and 1982. A rather high complication rate was observed by Lehmann and colleagues[33] in a 10-year follow-up of patients with fusions performed prior to 1964. These involved an increase in both spinal stenosis and instability as high as two levels above the arthrodesis. A few of the other clinical complications involved with fusion include the following: pseudoarthrosis, inadequate mechanical support, spondylolysis acquisita, spondylolisthesis, pain at donor site, wire breakage and dislodgment, neurologic deficit, Harrington rod metal–bone interface failures, cancellous bone graft failures and displacements, hematoma, sexual dysfunction, and facet degeneration.[24, 25, 42] Thus, one of the adverse effects of fusion is a significantly high rate of complications.

IN VITRO EXPERIMENTAL INVESTIGATIONS

The need for the biomechanical evaluations of the fixation systems is evident, in view of the uncertainties described above. The in vitro experimental investigations reported in the literature may best be discussed under three categories. The studies in the first category pertain to the component design of the system itself, for example, the shape and size of the screws and the dimensions of the plate constituting the Steffee plate system. This requires a thorough knowledge of (1) morphology and functional spinal anatomy, and (2) mechanical testing of the individual components of the system once those have been fabricated out of an appropriate material. Krag and associates, Liu and colleagues, and a few other investigators have published detailed experimental protocols that were developed and used by the authors to evaluate various fixation systems.[2, 6, 30, 36, 49]

The second category consists of investigations related to the overall strength afforded by the use of a particular instrumentation.[4, 18, 23, 54] In these studies, ligamentous spine segments (say T12–sacrum) are biomechanically evaluated, injured to mimic a clinically relevant injury, and then stabilized with instrumentation. The stabilized spinal segments are subjected to flexion, extension, lateral bending, or axial twist loads to the point of failure. The load and resulting overall displacement at failure, for example, are compared with similar data obtained for a group of intact spines. This helps to characterize the overall stiffness of the stabilized spines. The results of such studies have shown that most of the devices currently in use are effective in restoring the stability to the injured specimens, although the degree of effectiveness varies among different devices. These studies do not, however, provide insights into the load displacement behavior of the injured/stabilized level and the adjacent levels. These comparisons are important from a clinical standpoint. Experiments elucidating these aspects constitute the last category.[7, 16, 17, 26, 31, 42, 43, 53] The characteristic and evaluation protocol, as undertaken by the authors,[14–17] is summarized below.

Fresh human cadaveric ligamentous spine segments (T12–sacrum) are potted at the sacrum, and clinically relevant loads are applied through a loading frame attached to the top vertebra of the specimen. A maximum of a 3.0 N•m moment (e.g., in flexion) achieved in four incremental loading steps is applied. The three-dimensional motion responses of each vertebra of the normal specimen, following each loading step application, are recorded with the help of a Selspot II system (see p. 201). To mimic a typical surgical decompression procedure used in treating patients with spinal stenosis, the specimen is injured at the L4–L5 motion segment and tested again. The decompressed motion segment is stabilized with a fixation device before the test protocol is repeated for the final time.

The six components of motion—three translations (T_{xH}, T_{yH}, and T_{zH} of point H) and three rotations (R_x, R_y, and R_z)—characterize the three-dimensional motion behavior of any vertebra with respect to the adjacent vertebra of the specimen. The data for the stabilized specimens are normalized with respect to the corresponding motion of the intact specimens using the following relationships:

$$NR_j = \frac{(R_j - R_o)}{R_o} \times 100$$

$$NT_j = \frac{(T_j - T_o)}{T_o} \times 100$$

where NR_j (NT_j) = normalized relative rotational angle (or translation) between two vertebrae about (or along) the j axis (x, y, or z) for the stabilized specimen at a specific load step; R_j (T_j) = relative rotational angle (or translation) between two vertebrae (R_x, R_y, or R_z) for the stabilized specimen at the corresponding load step; and R_o (T_o) = the corresponding relative rotational angle (or translation) for the intact specimen.

Normalizations were carried out to make each specimen serve as its own control. Comparisons are thereby made more meaningful, that is, the change, if any, in the motion behavior after stabilization would be highlighted. If NR_j and NT_j were greater than zero there would be an increase in motion after stabilization. In other words, for values of NR_j and/or NT_j less than zero, the rigidity would be greater compared with the intact case. Student *t*-tests are performed to evaluate the significance levels (using one-tailed *t*-test) of the changes in the load-displacement behavior with respect to the corresponding intact state.

Using the above protocol, the three-dimensional load displacement behaviors of intact specimens in flexion, extension, right and left lateral bending, and left and right axial rotation were recorded. The specimens were then divided into four randomly assigned groups of 10 specimens each for further testing as described below.

Group I. The specimens were destabilized at the L4–L5 level to simulate bilateral nerve root decompression clinically indicated for central and lateral spinal stenosis (Fig. 1). The supraspinous and interspinous ligaments were transected at the L3-L4 and L5-S1 levels and two 19-gauge stainless steel wires were placed on both sides of the midline from the L3–L4 to the L4–L5 interspace and similarly from the L4–L5 to the L5–S1 interspace. A small amount of the ligamentum flavum was also removed at the median raphe to allow passage of the wires. The specimens were stabilized with the Luque loops, shown schematically in Figure 2C, of appropriate sizes.

Group II. The specimens in this group were injured by creating bilateral laminectomy, bilateral facetectomy, and total discectomy across the L4–L5 motion segment (Fig. 2A). The injury model is an extension of the Group I with the addition of total discectomy. A bone graft was inserted into the disc space and further stabilized sequen-

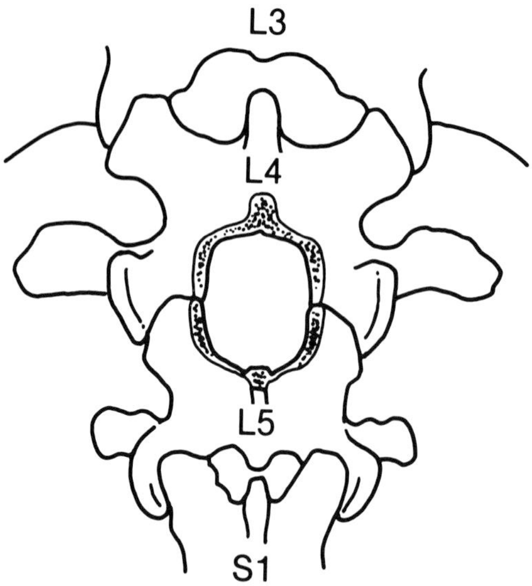

Figure 1 □ Schematics of the spinal decompression surgery. It involves cutting the supraspinous and interspinous ligaments, and the ligamentum flavum. Bilateral laminectomy and facetectomy complete the procedure.

tially, by use of the Steffee plates and then the Luque loop (Figs. 2*B*, and *C*). This group provided a comparison between the two fixation devices (Luque and Steffee) for the same injury model.

Group III. The specimens in this group were used to assess the efficacies of the Luque loop and Steffee plates while the L5–S1 level was stabilized in place of the L4–L5 level. The injury model was similar to that of Group II.

Group IV. In this group, the injuries and stabilizations of Groups II and III were combined to determine the stabilization characteristics of the Luque loop and the Steffee plates used to stabilize the L4–L5–S1 segments, instead of one segment only.

The specimens were tested, after each injury and after each stabilization procedure, in a manner entirely analogous to that of the intact state: the positional information of all the light emitting diodes (LEDs) was stored. The LED spatial location data of the intact, injured, and stabilized specimens were reduced further to yield the percentage of change in displacements. Comparisons with respect to the intact cases as functions of load magnitude, load type, and all vertebral levels (i.e., stabilized and adjacent segments) were undertaken.

Group I—Luque Loop Across the L4–L5 Motion Segment

In the flexion mode the relevant primary motions involved are the flexion rotation (R_x) and the anterior translation (T_z). At the L4–L5 motion segment (Fig. 3) the flexural rotation decreased after stabilization (−39.6%, $p < 0.01$). The translation demonstrated decreasing trends but not at a significant level, decreasing after stabilization (−10.0%, $p < 0.20$). Above the injured-stabilized level at the L3–L4 (Fig. 4), the rotation increased after stabilization (25%, $p < 0.05$). No sig-

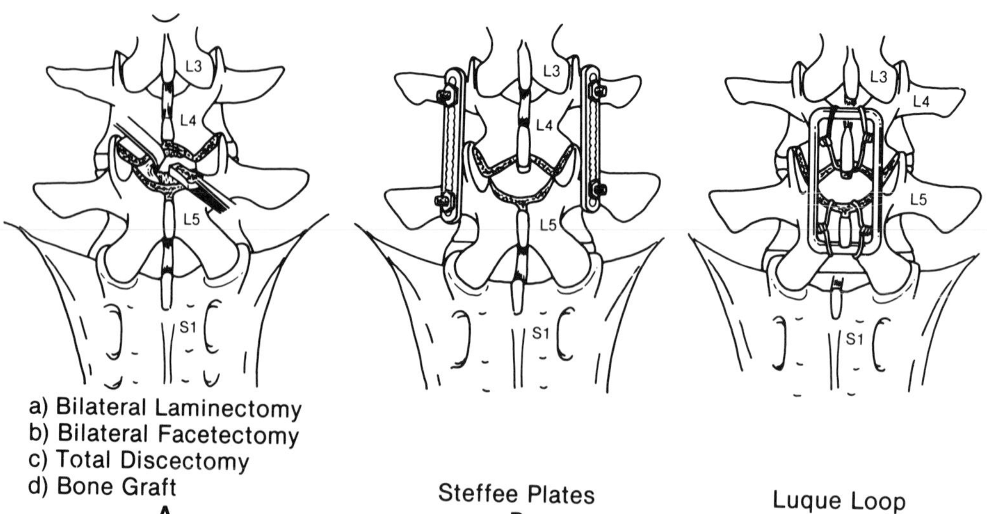

Figure 2 □ The injury to achieve spinal decompression is shown. The injured specimen is stabilized sequentially using Steffee plates (*B*) and then the Luque loop (*C*).

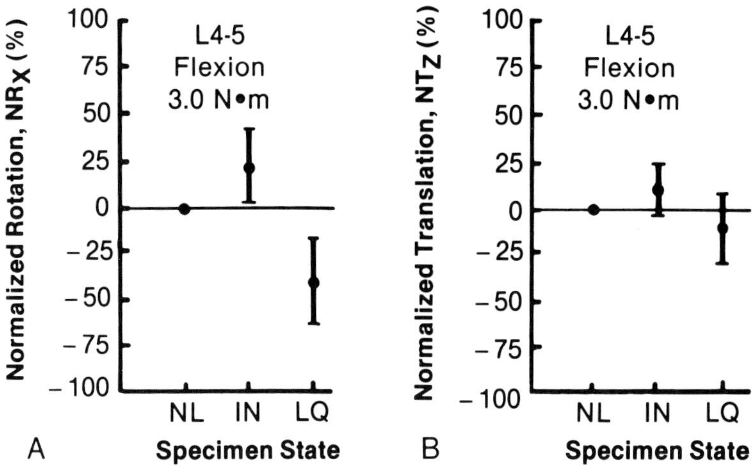

Figure 3 □ Normalized primary motion components at the L4–L5 corresponding to 3.0 N•m of flexion moment as a function of a specimen state. (NL = normal state; IN = injured state, and LQ = Luque closed-loop state.) *A* shows normalized rotation NR_x, and *B* shows normalized translation NT_z. (Modified from Goel, V.K., Nye, T.A., et al.: A technique to evaluate an internal spinal device by use of the Selspot system—An application to the Luque closed loop. Spine 12:150, 1987.)

nificant changes were observed in translation. Below the injury level at L5–S1, the rotation increased after stabilization (39%, $p < 0.2$) but not significantly. At the L4–L5 motion segment (Fig. 5), the rotation in extension decreased after stabilization (-36.0%, $p < 0.05$). The use of closed loop to stabilize the segment restored the translation motion to normal (no significant change).

In left and right lateral bending, the

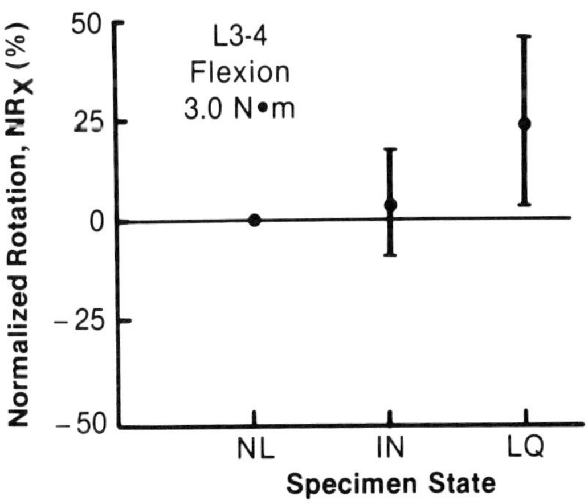

Figure 4 □ Normalized primary rotation, NR_x, at L3–L4, corresponds to 3.0 N•m of flexion moment as a function of specimen state. (NL = normal state; IN = injured state, and LQ = Luque closed-loop state.) (Modified from Goel, V.K., Nye, T.A., et al.: A technique to evaluate an internal spinal device by use of the Selspot system—An application to the Luque closed loop. Spine 12:150, 1987.)

changes in primary motion components at the stabilized level (L4–L5), as well as at adjacent levels, were found to be less than 10%. Thus, no definite conclusions can be made regarding the degree of instability induced after injury or the effectiveness of the closed loop. This was also found to be the case in the axial rotation mode.

A summary of the above results in terms of levels of significant changes in the primary motion parameters is given in Table 1. An arrow represents a change (up for increase and down for decrease) at $p < 0.05$. A dash (–) is used to denote no significant change with regard to the normal state. "WI" indicates an increase in motion at a very weak significance level ($p < 0.1$ or $p < 0.2$). The primary rotation components in flexion at the L4–L5 motion segment, for example, were significantly reduced after stabilization.

After stabilization with closed loop, the motion at the L3–L4 motion segment (i.e., the level above the injured-stabilized level) increased significantly in flexion. This increase in motion may be due to the use of the closed loop at the L4–L5 and/or the cutting of the supraspinous and interspinous ligaments and, to some extent, the ligamentum flavum at the L3–L4 to install the closed loop appropriately. In extension, the closed loop impinged against the L3 spinous process upon loading. Obviously, this interfer-

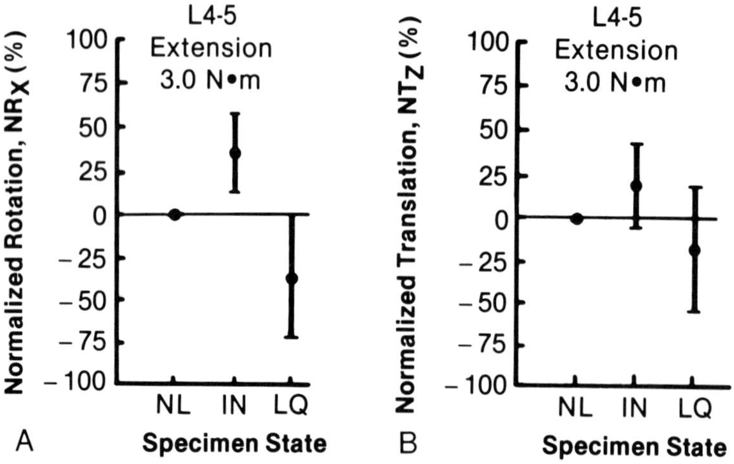

Figure 5 □ Normalized primary motion components at L4–L5, correspond to 3.0 N•m of extension moment as a function of specimen state. (NL = normal state; IN = injured state, and LQ = Luque closed-loop state.) (Modified from Goel, V.K., Nye, T.A., et al.: A technique to evaluate an internal spinal device by use of the Selspot system—An application to the Luque closed loop. Spine 12:150, 1987.)

ence would lead to a decrease in motion at the L3–L4 level in the extension mode, as observed.

The supraspinous and interspinous ligaments at L5–S1 were also transected to accommodate the closed loop, but the increase in the motion after stabilization was marginal, suggesting that these ligaments do not play a significant role in resisting flexion. We believe this is primarily the result of differences in the orientation of facets across the L3–L4 and L5–S1 segments. The facets exhibit a more sagittal disposition at the L3–L4 level, whereas an almost coronal placement exists at the lumbosacral junction. The facet orientation at L5–S1 is thus better suited to resist flexion–extension loads.

Table 1 □ Level of Significant Changes in Motion at Various Motion Segments (with Respect to Normal Specimen Behavior)

LOAD TYPE	PRIMARY MOTION	AFTER STABILIZATION OF L4–L5		
		L3–L4	L4–L5	L5–S1
FLX	R_x	↑	↓	WI
	T_z	—	—	—
EXT	R_x	↓	↓	—
	T_z	↓	—	—
RLB	R_z	—	—	—
	T_x	—	—	—
LLB	R_z	—	—	—
	T_x	—	—	—
LAR	R_y	—	—	—
RAR	R_y	—	—	—

Note: Up arrow means an increase in motion at $p < 0.05$ (down arrow a similar decrease). A dash means that no significant change in motion could be seen. WI stands for a weak increase in motion at $p < 0.1$ or $p < 0.2$.
FLX = flexion; EXT = extension; RLB = right lateral bending; LLB = left lateral bending; LAR = left axial rotation moment; RAR = right axial rotation moment.

Based on the above results, the closed loop system seems to provide stability based on the following principles. In flexion–extension the tension induced in the wire during twisting helps to transmit loads from L4 to the closed loop and then to the L5 vertebra. The stability provided against the axial rotation and lateral bending loads is primarily attributable to frictional force between the loop and the laminae of L4 and L5. This frictional force is a function of the normal force component resulting from the tension in the wires. In vivo, the wires would become loose with time, and the stabilizing effect would be compromised. The smallness of the frictional force would help explain the lack of stability in the axial rotation and/or lateral bending modes.

Groups II—IV Results

The inability of the closed loop to provide significant fixation in the Group I model in axial rotation and lateral bending raises questions about its ability to impart a definite stability in cases of spinal decompression when rigidity in response to lateral bending loads is also required. Relevant sample cases include the application of the closed loop for patients suffering from disc herniation, spinal stenosis, and/or facet disorders. The situation may be further compromised if more than one motion segment needs to be stabilized, because solid fusion may be even more difficult to achieve in such cases. The studies in Groups II, III, and IV were designed with these questions in mind. Data analyses, similar to the ones undertaken for Group I, were also undertaken for the specimens tested in these groups. The effectiveness of the Luque loop in stabilizing the injured models in all groups seems to be similar to that observed for the Group I model. The rigidity of the injured specimens stabilized with Luque loop in flexion increased by about 60%. No significant increase in rigidity was observed in other load types. The use of Steffee plates increased the rigidity of the injured specimen by 70% to 80% for all loading modes. Results similar to those we reported, in which the Steffee plates were used, may be expected of the other screw plate devices.

TECHNIQUE USED FOR TESTING WHOLE SPINE SEGMENTS

The spinal elements of a motion segment impart the much needed stability/flexibility to the segment. Their relative contributions in resisting various load types can be estimated by determining the load-displacement behaviors of intact specimens and specimens in which a particular element (e.g., facet) is dissected. A number of experimental protocols have been developed with these objectives in mind. These techniques make it possible to investigate changes in the relative motion between the two adjacent vertebrae as a function of injury/stabilization. However, the effects of induced injury/stabilization on the adjacent levels cannot be investigated. For this purpose, multilevel spine segment studies are mandated. A technique, based on the Selspot II system (Selcom Selective Electronic, Inc., Valdese, North Carolina) developed by the authors, is described below.[14–16]

Materials

Whole ligamentous lumbar spine specimens (T12–sacrum) are procured, screened, and frozen. A loading frame and a base are also attached to the topmost vertebra (T12 or L1) and the sacrum, respectively (Fig. 6). Knowledge of the locations of three noncolinear points on a vertebra (considered to be rigid) is necessary and sufficient to specify uniquely the position of the vertebra in space. For this purpose three points are identified in the following manner on each of the five vertebral bodies (Fig. 6C). A pilot hole is drilled laterally through the vertebral body. Then epoxy is injected and an 8-32 threaded rod, 100 mm long, is screwed into it. The rod is further tightened by nuts. The outline of the spinous process is identified and a hole punched into it using a small nail. Epoxy is injected, and a rod is screwed into the hole. Infrared light-emitting diodes (LEDs) are attached to the free ends of the rods. Altogether, 15 LEDs are identified on the five vertebrae (L1–L5). Three more LEDs (nos. 16, 17, and 18) are used to define a fixed coordinate system on the specimen (Fig. 6*A*). These are secured to the base of the specimen through a 25.4-mm (1-inch) thick Plexiglas plate referred to as the base plate. The x-axis is in a frontal plane about 25.4 mm anterior to the L5 vertebral body, and its positive direction stretched out towards the left of the specimen. The z axis is in the midsagittal plane with its positive direction stretching out anteriorly, and the x–z plane is parallel to the base. The y axis, obtained as a cross product of the x and z axes, is vertically upward from this plane.

Three-dimensional (3-D) Motion Measurement Technique

The 3-D motion of the specimen is monitored using the Selspot II system. It is an optoelectronic motion analysis system and is based on the principles of stereophotogrammetry. In practical terms, stereophotogrammetry is a method of determining the spatial coordinates of a definable point from a set of photographs of that point taken from different camera positions. The transformation coefficients relating the coordinates of a point from the photographs to the spatial coordinates of that point are obtained by first photographing an object (calibration frame) having at least four distinguishable points whose spatial coordinates with respect to a global axes system are known. The entire time-consuming process of taking photographs and then computing the spatial coordinates has been fully automated in the Selspot II system. The infrared LEDs, attached rigidly to the object, are used as definable points. The 3-D Cartesian coordinates of the light source are constructed by premultiplying the positional information by the calibration matrix. Mann and Antonsson[39] reported an accuracy of 1 mm in translation and 20 milliradians (1 degree) in rotation, using the Selspot I system for a 2-m-cube viewing volume. These estimates

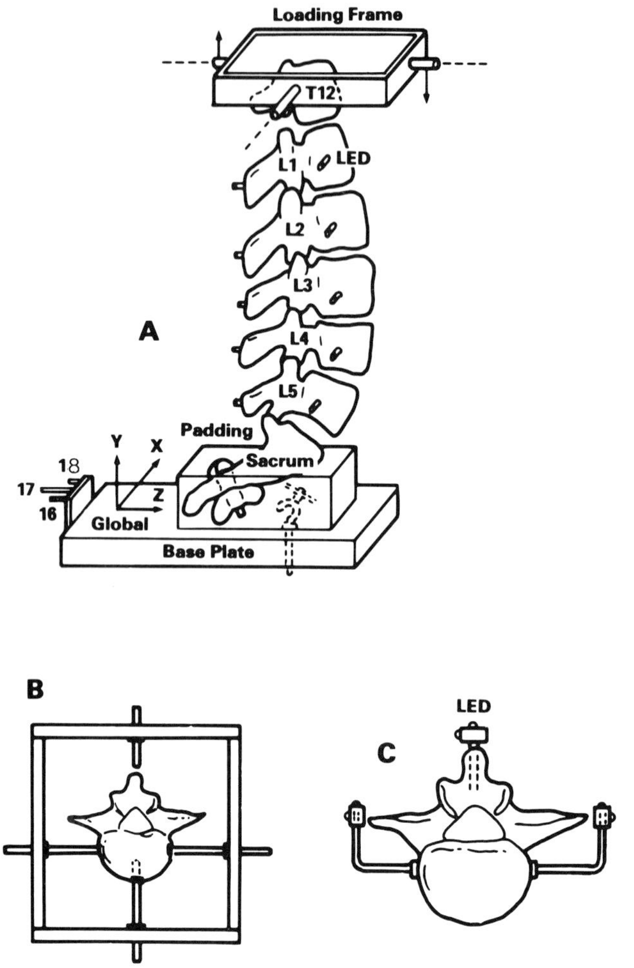

Figure 6 □ The steps involved in preparing a specimen for testing are schematically shown. *A*, The relative positions of the loading frame, LEDs, plastic padding base plate, and the directions of the global axes are shown. The arrows at the loading rods indicate arrangement of load lines to apply flexion moment to the specimen. *B*, Details of the loading frame and rods are illustrated. *C*, Method to attach three LEDs to a vertebra is shown.

of accuracy markedly improve as the viewing volume is reduced.[11] Calibration and verification studies undertaken by us[13, 15] to estimate the accuracy of the Selspot II system for 0.2 m × 0.25 m × 0.2 m (0.25-m cube) viewing volume have further corroborated the previous results. The accuracy we observed was <0.5 mm in translation (and <10 milliradians in rotation). Accuracy of this order is more than adequate for in vitro 3-D spinal studies.

Testing of Specimen

A specimen mounted in the Selspot II system and ready for testing is shown in Figure 7. A maximum moment of 3.0 N•m, achieved in six steps of 0.0 N•m (no load position), 0.5 N•m, 1.0 N•m, 2.0 N•m, 3.0 N•m, and 0.0 N•m (all loads removed), is applied. The moments are applied through various positional arrangements of nylon strings, pulleys, and dead weights. For example, the strings are arranged parallel to the *y* axis and in the *y–z* plane, and dead weights are applied in appropriate directions to achieve flexion bending (moment about the positive *x* axis) (Fig. 7*A*). Because the lever arm between the two forces is fixed at 500 mm, the corresponding dead weights applied to achieve the six moment steps are 0 g, 100 g, 400 g, 600 g, and 0 g.

Before beginning the experiment, the specimen is loaded twice through the six load steps in a particular load type. This "preconditioning" has been found to be extremely relevant in achieving repeatability in biomechanical experiments. The sequence of the load types followed during specimen testing and data collection is flexion followed by extension, right lateral bending, left lateral bending, left axial rotation moment, and right axial rotation moment. The Selspot II system is activated during the

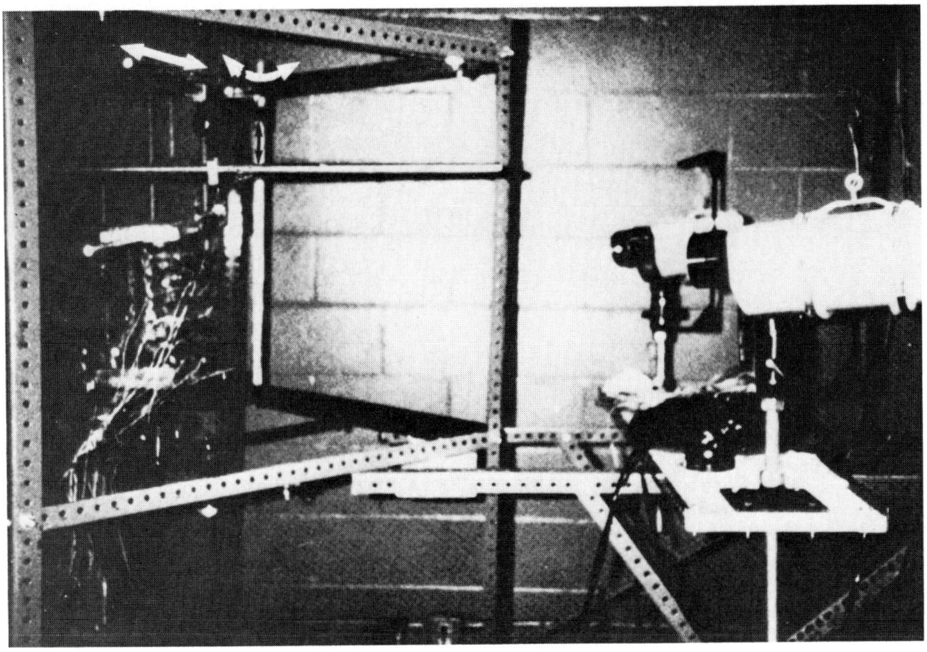

Figure 7 □ Prepared specimen housed in the testing rig. Two Selspot II cameras are visible. The specimen was subjected to various loads through pulleys, which could be moved in space with the aid of horizontal and vertical rods (shown).

third load cycle after each load step, and the positions of the 18 LEDs are recorded. An average of 50 frames is used to define the spatial position of the LEDs after each load step. The intact specimen is tested twice to ensure test-retest repeatability.

Disc Center

If the position of any point on the vertebra is known with respect to the coordinate system that is defined by the three LEDs used to monitor vertebral motion, then its position could be calculated in any monitored orientation of the lumbar spine (i.e., after the application of any load step in any load type), with respect to the global axes system, through the principles of rigid body mechanics. On the Selspot II system, the disc centers, after dissecting the vertebrae, are digitized by holding each of the vertebra in a fixture with the three LEDs, already attached, facing the cameras and a fourth LED held against the disc center.

Data Analysis

The LED locations are all converted to spatial positions with respect to the global axes system. The principles of rigid body motion are used to express the motion of each vertebra, in terms of six displacement components, after the load application and with respect to the starting position of the specimen at the beginning of a particular load type.[44] The six displacement components are as follows: three Bryant angles, R_x, R_y, and R_z; and three translational components, T_{xH}, T_{yH}, and T_{zH}, of a point on the superior vertebra (H) about and along the x, y, and z axes, respectively. The Bryant angles define the rotation in the sagittal plane (flexion—R_x) followed by a rotation in a transverse plane (axial—R_y) and lastly in the frontal plane (lateral bending—R_z). The load-displacement curves are highly nonlinear in nature and are sometimes referred to as flexibility curves as well (Fig. 8*A*). The motion parameters show a dramatic decrease in their magnitude in the flexion mode after stabilization (Fig. 8*B*). It is generally observed, that significant components of the motion occur in the plane of the applied load.[13]

For example, in flexion the primary (major/main/principal) motion components are a rotation about the x axis (R_x) and a translation along the z axis (T_{zH}). The remaining

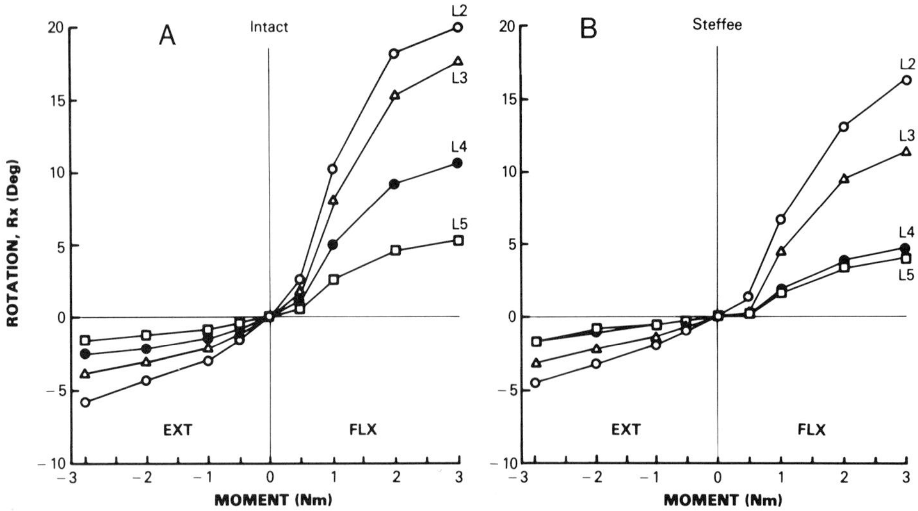

Figure 8 □ The flexion rotation component of motion of Point H in flexion. *A* is the intact specimen, and *B* is the stabilized specimen.

four components, termed secondary (minor/coupled) components, are an order of magnitude smaller than the corresponding primary motion components. The primary motion components are the responses of the specimen in the plane of loading, whereas the other components signify the out-of-plane motion, or the coupling effect.

ANALYTIC INVESTIGATIONS

Experimental investigations such as the ones described above have enabled investigators to understand the effects of instrumentation on the levels adjacent to the stabilized levels during the physiologic range of motion of the spine. This is an important contribution, from a clinical viewpoint. However, it is almost impossible to address all the parameters that can be varied within a given system, not to mention the number of fixation systems available.

A number of other clinical issues still need to be addressed, such as the loosening/breaking of screws, redistribution of loads, and stresses and strains within both the stabilized and the adjacent segments. An investigation of these factors will not only advance our understanding of the interaction between the spine and the instrumentation but may afford us an opportunity to improve the designs. This mandates developing analytic models. The authors have developed extensive three-dimensional nonlinear finite element models of the lumbar spinal segments (one segment, and two-motion segments) to investigate the effects of an interbody bone graft and a fixation device like the Steffee screw plate system on the spine.[15, 26] The description of the intact, injured, and stabilized finite element models are provided on page 208. The following paragraphs describe only the responses of the stabilized model (Steffee system) in compression, flexion, and extension.

Response in Axial Compression Mode

The injury and subsequent stabilization of the model using the interbody bone graft and the Steffee plates resulted in a localized increase in stresses (von-Mises) in the cortical bone region immediately below the screws (Fig. 9 and Table 2). The maximum stresses in the cortical bone for the stabilized and intact cases were 4.98 MPa and 2.21 MPa respectively. These figures correspond to an axial load of 405 N. This represented an increase of 125% with respect to the intact case. However, the overall stress level in the cortical shell of an entire cross section below the screws showed a very small increase in magnitude compared with the intact case. In the cancellous bone region, the corresponding maximum stresses were 0.14 MPa and 0.22 MPa. A decrease of about 36% was thus observed in the stresses of the cancellous bone following stabilization (Fig. 9). The average stress in the bone graft was 1.12 MPa. The load transmitted across the

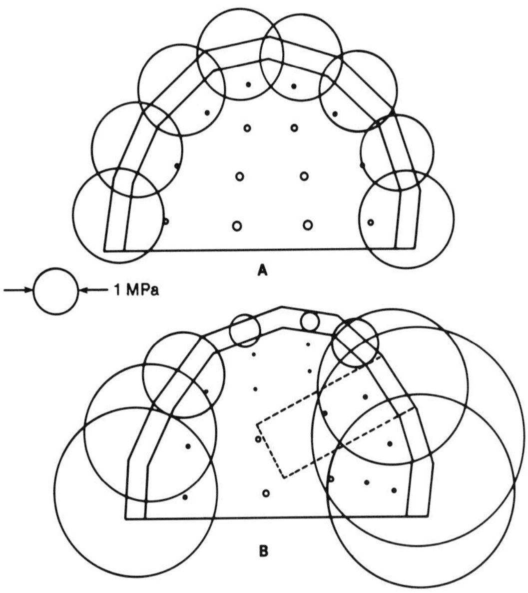

Figure 9 □ The distribution of stresses (von-Mises) in the cortical and cancellous bone regions below the screw for *A*, the intact model, and *B*, the stabilized model. The stresses in the cancellous bone show a decrease in the stabilized model. The increase in the stresses in the cortical region is a localized effect. The response is for the axial compressive load. (Modified from Goel, V.K., Kim, Y.E., Lim, T.H., and Weinstein, J.N.: An analytic investigation of the mechanics of spinal instrumentation. Spine 13:1003, 1988.)

bone graft (compressive stress × area of cross section) was 320 N and constituted 80% of the applied load. In contrast, 96% of the load was transmitted by the disc in the intact model. Thus, the plates transmitted 20% of the applied load, as opposed to 4% transmitted by the facets in the intact model. The load transmission path in the stabilized model with the bone graft totally removed would pass entirely through the screws and the plates. In this case the screws would be loaded as cantilever beams. Consequently, it is possible to compute theoretic stresses in the screw. The model computed stresses in the screw (223 MPa) compared favorably with the theoretic calculated value of 262 MPa. This further validated our model to some extent and also suggested that, in the absence of bone graft, the screws may experience stresses very close to their failure limit. The disc annulus was found to experience a negligible stress.

Response in Flexion and Extension Modes

The trend in stresses in the cortical bone region in flexion and extension modes was similar to that in the axial compression case (Table 2). The stresses in the cancellous bone region for the stabilized model showed an increase. However, these magnitudes are lower than those for the compression case. The average stress in the bone graft was about 1.0 MPa in both cases. The stresses in the plates and screws for the three load types analyzed are also shown in Table 2.

Discussion

To interpret the above results properly, the following should be noted.

The model has been developed using the Steffee plates. However, the results presented will be true for any of the screw plate devices currently available on the market. For the purpose of this analysis a perfect bond has been assumed at the bone–screw interface, and also across the screw–plate interface. This represents an idealized situation. In reality, some motion is always present, especially at the bone–screw interface. The amount of motion will depend on the quality of the bone, the characteristics of a particular device, and the technique used for implanting the device. The presence of

Table 2 □ Stresses for the Three Load Types

LOAD TYPE (MAGNITUDE)		CORTICAL BONE Stab.	CORTICAL BONE Intact	CANCELLOUS BONE Stab.	CANCELLOUS BONE Intact	BONE GRAFT Stab.	PLATE Stab.	SCREW Stab.
Axial Comp (405 N)	Max.	4.98	2.21	0.137	0.22	2.58	3.57	1.52
	Ave.	2.18	1.98	0.104	0.12	1.12	1.53	0.89
Flexion (2.05 N•m)	Max.	3.37	1.1	0.11	0.024	1.62	3.07	1.58
	Ave.	0.67	0.86	0.018	0.017	0.96	2.02	0.98
Extension (2.05 N•m)	Max.	3.01	1.62	0.059	0.034	2.26	3.53	1.68
	Ave.	0.95	1.09	0.032	0.02	1.04	2.3	1.02

Stab. = stable; Max. = maximum; Ave. = average.

motion is likely to alter the load transfer mechanism across the stabilized motion segment.

The stabilized model may be treated as a linear model because of the absence of soft tissues and small motions exhibited during analysis. The response of the model to loads other than the ones used here can be obtained by a linear superposition of the stresses for the load magnitudes reported here. Similarly, the response of the stabilized model to complex loads would be a linear combination of the cases analyzed. For example, the stress distributions within the structures for 2.05 N•m of flexion moment and a preload of 405 N can be obtained by adding the stress values for the 405 N axial case and 2.05 N•m flexion case from Table 2. Finally, it is essential to estimate the loads experienced by a stabilized spine in order to identify, in conjunction with the stresses, the structures most likely to experience failure over time.

Present knowledge of the forces within the trunk muscles and spinal elements of a motion segment of a normal subject is primarily based on the semiquantitative biomechanical models of the human spine.[38, 48] Most of the in vivo experimental data have been accumulated by monitoring loads on the spinal instrumentation used to stabilize an injured lumbar spine.[30] The results of the biomechanical models suggest that a motion segment may experience axial compressive loads ranging from 400 N (during quiet standing) to as high as 7,000 N (during lifting).[38, 48] The flexion moment acting across a motion segment during lifting, according to the above publications, is primarily balanced by the restorative moments generated by the back muscles. Thus, the disc, per se, in a normal subject does not generate flexion moment in resisting the external bending moment. The in vivo measurement of loads on an external fixation device used for human lumbar spine fractures indicates that the implant is also very largely shielded from bending moments by the trunk muscles.[30] In vivo bending of spinal plates has not been reported to be a problem. Mechanical testing in vitro has shown that a plastic deformation of the Roy-Camille plates occurs at 11.3 N•m.[30] Thus, the bending moment across a stabilized motion segment in vivo must be lower than this value. Keeping in mind that (1) the stabilized segment may be protected further by the use of braces following surgery and (2) the patients are not expected to undertake strenuous activities immediately after surgery, the stabilized motion segment may experience about 400 N of preload and a bending moment less than 10 N•m. It is also evident as the patients recover from surgery that, with time, the primary load on the spine would be the axial component.

The stress results of Table 2, when linearly extrapolated to 10 N•m of flexion bending and a preload of 405 N, show that none of the structures experiences high stresses in comparison with the corresponding failure strength (Table 3). The results of Table 2 also show, for the first time, that the average stresses in the cancellous bone below the screw level in the stabilized model for the compression, flexion, and extension cases are lower than the corresponding values in the intact case. The finding that compressive load is the main component of the load exerted on the spine suggests that the bone is stress-shielded by the screw plate system and more load is being transmitted through the fixation device as compared with the posterior elements in an intact model (20% versus 4%, as stated earlier). The use of interbody bone graft is essential, although it transmits a lower percentage of applied load in comparison with the intact case and, therefore, plays an active role in transmitting the applied loads. This is further corroborated by the results of the model in which the disc space between the vertebrae was kept void. The stresses in the screws in that case increased greatly in the absence of the bone graft.

The decrease in stresses in the cancellous bone region and the localized increase in stresses in the cortical shell (pedicles) around the screw support the clinical observation that screws may become loose with time. It is hypothesized that, once the screws

Table 3 □ Failure Strengths

	COMPUTED STRESS (MPa)	YIELD STRESS (MPa)	REFERENCES
Cortical bone	21.42	138	15
Cancellous bone	0.67	1–10	15
Bone graft	10.5	—	—
Plate	18.54	698	15
Screw	9.22	698	15

become loose, the structures may interact to increase stresses on the screws. This may, in turn, lead to pedicle screw breakage because of the cumulative effects of high stresses, stress concentrations resulting from the screw threads, and fatigue loading in the presence of body fluids. However, our finding that the bone graft is a weight-bearing structure from the time of its implantation tends to suggest that the bone healing may already have taken place by the time screws become loose or break. Clinical follow-ups are generally supportive of this observation, since few neurologic sequelae have been encountered when screw breakage has occurred. Nevertheless, the longer the fatigue life of the pedicle screws, the lower is the risk of screw breakage before complete fusion. Nitrogen-ion implantation, used by our group[36] as a surface treatment to inhibit cracks from forming in screws, showed doubling of the fatigue life near the endurance limit of the untreated "as-received" screws.

The use of the two-motion–segments (three-vertebrae) stabilized model may provide invaluable data regarding the biomechanical effects across levels adjacent to the stabilized segment. The development of multisegment finite element models and their execution is potentially very time consuming and expensive. For this reason, the effects of injury or disc degeneration (induced at the L4–L5 segment) on the adjacent L3–L4 motion segment only have been investigated so far.[26] However, these initial results have suggested that the further away the segment is from the injured and stabilized segment, the lower is the change in the biomechanical behavior. This is in accordance with St. Venant's principle.

The results of the finite element model with disc degeneration simulated at the L4–L5 level indicate that the nucleus pressure in the L3–L4 disc, compared with the case in which the L4–L5 disc was also normal, showed an 8% to 10% increase. The replacement of the intact L4–L5 disc nucleus with a fibrous material to simulate disc degeneration leads to stiffening of the segment. The use of bone graft and plates to stabilize the L4–L5 motion segment, from a mechanical viewpoint, also increases the stiffness and/or rigidity of the segment. The increase would be more than that obtained by replacing the disc nucleus with a fibrous material. The stiffness is also higher in cases in which the bone graft has healed and the plates have been removed—stabilization without instrumentation. The findings of our disc degeneration model suggest that the adjacent discs are likely to experience higher stresses as a result of stabilization. Furthermore, the use of the bone graft alone for restoring spinal stability may, upon its fusion, also have similar adverse effects on the adjacent segments. We believe, based on the above results, that the adverse iatrogenic effects seen clinically are not entirely attributable to the use of instrumentation itself. The healed bone graft alone may also induce similar effects. Consequently, efforts may be directed toward the development and use of more compliant materials in place of the bone graft and the plates. More specifically, it would be advantageous to create an internal fixation system that is highly rigid at first but begins to deteriorate (i.e., loosen) with time. Also, to prevent screw breakage over time our group recommends nitrogen-ion surface treatment to increase the endurance limit of the screws.

In summary, our results indicate that the interbody bone graft is a weight-bearing structure from the day of its implantation. The use of a fixation device stress-shields the vertebral bodies. A greater load is transmitted through the screw plate system, as compared with the load through the posterior elements in the intact case. As a result of this load bearing, the screws are also likely to loosen with time. The use of an interbody bone graft alone or in combination with any of the currently available fixation devices is likely to induce higher stresses across the adjacent segments. This stress augmentation, in turn, may trigger disc degeneration and other adverse iatrogenic effects as seen in clinical follow-ups.

DEVELOPMENT OF FINITE ELEMENT MODELS—INTACT, INJURED, AND STABILIZED

The following describes the steps involved in preparing a 3-D finite element model of an intact lumbar spine segment, and modifications thereof, to simulate injury and stabilization.[15, 26]

Geometric Data

In order to formulate 3-D finite element models of intact, injured, and stabilized lumbar motion segments, the geometric data of the

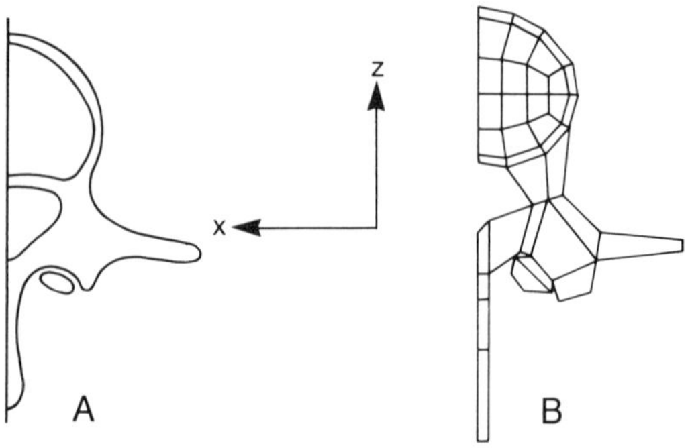

Figure 10 □ Steps involved in preparing a three-dimensional finite element mesh. *A* shows the enlarged view of a transverse slice from a CT scan. The *y* coordinate for all the points on this is equal. *B* represents different regions with quadrilateral elements. (Modified from Goel, V.K., Kim, Y.E., Lim, T.H., and Weinstein, J.N.: An analytic investigation of the mechanics of spinal instrumentation. Spine 13:1003, 1988.)

L3–L4 motion segment were acquired from 1-mm thick computed tomographic (CT) scans (transverse slices) of a cadaveric ligamentous spine specimen. Each CT slice was enlarged in order to facilitate identification of the different regions (Fig. 10*A*). Each region was then divided into several quadrilateral-shaped elements (Fig. 10*B*). The four nodes characterizing a particular element were digitized to obtain their x and z coordinates with respect to the global axes system. The *y* coordinate of these nodes was equal to the depth of the corresponding transverse slice on the CT film. For all practical purposes, the transverse cross-sectional shape of an intact "normal" specimen may be assumed to be symmetric about the midsagittal plane. This observation enabled us to digitize only one half of each section and to have the other half automatically simulated in the computer. The coordinate data of elements from different cross sections were then assembled to generate three-dimensional meshes for a number of finite element models (Fig. 11). The midtransverse disc plane of all one-motion segment models was horizontal. For the intact half two-motion segments model (INH2S), the L5 vertebral body was rotated in the sagittal plane by 9 degrees to create lordosis in the model. Thus for the two-motion segments model the L4–L5 mid-disc plane was inclined, rather than horizontal (Fig. 11*B*). For the sake of convenience in preparing the computer models, the differences in the overall dimensions between the L4 and L5 vertebral bodies were neglected.

Material Properties and Element Types Used

The elements chosen for the formulation of the models are described below. The material properties assigned were obtained from literature.[15]

Vertebral Body

The cortical shell and the cancellous bone core of the vertebral body, and the posterior

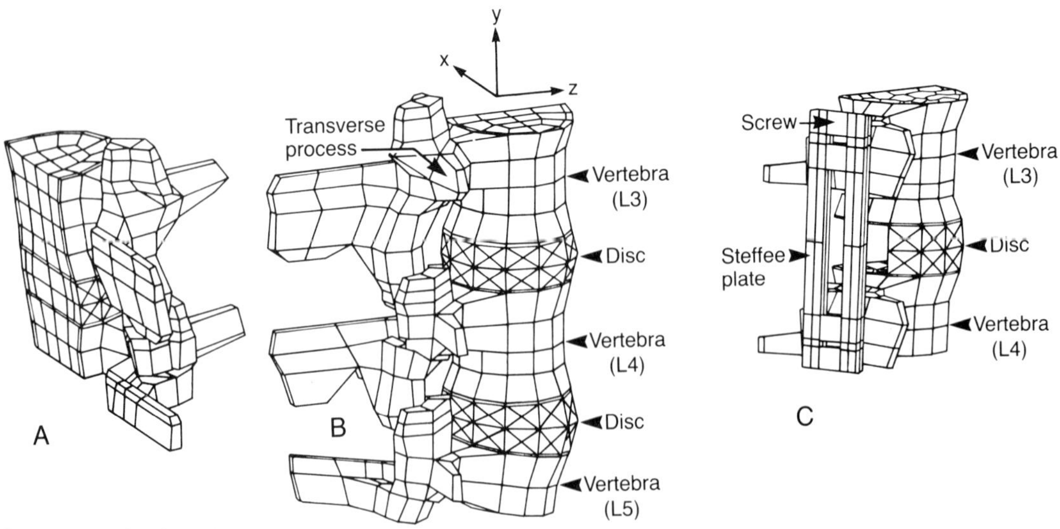

Figure 11. □ The three-dimensional finite element models. *A* shows an intact half one-motion segment model (INH1S). *B* illustrates an intact half two-motion segments model (INH2S). *C* shows a stabilized half one-motion segment model (SPH1S). The bone graft is not shown, for the sake of clarity.

bony elements, were modeled as 3-D isoparametric 8-nodal (brick) elements. The material properties were assumed to be homogenous and isotropic.

Disc

The annulus fibrosus was modeled as a composite material consisting of a series of fiber bands (lamellae) imbedded in the ground substance around the nucleus. The fibers in each of the six layers were arranged at 38 degrees to the horizontal in a crisscross pattern. The fibers were modeled as "tension-only" 3-D linear spar elements (cable elements). This combination of assumed material properties and the fiber angle produced a load-deformation behavior of the annulus composite, in tension, that was similar to the experimental behavior reported by Wu and Yao.[52] The fact that these elements are active in tension, and not in compression, allowed an appropriate simulation of the role of fibers in the disc. The ground substance of the annulus was modeled as 3-D isotropic 8-nodal elements. The hydrostatic characteristics of the nucleus pulposus were simulated with a 3-D incompressible fluid element, represented by its bulk modulus.

Facet Articulation

A 3-D interface element (gap element), capable only of supporting a compressive load normal to its surface and a shear force (force of friction, for example) along the surface, was used for this purpose. In all, six gap elements were assigned for each facet articulation. The average initial gap between the articulating surfaces, based on the CT film, was considered to be 0.45.

Ligaments

The ligaments, being active in tension only, were also modeled as bilinear cable elements, much as were the fibers in the annulus. These elements were assumed to carry no pretension and were oriented along the respective ligament fiber directions.

Intact Models

A total of four 3-D nonlinear (geometric) finite element models, based on the geometric and material property data described above, were developed for the present study. Models INH1S (intact, half model of one-motion segment—L3–L4), INF1S (intact, full model of one-motion segment-L3–L4), and INH2S (intact, half model of two-motion segments—L3–L5) were used to study the response of an intact spine to various loading modalities.

Injury Models

The 3-D mesh of the intact models was modified to simulate the following clinically relevant injuries. The elements corresponding to the nucleus were removed to simulate chymonucleolysis (CHM). The mesh was further modified for the bilateral total discectomy model (TDS). The part of the mesh representing the laminae, facets, capsular ligaments, ligamentum flavum, and posterior longitudinal ligament was removed. The effects of disc degeneration, mimicked across the L4–L5 disc space on the stress distribution at the L3–L4 segment, were investigated by replacing the L4–L5 disc nucleus with a fibrous material in the INH2S model. The replacement of disc nucleus with a fibrous material increased the stiffness (or the rigidity) of the L4–L5 motion segment.

Stabilized Spine Model

The 3-D mesh of the INH1S model was modified to simulate a bilateral nerve root decompression and total discectomy surgery as indicated for spinal stenosis; it was then stabilized using a bone graft and a Steffee plate system. The resulting model for the stabilized spine (SPH1S) is shown in Figure 11C. The procedure adopted is as follows: The mesh representing the supraspinous, interspinous, capsular, and posterior longitudinal ligaments, ligamentum flavum, part of the annulus in the posterior region, facets, part of the laminae, and the nucleus were removed from the intact model. An interbody bone graft comprising the cortical as well as cancellous bone tissues was simulated between the two vertebral end plates, using 3-D isoparametric 8-nodal elements. Because it was not practical to identify properly the elements in the cortical and cancellous regions, the graft was assumed to be made of a homogenous material having properties between those of the cortical and cancellous bone tissues. The area of cross section of the bone graft was 415 mm². The bone graft can transmit loads through compression only in the absence of a bony healing. At a given load step, therefore, the stress distributions within the model were determined while assuming that the bone graft can transmit loads in compression as well as in tension. The elements found in tension were then disconnected from the corresponding elements of the end plate to find a new solution. The procedure was repeated until elements in compression only were present in the model. Thus, solutions were obtained in an iterative manner. Screws of 6.5 mm in diameter and 38 mm in length were placed in the pedicles and the cancellous bone regions of the vertebral bodies. The screws were modeled as squares in cross section (in place of the circular shape) to avoid excessive distortion of the element mesh around screws. However, the moment of inertia of the assumed shape in bending was made equal to that of the actual screw by adjusting the dimensions appropriately. The element mesh, as shown in Figure 11C, used to simulate Steffee plates was generated around the screws. Perfect connections were assumed at the screw–plate and bone–screw interfaces. The stabilized model was further modified by completely removing the bone graft and the disc annulus. It helped to validate the response of the model, in axial compression, by comparing stresses in the screw with the theoretic calculations.

The half models were used to investigate the segment behavior in the flexion and extension modes only. The use of half models saved computer resources without sacrificing the accuracy of the results. The full models were used for the lateral bending and axial twist load types because of the absence of the symmetric behavior that is present in the flexion–extension modes.

Boundary and Loading Conditions

The inferior surface of the most inferior vertebral body and its inferior facets were not allowed to move in any direction. In the half models (INH1S and INH2S), all nodes located on the midsagittal plane were restricted in the x direction because of the sagittal symmetry.

The axial compressive loads (maximum of 405 N) were simulated by applying uniform pressures on the surface of the most superior vertebral body. The sagittal-plane bending (flexion–extension) moments (maximum 11.6 N•m) were represented by a linearly varying distribution of the loads in the appropriate loading plane. The pure bending moments were generated by zeroing the net compressive force acting on the surface. Complex load cases, such as flexion bending with an axial compressive preload, were also analyzed. The main consideration during the selection of these loads was to simulate situations that have been analyzed through experimental in vitro studies. This permitted us to validate the output of the intact finite element models.

The finite element models described above were executed using the nonlinear finite element program. The maximum loads were achieved in five load steps, and the solution at each step with respect to the zero load step was obtained in an iterative manner. The iteration process was stopped when the difference in the displacement field at the most recent iteration was found to be less than 0.01 mm, compared with the preceding iteration; at this point, the solution was considered to have converged. The output was processed further to yield load-displacement curves, changes in the nucleus pressure, disc bulge, forces in various spinal structures (including the forces across the facets), strains in the ligaments and the annulus fibers, and stress fields within the bony elements and ground substance of the annulus. The stress results presented are expressed in terms of von-Mises stresses using the equation

$$\sigma = 1/\sqrt{2}[(\sigma 1 - \sigma 2)^2 + (\sigma 2 - \sigma 3)^2 + (\sigma 3 - \sigma 1)^2]^{1/2}$$

where σ1, σ2, and σ3 are the three principal stresses at a point. As can be seen from the equation, it is an equivalent stress value whose comparison with the failure strength of the structure can suggest whether or not the component is likely to fail.

Comparison of the predicted gross response characteristics of the intact one-motion segment models (like load-displacement behavior, intradiscal pressure, strains in ligaments), with available experimental measurements, indicated satisfactory agreements.[16] The effects of a fixation device on the mechanics of a spine segment have been described.

Acknowledgments

Research supported in part by an NIH grant (AM 32954-5) and contracts from AcroMed Corp., Cleveland, Ohio. The authors express their gratitude to the following individuals who have helped in undertaking a number of projects that formed the basis of this chapter: Drs. K. Nishiyama, G. Njus, and T. Okuma; and Messrs. P. Bahr, P. Geng, S. Goyal, T. Nye, D. Rippe, L. M. Voo, and W. Du.

References

1. Bogduk, N., The innervation of the lumbar spine, Spine 8:286, 1983.
2. Brunski, J. B., Hill, D. C., and Moskowitz, A.: Stresses in a Harrington distraction rod: their origin and relationship to fatigue fractures in vivo. J. Biomech. Engr. 105:101, 1983.
3. Callahan, R. A., Johnson, R. M., Margolis, R. N., et al.: Cervical facet fusion for control of instability following laminectomy, J. Bone Joint Surg. 59A:991, 1977.
4. Casey, M. P., and Jacobs, R. R.: Internal fixation of the lumbosacral spine: A biomechanical evaluation. 12th Proceedings of International Society for the Study of the Lumbar Spine. Montreal, Canada, Jun. 3–7, 1984.
5. Cloward, R. B.: Posterior lumbar interbody fusion updated. Clin. Rel. Res. 193:38, 1985.
6. Cook, S. D., Barrack, R. L., Georgettee, F. S., et al.: An analysis of failed Harrington rods. Spine 10:313, 1985.
7. Du, W.: Biomechanics of Spinal Instrumentation—An Experimental Investigation. M.S. Thesis, University of Iowa, Iowa City, 1988.
8. Deorio, J. K., and Bianco, A. J.: Lumbar disc excision in children and adolescents. J. Bone Joint Surg., 64A:991, 1982.
9. Eie, N., Solgaard, T., and Kopple, H.: The knee-elbow position in lumbar disc surgery: A review of complications, Spine 8:897, 1983.
10. Feffer, H. L., Wiesel, S. W., Auckler, J. M., and Rothman, R. H.: Degenerative spondylolisthesis: To fuse or not to fuse. Spine 10:287, 1985.
11. Fioretti, S., Germani, A., and Leo, T.: Stereometry in very close range stereophotogrammetry with non-metric cameras for human movement analysis. J. Biomech. 18:831, 1985.
12. Frymoyer, J. W.: The role of spine fusion. Spine 6:289, 1981.
13. Goel, V. K.: Three-dimensional motion behavior of the human spine—A question of terminology. J. Biomech. Engr. 109:353, 1987.
14. Goel, V. K., Goyal, S., Clark, C., et al.: Kinematics of the whole lumbar spine—effect of discectomy. Spine 10:543, 1985.
15. Goel, V. K., Kim, Y. E., Lim, T. H., and Weinstein, J. N.: An analytic investigation of the mechanics of spinal instrumentation. Spine 13:1003, 1988.
16. Goel, V. K., Nye, T. A., Clark, C. R., et. al.: A technique to evaluate an internal spinal device by use of the Selspot system—An application to the Luque closed loop, Spine, 12:150, 1987.
17. Goel, V. K., Weinstein, J., Liu, Y. K., Okuma, T., et al.: Comparative biomechanical evaluation of the Steffee and Luque loop systems. XIV Proceedings of International Society for the Study of the Lumbar Spine. Rome, Italy, May 24–28, 1987.
18. Guyer, D. W., Yuan, H. A., Werner, F., et al.: Biomechanical comparison of seven internal fixation devices for the lumbosacral junction. Spine 12:569, 1987.
19. Harris, R. I., and Wiley, J. J.: Acquired spondylolysis as a sequel to spine fusion. J. Bone Joint Surg. 45A:1159, 1963.
20. Hirabayashi, K., Maruyama, T., Wakano, K., et al.: Postoperative lumbar canal stenosis due to anterior spinal fusion. Keio J. Med. 30:133, 1981.
21. Hutter, C. G.: Spinal stenosis and posterior lumbar interbody fusion. Clin. Rel. Res. 193:103, 1985.
22. Inoue, S., Watanabe, T., Hirose, A., et al.: Anterior discectomy and interbody fusion for lumbar disc herniation. Clin. Rel. Res. 183:22, 1984.
23. Jacobs, R. R., Nordwall, A., and Nachemson, A.: Reduction, stability and strength provided by internal fixation systems for thoraco-lumbar spinal injuries. Clin. Rel. Res. 171:300, 1982.
24. Kahanovitz, N., Arnoczky, S. P., Levine, D. B., and Otis, J. P.: The effects of internal fixation on articular cartilage of unfused canine facet joint cartilage. Spine 9:268, 1984.
25. Kahanovitz, N., Bullough, P., and Jacobs, R. R.: The effect of internal fixation without arthrodesis on human facet joint cartilage. Clin. Rel. Res. 189:204, 1984.
26. Kim, Y. E.: An Analytical Investigation of the Biomechanics of a Human Lumbar Motion Segment. Ph.D. Dissertation, University of Iowa, Iowa City, 1988.
27. Kim, Y. E., Goel, V. K., and Weinstein, J.: Biomechanical basis for the effectiveness of chymonucolysis. XV Proceedings of International Society for the Study of the Lumbar Spine. Miami, April. 13–17, 1988.
28. Kim, Y. E., Goel, V. K., and Weinstein, J.: The role of facets in denucleated discs—an analytical biomechanical study. Proceedings of 34th Orthopedic Research Society, Atlanta, Feb. 1–4, 1988.
29. Kornblatt, M. D., and Jacobs, R. R.: The effect of bracing and internal fixation on lumbar spine fusion in 100 consecutive cases: A preliminary report. 12th Proceedings of International Society for the Study of the Lumbar Spine. Sydney, Australia, Apr 14–19, 1985.
30. Krag, M. H., Beynnon, B. D., Pope, M. H., and Frymoyer, J. W.: An internal fixator for posterior application to short segments of thoracic, lumbar, or lumbosacral spine. Clin. Rel. Res. 203:75, 1986.
31. Lee, C. K., Langrana, N. A., and Yang, S. W.: Lumbosacral spinal fusion: A biomechanical study. Spine 6:574, 1984.
32. Lee, C. K.: Lumbar spinal instability (olisthesis) after extensive posterior spinal decompression. Spine 8:429, 1983.
33. Lehmann, T. R., Tozzi, J. E., Weinstein, J. N., et al.: Long term follow up of lower lumbar fusion patients. Spine 12:97, 1987.
34. Leong, J. C., Chun, S. Y., Grange, W. J., and Fang, D.: Long term results of lumbar intervertebral disc prolapse. Spine 8:793, 1983.
35. Lipson, S. J., Degenerative spinal stenosis following old lumbosacral fusions. Orthop. Transact. 7:143, 1983.
36. Liu, Y. K., Njus, G. O., Bahr, P. O., and Geng, P.:

Fatigue life improvement of nitrogen-ion implanted pedicle screws. Spine (in press), 1988.
37. Louis, R.: Single-staged posterior lumbo-sacral fusion by internal fixation with screw plates. Proceedings of the International Society for the Study of the Lumbar Spine. Sydney, Australia, Apr. 14–19, 1985.
38. McGill, S. M., and Norman, R. W.: Partitioning of the L4–L5 dynamic moment into disc, ligamentous, and muscular components during lifting. Spine 11:666, 1986.
39. Mann, R. W., and Antonsson, E. K.: Gait analysis—precise, rapid, automatic, 3-D position and orientation kinematics and dynamics. Bull. Hosp. Joint Dis. 43:137, 1983.
40. Mooney, V.: The role of spinal fusion. Spine 6:304, 1981.
41. Nachemson, A.: The role of spine fusion. Spine 6:306, 1981.
42. Nye, T. A.: The Effect of Stabilization upon the Kinematics and Ligamentous Strains of the Entire Lumbar Spine. M.S. Thesis, University of Iowa, Iowa City, 1985.
43. Panjabi, M. M., Abumi, K., and Duranceau, J. S.: Three-dimensional stability of thoraco-lumbar fractures stabilized with eight different instrumentations. Proceedings of 33rd Annual Orthopaedic Research Society, Jan. 19–22, San Francisco, 1987, pp. 458.
44. Panjabi, M. M., Krag, M. H., and Goel, V. K.: A technique for measurement and description of three-dimensional six degree-of-freedom motion of a body with an application to the human spine. J. Biomech. 14:447, 1981.
45. Rish, B. L.: Critique of the surgical management of lumbar disc disease in a private neurosurgical practice. Spine 9:500, 1984.
46. Rothman, S. L. G., and Glen, W. V.: CT evaluation of interbody fusion. Clin. Res. Rel. 193:47, 1985. (See other articles of the symposium: Posterior lumbar interbody fusion [in this issue].)
47. Schneck, C. D.: The anatomy of lumbar spondylosis. Clin. Rel. Res. 193:20, 1985.
48. Schultz, A. B.: Loads on the lumbar spine. *In* Jayson, M. I. V. (ed.): The Lumbar Spine and Back Pain. New York, Churchill Livingstone, 1987, p. 204.
49. Skinner, R., Maybee, J., Venter, R., and Chalmers, W.: Experimental testing and comparison of variables in transpedicular screw fixation: A biomechanical study. Personal communication, 1986.
50. Sypert, G. W.: Low back pain disorders—lumbar fusion, Clin. Neurosurg. 33:457, 1986.
51. Tile, M.: The role of surgery in nerve root compression. Spine 9:57, 1984.
52. Wu, H. C., and Yao, P. F.: Mechanical behavior of the human annulus fibrosus. J. Biomech. 9:1, 1976.
53. Yang, S. W., Langrana, N. A., and Lee, C. K.: Biomechanics of lumbo-sacral spinal fusion in combined compression torsion loads, Spine 11:137, 1986.
54. Zindrick, M. R., Wiltse, L. L., Holland, R. R., et al.: A biomechanical study of intrapedicular screw fixation in the lumbosacral spine. XII Proceedings of International Society for the Study of the Lumbar Spine. Sydney, Australia, Apr. 14–19, 1985, p. 50.

OCCUPATIONAL BIOMECHANICS

Gunnar B. J. Andersson

Other chapters in this book have addressed the biomechanics of the spine in a general context. The purpose of this chapter is to discuss the biomechanics of the spine from an occupational standpoint, particularly as it relates to posture and manual handling. Vibration, which is another occupational concern with respect to back pain, is discussed in Chapter 4. This chapter is intended to be an introduction and so presents a conceptual framework. Those interested are referred to other authors such as Andersson and Chaffin[4] and Pope and colleagues.[27]

Occupational biomechanics is important because of the injury mechanisms believed to result in low back pain and also because of the close relationship between work and low back disability.[4, 27] As an introduction to the biomechanical discussion, therefore, a brief section on possible mechanical injury mechanisms leading to low back pain in the occupational environment is presented. An understanding of these issues should facilitate discussions of etiology, treatment, and prevention.

INJURY MECHANISMS

At least three mechanically based injury models present themselves as possible causes of occupational low back pain: single overloads, repetitive loading, and static loading. Direct trauma (extrinsic overload), such as from a fall or a blow to the back, are uncommon causes of low back pain in industry. Overexertion (intrinsic overload), on the other hand, is quite common. In the United States, for example, official statistics indicate that overexertion causes low back pain in 60% of all low back pain patients and that almost 500,000 workers are injured by overexertion each year.[27, 34] Single overexertion is probably a less frequent cause of injury than repetitive loading. However, statistical information does not allow sufficient differentiation to estimate the relative importance of either one. It is generally believed that repetitive loading causes failure because of fatigue of the various tissues. Fatigue can be defined as a loss of strength because of intermittent stresses over time leading to material failure. This type of failure can occur with quite small stresses, compared with those required for single stress failure (Fig. 1). Fatigue failure is believed to occur through crack propagation. In most materials these cracks continue to propagate until failure occurs, if they are not repaired. However, in biologic tissue, under the right circumstances, these cracks can heal spontaneously instead of propagating. If the tissue is not continuously stressed at a level causing the crack to continue to spread, the healing processes will close the crack and the tissue will regain its strength. Therefore, fatigue failure can be influenced by the rest-work relationship. Biologic tissue probably heals continuously, possibly without the formation of any significant residual scar.

The risk of overexertion injuries is influenced by age, fatigue, and concomitant diseases, but the degree of their effects is unknown. This means that the load level at which an injury may occur is individual and can vary over a wide range.

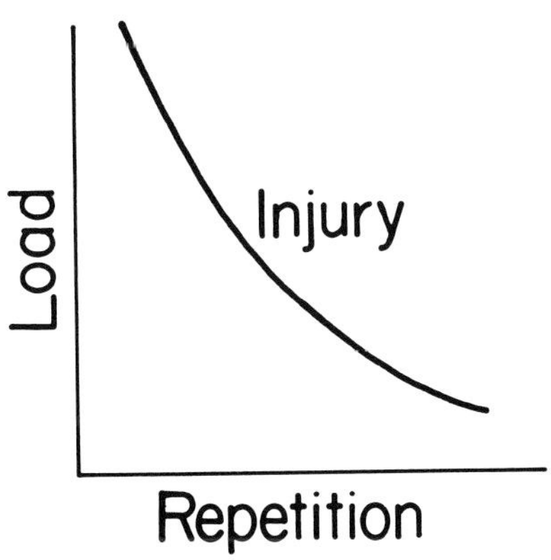

Figure 1 □ A fatigue curve illustrates the importance of repetition and load to fatigue failure. (Modified from Frankel, V.H., and Nordin, M.: Basic Biomechanics of the Skeletal System. Philadelphia, Lea & Febiger, 1980.)

The tissues involved in overexertion injuries are usually unknown. Dics have frequently been considered and it is known that degenerative changes occur with age and can be accelerated by mechanical loading. Annular cracks can be examples of fatigue crack propagation, although again we lack complete understanding. The vertebral bodies can also be involved. The fatigue, creep, and damage accumulation characteristics of bone are poorly understood. Trabecular microfractures from cyclic overloading have been observed. Fatigue fractures of bone would most likely be a frequent cause of injury in older subjects with osteoporosis.

The importance of muscle strain in low back disorders is not known. Clinically, "low back sprain" and muscle strains in the extremities have many similarities. Because "muscle injuries" to the back are seldom explored surgically, pathologic correlates of low back sprain do not exist. Experimental studies show that strain injuries to muscle occur in the myotendinous junction, regardless of whether the muscle is strained passively or actively and regardless of the strain rate.[14, 15] Muscle injuries have not been produced experimentally by either isometric or concentric contractions.

Lumbosacral sprain also implies that a ligamentous injury can be responsible. As with muscle injuries, most information comes from the extremities rather than from the spine.[1] Ligamentous structures are rich in nociceptors, so that any type of mechanical failure can be expected to be painful. Knee sprains have traditionally been divided into Grades I (mild), II (moderate) and III (severe, complete disruption). Whether this classification system would be applicable to the spine is not known.

Static loading influences collagen tissue as well as muscles. It is a well-known fact that the nutrition provided to the intervertebral disc is influenced by the mechanical stress placed on that disc and that at low levels of stress there is an inflow of fluid, and at high levels an outflow.[20] Animal experiments indicate that moderate activity beneficially effects the nutrition of disc tissue, compared with a static situation.[17, 18] Local ischemia is believed to cause disorders at the insertion site of tendon, ligaments, and articular capsules into the bone. Such ischemia can result from continuous loading of those insertion areas and may produce degeneration with microruptures, inflammation, and pain. This disorder has been named insertion disorder, or enthesopathy. The degree to which enthesopathies play a role in low back disorders is unknown. Ischemia can also affect statically loaded tendons, causing microruptures and focal cell death. Muscles are also negatively influenced by static loading. When contracting above a certain level, the circulation is impaired, resulting in an accumulation of metabolites such as lactate and an associated drop in intramuscular pH. Ultimately, this can lead to abnormal muscle enzyme function and inhibition of adenosine triphosphate (ATP) production and of the contraction. Energy depletion of muscle can also occur with continuous static loading. Negative effects from sustained contractions can occur at contraction levels as low as 4% of maximum voluntary contraction.[28]

BIOMECHANICS OF POSTURE

When discussing the occupational biomechanics of posture, the basic work posture needs to be considered, as well as the ability of an individual to change that posture. Furthermore, we need to consider additional postures that may have to be adopted for longer or shorter periods of time in order to perform a certain job. Sometimes force has be exerted in a given posture. Obviously, this further increases the load. These situations are considered under Manual Handling.

At work, standing and sitting postures are the two main basic postures. Standing offers advantages in terms of mobility, reach, exertion of force, and space requirements. Sitting, on the other hand, is less stressful for the legs, less energy consuming, less demanding on the circulation of the lower extremities, and more suitable when a precision job is performed. Variations of standing postures such as bending forward or to the side, or twisting the trunk, are more infrequently obtained postures that in some work situations, however, may be required for substantial periods of time. To maintain a posture, gravity must be opposed by muscle activity and tension in soft tissues. No posture should be maintained for a long period of time without the opportunity for a change. This is because of the negative effects of static loading on muscles and joint tissues, and it is an important consideration requiring attention—not only to the workplace design but also to the design of the work performance.

Standing Postures

Upright standing is a very stable posture requiring little muscle activity in the back muscles and in the abdominal muscles.[1, 3] A slight postural sway normally occurs. Shifting the center of gravity of the trunk, such as by bending forward or sideways, or simply by moving an arm, requires muscle forces to counterbalance the moment created by that body segment mass and its moment arm. These forces, which, for the spine, are primarily supplied by the trunk muscles, will create internal compression and shear forces in the spinal motion segment. The simple situation of bending forward is illustrated in Figure 2, in which a completely symmetric flexed posture is assumed. The situation becomes substantially more complex when asymmetry prevails. In asymmetric postures, asymmetric muscle contractions occur. These can result in unequal stress concentrations on different component structures of the spine and, therefore, should be avoided. Twisting, which in the lumbar spine is resisted by the facet joints, carries the additional negative effect of straining those joints. Further, the disc is more sensitive to rotational strain than to compression, tension, and shear.[13] The asymmetry of muscle forces occurring in lateral bending is illustrated in Figure 3. As expected, the activity levels on the side contralateral to the direction of bending are substantial, whereas there is little reason for activity on the side of the bending except at the beginning of the movement. To maintain low muscle forces and, consequently, low stresses on the spinal structures, upright symmetric postures are always preferred. Restrictions on bending and twisting are therefore indicated in patients with low back pain.

Sitting Postures

During sitting, the pelvis rotates backward and the lumbar spine flattens (Fig. 4). Radiographic studies show that this rotation of the pelvis and flattening of the lumbar spine

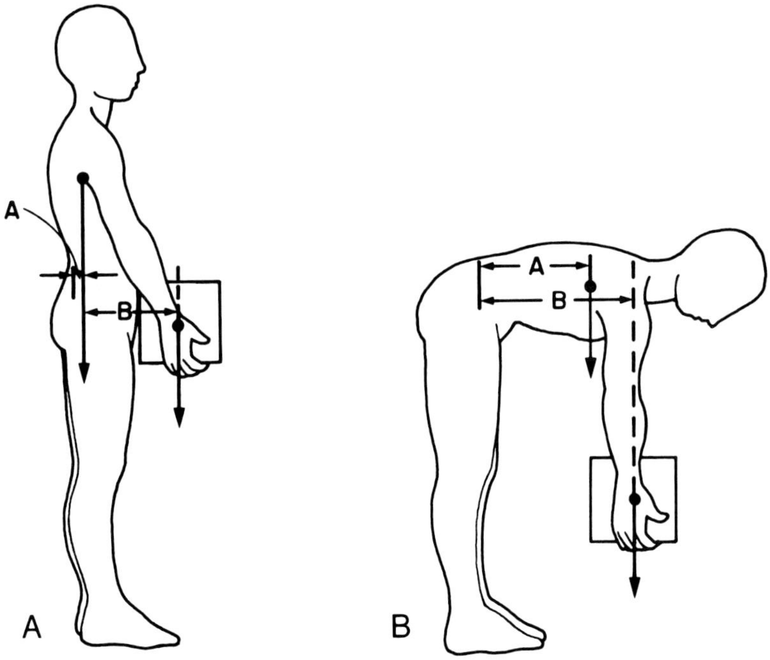

Figure 2 □ During bending forward, the center of gravity of the trunk moves forward relative to the lumbar spine. Therefore, the moment arm (A) increases. Assume A to be 0.02 m during standing, and 0.22 m during bending. The weight of the upper body is estimated to be 450 N. The forward bending moment resulting from the posture of the trunk is 9 N•m in upright standing (*A*), and 99 N•m during bending (*B*). To the trunk moment should be added the moment created by the weight of the box (100 N) and its moment arm (B) (0.18 m in upright standing, 0.31 m during bending). The moment attributable to the external load changes only slightly from 18 N•m (*A*) to 31 N•m (*B*).

Figure 3 □ During bending to the right, substantial muscle activity is recorded on the left side of the trunk. This activity is needed to maintain equilibrium. (From Andersson, G.B.J., Örtengren, R., Herberts, P.: Quantitative electromyographic studies of back muscle activity related to posture and loading. Orthop. Clin. North Am. 8:85–96, 1977.)

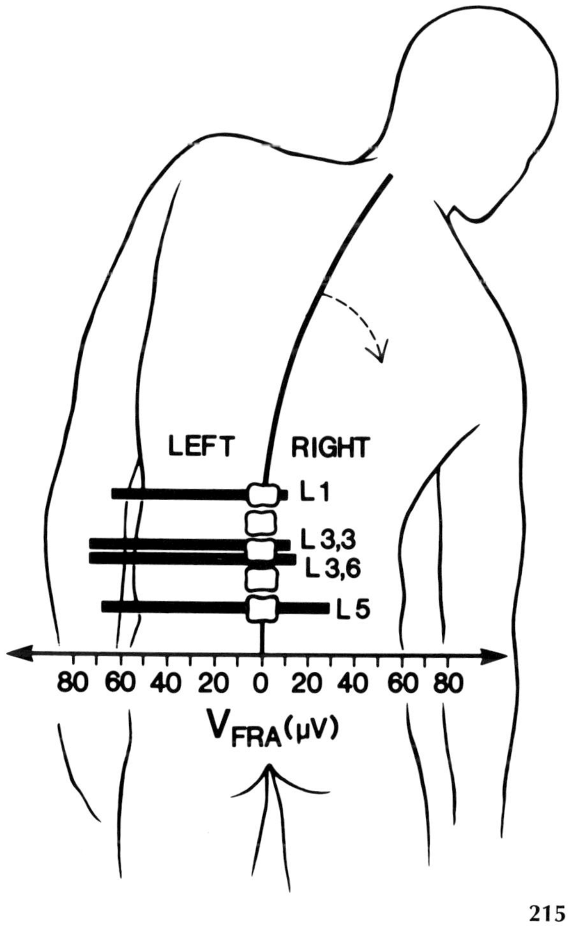

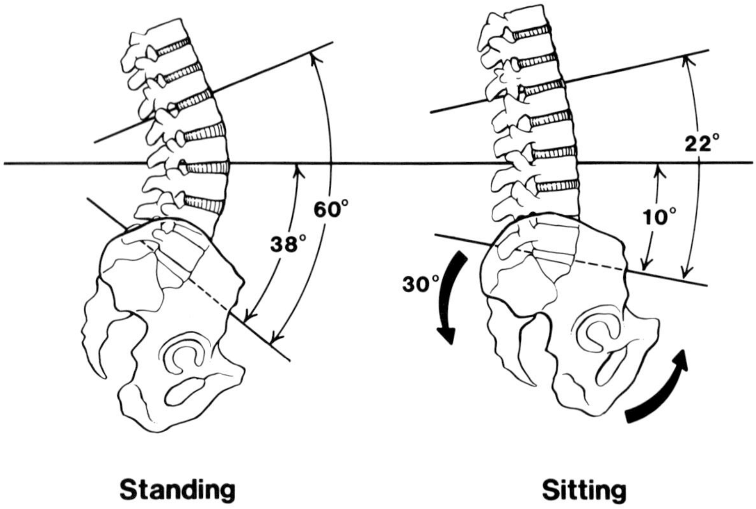

Figure 4 □ When sitting down the pelvis rotates backward and the lumbar spine flattens. (From Andersson, G.B.J., Murphy, R.W., Örtengren, R., and Nachemson, A.: The influence of backrest inclination and lumbar support on the lumbar lordosis in sitting. Spine 4:52–58, 1978.)

can be influenced by the use of backrests, particularly if they are fitted with lumbar supports.[6, 30] Indeed, Andersson and colleagues[6] found that the shape of the spine during sitting with a backrest at 110 degrees to the seat and a lumbar support of 4 cm was similar to that during standing. Pelvic rotation and flattening can also, although to a lesser degree, be influenced by forward sloping of the seat surface.[9, 23] The shape of the lumbar spine and the support of the lumbar spine are quite important biomechanical considerations, because they influence muscle contractions and load on the spine. Measurements of muscle activity in the lower back show that the activity decreases with an increase in backrest inclination (Fig. 5). The addition of a lumbar support to the backrest seems to further reduce the activity of the lumbar muscles, at least up to 5 cm of lumbar support.[7, 19] Similarly, in vivo pressure measurements in lumbar discs have confirmed the importance of proper support to the spine. Indeed, during sitting on a stool without a backrest, the pressure in the lumbar disc, and therefore the load on the lumbar spine, increases compared with during standing (Fig. 6). The reason for this increase is the increase in trunk moment that occurs when the pelvis is rotated backward and the lumbar spine and trunk are rotated forward, and also the deformation of the disc itself caused by the lumbar spine flattening. Therefore, when the chair is fitted with a backrest, the inclination of this support and any additional lumbar support are both important to reduce the load on the lumbar spine.[7] Figure 7 illustrates that when the backrest inclination increases, the disc pressure decreases, and that the same is true when a lumbar support is fitted to the backrest—at least for up to 5 cm.

The muscle activity and disc pressure measurements can be interpreted as follows. When backrests are used, part of the body weight above the lumbar spine is transferred to that backrest, thus reducing the load on

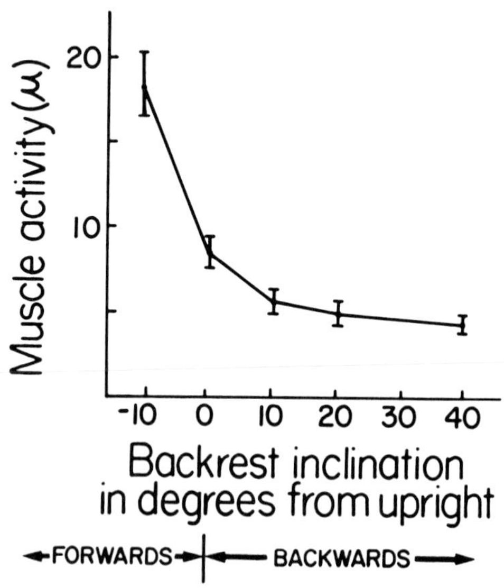

Figure 5 □ The muscle activity of the lumbar erector spinae muscles decreases as the back rest inclination increases. (From Andersson, G.B.J., Örtengren, R., Nachemson, A., and Elfstrom, G.: Lumbar disc pressure and myoelectric back muscle activity during sitting. Scand. J. Rehab. Med. 6:104–114, 1974.)

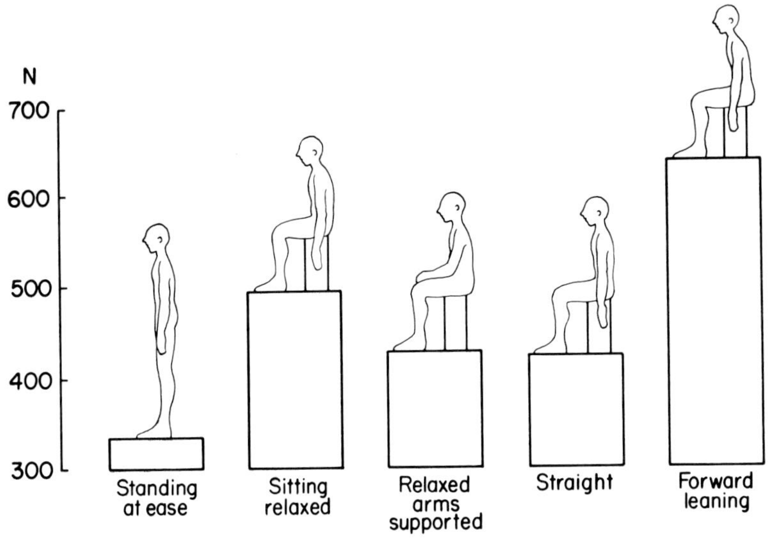

Figure 6 □ The load on the L3 disc in unsupported sitting is higher than the load during standing. (From Andersson, G.B.J., Örtengren, R., Nachemson, A., and Elfstrom G.: Lumbar disc pressure and myoelectric back muscle activity during sitting. Scand. J. Rehab. Med. 6:104–114, 1974.)

the lower back caused by the weight of the upper body. The more the backrest is inclined backward, the more body weight is transferred to it. By adding a lumbar support to the backrest, the deformation of the lumbar spine is also reduced and a shape similar to that of a standing person is obtained (Fig. 8). Similarly, the load on the spine can be reduced by fitting the chair with armrests, which removes the upper body weight because the arms are supported and, therefore, reduces the load on the spine. If the backrest of the chair slopes substantially backward, this effect is minor because the body weight is already supported.

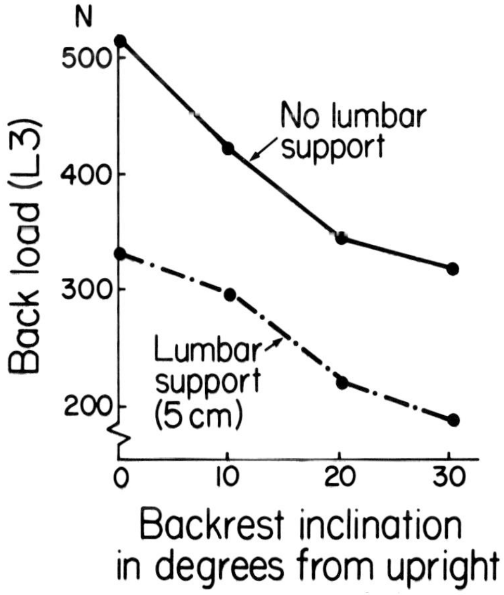

Figure 7 □ The load on the L3 disc decreases as the back rest inclination increases. When a lumbar support is added, the load decreases further. Calculations are based on disc pressure measurements. (From Andersson, G.B.J., Örtengren, R., Nachemson, A., and Elfstrom, G.: Lumbar disc pressure and myoelectric back muscle activity during sitting. Scand. J. Rehab. Med. 6:104–114, 1974.)

When one performs work while sitting, the posture is influenced not only by the seat but also by the design of the entire workplace and by the task at hand. In a car, for example, the ability to see the road and to reach instruments and pedals restricts the options, as do the dimensions of the car. In the office and factory, the height of the seat and table is important to the load on the spine during sitting. Leg support is critical to reduce and properly distribute the load on the buttocks and on the back of the thighs. When a chair is too high, the feet do not reach the floor, and uncomfortable pressure is therefore exerted on the back of the thighs, requiring the subject to slide forward on the seat and to no longer be able to use the backrest properly. On the other hand, if the chair is too low, then very acute angles occur at the hip and knee joints, making the posture uncomfortable. The relationship of chair height to table height is important, not only from the viewpoint of low back biomechanics, but also in regard to neck and shoulder biomechanics. Generally, a table that is too high requires a more upright

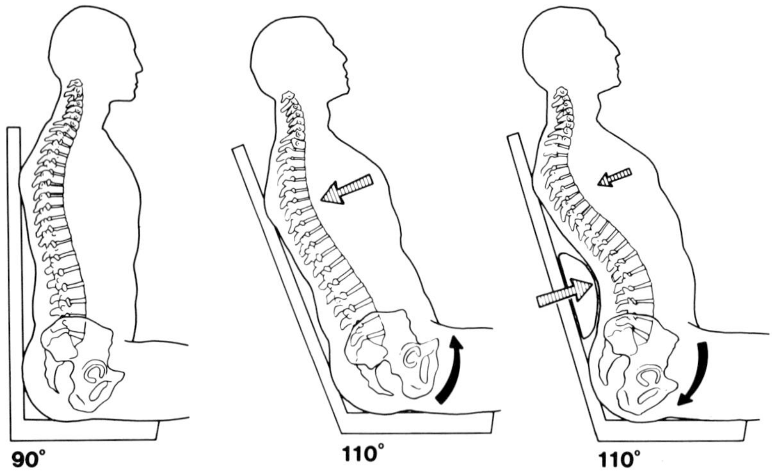

Figure 8 □ When the back rest inclination increases, a greater part of the body weight is transferred directly to the back rest, and therefore does not load the spine. A lumbar support maintains the lumbar lordosis.

posture in which the arms are abducted, whereas a table that is too low requires some degree of forward bending.

Regardless of how well the workspace is designed, it is important that the posture not remain the same for long periods of time. As discussed above, this has negative effects on muscles, ligaments, and discs. In the era of video display terminal (VDT) work, this becomes even more important, since many people now work in areas in which very few movements are required to perform the job.[2] Consequently, in this situation carefully designed break periods have to be introduced. These need not be excessively long and should probably be active, including some kind of exercise. Frequent short breaks are preferable to long breaks. Because of the problems of postural fixations, some countries and some of the United States actually introduced limitations in the time period a VDT worker is allowed to sit in front of the screen continuously. The National Institute of Occupational Safety and Health (NIOSH)[24] recommends a 15-minute break after 1 or 2 hours of VDT work, and a Swedish recommendation[8] is an upper limit of 1 to 2 hours of continuous work. In general, work in sitting workplaces should include fixed breaks at least every hour. This has actually been found to increase productivity as well as worker health.

Recumbent Posture

Although the recumbent posture is a very rare occupational posture, it is often a posture that a back patient discusses with his or her physician. It is not known which type of bed prevents back pain and allows back patients to recover more quickly and sleep better. The usual advice has been to use a relatively firm bedding surface with good overall support while avoiding excessive local pressure on bony prominences. Usually, the most comfortable position for people with back pain is lying prone with pillows under the legs so that the hips and the knees are in an almost 90-90–degree position; this is, of course, not always the case. In the treatment of any back problem individual differences exist. Generally, patients should be advised to sleep in the position that is most comfortable. The firmness of the mattress is another issue that has been discussed frequently over the years, without any scientific evidence pointing one way or another. Commercial interests have led to promotion of many different sleeping surfaces, including the water bed. One Swedish study shows that back patients generally prefer softer mattresses to harder ones and that their rapid-eye-movement (REM) sleep increases on a softer sleeping surface.[12] Some patients say they sleep better on the floor or when they introduce a hardboard under the mattress. The most important feature, probably, is evenness of the sleep surface that provides uniform body support and does not force an individual into an abnormal posture.

MANUAL MATERIAL HANDLING

Manual material handling still occurs very commonly in industry, in spite of increasing automation.[25, 33] From a biomechanical standpoint, four factors are important to consider in a discussion of manual material handling. The first is the posture of the subject when the lift, push, or pull is performed. The second is the weight of the object to be handled and its location relative to the body. The third is the origin and end point of the material handling maneuver, and the fourth is the speed at which the object is being moved from origin to end point.

Other aspects to be considered include the symmetry of the lifting activity and the time period during which lifting is performed. The bulk and size of the object are also important as are its mass distribution and the ability to grip it properly.

Lifting

The load on the spine created by a manual handling activity is proportional to the external moment acting on the spine. This external moment is produced not only by the weight of the object being lifted and its distance to the spine, but also by the weight and location of the person's body segments. These external moments can be calculated quite easily using a free body technique (Fig. 9).[31, 32] In those calculations, the moment caused by the weight of the object and its moment arm to the lumbar spine (the perpendicular distance from the center of mass of the object to the center of rotation of the spine) are added to the moment caused by the various body segments and their perpendicular distances to the center of rotation of the spine. The mass center locations of the body segments are used for these calculations. As illustrated in Figure 10, those body segments are mainly the trunk, the head, and the arms. In order for the body to be in equilibrium, the external moments must be counterbalanced by internal forces, creating internal moments, so that the sum of the moments acting on the lumbar spine is zero. These internal moments are primarily created by the muscle contractions, but contributions are also made by tensions in the ligamentous structures and resistances of the motion segment itself. Pressures in the thoracic and primarily abdominal cavities can, under some circumstances, aid in creating the counteracting moments (Fig. 11). From a mechanical standpoint, the muscles are

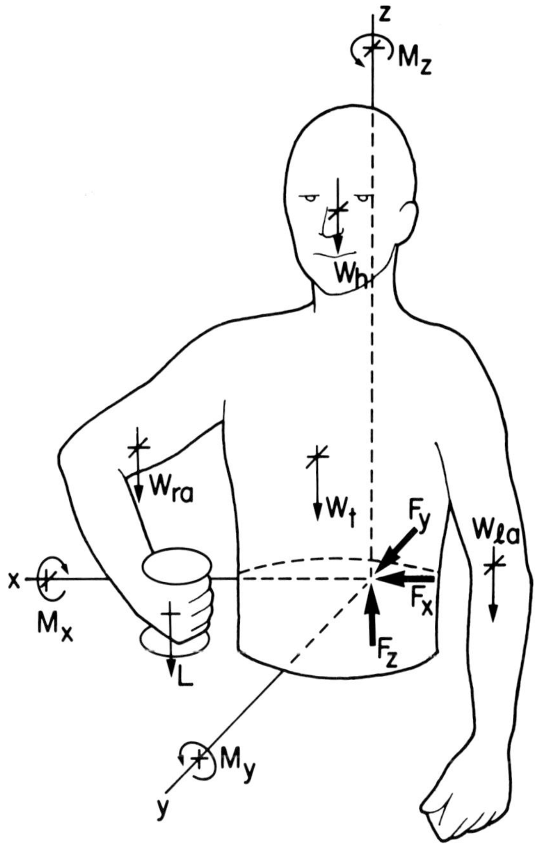

Figure 9 □ External forces and net reaction forces and moments act on the lumbar spine when a weight is held in the right hand. (From Schultz, A.B., and Andersson, G.B.J.: Analysis of loads on the lumbar spine. Spine 6:76–84, 1981.)

unfortunately placed relatively close to the spine. Therefore, they act with small moment arms and have to produce large forces, which in turn creates large compression and shear forces on the lumbar spine.

Based on this discussion, it is obvious why the posture of the individual is important. Large internal forces and moments are created simply from the act of maintaining, for example, a forward bending posture. In addition, forces and moments are created by the weight of the object to be handled and by the location of the object relative to the spine. Given the same object weight, these latter forces and moments are largely determined by the origin and end point of the material handling maneuver. In symmetric lifting activities, the horizontal and vertical locations of a load at the start of a lift and at its end point will also determine the travel distance and therefore, to some degree, the duration of the lifting activity (Fig. 12).

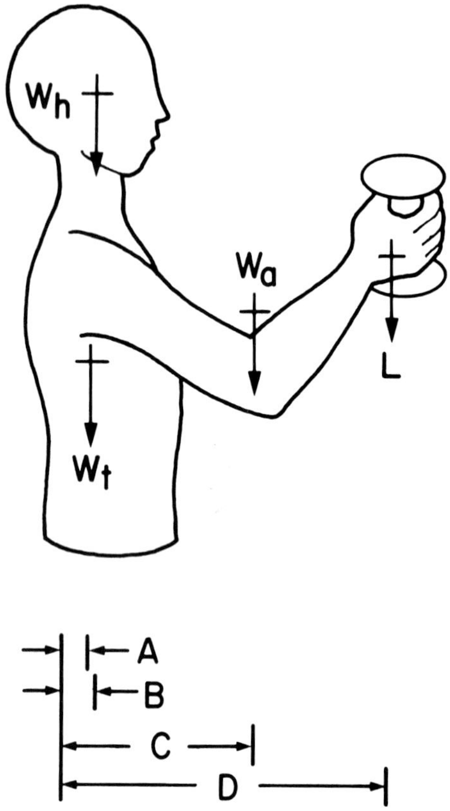

Figure 10 □ The moments created by the upper body segments and their perpendicular distances to the center of rotation of the spine, as well as the moment created by the external load and its moment arm, together create the external moments acting on the lumbar spine. (From Schultz, A.B., and Andersson, G.B.J.: Analysis of loads on the lumbar spine. Spine 6:76–84, 1981.)

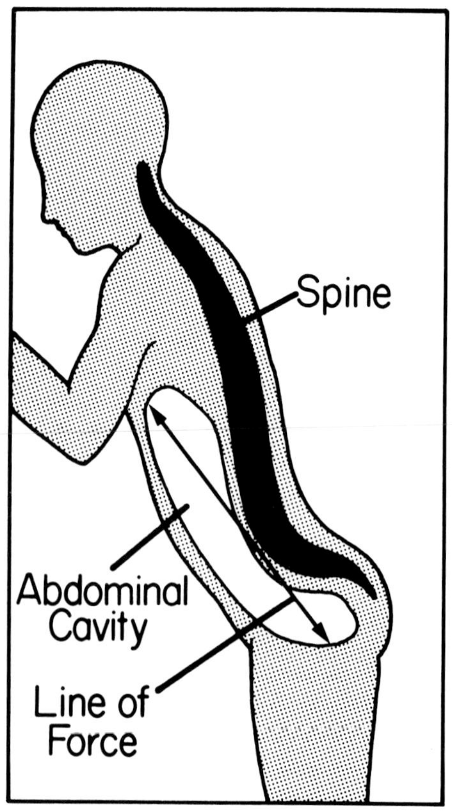

Figure 11 □ Intra-abdominal pressure supports the extensor mechanism. (Redrawn after Troup, J.D.G., and Edwards, F.C.: Manual Handling. A Review Paper. London, Her Majesty's Stationery Office, 1985.)

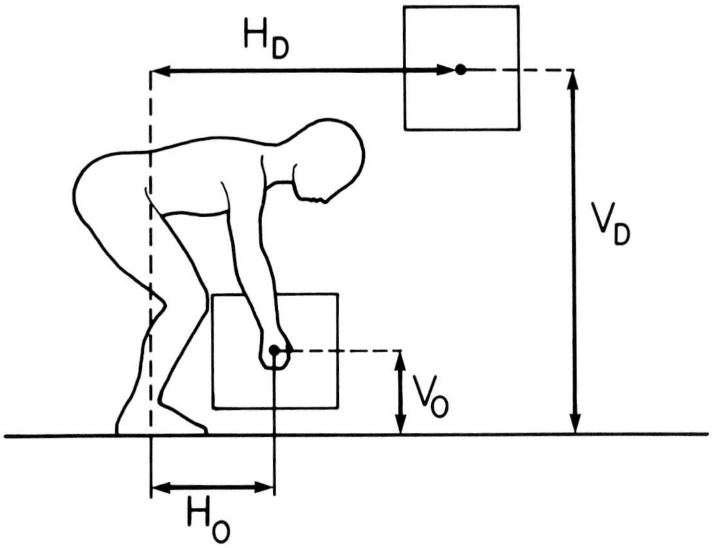

Figure 12 □ Example of a lift. The origin and destination is determined both in the horizontal and vertical directions. The motion from origin to destination is the travel distance of the weight. (H_O = horizontal origin; H_D = horizontal destination; V_O = vertical origin; V_D = vertical destination.)

Symmetric lifting, holding the load with both hands in front of the body, is believed to be the most common method of manual material handling. In that situation, the muscles can be used most efficiently and the stresses are bilaterally equalized. However, asymmetric lifting is not entirely uncommon. In these situations, there is not only a forward bending moment as illustrated on previous figures, but also a lateral bending and sometimes a twisting moment. Unfortunate stress concentrations can occur from asymmetric lifting maneuvers, which in general should be avoided. In addition, the strength of the arm and shoulder is not developed well enough to permit lifting heavy weights in asymmetric fashions.[4, 25, 27]

The fourth consideration is the speed with which lifting is performed. As illustrated in Figure 13, the external moment during a dynamic lifting activity is proportional to the speed of the lift.[11] In the calculation of the external moments acting on the spine in our previous examples, the inertial forces have been ignored. This means that the actual moments were underestimated. Comparison of static and biomechanical analyses of lifting show that inertial forces can increase the moment by as much as 33% to 60%.[21, 22]

Based on these facts, a simple set of guidelines for lifting can be created. These guidelines include maintaining a symmetric, upright posture, thereby avoiding forward flexion, lateral bending, and twisting; lifting the object as close to the body as possible; keeping the weight of the object as low as possible; whenever possible, lifting symmetrically, using both hands; and lifting smoothly without major jerks and at moderate lifting speed. Notably absent from these suggestions is the often repeated advice to lift with bent knees. This method, sometimes referred to as squat lifting or leg lifting, has been advocated over the years as a less stressful alternative to back lifting or stoop lifting in which the knees are kept comparatively straight and the trunk is flexed. Although many of the above recommendations can best be obtained by using the leg lifting technique, particularly when the load is to

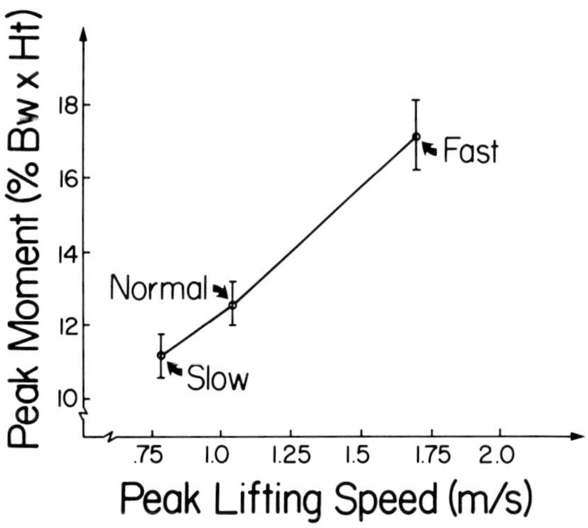

Figure 13 □ The moment at the lumbar spine increases as the lifting speed increases. The subjects were asked to lift at slow, normal, and fast paces. (From Bush-Joseph, C., Schipplein, O.D., Andersson, G.B.J., and Andriacchi, T.P.: Influence of dynamic factors on the lumbar spine movement in lifting. Ergonomics 31:211–216, 1988.)

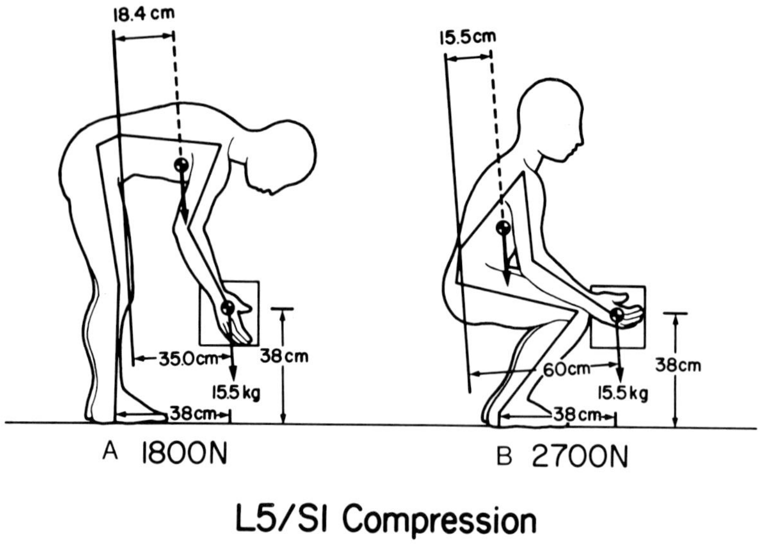

Figure 14 □ Biomechanical analysis of two methods of lifting a box, which because of its dimensions cannot be moved in between the legs. The bent knee method (*B*) produces a greater moment than the bent back method (*A*), because of the longer moment arm to the load. (Reprinted from *IIE Transactions* 6:105–113, 1974. Copyright Institute of Industrial Engineers, 25 Technology Park/Atlanta, Norcross, Georgia 30092.)

be lifted from the floor, bending the knees in itself is not the goal and is not what reduces the load. Rather, squatting is a means by which a more upright body posture can be achieved and by which the load can be moved in closer to the body. This requires that the object fit between the legs. If it is too large to be brought between the legs, the squat lifting method is actually a more stressful method of lifting than the stoop lifting method (Fig. 14). This is because, in order to lift in front of the knees, the moment arm to the spine increases in squat lifting.[26] A further disadvantage of the squat lifting method is the increased load on the knee joints and the increased demand on the quadriceps muscles created by that technique. This is a limitation during lifting of heavy weights, which actually forces the subjects to change the technique from a crouch lift to more of a stoop lift.[29] The leg lifting technique is also more energy demanding, as illustrated in Figure 15. An alternative to these techniques is the free-style technique, in which the individuals lift as they please. In analyzing this technique, it becomes apparent that it is an intermediate technique, between pure stoop lifting and pure squat lifting. Controlled field studies indicate that workers often adopt this technique, even when instructed otherwise.[25–27]

Lifting Limitations and Regulations

It is clear from the preceding discussion that any legislation related to lifting must take into account more than the weight of the object to be lifted; it also needs to consider a host of other factors. A general weight recommendation, such as 50 pounds (25 kg) or, as suggested by ILO (International Labour Conference) in 1967, 55 kg (110 pounds) for adult men and "substantially" less for women and younger workers, is as meaningful as a general speed limit without concern for the driving environment. In 1981 NIOSH published guidelines suggesting two limits and defining them by (1) the horizontal location of the load relative to the body at the start of the lift; (2) the vertical location of the load at the origin of the lift; (3) the vertical displacement of the load during the lift; and (4) the frequency of the lift. In

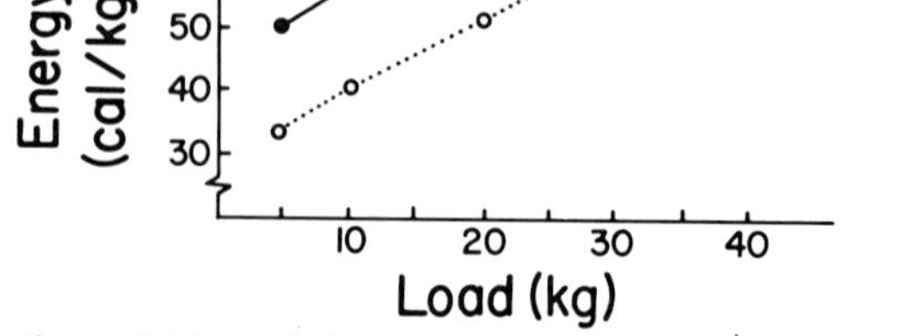

Figure 15 □ Metabolic rates for different types of lifting are shown. (Redrawn after Brown, J.R.: Lifting as an Industrial Hazard. Labour Safety Council of Ontario, Ontario Department of Labour, Ontario, Canada, 1971.)

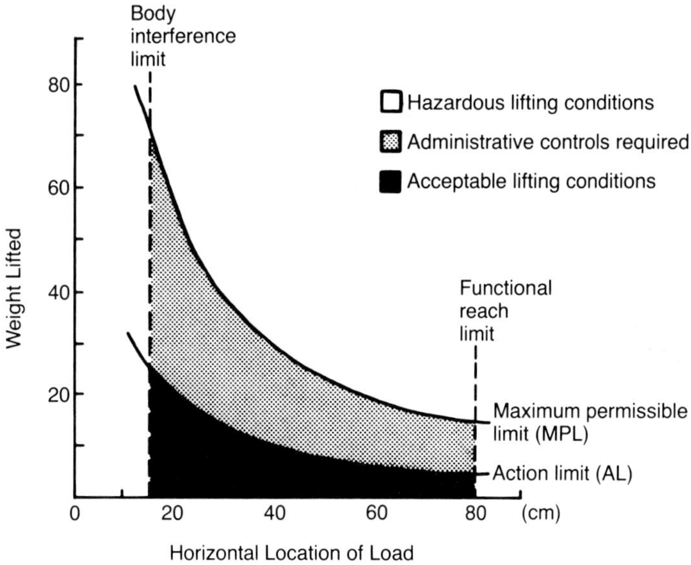

Figure 16 □ The NIOSH guidelines for symmetric lifting are shown. (See text for details). (From Posner, I., White, A., Edwards, W., and Wilson, C.: A biomechanical analysis of the clinical stability of the lumbar and lumbosacral spine. Spine 7:374–389, 1982; Waters, R. L., and Morris, J. M.: Effects of spinal supports on the electrical activity of muscles of the trunk. J. Bone Joint Surg. 52A:51–60, 1970.)

addition, the weight of the object is always considered. The lower of the two limits was termed the *action limit*. Below that limit the risk of injury from overexertion was considered minimal. The upper limit was termed the *maximum permissible limit*, above which any load could be hazardous. Between the two limits, ergonomic redesign or administrative control (such as worker selection, training, limiting frequency of lifts) was suggested. Figure 16 illustrates the relationship of the limits to the weight lifted and the horizontal distance of load. Although the NIOSH guidelines are not perfect and cover only symmetric lifting, they are a giant step ahead of the simple weight restrictions used in the past.

Pulling and Pushing

Pulling and pushing of loads are also important manual material handling tasks. Although approximately 20% of the overexertion injuries have been associated with such activities,[25] they have been analyzed comparatively less often than lifting. When pulling and pushing, the effect of friction is critical. This means that appropriate footing and floor conditions are important considerations.

If the foot slips, falls can occur that cause severe injury, and not only to the spine. The vertical height of the place (handle) at which one pushes and pulls is important. By lowering the body, one can use the body weight more effectively (by leaning forward when pushing, and backward when pulling). This is advantageous for generating force but increases the risk of falling.

CONCLUSIONS

Occupational back injuries are common, presenting problems to workers, employers, physicians, and society. Adherence to some basic biomechanical principles may reduce the magnitude of the problem but will not completely eliminate it. Optimization of work postures, provision of ergonomically sound work benches, tables, chairs, tools and other workplace materials, and proper instruction in work methods are cornerstones in back pain prevention and in rehabilitation of the injured worker.

References

1. American Academy of Orthopaedic Surgeons Symposium: Injury and Repair of the Musculoskeletal Soft Tissues. A.A.O.S., Park Ridge, Illinois, 1988.
2. Andersson, G. B. J.: Biomechanical aspects of sitting: An application to VDT terminals. Behav. Info. Tech. 6:251–269, 1987.
3. Andersson, G. B. J.: Measurements of load on the lumbar spine. *In* White, A. A. III, and Gordon, S. L. (eds.): Symposium on Low Back Pain. St. Louis, C. V. Mosby, 1982, pp. 220–251.
4. Andersson, G. B. J., and Chaffin, D. B.: Occupational Biomechanics. New York, John Wiley & Sons, 1984.
5. Andersson, G. B. J., Örtengren, R., and Herberts, P.: Quantitative electromyographic studies of back muscle activity related to posture and loading. Orthop. Clin. North Am. 8:85–96, 1977.

6. Andersson, G. B. J., Murphy, R. W., Örtengren, R. and Nachemson, A.: The influence of backrest inclination and lumbar support on the lumbar lordosis in sitting. Spine 4:52–58, 1978.
7. Andersson, G. B. J., Örtengren, R., Nachemson, A., and Elfström, G.: Lumbar disc pressure and myoelectric back muscle activity during sitting. Scand. J. Rehab. Med. 6:104–114, 1974.
8. A.S.F.: Ordinance concerning work with VDUs. National Board of Occupational Safety and Health. Stockholm, Sweden, 1985.
9. Bendix, T.: Posture of the trunk when sitting on forward-inclining seats. Scand. J. Rehab. Med. 15:197–203, 1984.
10. Brown, J. R.: Lifting as an Industrial Hazard. Labour Safety Council of Ontario, Ontario Department of Labour, 1971.
11. Bush-Joseph, C., Schipplein, O. D., Andersson, G. B. J., and Andriacchi, T. P.: Influence of dynamic factors on the lumbar spine moment in lifting. Ergonomics 31:211–216, 1988.
12. Engdal, S.: The importance of the bed surface to back pain, sleep and circulation [Manuscript]. Stockholm, Werner-Gren Research Center, 1983.
13. Farfan, H.: Mechanical disorders of the low back. Philadelphia, Lea & Febiger, 1973.
14. Garrett, W. E., Jr., Nikolaou, P. K., Ribbeck, B. M., et al.: The effect of muscle architecture on the biomechanical failure properties of skeletal muscle under passive extension. Am. J. Sports Med. (in press, 1989).
15. Garrett, W. E., Jr., Safran, M. R., Seaber, A. V., et al.: Biomechanical comparison of stimulated and skeletal muscle pulled to failure. Am. J. Sports Med. (in press, 1989).
16. International Labour Organization (I.L.O.): Maximum permissible weight to be carried by one worker. Geneva, I.L.O. Office, 1964–1967.
17. Holm, S., and Nachemson, A.: Nutritional changes in canine intervertebral disc after spinal fusion. J. Clin. Orthop. 169:243–258, 1982.
18. Holm, S., and Nachemson, A.: Variations in the nutrition of the canine intervertebral disc induced by motion. Spine 8:866–874, 1983.
19. Hosea, T. M., Simon, S. R., Delatizky, J., et al.: Myoelectric analysis of the paraspinal musculature while driving. Spine 11:928–936, 1986.
20. Kramer, J.: Pressure dependent shifts in the intervertebral disc. Orthop. Clin. North Am. 8:211–216, 1977.
21. Leskinen, T. P. J., Stalhammar, H. R., Kuorinka, I. A. A., and Troup, J. D. G.: A dynamic analysis of spinal compression with different lifting techniques. Ergonomics 26:595–604, 1983(a).
22. Leskinen, T. P. J., Stalhammar, H. R., Kuorinka, I. A. A., and Troup, J. D. G.: The effect of inertial factors on spinal stress when lifting. Engineer. Med. 12:87–89, 1983(b).
23. Mandal, A. C.: Workchair with tilted seat. Ergonomics 19:157–164, 1976.
24. N.I.O.S.H. (National Institute of Occupational Safety and Health): Potential Health Hazards of Video Display Terminals. D.H.H.S. Publication No. 81–129, Cincinnati, 1981.
25. N.I.O.S.H. Technical Report: Work Practices Guide for Manual Lifting. D.H.H.S. (N.I.O.S.H.) Publication No. 81–122, Cincinnati, 1981.
26. Park, K., and Chaffin, D. B.: A biomechanical evaluation of two methods of load lifting. A.I.I.E. Trans. 6:105–113, 1974.
27. Pope, M. H., Frymoyer, J. F., and Andersson, G. B. J.: Occupational low back pain. New York, Praeger Press, 1984.
28. Sato, H., Ohashi, J., Iwanaga, K., et al.: Endurance time and fatigue in static contractions. J. Human Ergol. 13:147–154, 1984.
29. Schipplein, O. D., Trafimow, J. H., Andersson, G. B. J., Andriacchi, T. P.: Relationship between moments at the L5/S1 level, hip and knee joint during lifting. J. Biomech. 1989. (Submitted for publication.)
30. Schoberth, H.: Sitzhaltung, Sitzschaden, Sitzmöbeln. Berlin, Springer-Verlag, 1962.
31. Schultz, A. B., and Andersson, G. B. J.: Analysis of loads on the lumbar spine. Spine 6:76–84, 1981.
32. Schultz, A., Haderspeck, K., Warwick, D., and Portillo, D.: Use of lumbar trunk muscles in isometric performance of mechanically complex standing tasks. J. Orthop. Res. 1:77–91, 1983.
33. Troup, J. D. G., and Edwards, F. C.: Manual handling. A review paper. London, Her Majesty's Stationery Office, 1985.
34. U.S. Department of Labor: Back injuries associated with lifting. Bureau of Labor Statistics Bulletin #2144, 1982.

LUMBAR ORTHOSIS (BRACE)

Casey K. Lee

Lumbosacral orthoses have been used for many types of disorders of the lumbosacral spine, such as idiopathic low back pain, spondylolysis, spondylolisthesis, disc herniation, degenerative instability, spinal stenosis, spondylitis, and other traumatic disorders of the spinal column. The popularity of the lumbosacral orthosis has been declining, while that of surgical treatment has rapidly increased. The authors present a review of the literature with regard to both the biomechanical and clinical effectiveness of various orthoses and the current status of their use.

HISTORY

Although initially utilized as women's foundations, lumbosacral corsets have historically been traced back approximately 2,000 years to the Minoan period.[4] Galen attempted to correct scoliotic curves using bandages around the chest in 200 BC, and crude spinal corsets fashioned from bark were recovered from the cliff dwellings of pre-Colombian Indians living, circa 900 AD, in the southwestern United States.[2, 27] The first lumbosacral corset, fabricated with the specific intention of supporting the lumbosacral spine, was made in 1530 for Catherine of Medici.[5] This support consisted of an iron corset that extended from the midthorax to over the iliac crests, with hinges on one side and a fastening clasp on the opposite side. In past centuries, lumbosacral orthoses were usually worn by persons with spinal deformities secondary to scoliosis or Pott's disease. C. F. Taylor, in 1863, described and designed a brace that hyperextended the spine using the now familiar principle of three point fixation.[2] This brace was originally prescribed for the treatment of Pott's disease. These same braces or variants of them are currently being used for an entirely different entity: the treatment of low back pain.

ANATOMY

The lumbosacral spine can be divided into two distinct anatomic and functional regions: L1–L4 and L4–sacrum–pelvis. The upper and middle lumbar spine (L1–L4) is anatomically different from the lower lumbosacral junction. The orientation of the facet joints progresses from a more sagittal to a coronal plane as the joints progress in a proximal to distal direction. These anatomic differences result in the very different biomechanical characteristics of these two regions.[24] The biomechanical characteristics of the L4–L5 motion segment depend upon its anatomic relationship to the iliac crests. If the L4–L5 motion segment is located below a horizontal line drawn between the iliac crests, it behaves more like the L5–S1 motion segment. Conversely, if it lies above the iliac crests line, the L4–L5 motion segment behaves like an upper lumbar segment. Because of the anatomic differences and the iliolumbar ligaments, which stabilize the segment to the pelvis, the shape and size of the disc changes from the upper to lower lumbar spine. The disc of the L5–S1 segment is oval and much larger than the more proximal segments.

BIOMECHANICS

A spinal motion segment consists of three joints: the intervertebral disc and the two posterior facet joints. There are six degrees of freedom of motion about three axes. Angular movement is the result of lateral bending, axial rotation, and flexion–extension. Most lumbosacral orthoses are designed to limit the motions that produce angular movements.

The biomechanical goals of external spinal supports are immobilization, stabilization, correction of deformity or maintenance of alignment, and decreased loading on the joints of the lumbosacral spine. In 1970, Perry, after reviewing the results of a questionnaire answered by 3,460 practicing orthopedic surgeons, reported that a lumbosacral orthosis was prescribed first with the expectation of restricting motion and second to obtain some degree of abdominal support.[23] Although the exact biomechanical principle of lumbosacral orthoses has yet to be elucidated, immobilization of the trunk, increased intra-abdominal pressure, modification or correction of posture and the modification of muscle functions have all been suggested possibilities.

Lumbosacral orthoses have varying degrees of rigidity or flexibility, posture control, and load relieving effect, depending on the physical design and materials used in the construction of the orthosis. Rigid orthoses utilize the principle of three point fixation, which consists of two counterforces applied at the upper and lower ends of the brace with an oppositely directed third force in the middle of these two. The proximal support is generally located just inferior to the xiphisternum and scapulae and the distal support is usually located at the pelvis, proximal to the greater trochanters at the level of the midsacrum.

A brace employing three point fixation can be constructed so that it maintains the lumbosacral spine in either an extended or a flexed posture. Three point fixation primarily limits movements in flexion and extension. Positioning the middle counterforce anteriorly at the midlumbar level produces a flexed posture of the lumbosacral spine;

an example of this is the Raney jacket. An extended posture results if the middle counterforce is placed posteriorly at the posterior midlumbar spine; an example is the Jewett hyperextension brace. More complete restriction of sagittal motion and production of an extended posture can be obtained with a custom-molded orthosis, which utilizes three point fixation with an anteriorly directed midlumbar counterforce.

Biomechanical studies were conducted to measure the intersegmental motion in flexion and extension, as well as to assess gross motion of the lumbosacral spine during the wearing of various orthoses. The effect of an orthosis on intersegmental motion was investigated by Norton and Brown[22] and Fidler and Plasmans.[6] The results of these two studies are contradictory. Norton and Brown, using Kirschner wires placed into the spinous processes, found little immobilization effect while an individual wore an orthosis; in fact, it actually increased in certain circumstances.[22] Conversely, Fidler and Plasmans found varying degrees of significant immobilization of intersegmental motion, depending on the type of orthosis tested (canvas jacket, Raney jacket, body jacket cast, and pantaloon-type cast).[6] Measured roentgenographically, the canvas jacket reduced motion by 30% at each level. The Raney body jacket and body jacket cast reduced motion in the midlumbar region by approximately 66%; however, neither was different from the corset in immobilizing the upper lumbar levels. Motion at the L4–L5 and L5–S1 levels was reduced by 92% with the pantaloon cast.[6] Lantz and Schultz studied the effect of a molded thoracolumbosacral orthosis (TLSO), chairback brace, and lumbosacral corset on gross body motion. Decreases of up to 20% in flexion and up to 45% in extension were noted with an orthosis.[8] Orthoses that are well-fixed to the thorax with inadequate pelvic fixation tend to produce a concentration of the forces at the T12–L1, L1–L2, and L2–L3 levels when the trunk is flexed, because the brace pulls away from the posterior aspect of the pelvis. Compensatory movements below these levels result. This has been noted to occur with the body jacket and Taylor brace. Braces that are better fixed at the pelvis than the chest, such as the corset or chairback brace, produce a concentration of restricting forces at the L4–L5 and L5–S1 levels; however, these restricting forces are relatively small.[22]

Limitation of lateral bending is usually accomplished with the addition of longitudinal lateral side bars that provide two point fixation. The degree of control depends on the rigidity of the side bars and the quality of the interface at the thorax and pelvis. In order to obtain rigid control of lateral bending, Norton and Brown designed an experimental brace that consisted of bilateral trochanteric pads added to a conventional chairback-type orthosis for three point immobilization. Although effective, the brace was poorly tolerated by patients.[22] A lumbosacral corset, chairback brace, and molded TLSO have all been shown to restrict lateral bending by 29%, 45%, and 49%, respectively.[8]

Axial rotation of the lumbosacral spine averages 6 degrees during standing and 1.5 degrees during walking.[11] Control of axial rotation by a lumbosacral orthosis relies on two point fixation and the inherent rigidity of the brace itself. Lumsden and Morris studied the effect of lumbosacral braces on axial rotation of the lumbosacral spine.[11] External immobilization with a corset or brace did not appear to decrease lumbosacral rotation during normal level walking, but actually increased in some subjects.[11]

Any brace, of rigid or flexible construction, depends on the topography of the body for fixation. The trunk and pelvis are analogous to an oval cylinder with the spine lending support. Fixation is best achieved by a fit between the orthotic and bony prominences. However, between the brace and the bone lies the skin and underlying soft tissue. These loose tissue layers between the skeletal superstructure and the brace force the brace to rely on friction for fixation. This is not a great problem proximally, because the thorax provides a relatively large surface area upon which the brace can act. However, the surface area of the pelvis is much smaller and provides much less adequate fixation. Incorporating the hip joint affords more complete fixation and markedly limits or eliminates hip motion, but it renders the patient more disabled or uncomfortable.

Almost all orthoses, rigid or flexible, have been found to increase intra-abdominal pressure.[7] Normally, the anterior abdominal muscles that are most active in the production of this pressure are the transverse and obliques.[7] The increase of intra-abdominal pressure that may occur with the use of a lumbosacral orthosis may have a load-relieving effect in the spinal motion segments. A reduction in the joint reaction force at the lumbosacral junction has been demonstrated secondary to this effect.[16] A 30% decrease in the intradiscal pressure has been recorded as intra-abdominal pressure was increased by the use of corsets or braces during sagittal-plane forward bending.[17, 18]

The type of orthosis prescribed depends on the degree or type of immobilization desired. Understanding the difference between segmental immobilization and gross immobilization is essential. Segmental immobilization is not the reduction but the elimination of motion of a particular motion segment. This requires a very rigid form of immobilization, which is probably most completely achieved with some form of internal fixation or external fixation (e.g., percutaneous pin fixation) or a very rigid orthosis. Pathologic conditions requiring segmental immobilization are fractures or fracture-dislocations, spondylitis, and degenerative or postoperative instability.

Gross restriction of motion is the term used to describe a decrease in the range of motion in one or more of the three planes that allow the patient to function without pain. Attenuated ligamentous, capsular, and annulus structures of a degenerated motion segment may become painful in certain extreme ranges of motion. An orthosis that provides restriction of gross motion will protect the patient from these painful movements.

Decreasing the load of the intervertebral joint may be one of the goals of bracing. A load-relieving effect may be the result of two mechanisms: increased intra-abdominal pressure and decreased trunk muscle activity. Although it is generally believed to be one of the most significant effects of an orthosis, the load-relieving mechanism of increased intra-abdominal pressure is not well understood. Some have demonstrated that intra-abdominal pressure is either unaffected[16] or inconsistently affected by an orthosis.[17] However, a corset or brace has been noted to decrease intradiscal pressure by approximately 30% in forward flexion.[17, 18, 20] Decreased trunk muscle activity may be a mechanism by which an orthosis decreases the intervertebral joint reaction forces. Myoelectric studies have demonstrated that orthoses (chairback, molded TLSO) inconsistently reduce the myoelectric activity of the erector spine and abdominal muscle.[9, 17, 25] Another consideration is that the brace (e.g., body jacket) itself may decrease the joint reaction force by transmitting a portion of the load from the upper trunk to pelvis, if it is rigid and well fixed proximally and distally.

CLINICAL APPLICATIONS

The clinical goals of the practitioner prescribing a lumbosacral orthosis are relief of pain, increased functional capacity, and reduced disability of the patient. A lumbosacral orthosis may be prescribed for idiopathic low back pain, fracture or fracture-dislocations, spondylolysis, spondylolisthesis, spinal stenosis, facet syndrome, instability, and spondylitis. The clinical usefulness of spinal orthoses may be secondary to the control of posture, stabilization of gross body motion, and/or rigid immobilization. Nachemson has reviewed the indications for orthoses in lumbosacral disorders with or without verifiable diagnosis.[19]

The control of posture can be effective in the treatment of spondylolysis, spondylolisthesis, and spinal stenosis. Limitation of gross body motion is the goal of bracing in both the acute lumbosacral sprain and degenerative instability. Although symptomatic relief may occur with the limitation of gross motion, correction of the actual instability requires segmental immobilization, which may necessitate internal fixation or fusion. In order to immobilize the thoracolumbar juntion, L1–L2 and L2–L3, a thoracolumbosacral flexion–extension orthosis (TLSO) would be appropriate. It has been demonstrated that angular movements at the L3–L4 level can be reduced to one-third of normal with either a Raney jacket, which is a flexion orthosis, or a body jacket cast.[6] However, in order to adequately immobilize the L4–L5, L5–S1 and sacroiliac joints, the hip must be immobilized. The body jacket with a thigh spica accomplishes this allowing only 2 degrees of angular movement (12% of normal) at the L4–L5 level and 1.4 degrees (8% of normal) at the L5–S1 level.[6]

Commonly prescribed spinal orthoses have been claimed to be effective in clinical use, but few controlled studies have been performed.[1, 15] Results of these studies indicate the clinical usefulness of spinal orthosis for low back pain, but controversy exists. Studies of patient populations who had low back pain of an unknown cause and were treated with orthoses yielded inconclusive results.[1, 14, 15] Studies that used specific spinal orthoses in patients who had a known pathologic condition such as spondylolisthesis and spondylolysis provided reliable, reproducible results.[10, 13, 27]

The most common indication for spinal bracing is idiopathic low back pain. Entities in this category include the acute lumbosacral sprain, myofascial syndrome, and internal disc derangements. Each of these entities is an individual disease process and probably requires a different approach and prescription. Accurate diagnosis and an understanding of the biomechanical needs of the patient are essential.

The orthosis usually prescribed for acute lumbosacral strain/sprain is a lumbosacral corset.[23] Corsets can be ordered with or without rigid stays. Those with a lumbar support have been reported to produce a lordosis and provide some pain relief. The rigidity and the configuration of the stays added to the corset determine its rigidity. Corsets without support are theorized to function by two mechanisms: greater intra-abdominal pressure and restriction of gross movement. Canvas corsets have been shown to reduce angular movements at each level to approximately 66% of normal,[6] however, axial rotation was not well controlled.[11] Corsets have also been reported to have both a massaging effect and a significant placebo effect.[7, 19] Molded and rigid frame orthoses have been utilized for this condition, although much less frequently.

Internal disc derangements and other causes of discogenic pain have been treated with lumbosacral corsets with or without stays, orthoses with a flexion or extension effect, or rigid orthoses that utilize three point fixation. The biomechanical goals in the treatment of these conditions are as follows: the relative unloading of the disc by transferring a portion of the load to the posterior elements, a limitation of gross motion, and postural modification. Flexion braces have had poor success in treating these patients,[13] whereas restoration of lumbar lordosis has been found to provide relief of pain in a significant number.[12]

Vertebral body fractures of the thoracolumbar and lumbar spine without neurologic deficit have been treated with bracing. Rigid lumbosacral orthoses such as the body cast or molded body jacket have been successfully employed in the treatment of compression and compression-burst–type fractures of the T12–L2 levels and burst-type fractures of L3–L5 levels. Posterior element fractures can be treated with either a body jacket cast or a molded body jacket. Immobilization of fractures requires a very rigid form of fixation; however, it has been demonstrated that no orthosis provides this level of rigidity. The orthosis provides both symptomatic relief and prevention of further deformity. An example of this is the treatment of compression fractures in the osteoporotic patient with a hyperextension brace. Fracture dislocations of the T12–L2 levels have also been successfully treated with a rigid orthosis applied postoperatively.

Back pain secondary to spondylolysis and spondylolisthesis, particularly in the adolescent, has been reported to respond to bracing in a rigid flexion brace (Boston brace), with good to excellent relief of pain in 100% and healing of the isthmic fracture in 16% of the patients studied.[13] Adults with isthmic spondylolisthesis with a documented 25% to 50% slip at the L5–S1 level were treated with a rigid thermoplastic flexion brace; 87% were noted to have complete pain relief, and the remainder had at least some pain relief.[27] The flexion orthosis for the treatment of these conditions should provide limitation of gross body motion, stabilization, and correction of posture. Patients with facet syndrome can also be treated effectively with a rigid flexion brace. The orthosis has the effect of transferring load from the facet joint to the intervertebral disc and limits torsional movement.

Bracing has been employed with some success in the treatment of spinal stenosis.[13, 27] The orthosis for this condition should provide stabilization and maintain a flexed posture. A flexed posture commonly provides relief from the pain and neurogenic claudication in the early stage of the disease process. Once the patient has severe symptoms from spinal stenosis, he or she does not become well; surgery seems to be the only solution.[28]

The treatment of spondylitis requires control of segmental motion at the involved levels. Rigid orthoses such as the TLSO, pantaloon cast, or body jacket are most effective in the initial 4 to 6 weeks when used in conjunction with appropriate medical treatment. Once the acute symptoms and paraspinal muscle spasm subside, a less rigid brace or corset can be used.

Orthoses can be prescribed for the patient who underwent an extensive decompression procedure during the early postoperative period. If postcompression instability is expected, owing to preoperative instability and/or extensive decompression, one should combine rigid internal fixation with decompression and fusion during surgery, rather than depend on postoperative bracing for stability.

NEGATIVE EFFECTS OF ORTHOSES

Orthoses must be comfortable during both standing and sitting. If the selected orthosis is unduly awkward or uncomfortable, compliance will suffer. Patients with a diaphragmatic hernia or pulmonary disease may be poor candidates for any type of orthosis that either restricts chest expansion or increases intra-abdominal pressure.

Although the added support afforded by a lumbosacral orthosis may satisfy the patients' biomechanical and clinical needs, this added support may allow the following negative effects to occur: atrophy; fibrosis and contractures of the paraspinal and anterior abdominal muscles, fascia and ligaments; skin irritation; and development of a psychologic dependence.[3, 19, 21]

SUMMARY AND FUTURE STUDIES

Spinal orthoses such as a lumbosacral corset with stays can be prescribed for lumbosacral strain/sprain, disc herniation, and other discogenic pain for a short duration (6 to 8 weeks). A more rigid brace can be prescribed for spondylolysis, spondylolisthesis, and early spinal stenosis during the acute exacerbation of symptoms. Very rigid immobilization using a TLSO or pantaloon cast is employed for spondylitis or the acute phase of traumatic conditions.

For spondylitis, fracture or fracture-dislocations, and certain types of spinal instability, a very rigid spinal orthosis, such as a TLSO or molded body jacket with or without extension to include hip joint, can be most effective. Patients who experience chronic persistent low back pain with an accurately diagnosed pathologic condition are more effectively treated surgically.

Future studies should include prospective controlled clinical studies of the effectiveness of a specific type of orthosis for a known pathologic condition. Future studies should also include the development of a functional lumbosacral orthosis that will allow painless function of the lumbosacral spine while limiting only painful movements. This will increase both patient acceptance and functional capacity.

Acknowledgment

The author wishes to thank Dr. Mark Hambly for his assistance in compiling this manuscript.

References

1. Ahlgren, S. A., and Hansen, T.: The use of lumbosacral corsets prescribed for low back pain. Prosthet. Orthot. Internat. 2:101–104, 1978.
2. American Academy of Orthopaedic Surgeons: Orthopaedic Appliances Atlas. Ann Arbor, Edwards, 1952, pps. 180–187.
3. American Academy of Orthopaedic Surgeons: Atlas of Orthotics, Biomechanical principles and application. St. Louis, C. V. Mosby, 1975, pp. 312–360.
4. Evans, A.: The Palace of Minos at Knossos, Vol. 1. London, MacMillan, 1921, p. 503.
5. Ewing, E.: Fashion in Underwear. Batsford, 1971, p. 13.
6. Fidler, M. W., and Plasmans, C. M. T.: The effect of four types of support on the segmental mobility of the lumbosacral spine. J. Bone Joint Surg. 65A:943–947, 1983.
7. Grew, N. D., and Deane, G.: The physical effect of lumbar spine supports. Prosthet. Orthot. Int. 6:79–87, 1982.
8. Lantz, S. A., and Schultz, A. B.: Lumbar spine orthosis wearing. 1. Restriction of gross body motions. Spine 11:834–837, 1986.
9. Lantz, S. A., and Schultz, A. B.: Lumbar spine orthosis wearing. 2. Effect on trunk muscle myoelectric activity. Spine 11:838–842, 1986.
10. Larsson U., Choler U., Lidstrom A., et al.: Autotraction for treatment of lumbagosciatica: A multicentre controlled investigation. Acta Orthop. Scand. 51:791–798, 1980.
11. Lumsden, R. M., and Morris, J. M.: An in vivo study of axial rotation and immobilization at the lumbosacral joint. J. Bone Joint Surg. 50A:1591–1602, 1968.
12. McKenzie, R. A.: Prophylaxis in recurrent low back pain. N. Z. Med. J. 89:22–23, 1979.
13. Micheli, L. J., Hall, J. E., and Miller, M. E.: Use of modified Boston brace for back injuries in athletes. Am. J. Sports Med. 8:351–356, 1980.
14. Million, R., Hall, W., Nilsen, K. H., et al.: Assessment of the progress of the back-pain patient. Spine 7:204–211, 1982.
15. Million R., Nilsen, K. H., Jayson, M. I. V., et al.: Evaluation of low back pain and assessment of lumbar corsets with and without back supports. Ann. Rheum. Dis. 40:449–454, 1981.
16. Morris, J. M., et al.: Role of the trunk in stability of the spine. J. Bone Joint Surg. 43A:327, 1961.

17. Nachemson, A., Schultz, A. B., and Anderson, G. B. J.: Mechanical effectiveness studies of lumbar spine orthoses. Scand. J. Rehab. Med. 9(Suppl.):139, 1983.
18. Nachemson A.: Advances in low back pain. Clin. Orthop. Rel. Res. No. 200:266–278, 1985.
19. Nachemson, A.: Orthotic treatment for injuries and diseases of the spinal column. Phys. Med. Rehab. 1:11–24, 1987.
20. Nachemson, A., and Morris, J.: In vivo measurements of intradiscal pressure. J. Bone Joint Surg., 46A:1077–1092, 1964.
21. Nash, C. L.: Current concepts review. Scoliosis bracing. J. Bone Joint Surg. 62A:848–852, 1981.
22. Norton, P. L., and Brown, T.: The immobilizing efficiency of back braces. Their effect on the posture and motion of the lumbosacral spine. J. Bone Joint Surg. 39A:111–138, 1957.
23. Perry, J.: The use of external support in the treatment of low back pain. Report of the Subcommittee on Orthotics of the Committee on Prosthetic-Orthotic Education. National Academy of Sciences, National Research Council. J. Bone Joint Surg. 52A:1440–1442, 1970.
24. Posner, I., White, A., Edwards, W., and Wilson, C.: A biomechanical analysis of the clinical stability of the lumbar and lumbosacral spine. Spine 7:374–389, 1982.
25. Waters, R. L., and Morris, J. M.: Effects of spinal supports on the electrical activity of muscles of the trunk. J. Bone Joint Surg. 52A:51–60, 1970.
26. White, A., and Panjabi, M.: Spinal braces: Functional analysis and clinical applications. *In* White, A., and Panjabi, M. (eds.): Clinical Biomechanics of the Spine. Philadelphia, J. B. Lippincott, 1978, pp. 345–363.
27. Willner, S.: Effect of a rigid brace on back pain. Acta Orthop. Scand. 56:40–42, 1985.
28. Wiltse, L. L., Kirkaldy-Willis, W. H., and McIvor, W. D.: The treatment of spinal stenosis. Clin. Orthop. Rel. Res. 115:83–91, 1977.

5 □ Biochemistry

Jill Urban
Sten H. Holm
Stephen J. Lipson

DISC BIOCHEMISTRY IN RELATION TO FUNCTION

Jill Urban

The intervertebral disc plays an important role in the mechanical functioning of the spinal column; hence, there have been numerous experimental and theoretical studies of its behavior under load.[48] The biologic and biochemical nature of the disc has been neglected by comparison, and yet ultimately the mechanical properties of the disc depend on the nature of the structural macromolecules that constitute the disc matrix and on the interplay among them. Here, the relevant aspects of disc and end-plate biochemistry are briefly reviewed and our present understanding of the function of the discal constituents is discussed. Disc biochemistry has been reviewed in detail by Eyre,[16] and more recently by Ayad and Weiss[4] and Johnstone.[26]

BROOM'S MODEL OF THE EXTRACELLULAR MATRIX

The function of the matrix constituents is well demonstrated in a physical model of cartilage developed by Broom and Marra,[11] shown in Figure 1. This model consists of a string network enclosing balloons; the balloons inflate the network and prevent it from collapsing. If a load is applied to this structure, it can be seen that the deformation of the network depends on a number of factors. Among these are the magnitude of the load and the manner of its application. However, the degree of deformation also depends on the nature of the structure, on the properties of string, on the weave of the string network, on the number of linkages and knots, and on how the network is anchored to its base. It depends too on the number of balloons and their degree of inflation. In general, if the balloons are highly inflated and the string network is tightly knotted and taut, the network deforms less than if the balloons are underinflated or do not completely fill the framework, and as a result the network is floppy.

In cartilaginous tissues, collagen makes up the structural framework of the tissue and anchors the cartilage to the bone. It thus fulfills the functions of string in the physical model; like string, collagen is strong in tension but cannot alone support a compressive load.[63] In cartilage, the proteoglycan (PG) solution inflates the collagen network and enables tissue to carry compressive load; similarly, compressive load can be carried by the string-balloon structure because of the air-filled balloons that inflate the string framework.

The string-balloon model of cartilage behavior is applicable only to constant volume deformation under load. The behavior of cartilage departs from that of the model if the load is maintained; under sustained load, cartilaginous tissues creep, partly because of fluid loss. In order to mimic the behavior of cartilage under these conditions, the balloons would have to leak air under load and be automatically self-filling as the load was removed. This behavior would be

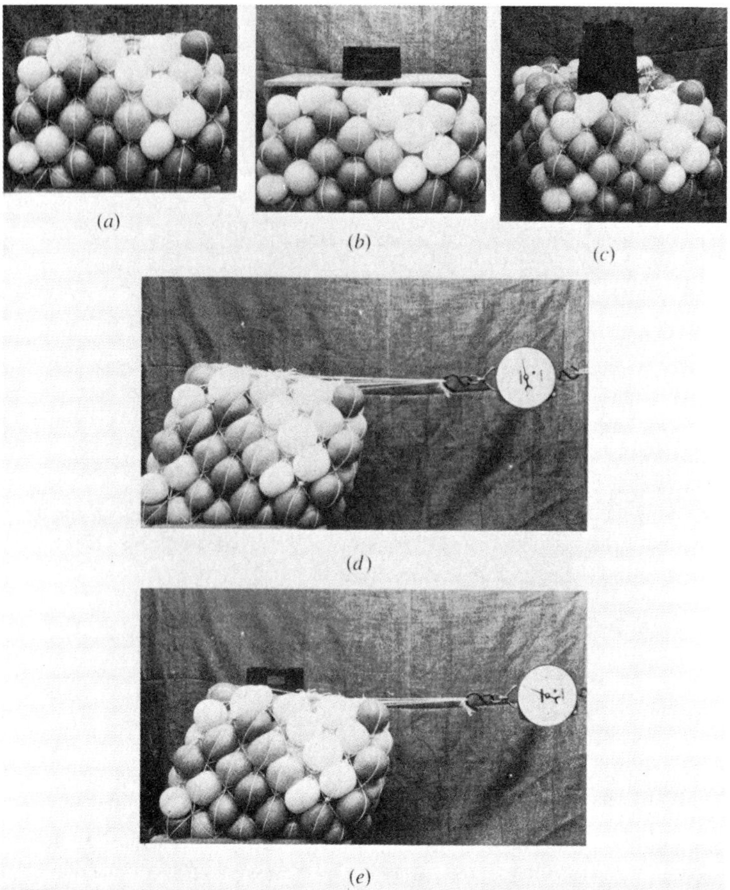

Figure 1 □ A model of articular cartilage has been constructed from a string network packed with air-filled balloons: *A*, details of the network; *B*, surface of the network; *C*, deformation of the network under a nonuniform compressive load; *D* and *E*, deformation of the network under a shear stress. (Adapted from Broom, N. D., and Marra, D. L.: New structural concepts of articular cartilage demonstrated with a physical model. Connect Tissue Res. 14:1–8, 1985. © 1985 by Gordon and Breach Science Publishers, Inc., London, England.)

analogous to that of the PGs, which lose fluid and reimbibe it as loading conditions change.

Because the mechanical properties of the disc are governed largely by the nature of collagen and of the network it forms and by the physical properties of the PGs, collagen and PGs are discussed in more detail below.

COLLAGEN

Collagen is the major structural protein of the body. In the disc, it accounts for about one half the dry weight of the annulus and about 20% to 30% of the nucleus dry weight.[1, 1a] The nature of the collagen molecule and the structure of the collagenous framework of the tissue determine the structural integrity and mechanical strength of the disc. Many aspects of collagen structure and function have been recently reviewed.[43]

Molecular Structure

The triple helix is common to all collagens. Here, three individual chains, themselves left-handed helices, coil around one another to form a right-handed superhelix, the tropocollagen molecule. Each individual chain of the major fibril-forming collagens consists of just over 1,000 amino acid residues; every third residue is glycine, and the other two are mainly proline and hydroxyproline.[44] Hydroxyproline helps stabilize the triple helix; because hydroxyproline occurs in very few other proteins, it is often used as a biochemical marker for collagen. Among the other amino acids that occur in the protein chain, the positions of lysine and hydroxylysine residues are of particular importance because they are the sites of formation of intermolecular cross-links, which impart stability to the collagen fibrils.[20]

Collagen is synthesized and secreted as procollagen. Procollagen is significantly larger than collagen; nonhelical regions, the propeptides, are found at either end of the triple helix. These propeptides are thought to play a role in the intracellular assembly of the triple helix. Once this assembly is completed and the triple helical molecule is secreted, the propeptides are enzymatically

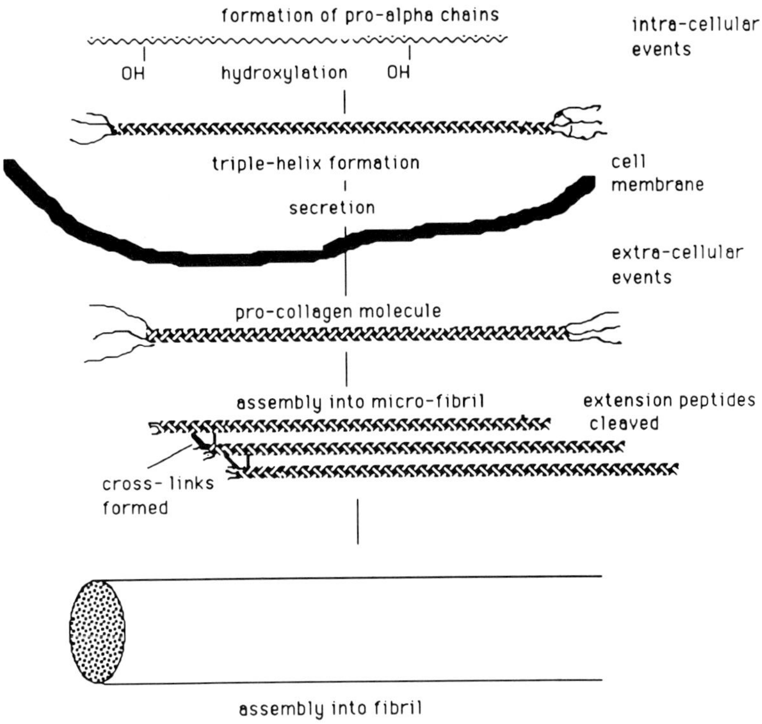

Figure 2 □ The banded structure of collagen fibrils, schematic view, and TEM of a collagen fibril are shown. (From Nimni, M. E., and Harkness, R. D.: Molecular structure and fraction of collagen. *In* Nimni, M. E. (ed.): Collagen, Vol. I. Copyright CRC Press, Boca Raton, FL, 1988).

removed from the remaining triple helical molecules.[44] The resulting tropocollagen molecules aggregate to form regular arrays of fibrils organized in a quarter stagger arrangement; this organization of the fibrils results in the characteristic collagen-banding pattern that is seen in electron micrographs (Fig. 2).

The diameter of the collagen fibril varies considerably among tissues and also varies with age.[46] Little is known, at present, about the factors that control fibril assembly and the final fibril diameter.[7] Work on fibril formation in vitro suggests that fibril diameter depends on collagen type,[8] and that the presence of other constituents of the matrix, especially PGs, may have a strong influence on fibril assembly.[65]

The collagen fibrils are stabilized by molecular cross-links, which form at specific lysine and hydroxylysine residues of the α-chain;[20] as a result of these cross-links, collagen fibrils have a high tensile strength and are very inextensible. The extent and type of cross-linking changes with maturation and age and are thought to affect the mechanical properties of the tissue. Cross-linking is mediated by the enzyme lysyl oxidase. If cross-linking is prevented by adding drugs that inhibit the activity of this enzyme, the collagen network that forms is very fragile. Inherited disorders of collagen in which cross-linking is affected also lead to a weak and fragile collagen network. The collagen of the disc, especially in the nucleus, has a high cross-link density.[20]

Collagen Types

Collagen is not a single protein. Rather, it describes a family of genetically distinct proteins, all of which have at least one triple helical region. Up until now, at least 12 different collagen types have been identified.[37] At least seven of these types have been identified in the intervertebral disc.[20a] Table 1 shows how these collagens are distributed in various tissues.

Table 1 □ Tissue Distribution of Collagen Types[4]

COLLAGEN TYPE	TISSUE DISTRIBUTION
I	Skin, tendon, bone, cornea
II	Cartilage, nucleus pulposus
III	Skin, blood vessels, tendon
IV	Basement membrane
V	Cornea
VI	Skin, blood vessels, disc, cartilage
VII	Sub-basal lamina
VIII	Cornea, growth plate, perichondrium, elastic cartilage, dura
IX	Cartilage, disc
X	Calcified cartilage, growth plate
XI	Cartilage
XII	Skin, tendon

The major collagens found in the disc are Types I and II.[17–19] Both fibril-forming collagens obviously have a mechanical role and are differently distributed as discussed below. Although the differences in the mechanical properties of these different collagen types are not yet understood, the fibrils of Type II collagen generally are much finer than those of Type I collagen. In keeping with this observation, the fibrils of the nucleus of the disc are finer than those of the annulus.[20a] Interactions with other components of the extracellular matrix may depend on collagen type; these interactions may also affect the mechanical properties of the tissue.[51]

Besides these major collagens, there are several minor collagens in the disc, existing in measurable concentrations. The function of these minor collagen types is unknown. However, Types IX and XI may be associated with Type II fibrils, and Types V and XII with Type I fibrils.[7, 61] Type VI collagen is particularly abundant in the disc; up to 20% of the collagen in the young disc nucleus is Type VI.[66] Type VI forms very fine fibrils and is unlikely to play a structural mechanical role.[29] Type VI is intimately associated with the PG fraction of the matrix; it may play a part in maintaining the position of other components in the tissue.[66] It has also been found directly around the cell and in contact with the chondrocyte membrane and may play some role in the interactions between the cell and matrix.[47]

Organization of the Collagen Network of the Disc and End Plate

The gross arrangement of the collagen network of the disc can be seen with the naked eye; one of the most notable features of the disc observed when it is sectioned horizontally is the series of concentric lamellae that encircle the disc and constitute the annulus fibrosus. These lamellae consist of bundles of collagen fibrils that run obliquely between the adjacent vertebral bodies and that are firmly anchored to them or to the cartilaginous end plates. The angle of the fiber bundles alternates in successive lamellae. The nucleus, in comparison, does not have an organized network; the fine fibrils of the nucleus form a loose irregular mesh. These fibrils are not connected to the cartilaginous end plates, but those at the boundary of the annulus merge with the fibrils of the inner lamellae.[25] The collagen fibrils of the end plate lie parallel to the surface of the vertebral body through the thickness of the cartilaginous end plate.[3] At the end plate–disc interface, the fibrils above the annulus change direction steeply to continue and merge with those of the annulus.[50]

The highly specialized weave provides the disc with the flexibility to act as a joint, yet enables it to withstand the pressures resulting from external loading; because of the nature of the network, the disc can deform considerably as the lamellae move relative to each other, even though collagen itself is relatively inextensible. There have been several theoretic models that relate the structure of this collagen network to disc deformation during compression, torsion, and flexion.[24] There is yet little experimental evidence to support any of these models.

PROTEOGLYCANS

PGs are the other major macromolecular constituent of the disc. PGs are a family of macromolecules consisting of carbohydrate (glycosaminoglycan [GAG] chains) covalently bonded to a central protein core. The structure and function of cartilage PGs have recently been reviewed.[14] The type of GAG and the number of chains bound to the protein core are widely variable. In cartilage there are at least two main subpopulations of PGs. The first are small PGs that have only one or two GAG chains. One of these PGs seems to be associated with the collagen fibrils,[51] but its function is unknown. Only a small fraction of the total PGs consists of these small PGs. The main PG found in cartilage is a large, aggregating PG with many GAG chains attached to the protein core. These two GAGs, chondroitin sulfate (CS) and keratin sulfate (KS), occupy different regions of the protein core—the KS-rich region and the CS-rich region of the monomer, respectively. Beyond the KS-rich region, the protein core ends in two globular domains. One of these globular domains, the hyaluronic acid–binding region, is so named because a proportion of the monomers are not free in the tissue but are attached through this domain to long chains of hyaluronic acid to form PG aggregates. The attachment is stabilized by link protein, which binds to both the hyaluronic acid chains and the

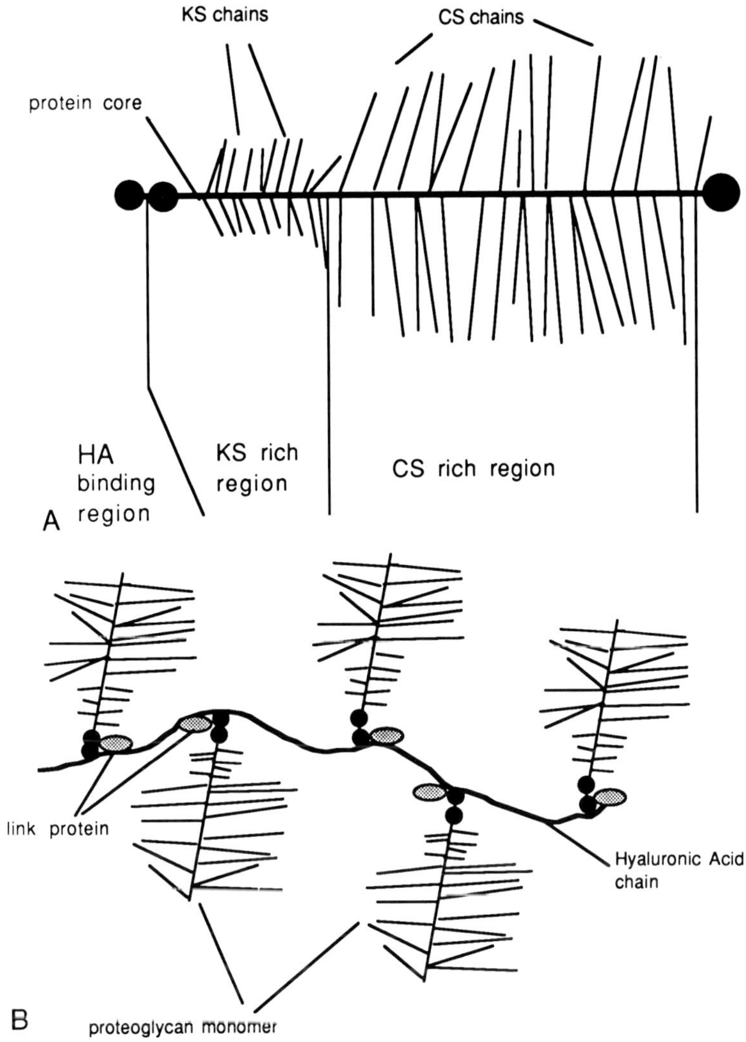

Figure 3 □ *A, B,* Schematic view shows the structure of the large aggregating proteoglycan of cartilage. (Modified from Carney, S. L., and Muir, H.: The structure and function of cartilage proteoglycans. Physiol. Rev. 68:858–910, 1988.)

hyaluronic acid–binding region of the PG. The structure of the PG is shown schematically in Figure 3.

Proteoglycans of the Disc

The large PGs of the disc, like those of cartilage, form a heterogeneous population. Many of the monomers appear to have lost their hyaluronic acid–binding region and thus are unable to form aggregates. The monomers tend to be smaller than those from hyaline cartilages. The GAG side chains also differ in size from those of hyaline cartilages; in particular, the CS chains are shorter and KS chains tend to be longer than those from other cartilages.[26, 38] The PGs of the nucleus differ from those of the annulus; the proportion of KS to CS is higher in the nucleus than in the annulus, and a smaller proportion of the nucleus monomers appears to exist as aggregates.[1] There are age-related changes in the proportion of monomers able to aggregate. About 40% of adult human annulus PGs and 15% of adult nucleus PGs can aggregate, whereas 60% and 25% of the monomers in the young disc are in the form of aggregates. This compares with about 80% of PGs able to form aggregates in hip articular cartilage.[26] There are indications that the disc PGs are able to form aggregates when they are newly synthesized[45] but that they are degraded in the tissue, and their hyaluronic acid–binding region disappears.[38] The functional significance of differences in degree of aggregation and of PG size is not yet understood. It has been suggested that aggregation helps keep the PGs in the tissue, because there is no evidence that these large PGs are held there by any form of binding. Recent work using monoclonal antibodies to various positions of the disc PG has suggested that the heterogeneity of disc PGs results from an accumulation of breakdown products.[27]

Fixed Charge Density

One important property of the GAGs is that they are charged. Both CS and KS contain charged sulfate and carboxyl groups, which import a net negative charge to the matrix. CS has two charges per disaccharide, whereas KS averages one. The concentration of fixed negative charges, the fixed charge density (FCD), thus does not depend only on the concentration of PG in the tissue but also on the ratio of CS to KS. The FCD confers important properties on the disc because it controls the distribution of charged solutes[35] and also the osmotic pressure of the matrix, as discussed later. The distribution of charged solutes may also have important effects on cell function.[55]

Proteoglycan Function

Osmotic Pressure of PG Solution

The high osmotic pressure of PG solution is attributable to two factors. The first results from the polyelectrolyte nature of the PGs, that is, from the fixed negative charges on the GAG side chains. Ions and other solutes distribute themselves between the plasma and the disc matrix in order to maintain electrochemical equilibrium for all species. The expression that describes this equilibrium distribution, the Gibbs-Donnan equation, shows that because of the net negative charge on the disc, the total number of ions in the disc is always greater than in the plasma. Because osmotic pressure results from the difference in the number of particles dissolved between the two phases, the excessive number of ions in the disc leads to a high osmotic pressure in the matrix.[57, 60] The second factor that contributes to the osmotic pressure of the disc results from excluded volume contributions of the polymer segments and depends on the size and shape of the PGs. This factor is much smaller in the disc than the Gibbs-Donnan or ionic contribution.[15] It is thus not surprising that PG size or the degree of aggregation has little influence on the osmotic properties of the disc, compared with the charge density. The relationship between osmotic pressure and PG concentration expressed as FCD is shown in Figure 4.

In the nucleus of adult discs removed post mortem, the FCD lies between 0.2 and 0.4 mEq/ml, depending on age. The resulting osmotic pressure expressed by PGs on these discs is consequently 0.1 to 0.3 mPa (1 to 3 atm).[58] The FCD of the annulus, and hence its osmotic pressure, is somewhat lower, although it is still considerable in comparison with that of non–weight-bearing tissues.

Proteoglycan Concentration and Pore Size Distribution

The matrix of the disc consists mainly of large PGs that are densely packed between collagen fibrils. The collagen fibrils are spaced at several hundred angstroms; however, the distance between the GAG chains is only 20 to 40 Å.[13] The PGs thus determine the fine structure of the matrix, as shown in Figure 5; the higher the concentration of PGs, the smaller is the effective diameter of the "pores" formed by the GAG chains. Because the pore size depends on PG concentration, any changes in hydration will affect the pore size. If the disc loses fluid and the PG concentration increases, the PGs become compressed as the same number of PG chains packs into a smaller volume of fluid. Consequently, the average pore diameter of the matrix decreases. Alternatively, if the disc swells, the PG concentration falls and the effective pore size increases.

The pore size distribution in the disc has important physiologic implications. First, it determines how fast fluid can flow into or out of the disc under a pressure gradient. Fluid flow can be described by Darcy's Law

$$J = k\, dP/dx$$

where J is the rate of fluid flow, k is the hydraulic permeability coefficient, and dP/dx is the pressure gradient causing flow.[41] The hydraulic permeability coefficient of the matrix is related to pore size, and it decreases as the radius of the pore decreases; based on theoretic considerations, the hydraulic permeability is related to the square of the radius and therefore falls off very steeply as pore size decreases.[6a]

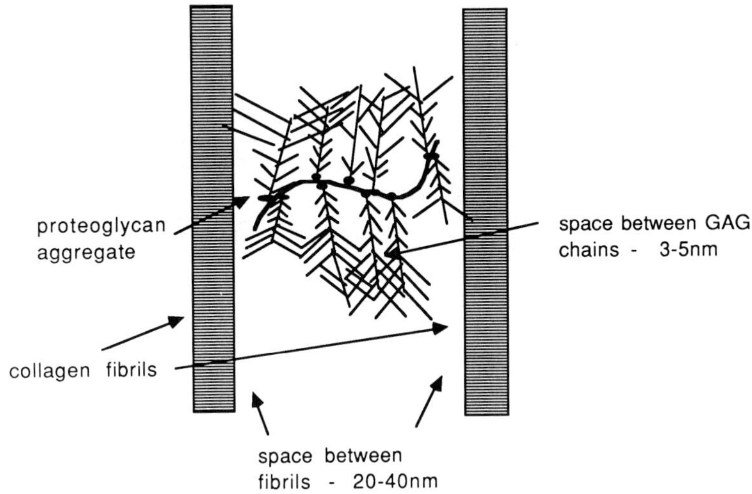

Figure 4 □ Schematic view of the organization of the disc matrix demonstrates that the fine pore structure depends on proteoglycan concentration, rather than on collagen. (Modified from Maroudas, A.: Physico-chemical properties of articular cartilage. *In* Freeman, N. A. R. (ed.): Adult Articular Cartilage, 2nd Ed. London, Pitman Medical, 1979.)

The pore size distribution and the FCD, both of which depend on the PG concentration of the disc, thus determine the maximum concentrations of solutes that can enter the disc and move through the matrix.

Ionic Solutes □ The concentration of ionic solutes is determined partly by the constraints of the Gibbs-Donnan equilibrium distribution. In general, cations have a higher concentration in the disc than in the plasma. The concentration of sodium in the plasma is around 150 mM, whereas that in the disc depends on the PG concentration, although it can rise to 300 to 400 mM, depending on the region and age of the disc. If water is expressed from the disc as the result of external loading, the concentration of sodium rises further.[30, 31] Divalent cations, such as calcium or magnesium, are even more sensitive to PG concentration, and their concentration may be as much as 10 times as great as that found in the plasma.[36] Small anions on the other hand are excluded from the disc matrix by the fixed negative charges that are present. The concentration of chloride, for instance, is less than half of that in the plasma, whereas divalent cations such as sulfate, an important substrate for manufacture of PGs, may have a value of only one fifth of that in the plasma.

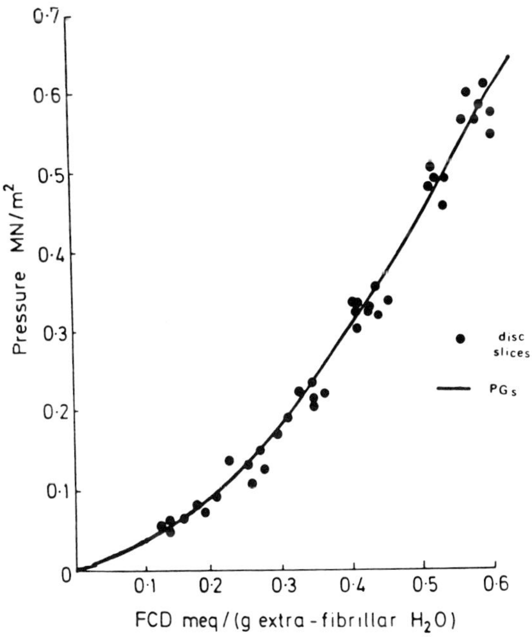

Figure 5 □ The relationship between proteoglycan osmotic pressure and proteoglycan concentration is expressed as fixed charge density (FCD). (From Urban, J. P. G., and McMullin, J. F.: Swelling pressure of the intervertebral discs: Influence of age, spinal level, composition, and degeneration. Spine 13:179–186, 1988.)

Macromolecular Solutes □ The solute distribution in the disc matrix is affected not only by the charge of the PGs but also by the pore size distribution. Very small solutes, such as amino acids, have a partition coefficient of unity; the partition coefficient is defined as the concentration on a molal basis in the disc matrix, relative to the concentration in the surrounding fluid or plasma. Thus, small solutes are not excluded from any of the fluid space of the matrix. As the molecular size of solutes increases, the partition coefficient falls. Even glucose, molecular weight 200, is partially excluded from the disc; its partition coefficient on a molal basis is only around 0.7 to 0.8 in the disc nucleus.[59] Larger solutes may have very low partition coefficients indeed. Solutes the size of bovine serum albumin are virtually excluded from the matrix of nondegenerate discs (unpublished observation); the partition coefficient of such solutes, which have a molecular weight of 60,000 to 70,000, is about .01 to .001. Although little work has been done on the relationship between molecular size and partition coefficient in the disc because of experimental problems associated with the disc swelling in solution, partition coefficients in relationship to solute molecular weight and FCD of the matrix have been extensively explored in articular cartilage.[35]

Physiologic Importance of the Partition Coefficient □ The movement and partition of solutes in the matrix concentration are of considerable physiologic importance. First, the concentration of ions determines the osmotic pressure of the disc (discussed above). Second, small nutrients such as O_2 glucose and substrates for synthesis of macromolecules must move through the matrix to reach the cells. The concentrations of nutrients and of larger molecules such as enzymes, hormones, and other active substances around the cell depend on their partition coefficient in the matrix. Products of synthesis must move away from the cell into the bulk of the extracellular matrix. Most of the assembly of the matrix depends on the physical properties of the secreted macromolecules, and the cell plays little direct part in matrix assembly.[14] The speed at which degraded macromolecules are lost from the tissue also depends on the way their breakdown products can pass through the disc. Because these products are still osmotically active,[60] it is obviously beneficial if they are not lost too rapidly from the disc.

Proteoglycans and Disc Hydration

Fluid is the major constituent of the disc, and it influences the mechanical response of the disc and other tissue properties. However, the fluid content of the disc is not constant. Fluid is expelled from the discs when they are placed under a sustained external load and is reimbibed when the load is removed.[2, 64] Discs also swell in vitro when placed in aqueous solution. The fluid content thus depends on the external load on the disc.

Fluid content of the disc is determined by the difference between the hydrostatic and osmotic pressures in the matrix. The hydrostatic pressure arises in vivo from the external loads that are applied to the disc via muscles and ligaments and by body weight and so varies with posture and movement.[42] The origin of osmotic pressure in the disc is primarily ionic and arises from the disc PGs, as discussed. Fluid movement in the disc also depends on the hydraulic permeability of the matrix, as this affects the rate of fluid loss or gain under any pressure gradient. A recent model suggests that, in vivo, the resistance to fluid loss at the boundary between the disc and the interstitium surrounding it also has a strong influence on fluid movement into and out of the disc.[53]

Diurnal Changes in Fluid Content of the Intervertebral Disc □ Because the disc is under constantly changing external loads, neither its shape nor its fluid content is constant. If the disc is loaded its height alters by means of two mechanisms. Initially the disc deforms through a rearrangement of the collagen network and the bulk movement of the disc matrix. The extent of this deformation varies among discs, but the factors that govern this deformation are not yet well understood. No consistent pattern related to age, sex, or degree of degeneration has been found. If the change in load is of short duration the deformation is virtually at constant volume. However, if the load is maintained the disc creeps; a substantial fraction of the creep deformation results from fluid loss.[28]

The relationship among change in load on the disc, disc swelling pressure, and fluid content of the disc is illustrated in Figure 6. The solid line represents the curve of applied pressure versus equilibrium hydration; a disc lying on this curve is at osmotic equilibrium and will experience no net fluid shifts. The line represents the swelling pressure–hydration curve. If one begins at point 1, where the disc is assumed to be at equilibrium, and then applies a pressure to the disc, it moves from that point on the equilibrium to the curve to point 2, which is well above it. At point 2, the hydrostatic pressure is greater than the osmotic pressure of the disc, since the hydration has remained

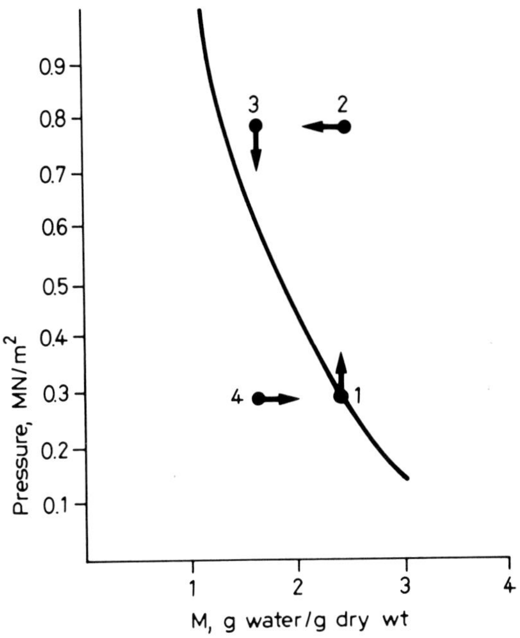

Figure 6 □ Schematic view shows the relationship between stress on the disc and fluid expression. At *1*, the swelling pressure is equal to the applied pressure, and this point lies on the equilibrium swelling pressure curve. There is no net fluid flow. At *2*, the applied pressure is greater than swelling pressure, so fluid tends to be expressed to increase the proteoglycan concentration and hence the swelling pressure.

constant. Because the disc is no longer at osmotic equilibrium, the pressure gradient tends to express fluid from the disc. The rate at which fluid is expressed from the disc depends partly on the pressure gradient and partly on the hydraulic permeability of the tissue. Fluid loss is therefore most rapid initially when both the pressure gradient and hydraulic permeability are maximum. As fluid is expressed, the PG concentration rises, the swelling pressure of the tissue increases, and the pressure gradient falls. As the PG content increases, the hydraulic permeability also falls. Both mechanisms help limit the amount of fluid lost to and from the disc. Fluid expression continues until the disc reaches the equilibrium curve. Because of the size of the disc and the slow rate of fluid flow, the osmotic equilibrium is unlikely to be reached during a normal day of loading. If the load on the disc is removed at point 3, the hydrostatic pressure falls and the disc now lies below the equilibrium curve at point 4. Here the pressure gradient is such that fluid is imbibed to dilute the PGs and reduce the swelling pressure of the tissue. During swelling the hydraulic permeability increases and swelling thus tends to occur more rapidly than fluid loss. The disc is therefore able to replace the fluid lost during 16 hours of activity within 8 hours of rest.

Influence of Disc Composition on Hydration Under Load □ Because the osmotic pressure of PGs depends not on size but on their charge density,[56] all discs will have the same PG concentration at equilibrium under equivalent pressures, as shown diagrammatically in Figure 7.

Of physiologic interest is the ratio of fluid to dry weight, which differs depending on the ratio of PG to collagen. Discs with a low PG-to-dry weight ratio have a low total hydration and appear thin and desiccated, whereas discs with a high PG-to-dry weight ratio have a high fluid content. Thus the overall fluid content of a disc depends on its composition and on the applied load. Equilibrium hydration can satisfactorily be estimated by using these parameters.[58]

DISC COMPOSITION

The major constituents of the disc are collagen PGs and water. Other uncharacterized glycoproteins and traces of elastin have also been found. In addition, about 2% to 5% of the matrix volume is occupied by cells.

The relative proportion of the matrix constituents varies with position changes in the disc and down the spine and with age changes. The proportion of the three main constituents of the disc (i.e., water, collagen, and PG) is shown in Table 2. The nucleus is hydrated more than the annulus and has a higher concentration of PGs. Conversely, the concentration of collagen is lower in the nucleus than in the annulus. There is a gradient in the composition of these components through the annulus; the outer annulus has the highest collagen content and the lowest water and PG content, whereas the composition of the inner annulus approaches that of the nucleus.[1, 1a, 34, 60]

The molecular forms of PG and collagen alter also with changing position. Toward the center of the disc the PGs become smaller and less aggregated and the KS-to-CS ratio increases.[1, 26] No collagen I is found in the nucleus; a small fraction is found in the inner annulus, and the proportion of colla-

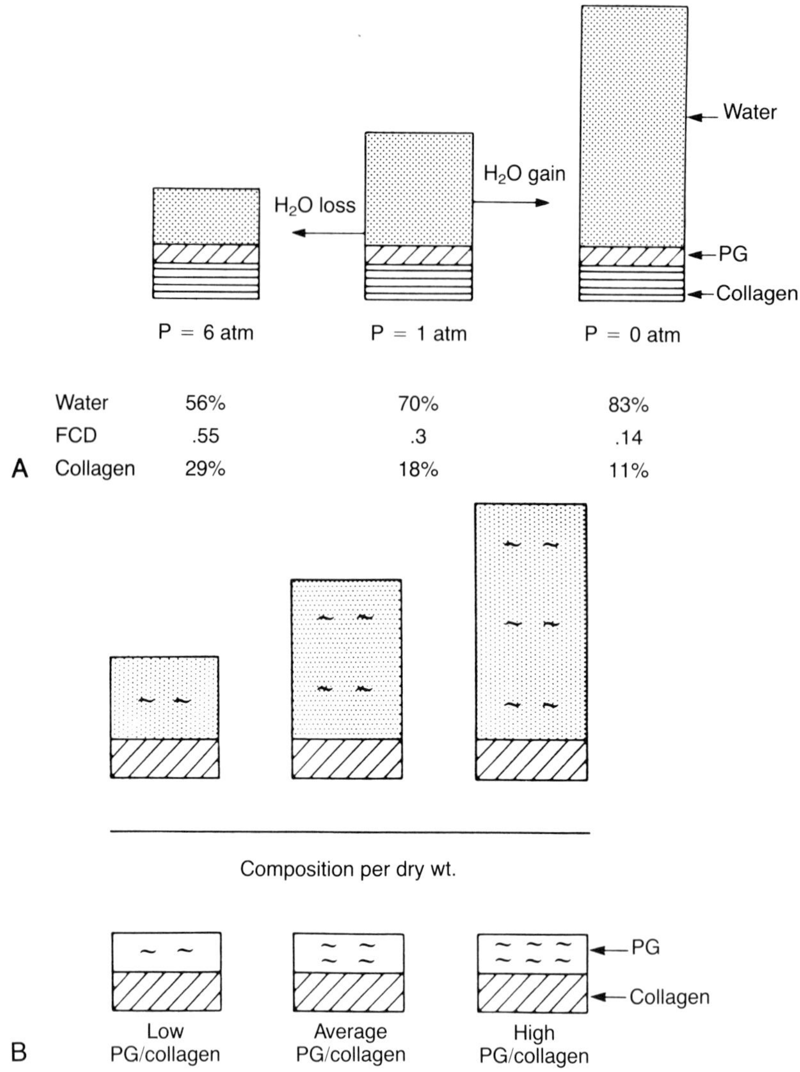

Figure 7 □ Schematic view shows the effect of proteoglycan concentration and of external pressures on disc hydration. *A,* For any one disc region, the amounts of proteoglycan and collagen remain constant, but the concentration changes as fluid is expressed under load or as the disc swells. *B,* The proteoglycan concentration is constant for all discs exposed to the same load. Discs with a high proteoglycan-to-collagen ratio will thus be more hydrated than discs with a low proteoglycan-to-collagen ratio. (From Urban J. P. G., and McMullin, J. F.: Swelling pressure of the intervertebral discs: Influence of age, spinal level, composition, and degeneration. Spine 13:179–186, 1988.)

Table 2 □ Composition of Adult Human Lumbar Intervertebral Disc[4, 50]

COMPONENT	ANNULUS		NUCLEUS	END PLATE
	OUTER	INNER		
Water (g/g dry wt)	1.0–2.0	2.0–3.0	3.0–5.0	1.0–1.5
Collagen (g/g dry wt)	0.5–0.6	0.15–0.3	0.15–0.25	0.5–0.7
GAG (g/g dry wt)	0.05	0.1–0.15	0.15–0.35	0.05–0.15

gen I increases through the annulus until in the outer annulus it is the predominant collagen. Conversely, little collagen II is found in the outer annulus, and the proportion of collagen II rises toward the nucleus; in the nucleus it is the major collagen.[19]

Change with Age

The composition of the disc changes with advancing age. The most noticeable change is loss of both water content and PGs in the nucleus.[21, 22] In juvenile discs over 85% of the nucleus volume consists of water. This decreases to around 70% to 75% water in adult discs and decreases even further with aging. The PG concentration also falls considerably with age, particularly in the nucleus. The composition of the monomer also changes with age; in general the degree of aggregation and the size of the monomer both fall, particularly in the nucleus.[1, 26] The proportion of KS consequently rises with age. Little systematic change consequent to aging has been seen in collagen content.[1a] However, one study suggests that the ratio of collagen I to collagen II changes with age in response to external loads.[10]

Changes in Composition of the Disc with Degeneration and Disease

Changes in the composition of the disc have been characterized for a few pathologic conditions. Scoliotic discs appear to have a lower PG content than normal discs of similar age. These changes appear to be greatest at the apex of the curve but are thought to result from changes in mechanical stress on the disc and are secondary to the curve rather than a primary factor in the etiology of scoliosis.[62] Abnormalities of collagen have not so far been found in scoliotic patients, although they have been searched for in many studies.[20] In disc degeneration and in spondylolisthesis, the principal change appears to be a loss of PGs.[40, 49] One study has found that in degenerate discs the remaining PGs were larger than those of normal size and were also more able to aggregate.[34] It is not clear whether turnover and synthesis of new large aggregating PGs are more rapid in such degenerate discs, as these authors suggest, or whether the large aggregating PGs are less able to escape from the degenerate discs.

Enzymes and the Disc

Enzymes capable of degrading the collagens of the extracellular matrix have been found in extracts from human discs.[52] Although there is no study of enzymes that are capable of degrading PGs, it seems that such enzymes must be in the disc.[39] PGs are synthesized as very large molecules capable of forming aggregates with hyaluronic acid,[45] but within 1 or 2 months after synthesis these PGs are degraded and may lose their aggregating capacity.[38]

Enzymes that degrade the matrix have been used clinically as an alternative to disc surgery for herniated discs. Chymopapain has been used clinically in tens of thousands of cases. Chymopapain degrades the protein core of the PG.[12] The GAG chains, which are much smaller than the PG, are thus able to diffuse out of the disc and into the blood vessels and surrounding tissue. With loss of GAG the FCD of the disc matrix falls, as does the osmotic pressure. The disc loses fluid under load because there is no compression-resisting component remaining in the tissue. It should be noted however that it is not the degradation of the PG itself that causes loss of disc turgor and height; the osmotic pressure of the PGs does not depend on their size but results mainly from the FCD of the disc.[15] Once the PGs have been degraded, the osmotic properties of the disc do not change until the GAG chains start disappearing from the matrix. Collagenase has also been used clinically to collapse the disc. Presumably the administration of collagenase destroys the cartilaginous framework of the disc, and this allows the PGs to escape from the tissue.

METABOLISM OF MATRIX CONSTITUENTS

Although the mechanical functioning of the intervertebral disc depends on the characteristics of the matrix, the cells of the disc are responsible for renewing and turning over the matrix constituents. Little is known about matrix synthesis in the disc, but several animal studies have shown that PGs are synthesized in vivo, even in mature adults. The turnover in young animals is relatively fast—in 6-week-old guinea pigs the half-life of the CS component was about 30 days and an even shorter half-life was found for PG turnover in 4-week-old rabbits.[33] However, in mature animals PG turnover is slow. Half-lives of greater than 120 days have been found for mature rabbits, whereas in adult dogs the total turnover time is between 2 and 4 years.[59]

There have been few in vitro studies of PG synthesis in discs, principally because of the difficulties of handling the tissue in vitro. If the disc tissue is incubated in vitro the slices swell and PGs leach out.[57] The resulting change in disc composition affects metabolism and it is difficult therefore to relate in vitro studies to the metabolism of the disc in vivo. However, a method has recently been developed for incubating the disc in vitro; for this technique the disc slices are enclosed in dialysis sacks and incubated in iso-osmotic solutions.[6] In this way swelling and leaching of PGs is prevented, and the environment of the disc cells remains similar to that found in vivo. Rates of PG synthesis in human annulus have been found with this technique to be around 2.0 to 3.1^{-6} mM/gm dry wt/hr.[5] The rate was found to vary with position in the disc and was highest in the mid-annulus region. This rate of synthesis is very low; it is only one third to one half the rate of synthesis in human articular cartilage. The average total turnover time in the annulus of the adult human disc is calculated from these results to be greater than 2 years.

Although these slow turnover times suggest that the possibility of repair is small, synthesis rate has been found to be influenced by a number of factors. The loss of PGs from the pericellular environment of the chondrocyte may stimulate synthesis; fluid content of the matrix has also been found to influence synthesis rate. Hormones and growth factors can increase the rate of PG synthesis in the disc and in other cartilages and would have greater access to the chondrocytes after PGs were lost because their partition coefficient would increase.[6, 45] Animal models suggest that some form of PG replacement is possible. When dog discs were treated with chymopapain and lost all PGs from the disc and end plate, it was observed that undamaged disc cells were able to resynthesize PGs and re-expand the disc within 3 to 4 months.[9] Even though some animal models suggest that PGs can be replaced to some extent, it is not clear whether such replacement is possible in degenerate adult human discs.

It is clear that PGs are synthesized in the disc throughout life, but very little is known about collagen synthesis. No studies have been reported on the rates of collagen synthesis in the disc. It is thought that once the collagen network is formed its turnover is very slow. One study investigated the nature of the cross-links in the intervertebral disc in relation to synthesis.[23] The nature of the cross-links is related to the maturity of the collagen; newly synthesized collagen tends to have reducible cross-links, whereas once the collagen fibrils mature the cross-links become irreducible.[20] Herbert[23] found that in the degenerate human disc and in the disc above it the proportion of reducible collagen cross-links increased, suggesting some form of collagen remodeling or synthesis. A recent study suggests that in some cases herniated disc is actually newly synthesized fibrocartilage;[32] from cross-link assays the maturity of the collagen in the herniated fragment was found to be less than that of the bulk disc tissue. These studies suggest that collagen can be laid down in the adult disc under some circumstances. Whether the collagen network ordinarily turns over or is capable of repair is still an unanswered question. It is clear, however, that if the disc and collagen network are injured full function cannot be restored without a renewal of this collagen framework. Until the collagen framework is restored the mechanical function of the disc will be impaired and the PGs will no longer be anchored in the tissue and will thus disappear.

References

1. Adams, P., and Muir, H.: Qualitative changes with age of human lumbar discs. Ann. Rheum. Dis. 35:289–296, 1976.

1a. Adams, P., Eyre, D.R., Muir, H.: Biochemical aspects of development and ageing of human lumbar intervertebral discs. Rheum. Rehab. 16:22–29, 1977.

2. Armstrong, J.R.: Lumbar Disc Lesions. Edinburgh, Churchill-Livingstone, 1958.

3. Aspden, R.M., Hickey, D.S., and Hukins, D.W.L.: Determination of collagen fibril orientation in the cartilage of the vertebral endplate. Conn. Tissue Res. 9:83–87, 1980.

4. Ayad, S., and Weiss, J.B.: Biochemistry of the intervertebral disc. *In* Jayson, M.I.V. (ed.): The Lumbar Spine and Back Pain. Edinburgh, Churchill-Livingstone, 1986, pp. 100–137.

5. Bayliss, M.T., Johnstone, B., and O'Brien, J.P.: Proteoglycan synthesis in the intervertebral disc: Var-

iation with age, region, and pathology. Spine 13:972–981, 1988.
6. Bayliss, M.T., Urban, J.P.G., Johnstone, B., and Holm, S.: A method for measuring 35S-sulphate incorporation rate in the intervertebral disc. J. Orthop. Sci. 4:10–17, 1986.
6a. Bert, J.L., and Fatt, I.: Relation of water transport to water content in swelling biological membranes. Surface chemistry of biological membranes. New York, Plenum Press, 1970.
7. Birk, D.E., and Trelstad, R.L.: Extracellular compartments in tendon morphogenesis: Collagen fibril bundle and macroaggregate formation. J. Cell. Biol. 103:231–240, 1986.
8. Birk, D.E., Fitch, J.M., Babiarz, J.P., and Linsenmeyer, T.F.: Collagen Type I and Type V are present in the same fibril in the avian corneal stroma. J. Cell. Biol. 106:999–1008, 1988.
9. Bradford, D.S., Cooper, K.M., and Oegema, T.R.: Chymopapain, chemonucleolysis and nucleus pulposus regeneration. J. Bone Joint Surg. 65A:1220, 1983.
10. Brickley-Parson, D., and Glimcher, M.: Is the chemistry of collagen in the intervertebral disc an expression of Wolff's law? A study of the human lumbar spine. Spine 9:146–163, 1984.
11. Broom, N.D., and Marra, D.L.: New structural concepts of articular cartilage demonstrated with a physical model. Conn. Tissue Res. 14:1, 1985.
12. Buttle, D.J., Abrahamson, M., and Barret, A.J.: The biochemistry of the action of chymopapain in the relief of sciatica. Spine 11:688–694, 1986.
13. Byers, P.D., Bayliss, M.T., and Maroudas, A.: Hypothesizing about joints. *In* Maroudas, A., and Holborow, E.J. (eds.): Studies in Joint Diseases 2. London, Pitman, 1983.
14. Carney, S.L., and Muir, H.: The structure and function of cartilage proteoglycans. Physiol. Rev. 68:858–910, 1988.
15. Comper, W.D., and Preston, B.N.: Model connective tissue systems: A study of polyion-mobile ion and of excluded-volume interactions of proteoglycans. Biochem. J. 143:1–9, 1974.
16. Eyre, D.R.: Biochemistry of the intervertebral disc. Int. Rev. Conn. Tissue Res. 8:227–291, 1979.
17. Eyre, D.R., and Muir, H.: Collagen polymorphism: Two molecular species in pig intervertebral discs. F.E.B.S. Lett. 42:192–196, 1974.
18. Eyre, D.R., and Muir, H.: Types I and II collagens in the intervertebral disc. Biochem. J. 157:267–270, 1976.
19. Eyre, D.R., and Muir, H.: Quantitative analysis of types I and II collagens in human intervertebral discs at various ages. Biochim. Biophys. Acta 492:29–42, 1977.
20. Eyre, D.R., Paz, M.A., and Gallop, P.M.: Crosslinking in collagen and elastin. Ann. Rev. Biochem. 53:717–748, 1984.
20a. Eyre, D.R., et al.: "The intervertebral disc" in new perspectives on low back pain. Am. Acad. Orthop. Surg., pp. 147–208, 1989.
21. Hallen, A.: Hexosamine and ester sulphate content of the human nucleus pulposus at different ages. Acta Chem. Scand. 12:1869–1872, 1958.
22. Hallen, A.: The collagen and ground substance of the human nucleus pulposus at different ages. Acta Chem. Scand. 16:705–709, 1962.
23. Herbert, C.M., Lindberg, K.A., Jayson, M.I.V., and Bailey, A.J.: Changes in the collagen of human intervertebral discs during ageing and degenerative disc disease. J. Mol. Med. 1:79–91, 1975.
24. Hickey, D.S., and Hukins, D.W.L.: Relation between the structure of the annulus fibrosus and the function and failure of the intervertebral disc. Spine 5:106–116, 1980.
25. Inoue, H., and Takeda, T.: Three dimensional observations of collagen framework of lumbar intervertebral discs. Acta Orthop. Scand. 46:949–956, 1975.
26. Johnstone, B.: Structure and biosynthesis of human intervertebral disc proteoglycans. Ph.D. Thesis, London University, 1987.
27. Johnstone, B., and Caterson, B.: Proteoglycans of the intervertebral disc: Heterogeneity results from breakdown products (abstr.). J. Cell. Biol., 1989.
28. Kazarian, L.: Creep characteristics of the human spinal column. Orthop. Clin. North Am. 6:3–18, 1975.
29. Keene, D.R., Engvall, E., and Glanville, R.W.: Ultrastructure of type VI collagen in human skin and cartilage suggests an anchoring function for this filamentous network. J. Cell. Biol. 107:1995–2006, 1988.
30. Kraemer, J., Kolditz, D., and Gowin, R.: Water and electrolyte content of human intervertebral discs under variable load. Spine 9:69–71, 1984.
31. Kraemer, J.: Intervertebral Disc Diseases. New York, Georg Thieme Verlag, 1981.
32. Lipson, S.J.: Metaplastic proliferative fibrocartilage as an alternative concept to herniated intervertebral disc. Spine 13:1055–1060, 1988.
33. Lohmander, S., Antonopolous, C.A., and Friberg, U.: Chemical and metabolic heterogeneity of chondroitin sulfate and keratan sulfate in guinea pig cartilage and nucleus pulposus. Biochim. Biophys. Acta 304:430–448, 1973.
34. Lyons, G., Eisenstein, S., and Sweet, B.M.: Biochemical changes in intervertebral disc degeneration. Biochim. Biophys. Acta 673:443–453.
35. Maroudas, A.: Physico-chemical properties of articular cartilage. *In* Freeman, N.A.R. (ed.): Adult Articular Cartilage, 2nd Ed. London, Pitman Medical, 1979.
36. Maroudas, A., and Evans, H.: A study of ionic equilibria in cartilage. Conn. Tissue Res. 1:69, 1972.
37. Mayne, R., and Burgeson, R. (eds.): Structure and Function of Collagen Types. New York, Academic Press, 1987.
38. McDevitt, C.A.: Proteoglycans of the intervertebral disc. *In* Ghosh, P. (ed.): Biology of the Intervertebral Disc. New York, C.R.C. Press, 1988.
39. Melrose, J., Ghosh, P., and Taylor, T.K.F.: The serine proteases and serine protease inhibitors of the human intervertebral disc. Tenth F.E.C.T. Meeting, Abstr. 426, 1986.
40. Mitchell, P.E.G., Hendry, N.G.C., and Billewicz, W.Z.: The chemical background of intervertebral disc prolapse. J. Bone Joint Surg. 43B:141–151, 1961.
41. Myers, E.R., Zhu, W., and Mow, V.C.: Viscoelastic properties of articular cartilage and meniscus. *In* Nimni, M.E. (ed.): Collagen, Vol. II. New York, C.R.C. Press, 1988.
42. Nachemson, A.: Lumbar interdiscal pressure. Acta Orthop. Scand. 43(suppl.):1–110, 1960.
43. Nimni, M.E. (ed.): Collagen, Vols. I, II, III. New York, C.R.C. Press, 1988.
44. Nimni, M.E., and Harkness, R.D.: Molecular struc-

ture and function of collagen. *In* Nimni, M.E. (ed.): Collagen, Vol. I. New York, C.R.C. Press, 1988.
45. Oegema, T.R., Bradford, D., and Cooper, K.: Aggregated proteoglycan synthesis in organ cultures of human nucleus pulposus. J. Biol. Chem. 245: 10579–10581, 1979.
46. Parry, D.A.D., Barnes, G.R.G., and Craig, A.S.: A comparison of the size distribution of collagen fibrils in connective tissue as a function of age and a possible relation between fibril size distribution. Proc. R. Soc. Lond. [Biol.] 203:305, 1978.
47. Poole, C.A., Ayad, S., and Schofield, J.R.: Chondrons from articular cartilage: 1. Immunolocalization of type VI collagen in the peri-cellular capsule of isolated canine tibial chondrocytes. J. Cell. Sci. 90:635–643, 1988.
48. Pope, M., Wilder, D., and Booth, J.: The biomechanics of low back pain. *In* White, A.A., and Gordon, S.L. (eds.): Idiopathic Low Back Pain. St. Louis, C.V. Mosby, 1982.
49. Roberts, S., Beard, H.K., and O'Brien, J.P.: Biochemical changes of the intervertebral discs in patients with spondylolisthesis or with tears of the posterior annulus fibrosus. Ann. Rheum. Dis. 41:78–85, 1982.
50. Roberts, S., Menage, J., and Urban, J.P.G.: Biochemical and structural properties of the cartilage endplate and its relation to the properties of the intervertebral disc. Spine 14:166–174, 1989.
51. Scott, J.E.: Proteoglycan-fibrillar collagen interactions. Biochem. J. 252:313–323, 1988.
52. Sedowofia, K.A., Tomlinson, I.W., Weiss, J.B., et al.: Collagenolytic enzyme systems in human intervertebral disc: Their control mechanism and their possible role in the initiation of biomechanical failure. Spine 7:213–221, 1982.
53. Simon, B., Wu, J.S.S., Carlton, M.W., et al.: Poroelastic dynamic structural models of rhesus spinal motion segments. Spine 10:494, 1985.
54. Thompson, J.P., Bradford, D.S., and Oegema, T.R.: Biosynthetic stimulation of adult canine intervertebral disc by growth factors. Trans. Orthop. Res. Soc. 14:259, 1989.
55. Urban, J.P.G., and Bayliss, M.T.: Regulation of proteoglycan synthesis in cartilage: Influence of inorganic ions. Biochim. Biophys. Acta (in press, 1989).
56. Urban, J.P.G., and Maroudas, A.: Measurement of fixed charge density and partition coefficients in the intervertebral disc. Biochim. Biophys. Acta 586:166–178, 1979.
57. Urban, J.P.G., and Maroudas, A.: Swelling of the intervertebral disc in vitro. Conn. Tissue Res. 9:1–10, 1981.
58. Urban, J.P.G., and McMullin, J.F.: Swelling pressure of the intervertebral discs: influence of age, spinal level, composition and degeneration. Spine 13: 179–186, 1988.
59. Urban, J.P.G., Holm, S., and Maroudas, A.: Diffusion of small solutes into the intervertebral disc: An in vivo study. Biorheology 16:447–464, 1978.
60. Urban, J.P.G., Maroudas, A., Bayliss, M.T., and Dillon, J.: Osmotic pressure of proteoglycans at the concentration found in cartilage. Biorheology 16:447–464, 1979.
61. Vaughan, L., Mendler, M., Huber, S., et al.: Periodic distribution of collagen IX along cartilage fibrils. J. Cell. Biol. 106:991–997, 1988.
62. Venn, G., Sims, T., and Mason, R.M.: Collagen stability and cross-linking in the normal and kyphoscoliotic mouse intervertebral discs. Biosci. Rep. 8:315–322, 1988.
63. Viidik, A.: Functional properties of collagenous tissues. *In* Hall, D., and Jackson, D.S. (eds.): International Review of Connective Tissue Research. New York, Academic Press, 1972.
64. Virgin, W.J.: Experimental investigations into the physical properties of the intervertebral disc. J. Bone Joint Surg. 33B:607, 1951.
65. Vogel, K.G., and Trotter, J.A.: The effect of proteoglycans on the morphology of collagen fibril formation in vitro. Coll. Rel. Res. 7:105–114, 1987.
66. Wu, J.-J., Eyre, D.R., and Slayter, H.S.: Type VI collagen of the intervertebral disc. Biochemical and electron-microscope characterisation of the native protein. Biochem. J. 248:373–381, 1987.

NUTRITION OF THE INTERVERTEBRAL DISC

Sten H. Holm

One of the most common, expensive, and important medical problems of today is low back pain. All over the world, the problem seems to increase.[4, 51, 54, 81] In general, our understanding of the patient's symptoms is poor, and many different parameters could influence the symptomatology of low back pain (Fig. 1). The enormous complexity of back pain ranges from basic biochemistry and cell metabolism to message transport systems in nerve fibers and translation to the cerebral cortex. To this are added social and psychologic contributions.

The spinal column is a complicated structure with shock-absorbing discs interposed between the vertebrae. Much low back pain is thought to originate from the intervertebral discs. In order to find relevant clues related to the etiology of disorders in the back, research has concentrated on examin-

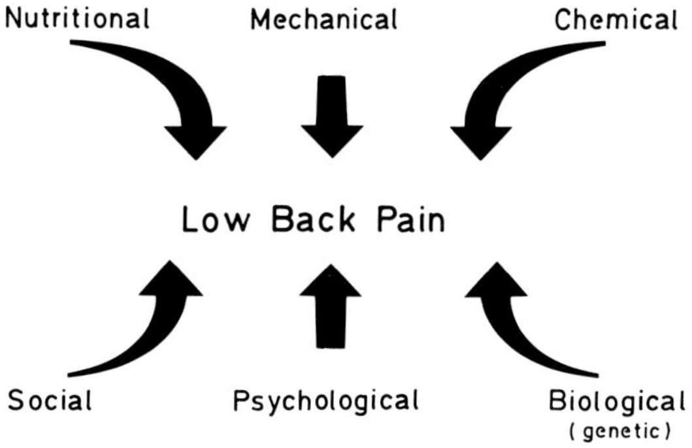

Figure 1 □ Schematic representation of parameters that affect the symptomatology of low back pain.

ing the behavior of healthy and degenerated intervertebral discs from both mechanical and biochemical points of view. Another area of interest has been the nutrition of the disc, particularly as it has been postulated that inadequate nutrition may cause degeneration of disc tissue.[32, 52, 53, 74, 75]

A high proportion of the cases of low back pain are idiopathic. Even among patients for whom a definite diagnosis has been established, the cause of the disorder is generally unknown, and the method of treatment is not always agreed upon.

"Disc failure" has been thought to be the result of some mechanical insult to the spine. Thus, there is an extensive body of work describing the mechanical properties of the disc and the spinal motion segment.[6, 62] Less work has been done on the biology of the disc, although it has now become clear that the health of a disc depends on the well-being of its cells, which renew and maintain the matrix of the disc itself. Recent work suggests that these cells respond to mechanical stimulation and that changes in the disc matrix affect its behavior.

COMPOSITION OF THE DISC

The intervertebral disc is a specialized connective structure, designed to provide strength and mobility. For its normal function it must possess viscoelastic properties. Any change in its structure is liable to interfere with properties that are needed for equalization and absorption of the various stresses exerted on the vertebral column (Fig. 2). The intervertebral discs occupy

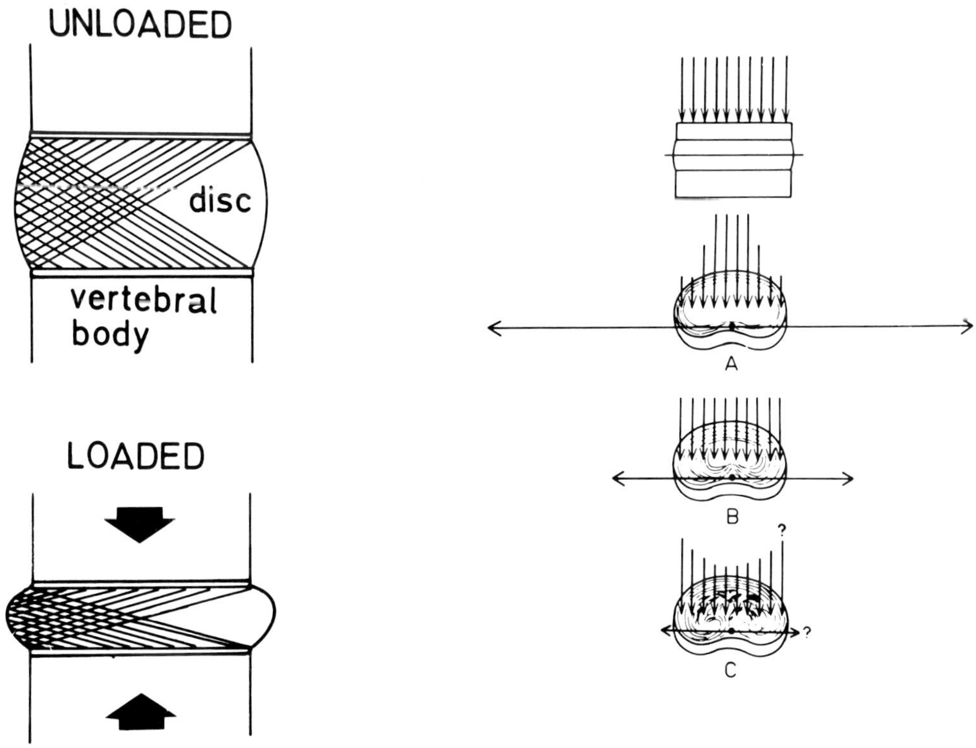

Figure 2 □ Changes in the crossing angle of the collagen bundles in an unloaded and in a loaded situation. Relative relationship between the load on the lumbar disc and the vertical and tangential stresses on the annulus fibrosus. (*A* = normal disc; *B* = moderately degenerated disc, *C* = severely degenerated disc. (From Nachemson, A.: Lumbar interdiscal pressure: Experimental studies on post-mortem material. Acta Orthop. Scand. 43 (Suppl.):1–104, 1960. © 1960 Munksgaard International Publishers Ltd., Copenhagen, Denmark.)

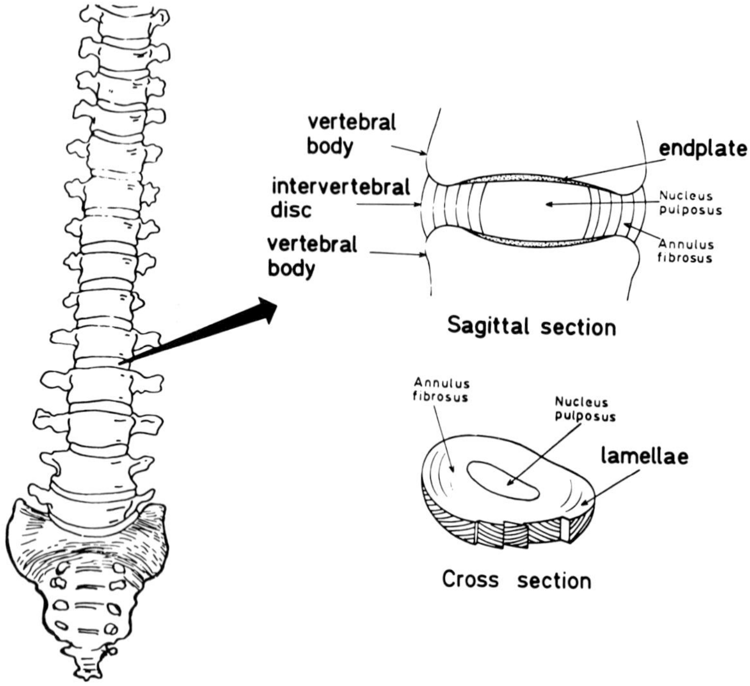

Figure 3 □ Schematic view of the spine and different regions of the intervertebral disc.

about one third of the spine. Because they provide the spinal column with its flexibility and act as shock absorbers between the vertebrae, their behavior has a great impact on the mechanics of the entire spine.[62]

The intervertebral disc may be considered as consisting of two separate regions, the inner soft pulp in nucleus pulposus and the outer firm annulus fibrosus. The cartilaginous end plates, which are interposed between the discs and the bony structure of the vertebral bodies, are generally not considered to be part of the discs themselves (Fig. 3). The nucleus pulposus occupies about 40% to 60% of the disc volume. The nucleus in young humans and in most animal discs is highly hydrated, soft, and translucent. It is surrounded by the firmer, less hydrated annulus fibrosus. When the human disc matures, hydration of the nucleus drops markedly, the nucleus loses its translucency and becomes firmer, and the boundary between the nucleus and the annulus becomes difficult to distinguish. Similar changes are seen in some animals, such as chondrodystrophoid dogs, but in other animals the discs remain translucent throughout life.[11, 24, 32, 34] The annulus consists of a series of concentric lamellae, which are visible to the naked eye when the disc is sectioned horizontally. The lamellae consist of bundles of collagen fibers, which run obliquely between the adjacent vertebral bodies and are firmly anchored to them or to the cartilaginous end plate.[28, 40, 71, 72]

The human disc degenerates early; by the age of 30 years, clefts and fissures are already visible in the annulus. There are also chemical changes and loss of disc height. It is not clear, however, whether these changes are regarded as part of the normal aging processes or whether they are degenerative.[10, 65]

The major structural macromolecules in the disc are collagen and proteoglycans.[9, 21] Other glycoproteins, elastin, and some serum proteins have all been reported in minor quantities. However, the disc acts mechanically as a concentrated proteoglycan solution held within the collagen network (Fig. 4).

Proteoglycans

Proteoglycans are a family of macromolecules consisting of glycosaminoglycan chains bound to a central protein core to form a brushlike structure (Fig. 5). These proteoglycan monomers are large polypeptide molecules with molecular weights of 50,000 to several million. The major glycosaminoglycans in the disc are chondroitin sulfate and keratan sulfate. These glycos-

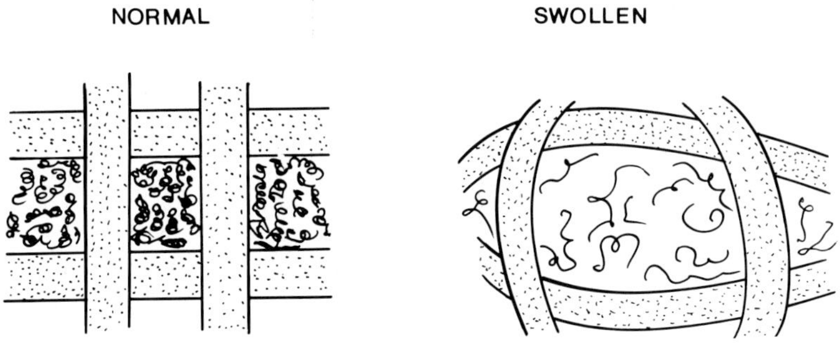

Figure 4 □ Schematic representation of a normal and a swollen collagen/proteoglycan matrix in the intervertebral disc. Changes in the osmotic pressure or mechanical properties may result in advanced swelling after imbibition of fluid, thus changing concentration gradients and transport properties of the tissue.

aminoglycans occupy different regions of the protein core. The keratan sulfate–rich region lies toward one end of the core, and beyond it the core ends in two globular regions, one of which is the hyaluronic acid–binding region, so called because a proportion of the proteoglycan monomers are attached to long chains of hyaluronic acid to form proteoglycan aggregates. The aggregates are stabilized by link protein. It has been suggested that aggregation helps to keep proteoglycans in tissue, but the function of aggregation is not yet understood.[29]

A large fraction of disc proteoglycans are not able to aggregate; this fraction increases with age. It has been suggested that this loss of aggregation results from enzymatic removal of the hyaluronic acid–binding region of the core protein.[1, 15, 49] Enzymatic attack on the disc proteoglycans could account for their small size and polydispersity, since it is noted that newly synthesized proteoglycans are much larger than those that are resident in the tissue; most can aggregate in the presence of hyaluronic acid and contain a much higher proportion of chondroitin sulfate.[1, 9, 19, 21, 48, 68, 69] In disc degeneration there is extensive loss of proteoglycans, particularly of the small chains, and thus the remaining proteoglycans are larger. In addition, a greater proportion are able to aggregate, as compared with normal age-matched discs. These proteoglycans are more representative of those found in young discs. Several authors suggest that the change in proteoglycan structure results from faster turnover of proteoglycans as an attempt at tissue repair.[15, 24, 49]

Collagen

The disc contains two major collagen types. The fine fibrils of the nucleus are virtually all Type II collagen, whereas the outer annulus is predominantly Type I collagen. The proportion of Type I collagen in an annulus

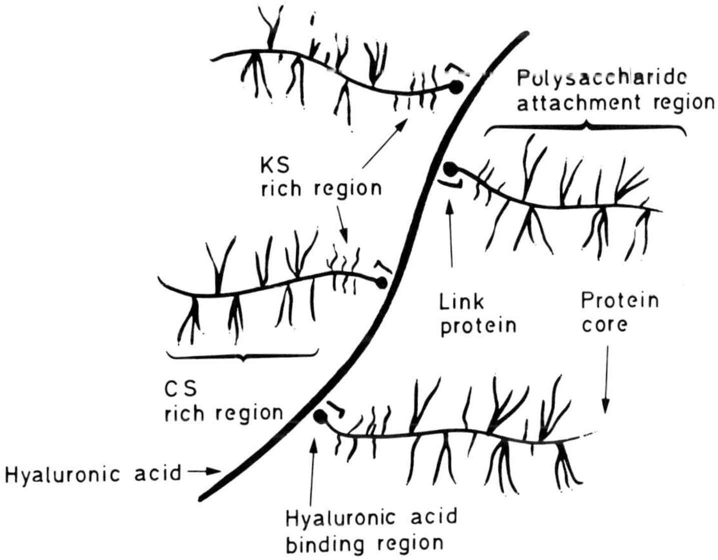

Figure 5 □ Model of the "brush-like" proteoglycan molecular system. (From Urban, J. P. G., and Maroudas, A.: The chemistry of the intervertebral disc in relation to its physiological functions and requirements. Clin. Rheum. Dis. 6:51–56, 1980.)

decreases toward the nucleus as the proportion of Type II collagen rises.[20, 21] It is not known whether the fibrils of the disc are of mixed collagen types or whether each collagen type forms its own fibril. Chemical evidence from staining with specific antibodies suggests the latter.[9]

The organization of collagen fibrils in the disc is highly specialized. The three-dimensional collagen framework has been described and illustrated by scanning electron micrographs.[40] In the annulus, collagen is arranged in 15 to 20 concentric lamellae made of parallel bundles. The fiber bundles of each lamella run obliquely between the adjacent vertebral bodies and are firmly anchored to them or to the cartilaginous end plate (Fig. 3).[28]

In the nucleus the collagen fibers are much finer than in the annulus and are arranged in a loose irregular mesh. However, the nucleus fibrils are not connected to the cartilaginous end plate at the boundary with the annulus; these fibrils merge with those of the inner concentric lamellae.

The arrangement of the collagen network in the disc has an important influence on how load is distributed. The fiber bundles of the adjacent lamellae are only loosely interconnected. Even the collagen is only slightly extensible; the fact that the lamellae can move separately provides the structure considerable extensibility, especially in the vertical direction. The annulus is thus able to move and bulge outward under the pressure evenly applied to it by the gel-like nucleus or to increase in height during extension by changing the cross angle of its fibers.[12, 30, 39, 40, 42, 44, 61, 71, 82]

Water

Water is the major constituent of the disc; 90% of the young nucleus is water. Although the water content decreases with age, the substance remains an important component of the old and degenerated disc. The water content of the disc is not constant but varies with applied load.[18] Because of the low cell content, most of this water is extracellular and is associated with the collagen and proteoglycans. A significant proportion of the water in aged or degenerated discs with low proteoglycan content may be intrafibrillar.[26] The intrafibrillar fraction of water is freely exchangeable, but is not available to the proteoglycans and other large macromolecules, which are sterically excluded from within the collagen fibrils.

Other Tissue Components

A considerable proportion of noncollagenous proteins have reportedly been found in the disc.[24, 28] These proteins have not been characterized. Glycoproteins, of which the biologic function is unknown, have been found, as have some serum proteins, particularly in aged and degenerated discs. A part of this fraction probably consists of proteoglycan core protein and minor collagens.

Extracellular Matrix

The disc composition changes with age and spinal level.[1] In any disc, the proportions of the three main components (i.e., collagen, proteoglycans, and water) vary with position. Concentrations of proteoglycans and water are highest in the nucleus and fall to low values in the outer annulus. The reverse profiles are shown for collagen.

Disc Cells

The cells of the annulus, like those of other cartilaginous tissues, are thought to arise from the mesenchyme. However, those of the nucleus come from the notochord. In humans the notochordal cells have disappeared by late childhood, but in some animals the notochordal cells of the nucleus persist into adulthood. The cells of the adult disc may be considered to be chondrocytes or chondrocyte-like cells (i.e., "disc cells"); some authors judge the cells of the outer annulus to be more like fibrocytes.[50, 63] The cells in the nucleus are rounded, whereas in the outer annulus they are more cigar shaped.[50]

The cell density in the intervertebral disc is relatively low. It is uniform across the disc, except toward the disc margins and in the outer annulus (Fig. 6).

MECHANICAL AND PHYSICOCHEMICAL FUNCTION OF TISSUE COMPONENTS

Proteoglycans

The mechanical properties of the intervertebral disc depend to a large extent on the hydration of the tissues.[2, 5] The proteoglycans

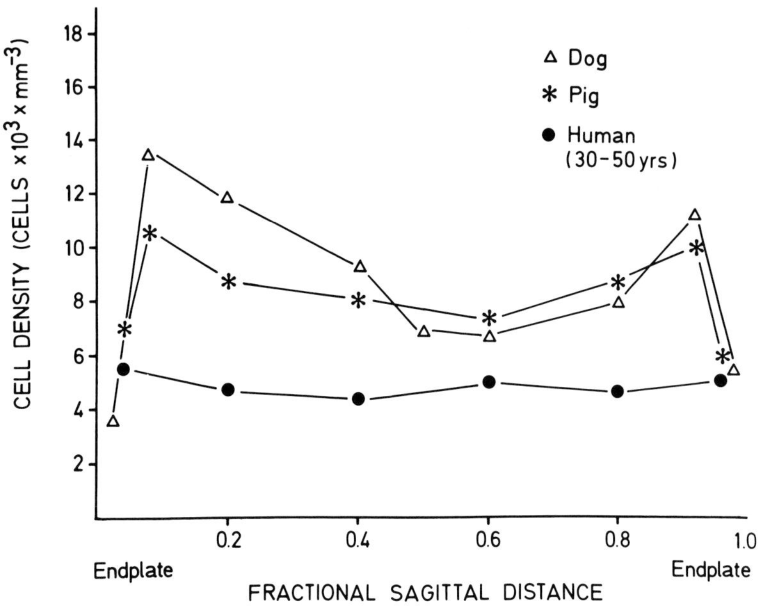

Figure 6 □ Profiles of cell densities across the intervertebral disc. The adult human profile is quite flat, whereas the profiles for the animals show variations close to the vertebral endplate.

are responsible for maintaining hydration of the disc under the high external loads placed upon it; both osmotic pressure and resistance of tissue to fluid loss under pressure are controlled by proteoglycans. The proteoglycans themselves are polyelectrolytes, that is, there are fixed negative charges on the glycosaminoglycans; hence the tissue acts as an ion exchanger, and its ion content is high compared with that of the surrounding plasma. Ions distribute themselves between the plasma and the disc in order to maintain an electrochemical equilibrium. Within the fixed-charge density of the disc, there is no evidence of ion binding, and the Gibbs-Donnan equilibrium appears to describe ion partitions between disc and plasma.[25, 60, 77] Because of the negative charge on the macromolecules, the total number of ions in the tissue is always greater than in the plasma. Osmotic pressure of the disc results from a difference in the number of soluble particles between the two phases; the excess number of ions in the tissue leads to the high osmotic pressure of the disc. Another factor contributing to the osmotic pressure of the disc depends on the excluded volume contributions of the macromolecule segments and, hence, on size and shape of the proteoglycans. In cartilaginous tissues this factor is insignificant, compared with that from the Gibbs-Donnan ionic contribution; therefore it is not surprising that neither proteoglycan size nor degree of aggregation influences osmotic pressure compared with the charge density.[25, 78]

Osmotic pressure depends on charge concentration rather than proteoglycan size or degree of aggregation. Because the proteoglycans are densely packed, there is a great deal of interweaving of the glycosaminoglycan chains. The chains effectively divide the matrix into small pores; the higher the glycosaminoglycan concentration, the more closely packed are the entangled glycosaminoglycan chains, and the smaller the effective pore size. The fine pore structure of the matrix is thus determined by proteoglycan concentration, rather than by the collagen network.

Fluid Transport in the Disc

The rate at which fluid can flow through the matrix is governed by the pore size and is described in terms of a hydraulic permeability coefficient. The larger the pores, the higher is the value of the hydraulic permeability coefficient, and the faster the rate of the fluid flow (Fig. 7). When the disc is at equilibrium, there is no fluid flow. However, in the vertebral disc the external loads constantly change as a result of variations in posture and activity. These changes in load disturb the balance between pore pressure and osmotic pressure; the result is fluid flow. Because osmotic pressure is related to proteoglycan content and therefore its hydraulic

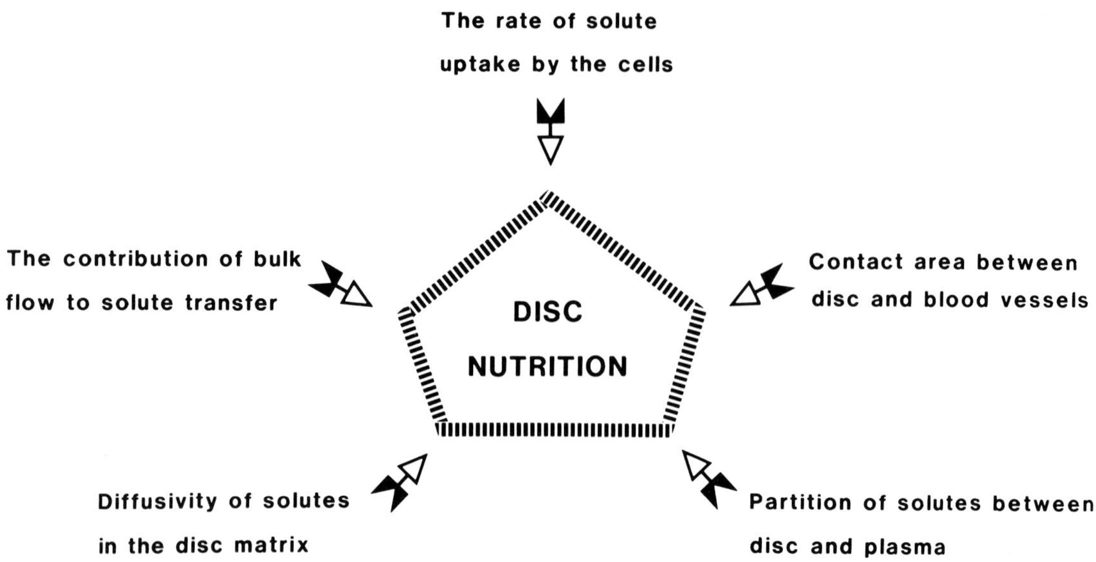

Figure 9 □ Summary of factors of specific importance when considering the nutrition of the intervertebral disc.

about 2% of the glucose used is oxidized to carbon dioxide, this pathway provides about 40% of the total energy produced. That is because per mole of glucose, complete oxidation gives rise to 36-mol adenosine triphosphate (ATP), whereas anaerobic glycolysis produces only 2-mol ATP. Lactic acid production is also dependent on oxygen tension levels; it increases to about 40% to 50% as the oxygen tension decreases from 70 to 7 mmHg.[32] The canine nucleus pulposus has a particularly high rate of lactic acid production, compared with other cartilaginous tissues. This rate becomes even more marked on a cellular basis because the cell density of the intervertebral disc is extremely low.

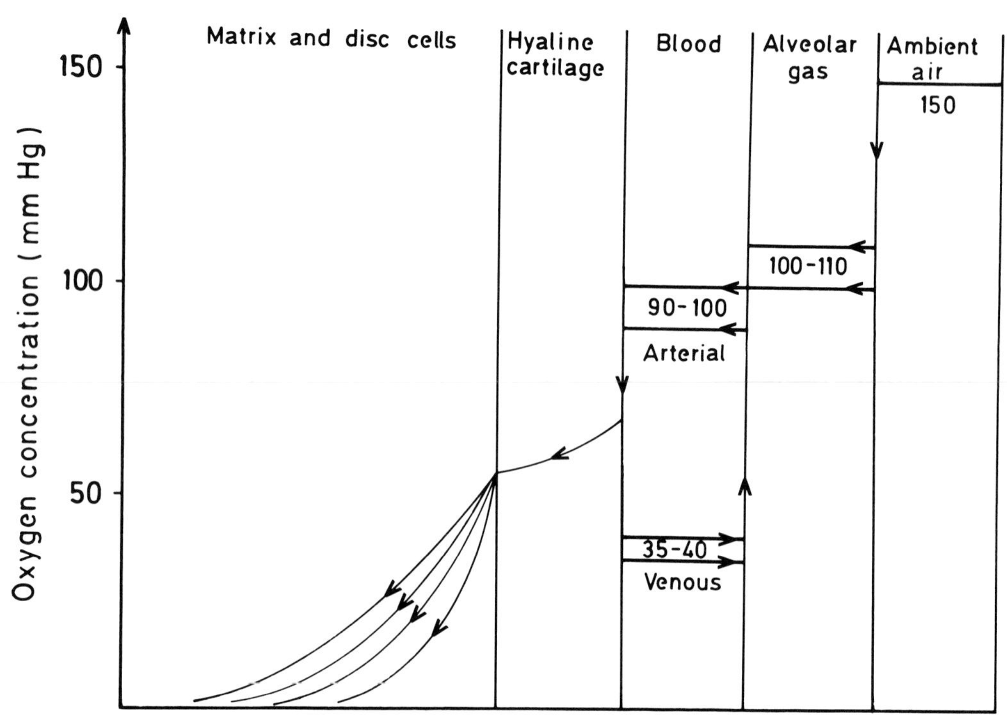

Figure 10 □ A schematic representation of the decrease in oxygen tension from the ambient air through the pulmonary system and the blood into the matrix of the intervertebral disc.

This high rate of lactic acid production could arise from the very low oxygen tension in the center of the disc.

Steep gradients in concentration across the disc exist for lactate. The lactate concentration profile in the center of the disc was 5 to 18 times higher than that found in blood, whereas the lactate concentration near the end plate was very similar to that found in the circulation.[32] The high lactate levels that are observed must be associated with the lowering of pH. It should be noted that pH values as low as 5.6 have been found in human discs that were removed at operation.

It is known that the intervertebral disc contains many proteases.[9, 57] More recently, collagenase—some in latent form—and elastase have also been found.[66] A system of protease inhibitors has also been extracted from human intervertebral disc.[43] It is evident from the degradation of newly formed proteoglycans that some degradative enzyme systems are present in the intervertebral disc matrix.[15, 58] In the healthy disc, there is likely to be a delicate balance between the active and latent forms of enzymes and the potency of the inhibitor present; this balance could be very pH-sensitive, and hence a change in disc metabolism, which decreases pH, could lead to a rapidly accelerating matrix breakdown.

Matrix Synthesis

Relatively little information is available on matrix synthesis in the intervertebral disc. In cartilage, however, matrix biochemistry has been studied extensively.[29] There have been some in vivo studies that show a proteoglycan turnover in the intervertebral disc;[17, 48, 76] several pools were found to turn over at different rates. It was shown that, in the disc, the transitional zone was most active in regard to protein synthesis,[67] and also that the rate of synthesis was not constant across the disc.[76] These studies indicate that proteoglycans of the disc are continuously but slowly synthesized by the disc cells; therefore the rate of repair is relatively slow.

FACTORS INFLUENCING NUTRITION

Anything that negatively disturbs the surrounding capillary network is a potential risk factor for adequate nutrition of the intervertebral disc (Fig. 9). Among all the possible functions that might alter the rheologic system, and thereby affect transport to and metabolism of the disc cells, various modes of exercise seem to be important. First, during prolonged exercise as well as under prolonged external load, the disc deforms through bulk movement and loses fluid.[44–46, 80] The change in disc dimension may affect the concentration of nutrients in the center of the disc. Exercise may also affect the peripheral circulation in several ways and hence alter the rate at which metabolites reach the disc interphase. Second, by introducing external factors that may disturb the circulation, such as smoking, vibration, or specific medical treatment, the nutrition of the disc may be affected. Finally, motion of the disc system itself changes the concentration of blood solutes such as lactic acid and glucose and may affect pH.[33, 34] These external changes may also influence the concentration of such substances in the disc itself. However, in the normal disc, these changes would be expected to be immediate and reversible. In degenerated discs, the transport function may be disturbed to such an extent that there is no adequate reversible transport function.

In contrast, a prolonged period of exercise, or alternatively of immobilization, of a disc segment appears to have a dramatic and permanent influence on the transport of nutrients into the disc.

Effects Induced by Exercise

Under various exercising regimes, groups of animals were exercised daily and were made to run and jog and to crawl under or jump over many obstacles.[34, 38] The idea was also to include exercise that involved much flexion and extension as well as lateral bending of the spine. The changes found in the thoracolumbar region were in direct contrast to those found in discs of the fused segments. There was an increase in the rate of solute transport to these discs and a higher rate of consumption by the cells (Figs. 11 and 12).[34] The differences between transport into discs that had been fused and into those of the exercised animals could result from long-term changes in the contact area between the disc tissue and the blood supply; exercise increased these contacts, thus improving nutrition, whereas fusion resulted in a diminution of these blood contacts. When

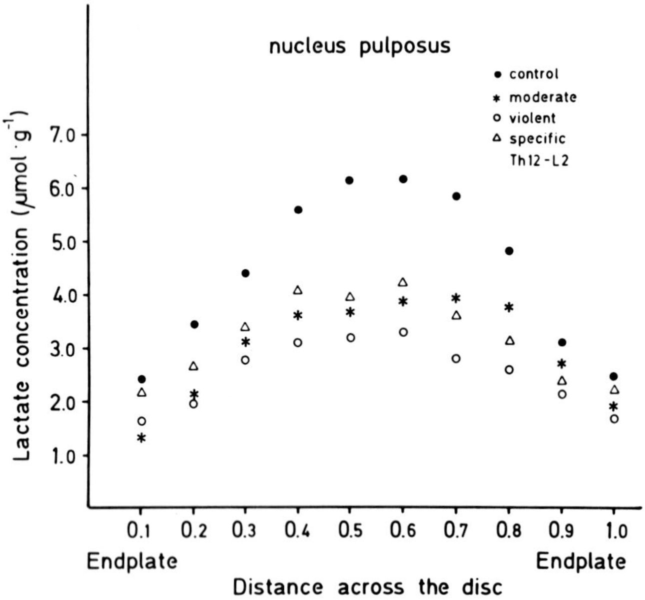

Figure 11 □ Lactate concentration profiles across the nucleus of the thoracolumbar discs. The control animals were kept in their cages, whereas three other groups of animals were exposed to either moderate, violent, or specific exercise. (From Holm, S., and Nachemson, A.: Variations in the nutrition of the canine intervertebral disc induced by motion. Spine 8:866–874, 1983.)

small animals were exercised on a horizontal treadmill, the transport into the disc and metabolism in the central portion of the disc appeared to be negatively affected after 2 months of such exercise.[38] The discs showed indications of degeneration. The mechanism of this change is unknown. However, it should be noted that exercise under these regimes was severe and involved a very high stress component compared with what the animals normally experienced.[37]

The results of these sets of experiments show that, under some circumstances, exercise may improve the nutrition of the disc, but under other circumstances exercise may be detrimental. At present it is difficult to predict the effect of exercise, but results suggest that moderate exercise regimes may be beneficial.

The synthesis of proteoglycans after various exercising regimes is difficult to interpret. The discs studied in the experiments in which jogging at a moderate speed was performed, as well as the discs adjacent to fused segments, showed no signs of proteoglycan degradation.[33, 34] In the experiments

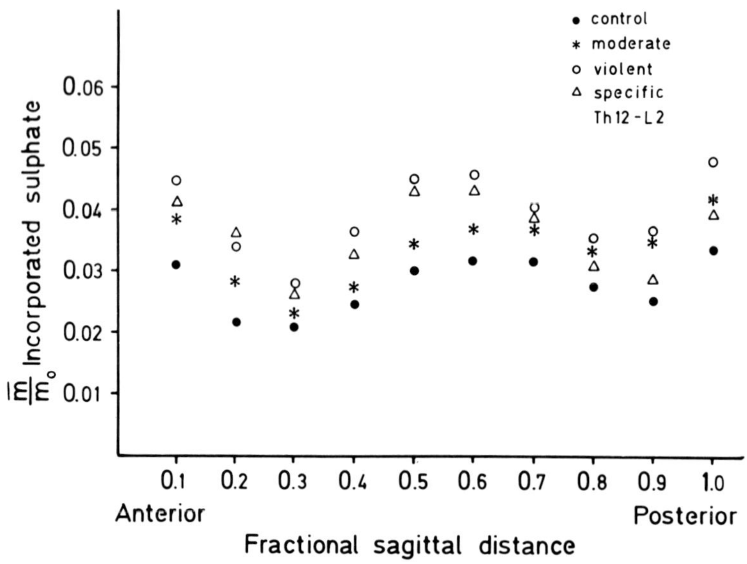

Figure 12 □ Incorporated sulfate across thoracolumbar intervertebral discs that have been exposed to various exercising regimens. (From Holm, S., and Nachemson, A.: Variations in the nutrition of the canine intervertebral disc induced by motion. Spine 8:866–874, 1983.)

in which small animals were exercised on a treadmill, severe degeneration was seen within 10 weeks.[38]

In studies using "experimental bipedal" animals, it was found that the adoption of an upright stance induced degenerative changes in the disc nuclei of these animals.[31, 83] A possible explanation for this is that the thickness of the calcified layer between the disc and the vertebral body may have increased, a situation also noticed in the treadmill experiments.[38] It is thus possible that the nutritional route through the end plate was interrupted by increased calcification or cellular hypertrophy. This interruption of the nutritional pathways led to disorders of the disc.

Fusion of Disc Segments

Fusion immobilizes the incorporated segments and changes mechanical stresses as well as composition in both the fused and adjacent discs.[22, 73] The concentration gradients of several solutes, as well as molecular synthesis and metabolism, are affected to a great extent even after a short period of immobilization. These changes indicate that the metabolic activity of disc cells decreases after fusion; possibly a portion of the cells have died. A significant increase of lactate concentration of the fused segment in the disc and a higher concentration of oxygen have been reported (Figs. 13 and 14).[33] A possible mechanism of this increase could be a lower rate of transport of lactate from the disc. Perhaps fusion gradually reduced blood supply to the end plate of the disc, thus partially closing one important route for movement of solutes out of the tissue and allowing the concentration of metabolic products to build up. It is of interest to note that in the discs adjacent to the fused segments, which presumably also underwent abnormal mechanical stresses, the changes seen were in a direction opposite to those seen in the fused segments. The adjacent discs showed similarities to the discs of moderately trained animals, in which one notices a stimulation of solute transport and metabolism.

Vibrations

High energy input to the spinal column and the disc system, including excessive loading patterns or specific movements, such as vibrations, is known to negatively affect the disc structure, cells, and macromolecules.[64] Furthermore, epidemiologic studies have demonstrated a higher incidence of back pain in human subjects exposed to vibrations.[64] Experimental studies have been performed in which nutritional factors have

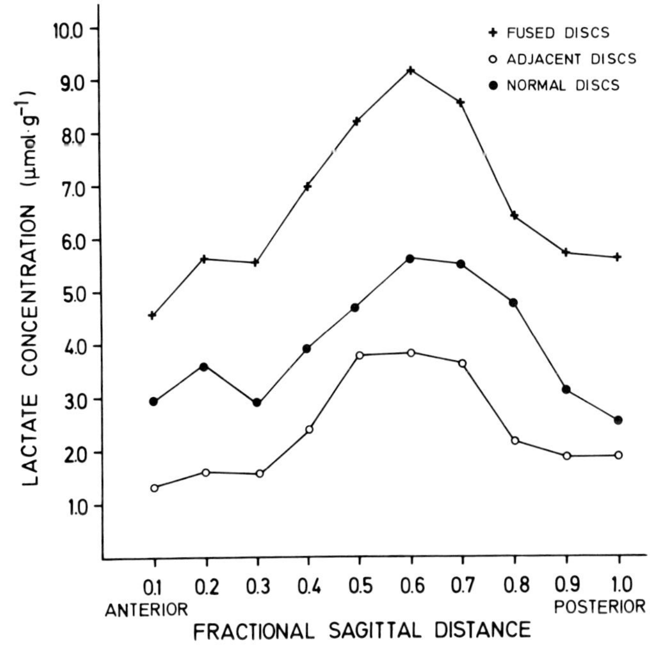

Figure 13 □ Lactate concentration profiles across normal discs and adjacent to the fused segments. (From Holm, S., and Nachemson, A.: Nutrition changes in the canine intervertebral disc after spinal fusion. Clin. Orthop. Rel. Res. 169:243–258, 1982.)

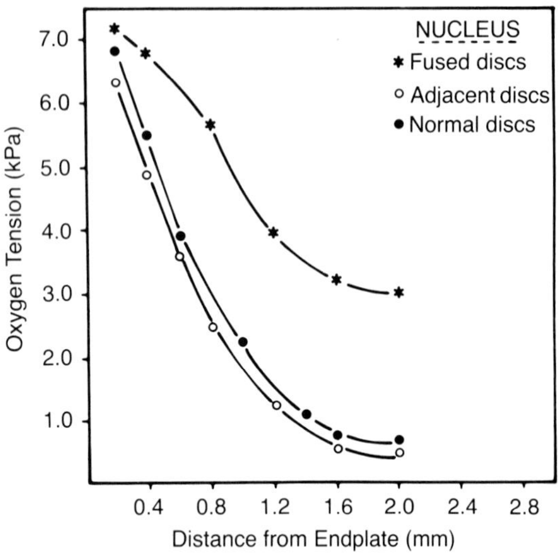

Figure 14 □ Oxygen tension gradients in canine nuclei pulposi of normal, fused, and adjacent discs, from the endplate to the center of the disc. (From Holm, S., and Nachemson, A.: Nutrition changes in the canine intervertebral disc after spinal fusion. Clin. Orthop. Rel. Res. 169:243–258, 1982.)

been investigated using low-frequency vibrations. Under anesthetic conditions, animals were placed in a vertical position on a vibrating platform.[36] Accelerometers registered the input forces, and the frequencies used were in the range of 5 Hz. The results show a significant reduction in intradiscal oxygen tension as well as in cellular activity. The uptake rates of sulfate decreased with an increasing vibration time, as did the water content of the disc, especially in the nucleus pulposus (Fig. 15).[36] Even the disc height decreased comparatively. The relatively rapid loss of water exceeded the diffusional transport capacity, indicating an additional pathway of solute flow and/or an increased diffusional efficiency. As vibrations are known to exert effects on different microvascular systems in the body, the relevance to nutrition of the lumbar intervertebral disc, which is critically dependent upon a highly efficient blood pool underneath the vertebral end plate and at the periphery of the annulus fibrosus, is obvious.

Smoking

The efficiency of solute delivery from the blood capillaries, solute diffusivity, cellular uptake rate, and the dimensions of the disc system are factors of specific importance, particularly in the case of large human discs, in which the balance between nutrient utilization and supply is precarious; a loss in blood vessel contact or a reduction in blood flow at the periphery of the disc could lead to inadequate nutrition and a build-up of waste products. Several factors can create a potential risk of blockage or constriction of blood capillaries and consequently can affect the blood flow. One such risk factor is cigarette smoking.[7, 8] Smoking has also been regarded as a potential risk factor for initiating low back pain.[23, 35, 41, 70] Unfortunately, these epidemiologic studies evaluated only the subjective symptoms of low back pain and no structural or nutritional changes; therefore, the conclusion of such studies can

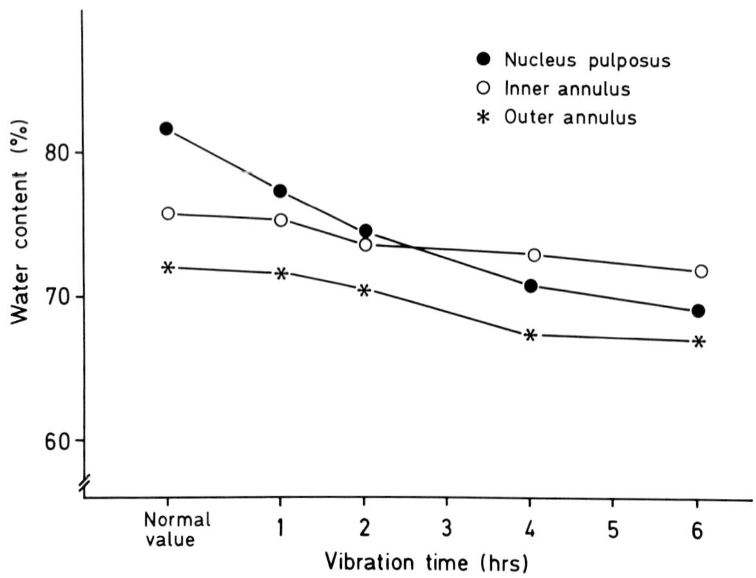

Figure 15 □ Variations in water content in discs from animals that have been exposed to vibration (5 Hz) for various periods.

EFFECTS (%) OF SMOKE ON SOLUTE TRANSPORT

Exposure time (minutes)	^{35}S	^{3}H	Oxygen
20 – 30	−27 ± 10	−18 ± 5	−42 ± 12
180	−46 ± 8	−42 ± 13	−48 ± 15

Figure 16 □ Effects of smoke on transport of sulphate (^{35}S), methyl glucose (^{3}H) and oxygen into the intervertebral disc. The reduction seen for all three parameters differed significantly compared with the unexposed group.

be controversial. In a recently performed experimental study, animals were exposed to cigarette smoke for a period of time ranging from 20 to 30 minutes to as long as 3 hours. The results show a reduced efficiency of blood vessels, and there was a considerable constriction of capillaries. Solute transport was already significantly reduced after 20 to 30 minutes of exposure (Fig. 16). An accumulation of metabolic waste products was also seen, which indicates a reduced transport efficiency away from the disc tissue (Fig. 17).[35]

The recovery time after smoke exposure was longer for charged molecules than for uncharged molecules, in regard to transport and metabolism. The cells reacted in an anaerobic direction, and the uptake rate of sulfate was reduced by some 35% after a short exposure time.[35]

The differences in transport efficiency suggest that the transport routes are differently affected between charged and uncharged molecules; pore size, molecular exclusion, and concentration gradients are parameters of potential importance. Furthermore, the cell reactions were rapid, indicating that the intervertebral discs are indeed sensitive to an affected rheologic surrounding.

When blood vessels are closed or constricted, the exchange area will be reduced, and the transport of nutrients to the cells as well as the disposal of waste products will not be adequate. Disc cells could either die or be unable to meet the energy demands required in, for example, the production of a functional matrix.

These findings demonstrate that cigarette smoke affects the circulatory system outside the intervertebral disc, as well as cellular uptake rates and metabolite production within the disc. By reducing the transport

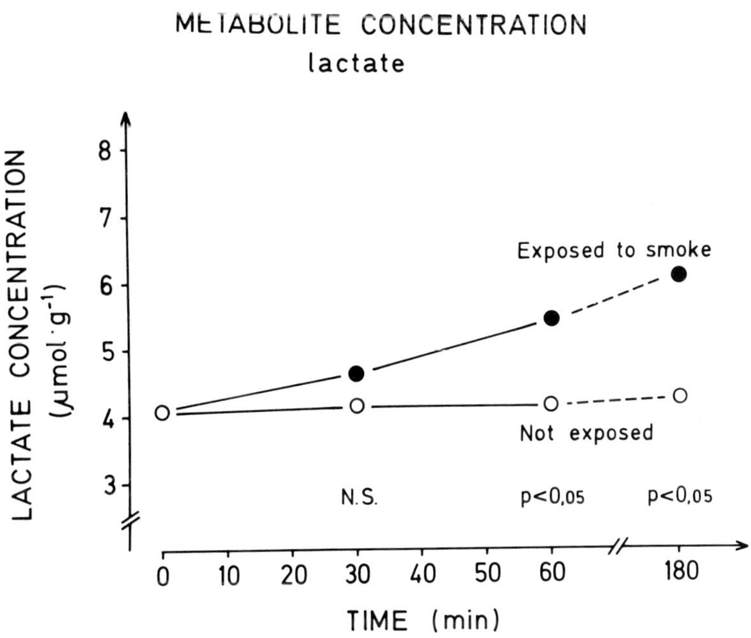

Figure 17 □ Lactate concentration in porcine nucleus pulposus. The accumulation of lactate, after 60 minutes and 3 hours of smoke exposure, is significantly higher compared with the control discs.

of substrates into the disc and of waste products out of the system, the inevitable consequence over a longer period of time will be a deficient nutrition, leading to cellular malfunction; an unhealthy cascade of events, including enzymatic degradation; instability; and probably back pain.

CONCLUSIONS

Various modes of exercise or lack of exercise have long-term effects on the disc matrix and cell metabolism. Segmental spinal fusions induce nutritional effects on the encased segment as well as on the adjacent motion segments. Disturbances of the external capillary network can lead to negative effects in the disc tissue. Although it is difficult to compare different exercise regimes, the results point to certain general trends; moderate exercise appears to improve solute transport and disc cell metabolism, providing optimal blood composition and overall rheologic functioning, and is probably necessary to a healthy and adequately functioning intervertebral disc. Removal of load from the disc can lead to deleterious changes. Axial vibrations and cigarette smoking impose significant transport disadvantages as well as changes in metabolism by affecting the surrounding capillary network and thereby reducing the transport efficiency into and out of the disc tissue.

It should be pointed out that results obtained in experimental investigations can be extrapolated and applied to the human situation only with extreme caution. Although it is established that exercise, vibration, and smoking influence nutrition of the intervertebral disc, too few studies have been conducted in this area to allow conclusions about the long-term effects on disc health. In order to understand the nutritional properties and function of the intervertebral disc and to find clues of relevance for spinal disorders and back pain, we need to know the type and magnitude of the exercise, the segmental load distribution and response, and the reversibility of blood vessel and disc cell reactions.

Practical Significance □ The aforementioned conclusions have the following practical significance:

1. The intervertebral discs need a well-developed and efficient vascular surrounding.
2. The chemical composition of blood and other mediating fluid pools must possess an optimal energy balance.
3. Solutes must at all times be available in a sufficient amount to the disc cells in order to fulfill development, maintenance, and repair of the structure.
4. The magnitude and distribution of the load and various exercising regimes are all vitally important factors that must be individually balanced against the inherent energy requirements in order to achieve an acceptable ergonomic situation.

References

1. Adams, P., and Muir, H.: Qualitative changes with age of proteoglycans of human lumbar discs. Ann. Rheum. Dis. 35:289–296, 1976.
2. Adams, M.A., and Hutton, W.C.: The effects of posture on the fluid control of the lumbar intervertebral disc. Spine 8:665–671, 1983.
3. Adams, M.A., and Hutton, W.C.: The effect of fatigue on the lumbar intervertebral disc. J. Bone Joint Surg. (Br.) 65:199–203, 1983.
4. Akeson, W.H., and Murphy, R.: Editorial comment: Low back pain. Clin. Orthop. Rel. Res. 129:2–3, 1977.
5. Andersson, G.B.J., and Schultz, A.B.: Effects of fluid injection on mechanical properties of intervertebral disc. J. Biomech. 12:453–458, 1979.
6. Anderson, G.B.J.: Measurements of load on the lumbar spine. *In* White, A.A., and Gordon, S.L. (eds.): Idiopathic Low Back Pain: Symposium, American Academy of Orthopaedic Surgeons. London, C.V. Mosby, 1982, pp. 220–251.
7. Asano, M., and Branemark, P.-I.: Cardiovascular and microvascular responses to smoking in man. Adv. Microcirc. 3:125–158, 1970.
8. Astrup, P., and Kjeldsen, R.: Carbon-monoxide smoking and arteriosclerosis. Med. Clin. North Am. 58:323–350, 1973.
9. Ayad, S., and Weiss, J.B.: Biochemistry of the intervertebral disc. *In* Jayson, M.I.V. (ed.): The Lumbar Spine and Back Pain, 3rd Ed. Edinburgh, Churchill Livingstone, 1986, pp. 407–436.
10. Beadle, O.A.: The intervertebral disc: Observations of the normal and morbid anatomy in relation to certain spinal deformations. Report 161, London M.R.C., 1931.
11. Braund, K.G., Gosh, P., Taylor, T.K.F., and Larsen, L.H.: Morphological studies of the canine intervertebral disc. The assignment of the beagle to the achondroplastic classification. Res. Vet. Sci. 19:167–172, 1975.
12. Brinckmann, P., Frobin, N., Hierholzer, E., and Horst, M.: Deformation of the vertebral end-plate under axial loading of the spine. Spine 8:851–856, 1983.
13. Brodin, H.: Paths of nutrition in articular cartilage and intervertebral discs. Acta Orthop. Scand. 24:177–180, 1955.

14. Brown, M.D., and Tsaltas, T.T.: Studies on the permeability of the intervertebral disc during skeletal maturation. Spine 1:240–244, 1976.
15. Cole, T.C., Burkhardt, D., Frost, L., and Ghosh, P.: The proteoglycans of the canine intervertebral disc. Biochim. Biophys. Acta 839:127–138, 1985.
16. Crock, H.W., and Goldwasser, M.: Anatomic studies of the circulation in the region of the vertebral endplate in adult greyhound dogs. Spine 9:702–706, 1984.
17. Davidson, E., and Small, W.: Metabolism in vivo of connective tissue mucopolysaccharides. Chondroitin sulphate C and keratan sulphate of nucleus pulposus. Biochim. Biophys. Acta 69:445–452, 1963.
18. Eklund, J.A., and Corlett, E.N.: Shrinkage as a measure of the effect of load on the spine. Spine 9:189–194, 1984.
19. Emes, J.H., and Pearce, R.H.: The proteoglycans of the human intervertebral disc. Biochem. J. 145:549–556, 1975.
20. Eyre, D.E., and Muir, H.: Quantitative analysis of types I and II collagens in human intervertebral disc at various ages. Biochim. Biophys. Acta 492:29–42, 1977.
21. Eyre, D.E.: Biochemistry of the intervertebral disc. Connect. Tissue Res. 8:227–290, 1979.
22. Frymoyer, J.W., Hanley, E.N., Howe, J., et al.: A comparison of radiographic findings in fusion and nonfusion patients ten or more years following lumbar disc surgery. Spine 4:435–440, 1979.
23. Frymoyer, J.W., Pope, M.H., Constanza, M.C., et al.: Epidemiologic studies of low-back pain. Spine 5:419–424, 1980.
24. Ghosh, P., Taylor, T.K.F., Braund, K.G., and Larsen, L.H.: The collagenous and non-collagenous proteins of the canine intervertebral disc and their variation with age, spinal level and breed. Gerontologia 22:124–132, 1975.
25. Grodzinsky, A.J.: Electromechanical and physicochemical properties of connective tissue. Crit. Rev. Biomed. Engineer. 9:133–199, 1983.
26. Grynpas, M.D., Eyre, D.S., and Kirschner, D.A.: Collagen of the intervertebral disc. X-ray diffraction evidence for difference in molecular packing of types I and II collagens. Biochim. Biophys. Acta 626:346–355, 1980.
27. Hansen, H.J., and Ullberg, S.: Uptake of ^{35}S in the intervertebral disc after injection of ^{35}S-sulphate. An autoradiographic study. Acta Orthop. Scand. 30:84–90, 1980.
28. Happey, M.: Studies of the structure of the human intervertebral disc in relation to its functional and ageing processes. *In* Sokoloff, L. (ed.): The Joints and Synovial Fluid. London, Academic Press, 1980, pp. 95–137.
29. Heinegård, D., and Paulsson, M.: Structure and metabolism of proteoglycans. *In* Piez, K.A., and Reddi, A.H. (eds.): Extracellular Matrix Biochemistry. New York, Elsevier, 1984.
30. Hickey, D.S., and Hukins, D.L.: The relationship between the structure of the annulus fibrosus and the function and failure of the intervertebral disc. Spine 5:105–116, 1986.
31. Hoerlein, B.F.: Canine Neurology—Diagnosis and Treatment. Philadelphia, W.B. Saunders, 1971.
32. Holm, S., Maroudas, A., Urban, J.P.G., et al.: Nutrition of the intervertebral disc. Connect. Tissue Res. 8:101–119, 1981.
33. Holm, S., and Nachemson, A.: Nutrition changes in the canine intervertebral disc after spinal fusion. Clin. Orthop. Rel. Res. 169:243–258, 1982.
34. Holm, S., and Nachemson, A.: Variations in the nutrition of the canine intervertebral disc induced by motion. Spine 8:866–874, 1983.
35. Holm, S., and Nachemson, A.: Immediate effects of cigarette smoke on nutrition of the intervertebral disc of the pig. Orthop. Transact. 8:380, 1984.
36. Holm, S., and Nachemson, A.: Nutrition of the intervertebral disc: Effects induced by vibrations. Orthop. Transact. 9:451, 1985.
37. Holm, S.: Nutritional variations in articular cartilage induced by exercise. Scand. J. Rheumatol. 60 (Suppl.):A116, 1986.
38. Hudlicka, O., and Tyler, K.R.: The effect of long-term high frequency stimulation on capillary density and fibre types in rabbit fast muscles. J. Physiol. (London) 353:435–445, 1984.
39. Inoue, H.: Three-dimensional observation of collagen framework of intervertebral discs in rats, dogs and humans. Arch. Histol. Jpn. 36:39–56, 1973.
40. Inoue, H., and Takeda, T.: Three-dimensional observations of collagen framework of lumbar intervertebral discs. Acta Orthop. Scand. 46:949–956, 1975.
41. Kelsey, J.L.: An epidemiological study of acute herniated lumbar intervertebral disc. J. Rheumatol. Rehab. 14:144–159, 1975.
42. Klein, J.A., Hickey, D.S., and Hukins, D.W.: Radial bulging of the annulus fibrosus during compression of the intervertebral disc. J. Biomech. 16:211–217, 1983.
43. Knight, J.A., Stephens, R.W., Bushell, G.R., et al.: Neutral protease inhibitors from human intervertebral disc and femoral head articular cartilage. Biochim. Biophys. Acta 584:304–310, 1979.
44. Koeller, W., Meier, W., and Hartmann, F.: Biomechanical properties of human intervertebral discs subjected to axial dynamic compression. A comparison of lumbar and thoracic discs. Spine 9:925–933, 1984.
45. Krämor, J.: Zur Biomechanik des lumbalen bewegungs-lements. *In* Junghans, H. (ed.): Die Wirbelsaule in Forschung und Praxis. Stuttgart, Hippokrates, 1971, pp. 19–63.
46. Krämer, J.: Pressure-dependent fluid shifts in the intervertebral disc. Orthop. Clin. North Am. 8:211 216, 1977.
47. Lewin, T.: Osteoarthritis in lumbar synovial joints—a morphological study. Acta Orthop. Scand. 73(Suppl.):5–108, 1964.
48. Lohmander, S., Antonopoulus, C.A., and Friberg, U.: Chemical and metabolic heterogeneity of chondroitin sulphate and keratan sulphate in guinea pig cartilage and nucleus pulposus. Biochim. Biophys. Acta 304:430–448, 1973.
49. Lyons, G., Eistenstein, S.M., and Sweet, M.B.E.: Biochemical changes in intervertebral disc degeneration. Biochim. Biophys. Acta 673:443–453, 1981.
50. Maroudas, A., Stockwell, R.A., Nachemson, A., and Urban, J.: Factors involved in the nutrition of the human lumbar intervertebral disc: Cellularity and diffusion of glucose in vitro. J. Anat. 120:113–130, 1975.
51. Nachemson, A.: Lumbar interdiscal pressure. Experimental studies on post-mortem material. Acta Orthop. Scand. 43(Suppl.):1–104, 1960.

52. Nachemson, A., Lewin, T., Maroudas, A., and Freeman, M.A.R.: In vitro diffusion of dye through the end-plates and the annulus fibrosus of human lumbar intervertebral discs. Acta Orthop. Scand. 41:589–607, 1970.
53. Nachemson, A.: The lumbar spine: An orthopedic challenge. Spine 1:59–71, 1976.
54. Nachemson, A.L., and Anderson, G.B.J.: Classification of low back pain. Scand. J. Work, Environ. Health 8:134–136, 1982.
55. Naylor, A.: The biophysical and biomechanical aspects of intervertebral disc herniation and degeneration. Ann. R. Coll. Surg. Engl. 31:91–114, 1962.
56. Naylor, A.: The structure and function of the intervertebral disc. Orthopaedics (Oxford) 3:7–22, 1970.
57. Naylor, A.: Late results of laminectomy for lumbar disc prolapse. A review after ten to twenty-five years. J. Bone Joint Surg. (Br.) 56:17–29, 1974.
58. Oegema, T.R., Bradford, D.S., and Cooper, K.M.: Aggregated proteoglycan synthesis in organ cultures of human nucleus pulposus. J. Biol. Chem. 254:10579–10581, 1979.
59. Ogata, K., and Whiteside, L.A.: Nutritional pathways of the intervertebral disc: An experimental study using hydrogen washout technique. Spine 6:211–216, 1981.
60. Parker, K., Maroudas, A., and Winlove, P.: Diffusivities and partitions of inorganic ions in CS and HA solutions. Biorheology (in press).
61. Pearcy, M., Portek, J., and Shepherd, J.: The effect of low back pain on lumbar spinal movements by three-dimensional x-ray analysis. Spine 10:150–153, 1985.
62. Pope, M., Wilder, D., and Booth, J.: The biomechanics of low back pain. *In* White, A.A., and Gordon, S.L. (eds.): Idiopathic Low Back Pain: Symposium, American Academy of Orthopaedic Surgeons. London, C.V. Mosby, 1982, pp. 252–295.
63. Postacchini, F., Bellocci, M., and Massobrio, M.: Morphologic changes in annulus fibrosus during ageing. Spine 9:596–603, 1984.
64. Sandover, J.: Vibration and people. Clin. Biomech. 1:150–159, 1986.
65. Schmorl, G., and Junghanns, H.: The Human Spine in Health and Disease. New York, Grune & Stratton, 1971.
66. Sedowofia, S.K.A, Tomlinson, I., Jayson, M.I.V., and Weiss, J.B.: Identification of collagenase and other neutral proteinases in human intervertebral discs. Ann. Rheum. Dis. 38:573–592, 1979.
67. Souter, W.A., and Taylor, T.K.F.: Sulphated acid mucopolysaccharide metabolism in the rabbit intervertebral disc. J. Bone Joint Surg. (Br.) 52:371–384, 1970.
68. Stevens, R.L., Dondi, P., and Muir, H.: Proteoglycans of the intervertebral disc. Biochem. J. 179:573–578, 1979.
69. Stevens, R.L., Ewans, R.J.F., Revell, P.A., and Muir, H.: Proteoglycans of the intervertebral disc. Biochem. J. 179:561–572, 1979.
70. Svensson, H.-O., Vedin, A., Wilhelmsson, C., and Andersson, G.: Low-back pain in relation to other diseases and cardiovascular risk factors. Spine 8:277–285, 1983.
71. Szirmai, J.A.: Structure of the intervertebral disc. *In* Balazs, E.A. (ed.): Chemistry and Molecular Biology of the Intracellular Matrix. New York, Academic Press, 1970, pp. 1279–1308.
72. Takeda, T.: Three dimensional observation of collagen framework of human lumbar disc. J. Jpn. Orthop. Assoc. 49:45–57, 1975.
73. Taylor, T.K.F, Ghosh, P., Braund, K.G., et al.: The effect of spinal fusion on intervertebral disc composition. An experimental study. J. Surg. Res. 21:91–104, 1976.
74. Urban, J.P.G.: Fluid and Solute Transport in the Intervertebral Disc. Ph.D. Thesis, London University, 1977.
75. Urban, J., Holm, S., Maroudas, A., and Nachemson, A.: Nutrition of the intervertebral disc. An in vivo study of solute transport. J. Clin. Orthop. 129:101–114, 1977.
76. Urban, J., Holm, S., and Maroudas, A.: Diffusion of small solutes in the intervertebral disc: An in vivo study. Biorheology 15:202–223, 1978.
77. Urban, J.P.G., and Maroudas, A.: Measurement of fixed charge density in the intervertebral disc. Biochim. Biophys. Acta 586:166–178, 1979.
78. Urban, J.P.G., Maroudas, A., Bayliss, M.T., and Dillon, J.: Swelling pressures of proteoglycans at the concentrations found in cartilaginous tissues. Biorheology 16:447–464, 1979.
79. Urban, J.P.G., and Maroudas, A.: The chemistry of the intervertebral disc in relation to its physiological functions and requirements. Clin. Rheum. Dis. 6:51–56, 1980.
80. Urban, J.P.G., and Maroudas, A.: Swelling of the intervertebral disc in vivo. Connect. Tissue Res. 9:1–10, 1981.
81. White, A.A., Edwards, T.W., Liberman, K., et al.: Biomechanics of lumbar spine and sacroiliac articulation: Relevance to idiopathic low back pain. *In* White, A.A., and Gordon, S.L. (eds.): Idiopathic Low Back Pain: Symposium, American Academy of Orthopaedic Surgeons. London, C.V. Mosby, 1982, pp. 296–322.
82. Wiidik, A.: Functional properties of collagenous tissues. Internat. Rev. Connect. Tissue Res. 6:127–215, 1973.
83. Yamada, K.: The dynamics of experimental posture. Experimental study of intervertebral disc herniation in bipedal animals. J. Exp. Med. 8:350–361, 1962.

AGING VERSUS DEGENERATION OF THE INTERVERTEBRAL DISC

Stephen J. Lipson

The aging of tissues implies an accumulation of changes over time. Degeneration, on the other hand, implies a deterioration of the physical properties of a tissue with retrogressive pathologic changes in the cells or tissue, the consequence of which is destruction or inhibition of function. As the intervertebral disc (IVD) ages, it undergoes degeneration. However, clinicians tend to distinguish between aging as a morphologic anatomic change and degeneration as that same change associated with a clinical complaint. Although IVD degeneration (IVDD) is often radiologically demonstrable in adults with low back pain,[26] a causal relationship between low back pain and degenerative changes is not established.[34] Common radiographic IVDD can be noted in the absence of low back disorders.[25] There is no distinction between the anatomic changes of degeneration through aging and those that may be called pathologic.[10, 22] This author takes the position that aging and degeneration are the same pathologic process and that some physiologic feature or features occurring during degeneration can cause a clinical complaint. The clinical features are not discussed, but rather the information on the tissue changes that occur as a result of degeneration through aging.

MACROSCOPIC DEGENERATION

IVDD can simply be defined as the loss of normal IVD architecture accompanied by progressive fibrosis. IVDD is denoted as the loss of the gelatinous nucleus pulposus (NP), gradual disappearance of the originally well-defined border between the NP and annulus fibrosus (AF), coarsening of the AF lamellae, progressive fibrosis, and later fissuring of the AF with the deposition of aging pigment.[10, 17, 22, 51] On the basis of these observations, IVDD has been graded by Nachemson[39] and Lewin[27] with essentially the same classification. Nachemson's classification divides IVDD into four grades denoting the range from young or normal IVD to severe IVDD by the progressive loss of the NP, the distinction of the NP–AF border, and the appearance of fibrosis and fissuring along with marginal osteophyte formation. In a collected autopsy series,[36] IVDD first appeared in the second decade in males and the third in females with 97% of the discs demonstrating degeneration by 50 years of age. L3–L4 and L4–L5 are usually the most degenerated discs.

HISTOLOGIC DEGENERATION

In the fetal and infant NP, notochordal cells are found as clusters of vacuolated cells floating in a basophilic matrix. Histochemically, the enzymes found in these cells are similar to those in perichordal cells.[52] There is a fine fibrillar structure in the matrix, and both fibroblasts and chondrocytes are noted along with the notochordal cells. The original peripheral portion of the nucleus is fibrous, finally blending with the fibers of the AF. This border becomes indistinct after the second decade.[9, 11] Gradual cavitation, apparent dessication, cellular degeneration, fibroblastic proliferation, and calcium salt deposition follow. The fibroblasts are not orderly, as they are in the AF, and more chondrocytes appear. As degeneration progresses, the AF and NP are indistinct, and fibrocartilage replaces the NP area.[9]

The lamellae of the AF become coarser and hyalinized with age. Fissures become apparent, and pigmentation may occur. Nests of chondrocytes can be noted by the fourth decade, as can the progression of fibrocartilaginous change. Vascular invasion also can be observed. The progression of IVDD is marked by further conversion to more disorganized fibrocartilage. In the aging AF, the pericellular area loses a periodic acid–Schiff (PAS) positive component, enhanced Alcian blue staining occurs, and the matrix becomes more granular.[51] While the AF lamellae become disordered, more random PAS reactive granules appear amid random arrays of Alcian blue reactive fibrous material, implying an alteration in the collagen-proteoglycan relationship. These are considered regressive changes that can alter the mechanical properties of the AF.[51]

As NP degeneration occurs, PAS positivity increases and corresponds to age pigment, whereas proteoglycan (PG) Alcian blue–staining decreases.[43] These changes are concomitants of AF fibrocartilaginous metaplasia in which chondrocytes and chondrons begin to appear in the inner AF; the Alcian blue territorial matrix appears, as the once-orderly AF lamellae becomes more random.

The fine structure of human IVD shown by electron microscopy has been extensively reviewed.[5] Cell activity, localization of collagen, PG and noncollagenous proteins can be accomplished. The collagen fibrils of the AF lamellae provide tensile strength and are architecturally organized in layers with an angle of 40 to 70 degrees between layers. Occasional granules are found adhering to the fibril surface. The fibrils are tightly packed and increase in diameter and variability with age. Near the NP–AF border, fibrils are less dense and less organized. In the NP they form a loose network with more varied diameters. PG and noncollagenous proteins coat the NP collagen fibrils. With age the fibrillar diameter increases and the fibrils of the NP become more dense.

PG provides resistance to compression in IVD as in other cartilaginous tissues. PG forms small granules in the extracellular matrix, often in association with collagen fibrils. Electron microscopy monolayer technique[6] demonstrates that infant PG forms aggregates with hyaluronic acid, but this occurs less extensively and the aggregates are smaller than in articular cartilage. It is believed that regional differences in PG structure and aggregate formation allow variation in the hydrodynamic, and therefore mechanical, properties of the tissue.

Histologic studies at the light and electron-microscopic level demonstrate that the biochemical constituents of IVD display an architectural array that reflects the gross structure of IVD, and therefore its properties. Alteration in the constituents with regard to content, structure, and array can be expected to parallel degenerative change. The factor, or factors, that provoke these degenerative alterations remains unknown.

BIOCHEMISTRY OF STRUCTURAL COMPONENTS

The major structural components of IVD are collagen, PG, and water, together making up 90% to 95% of the volume of normal IVD. The collagen network provides the intervertebral connection, while its lamellar structure permits motion. PG provides hydration of the IVD tissue and, via its osmotic properties, imbibes water, swells the IVD, and maintains tissue turgor. Through high concentrations, with its hydrodynamic and electrostatic properties, PG regulates fluid loss.

Water

The IVD is normally highly hydrated. The NP consists of about 85% water, and the AF 78%. In both tissues, water content falls to about 70% with degeneration.[16, 18, 24, 41, 44] PG content and hydration decrease with age, especially in the NP.[31, 37] An investigation of water content with regard to PG content, age, spinal level, and degeneration[50] demonstrated that PG content and hydration fell with age and varied with spinal level. The relationship of swelling pressure and hydration, however, was dependent on IVD PG: collagen, rather than on age or degeneration.

Collagen

IVD contains Type I and Type II collagen.[14] In human AF, overall, it is about 60% Type II and 40% Type I. In AF there is an interchanging radial distribution of collagen types with, exclusively, Type II in the NP.[15, 23] Type II fibrils from NP exhibit greater intermolecular spacing than Type I when examined by x-ray diffraction.[19] It is a feature associated with increased water content, implying that highly hydrated Type II fibrils may better deform and absorb compressive forces.

In both young and old human IVD, collagen content in outer AF is higher than that in inner AF and NP.[2, 4] In younger spines, total collagen content varies little, but in older spines, the AF collagen content increases down the spine as well as outward in the AF. Total collagen content undergoes alteration with age and topographically increases by a small amount.[4] This change also occurs in the NP. There is, however, an alteration in the proportion of Type I to Type II; with age, Type I increases in content.[4] This pattern is noted in both pigs and humans.[12]

Irreducible cross-linking in collagen accumulates with age and in IVD reducible cross-links are absent by age 25.[23] A study of

IVD above degenerated IVD demonstrated reducible cross-links along with the appearance of Type I collagen.[23] This finding indicates the new synthesis of collagen. Reducible cross-links were found with topographic variation in IVD and although the content is lower with age, new synthesis can be found if IVD is sampled regionally.[4] Hydroxypyridinium (HP) is the major irreducible cross-link in adult collagen, and IVD and articular cartilage are the tissues most rich in HP.[13] HP increases with age,[38] and Type II collagen contains more HP than does Type I.[13] A study of HP in human herniated IVD tissue has shown a decrease in HP content relative to endogenous AF, indicating a new synthesis of collagen.[28]

Immunofluorescent studies of human IVD have shown no qualitative difference in collagen types in surgical and postmortem tissue, but Type III collagen, associated with fibril formation in reticular networks, was found in pericellular areas along with PG.[48] Similar studies in spondylolisthesis IVD showed a reduction in Types I and III, but no change in patients with posterior annular tears.[45] Type III collagen, therefore, appears to arise regionally during IVDD.

Current information in collagen biochemistry indicates, in summary, that IVDD is accompanied by an alteration in the array of collagen subtypes; Type I replaces Type II, Type III appears, and there is an overall accumulation of irreducible cross-links, but a regional appearance of newly synthesized collagen. The regional changes imply that new synthesis reflects areas of tensile versus compressive loads and is a cellular response to these mechanical loads.[4]

Proteoglycans

PGs of IVD are homologous to those from articular cartilage.[47] They contain a core protein, glycosaminoglycans of chondroitin sulfate (CS), and keratan sulfate (KS) attached to the core, and they are able to aggregate with hyaluronic acid (HA), stabilized by link protein. They have shorter KS and CS chains than do cartilage PGs, and a shorter core protein. A higher proportion of aggregating PGs are found in AF than in NP. The smaller size of PGs from IVD is an intrinsic property.[46]

The NP is richer in PGs than the AF.[2, 24, 35, 49] As age and degeneration advance, the total PG content decreases,[20, 24, 37, 40, 50] KS:CS increases,[3, 18, 20, 32, 33] extractability increases, and aggregation decreases,[3] although the HA content of the IVD is in excess of that needed for maximum aggregation.[21] A study of PG content in IVDD graded by the Lewin method[27] demonstrated a decreasing PG content with increasing grades of IVDD.[42] Regional studies of the IVD show that water and PG content are lost with degeneration, most especially in the NP, and that the loss of the ability of PGs to aggregate is associated with a decrease in the size of the core.[31] It is suggested that degradation occurs in the HA binding region and that PG synthesis is slower in IVDD. A study of surgical and postmortem tissues showed that, except in the youngest patients, PGs were of similar size in all patients and a wide range of aggregating PGs was present.[48] No correlations could be made with a clinical diagnosis.

Biochemical Changes in Animal Models

Animal modeling has allowed some insight into biochemical changes in the IVD. A rabbit model of surgically induced ventral herniation has been studied.[29, 30] In this model, progressive fibrocartilaginous metaplasia occurs with the proliferation of tissue altering the IVD architecture. Morphologically, an end-stage IVDD is reached. Water content is acutely lost and regained by the fourth day after injury, parallel to the initial loss and apparent rapid synthesis of PGs. The progressive loss of water and PG content then follows. The aggregating population of PGs, initially lost, was repleted at about 3 weeks after injury, but then lost by 6 to 7 weeks. The size of the monomeric PGs did not change with degeneration, but newly synthesized PG monomers were always larger than the average population. This model postulates an acute response of inner AF cells to the surgical injury and raises the possibility of the tissue attempting to repair itself.

PGs have been studied in fused canine spines.[7, 8] In chondrodystrophic dogs, IVD in the fused and parafusion area was studied.[7] Isolated PGs had less ability to aggregate and a slightly smaller hydrodynamic size at 6 months, although they were larger at 12 months after fusion. CS increased proportionately. These studies concluded that a new PG population is synthesized, a type seen in younger, less mature tissues. A similar study was performed in nonchondrodystrophic dogs.[8] PGs increased in content, extractability, and size. The ability to aggregate was greater. There was no change in CS:KS. The difference in behavior of these two breeds under the same conditions of experimental fusion is hypothesized to result from genetically determined differences in the matrices and cells.

CONCLUSIONS

The usual concept of IVDD is that it is morphologically defined and represents a tissue change that includes a loss of components. Histologic and fine structure studies indicate that tissue is progressively remodeled; a loss of the normal array of matrix components is seen. Biochemical studies indicate that IVDD is not simply progressive fibrosis of the IVD, but a remodeling process on a regional basis with the replacement of Type II collagen by Type I and the appearance of Type III collagen. Qualitative changes occur in the PG component. Animal studies indicate that IVD cells are responsive to mechanical alteration but may be governed by constitutional factors. IVDD should not be viewed as simply a deteriorative, destructive process, but rather as a remodeling process. Improving our understanding of cell regulation and expression may lead to further insight into IVDD.

References

1. Adam, M., and Deyl, Z.: Degenerated annulus fibrosus of the intervertebral disc contain collagen Type III. Ann. Rheum. Dis. 43:258–263, 1984.
2. Adams, P., Eyre, D.R., and Muir, H.: Biochemical aspects of development and ageing of human lumbar intervertebral discs. Rheumatol. Rehab. 16:22–29, 1977.
3. Adams, P., and Muir, H.: Qualitative changes with age of proteoglycans of human lumbar disc. Ann. Rheum. Dis. 35:289–295, 1976.
4. Brickley-Parsons, D., and Glimcher, M.J.: Is the chemistry of collagen in intervertebral discs an expression of Wolff's law? A study of the human lumbar spine. Spine 9:148–163, 1984.
5. Buckwalter, J.A.: The fine structure of human intervertebral disc. *In* White, A.A. III, and Gordon, S.L.: Symposium on Idiopathic Low Back Pain. St. Louis, C.V. Mosby, 1982, pp. 108–143.
6. Buckwalter, J.A., Pedrini-Mille, A., Pedrini, V., and Tudisco, C.: Proteoglycans of human infant intervertebral disc. Electron microscopic and biochemical studies. J. Bone Joint Surg. 67A:284–294, 1985.
7. Cole, T.-C., Burkhardt, D., Ghosh, P., and Taylor, T.: Effects of spinal fusion on the proteoglycans of the canine intervertebral disc. J. Orthop. Res. 3:277–291, 1985.
8. Cole, T.-C., Ghosh, P., Hannan, N.J., et al.: The response of canine intervertebral disc to immobilization produced by spinal arthrodesis is dependent on constitutional factors. J. Orthop. Res. 5:337–347, 1987.
9. Coventry, M.B., Ghormley, R.K., and Kernohan, J.W.: The intervertebral disc: Its microscopic anatomy and pathology. Part II. Changes in the intervertebral disc concomitant with age. J. Bone Joint Surg. 27A:233–247, 1945.
10. Coventry, M.B., Ghormley, R.K., and Kernohan, J.W.: The intervertebral disc: Its microscopic anatomy and pathology. Part III. Pathologic changes in the intervertebral disc. J. Bone Joint Surg. 27A:460–474, 1945.
11. Eckert, C., and Decker, A.: Pathological studies of intervertebral discs. J. Bone Joint Surg. 29A:447–454, 1947.
12. Eyre, D.R.: Biochemistry of the intervertebral disc. Internat. Rev. Connect. Tissue Res. 8:227–291, 1979.
13. Eyre, D.R., Koob, T.J., and van Ness, K.P.: Quantitation of hydroxypyridinium cross links in collagen by high-performance liquid chromatography. Analyt. Biochem. 137:380–388, 1984.
14. Eyre, D.R., and Muir, H.: Collagen polymorphism: Two molecular species in pig intervertebral disc. F.E.B.S. Letters 42:192–196, 1974.
15. Eyre, D.R., and Muir, H.: Types I and II collagens in intervertebral disc. Interchanging radial distributions in annulus fibrosus. Biochem. J. 157:267–270, 1976.
16. Eyring, E.J.: The biochemistry and physiology of intervertebral disk. Clin. Orthop. Rel. Res. 67:16–28, 1969.
17. Friberg, S., and Hirsch, C.: Anatomical and clinical studies on lumbar disc degeneration. Acta Orthop. Scand. 19:222–242, 1949.
18. Gower, W.E., and Pedrini, V.: Age related variations in protein-polysaccharides from human nucleus pulposus, annulus fibrosus and costal cartilage. J. Bone Joint Surg. 51A:1154–1162, 1969.
19. Grynpas, M.D., Eyre, D.R., and Kirschner, D.A.: Collagen Type II differs from Type I in native molecular packing. Biochim. Biophys. Acta 626:346–355, 1980.
20. Hallen, A.: Hexosamine and ester sulphate content of the human nucleus pulposus in different ages. Acta Chim. Scand. Vol. 12, 1958.
21. Hardingham, T.E., and Adams, P.: A method for the determination of hyaluronate in the presence of other glycosaminoglycans and its application to human intervertebral discs. Biochem. J. 159:143–147, 1976.
22. Harris, R.I., and Macnab, I.: Structural changes in the lumbar intervertebral discs. Their relationship to low back pain and sciatica. J. Bone Joint Surg. 36B:304–322, 1954.
23. Herbert, C.M., Lindberg, K.A., Jayson, M.I.V., and Bailey, A.J.: Changes in the collagen of human intervertebral discs during ageing and degenerative disc disease. J. Molec. Med. 1:79–81, 1975.

24. Hirsch, C., Paulson, S., Sylven, B., and Snellman, O.: Biophysical and physiological investigations on cartilage and other mesenchymal tissues. Acta Orthop. Scand. 22:175–181, 1952.
25. Hult, L.: Cervical, dorsal and lumbar spine syndromes. Acta Orthop. Scand. 17(Suppl.):65–73, 1954.
26. Kellgren, J.H., and Lawrence, J.S.: Osteoarthrosis and disc degeneration in an urban population. Ann. Rheum. Dis. 17:388–397, 1958.
27. Lewin, T.: Osteoarthritis in lumbar synovial joints. Acta Orthop. Scand. 73(Suppl.):31, 1964.
28. Lipson, S.J.: Metaplastic proliferative fibrocartilage as an alternative concept to herniated intervertebral disc. Spine 13:1055–1060, 1988.
29. Lipson, S.J., and Muir, H.: Experimental intervertebral disc degeneration. Morphologic and proteoglycan changes over time. Arth. Rheum. 24:12–21, 1981.
30. Lipson, S.J., and Muir, H.: Proteoglycans in experimental disc degeneration. Spine 6:194–210, 1981.
31. Lyons, G., Eisenstein, S.M., and Sweet, M.B.E.: Biochemical changes in intervertebral disc degeneration. Biochim. Biophys. Acta 673:443–453, 1981.
32. Lyons, H., Jones, E., Quinn, F.E., and Sprunt, D.H.: Protein-polysaccharide complexes of normal and herniated intervertebral discs. Proc. Soc. Exp. Biol. 115:610–614, 1964.
33. Lyons, H., Jones, E., Quinn, F.E., and Sprunt, D.H.: Changes in the protein-polysaccharide fractions of nucleus pulposus from human intervertebral disc with age and disc herniation. J. Lab. Clin. Med. 68:930–939, 1966.
34. Magora, A., and Schwartz, A.: Relation between the low back pain syndrome and x-ray findings. 1. Degenerative osteoarthritis. Scand. J. Rehab. Med. 8:115–125, 1976.
35. Malinsky, J.: Histochemical demonstration of carbohydrates in human intervertebral discs during postnatal development. Acta Histochem. 5:120–128, 1958.
36. Miller, J.A.A., Schmatz, C., and Schultz, A.B.: Lumbar disc degeneration: Correlation with age, sex, and spine level in 600 autopsy specimens. Spine 13:173–178, 1988.
37. Mitchell, P.E.G., Hendry, N., and Billewicz, W.T.: The chemical background of intervertebral disc prolapse. J. Bone Joint Surg. 43B:141–151, 1961.
38. Moriguchi, T., and Fujimoto, D.: Age related changes of the collagen cross-link, pyridinoline. J. Biochem.. (Tokyo). 84:933–935, 1978.
39. Nachemson, A.: Lumbar intradiscal pressure. Acta Orthop. Scand. 43(Suppl.):43–44, 1960.
40. Naylor, A.: The biophysical and biochemical aspects of intervertebral disc herniations and degeneration. Ann. R. Coll. Surg. Engl. 31:91–114, 1962.
41. Naylor, A., and Horton, W.G.: The hydrophilic properties of the nucleus pulposus of the intervertebral disc. Rheumatism. 11:32–35, 1955.
42. Pearce, R.H., Grimmer, B.J., and Adams, M.E.: Degeneration and the chemical composition of the human lumbar intervertebral disc. J. Orthop. Res. 5:198–205, 1987.
43. Pritzker, K.P.H.: Aging and degeneration in the lumbar intervertebral disc. Orthop. Clin. North Am. 8:65–77, 1977.
44. Puschel, J.: Der Wassergehalt Normaler und Degenerierter Zwischenwirbelscheiben. Beitr. Pathol. Anat. 84:123–130, 1930.
45. Roberts, S., Beard, H.K., and O'Brien, J.P.: Biochemical changes of intervertebral discs in patients with spondylolisthesis or with tears of the posterior annulus fibrosus. Ann. Rheum. Dis. 41:78–85, 1982.
46. Stevens, R.L., Dondi, P.G., and Muir, H.: Proteoglycans of intervertebral disc. Absence of degradation during isolation of proteoglycans from the intervertebral disc. Biochem. J. 179:573–578, 1979.
47. Stevens, R.L., Ewins, R.J.F., Revell, P.A., and Muir, H.: Proteoglycans of the intervertebral disc. Biochem. J. 179:561–572, 1979.
48. Stevens, R.L., Ryvar, R., Robertson, W.R., et al.: Biological changes in the annulus fibrosus in patients with low-back pain. Spine 7:223–233, 1982.
49. Sylven, B.: On the biology of the nucleus pulposus. Acta Orthop. Scand. 20:275–279, 1951.
50. Urban, J.P.G., and McMullin, J.F.: Swelling pressure of the lumbar intervertebral discs: Influence of age, spinal level, composition, and degeneration. Spine 13:179–187, 1988.
51. van den Hoof, A.: Histological age changes in the anulus fibrosus of the human intervertebral disk. Gerontologia 9:136–149, 1964.
52. Wolfe, H.J., Putchar, G.J., and Vickery, A.L.: Role of the notochord in human intervertebral disk. I. Fetus and infant. Clin. Orthop. Rel. Res. 39:205–212, 1965.

6 □ Radiology

Wolfgang Rauschning
Kenneth B. Heithoff
David W. Stoller
Harry K. Genant
Ian A. F. Stokes
Roger P. Jackson
Rae R. Jacobs

■ IMAGING ANATOMY OF THE LUMBAR SPINE

Wolfgang Rauschning

Multiplanar sectional imaging modalities such as polytomography, x-ray computed tomography (CT), magnetic resonance imaging (MRI), and to some extent ultrasonography are routinely used to assess disorders of the lumbosacral spine. Dramatic improvements of both spatial and contrast resolution have been achieved in recent years, and further improvement of the computerized modalities is anticipated. CT and MRI are already the primary techniques used by many diagnosticians, while the use of invasive techniques, such as myelography, has decreased. The use of these techniques to image the lumbosacral spine has been documented in a great number of scientific papers and textbooks.[4, 11, 13, 14, 17, 20, 23, 24, 27] CT normally images the lumbosacral spine in the axial plane in a slice-by-slice fashion. Computer reconstruction of the image data allows the display of the spine in other planes such as the coronal and sagittal planes and also in nonorthogonal, oblique planes. For special studies, reconstruction in curved planes, following the lumbosacral curvatures, is possible. In contrast to CT, MRI allows the simultaneous acquisition of a series of images in any optional imaging plane; depending on the imaging technique used, it is also possible to obtain functional metabolic data on blood circulation, inflammatory changes, and neoplastic lesions. In this sense, MRI has the promising potential to disclose such lesions of the lumbar spine with exquisite resolution and depiction of the spinal soft tissues. With currently used scanners, CT is usually superior in defining detail of the bony elements of the vertebral column. Both CT and MRI allow the accurate measurement of spinal dimensions to be taken directly from the films, whereas conventional polytomography appreciably magnifies the bony structures.

Segmental image interpretation in various anatomic planes is difficult because the diagnostician has to know highly complex three-dimensional topographic-anatomic relationships and their normal variations in two-dimensional images in order to be able to assess disorders and abnormalities. Conventional descriptive texts and atlases are of limited value for the assessment of diagnostic scans; very few diagnosticians are able to mentally transform descriptive anatomic data into two-dimensional topographic relationships. Consequently, a great number of sectional-anatomic atlases have been published in the past decade, most of them by clinicians, and notably radiologists.[3, 5, 6, 9, 10, 15, 16, 19, 21, 22, 29] As imaging technology improves, a regionally specialized anatomic imaging reference material is needed. The normal and pathologic anatomy of the lumbar spine has been described in authoritative articles and textbooks.[1, 2, 7, 8, 12, 18, 25, 26, 28, 30] This brief textbook chapter can neither substitute for a detailed imaging atlas nor describe normal and pathologic anatomy at large. It can only serve as a pictorial reference for commonly used diagnostic techniques for the lumbosacral spine.

AXIAL PLANE (Figs. 1 to 5)

The segmentally repetitive arrangement of bony vertebrae and intervening soft tissues allows the description of anatomic features that can be distinguished at given levels. The upper and lower borders of the pedicles and the vertebral end plates can serve as anatomic reference marks. Such a simplistic approach does not take into account the morphologic differences between different lumbar vertebral levels; the lumbosacral segment, especially, displays a number of important anatomic differences from higher lumbar levels (Fig. 4). The intervertebral discs are oval with a transverse diameter wider than the sagittal diameter. The discs are slightly larger than the adjacent end plates, especially in the lower lumbar spine. The annulus fibrosus blends with the strong fibers of the anterior longitudinal ligament and the considerably thinner posterior longitudinal ligament (Fig. 1). The posterior disc margin is slightly concave toward the vertebral canal; an exception is the lumbosacral disc, in which the margin is straight or slightly convex. The thecal sac (dura) is firmly attached to the posterior disc circumference, and the posterior longitudinal ligament fans out and is firmly interwoven with the annulus fibrosus; the dura is attached to this ligament, except at the lumbosacral level, where adipose epidural tissue intermingled with epidural veins is occasionally interposed between the disc and the dura. This tissue layer continues into the anterior portion of the sacral canal. The annulus fibrosus of most discs is thick at the anterior and lateral circumference of the disc and considerably thinner at the posterolateral aspect. The nucleus pulposus lies slightly posterior to the geometric center of the disc, surrounded by light fibrocartilaginous layers of the inner annulus. The nucleus and the inner annular portion together account for the high signal in T1-weighted MR scans. Toward the disc periphery, the annular lamellae contain increasingly larger proportions of dense collagen, which renders these layers increasingly dark on MR images. The outer annular portions are displayed as a dark "capsular" layer on sectional anatomic images. The thecal sac is typically round or slightly triangular (Figs. 1 and 3). At the disc level, it is surrounded by epidural fat, which contains relatively few epidural veins. A vein constantly seen on both CT scans and MR images is the longitudinal vein of the anterior internal venous plexus, which connects the voluminous vein convolutions behind the posteriorly concave vertebral bodies. This longitudinal vein lies in an angle between the dura and the disc about 1 cm lateral to the midline (Figs. 1 and 3*A*). Toward the lower portion of the disc, the intervertebral foramen has a smaller sagittal diameter because the ligamentum flavum attaches to the anterior aspect of the superior articular process. At this retrodiscal level, the nerve root lies outside the foraminal outlet. Toward the pedicle, the foramen widens considerably in the sagittal plane. Most of this subpedicular space is occupied by the dorsal root ganglion (Fig. 3*A*). Most veins and the segmental artery traverse the subpedicular portion of the foramen. At the disc level, the thecal sac is bounded by the interlaminar ligamentum flavum posterolaterally (Figs. 1*B* and 3*A*). In extension and in disc degeneration with loss of intervertebral disc height, the infolding of the ligamentum flavum in combination with bulging of the disc accounts for the hourglass-shaped segmental indentations of the thecal sac that are demonstrated on myelograms. Posterior to the thecal sac, a poorly vascularized fat pad occupies the space between the right and left ligamentum flavum (Figs. 1 and 3). The interlaminar ligamentum flavum is laterally continuous with the capsular ligamentum flavum. Owing to the ligamentum flavum, which covers most of the laminae and facet joints, the nerve roots encounter no contact with bony vertebral elements posteriorly; the thecal sac abuts a bony portion of the lamina at the upper laminar border. Interposed between the lamina and the dura are some fat and epidural veins of the posterior internal venous plexus (sublaminar plexus) (Figs. 2 and 4). Few veins cover the vertebral canal aspect of the ligamentum flavum. The ligamentum flavum with its high content of elastin fibers renders a higher MR signal than do the annulus fibrosus and collagenous vertebral column ligaments. At the inferior border of the pedicle (Fig. 2), the cauda equina nerve roots have pierced the thecal envelope and lie close to the medial and

Text continued on page 277

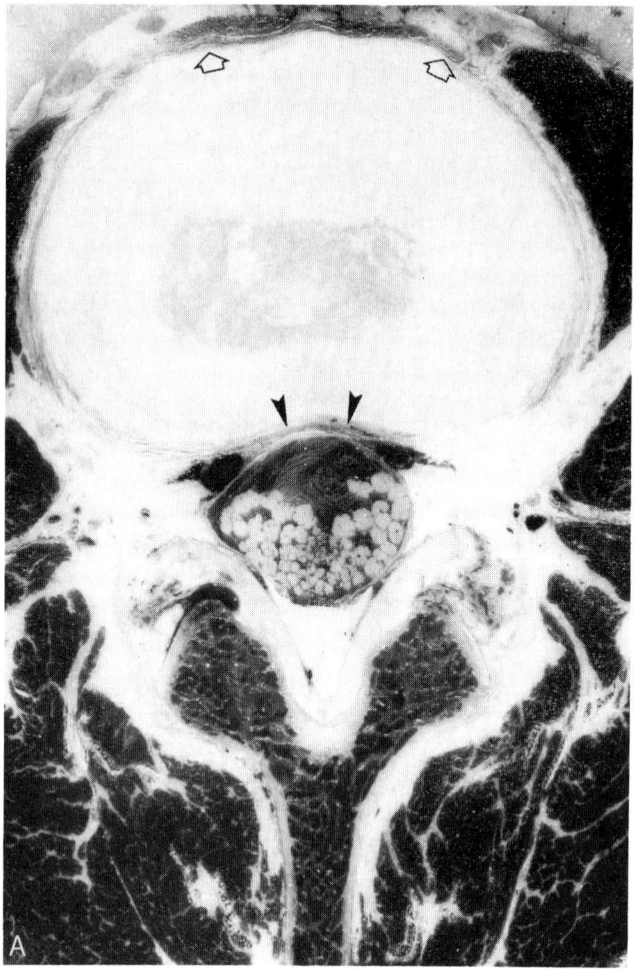

Figure 1 □ *A,* This is an axial section through the upper central portion of a normal L4–L5 intervertebral disc from a young male adult. The disc is oval and its transverse diameter is greater than its sagittal diameter. Its posterior margin is markedly concave. Darker circumferential fibers of the annulus fibrosus are blending anteriorly with the thick anterior longitudinal ligament (*open arrows*) and posteriorly with the posterior longitudinal ligament (*closed arrows*). The nucleus pulposus is in the posterior central portion of the disc and is surrounded by homogeneous fibrocartilaginous inner annular material. This material, together with the nucleus, accounts for the high MR signal in the normal disc. The cross section of the lamina displays a Y shape. The ligamentum flavum covers the entire vertebral canal aspect of the lamina (only a narrow portion of the upper lamina is devoid of this ligament insertion; for reference see sagittal sections in Figures 8 and 9). The paraspinal muscles cover the spine.

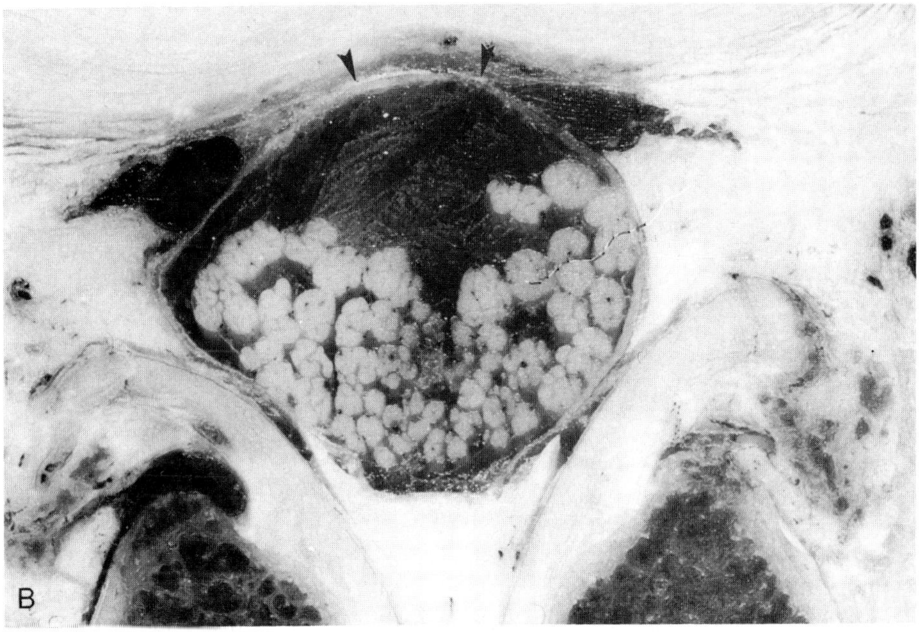

Figure 1 *Continued B,* Close-up photograph shows the vertebral canal, displaying the lumbar and sacral cauda equina nerve roots layered slightly posterior in the thecal sac. The dura is firmly attached to the posterior longitudinal ligament and posterior disc margin (*arrows*) and also abuts the ligamentum flavum. At the posterior aspect of the dura, a poorly vascularized triangular fat pad occupies the space between the dura and the laminar ligamentum flavum. This fat pad, as well as the fat lateral to the dura, renders a high MR signal and has low density on a CT scan. The longitudinal veins of the anterior internal venous plexus are located in an angle between the dura and the posterior disc margin.

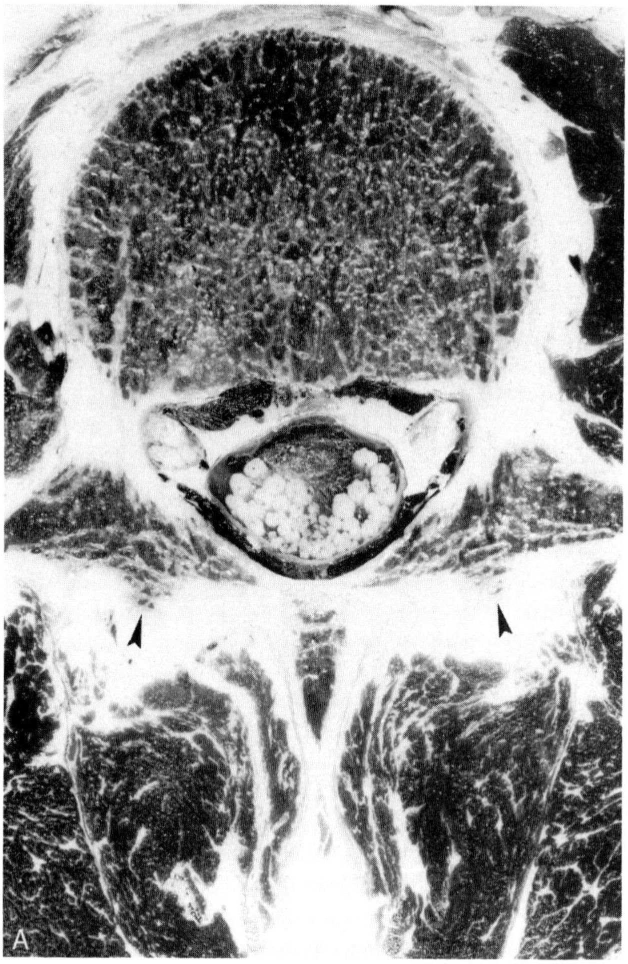

Figure 2 □ *A,* Axial section through the L4 vertebral body (same specimen as in Fig. 1), at the level of the lower pedicle. The vertebral body is covered anteriorly by the thick and broad anterior longitudinal ligament. The texture of the cancellous bone is coarse. Nerve trunks and blood vessels lie close to the lateral aspect of the vertebra deep under the psoas muscle. The transverse processes lie posterior to the lower cortical margin of the pedicles and carry, at their posterior aspect, the accessory processes (*arrows*). The thin (upper) margin of the lamina is not covered with ligamentum flavum. Posteriorly, the various layers of the erector trunci muscle can be distinguished.

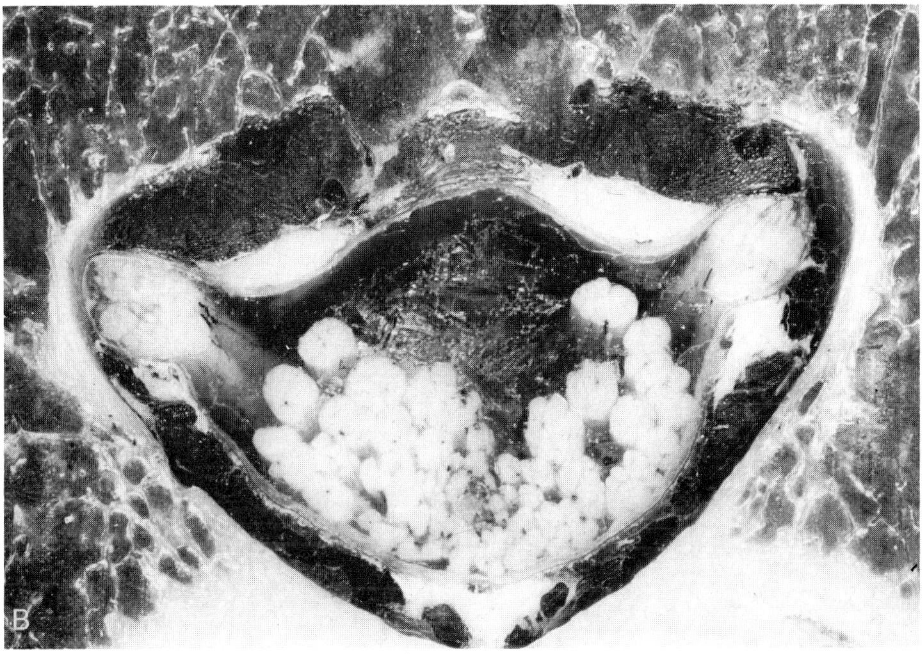

Figure 2 *Continued B,* Close up photograph of the vertebral canal of the same specimen at a slightly higher level through the inferior portion of the pedicle and upper margin of the lamina. The purely osseous boundaries of the canal are covered with the anterior and posterior internal venous plexus (*dark areas*), which surround the thecal sac. Laterally and slightly anteriorly, the root sleeves of the L4 root form axillary outpouchings that track toward the inner aspect of the pedicles. The number of cauda equina roots in each root sleeve varies. Through the frozen cerebrospinal fluid (CSF), the epineurial blood vessels can be seen. Anteriorly, the thecal sac is affixed to the posterior longitudinal ligament (PLL), which has small sagittal and transverse diameters and lies posterior to the bony margin of the vertebra. This distance is caused by the posterior bulge of the disc; the PLL stretches from disc to disc in a bowstring fashion, leaving a retrovertebral space which is occupied by a venous plexus and fat. Anterior to the PLL, the bony foramina of the basivertebral vein outlet are seen.

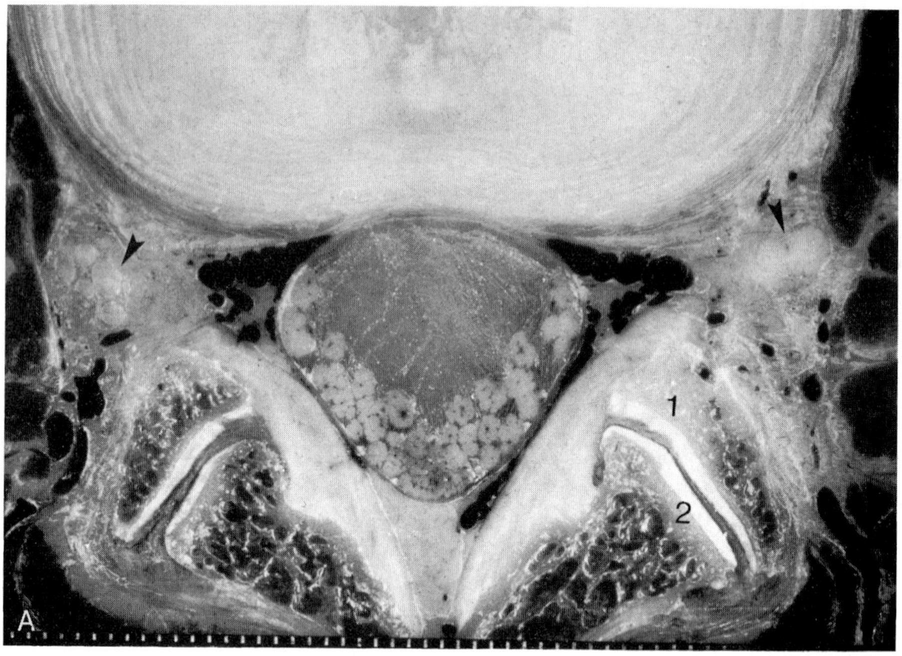

Figure 3 □ *A,* Axial cross-sectional photograph of the vertebral canal at the lower disc level of L3–L4. The disc in this specimen is less concave than the one in Figure 1. The nucleus pulposus has a cloudy appearance, and the layers of the annulus fibrosus are thicker laterally than at the posterolateral aspect, becoming increasingly dense and dark toward the periphery of the disc. The L3 nerves lie in the central portion of the foraminal outlet at some distance from the disc margin (*arrows*). The thecal sac is large; the comparatively thin cauda equina roots are layered posteriorly. Lateral to the dura, a rete of internal vertebral veins is found. The ligamentum flavum is thick and forms the joint capsule between the superior (*1*) and inferior (*2*) articular processes.

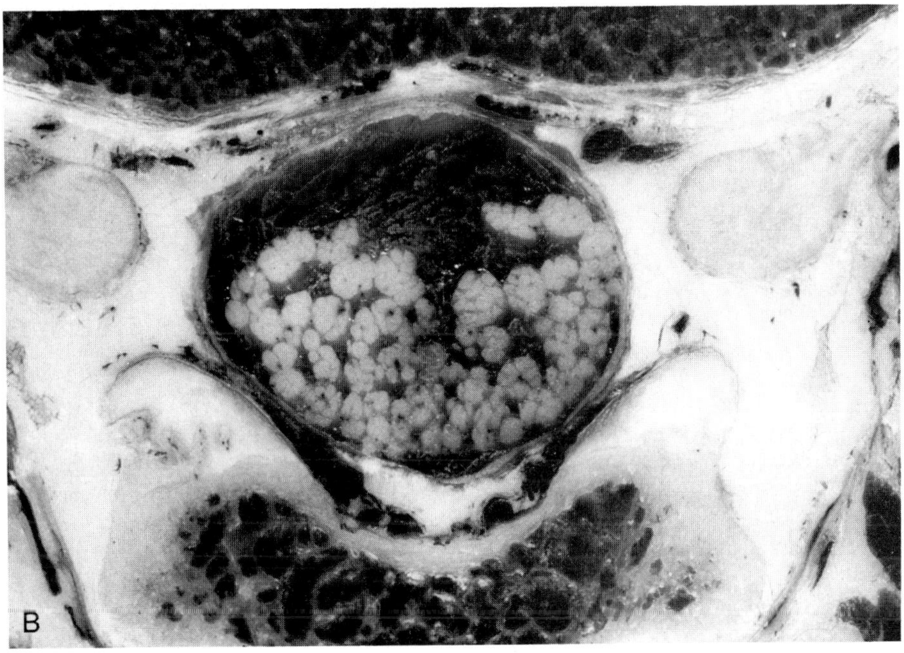

Figure 3 *Continued B,* Close-up photograph of the L3–L4 foramen 5 mm below the pedicle of L3. The vertebral body has a slightly concave posterior contour. The posterior longitudinal ligament is interposed between the dura and the vertebra. In the center of the foramen, the dorsal root ganglia of L3, surrounded by fat, are interspersed with few thin blood vessels. Posteriorly, the upper portion of the ligamentum flavum is attached to the lamina.

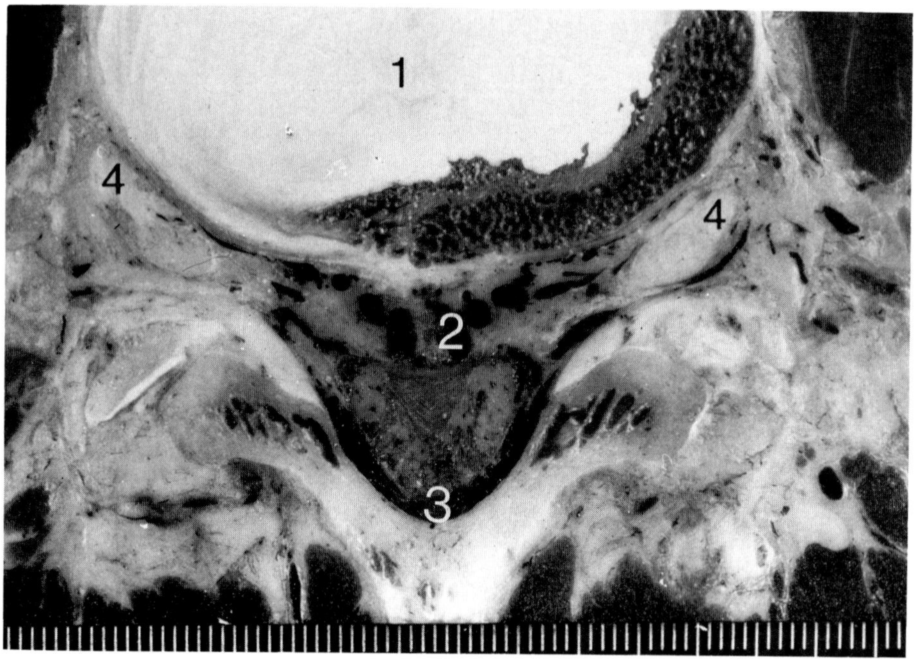

Figure 4 □ Axial photograph through the lower portion of the L5 vertebra, showing the entire length of the L5–S1 root canal. The lower end plate of L5 is oval with a convex posterior margin. The end plate is cut slightly obliquely to display the insertion of the cartilaginous end plate (*1*) into the bony end plate, which is a condensation of the cancellous bone having a honeycomb surface pattern. The triangular thecal sac lies posteriorly in the vertebral canal. The L5 root canal is longer than the canals at higher levels and tracks more anteriorly. The L5 roots follow a more horizontal course than the roots at higher lumbar levels. The layer of fat between the dura and the L5 vertebra and the upper sacrum typically carries thick veins (*2*). Veins are also seen between the dura and the lamina of L5 (*3*). At L5, the root and the dorsal root ganglion sweep around the posterolateral margin of the disc and vertebral body (*4*).

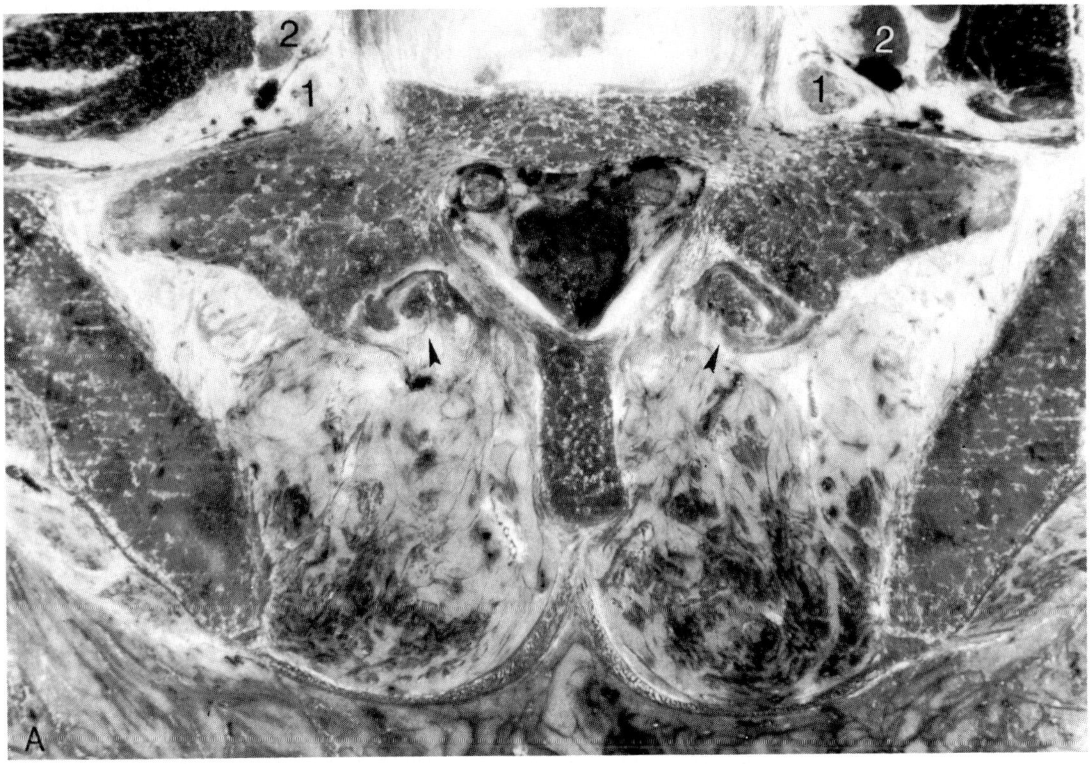

Figure 5 □ *A,* Axial section through the upper sacrum and the L5–S1 disc displays a roughly triangular upper sacral canal in which the thecal sac is located posteriorly. The S1 root sheaths lie in the anterolateral corners of the canal. The lower tips of the inferior articular processes of L5 are marked with arrows. L5 nerves are in the angle between the disc and the heavy alar portion of the sacrum, slightly anteriorly and laterally; the thick lumbosacral nerve trunk tracks are seen inferiorly (*2*). Posteriorly, the erector muscles show fatty degeneration. The muscles are covered by the thick and coarse lumbosacral fascia, which attaches to the supraspinous ligament and the posterior sacral crest. *B,* Section through the vestige of the S1–2 disc (*1*) shows dense cancellous bone in the "body" of S1 and the lamina (*2*), whereas the lateral portion of the sacrum contains bone marrow and fat and little bone. The large sacral foramina carry the S1 roots. The posterior crest of the ilium is markedly curved medially and articulates with the sacrum on the viewer's right (*3*). Sagittal placement of fixation pins would endanger the first sacral roots, in this case. The upper portion of the sacroiliac joints is marked with arrows. The fascicles of the lumbar nerves lie immediately anterior to the sacrum. *C,* Axial section through the lower sacrum and sacroiliac joints. Note the location of the sacral roots and ganglia (marked as S1–S3) and the poor quality of the cancellous bone in the lateral alar portion of the sacrum.

Illustration continued on following page

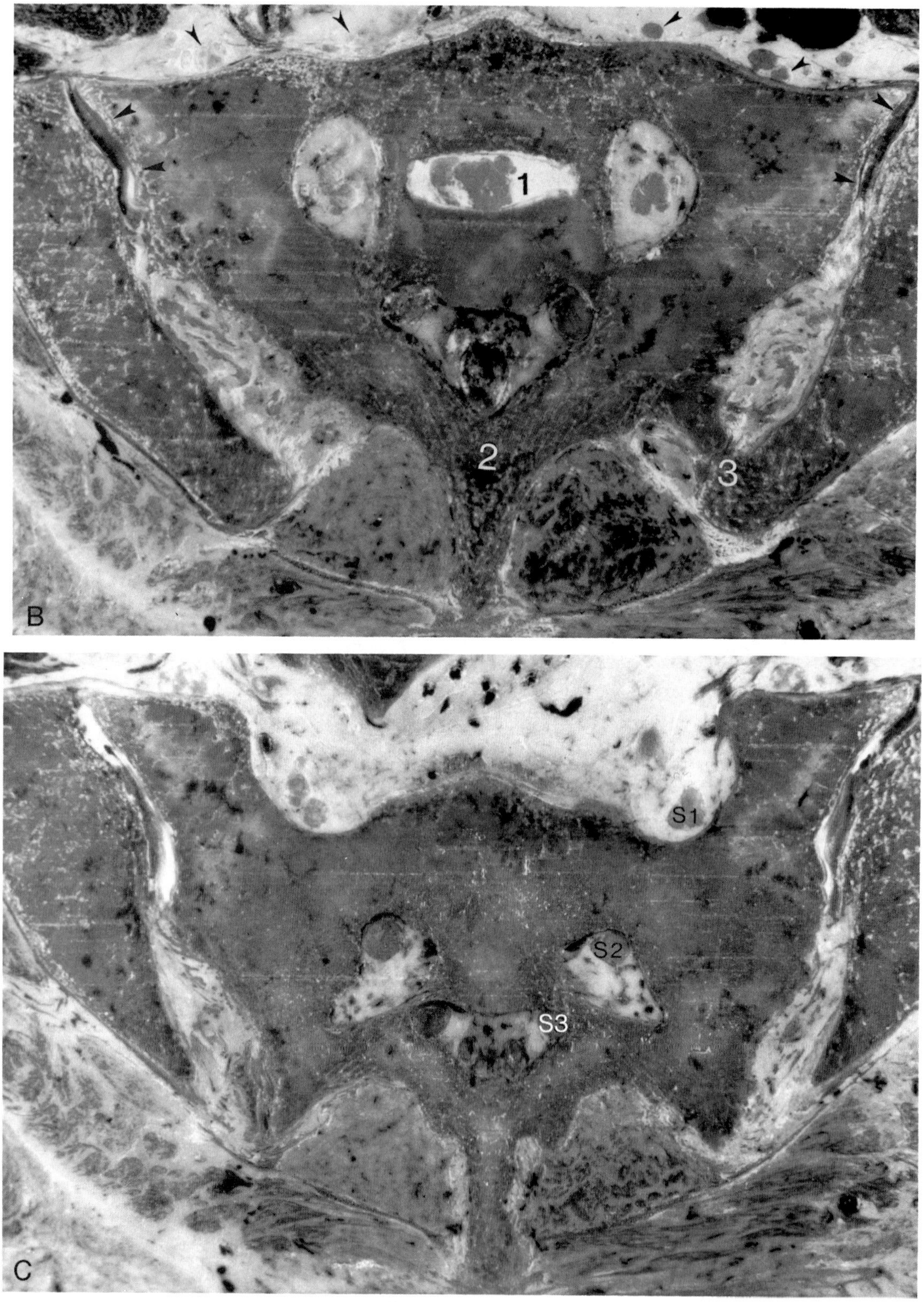

Figure 5 *Continued*

anterior aspect of the pedicle border, contained in the root sleeve. The root sleeves are continuous with the thick lumbar dorsal root ganglia, which are located immediately under the pedicles. The lumbar roots (except for the fifth lumbar root) track laterally and steeply caudally around the inner aspect of the pedicle and posterior aspect of the disc; at the infrajacent pedicle level, the lumbar nerve curves around the lateral aspect of the pedicle and the anterior base of the transverse process. The fifth lumbar root and nerve run in a long tunnel between the heavy transverse process of L5 and the ala of the sacrum. The course of this canal is more horizontal here than at higher lumbar levels (Fig. 4). Axial sections through the sacrum at different levels display dramatic changes of the cross-sectional shape of the sacrum (Fig. 5). The sacral canal is roughly triangular; the thecal sac lies in the posterior portion of the upper sacrum. Thick sacral roots and ganglia occupy a large proportion of the pelvic foramina, whereas the dorsal roots are very small. Numerous fascicles of the sacral plexus, together with veins and arteries, lie immediately anterior to the sacrum. In many cases, the alar portion of the sacrum contains much less cancellous bone than the body portion and the posterior processes of the sacrum (Fig. 5*B*, *C*).

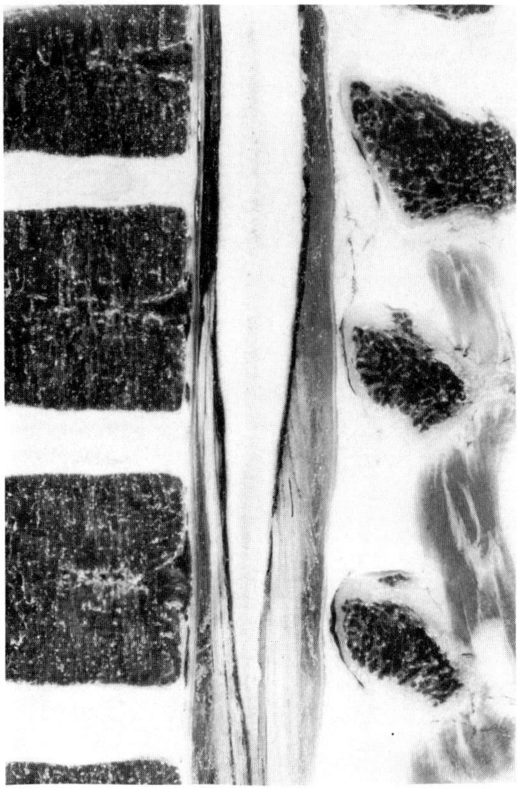

Figure 6 □ Sagittal section through the thoracolumbar region in the midline. The conus medullaris and the root bundles of the cauda equina occupy a large proportion of the subarachnoid space. The anterior wall of the vertebral canal is straight, and there is no marked bulging of the intervertebral discs. The disc height increases from T11 to L1. The thickest intumescence of the medulla is at the T11 and T12 levels; the tips of the conus usually lie at the level of the L1–L2 disc. Note that the strong periosteum at the posterior aspect of the vertebrae is continuous with the annular margin of the discs. In the epidural space, small amounts of fat and veins are seen.

SAGITTAL PLANE

In the upper lumbar spine and thoracolumbar junction, midline images display the conus medullaris together with the anterior and posterior bundles of cauda equina nerve roots, which emerge directly from the conus (contrary to the cervical and thoracic roots that form by the merging of a number of rootlets). The vertebral canal is tubular with straight anterior and posterior walls. Although the posterior vertebral and disc margins are markedly concave on axial cross sections, the vertebral body and disc contours are straight in sagittal sections (Fig. 6). A narrow band of the lamina abuts the thecal sac, and most of its posterior aspect is covered by the triangular fat pad between the right and left ligamenta flava, which fuse in the midline with a concave margin toward the vertebral canal; posteriorly, the ligamenta flava are continuous with the interspinous ligament and the supraspinous ligament complex. Toward the midlumbar and lumbosacral portion of the spine, midline sections invariably display concave vertebral body contours and the convex posterior contour of the intervertebral discs. Axial loading and extension accentuate a posteriorly convex bulge of the disc. Figure 7, *A* and *B*, demonstrates considerable interindividual differences of the vertebral column and vertebral canal. The length of the pedicles is important for the sagittal diameter of the vertebral canal. A similar pleomorphology is encountered in the lateral portion of the vertebral canal and in the foramina (root canals). Whereas most blood vessels traverse these osseoligamentous tunnels horizontally, the root complex (root sleeve, ganglion, lumbar nerve) runs in a steeply oblique di-

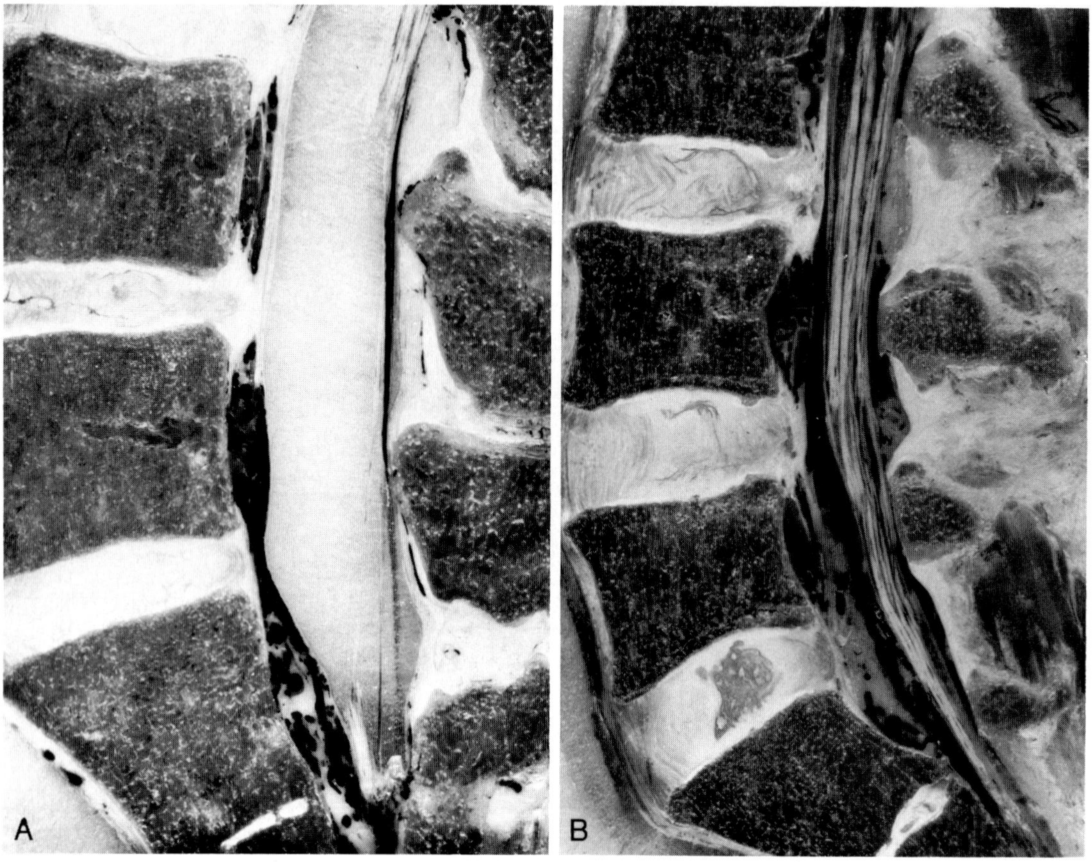

Figure 7 □ *A,* Sagittal section through a lower lumbar spine and upper sacrum in the midline, displaying a very wide vertebral canal and thecal sac. The vertebral bodies are high, and the discs are thin. The subarachnoid space shows few roots, which are located more laterally. Note the marked bulge of the L3 and L4 discs; the posterior longitudinal ligament bridges over the retrovertebral concavity in a bowstring fashion, creating a space for the anterior internal venous plexus. This venoadipose layer is thicker in the lower lumbar spine and the sacrum. The spinous processes are heavy and thick with a nearthrosis forming at L4–L5 (kissing spines). *B,* Sagittal section through a lower lumbar spine and upper sacrum in the midline showing markedly bulging thick discs and comparatively low vertebral bodies. The short pedicles in this specimen account for the small sagittal diameter of the vertebral canal. Slight disruption of annular lamellae is noted in the L3 and L4 discs, whereas the L5 disc is macroscopically normal. The congested ventral internal venous plexus occupies the retrovertebral space; the cauda equina roots are "crowded" in the small thecal sac, which is located in the posterior portion of the canal. Compared with *A,* the spinous processes are slender. Some buckling of the ligamentum flavum is noted at L4–L5.

rection, laterally and downward (Fig. 8). Because the root is the most important structure, no single imaging plane ideally displays the relationships of the root to its adjacent anatomic structures. After the offset of the root sheath from the dura immediately medial to the pedicle, the root runs through a short shallow space that is found at the inferomedial aspect of the pedicle and anterior to the medial portion of the facet joint, a space commonly referred to as the lateral recess or subarticular gutter. This space is normally deep at the lumbosacral level and very shallow or nonexistent at higher levels. In pathologic conditions in which the vertebral canal cross-sectional shape is becoming increasingly trifoliate owing to facet joint degenerative hypertrophy, lateral recesses are seen above the lumbosacral segment. The root crossing through this space is bounded laterally by the pedicle, posteriorly by the facet joint and ligamentum flavum capsule, and anteriorly by the disc. In degenerative collapse of the motion segment, the encroachment of the root by bulging disc and infolding ligamentum flavum may cause radicular compression symptoms. Venous congestion has been observed in most spec-

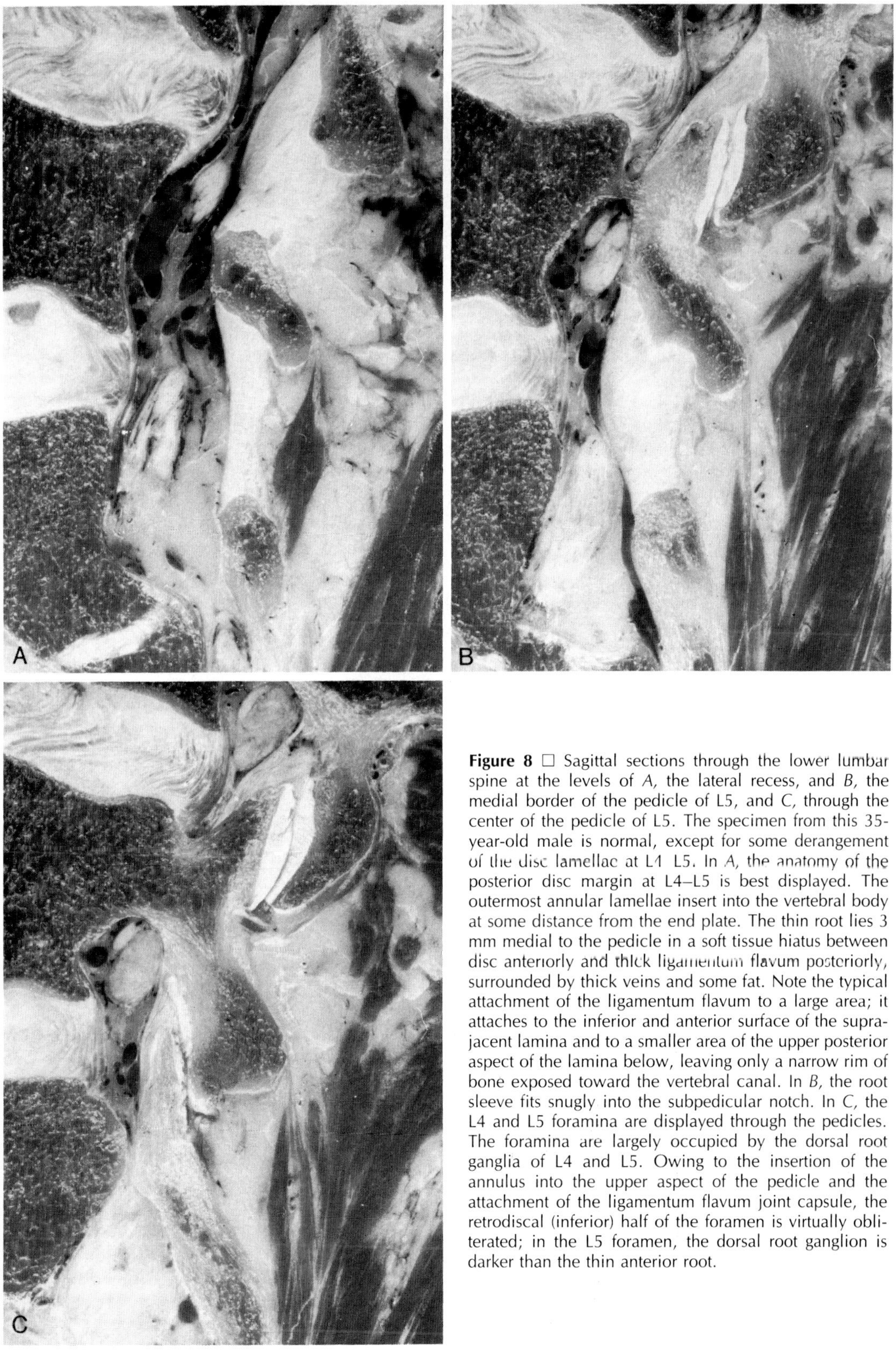

Figure 8 □ Sagittal sections through the lower lumbar spine at the levels of *A*, the lateral recess, and *B*, the medial border of the pedicle of L5, and *C*, through the center of the pedicle of L5. The specimen from this 35-year-old male is normal, except for some derangement of the disc lamellae at L4–L5. In *A*, the anatomy of the posterior disc margin at L4–L5 is best displayed. The outermost annular lamellae insert into the vertebral body at some distance from the end plate. The thin root lies 3 mm medial to the pedicle in a soft tissue hiatus between disc anteriorly and thick ligamentum flavum posteriorly, surrounded by thick veins and some fat. Note the typical attachment of the ligamentum flavum to a large area; it attaches to the inferior and anterior surface of the suprajacent lamina and to a smaller area of the upper posterior aspect of the lamina below, leaving only a narrow rim of bone exposed toward the vertebral canal. In *B*, the root sleeve fits snugly into the subpedicular notch. In *C*, the L4 and L5 foramina are displayed through the pedicles. The foramina are largely occupied by the dorsal root ganglia of L4 and L5. Owing to the insertion of the annulus into the upper aspect of the pedicle and the attachment of the ligamentum flavum joint capsule, the retrodiscal (inferior) half of the foramen is virtually obliterated; in the L5 foramen, the dorsal root ganglion is darker than the thin anterior root.

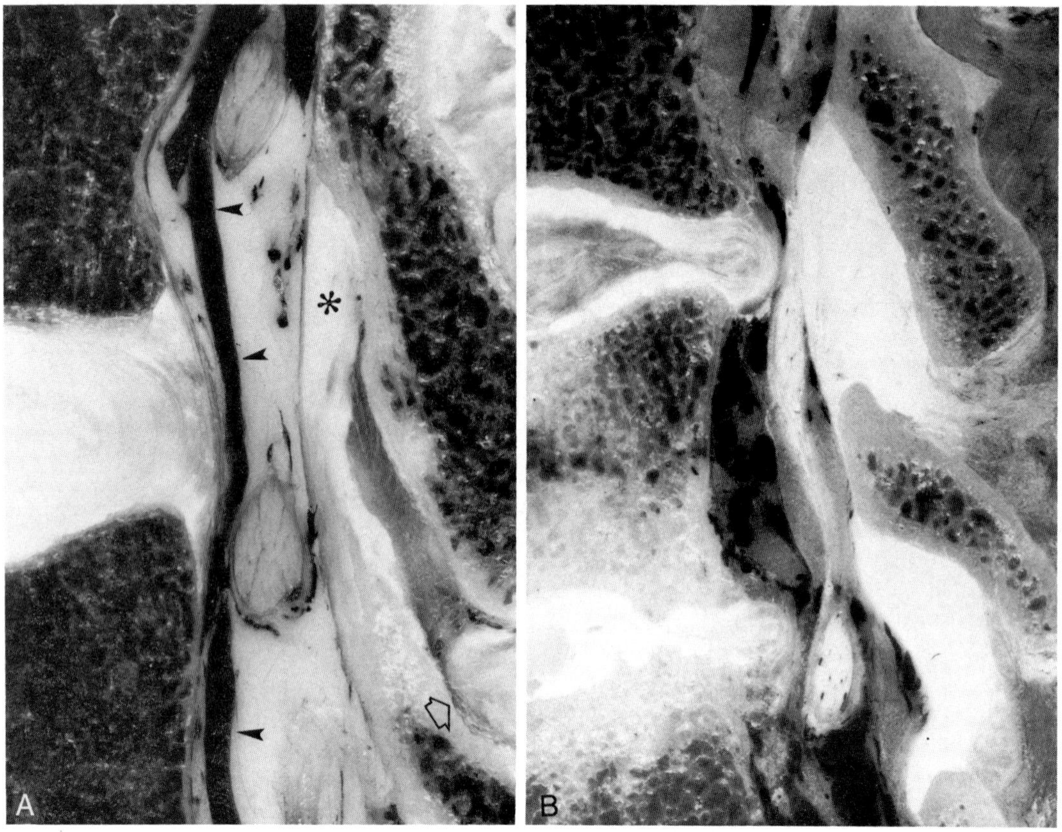

Figure 9 □ *A*, Lateral recess anatomy in the sagittal plane in a normal specimen, and *B*, a specimen with severe two-level disc degeneration. In the normal specimen, the concavity of the vertebral body and the bulge of the disc margin follow a sinusoid curvature. This is also reflected in the undulating course taken by the longitudinal ventral internal vein (which connects the retrovertebral veins of the ventral internal plexus), marked by arrowheads. The posterior boundary of the vertebral canal is osseoligamentous with a straight laminar bony wall and a soft tissue component of the interlaminar and articular ligamentum flavum (*asterisk*). Note the typical insertion of the ligamentum flavum and the slight gaping of the facet joint space, which also displays a meniscoid fold inferiorly (*open arrow*). In *B*, the L4–L5 disc is severely degenerated; at L5–S1, the total resorption of the disc with fusion of the cartilaginous end plates is associated with sclerosis adjacent to the end plates. At both levels, a sharp and marked posterior disc bulge causes infolding of the peripheral annular layers into the vertebral canal. At the L4–L5 level this infolding is accompanied by the anterior bulging of the retracted (shortened) ligamentum flavum, catching the L5 root in a soft tissue hiatus.

imens with appreciable degenerative disc disease (Fig. 9). In severe cases, the collapse of a lumbar motion segment causes severe compromise of the root at a considerable length because the superior articular process migrates anteriorly and superiorly into the subpedicular notch, pushing the retracted ligamentum flavum capsule against the root and foraminal blood vessels (Fig. 10).

CORONAL PLANE

Owing to the lordotic curvature of the lumbar spine, coronal images cannot display all segments in a true coronal plane. Curved coronal reconstructed CT scans may be used to visualize the anterior wall of the vertebral canal in its entirety. For MR imaging, the coronal plane almost ideally displays the course of the intrathecal and foraminal roots and their relationships to the pedicles. This plane also renders valuable information about the segmental arterial blood supply and venous drainage. The internal and external veins of the spine communicate not only through the foramina and vertebral bodies, but also through venous channels that run through the pedicles (Fig. 11). The very close relationship of the intrathecal cauda equina roots, as well as the root sleeves and ganglia, to the pedicles is illustrated in Figure 11. Improved MR resolution is expected

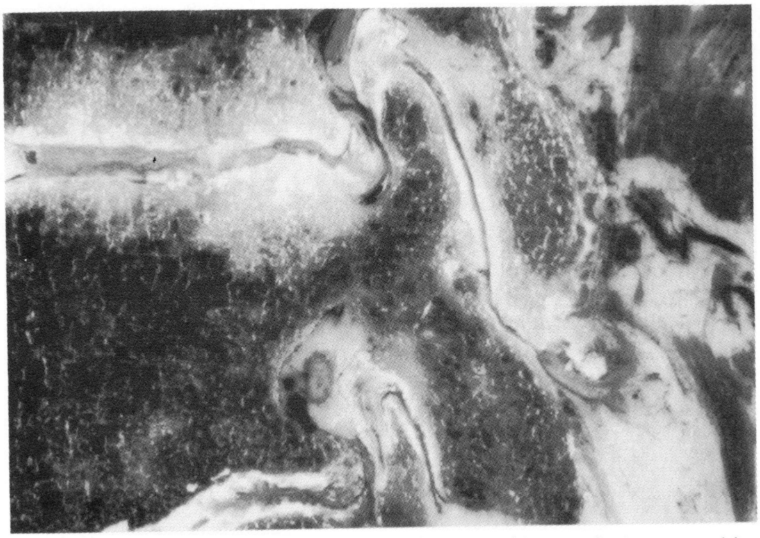

Figure 10 □ Sagittal section photograph through the L4 and L5 foramina of a severely degenerated lumbar spine. At L4–L5, severe disc degeneration is associated with end plate sclerosis; the L5 disc is subtotally resorbed. The marked bulge of both discs and the subluxation of the facet joints caused by the disc-height collapse completely obliterate the lower portion of the foramina and also cause sharp infolding of the capsular ligamentum flavum into the subpedicular notch, compressing the L4 root from the posterior direction.

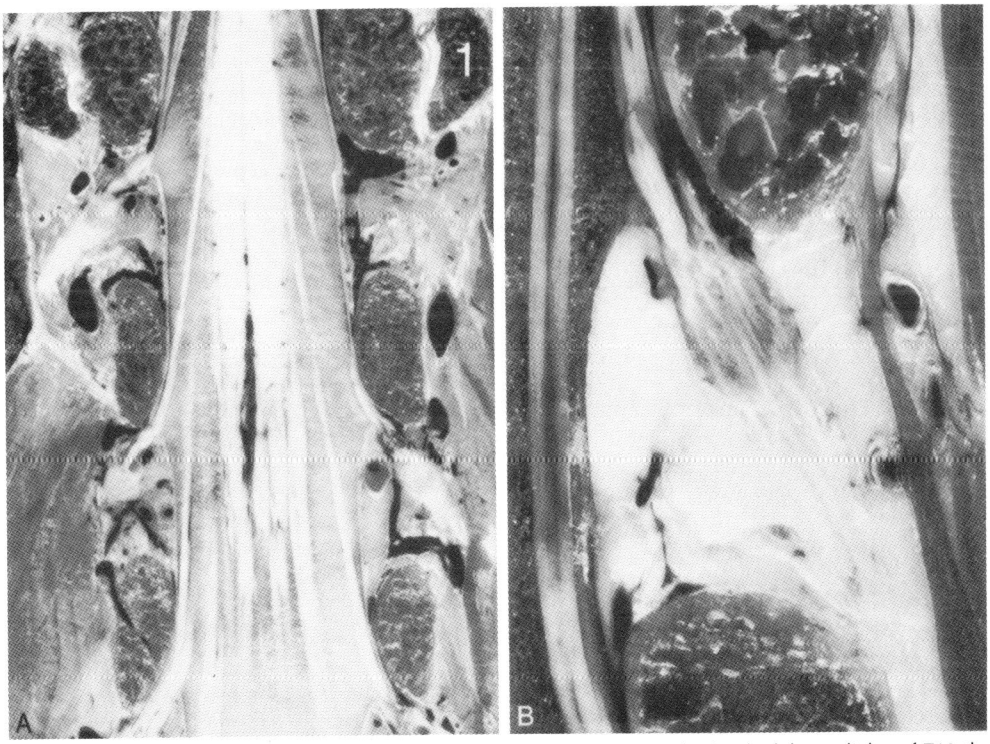

Figure 11 □ *A,* This is a coronal section through the thoracolumbar junction at the level of the pedicles of T12 through L2. Note the twelfth ribs (1). The craniocaudal diameter of the pedicles is greater than their transverse diameter. The anterior portion of the conus medullaris is displayed, together with the ventral roots, which take a steep course toward their foramen. The thecal sac is wide and snugly follows the inner contour of the pedicles, rendering shallow the axillary pouches at the inferomedial aspect of each pedicle that is pierced by the roots. The roots lie in close contact with the medial and lower aspect of the pedicles. The dorsal root ganglia are located halfway between the pedicles and almost outside the foramina, surrounded by large bodies of fat intermingled with blood vessels. *B,* Close-up photograph of a typical upper lumbar foramen in the coronal plane shows a cylindric dorsal root ganglion lying obliquely between the pedicles. The postganglionic lumbar nerve tracks steeply downward and sweeps around the superolateral aspect of the infrajacent pedicle.

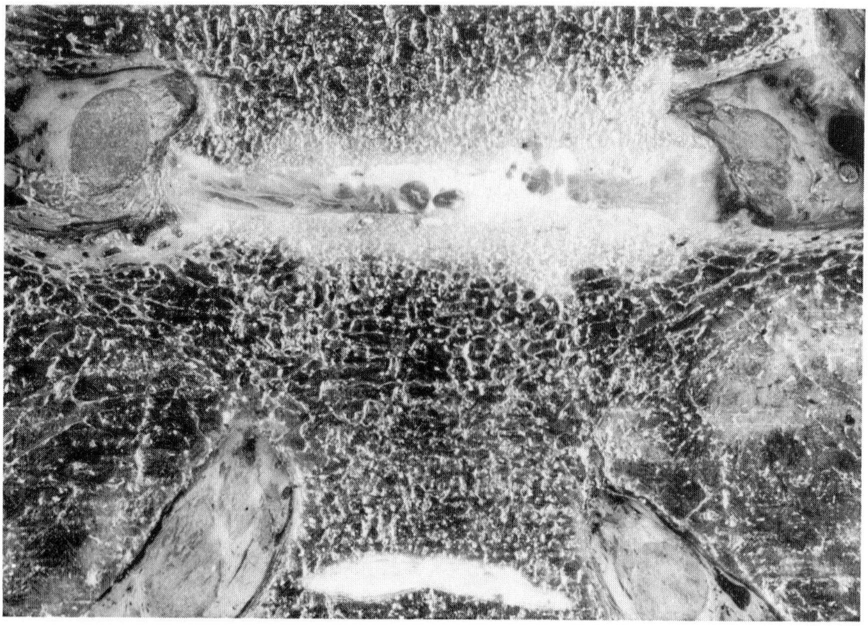

Figure 12 □ Coronal section through the lumbosacral segment and the sacral foramina of S1. The lumbosacral disc is subtotally resorbed with partial fusion of the cartilaginous end plates and accentuated sclerosis of the end plates, also causing the formation of circumferential (spondylotic) end plate ridges. The L5 nerves lie under the heavy transverse process of L5 and the ala of the sacrum, and they are stretched around the hypertrophic end plates.

to demonstrate circulatory disturbances as well as inflammatory changes in the vulnerable neurovascular elements; the coronal plane displays these structures on two sides, thereby allowing a comparative assessment on MR scans. Sections through the lamina and the facet joints display the articular processes and the transverse processes. Images through the posterior portion of the L5 vertebral body show the relationships of the fifth lumbar nerves to the transverse process of L5 and the ala of the sacrum outside the foramen. This space may be critically narrow in disc height collapse, in combination with scoliotic deformity (Fig. 12).

References

1. Batson, O.V.: The vertebral vein system. Am. J. Roentgenol. 78:195–200, 1957.
2. Breig, A.: Adverse Mechanical Tension in the Central Nervous System. An Analysis of Cause and Effect. Relief by Functional Neurosurgery. New York, Almqvist & Wiksell International (Stockholm) and John Wiley & Sons, 1978.
3. Bo, W.J., Meschan, J., and Krueger, W.A.: Basic Atlas of Cross-Sectional Anatomy. Philadelphia, W.B. Saunders, 1980.
4. Burton, C.V., Heithoff, K.B., Kirkaldy-Willis, W., and Ray, D.C.: Computed tomographic scanning and the lumbar spine. II. Clinical considerations. Spine 4:356–368, 1979.
5. Cahill, D.R., and Orland, M.J.: Atlas of Human Cross-Sectional Anatomy. Philadelphia, Lea & Febiger, 1984.
6. Carter, B.L.: Cross-Sectional Anatomy, Computed Tomography and Ultrasound Correlation. Adopted from the Eyclesheimer-Schoemaker Atlas of 1911. New York, Appleton-Century-Crofts, 1977.
7. Crock, H.V., and Yoshizawa, H.: The Blood Supply of the Vertebral Column and Spinal Cord in Man. New York, Springer-Verlag, 1977.
8. Eisenstein, S.: The trefoil configuration of the lumbar vertebral canal. A study of South African skeletal material. J. Bone Joint Surg. 62B:73–76, 1980.
9. Eyclesheimer, A.C., and Schoemaker, D.M.: A Cross-Section Anatomy. New York, Appleton-Century-Crofts, 1911, reedited 1970.
10. Gambarelli, J., Guérinel, G., Chevrot, L., and Mattèi, M.: Computerized Axial Tomography. An Anatomic Atlas of Serial Sections of the Human Body. Anatomy-Radiology Scanner. New York, Springer-Verlag, 1977.
11. Genant, H.K., Chafetz, N., and Helms, C.A.: Computed Tomography of the Lumbar Spine. San Francisco, Department of Radiology, University of California, 1982.
12. Hadley, L.A.: Anatomical-roentgenographic studies of the posterior spinal articulations. Am. J. Roentgenol. 86:270–276, 1961.
13. Haughton, V.M., and Williams, A.L.: Computed Tomography of the Spine. St. Louis, C.V. Mosby, 1982.
14. Heithoff, K.B., and Ray, C.D.: Principles of the computed tomographic assessment of lateral spinal stenosis. *In* Genant, H.K. (ed.): Spine Update. San Francisco, Radiology Research and Educational Foundation, 1984.

15. Hollingshead, W.H.: The Back and Limbs. Anatomy for Surgeons, Vol. III. New York, Harper & Row, 1982.
16. Kieffer, S.A., and Heitzman, E.R.: An Atlas of Cross-Sectional Anatomy. Computed Tomography, Ultrasound, Radiography, Gross Anatomy. New York, Harper & Row, 1979.
17. Lancourt, J.E., Glenn, W.V., and Wiltse, L.L.: Multiplanar computerized tomography in the normal spine and in the diagnosis of spinal stenosis. A gross anatomic computerized tomographic correlation. Spine 4:379–390, 1979.
18. Lang, J., and Wachsmuth, W.: Praktische Anatomie. Ein Lehr- und Hilfsbuch der Anatomischen Grundlagen arztlichen Handelns. New York, Springer-Verlag, 1972.
19. Ledley, R.S., Huang, H.K., and Mazziotta, J.C.: Cross-Sectional Anatomy. An Atlas for Computed Tomography. Baltimore, Williams & Wilkins, 1977.
20. Lee, B.C.P., Kazam, E., and Newman, A.D.: Computed tomography of the spine and spinal cord. Radiology 128:95–102, 1978.
21. Lyons, E.A.: A Color Atlas of Sectional Anatomy. Chest, Abdomen and Pelvis. St. Louis, C.V. Mosby, 1978.
22. Peterson, R.R.: A Cross-Sectional Approach to Anatomy. Chicago, Year Book Medical Publishers, 1980.
23. Post, M.J.D.: Computed Tomography of the Spine. Baltimore, Williams & Wilkins, 1984.
24. Rauschning, W.: Detailed sectional anatomy of the spine. *In* Rothman S.L.G., and Glenn, W.V. (eds.): Multiplanar CT of the Spine. Baltimore, University Park Press, 1985.
25. Resnick, D., and Niwayama, G.: Degenerative Disease of the Spine. Diagnosis of Bone and Joint Disorders. Philadelphia, W.B. Saunders, 1981.
26. Rosse, C., and Clawson, D.K.: The Musculoskeletal System in Health and Disease. New York, Harper & Row, 1980.
27. Rothman, S.L.G., and Glenn, W.V. (eds.): Multiplanar CT of the Spine. Baltimore, University Park Press, 1985.
28. Schmorl, G., and Junghanns, H.: The Human Spine in Health and Disease. New York, Grune & Stratton, 1971.
29. Schnitzlein, H.N., Hartley, E.W., Murtagh, F.R., et al.: Computed Tomography of the Head and Spine. A Photographic Color Atlas of CT, Gross, and Microscopic Anatomy. Baltimore, Urban & Schwarzenberg, 1983.
30. Yong-Hing, K., Reilly, J., and Kirkaldy-Willis, W.H.: The ligamentum flavum. Spine 1:226–234, 1976.

■ COMPUTED TOMOGRAPHY AND PLAIN FILM DIAGNOSIS OF THE LUMBAR SPINE

Kenneth B. Heithoff

Computed tomography (CT) is but one method of imaging the lumbar spine. The advent of magnetic resonance imaging (MRI) raises many questions about which test is most appropriate for each individual and whether any definable areas exist in which MRI has replaced and/or should replace CT.

In this chapter, I will indicate how CT is currently utilized in our lumbar spine practice and how it interdigitates with the plethora of other imaging modalities and tests available (i.e., MRI, myelography, plain films, contrast-enhanced CT [intravenous and intrathecal], discography, and disco-CT). In our increasingly cost-conscious but more complex world of imaging, assisting the clinician in the appropriate selection and sequencing of tests in order to obtain the most information for the least cost is becoming a more vital role for the consulting radiologist. Our experience is drawn from the more than 80,000 CT scans of the lumbar spine we have performed since 1976 and 15,000 MR scans of the lumbar spine performed from 1986 to 1989.

CT continues to be our procedure of choice for lumbar spine imaging of nonoperated patients. In our environment, CT is approximately one half the cost of MR and is a complete screening examination for degenerative spine disease, including disc herniation (herniated nucleus pulposus, or HNP) and stenosis.

In our tertiary referral practice, anteroposterior (AP) and lateral CT scout images are obtained in every case and serve as our plain films. They are essential for orientation and correlation of the findings noted on axial images. They are adequate for detecting abnormalities of spinal alignment, loss of disc height, gross degenerative changes, and/or bony destruction. We rarely, if ever, require additional plain films.

In each case, the AP and lateral computed radiographs are reviewed for disc space narrowing, end-plate changes, and degenerative spurring. The AP computed radiograph is utilized to determine the number of lumbar vertebrae and the presence of any transitional vertebrae and/or other congenital anomalies.

Abnormalities of bony alignment such as lytic or degenerative spondylolisthesis, retrolisthesis, scoliosis, and kyphosis are noted. Hyperlordosis, increased lumbosacral angulation, and the level of the intracristal line are noted on the lateral computed radiograph. Comment is also made regarding the hip joints and sacroiliac (SI) joints, which are routinely included on the AP computed radiograph.

Routine, 5-mm axial nonangled images are obtained from the anterosuperior margin of the S1 vertebra to the midpedicle of L3. Axial images are spaced at 3-mm increments at L5–S1 for improved resolution of the reformatted images. Survey images are obtained at L1–L2 and L2–L3 if the lateral computed radiographs demonstrate abnormalities at those levels, or if the patient's pain drawing indicates groin or anterior thigh pain (each patient is asked to fill out a detailed history of lumbar spine symptoms, including a pain drawing). This routine has been successful in detecting a number of lateral L2–L3 disc herniations and a very occasional L1–L2 herniation (Fig. 1).

Sagittal reformatted images are a necessary part of every CT examination of the lumbar spine. We utilize a General Electric reformatting program on a remote console that reformats the images in background. A complete set of reformatted images is obtained through both entire nerve root canals and the central spinal canal, beginning on the right and extending to the left at 3-mm intervals; an axial image of the L5–S1 intervertebral canals is used as a reference. Other off-site programs are available for reformatting. However, the advantage of on-site reformatting is that axial and reformatted images are available for interpretation within minutes after completion of the examination, expediting interpretation and consultation with referring physicians. We have not found coronal images to add significant information to lumbar spine imaging and, as with MRI, routinely utilize only axial and sagittal images.

Three-dimensional (3-D) imaging has not been accepted by our clinicians, nor is it believed in our practice to add essential diagnostic information; therefore, it is infrequently used in our practice. I believe that it could, however, play a significant role in helping to plan the surgical approach for a patient with lateral stenosis by better defining the exact size and location of the osteo-

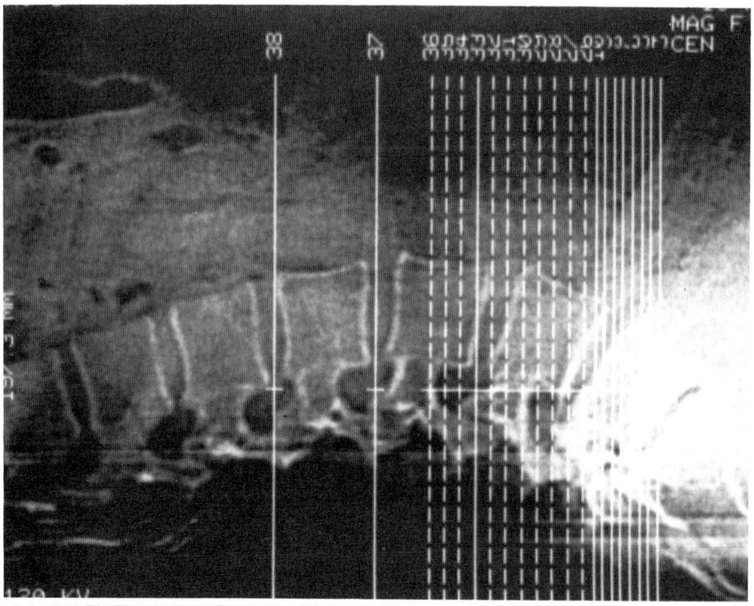

Figure 1 □ Lateral computed radiograph of the lumbar spine showing our scanning technique. Note that the scans obtained at L5–S1 are 3-mm adjacent images and/or 5-mm images with 3 mm of table incrementation. Scans of 5 mm are obtained from the midpedicle of L5 to the L3 pedicle, and survey images were obtained at L1–L2 and L2–L3. Survey images are obtained at L1–L2 and L2–L3 when there is evidence of degenerative disc disease on the lateral computed radiograph or when the patient has symptoms referable to the upper lumbar region (i.e., groin or anterior thigh pain). Axial adjacent images from L3 to S1 are obtained to provide continuous imaging of the lumbar anatomy and to allow sagittal reformatted images of the lower spine for quantification of lateral spinal stenosis.

phytic spur and its relationship to other bony structures. In other words, it does not add additional diagnostic information for the skilled spine radiologist, but it can be useful for communicating the 2-D information to his or her surgical colleagues, as a teaching device for learning radiologists, and for those unfamiliar with or unaccepting of the concept of lateral spinal stenosis. In my experience, the most common surgical error is failing to extend the decompression of the intervertebral nerve root canal sufficiently laterally at L5–S1 when the caudal surface of the pedicle is causing compression of the ganglia beyond the superior articular process, which results in residual far-lateral stenosis. A 3-D representation makes it much easier to visualize this lesion and to understand the necessary surgical approach.

LATERAL ENTRAPMENT SYNDROMES

Lateral stenosis is much more common than recognized prior to the advent of the cross-sectional imaging modalities of CT and MRI. In our experience, it is the most common cause of failed lumbar spinal surgery. Therefore, a thorough understanding of the types and location of stenosis, as well as the appropriate surgical approaches for correction, is essential. I will discuss our concepts in considerable detail.

The pathogenesis of lumbar spondylosis and stenosis is believed to be recurrent rotational strains that result in simultaneous disc resorption, loss of disc height, formation of osteophytes (uncinate spurs), and degenerative enlargement of facets. [1–10] Repeated rotational strains and other insults and injuries, combined with normal aging, accelerate degenerative disc disease and produce degenerative changes in the posterior zygapophyseal joints.[6–7] Changes in the disc are inevitably associated with degenerative changes in the posterior zygapophyseal joints and vice versa. This concept of a three-joint complex, proposed by Farfan and popularized by Kirkaldy-Willis, is well supported by experimental and clinical evidence.[2–5]

Loss of disc height is caused by internal disruption, resorption, chemonucleolysis, infection, and the sequelae of discectomy.[6, 9] Pathologic conditions of the posterior zygapophyseal joint accompanying disc degeneration and loss of disc volume are capsular laxity, ligamentous instability, and posterior joint strain with subsequent overriding and subluxation of the posterior joints.

Later changes in the superior and inferior articular processes include hypertrophy and osteophyte formation, which reflects subperiosteal bone deposition. Enlargement of the inferior articular facets by those pathologic processes may result in central stenosis (Fig. 2). Compression of a spinal nerve may occur either within the subarticular recess of the central spinal canal or more distally within the nerve root canal; that is, the L5 nerve root may be compressed proximally at the L4–L5 level or distally within the L5–S1 intervertebral nerve root canal. The subarticular recess is a pathologic narrowing of the spinal recess of the central canal. It is not to be confused with stenosis of the intervertebral nerve root canal (lateral stenosis). Subarticular stenosis is a central phenomenon and results in compression of the traversing nerve root (i.e., L5 at L4–L5), rather than the exiting nerve root (see Fig. 6*A*). The zygapophyseal joints may become widened or narrowed, and the joint surface may be irregular or frayed. Hypertrophic overgrowth of the superior and inferior articular facets, as well as osteophytes, is common evidence of these degenerative changes.

Asymmetric orientation of the zygapophyseal joints (tropism) and asymmetric failure of formation, or maldevelopment, are believed by some to be predisposing factors in degenerative spondylosis because of the unequal stress loading of the spine.[5] Asymmetry of the transitional vertebrae, such as partial, unilateral lumbarization of the first sacral segment (present in nearly one half of a large series of transitional vertebrae that we recently studied), may also contribute to unequal stress loading and a higher incidence of low back pain. We have found a significant number of cases of lateral spinal stenosis at the transitional level (i.e., S1–S2 in cases of lumbarization of S1) on the side of the lumbarization, owing to unilateral motion, with degenerative facet hypertrophy and osteophytes at the margin of the transitional disc. We have also noted a greater incidence of disc herniation at the level above the immobile, persistently sacralized side, apparently placing increased stress on the disc above. Bony entrapment of lumbar nerve roots may be produced by the follow-

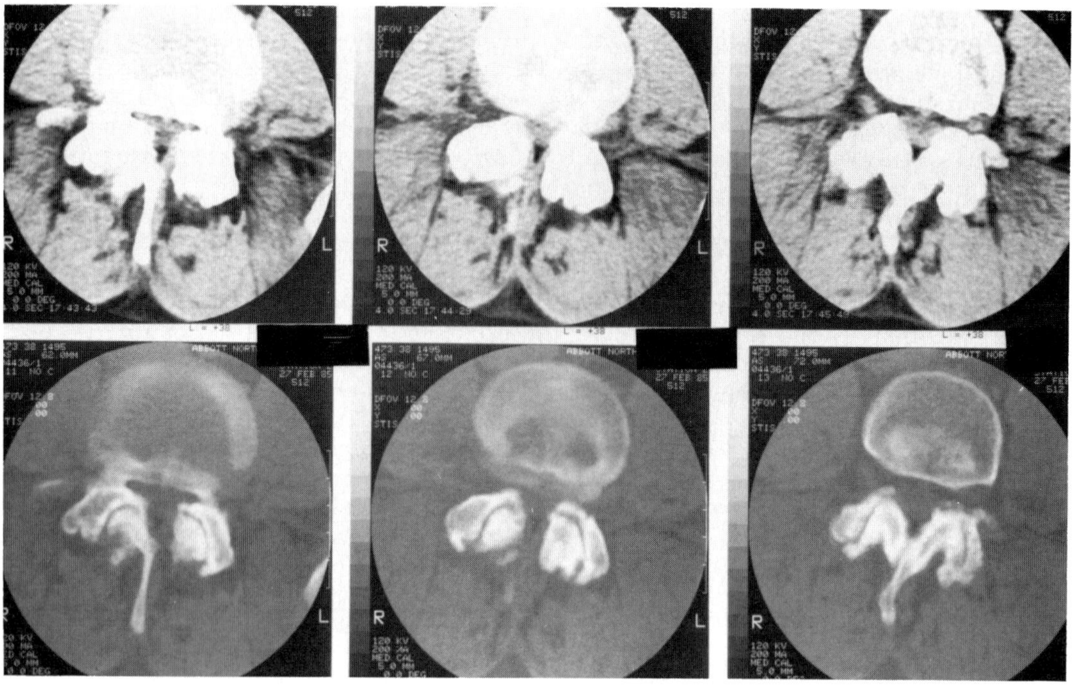

Figure 2 □ Axial soft tissue and bone images at the L4 level in a patient with degenerative spondylolisthesis at L4–L5. Note the severe degenerative facet disease with erosive narrowing of the facet joints and erosion of the anteromedial aspect of the superior articular process, allowing forward subluxation of the intact neural arch of L4 on L5. The medial hypertrophy of the thinned anterior aspects of the superior articular processes and hypertrophy of the inferior articular processes are impinging on the dorsolateral aspect of the central spinal canal and, in conjunction with thickening of the ligamentum flavum, are producing a moderate to moderately severe central spinal stenosis and bilateral subarticular recess stenoses. Note the associated central disc bulge, which contributes to narrowing of the central spinal canal and more prominent left-sided subarticular recess impingement. In most patients, the spondylolisthesis is responsible for the greatest portion of the visualization of the central portion of the involved L4–L5 disc; mild degenerative central bulging of the disc annulus is present in most patients and, not uncommonly, any associated contained central disc herniation. Central disc herniation as is present in this case is denoted by the asymmetry of the disc. In many patients, the exiting L4 nerve roots are compressed by lateral bulging of the disc, which produces a homogeneous appearance of the intervertebral nerve root canals, which is not present in this patient.

ing separate processes, which occur singly or in combination: (1) degenerative hypertrophy and instability, (2) developmental stenosis, usually with superimposed degeneration, and (3) lesions, such as trauma or lytic spondylolisthesis, that produce direct entrapment of the spinal nerves.[6, 15–17]

Central and lateral spinal stenoses are not separate entities but rather are sequelae of the spectrum of spondylosis that occur during the course of the above three pathologic processes. Developmental stenosis is ordinarily asymptomatic until the secondary development of degenerative spondylosis or disc protrusion causes a critical narrowing of the central canal or subarticular recess. Spondylosis and stenosis are not synonymous, however, and degenerative changes may produce an enlargement of the articular processes without a narrowing of the central spinal canal or lateral nerve root canals. Fixed lateral spinal stenosis with nerve root entrapment within the intervertebral nerve root canal is more common in the patient population we examine than is either subarticular recess or central spinal stenosis. Anatomically severe lateral stenosis may be present without associated symptoms, apparently as a result of the lumbar nerve root and ganglia adapting to gradually increasing compression. In such cases, cadaver studies show a marked attenuation of the nerve roots with intact microvascularity.

In most cases of lumbar lateral spinal stenosis, the pathologic anatomy can accurately be diagnosed only through the use of CT or MR scanning. The severity of lateral stenosis, however, is not well demonstrated with only transaxial CT scans but requires additional sagittal reconstruction of the axial images (reformatting). Such reformatting has significantly helped to identify three types of lateral spinal stenoses as first described by Charles Ray: up-down (cephalocaudal), front-back (ventrodorsal), and pinhole (combined) (Fig. 3). The reformatted images are also important in planning the surgical approach to stenotic lesions. Recently developed 3-D reconstruction techniques are particularly useful in defining these types of stenoses and for surgical planning, as they present the lesion in a topographic format that defines for the surgeon the position, extent, and morphology of the stenosis more clearly than do axial images (Fig. 4).

Enlargement of the superior articular process (SAP) in conjunction with loss of disc height *was* thought to be the most common cause of lateral stenosis. Theoretically, as the disc loses volume, concomitant ligamentous laxity results in anterior and superior subluxation of the SAP of the vertebra below. As the disc space narrows more markedly, the superior articular process underrides the pedicle above, and the nerve root exiting at that level may become entrapped.

Although entrapment or pressing of a root or ganglion cephalad against the pedicle by the superior tip of a hypertrophic superior facet has been thought to be common, actually it is not. The lateral stenosis occurring most frequently is the up-down type. Narrowing of the neural foramen in the cephalocaudal or vertical axis is usually associated with a collapse of the disc space and osteophyte formation. The most common osteophyte is the uncinate spur, which is anatomically analogous to the spur often seen in the cervical spine (Fig. 5). Front-back stenosis, a narrowing in the anteroposterior plane, is usually caused by hypertrophy of the superior facet, compressing the nerve root against an uncinate spur that arises from the vertebral body just caudal to the pedicle, and sometimes against an osteophytic disc bar as well (see Fig. 3*D*, *E*). This type of stenosis is seen less frequently, as is the pinhole or combined stenosis, which results from a confluent compression of the nerve structure by pedicle, facet, vertebral body, and spur.

Because of considerable variation in the nomenclature used to describe stenosis and in the appreciation of the underlying pathologic conditions and appropriate surgical treatment, we support the suggestion that the major classes of spinal stenosis be designated as *central, subarticular* (or spinal recess, as proposed by the 1988 Nomenclature Committee of the North American Spine Society), and *lateral* (Fig. 6*A*). Burton suggests the following classification: central zone, foraminal zone, and extraforaminal zone. It should be noted that the term "extraforaminal" is a misnomer and actually refers to the type of lateral stenosis at L5–S1 that involves compression of the L5 nerve ganglion between the inferior margin of the pedicle of L5 and the sacrum lateral to the SAP of S1. The L5–S1 nerve root "canal" is a complex structure and is not truly a canal throughout its entire length, since the posterior wall of the lateral third of the canal lying between the lateral aspect of the SAP of S1 and the inferolateral margin of the pedicle is open. The term extraforaminal stenosis arises out of a misunderstanding of the configuration and length of the canal. Surgeons who believe that stenosis and nerve root compression occurring lateral to the facets are extraforaminal fail to realize that the SAP of S1 is not the lateral border of the canal at L5–S1, as it is at other levels, because the pedicle of L5 flares laterally and lies considerably lateral to the SAP. Approximately one third of the L5–S1 intervertebral nerve root canal lies between the lateral aspect of the SAP of S1 and the inferolateral border of the pedicle of L5, which is the true lateral border of the L5–S1 nerve root canal (Figs. 5 and 6*B*). By definition, if the nerve root is extraforaminal, it cannot be compressed, only displaced, because it is outside the nerve root canal. Another familiar term for this type of lateral stenosis is the "far-out" stenosis of Wiltse. Again, the L5 ganglia are compressed by the pedicle of L5, not the transverse process as reported, because the L5 nerve root emerges from the canal immediately adjacent to the vertebral body.[45] None of these classifications, however, addresses pathoanatomy and structural etiology; they consider only gross location.

In review, the principal structures associated with stenosis that may be affected by pathologic changes in the low back are as follows: internal disc tissue, annulus disc end-plate margins, facet joints, vertebral bodies, laminae (neural arch and ligamentum flavum). In general, lateral stenoses usually result from a multiplicity of degenerative and proliferative processes causing the

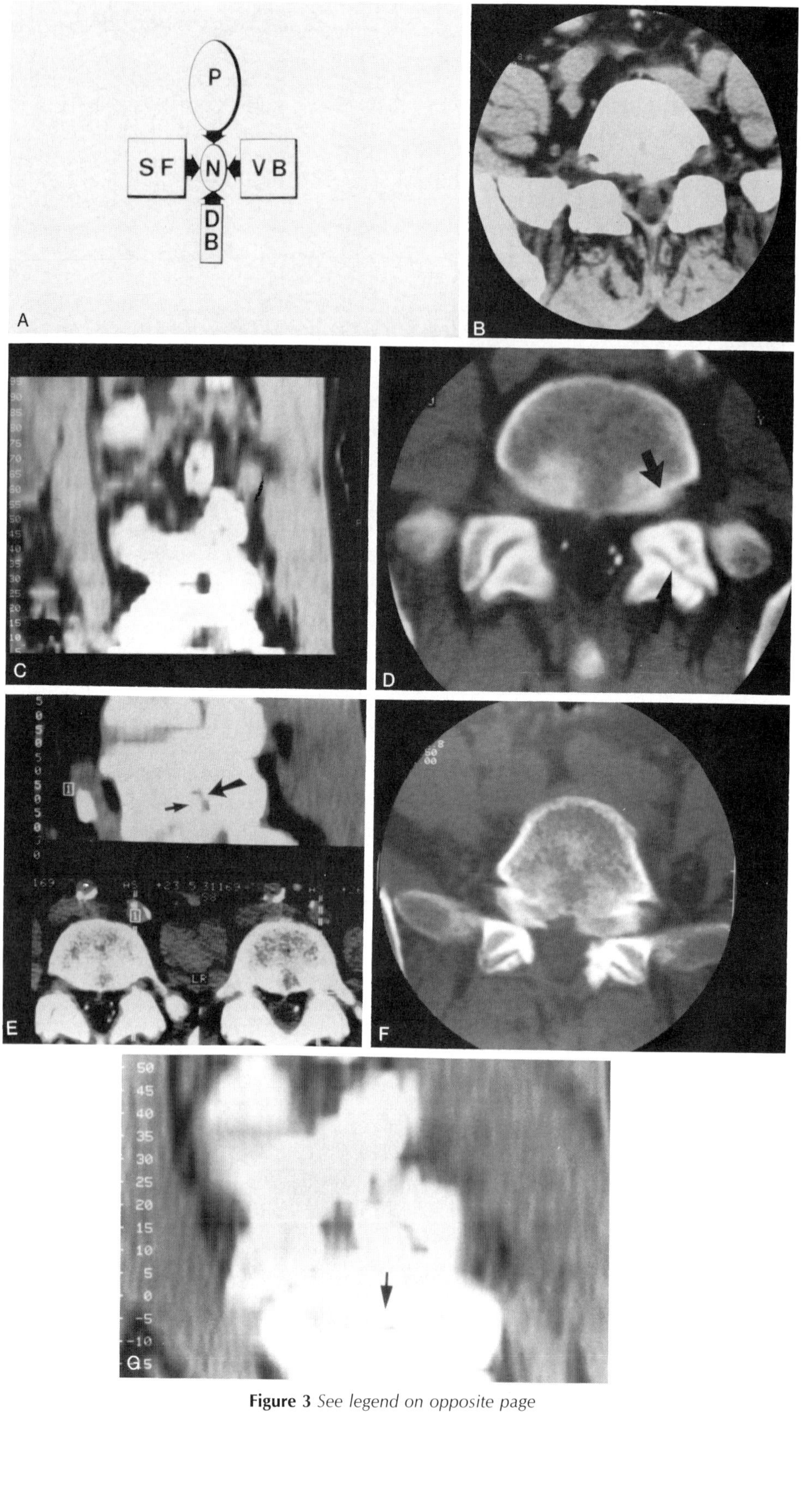

Figure 3 *See legend on opposite page*

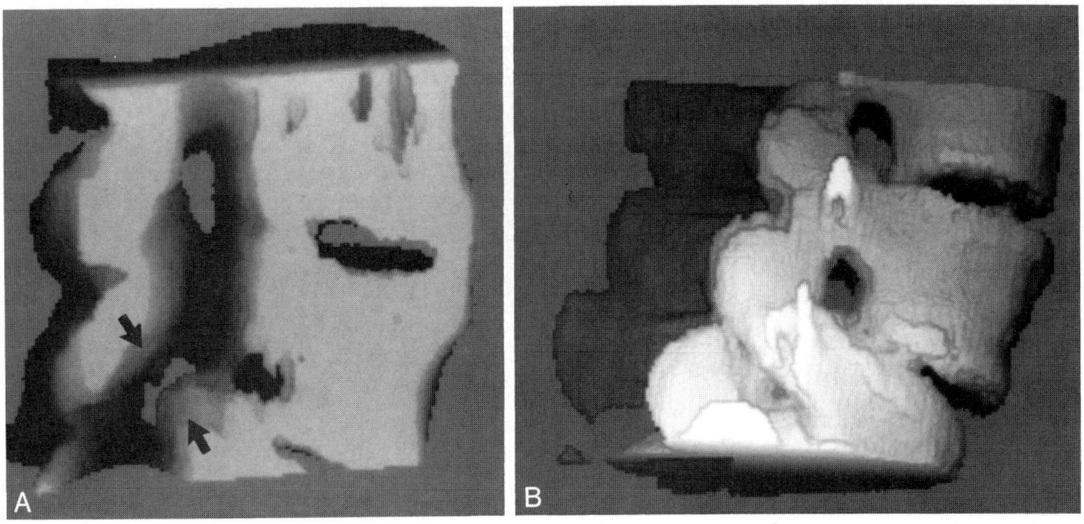

Figure 4 □ *A,* Three-dimensional image of this patient shows the narrowing of the intervertebral nerve root canal due to the large osteophytes arising from the posterior margin of the L5–S1 vertebra. The L5–S1 nerve root canal shows moderately severe narrowing in the AP dimension (*arrows*). *B,* Three-dimensional image of this patient shows the narrowing of the intervertebral nerve root canal due to the large osteophytes arising from the posterior margin of the L5–S1 vertebra. The L5–S1 nerve root canal shows moderately severe narrowing in the AP dimension.

Figure 3 □ *A,* Diagram representing the different forms of bony lateral spinal stenosis. N = intervertebral nerve root canal, P = pedicle, SF = superior articular process or facets, DB = disc bar, and VB = vertebral bodies. Up-down stenosis is caused by prominence of the disc bar and/or posterolateral osteophytes, whereas loss of disc height causes the descent of the pedicle to produce up-down stenosis. Front-back stenosis is caused by one or more of the following: hypertrophic overgrowth of the superior articular process, ligamentous laxity that allows the forward subluxation of the superior articular process, or, commonly, osteophytic or uncinate spurring arising from the posterior margin of the L5 vertebral body, which contributes to the front-back narrowing. In fact, front-back narrowing rarely occurs without associated osteophytic spurring (uncinate) arising from the dorsolateral aspect of the vertebral body. *B,* Axial computed tomographic (CT) image showing a focal osteophytic spur arising from the dorsolateral aspect of the L5 vertebral body. Note the ventral location of the L5 nerve root ganglia as they lie within the intervertebral nerve root canal. They lie immediately adjacent to the vertebral body, allowing direct impingement on the ganglia by an osteophytic spur arising from the vertebral body. Note that the ganglia are separated from the superior articular process with a considerable amount of fat lying between the dorsal aspect of the ganglia and the superior articular process. This type of uncinate spur produces an up-down stenosis with compression of the ganglia between the osteophytic spur on its caudal surface and the pedicle of L5 on its cranial surface. Note the normal anteroposterior (AP) dimension of the intervertebral nerve root canal and the intimate contact of the spur with the medial aspect of the ganglia. *C,* Sagittal reformatted image of the right L5–S1 intervertebral nerve root canal in the same patient as in *B.* Note that the osteophytic spur is producing severe compression of the exiting L5 nerve root ganglia, causing a severe up-down lateral spinal stenosis. Note the apparently normal fat-filled foramen, which actually represents the dorsal half of the intervertebral nerve root canal. The nerve root never lies within the dorsal half of the intervertebral nerve root canal. This is because of its constant ventral position related to ligamentous attachments to the nerve and the trochlear effect of the nerve as it exits in close proximity to the vertebral body ventrally. Many radiologists and surgeons fixate on the presence of epidural fat in the intervertebral nerve root canal as a sign of normalcy. This has caused failure to recognize this severe and significant type of lateral spinal stenosis. The only soft tissue structure normally lying in the dorsal aspect of the intervertebral nerve root canal is the ligamentum flavum. Masses arising from the dorsal aspect of the nerve root canal represent unusually positioned synovial cysts and/or chondromas. *D,* Axial CT image at L5–S1 depicts moderately severe front-back bony lateral spinal stenosis caused by moderate hypertrophic overgrowth of the superior articular process of S1 on the left (*long arrow*) and a moderate-sized uncinate spur (*short arrow*). *E,* Sagittal reformatted image of this patient shows the moderate front-back bony lateral spinal stenosis resulting from the uncinate spur ventrally (*small arrow*) and the overgrowth of the superior articular process dorsally (*large arrow*). *F,* Axial CT image showing large irregular osteophytic spurs arising from both the posterolateral aspect of the L5 vertebral body and the posterosuperior aspect of S1. These osteophytes are to be distinguished from uncinate spurs in that they arise on either side of the L5–S1 disc and are more generalized. *G,* Sagittal reformatted CT image showing very severe pinhole stenosis of the L5–S1 intervertebral nerve root canal. Note the marked circumferential constriction of the intervertebral nerve root canal, attributable to a combination of loss of disc height, hypertrophy of the superior articular process, and posterolateral uncinate spurring arising from the L5 vertebra.

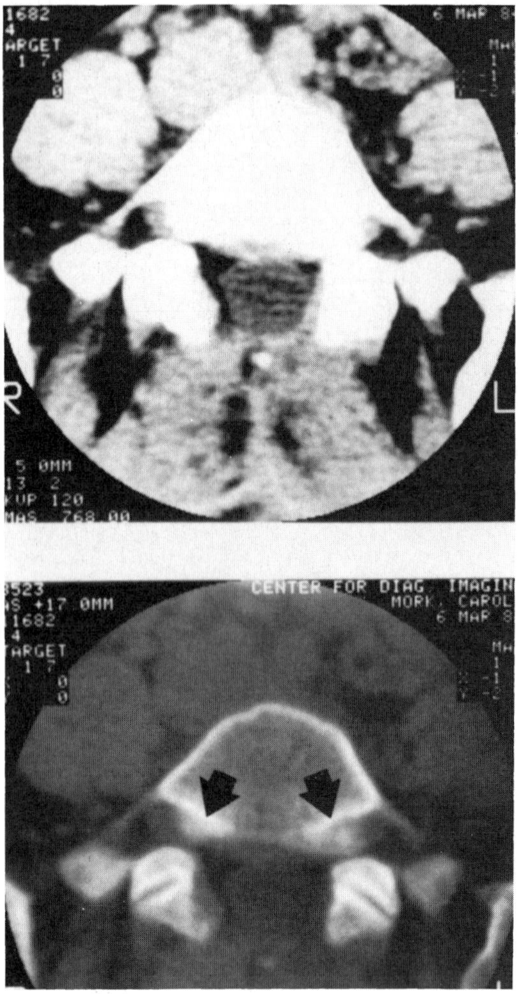

Figure 5 □ Note the large bilateral osteophytic spurs arising from the dorsolateral aspects of the L5 vertebra bilaterally (*arrows*). The very large uncinate spur on the left is producing severe cephalocaudal compression of the exiting L5 nerve root ganglia, which lie directly cranial to it. The compression of the ganglia is between the uncinate spur on its caudal margin and the undersurface of the pedicle of L5 and its cranial margin. Note the visualization of the very far lateral and inferior aspect of the L5 pedicle bilaterally.

neural foramen to become narrow in one or several of its dimensions.[20–21, 27–29] Because osteophytosis is a part of the process of autostabilization, the location of these excrescences must provide clues as to the natural dynamics of instability in given patients.[21–22, 26, 30, 31] Nonetheless, the key structures participate in the formation of lateral stenoses in a remarkably limited number of locations and variations; how they do so constitutes the basis of our highly functional, simple pathoanatomic classification.[37] Further, this scheme is eminently useful for the clinician and surgeon in planning treatment, especially decompressive surgery.

UP-DOWN STENOSIS

In contrast to central stenoses, which are usually seen at one or more lumbar spinal levels, typically L4–L5 and above, bony lateral spinal stenosis occurs about 90% of the time at the lumbosacral space.[21–22, 28, 32] In addition to their frequent occurrence at this level, they usually are more complex here than at any other spinal segment. This is because of the more complex composition of the lumbosacral nerve root canals relating to the anatomic configuration of the sacrum. Furthermore, once the principles are appreciated, they are easily extrapolated to the higher lumbar motion segments.

We initially considered hypertrophy of the superior articular facet to be the major cause of lateral stenosis.[23, 24, 29, 33–39] Indeed, it seems plausible that as the disc space collapses, the tip of the superior facet "rises up" in the foramen and presses the nerve cephalad against the pedicle. Although this is an uncommon occurrence, most authors still hold to this concept. In our sample survey of patients, we found that among the scans interpreted as showing lateral stenosis, 92% had predominantly up-down stenosis, and 4% each had front-back or pinhole stenosis.[32]

Instead, in the clear majority of patients, the nerve structure is compressed (or trapped) against its own pedicle (i.e., the nerve corresponding to or emerging at that same vertebral level) by an osteophytic process arising caudad or below the nerve. Far less often, the ganglion is forced against its vertebral body from behind by a hypertrophic facet or by a rather rare benign synovial chondroma (or cyst) arising from the ventral aspect of the facet joint. In most cases, the lateral spinal stenotic process begins with a narrowing or collapse of the disc space, reducing the cephalocaudal height of the intervertebral nerve root canal.[18, 21, 23–24, 38, 40] When this process occurs together with the development of posterolateral osteophytes arising from the disc end plate or uncinate process on the L5 vertebral body or the superior margin of S1 (Fig. 7), the typical up-down stenosis is found. This osteophytosis, occurring as a result of annular bulging, instability, and tearing of outer annular (or Sharpey's) fibers from the vertebral end plate and vestigial uncinate processes of L5, represents the final blow leading to up-down lateral nerve root entrapment.

These compressing spurs appear in standard axial CT images as dense, rounded, or sharp bony structures that project dorsally and superiorly into the intervertebral nerve root canal from below; the compressed ganglion often appears enlarged on axial images owing to cephalocaudal compression. The AP dimension of the cranial portion of the canal may appear normal (Fig. 8). This appearance is quite misleading in that one may interpret it as showing an adequate foramen; in fact, the cephalocaudal dimension of the foramen is not at all well appreciated in standard CT axial images. The location of these spurs correlates anatomically with the uncinate process of vertebral bodies seen at all levels of the spine, at all (including fetal) stages of life. The uncinate process is itself related to intervertebral stabilization. Hypertrophic changes lead to the cephalic encroachment of these processes into the nerve root canal, constricting the ganglion. These spurs often appear as easily identified dense bony processes on CT and MR images, but they are actually covered by tough, smooth tissue made of ligaments and outer fibers of the annulus fibrosus, when seen at surgery. Therefore, unless one is made aware of these spurs by preoperative imaging, they are easily overlooked at surgery. They are, in fact,

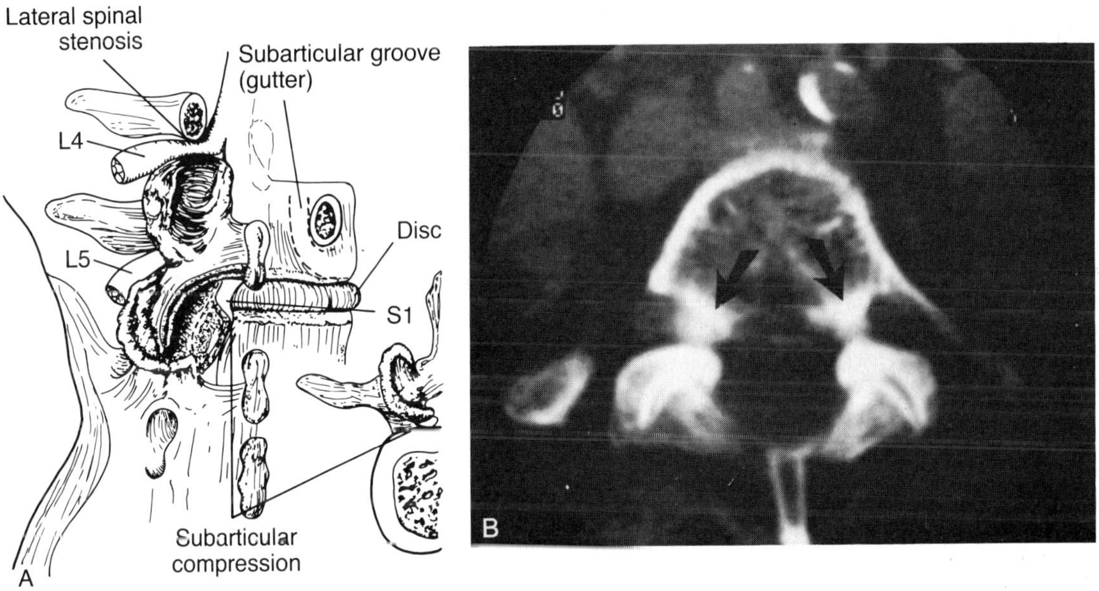

Figure 6 □ *A,* A line drawing depicting both lateral spinal stenosis and subarticular recess stenosis. The depicted lateral spinal stenosis is the classic stenosis of Kirkaldy-Willis with impingement of the exiting L4 nerve root between the hypertrophied superior articular process of L5 and the undersurface of the pedicle of L5. Lateral spinal stenosis affects the exiting nerve root within the intervertebral nerve root canal, whereas subarticular recess stenosis involves the nerve root traversing the disc within the central spinal canal. The subarticular recess is a pathologic entity when caused by medial hypertrophy of the base of the superior articular process, as is shown in this drawing. Subarticular recess impingement of the nerve root crossing the disc may also occur in patients with a trefoil configuration of the central spinal canal and a laterally bulging disc. *B,* Bilateral uncinate spurs. This axial CT scan shows bilateral uncinate spurring. Notice the symmetry and typical location of the osteophytic spurs. Spurs occlude the entire AP dimension of the intervertebral nerve root canal. The large size of the spurs indicates significant up-down bony lateral spinal stenosis with compression of both L5 nerve root ganglia (*arrows*). Note the considerable lateral extension of the intervertebral nerve root canal between the lateral aspect of the uncinate spur and superior articular process and the undersurface of the L5 pedicle on the left. Foraminal stenosis occurring within this lateral one half to one third of the intervertebral nerve root canal has been called "far lateral stenosis" and "extraforaminal stenosis," which are misnomers. If one accepts the width of the pedicle as the width of the intervertebral nerve root canal, as one does at other levels, the intervertebral nerve root canal at L5–S1 extends to the far lateral and inferior aspect of the pedicle. Note that the exiting L5 nerve root ganglia on the left exit under the pedicle adjacent to the vertebral body, rather than the transverse process, of L5. Therefore, the far-out stenosis of Wiltse is caused by compression of the nerve root ganglia by the pedicle of L5, which flares into the transverse process, rather than by the transverse process itself.

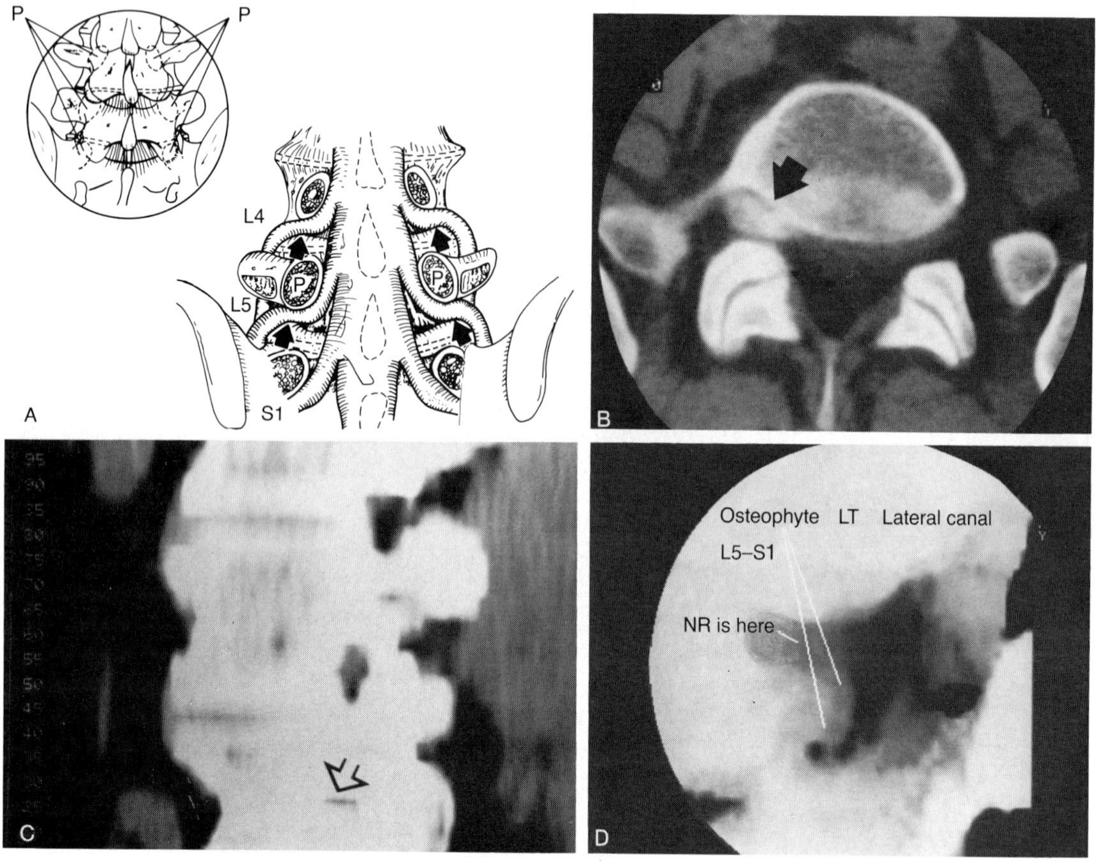

Figure 7 □ Uncinate spurring. *A,* A diagram prepared by Dr. Charles Ray shows the cephalocaudal compression of the exiting L4 and L5 nerve roots by uncinate spurs arising from the posterior aspect of the L4 and L5 vertebral bodies, respectively. The diagram shows the L5 pedicles as rounded rather than having a concave undersurface with a more caudal extension of the lateral margin of the interior surface of the pedicle, which would be more anatomically correct. Note the typical position of the uncinate spur as it rises from the dorsolateral aspect of L5. Note also the illustrative descent of the pedicle of L5 resulting from severe narrowing of the disc space at the involved levels. A combination of loss of disc height, descent of the pedicle, and growth of the uncinate spur is responsible for the up-down bony lateral spinal stenosis. *B,* Unilateral uncinate spur. Note the large size of the right-sided L5–S1 uncinate spur and the marked occlusion of the intervertebral nerve root canal caused by it. Note that a low density demarcates the attachment of the uncinate spur to the posterior aspect of the vertebra. In most patients, the uncinate spur can be delineated from the normal initial configuration of the vertebral body (*large arrow*). Note the associated degenerative hypertrophic overgrowth of the superior articular process causing front-back stenosis. Also note the up-down stenosis caused by the uncinate spurs (*small arrow*). *C,* This sagittal reformatted image of the right side of the L5–S1 intervertebral nerve root canal of the patient in *B* shows the marked up-down stenosis caused by the large uncinate spur. The exiting right L5 nerve root ganglia are severely compressed in the cephalocaudal plane between the pedicle above and the uncinate spur below (*open arrow*). *D,* Lateral 3-D image of an uncinate spur at L5–S1. Note the uncinate spur arising from the posterior aspect of the L5 vertebral body just above the degenerated and narrowed L5–S1 disc. This 3-D study was performed following the intrathecal injection of iohexol (Omnipaque). This opacified the L5 nerve root sheath and provided an image of the position of the L5 nerve root ganglia in the ventral half of the intervertebral nerve root canal. Note the large size of the dorsal half of the intervertebral nerve root canal, which contains only epidural fat. This space may be very large in the presence of severe cephalocaudal compression of the L5 nerve root ganglia, which always reside in the ventral half of the intervertebral nerve root canal as defined here. Therefore, radiographic definition of the uncinate spur is critical; without previous knowledge of the presence of this spur, the surgeon may probe the dorsal aspect of the intervertebral nerve root canal and wrongly assume that the canal is patent and that nerve root compression is absent. Additionally, these spurs are covered with cartilage and glistening soft tissue, owing to the attachment of Sharpey's fibers, and are more easily palpated at surgery than are visualized.

easier to palpate than to see, which explains why they were not recognized earlier.

The intraforaminal nerve structures normally have relatively little freedom of movement, save for a few millimeters of in-and-out sliding. The sheath within which the root and ganglion lie as they traverse the intervertebral canal to leave the foramen is anchored by various filamentous extradural ligaments and lateral reflections of the ligamentum flavum in close proximity to the inferior aspect of the pedicle and the posterior margin of the vertebral body. In addition, the neurovascular bundle containing Luschka's nerve emerges ventrally from the ganglion to penetrate and anchor into the posterolateral annulus along with Hofmann's ligaments.

These structures tether the ganglion in a predictable intraforaminal location.[22] Further, there is normally a weak outward elastic traction on the spinal nerves. All these structures and actions cause the laterally passing neural elements (root, ganglion, and spinal nerve) to remain relatively fixed in the superior, ventral portion of the foramen; the root, ganglion, and spinal nerve circle immediately caudal to the pedicle, almost as a rope passes around a pulley.

One can easily appreciate that the posterolateral osteophytic (uncinate) spurs cause a narrowing of the only space in which the nerve structures can normally lie, that is, the space bounded by the spur caudally and the pedicle cranially. The ganglion can move away neither dorsally nor cranially; it cannot become displaced elsewhere. This up-down compressive situation has been demonstrated and confirmed both in pathologic specimens and many times during surgical decompression. This up-down stenotic encroachment occurs in the superior, ventral half of the intervertebral nerve root canal. Reformatted CT and sagittal MR images may show severe compression of root or ganglion in this more ventral location; yet the dorsal portion of the canal remains filled with epidural fat. The uninitiated may focus on the epidural fat in the dorsal part of the canal and assume that there must be space enough for the nerve or ganglion in the canal, thus entirely missing the necessarily ventral location of the typical entrapment (Figs. 8C and 9). In contrast, sagittal reformatted images of the normal foramen usually adequately display the exiting nerve roots and ganglia surrounded on all sides by a thin layer of fat. Sagittal MRI provides the best delineation of various soft tissue structures within the intervertebral nerve root canals (ganglia, lateral disc, veins, ligamentum flavum, and fibrosis), which are isodense on sagittal reformatted CT images but have clearly defined differing signal intensities on MR scans.

On axial images, the typical uncinate spur appears as a rounded, oval, bony overgrowth projecting into the middle third of the intervertebral nerve root canal (Fig. 10*A*). The uncinate spur lies directly caudal to the exiting L5 nerve root ganglion within the ventral half of the nerve root canal. Axial images may be difficult to interpret with respect to compression of the ganglion, because the thin slices obtained at the L5–S1 level often show the ganglion on one image and the uncinate spur on the image immediately caudal, without showing the nerve root compression. However, a ganglion compressed in the cephalocaudal direction appears enlarged in the axial plane. When uncinate spurring is noted, this asymmetry of the affected ganglion should be looked for on the axial images. The presence and degree of nerve root compression by uncinate spurring are, however, best quantified by examining sagittal reformatted images. For these reasons, we find that sagittal reformatted CT and sagittal MRI are critical in the evaluation of lateral spinal stenosis (Fig. 10*B*).

Aging vertebral bodies are frequently reduced in height and become wider at the end-plate margins. The pedicle, in contrast, increases slightly in diameter and may alter its normally oval configuration to become larger and more rounded. These changes are best appreciated on plain films of the lumbar spine or by coronal reformatting of the CT scan. In effect, this finding represents a relative descent of the pedicle down the vertebral body. The pedicles of L5 and S1 begin to approach each other from above and downward, further restricting the cephalocaudal (up-down) diameter of the foramen. Disc margins, especially those along the most mobile quadrants in which the annulus may be slowly tearing and healing, become more prominent and calcified. These disc margin bars, in addition to the uncinate spur, may contribute to the up-down narrowing, as discussed earlier. The uncinate spurs, which are exceptionally important in

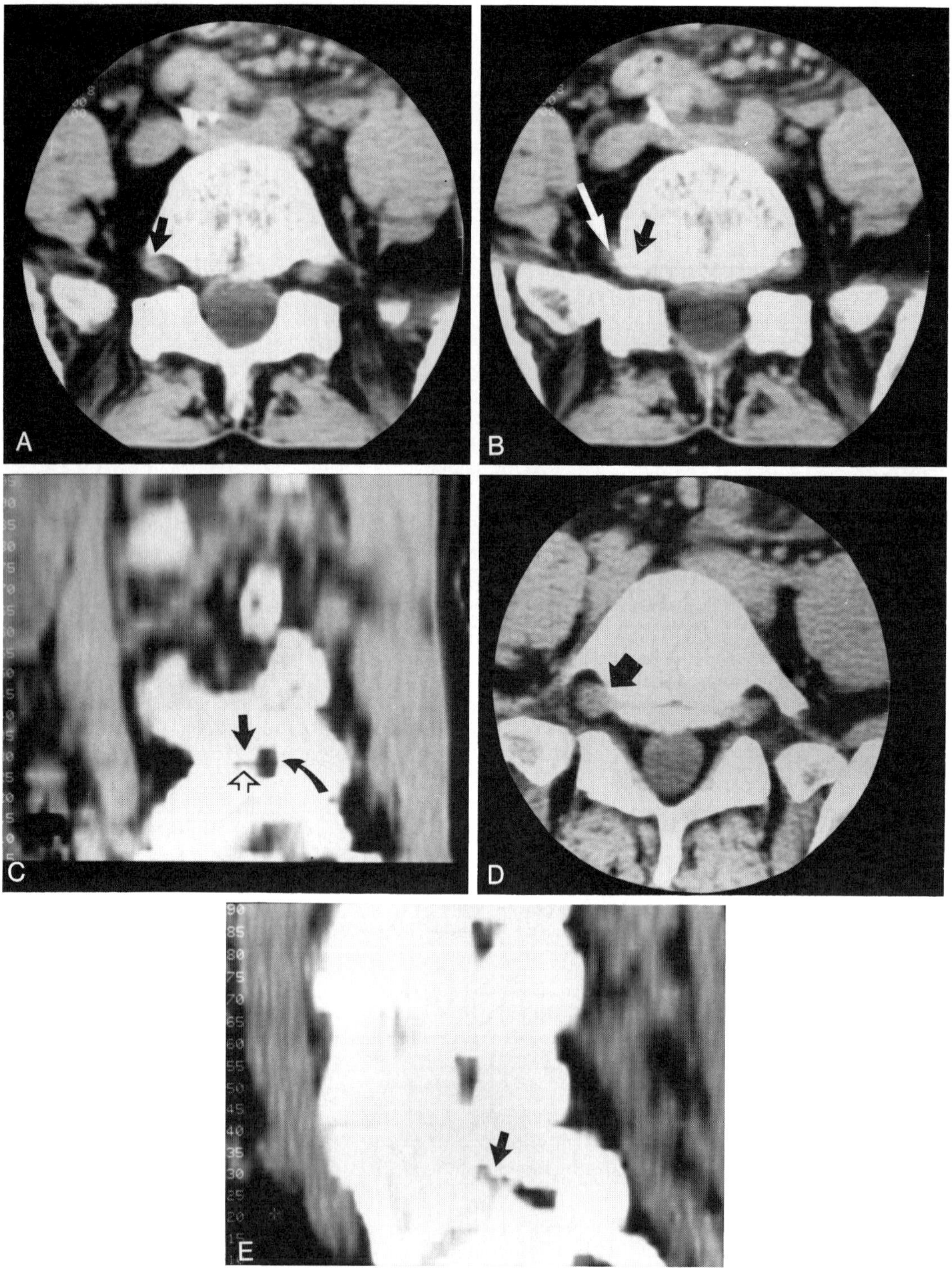

Figure 8 □ Uncinate spurring and lateral spinal stenosis. *A,* Axial CT image shows mild enlargement of the right L5 nerve root ganglion in the axial plane. There is partial volume imaging of the cranial aspect of the uncinate spur, which is producing up-down compression of the ganglion (*arrow*). *B,* This axial image was obtained 3-mm slices caudal to the image depicted in *A*. This shows a moderately large uncinate spur that directly underlies the ganglion. Note the displaced L5 nerve root ganglion as it passes laterally and caudal to this osteophyte (*white arrow*). *C,* Sagittal reformatted image shows that the ventral half of the L5–S1 intervertebral nerve root canal is slitlike, and there is compression of the L5 nerve root ganglion between the osteophyte caudally (*open arrowhead*) and the undersurface of the pedicle cranially (*arrow*).

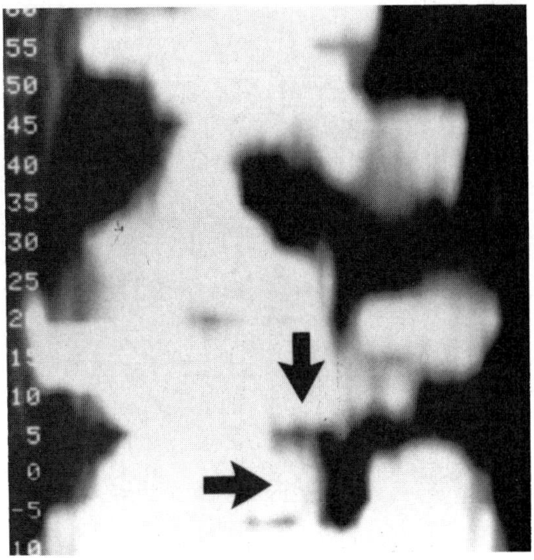

Figure 9 □ Uncinate spurring with severe lateral spinal stenosis. This sagittal reformatted image of the L5–S1 intervertebral nerve root canal shows a large uncinate spur (*horizontal arrow*), which is producing marked up-down (cephalocaudal) compression of the L5 nerve root (*vertical arrow*). Note the fat-containing dorsal half of the intervertebral nerve root canal. To the uninitiated, this could be read as a normal canal because of the myopic focus on fat within the intervertebral nerve root canal as a sign of normalcy, an error that is found throughout the radiologic literature. Therefore, direct visualization of the ganglion and its relationship to any osteophytic spurs within the intervertebral nerve root canal is essential.

stenosis formation, arise from the dorsolateral margin of the vertebra at the end plate in closest proximity to the pedicle. Lumbar uncinate processes, like those in the cervical spine, are vestigial in normal spines but become enlarged and osteophytic with a tearing of Sharpey's fibers at the annulus of the disc. The location and appearance of these spurs are constant in all patients in whom they are seen, reliably indicating a pathologic, hypertrophic change in the uncinate process (Figs. 6 to 10). Uncinate spurs are to be distinguished from the more widespread, irregular, and highly variable end-plate spurs or bars. These bars are more lateral in position and more variable and linear in appearance as they extend laterally to parallel the end plate.

In contrast to the uncinate spurs, the common or ventral annular disc plate osteophytes are less commonly the sole cause of significant nerve root entrapment. When they are, they tend to involve the ganglia far laterally with compression between the osteophyte and the caudal and lateral margin of the pedicle of L5, a stenosis sometimes inaccurately referred to as extraforaminal, or more accurately as far out. However, these spurs may elevate the nerve and therefore effectively compress it (Fig. 11).

LATERAL SPINAL STENOSIS AND LYTIC SPONDYLOLISTHESIS

Lytic spondylolisthesis at L5–S1 is often associated with bony lateral spinal stenosis when there is concomitant degenerative narrowing of the L5–S1 disc. In fact, the lateral scout view and/or plain radiographs of the lumbar spine are highly predictive of lateral stenosis in this disease entity. That is, most patients with lytic spondylolisthesis and degenerative disc space narrowing at L5–S1 are found to have bony lateral spinal stenosis and compression of the L5 nerve root ganglion when studied by axial CT and sagittal reformatted images, whereas those with lytic

---

Figure 8 *Continued* What appears to be a small normal intervertebral nerve root canal dorsal to this stenosis is the dorsal half of the nerve root canal, which is always vacant and contains only fat and the ligamentum flavum as it courses over the ventral surface of the superior articular process (*curved arrow*). *E,* The sagittal reformatted image of the right L5–S1 nerve root canal shows severe cephalocaudal constriction of the distorted intervertebral nerve root canal. The elongation of the nerve root canal results from the forward subluxation of L5 on S1. The cephalocaudal, or up-down, stenosis is caused by loss of disc height and descent of the pedicle and pars superior of L5 onto the L5 nerve root ganglion and L5–S1 disc plate (*arrow*). Again, the dorsal half of the nerve root canal is vacant and contains fat. Therefore, this is not the sign of a normal canal but might be probed at surgery based on the erroneous assumption that the canal was patent. *D,* Axial CT scan illustrating the "too-large" nerve root sign present in patients with cephalocaudal compression of the L5 nerve root ganglion. The nerve root ganglion on the right is large and irregular when compared with the L5 nerve root on the left, owing to cephalocaudal compression by the pedicle of L5 above and the L5–S1 disc plate below (*arrow*).

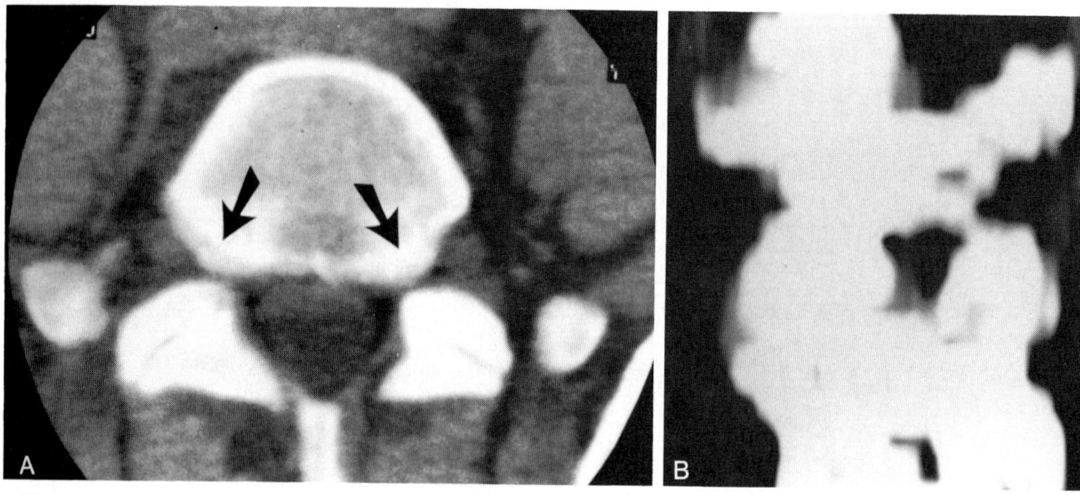

Figure 10 □ *A*, Axial CT image showing symmetric moderate-size bilateral uncinate spurs. Again, notice the typical appearance and position of these osteophytic spurs as they encroach upon the medial half of the intervertebral nerve root canal, directly ventral to the medial aspect of the superior articular process (SAP). Note also that the L5 nerve root ganglia lie lateral to the uncinate spurs *(arrows)* at the level of this scan, which is caudal to the impingement that is occurring in the more cranial and medial aspects of the canal as the nerve root descends caudally and laterally through the canal. The lateral margin of the canal is often defined by the iliolumbar ligament, which extends caudally from the inferior margin of the pedicle of L5. Therefore, the triangular space lateral to the uncinate spur and the SAP (in this case), which are filled by the ganglia, represent the lateral one half to one third of the intervertebral nerve root canal; that is, the ganglia in this image are still within the intervertebral nerve root canal and are not "extraforaminal," since they lie medial to the plane of the lateral aspect of the pedicle of L5. *B*, Sagittal reformatted image of the patient in *A*. Note the moderately severe cephalocaudal bony lateral spinal stenosis of the ventral half of the intervertebral nerve root canal and marked compression of the ganglia, which lie between the cranial margin of the spur and the undersurface of the pedicle. Again, note the presence of fat within the dorsal aspect of the canal, which never contains neural elements.

listhesis and a normal disc rarely have stenosis.

The mechanism of lateral spinal stenosis in lytic spondylosthesis is a caudal and ventral migration of the pars superior and pedicle of L5 with entrapment of the L5 nerve root ganglion by the undersurface of the pedicle and pars superior as it settles onto the L5–S1 disc and S1 vertebral body and sacral alae. The L5 nerve root travels ventrally with the L5 vertebral body and is compressed within the ventral aspect of the deformed intervertebral nerve root canals, which become elongated in the AP dimension. Axial images alone may be deceptive, because the AP dimension of the canal on them appears completely normal or elongated, and the ganglia may be well visualized without apparent bony entrapment. Only on reformatted CT or sagittal MR images is the very narrowed cephalocaudal dimension of the nerve root canal easily appreciated. Pre-impingement and post-impingement swelling of the nerve root and postganglionic portion, respectively, may occur (Fig. 12).

Because the posterior L5–S1 disc surface becomes axial in its orientation owing to the ventral subluxation of L5 on S1, any protrusion arising from this disc projects craniad, rather than dorsally. Therefore, focal disc protrusions extend either craniad into the central spinal canal or, more commonly, craniad and laterally into the intervertebral nerve root canal. This presents a diagnostic dilemma in a patient with unilateral sciatica and lytic spondylolisthesis with bony lateral spinal stenosis. The attenuation values of the nerve root ganglia and a possible lateral disc protrusion are indistinguishable within the stenotic canal in most patients studied by axial and sagittal reformatted high-resolution computed tomography (HRCT) images. One cannot be sure whether the compression of the ganglia is strictly bony or whether there is an associated lateral disc herniation (Fig. 13*A*).

MRI, however, has proved useful in identifying lateral disc herniation, in general, and lateral disc herniation associated with spondylolisthesis, in particular (Fig. 13*B*, *C*). A contained lateral disc herniation with an-

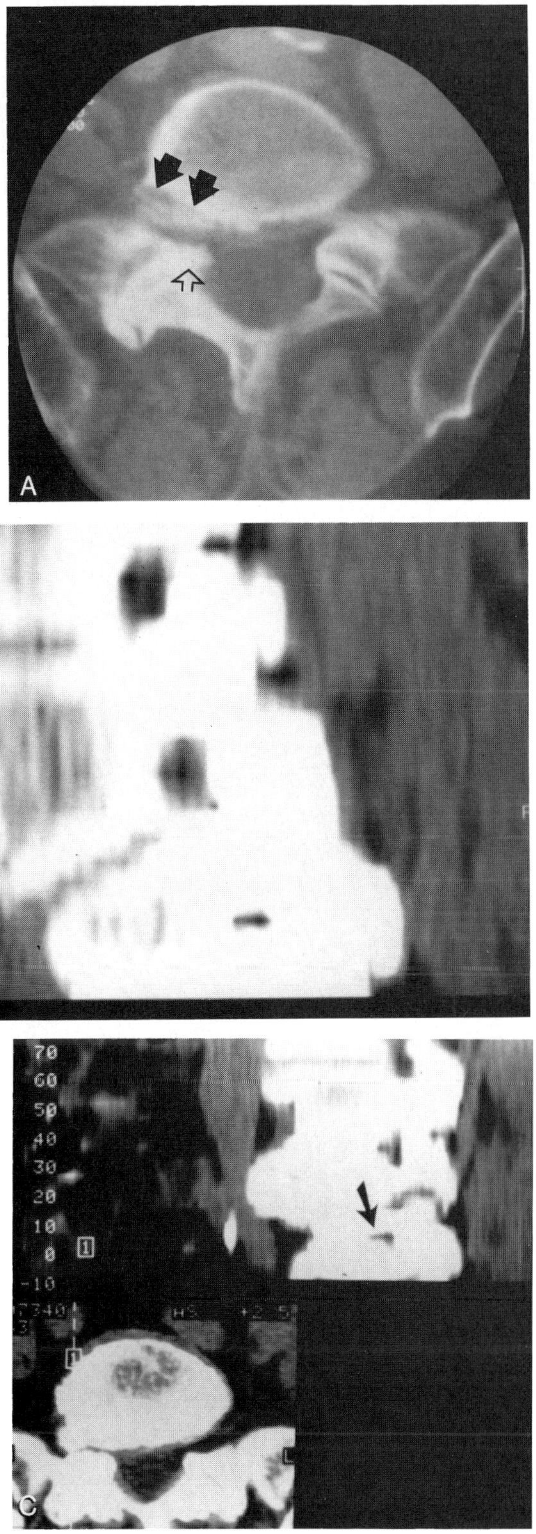

Figure 11 □ *A,* Severe lateral spinal stenosis at L5–S1 on the right. Note the diffuse osteophytic spurring at the margins of the L5-S1 disc. These are more diffuse spurs and are to be distinguished from uncinate spurs. These osteophytes arise at the very margin of the vertebral bodies on either side of the disc and project in a cranial direction into the intervertebral nerve root canal. They are very often associated with severe loss of disc height, which is unilaterally more severe on the side of the osteophytes, as is true in this case (*dark arrows*). Note also the hypertrophic overgrowth of the base of the superior articular process of S1 on the right (*open arrowhead*), which is producing moderate narrowing of the bony subarticular recess and of the medial aspect of the right L5–S1 intervertebral nerve root canal. *B,* Sagittal reformatted image of the patient in *A.* Moderate cephalocaudal bony lateral spinal stenosis is caused by the osteophytic spurs arising at the margin of the L5 and S1 vertebrae at the margin of the L5–S1 disc. Note that these spurs are different from uncinate spurs in that they are more generalized and linear and typically cause less severe cephalocaudal stenosis. This is because they arise from the margin of the vertebra rather than on the more cranial dorsolateral aspect of the L5 vertebra at the attachment of Sharpey's fibers. Because of their parallel ridgelike appearance, I have called these types of spurs "tramtrack" osteophytes. However, the mechanism of nerve root impingement is comparable to that of uncinate spurring in that significant lateral stenosis and nerve root compression, when present, are always associated with loss of disc height, which causes a concomitant descent of the pedicle of L5. *C,* Axial and sagittal reformatted image of a patient with an irregular far-lateral osteophytic spur. Note the far-lateral position of the osteophytic spur and its irregular configuration. This is to be distinguished from an uncinate spur by its position and irregular appearance. The spurs are uniformly associated with prominent lateral osteophytes, which continue to extend along the lateral margin of the vertebral body and disc beyond the intervertebral nerve root canal. They can produce very-far-lateral lateral stenosis. The surgeon must be aware that in this type of osteophytic spur the decompression needs to be extended to the far-lateral aspect of the intervertebral nerve root canal, as defined by the lateral aspect of the pedicle of L5.

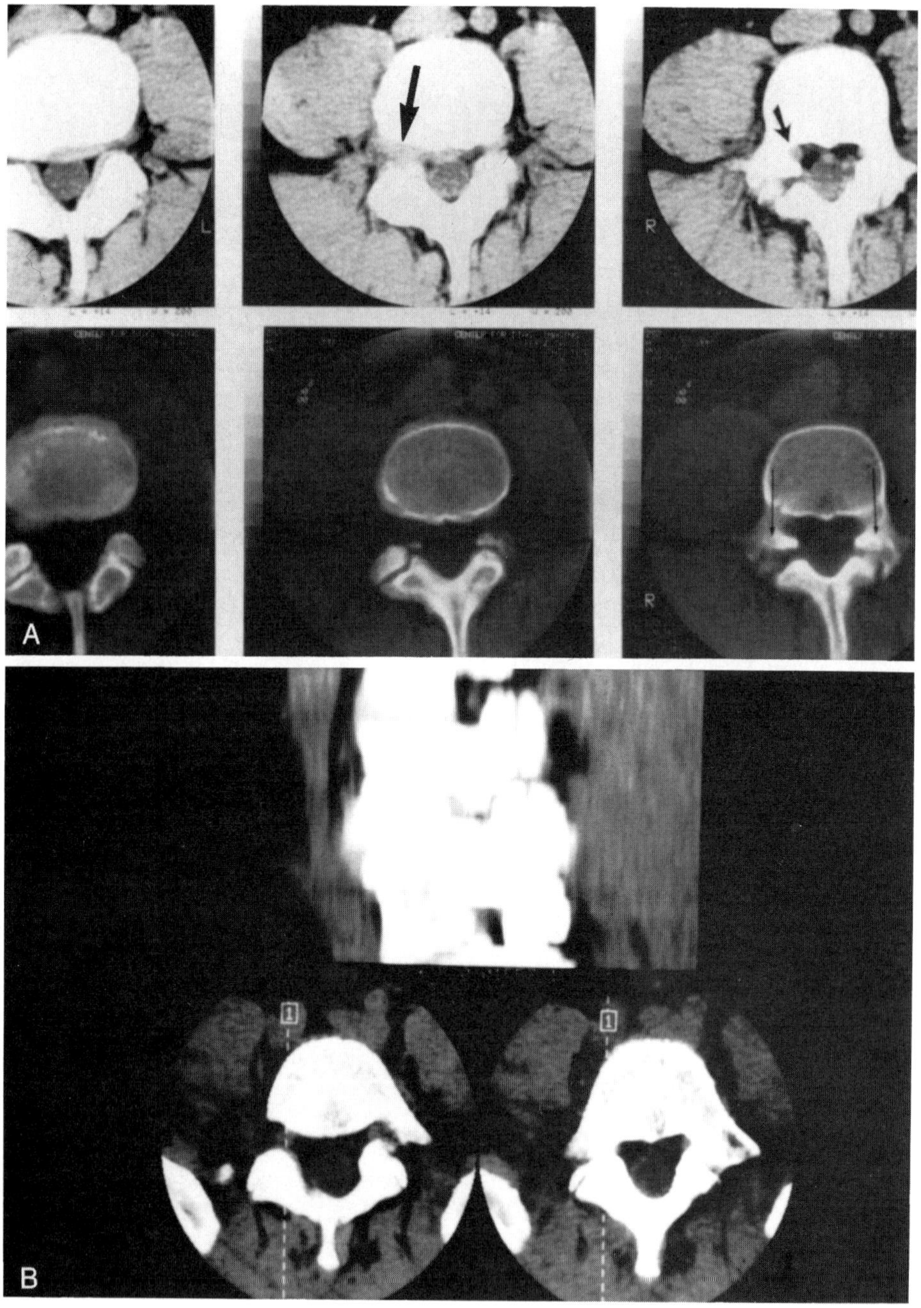

Figure 12 □ *A,* Composite axial images of the L4–L5 level in a patient with Grade-1 lytic spondylolisthesis. Note the pre-impingement swelling of the L4 nerve root as it enters the stenotic right L4–L5 intervertebral nerve root canal (*small arrow*). The canal is opacified by soft tissue. This consists of a combination of a lateral disc herniation and the compressed right L4 nerve root ganglia within the canal (*large arrow*). On the basis of this image, without reformatting, one cannot determine whether the soft tissue in the canal is attributable to cephalocaudal compression of the ganglia alone, whether it is caused by lateral disc herniation, or whether there is a coexistent cephalocaudal lateral stenosis, which is often noted in patients with lytic spondylolisthesis. *B,* Sagittal reformatted image of the patient in *A.* Note the moderate cephalocaudal bony lateral spinal stenosis caused by loss of disc height and overgrowth of the margin of the defect in the pars superior of L4. Because there is cephalocaudal lateral spinal stenosis, CT is not capable of excluding the possibility of a concomitant lateral disc herniation. However, this is now possible with magnetic resonance imaging (MRI), which can easily distinguish between the soft tissue density of ganglia and lateral disc herniation in such patients. Surgically, this patient had both focal lateral disc herniation and moderately severe cephalocaudal lateral stenosis.

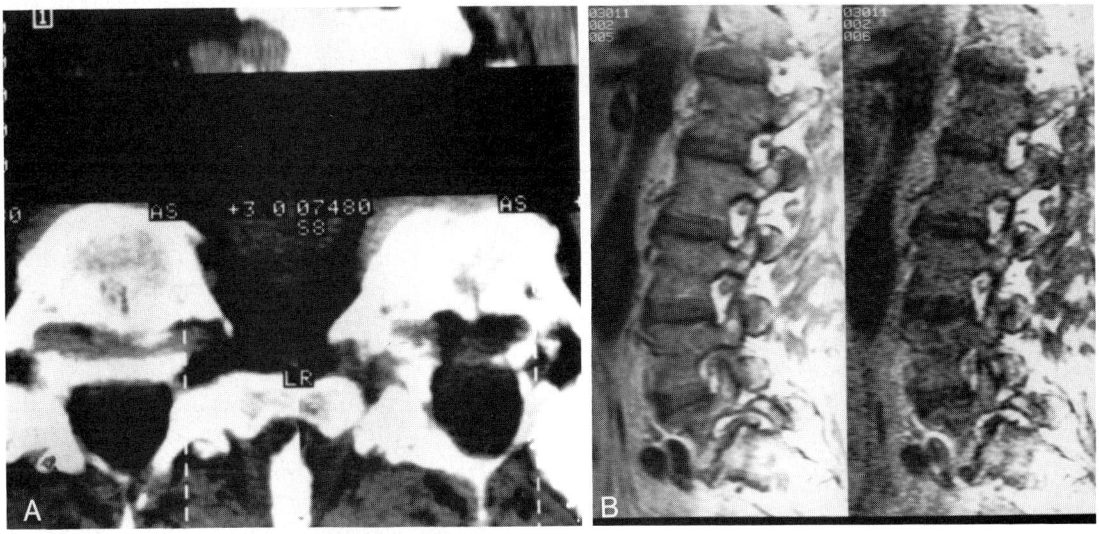

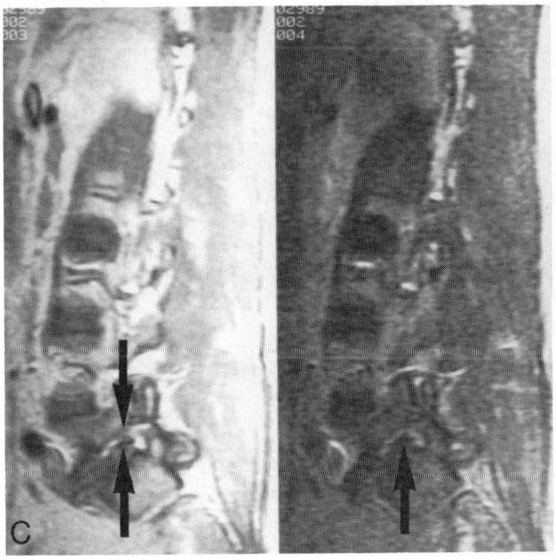

Figure 13 □ *A,* Lytic spondylolisthesis and lateral spinal stenosis. This scan shows axial images at L5–S1 and the sagittal reformatted image through the left L5–S1 intervertebral nerve root canal. Note the fragmentation and hypertrophic overgrowth of the pars superior on the left-hand axial image. Note the compression of the exiting left L5 nerve root ganglia by the lateral aspect of the L5–S1 disc bar on the image immediately caudal to it on the left. The sagittal reformatted image at the top of the scan obtained along the parasagittal line through the L5–S1 intervertebral nerve root canal shows a severe cephalocaudal compression of the exiting L5 nerve root ganglia. This can be predicted from plain films and the lateral computed radiographs in a percentage of patients when severe loss of disc height is present. This type of lateral spinal stenosis is the most common cause of sciatica in patients with lytic spondylolisthesis at L5–S1. It is much more common than disc herniation either at L4–L5 or at L5–S1. *B,* MRI of lytic spondylolisthesis and lateral spinal stenosis. Note the severe cephalocaudal narrowing of the L5–S1 intervertebral nerve root canal resulting from severe loss of disc height. The L5 nerve root ganglion is severely compressed between the pedicle and pars superior cranially, and the degenerated L5–S1 disc plate and S1 vertebra caudally. The ganglion is so compressed that it is virtually obscured by the compressive disc. *C,* MRI of lateral stenosis due to lateral disc herniation. Note the severe lateral spinal stenosis caused by an irregular, lateral low-density disc herniation, which projects craniad into the intervertebral nerve root canal. This is a patient with lytic spondylolisthesis and moderate cephalocaudal narrowing of the intervertebral nerve root canal due to loss of disc height. Axial and sagittal reformatted images show opacification of the intervertebral nerve root canal. Because the disc and ganglia show essentially the same density on CT, a lateral disc herniation could not be excluded. The MR scan shows an irregular low-signal-intensity annular disc fragment within the intervertebral nerve root canal, causing severe cephalocaudal compression of the ganglia. The position of the ganglia is defined by the opposing arrows in the left-hand proton density image. The lateral disc herniation is visualized by the cranially directed arrow in the right-hand image.

nular deformity can be easily differentiated from the ganglion because the annulus is of low signal intensity, whereas the nuclear material and ganglia are of intermediate signal intensity. An asymmetric lateral disc herniation is not an uncommon cause of sciatica in lytic spondylolisthesis. In affected patients, the bony lateral spinal stenosis is often symmetric and lateral disc protrusion is the cause of the sciatica. This is best studied by sagittal MRI with 3-mm sections. A central or posterolateral disc bulge or herniation at the L4–L5 level is said to be the most common herniation associated with lytic spondylolisthesis; however, these do not commonly produce L5 nerve root compression because there is a large epidural space between the thecal sac and the L4–L5 intervertebral disc resulting from the forward listhesis of the L5 vertebral body. In our experience, the most common cause of sciatica in a patient with lytic spondylolisthesis is first lateral stenosis at L5–S1 and then lateral herniation at L5–S1.

DEGENERATIVE SPONDYLOLISTHESIS

Degenerative spondylolisthesis, a relatively common cause of central and subarticular (spinal recess) stenosis, is characterized by a distinctive CT appearance; this consists of marked degenerative hypertrophic overgrowth of the facets and thickening of the ligamentum flavum, which is often marked, and is associated with ligamentous laxity and erosion of the medial aspect of the SAP (Fig. 14). This marked erosion of the supportive SAP of the caudal vertebral body allows ventral subluxation of the intact neural arch of the cephalic vertebral body with a resulting constriction of the central spinal canal and thecal sac. The compression of the thecal sac and nerve roots occurs between the lamina and hypertrophied inferior articular processes (IAPs) dorsally and the posterior aspect of the involved disc and caudal vertebral body ventrally. Bulging or herniation of the involved disc and marked thickening of the ligamentum flavum produce most of the neural compression in the majority of patients. Therefore, degenerative spondylolisthesis typically produces central spinal stenosis as well as subarticular recess stenosis with compression of the traversing nerve roots (e.g., L5 nerve roots at the L4–L5 level) (Fig. 14*B*).

Degenerative spondylolisthesis occurs most commonly at the L4–L5 level. The typical patient is an overweight middle-aged to elderly female with hyperlordosis. The lateral computed radiographs usually show degenerative disc space narrowing at the involved level and, frequently, moderate hyperlordosis. The association of diabetes (reported in up to 30% of these patients), marked degenerative overgrowth of these facets, and the paucity of significant back pain and sciatica before the onset of symptoms of spinal claudication raise the question of a lack of pain sensitivity of the involved joints (i.e., a Charcot-like joint degeneration).

Lateral spinal stenosis is relatively unusual in these patients because the pedicles of L4 arise relatively more cephalad on the vertebral body than the pedicles of L5. Therefore, loss of disc height alone at L3–L4 and L4–L5 does not ordinarily produce a cephalocaudal bony lateral spinal stenosis. Lateral spinal stenosis, when it does occur, is almost always secondary to a rotary component of the subluxation. The lateral spinal stenosis then occurs on the side with anterior subluxation of the SAP that rotates into the intervertebral nerve root canal, producing bony lateral impingement of the exiting nerve root ganglion (i.e., L4 at L4–L5). The compression occurs between the ventral or cephalic margin of the hypertrophied SAP and the undersurface of the pedicle above (Fig. 14*C*).

Patients with degenerative spondylolisthesis exhibit significant degenerative soft tissue abnormalities related to their longstanding instability. A significant fibrocartilaginous build-up nearly always occurs at the posterior margin of the disc and projects dorsally into the central spinal canal and laterally into the intervertebral nerve root canals. The build-up produces an opacification of the nerve root canals and an indistinct visualization of exiting nerve roots. On CT examinations this appears to represent fibrosis around the nerve roots. However, sagittal MR images show this to be due to the up-down compression of the ganglia resulting from prominent lateral bulging of the annulus of the disc in most cases and lateral herniation in a few. However, much of the *apparent* prominence of the disc extending

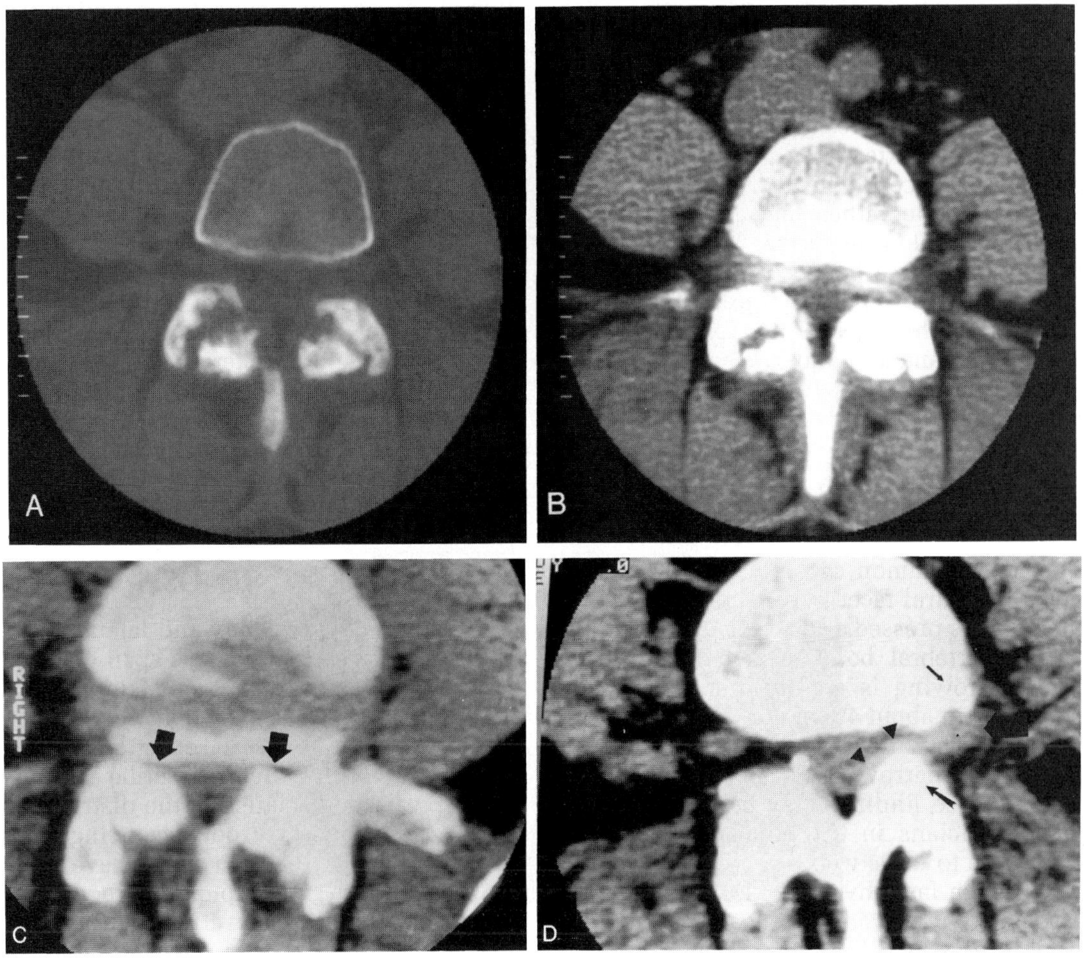

Figure 14 □ *A,* Degenerative spondylolisthesis. Axial CT scan with bone level and window shows typical marked erosive degenerative zygapophyseal joint disease of the L4–L5 facets. Notice the marked cystic erosion of facet joints. Also note the marked erosion of the facets themselves. There is a concomitant moderate thickening of the ligamentum flavum. *B,* Degenerative spondylolisthesis. This axial CT scan was filmed with a soft tissue window and level to show the central stenosis and bilateral subarticular recess stenosis caused by the forward subluxation of the intact neural arch of L4 as well as the thickened ligamentum flavum. The forward subluxation of L4 is defined by the width of the L4–L5 disc behind the L4 vertebral body. This is not due to pathologic disc protrusion, but merely to partial volume imaging of the disc and the vertebral body because of the forward subluxation of L4. Note the opacification of the intervertebral nerve root canals bilaterally. MRI has shown this to be attributable to posterolateral bulging of the disc in most patients, rather than to a fibrotic reaction resulting from chronic instability, as was initially thought on the basis of CT. *C,* Degenerative spondylolisthesis with moderate central stenosis and severe bilateral subarticular recess stenosis. This axial CT image at the L4–L5 level in a patient with Grade 1 spondylolisthesis shows complete erosion of the anteromedial aspect of the superior articular processes with marked ventral subluxation of the inferior articular processes into the central spinal canal. This is causing severe bilateral subarticular recess stenosis and marked compression of the traversing L5 nerve roots, which directly underlie the inferior articular processes (*arrows*). There are mild to moderate thickening of the ligamentum flavum and mild central bulging of the disc annulus, which contribute to the prominent constriction of the thecal sac. In most cases of degenerative spondylolisthesis, the central stenosis is predominantly soft tissue stenosis and results from marked thickening of the ligamentum flavum and degenerative central bulging of the L4–L5 disc; the bony stenosis is relatively mild. *D,* Degenerative spondylolisthesis with lateral spinal stenosis. This axial CT scan at the L4–L5 level shows a rotatory subluxation of the left SAP into the left L4–L5 intervertebral nerve root canal (*large arrow*). Associated focal dorsolateral osteophytic spurring arises from the inferolateral aspect of the L4 vertebral body (*small arrow*), and there is moderate thickening of the ligamentum flavum (*arrowheads*). Note that the inferior articular processes have overridden and eroded the medial aspect of the SAP and, along with the ligamentum flavum, are forming the posterior border of the left L4–L5 intervertebral nerve root canal. Note the moderately severe edema of the compressed L4 nerve root ganglion (*largest arrow*), which is twice the size of the right L4 nerve root ganglion. It is unusual for lateral spinal stenosis to be present at the level of degenerative spondylolisthesis, unless there is associated rotatory subluxation.

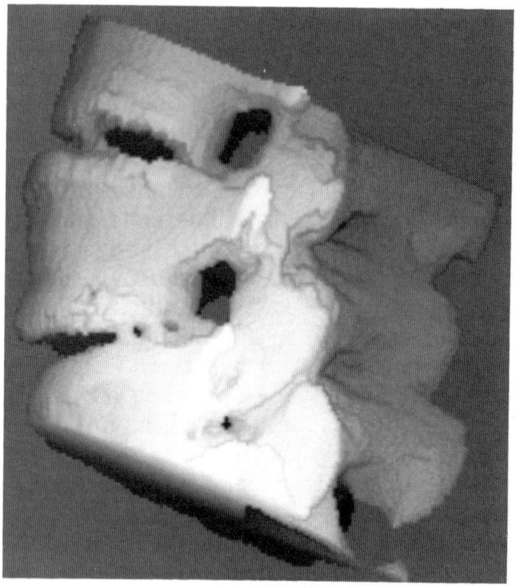

Figure 16 □ Pinhole stenosis. This lateral view of a 3-D reconstruction of the lumbar spine shows severe concentric stenosis of the left L5–S1 intervertebral nerve root canal resulting from a combination of uncinate spurring, spurring at the margin of the L5–S1 disc, loss of disc height, and hypertrophic overgrowth of the SAP.

LATERAL, EXTRAFORAMINAL LESIONS, INCLUDING FAR-OUT STENOSIS

Wiltse and colleagues[29] describe a "far-out" syndrome characterized by the entrapment of the L5 nerve between a deeply descending transverse process of L5 and the superior portion of the medial sacral ala. As previously discussed, this actually involves the pedicle of L5 (not the transverse process) and is merely a form of lateral stenosis occurring at the far lateral aspect of the L5–S1 nerve root canal. This has been seen in about 6% of our patients diagnosed as having stenosis. Another type of far-out stenosis appears to be more common and is frequently the cause of failed lateral stenosis surgery, as was noted in our study of 100 consecutive laminectomies performed in 1984 at the Institute for Low Back Care. This type occurs in patients having a high medial segment of the sacra ala, a relatively low posterolateral S1 disc margin with a prominent osteophytic bar formation, and a lateral bulging of that disc.[26] In this situation, the L5 nerve passes dorsal to and is compressed by the disc bar against the lateral and caudal aspect of the pedicle of L5 as it descends (Fig. 17*A*). Far-lateral stenosis can be easily missed at surgery at the L5–S1 level, owing to the complex anatomic configuration of the nerve root canal. At other levels of the lumbar spine, the superior articular facet marks the lateral boundary of the nerve root canal. However, at L5–S1 the lateral margin of the pedicle of L5 lies considerably lateral to the facet joint and commonly causes cephalocaudal compression of the exiting L5 nerve root ganglia in patients who have significant degenerative loss of disc height of the L5–S1 disc. Also, importantly, the undersurface of the L5 pedicle is concave, and the lateral margin is most caudal as it flares to form the transverse process. A loss of disc height can result in the most severe stenosis being at the very far lateral border of the intervertebral nerve root canal; this is caused by the linear, sharply demarcated inferior border of the L5 pedicle, which may be only millimeters wide (Fig. 17*B*). Therefore, the extent and type of the stenosis must be clearly described preoperatively so that decompression sufficient to completely eliminate the stenosis can be planned.

In a recent survey of 100 postoperative patients at the Institute for Low Back Care, five had residual far-lateral stenosis, despite the attempted surgical correction of L5–S1 lateral spinal stenosis that was clearly identified by HRCT and understood by the surgeon before the operation.[42] The stenosis resulting from approximation of the lateral aspect of the L5 pedicle and the L5–S1 disc and the sacral alae is a far-lateral, far-out stenosis that is cephalocaudal in orientation. This can be completely overlooked if the HRCT examination consists of axial images alone without benefit of the sagittal reformatted images. Stenosis can occur focally anywhere within the intervertebral nerve root canal, as in the instance of stenosis caused by the lateral aspect of the pedicle of L5. Therefore, multiple, closely spaced reformatted CT and/or MR images of the *entire* nerve root canal are necessary. Not infrequently, when we are suspicious of far-lateral stenosis on axial images that is not shown by sagittal reformatted images, the reformatting was not extended laterally enough. In patients with a severe loss of disc height and descent of the pedicle onto the L5–S1 disc and sacral alae (i.e., patients with lytic spondylolisthesis), the necessity for sagittal reformatted images becomes clear. In some patients, oblique reformatted

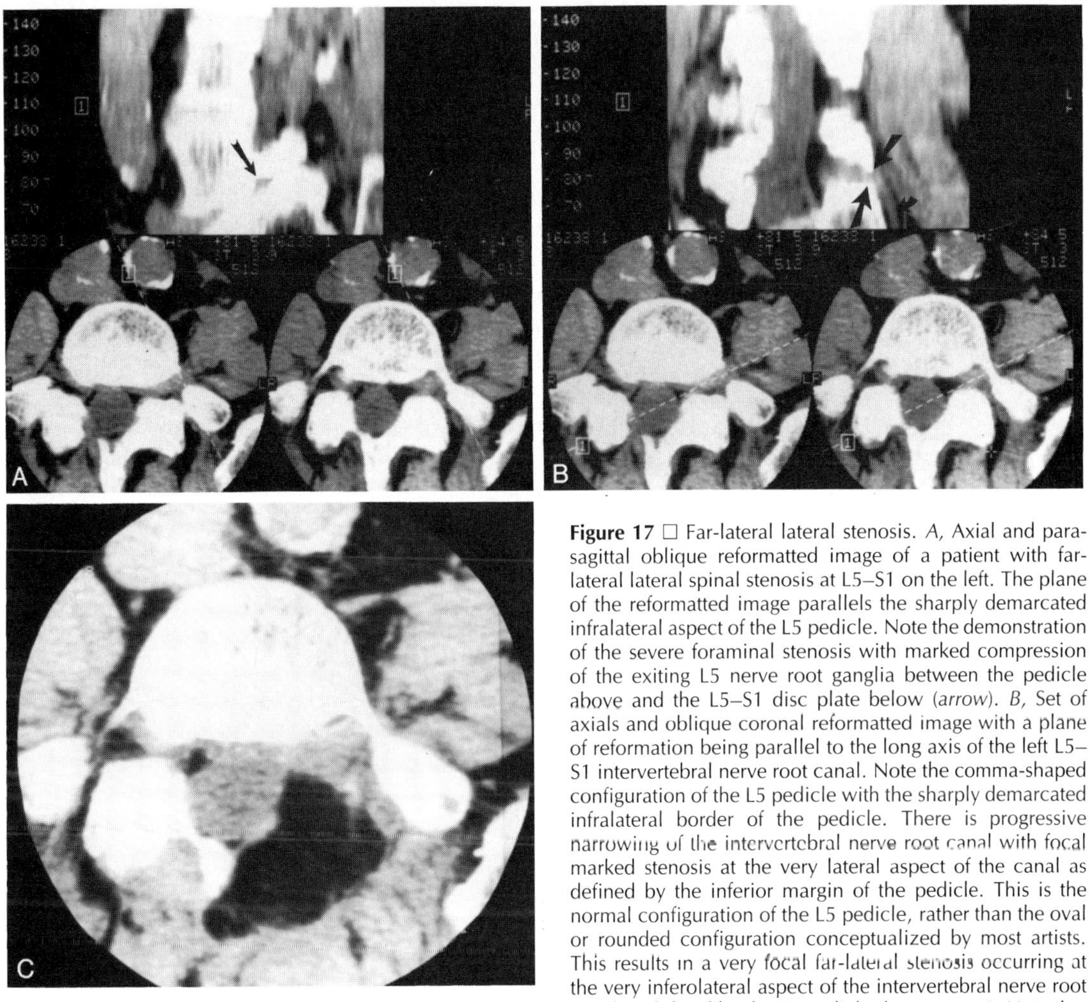

Figure 17 □ Far-lateral lateral stenosis. *A,* Axial and parasagittal oblique reformatted image of a patient with far-lateral lateral spinal stenosis at L5–S1 on the left. The plane of the reformatted image parallels the sharply demarcated infralateral aspect of the L5 pedicle. Note the demonstration of the severe foraminal stenosis with marked compression of the exiting L5 nerve root ganglia between the pedicle above and the L5–S1 disc plate below (*arrow*). *B,* Set of axials and oblique coronal reformatted image with a plane of reformation being parallel to the long axis of the left L5–S1 intervertebral nerve root canal. Note the comma-shaped configuration of the L5 pedicle with the sharply demarcated infralateral border of the pedicle. There is progressive narrowing of the intervertebral nerve root canal with focal marked stenosis at the very lateral aspect of the canal as defined by the inferior margin of the pedicle. This is the normal configuration of the L5 pedicle, rather than the oval or rounded configuration conceptualized by most artists. This results in a very focal far-lateral stenosis occurring at the very inferolateral aspect of the intervertebral nerve root canal as defined by the L5 pedicle (*large arrows*). Note that this stenosis is considerably lateral to the entire SAP of S1, requiring extension of decompressive foraminotomy beyond the SAP to the infralateral lateral aspect of the pedicle of L5 itself, in order to effect surgical relief of this form of stenosis. *C,* Postoperative axial CT in the same patient shown in *A* and *B.* Note that there has been a complete facetectomy and left-sided hemilaminotomy with placement of a fat graft. Note also that this has not addressed the far-lateral lateral stenosis, which is still present 1 cm distal to the surgical decompression. Oblique reformatted images through the pedicle showed the stenosis to be unchanged from the preoperative study. The patient had significant persistent L5 radiculopathy. Repeat surgery with removal of the undersurface of the pedicle of L5 resulted in complete cessation of the patient's symptoms. In our experience, the failure to recognize this type of far-lateral up-down stenosis is the most common missed lesion even in the hands of skilled spine surgeons familiar with lateral spinal stenosis. This failure occurs because of the concept of the foramen being defined by the SAP and the difficulty in visualizing the stenotic lesion, which is very far lateral and ventral and is difficult to approach surgically.

images paralleling the plane of the L5 pedicle may be necessary to adequately define the stenosis (Fig. 17*A*, *B*).

Two unexpected benefits of MRI have been the clear depiction of lateral spinal stenosis and the excellent correlation between sagittal MR and sagittal reformatted CT images. Both modalities clearly depict bony lateral spinal stenosis within the intervertebral nerve root canal. Superior soft tissue contrast resolution makes MRI a valuable adjunct in the study of lateral nerve root entrapment, because MRI presents definably different signal intensities for the nerve root ganglion, lateral disc herniation, postoperative fibrosis, conjoined nerve root, and inflammation and/or edema. By comparison, CT shows these various anatomic entities within the intervertebral nerve root canal as homogeneous, nondiscrete soft tissue abnormalities opacifying the intervertebral nerve root canal.

DYNAMIC STENOSIS

Lateral stenosis may be either fixed or dynamic. Dynamic stenosis is thought to occur in patients with ligamentous laxity in whom rotary motion and weight loading of the spine cause anterior and superior subluxation of the superior articular facet. This produces impingement of the nerve root, either in the subarticular recess or the intervertebral nerve root canal. To demonstrate this lesion with HRCT, extension–rotation views of the lumbar spine are obtained following a routine study of the spine in flexion. By positioning the patient with the shoulders flat on the table and the ipsilateral hip elevated, the patient's pain may be reproduced, and ligamentous laxity with widening of the zygopophyseal joints and dynamic narrowing of the lateral nerve root canal on the elevated side may be demonstrated. Impingement of the nerve root ganglion is seen as a flattening of the posterior aspect of the ganglion by the SAP (Fig. 18). Because this procedure is time consuming and the demonstrated ligamentous laxity has been both minimal and subtle, it is performed sparingly.

NERVE SWELLING AND OTHER MEANS OF ENTRAPMENT

Post-impingement swelling of a spinal nerve, as it leaves the canal and passes downward (along the ventral surface of the sacral ala, in the case of L5), and pre-impingement swelling (seen less often) are also important direct signs of root, ganglion, or nerve entrapment. One does not always see these in patients having definitive bony stenosis. However, when present, such swelling is a reliable radiographic sign, virtually always correlating well with clinical symptoms (Fig. 19). Such swelling is probably due to a combination of hydrodynamic factors, that is, interference with lymphatic and vascular circulation around or in the nerve sheath or a blockage of axoplasmic transport deep inside the nerve or ganglion. The hollow, microscopic nerve axons transport a remarkable "soup" of substances, such as nerve growth factor, neurotransmitters, hormones, electrolytes, and water.[26] These substances are transported in both directions within the exoplasm. Obstruction of the flow of these materials causes the nerve to swell on both sides of the blockage. This hourglass configuration of the nerve structure is often seen at the time of surgical decompression. Incidentally, obstruction or delayed delivery of some of the axoplasmic substances may have marked effects on the distal nerve terminals and neuromotor junctions; therein lies the cause of many of the symptoms (e.g., neurogenic claudication, pain, and weakness) found in patients with stenosis.[18]

A question often arises: How it is possible to have a symptomatic compression of a nerve or ganglion when it rests within a canal composed of bony structures that do not move relative to one another? Such is the situation in which an uncinate spur arising from the inferior disc margin at a given lumbar segment entraps the ganglion by pressing it against its own pedicle. Such entrapment can occur in other body locations (e.g., in the cranial vault and in the lower leg as part of anterior compartment syndrome). To solve this seeming conundrum, one must consider the swelling. The nerve structure passing through a tight but adequate bone passage becomes "choked" when, because of local trauma, torsional injury, traction, inflammation, and so forth, the nerve begins to swell, leading to a sequence of edema, swelling, and entrapment. The reduction of such swelling by corticoids is one confirmation of this process. This autoentrapment sequence is probably the main event in patients with long-standing lateral stenosis (and lateral recess stenosis,

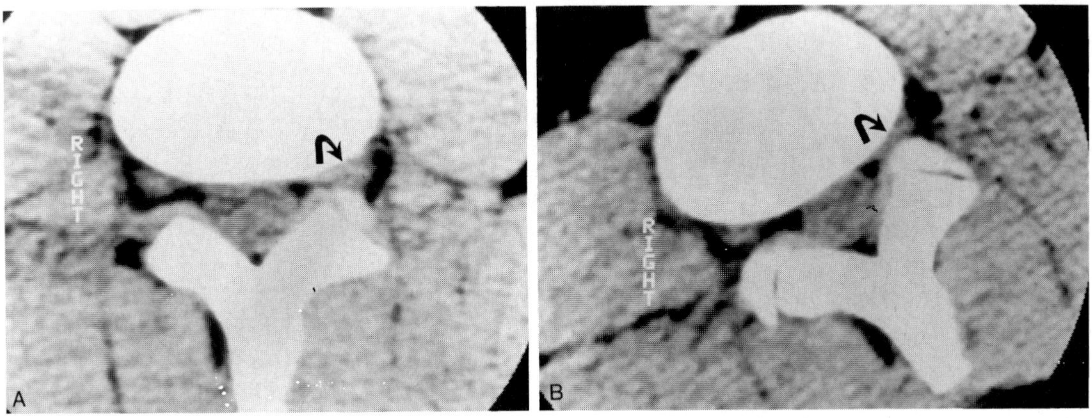

Figure 18 □ Dynamic stenosis. *A,* An axial CT image at the L4–L5 level shows narrowing of the AP dimension of the left L4–L5 intervertebral nerve root canal, attributable to mild thickening of the ligamentum flavum. Note the enlargement of the left L4 nerve root ganglia (*curved arrow*) and the lack of fat within the intervertebral nerve root canal. The patient had a left L4 radiculopathy with an increase in symptoms during extension and rotation. Dynamic impingement of the ganglia was suspected. *B,* This axial CT scan was obtained in both left anterior rotation of the pelvis and extension. There is dynamic narrowing of the left L4–L5 nerve root canal and flattening of the left L4 nerve root ganglia, consistent with dynamic stenosis (*curved arrow*).

as well) of low clinical importance which suddenly decompensates, resulting in pain and disability. Many patients with borderline lateral stenosis and a frankly herniated disc develop a postdiscectomy swelling of the nerve that renders the lateral stenosis symptomatic, producing failed back surgery syndrome (FBSS).

MRI IN LATERAL STENOSIS

MRI, thoroughly discussed elsewhere in this book, has proved to be a valuable adjunct to CT and other diagnostic radiographic tests of the lumbar spine. When used in conjunction with CT it provides markedly improved soft tissue contrast resolution of lumbar disc and neural elements and allows imaging directly in multiple planes, including coronal, sagittal, and axial planes. The improved soft tissue resolution allows clear differentiation between soft tissue structures (disc material, neural elements, intraspinal hematomas, spinal tumors, and postoperative recurrent herniations) and fibrosis, which are often isodense on CT (Fig. 20). Spatial

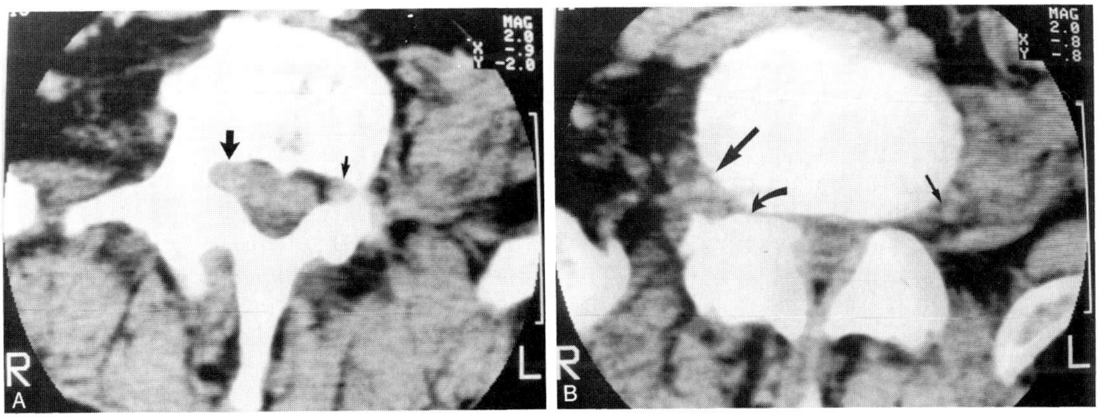

Figure 19 □ Compressive nerve root edema. *A,* This axial image of the lumbar spine is just cranial to the L5–S1 intervertebral nerve root canals. Note the enlargement of the right L5 nerve root ganglia (*large arrow*) as compared with the normal left L5 nerve root (*small arrow*). This represents pre-impingement swelling of the L5 nerve root as it enters the stenotic L5–S1 nerve root canal seen in *B. B,* Axial CT image of the intervertebral nerve root canals at L5–S1 shows severe front-back bony lateral spinal stenosis at L5–S1 on the right (*curved arrow*). There is marked edema of the right L5 nerve root ganglia (*large arrow*) and an indistinct margin of the ganglia, consistent with edema. Compare this with the normal left L5 nerve root ganglia (*small arrow*). Bony stenosis may exist without symptoms when the nerve root accommodates to the slowly progressive stenosis; however, when nerve root edema is present, there is a positive correlation between the CT scan and the clinical symptoms in virtually every case.

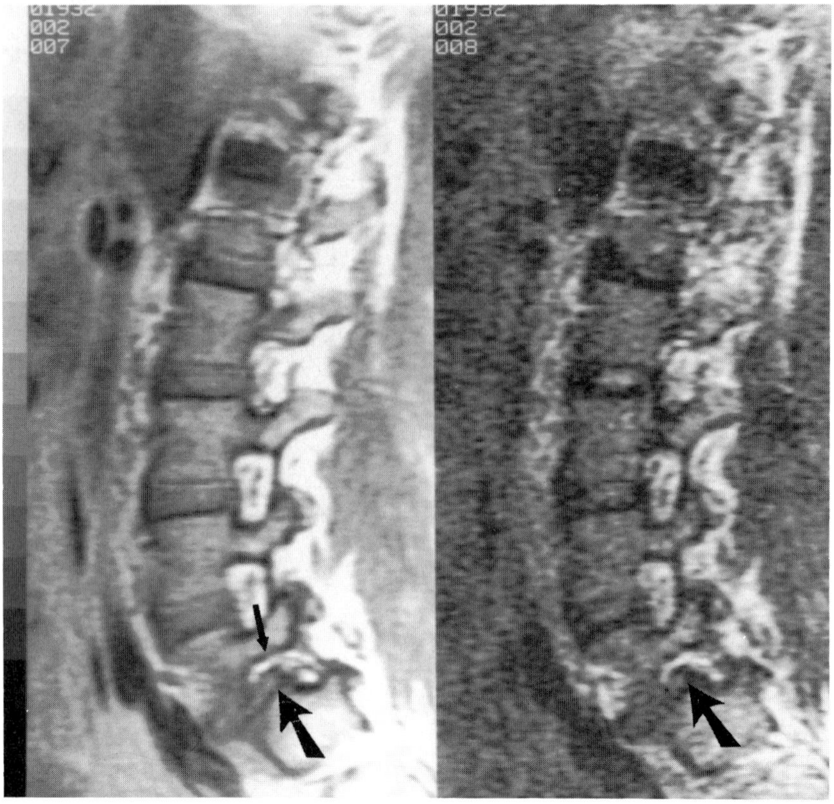

Figure 20 □ MRI of lateral disc herniation. The sagittal MRI clearly demonstrates a low-signal-intensity lateral disc herniation (*large arrow*), which is producing severe cephalocaudal compression of the L5 nerve root ganglia (*small arrow*) against the L5 pedicle. The CT in this case showed mild to moderate cephalocaudal narrowing of the intervertebral nerve root canal and opacification of the nerve root canal with an inability to distinguish between ganglia and underlying disc. The MR scan was diagnostic of the lateral disc herniation in the face of bony stenosis.

resolution is also nearly equal to that of CT, and sagittal images have a resolution considerably better than that of reformatted CT images. Unlike CT images, which reflect only a single parameter (attenuation values), MR images are a composite of T1 and T2 information, proton density, and vascular flow. Because the parameters of MRI (echo time [TE] and repetition time [TR]) and thus T1 and T2 weighting can be altered, widely varying appearances of signal intensity and depictions of normal and pathologic anatomy can be produced. The selection of the parameters that most clearly depict the disease present is both challenging and essential.

CT IN DEGENERATIVE DISC DISEASE

In our hands, CT has been a highly accurate tool in the diagnosis of frank disc herniation with nerve root compression as the cause of sciatica. Our criteria are very specific for a definitive diagnosis of herniation: first, the disc protrusion *must be focal and asymmetric,* often dorsolateral in position, and directly underlying the nerve root traversing that disc; second, there should be demonstrable nerve root compression and/or displacement; third, there is often post-impingement swelling of the affected nerve root caudal to the herniation with enlargement of the nerve, and indistinctness of its margin owing to edema, inflammatory exudate, or prominence of adjacent epidural veins (Fig. 21). When these findings are present, the diagnostic accuracy of CT is high (Table 1). Problems arise, however, in accurately diagnosing more diffusely bulging or herniated discs and differentiating these from the normal contours of the L5–S1 disc. The L5–S1 disc *normally* has a posterior convex configuration on axial CT images because of the normal rounded posterior margin of L5 and the sacrum in most patients and the oblique angle of the L5–S1

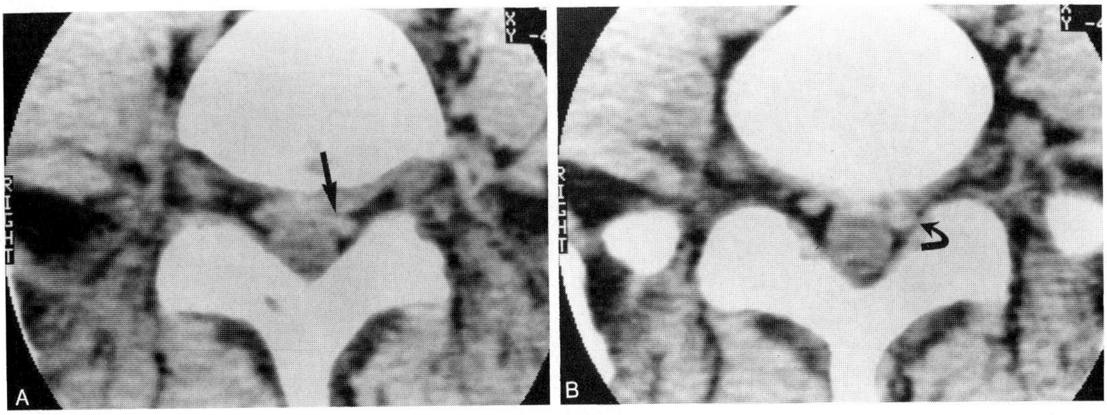

Figure 21 □ Classic herniated lumbar disc. *A,* This axial CT scan shows a moderate-sized, smoothly marginated, asymmetric, left-sided L5–S1 disc herniation with dorsal displacement of the left S1 nerve root (*arrow*). The asymmetry and nerve root displacement are the hallmarks of disc herniation and differentiate it from simple annular bulging. The dorsal displacement of the nerve root is also a very strong radiographic sign of disc herniation, since I have never seen an asymmetric positioning of the nerve roots as they merge from the thecal sac, with respect to the posterior aspect of the vertebral body in the AP plane, in the absence of an underlying mass (herniated disc is the most common of these). In order to apply this sign in every case, one must take into account any rotation of the vertebral bodies in patients with scoliosis. Therefore, if one is questioning whether a disc herniation is present, the observation of dorsal displacement of the nerve root is a very strong indication that the soft tissue density in question is an underlying disc herniation. A secondary sign may be found by a review of the scan immediately caudal to the questioned disc herniation. If the involved nerve root is separated from the posterior margin of the S1 vertebra, with epidural fat lying between it and the vertebra while the normal opposite side is tightly opposed to the vertebra, that finding is also an excellent sign of nerve root displacement by an underlying disc herniation. *B,* Axial CT scan one slice caudal to that in *A.* Note both the persistent dorsal displacement of the edematous, enlarged, left S1 nerve root (*curved arrow*) as well as the indistinctness of the margin of the ganglia and the infiltration of the perineural fat by engorged veins and/or edema. Nerve root edema in association with a compressive lesion such as disc herniation or stenosis is again a very strong sign of symptomatic nerve root impingement.

disc with the plane of the nonangled axial CT scan. Because of the lumbosacral angulation, the normal L5–S1 disc has an oblique course from its attachment to L5 *posteriorly* as well as to its attachment to S1 *inferiorly.* Therefore, an axial image obtained partially through the inferior margin of L5 and partially through the L5–S1 disc will show an apparent bulge. This is normal. Similarly, minor, *symmetric* bulges at L5–S1 are very common and should not be construed as herniations. These disc margins are widely separate from the S1 nerve roots and should *never* be considered as herniations or a cause of sciatica. Overcalling these minor changes, I believe, represents the most common error in CT lumbar spine scanning, and the purported high incidence of false-positive diagnoses of disc herniation attributed to CT. We use midline sagittal reformatted images to differentiate between true disc bulges at L5–S1 and apparent bulging due to lumbosacral angulation.

Table 1 □ CT Diagnosis of Herniated Discs: February—May, 1980 (78 Patients)

SURGICAL CONFIRMATION	NUMBER OF PATIENTS	PERCENTAGE OF PATIENTS
Surgical—HRCT agreement	40	91
False positive	3*	7
False negative	1†	2

*All false-positive examinations occurred in patients previously operated upon, with postoperative epidural fibrosis.
†Soft disc missed because of wide window width setting.

There is one condition in which a "bulging disc" or symmetric contained herniation can cause nerve root entrapment; that is in patients with trefoil central canals and narrowed bony lateral recesses or pathologically narrowed subarticular recesses resulting from degenerative facet hypertrophy. In these patients a combination of widely bulging disc and bony hypertrophy can cause subarticular stenosis and nerve root compression with sciatica (Fig. 22).

Because CT cannot differentiate annulus from nucleus as MRI can, it is difficult to differentiate accurately between a contained herniation (intact outer annulus and posterior longitudinal ligament) and a noncontained herniation. If the disc herniation is either large, large and irregular, or extending significantly craniad or caudally to the disc, one can assume, usually correctly, that it is

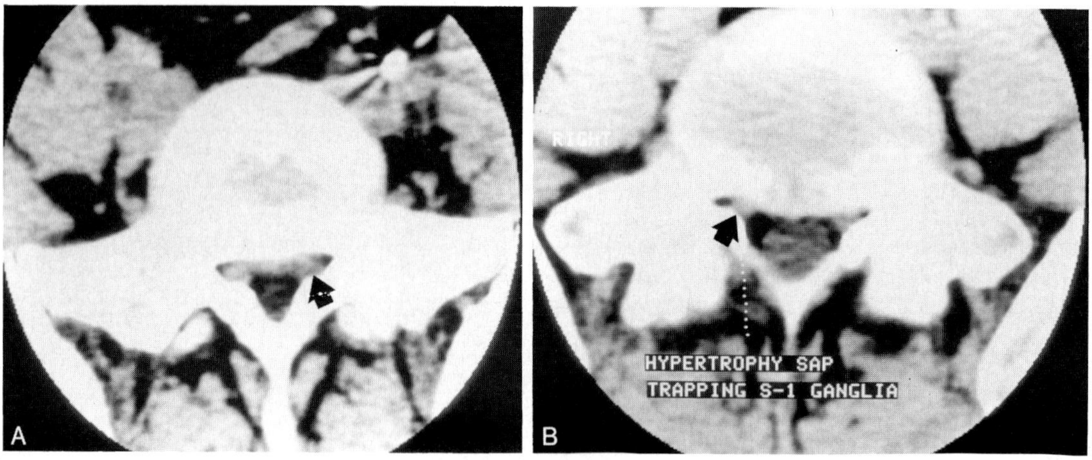

Figure 22 □ Subarticular recess stenosis. *A,* The axial CT image obtained just caudal to the L5–S1 disc shows bilateral subarticular recess compression of the S1 nerve roots by a combination of a broad-based central bulging disc in conjunction with a congenitally small trefoil configuration of the central spinal canal with narrowed bony lateral recesses. There is more compression of the left S1 nerve root with dorsal displacement of that nerve root, which merges with the posterior margin of the disc (*arrow*). *B,* Axial CT scan shows right-sided L5–S1 subarticular recess stenosis caused by mild hypertrophic spurring of the base of the SAP of S1 on the right with associated thickening of the lamina. There is moderate flattening of the dorsal aspect of the right S1 ganglia (*arrow*) in this patient with a right S1 radiculopathy. Surgery confirmed significant compression of the right S1 nerve root ganglia, which appeared edematous at the time of surgery.

noncontained. However, if the disc is small or moderate in size and smoothly marginated, any attempts to differentiate contained from noncontained herniation by means of CT are guesswork. If this distinction is necessary (e.g., in the case of percutaneous discectomy in which contained herniations are said to have improved results) preoperative MRI evaluation is necessary. MRI has enhanced our understanding of disc pathology and lends itself to a very specific and accurate nomenclature of degenerative disc disease. That is, it is now possible to clearly differentiate thickened redundant annuli from diffuse contained central disc herniations and to visualize complete and incomplete annular tears (both radial and circumferential) and inflammatory fluid within annular tears, which may be significant in predicting symptomatic disc lesions (19 of 20 patients with fluid within annular tears had positive symptomatic discograms, which reproduced their typical pain).*

MRI has shown us that many of the nonspecific symmetric central disc protrusions, which, based on CT, we previously and conservatively called "annular bulges," are actually contained central herniations with a dorsal migration of nuclear material beyond the posterior margin of the vertebral body.

This finding presents a challenge under our current worker's compensation system, because the mention of the term herniation, as opposed to bulging annulus, can lead to a significantly higher financial settlement. The situation is unfortunate, because this is new diagnostic information that is visualizable with MRI only, and we have no correlative clinical research yet available to indicate that the clinical symptoms or responses to treatment are different for simple degenerative thickening of the annulus, incomplete annular tears, and contained herniations. However, now that we can accurately differentiate among them using MRI, clinical research can decide the issue. We hope that this added information will lead to more specific treatment modalities and rational compensation schemes.

CT VERSUS MYELOGRAPHY IN DISC HERNIATION AND STENOSIS

In an attempt to determine the specificity and sensitivity of CT and compare them with those of myelography in the assessment of degenerative disc disease and stenosis (central, subarticular, and lateral), we performed

*Charles April: San Antonio, Challenge of Lumbar Spine. Personal communication, 1988.

a computer search of 20,000 examinations of the lumbar spine. Records of patients with herniated disc and/or stenosis (4,990 codes) were retrieved from the computer, and 1,120 charts were reviewed. Of these, 84 patients who had preoperative CT and myelographic examinations had surgically confirmed disc herniation and/or stenosis. (The myelographic studies were performed and interpreted at other institutions because outpatient myelography was not performed in our clinic.) Preoperative myelography was the factor that limited the number of patients qualifying for the study. The low number reflects the diminished role of preoperative lumbar myelography in our practice in 1984.

The study included a retrospective comparison of the reported interpretation of the myelograms performed elsewhere and our interpretation of the preoperative CT images of the lumbar spine. The interpretations of the myelograms were obtained from the radiologists' reports. No effort was made to discern whether information from a prior CT study of the spine was available to those radiologists at the time they interpreted the myelograms.

The double-blinded prospective portion of the study was performed by two spine radiologists using myelographic films and hard-copy films of CT examinations. Both the myelograms and CT images were independently interpreted without knowledge of the previous interpretations or clinical information. The myelographic and CT films were placed separately in unlabeled jackets, and the patient name and clinical information were obscured. No evaluation of the digital console images was performed.

All studies were analyzed for the presence of stenosis (lateral, subarticular, and central) and disc herniation. Positive correlations between surgery and CT and myelography were determined to be present only when a precise anatomic location existed (i.e., when the lesion was site specific as to level, side, and degree of severity). Examinations were categorized as normal or as indicating mild, moderate, or severe disease. Surgical confirmation was obtained in all 84 patients. An additional 10 normal CT examinations were included in the CT portion of the study to assess the incidence of false-positive CT interpretation of stenosis and disc herniation in the normal population.

Retrospective Analysis

We conducted a retrospective analysis of CT performed at our institution and myelography performed elsewhere in 78 patients with disc herniations. Preoperative CT was 97% accurate in the evaluation of disc herniation: true positive, 92% (72 patients); true negative, 5% (four patients); false negative, 1.5% (one patient); and false positive, 1.5% (one patient). The accuracy of preoperative myelography performed by radiologists at other institutions was true positive, 86% (65 patients); true negative, 3% (two patients); false negative, 6% (five patients); and false positive, 5% (four patients). Two myelograms were technically inadequate.

We also conducted a retrospective analysis of the accuracy of these modalities in assessing 19 patients with surgically proven lateral spinal stenosis. Preoperative CT performed at our institution was 100% accurate in detecting the presence of lateral stenosis in these 19 patients. There were no false-positive or false-negative examinations in the 84 patients evaluated by CT. By contrast, myelography performed elsewhere was negative in all cases, representing a 100% false-negative rate.

We also performed a retrospective analysis of the efficacy of CT and myelography in the diagnosis of central stenosis. The true-positive rate was 100% for both CT and myelography in nine patients with central stenosis. No myelograms were specifically interpreted as showing subarticular recess stenosis. Nonetheless, abnormalities were noted and described in language generally denoting subarticular stenosis, and these myelograms were considered to be correctly interpreted. However, the specific observation of selective nerve root entrapment (i.e., L5 nerve root at the L4–L5 level) was never made by the myelographers. All cases of subarticular stenosis were correctly interpreted on the initial CT reading.

Blinded Prospective Analysis

Ninety-four patients were included in the prospective comparison of CT and myelography. Of these, 84 had surgically documented lumbar disc herniation and/or stenosis; 10 were normal, included for the purpose of evaluating the incidence of false-positive CT interpretations in the normal

Table 2 □ Retrospective Independent Analysis of CT and Myelography

CT	NUMBER OF PATIENTS	PERCENTAGE OF PATIENTS	MYELOGRAPHY*	NUMBER OF PATIENTS	PERCENTAGE OF PATIENTS
HERNIATED DISC					
True positive	72	92	True positive	65	86
True negative	4	5	True negative	2	3
False negative	1	1.5	False negative	5	6
False positive	1	1.5	False positive	4	5
	78	100		76	100
LATERAL STENOSIS					
True positive	19	100	True positive	0	0
False negative	0	0	False negative	19	100
False positive	0	0	False positive	0	0
	19	100		19	100
CENTRAL STENOSIS AND SUBARTICULAR STENOSIS					
True positive	9	100	True positive	9	100
False positive	0	0	False negative	0	0
False positive	0	0	False positive	0	0
	9	100		9	100

population. The CT studies of all 10 normal patients were interpreted correctly by both radiologists, resulting in a true-negative accuracy of 100% with no false-positive diagnoses of disc herniation or stenosis. The results are tabulated in Tables 2 and 3.

Disc Herniation

In the blinded prospective study, 60 patients had surgically confirmed disc herniations. The prospective accuracy of CT and myelography in this patient population was as follows. Reader 1 was 91% accurate in interpreting herniation from CT images and 80% accurate in interpreting it from myelograms. The false-negative rate with CT was 7% (four patients), whereas the false-negative rate with myelography was 12% (seven patients). CT was falsely positive in 2% of cases (one patient), whereas myelography was falsely positive in 7% (four patients).

In interpreting disc herniation from CT images, Reader 2 achieved a true-positive rate of 87% (52 patients); interpreting myelograms, the same reader achieved a true-positive rate of 85% (51 patients). The false-negative rate was 11% (seven patients) with CT, and 13% (eight patients) with myelography. The false-positive rate was 2% (one patient) for both CT and myelography.

Central Stenosis

When the studies were used to evaluate central spinal stenosis, the results were as follows. Interpreting CT images, Reader 1 achieved a true-positive rate of 100% (nine patients). Interpreting myelograms, the same reader achieved a true-positive rate of 88% (seven patients), and made an erroneous but positive diagnosis of central disc herniation producing central stenosis in one patient (12%). (Central stenosis was diagnosed; the disc herniation was not.)

Interpreting CT images, Reader 2 achieved an accuracy rate of 100% (nine patients). Interpreting myelograms, he achieved a true-positive rate of 89% (eight patients) and a false-negative rate of 11% (one patient).

Subarticular Stenosis

Evaluating subarticular stenosis from CT images, Reader 1 achieved a true-positive rate of 91% (10 patients) and a false-negative rate of 9% (one patient). Evaluating myelograms, he achieved a true-positive rate of 45% (five patients) and a false-positive rate of 10% (one patient). In the false-negative CT examination, a small free-fragment disc herniation was misinterpreted as a swollen L5 nerve root due to bony subarticular recess impingement. Reader 2 correctly interpreted all 11 (100%) CT studies showing subarticular stenosis. With myelography, the true-positive rate was 55% (six patients) and the false-negative rate was 45% (five patients).

Lateral Stenosis

Reader 1 correctly interpreted the CT examinations of the 12 patients (100%) with

Table 3 □ Double-Blind Comparison of CT and Myelography

	READER 1		READER 2	
	Number of Patients	Percentage of Patients	Number of Patients	Percentage of Patients
HERNIATED DISC				
CT				
True positive	55	91	52	87
False negative	4	7	7	11
False positive	1	2	1	2
Total	60	100	60	100
Myelography				
True positive	48	80	51	85
Equivocal	– 1	1	—	—
False negative	7	12	8	13
False positive	4	7	1	2
Total	60	100	60	100
CENTRAL STENOSIS				
CT				
True positive	9	100	9	100
False negative	0	0	0	0
False positive	0	0	0	0
Total	9	100	9	100
Myelography*				
True positive	7	88	8	89
Positive-error	1	12	—	—
(HNP)	0	0	1	11
False negative	0	0	0	0
False positive	8	100	9	100
Total				
LATERAL STENOSIS				
CT				
True positive	12	100	12	100
False negative	0	0	0	0
False positive	0	0	0	0
Total	12	100	12	100
Myelography				
True positive	—	—	1	8
Definite	0	0	—	—
Equivocal	4	36	—	—
False negative†	8	64	11	92
False positive	—	—	0	0
Total	12	100	12	100
SUBARTICULAR STENOSIS				
CT				
True positive	10	91	11	100
False negative	—	—	0	0
False positive	1	9	0	0
Total	11	100	11	100
Myelography				
True positive	5	45	6	55
False negative	5	45	5	45
False positive	1‡	10	0	0
Total	11	100	11	100

*Myelogram technically inadequate.
†Stenosis missed at L4–L5 and L5–S1 because of block at L3–L4.
‡Positive but mistaken for HNP.

lateral stenosis and made no false-positive or false-negative interpretations. Interpreting myelograms, the same reader achieved a true-positive rate of 0% and made an equivocal diagnosis in four patients (36%) and a false-negative diagnosis in seven patients (65%). Reader 2 also achieved 100% accuracy (12 patients) with CT; myelographic interpretation resulted in a true-positive diagnosis in one patient (8%) and false-negative diagnoses in 11 patients (92%).

Retrospective Analysis of 100 Consecutive Lumbar Laminectomies

A large number of surgeons in many practices provided the surgical confirmation in the retrospective and blinded prospective portion of the study. When the studies were being designed, the diversity of this group raised the possibility of the study being flawed by the nonhomogeneity of surgical beliefs, approaches, and reporting with respect to lateral and subarticular stenosis. Consequently, to determine the relative incidence of disc herniation and lateral stenosis (as well as the accuracy of CT in delineating these entities in a more homogeneous population), we performed a retrospective analysis of the diagnostic accuracy of preoperative CT in 100 consecutive cases of lumbar laminectomies performed at the Institute for Low Back Care (ILBC) in 1984. In that year, only three lumbar myelograms were requested by ILBC physicians, whereas over 2,000 CT scans were performed (197 of these were contrast-enhanced CT studies that had supplanted myelography).

Results

Surgery confirmed herniated discs in 73% of these patients, lateral stenosis in 62%, and a combination of herniation and stenosis in 37%. Many patients had had previous operations. Patients were studied with both plain CT and metrizamide-enhanced CT. CT interpretation for these patients resulted in a 96% composite accuracy in the diagnosis of both herniated disc and lateral stenosis.

The errors were as follows. One error was a CT diagnosis of herniated disc that, at surgery, proved to be a bulging disc with nerve root compression within the subarticular recess. Review of the case revealed a tight subarticular recess in which differentiation of the disc and the swollen nerve root was not possible. Surgery consisted of hemilaminotomy without discectomy and resulted in 100% improvement. Therefore, although not anatomically precise, the CT diagnosis was site specific and led to correct surgical management of the case. In a second patient, a CT diagnosis of herniated disc was made, and both herniated disc and lateral stenosis were found at surgery. A third patient was diagnosed by means of CT as having a subarticular stenosis. Both stenosis and a very small free-fragment disc herniation were found at surgery. In this patient, the bony stenosis was severe, and the soft tissue density was believed to represent a swollen nerve root. At surgery, a small free-fragment disc herniation underlying the swollen nerve root was found. The fourth error was a CT interpretation of a small disc herniation that was found to be a large free fragment. On retrospective review, the herniation appeared small. Additional extrusion of the disc material might have occurred between the time of the CT examination and surgery, since the patient's symptoms worsened during that time.

Postoperative Results

To determine whether the improved diagnostic accuracy of CT led to better patient care and surgical results, we compared our patient group to patients, previously operated upon, who were described in the literature. Our patients were graded as to postoperative improvement according to (1) abatement of clinical signs and symptoms, (2) decreased use of medication, (3) ability to return to work, (4) subjective evaluation by the patient, and (5) physician evaluation. There was a 6-month or longer period of follow-up for all patients.

Sixty-five patients had had no prior surgery. Of these, 93% showed a 50% or greater improvement, and 71% showed 80% to 100% improvement. Of the 35 patients who had previous surgery, 91% showed 50% or greater improvement, and 40% showed 80% to 100% improvement (see Table 1). Of these, 23 had had two prior surgical procedures; 75% of this group showed 60% or greater improvement. Seven patients in this study showed either no improvement or 20% to 30% improvement. All seven were making workmen's compensation claims.

In this review of 100 consecutive laminectomies, five patients had residual postoperative far-out lateral spinal stenosis (all at L5–S1). Surgery had been performed to relieve lateral spinal stenosis diagnosed by CT and clinical examination. All five were only 40% to 50% improved following their surgery. Two underwent subsequent operations on the basis of CT demonstration of residual far-lateral stenosis, and both were then 100% improved.

This retrospective and prospective study of CT and myelography conclusively demonstrates the inability of myelography to delineate lateral entrapment of lumbosacral nerve roots. All 19 cases of lateral stenosis and lateral (foraminal) disc herniation were missed by the initial myelographers, and essentially all were missed by us upon review of the myelograms. Anatomically, lateral entrapment most often involves the ganglia within the intervertebral nerve root canal distal to the termination of the nerve root sheath. Therefore, one has no hope of demonstrating these lesions on myelography. A defect demonstrated by myelography is nonspecific and may be due to disc herniation, subarticular stenosis, or lateral stenosis.

CT was found to be more sensitive and specific for the evaluation of both disc herniation and stenosis. CT allows more precise depiction of the pathologic anatomy because one can directly visualize the bony and soft tissue abnormalities. In contrast, myelography depicts only indirect, nonspecific mass effects. As a result, CT allows not only more precise and complete radiologic diagnosis but also improved surgical planning.

At the heart of all diagnostic endeavors is the desire to improve patient care and surgical results. The surgical results we achieved in patients who underwent operations again—75% significant improvement (60% or more) in 23 patients with two previous surgeries and 56% improvement in patients with three previous surgeries—far exceed the ordinarily expected results (i.e., the often-quoted statistics of 70% expected improvement following the first surgical procedure, 30% following the second, and 5% following the third).

Because modern imaging modalities allow diagnoses that are not possible with myelography and improved surgical techniques, one should expect more favorable results in patients with a failed back surgery syndrome who have CT-proven and surgically proven nerve root compression lesions undiagnosed on previous imaging and missed at prior surgery. In fact, this is occurring, as documented by our results. We believe this improvement is largely attributable to the increasing use of CT and MR, which have enhanced our understanding of degenerative spine disease by improving the imaging of both herniated discs and stenosis. The significant difference between these modalities and myelography is their ability to depict lateral nerve root entrapment. In 60% of our patients with failed back surgery syndrome, missed lateral stenosis was the cause of symptoms. For this reason, CT and MRI are essential in the preoperative work-up of low back pain and sciatica. Myelography, because of its inherent inability to depict lateral spinal nerve root entrapment, is an inadequate preoperative screening procedure and, if performed, must be supplemented by CT.

As evidenced by the few preoperative myelograms performed in the large group of patients surveyed (84 out of the 1,120 chart reviews), the use of myelography is on the wane. Outpatient metrizamide-enhanced CT had largely replaced myelography in the evaluation of suspected postoperative recurrent disc herniation. Now MRI is largely supplanting intrathecal contrast-enhanced CT as the procedure of choice in the evaluation of postoperative lumbar spine patients with recurrent symptoms.

Many surgeons have justified ordering a preoperative myelogram by raising the possibility of missing a conus tumor. Love's paper[46] on conus tumors is cited frequently in this regard, but the paper is often misinterpreted. Love states that 5% of patients with conus tumors present with sciatica–*not* that 5% of patients with sciatica have conus tumors.

In our experience with over 80,000 CT examinations of the spine, only five cases of conus or nerve root tumor lying proximal to the levels scanned by CT have been subsequently detected (four by myelography and one by MRI) in patients with sciatica. All were diagnosed within the same diagnostic work-up because of the presence of signs and symptoms other than sciatica that suggested a more proximal lesion.

Ten normal patients were included in the patient population. All were diagnosed as normal by both spine radiologists in the blinded prospective portion of the study. Therefore, in this study, there was no observed propensity for CT to be associated with a high incidence of false-positive interpretation of disc herniation in the normal population as was reported by Bell and coworkers.[47] In this study of normals, a complete examination of the lumbar spine with axial scans from L3 to S1 and sagittal reformatting was performed, whereas Bell and colleagues obtained only a single slice at each disc level in their study of normal patients. We believe that this difference is largely responsible for their high incidence of false-positive diagnosis of disc herniation in a normal population and for their high rate of interobserver variability.

There was an observed decrease in the accuracy of interpretation of both CT and myelography in the prospective study as compared with the retrospective analysis of the original CT and myelographic reports. Our somewhat lower accuracy in myelographic interpretation as compared with the initial readings (80% and 85% versus 89%) can be attributed, in part, to the infrequent use of myelography in our practice and the lack of recent experience, as well as to our not having performed the procedure and therefore not visualizing the anatomy fluoroscopically.

We believe the use of only hard-copy film images in research studies leads to a less accurate interpretation of digital examinations such as CT and MR. In actual practice, difficult spine cases are routinely evaluated from digital console images, with the ability to use differing window and level settings to highlight disease. We believe that the use of only film images in the prospective study directly led to greater uncertainty and inaccuracy in the identification of subtle soft tissue abnormalities. Researchers designing studies comparing the digital modalities of CT and MR versus myelography must take into account that they cannot obtain a true measure of the accuracy of CT unless digital images are evaluated in addition to plain film images.

Myelographic studies of the postoperative patient with fibrosis and recurrent sciatica are difficult to interpret. Our results indicate that when intrathecal contrast is required, myelography should be replaced or aug-

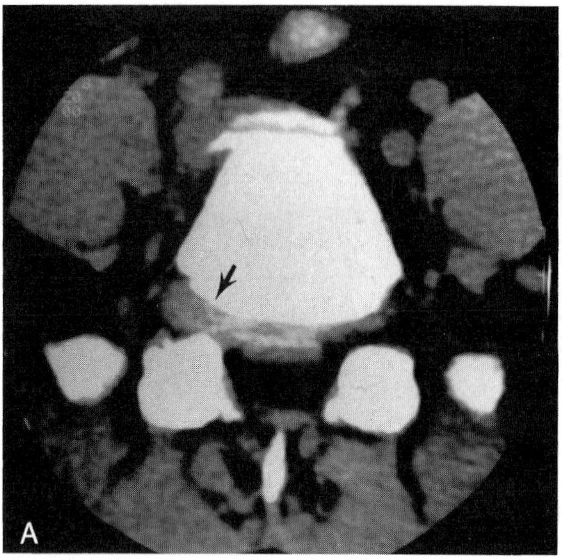

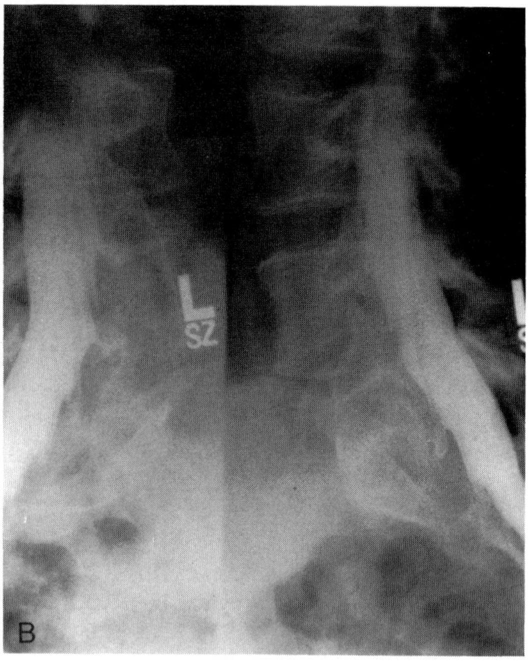

Figure 23 □ CT versus myelography in lateral disc herniation. *A,* The axial CT image shows a large lateral disc herniation at L5–S1 on the right (*arrow*), which is presenting as a large soft tissue mass within the intervertebral nerve root canal and is producing severe compression of the right L5 nerve root ganglia. *B,* Myelogram of the same patient was interpreted as normal and was unable to detect the lateral disc herniation. This is expected because the herniation is compressing the ganglia beyond the nerve root sheath. This finding illustrates the inability of myelography to adequately detect lateral nerve root impingement by disc herniation or bony stenosis.

mented by contrast-enhanced CT to increase accuracy. A prospective study of 43 postoperative patients with symptoms of recurrent disc herniation who were reoperated upon after contrast-enhanced CT determined an accuracy of 95% in differentiating postoperative fibrosis from recurrent or residual herniated nucleus pulposus (85% true positive, 10% true negative; 2.5% false positive, 2.5% false negative).

In 1984, we performed only three myelograms. MRI is now supplanting contrast-enhanced CT in the evaluation of the postoperative patient because it is noninvasive, has better soft tissue and low-contrast resolution, and improves the depiction of disease and postoperative changes within the intervertebral nerve root canals and thecal sac. The most common use of myelography has been in the evaluation of arachnoiditis, which now can be accomplished in most cases with axial T2-weighted MRI, as reported by Ross and colleagues.[43]

Disc abnormalities missed on myelograms and detected on CT images in this study were as follows: (1) lateral disc herniations (Fig. 23), (2) a large free-fragment L5–S1 disc herniation in a patient with a large epidural space, (3) lateral bulging disc producing L5 nerve root entrapment within the L5–S1 nerve root canal in a patient with cephalocaudal lateral stenosis due to lytic spondylolisthesis, and (4) disc herniation and lateral stenosis caudal to a complete block caused by postoperative arachnoiditis.

Iophendylate (Pantopaque) myelography is mentioned only to decry its continued use in the evaluation of lumbar spine disease. Irrefutable evidence is now available that iophendylate causes arachnoiditis. CT often demonstrates focal clumping of lumbosacral nerve roots around droplets of iophendylate in cases subsequently studied with water-soluble contrast-enhanced CT. Many of these patients have not had surgery. We have studied three patients who developed clinical and CT evidence of adhesive arachnoiditis following lumbar injection of iophendylate for evaluation of cervical spine disease. They had no history of lumbar spine disease before the injection, and the films of the lumbar spine during the cervical study were normal. Given the availability of water-soluble contrast materials, CT, and MR, I cannot think of an instance in which the use of intrathecal iophendylate can be justified, given its demonstrated ability to produce an incurable disease state.

This study indicates the superiority of CT over myelography in the evaluation of degenerative disc disease and its striking superiority in the evaluation of lateral spinal stenosis and lateral nerve root entrapment. Our results indicate that the preoperative use of CT improves surgical success rates both in patients previously not operated on and in those with FBSS. We partially attribute this improvement to the better understanding of spine pathology in general, and lateral nerve root entrapment in particular, made possible by CT, and more recently by MRI. Finally, it is essential that the imager and surgeon adopt a close, cooperative team approach and a precise and common nomenclature to obtain the best results. Classification of anatomy appreciated by radiology may well aid the radiologist in his or her understanding of the various disorders, but such classifications must primarily provide therapeutic guidance to the clinician and surgeon if they are to be of any intrinsic value to the patient.

SUMMARY

High-resolution CT of the lumbar spine has led to a dramatic expansion of the understanding and knowledge of the normal and pathologic anatomy of the lumbar spine. In our practice, it remains the diagnostic radiologic procedure of choice in the initial evaluation of nonoperated patients with low

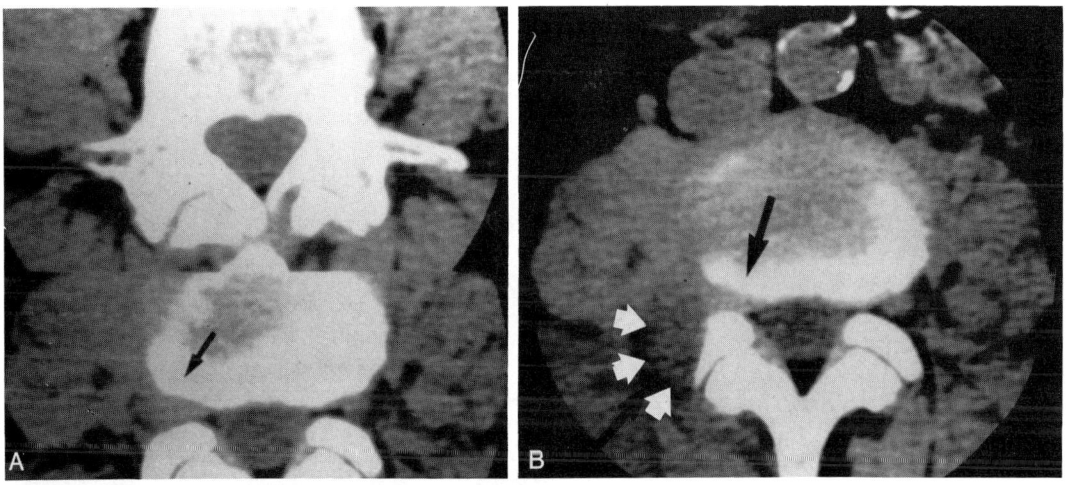

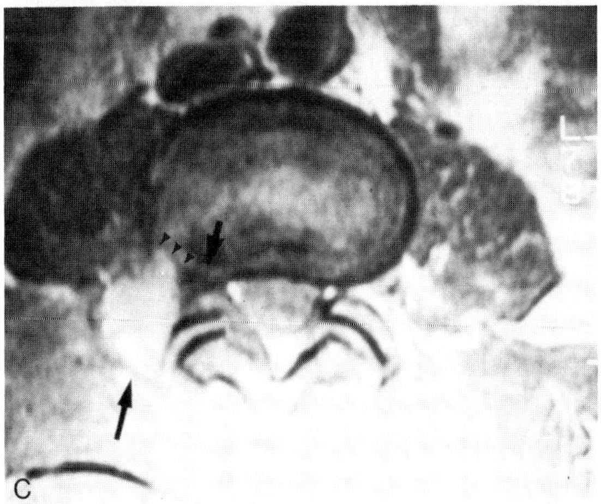

Figure 24 □ MRI and CT evaluation of lateral nerve root entrapment in the postoperative patient. *A,* Preoperative CT scan of the lumbar spine at L4–L5 shows a lateral disc herniation (*arrow*), which is opacifying the nerve root canal and compressing normal appearance of the left L4 nerve root ganglia. *B,* This postoperative CT scan of the lumbar spine was obtained 5 days following a discectomy with a paralateral approach. The patient had sudden, acute, recurrent right L4 radiculopathy. Note the surgical resection of the lateral aspect of the SAP and the paraspinous soft tissue mass adjacent to the articular process (*white arrowheads*). The right L4–L5 intervertebral nerve root canal remains opacified, and the soft tissue is of a density higher than that of the paraspinous mass (*large arrow*). Although differing densities were identified, CT was unable to differentiate postoperative edema, edematous ganglia, and a recurrent disc herniation from hematoma within the intervertebral nerve root canal in the paraspinous region. *C,* Postoperative MRI in this patient showed the large paraspinous soft tissue mass to represent postoperative hematoma (*large arrow*). It also showed that the intervertebral nerve root canal was filled with an abnormal low-signal-intensity lesion, on both axial and sagittal MR images, which was of the same density as the annulus; discontinuity of the annulus was seen lateral to this (*arrowheads*). A diagnosis of recurrent lateral annular disc herniation was possible on the basis of the MRI. Surgery confirmed this diagnosis.

back pain and sciatica. We find it to be highly accurate in the diagnosis of disc herniation (95%) and to best evaluate bony entrapment syndromes.

MRI has become an invaluable diagnostic adjunct to CT and is used when high-resolution CT has not provided a clear diagnosis or when CT findings and clinical symptoms conflict. MRI is the procedure of choice in the differentiation of soft tissue abnormalities, such as spinal neoplasm, infection, and hematoma; it is also preferred in the evaluation of the postoperative patient with recurrent sciatica (i.e., in differentiating recurrent disorders in discs and other soft tissue structures, such as hemorrhage, fibrosis, infection, conjoined nerve root, and enlargement of the ganglia due to edema).

It is particularly valuable in the evaluation of the postoperative patient with laterally situated disease within the nerve root canal. This is because no other modality can differentiate between postoperative fibrosis and other normal and pathologic structures within the nerve root canal, as they are isodense on CT and intrathecal contrast cannot extend laterally beyond the nerve root sheath (Fig. 24).

It has been stated that the most common cause of FBSS has been the lack of a proper diagnosis before the first surgical procedure. High-resolution CT and MRI provide very accurate means of preoperatively assessing both bony and soft tissue disease of the spine. High-resolution CT and MRI allow the direct visualization of not only the pathologic processes affecting the spine, but also the compressive effects these lesions may have on the nerve roots and thecal sac. Both provide direct evidence of nerve root involvement by bony stenosis, herniated disc, and postoperative perineural fibrosis. Together they do the following more accurately than did previous imaging modalities: provide clear images of the bony spinal canal and intervertebral nerve root canal as well as the soft tissues occupying those spaces; identify herniated and sequestered discs; differentiate the various causes of FBSS (e.g., recurrent disc, fibrosis, stenosis, fusion overgrowth, and arachnoiditis); and define nerve root entrapment. CT and MR are both accurate and complete examinations; MRI is preferred in the postoperative patient because it is noninvasive, can most accurately differentiate recurrent disc herniation from fibrosis,[44] can contribute additional valuable information in the lateral areas of the spine, and can now accurately assess arachnoiditis.

References

1. Crock, H.V.: A Reappraisal of intervertebral disc lesions. Med. J. Aust. 1:983, 1970.
2. Farfan, H.F.: Effects of torsion on the intervertebral joints. Can. J. Surg. 12:336, 1969.
3. Farfan, H.F.: Mechanical Disorders of the Low Back. Philadelphia, Lea & Febiger, 1973.
4. Farfan, H.F.: The pathological anatomy of degenerative spondylolisthesis: A cadaver study. Spine 5:412, 1980.
5. Farfan, H.F., and Sullivan, J.D.: The relation of facet orientation to intervertebral disc failure. Can. J. Surg. 10:179, 1967.
6. Kirkaldy-Willis, W.H., Heithoff, K.B., Bowen, C.V.A., and Shannon, R.: Pathological anatomy of lumbar spondylosis and stenosis, correlated with the CT scan, radiographic evaluation of the spine. *In* Post, M.J.D. (ed.): Current Advances with Emphasis on Computed Tomography. New York, Masson Publishing, 1980.
7. Kirkaldy-Willis, W.H., and McIvor, G.W.D.: Spinal stenosis. Clin. Orthop. 115:2, 1976.
8. Kirkaldy-Willis, W.H., Paine, K.W.E., Cauchoix, J., et al.: Lumbar spinal stenosis. Clin. Orthop. 99:30, 1974.
9. Kirkaldy-Willis, W.H., Wedge, J.H., Yong-Hing, K., and Reilly, J.: Pathology and pathogenesis of lumbar spondylosis and stenosis. Spine 3:319, 1978.
10. Keim, H.A., and Kirkaldy-Willis, W.H.: Low Back Pain. Clinical Symposia, Vol. 32. Summit, New Jersey, Ciba Pharmaceutical, 1980.
11. Jacobson, R.E., Gargano, F.P., and Rosomoff, H.L.: Transverse axial tomography of the spine, Parts 1 and 2. J. Neurosurg. 42:406, 1975.
12. Keller, J.T., Dunsker, S.B., McWhorter, J.M., et al.: The fate of autogenous grafts to the spinal dura. J. Neurosurg. 49:412, 1978.
13. Kestler, O.C.: Overgrowth (hypertrophy) of lumbosacral grafts causing a complete block. Bull. Hosp. Joint Dis. 27:51, 1966.
14. Crock, H.V.: Isolated lumbar disc resorption as a cause of nerve root canal stenosis. Clin. Orthop. 115:109, 1976.
15. Nelson, M.A.: Lumbar spinal stenosis. J. Bone Joint Surg. 55:506, 1973.
16. Post, M.J.D., Gargano, F.P., Vining, D.Q., and Rosomoff, H.L.: A comparison of radiographic methods of diagnosing constrictive lesions of the spinal canal (Toshiba unit versus CT scanner). J. Neurosurg. 48:360, 1978.
17. Sheldon, J.J., Russin, L.A., and Gargano, F.P.: Lumbar spinal stenosis: Radiographic diagnosis with special reference to transverse axial tomography. Clin. Orthop. 115:53, 1976.
18. Bell, G.R., Rothman, R.H., Booth, R.E., et al.: A study of computer-assisted tomography. II. Comparison of metrizamide myelography and computer tomography in the diagnosis of herniated lumbar disc and spinal stenosis. Spine 9:552, 1984.
19. Chafetz, N., and Genant, H.K.: Computed tomography of the lumbar spine. Orthop. Clin. North Am. 14:147, 1983.

20. Kornberg, M., and Rechtine, G.R.: Quantitative assessment of the fifth lumbar spinal canal by computed tomography in symptomatic L4–L5 disc disease. Spine 10:328, 1985.
21. Lifson, A., Heithoff, K.B., Burton, C.V., and Ray, C.D.: High resolution computed tomographic scanning of the lumbosacral spine. Mod. Neurosurg. 1:31, 1982.
22. Postacchini, F.: Lumbar spinal stenosis and pseudostenosis. Ital. J. Orthop. Traumatol. 9:339, 1983.
23. Robertson, G.H., Llewellyn, H.T., and Taveras, J.M.: The narrow lumbar spinal canal syndrome. Radiology 107:89, 1973.
24. Simeon, F.A., and Rothman, R.H.: Clinical usefulness of CT scanning in the diagnosis and treatment of lumbar spine disease. Radiol. Clin. North Am. 21:197, 1983.
25. Bolender, N.F., Schonstrom, N.S., and Spengler, D.M.: Role of computed tomography and myelography in the diagnosis of central spinal stenosis. J. Bone Joint Surg. (Am.) 67:240, 1985.
26. Verbiest, H.: Further experiences on the pathological influences of a developmental narrowness of a bony lumbar vertebral canal. J. Bone Joint Surg. (Br.) 37:576, 1955.
27. Beers, G.H., Carter, A.P., Leiter, B.E., et al.: Interobserver discrepancies in distance measurements from lumbar spine CT scans. A.J.R. 144:395, 1985.
28. Schornstrom, N.S., Bolender, N.F., and Spengler, D.M.: The pathomorphology of spinal stenosis as seen on CT scans of the lumbar spine. Spine 10:806, 1985.
29. Wiltse, L.L., et al.: Alar transverse process impingement of the L5 spinal nerve: The far-out syndrome. Spine 9:31, 1984.
30. Rothman, S.L., and Glenn, W.V., Jr.: CT multiplanar reconstruction: 253 cases of lumbar spondylosis. A.J.N.R. 5:81, 1984.
31. Stewart, J.R., and Thorne, R.P.: Lumbar spinal stenosis. Orthop. Nurs. 2:35, 1983.
32. Ray, C.D.: Far lateral decompressions for stenosis: The paralateral approach. *In* White, A.H., Rothman, R.H., and Ray, C.D. (eds.): Lumbar Spine Surgery: Techniques and Complications. St. Louis, C.V. Mosby, 1986.
33. Arnoldi, C., Brodsky, A.E., Cauchoix, J., et al: Lumbar spinal stenosis and nerve root entrapment syndromes. Definition and classification. Clin. Orthop. 115:4, 1976.
34. Brodsky, A.E.: Low back pain syndromes due to spinal stenosis and posterior cauda equina compression. Bull. Hosp. Joint Dis. 30:66, 1969.
35. Lancourt, J.E., Glen, W.V., and Wiltse, L.L.: Multiplanar computerized tomography in the normal spine and in the diagnosis of spinal stenosis: A gross anatomic-computerized tomographic correlation. Spine 4:379, 1979.
36. Lee, B.C.P., Kazam, E., and Newman, A.P.: Computed tomography of the spine and spinal cord. Radiology 128:95, 1978.
37. Ray, C.D.: Methods of resection of bone spurs, osteophytes, and bony encroachment. *In* White, A.H., Rothman, R.H., and Ray, C.D. (eds.): Lumbar Spine Surgery: Techniques and Complications. St. Louis, C.V. Mosby, 1986.
38. Weisz, G.M., and Lee, P.: Spinal canal stenosis. Concept of spinal reserve capacity: Radiologic measurements and clinical applications. Clin. Orthop. 179:134, 1983.
39. Wright, A.: Symposium: The role of spinal fusion. Spine 6:292, 1981.
40. Wiltse, L.L., Kirkaldy-Willis, W.H., and McIvor, G.W.D.: The treatment of spinal stenosis. Clin. Orthop. 115:83, 1979.
41. Weinstein, P.R.: Diagnosis and management of lumbar spinal stenosis. Clin. Neurosurg. 30:677, 1983.
42. Heithoff, K.B.: Cooperative study of the efficacy of metrizamide myelography and CT in the study of lumbar disc disease and spinal stenosis. 71st Scientific Assembly, Radiological Society of North America. Chicago, November 17–22, 1985.
43. Ross, J.S., et al.: MR imaging of lumbar arachnoiditis. A.J.N.R. 8:885, 1987.
44. Heithoff, K.B.: Comparison of MRI and metrizamide-enhanced CT scanning in the evaluation of post-operative recurrent disc herniation versus fibrosis. Annual Meeting of the I.S.S.L.S., Dallas, May, 1986.
45. Burton, C.V.: Spinal imaging: A modern inconvenience? Spinal Update 10:83, 1987.
46. Love, J.G.: The differential diagnosis of intraspinal tumors and protruded intervertebral discs. J. Neurosurg. 1:275, 1944.
47. Bell, G.R., Rothman, R.H., Booth, R.E., et al.: A study of computer-assisted tomography. II. Comparison of metrizamide myelography and computed tomography in the diagnosis of herniated lumbar disc and spinal stenosis. Spine 9:552, 1984.
48. Mooney, V.: Symposium: Spine fusion. Seventh Annual Meeting of the I.S.S.L.S., New Orleans, May 27, 1980.

MAGNETIC RESONANCE IMAGING OF THE LUMBAR SPINE*

David W. Stoller
Harry K. Genant

Accurate diagnosis and evaluation of the lumbar spine are necessary in the specialties of orthopedics, rheumatology, neurology, and neurosurgery. At best, standard radiographs of the spine provide a limited interpretation of nonosseous events occurring in the discs, cord, cerebrospinal fluid (CSF), and ligaments (structures not directly visualized on plain film studies). Myelography, an invasive procedure, indirectly evaluates the disc by visualizing the contour of the thecal sac and nerve root sleeves. Computed tomography (CT) is useful in delineating bone detail, and direct axial scans of the spine provide soft tissue discrimination of the disc, nerve roots, and thecal sac.[7, 11, 21, 59, 60] However, sagittal, coronal, or oblique views cannot directly be acquired, and they require reformations. CT is excellent for assessing postoperative pseudoarthrosis, but fibrosis and scarring may be difficult to differentiate from disc material, especially in the absence of contrast enhancement. Magnetic resonance imaging (MRI) complements CT and myelography in the routine evaluation of the spine for degenerative disc disease, trauma, infection, neoplasia, and intrinsic cord disease.[3, 8, 14–16, 19, 20, 29, 32, 36, 39, 44, 46, 50, 53]

MRI makes it possible to distinguish and assess the separate components of the disc, including the nucleus pulposus and annulus fibrosus, in early degenerative disc disease. The disc–thecal sac interface is defined without the administration of a contrast agent; the structure of the cord is visualized by contrast with the surrounding CSF; and the dura and supporting ligaments of the spine are demonstrated in either sagittal or axial images. MRI has the unique advantage of providing direct marrow imaging in the study of patients with marrow infiltrative diseases, metastasis, infection, or reactive end-plate changes.[24, 31, 40, 41]

IMAGING PROTOCOLS FOR THE LUMBAR SPINE

Advances in MRI of the lumbar spine have paralleled the development of improved surface coil technology. An increased signal-to-noise ratio with excellent contrast and spatial resolution has made it possible to delineate spinal anatomy in sagittal and axial planes.[22, 26, 27, 54, 55] The lumbar spine is imaged using a planar surface coil with its long axis oriented parallel to the spine. This permits acquisition with a field of view (FOV) approximating the anatomic region of interest. When the area of interest is restricted to one or two vertebral levels, a 5-inch circular spine coil may be used to provide a higher signal-to-noise ratio.

High-resolution T1-weighted (TR [repetition time] = 1,000 msec and TE [echo time] = 20 msec) images acquired with a 256 × 256 matrix, a 20- to 24-cm sagittal FOV, or a 16-cm axial FOV at four excitations require a 17-minute acquisition time per imaging plane. T2-weighted sequences complement a partial saturation protocol in differentiating the bright CSF subarachnoid space from low-spin-density ligaments and cortical bone. Intrinsic cord lesions frequently require T2 weighting so that they can be differentiated from isointense CSF or cord. The nucleus pulposus and the disc–thecal sac interface are best defined on T2-weighted sequences. Adequate T2 weighting with prolonged TR settings (TR = 2,000 msec and TE = 20.6 msec) requires an additional 17 minutes of imaging time at a 256 × 256 matrix using four excitations. The trade-off in using two excitations to limit imaging time is that the signal-to-noise ratio substantially decreases.

Gradient-echo techniques have made it possible to achieve multiplanar T2 (T2*)

*Portions of this chapter were previously published in Stoller, D.W., et al.: Magnetic Resonance Imaging of Orthopedics and Rheumatology. Philadelphia, J.B. Lippincott, 1989.

images using flip angle pulse sequences (TR = 400 msec and TE = 15 msec) with θ values of less than 90 degrees. This is significant in providing T2-weighted contrast without the time restrictions inherent in conventional spin-echo techniques using a 90- to 180-degree pulse pair. Instead of conventional T2 weighting, a T2* gradient-echo sequence can be used to supplement the T1-weighted acquisition. Even though T2* gradient-echo contrast may be substituted for conventional T2 weighting, it should be noted that their contrast properties are not equivalent. For instance, desiccated discs that image with low signal intensity on T2-weighted images may remain isointense with intact intervertebral discs on T2* gradient refocused images.

NORMAL MRI ANATOMY OF THE LUMBAR SPINE

Sagittal Images

T1-Weighted Images

CSF within the subarachnoid space is visualized with a low signal intensity, in contrast to the brighter (intermediate) signal intensity of the cord, and posterior epidural fat images with a high signal intensity. Anterior epidural fat is prominent in the L5–S1 region. Yellow or fatty marrow within the vertebral bodies of the thoracic and lumbar spine images with a high signal intensity, in contrast to the intermediate signal intensity of intervertebral discs. Nuclear–annular differentiation is not precisely defined on T1-weighted images (Fig. 1). The cord is of uniform intermediate signal intensity. The conus medullaris is tapered and terminates posteriorly at the level of L1. Sagittal images of the lumbar spine with a 24-cm FOV demonstrate the conus medullaris. The cauda equina is of a signal intensity lower than that of the conus medullaris, secondary to greater surface contact with surrounding CSF. On T1-weighted images, anterior and posterior longitudinal ligaments are difficult to distinguish from low-signal-intensity cortical bone. The exiting nerve roots are visualized with intermediate signal intensity within the teardrop-shaped intervertebral foramina and are surrounded by high-signal-intensity fat (Fig. 2). On parasagittal images, the low-signal-intensity radicular vein and intermediate-signal dorsal root are demarcated by abundant high-signal-intensity fat within the lumbar neural foramina.

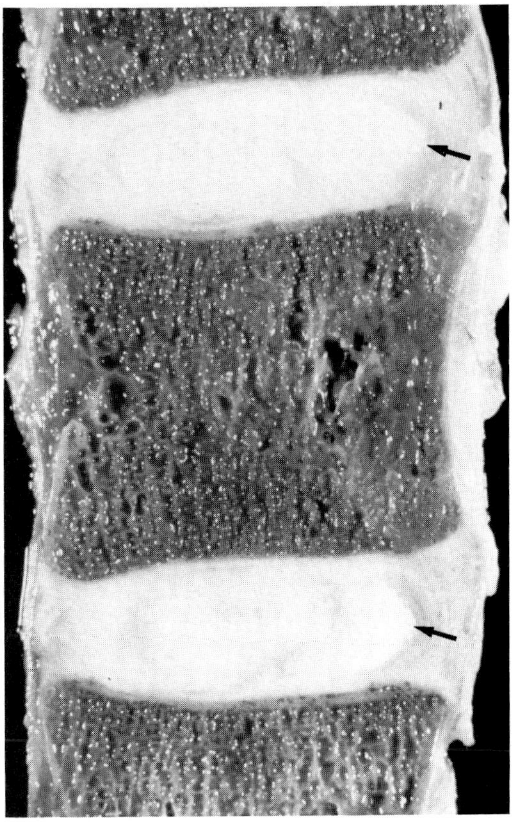

Figure 1 □ Gross sagittal specimen of the lumbar spine demonstrates nuclear-annular separation (*arrows*).

T2-Weighted Images

Intervertebral discs image with bright signal intensity on T2- and T2*-weighted images. Epidural fat is visualized with an intermediate signal intensity (see Fig. 2). Vertebral body marrow demonstrates intermediate signal intensity on T2-weighted images and low signal intensity on T2*-weighted images. On T2-weighted images, the conus medullaris demonstrates signal intensity lower than that of the surrounding bright CSF. The nucleus pulposus and inner annular fibers image with increased signal intensity on T2-weighted images, whereas peripheral annular fibers maintain low signal intensity. A low-signal-intensity band in the midportion of the intervertebral disc is thought to represent an invagination of annular fibers, although an anatomic correlate has not yet been found. The basivertebral vein is identified as a high-signal-intensity segment in

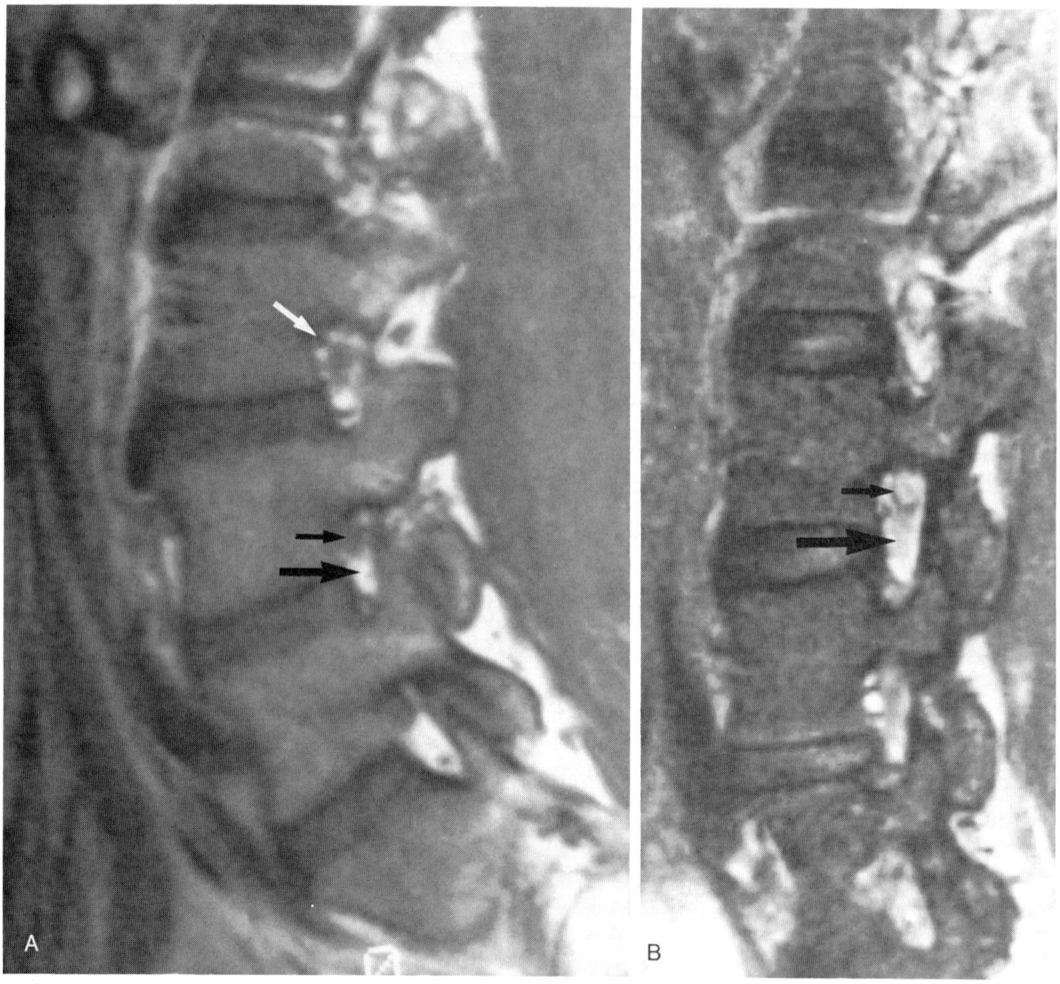

Figure 2 □ Intervertebral foramina. *A,* Parasagittal T1-weighted image demonstrates high-signal-intensity epidural fat (*large black arrow*), intermediate-signal-intensity dorsal root ganglion (*small black arrow*), and low-signal-intensity radicular vein (*white arrow*). (TR = 600 msec, TE = 20 msec.) *B,* Intermediate-signal-intensity foraminal fat (*large arrow*) has poor contrast compared with the intermediate-signal-intensity dorsal root ganglion (*small arrow*) on a conventional T2-weighted parasagittal image. (TR = 2,000 msec, TE = 60 msec.)

the midposterior aspect of the vertebral body.

Axial Images

T1-Weighted Images

High intensity signal from fatty marrow is visualized in the body, pedicle, lamina, and transverse and spinous processes of the vertebra. The intraforaminal vein (of low signal intensity) can be seen anterior to the dorsal root ganglion (of intermediate signal intensity). The budding and exiting nerve roots of the dorsal root ganglion are well defined, and they image with an intermediate signal intensity, being surrounded by high-signal-intensity fat. Nerve roots are often identified within the lower-signal-intensity thecal sac. Posterior epidural fat is identified behind the low-signal-intensity subarachnoid space. The basivertebral vein, retrovertebral plexus, and anterior epidural veins are displayed as low-signal-intensity structures. The ligamentum flavum parallels the inner surface of the lamina and demonstrates intermediate signal intensity.

T2-Weighted Images

An axial myelographic effect can be generated with gradient refocused images in a fraction of the time required for conventional spin-echo techniques (Fig. 3). On T2*-

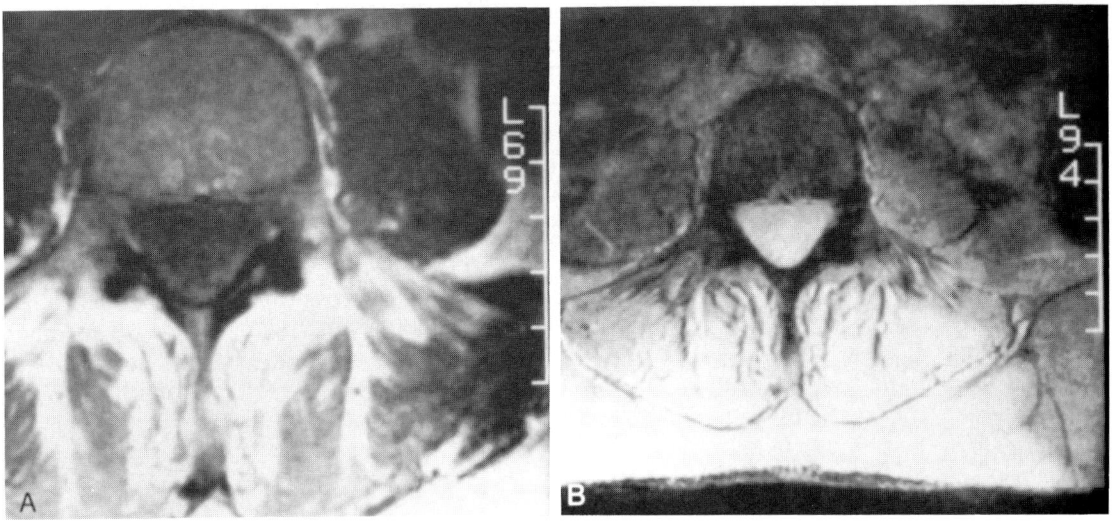

Figure 3 □ Axial myelographic contrast. *A,* T1-weighted axial image, and *B,* T2* gradient-echo axial image are shown at midlumbar body level. The thecal sac demonstrates bright signal intensity with T2* contrast.

weighted images, the lumbar cauda equina is visualized with low signal intensity, in contrast to the high signal intensity of CSF (Fig. 4). Facet cartilage images with high signal intensity on gradient-echo images and intermediate signal intensity on conventional T2-weighted images. High-signal-intensity nuclear material and inner annular fibers are distinguished from low-signal-intensity peripheral collagen fibers of the annulus. Anterior-signal void within the thecal sac is more frequent with long TR/TE sequences that accentuate CSF pulsation artifacts.

PATHOLOGY OF THE SPINE

MRI can be used to evaluate infection, trauma, and neoplasia involving osseous structures, soft tissue, and the spinal cord.[3, 8, 14–16, 19, 20, 24, 29, 31, 32, 36, 39, 40, 41, 44, 46, 50, 53] Direct marrow imaging facilitates early detection of marrow replacement disorders such as leukemia, multiple myeloma, and metastasis. Atlantoaxial instability can be functionally imaged using separate acquisitions with the patient positioned in flexion and extension. Signal characteristics of cystic lesions (syringomyelia and hydromyelia)

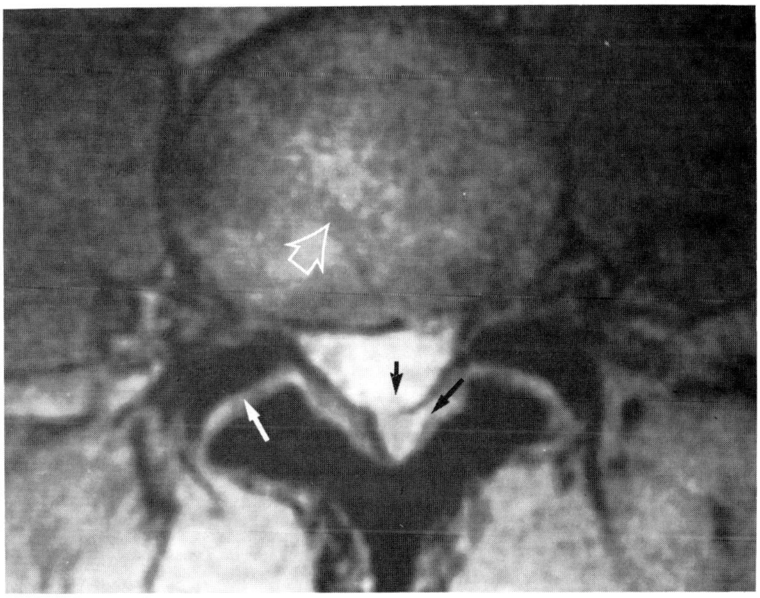

Figure 4 □ T2* gradient-echo axial image of lumbar intervertebral disc identifies high-signal-intensity disc (*open white arrow*), articular cartilage (*solid white arrow*), ligamentum flavum (*solid black arrow*), and low-signal-intensity cauda equina (*short black arrow*). (TR = 400 msec, TE = 15 msec; flip angle = 30 degrees.)

are similar to those of CSF. Intramedullary lipomas image with high signal intensity on T1-weighted images and with intermediate- to high-signal-intensity on T2-weighted images; they are dark on short T1 inversion recovery (STIR) sequences. Lipomas can sometimes be confused with subacute hemorrhage (also bright on T1-weighted images), but hemorrhage shows increased signal intensity on long TR/TE (T2-weighted) sequences. The detection of neurofibromas[6] and meningiomas, common intradural extramedullary tumors, may require the use of intravenous gadolinium diethylenetriamine penta-acetic acid (DTPA) (a paramagnetic contrast agent) to improve their visualization.

Degenerative Disc Disease

The accuracy of MRI has been shown to be equivalent to CT and myelography in the assessment of lumbar disc herniations.[4, 8, 12, 15, 16, 32, 34, 39, 44–46, 53] Herniations identified in the sagittal plane should be confirmed on axial images, and thin (3-mm) sections are only rarely necessary to characterize the disc abnormality (Fig. 5). Associated Schmorl's nodes and decreased intervertebral signal intensity can be seen on T2-weighted images. Marginal osteophytes contribute to extrinsic (extradural) impression on the thecal sac. Flow artifacts in the lumbar spine should not be mistaken for intrinsic pathologic conditions and may be accentuated around areas of stenosis.

In early lumbar degenerative disc disease there may be a loss of hydropic integrity or intradiscal desiccation, characterized by decreased signal intensity on conventional T2-weighted images (Fig. 6). Inhomogeneity and areas of decreased signal intensity on T2* gradient-echo images are usually associated with severe degenerative disc disease. Disc–CSF separation may be difficult on T1-weighted images because the posterior disc margin and thecal sac both image with low signal intensity. Most herniated discs are depicted as degenerative or desiccated on conventional T2-weighted images in contrast to T2* gradient refocused images (Figs. 7 and 8). Lateral disc herniations can efface the bright-signal-intensity neural foraminal fat, without compromising the thecal sac. Large posterolateral disc herniations may compromise both the thecal sac and exiting nerve root. The sagittal imaging plane may be more sensitive for defining deformities of the thecal sac at the disc–thecal sac interface. T2-weighted images are effective in increasing contrast discrimination between high-signal-intensity CSF and low-signal-in-

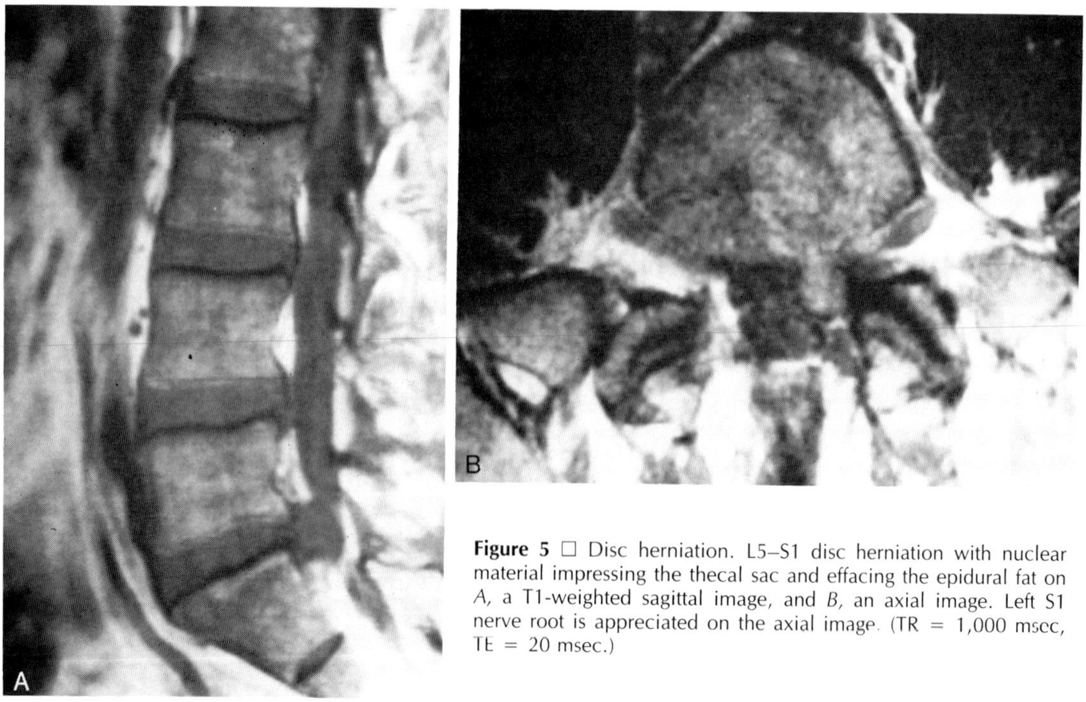

Figure 5 □ Disc herniation. L5–S1 disc herniation with nuclear material impressing the thecal sac and effacing the epidural fat on *A*, a T1-weighted sagittal image, and *B*, an axial image. Left S1 nerve root is appreciated on the axial image. (TR = 1,000 msec, TE = 20 msec.)

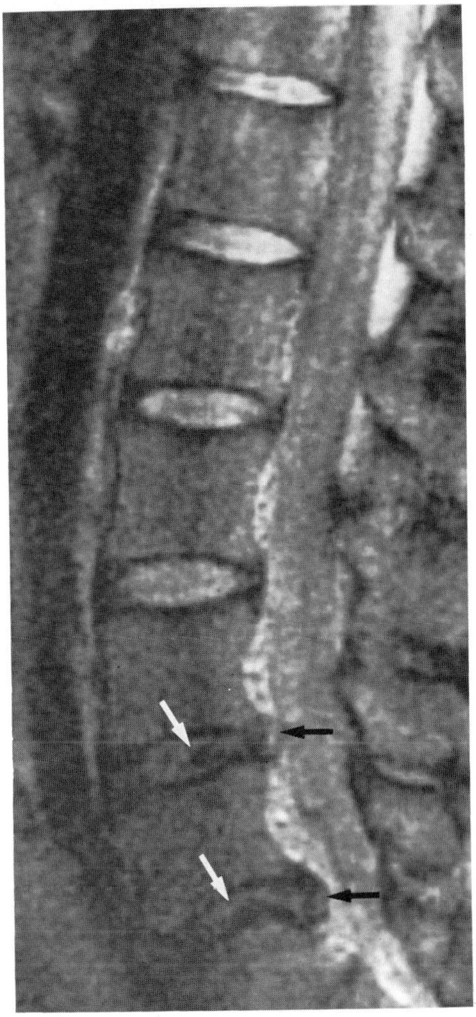

Figure 6 □ Low-signal-intensity desiccated discs (*white arrows*) and herniated discs (*black arrows*) at L4–L5 and L5–S1 are visible on conventional T2-weighted sagittal images. (TR = 2000 msec, TE = 60 msec.)

tensity annular fibers at the disc–thecal sac boundary. Acute herniations may be associated with increased signal intensity on conventional T1- or T2-weighted images. On gradient-echo images, the posterior annular fibers and longitudinal ligament image with low signal intensity (Fig. 9), facilitating differentiation of the disc and CSF. Gradient-echo images also display the black line of the dura in the lumbar spine, which may be displaced in posterior disc herniations. Nuclear material extruded from the disc usually images with low signal intensity on conventional T1- and T2-weighted images and with high signal intensity on gradient-echo sequences.

Axial images are important in evaluating neural foramina and nerve root effacement in cases of lateral and posterolateral disc herniations. Axial gradient-echo images help distinguish herniated disc material from higher-signal-intensity CSF. The path of extruded nuclear material may be outlined on axial T2*-weighted images (discogram-like effect) (Fig. 10). Disc material or fragments superior or inferior to the intervertebral disc level may represent free fragments (Fig. 11). Calcified cysts of the facet joint may mimic a calcified free fragment.

A decrease or effacement of epidural fat is seen with *lumbar canal stenosis*.[46] Indentations of the thecal sac are caused by both disc and osteophytic impingement. Facet and ligamentum flavum hypertrophy contributes to neural foraminal and central canal stenosis (Fig. 12). Canal dimensions in

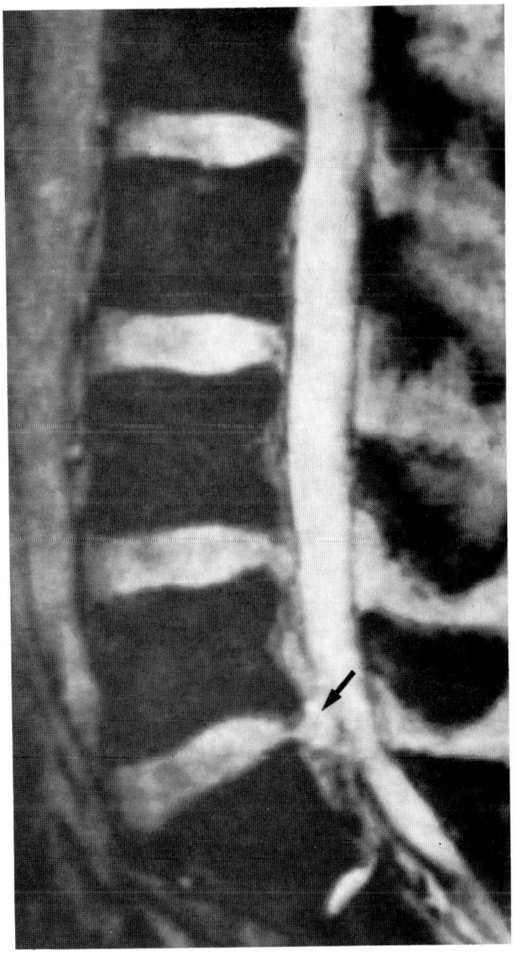

Figure 7 □ T2* gradient-echo sagittal image shows L5–S1 disc herniation with high-signal-intensity extruded nuclear material (*arrow*) that is isointense with adjacent intervertebral disc.

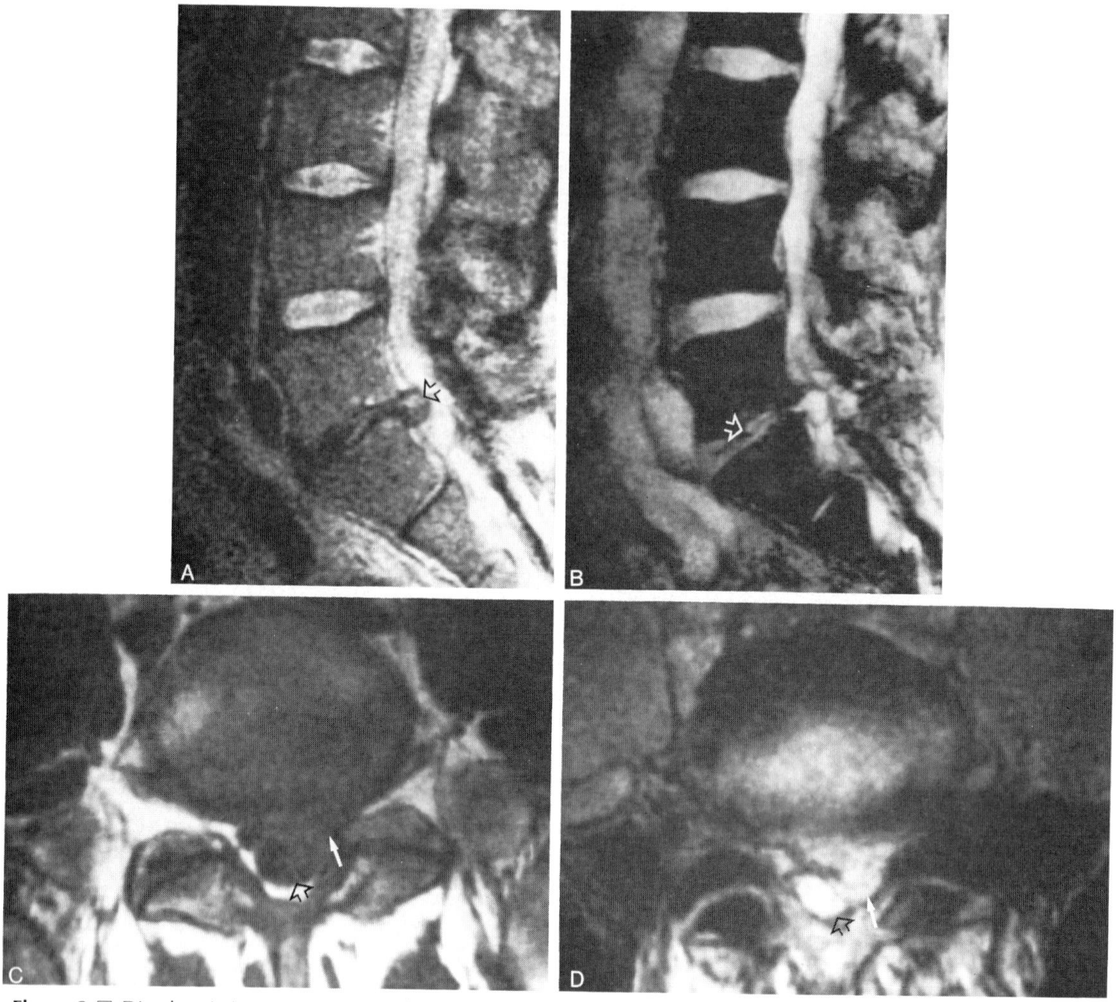

Figure 8 □ Disc herniation on conventional spin-echo and gradient-echo techniques. *A,* T2-weighted image and *B,* T2* gradient-echo image demonstrate herniated and extruded L5–S1 nuclear material. Intervertebral disc contents (*arrow*) remain low in signal intensity on a conventional T2-weighted sequence (*A*). On the T2* gradient-echo image, nuclear material generates high signal intensity, whereas the adjacent desiccated disc is visualized with signal inhomogeneity and low-signal-intensity clefting (*B, arrow*). *C,* Corresponding T1-weighted axial image and *D,* T2*-weighted axial image display superior contrast definition of herniated nuclear material (*solid arrow*) and deformed thecal sac (*open arrow*) on gradient-echo sequence (*D*).

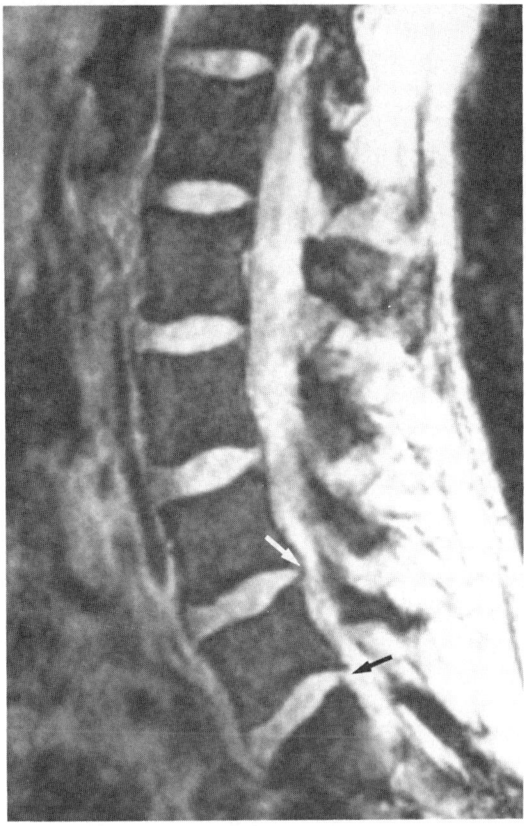

Figure 9 □ Intact (*white arrow*) and disrupted (*black arrow*) annular complex is demonstrated on a T2* gradient-refocused sagittal image. (TR = 400 msec, TE = 15 msec; flip angle = 30 degrees.)

stenosis are most accurately assessed on T2-weighted images, in which there is a bright CSF–extradural interface.

Pars defects and grades of spondylolisthesis can be assessed on sagittal and axial images. The sclerosis associated with a pars interarticularis defect is imaged as low signal intensity on T1- and T2-weighted images.

The Postoperative Spine

Computed tomography plays an important role in assessing postoperative bony detail, especially in evaluating pseudoarthrosis in lumbar spine fusions.[56] MRI, however, is also useful in characterizing end-plate and associated marrow changes.[35] Preliminary work indicates that stable *fusions of the lumbar spine* are associated with fatty marrow conversion at the end plates of the corresponding levels.[30] This yellow or fatty marrow conversion images with increased signal intensity on T1-weighted images and becomes isointense with adjacent marrow on T2-weighted images. On T1-weighted images, fusion instability frequently demonstrates low signal intensity adjacent to the end plates, which increases with progressive T2 weighting. Focal fatty marrow conversion has also been documented in patients with degenerated discs (Fig. 13).[35] End-plate scle-

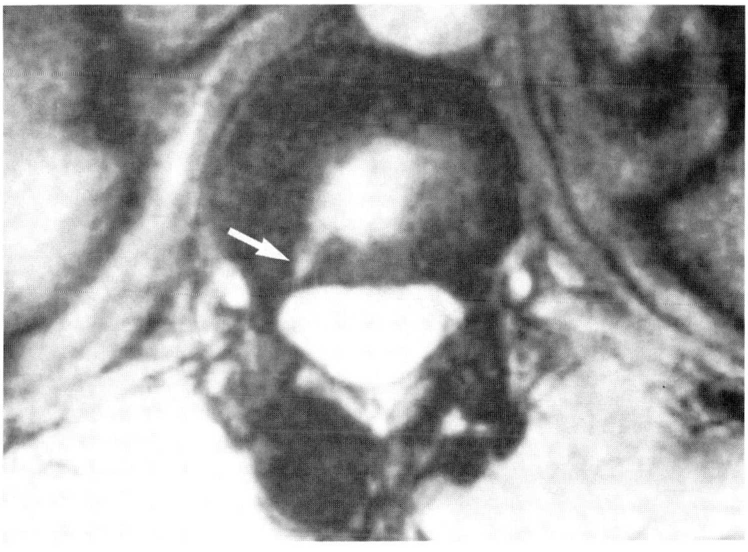

Figure 10 □ Discogram-like effect shows the path of extruded nuclear material (*arrow*) on T2* gradient-echo axial image. (TR = 400 msec, TE = 15 msec; flip angle = 30 degrees.)

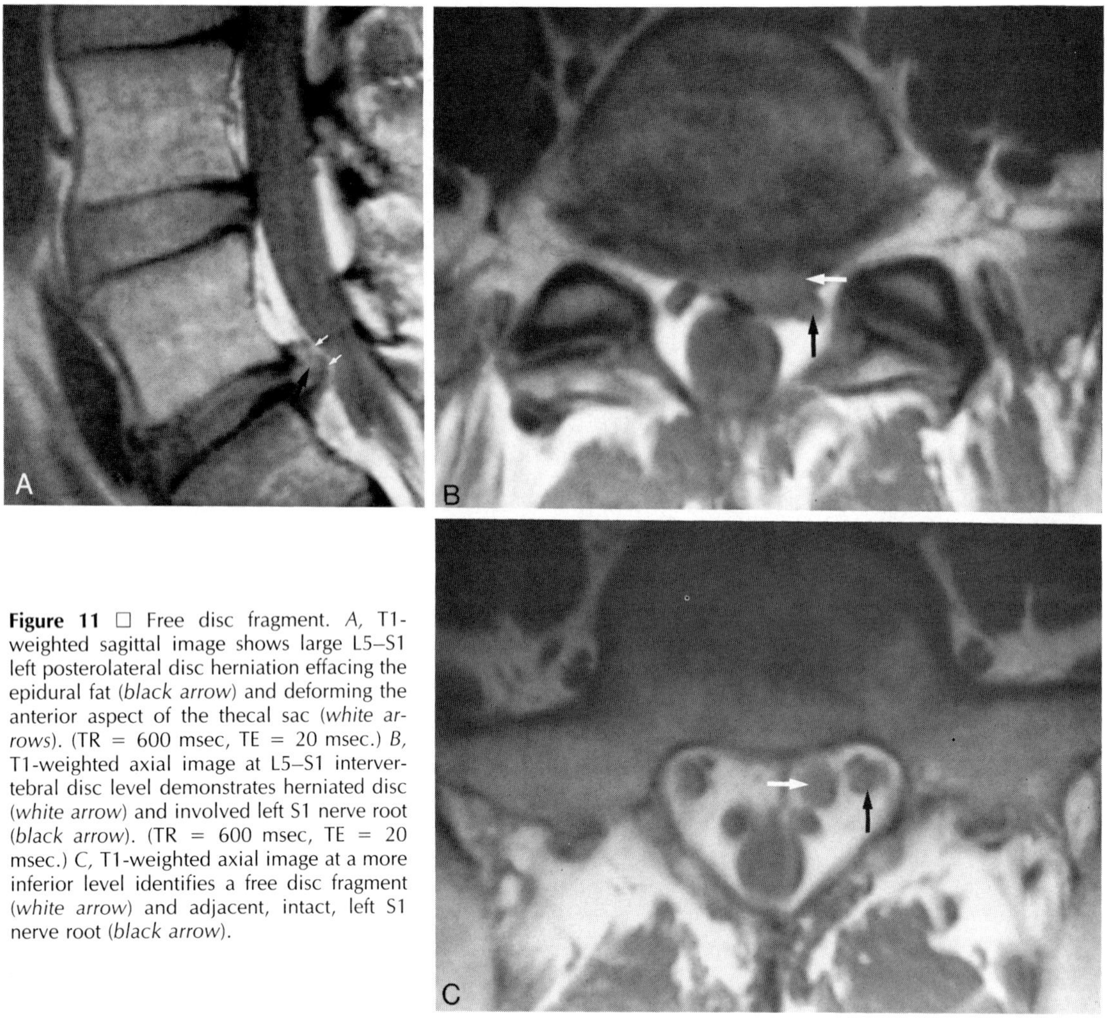

Figure 11 □ Free disc fragment. *A,* T1-weighted sagittal image shows large L5–S1 left posterolateral disc herniation effacing the epidural fat (*black arrow*) and deforming the anterior aspect of the thecal sac (*white arrows*). (TR = 600 msec, TE = 20 msec.) *B,* T1-weighted axial image at L5–S1 intervertebral disc level demonstrates herniated disc (*white arrow*) and involved left S1 nerve root (*black arrow*). (TR = 600 msec, TE = 20 msec.) *C,* T1-weighted axial image at a more inferior level identifies a free disc fragment (*white arrow*) and adjacent, intact, left S1 nerve root (*black arrow*).

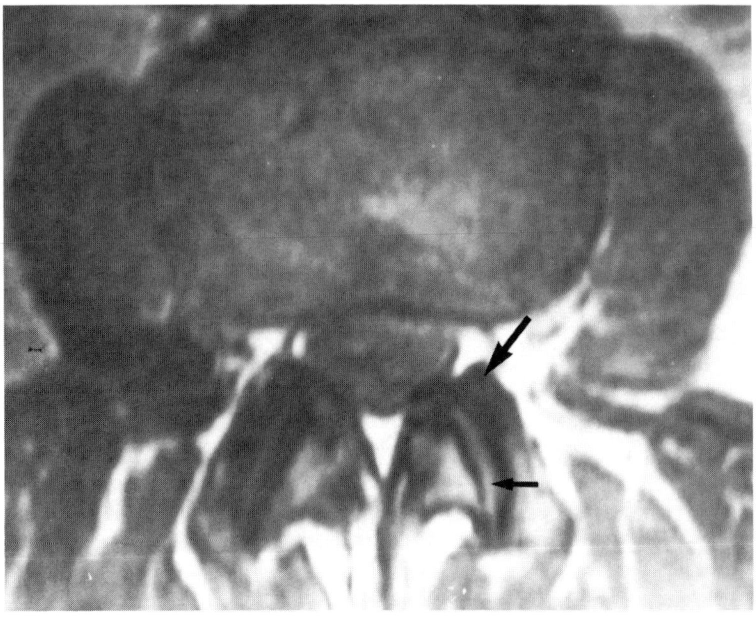

Figure 12 □ Hypertrophied apophyseal joints (*large arrow*) visualized on T1-weighted axial image. Intermediate-signal-intensity articular cartilage is identified (*small arrow*). (TR = 1,000 msec, TE = 20 msec.)

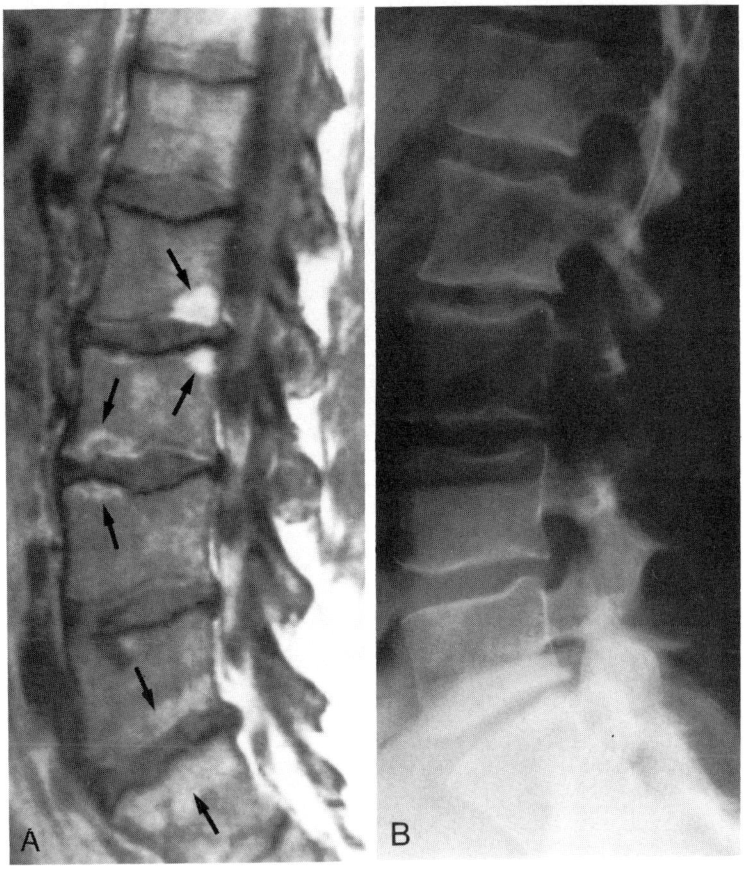

Figure 13 □ End-plate changes in degenerative disease. *A,* Focal areas of developing end-plate yellow marrow (*arrows*) in the degenerative spine. (T1-weighted sagittal image; TR = 600 msec, TE = 20 msec.) *B,* Conventional radiograph for comparison.

rosis is visualized with low signal intensity on T1- and T2-weighted images.

MRI has also been used to assess postoperative changes in *fusion* and *laminectomy* and in *chymopapain and percutaneous nuclectomy* (Fig. 14).[23, 38] The sensitivity and specificity of MRI have been shown to be equal to those of intravenous contrast CT in distinguishing recurrent disc herniations from scar or fibrosis. Scar tissue demonstrates low to intermediate signal intensity on T1-weighted images and intermediate to increased signal intensity without mass effect on T2-weighted images. Gadolinium contrast has been shown to have a role in defining and enhancing epidural fibrosis.[47] Disc herniations (protrusions and extrusions) demonstrate mass effect and do not increase in signal on conventional T2-weighted images. On gradient-echo images, herniated disc material may generate signal higher than that of adjacent fibrosis or scar tissue. When one is interpreting MRI studies of the spine with metallic artifacts, the increased sensitivity to magnetic susceptibility with gradient echoes must be considered.

Clumping and irregular separation of the nerve roots are characteristic of *arachnoiditis,*[48] which often requires T2-weighted axial images to display the distortion of thecal sac and roots. A postoperative fluid collection or *pseudomeningocele* images with signal characteristics analogous to those of CSF, that is, low signal intensity on T1-weighted images and high signal intensity on T2-weighted images (Fig. 15). Focal collections of iophendylate (Pantopaque) in the thecal sac have a characteristic appearance on MR scans, and they image with high signal intensity on T1-weighted images and low signal intensity on T2-weighted images (Fig. 16).[17] Lipomas also image with higher signal intensity on T1-weighted images and may be confused with residual iophendylate. Associated spinal dysraphism or nulled signal intensity on short STIR sequences is characteristic of a lipomatous lesion and helps to distinguish the two.[1]

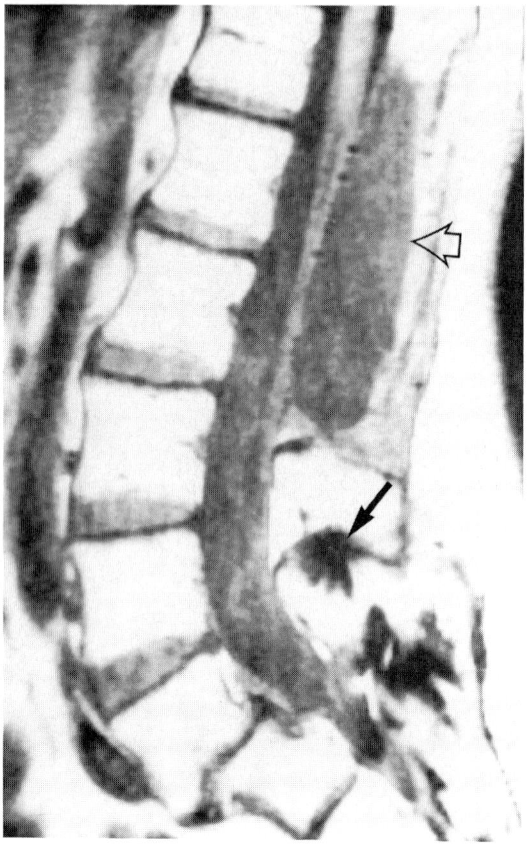

Figure 14 □ Postoperative fusion with signal void in metallic artifact (*solid arrow*) on a T1-weighted image. Postoperative fluid collection is indicated (*open arrow*). (TR = 600 msec, TE = 20 msec.)

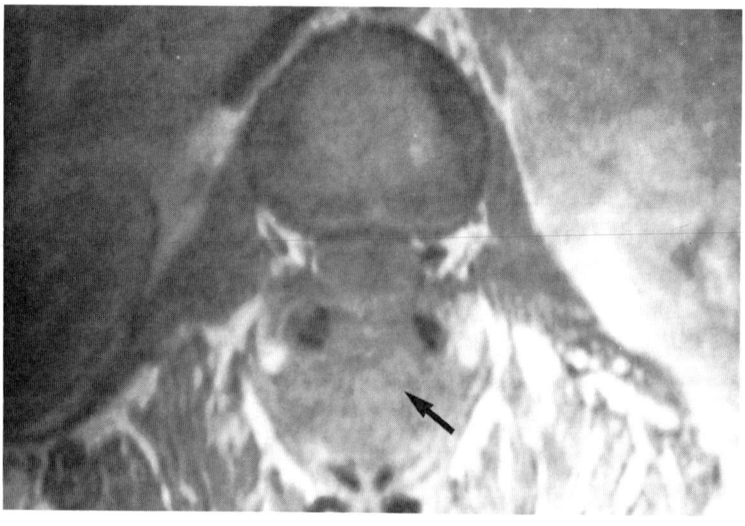

Figure 15 □ Postoperative pseudomeningocele (*arrow*) is visualized with low signal intensity on an intermediately weighted image. (TR = 2,000 msec, TE = 20 msec.)

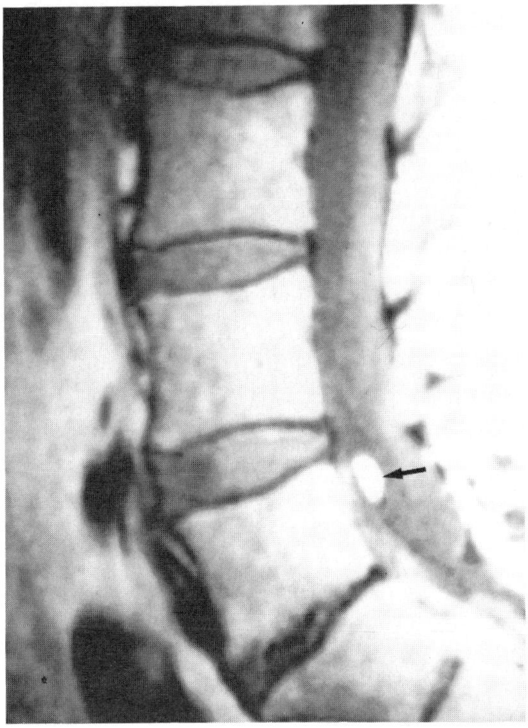

Figure 16 □ High-signal-intensity iophendylate (Pantopaque, *arrow*) on T1-weighted sagittal image. (TR = 1,000 msec, TE = 20 msec.)

Fractures

MRI has been used in the assessment of traumatic and nontraumatic vertebral body fractures.[25, 34, 52] In *traumatic fractures*, retropulsed fracture fragments are identified relative to the cord, thecal sac, and neural foramina (Fig. 17). In the acute and subacute stages, hemorrhage and/or edema image with low signal intensity on T1-weighted images and high signal intensity on T2-weighted images. A chronic fracture does not demonstrate increased signal intensity on long TR/TE sequences. *Osteoporotic* or *nontraumatic compression fractures* may be characterized on T1-weighted images by low-signal-intensity bands parallel to the end plates, which increase in signal intensity on T2-weighted images (Fig. 18). In some cases, compression fractures cannot be differentiated from metastatic disease, although associated convexity or bulging of the posterior vertebral body margin suggests neoplastic disease and a pathologic fracture. On T2-weighted images, the branching pattern of the high-signal-intensity basivertebral plexus may simulate fracture.

Infection

MRI is more sensitive in the detection of vertebral *osteomyelitis* than either conventional radiography or CT.[33] Specificity rates of MRI are also superior to those of corresponding nuclear scintigraphic studies. Infection of vertebral bodies and adjacent intervertebral disc spaces is visualized on T1-weighted images as areas of low signal intensity (Fig. 19). On T2-weighted images, high signal intensity is observed crossing the involved bone and disc space, and an irregularity of cortical margins is seen. In advanced stages of infection such as tuberculous spondylitis, a soft tissue mass (of low signal intensity on T1-weighted images and high signal intensity on T2-weighted images) is frequently observed.[10] Unlike neoplastic disease, infection is associated with a loss of disc space height and the low-signal-intensity intranuclear cleft normally seen on T2-weighted images.

Metastatic and Marrow Disease

MRI directly images fatty or yellow marrow with high signal intensity, and it images erythropoietic or red marrow with low signal intensity in normal and pathologic states.[2, 9, 18, 28, 37, 57, 58] T1, T2, T2* gradient-echo, and STIR sequences have complementary roles in visualizing replacement of normal marrow in primary,[49] metastatic, and infiltrative disease processes. MRI is also useful in differentiating benign processes that may mimic malignancy on conventional radiography.

Because most *metastatic tumors* are characterized by long T1 and T2 values, there is good contrast between normal adult marrow and marrow infiltrated by metastatic processes.[51] On STIR images, signal from normal yellow marrow is suppressed, and T1 and T2 prolongation effects are additive. Metastatic lesions from carcinoma of the breast (Fig. 20), prostate (Fig. 21), lung, colon, and testes; from Ewing sarcoma; and from multiple myeloma have been visualized with increased signal intensity on conventional T2-weighted images, on T2*-weighted images, and on STIR images—even in patients for whom nuclear scintigraphic findings were equivocal. Blastic lesions generally image with low signal intensity, regardless of the selected pulse parameters. With STIR

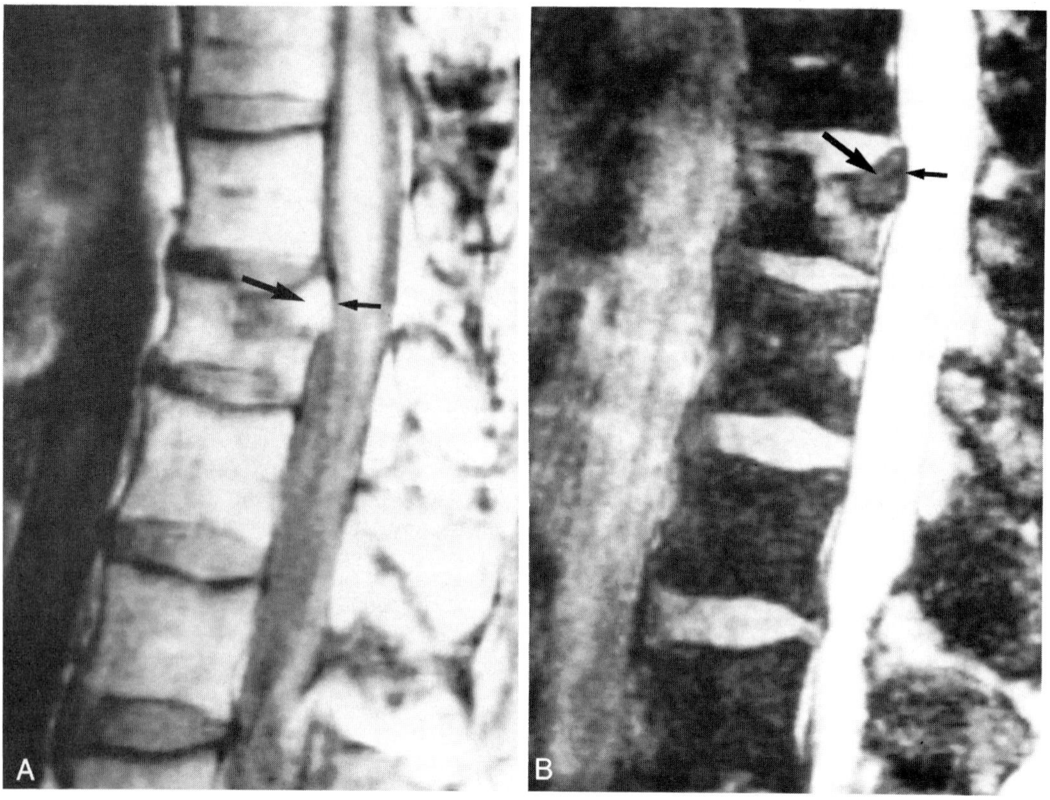

Figure 17 □ Post-traumatic L1 vertebral body fracture. Fracture (*large arrow*) images show *A,* low-signal-intensity hemorrhagic marrow on a T1-weighted image, and *B,* increased signal intensity on a T2* gradient-echo image. Retropulsed fracture segment (*small arrow*) is identified impressing on the thecal sac.

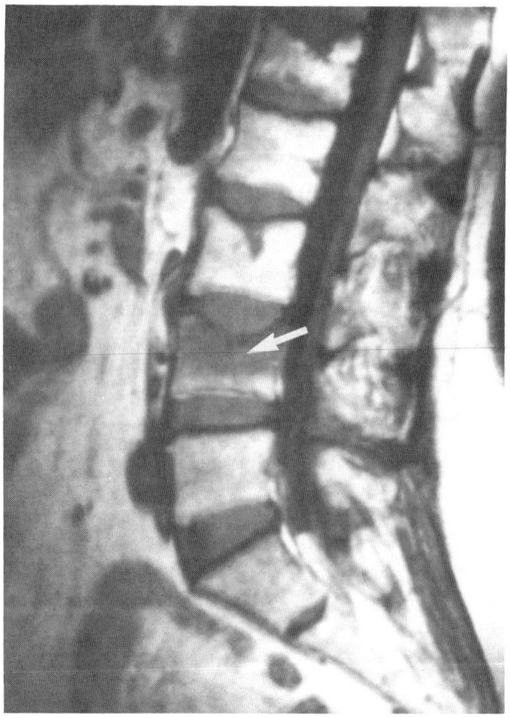

Figure 18 □ Low-signal-intensity band of marrow edema (*arrow*) is seen in association with L4 osteoporotic compression fracture on T1-weighted sagittal image. (TR = 600 msec, TE = 20 msec.)

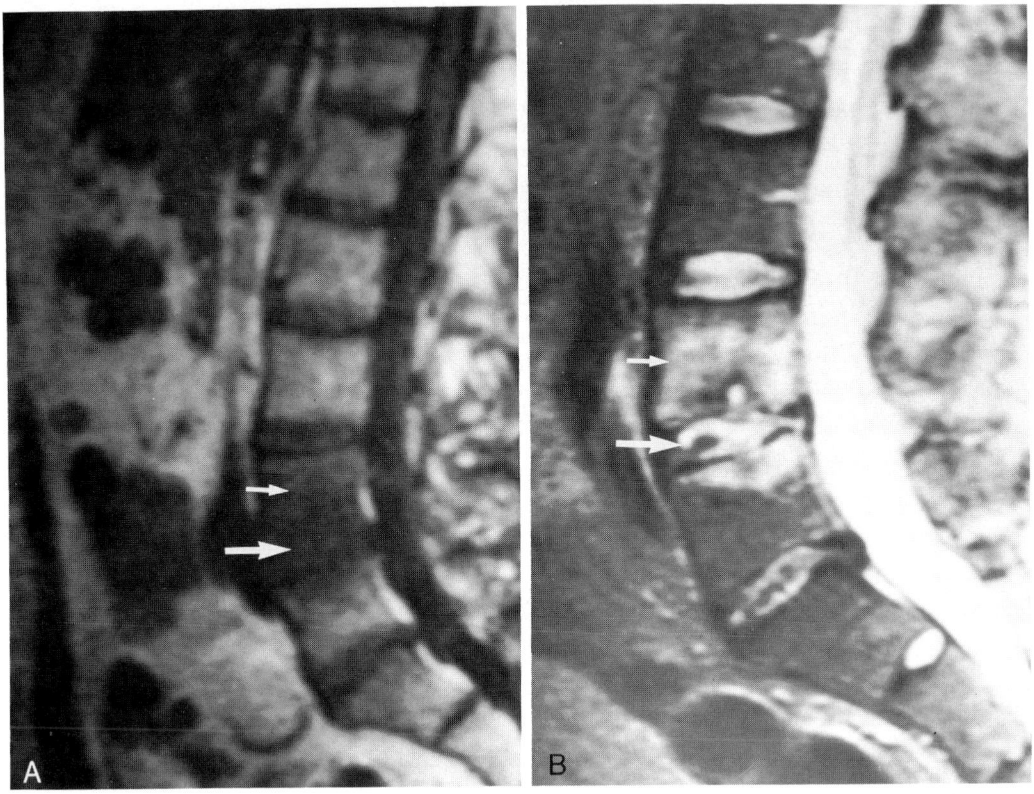

Figure 19 □ Staphylococcal osteomyelitis. Low-signal-intensity marrow involvement (*small arrow*) of L4 and L5 is seen crossing the discovertebral junction (*large arrow*). *A,* It has low signal intensity on the T1-weighted image, and in *B,* it shows high signal intensity on the T2-weighted image.

images, however, metastatic foci within blastic lesions have been observed with increased signal intensity.[42] Epidural involvement, with posterior cortical disruption, is best appreciated on T2, T2*, STIR, or gadolinium-enhanced studies.[5, 13] Gadolinium generates a higher signal intensity in neoplastic tissue on short TR/TE sequences (the effect of T1 and T2 shortening), whereas the adjacent CSF remains dark. This precisely defines the boundary between the tumor and thecal sac, which is not possible by means of conventional T2 weighting or even by STIR images in which both CSF and tumor image with high signal intensity.

MRI is also sensitive to the replacement of marrow fat with tumor cell populations that have T1 values significantly longer than those of normal yellow marrow.[37, 42] Marrow infiltrates from *leukemia* and *lymphoma* have been successfully identified on STIR sequences as areas of high signal intensity within a black or gray background of nulled fat signal from uninvolved marrow. Because marrow lymphoma may present with a patchy or nodular involvement of the spine and pelvis, MRI localization before biopsy reduces the number of false negatives resulting from sampling error.

Fatty replacement of the affected marrow in patients undergoing *radiation* and *chemotherapy* can be imaged on T1, T2, and STIR sequences.[43]

PERSPECTIVE ON MRI OF THE SPINE

MRI affords a unique perspective for noninvasive imaging of the spine in degenerative disc disease affecting both osseous and disc structures. The ability to image directly the nucleus pulposus, CSF, and spinal cord facilitates the discrimination of the disc–thecal sac interface without the use of CT or myelography. In studies comparing MRI with conventional diagnostic imaging modalities, a greater potential for MRI in the

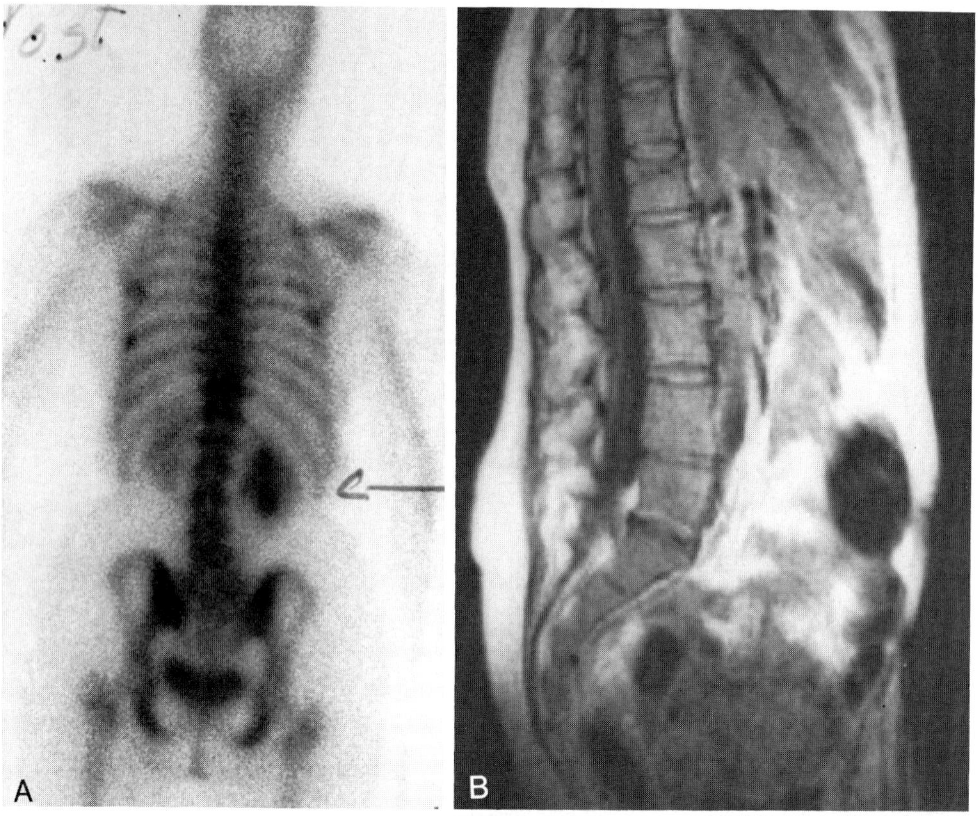

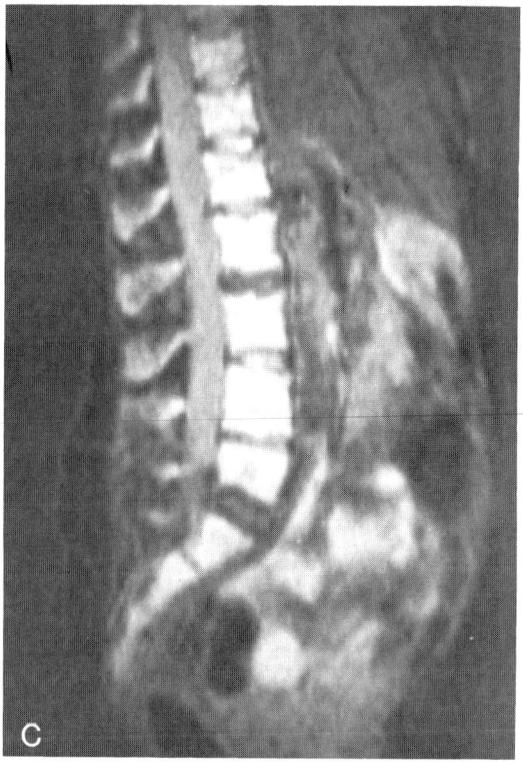

Figure 20 □ Metastatic breast carcinoma. *A,* Unremarkable bone scan was obtained from a patient with aggressive metastatic breast carcinoma. *B,* T1-weighted image and *C,* short T1 inversion recovery (STIR) image show low and high signal intensities, respectively, in diffuse marrow involvement of the entire thoracic and lumbar spines.

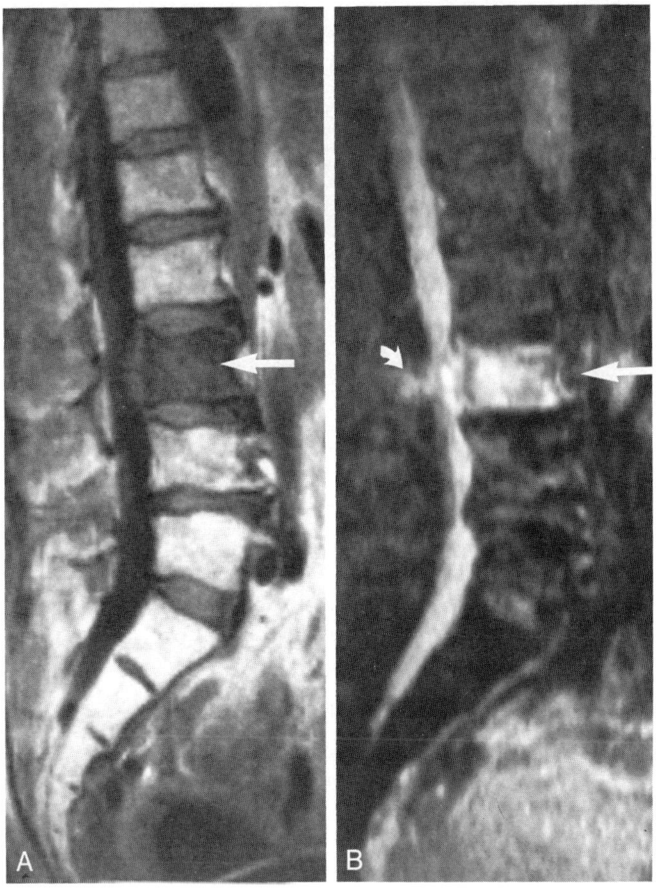

Figure 21 □ Metastatic prostate carcinoma. Carcinoma (*straight arrow*) is visualized in *A*, with low signal intensity on a T1-weighted sagittal image, and in *B*, with high signal intensity on STIR sequence. In addition, posterior element involvement (*curved arrow*) is uniquely demonstrated on the STIR image (*B*).

characterization of trauma, infection, and neoplasia has been documented. Direct marrow imaging has expanded the application of MRI in identifying and monitoring patients with leukemia, lymphoma, and metastatic disease involving the spine. The postoperative spine presents a unique clinical and radiologic challenge to which MRI can contribute valuable information regarding postoperative scarring, recurrent disc disease, and fusion stability.

References

1. Altman, N.R., and Altman, D.H.: MR imaging of spinal dysraphism. A.J.N.R. 8:533, 1987.
2. Beltran, J., et al.: Tumors of the osseous spine: Staging with MR imaging versus CT. Radiology 162:565, 1987.
3. Berger, P.E., et al.: High resolution surface coil magnetic resonance imaging of the spine: Normal and pathologic anatomy. RadioGraphics 6:573, 1986.
4. Berger, P.E., et al.: High resolution surface coil magnetic resonance imaging of the spine: Normal and pathologic anatomy. RadioGraphics 6:573, 1986.
5. Berry, I., et al.: Gd-DPTA enhancement of cerebral and spinal tumors on MR imaging. Radiology 165P:38, 1987.
6. Burk, D.L., et al.: Spinal and paraspinal neurofibromatosis: Surface coil MR imaging at 1.5 T. Radiology 162:797, 1987.
7. Braun, I.F., et al.: Contrast enhancement in CT differentiation between recurrent disk herniation and postoperative scar: Prospective study. A.J.N.R. 6:607, 1985.
8. Chafetz, N.I., et al.: Recognition of lumbar disk herniation with NMR. A.J.R. 141:1153, 1983.
9. Daffner, R.H., et al.: MRI in the detection of malignant infiltration of bone marrow. A.J.R. 146:353, 1986.
10. deRoss, A., et al.: MRI of tuberculous spondylitis. A.J.R. 146:79, 1986.
11. Dixon, A.K., and Bannon, R.P.: Computed tomography of the postoperative lumbar spine: The need for, and optimal dose of, intravenous contrast medium. Br. J. Radiol. 60:215, 1987.
12. Edelman, R.R., et al.: High-resolution MRI: Imaging anatomy of the lumbosacral spine. Magn. Reson. Imaging 4:515, 1986.
13. Emory, T.H., et al.: Comparison of Gd-DPTA MR imaging and radionuclide bone scans (WIP). Radiology 165P:342, 1987.
14. Glenn, W.V., Burnett, K., and Rauschning, W.: Magnetic Resonance Imaging of the Lumbar Spine: Nerve Root Canals, Disc Abnormalities, Anatomic

Correlations, and Case Examples. Milwaukee, GE Medical Systems, 1986.
15. Grenier, N., et al.: Degenerative lumbar disk disease: Pitfalls and usefulness of MR imaging in detection of vacuum phenomenon. Radiology 164:861, 1987.
16. Grenier, N., et al.: Normal and degenerative posterior spinal structures: MR imaging. Radiology 165:517, 1987.
17. Hackney, D.B., et al.: MR characteristics of iophendylate (Pantopaque). J. Comput. Assist. Tomogr. 10:401, 1986.
18. Hajek, P.C., et al.: Focal fat deposition in axial bone marrow: MR characteristics. Radiology 162:245, 1987.
19. Haughton, V.M.: MR imaging of the spine. Radiology 166:297, 1988.
20. Heithoff, K.B.: Spontaneous Lumbar Epidural Hematoma. Milwaukee, G.E. Medical Systems, M.R. Clinical Symposium, Vol. 3, No. 3, 1987.
21. Helms, C.A., Vogler, J.B., III, and Hardy, D.C.: CT of the lumbar spine: Normal variants and pitfalls. RadioGraphics 7:447, 1987.
22. Hoult, D.I., Chen, C.-N., and Sank, V.J.: The field dependence of NMR imaging. Magn. Reson. Med. 3:730, 1986.
23. Huckman, M.S., et al.: Chemonucleation and changes observed on lumbar MR scan: Preliminary report. A.J.R.N. 8:1, 1987.
24. Kaplan, P.A., et al.: Bone marrow patterns in aplastic anemia: Observations with 1.5 T MR imaging. Radiology 164:441, 1987.
25. Kaplan, P.A., Orton, D.F., and Russell, J.A.: Osteoporosis with vertebral compression fractures, retropulsed fragments, and neurologic compromise. Radiology 165:533, 1987.
26. Kaufman, L., and Crooks, L.E.: Technical advances in magnetic resonance imaging. *In* Goldberg, H., Higgins, C.B., and Ring, E.J. (eds.): Contemporary Imaging. San Francisco, University of California Press, 1985.
27. Kaufman, L.: Optimal field strength in proton MRI. Toshiba Med. Rev. (Int.). 16:5, 1986.
28. Kricun, M.E.: Red-yellow marrow conversion: Its effect on the location of some solitary bone lesions. Skeletal Radiol. 14:10, 1985.
29. Kulkarni, M.V., et al.: Acute spinal cord injury: MR imaging at 1.5 T. Radiology 164:837, 1987.
30. Lang, P., et al.: Magnetic resonance imaging in the assessment of functional lumbar spinal stability (abstr.). New York City, Sixth Annual Meeting and Exhibition of the Society of Magnetic Resonance in Medicine, Aug. 17–21, 1987, p. 149.
31. McKinstry, C.S., et al.: Bone marrow in leukemia and aplastic anemia: MR imaging before, during, and after treatment. Radiology 162:701, 1987.
32. Modic, M.T., et al.: Magnetic resonance imaging of intervertebral disk disease: Clinical and pulse sequence considerations. Radiology 152:103, 1984.
33. Modic, M.T., et al.: Vertebral osteomyelitis: Assessment using MR. Radiology 157:157, 1985.
34. Modic, M.T., et al.: Magnetic resonance imaging of the spine. Radiol. Clin. North Am. 24:229, 1986.
35. Modic, M.T., et al.: Degenerative disk disease. Assessment of changes in vertebral body marrow with MR imaging. Radiology 166:193, 1988.
36. Nokes, S.R., et al.: Childhood scoliosis: MR imaging. Radiology 164:791, 1987.
37. Olson, D., et al.: Magnetic resonance imaging of the bone marrow in patients with leukemia, aplastic anemia, and lymphoma. Invest. Radiol. 21:540, 1986.
38. Onik, G., et al.: Percutaneous lumbar diskectomy using a new aspiration probe. A.J.R.N. 6:290, 1985.
39. Pech, P., and Haughton, V.M.: Lumbar intervertebral disk: Correlative MR and anatomic study. Radiology 156:699, 1985.
40. Porter, B.A.: MR may become routine for imaging bone marrow. Diagn. Imaging, February, 1987.
41. Porter, B.A., Shields, A.F., and Olson, D.O.: Magnetic resonance imaging of bone marrow disorders. Radiol. Clin. North Am. 24:269, 1986.
42. Porter, B.A., et al.: Low-field STIR imaging of marrow malignancies. Radiology 165P:275, 1987.
43. Ramsey, R.G., and Zacharias, C.E.: MR imaging of the spine after radiation therapy: Easily recognizable effects. J.N.R. 6:247, 1985.
44. Ramsey, R.G.: MRI's reputation grows in herniated disk evaluation. Diagn. Imaging, June:120, 1987.
45. Reicher, M.A., et al.: MR imaging of the lumbar spine: Anatomic correlations and the effects of technical variations. A.J.R. 147:891, 1986.
46. Ross, J.S., et al.: Lumbar spine: Postoperative assessment with surface-coil MR imaging. Radiology 164:851, 1987.
47. Ross, J.S., et al.: MR enhancement of epidural fibrosis by Gd-DPTA: Biodistribution and mechanism. Radiology 165P:142, 1987.
48. Ross, J.S., et al.: MR imaging of lumbar arachnoiditis. A.J.R. 149:1025, 1987.
49. Ross, J.S., et al.: Vertebral hemangiomas: MR imaging. Radiology 165:165, 1987.
50. Rubin, J.B., and Enzmann, D.R.: Optimizing conventional MR imaging of the spine. Radiology 163:777, 1987.
51. Sarpel, S., et al.: Early diagnosis of spinal-epidural metastasis by magnetic resonance imaging. Radiology 164:887, 1987.
52. Sartoris, D.J., et al.: Vertebral-body collapse in focal and diffuse disease: Patterns of pathologic processes. Radiology 160:479, 1986.
53. Schellinger, D., et al.: Facet joint disorders and their role in the production of back pain and sciatica. RadioGraphics 7:923, 1987.
54. Stoller, D.W., and Genant, H.K.: MRI helps characterize disorders of the spine. Diagn. Imag. 9:128, 1987.
55. Stoller, D.W., and Genant, H.K.: Fast imaging of the spine. *In* Genant, H.K. (ed.): Spine Update 1987. San Francisco, Radiology Research and Education Foundation, 1987, pp. 47–54.
56. Stoller, D.W., et al.: Applications of computed tomography in the musculoskeletal system. Curr. Orthop. 1:219, 1987.
57. Sugimura, K., et al.: Bone marrow diseases of the spine: Differentiation with T1 and T2 relaxation times in MR imaging. Radiology 165:541, 1987.
58. Weaver, G.R., and Sandler, M.P.: Increased sensitivity of magnetic resonance imaging compared to radionuclide bone scintigraphy in the detection of lymphoma of the spine. Clin. Nucl. Med. 12:333, 1987.
59. Weiss, T., et al.: CT of the postoperative lumbar spine: Value of intravenous contrast. Neuroradiology 28:241, 1986.
60. Zinreich, S.J., et al.: CT myelography for outpatients: An inpatient/outpatient pilot study to assess methodology. Radiology 157:387, 1985.

RELIABILITY OF RADIOGRAPHIC STUDIES

Ian A. F. Stokes

The inaccessibility of the lumbar spine to noninvasive clinical examination has resulted in a heavy reliance being placed on radiography and other imaging techniques. Radiology is rapidly approaching its first 100 years and new imaging technologies have recently been developed. However, *plain* radiography is still the type most widely used in the lumbar spine. Radiography is used to show the form and alignment of the spine (i.e., its curvatures in various planes), the form of the vertebrae (e.g., the presence of fractures and congenital defects, alignment of facets, canal dimensions), the motion of the spine, the quality of bone and of joint spaces, and, by means of contrast medium techniques, the geometric configuration of certain soft tissues. This chapter addresses the reliability with which radiologic methods can demonstrate objective signs (bony dimensions, motion, and spinal degeneration) as well as their diagnostic accuracy.

The reliability of continuous measurements such as bony dimensions or ranges of movement is described by error estimates (e.g., standard error, technical error, precision). *Technical error* is the square root of the sum of squared differences between pairs of repeated measurements divided by twice the number of observations. It can be used to measure both the extent to which different observers agree on a measurement and the ability of each observer to repeat his or her measurement reliably. Reliability is described by indices of diagnostic power when one is estimating the accuracy of the detection of certain signs or confirming a diagnosis. Sensitivity is the probability of obtaining a correct diagnosis for patients who have the condition, and specificity is the probability of obtaining a correct diagnosis in patients who do not have the condition.[83] Unfortunately, the rigorous quantification of the reliability of radiographic studies is often difficult or impossible because of ethical considerations. For instance, in order to establish the precision of a particular examination, it might be necessary to take several repeat films of the same patient. To establish the diagnostic power of a particular technique, a large healthy or unaffected population needs to be examined in order to establish the false-positive and true-negative rates. The independent confirmation of many radiologic observations requires direct observation at surgery or necropsy. Therefore, much of the scientific basis for the clinical use of radiology has been established indirectly by observing statistical associations of radiologic signs with clinical findings or reported symptoms.

NATURE OF THE RADIOGRAPHIC IMAGE

X-rays can pass through biologic tissues but tend to be absorbed by heavier elements, especially those that mineralize bone. The degree of absorption depends on the spectrum of x-ray wave lengths. The spectrum is controlled by the voltage applied to the x-ray tube, by the filtration added to the exit port, and, to some extent, by the air gap between the tube and the patient. X-rays are absorbed and scattered, by tissues, within the patient. After exiting the patient, they may be further scattered or filtered by the air gap and by a Potter-Bucky diaphragm (designed to absorb scattered radiation) placed in front of film. The image on the film is produced by light emitted from scintillation screens placed on either side of it. Therefore, the resulting image also depends on the properties of the scintillation screen. For instance, highly sensitive screens tend to have a larger grain size and a nonlinear response to the intensity of irradiation. The same principles also apply to newer techniques (i.e., image intensifiers, digital radiography and computed tomography [CT]), in which an electronic detector is used in place of the conventional intensifying screen and silver emulsion film.

The resulting image can therefore be considered as a gray scale, showing the accumulated attenuation of x-rays by the tissues and air gap through which they have passed, superimposed over a "noise" or background intensity created by scattered x-rays. The great advantage of CT is that it generates, instead, an image from a uniformly thin plane of the patient. It also has a more uniform geometric scaling. In the case of plane radiography, the divergent beam from the x-ray source causes geometric magnification. Parts of the body that are close to the x-ray film are magnified less than those at a greater distance from the film. Greater distance from the film also causes image degradation because of image scattering and the finite size of the x-ray source within the tube.

CLINICAL USES OF RADIOGRAPHIC STUDIES

Park[55] surveyed radiology departments in British hospitals and estimated that 4% of the workload was related to lumbar spinal examinations. In most patients, a specific disease process (such as fracture, neoplasm, or prolapsed intervertebral disc) was not suspected. Most of the requests were to examine patients with nonspecific low back pain. Most of the resulting films were classified either as normal or as having nonspecific changes commensurate with the age of the patient. It appeared that the radiologic examination was being used as a routine screening examination for patients with nonspecific backache. Similarly, Nachemson[50] estimated that clinically unsuspected positive findings were found only about once in every 2,500 x-ray examinations of the lumbar spines of patients aged 20 to 50 years. The clinical interpretation of objective radiologic findings is tremendously complicated because most objective findings occur in asymptomatic populations almost as frequently as they do among those with low back pain. Essentially equal prevalences of "abnormal" findings are reported for disc height and degenerative changes,[17, 30, 34, 72, 77] sacral angle and degree of lordosis,[23, 72] deep-seated sacrum,[16] congenital anomalies,[16, 17, 72] and posterior displacement of the L5 body.[17] Among those radiologic findings that are known to have a higher prevalence in a low back pain population, some factors, such as lumbar lordosis and restricted motion,[2, 46] could simply be acute spinal modifications resulting from the painful symptoms. About half of 58 asymptomatic subjects studied by Wiesel and associates[81] were found to have abnormalities on CT scans. Abnormal discograms were found by Holt[29] in 37% of the intervertebral discs of 30 asymptomatic young male volunteers. It is this background of false-positive findings that necessitates a cautious interpretation of any positive radiologic findings.

RELIABILITY OF MEASUREMENTS OF SHAPE AND MOTION

Curvature of the spine can be measured by evaluating the difference between the inclination of two specified vertebrae. Thus, the measurement of spinal curvature is considerably more repeatable if the same vertebrae are selected in repeated measurements of Cobb angle.[51, 71] However, even if this factor is held constant, the within- and between-observer variability of measurement is between 5 degrees and 10 degrees, which corresponds to the threshold of change frequently cited as an indication for modifying a treatment.[51] Probably, lordosis and kyphosis can be measured more reliably, since the vertebral end plates are often visualized more easily in lateral than in anteroposterior (AP) films.

The shape of vertebrae, and especially of the neural canal, is measured in order to identify patients at risk of spinal stenosis. In a comparison between radiographic and direct measurements of cadaveric lumbar spinal canals, Leiviskä and colleagues[35] found that the technical error was between 1 mm and 3 mm for measurements in the frontal and sagittal planes. These errors corresponded to percentage errors of between 6% and 20%. They concluded that their study validated these measurements from plane films as a reasonable alternative to those from CT scans. Porter and coworkers[63] reported measurements, by ultrasound, of the oblique diameter (from lamina to vertebral body) with an accuracy of ±1.5%.

Motion within the spine, or within parts of it, is measured by determining the position or angulation of two vertebrae in each of two or more radiographic exposures (Fig. 1). The motion is calculated as the differences of these four or more measurements. Taking differences is a method notorious for producing large measurement errors, since the errors are accumulated and can become a large proportion of the quantity being measured. Thus, the measurement of the small angular and linear motions that occur in the spinal articulations is a difficult challenge.

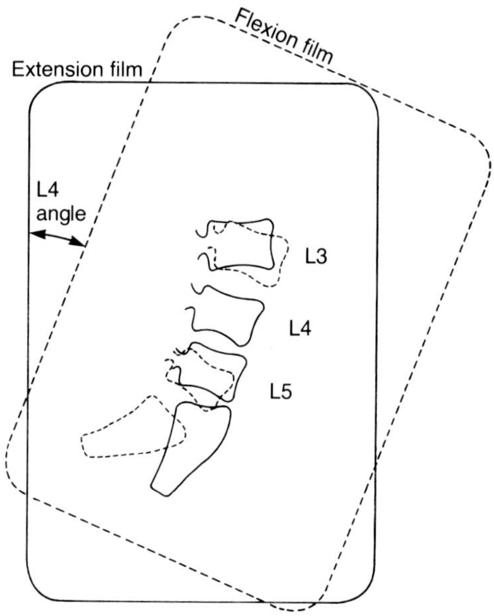

Figure 1 □ Method of measuring intervertebral motion by film overlay method. The intervertebral motion is calculated by subtracting the angle measured as shown from the corresponding angle for the adjacent vertebra. This subtraction can lead to errors that are large compared with the motion being measured. (From Stokes, I.A.F., Bevins, T.M., and Lunn, R.A.: Back surface curvature and measurement of lumbar spinal motion. Spine 12:357, 1987.)

The motion of the spine takes place in three dimensions with 6 degrees of freedom (three rotations and three translations). Therefore, motion occurring in any plane other than that parallel to the x-ray film can contaminate the measurements in the film plane. Biplanar radiography is used to measure the full three-dimensional motion.[5, 52, 56–58, 67, 74–76] The positions of landmarks that can be identified in the two radiographic views are digitized relative to a fixed-axis system. A computer program is then used to calculate the three-dimensional coordinates of each landmark at its position at the time of radiography. This technique can therefore compensate for magnification of the x-ray image. If there are at least three landmarks on each moving body (vertebra), then the motion of each vertebra and the relative motion at each intervertebral articulation can be calculated. Experimental studies have shown that landmarks can be identified with a precision of between 1 mm and 2 mm in each of the three principal axis directions.[67, 75] This means that when the landmarks on two adjacent vertebrae recorded in two successive pairs of biplanar films are combined, the accuracy of measurement is between 2 and 3 degrees for relative angular motion, and between 2 and 3 mm for translation motion.[75] Therefore, for an angular motion of 10 degrees (typical range of intervertebral motion), the measurement precision is about 25% of the expected measurement. In the case of translation measurements, the precision of the measurement is comparable to, or greater than, expected values of the linear components of intervertebral motion.

For a given intervertebral motion, the measured values of each of the six components of motion depend on the placement of the measurement axis system. For instance, if the origin of the axes were placed at the center of the intervertebral disc and the axis for intervertebral motion passed through the origin, no translation motion would be recorded. If, instead, the origin of axes for measurement were placed at the center of the vertebral body, then the angular motion about the axis passing through the disc would appear partly as a rotation and partly as a translation occurring at the new origin of axes. It is important, therefore, to record the location of the axis of motion as well as the rotations about this axis. The instantaneous screw axis provides a method of describing intervertebral motion in cadaver specimens[54] and of providing the magnitude of rotation, the axis about which it occurs, and the relative translation. Unfortunately, determining the instantaneous axis of rotation is extremely sensitive to measurement errors[53] and has not been adopted for in vivo studies. If all the motion is occurring in a plane parallel to that of the x-ray film, then axes of rotation are perpendicular to the film plane and can be identified as a center of rotation, where the axis transects the film. Determining the center of rotation is also very sensitive to measurement error, but it has been adopted as a technique to characterize flexion and extension motion.[61, 70] A center of rotation within the disc applies pure flexion and extension, whereas, if the center of rotation lies below the intervertebral disc, shearing of the disc must accompany flexion and extension (Fig. 2).

SURFACE MEASUREMENTS OF SPINAL MOTION

To avoid the hazards of ionizing radiation, a number of noninvasive techniques have been proposed. One of the following meas-

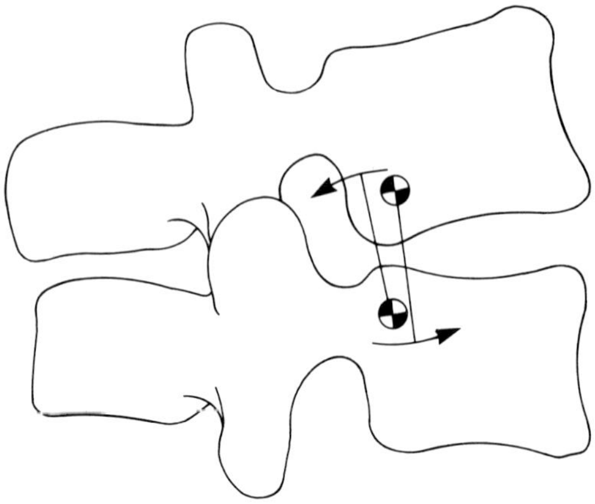

Figure 2 □ The position of the axis (or center) of rotation determines the magnitude and the direction of shear or translation motion accompanying an angular motion.

urement principles is adopted: (1) measurement of the change in the separation of two surface landmarks[40, 48] and (2) measurement of the change of relative inclination of two points on the back surface, measured either directly by inclinometers[37] or indirectly from tracings of the back profile made by a pantograph or a flexible ruler.[6, 25, 73] Comparative studies have shown that these measurements correlate with radiographic measurements (Pearson correlation coefficient between 0.6 and 0.8).[40, 62, 73] Sources of error include systematic effects resulting from the differing anatomy of various subjects, observer bias in selecting reference points, for example, and random measurement errors. The total range of flexion and extension of the lumbar spine is about 80 degrees, so an expected surface measurement error of 11 degrees[73] corresponds to a measurement error of 14%. Surface measurement techniques are not suitable for measuring intervertebral motion because of their lack of precision.[73] Manual palpation and the subjective assessment of segmental range of motion was characterized by large interobserver variability in a study in which healthy subjects were examined.[20] Noninvasive measurement of spinal motion continues to be a technical challenge to researchers and clinicians.

RELIABILITY OF RADIOLOGIC ASSESSMENT OF DEGENERATIVE CHANGE

Because x-ray images primarily demonstrate the quality and quantity of bone tissue, they can show degenerative changes affecting bone. Loss of bone mineral can be demonstrated by x-ray studies,[22] and these measurements correlate with a loss of strength.[44] Other accepted signs of spinal degeneration include sclerotic bone, facet hypertrophy, claw spurs, traction spurs, and Schmorl's nodes. Nonosseous signs of spinal degeneration visible on plane films include disc space narrowing and the vacuum sign, which is thought to indicate internal fissuring of the disc. Plane radiographs can demonstrate further degenerative changes of soft tissue when contrast media are employed. The discogram, myelogram, radiculogram, and facet arthrogram are commonly accepted techniques for demonstrating the shape and condition of the corresponding soft tissue structures.

The reliability of these techniques to demonstrate degenerative changes has been evaluated by comparing the radiographic images with gross examination of cadaveric specimens. Friberg and Hirsch[12] examined 100 spines of all ages and found that only 46% had normal radiographs. Gross examination showed that disc degeneration could be present without radiographic changes. However, when they obtained flexion and extension radiographs, they found that 16 of 17 cases with "instability" had severe disc changes. A similar correspondence between disc degeneration and abnormal motion in cadaveric specimens was found by Harris and MacNab.[24] Malmivaara[42] reported a poor relationship between disc narrowing and the size of marginal osteophytes, compared with the degree of disc degeneration assessed from discograms of the thorocolumbar region of 37 cadaver spines. He concluded that the assessment of disc degeneration from conventional radiographs was unreliable. Furthermore, in the thoracolumbar region, Malmivaara and colleagues[41] detected Schmorl's nodes in 19 of 24 cadaver spines studied by direct observation of sections, whereas previously made plane radiographs and discograms of these specimens demonstrated about half of the nodes having an aperture area exceeding 0.5 cm and only about 25% of those with a smaller aperture area. Therefore, many cases of Schmorl's nodes are presumably missed in routine clinical radiographs. The integrity of the nucleus pulposus of the intervertebral disc can accurately be assessed by means of discography when compared with direct observation of subsequently sectioned cadaveric specimens.[1, 9] However, false-negative discogram findings were obtained in a substantial number of cadaver specimens and in patients who underwent operation by Yasuma for disc herniation.[82] These appeared to result from degenerative changes in the annulus that did not correspond to nucleus disruption. Furthermore, disc degeneration as shown by an abnormal discogram does not always correlate with painful symptoms, as is evident in the 37% false-positive rate reported in 30 asymptomatic male volunteers (21 to 41 years of age) studied by Holt.[29] Quinnell and Stockdale[65] considered that false-positive discograms may be attributable to artifacts resulting from needle misplacement.

The determination of an exact correlation between radiographic changes and disc degeneration is handicapped by the lack of an adequate definition of the "gold standard" of degenerative change to serve as the basis for comparison. After adopting an abnormal discogram as their standard of disc degeneration, Quinnell and Stockdale[64] compared static and dynamic (flexion and extension) findings from plane films in 111 discs in 30 patients, and they obtained false-positive rates and false-negative rates that ranged between 21% and 42%. These values are close to those that would result from an entirely random association. The exception was in measuring disc shear motion accompanying flexion; in this instance, the assessment yielded no false-positive findings of degeneration but did produce a significant false-negative rate. In an earlier study[66] the same authors found a poor correlation between abnormal discograms and the presence of osteophytes.

RELIABILITY OF RADIOGRAPHIC STUDIES FOR DETERMINING ORIGIN OF PAIN

Although signs of disc degeneration increase with age[16, 30, 34] and severe changes tend to occur more commonly in subjects with a history of low back pain,[4, 30, 34] plane radiographs alone are generally accepted as being of little value in making a diagnosis for a particular patient. Instead, they are used more commonly for confirming a clinical suspicion of organic disease or, in rare cases, demonstrating clinically unsuspected findings.[45, 50, 55] However, a heavy reliance is placed on radiology to confirm the level of the spine at which surgical intervention is planned for patients with spinal fracture, metastatic disease, or disc herniation. There is a correlation between levels of the spine at which degenerative signs are most prevalent and the levels to which painful symptoms are attributed.[34] Despite this association, Park[55] examined the correspondence between standardized radiographic criteria of disc degeneration and complaints of low back pain and sciatica from the data published by Lawrence[34] and deduced that the sensitivity of the radiographic assessment was only 59%, and the specificity only 55% (that is, the false-negative rate was 41% and the false-positive rate 45%). LaRocca and MacNab[33] determined that the radiographic appearance of subjects with and without low back pain was sufficiently similar that spinal radiographs should not be used in pre-employment screening, because they would have extremely poor predictive value.

Studies with contrast media (myelogram and discogram) and CT have a greater reliability for determining the level of the spine responsible for painful symptoms in patients undergoing surgical disc excision. Bell and coworkers[3] assessed 122 patients by CT and myelography prior to surgery and found myelography to be more accurate than CT in diagnosing herniated lumbar disc (83% correct for myelography, 72% for CT) and stenosis (93% and 89% correct for myelography and CT, respectively). Haughton and coworkers[27] prospectively studied 107 patients by both CT and myelogram. Of these, 52 proceeded to surgical exploration. In 46 cases, the CT scan showed a perfect agreement with surgical findings; 44 showed perfect agreement of myelographic and surgical findings. There were eight false positives by CT and nine false positives by myelography. The number of false negatives was one for the CT examination and two by myelographic examination. In another study, determining the presence and level of a disc herniation by a CT scanner was slightly more accurate than by myelography.[77] Similar findings were obtained by Troisier and Gozlan.[79] False-positive findings appear to be the greater problem. Wiesel and colleagues[81] found an approximately 50% false-positive rate in CT examination of 58 normal volunteers. MacNab[39] found approximately 8% of negative findings at surgery in patients with positive myelographic indications for surgery. He attributed this finding to inadequate surgical exploration, rather than to false-positive findings preoperatively. Penning and Wilmink[60] have shown how the myelographic appearance can be affected by the degree of flexion or extension of the lumbar spine. They reported that posture-dependent bilateral nerve root compression syndrome could be demonstrated by CT and myelography performed in flexion and extension. It was especially common in the presence of facet hypertrophy. These and other studies addressing the relative diagnostic power of the developing imaging technologies, together with the developing technology of magnetic resonance imaging (MRI),[7, 19, 47, 69, 84] signify a continuing evolution in the use of radiology to assess patients with low back pain. These new techniques are addressed in greater detail elsewhere in this book.

The diagnostic value of discography has been controversial because of false-positive[29] and false-negative[82] findings. Sachs and colleagues[68] developed a scheme for classifying discograms that distinguished between degeneration and disruption of the annulus and took into account whether the injection of contrast medium provoked a painful response. The reproducibility of grading by three observers was 91% for degeneration, and 88% for annular disruption. Transverse CT was used in the classification scheme to provide an additional axial view. The North American Spine Society[10] published a position statement proposing that discography can be appropriate as a preoperative examination, provided that observations at the time of injection are considered in interpreting the results. They emphasized the pain response to injection, the volume of medium injected, and the resistance to injection.

MEASUREMENTS OF MOTION AND PAINFUL SYMPTOMS

Although plane radiographs can demonstrate certain characteristics of the lumbar spine in a passive state, radiography also provides the opportunity to measure motion of the spine and correlate this with painful symptoms. Mensor and Duvall[46] reported that increased intervertebral motion at the L4–L5 interspace was more commonly present in patients with low back pain than in asymptomatic subjects. Conversely, after laminectomy and fusion, Froning and Frohman[13] reported that postoperative relief of pain was greater in the patients who had restricted intersegmental motion. However, Frymoyer and coworkers[14] found similar degrees of segmental mobility at levels of disc surgery without fusion in those with good and poor clinical results. Pearcy and colleagues[56] used biplanar radiography to compare an asymptomatic group of subjects, a group having low back pain and no nerve tension signs, and a third group with back pain and sciatica. Restricted motion was found in both low back pain groups. The group without nerve tension signs showed out-of-plane motion accompanying flexion, which was attributed to asymmetric muscle actions. The group with neurologic involvement showed evidence of segmental splinting of a painful level. However, these findings were not observed consistently enough to be of diagnostic value. Restriction of motion at a painful segmental level was reported by Duncan and Hoen,[8] especially in lateral bending of the spine. They proposed that this sign could help to diagnose herniated discs. Weitz[80] named this phenomenon the *lateral bending sign* and reported on 144 patients in whom 36 had abnormal bending that could often pinpoint the anatomic level of lumbar disc herniation. A similar finding was reported in 18 patients with lumbar disc herniation studied by biplanar radiography in lateral bending.[74]

Hypermobility and excessive forward–backward motion in intervertebral joints was considered to be an early sign of degeneration by Harris and MacNab[24] and by Friberg and Hirsch,[12] based on observations of cadaver specimens. A similar phenomenon has been reported in clinical series.[2, 18, 21, 26, 32, 49] The abnormal motion is associated with "traction" spurs.[38] This led to the concept of "segmental instability" and its treatment by segmental fusion,[15, 31, 36] although there is little agreement among clinicians about how to define this syndrome.[11] Morgan and King[49] reported the instability phenomenon in flexion and extension radiographs. In 28.6% of 500 consecutive cases examined for lumbosacral pain, the films were made with the patient seated and with the arms supporting the weight of the trunk. The "instability" was most common at L4–L5. Abnormality of motion in flexion and extension was demonstrated by an abnormal position of the "motion point"[59] and an abnormal location of the axis of rotation in flexion and extension of cadaver specimens.[70] However, in 10 patients with spondylolisthesis studied by Pearcy and Shepherd[57] and in 24 patients studied by Penning and Blickman,[61] no evidence of abnormal forward–backward motion of the affected vertebral bodies was observed. Furthermore, the axis of motion in the latter series was not abnormally displaced. These authors reject the idea of instability in the spine with spondylolisthesis. Stokes and Frymoyer[76] reported on 78 patients who had a clinical diagnosis of segmental instability and found that the forward–backward translation movement in intervertebral discs did not differ significantly at affected levels from those at unaffected levels, although the ratio between translation motion and angular motion was somewhat elevated in the affected levels. It was concluded that flexion and extension radiography was not useful in the diagnosis of lumbar instability. The amount of translation motion depends on the measurement technique adopted. This is because a combination of rotation and translation (as typically occurs in intervertebral motion) appears as different amounts of translation motion between different pairs of points on the adjacent vertebrae.

The degree to which translation motion accompanies angular motion in intervertebral joints probably depends on a number of factors, including the conditions at the time of radiography. The position of the axis of rotation determines the relative amount of rotation and shear that occurs at the intervertebral disc. Instability, characterized by abnormal or erratic motion, may occur in some patients during the locus of motion from flexion to extension, but it would only be detected radiographically if it were manifested at the static end points of the motion. This inherent difficulty in recording motion could be overcome by using motion radiography, but at the expense of much greater radiation exposure. The locus of motion must also depend on the exact balance of muscular activity accompanying the motion, which in turn could be responsible for large variability within the same patient. Therefore, the degree to which the measurement of segmental motion can be used in the diagnosis of lumbar spinal disorder remains unclear, mainly because of the technical difficulties of recording and measuring the motion.

CONCLUSIONS

Radiology has always held an important position in the examination of the lumbar spine because of the inaccessibility of this part of the body to other noninvasive examinations. Conventional radiography primarily demonstrates ossified parts of the spine. This may be responsible in part for the failure of positive radiologic signs to correspond consistently with painful symptoms. As long as the exact mechanisms of pain production in the lumbar spine remain obscure, we will probably continue to see that radiology alone has generally poor diagnostic power. Currently, rates of false-positive findings are high for most radiographic signs considered to be related to spinal degeneration. A major problem is the lack of a gold standard of degeneration of connective tissues against which to measure correlations with radiologic findings. There appears to be a great need for clinicians and researchers to agree on terminology in this area.

Radiologic images are essentially static. This limits their ability to provide information about painful symptoms, which are often elicited by movement or loading of spinal structures and are relieved under static conditions. Unfortunately, most imaging techniques are technically difficult under dynamic conditions. These technical problems may be part of the reason for disappointing results from motion studies of the spine. Most of the new technology further restricts the ability to perform dynamic imaging or imaging at the end of the range of movements. Other methods of pain provocation, such as the injection of contrast medium, have shown greater promise for improving diagnostic accuracy.

There is no doubt that x-ray imaging has contributed tremendously to the understanding of lumbar spinal function and pathology and of mechanisms of pain production. Diagnostic imaging will always be an important one of the tools for examining the otherwise very inaccessible components of the lumbar spine.

Acknowledgments

The author was supported by the National Institutes of Health through awards NIH RO1 AM 30165 and NIH RO1 AR 38507.

References

1. Adams, M.A., Dolan, P., and Hutton, W.C.: The stages of disc degeneration as revealed by discograms. J. Bone Joint Surg. 68B:36–41, 1986.
2. Aho, A., Vartiainen, O., and Salo, O.: Segmental mobility of the lumbar spine in antero-posterior flexion. Ann. Med. Int. Fenniae 44:275–285, 1955.
3. Bell, G.R., Rothman, R.H., Booth, R.E., et al.: A study of computer-assisted tomography. II. Comparison of metrizamide myelography and computed tomography in the diagnosis of herniated lumbar disc and spinal stenosis. Spine 9:552–556, 1984.
4. Biering-Sorenson, F., Hansen, F.R., Schroll, M., and Runeborg, O.: The relation of spinal x-ray to low-back pain and physical activity among 60-year-old men and women. Spine 10:445–451, 1985.
5. Brown, R.H., Burstein, A.H., Nash, C.L., and Schock, C.C.: Spinal analysis using a three dimensional radiographic technique. J. Biomech. 9:355–365, 1976.
6. Burton, A.K.: Regional lumbar sagittal mobility: Measurement by flexicurves. Clin. Biomech. 1:20–26, 1986.
7. Chafetz, N.I., Genant, H.K., Moon, K.L., et al.: Recognition of lumbar disk herniation with NMR. A.J.R. 141:1153–1156, 1983.
8. Duncan, W., and Hoen, T.I.: A new approach to the diagnosis of herniation of the intervertebral disc. Surg. Gynecol. Obstet. 75:257–267, 1942.
9. Erlacher, P.R.: Nucleography. J. Bone Joint Surg. 34B:204–210, 1952.
10. Executive Committee of the North American Spine Society: Position statement on discography. Spine 13:1343, 1988.
11. Fidler, M.W., cited by Nachemson, A.: The role of spine fusion. Question 8. Spine 6:306–307, 1981.
12. Friberg, S., and Hirsch, C.: Anatomical and clinical studies on lumbar disc degeneration. Acta Orthop. Scand. 19:222–242, 1949.
13. Froning, E.C., and Frohman, B.: Motion of the lumbosacral spine after laminectomy and spine fusion. J. Bone Joint Surg. 50A:897–918, 1968.
14. Frymoyer, J.W., Hanley, E.N., Howe, J., et al.: A comparison of radiographic findings in fusion and nonfusion patients ten or more years following lumbar disc surgery. Spine 4:435–440, 1979.
15. Frymoyer, J.W., and Selby, D.K.: Segmental instability. Rationale for treatment. Spine 10:280–286, 1985.
16. Frymoyer, J.W., Newberg, A., Pope, M.H., et al.: Spine radiographs in patients with low-back pain. An epidemiological study in men. J. Bone Joint Surg. 66A:1048–1055, 1984.
17. Fullenlove, T.M., and Williams, A.J.: Comparative roentgen findings in symptomatic and asymptomatic backs. Radiology 68:572–574, 1957.
18. Gianturco, C.: A roentgen analysis of the motion of the lower lumbar vertebrae in normal individuals and in patients with low back pain. Am. J. Roentgenol. Rad. Ther. 52:261–268, 1944.
19. Gibson, M.J., Buckley, J., Mawhinney, R., et al.: Magnetic resonance imaging and discography in the diagnosis of disc degeneration. J. Bone Joint Surg. 68B:369–373, 1986.
20. Gonella, C., Paris, S.V., and Kutner, M.: Reliability in evaluating passive intervertebral motion. Phys. Ther. 62:436–444, 1982.
21. Hagelstam, L.: Retroposition as an early sign of tuberculous spondylitis of the lumbar spine vertebrae. Acta Chirurg. Scand. 143(Suppl.):31–49, 1949.
22. Hansson, T., Sandstrom, J., Roos, B., et al.: The bone mineral content of the lumbar spine in patients with chronic low back pain. Spine 10:158–160, 1985.
23. Hansson, T., Bigos, S., Beecher, P., and Wortley, M.: The lumbar lordosis in acute and chronic low-back pain. Spine 10:154–155, 1985.
24. Harris, R.I., MacNab, I.: Structural changes in the lumbar intervertebral discs. J. Bone Joint Surg. 36B:304–322, 1954.
25. Hart, D.L., and Rose, S.J.: Reliability of noninvasive method for measuring the lumbar curve. J. Orthop. Sports Phys. Ther. 8:180–184, 1986.
26. Hasner, E., Schalimtzek, M., and Snorrason, E.: Roentgenological examination of the function of the lumbar spine. Acta Radiol. 37:141–149, 1952.
27. Haughton, V.M., Eldevik, O.P., Magnaes, B., and Amundsen, P.: A prospective comparison of computed tomography and myelography in diagnosis of herniated lumbar discs. Radiology 142:103–110, 1982.
28. Hirsch, C., Jonsson, B., and Lewin, T.: Low-back symptoms in a Swedish female population. Clin. Orthop. 63:171–176, 1969.
29. Holt, E.P.: The question of lumbar discography. J. Bone Joint Surg. 50A:720–726, 1968.
30. Horal, J.: The clinical appearance of low back disorders in the city of Gothemburg, Sweden. Acta Orthop. Scand. 118(Suppl.):51–68, 1969.
31. Kirkaldy-Willis, W.H., and Farfan, H.F.: Instability of the lumbar spine. Clin. Orthop. 165:110–123, 1982.
32. Knutsson, F.: The instability associated with disc degeneration in the lumbar spine. Acta Radiol. 25:593–609, 1944.
33. LaRocca, H., and MacNab, I.: Value of pre-employment radiographic assessment of the lumbar spine. Can. Med. Assoc. J. 101:383–388, 1969.
34. Lawrence, J.S.: Disc degeneration. Its frequency and relationship to symptoms. Ann. Rheum. Dis. 28:121–138, 1969.
35. Leiviskä, T., Videman, T., Nurminen, T., and Troup, J.D.G.: Radiographic versus direct measurements of the spinal canal at lumbar vertebrae L3–L5 and their relations to age and body stature. Acta Radiol. (Diagn.) 26:403–411, 1985.
36. Lettin, A.W.F.: Diagnosis and treatment of lumbar instability. J. Bone Joint Surg. 49B:520–529, 1967.
37. Loebl, W.Y.: Measurement of spinal posture and range of spinal movement. Ann. Phys. Med. 9:103–110, 1967.
38. MacNab, I.: The traction spur—An indicator of segmental instability. J. Bone Joint Surg. 53A:663–670, 1971.
39. MacNab, I.: Negative disc exploration. An analysis of the causes of nerve root involvement in 68 patients. J. Bone Joint Surg. 53A:891–903, 1971.

40. Macrae, I.F., and Wright, V.: Measurement of back movement. Ann. Rheum. Dis. 28:584–589, 1969.
41. Malmivaara, A., Videman, T., Kuosma, E., and Troup, J.D.G.: Plain radiographic, discographic, and direct observations of Schmorl's nodes in the thoracolumbar junctional region of the cadaveric spine. Spine 12:453–457, 1987.
42. Malmivaara, A.: Disc degeneration in the thoracolumbar junctional region. Evaluation by radiography and discography in autopsy. Acta Radiol. Diagn. 28:755–760, 1987.
43. Malmivaara, A., Videman, T., Kuosma, E., and Troup, J.D.G.: Radiographic vs. direct measurements of the spinal canal of the thoracolumbar junctional region (T10–L1) of the spine. Spine 11:574–578, 1986.
44. McBroom, R.J., Hayes, W.C., Edwards, W.T., et al.: Prediction of vertebral body compressive fracture using quantitative computed tomography. J. Bone Joint Surg. 67A:1206–1214, 1985.
45. McCall, I.W.: Radiologic assessment of back pain. Semin. Orthop. 1:71–85, 1986.
46. Mensor, M.C., and Duvall, G.: Absence of motion at the 4th and 5th lumbar interspaces in patients with and without low back pain. J. Bone Joint Surg. 41A:1047–1054, 1959.
47. Modic, M.T., Pavlicek, W., Weinstein, M.A., et al.: Magnetic resonance imaging of intervertebral disk disease. Radiology 152:103–111, 1984.
48. Moll, J.M.H., and Wright, V.: Normal range of spinal mobility. An objective clinical study. Ann. Rheum. Dis. 30:381–386, 1971.
49. Morgan, F.P., and King, T.: Primary instability of lumbar vertebrae as a common cause of low back pain. J. Bone Joint Surg. 39B:6–22, 1957.
50. Nachemson, A.L.: The lumbar spine. An orthopaedic challenge. Spine 1:59–71, 1976.
51. Oda, M., Rauh, S., Gregory, P.B., et al.: The significance of roentgenographic measurement in scoliosis. J. Pediatr. Orthop. 2:378–382, 1982.
52. Olsson, T.H., Selvik, G., and Willner, S.: Mobility in the lumbosacral spine after fusion studied with the aid of roentgen stereophotogrammetry. Clin. Orthop. 129:181–190, 1977.
53. Panjabi, M.M., Goel, V.K., Walter, S.D., and Schick, S.: Errors in the center and angle of rotation of a joint. An experimental study. J. Biomech. Engineer. 104:232–237, 1982.
54. Panjabi, M.M., Krag, M.H., and Goel, V.K.: A technique for measurement and description of three-dimensional six degree-of-freedom motion of a body joint with an application to the human spine. J. Biomech. 14:447–460, 1981.
55. Park, W.M.: The place of radiology in the investigation of low back pain. Clin. Rheum. Dis. 6:93–132, 1980.
56. Pearcy, M., Portek, I., and Shepherd, J.: The effect of low-back pain on lumbar spinal movements measured by three-dimensional x-ray analysis. Spine 10:150–153, 1985.
57. Pearcy, M., and Shepherd, J.: Is there instability in spondylolisthesis? Spine 10:175–177, 1985.
58. Pearcy, M., and Burrough, S.: Assessment of bony union after interbody fusion of the lumbar spine using a biplanar radiographic technique. J. Bone Joint Surg. 64B:228–232, 1982.
59. Pennal, G.F., Conn, G.S., McDonald, G., et al.: Motion studies of the lumbar spine. A preliminary report. J. Bone Joint Surg. 54B:442–452, 1972.
60. Penning, L., and Wilmink, J.T.: Posture-dependent bilateral compression of L4 or L5 nerve roots in facet hypertrophy. A dynamic CT myelographic study. Spine 12:488–500, 1987.
61. Penning, L., and Blickman, J.R.: Instability in lumbar spondylolisthesis: A radiologic study of several concepts. A.J.R. 134:293–301, 1980.
62. Portek, I., Pearcy, M.J., Reader, G.P., and Mowat, A.G.: Correlation between radiographic and clinical measurement of lumbar spine movement. Br. J. Rheumatol. 22:197–205, 1983.
63. Porter, R.W., Wicks, M. and Ottewell, D.: Measurement of the spinal canal by diagnostic ultrasound. J. Bone Joint Surg. 60B:481–484, 1978.
64. Quinnell, R.C., and Stockdale, H.R.: Flexion and extension radiography of the lumbar spine: A comparison with lumbar discography. Clin. Radiol. 34:405–411, 1983.
65. Quinnell, R.C., and Stockdale, H.R.: An investigation of artifacts in lumbar discography. Br. J. Radiol. 53:831–839, 1980.
66. Quinnell, R.C., and Stockdale, H.R.: The significance of osteophytes on lumbar vertebral bodies in relation to discographic findings. Clin. Radiol. 33:197–203, 1982.
67. Rab, G.T., and Chao, E.Y.: Verification of roentgenographic landmarks in the lumbar spine. Spine 2:287–293, 1977.
68. Sachs, B.L., Vanharanta, H., Spivey, M.A., et al.: Dallas discogram description. A new classification of CT/discography in low-back disorders. Spine 12:287–294, 1987.
69. Schneiderman, G., Flannigan, B., Kingston, S., et al.: Magnetic resonance imaging in the diagnosis of disc degeneration: Correlation with discography. Spine 12:276–281, 1987.
70. Seligman, J.V., Gertzbein, S.D., Tile, M., and Kapasouri, A.: Computer analysis of spinal segment motion in degenerative disc disease with and without axial loading. Spine 9:566–573, 1984.
71. Sevastikoglou, J.A., and Bergquist, E.: Evaluation of the reliability of radiographic methods for registration of scoliosis. Acta Orthop. Scand. 40:608–613, 1969.
72. Splithoff, G.A.: Lumbosacral junction: Roentgenographic comparison of patients with and without backache. J.A.M.A. 152:1610–1613, 1953.
73. Stokes, I.A.F., Bevins, T.M., and Lunn, R.A.: Back surface curvature and measurement of lumbar spinal motion. Spine 12:355–361, 1987.
74. Stokes, I.A.F., Wilder, D.G., Frymoyer, J.W., and Pope, M.H.: Assessment of patients with low-back pain by biplanar radiographic measurement of intervertebral motion. Spine 6:233–240, 1981.
75. Stokes, I.A.F., Medlicott, P.A., and Wilder, D.G.: Measurement of motion in painful intervertebral joints. Med. Biol. Engineer. Comput. 18:694–700, 1980.
76. Stokes, I.A.F., and Frymoyer, J.W.: Segmental motion and instability. Spine 12:688–691, 1987.
77. Teplick, J.G., and Haskin, M.E.: CT and lumbar disc herniation. Radiol. Clin. North Am. 21:259–288, 1983.
78. Torgerson, W.R., and Dotter, W.E.: Comparative roentgenographic study of the asymptomatic and

symptomatic lumbar spine. J. Bone Joint Surg. 58A:850–853, 1976.
79. Troisier, O., and Gozlan, E.: Mesure comparative des hernies discales sur la discographie et le scanner. Ann. Readapt. Med. Phys. 30:247–254, 1987.
80. Weitz, E.M.: The lateral bending sign. Spine 6:388–397, 1981.
81. Wiesel, S.W., Tsourmas, N., Feffer, H.L., et al.: A study of computer-assisted tomography. I. The incidence of positive CAT scans in an asymptomatic group of patients. Spine 9:549–551, 1984.
82. Yasuma, T., Ohno, R., and Yamuchi, Y.: False-negative lumbar discograms. Correlation of discographic and histological findings in postmortem and surgical specimens. J. Bone Joint Surg. 70A:1279–1290, 1988.
83. Yerushalmy, J.: Statistical problems in assessing methods of medical diagnosis, with special reference to x-ray techniques. Pub. Health Rep. 62:1432–1449, 1947.
84. Zindrick, M.R., Lorenz, M.A., Noonan, C., and Montegrano, V.C.: The correlation between MRI, discogram and pain reproduction. Presented at the 14th annual meeting of International Society for Study of the Lumbar Spine, Rome, Italy, 1987. Orthop. Transact. 12:65, 1988.

COMPUTED TOMOGRAPHY-DISCOGRAPHY

Roger P. Jackson
Rae R. Jacobs

Myelography has long been considered the bench mark against which other diagnostic tests are measured. It has proven reliability in the diagnosis of lumbar herniated nucleus pulposus[1, 17] and is a study that may be easily interpreted and readily obtained in most all radiology departments throughout the world. Computed tomography (CT) has challenged the diagnostic utility of myelography by matching its accuracy,[4, 11, 17, 43, 49, 53] exposing the patient to less radiation, and lowering the complication rate.[49] CT has been demonstrated to be superior to myelography in the diagnosis of lateral lumbar disc herniations.[3, 14, 17, 27, 36, 38, 40, 43, 44] The combination of the two techniques has resulted in further refinement of imaging, especially of a widened anterior epidural space at the L5–S1 level.[26] Discography has remained somewhat controversial as a clinical diagnostic tool. High diagnostic accuracy has been reported.[33, 47, 50] In addition, this test has been shown to reproduce accurately the patient's pain pattern[33, 47] and to demonstrate lateral disc herniations.[29, 31] The combination of discography and CT has been recently recognized as an accurate tool for diagnosing disc disease,[21, 45, 51, 52] especially foraminal lumbar disc herniations.[2, 20, 35]

A review of the literature finds many studies reporting a diagnostic accuracy for CT ranging from 48% to 100% and for myelography ranging from 60% to 100% in the diagnosis of lumbar disc disease.[3, 8, 16, 17, 23, 25, 26, 37, 48, 49, 53] The sensitivity and specificity of myelography have been reported to be 97% and 100%, respectively.[18] Low false-negative and false-positive rates of 4% and 6% have been published.[17] Other studies have also published low false-negative rates of 6.3%[43] and 7.6%.[39]

It is difficult to obtain good statistics for comparison because most studies, by virtue of their design, tend to be biased toward the test that is a major factor supporting surgery in the first place. In addition, most studies do not contain significant numbers of patients (or discs) who have undergone explorations with the negative results that are necessary to allow for calculations of more accurate false-positive and false-negative rates.

We have now evaluated over 1,000 patients by means of CT-discography. Our interest in this area has led us more recently to study a number of patients prospectively in order to better compare the relative accuracies of CT, myelography, CT-myelography, discography, and CT-discography in the diagnosis of lumbar herniated nucleus pulposus. In order to calculate more accurate false-positive and false-negative rates, during our prospective comparative studies efforts were made at the time of surgery to explore as many discs as possible. Our findings were carefully recorded so that they could be correlated with the readings of the preoperative radiographic tests, as interpreted by four different observers. All operative findings, negative or positive, at each explored site were recorded and correlated accordingly. This also allowed us to calculate more reliable sensitivities and specificities for these tests. We also studied the effect of prior laminectomy surgery and foraminal disc herniation upon the accuracies of these various tests. The level of confidence and the percentage of equivocal results for each test were also determined. In addition, we prospectively studied the diagnostic accuracy of disc injection pain in patients proved at surgery to have lumbar disc herniations.

During 1985 and part of 1986, 124 patients with suspected lumbar herniated nucleus pulposus that was refractory to conservative management were studied with five diagnostic tests consisting of CT, metrizamide myelography, CT-myelography, three-level lumbar discography, and CT-discography. All patients completed all five tests and came to surgical exploration of at least one side of one disc space. It has been our procedure to perform myelography and discography during the course of a hospital admission. These two tests are generally carried out on consecutive days, although some patients have undergone both procedures during the same day. CT is routinely performed from L3 to S1 with 5-mm sections overlapping 1 mm. Both bone and soft tissue window settings are obtained. The gantry is angled, and lumbar lordisis is adjusted by hip and knee flexion such that sections are made parallel to each disc and no areas are skipped. The time required to complete a CT study has averaged 30 minutes, with an average of approximately 30 sections per study.

Myelography is performed by lumbar puncture at various levels from L2 to S1 with a 22-gauge spinal needle and, during this period of time, infusion of 14 cc of metrizamide in a concentration of 180 mg iodine/cc. We are now using iohexol and prefer it. Patients undergo complete myelographic radiography with visualization of the conus medullaris followed by CT within an hour or two. CT is routinely performed from L3 to S1 as just described.

For the purpose of our comparative studies, all patients had discography performed at the three most caudal disc levels, typically L3–4, L4–5, and L5–S1. In patients with transitional lumbosacral vertebra, the three most caudal open disc spaces were studied. In this procedure, the patient's back is scrubbed with chlorhexidine (Hibiclens) on the evening before and on the morning of testing. The patients are given medication for sedation. A surgical mask and sterile gloves are used by the physician performing the test, and a strict sterile technique must be followed. Local anesthetic in the skin is first injected. A two-needle technique is utilized, in which 3.5-inch-long 19-gauge styletted spinal needles are advanced, under fluoroscopic control, in either a posterior or lateral approach toward the disc space. We have found a posterior transdural approach to be more reliable and less painful, especially at the L5–S1 level. Puncture of the dura with the 19-gauge needles is carefully avoided. Six-inch-long 26-gauge styletted spinal needles are directed through the larger-diameter needles and into the center of the disc. It is generally necessary to put some degree of curvature on these needles before inserting them, especially at the L5–S1 level.

Up to 4 cc of water-soluble contrast is injected slowly at each level studied. A minimum of 2.5 to 3 cc of contrast medium is believed necessary for an adequate evaluation of a pathologic disc. Intact discs rarely accept more than 2.5 cc of contrast medium. The contrast agents presently approved by the Food and Drug Administration (FDA) for intradiscal injection include diatrizoate meglumine injection USP 60% (Reno-M-60, Hypaque-60); diatrizoate meglumine 52% and diatrizoate sodium 8% (Renografin-60); and diatrizoate meglumine 52%, diatrizoate sodium 8%, and iodine 29.2% (MD-60, Angio-Vist 292).

After the injection of each disc, the patient's pain response is recorded. Posteroanterior (PA), lateral, and oblique radiographs of the injected discs are obtained. The gantry on the fluoroscopy table is angled to provide better tangential views of the injected discs. Three-level discography is generally accomplished within 30 minutes in most patients.

CT scanning is delayed 3 to 4 hours following disc injections, especially if there has been any epidural or paralumbar extravasation of contrast material. Such a time delay is necessary to allow for all extravasation of contrast to dissipate. Standard CT scanning with angling of the gantry is carried out through the injected discs. Bone and soft tissue window settings are again utilized.

During our protocol studies, each of the five preoperative radiographic tests was read without knowledge of the results of other tests or of the patient's history and physical examination. The radiographs were evaluated independently by a spine surgeon, a spine fellow, and two radiologists skilled in neuroradiologic diagnosis. All four evaluators examined all three disc spaces from one neural foramen across to the other, in all five studies. The location of a so-called herniated disc was recorded as posterolateral and right or left, or as foraminal and right or left. Central herniations usually favored one side and were recorded as such. The level of confidence in each diagnosis was recorded as "definitely herniated," "most probably herniated," "possibly herniated," "probably not herniated," or "definitely not herniated." The type of herniated nucleus pulposus suspected was described as protruded, extruded, or sequestered by the observers.

The gold standard for comparison was proven disc disease, or its absence, at surgery. Again, every patient had surgical exploration of at least one side of one disc space. Most of the patients (113) in this protocol study had disc herniations. Eleven patients were also studied who had explorations for reasons other than herniated nucleus pulposus (e.g., placement of screws during a fusion procedure for lumbar instability of a degenerative nature). This was done to more accurately determine false-positive and false-negative rates. The surgical findings were documented precisely regarding the location and type of herniation. For the calculations, protruded, extruded, and sequestered discs were considered to be herniated. Patients with spinal stenosis were excluded from this prospective part of our studies.

The data were compiled and entered for computer analysis. Accuracies, false-positive and false-negative rates, percentages of equivocal results (possibly herniated), sensitivities, and specificities were calculated. For the determination of results, a radiographic reading of "definitely herniated," "most probably herniated," or "possibly herniated" was considered to be a correct response if a herniation was surgically discovered at a specific site. Statistical testing was performed using analysis of variance with repeated measures on ranked data followed by Duncan's multiple comparisons test.

A separate analysis of the complications and side effects of myelography and discography during our protocol studies was performed. Because many of the patients had surgery within 24 hours of completion of the testing and some side effects were thus masked, charts of all patients who underwent myelography and discography within a 72-hour period during the time of our protocol study were reviewed. Complications were defined as serious or life-threatening sequelae such as death, seizures, anaphylactic reactions, disc space infections, disc herniations, or extension of herniations. Side effects were less serious reactions such as nausea, vomiting, headache, or neck stiffness. Delays in hospital discharge were noted and an attempt was made, based upon the temporal sequence, to attribute each side effect to myelography, discography, or both.

The 124 patients operated on during this protocol had a mean age of 42.7 years (range 21 to 76 years). There were 87 males (70.2%) and 37 females (29.8%). A group of 111 patients had no prior disc surgery, and 13 patients had one or more previous discectomies. Surgical exploration of 231 sites (level and side) was performed. Disc herniation was found in 113 patients; 12 patients had two-level herniations, so 125 discs were removed in all. The most frequent level of herniation was L5–S1 (51.2%), followed by L4–L5 (43.2%) and L3–L4 (5.6%) (Table 1). Overall, about half of the herniations (49.6%) were disc extrusions, 27.2% sequestrations, and 20.8% protrusions. Foraminal or extraforaminal herniations were found in 17 patients. This included 3 lateral herniations with extension into the neural foramina, 12 intraforaminal herniations, and 2 extraforaminal herniations. The mean age of this group, 56.1 years, was significantly higher than that of the entire group ($p < .01$). We reported a previous study of patients with foraminal and extraforaminal lumbar disc herniations with this same finding.[20]

The radiographic diagnoses for the 231 sites surgically explored are listed in Table 2. The third column indicates the percentage of discs thought by the four observers to be

Table 1 □ Type of Lumbar HNP by Level

TYPE	L3–L4 N	L3–L4 %	L4–L5 N	L4–L5 %	L5–S1 N	L5–S1 %	TOTAL N	TOTAL %
Bulge	0	0.0	2	3.7	1	1.6	3	2.4
Protrusion	1	14.3	13	24.1	12	18.8	26	20.8
Extrusion	5	71.4	24	44.4	33	51.6	62	49.6
Sequestration	1	14.3	15	23.4	18	28.1	34	27.2
Total	7	5.6	54	43.2	64	51.2	125	100.0

HNP = herniated nucleus pulposus.

"possibly herniated," as opposed to the more confident diagnoses of "definitely herniated" or "most probably herniated" listed in the first two columns. It can be seen that CT-discography provided the fewest (7.8%) equivocal diagnoses, compared with myelography (15.6%), CT-myelography (18.3%), CT (22.5%), and discography (71.1%). CT-discography also provided the highest percentage of "definite" diagnoses (35.0%) compared with CT-myelography (17.1%), myelography (15.1%), CT (11.6%), and discography (0.1%).

Table 3 collapses the first three columns of Table 2 (diagnoses of definitely, most probably, and possibly herniated) into a diagnosis of "herniated" and the last two columns (diagnoses of probably not and definitely not herniated) into a diagnosis of "not herniated." This demonstrates that the plain discogram radiograph is too sensitive a study in that 75.5% of the sites were thought to be herniated, as compared with the 54.1% found surgically. On the other hand, disc injection pain was not sufficiently sensitive, in that only 28.6% of the sites were believed to be herniated on the basis of pain pattern reproduction. CT, myelography, CT myelography, and CT-discography provided a diagnosis of disc herniation that approximated the percentage found at surgery.

In order to define more precisely the relative merit of each test, formal calculations of accuracy, false-negativity, false-positivity, sensitivity, and specificity were performed. These are reported in Table 4. The most accurate test was CT-discography (86.8%) compared with 77.1% for CT-myelography ($p < .05$), 73.5% for CT ($p < .01$), 70.2% for myelography ($p < .01$), and 58.4% for discography ($p < .01$). The accuracy of disc injection pain in the diagnosis of disc herniation was 64.1%. No statistical comparison was made because of the differences in the methodology of rating this test and the radiographic tests. Interobserver reliability for accuracy was very good, as the standard deviation was less than 4% among the four observers for all five studies. There was no statistical difference between the accuracy of CT and myelography. CT-discography had the lowest false-positive rate (19.3%), compared with 24.1% for CT (n.s.), 29.9% for myelography ($p < .01$), and 24.3% for CT-myelography (n.s.). The 8.0% false-negative rate for CT-discography was also significantly less than 28.5% for CT ($p < .01$) and 29.8% for myelography ($p < .01$). There was no significant difference in the false-negative rates among CT, myelography, and CT-myelography.

CT-discography ranked highest in sensitivity for lumbar disc herniations (92.0%), compared with 78.2% for CT-myelography

Table 2 □ Radiographic Diagnosis at the 231 Sites Explored by Individual Test

TEST	DEFINITELY HNP (%)	PROBABLY HNP (%)	POSSIBLY HNP (%)	PROBABLY NOT HNP (%)	DEFINITELY NOT HNP (%)
CT	11.6	15.8	22.5	44.0	6.1
Myelography	15.1	21.0	15.6	40.7	7.6
Myelography-CT	17.1	17.9	18.3	37.1	9.7
Discography	0.1	4.2	71.1	20.5	4.0
Discography-CT	35.0	15.7	7.8	33.0	8.6

HNP = herniated nucleus pulposus.

Table 3 □ Disc Herniations Found, by Test, Compared with Surgery

TEST	HNP (%)	NO HNP (%)
CT	49.9	50.1
Myelography	51.7	48.3
Myelography-CT	53.3	46.7
Discography	75.5	24.5
Discography-CT	58.4	41.6
Disc Injection Pain	28.6	71.4
Surgery	54.1	45.9

HNP = herniated nucleus pulposus.

($p < .05$), 71.5% for CT ($p < .01$), 70.2% for myelography ($p < .01$), and 81.4% for discography (n.s.). There was no significant difference in the sensitivity rates among CT, myelography, and CT-myelography. CT-discography had an 80.7% specificity, compared with 75.9% for CT (n.s.), 75.7% for CT-myelography (n.s.), 70.1% for myelography (n.s.), and 31.4% for discography ($p < .01$). All other tests were more specific than discography ($p < .01$). Disc injection pain as a diagnostic test was fairly specific, in fact the most specific, for lumbar disc herniation (88.7%), but was not very sensitive (43.2%). Correspondingly, the false-negative and false-positive rates for this test were 56.8% and 11.3%, respectively.

The accuracy of diagnosis of lumbar disc herniation for the five tests was examined for various subgroups of the total population, including those who had foraminal disc herniations and those who had previous disc surgery with recurrent disc herniations. The results are shown in Table 5. CT-discography was the most accurate test in patients with recurrent herniations (94.0%), compared with 81.0% for CT-myelography ($p < .05$), 80.0% for CT ($p < .01$), 73.7% for myelography and 62.0% for discography ($p < .01$). Discography was significantly less accurate than the other tests. No other comparisons were significantly different. None of the tests was significantly less accurate for such patients than for the rest of the population. CT-discography was also the most accurate test for foraminal herniations (91.1%), compared with 71.2% for CT, 65.1% for CT-myelography, 57.8% for myelography, and 47.4% for discography ($p < .01$ for all tests). CT was superior to myelography for the diagnosis of foraminal disc herniation ($p < .01$), and all tests were superior to discography. Myelography, CT-myelography, and discography were significantly less accurate in the diagnosis of foraminal disc herniation, compared with other types of herniation ($p < .005$). The sensitivity of CT-discography for diagnosis in patients with recurrent disc herniations was 100%, compared with 88.5% for CT-myelography, 86.5% for CT and discography, and 78.8% for myelography. CT-discography was also more specific (87.5%) compared with 72.9% for CT and CT-myelography, 68.1% for myelography, and 35.4% for discography. CT-discography was more sensitive for foraminal disc herniation (97.5%), compared with 81.3% for discography, 63.7% for CT, 61.2% for CT-myelography, and 45% for myelography. Similarly CT-discography was more specific (86.6%) compared with 76.6% for CT, 67.9% for CT-myelography, 67.0% for myelography, and 23.2% for discography. Thus, CT-discography is highly sensitive and specific for these types of herniations in contrast to discography, which is sensitive but not specific.

The diagnostic accuracies of the five radiographic studies were examined for the L3–L4, L4–L5, and L5–S1 levels. CT-discography was the most accurate test at all levels, ranging from 84.8% at L4–L5 to 95.6% at L3–L4. The accuracy of CT ranged from 70.6% at L4–L5 to 76.5% at L5–S1, whereas the accuracy of myelography conversely decreased from 82.4% at L3–L4 to 65.8% at L4–L5 and 72.3% at L5–S1. The presence of a widened anterior epidural space favors CT over myelography at the L5–S1 level, whereas the narrower canal at the L3–L4 level favors myelography. The combination of CT with myelography increases the accuracy at L3–L4 to 81.8%, and at L5–S1 to 82.2%.

Pain with disc injection was noted in most patients and classified into localized back pain, which was considered to be not significant, and radicular pain similar in quality and location to the patient's usual pain, which was considered significant. Disc injection in 46 patients reproduced their usual pain patterns. In four of these patients, disc injection at two levels reproduced their clinical pain. Therefore, the injection of 50 discs in all reproduced the patients' clinical pain patterns. Of these discs, six were radiographically normal and not able to be explored. Only 44 of 122 (36.1%) protruded, extruded, or sequestered discs produced radicular pain

Table 4 □ Comparison of Tests

TEST	ACCURACY (%)	FALSE NEGATIVE (%)	FALSE POSITIVE (%)	SENSITIVITY (%)	SPECIFICITY (%)
CT	73.5 ± 4.0	28.5 ± 14.3	24.1 ± 10.1	71.5 ± 14.3	75.9 ± 10.1
Myelography	70.2 ± 0.6	29.8 ± 2.8	29.9 ± 2.6	70.2 ± 2.8	70.1 ± 2.6
Myelography-CT	77.1 ± 2.9	21.8 ± 9.8	24.3 ± 8.6	78.2 ± 9.8	75.7 ± 8.6
Discography	58.4 ± 2.1	18.6 ± 20.6	68.6 ± 25.4	81.4 ± 20.6	31.4 ± 25.4
Discography-CT	86.8 ± 2.6	8.0 ± 2.4	19.3 ± 7.3	92.0 ± 2.4	80.7 ± 7.3
Disc Injection Pain	64.1	56.8	11.3	43.2	88.7

on injection. Pain was most frequently reproduced in protruded (44.0%) discs, compared with extruded (37.1%) and sequestered (30.3%) discs.

During the time of this protocol study, a total of 253 patients underwent both myelography and discography within a period of 72 hours. Of these patients, 149 (58.9%) were discharged after testing. The remainder had surgery during the same hospital admission. There were no serious complications as defined previously in this group of patients; 48.6% had no side effects from the testing. The remaining 51.4% of patients had one or more side effects as listed here. The most common was headache (40.7%), followed by nausea and vomiting (15.4%), nausea alone (4.7%), and neck stiffness (5.5%). Three of the 103 patients (2.9%) who had headaches required a blood patch, which resolved the symptoms completely within 24 hours. Discharge from hospital generally occurred 1 to 2 days after myelography and discography, unless the patient had surgery during the same hospitalization. Surgery was not delayed in any patient because of side effects from those tests. Discharge was delayed in 3.9% of patients who did not have surgery, owing to side effects. Two patients (0.8%) required readmission for treatment of severe headache and/or nausea and vomiting.

Of all side effects, 55.4% were attributed to myelography, as the symptoms occurred and usually resolved prior to discography. Nausea and vomiting were very common, but they have become much less frequent since we have been using iohexol instead of metrizamide. Twenty percent of side effects were attributed to discography alone, and 24.6% to both tests. The subgroup of patients who underwent both tests during the same day did not fare any more poorly than the remaining patients.

Diagnostic tests should be as accurate as possible, with high sensitivity to detect all positive findings and high specificity to exclude all negative and unrelated diagnoses. These rates will be affected by the diagnostic criteria used, which, in turn, are related to the desired level of confidence in the diagnosis. We have attempted to determine the true value of each test studied by demanding rigid diagnostic criteria. Each study was read without knowledge of clinical data, surgical pathologic findings, or other test results. The exact locations (level and side) of any herniations had to be noted, and the absence of disease at the other sites also had to be properly diagnosed. In addition, each evaluator was required to express a level of confidence in each diagnosis. The 106 (45.9%) sites explored and found to be free of disc herniation provided good numbers

Table 5 □ Accuracy of Tests for Patients with Prior Surgery and Foraminal HNP

TEST	PATIENTS WHO HAD PRIOR SURGERY (%)	PATIENTS WHO HAD FORAMINAL HNP (%)	ALL PATIENTS (%)
CT	80.0	71.2	73.5
Myelography	73.7	57.8	70.2($p < .005$)
Myelography-CT	81.0	65.1	77.1($p < .005$)
Discography	62.0	47.4	58.4($p < .005$)
Discography-CT	94.0	91.1	86.8

HNP = herniated nucleus pulposus.

to determine fairly accurate false-positive and false-negative rates for each diagnostic test. An ideal study would demand an exploration of each level and side in every patient evaluated by the radiographic studies in order to calculate more accurate false-positive and false-negative rates. For obvious reasons, however, this is not possible in clinical practice.

Because many patients in our protocol study were referred from other specialists and surgeons who could not make a diagnosis based upon the initial work-up, this population is perhaps skewed somewhat toward more complex and subtle disorders. Consequently, a considerable number of foraminal disc herniations were found. These factors contribute to the lower accuracy rates presented here, compared with those reported in the literature.[1, 4, 16, 17, 25, 26, 43, 46, 49, 53] Lower diagnostic accuracies have been reported when more strict criteria were demanded.[3] Carrera and associates[7] reported 60.7% accuracy for myelography, and Moufarrij and colleagues[37] reported 48.0% accuracy for CT when strict criteria were used. We believe our results accurately assess the relative value of each test in such a worst-case scenario. In clinical practice, it is never necessary to make decisions on the basis of one test only, but it is valuable to know the relative accuracy and confidence of these tests. Kratzer and Hipp[28] reported that more than one radiographic study was required to establish a diagnosis in 22.0% of patients defined as having problem cases. Depending on the population, various percentages of patients will need to undergo multiple studies to arrive at an accurate diagnosis.

We have frequently noted the extravasation of contrast material epidurally into the spinal canal or out into the neural foramina, which is associated with degenerated but not necessarily herniated discs. CT performed within a short time following disc injection will produce artifacts resulting from this extravasated material. We recommend waiting at least 3 to 4 hours to allow for dissipation of the contrast material. Our in vitro studies have found nuclear disc material to have an affinity for water-soluble contrast media,[19, 20] which allows for its enhancement with CT. The radiographs of tissues removed at surgery and exposed to such contrast media have shown uniform enhancement of the nucleus pulposus, enhancement of only the fine septa in fat, only moderate enhancement of epidural scar tissue, and essentially no enhancement of annulus, compared with controls.[19]

The leakage of contrast medium through a needle puncture in the disc has been demonstrated by McCutcheon and Thompson.[35] Such an artifact may be confused with an annular pathologic condition. When we have used 26-gauge needles and allowed at least 3 to 4 hours for dissipation of extravasated contrast media, we have not found this to be a problem. Many degenerated but nonherniated discs seen by CT-discography reveal radial fissures extending in a posterolateral direction, either unilaterally or bilaterally (Fig. 1*A*). This finding is interesting and raises the question of whether these patients may be at risk for subsequent herniation.

The differentiation between recurrent disc herniation and postoperative scar formation is usually difficult. The accuracy of CT has been reported to be 43.0% without contrast enhancement[5] and 70% to 74% with intravenous contrast enhancement.[5, 41] We have noted a 94.0% accuracy rate with CT-discography, compared with 80.0% for CT and 73.7% for myelography (Figs. 2 and 3). More importantly, it is desirable for a test used in the diagnosis of recurrent disc herniation to be highly specific. CT, myelography, CT-myelography, and CT-discography are all very sensitive, but CT-discography is the most specific study. Again, our studies have demonstrated herniated nuclear material to have an affinity for water-soluble contrast media greater than that of epidural scar tissue. The enhancement of recurrent herniated disc material affords CT-discography greater accuracy, sensitivity, and specificity (Fig. 3*A*, *B*).

Myelography and CT, alone or in combination, are both significantly less accurate than CT-discography in the diagnosis of foraminal disc herniations. This is related to both sensitivity and specificity. Foraminal disc herniations are often missed by these tests.[20, 29, 38] In order to diagnose these herniations, it is desirable to employ a test that is very sensitive. CT-discography provides 98.0% sensitivity, compared with 77.0% for CT and 67.0% for myelography. Discography has 81.0% sensitivity, but only 23.0% specificity. Among these five tests for the diagnosis of foraminal lumbar disc herniation,

CT-discography is the study of choice because of its demonstrated high accuracy, sensitivity, and specificity for this suspected lesion (Fig. 1*B*). Magnetic resonance imaging (MRI) may prove to be more accurate, sensitive, and specific for these types of herniations and to have obvious other advantages as well, but a sufficient number of studies are not reported at this time.

Our data demonstrate a fairly high sensitivity (81%), but a low specificity (31%) for discography in the diagnosis of lumbar disc herniation. This test is unable to discriminate adequately between degenerated and herniated discs (Figs. 1 and 4). On the other hand, disc injection pain is specific (89%) but not very sensitive (43%). These two components of the procedure complement each other and probably account for the continued use of this test.

The incidence of side effects in our studies (48.6%) corresponds well to the 46% to 72% reported for metrizamide myelography alone.[18, 30, 55] Piepgras and associates[42] reported that discography and myelography have the same risks but that the side effects of discography are less. An animal study by Kahanovitz and colleagues[24] revealed that intradiscal injection of metrizamide results in no gross or histologic damage to the disc.

Our experience with discography includes over 3,350 disc injections in more than 1,300 patients. Discitis has been observed in 0.35% of discs injected, or in 0.77% of the patients studied. Others have reported an incidence of 0.1% to 2.7%.[6, 9, 10, 12, 15, 32, 34, 47]

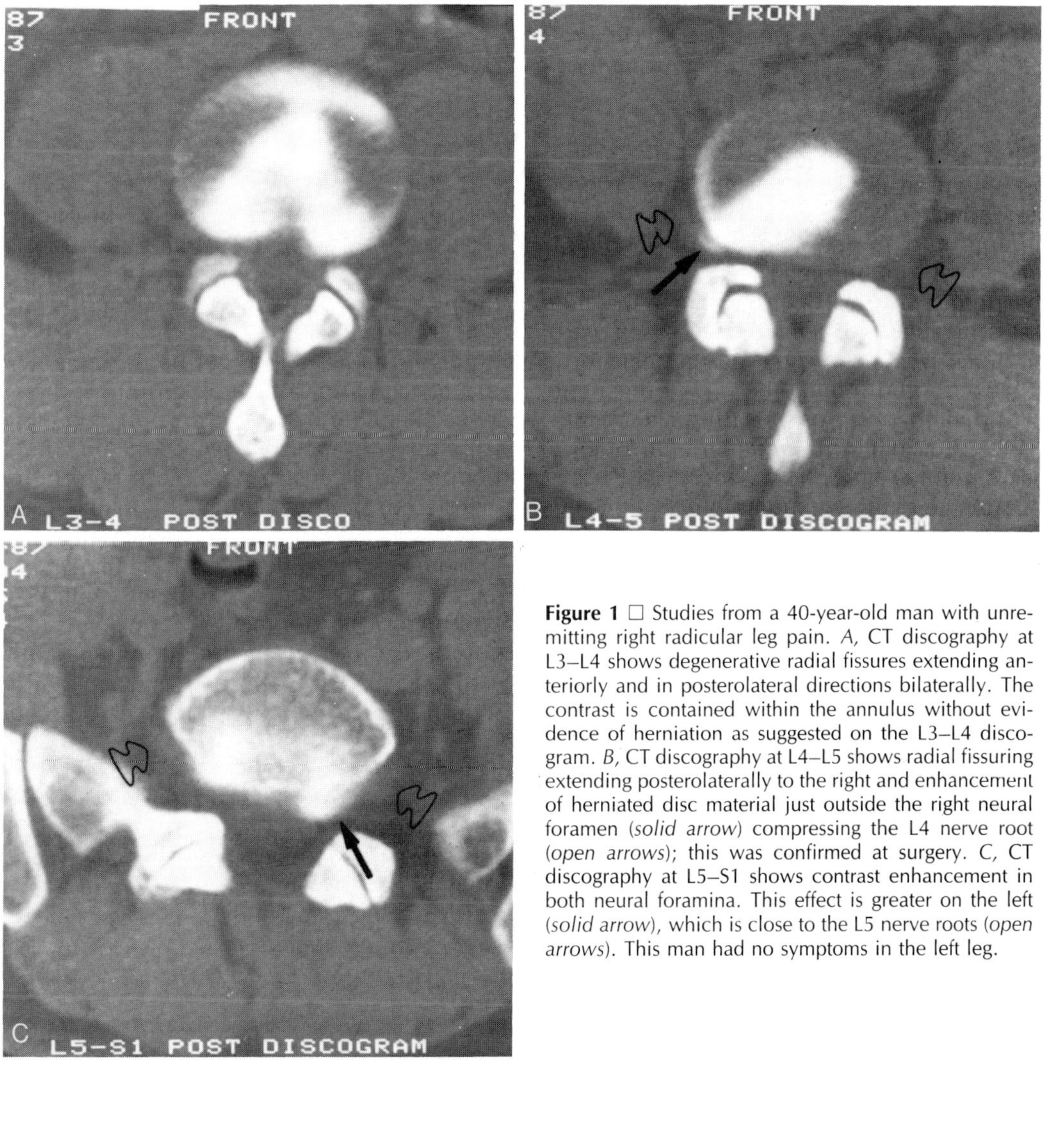

Figure 1 □ Studies from a 40-year-old man with unremitting right radicular leg pain. *A,* CT discography at L3–L4 shows degenerative radial fissures extending anteriorly and in posterolateral directions bilaterally. The contrast is contained within the annulus without evidence of herniation as suggested on the L3–L4 discogram. *B,* CT discography at L4–L5 shows radial fissuring extending posterolaterally to the right and enhancement of herniated disc material just outside the right neural foramen (*solid arrow*) compressing the L4 nerve root (*open arrows*); this was confirmed at surgery. *C,* CT discography at L5–S1 shows contrast enhancement in both neural foramina. This effect is greater on the left (*solid arrow*), which is close to the L5 nerve roots (*open arrows*). This man had no symptoms in the left leg.

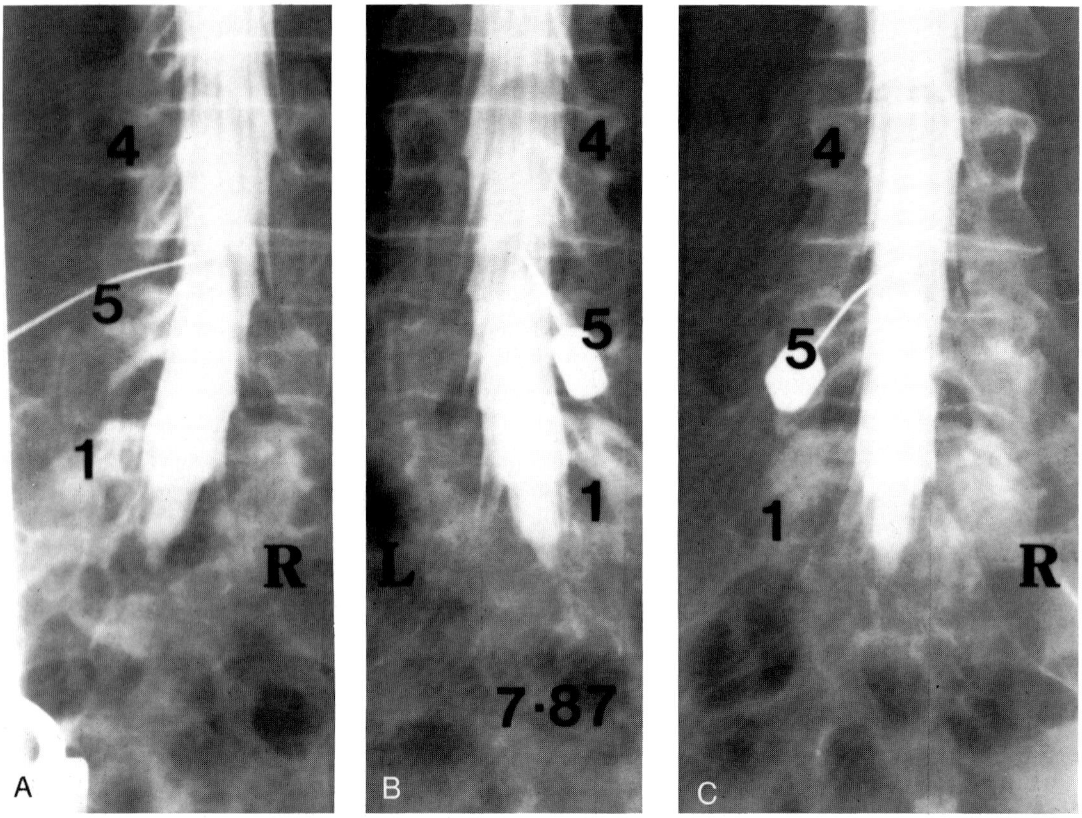

Figure 2 □ *A–C,* Right and left oblique and PA radiographs of the lumbar myelogram from a 45-year-old woman with recurrent right radicular leg pain show no extradural defects and only slightly less filling of the right S1 nerve root sleeve.

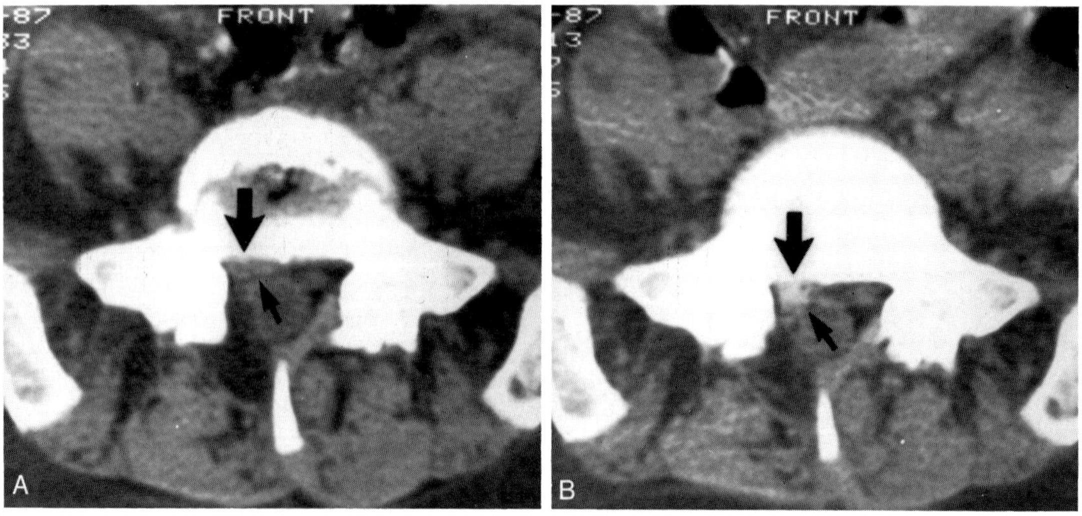

Figure 3 □ Studies from the same woman shown in Figure 2. Plain CT and CT discography studies at the same levels for comparison show enhancement of disc material (*arrows*) and differentiation from epidural scar tissue confirming the diagnosis of recurrent right L5–S1 herniated nucleus pulposus. This condition was confirmed at surgery.

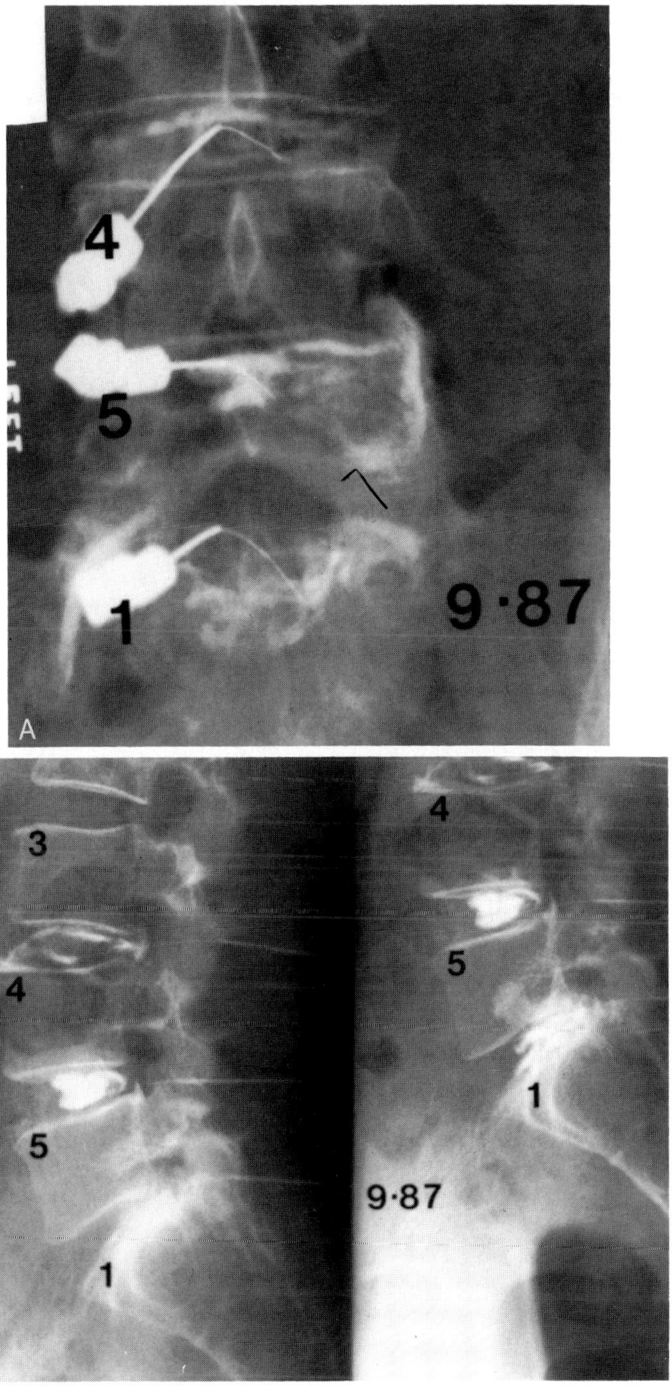

Figure 4 □ *A, B,* PA and lateral radiographs of the discograms from a 40-year-old man with unremitting right radicular leg pain show degenerative changes in all three discs. Lateral view suggests posterior disc protrusion at L3–L4. Plain CT, myelography, and CT myelography studies conducted prior to CT discography were all interpreted as negative.

The risks of any test must be weighed against the potential benefits. Although the data presented here clearly demonstrate that CT-discography is more accurate, sensitive, and specific than myelography and CT in the diagnosis of lumbar disc herniation, we recommend that less invasive studies be carried out first. CT-discography should be reserved for patients who have negative or equivocal diagnoses based on other studies. The sensitivity of CT-discography for foraminal disc herniation (97.5%) and the specificity for recurrent disc herniation (87.5%) provide further indications for the use of this test.

We have recently studied the diagnostic accuracy, sensitivity, and specificity of MRI in the diagnosis of lumbar disc herniations with results similar to those of CT, myelography, and CT-myelography reported here.[22] Further refinement and experience may soon make MRI the procedure of choice for the diagnosis of suspected lumbar herniated nucleus pulposus.

CT-discography appears to be a fairly safe and highly accurate test for the diagnosis of a lumbar disc herniation. It has both high sensitivity and specificity and the lowest false-positive and false-negative rates. More importantly, it provides a higher level of confidence and fewer equivocal results than do myelography and CT. It is recommended in selected patients with suspected lumbar disc herniations whose other tests are nondiagnostic, especially in patients with possible foraminal or recurrent disc herniations.

References

1. Aejmelaeus, R., Hiltunen, H., Harkonen, M., et al.: Myelographic versus clinical diagnostics in lumbar disc disease. Arch. Orthop. Traumat. Surg. 103:18–25, 1984.
2. Angtuaco, E. J., Holder, J. C., Boop, W. C., and Binet, E. F.: Computed tomographic discography in the evaluation of extreme lateral disc herniation. Neurosurgery 14:350–351, 1984.
3. Bell, G. R., Rothman, R. H., Booth, R. E., et al.: A study of computer-assisted tomography: A comparison of metrizamide myelography and computed tomography in the diagnosis of herniated lumbar disc and spinal stenosis. Spine 9:552–556, 1984.
4. Bosacco, S. J., Berman, A. T., Garbarino, J. L., et al.: A comparison of CT scanning and myelography in the diagnosis of lumbar disc herniation. Clin. Orthop. Rel. Res. 190:124–128, 1984.
5. Braun, I. F., Hoffman, J. C., Jr., Davis, P. C., et al.: Contrast enhancement in CT differentiation between recurrent disc herniation and postoperative scar: Prospective study. A.J.R. 45:785–790, 1985.
6. Brodsky, A. E., and Binder, W. F.: Lumbar discography: Its value in diagnosis and treatment of lumbar disc lesions. Spine 4:110–120, 1979.
7. Carrera, C., Williams, A., and Haughton, V.: Computed tomography in sciatica. Radiology 137:443–437, 1980.
8. Claussen, C., Grumme, T., and Treisch, J.: The diagnosis of lumbar disc prolapse—Computed tomographic and myelographic findings. R.O.F.O. 136:1–8, 1982.
9. Collis, J. S., Jr., and Gardner, W. J.: Lumbar discography: An analysis of one thousand cases. J. Neurosurg. 19:452–461, 1962.
10. Crock, H. V.: Practice of Spinal Surgery. New York, Springer-Verlag, 1983.
11. Demichev, N. P.: Traumatic suppurative intervertebral osteochondritis. Vestn.-Khir. 135:75–79, 1985.
12. Fraser, R. D., Osti, O. L., and Vernon-Roberts, B.: Discitis after discography. J. Bone Joint Surg. [Br.] 69:26–35, 1987.
13. Fries, J. W., Abodeely, D. A., Vijungco, J. G., et al.: Computed tomography of herniated and extruded nucleus pulposus. J. Comput. Assist. Tomogr. 6:874–887, 1982.
14. Godersky, J. C., Erickson, D. L., and Seljeskog, E. L.: Extreme lateral disc herniation: Diagnosis by computed tomographic scanning. Neurosurgery 14:549–552, 1984.
15. Gresham, J. L., and Miller, R.: Evaluation of the lumbar spine by diskography and its use in selection of proper treatment of the herniated disk syndrome. Clin. Orthop. Rel. Res. 67:29–41, 1969.
16. Gulati, A., Weinstein, R., and Studdard, E.: CT scan of the spine for herniated discs. Neuroradiology 22:57–60, 1981.
17. Haughton, V., Eldevik, O., Magnaes, B., and Amundsen, P.: A prospective comparison of computed tomography and myelography in the diagnosis of herniated lumbar discs. Radiology 142:103–110, 1982.
18. Herkowitz, H. N., Romeyn, R. L., and Rothman, R. H.: The indications for metrizamide myelography. Relationship with complications after myelography. J. Bone Joint Surg. 65A:1144–1149, 1983.
19. Jackson, R. P.: Unpublished data, 1985.
20. Jackson, R. P., and Glah, J. J.: Foraminal and extraforaminal lumbar disc herniation: diagnosis and treatment. Spine 12:577–585, 1987.
21. Jackson, R. P., Becker, G. J., Jacobs, R. R., et al.: The neuroradiographic diagnosis of lumbar herniated nucleus pulposus (I): A comparison of computed tomography (CT), myelography, CT-myelography, discography and CT-discography (submitted to Spine).
22. Jackson, R. P., Cain, J. E., Jr., Jacobs, R. R., et al.: The neuroradiographic diagnosis of lumbar herniated nucleus pulposus (II): A comparison of computed tomography (CT), myelography, CT-myelography and magnetic resonance imaging (submitted to Spine).
23. Jenkinson, D.: CT beats myelography for lumbar spine diagnoses. J. Am. Med. Assoc. 246:2112–2113, 1981.
24. Kahanovitz, N., Arnoczky, S. P., Sissons, H. A., et al.: The effect of discography on the canine intervertebral disc. Spine 11:26–27, 1986.
25. Kampmann, H., Schroedl, P., and Spranger, M.: Diagnosis of lumbar intervertebral disk prolapse by computed tomography. A comparative clinical

study between myelographic, computed tomographic, and the surgical research results with 158 patients. Rontgenblatter 38:387–391, 1985.
26. Ketonen, L., and Gyldensted, C.: Lumbar disc disease evaluated by myelography and postmyelography spinal computed tomography. Neuroradiology 28:144–149, 1986.
27. Kornberg, M.: Extreme lateral lumbar disc herniations. Spine 12:586–589, 1987.
28. Kratzer, M., and Hipp, E.: Value of myelography and computed tomography in problem cases of lumbar intervertebral disk diagnosis. Z. Orthop. 124:107–111, 1986.
29. Kurobane, Y., Takahashi, T., Tajima, T., et al.: Extraforaminal disc herniation. Spine 11:260–268, 1986.
30. Laasonen, E. M.: Iohexol and metrizamide in lumbar myelography. Comparison of side effects. Acta Radiol. Diagn. 26:761–765, 1985.
31. Massare, C.: Lumbar discography. Rontgenblatter 29:184–192, 1976.
32. Massie, W. K., and Stevens, D. B.: A critical evaluation of discography. J. Bone Joint Surg. [Am.] 49A:1243–1244, 1967.
33. Milette, P. G., and Melanson, D.: A reappraisal of lumbar discography. J. Can. Assoc. Radiol. 33:176–182, 1982.
34. McCullough, J. A., and Waddell, G.: Lateral lumbar discography. Br. J. Radiol. 51:498–502, 1978.
35. McCutcheon, M. E., and Thompson, W. C., III: CT scanning of lumbar discography. A useful diagnostic adjunct. Spine 11:257–259, 1986.
36. Motateanu, M., Fankhauser, H., Mansouri, B., and de Tribolet, N.: Extreme lateral lumbar disc herniation. Apropos of a series of 25 cases. Neurochirurgia 32:74–80, 1986.
37. Moufarrij, N., Hardy, R., and Weinstein, M.: Computed tomographic, myelographic, and operative findings in patients with suspected herniated lumbar discs. Neurosurgery 12:184–188, 1983.
38. Osborne, D. R., Heinz, E. R., Bullard, D., and Friedman, A.: Role of computed tomography in the radiological evaluation of painful radiculopathy after negative myelography: Foraminal neural entrapment. Neurosurgery 14:147–153, 1984.
39. Pasariello, R., Trecco, F., Cerone, G., et al.: Computerized axial tomography and electromyography in vertebral and spinal cord pathology. Radiol. Med. (Torino) 70:498–500, 1984.
40. Patrick, B. S.: Extreme lateral ruptures of lumbar intervertebral discs. Surg. Neurol. 3:301–304, 1975.
41. Pfadenhauer, K., Ebeling, U., Bergleiter, R., and Stoeter, P.: The reliability of computed tomography in the diagnosis of recurrent symptoms after lumbar disc operations. R.O.F.O. 139:127–131, 1983.
42. Piepgras, U., Kammerer, V., and Huber, G.: Comparison between myelography and discography for lumbar prolapsed intervertebral discs. Rontgenblatter 29:193–200, 1976.
43. Raskin, S., and Keating, J.: Recognition of lumbar disc disease: Comparison of myelography and computed tomography. Am. J. Neuroradiol. 3:215–221, 1982.
44. Recoules, D., Baron, J. J., Gayet, A., and Pouchat, J. M.: Lumbar disc hernia through the intervertebral foramen. Apropos of 37 surgically treated hernia. Neurochirurgia 30:301–307, 1984.
45. Sachs, B. L., Vanharanta, H., Spicey, M. A., et al.: Dallas discogram description. A new classification of CT/discography in low back disorders. Spine 12:287–294, 1987.
46. Sachsenheimer, W., Hamer, J., and Muller, H.: The value of spinal computed tomography in diagnosis of herniated lumbar discs. Acta Neurochir. 60:107–114, 1982.
47. Simmons, E. H., and Segil, C. M.: An evaluation of discography in the localization of symptomatic levels in discogenic disease of the spine. Clin. Orthop. Rel. Res. 108:57–69, 1975.
48. Stoeter, P., Schneider, I., Bergleiter, R., and Ebeling, U.: Diagnostic importance of CT examination of the lumbosacral region of patients with lumbo-sciatica. R.O.F.O. 136:515–524, 1982.
49. Tchang, S., Howie, J., Kirkaldy-Willis, W., et al.: Computed tomography versus myelography in diagnosis of lumbar disc herniation. J. Can. Assoc. Radiol. 33:15–20, 1982.
50. Troisier, G., and Cypel, D.: Discography: An element of decision. Surgery versus chemonucleolysis. Clin. Orthop. Rel. Res. 206:70–78, 1986.
51. Vanharanta, H., Sachs, B. L., Spivey, M. A., et al.: The relationship of pain provocation to lumbar disc deterioration as seen by CT/discography. Spine 12:295–298, 1987.
52. Videman, T., Malamivaara, A., and Mooney, V.: The value of the axial view in assessing discograms. An experimental study with cadavers. Spine 12:299–304, 1987.
53. Williams, A., Haughton, V., and Syvertsen, A.: Computed tomography in the diagnosis of herniated nucleus pulposus. Radiol. Med. (Torino) 135:95–99, 1980.
54. Wiltse, L., Widell, E. H., Jr., and Yuan, H. A.: Chymopapain chemonucleolysis in lumbar disc disease. J.A.M.A. 231:474–479, 1975.
55. Witwer, G., Cacayorin, E. D., Bernstein, A. D., et al.: Iopamidol and metrizamide for myelography: Prospective double-blind clinical trial. A.J.R. 143:869–873, 1984.

7 □ Clinical Entities

Sam W. Wiesel
Henry L. Feffer
Richard H. Rothman
Steven R. Garfin
Harry N. Herkowitz
Henrik Weber
John A. McCullough
Shun-ichi Inoue
Hideshige Moriya
Kazuhisa Takahashi
Keiichi Takata
Vert Mooney
Mark D. Brown
Bradford L. Currier
Thomas W. McNeill
David K. Selby

A LUMBAR SPINE ALGORITHM

Sam W. Wiesel
Henry L. Feffer
Richard H. Rothman

Patients who have low back pain present with a set of symptoms that are not labeled with a specific diagnosis. The task confronting the examining physician is to integrate their symptoms, physical findings, and diagnostic test results into a logical diagnosis and then to develop a treatment plan. The physician's capacity to achieve this goal is determined by the accuracy of his or her thought processes. To standardize and organize decision-making, a systematized approach to patients presenting with low back pain has been developed.

The plan is presented in the form of an algorithm, which Webster's dictionary defines as "a set of rules for solving a particular problem within a finite number of steps." In this case the problem is the universe of low back pain patients, and the rules are derived from a large body of existing information. The algorithm can be followed in sequence (Fig. 1); it can also be presented in tabular form (Table 1).

EVALUATION GOALS

The algorithm was developed with four major goals in mind. The first and most important is the early return of patients to their normal activities. Unfortunately, complete relief of pain is not always achieved. Patients with residual pain must be encouraged to return to as much activity as possible. Patient education is germane to this goal. Many people refrain from work, recreation, or household chores simply because increasing their activity produces mild discomfort. In their minds, pain is a signal that they are causing damage to their backs. These patients need to be reassured that the diagnosis of lumbar disc disease does not herald the onset of a progressive crippling disorder and that disc degeneration is a normal pattern of aging. In many cases this information will keep patients functioning and prevent psychologic impairment as well.

The second goal is to avoid unnecessary surgery. Surgical intervention has definite indications that must be adhered to. There is no excuse, today, for exploratory surgery in the lumbar spine. The sorrowful saga of the thousands of patients who have undergone multiple spine operations with poor results bears witness to the disastrous overuse of spine surgery in the past. As evidence, one need only look at the review published

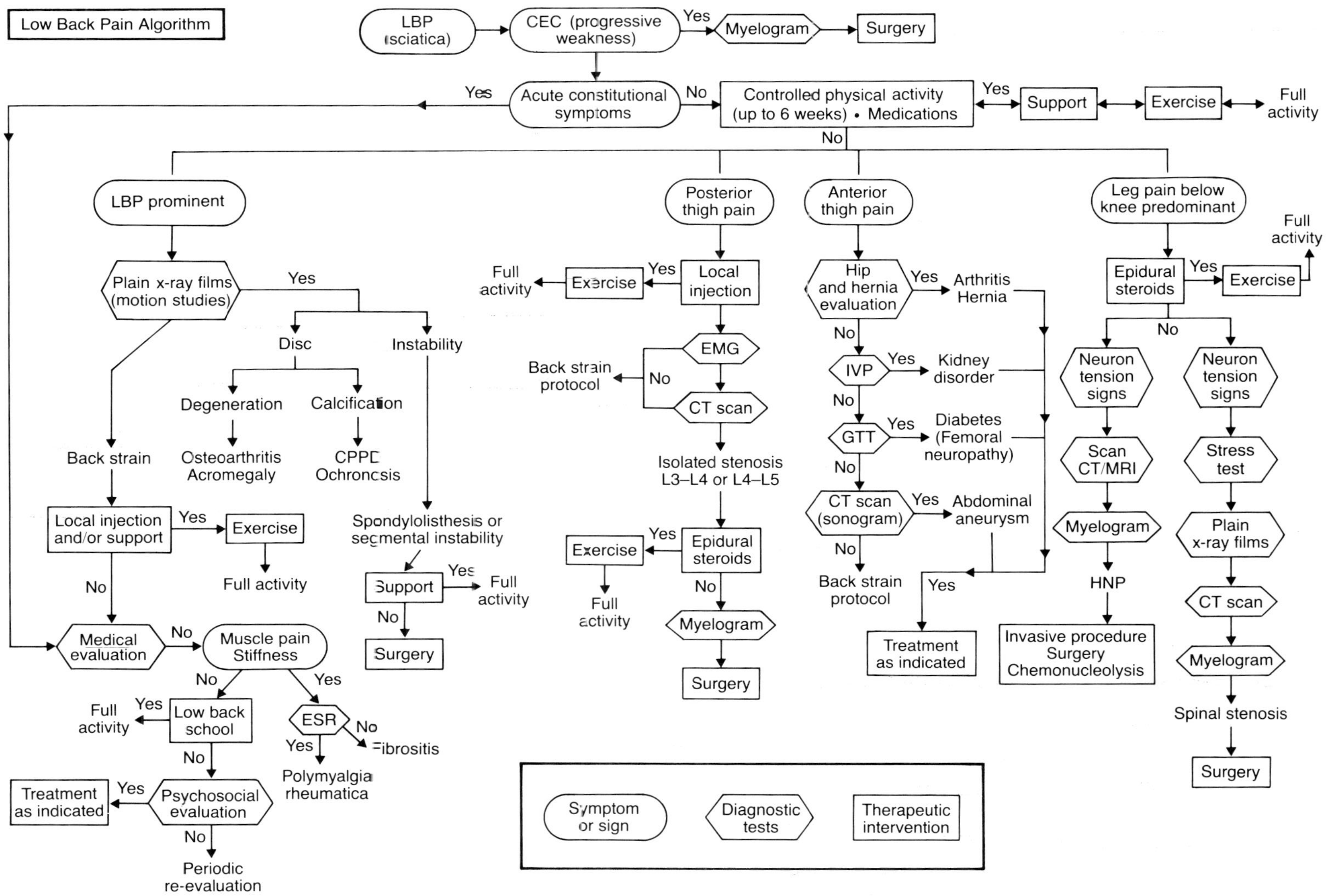

Figure 1 □ This diagram shows an algorithm for treatment of patients with low back pain. It is presented in a sequential form.

Table 1 □ Differential Diagnosis of Low Back Pain

EVALUATION	BACK STRAIN	HNP	SPINAL STENOSIS	SPONDYLO-LISTHESIS/ INSTABILITY	TUMOR	SPONDYLO-ARTHROPATHY	METABOLIC	INFECTION
Predominant pain (leg versus back)	Back	Leg	Leg	Back	Back	Back	Back	Back
Constitutional symptoms					+	+		+
Tension sign		+						
Neurologic examination		+	+ after stress					
Plain x-ray studies			+	+	±	+	+	±
Lateral motion x-ray studies				+				
CT scan		+	+		+			+
Myelogram		+	+					
Bone scan					+	+	+	+
ESR					+	+		+
Ca/P/alk phos					+		+	

by Aitken and Bradford in 1947.[1] They investigated 170 surgical cases from the files of a large national compensation carrier and found that only 17% of the patients had good results; 45% were judged as poor or bad results. Discs were removed at levels that did not correlate with the neurologic examination or myelogram findings, and complications such as postoperative foot drop or paralysis of the quadriceps muscles occurred in 5% of the group.

Fortunately, with adherence to strict criteria, the results of spine surgery have become much better. In a recent review of 800 patients selected for lumbar spine surgery using the algorithmic indications for surgery, 90% to 95% had good results.[8] It cannot be overemphasized that objective criteria for surgery must be present.

Conversely, when conservative management has failed and the patient demonstrates a pathologic condition that lends itself to surgical treatment, the operation should not be unduly delayed. Surgery to relieve a ruptured disc becomes less effective when it is delayed for more than 3 months. The optimal time for surgical intervention must be clearly defined and understood.[15]

The third goal is the efficient and precise use of diagnostic studies. With the availability of computed tomography (CT), magnetic resonance imaging (MRI), psychologic profiles, and specialty consultants—each with a particular battery of tests—the physician must resist the impulse to use every test available and to acquiesce to the patient's often insistent demands for "the latest study." There is a proper time and indication for each of these diagnostic measures. Decision-making can actually be more difficult and less beneficial when too many data are made available too early in the treatment process.

The final objective should be to devise a treatment format that will make therapy available at an acceptable cost to society. When a disease has the enormous economic impact that low back pain does, it is vital that the individual and society are able to afford the diagnostic tests and treatment. In this day of the $600 body scan and the $6,000 surgical procedure, one must take care to avoid unnecessary and cost-ineffective measures.

PATIENT EVALUATION

The information necessary to use the algorithm is initially obtained through the history and physical examination. The aim of the history is to allow the physician to develop a precise subjective assessment of the patient's pain syndrome. It is particularly important to differentiate mechanical back pain from nonmechanical pain that is present at rest. Locating the pain; determining whether it is sharp, dull, aching, burning, or dysesthetic; and ascertaining whether there are exacerbating or ameliorating events are some of the variables that help to define the cause of the pain.

One must also question patients about their general health and obtain a thorough systems review. It is particularly important to find out whether the patient has noticed any change in bowel or bladder habits and/or experienced constitutional symptoms such as fever, chills, or weight loss. Many systemic illnesses may present as low back pain.

The physical examination is oriented toward gathering objective data about the patient's condition. The attitude of the back, areas of tenderness, neurologic findings, and tension signs are the significant items of information. Routinely, one should examine the patient's abdomen, check the hips, and palpate for peripheral pulses. If there is any suggestion of other medical problems, the appropriate examination should also be performed.

Finally, in the process of taking the history and performing the physical examination, one should observe the patient to detect any nonorganic signs. Waddell's standardized group of tests has proven helpful in uncovering psychosocial problems contributing to patient symptoms.[14] One must appreciate that underlying psychosocial disorders can aggravate and/or actually present as low back pain.

THE ALGORITHM

The aim of the algorithm is to select the correct diagnostic category and proper treatment avenues for each patient with low back pain. Good decision-making depends on the physician having a thorough knowledge of the pathophysiology of the disorders involved. A specific patient may fall outside the limits of the algorithm and require a different approach. The algorithm is only an aid in stratifying these patients, and the physician must constantly be on the alert for exceptions.

Cauda Equina Compression Syndrome

When presented with the broad range of patients with low back pain, the physician must initially make a ruling on the presence or absence of cauda equina compression (CEC) syndrome.[6] Mechanical compression of the cauda equina is the only surgical emergency in lumbar spine disease. This usually is the result of pressure on the caudal sac, through which the nerves pass to the lower extremities, bowel, and bladder. The signs and symptoms are a complex mixture of low back pain, bilateral motor weakness of the lower extremities, bilateral sciatica, saddle anesthesia, and even frank paraplegia with bowel and bladder incontinence. Major progressive motor weakness should also cause suspicion. CEC can be caused by either bone or soft tissue damage, the latter generally a ruptured or herniated disc in the midline.

Once this diagnosis is suspected, the patient should immediately undergo myelography and, if the results are positive, emergency surgical decompression. The major need for prompt surgical intervention is to arrest the progression of neurologic loss; the chance of an actual return of neurologic function after operation is slight. Although the incidence of CEC syndrome in the total population of low back pain patients is very low, it is the one entity that requires immediate attention; if its diagnosis is missed, the consequences can be disastrous.

Conservative Care

The remaining patients constitute the overwhelming majority. They should be started on a course of conservative (nonoperative) therapy, regardless of the diagnosis. At this stage, the specific diagnosis, regardless of whether it is a herniated disc or a simple back strain, is not important to the therapy because the entire population is treated the same way. A few of these patients eventually will need an invasive procedure (surgery), but at this point there is no way to predict which individuals will respond to conservative therapy and which ones will not.

The early treatment of low back pain is a waiting game. The passage of time, the judicious use of medication, and controlled physical activity are the modalities that have proved safest and most effective. Most patients respond to this approach. Because of today's emphasis on quick solutions and high technology, many patients are pushed toward more complex (i.e., more invasive) treatment. This "quick fix" has no place in the treatment of patients with low back pain. In most cases, surgical treatment does not return the patient to heavy work, and in the long run the best chance of getting a patient back to full activity is the nonoperative approach.

Rest (Controlled Physical Activity)

Over the years, rest has evolved as one of the most important elements in the treatment of low back pain. The purpose of rest is to allow injured tissue to heal. The relief may or may not be permanent. The amount of rest prescribed varies for each patient.

When patients first present with acute symptoms, they may require a short period of total bed rest (i.e., 2 to 7 days).[5, 19] As their discomfort eases, they should be strongly encouraged to take short walks but to do as little sitting as possible. As time passes, each patient's physical activity is tailored to increase movement without incurring a return of symptoms. Complete bed rest for long periods (more than 2 weeks) has a deleterious effect on the body in general and should be closely monitored. Thus, the physician must strictly control the patient's physical activity during the course of treatment.

Drug Therapy

The judicious use of medication is an important adjunct to the treatment of low back pain. Anti-inflammatories, analgesics, and muscle relaxants are the three main categories of drugs commonly used.

Anti-inflammatory agents are employed because of the belief that inflammation within the affected tissues may be a major cause of pain in the low back. This is certainly true for patients whose symptoms are secondary to a herniated disc. The leg pain these people experience is a result not only of mechanical pressure from the ruptured disc but also of the inflammation around the involved nerve roots. If the inflammation can be dispelled, the patient's pain usually subsides.[11]

A variety of anti-inflammatory agents are available. Based on several scientific studies, none appears to be superior to the others. The patient should be started on adequate doses of aspirin, which is both effective and inexpensive. If the response is not satisfactory, other anti-inflammatory agents such as naproxen, ibuprofen, or indomethacin can be tried. Any of these medications should be used in conjunction with controlled physical activity to relieve pain; drugs do not replace adequate rest. In some cases, after initial recovery patients experience intermittent recurrent attacks or complain of chronic symptoms; in some instances these people are relieved by a maintenance dose of an anti-inflammatory drug.

Analgesic medication must be prescribed with great care for the patient with low back pain. The treating physician should maintain control of the patient's drug intake at all times; there are too many instances of patients taking undue advantage of the situation. Finally, addicting narcotics have no place in the treatment regimen of patients with chronic low back problems.

Muscle relaxants are generally not recommended for treatment of low back pain. In most cases, muscle spasm is secondary to a primary problem such as a herniated disc. If the pain from the ruptured disc can be controlled, the muscle spasm subsides. Occasionally, the muscle spasm is so severe that some type of treatment is required; methocarbamol and carisoprodol are the recommended drugs. The use of diazepam should be discouraged because it is actually a physiologic depressant, and depression often is an integral feature of back pain syndromes. Administering diazepam to depressed patients only increases their problems. If anxiety is prominent and a sedative is needed, phenobarbital will alleviate the symptoms.

In summary, drug therapy should be viewed as an adjunct to adequately controlled physical activity. Anti-inflammatory medication should be the primary agent employed. Analgesics should be used selectively in a controlled environment and should not be used for extended periods. Muscle relaxants generally are not recommended and, if prescribed, should be carefully monitored.

Braces and Corsets

Once patients have achieved approximately 80% relief, they should be mobilized with the help of a lightweight, flexible corset. External support with a corset or brace is needed only briefly during the average patient's recovery period. As the acute symptoms subside, a properly fitted corset helps the patient regain mobility more quickly. With continued long-term use of a brace, however, soft tissue contractures and muscle atrophy will occur. The young patient should rely on a brace only to hasten ambulation. Theory holds that the strong, flexible lumbar and abdominal muscles function as an excellent "internal brace" because they are adjacent to the structure they are supporting—the vertebral column.

There are two situations in which long-term bracing is reasonable. For the obese patient with weak abdominal muscles, a firm corset with flexible metal stays reinforces the abdominal muscles. It has been shown that if a lumbosacral corset is properly applied, intradiscal pressure in the lumbar area decreases by approximately 30%.[10]

The aging patient with multilevel degenerative disease of the lumbar spine is the second type who may benefit from long-term bracing. These older people do not tolerate exercise very well, and exercise may aggravate their back conditions. A well fitted brace may provide significant relief of pain.

Exercise

As patients increase their activity level, they should begin a program of exercise. Some form of exercise probably is the most commonly prescribed therapy for patients recovering from low back pain. Two regimens are commonly advocated: isometric flexion exercises and hyperextension exercises. Both programs are purported to reduce the frequency and intensity of low back pain episodes, although there is no scientific evidence to support this contention.

The isometric flexion exercises are the most popular ones. These are based on Williams' theory that by reducing the lumbar lordosis, back pain is decreased. This goal is achieved by strengthening both abdominal and lumbar muscles, thus creating a "corset of muscles" to support the lumbar spine.

Hyperextension exercises strengthen the paravertebral muscles. These exercises generally are begun after a patient has satisfactorily completed a course of isometric flexion exercise. The strengthened paravertebrals can then be used as internal support for the lumbar spine. It should be stressed that there is no objective proof that exercises reduce the recovery time or the frequency of recurrences. Empirically, they appear to have a positive psychologic effect and allow patients to take an active part in their own treatment programs.

The pathway along this section of the algorithm is a two-way street; if regression and exacerbation of symptoms occur, the physician can resort to more stringent conservative measures. Most acute low back pain patients will proceed along this pathway, returning to their normal life patterns within 6 weeks of the onset of symptoms.

Back Pain Versus Leg Pain

If the initial conservative treatment regimen fails after 6 weeks, symptomatic patients are sorted into four groups. The first consists of people in whom low back pain predominates. The second group complain mainly of leg pain, defined as pain radiating below the knee (commonly referred to as sciatica). The third group have posterior thigh pain. The fourth group have anterior thigh pain. Each group follows a separate diagnostic path.

Low Back Pain

In patients who have predominantly low back pain and persistent symptoms after 6 weeks of conservative care, the plain x-rays should be carefully examined for abnormalities. Spondylolysis—with or without spondylolisthesis—is the most common structural cause of significant low back pain. Approximately 5% of the population has this defect, which is thought to be caused by a combination of genetics and mechanical stress.[11] In spite of it, most of the patients are able to perform activities of daily living with little or no discomfort. When symptoms are present, they usually respond to nonoperative measures, including a thorough explanation of the problem, a back support, and exercises. In a small percentage of patients, symptoms persist and conservative treatment fails; in these cases, a fusion of the involved spinal segments becomes necessary. This is one of the few situations in which primary fusion of the lumbar spine is indicated.

Weight-bearing, lateral flexion–extension x-ray films should be scrutinized for evidence of instability. Predicating a need for fusion on the basis of these findings is surrounded by ambiguity. Each region of the vertebral column has an upper limit of what may be considered normal angulation and/or translational motion.[16] In a normal state, a small amount of angulation occurs but with very little translational movement. With degenerative disc disease, the angulatory and translational motion changes in flexion and extension can be considerable, creating pronounced sheering forces parallel to the plane of the disc as well as abnormal tensile stresses at the points of ligamentous attachment. This process has been termed "segmental instability."

Unfortunately, little information is available to explain why some patients with segmental instability develop back pain and others do not. In contrast to our ability precisely to define nerve root compression, it is nearly impossible to so define the anatomic origin of back pain in the presence of roentgenographic instability. The guidelines currently being followed were developed by White and associates. Relative flexion–sagittal plane translation of more than 12% of the anteroposterior diameter of the vertebral body, or a relative flexion–sagittal plane rotation of more than 11 degrees, is accepted as evidence of instability in the lumbar spine.[16] At the lumbosacral junction, the criteria are slightly different: relative flexion–sagittal plane translation of more than 25% or extension–sagittal plane rotation of more than 19 degrees is significant.

If these roentgenographic stigmas of instability are present on weight-bearing lateral flexion–extension views of the lumbosacral spine, spinal fusion may be considered. The surgeon and patient must both realize that the rate for good or excellent results from a fusion of back pain is 75% at best.[4] Further confirmatory evidence to determine the precise level of origin of the patient's symptoms may be gathered from facet injections and discography; unfortunately, these tests have a high rate of false-positive results.

Actually, most patients with evidence of instability are *not* operated on; they improve with conservative measures, their symptoms are found to have nonorthopedic causes, or they have a psychosocial disturbance. More scientific work must be carried out to better define the exact indications for spine fusions for low back pain. It should be emphasized that the results are unpredictable and that fusion should be undertaken only as a last step in treatment of the well-motivated and fully informed patient.

The vast majority of patients with low back pain predominating have normal plain x-ray findings. Their diagnosis is back strain. Before an additional work-up is done, a local injection of steroids and lidocaine (Xylocaine) may be used at the point of maximum tenderness. This can be quite successful, and, if the response is good, the patient may be started on exercises with a gradual resumption of normal activities. In some patients, if objective findings are absent, a trigger-point injection may be considered as early as the third week after onset of symptoms.

If the patient does not respond to a local injection, other pathologic conditions must be seriously considered. A technetium diphosphorate bone scan, along with a general medical evaluation, should be obtained. The bone scan is an excellent tool, often identifying early bone tumors or infections that are not visible on routine radiographs. It is particularly important to obtain this study in the patient with nonmechanical back pain. If the pain is constant, unremitting, and unrelieved by postural adjustments, more often than not the correct diagnosis will be of an occult neoplasm or metabolic disorder not readily apparent from other testing.

A thorough medical search also frequently reveals problems missed earlier such as a posterior penetrating ulcer, pancreatitis, renal disease, or an abdominal aneurysm. The medical evaluation often is directed by an internist, rheumatologist, or neurologist, depending on the patient's particular symptom complex. Approximately 3% of cases of apparent low back pain that present at orthopedic clinics are attributable to extraspinal causes.[18] Before referring these cases to a consultant, several laboratory tests should be performed. An erythrocyte sedimentation rate is a quick and inexpensive assay with a reported sensitivity of 59% in detecting occult pathologic disorders such as infection, tumor, and many of the systemic arthritides.

In the older patient, laboratory investigation routinely includes tests for serum protein electrophoresis, alkaline phosphatase, calcium, complete blood count with differential, antinuclear antibody titer, routine urinalysis, and acid phosphatase. In the younger patient with decreased lumbar flexion or x-ray evidence of sacroiliac disorders, histocompatibility testing (HLA-B27) is obtained to check for ankylosing spondylitis. If any of these studies is positive, the patient should be transferred into a nonorthopedic treatment program.

BACK SCHOOL

If the patient is not found to have any medical abnormality, he or she is referred to the low back school. It is believed that many of these patients are suffering from discogenic pain or facet joint pain syndrome. In most cases, with the passage of time, reassurance, and an exercise program under the guidance of the low back school educators, the patient will gradually improve.

The concept of a back school was originated in 1970 by Zachrissen in Sweden.[20] The concept is that patients who understand the anatomic, epidemiologic, and biomechanical factors that give rise to low back pain can handle their own problems better than those without that knowledge. An audiovisual approach was developed, through which the patient first is introduced to the goals of the program. Then, the basic anatomy and physiology of various back disorders are presented in a classroom setting so that the patients realize their problem is not unique. The patients are taught proper biomechanics of the spine and how to apply these to their daily activities so as to reduce the forces applied to the spine. Finally, an exercise program is outlined for each patient. This multifaceted approach has been quite successful.

The program outlined above has had many variations. Some back school programs are complex and costly, involving as many as 15 hours of classroom time. The authors believe that the simpler the program, the more readily the patient will accept it. There is no proof that back school can prevent or even decrease the incidence of low back pain; its aim is to provide the patients with a basic understanding of the problem so that they will not be afraid of hurting their backs in everyday situations.

PSYCHOSOCIAL EVALUATION

If the low back school is not successful, the patient should undergo a thorough psychosocial evaluation in an effort to explain the failure of the previous courses of treatment.[14] This assessment is predicated on the belief that a patient's disability is related not only to the pathologic anatomy but also to the individual's perception of pain and his or her stability in relation to the social environment. It is quite common to see a patient with a frank herniated disc continue working—regarding the disability as only a minor problem—while a hysterical patient takes to bed at the slightest twinge of low back discomfort.

Psychologically distressed patients often complain of symptoms that are vague, poorly localized, and lack a normal relationship to time, physical activity, and anatomy. The seven symptoms that have the highest degree of association with this category are tailbone pain, whole-leg pain, whole-leg numbness, whole-leg giving way, absence of pain-free intervals, intolerance of or inappropriate reaction to treatment, and a past history of emergency admission to the hospital for low back pain.

Drug habituation, depression, and alcoholism are frequently found in association with back pain. If the evaluation suggests any of these problems, proper measures should be instituted to overcome the disability. A surprising number of ambulatory patients are addicted to commonly prescribed medications, using complaints of back pain as an excuse to obtain these drugs. Oxycodone hydrochloride (Percodan) and diazepam (Valium), alone or in combination, are two of the most popular offenders. Oxycodone hydrochloride is truly addictive. Diazepam is both habituating and depressing. Since the complaint of low back pain may be a common manifestation of depression, prescribing these drugs is counterproductive.

PERSISTENT PAIN WITHOUT PSYCHOSOCIAL ABNORMALITY

Approximately 2% of patients who initially present with low back pain will fail treatment and elude any diagnosis.[18] There will be no evidence of any structural problem in the back or criteria for underlying medical disease or psychiatric disorder. This is a very difficult group to manage.

The authors' strategy has been to discontinue narcotics, provide reassurance, and periodically re-evaluate the patient. Over time, one third of these patients will be found to have an underlying medical disease; thus, one cannot abandon this group and discontinue treatment. The remaining two-thirds should be encouraged to engage in as much physical activity as possible.

Sciatica

The next group consists of patients with sciatica—pain radiating below the knee. For these people, symptoms are usually secondary to mechanical pressure and inflammation of the nerve roots originating in the back and extending down the leg. The cause of the mechanical pressure may be soft tissue (herniated disc) or bone, or a combination of the two.

At this point in the algorithm, the patient has had up to 6 weeks of controlled physical activity and medication but still has symptoms. The next therapeutic step is an epidural steroid injection performed on an outpatient basis. The theory is that anti-inflammatory medication (steroids) directed into the epidural space will be more effective than oral medication in reducing inflammation. However, a recent double-blind study showed that steroids plus procaine (Novocain) worked no better than procaine alone to relieve symptoms.[2] In both study groups, 40% of the population had a significant decrease in symptoms. Nevertheless, an epidural injection is worth trying: the chance of success is 40% and morbidity is low, particularly compared with either of the next treatment steps—chemonucleolytic injection or surgery.

If the infection is effective in alleviating the patient's leg pain, a program of exercises is begun, with the patient encouraged to return to a lifestyle as normal as is possible. In most cases, heavy work (i.e., lifting more than 25 kg repetitively) is not recommended, since these patients will be prone to recurrences. This treatment regimen usually is complete in less than 3 months. Most patients with an acute radiculopathy will respond and need not undergo any major invasive treatment.

If the epidural injections prove ineffective, more potent invasive treatment should be considered. The physician now must carefully re-evaluate the patient for a neurologic deficit and a positive tension sign; either finding (along with continued leg pain) warrants obtaining a metrizamide myelogram. If the myelogram is clearly positive, an invasive procedure is a viable option. Computed tomography (CT) and magnetic resonance imaging (MRI) both can be helpful in this situation. If the neurologic examination and tension sign are positive and consistent with the findings on either the CT scan or the MR image, myelography need not be performed because it is invasive. If there is any question about the findings, one should proceed with the myelogram. If all criteria are present and an invasive procedure is indicated, the physician must choose between chemonucleolysis and standard surgical removal of the herniated disc.

Chemonucleolysis

Chemonucleolysis is the injection of a substance into the nucleus pulposus to dissolve it and thus relieve the pressure on the neural elements. For this process, which has been used for several years, two types of drugs are currently available: chymopapain and collagenase. Each dissolves a different material within the nucleus pulposus. Chymopapain dissolves the proteoglycans, whereas collagenase works on the collagen. The technique has been refined, and currently the procedure is performed under local anesthesia without discography. Skin testing for allergy should be performed. The indications for chemonucleolysis are the same as those for surgery; this procedure should not be carried out by anyone who does not perform routine spine surgery such as laminectomy for a herniated disc. Chemonucleolysis is not indicated when a bony lesion is present or in the patient who has undergone multiple spine operations.

The results of chemonucleolysis have been controversial. Surgical treatment for an acute soft herniated disc provides good to excellent results in 90% to 95% of patients.[8] In a recent prospective double-blind study, 77% of patients treated with chymopapain were assessed as moderately improved, compared with 47% of saline-treated patients.[7] Chymopapain yields better results than a placebo but poorer results than surgery. The exact indications for chemonucleolysis are not clear, and questions about its safety remain. Its role will not be determined until more surgeons gain experience in its use.

There is no question that use of chemonucleolysis should be approached with the same seriousness as surgery. The complications can be grave (i.e., paralysis and death), and the technique is challenging. One of the more serious errors is failure to meet the strict criteria for its use, which are leg pain, a positive tension sign or neurologic deficit, and a positive contrast study. In other words, indications for the use of chemonucleolysis should be the same as those for a major surgical procedure.

Surgery

Surgery has proved to be safe and efficient in treating patients who have herniated discs and have failed to respond to conservative therapy. The indications are the complaint of leg pain, a positive tension sign and/or neurologic deficit, and a positive contrast study. There is repeated documentation that for surgery to be effective in treatment of a herniated disc, the surgeon must find unequivocal operative evidence of a nerve root compression. Mechanical nerve root compression must be firmly substantiated, not only by neurologic examination but by radiographic data, before a laminectomy. There is no place for "exploratory" back surgery. If the patient has neither a neurologic deficit nor a positive straight leg raising test, then regardless of the radiographic findings, the evidence of nerve root compression is not sufficient to warrant surgery. Twenty-five per cent of asymptomatic patients have positive myelograms;[9] 35% have positive CT scans.[17] Patients without objective physical findings have poor results from surgery. Those who meet the criteria for lumbar laminectomy will have a satisfactory outcome; 95% can expect good to excellent results.

The second group of patients whose symptoms are based on mechanical pressure on the neural elements are those with spinal stenosis.[12] This is a narrowing of the spinal canal secondary to increased bone formation and degeneration, which is a natural occurrence with aging. However, if the spinal canal is small to begin with and continues to decrease, pressure develops on the nerve and may cause radiation of pain into the leg. These patients may or may not have a positive neurologic examination or straight-leg raising test. If they are ambulated until their symptoms can be reproduced, this "stress test" can cause the initially negative neurologic and tension signs to become positive.[3] Patients over sixty years of age are those most affected by spinal stenosis.

The diagnosis of spinal stenosis can usually be made from the plain x-ray films, which will demonstrate facet degeneration, disc degeneration, and decreased interpedicular and sagittal canal diameters. A CT scan or myelogram will more clearly define the involved areas. If symptoms are severe and spinal stenosis is radiographically evident, surgery is appropriate. Chemonucleolysis is not indicated because the chemicals do not dissolve the bone that is the major offending agent in stenosis. Age alone is no deterrent to surgery; many elderly people who are in good health, except for a narrow spinal canal, benefit greatly from adequate decompression of the lumbar spine.

Anterior Thigh Pain

A small percentage of patients have pain that radiates from the back into the anterior thigh. This usually is relieved by rest and anti-inflammatory medication. If the discomfort persists after 6 weeks of treatment, a work-up should be initiated to search for underlying pathologic conditions. Several entities must be considered.

A hip problem or a hernia can be ruled out with a thorough physical examination. If the hip examination is positive, x-ray studies should be obtained. An intravenous pyelogram (IVP) is useful to evaluate the urinary tract, because kidney stones often may present as anterior thigh pain. Peripheral neuropathy, most commonly secondary to diabetes, also can present with anterior thigh pain; a glucose tolerance test, as well as an electromyogram (EMG), will reveal this underlying problem.

Finally, a retroperitoneal tumor can cause symptoms by mechanically pressing on the nerves that innervate the anterior thigh. A CT scan or MR image of the retroperitoneal area will eliminate or confirm this possibility.

If any of the entities reviewed above is revealed, the patient is treated accordingly. If no physical cause can be found for the anterior thigh pain, the patient is treated for recalcitrant back strain by the method already outlined.

Posterior Thigh Pain

This final group of patients will complain of back pain with radiation into the buttocks and posterior thigh.[11] Most will feel relief of symptoms with 6 weeks of conservative therapy. However, those whose pain persists after that period should be considered to have back strain and given a trigger-point injection of steroids and lidocaine. If the injection is unsuccessful, it is necessary to distinguish between referred and radicular pain.

Referred pain is pain in mesodermal tissues of the same embryologic origin. The muscles, tendons, and ligaments of the buttocks and posterior thighs have the same embryologic origin as those of the low back. When the low back is injured, pain may be referred to the posterior thigh, where it is perceived by the patient. Referred pain cannot be cured with a surgical procedure.

Radicular pain is caused by compression of an inflamed nerve root along the anatomic course of the nerve. A herniated disc or spinal stenosis in the high lumbar area (L2–L3 or L3–L4 interspace) can cause radiation of pain into the posterior thigh. An MR and/or CT scan may be used in this situation. If the studies are within normal limits, the patient is considered to have back strain and treated according to the algorithm. If an abnormality is found, the patient is diagnosed as having mechanical pressure on the neural elements, either from a herniated disc or spinal stenosis. Epidural steroids should be tried first; if these do not provide adequate relief, surgery should be contemplated.

This group of patients is very difficult to treat. The biggest mistake occurs when surgery is performed on people thought to have radicular pain who actually have referred pain. Again, referred pain is not responsive to surgery.

SUMMARY

In most instances, the treatment of low back pain is no longer a mystery. The algorithm presents a series of easy-to-follow and clearly defined decision-making processes. Use of this algorithm provides patients with the most helpful diagnostic and therapeutic measures at the optimal time. It neither denies them beneficial surgery nor subjects them to procedures that are useless technical exercises.

The algorithm is an overview of a multitude of subjects that includes diagnostic tests and therapeutic entities. The ensuing chapters discuss each step on the pathway in detail. It should be pointed out that the algorithm itself is merely a frame into which new knowledge can be fitted to keep the physician abreast of the most effective methods of diagnosing and treating low back pain.

References

1. Aitken, A. P., and Bradford, C. H.: End results of ruptured intervertebral discs in industry. Am. J. Surg. 73:365, 1947.
2. Cuckler, J. M., Bernini, P. A., Wiesel, S. W., et al.: A prospective, randomized, double-blind study of the use of epidural steroids in the treatment of lumbar radicular pain. J. Bone Joint Surg. 67A:63, 1985.
3. DePalma, A., and Rothman, R. H.: The Intervertebral Disc. Philadelphia, W. B. Saunders, 1970.
4. DePalma, A., and Rothman, R. H.: Surgery of the lumbar spine. Clin. Orthop. 63:162–170, 1969.
5. Deyo, R. A.: Conservative therapy for low back pain: Distinguishing useful from useless therapy. J.A.M.A. 250:1057, 1983.
6. Floman, Y., Wiesel, S. W., and Rothman, R. H.: Cauda equina presenting as a herniated lumbar disk. Clin. Orthop. 147:234–237, 1980.
7. Fraser, R. D.: Chymopapain for the treatment of intervertebral disc herniation: The final report of a double-blind study. Spine 9:815–818, 1984.
8. Garfin, S. K., Booth, R. E., Simeone, F. A., and Rothman, R. H.: Results of Surgical Decompression for Lumbar Nerve Root Compression. Presented to the Spine Study Group, Mar., 1986.
9. Hitselberger, W. E., and Witten, R. M.: Abnormal myelograms in asymptomatic patients. J. Neurosurg. 28:204–206, 1968.
10. Nachemson, A., and Morris, J. M.: In vivo measurements of intradiscal pressure: Discometry, a method for determination of pressure in the lower lumbar disc. J. Bone Joint Surg. 46A:1077, 1964.
11. Rothman, R. H., and Simeone, F. A.: The Spine, 2nd Ed. Philadelphia, W. B. Saunders, 1982.
12. Verbiest, H.: Results of surgical treatment of idiopathic developmental stenosis of the lumbar vertebral canal: A review of twenty-seven years' experience. J. Bone Joint Surg. 59B:181, 1977.
13. Waddell, G., Main, C., Morris, E., et al.: Chronic low-back pain, psychologic distress, and illness behavior. Spine 9:209, 1984.
14. Waddell, G., McCulloch, J. A., Kummel, E., and Venner, R. M.: Nonorganic physical signs in low back pain. Spine 5:117, 1980.
15. Weber, H.: Lumbar disc herniation: A controlled, prospective study with ten years of observation. Spine 8:131, 1983.
16. White, A. A., Panjabi, M. M., Posner, I., et al.: Spinal stability: Evaluation and treatment. *In* The American Academy of Orthopaedic Surgeons: Instructional Course Lectures XXX. St. Louis, C. V. Mosby, 1981, p. 457.
17. Wiesel, S. W., Bell, G. R., Feffer, H. L., et al.: A study of computer assisted tomography: Part I. The incidence of positive CAT scans in an asymptomatic group of patients. Spine 9:549, 1984.
18. Wiesel, S. W., and Borenstein, D.: Back pain of unknown etiology. Presented at The American Academy of Orthopaedic Surgeons' annual meeting, New Orleans, 1985.
19. Wiesel, S. W., Cuckler, J. M., DeLuca, F., et al.: Acute low back pain: An objective analysis of conservative therapy. Spine 5:324, 1980.
20. Zachrissen, M.: The Low Back School. Danderyd, Sweden, Danderyd's Hospital, 1972.

THE INTERVERTEBRAL DISC

Disc Disease—Does It Exist?

Steven R. Garfin
Harry N. Herkowitz

"When I use a word," Humpty Dumpty said, in rather a scornful tone, "it means just what I choose it to mean—neither more nor less."

"The question is," said Alice, "whether you can make words mean so many different things."

"The question is," said Humpty Dumpty, "which is to be master—that's all."

LEWIS CARROLL IN
Through The Looking Glass,
1872

Degenerative changes in discs are ubiquitous among humans. The slow, unrelenting changes that are associated with disc degeneration begin in individuals in their twenties. In fact, for the lower lumbar discs, the alterations associated with degeneration are usually present for a greater part of one's life than is the so-called normal state.

One dictionary definition of *disease* is "an abnormal condition of an organism or part, especially as a consequence of infection, inherent weakness, or environmental stress, that impairs normal physiological functioning."[193] Is disc degeneration a disease according to this definition? The biologic definition of *degeneration* is "the usually irreversible deterioration of specific cells or organs with corresponding functional impairment, caused by injury or disease, and often resulting in necrosis or death."[193] This definition uses the terms disease and injury, but are they appropriately applied to the so-called degenerative disc changes?[72] More importantly, do these changes lead to pain, are they irreversible, or are they just coincidental findings that, because they are ubiquitous (as is low back pain), are frequently implicated as a cause of low back pain?[12, 70]

The changes seen in discs and often associated with low back pain are functions of aging and are a combination of primary and secondary aging.[124] Primary aging has been defined as being inherent, programmed, genetic, and unavoidable. Secondary aging, on the other hand, is associated with the physical stresses and the recurrent, cumulative injuries associated with activities of daily living.[169]

There are two major theories of the aging mechanism, each of which has many subsets. One theory is concerned with the programmed limit on life span resulting from differentiation that is predetermined by a genetic process. A definite limit in the viability of cells is set at the time of the cell's origin.[76, 77, 146b] The other theory suggests an accumulation of multiple errors, as life proceeds, to a catastrophic level.[79a, 86a, 86b, 145, 146] Apart from these theories, it is known that (1) there is a maximum life span for each species; (2) human cells have a limited replicative life span in tissue culture, which is inversely related to the age of the donor; (3) pacemaker cells have been invoked as the controls in the aging system;[27] (4) changes in proteins and their synthesis,[6, 14a] DNA structure,[146a] and enzyme activity[90, 91] have been described in aging cell populations; and (5) cells from Werner's syndrome, a genetic disease that causes premature aging, display an increased amount of altered protein compared with their normal counterparts.[86a] Changes seen in the disc, therefore, must be separated from alterations related to age before they can be considered characteristics of a disease process.

The above factors associated with primary aging are inescapable, and the longevity of the discs is established at birth. However, the secondary factors may be alterable, and their effects possible to delay, although it is unlikely that they can completely be avoided. If aging is a disease, then degenerative discs are part of that disease state. For most of us, however, adding the modifier *disease* to the condition of degenerative discs is probably a misnomer.

IS DEGENERATIVE DISC DISEASE THE CAUSE OF LOW BACK PAIN?

If the degenerative changes in intervertebral discs cause low back pain, disability, and dysfunction, then they would qualify as a disease state. However, the etiologic conditions and mechanisms underlying or causing low back/spinal pain syndromes are, for the most part, unknown.[100, 129, 134, 149, 194] Several structures in the lumbar spine have been implicated in low back pain. These include the intervertebral disc, vertebral bodies, microcirculation within the vertebral column, facet joints, ligaments, muscles, and nerves.* It can be argued that changes in the intervertebral disc precede most of the other "pathologic" changes in the lumbar spine, and therefore that all sources of low back pain are intimately, or ultimately, related to the degenerative process that occurs first in the disc.[35, 36, 37, 38] However, Mooney and colleagues have recently documented that facet arthropathy can occur before or independently of degenerative disc changes, implying that in many cases pathoanatomic alterations in the disc need not be the factor initiating low back pain. Nevertheless, the pathoanatomic changes implicated in low back pain focus, in most instances, on the intervertebral disc.[129, 137, 180]

Although no definitive cause–effect relationship for all back pain disorders has been established, a direct relationship between changes in the intervertebral disc and the occurrence of low back pain and sciatic pain has been established for disc herniation, which is preceded by degenerative changes in the disc. The pain associated with disc herniation is presumably related to changes induced by direct pressure on the nerve root.[40, 120] However, because it is known that not all instances of spinal nerve root compression cause leg pain[85, 191, 192, 195] or disability, the "disease" of sciatica caused by a herniated disc may be as closely related to the nerve root and associated pain-causing mechanisms as to the degenerative disc itself.

The cause of low back pain in most patients is unknown.[51] A survey of 157 members of the North American Spine Society listed 149 different terms that the physicians use as their principal diagnosis for a typical patient evaluated for low back pain.[55] Although most of these terms reflect the physician's focus on intervertebral disc pathology, a significant number of respondents believed that low back pain was related to strains and/or sprains, facet arthritis, inflammatory diseases, and other non–disc-related pathologic conditions. Similarly, in a recent report by the Quebec Task Force on Spinal Disorders,[149] the panel members reviewed all available literature related to low back pain and were unable to develop a consensus concerning the precise origin of low back pain. They, therefore, classified back pain into "activity-related spinal disorders" and pain symptoms, and used clinical parameters of pain to diagnose the patient's condition. Although their literature review and treatment recommendations imply the authors' belief in a primary intervertebral disc focus, incontrovertible evidence of relationships between degenerative changes in the intervertebral disc and low back pain is not available. The changes in the disc should not, according to the multiplicity of diagnoses and treatments that exist, be assumed to be a disease state, at this time.

PATHOANATOMY OF DEGENERATIVE ALTERATIONS

Kirkaldy-Willis and associates have described a three-joint complex of the spinal column consisting of the intervertebral disc and the two posterior facet joints.[103, 104] In the intervertebral disc, pathoanatomic changes occur in stages.[184, 187] They progress from circumferential tears to radial tears in the annulus, which then may progress to internal disruption or disc herniation through the tears. Disc height is lost and disc resorption and degeneration follow.

Concomitantly, or in relation to these changes, a synovial reaction in the facet joints occurs. Facet cartilage disruption/destruction takes place, and osteophytes develop along the facet joints. Associated changes include buckling of the ligamentum flavum, over-riding or enlargement of the articular processes, formation of anterior and posterior osteophytes, narrowing of the neuroforamina, and central (as well as lateral) stenosis. Furthermore, end-plate sclerosis, vertebral and facet subluxations, and facet capsular laxity can all occur.[154] Descriptively, these are the changes of degenerative

*References 1, 2, 10, 14–16, 28, 35–37, 39, 43, 47, 52, 53, 71, 81, 84, 86, 94, 99, 100, 103, 106, 107, 109, 112, 113, 120–122, 129–131, 135, 144, 149, 150, 152, 154, 156–158, 160–164, 166, 168, 174, 185, 186, 188–190, 194, 200.

disc "disease." These findings can be seen on radiographs as well as on CT scans, discograms, and MR scans of individuals with low back pain. Vernon-Roberts, however, has shown that these changes are present in nearly all individuals of middle age (i.e., 55 years of age) and that they are associated with age[188, 189] but not necessarily with low back pain. Similarly, Wiesel and colleagues and others have shown on CT scans, as well as on other imaging studies in asymptomatic individuals, that changes attributed to degenerative disc disease need not be painful.[154, 189, 195]

If changes associated with degenerative discs are a disease, then the cause of back pain could be any one of a number of associated pathoanatomic conditions. The pain may have its source within the disc itself or in the nociceptors of associated structures. Nociceptive receptor systems have been identified in myofascial structures of the low back, in the articular joints, in the ligaments along the osseous structures, and along the vascular channels, as well as along the dura, meninges, and dorsal root ganglia.[93, 94, 99, 109, 164, 200] Pain perception may be related to one or more of the following causes of pressure on associated structures: osteophytes, bulging discs, disc herniation, arthritic changes along the intervertebral disc or facet joints, bony changes associated with disc disruption/protrusion (e.g., vertebral sclerosis, Schmorl's nodes, osteoporosis, etc.) and/or compression as in spinal stenosis.

BIOCHEMICAL CHANGES

Chemical, as well as mechanical, factors may be involved in producing inflammation and pain.[50, 102, 175] Marshall and others have proposed that breakdown products from a degenerating nucleus pulposus might leak out and induce a "chemical radiculitis."[116, 117] Intraoperative measurements of pH in the nucleus pulposus at the level of disc herniation have demonstrated low pH values, particularly in patients who develop extensive adhesions around nearby nerve roots.[125, 136] These findings might indicate a chemical interaction between the degenerating intervertebral disc and the nerve root that courses over it, leading to a radiculitis and pain syndrome. This may be initiated by a direct irritating effect of proteoglycans from the discs and/or by an autoimmune reaction from exposure to disc tissues.[20, 21, 49, 64–66, 118, 143, 146a] These latter conditions, particularly if they are induced by degenerative changes and a reaction of the body toward these internally exposed chemicals, are consistent with a disease state, as opposed to a pure aging phenomenon. The major measured chemical components of intervertebral discs are collagen and proteoglycans.* With aging, there appears to be no significant alteration in the type of collagen.[4, 44, 74, 79] As with most tissues, there is an increase in reducible collagen crosslinks during the growth period. However, after maturity is reached, the amount of stable nonreducible crosslinks does not change significantly.[79]

On the other hand, the proteoglycan content of the nucleus and annulus do alter with age.[4, 75, 108, 119] Naylor and others have described an increase in keratan sulfate relative to chondroitin sulfate in older populations.[140, 141] Lyons and associates observed a decrease in molecular weight of proteoglycans with increasing age.[110] There also are differences in the degree of binding of proteoglycans to collagen in the disc and a decrease in aggregation of these proteoglycans with advancing age.[5] This alteration in aggregation ability with age may affect orientation of the various biochemicals and affect the biomechanical properties of these tissues.

If the chemical components of the aging disc are compared with those of a herniated disc, a difference may be noted in the latter, which represents a more purely degenerative state. Disc herniations, at least surgically treated ones, occur frequently in the 35- to 45-year-old group.[168] The biochemistry of the disc fragments in this younger group resembles that found in a more aged disc.[41, 79, 110, 119] This may suggest an accelerated "aging" process that could be considered more like a disease. Mitchell and associates have demonstrated higher collagen content in herniated discs, which was out of proportion to that found in aging discs.[119]

In young individuals, chondrocytes have been identified in both the nucleus and the annulus. Chondrocytes are not known to synthesize collagenase.[172a] However, electron-microscopic studies of disc fragments have demonstrated lysosomes in chondro-

*References 4, 6, 7, 11, 19, 22–24, 27, 29, 30, 33, 41, 44, 66, 74, 177, 178.

cytes associated with partially degraded collagen within the fragment.[176] Collagenase itself, however, has not been identified in normal disc tissue. Separately, in older individuals, fibroblasts have been identified in the annulus. This finding suggests, along with the observation of vascular intrusions into the disc, that healing (following disruption-"degeneration") is taking place, which implies that these may not be the normal changes accepted by the body.

The hydration state of the disc changes with aging and may also reflect significant pathologic alterations within a degenerating or "symptomatic" disc.[26, 98] Most of the changes appear to be physiologic ones, although some of these alterations may progress and become expressible as apparent disease states in the fourth and fifth decades of life, or later. The water content of a disc, which approximates 90% in childhood, decreases to approximately 70% by the sixth decade.[31, 69, 78, 82, 148, 182] However, these changes occur predominantly within the nucleus, and only limited alterations in the water content are observed in the annulus as age increases. The hydration of a disc is probably maintained by the gel-like lattice of the collagen/proteoglycan aggregations. Advancing age and the changes seen in proteoglycan composition in the nucleus, along with decreases in binding capacity, are accompanied by less ability to maintain water within the nucleus. Naylor and Smare have suggested a molecular breakdown in the degenerating disc, and the deterioration of complex structures that form the gel into simpler but more numerous molecules.[141] This could increase the osmotic pressure, possibly attracting (at least temporarily) more water into the disc, leading to a state of "hyperhydration." The resultant increased intradiscal pressure could then lead to disc rupture, particularly if pre-existing degenerative tears in the annulus were present. Naylor postulated that the changes in the polymers were "due to an endocrine or metabolic factor," which would be consistent with a so-called disease state and separate from the normal age-related changes that are observed, and that they do not necessarily cause disc herniation, sciatica, or chronic back pain.

Nachemson and coworkers have also extensively studied hydration effects on the disc.[126–128, 131, 132, 134, 138, 139] They have shown that alterations in intradiscal pressure can be affected by activity, position, and exercise.[3] Perhaps, by correctly prescribing exercise and aerobic activities, secondary aging changes on the disc can be decreased and pathologic disease states avoided or at least delayed.

ANATOMIC STUDIES

In order to determine whether disc degeneration is a disease, both the basic and clinical sciences must be evaluated. From a review of the basic science of the degenerative intervertebral disc, there is little doubt that this is a primary aging process and that secondary factors influence the rapidity with which it occurs. Does this normal aging process produce the clinical symptoms of low back pain? What factors can be analyzed to determine whether the attribution of the word *disease* to disc degeneration is valid? Questions that can be asked are (1) Does disc degeneration lead to abnormal movement of the motion segment? (2) Does disc degeneration precipitate degenerative changes in other structures within the motion segment? (3) Can low back pain symptoms be unequivocally correlated with the radiographic appearance of disc space narrowing? (4) Can discography and volumetric studies correlate patterns of disc degeneration with clinical symptomatology?

Pathoanatomic Changes

In cadaveric spines, instability due to degeneration of the intervertebral disc has been studied by Seligman and associates using the L4–L5 motion segment.[159] They developed a computer program to analyze the centers of rotation in the lumbar vertebrae. The advantage of this method over standard flexion–extension radiographic studies is that it can measure much smaller angles of rotation than can standard radiographs and, therefore, is considerably more sensitive to motion changes.[63] They divided their specimens into normal and degenerative discs. The degenerative discs were classified as having minor, mild, moderate, or severe degeneration. Normal disc segments produced loci in the posterior half of the disc. As the amount of disc degeneration increased, the loci lengthened and widened, indicating erratic and/or translational movement. The only exception to this was in the severely degenerative discs, which produced stiffer segments leading to reduced mobility. The question to consider concerns whether this erratic movement produced by the degenerative disc is responsible for the development of low back pain.

The process of degenerative disc "disease" begins with circumferential tears in the annulus.[104, 190] This may lead to frank disc herniation or, more commonly, degeneration of the disc or internal disc disruption. The instability that may develop leads to arthritis of the facet joint, an anatomic structure that itself may be responsible for low back pain.[122]

Dunlop and associates performed pressure measurements across facet joints in twelve cadaveric normal and degenerative disc motion segments.[45] They found that narrowing of the disc space significantly increased pressure recordings across the facet joints, especially when the spine was placed in extension. This provides a possible explanation for the development of facet joint arthritis and/or the etiology of pain associated with degeneration of the intervertebral disc.

If motion segment instability and degeneration of the structures within the motion segment are the cause of back pain, it seems logical that spinal fusion would alleviate the back pain associated with these changes.[53, 54, 96, 153] The results of surgery for this condition must be judged against the natural history of nonoperative management. The success of posterolateral fusion for low back pain related to several disorders, including degenerative disc disease, has been reported by Jackson and colleagues as well as others.[42, 97, 172] Of 129 patients who underwent fusion by Jackson and colleagues, 20 of 33 (60%) of those treated for "degenerative disc disease" had good results. Similarly, the results of anterior interbody fusion for lumbar degenerative disc disease have been reported by many different authors.* Sorenson, reporting on 98 patients, noted improvement in 73%. However, 31 patients had constant pain after surgery.[167] A review of the Mayo Clinic experience by Stauffer and Coventry revealed good results in 36%, fair in 20%, and poor in 44%.[171] There were, however, only three patients with primary degenerative disc disease, two of whom had a good clinical result. Flynn and Hoque reported on 50 patients who had undergone anterior interbody fusion.[56] Twenty-six patients were categorized as successful (52%), whereas 24 patients had a poor result (48%). Of those with primary degenerative disc disease, good results were noted in two patients, fair results in one, and poor results in four.

*References 34, 39, 54, 56, 68, 95, 144, 151, 167, 171.

The results from these various series do not appear to exceed, or even to approach, the results observed by following the natural history of low back pain. Hakelius studied 583 patients with back and leg pain. Both surgical and nonsurgical patients were followed for an average of 7 years. Back pain symptoms related to disc degeneration were reported to be minimal in 85% of the patients at the end of the 7 years.[73] Similar results have been shown by other nonoperative studies of low back pain. It is obvious that factors besides the appearance of a degenerative disc play an important role in the production of pain and disability.

Radiographic Changes

It is not unusual to see, in a patient with low back pain, radiographs demonstrating disc degeneration in the lumbar spine. Can it be assumed that the cause of the patient's pain is the degenerative disc? There are certain well-described radiographic changes that occur in association with degenerative discs.[25, 40, 48, 57, 59, 154] These include loss of height of the disc space anteriorly or uniformly, with a slight associated loss of lumbar lordosis. There may be anteroposterior subluxation or lateral subluxation of one vertebra on the other.[105, 111, 112] Late changes include a vacuum phenomenon within the disc, osteophytes, vertebral sclerosis, apophyseal joint malalignment, facet hypertrophy, narrowing of the interlaminar space, and thickening of spinous processes.[9] These changes are consistent with degenerative disc disease and correspond to anatomic changes seen on postmortem examinations. However, they are not always associated with pain* and in that sense cannot be considered a disease, since they are asymptomatic, do not alone lead to disability or dysfunction, and cannot be shown to be

*References 67, 85, 114, 115, 188, 189, 195, 198, 199.

related to injury, environmental stresses, and/or other external relationships.[18, 90, 91, 199]

Splithoff reported on two groups of patients, one asymptomatic and one symptomatic with low back pain.[170] The conclusion of that study maintained that routine radiographs of the lumbosacral spine were of little value in identifying the cause of the patient's pain. A similar conclusion was obtained by Horal in a study of workers in Scandinavia, in which no relationship between plain radiographic findings and back pain was found.[89] Torgerson and Dotter compared the radiographs of 217 asymptomatic patients taken from intravenous pyelograms against 387 patients seen for low back pain.[184] In the asymptomatic group, 48 patients (22%) demonstrated a narrowing of a lumbar disc. Of the 387 patients with low back pain, 218 (56%) had evidence of disc degeneration. Of asymptomatic patients in their forties, only 4 of 64 (6%) showed evidence of disc degeneration, whereas 70 of 146 symptomatic patients (48%) in the same decade of life showed evidence of disc degeneration. A statistically significant increase in degenerative discs was noted in the symptomatic group through the eighth decade. However, the incidence of disc degeneration in asymptomatic patients increased with each decade, which is indicative of physiologic aging of the intervertebral disc. This study concluded that disc degeneration was a cause of low back pain, at least in patients under forty years of age. Similar findings were reported by Frymoyer and associates in 292 individuals.[57] In their study, 96 individuals were asymptomatic, 134 had experienced moderate low back pain, and 62 had a history of severe low back pain. Radiographically, disc space narrowing between L4 and L5 significantly correlated with complaints of low back and leg pain.

Discographic Changes

If the degenerative disc is the cause of low back pain, stimulation of the disc space by fluid injection, and/or degenerative changes seen on discography should correlate with the patient's symptoms.[160, 196] However, discography has remained a controversial diagnostic procedure. It is difficult to correlate clinical symptoms with the discographic appearance because normal aging produces degenerative patterns, irrespective of symptoms. In addition, the subjective pain response to fluid injection into the disc is of questionable value. Holt studied, by means of discography, 30 individuals who had no history of back pain.[88] A total of 72 discs were injected. At each interspace, a significant number of discs appeared to be degenerative or ruptured. In 11 discs (15%), severe pain was reported when a degenerative pattern extending to the annulus was noted. In 16 discs (22%) dye leakage into the epidural space was associated with back pain or leg pain. The conclusion reached by the author indicated that the pain was related to the dye contacting tissues that had sensory fiber innervation. The results, demonstrating a 37% false-positive rate for discography, suggest that degenerative discs do not routinely cause low back pain, and vice versa. Van-Haranta and associates studied the pain response elicited after the injection of contrast material into the disc and correlated it with the pattern of degeneration seen on a CT scan/discogram.[184] The pain production by injection was different from the patient's back complaints, or no pain was elicited on injection, in 70% of patients with slight annular disruption, 46% of patients with moderate disruption, and 25% of patients with severe annular disruption. This study, resembling Holt's study, also indicates that the cause of the low back pain in a significant number of patients may not be related directly to the degenerative disc itself; or, conversely, the degenerative disc does not always cause pain, or indicate a disease state, even though degenerative changes exist.

Conclusion/Summation

After answering the questions posed previously, can it be said that disc degeneration is a disease? The answer appears to be "yes and no."

Degeneration of the intervertebral disc leads to excessive and perhaps erratic movement of the motion segment in vitro.[53] However, does this also apply to the in vivo situation when the effect of muscular support of the vertebral column is taken into account? In addition, if erratic movement of the degenerative motion segment occurs in vivo, does it produce low back pain?

Deterioration of the intervertebral disc leads to degeneration of other structures in the motion segment, resulting in lumbar spondylosis, or the process of primary aging of the lumbar spine, and should not be classified as a disease. However, radiographic studies of asymptomatic and symptomatic patients with low back pain document a statistically higher incidence of disc degeneration at L4–L5 in younger adult patients (under 40 years of age) with low back pain, suggesting a cause–effect relationship between the subjective complaint of low back pain and the radiographic findings of disc degeneration, at least in this age group.[57, 179]

In reviewing the role of discography and volumetric studies for identification of a symptomatic degenerative disc, it behooves us to note the low sensitivity and specificity of this procedure in isolating symptomatic disc degeneration.[88] Again, we are led to question the source of the pain in a patient with disc degeneration. Theoretically, if the degenerative disc is the sole source of the patient's low back pain, then spinal fusion should alleviate the painful condition. The poor results of spinal fusion for low back pain, whether it be anterior interbody, posterolateral or posterior fusion, cast doubt on the aging disc as the sole source of low back pain.

Radicular symptoms frequently develop 5 to 6 years after low back pain, as do associated changes that follow or occur concomitantly with disc degeneration.[12, 22, 101, 154] Authors of many studies have noted, particularly in patients with sciatica, that, with or without surgery, improvement in the symptom complaint of leg pain is likely, although back pain is generally a more recalcitrant complaint.[73] The degenerative disc, if it causes back pain or sciatica, can in this setting be considered to be a disease, since it causes disability and dysfunction. However, it is self-limited in most of the cases in which it does create a symptomatic problem.* The peak onset of symptoms appears to be in the fourth and fifth decades of life, coincident with the greatest decrease in hydration of the disc, but not consistent with the more dramatic alterations seen radiographically and morphologically in the more aged population.

Disc degeneration is part of the primary aging process. Its role in the production of low back pain may be related to exaggerated movement of the motion segment with the resultant deterioration of the facet joints and other supporting structures of the motion segment. Regardless of whether the condition is physiologic aging or pathologic degeneration, each patient's complaints of low back pain must be evaluated carefully. Although the disc is the likely source in many, it may not be the primary source in all individuals.

Degeneration of the lumbar intervertebral disc is a progressive and relentless process. It occurs in most discs of the body, in all individuals. The characteristic morphologic, chemical, radiographic, and clinical pictures are similar in symptomatic and asymptomatic individuals. The alterations occur with aging and do not strictly meet the definition of *disease*. However, most scientific attention has been focused on the disc, as opposed to the myofascial structures, and therefore the relationship to pain-related complaints has centered upon the disc and degenerative processes.

Is it really a disease? It would not appear that the degenerative process is in fact a disease, but that it is more like a primary aging phenomenon that, in some people, is accompanied by accelerated secondary aging components. If a single disc was usually the primary cause of low back pain, then removing the disc or fusing that segment should provide symptomatic relief in most individuals. The plethora of procedures that have been described to "attack" the disc, or to remove it, suggests it is not the sole culprit in back pain and that its eradication may not be the answer to this "epidemic."

*References 8, 13, 15, 32, 90, 91, 134, 168, 173, 191, 192.

References

1. Adams, M. A., and Hutton, W. C.: The effect of posture on the role of the apophyseal joints in resisting intervertebral compressive forces. J. Bone Joint Surg. 62B:358–362, 1980.
2. Adams, M. A., and Hutton, W. C.: The mechanical function of the lumbar apophyseal joints. Spine 8:327–330, 1983.
3. Adams, M. A., and Hutton, W. C.: The effect of posture on the fluid content of the lumbar intervertebral discs. Spine 8:665–671, 1983.
4. Adams, P., Eyre, D. R., and Muir, H.: Biochemical aspects of development and aging of human lumbar intervertebral discs. Rheumatol. Rehabil. 16:22–29, 1977.
5. Adams, P., and Muir, H.: Qualitative changes with

age of proteoglycans of human lumbar discs. Ann. Rheum. Dis. 35:289, 1976.

6. Adelman, R. C.: Age-dependent effects in enzyme induction—a biomechanical expression of aging. Exp. Gerontol. 6:75–87, 1971.
7. Akeson, W. H., Woo, S. L. -Y., Taylor, T. K., et al: Biomechanics and biochemistry of the intervertebral disks: The need for correlation studies. Clin. Orthop. 129:133–140, 1977.
8. Anderson, J. A. D.: Rheumatism in industry: A review. Br. J. Indust. Med. 28:103–121, 1971.
9. Andersson, G. B. J., Schultz, A., Nathan, A., and Irstam, L.: Roentgenographic measurement of lumbar intervertebral disc height. Spine 6:154–158, 1981.
10. Arnoldi, C. C., Brodsky, A. E., Cauchoix, J., et al.: Lumbar spinal stenosis and nerve root entrapment syndromes: Definition and classification. Clin. Orthop. 115:4–5, 1976.
11. Barnes, M. J., Cornstable, B. J., Morton, C. F., and Royce, P. M.: The influence of dietary calcium deficiency and parathyroidectomy on bone collagen structure. Biochem. J. 39:461, 1974.
12. Benn, R. T., and Wood, P. H. N.: Pain in the back: An attempt to estimate the size of the problem. Rheumatol. Rehabil. 14:121–128, 1975.
13. Benn, R. T., and Wood, P. H. N.: Statistical appendix—digest of data on the rheumatic diseases: 4 morbidity and mortality, and hospital services for rheumatism sufferers. Ann. Rheum. Dis. 31:522–529, 1972.
14. Benner, B., and Ehni, G.: Spinal arachnoiditis: The postoperative variety in particular. Spine 3:4–44, 1978.

14a. Bick, M. D., and Strehler, B. L.: Leucyl transfer RNA synthetase changes during soybean cotyledon senescence. Proc. Natl. Acad. Sci. U.S.A. 68:224, 1971.

15. Biering-Sorensen, F.: Low back trouble in a general population of 30-, 40-, 50-, and 60-year-old men and women: Study design, representativeness and basic results. Dan. Med. Bull. 29:289–299, 1982.
16. Biering-Sorensen, F.: A prospective study of low back pain in a general population: I. Occurrence, recurrence, and aetiology. Scand. J. Rehabil. Med. 15:71–79, 1983.
17. Biering-Sorensen, F.: A prospective study of low back pain in a general population: II. Location, character, aggravating and relieving factors. Scand. J. Rehabil. Med. 15:81–88, 1983.
18. Biering-Sorensen, F.: The relation of spinal x-ray to low-back pain and physical activity among 60-year-old men and women. Spine 10:451–455, 1985.
19. Bijlsma, F., and Peereboom, J. W.: The ageing pattern of human intervertebral disc. Gerontologia 18:157–168, 1972.
20. Bisla, R. S., Marchisello, P. J., Lockshin, M. D., et al.: Auto-immunological basis of disk degeneration. Clin. Orthop. 121:205–211, 1976.
21. Bobechko, W. T., and Hirsh, C.: Auto-immune response to nucleus pulposus in the rabbit. J. Bone Joint Surg. 47B:574, 1965.
22. Bornstein, P.: The nature of the intramolecular cross-links in collagen. The separation and characterization of peptides from the cross-link region of rat skin collagen. Biochemistry 6:3460–3473, 1967.
23. Bornstein, P.: Comparative sequence studies of rat skin and tendon collagen. The absence of a short sequence at the amino terminus of the skin alpha-1 chain. Biochemistry 8:63–71, 1969.
24. Bornstein, P.: The cross-linking of collagen and elastin and its inhibition in osteolathyrism. Am. J. Med. 49:429, 1970.
25. Brekkan, A.: Radiographic examination of the lumbosacral spine: An age-stratified study. Clin. Radiol. 34:321–324, 1983.
26. Brown, M. D., and Tsaltas, T. T.: Studies on the permeability of the intervertebral disc during skeletal maturation. Spine 1:240–244, 1976.
27. Bullough, W. S.: Aging of mammals. Nature 229:608, 1971.
28. Burton, C. V.: Lumbosacral arachnoiditis. Spine 3:24–30, 1978.
29. Bushell, G. R., Ghosh, P., Taylor, T. F. K., and Akeson, W. H.: Proteoglycan chemistry of the intervertebral disks. Clin. Orthop. 129:115–123, 1977.
30. Butler, W. T.: The structure of α1-CB3, a cyanogen bromide fragment from the central portion of the α1 chain of rat collagen. The tryptic peptides from skin and dentin collagens. Biochem. Biophys. Res. Comm. 48:1540, 1972.
31. Butler, W. T., and Wels, C. M.: Glycosaminoglycans of cat intervertebral disc. J. Biochem. 122:647, 1971.
32. Cady, L. D., Bischoff, D. P., O'Connell, et al.: Strength and fitness and subsequent back injuries in firefighters. J. Occup. Med. 21:269–272, 1979.
33. Cannon, D. J., and Davison, P. F.: Cross-linking and aging in rat tendon collagen. Exp. Gerontol. 8:51, 1973.
34. Chow, S. P., Leong, J. C. Y., Ma, A., and Yau, A. C. M. C.: Anterior spinal fusion for deranged lumbar intervertebral disc: A review of 97 cases. Spine 5:452–458, 1980.
35. Coventry, M. B., Ghormley, R. K., and Kernohan, J. W.: The intervertebral disk: Its microscopic anatomy and pathology, Part I. Anatomy, Development and Physiology. J. Bone Joint Surg. 27:105, 1945.
36. Coventry, M. B., Ghormley, R. K., and Kernohan, J. W.: The intervertebral disk: Its microscopic anatomy and pathology, Part II. Changes in the intervertebral disk concomitant with age. J. Bone Joint Surg. 27:233, 1945.
37. Coventry, M. B., Ghormley, R. K., and Kernohan, J. W.: The intervertebral disk: Its microscopic anatomy and pathology, Part III. Pathological changes in the intervertebral disk. J. Bone Joint Surg. 27:460, 1945.
38. Coventry, M. B.: Anatomy of the intervertebral disk. Clin. Orthop. 67:9, 1969.
39. Crock, H. V.: Isolated lumbar disc resorption as a cause of nerve root canal stenosis. Clin. Orthop. 115:109–115, 1975.
40. Dandy, W. E.: Loose cartilage from intervertebral disk stimulating tumor of the spinal cord. Arch. Surg. 19:660, 1929.
41. Davidson, E. A., and Woodhall, B.: Biochemical alterations in herniated intervertebral disks. J. Biol. Chem. 234:2951, 1959.
42. Dawson, E. G., Lotysh, M., Urist, M. R.: Intertransverse process lumbar arthrodesis with autogenous bone graft. Clin. Orthop. 154:90–96, 1981.
43. DePalma, A. F., and Rothman, R. H.: The Inter-

vertebral Disk. Philadelphia, W. B. Saunders, 1970.
44. Deleted in press.
45. Dunlop, R. B., Adams, M. A., and Hutton, W. C.: Disc space narrowing and the lumbar facet joints. J. Bone Joint Surg. 66B:706–710, 1984.
46. Dupuis, P. R., Yong-Hing, K., Cassidy, J. D., and Kirkaldy-Willis, W. H.: Radiologic diagnosis of degenerative lumbar spinal instability. Spine 10:262–276, 1985.
47. Edgar, M. A., and Nundy, S.: Innervation of the spinal dura mater. J. Neurol. Neurosurg. Psychiatry 29:530, 1966.
48. Eisenberg, R. L., Hedgcock, M. W., Gooding, G. A. W., et al.: Compensation examination of the cervical and lumbar spines: critical disagreement in radiographic interpretation. A.J.R. 134:519–522, 1980.
49. Elves, M. W., Bucknill, T., and Sullivan, M.: In vitro inhibition of leukocyte migration in patients with intervertebral disks lesions. Orthop. Clin. North Am. 6:59, 1975.
50. Eyring, E. J.: The biochemistry and physiology of the intervertebral disk. Clin. Orthop. 67:16, 1969.
51. Fager, C. A.: The age-old back problem: New fad, same fallacies. Spine 9:326–328, 1984.
52. Falconer, M. A., et al.: Observations on the causes and mechanics of symptom production in low back pain and sciatica. J. Neurol. Neurosurg. Psychiatry 11:13–26, 1948.
53. Farfan, H. F.: Mechanical Disorders of the Low Back. Philadelphia, Lea & Febiger, 1973.
54. Farfan, H. F., and Kirkaldy-Willis, W. H.: The present status of spinal fusion in the treatment of lumbar intervertebral joint disorders. Clin. Orthop. 158:198–214, 1980.
55. Fardon, D. F., White, A. H., and Wiesel, S.: Diagnostic Terms and Conservative Treatments Favored for Lumbar Disorders by Spine Surgeons in North America. Presented at North American Spine Society First Annual Meeting, Laguna Beach, California, 1985.
56. Flynn, J. C., and Hoque, M. A.: Anterior fusion of the lumbar spine: End-result study with long-term follow-up. J. Bone Joint Surg. 61A:1143–1150, 1979.
57. Frymoyer, J. W., Newberg, A., Pope, M. H., et al.: Spine radiographs in patients with low back pain: An epidemiological study in men. J. Bone Joint Surg. 66A:1048–1055, 1984.
58. Fujimakel, A., Crock, H., and Bedbrook, G.: The results of 150 anterior lumbar interbody fusion operations performed by two surgeons in Australia. Clin. Orthop. 165:164–167, 1982.
59. Gehweiler, J. A., and Daffner, R. H.: Low back pain: The controversy of radiologic evaluation. A.J.R. 140:109–112, 1983.
60. Gershon, H., and Gershon, D.: Inactive enzyme molecules in aging mice: Liver aldolase. Proc. Natl. Acad. Sci. U.S.A. 70:909, 1973.
61. Gershon, D., and Gershon, H.: An evaluation of the "error catastrophe" theory of aging in the light of recent experimental results. Gerontology 22:212, 1976.
62. Gertzbein, S. D.: Degenerative disk disease of the lumbar spine—immunological implications. Clin. Orthop. 129:68–71, 1977.
63. Gertzbein, S., Seligman, J., Holtby, R., et al.: Centrode patterns and segmental instability in degenerative disc disease. Spine 10:257–261, 1985.
64. Gertzbein, S. D., Tait, J. H., and Devlin, S. R.: The stimulation of lymphocytes by nucleus pulposus in patients with degenerative disk disease of the lumbar spine. Clin. Orthop. 123:149–154, 1977.
65. Gertzbein, S. D., Tile, M., Gross, A., and Falk, R.: Autoimmunity in degenerative disk disease of the lumbar spine. Orthop. Clin. North Am. 6:67, 1975.
66. Ghosh, P., Bushell, G. R., Taylor, T. F. K., and Akeson, W. H.: Collagens, elastin and noncollagenous protein of the intervertebral disk. Clin. Orthop. 129:124–132, 1977.
67. Gibson, E. S., Martin, R. H., and Terry, C. W.: Incidence of low back pain and pre-placement x-ray screening. J. Occup. Med. 22:515–519, 1980.
68. Goldner, J. L., Urbaniak, J. R., and McCollum, D. E.: Anterior disc excision and interbody spinal fusion for chronic low back pain. Orthop. Clin. North Am. 2:543–568, 1971.
69. Gower, W. E., and Pedrini, V.: Age-related variations in protein polysaccharides from human nucleus pulposus, annulus fibrosis, and costal cartilage. J. Bone Joint Surg. 51A:1154, 1969.
70. Grazier, K. L., Holbrook, T. L., Kelsey, J., and Stauffer, R. N.: The Frequency of Occurrence, Impact, and Cost of Musculoskeletal Conditions in the United States. Chicago, American Academy of Orthopaedic Surgeons, 1984.
71. Gunn, C. C., and Milbrandt, W. E.: Early and subtle signs in low-back sprain. Spine 3:267–281, 1978.
72. Hadler, N. M.: Legal ramifications of the medical definition of back disease. Ann. Intern. Med. 89:992–999, 1978.
73. Hakelius, A.: Prognosis in sciatica: A clinical follow-up of surgical and non-surgical treatment. Acta Orthop. Scand. (Suppl.):129, 1970.
74. Hallen, A.: The collagen and ground substance of human intervertebral disk at different ages. Acta Chem. Scand. 16:705, 1962.
75. Deleted in press.
76. Hayflick, L.: The limited in vitro lifetime of human diploid cell strains. Exp. Cell Res. 37:614, 1965.
77. Hayflick, L., and Moorhead, P. S.: The serial cultivation of human diploid cell strains. Exp. Cell Res. 25:585, 1961.
78. Hendry, N. G.: The hydration of the nucleus pulposus and its relation to the intervertebral disk derangement. J. Bone Joint Surg. 40B:132, 1958.
79. Herbert, C. M., Lindberg, K. A., Jayson, M. I. V., and Bailey, A. J.: Changes in the collagen of human intervertebral discs during aging and degenerative disc disease. J. Mol. Med. 1:79, 1975.
79a. Hill, B. T.: Influence of age on chromatin transcription in marine tissues using an heterologous and an homologous RNA. Gerontology 22:111, 1976.
80. Hirsch, C.: Studies on the pathology of low back pain. J. Bone Joint Surg. 41B:237–243, 1959.
81. Hirsch, C.: Etiology and pathogenesis of low back pain. Isr. J. Med. Sci. 2:362–370, 1966.
82. Hirsch, C., Paulson, S., Sylven, B., and Snellman, O.: Arthroplastique polymerase cartilagineuse de la hanche. Acta Orthop. Scand. 22:175, 1952.
83. Hirsch, C., Paulson, S., Sylven, B., and Snellman, O.: New observations on the mechanical behavior of lumbar discs. Acta Orthop. Scand. 23:254, 1954.
84. Hirsch, C., and Schajowicz, F.: Studies on struc-

tural changes in the lumbar annulus fibrosus. Acta Orthop. Scand. 22:184–231, 1952.
85. Hitselberger, W. E., and Witten, R.: Abnormal myelograms in asymptomatic patients. J. Neurosurg. 28:204, 1968.
86. Hockaday, J. M., and Whitty, C. W. M.: Patterns of referred pain in the normal subject. Brain 90:481–496, 1967.
86a. Holliday, R., Porterfield, J. S., and Gibbs, D. D.: Premature aging and occurrence of altered enzyme in Werner's syndrome fibroblasts. Nature 248:762, 1974.
86b. Holliday, R., and Tarrant, G. M.: Biochemical measure of the time and frequency of radiation-inducod allolic rccombination in *Ustilago*. Nature 238:26, 1972.
87. Holm, S., and Rydevik, B.: Nutritional supply to nerve roots. (Manuscript in preparation.)
88. Holt, A. P.: The question of lumbar discography. J. Bone Joint Surg. 50A:720–725, 1968.
89. Horal, J.: The clinical appearance of low back disorders in the city of Gothenberg, Sweden: Comparisons of incapacitated probands with matched controls. Acta Orthop. Scand. (Suppl.):118, 1969.
90. Hult, L.: The Munkfors investigation: A study of the frequency and causes of the stiff neck—brachialgia and lumbago—sciatica syndromes, as well as observations on certain signs and symptoms from the dorsal spine and the joints of the extremities in industrial and forest workers. Acta Orthop. Scand. (Suppl.):16, 1954.
91. Hult, L.: Cervical dorsal and lumbar spinal syndromes: A field investigation of a non-selected material of 1200 workers in different occupations with special reference to disc degeneration and so-called muscular rheumatism. Acta Orthop. Scand. (Suppl.):17, 1954.
92. Hutter, C.: Posterior intervertebral body fusion. Clin. Orthop. 179:86–96, 1983.
93. Hyyppa, M. T., Scheinin, H., Alaranta, H., et al.: Neurotransmission and the experience of low back pain: No association between CSF monoamine metabolites and pain. Pain 21:57–65, 1985.
94. Inman, V. T., and Saunders, J. B.: Referred pain from skeletal structures. J. Nerv. Ment. Dis. 99:660–667, 1944.
95. Inoue, S., Watanabe, T., Hirose, A., et al.: Anterior discectomy and interbody fusion for lumbar disc herniations: A review of 350 cases. Clin. Orthop. 183:22–31, 1984.
96. International Society for the Study of the Lumbar Spine: Symposium on the role of spine fusion for low-back pain. Spine 6:278–314, 1981.
97. Jackson, R. K., Boston, D. A., and Edge, A. J.: Lateral mass fusion: A prospective study of a consecutive series with long term follow-up. Spine 10:828–832, 1985.
98. Jayson, M. I. V., Herbert, C. M., and Barks, J. S.: Intervertebral discs: Nuclear morphology and bursting pressures. Ann. Rheum. Dis. 32:308, 1973.
99. Kellgren, J. H.: On the distribution of pain arising from deep somatic structures with charts of segmental pain areas. Clin. Sci. Mol. Med. 3:175–190, 1938.
100. Kellgren, J. H.: The anatomical source of back pain. Rheumatol. Rehabil. 16:3–12, 1977.
101. Kelsey, J. L.: An epidemiological study of acute herniated lumbar intervertebral discs. Rheumatol. Rehabil. 14:144–159, 1976.
102. Keyes, D. C., and Compere, E. L.: The normal and pathological physiology of the nucleus pulposus of the intervertebral disk. J. Bone Joint Surg. 14:897, 1932.
103. Kirkaldy-Willis, W. H.: A more precise diagnosis for low-back pain. Spine 4:102–109, 1979.
104. Kirkaldy-Willis, W. H., Wedge, J. H., Yong-Hing, K., and Reilly, J.: Pathology and pathogenesis of lumbar spondylosis and stenosis. Spine 3:319–328, 1978.
105. Knuttson, F.: The instability associated with disc degeneration in the lumbar spine. Acta Radiol. 25:593–609, 1944.
106. Lawrence, J. S.: Disc degeneration: Its frequency and relationship to symptoms. Ann. Rheum. Dis. 28:121–136, 1969.
107. Lippitt, A. B.: The facet joint and its role in spine pain: Management with facet joint injections. Spine 9:746–750, 1984.
108. Lipson, S. J., and Muir, H.: Vertebral osteophyte formation in experimental disk degeneration: Morphologic and proteoglycan changes over time. Arthritis Rheum. 23:319, 1980.
109. Loeser, J. D.: Pain due to nerve injury. Spine 10:232–235, 1985.
110. Lyons, H., Jones, E., Quinn, F. E., et al.: Changes in the protein-polysaccharide fractions of nucleus pulposus from human intervertebral disc with age and disc herniation. J. Lab. Clin. Med. 68:930, 1966.
111. MacNab, I.: Negative disc exploration: An analysis of the causes of nerve root involvement in sixty-eight patients. J. Bone Joint Surg. 53A:891–903, 1971.
112. MacNab, I.: The traction spur: An indicator of segmental instability. J. Bone Joint Surg. 53A:663–670, 1971.
113. MacNab, I.: The mechanism of spondylogenic pain. *In* Hirsch, C., and Zotterman, Y. (eds.): Cervical Pain. New York, Pergamon Press, 1972, pp. 89–95.
114. Magora, A., and Schwartz, A.: Relation between the low back pain syndrome and x-ray findings: I. Degenerative osteoarthritis. Scand. J. Rehabil. Med. 8:115–125, 1976.
115. Magora, A., and Schwartz, A.: Relation between low back pain and x-ray changes. Scand. J. Rehabil. Med. 12:47–52, 1980.
116. Marshall, L. L., and Trethewie, E. R.: Chemical irritation of nerve root in disc prolapse. Lancet 2:320, 1973.
117. Marshall, L. L., Trethewie, E. R., and Curtain, C. C.: Chemical radiculitis—a clinical, physiological and immunological study. Clin. Orthop. Rel. Res. 129:61–67, 1977.
118. Merlini, L., and Donati, U.: Auto-immunity and intervertebral disc disease. Ital. J. Orthop. Traumatol. 6:427–432, 1980.
119. Mitchell, P. E., Hendry, M. G., and Billewicz, W. Z.: The chemical background of intervertebral disk prolapse. J. Bone Joint Surg. 43B:141, 1961.
120. Mixter, W. J., and Barr, J. S.: Rupture of the intervertebral disc with involvement of the spinal canal. N. Engl. J. Med. 2A:210–215, 1934.
121. Mooney, V.: The syndromes of low back disease: Symposium on evaluation and care of lumbar

spine problems. Orthop. Clin. North Am. 14:505–515, 1983.

122. Mooney, V., and Robertson, J.: The facet syndrome. Clin. Orthop. Rel. Res. 115:149–156, 1976.

123. Zideman, P., Malmivaara, A., and Mooney, V.: Value of the axial view in assessing discograms and experimental study with cadavers. Spine 12:299–303, 1987.

124. Murphy, T. F.: A cure for aging? J. Med. Philos. 11:237–255, 1986.

125. Nachemson, A.: Intradiscal measurements of pH in patients with lumbar rhizopathies. Acta Orthop. Scand. 40:23, 1967.

126. Nachemson, A.: Lumbar intradiskal pressure. Experimental studies on postmortem material. Acta Orthop. Scand. (Suppl.)43:9, 1960.

127. Nachemson, A.: The influence of spinal movements on the lumbar intradiskal pressure and on the tensile stresses in the annulus fibrosis. Acta Orthop. Scand., 33:183, 1963.

128. Nachemson, A.: The load on lumbar discs in different positions of the body. Clin. Orthop. 45:107, 1966.

129. Nachemson, A.: The lumbar spine, an orthopaedic challenge. Spine 1:59, 1976.

130. Nachemson, A.: Towards a better understanding of low-back pain: A review of the mechanics of the lumbar disc. Rheumatol. Rehabil. 14:129–143, 1975.

131. Nachemson, A.: Recent advances in the treatment of low back pain. Intern. Orthop. 9:1–10, 1985.

132. Nachemson, A. L.: Disc pressure measurements. Spine 6:93–97, 1981.

134. Nachemson, A. L.: The natural course of low-back pain. *In* White, A. A., and Gordon, S. L. (eds.): Symposium on Idiopathic Low-Back Pain. St. Louis, C. V. Mosby, 1982, pp. 46–51.

135. Nachemson, A. L., and Anderson, G. B. J.: Classification of low-back pain. Scand. J. Work Environ. Health 8:134–136, 1982.

136. Nachemson, A., Diamant, B., and Karlsson, J.: Correlation between lactate levels and pH in discs of patients with lumbar rhizopathies. Experientia 24:1195, 1968.

137. Nachemson, A., and Elfstrom, G.: Intravital dynamic pressure measurements in lumbar discs. Scand. J. Rehab. Med. (Suppl.):1, 1970.

138. Nachemson, A., Lewin, T., Maroudas, A., and Freeman, M. A. R.: In vitro diffusion of dye through the end-plates and the annulus fibrosus of human combination-vertebral discs. Acta Orthop. 41:589, 1970.

139. Nachemson, A., and Morris, J. M.: In vivo measurements of intradiscal pressure. Discometry, a method for the determination of pressure in the lower lumbar discs. J. Bone Joint Surg. 46A:1077, 1964.

140. Naylor, A.: Biochemical changes in human intervertebral disk degeneration and prolapse. Orthop. Clin. North Am. 2:343, 1971.

141. Naylor, A., and Smare, D. L.: Fluid content of the nucleus pulposus as a factor in the disk syndrome. Br. Med. J. 2:975, 1953.

142. Naylor, A.: The biophysical and biochemical aspects of intervertebral disk herniation and degeneration. Ann. R. Coll. Surg. Engl. 31:91, 1962.

143. Naylor, A., Happey, F., Turner, R. L., et al.: Enzymic and immunological activity in the intervertebral disk. Orthop. Clin. North Am. 6:51, 1975.

144. O'Brien, J. P.: The role of fusion for chronic low-back pain. Orthop. Clin. North Am. 14:639–647, 1983.

145. Orgel, L. E.: The maintenance of the accuracy of protein synthesis and its relevance to aging. Proc. Natl. Acad. Sci. U.S.A. 49:517, 1963.

146. Orgel, L. E.: Aging of clones of mammalian cells. Nature 243:441, 1973.

146a. Pearson, C. H., Happey, F., and Naylor, A.: Lysosomal enzymes and degradation of the proteoglycans of the human intervertebral disc. Biochem. J. 129:44–45, 1972.

146b. Price, G. B., Modak, S. P., and Makinodan, T.: Age-associated changes in the DNA of mouse tissue. Science 171:917, 1971.

147. Pritzker, K. P. H.: Aging and degeneration in the lumbar intervertebral disc. Orthop. Clin. North Am. 8:65–76, 1977.

148. Puschel, J.: Der wassengehalf normaler und degenerierter zurachenwirbelscheiben. Beitr. Path. Anat. 84:123, 1930.

149. Quebec Task Force on Spinal Disorders: Scientific approach to the assessment and management of activity related spinal disorders—a monograph for clinicians. Spine 12:S1–S59, 1987.

150. Rashbaum, R. F.: Radiofrequency facet denervation: A treatment alternative in refractory low-back pain with or without leg pain. Orthop. Clin. North Am. 14:569–575, 1983.

151. Raugstad, T., Harbo, K., Hogberg, A., and Skeie, S.: Anterior interbody fusion of the lumbar spine. Acta Orthop. Scand. 53:561–565, 1982.

152. Raynor, R. B.: Disc herniation into a vertebral body. Surg. Neurol. 23:621–625, 1985.

153. Rothman, R. H., and Booth, R.: Failures of spinal fusion. Orthop. Clin. North Am. 6:299–304, 1975.

154. Rothman, R. H., Simeone, F. A., and Bernini, P. M.: Lumbar disc disease. *In* Rothman, R. H., and Simeone, F. A. (eds.): The Spine, Philadelphia, W. B. Saunders, 1982.

155. Sachs, B., et. al.: Dallas discogram description. Spine 12:287–297, 1987.

156. Saunders, J. B., and Inman, V. T.: Pathology of the intervertebral disk. Arch. Surg. 40:389, 1940.

157. Schaerer, J. P.: Radiofrequency facet rhizotomy in the treatment of chronic neck and low-back pain. Int. Surg. 63:53–59, 1978.

158. Schmorl, G., and Junghanns, H.: The human spine in health and disease, 2nd Am. Edn. (transl. from 5th German Ed. by Besemann, E. F.). New York, Grune & Stratton, 1971.

159. Seligman, J., Gertzbein, S., Tile, M., and Kapasouri, A.: Computer analysis of spinal segment motion in degenerative disc disease, with and without axial loading. Spine 9:566–573, 1984.

160. Simmons, E. H., and Segil, C. M.: An evaluation of discography in the localization of symptomatic levels in discogenic disease of the spine. Clin. Orthop. Rel. Res. 108:57–69, 1975.

161. Simons, D. G., and Travell, J. G.: Myofascial origins of low-back pain: 1. Principles of the diagnosis and treatment. Postgrad. Med. 73:66–70, 1983.

162. Simons, D. G., and Travell, J. G.: Myofascial origins of low-back pain: 2. Torso muscles. Postgrad. Med. 73:81–91, 1983.

163. Sims-Williams, H., Jayson, M. I. V., and Baddeley, H.: Small spinal fractures in back pain patients. Ann. Rheum. Dis. 37:262, 1978.

164. Sinclair, D. C., Feindel, W. H., Waddell, G., and Falconer, M. A.: The intervertebral ligaments as a source of segmental pain. J. Bone Joint Surg. 30B:515–521, 1948.
165. Smith, F. P.: Experimental biomechanics of intervertebral disc rupture through a vertebral body. J. Neurosurg. 30:134, 1969.
166. Smyth, M. J., and Wright, V. J.: Sciatica and the intervertebral disc. An experimental study. J. Bone Joint Surg. 40A:1401, 1958.
167. Sorenson, K.: Anterior interbody lumbar spine fusion for incapacitating disc degeneration and spondylolisthesis. Acta Orthop. Scand. 49:269–277, 1978.
168. Spangfort, E. V.: The lumbar disc herniation: A computer-aided analysis of 2,504 operations. Acta Orthop. Scand. (Suppl.)142:1–95, 1972.
169. Spiro, H. M.: Old doctors and old patients. Pharos 51:19–23, 1988.
170. Splithoff, C. A.: Lumbosacral junction roentgenographic comparison of patients with and without backache. J.A.M.A. 152:1610–1613, 1953.
171. Stauffer, R. N., and Coventry, M. B.: Anterior interbody lumbar spine fusion: Analysis of Mayo Clinic series. J. Bone Joint Surg. 54A:756–768, 1972.
172. Stauffer, R. N., and Coventry, M. B.: Posterolateral lumbar-spine fusion: Analysis of Mayo Clinic series. J. Bone Joint Surg. 54A:1195–1204, 1972.
172a. Stockwell, R. A., and Meachim, G.: The chondrocytes. *In* Freeman, M. A. R. (ed.): Adult Articular Cartilage. London, Pittman Medical Publishers, 1973, pp. 51–100.
173. Svensson, H. O., and Andersson, G. B. J.: Low back pain in 40–47-year-old men: Frequency of occurrence and impact on medical services. Scand. J. Rehabil. Med. 14:47–53, 1982.
174. Sweetman, B. J., and Anderson, J. A. D.: Capillary resistance and back pain. Rheumatol. Rehabil. 14:1–6, 1975.
175. Sylven, B.: On the biology of nucleus pulposus. Acta Orthop. Scand. 20:275, 1951.
176. Sylvest, J., Hentzer, B., and Kobayashi, T.: Ultrastructure of prolapsed disc. Acta Orthop. Scand. 48:32, 1977.
177. Szirmai, J. A.: Structure of the intervertebral disc. *In* Balazs, E.A. (ed.): Chemistry and Molecular Biology of the Intercellular Matrix. Vol. 3. London, Academic Press, 1970, pp. 1279–1308.
178. Taylor, T. F. K., and Akeson, W. H.: Intervertebral disc prolapse: A review of morphologic and biochemic knowledge concerning the nature of prolapse. Clin. Orthop. 76:54–79, 1971.
179. Torgerson, W., and Dotter, W.: Comparative roentgenographic study of the asymptomatic and symptomatic lumbar spine. J. Bone Joint Surg. 58A:850–853, 1976.
180. Urban, J. P. G., Holm, S., Maroudas, A., and Nachemson, A.: Nutrition of the intervertebral disc. An in vivo study of solute transport. J. Clin. Orthop. 129:101, 1977.
181. Deleted in press.
182. Urban, J. P. C., Holm, S., Maroudas, A., and Nachemson, A.: Nutrition of the intervertebral disc: Effect of fluid flow on solute transport. Clin. Orthop. 170:296–302, 1982.
183. Van den Hoof, A.: Histological age changes in the annulus fibrosus of the human intervertebral disk. Gerontologia 9:136, 1964.
184. VanHaranta, H., et al.: The relationship of pain provocation to lumbar disc deterioration as seen by CT/Discography. Spine 12:295–298, 1987.
185. Venner, R. M., and Crock, H. V.: Clinical studies of isolated disc resorption in the lumbar spine. J. Bone Joint Surg. 63B:491–494, 1981.
186. Verbiest, H.: Radicular syndrome from developmental narrowing of lumbar vertebral canal. J. Bone Joint Surg. 36B:230–237, 1954.
187. Verbiest, H.: Pathomorphologic aspects of developmental lumbar stenosis. Orthop. Clin. North Am. 6:177–196, 1975.
188. Vernon-Roberts, B.: The pathology and interrelation of intervertebral disc lesions, osteoarthrosis of the apophyseal joints, lumbar spondylosis and low back pain. *In* Jayson, M. I. V. (ed.): The Lumbar Spine and Back Pain. London, Pitman Publishing Limited, 1976.
189. Vernon-Roberts, B.: Degenerative changes in the intervertebral discs and their sequelae. Rheumatol. Rehabil. 16:13, 1977.
190. Vernon-Roberts, B., and Pirie, C. J.: Healing trabecular microfractures in the bodies of lumbar vertebrae. Ann. Rheum. Dis. 32:406, 1973.
191. Weber, H.: Lumbar disc herniation: A prospective study of prognostic factors including a controlled trial: J. Oslo City Hosp. 28:33–64, 1978.
192. Weber, H.: Lumbar disc herniation: A controlled, prospective study with ten years of observation. Spine 8:131–140, 1983.
193. Webster's II: New Riverside University Dictionary. Boston, Houghton-Mifflin, 1984.
194. White, A. A., and Gordon, S. L.: Symposium on Idiopathic Low Back Pain. St. Louis, C. V. Mosby, 1982.
195. Wiesel, S. W., Tsourmas, N., Feffer, H. L., Citrin, C. M., and Patronas, N.: A study of computer-assisted tomography: 1. The incidence of positive CAT scans in an asymptomatic group of patients. Spine 9:549–551, 1984.
196. Wiley, J. J., MacNab, I., and Wortzman, G.: Lumbar discography and its clinical applications. Can. J. Surg. 11:280, 1968.
197. Wiltse, L.: Surgery for intervertebral disc disease of the lumbar spine. Clin. Orthop. 129:22–45, 1977.
198. Witt, I., Vestergaard, A., and Rosenklint, A.: A comparative analysis of x-ray findings of the lumbar spine in patients with and without lumbar pain. Spine 9:298–300, 1984.
199. Wood, P. H. N.: Radiology in the diagnosis of arthritis and rheumatism. Transact. Soc. Occup. Med. 22:69–73, 1972.
200. Wyke, B.: The neurology of low back pain. *In* Jayson, M. I. V. (ed.): The Lumbar Spine and Back Pain, 2nd Ed. London, Pitman Publishing Limited, 1976.

Natural History of the Herniated Disc

Henrik Weber

Low back pain and sciatica have been with us since antiquity. The diagnostic and therapeutic advances through the years have been presented by Schiötz and by Wiltse in their interesting and thorough historical reviews.[57, 79]

The 1934 report of Mixter and Barr is the most important milestone in the history of herniated discs.[44] Recognizing the correlation between sciatic pain and disc protrusion was the first step toward understanding the numerous and obscure clinical spinal pain problems. The discovery of the clinical importance of disc prolapse resulted in a tremendous increase in operative activities to treat patients with any sort of back complaints, often based on vague and doubtful indications. A sufficient number of failures led to the adoption of a more adequate and sensible attitude toward surgery. The importance of evaluating patients with back trouble from several angles was first acknowledged many years later.

The next epoch making step was the comprehension of the clinical importance of the size and shape of the spinal canal.[67, 56, 50] In addition, the discovery and development of improved diagnostic methods and materials, such as less noxious water-soluble contrast media, computed tomography (CT), and magnetic resonance imaging (MRI), have increased the possibilities for evaluation of patients with spinal disorders. Paradoxically, the technologic advances have resulted in a tendency to overdiagnose and misinterpret the findings yielded by these sophisticated methods. To quote Waddell: "The diagnosis of disc prolapse is overused, misused, and abused by both patients and physicians."[69] However, the increased knowledge of the biomechanical, biochemical, and psychologic factors and their relation to the patient's symptoms and signs provides us with more opportunities to understand the clinical picture.

The degenerating process of the intervertebral lumbar disc, resulting in a complete or incomplete herniation, has been studied and described by many authors.[5, 9, 51, 53] Herniations with clinical consequences are most frequent between the ages of 30 and 50 years, probably because of the disappearance of the elastic properties of the nucleus in many elderly individuals in whom the nucleus is desiccated and fibrotic. Mechanical forces, nutritional conditions, chemical changes, constitutional factors, and other more or less unknown components are involved.

The speed of disc protrusion is a variable factor. A disc may bulge after disruption of the inner annular fibers, may be reduced in size for a while, and then may eventually extrude years later. In other individuals, the nucleus of a disc may rapidly break through the weakened annulus, resulting in irreparable damage to the nerve roots. In rare cases, the prolapse may even penetrate the anterior wall of the dura. The clinical picture may vary, from a condition with quiet onset that develops into a long-lasting and disabling condition, to an acute painful attack of sciatica that may present severe neurologic signs or may spontaneously improve without sequelae.

Predisposing factors that are associated with low back pain may be the same as those responsible for the development of disc herniations. Our knowledge of these factors is limited.

A varying number of presacral vertebrae (23 or 25), the presence of symmetric or asymmetric transitional vertebrae, and a particular type and configuration of the lumbar spine have been suggested as possible factors,[56] although these have not been confirmed. The number of presacral vertebrae with cranial or caudal shift and the number of transitional vertebrae in patients with a herniated disc correspond to the distribution of these conditions in a normal population.[78] A narrow spinal canal predisposes one to radicular symptoms in case of a prolapse. Different shapes of the spinal canal seem to be without significance, but a lateral bulging of the disc is more likely to cause symptoms in a trefoil-shaped canal. Nerve roots tethered by dural ligaments, and anomalous roots will more readily be affected by a disc protrusion than will mobile roots.[63]

A greater-than-average height (in men and women) and greater body mass index are found among persons who develop disc prolapse.[25, 34] Although the number of males operated on because of prolapsed discs is twice that of females, there are only slightly more males than females among nonsurgical, probable, and possible cases of prolapse.[30, 33, 37, 61] Occupational risk factors are motor vehicle driving and sedentary work.[35] Smoking and previous full-term pregnancies are also reported risk factors. No particular psychologic features are related to the appearance of the symptomatic disc prolapse.[68]

The underlying mechanism of the back symptoms preceding the radicular pain is unexplained. Pressure on the outer annulus fibers, on the posterior longitudinal ligament, and on the anterior wall of the dural sac may produce pain.[14] Metabolic disturbances in the tissue may be present. An affliction of the fibers from the posterior ramus of the spinal nerve has been suggested. The lesion of the annulus fibrosus may lead to an inflammatory reaction. The role of granulation tissue in the production of pain remains unclear.

DEFINITIONS

Disc herniations are traditionally divided into the following stages:

1. *The protruded or bulging soft disc.* The central mass of the disc has intruding fissures in the ruptured inner fibers of the annulus. The peripheral fibers are still intact.
2. *The extruded disc.* The nuclear material has also penetrated the outer fibers of the annulus, but the prolapsed tissue is connected to the central part of the disc.
3. *The sequestered disc.* One or more free fragments of the herniated mass have escaped into the spinal canal. They may migrate caudally, cranially, or laterally into the intervertebral foramen.

Stage 1 is called an incomplete herniation, whereas Stages 2 and 3 are referred to as complete herniations.[38] Both the size of the prolapse and the direction of the protrusion determine its clinical significance. The symptomatology varies from an asymptomatic condition to a disastrous compression of cauda equina.

DIAGNOSTIC CRITERIA AND TECHNIQUES

The clinical diagnosis is based on the history of the disease, the intensity of pain, characteristics and localization, changes in the spinal posture and mobility, a positive straight-leg raising test (SLR), loss of motor and sensory functions, and reflex abnormalities. A spinal fluid examination may help. Radiologic investigations have decisive value when operative treatment is being considered.

Case History

Most patients who present with symptoms and signs resulting from a ruptured disc have their first attacks of acute low back pain when they are in their twenties.[31, 37, 70, 71] Lifting, falling, slipping, abrupt movement, and heavy work are usually reported as causative factors. Approximately 10 years may pass before the first radicular symptoms appear; they are commonly preceded by back pain for a period of days or weeks. Precipitating factors are rarely observed at this stage. The long interval between the first attack of lumbago and the onset of radiating pain is probably attributable to intradiscal degeneration and regeneration forces, resulting in a maximal risk of disabling sciatica at around the age of 40 years.[61, 70, 71] However, symptomatic disc herniations are also seen in adolescents and people over 50 years of age.[10, 42]

It would be of clinical interest to differentiate between a transitory attack of low back pain and low back pain that is the forerunner of sciatica. Except for the insidious onset without precipitating that is characteristic of the first category, no identifying factors are known. Consequently, any attack of low back pain has to be regarded as a possible first symptom of a disc herniation, particularly in the group between 30 and 50 years of age. This is a problem when manipulation therapy is being considered in patients with lumbago of unknown origin.

More than 90% of the herniated lumbar discs are localized in the fourth and fifth interspaces. Herniations above the fourth level are relatively rare (5% to 10%) but are important to bear in mind. The pain from the fourth lumbar root radiates to the anterior aspect of the thigh. The L5 root pain is felt in the lateral part of the lower leg, in the dorsum of the foot, and toward the big toe. First sacral root pain is localized in the posterior aspect of the thigh, the popliteal space, the calf, the heel, and the lateral aspect of the foot in the fifth toe. Pain resulting from an affliction of the S2 to S4 roots is more inconsistent in its distribution and intensity, although sensory and motor deficits dominate. This alarming clinical condition resulting from cauda equina compression is discussed elsewhere.

As a rule, the root having the same number as the disc in question is not compressed because the lower margin of the vertebral arch lies above the disc in the lumbar region. The extruded mass thus compresses the root of the next number; for example, the L5 root is compressed when the L4–L5 disc is ruptured, and the S1 root is compressed from L5–S1 disc involvement. In rare cases of extreme lateral localization of the prolapse, compression of the root of the corresponding level may occur. Occasionally, a large midline disc herniation may compress several roots of the cauda equina, provoking symptoms and signs distally to the affected level. Polyradicular signs may also be produced by a moderate-size prolapse combined with degenerative hypertrophic bone formation and/or spondylolisthesis. The rare occurrence of a double root at one level and a missing root at a neighboring level may cause diagnostic difficulties.

Pain is the dominating and most disabling symptom in patients suffering from sciatica due to a ruptured disc. The pain intensity influences our attitude toward and management of the situation. However, the description of pain by the patient is not a reliable indication of damage to the nerve root, nor is it a reliable basis for prognosis. Psychologic mechanisms play a great role. Relief from pain in a recumbent position may indicate a favorable prognosis after the operation. The differentiation between referred pain elicited from mesodermal tissue—ligaments, joint capsule, periosteum, and annulus—and root pain may be difficult. Pain localized to the buttock, groin, pelvis, hip and thigh represents such a problem. Injection of local anesthetics under radiographic control, into the relevant facet joint(s) may sometimes clarify the origin of pain. Referred pain is usually poorly localized, dull, and less superficial than root pain. This has been confirmed recently by a detailed study of pain characteristics in patients with operatively verified disc prolapse.[41]

Coughing, sneezing, and pressure under defecation, as a rule, aggravate the radiating pain. The patient sometimes reports a feeling of coldness in the afflicted leg.[23] Other sensory symptoms are tingling, pins and needles, and numbness corresponding to the distribution of the nerve fibers. The patient is often not aware of muscle weakness but usually reports bladder and rectal disturbances.

A neurogenic claudication syndrome may be seen in patients with combined disc herniation and hypertrophic changes of the facet joint.

General Physical Examination

A complete physical examination of the patient is mandatory in patients with back pain and sciatica in order to exclude other causes, such as infections, malignancy, rheumatic diseases, and metabolic disturbances. Rectal examination and palpation of peripheral pulse should always be performed. The patient's mental state and social background are of importance.

The Spine

The spine should be examined in both recumbent and standing positions. The normal lumbar lordosis is often converted to a "straight spine" or even a kyphotic curvature in patients with sciatica. Scoliosis is also present in many cases. These postural changes are of reflex origin and reduce the pain produced by pressure on the nerve root. Contraction of the psoas muscle is partly responsible for the list.[22] In some patients an alternating scoliosis may be demonstrated.

The mobility of the lumbar spine is, as a rule, reduced in patients suffering from sciatica, the reduction being more pronounced in the sagittal plane than in the frontal plane.[70] Restricted spinal mobility is a common sign in low back syndromes of different causes, and its diagnostic value is limited. In disc herniations muscle tenderness in the lumbar region is common, partly because of the spastic contraction of the paraspinal muscles. A deep pressure in the intervertebral space just lateral to the midline may provoke or intensify radicular pain, owing to the increased compression of the underlying root.

Straight-Leg Raising Test (SLR)

This test was described by the French physician E. C. Lasègue (1816 to 1883) and is performed when the patient is supine. The extended leg is slowly elevated until radicular pain is elicited, as a result of the tension on the L5 or S1 nerve root. A positive test result at an angle of 15 to 30 degrees is a reliable sign of a disc prolapse. Pain elicited above 60 degrees elevation is of minor significance.

If the elevation of the leg provokes pain in only the back, buttock or thigh, no definite conclusions can be drawn. A positive SLR test result is often the only consistent finding in adolescents with herniated discs; neurologic deficits are rarer at that age.[19] In older patients, the significance of the test decreases, and a negative result never excludes a prolapse. A crossed positive SLR test result, that is, elevation of the contralateral leg provoking pain in the affected leg, is almost pathognomonic for a herniation.

If the foot is dorsiflexed during elevation of the leg, the pain may be elicited at a lesser angle. The bowstring test is another variant. The leg is raised until pain is elicited. The knee is then flexed, reducing the pain, which again is reinforced by pressure with the finger in the popliteal space.

If the patient is suspected of malingering, one may flex both knee and the hip to 90 degrees and then extend the knee gradually. Alternatively, the knee may be extended while the patient is in the sitting position. A malingering patient will then not report pain, although pain is apparently provoked by elevating the leg in the supine position. Patients with acute lumbago often complain of pain in the back when the examiner elevates the leg a few degrees only.

Motor Deficits

Among the root compression signs, motor deficits require attention because they are of diagnostic and prognostic importance. Figures 1 and 2 show the distribution of muscle groups with paresis registered in 280 hospitalized patients with sciatica resulting from a proven herniation in the 4th and 5th lumbar discs.[70, 72] In L5 root affliction, the weakness was mainly localized in the dorsiflexors of the foot, but in 30% to 40% of the patients other muscle groups were also involved. Similarly, in addition to the weakness of knee flexors and plantar flexor muscles in the S1 root affliction, other muscle groups are also affected in a certain percentage of patients. Slight weakness of the foot may best be discovered when the patient is trying to stand or walk on tiptoe or on heels. The examination of the gluteal muscles should be done in both the recumbent and the standing positions. Palpation of the muscles is important in detecting hypotonia of the gluteus medius in L5 involvement and the gluteus maximus in S1 root affliction.

The muscle weakness may be difficult to demonstrate in cases of severe pain. In our study, the involved muscle groups were

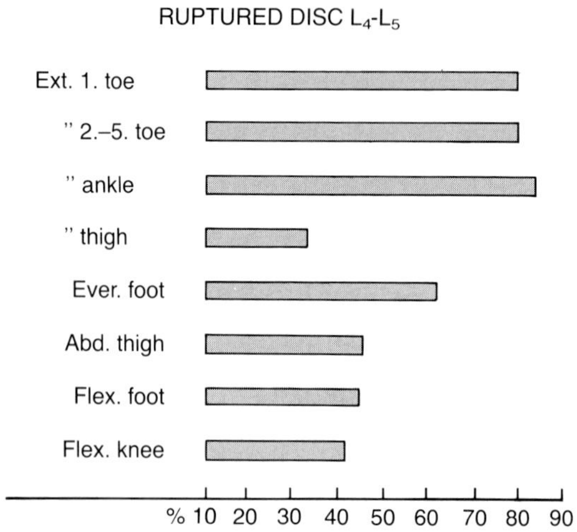

Figure 1 □ The distribution of paretic muscle groups in case of herniation corresponding to the second lowest lumbar disc.

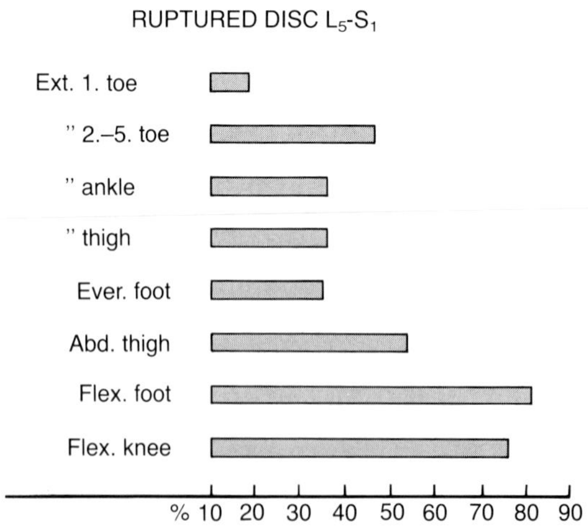

Figure 2 □ The distribution of paretic muscle groups in case of herniation corresponding to the lowest lumbar disc.

tested daily by a conventional manual technique. After 2 weeks with bed rest and, if necessary, analgesic medication, the pain no longer prohibited the performance of quantitative tests.

The maximal isometric strength of the muscle groups of the lower limb was registered with the patient in the horizontal position on an examination couch. The foot was fixed by an inelastic strap to a measurement beam with a built-in strain gauge. The signals were recorded on a moving paper strip. Corresponding muscle groups were examined alternately in the healthy and the afflicted legs. Based on control measurements in healthy persons, the difference in strength between the two legs may normally amount to 20%. Taking this into account, paresis was registered in 537 muscle groups in 133 patients.

In attacks of herniated disc the patient may suddenly note a complete paralysis, for example, of the dorsiflexors of the foot, and the pain may disappear. This symptomatology is a part of the syndrome called *acute back* and requires immediate admission to a neurosurgical department.[39]

Sensory Disturbance

Diminution or loss of cutaneous sensation corresponds to the peripheral distribution of the root fibers. A detailed examination of the different sensory qualities is of help in determining the level of the root lesion. Loss of pain sensation to pin prick (i.e., hypoalgesia or analgesia) should be mapped. In rare cases, a hyperesthesia may be present. In L5 root compression, analgesia or hypoesthesia on the medial portion of the dorsum of the foot and the big toe is most commonly found; in S1 compression, lesions on the lateral aspect of the foot and heel are most common. During the initial stage of sciatica the patients are more concerned about sensory dysfunction and sometimes may not even notice motor deficits as previously mentioned. Loss of joint sensation in the big toe may accompany L5 lesions.

Reflex Changes

Abolished or diminished ankle jerk is often a sign of S1 root compression. An affliction of L5 does not produce any change in reflex, but the knee jerk is reduced in herniation of the L2 and L3 discs.

Autonomic Nervous System

Abnormalities in the bladder function are common in patients with herniated discs. Urologic investigation with cystometry and flow measurements is necessary in many cases. Particularly in the cauda equina compression syndrome, the disorders of micturition and bladder paralysis, together with weakness of sphincter ani, may dominate the clinical picture.

Sensory Evoked Potentials (SEPs)

SEPs have proved to be of clinical value. By means of specific techniques this method can be used to identify the level of affliction and also to distinguish between root pain and referred pain.[15, 32]

Spinal Fluid Examination

A slightly increased protein content may be found as a sign in herniated disc patients. In 200 patients with verified herniated lumbar disc, the mean value was 600 mg/l with a variation of from 200 to 1,500 mg/l.[71] The upper normal limit of cerebrospinal fluid (CSF) protein is 500 mg/l.

Radiologic Examination

Roentgenographic examination of the lumbosacral spine and pelvis is indicated in patients with sciatica of extended duration. Usually, the findings provide no clue to the diagnosis, but may be of help in excluding other diseases of the spine. Myelography, CT, or MRI is necessary if an operation is being considered, in order to confirm the level of a herniation.[1, 12, 19] Because of the availability of modern water-soluble contrast media, the possibility of complications with myelography are remote.[58] Lateral herniations and prolapses in the fifth interspace may, in some patients, be difficult to disclose by means of ordinary myelography. CT combined with a contrast medium may be used in these individuals. Discography has not been applied in our patients.

In patients without actual sciatic pain or other signs, a radiculogram may show contrast defects that indicate a prolapsed disc.[28, 43]

CURRENT TREATMENT OPTIONS VERSUS NATURAL HISTORY

The diversified symptomatology and the unpredictable course of lumbar disc herniations should warn one against a hasty and uncritical acceptance or interpretation of the results of treatment. The duration of an attack, the intensity of the pain, and the number of relapses vary considerably, whereas the size and shape of the prolapse apparently are unchanged. Some patients, according to general consensus, require surgical intervention—as do, for instance, those with cauda equina compression syndrome, progressive pareses, an acute paralysis (drop foot) and intractable pain—provided that the radiologic findings correspond with the symptoms and signs. In numerous patients, on the other hand, bed rest, analgesic tablets, and loving care are efficient therapeutic measures.

The dilemma connected with the choice of treatment arises when symptoms and signs disable the patient for weeks and months, either continuously or frequently recurrent. A great number of therapeutic regimes are available, and many of them are advertised in daily papers, in the weekly press, and on radio and television. So-called alternative medicine flourishes, and the scientific basis of accepted physiotherapy is equivocal or unconfirmed. When the general practitioner, the neurologist, and the specialist in physical medicine are unsuccessful in their attempts to help the patient with a chronic ailment, the patient is easy prey for nonmedical "healers" offering cures such as bone setting, acupuncture, special diets, or herbs.

Patients who for a long period of time are incapacitated with back pain and/or sciatica due to a herniated disc tend to develop mental distress that may increase the disability and create social disturbances.[68, 69]

Most patients with lumbar disc herniations benefit from conservative treatment.

Conservative Treatment

Bed Rest

Pain relief is usually experienced by a patient confined to bed; presumably, relief occurs because of the reduction of intradiscal pressure and reduced activities in the back and abdominal muscles. Immobilization also diminishes the irritation of the nerve root and may improve the intraneural blood flow.[29, 47, 54]

Any position in bed is acceptable if it provides satisfactory pain relief. A supine position with the knees and hip flexed is probably the optimal one. The mattress should be firm but not hard. A board may be placed under a too-soft mattress. The duration of strict bed rest is a matter for discussion. One week is probably the shortest recommended time, and 2 weeks the longest. Toilet visits should be allowed, partly because many patients have problems with bladder and bowel function in bed and partly because motor weakness may thereby be more easily diagnosed.

The negative side effects of inactivity are obvious. Some patients complain of a temporary increase in back and radicular pain when confined to bed. In these instances, alternative rest and ambulation are an acceptable solution.

Back School

In 1972, Marianne Zachrisson-Forsell in Sweden introduced the idea of giving structured information to patients with low back pain and sciatica—the so-called "back school."[81] There is no doubt that a greater knowledge of etiology, symptomatology, and therapeutic methods is a supportive measure in the treatment program and may change the patient's attitude toward the illness. However, this presentation of medical facts is a difficult task and requires preparation and skill on the part of the teacher.

Medication

The relief of pain in the initial acute stage is important both for the comfort of the patient and for the physical and neurologic examination. Habit-forming drugs should not be used. The following drugs may be considered:

- Analgesics
- Psychoactive drugs
- Steroids
- Nonsteroidal anti-inflammatory drugs (NSAID)

Acetylsalicylic acid and paracetamol are the first drugs of choice. A combination with codeine is often used, but the small quantities of codeine have hardly any effect. In cases of severe pain, an addition of neuroleptic or psychoactive drugs may be efficient. Diazepam and levomepromazine have been compared in patients with severe radicular pain.[74] The effect was similar, but diazepam produced more side effects. In the author's experience, a combination of paracetamol and levomepromazine provides sufficient relief from pain in most patients. Levomepromazine has a sedative, muscle-relaxing, and analgesic effect and is not habit forming. Individual determinations of dosage are necessary.

Antidepressive drugs are not indicated in acute attacks, but they may reduce the need for analgesics in patients who have chronic pain.[49]

No study has convincingly shown any effect of systemic use of steroids on nerve root pain. The effect of an epidural injection of steroids in patients with herniated discs is a matter of dispute.[7, 60] A combination of steroids and morphine injected extradurally has also been suggested in cases of intractable pain, but the pain relief is short and complications may occur.[11, 52]

The effects of NSAID such as diflunisal, oxyphenbutazone, and phenylbutazone have been evaluated in controlled studies, with questionable results.[64, 75, 76]

Physiotherapy

Numerous physiotherapeutic methods are available for patients with sciatica resulting from a herniated lumbar disc. A horniated nucleus pulposus from a ruptured disc can never be pushed back into place.[1]

Traction therapy is frequently recommended and prescribed. There are several techniques, both passive and active, by which a traction force can be applied on the lumbar spine. Traction is used in acute as well as chronic cases. Bed rest for a few hours after the treatment has been suggested. If pain is provoked or aggravated during traction, the procedure should immediately be discontinued.

Manipulation is defined as an attempt to achieve specific spinal adjustment by means of a manual thrust directed at any bony spinal process. This method is contraindicated in patients who have root afflictions. No study has convincingly shown any effect of this treatment, except for a temporary relief in some patients with acute lumbago. We have registered too many patients admitted into the hospital with radicular symptoms and signs provoked or aggravated in connection with a manipulative thrust. Several reports have been published about root damage, even cauda equina lesions, after such treatment.[40, 57] The lack of evidence of positive effects, in addition to the risk of damage, should be reason enough to avoid manipulation in patients with suspected herniated discs.

Exercises, in the acute stage of sciatica, do more harm than good. Even isometric muscle contractions of the abdominal and paraspinal muscles increase the intradiscal pressure. In the rehabilitation period or in cases of long-lasting sciatica, exercises performed within the limit of tolerable root pain may be indicated for psychologic reasons and in order to improve the physical fitness. Swimming, moderate dancing (not rock!), skiing, and hiking in the woods may be beneficial. Physical activity does not prevent relapses of radicular symptoms in patients with herniated discs but may improve the results after conservative or surgical therapy.[70]

Massage can be performed in many ways. Some muscle relaxation may be achieved, but many patients admitted to our hospital complain about increased pain after such treatment.

Thermotherapy is also of modest importance. An ordinary hot bath usually produces a comfortable feeling, but heat may also exacerbate the pain. In chronic cases of herniated disc, both ice and heat application may be adjuvant therapies and may reduce the consumption of analgesics.

Electrotherapy, short-wave treatment, and ultrasound treatment are contraindicated.

Injections of local anesthetics, alone or in combination with steroids, in tender spots in the gluteal or trochanter regions have been used without any proof of a lasting effect.

Acupuncture may provide temporary pain relief in some patients, but it has not been used in our department.

Supporting appliances such as corsets, belts, or braces are also used in acute cases but are more useful in instances of chronic low back pain. Most patients with sciatica report relief, but some patients complain of increased pain.

Surgical Therapy

Absolute indications for operative intervention are mentioned in the introduction of this chapter.

The attitude with regard to surgical treatment of herniated discs varies considerably around the world, within the same country, and among departments of different specialties. This discrepancy shows that indications for surgical therapy are not based on scientific observation. In a prospective, controlled trial of a large series of patients with herniated L4–L5 and L5–S1 discs some years ago, this author discussed important variables to be considered in making the decision to operate.[73]

Chemonucleolysis

This method, which may be characterized as semiconservative, was introduced by Lyman Smith in 1963.[59] The enzyme chymopapain is injected percutaneously into the center of the disc in patients with bulging disc herniations. In cooperation with the Neuroradiological Department of Ullevål Hospital, a group of patients has been treated with this technique during the last 2 years (see Results, below).

THE RESULTS OF TREATMENT

Results of treatment for herniated discs are difficult to evaluate. The selection of patients always depends on the attitude and personal experience of the physician or surgeon. A number of variables in the somatic and mental constitution of the patients and in the social context have important effects on the results. The dominant symptom, pain, is difficult to measure. The natural history of the disease varies widely. The duration of symptoms before the beginning of treatment is significant. Directing different questionnaires to the same group of patients may influence the replies. Results are also dependent on the length of the observation period. The choice of control groups and control therapy may be problematic, owing to ethical and practical reasons. In spite of all the difficulties, objective evaluation is possible if we follow the guidelines described in the editorial in Spine, 1987.[8, 45]

Conservative therapy, including bed rest, information (back school), and analgesic drugs, is generally accepted as adequate treatment in the beginning of an attack of sciatica.

No convincing proof exists that any physiotherapeutic method may change the natural course of a herniated disc disease in a positive way. Traction therapy has been recommended and used for years, and favorable results are reported. However, no controlled study is published showing any definite ameliorative effect of the treatment. On the contrary, four controlled studies on patients with proven herniated disc, performed with four different traction methods, could not demonstrate any effect compared with the results in the control group.[77] The only useful information was that patients who experienced pain relief during traction seemed to have a greater chance of avoiding surgery. A few patients deteriorated temporarily during the treatment. Complications after traction therapy are reported.[17]

A temporary symptomatic effect may be achieved by numerous therapeutic methods, including placebo.[6]

The effect of NSAID and epidural injections of steroids are doubtful.

Several authors have published their results of conservative therapy; as a rule, these are retrospective studies.[21, 26, 48, 61] No uniform conclusion can be drawn.

A retrospective comparison of long-term results of conservative and surgical treatment has failed to show any significant difference.[24, 46] Presumably, patients with the most severe cases in these series have been submitted to surgery, thus invalidating an unbiased evaluation.

Some authors have compared the effects of chemonucleolysis and surgical treatment, but the series are relatively small. In prospective controlled studies, Crawshaw and colleagues and Ejeskär and Nachemson reported much better results in patients who underwent operation than in patients treated with intradiscal injections of chymopapain.[13, 18] Patients operated on after failure of chemonucleolysis have a less satisfactory outcome than was expected compared with a group of patients who underwent operation as a primary treatment. If a discography with water-soluble contrast is performed before the chymopapain injection, it seems that a high concentration of the contrast agent within the prolapse improves the results.[16]

Ahchong and colleagues have studied prognostic factors for low back pain with sciatica in 107 patients.[2] Of them, 62 were supposed to have a 91% chance of being successfully treated with conservative measures, whereas 18 other patients had an 89% chance of cure with a surgical intervention. Nine discriminating factors were listed; among them were duration of severe symptoms of more than 2 months, recognizable pain pattern, and presence of scoliosis.

The authors concluded that no single factor can be relied upon in clinical practice. However, the more adverse factors a patient possessed, the higher was the probability of the need for surgery.

Four other studies have shown that the results of surgery deteriorate if the radicular symptoms have lasted for 2 or 3 months.[27, 55, 65, 70]

The author's experience with prospective, controlled investigations will be briefly summarized.[70, 73] In 1970 to 1971, 280 patients with symptomatic herniated discs were consecutively admitted to the Neurological Department, Ullevål Hospital. After 14 days of observation, the majority of the patients were divided into three groups. A few required immediate operation because of severe neurologic signs. One group of 126 patients presented doubtful or uncertain indications for surgical treatment. All these patients consented to participate in a controlled study. The therapy was decided by randomization to either a conservative group or a surgical treatment group. This series of patients have been followed for 10 years.

Another group comprising 67 patients, including those with "acute back" and those operated on immediately, required surgical therapy. The third group with 87 patients had no indication for operative intervention and was treated conservatively. All groups were re-examined after 1 and 4 years.

The controlled study was shown that surgery is superior to conservative therapy if the results are evaluated after 1 year. During the following 9 years, the conservatively treated patients improved, and after 10 years no difference between the results of the operated group and the conservatively treated group could be observed. However, 17 patients within the group allotted to conservative therapy had to be operated on within the first year of observation because of intolerable pain. Thus, only if patients with unsatisfactory improvement by conservative therapy are operated on, may the ultimate results of conservative and operative treatment be characterized as equal.

The number of relapses during the first 4 years of observation was less among the operated patients than among the conservatively treated group. During 10 years of observation, approximately 20% of all the patients had reported relapses with a large variation in duration, although they were mainly temporary.

An analysis of 23 variables provided no information that could be used as guidelines for choosing therapy. The patients with good results from conservative therapy improved within 3 months, which may be regarded as a suitable period of time for observation in doubtful cases before surgery.

Pareses were observed in 32 patients who were operated on and in 31 who had conservative therapy. At the follow-up examination after 1 year, the restitution of muscle strength was unrelated to type of treatment. The improvement of muscle strength continued during the next 9 years of observation, at the end of which pareses were demonstrable in only five patients. No patient was made unable to work by muscle weakness during the observation period. Therefore, the prognosis of motor deficits is good and unrelated to type of treatment, and moderate pareses are not an indication for surgery.

In the total group of 280 female patients over 50 years of age, psychosocial problems, physical inactivity at leisure, a narrow spinal canal, and a duration of incapacity of more than 3 months are factors related to poor results. These findings are partly confirmed by other authors.[36, 38, 66, 80]

The author has also recorded the results after 1 year of chymopapain injections in 85 patients with sciatica due to verified herniated discs. The patients were below the age of 50, only one disc was affected, there were no psychosocial problems and no cauda equina compression symptoms. The duration of radicular pain was less than 6 months. All were examined by CT and radiculography with water-soluble contrast media. A satisfactory result was obtained in approximately two thirds of the patients, a result that had also been achieved by conservative treatment in the previously referred-to study. But the two series are not comparable. Twenty-two cases were operated on within 6 to 8 weeks after failure of the chymopapain treatment, with satisfactory results in only 60%, compared with 90% in an analogous group of patients who underwent operation as a primary treatment. In the author's limited experience, the results of chemonucleolysis are not very encouraging, compared with traditional methods.

THE AUTHOR'S CURRENT APPROACH

The author's opinion regarding the main points in the case history and the general physical and neurologic examination has been expressed in the previous discussions.

In order to better evaluate the localization and character of the pain, a visual analog scale and pain drawings are used. It should be emphasized that the examination of the spine and the nervous system requires that the patient be undressed.

When the indications for immediate surgical intervention are excluded, strict bed rest for 1 week is recommended, but the patient is allowed to use the toilet. Information about the disease is given. During the next week, mobilization is started slowly and cautiously. If necessary, salicylates or paracetamol are prescribed, occasionally in combination with psychoactive drugs such as levomepromazine or diazepam. An antiobstipation regimen is often necessary. Assistive appliances such as crutches, belts, or corsets may be needed.

No further investigation is done at this stage. Regular telephone contact is obligatory if the patient is treated as an outpatient. A second examination takes place after 2 weeks, and if the improvement is satisfactory a physiotherapist may take over the instruction and control.

During the period of bed rest, light isometric exercises may be performed within the pain limit. Any subsequent increase in physical activity will depend on a reduction of the radiating pain. The radiating pain should have disappeared before the patient returns to work; in the beginning, the return should be only part time. Manual traction may be considered in the acute stage in order to relieve pain temporarily. Other physiotherapy is of no avail.

If the conservative regimen does not provide satisfactory improvement within 3 to 4 weeks, supplementary investigations such as x-ray examination and tests to exclude rheumatologic, malignant, and infectious diseases are indicated. Skeletal scintigraphy may be useful. In patients below the age of 25 to 30 years with a single root affliction, CT is recommended as the first additional neuroradiologic investigation. This method provides sufficient confirmation of a clinically suspected prolapse. In patients above this age, radiculography is, as a rule, necessary before surgical intervention and may also be performed in outpatients. If the result is equivocal, contrast-enhanced CT may supply the final answer. The spinal fluid sample should also be analyzed in obscure cases for virus and *Borrelia* infections. The combination of CT with discography has been introduced and may be included in our armamentarium.

Sensory evoked potentials (SEP) may distinguish between root affliction and referred pain.

Surgical treatment or chemonucleolysis is considered if the symptoms and signs persist for several weeks and especially when the pain is intolerable. The decision to operate is made in cooperation with the neurosurgeon, the neuroradiologist, and the physiotherapist. After presentation of the findings at the conference, the situation is explained to the patient, who has to make the final decision. When chemonucleolysis has been considered, the same procedure is used. A shorter period of preoperative observation is recommended for patients with psychosocial problems.

There is no age limit for surgery, and even patients above 70 years of age have been operated on with good results. Chemonucleolysis is never performed in patients over 50 years of age. An increasing number and duration of recurrences speak in favor of operative treatment. Patients with chronic sciatica after an unsuccessful operation are treated in accordance with the principles suggested by Waddell and associates.[68]

WHAT DOES THE FUTURE HOLD, AND WHAT STUDIES ARE NEEDED?

For the future, we may rely upon a deeper knowledge of spinal diseases derived from basic research. The normal structural and biophysical properties of the cartilage in general, and of the intervertebral disc in particular; the immunologic processes; and the metabolic reactions are all fruitful fields of investigation. More elaborate biomechanical models and methods of recording will be developed. The relationship of so-called instability of the spine to the herniation of the nucleus pulposus is important.

In regard to clinical research, we need a more reliable foundation for the choice of treatment. That goal can be attained only by controlled, prospective studies with which no element of economic interest should be allowed to interfere. The methods of imaging are steadily improving and may perhaps bring us to a stage when a herniation will be predicted and prevented.

References

1. Adams, M. A., and Hutton, W. C.: Prolapsed intervertebral disc. A hyperflexion injury. Spine 7:184–191, 1981.
2. Ahchong, A. K., Teather, D., and Quinell, R. C.: Prognostic indicators for low back pain with sciatica. (Unpublished data.)
3. Amundsen, P., Helsingen, P., and Kristiansen, K.: Evaluation of lumbar radiculography ("myelography") with water-soluble contrast media. Acta Radiol. 1:659–665, 1963.
4. Andersson, J. G., Örtengren, R., and Nachemson, A.: Intradiscal pressure, intra-abdominal pressure and myoelectric back muscle activity related to posture and loading. Clin. Orthop. Rel. Res. 129:156–164, 1977.
5. Armstrong, J. R.: Lumbar Disc Lesions. Baltimore, Williams & Wilkins, 1965.
6. Beecher, H. K.: Surgery as placebo. J.A.M.A. 176:1102–1107, 1961.
7. Benzon, H. T.: Epidural steroid injection for low back pain and lumbo-sacral radiculopathy. Pain 24:277–295, 1986.
8. Bloch, M. D.: Methodology in clinical back pain trials. Spine 12:430–432, 1987.
9. Brown, M. D.: Intradiscal Therapy. Chymopapain or Collagenase. Chicago, Year Book Medical Publishers, 1983.
10. Cartier Giroux, J., and Leclercq, T. A.: Lumbar disc excision in the second decade. Spine 7:168–170, 1982.
11. Cohn, M. L., Huntington, C. T., Byrd, S. E., et al.: Epidural morphine and methylprednisolone. New therapy for recurrent low-back pain. Spine 11:960–963, 1986.
12. Cook, P. L., and Wise, K.: A correlation of the surgical and radiographic findings in lumbar disc herniation. Clin. Radiol. 30:671–682, 1979.
13. Crawshaw, C., Frazer, A. M., Merriam, W. F., et al.: A comparison of surgery and chemonucleolysis in the treatment of sciatica: A prospective randomized trial. Spine 9:194–196, 1984.
14. Cyriax, J.: Dural pain. Lancet 1:919–921, 1978.
15. Dvonch, V., Scharff, T., Wilton, H. B., et al.: Dermatomal somatosensory evoked potentials: Their use in lumbar radiculopathy. Spine 9:291–293, 1984.
16. Edwards, W. C., Orme, T. J., and Orr-Edwards, G.: CT-discography: prognostic value in the selection of patients for chemonucleolysis. Spine 12:792–795, 1987.
17. Eie, N., and Kristiansen, K.: Complications and hazards of traction in the treatment of ruptured lumbar intervertebral disks. J. Oslo City Hosp. 12:5–12, 1962.
18. Ejeskär, A., and Nachemson, A.: Surgery versus chemonucleolysis for herniated lumbar discs. Clin. Orthop. Rel. Res. 174:236–242, 1983.
19. Epstein, J. A., Epstein, N., Marc, J., et al.: Lumbar intervertebral disk herniation in teenage children: Recognition and management of associated anomalies. Spine 9:427–432, 1984.
20. Espersen, J. O., Kosteljanetz, M., Halaburt, H., and Miletic, T.: Predictive value of radiculography in patients with lumbago-sciatica. A prospective study (Part II). Acta Neurochir. 73:213–221, 1984.
21. Frantzen, E., and Zacharie, L.: The effect of conservative treatment of lumbago-sciatica. Nord. Med. 69:1509–1512, 1959.
22. Grieve, G. P.: Treating backache—a topical comment. Physiotherapy 69:316, 1983.
23. Hakelius, A., Nilsonne, U., Pernow, B., and Zetterqvist, S.: The cold sciatic leg. Acta Orthop. Scand. 40:614–623, 1969.
24. Hakelius, A.: Diagnosis in sciatica. A clinical follow up of surgical and non-surgical treatment. Acta Orthop. Scand. (Suppl.)129:1–51, 1970.
25. Heliövaara, M.: Body height, obesity, and risk of herniated lumbar intervertebral disc. Spine 12:469–472, 1987.
26. Henderson, R. S.: The treatment of lumbar intervertebral disk protrusion. An assessment of conservative measures. Br. Med. J. 2:597–598, 1952.
27. Hentzner, L. A.: Conservative and operative treatment for disk prolapse. A follow-up examination of 152 patients. Ugeskrift Laeger 135:2258–2262, 1973.
28. Hitselberger, W. E., and Wetten, R. M.: Abnormal myelograms in asymptomatic patients. J. Neurosurg. 28:204–206, 1968.
29. Howe, J. F., Loeser, J. D., and Calvin, W. H.: Mechanosensitivity of dorsal root ganglia and chronically injured axons: A physiological basis for the radicular pain of nerve root compression. Pain 3:25–41, 1977.
30. Hudgins, W. R.: Computer-aided diagnosis of lumbar disc herniation. Spine 8:604–615, 1983.
31. Hult, L.: The "Munckfors Investigation." Acta Orthop. Scand. (Suppl)16, 17:1954.
32. Keim, H. A., Hajdu, M., Gonzales, E. G., et al.: Somatosensory evoked potentials as an aid in the diagnosis and intraoperative management of spinal stenosis. Spine 10:338–344, 1985.
33. Kelsey, J. L.: An epidemiological study of acute herniated lumbar intervertebral disc. Rheumatol. Rehabil. 14:144–159, 1975.
34. Kelsey, J. L., and Ostfeld, A. M.: Demographic characteristics of persons with acute herniated lumbar intervertebral disc. J. Chron. Dis. 28:37–50, 1975.
35. Kelsey, J. L.: An epidemiological study of the relationship between occupations and acute herniated lumbar intervertebral discs. Int. J. Epidemiol. 4:197–204, 1975.
36. Kogstad, O., and Pedersen, B. B.: Operasjon eller konservativ behandling av lumbalt skiveprolaps? Tidsskr. Nor. Laegeforen. 98:1381–1383, 1978.
37. Kogstad, O., and Gudmundsen, J.: Low back pain.

An epidemiological study. Tidsskr. Nor. Laegeforen. 98:1076–1079, 1978.
38. Kosteljanetz, M., Espersen, J. O., Halaburt, H., and Miletic, T.: Predictive value of clinical and surgical findings in patients with lumbago-sciatica. A prospective study (Part I). Acta Neurochir. 73:67–76, 1984.
39. Kristiansen, K.: "Akutt rygg." Nord. Med. 52:1449–1450, 1984.
40. Ladermann, J. P.: Accidents of spinal manipulation. Ann. Swiss Chiropract. Assoc. (Neuchatel) 7:161–169, 1981.
41. Ljunggren, A. E., Jacobsen, T., and Osvik, A.: Pain descriptions as diagnostic predictors verified by surgical findings on removal of herniated lumbar intervertebral discs. Pain 16:265–276, 1983.
42. Maistrelli, G. L., Vaughan, P. A., Evans, D. C., and Barrington, T. W.: Lumbar disc herniation in the elderly. Spine 12:63–66, 1987.
43. McRae, D. L.: Asymptomatic intervertebral disc protrusions. Acta Radiol. 46:9–27, 1986.
44. Mixter, W. J., and Barr, J. S.: Rupture of the intervertebral disc with involvement of the spinal canal. N. Engl. J. Med. 211:210, 1934.
45. Nachemson, A. L., and LaRocca, H.: Editorial. Spine 12:427–429, 1987.
46. Nashold, B. S., and Hrubec, Z.: Lumbar Disc Disease. A Twenty-Year Follow-Up Study. St. Louis, C. V. Mosby, 1971.
47. Parke, W. W., and Watanabe, R.: The intrinsic vasculature of the lumbosacral spinal nerve roots. Spine 10:508–515, 1985.
48. Pearce, J., and Moll, J. M. H.: Conservative treatment and natural history of acute lumbar disc lesions. J. Neurol. Neurosurg. Psychiatr. 30:3–17, 1967.
49. Pheasant, H., Bursk, A., Goldfarb, J., et al.: Amitriptyline and chronic low-back pain. A randomized double-blind, crossover study. Spine 8:552–557, 1983.
50. Porter, R. W., Hibbert, C., and Wellman, P.: Backache and the lumbar spinal canal. Spine 5:99–105, 1980.
51. Porter, R. W.: Management of Back Pain. New York, Churchill Livingstone, 1986.
52. Rocco, A., Frank, E., Reisman, R., et al.: A Double-Blind Comparison of Epidural Steroids and Epidural Steroids Combined with Morphine in the Treatment of Recurrent Low Back Pain. Department of Anaesthesia, Brigham and Women's Hospital, Harvard Medical School. Boston, Massachusetts, 1987.
53. Rothman, R. H., and Simeone, F. A.: The Spine, 2nd Ed. Philadelphia, W. B. Saunders, 1982.
54. Rydevik, B., Brown, M. D., and Lundborg, G.: Pathoanatomy and pathophysiology of nerve root compression. Spine 9:7–15, 1984.
55. Salenius, P., and Laurent, L. E.: Results of operative treatment of lumbar disc herniation. Acta Orthop. Scand. 48:630–634, 1977.
56. Sand, P. G.: The Human Lumbo-Sacral Vertebral Column. An Osteometric Study (Thesis). Universitetsforlaget, Oslo, 1970.
57. Schiötz, E. H., and Cyriax, J.: Manipulation. Past and Present. London, William Heinemann Medical Books Ltd., 1975.
58. Skalpe, I. O., and Amundsen, P.: Lumbar radiculography with metrizamide. Radiology 115:91–95, 1975.
59. Smith, L., Garvin, P. J., and Jennings, R. B.: Enzyme dissolution of the nucleus pulposus. Nature 198:1311, 1963.
60. Snoek, W., Weber, H., and Jörgensen, B.: Double blind evaluation of extradural methyl prednisolone for herniated lumbar discs. Acta Orthop. Scand. 48:635–641, 1977.
61. Spangfort, E. V.: The lumbar disc herniation. A computer-aided analysis of 2,504 Operations. Acta Orthop. Scand. (Suppl.)142:61–77, 1972.
62. Sparup, K. H.: Late prognosis in lumbar disc herniation (Thesis). Copenhagen, 1960.
63. Spencer, D. L., Irwin, G. S., and Miller, J. A. A.: Anatomy and significance of fixation of the lumbosacral nerve roots in sciatica. Spine 8:672–679, 1983.
64. Standnes, B., and Weber, H.: Evaluation of the analgetic effect of diflunisal on patients with severe radicular pain. J. Oslo City Hosp. 31:137–139, 1981.
65. Surin, V.: Duration of disability following lumbar disc surgery. Acta Orthop. Scand. 48:466–471, 1977.
66. Thomas, M., Marshall, J., Grant, N., and Stevens, J.: Surgical treatment of low backache and sciatica. Lancet Dec. 24–31:1437–1439, 1983.
67. Verbiest, H.: A radicular syndrome from developmment narrowing of the lumbar vertebral canal. J. Bone Joint Surg. 36B:230–237, 1954.
68. Waddell, G., Main, C. J., Morris, E. W., et al.: Normality and reliability in the clinical assessment of backache. Br. Med. J. 284:1519–1523, 1982.
69. Waddell, G.: Clinical assessment of lumbar impairment. Clin. Orthop. Rel. Res. 221:110–120, 1987.
70. Weber, H.: Lumbar disc herniation. A prospective study of prognostic factors including a controlled trial (Thesis). Oslo, 1978.
71. Weber, H.: An evaluation of conservative and surgical treatment of lumbar disc protrusion. J. Oslo City Hosp. 20:81–93, 1970.
72. Weber, H.: The effect of delayed disc surgery on muscular pareses. Acta Orthop. Scand. 46:631–642, 1975.
73. Weber, H.: Lumbar disc herniation. A controlled, prospective study with ten years of observation. Spine 8:131–140, 1983.
74. Weber, H.: Comparison of the effect of diazepam and levomepromazine on pain in patients with acute lumbago-sciatica. J. Oslo City Hosp. 30:65–80, 1980.
75. Weber, H., and Aasand, G.: The effect of phenylbutazone on patients with acute lumbago-sciatica. J. Oslo City Hosp. 30:69–72, 1980.
76. Weber, H., and Økseter, K.: Antiflogistikabehandling av Pasien med Skivebetinget Ischias. Informa Geigy, 1978, pp. 41–44.
77. Weber, H., Ljunggren, A. E., and Walker, L.: Traction therapy in patients with herniated intervertebral lumbar disc. J. Oslo City Hosp. 34:61–70, 1984.
78. Wigh, R. E., and Anthony, H. F.: Transitional lumbosacral discs. Probability of herniation. Spine 6:168–171, 1981.
79. Wiltse, L. L.: History of surgery of the lumbar spine. Personal communication, 1986.
80. Wiltse, L. L., and Rocchio, P. D.: Preoperative psychologic tests as predictors of success of chemonucleolysis in the treatment of the low-back syndrome. J. Bone Joint Surg. 57A:478–483, 1975.
81. Zachrisson, M.: The low back pain school. Danderyd Hospital. Danderyd, Sweden, 1972.

☐ Surgical Indications and Techniques

John A. McCulloch
Shun-ichi Inoue
Hideshige Moriya
Kazuhisa Takahashi
Keiichi Takata

Sciatica, as a symptom, had been around for centuries before Mixter and Barr[29] published their now famous paper describing a "ruptured intervertebral disc" as its cause. Numerous authors before proposed various causes of sciatica,[5] but it was the article of Mixter and Barr that established the so-called dynasty of the disc (Table 1). To the unsophisticated, all leg pain was considered to be sciatica due to a ruptured disc, and the rush was on to excise the offending disc. Myelography with its false-negative rate (low sensitivity) at L5–S1 and its false-positive rate (low specificity) at L4–L5 did little to help sort out the various causes of sciatica. It took Verbiest,[42] rejected by his neurosurgical colleagues, but persistent to the point of publishing in the *Journal of Bone and Joint Surgery*, to call our attention to bony encroachment of nerve roots as a source of sciatic discomfort. The recent advances in computed tomography (CT) and magnetic resonance imaging (MRI) and a better understanding of the causes of leg pain have presented spinal surgeons with the opportunity to make consistently accurate diagnosis of the patient's symptom-producing disorders. Now it is truly within the surgeon's control to deliver consistently good results with surgical intervention. We are entering the age of a new standard for surgery used to treat patients with a herniated nucleus pulposus (HNP), which is characterized by the following:

Table 1 ☐ Historical Stages in Development of Lumbar Disc Surgery

STAGE I: CLINICAL DESCRIPTION OF SCIATICA	
Hippocrates (400 BC)— (Athens)	early description of sciatica
Cotugno (1764)[4]— (Italy)	accurate description of sciatica versus hip disease
Lasègue (1864)[25]— (France)	first description of tension signs
Goldthwait (1911)[12]— (Harvard, United States)	proposed that sciatica was due to an HNP
STAGE II: SURGICAL DESCRIPTION OF HNP	
Mixter and Barr (1934)[29]— (Harvard, United States)	described the surgical removal of an HNP
STAGE III: REFINEMENT OF SURGICAL TECHNIQUE	
Love (1934, 1939)[27]— (Mayo, United States)	described extradural removal of HNP, proposed limited surgical exposure
Lane and Moore (1948)[23]— (United States)	anterior approach to lumbar spine
Yasargil (1977)[48]— (Switzerland)	microsurgical lumbar discectomy
Williams (1978)[45]— (United States)	microsurgical lumbar discectomy
Caspar (1977)[3]— (West Germany)	microsurgical lumbar discectomy
STAGE IV: THE ERA OF MORE ACCURATE DIAGNOSES	
Verbiest (1977)[42]— (Holland)	bony encroachment of the nerve root
STAGE V: THE DECADE OF THE 1980s—Refinement in CT and MRI	

1. An accurate diagnosis of the pathologic condition as well as of its exact location.
2. Limited surgical intervention.
3. Limited complications.
4. An 85% success rate.
5. A return-to-work rate of 95%.

Against this background, the following section is written. Table 1 summarizes the historical stages in the development of lumbar disc surgery.

TERMINOLOGY

A normal disc is nonpainful. Motion can occur through the disc space, its outer annular rim can be touched with a needle at the time of discography, and it can be distended by discographic testing, without the production of pain. Abnormal discs are not necessarily painful. Many patients with disc degeneration can move their lumbar spines without pain and do not necessarily complain of pain at the time of discography. What causes pain to radiate down the sciatic nerve is truly an enigma.

Two basic syndromes occur in lumbar degenerative disc disease. The first, *instability*, is covered elsewhere in this book (see Posterior Spine Fusion, later in this chapter). The second, *encroachment*, is the topic of this chapter.

Encroachment of a lumbar nerve root implies the following:

1. Distortion of the normal anatomy exists, such that the contours of the spinal canal are altered by a disc herniation, an osteophyte, or ligamentum hypertrophy.
2. Contact occurs between the distorted anatomy and the neurologic contents of the spinal canal.
3. The encroachment on nerve root territory is chronic; that is, it occurs continuously over days, weeks, or months, rather than momentarily.
4. The segment in which these phenomena are present is mobile; encroachment syndromes do not occur at nonmobile levels.

The distortion of the annular contour that occurs because of a disc herniation may be as follows:

1. Contained. This is a simple disc protrusion in which the annular fibers are intact and contain the protruded nuclear material (Fig. 1).
2. Noncontained. Disc material has ruptured through the annulus and is no longer contained. The following two varieties occur:

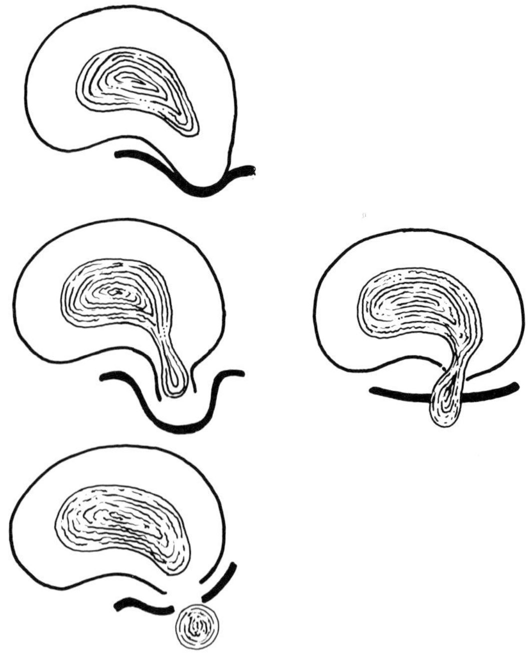

Figure 1 □ Top shows a contained disc protrusion. The middle left shows a noncontained subligamentous disc extrusion. On the middle right is a noncontained transligamentous disc extrusion. A noncontained disc sequestration is shown at the bottom.

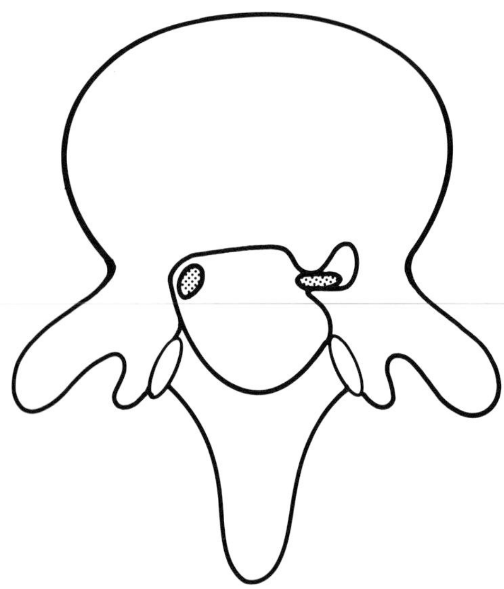

Figure 2 □ Schematic illustration of an axial computed tomographic (CT) scan showing a nerve root as the "sandwich filler" between a herniated nucleus pulposus (HNP) anteriorly and osteophyte posteriorly.

Table 2 □ Criteria for the Diagnosis of the Acute Radicular Syndrome (Sciatica due to an HNP)

1. Leg pain (including buttock) is the dominant complaint, rather than back pain.
2. Neurologic symptoms are specific (e.g., paresthesia in a typical dermatomal distribution).
3. Significant straight-leg raising (SLR) changes occur: (a) SLR less than 50% of normal, (b) Bowstring discomfort, (c)Crossover pain (any one or a combination of these).
4. Neurologic signs: 2 out of 4 of weakness, wasting, sensory loss, or reflex alteration.

Three or four of these criteria must be present, the only exception being the young patients who are very resistant to the effects of nerve root compression and thus may not have neurologic symptoms (Criterion 2) or signs (Criterion 4).

a. Extruded disc material—subligamentous (subannular) or transligamentous.
b. Sequestered—free fragment of disc material in the spinal canal.

The effect of a disc herniation on a nerve root can be magnified if subarticular stenosis is present. The nerve root then becomes the "sandwich filler" between the disc herniation in front and the subarticular stenosis behind (Fig. 2).

The symptoms of nerve root encroachment are tremendously variable. They depend on the patient's age, the degree of root compression, the place on the nerve root/dorsal root ganglion complex at which the pressure is occurring, and the types of resultant pathologic changes around and within the nerve root (see Etiology of Sciatica in Chapter 3).

In spite of the tremendous variability in sciatic symptoms and signs, a common thread exists for the diagnosis of acute radicular syndrome from a disc herniation. Table 2 outlines this syndrome (see also Fig. 3).

STAGING OF A DISC HERNIATION

As outlined in the Terminology section, disc herniations may be contained or noncontained. A brief review of surgical anatomy will help in understanding other methods of staging a disc herniation.

Surgical Anatomy

A vertebral body can be divided into upper and lower halves by a line drawn along the inferior borders of the pedicles (Fig. 4). If a disc space is added below (Fig. 5), an anatomic segment results. A nerve root is then added and assigned the same number as the pedicle beneath which it passes (Fig. 6).

There are six named posterior elements. Three of those posterior elements are above the line drawn along the inferior border of the pedicles (Fig. 7). Three of the posterior elements are below this line, and the junction between these two groups of posterior elements is the pars interarticularis (Fig. 8).

The posterior elements are joined, one anatomic segment to another, presenting "windows of opportunity" for entry into the spinal canal (Fig. 9). The most common window of entry used is the interlaminar space. The intertransverse interval is also a window for entry into the lateral reaches of the spinal canal, and its use is described later in the chapter.

To extend further the analogy of the windows of opportunity, each anatomic segment has been divided into a three-story "house" (Fig. 10). Now we are ready to provide further staging for the herniated nucleus pulposus (HNP).

Additional Staging for HNP

Contained disc protrusions are opposite the disc space and located in the first story (Fig. 11). Disc extrusions and sequestrations can be classified according to the size, shape, and location of the disc fragment. Figures

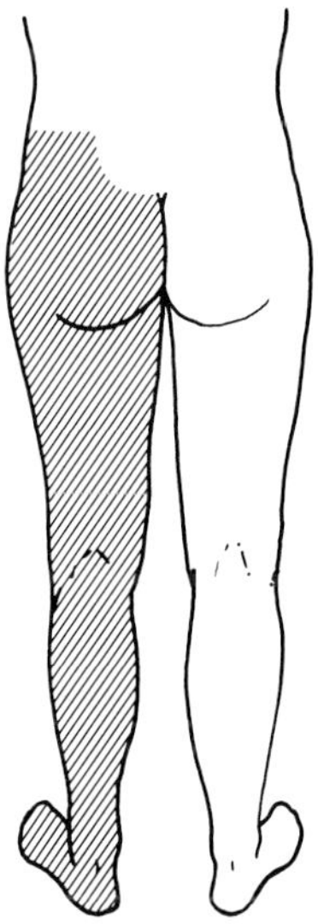

Figure 3 □ In regard to the location of pain in sciatica, the leg is considered to include the buttock.

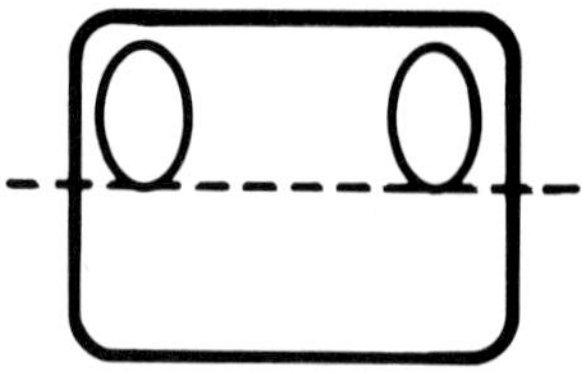

Figure 4 □ Vertebral body and its pedicles are shown. The pedicles lie mostly above the middle portion of the vertebral body.

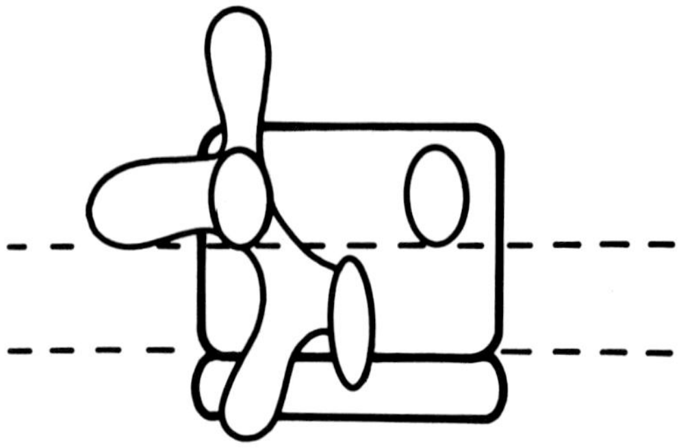

Figure 5 □ Anatomic segment is shown, with its six posterior elements and a disc inferiorly.

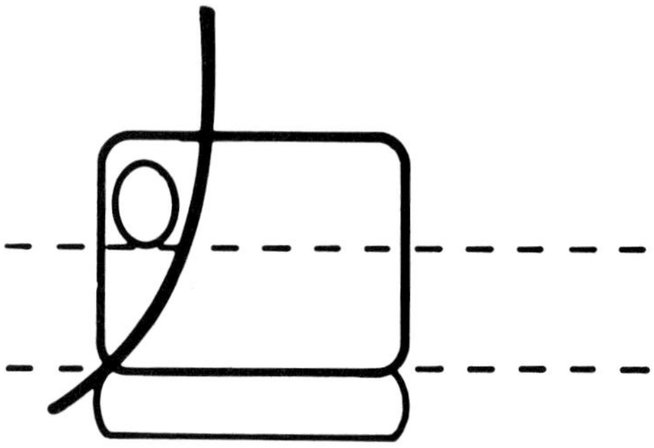

Figure 6 □ Nerve root as it courses through an anatomic segment. Nerve roots are numbered according to the pedicle beneath which they pass. If this is the fourth lumbar segment, with its attached fourth pedicle, then the root represented is L4.

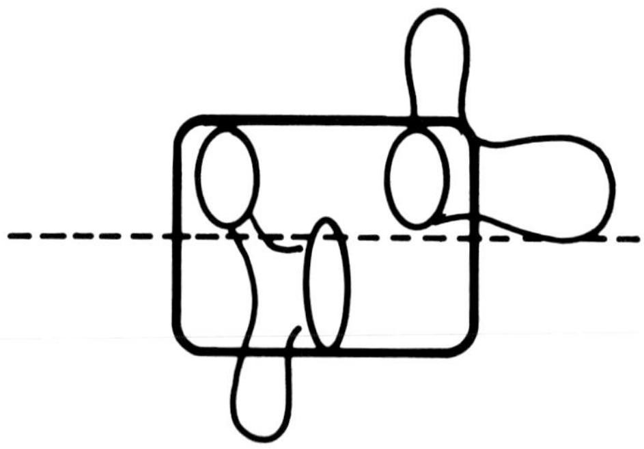

Figure 7 □ Six posterior elements are illustrated, three above the midvertebral dotted line, and three below the midvertebral dotted line.

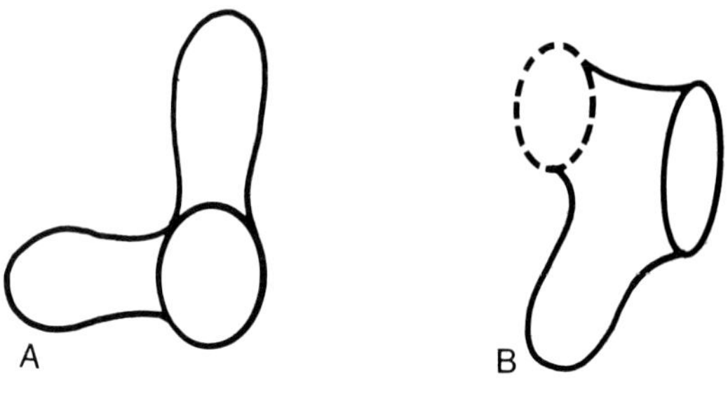

Figure 8 □ *A,* Three superior elements are shown: pedicle, superior facet, and transverse process. *B,* Three inferior elements are shown: spinous process, inferior facet, and lamina.

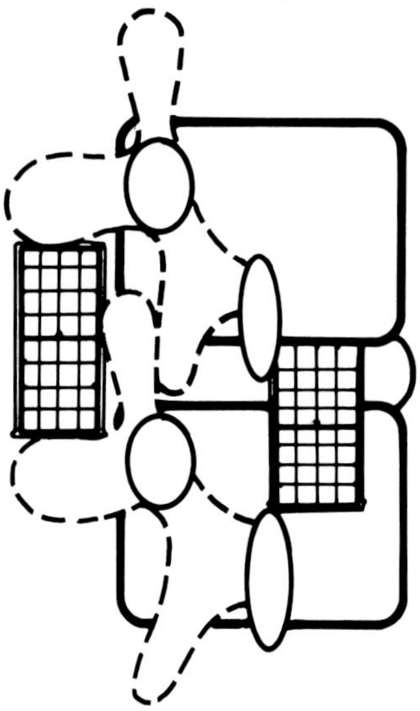

Figure 9 □ "Windows of opportunity" into the spinal canal are the medial interlaminar window and the more lateral intertransverse window.

12, 13, and 14 outline the basis of this classification.

Finally, artifactual changes in a disc herniation are important to note. Figure 15 shows significant artifactual change that can bear on the choice of treatment intervention.

INDICATIONS FOR SURGERY

General Statement

One has only to review the natural history of lumbar disc disease to realize that spinal surgeons play a palliative role in its management. The most outstanding study on the natural history of lumbar disc disease was carried out by Weber.[44] He randomly assigned large groups of patients with un-

Table 3 □ Weber's Results for Treatment of HNP

LENGTH OF FOLLOW-UP	NONSURGICAL RESULTS	SURGICAL RESULTS
1 year	60% better	92% better
4 years	No statistical difference between the two groups	
10 years	No difference between 4-year and 10-year follow-up	

equivocal signs of a disc herniation to surgical and nonsurgical groups. Table 3 summarizes his results. Weber has shown that, although surgery initially increases the number of good results, its advantages disappear with longer follow-up.

Hakelius[13] also completed a retrospective study of 583 patients with unilateral (L5 or S1) sciatica. His results were similar to Weber's in that the surgically treated patients initially had a better result, but by 6 months there was no difference between the two groups of patients. He did show that at a 7-year follow-up, the conservatively treated group had more low back pain, more sciatic discomfort, more recurrences, and more time lost from work.

One can only conclude from these and other studies on the natural history of sciatica due to a disc herniation that it is a transient, self-limiting condition. Satisfactory resolution over time is likely to occur, regardless of the method of treatment intervention, regardless of whether it is surgery or conservative treatment. If one is proposing surgical intervention,[37] then it is essential to prove that surgery carries a high rate of initial success with limited risk to the patient and at the least possible expense to those paying for the service.

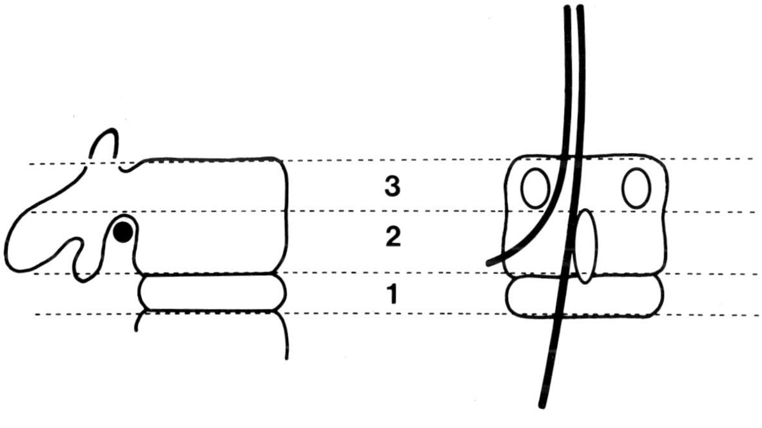

Figure 10 □ Once through the "windows of opportunity," each anatomic segment can be viewed as a three-story house: (1) first story—disc space level; second story—foraminal level; third story—pedicle level.

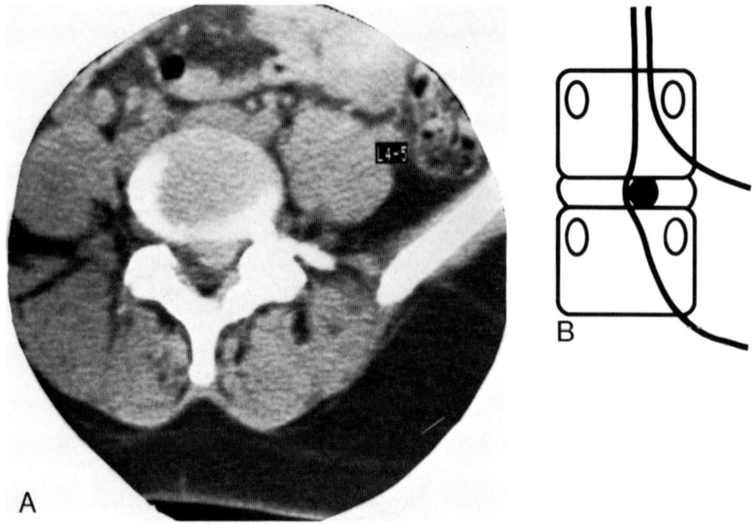

Figure 11 □ *A,* "First-story" disc herniation is exactly opposite the disc space. It has a reasonable chance of being a disc protrusion. *B,* This is a schematic illustration of a first-story HNP.

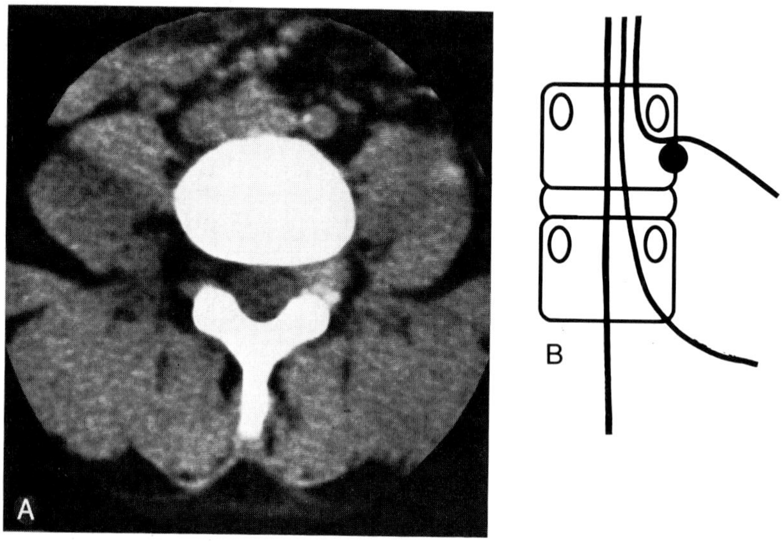

Figure 12 □ *A,* Second-story disc herniation. The disc has migrated superiorly to lie laterally in the foramen, opposite the second story. These are usually sequestered discs, but they may be subligamentous extrusions. *B,* Schematic drawing shows a second-story (foraminal) HNP.

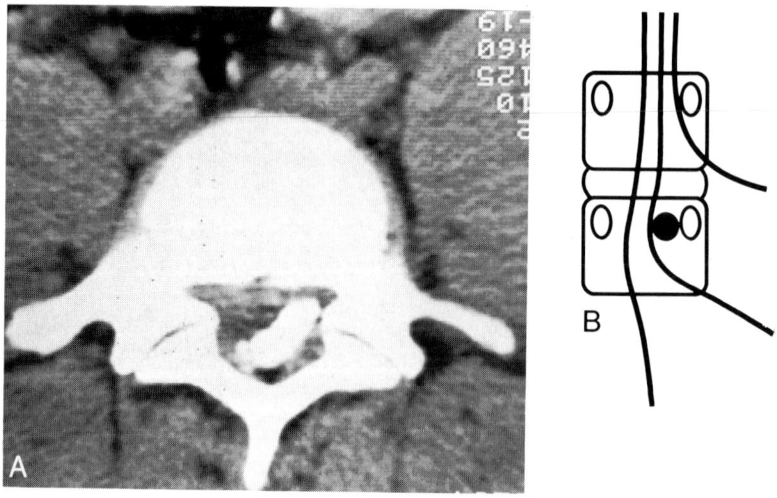

Figure 13 □ *A,* In the third-story disc herniation, the disc has migrated from the first story of the anatomic segment above (L4) into the third story of the segment below (L5). These are usually subligamentous extrusions, but on occasion they are sequestered discs. *B,* Schematic drawing shows a third-story (pedicle) HNP.

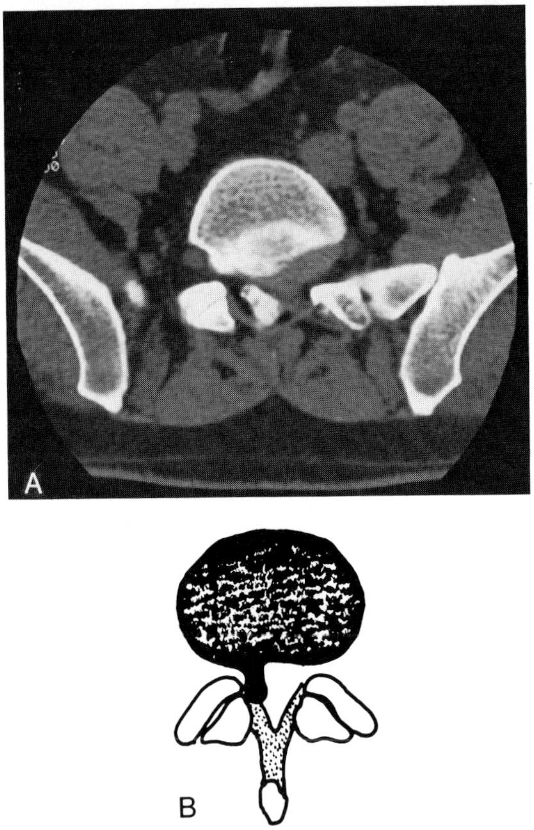

Figure 14 □ *A,* CT scan shows a disc herniation with a long sagittal dimension (also up in the second story). *B,* Schematic drawing of a pedunculated HNP with a long sagittal dimension and a narrow coronal dimension. These are almost always sequestered fragments.

Indications for Surgery in HNP

Surgery for the treatment of HNP is indicated under the conditions described below.

Increasing Neurologic Deficit □ In the face of progressing weakness, it is wise to intervene early with surgical excision of the disc rupture. Weber has shown that patients with a significant neurologic lesion eventually made as much recovery with nonsurgical treatment as they did with surgical treatment.

Significant Neurologic Deficit with Significant Straight-Leg Raising Reduction □ This is a relative indication for surgical intervention for an HNP. Again, Weber has shown that these patients eventually recovered just as well with nonsurgical intervention.

Bladder and Bowel Involvement. □ The acute massive disc herniation that causes bladder and bowel paralysis is usually a sequestered disc that requires immediate surgical excision for the best prognosis (see Pelvic Visceral Dysfunction—Cauda Equina Syndrome, later in this chapter).

Failure of Conservative Treatment □ This is the most common reason for surgical intervention in the presence of an HNP. Ideal conservative treatment is treatment that occurs over at least 6 weeks and not more than three months, and that results in improvement in the patient's symptoms and signs. During that time, the amount of complete bed rest that should be prescribed is 3 to 5 days. Other conservative measures[2] such as medication (pain, anti-inflammatory, muscle relaxant), modalities (heat and cold), and exercises may be used. The key to measuring the success of conservative treatment is not only the patient's relief of pain, but also the improvement in straight-leg raising ability. If a patient goes to bed with appropriate medication for 3 to 5 days and there is no improvement in straight-leg raising ability, then it is likely that the patient is going to follow a protracted conservative course and surgical intervention is indicated. It is proposed that surgical intervention in the acute radicular syndrome occur before 3 months of symptoms to try to avoid the chronic pathologic changes that can occur within a nerve root. Conservative treatment can also fail because the patient experiences recurrences of the sciatic syndrome. Table 4 out-

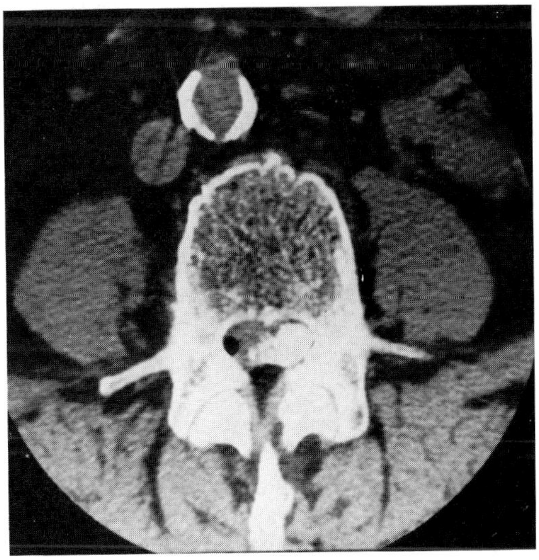

Figure 15 □ CT scan shows a third-story HNP containing air. This is usually a sequestered disc.

Table 4 □ Recurrent Sciatica*—Indications for Surgery

First episode of sciatica:	90% of patients will get better and stay better.
Second episode of sciatica:	90% of patients will get better, but 50% of the patients will have a recurrence of symptoms. Consider surgery.
Third episode of sciatica:	90% of the patients will get better, but almost all will have recurrent episodes of sciatica. Propose surgery.

*This condition is to be distinguished from recurrent HNP (disc herniation recurring after previous surgery).

lines the use of "recurrences of sciatica" as an indication for surgical intervention.

CONTRAINDICATIONS TO SURGICAL INTERVENTION

Before intervening surgically for the acute radicular syndrome resulting from a lumbar disc herniation, it is essential to have an accurate clinical diagnosis of the cause of the sciatica, an anatomic level of the lesion, and support for both clinical impressions by some form of investigation. If there is not a perfect union of the patient's clinical presentation, the anatomic level, and the structural lesion as demonstrated on myelography, CT scanning, or MRI, then the potential for a poor result increases dramatically.

Disabilities with significant nonorganic components[42] are usually a contraindication to surgical intervention. A nonorganic component does not "immunize" a patient against a disc herniation. On the other hand, few patients whose disability has a significant nonorganic component have a disc rupture as part of their causative pathologic condition.

Further contraindications to surgical intervention for a lumbar disc herniation are listed in Table 5. Table 6 outlines the differential diagnosis of sciatica.

Table 5 □ Contraindications to Surgery for an HNP

Wrong patient— one who has poor potential for recovery; for example, a workmen's compensation patient who is off work for more than 3 years.

Wrong diagnosis—e.g., other pathology causing the leg symptoms (see Table 4).

Wrong level (see section on complications).

A *painless* HNP—do not operate for primary complaint of weakness or paresthesias, in absence of pain.

An inexperienced surgeon applying poor technical skills.

Lack of adequate instruments.

Table 6 □ Differential Diagnosis of Sciatica

INTRASPINAL CAUSES

Proximal to Disc

- Conus and cauda equina lesions (e.g., neurofibroma, ependymoma)

Disc Level

- HNP
- Stenosis (canal or recess)
- Infection—osteomyelitis or discitis (with nerve root pressure)
- Inflammation—arachnoiditis
- Neoplasm—benign or malignant with nerve root pressure

EXTRASPINAL CAUSES

Pelvis

- Cardiovascular conditions (e.g., peripheral vascular disease)
- Gynecologic conditions
- Orthopedic conditions (e.g., osteoarthritis of hip)
- SI joint disease
- Neoplasms (invading or compressing lumbosacral plexus)

Peripheral Nerve Lesions

- Neuropathy (diabetic, tumor, alcohol)
- Local sciatic nerve conditions (trauma, tumor)
- Inflammation (herpes zoster)

INVESTIGATION OF A PATIENT PRIOR TO SURGERY FOR HNP

As this book is being written, we are at the crossroad in the development of investigative procedures for lumbar disc disease (see Chapter 6). The gold standard is still the water-soluble myelogram. However, many centers are gathering tremendous experience with plain CT, and, more recently, MRI, in the diagnosis of all forms of lumbar disc disease. This experience is developing to the exclusion of myelography, and within the next 5 years the gold standard for investigating a patient with lumbar disc disease will become CT scanning and/or MRI, with few indications for myelography. As this trend develops, it is prudent to recognize the pitfalls of CT scanning and MRI outlined in Table 7.

It is the author's (J.A.M.) opinion that electromyogram (EMG) examination and discogram assessment play little role in the evaluation of a patient with an HNP.

One final word of caution: It is essential that there be a marriage between the pa-

Table 7 □ Limitations of Newer Imaging Techniques

CT	The only areas of the spine seen are the areas scanned. Higher lumbar areas not scanned may harbor disease.
MRI	Exaggerates pathologic conditions, and there will be a phase of over-calling lesions before recognizing what is significant and what is not significant. Will show higher lumbar areas on sagittal sections.

tient's clinical syndrome and the structural lesion demonstrated by x-ray. Figure 16 demonstrates a patient with a spondylolisthesis at L4–L5, who presented with an acute radicular syndrome.

SURGICAL OPTIONS

The principle of surgical intervention is to relieve neural compression without complications and, specifically, without creating instability.

Choices include

1. The posterior approaches: the standard laminectomy; microlaminectomy—posterior; and microlaminectomy—lateral
2. The anterior approach
3. The percutaneous discectomy approach

SURGICAL TECHNIQUES

Posterior Approach

Surgery for a lumbar disc herniation can be carried out under general, spinal, or local anesthesia. The most expedient anesthetic agent is general, although there are surgeons who believe that the procedure is best accomplished under either spinal or local anesthesia.

Most surgeons agree that the kneeling position (Fig. 17) is the best for the surgeon and the patient. It allows for a free abdomen, removing pressure from the inferior vena cava, and decreasing venous flow through Batson's plexus, in turn reducing bleeding during surgery. In the kneeling position, one has to be mindful of a number of pitfalls, outlined in Table 8.

Whether one does or does not use magnification (loupes or microscope) to accomplish the disc excision is an unresolved issue. As long as the root is decompressed and the patient is relieved of symptoms, the

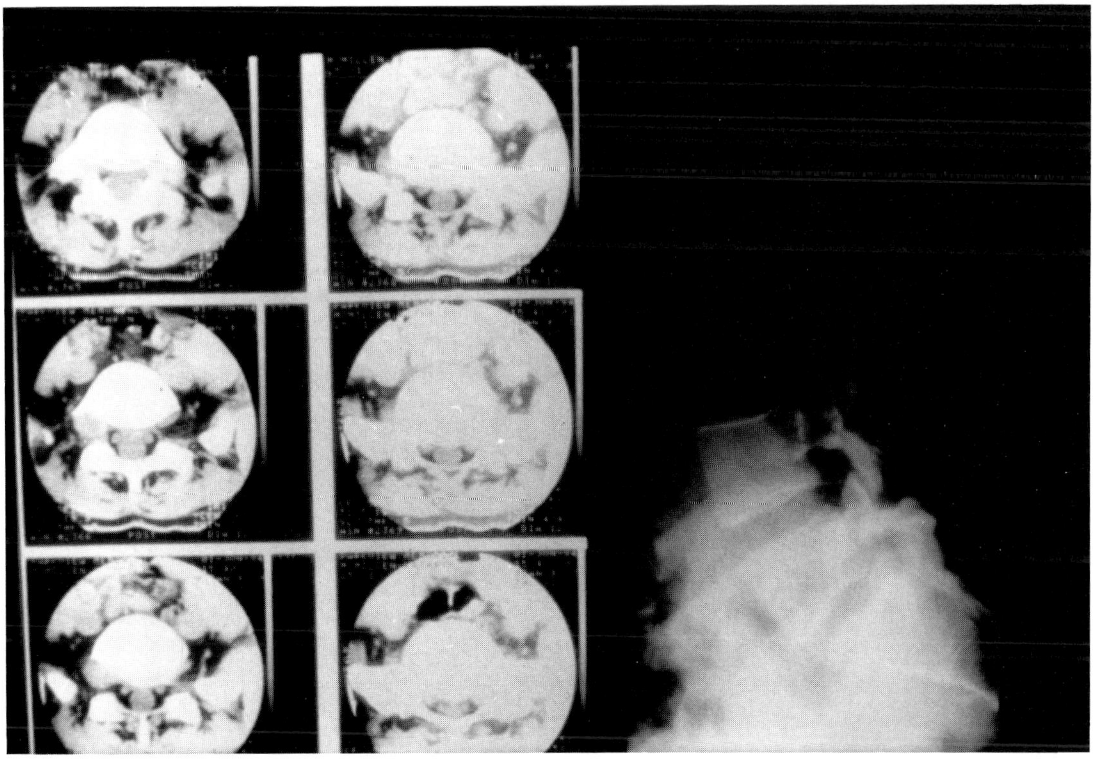

Figure 16 □ CT axials and plain lateral radiograph showing a spondylolisthesis (L5–S1) and an HNP foraminal, right (best seen in the bottom left-hand axial CT).

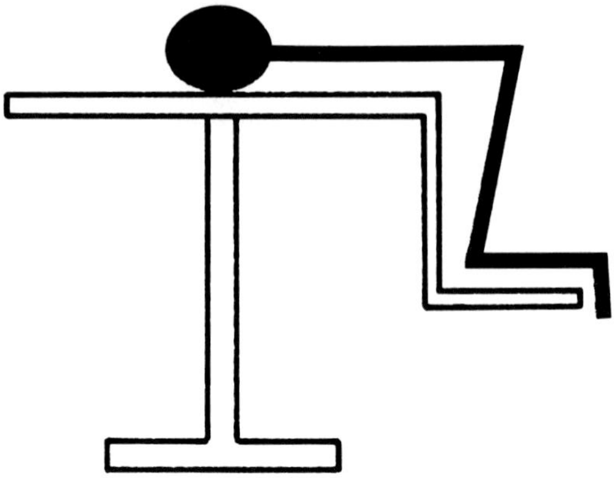

Figure 17 □ The kneeling position for spine surgery is illustrated.

mission has been accomplished. The microsurgeons believe this can be better accomplished with the assistance of the magnification and illumination of the microscope. The jury is still out.

The standard surgical approach for a laminectomy or a microdiscectomy has been outlined in many articles.[36] It is important to open the correct disc space. Once within the laminar opening, it is necessary to find the lateral border of the nerve root and reflect the nerve root and cauda equina sheath medially to expose the lesion. It is necessary to remove enough bone to see the lateral border of the nerve root. This may require removal of the medial edge of the superior facet of the anatomic segment below. The attempt to find the lateral border of the lumbar nerve root has a few potential pitfalls. The first problem is a nerve root that has been displaced laterally by an axillary disc herniation. A second pitfall is the posterior displacement of a nerve root that occurs because of the location of the disc herniation, placing the nerve root at jeopardy when the ligamentum flavum is being opened (Fig. 18*A*, *B*). It is important to remove all the offending lesion, not miss any extruded or migrated disc fragments, and not leave behind bony nerve root encroachment. (See Complication section.)

Table 8 □ Pitfalls of the Kneeling Position

Avoid pressure on the eyes.
Avoid neck extension, especially in the older patient.
Avoid abduction of the shoulders, which can cause a brachial plexus lesion.
Watch pressure points, especially around the ulnar nerve at the elbow.

Ninety-five percent of exposures for lumbar disc herniations occur at either L4–L5 or L5–S1, with the former tending to be in the older patient and the latter tending to be in the younger. Five percent of exposures occur at other levels (laterally at the L4–L5 level and at higher lumbar levels, such as L3–L4 and L2–L3).

It is important to be aware of root anomalies,[15, 22, 31, 33] which, by their nature, reduce nerve root mobility. Very small disc herniations can cause major sciatica symptoms in a patient with root anomalies. At the time of surgery, root anomalies lead to a very immobile nerve root and difficulty in reaching the more anterior lesions.

There is no uniform agreement on how much disc to remove. Williams[45] proposes that only the ruptured portion be removed; Spengler[38] and Hudgins[19] suggest a limited disc removal; the classic teaching is to remove all the ruptured disc and as much intradiscal material as possible, which includes curettage of the end plates. The author (J.A.M.) prefers the middle road of Spengler and Hudgins.

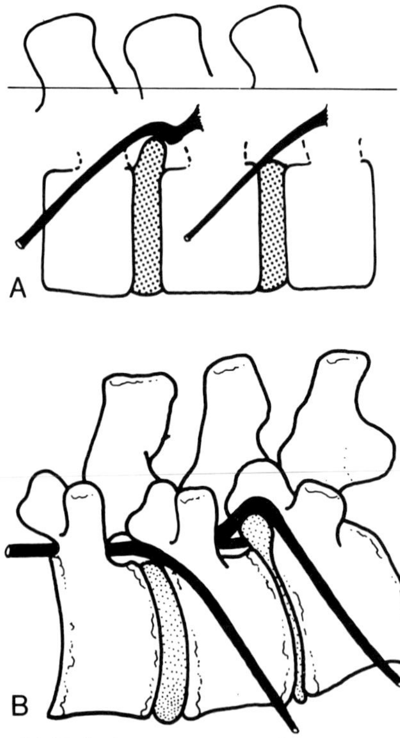

Figure 18 □ *A*, A nerve root may be pushed posteriorly into the lamina by the ruptured fragment of disc material. *B*, A more complete schematic illustration of *A*, shows the lamina removed to reveal the posterior displacement of the root.

Most surgeons are now using prophylactic antibiotics at the time of, and immediately after, lumbar disc surgery. This is a carry-over from implant surgery in orthopedics and, to date, there are no statistically valid studies in the literature to support the use of prophylactic antibiotics at the time of lumbar disc surgery.

The aim of all surgical intervention is to minimize scar formation. To this end, proposals have been made for the use of Gelfoam,[24] fat graft, and other materials.[49] The author (J.A.M.) does not use any of these materials, but rather relies on the very limited microsurgical exposure and early mobilization to reduce scar tissue formation (Fig. 19).

Results of Posterior Microdiscectomy

A study of 257 patients undergoing microsurgery for lumbar disc disease[10] (Table 9) has revealed an 84% success rate and a 95% return-to-work rate in patients undergoing surgery for virgin lumbar disc herniations. Less successful, but acceptable, results were obtained in patients with an HNP who made compensation claims and in patients with previous spine surgery procedures (Table 10). Less acceptable results were obtained in

Table 9 □ Follow-Up of Patients Undergoing Microsurgery for Lumbar Disc Disease[10]

Number of patients operated on		257
Average length of follow-up		19 mos
Number of patients followed		249 (97%)
Case distribution		
Virgin HNP	119	
Lateral zone stenosis	24	
Previous procedure		
Chymopapain	70	
Laminectomy	10	
Fusion added to microdiscectomy	26	
	249	

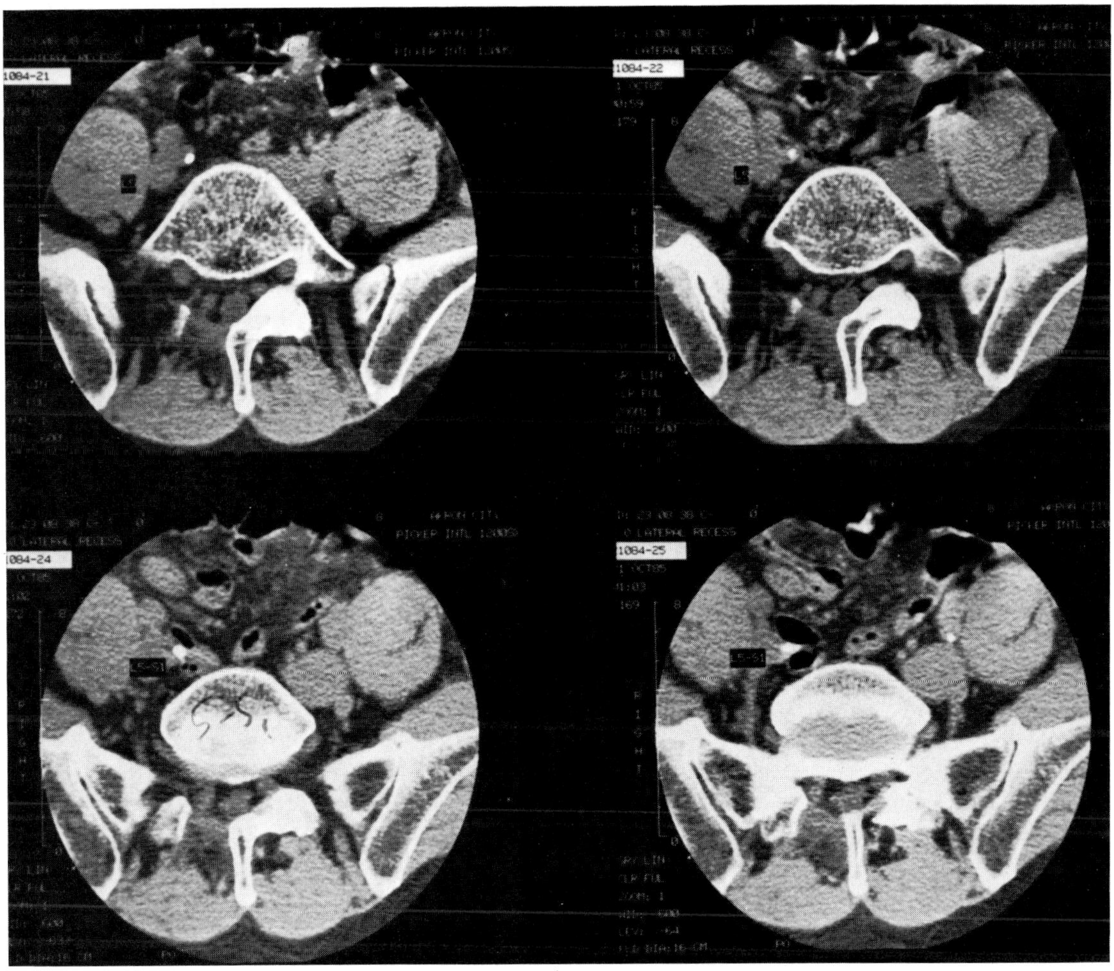

Figure 19 □ A "laminectomy membrane" following microdiscectomy, L5–S1, right. No fat or Gelfoam was used.

Table 10 □ Results in Compensation Patients and Patients with Previous Surgery

RESULT	COMPENSATION	PREVIOUS SURGERY*
Satisfactory	66% (27)	69.7% (46)
Unsatisfactory	34% (14)	30.3% (20)

*Excluding patients with lateral zone stenosis.

Table 11 □ Results in Lateral Zone Stenosis

RESULT	DECOMPRESSION	DECOMPRESSION WITH FUSION
Satisfactory	12 (50%)	9 (90%)
Unsatisfactory	12 (50%)	1 (10%)

lateral zone decompressions (Table 11) unless accompanied by a fusion. Analysis of a complication rate of 10% (Table 12) revealed relatively minor problems that did not affect outcomes and a decreasing incidence of complications as experience with the procedure grew. The short-term success rate in this series compared favorably with standard laminectomy–discectomy. Along with the reduction of hospital stay (average 2.3 days), microsurgery delivered acceptable results in patients with lumbar disc herniations.

Complications of Microsurgery for Lumbar HNP

More can be learned from complications than from successes. Although many are using microsurgical intervention for lumbar disc disease, there are also many critics. Fager[18] believes that microsurgery is associated with several disadvantages and many additional risks. He has stated that inherent to the procedure are inadequate exposure of the nerve root and incomplete decompression of the encroaching lesion.

A general review of the literature reveals complications associated with any spine-invasive procedure, as listed in Table 13.

COMPLICATIONS SPECIFIC TO MICROSURGERY

Some complications are specific to microsurgical intervention.

Wrong Level □ Anyone doing any volume of microsurgery will admit that at one time or another, they have exposed the wrong level. Figure 20 outlines the author's (J.A.M.) method of trying to avoid the wrong level exposure.

Missed Pathology □ Many critics of microsurgery state that because of the limited operative field, it is easy to miss a fragment of disc material that has migrated away from the disc space or to miss bony encroachment. Microsurgery for lumbar disc disease is not seek-and-find surgery; rather, by careful examination during the preoperative investigation, which includes CT and/or MRI, the surgeon will know exactly what disorder is causing the symptoms and where the lesion is located (Fig. 21).

Intraoperative Bleeding □ Because of the very small incision and the limited operative field, a small amount of bleeding under the microscope appears as a major hemorrhage. It is important to take steps to prevent excessive bleeding during microsurgery, such

Table 12 □ Complications

TYPE OF COMPLICATION	PATIENTS NUMBER/PERCENTAGE	OUTCOME
Dural tear (minor)	6 (2.70%)	Only one required repair, no problems
Wrong level exploration	6 (2.70%)	Recognized and corrected at time of surgery
Hemorrhage requiring transfusion	3 (1.35%)	
Superficial wound infection	2 (0.90%)	Resolved on antibiotics
Disc space infection	2 (0.90%)	Resolved on antibiotics
Increased neurodeficit	2 (0.90%)	Recovered quickly
Hematoma	1 (0.45%)	Resolved spontaneously
Gastritis	1 (0.45%)	Resolved
Urinary retention	1 (0.45%)	Resolved
	24 (10.8%)	

Table 13 □ Complications of Lumbar Spine Surgery[28]

Neurologic damage with increased neurologic deficit
Wound infection—superficial or deep
CSF fistula
Hematoma with or without cauda equina compression
Fatalities—pulmonary embolus; great vessel injury
Late complications—spinal stenosis; instability resulting in vertebral body translation; scarring, with or without arachnoiditis

as by taking the patients off anti-inflammatory medications before the surgery, properly positioning the patient on the table so that there is no abdominal compression, and using hypotensive anesthesia. During the surgical exercise, all bleeders should be stopped at the moment they occur, using regular cautery outside the spinal canal and bipolar cautery within the spinal canal.

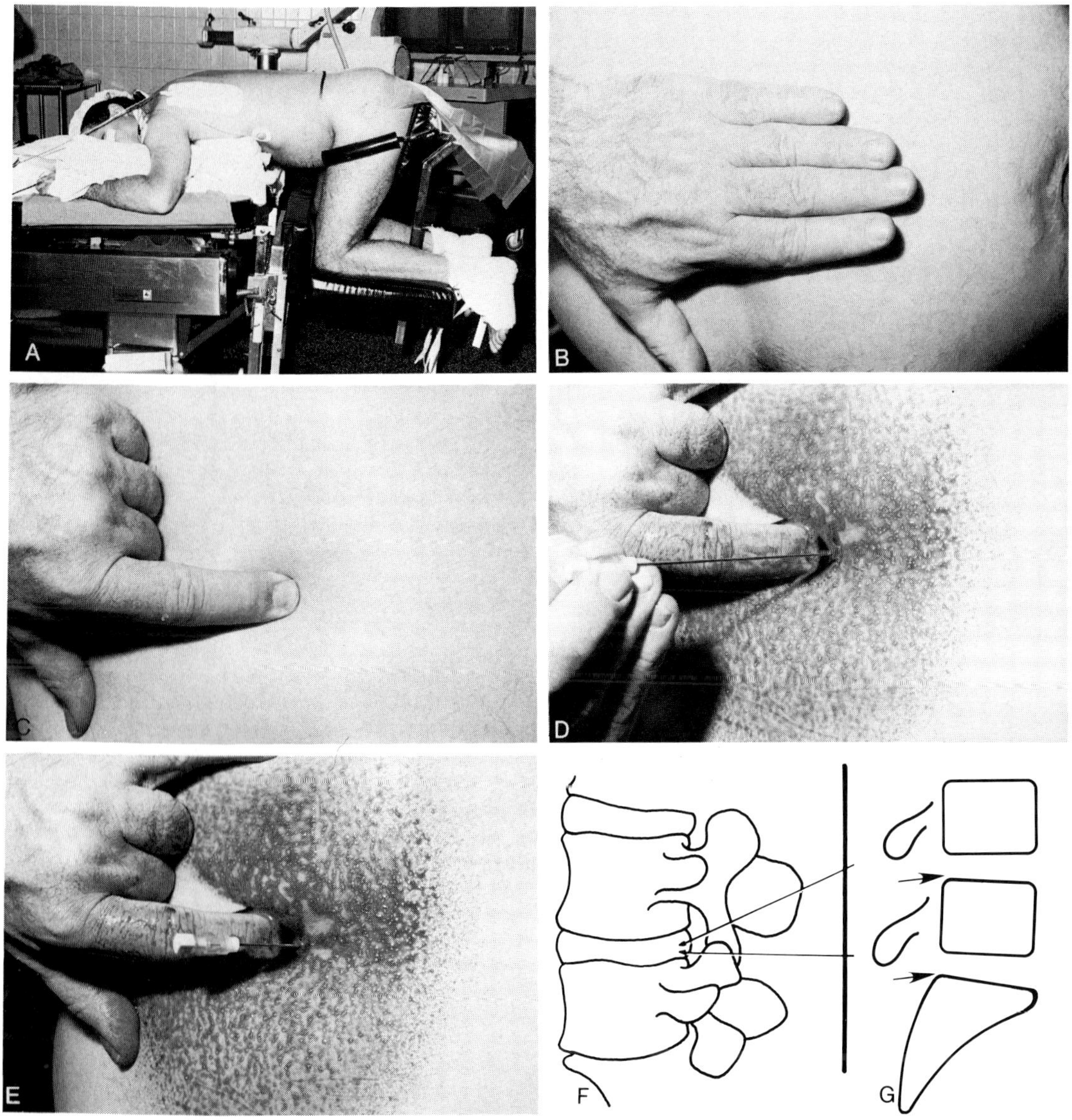

Figure 20 □ *A,* The patient is in the kneeling position with the image intensifier in position for marking. *B,* Before the image intensifier is in position, the interspinous interval one hand's breadth above the gluteal cleft is identified. This is usually the L5–S1 interspinous space, and it lies opposite or slightly above the posterior iliac spine *(C). D,* The skin is prepared, and *E,* the needle is inserted. *F,* The needle should be at the inferior edge of the disc space and in the interspinous interval. The needle should not be placed opposite the spinous process *(top arrow). G,* Arrows point to the needle, marking the position as depicted in *H.*

Illustration continued on following page

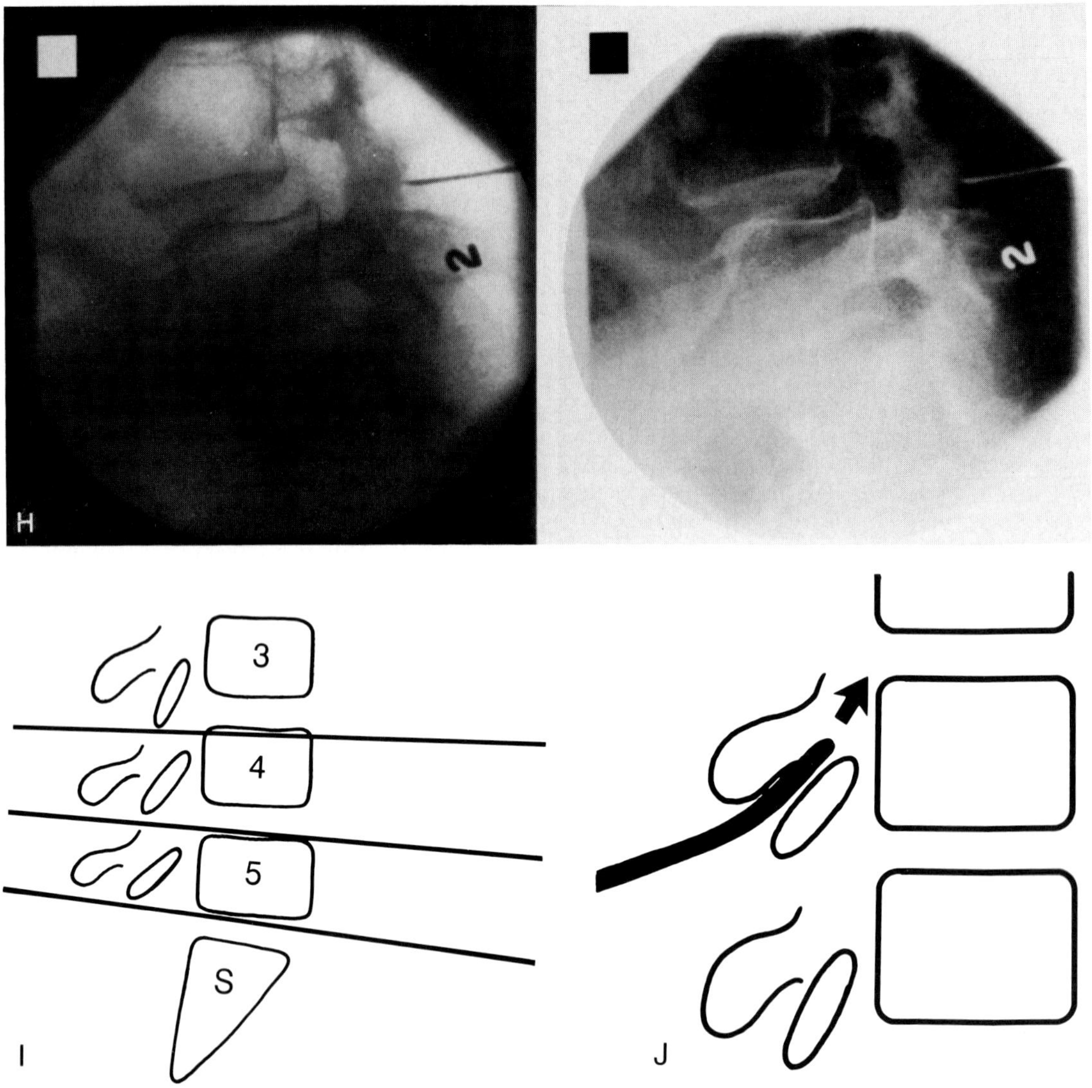

Figure 20 *Continued I,* The "laminar trap" is shown. As one ascends in the lumbar spine, the inferior edge of the lamina overlaps more of the disc space—a fact that is accentuated by placing the patient in the lordotic position. *J,* Marking the disc space too superiorly may shift the limited incision slightly higher, allowing the subperiosteal dissector to slide up the lamina and exposing the wrong level above.

Dural Injury □ The inexperienced surgeon with poor equipment is the one who causes neurologic damage during microsurgical intervention. It is essential to train oneself in the technique and to have the proper instrumentation available to reduce dural injury to a minimum. In fact, under the microscope, the nerve root can be seen so well that an experienced microsurgeon will have a lower rate of neurologic complication rate than someone using a standard laminectomy approach without magnification.

Disc Space Infection □ Wilson and Harbaugh[46] reported an increased incidence of disc space infection following microsurgery. They proposed that manipulation of the microscope over the wound was the source of this increased infection rate. This occurred in spite of surgical draping of the microscope, which leaves exposed eye pieces that are not sterile. This problem has led to the use of prophylactic antibiotics and the proposal that manipulation of the microscope over the open wound be kept to a minimum.

Anterior Approach

Anterior discectomy and interbody fusion for the lumbar spine was first reported by Lane and Moore in 1948.[23] In 1963, Harmon reported good clinical results of anterior fusion based on his study of 244 patients.[14] In 1965, Sacks reported on the clinical results of 150 patients treated by the transperitoneal approach to the lumbar spine.[34] He concluded that this procedure is indicated for patients with chronic backache due to intervertebral disc degeneration, patients with previous unsuccessful laminectomy or posterior fusion, and patients with spondylolisthesis that is less than one third forward-slipping. Hodgson and Wong also reported their clinical results of the extraperitoneal approach to lumbar disc degeneration.[18] Stauffer and Coventry reported on 83 patients who underwent anterior lumbar spine fusion.[39] They claimed that this procedure had a low rate of bony union (56%) and unsatisfactory clinical results.

In Japan, Suzuki and coworkers in 1958 were the first to report interbody fusion for lumbar disc herniation (30 cases).[40] Subsequently, other surgeons in Japan performed this surgery for lumbar disc herniation; these included Inoue and colleagues,[20] Hirabayashi,[16] Nakano,[30] and Tsuchiya.[41] More than 900 patients underwent this procedure, because of various lumbar disorders, at our institution since 1955, and satisfactory results were obtained after the long-term follow-up study.[21] The surgical indications and actual surgical procedures are presented in this section of the chapter.

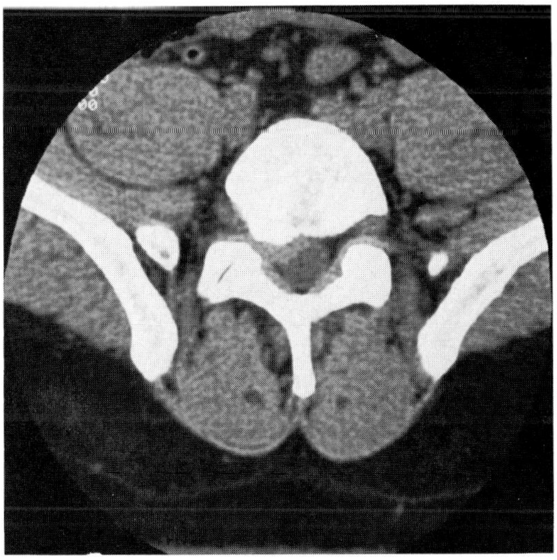

Figure 21 □ HNP, L5, right. This disc herniation with its osteophyte is in the second story of L5 and extends into the foramen. Complete exposure will necessitate removal of the inferior half of the lamina of L5.

Surgical Indications

Anterior discectomy with interbody fusion is indicated for various lumbar disorders, including lumbar disc herniation, spondylolytic spondylolisthesis, degenerative spondylolisthesis, spondylolysis, ring apophysis fracture, unstable spine, tuberculous spondylitis, and salvage surgery of the cases with previous posterior surgery. It is not indicated for spinal canal stenosis with multilevel involvement, sequestered lumbar disc herniation, or nerve compression that is mainly from the posterior direction, such as ossification of yellow ligament.

The advantages of the anterior procedure are as follows. Nerve decompression is achieved without damaging back muscles and without surgical maneuvers in the spinal canal. Disc height is regained by complete removal of the degenerated disc. Rigid fixation is assured by rigid interbody fusion. Disadvantages are relatively more extensive surgery and a longer postoperative course than found with the posterior approach. This procedure is especially indicated for young adults and physical laborers who have large central or lateral herniations, as well as for patients who have spondylolytic or degenerative spondylolisthesis, or combined stenosis caused mainly by disc herniation.

Figure 22 shows the myelograms and CT scans taken before and after the anterior lumbar surgery in a 43-year-old man with L4–L5 lumbar disc herniation. The neural structure was well-decompressed, and the disc height was normalized postoperatively. The patient became completely symptom-free after the surgery.

Figure 23 shows the preoperative and postoperative myelograms of a 49-year-old woman with L4 degenerative spondylolisthesis. A preoperative myelogram showed segmental spinal canal stenosis at the level of slippage. Note the normalization of the disc height and the reduction of the spondylolisthesis. Her preoperative symptoms, including intermittent claudication, were completely relieved.

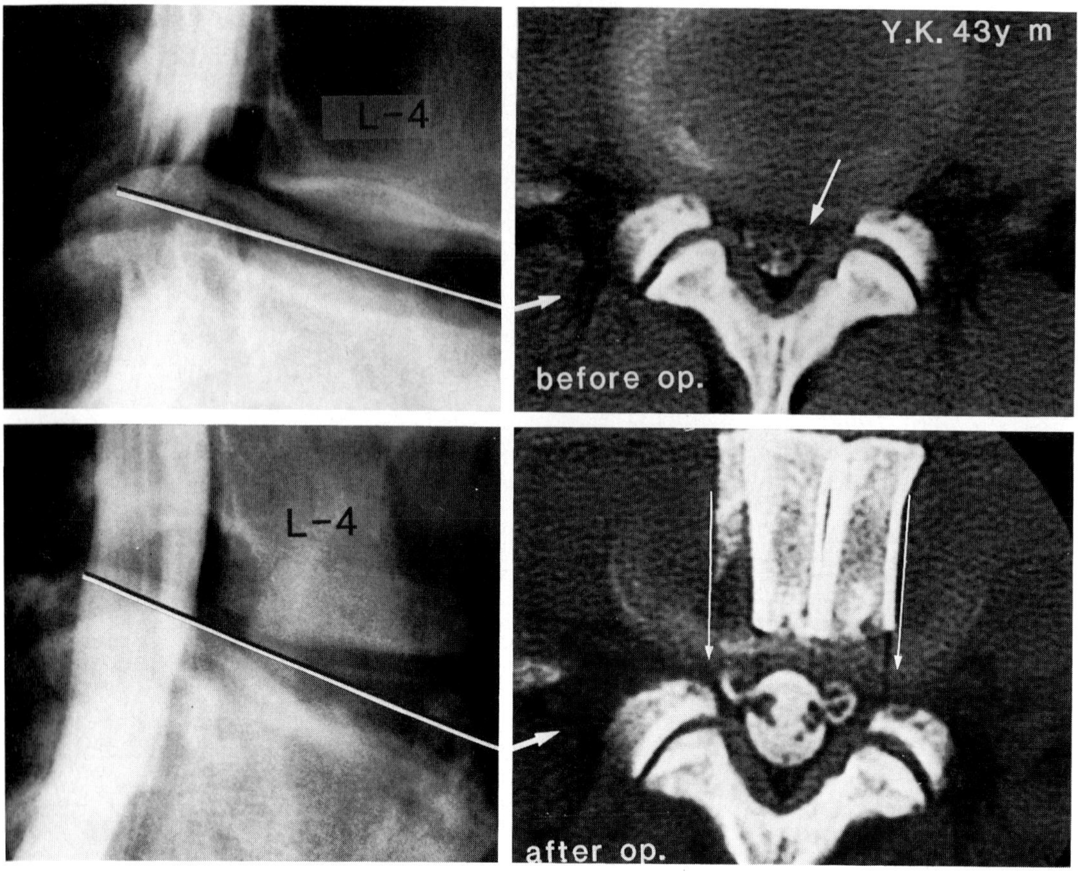

Figure 22 □ Preoperative and postoperative myelograms and CT myelograms in a 43-year-old man with L4–L5 disc herniation, who underwent anterior discectomy and interbody fusion. Note the satisfactory decompression after the surgery.

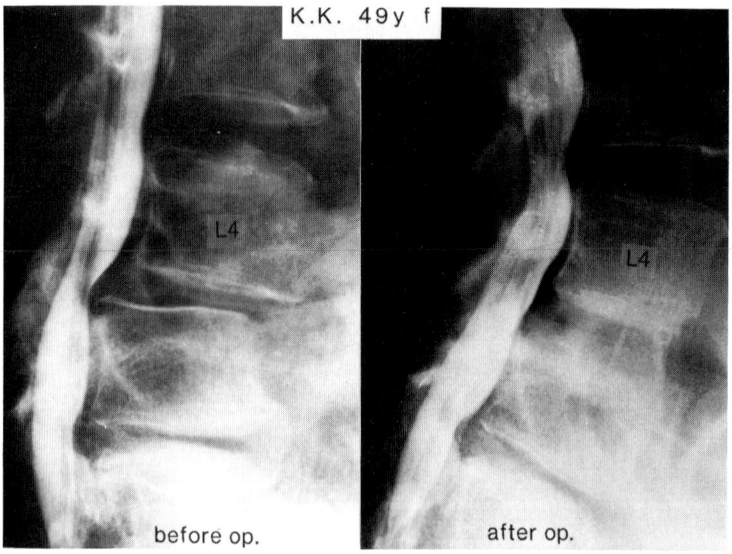

Figure 23 □ Preoperative and postoperative myelograms in a 49-year-old woman with L4 degenerative spondylolisthesis. The disc space was normalized and the slipping was reduced after the anterior lumbar surgery.

Surgically Relevant Anatomy

The abdominal wall is formed anteriorly by the rectus abdominis muscles, and laterally by the obliquus externus, obliquus internus, and transversus abdominis muscles (Fig. 24). The rectus muscles are enveloped by the rectus sheath. The anterior and posterior portions of the sheath fuse to form the linea alba. Because the linea alba is narrow in the lower abdomen, it should be initially cut on the side of the umbilicus when the abdominal cavity is opened. The peritoneum is located behind the posterior rectus sheath. Because the posterior sheath does not extend below the arcuate line, care must be taken not to rupture the peritoneum when the extraperitoneal approach is undertaken.

The large vessels are located immediately behind the posterior parietal peritoneum in front of the lumbar spine. The aorta lies anteriorly and to the left of the vena cava (Fig. 25). The aortic bifurcation is usually at the level of the L4–L5 intervertebral disc, and the common iliac veins join together just distal to this point. However, because there can be a great variation concerning the topography of the large vessels, preoperative evaluation of the anatomy of the large vessels by CT scan is essential for the anterior lumbar surgery. The superior hypogastric plexus lies between the right and left iliac arteries and anterior to the left common iliac vein, the L5 vertebral body, and L5–S1 intervertebral disc (Fig. 26). Injury of this plexus may result in dry ejaculation; therefore, care must be taken during the approach to the lumbosacral region.

Surgical Procedure

ANTERIOR TRANSPERITONEAL APPROACH

Preparation is the same as for ordinary abdominal surgery. The patient is given laxatives and enemas prior to the procedure. The operative field, including abdomen and pubis, is completely shaved. The surgery is performed under general anesthesia. Elastic stockings are applied during surgery for prevention of thrombophlebitis. In the supine position, the right arm of the patient is placed on the arm support over the chest. This facilitates obtaining bone graft from the right iliac crest.

The operation begins with a 15-cm midline abdominal incision while the umbilicus is pulled to the right side to avoid its penetration. The umbilicus should be at the center of the incision for the approach of the L4–L5 disc. For the L5–S1 disc, a subumbilical 15-cm incision is made (Fig. 27). The incision is deepened through the subcutaneous tissue down to the linea alba. The linea alba and peritoneum are pulled up and cut at a site near the umbilicus. Then the incision is continued upward with scissors and downward with a scalpel; one should

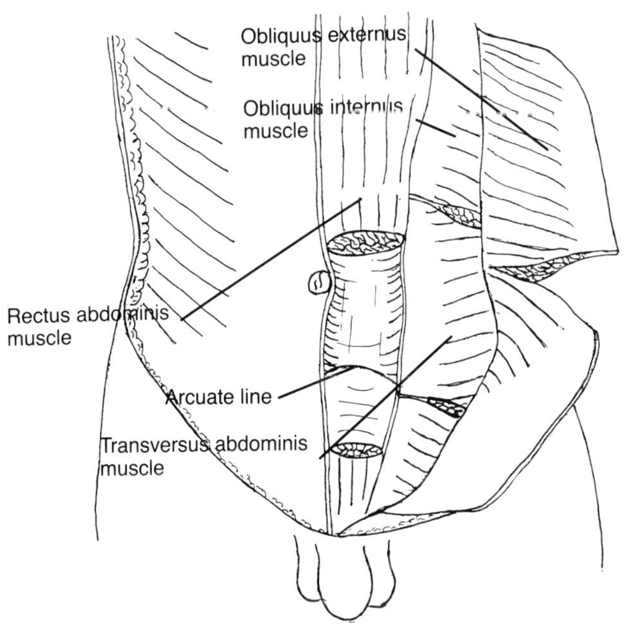

Figure 24 □ Topography of the abdominal wall.

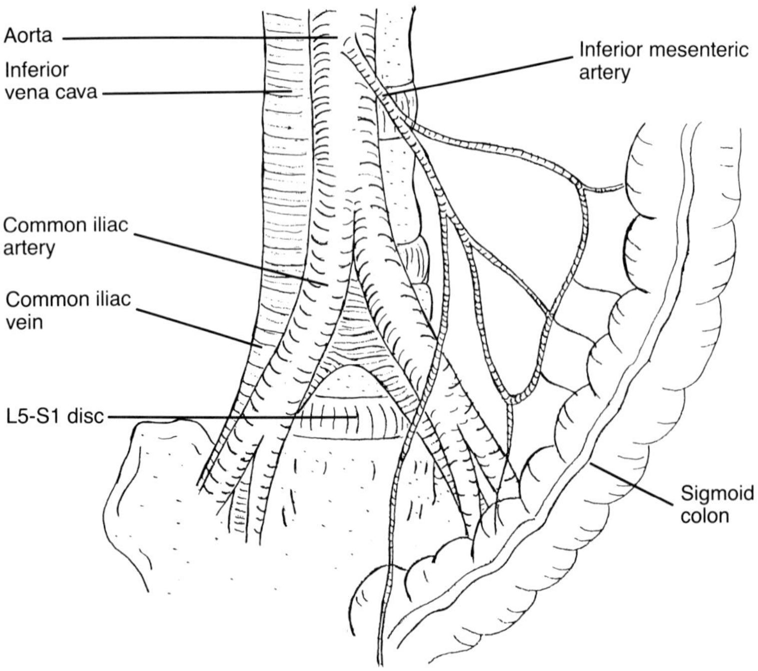

Figure 25 □ Location of the large vessels. The aortic bifurcation is usually at the level of the L4–L5 intervertebral disc, and the common iliac veins join slightly distal to this point. However, their position can vary greatly. When the anterior transperitoneal approach is undertaken, the inferior mesenteric artery is retracted to the left side.

avoid cutting the rectus sheath. Care must be taken not to damage the underlying viscera.

While commissures are protected by moist compression, an abdominal retractor is applied. The patient is slightly tilted with the head down. Using two rolls of large gauze, the intestines are pushed into the superior abdominal cavity, with the sigmoid colon being pulled to the left side. Here, the posterior parietal peritoneum is fully exposed.

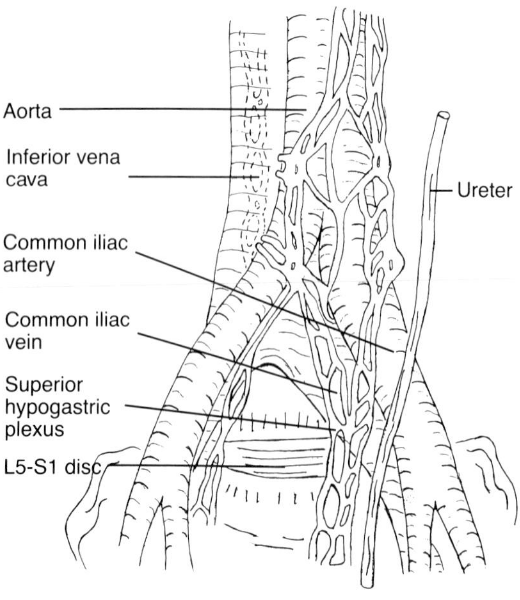

Figure 26 □ The superior hypogastric plexus is shown.

The promontorium, the aorta, and the bifurcation are identified by palpation. Grasped with toothless discectomy forceps, the posterior peritoneum is incised obliquely along the left side of the aorta and common iliac vessels. When necessary, palpation is repeated to obtain the correct orientation. Retroperitoneal tissue is carefully cleared by blunt dissection. The presacral plexus must be carefully identified and moved to the side. Generally speaking, L4–L5 disc is approached by displacing the aorta and vena cava to the right side (Fig. 28). If necessary, vertebral segmental vessels and the iliolumbar vein should be ligated and cut to facilitate further displacement of the large vessels. The L5–S1 disc can be approached through the space between the common iliac vessels (Fig. 29). When the level of the disc space is uncertain, an x-ray film should be taken to determine the level.

After the intervertebral disc is exposed, vascular retractors are inserted into the upper and lower vertebral bodies to clarify the operation field. The anterior longitudinal ligament is dissected by an H-shaped incision. Then the disc is resected by means of a long scalpel and longeurs. A disc spreader is used to extend the disc space to facilitate disc removal. The disc material should be

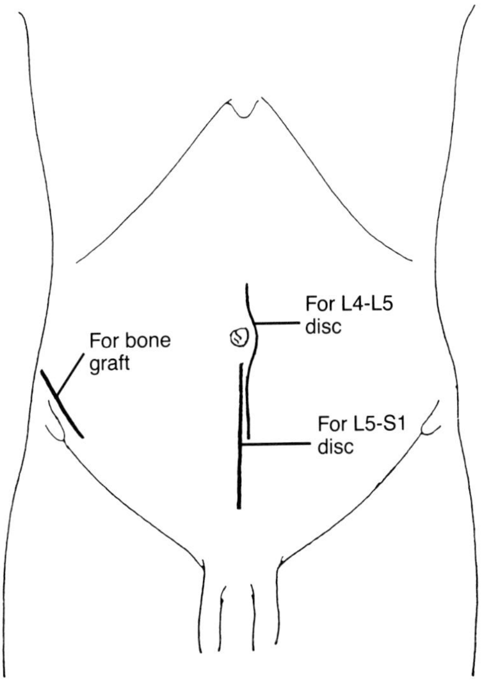

Figure 27 □ Skin incisions for anterior transperitoneal approach. For the L4–L5 disc, the umbilicus should be at the center of the incision. For the L5–S1 disc, a subumbilical incision is made.

removed as completely as possible to expose the end plates clearly.

Next, the end plates are chiseled away as far as the posterior limbus. This should be continued until the cancellous bone is exposed. Usually, the removal of about 1 to 2 mm of the end plates is necessary; the remaining disc material is removed completely. The width, depth, and height of the dissected disc space are measured using a ruler and calipers. When bone graft is obtained from the iliac crest, care must be taken not to damage the lateral femoral cutaneous nerve. Two pieces of well-shaped cortical–cancellous iliac bone grafts are prepared. The size of the graft is approximately three quarters of the anteroposterior (AP) diameter of the disc space. The disc space is spread by the disc spreader, and the bone grafts are tightly tapped into the position (Fig. 30). Bleeding is easily stopped by applying pressure with saline gauze.

Next, the anterior longitudinal ligament is sutured. The vascular retractors are then removed. The common iliac vessels are restored to the normal position. After complete hemostasis is confirmed, retroperitoneal closure is undertaken by a continuous seroserous suture; slowly absorbable string is used. The peritoneum and abdominal viscera should be kept moist by using warm saline throughout the surgical procedure. Coagulated blood should be thoroughly removed from the peritoneal cavity by using moist gauze. The abdominal retractors are then removed. Next, the two gauze rolls are removed from the abdominal cavity, and the bowel loops are anatomically repositioned. The greater omentum is then placed over the intestinum.

Finally, the abdominal wall is closed in three layers; the peritoneum, rectus abdom-

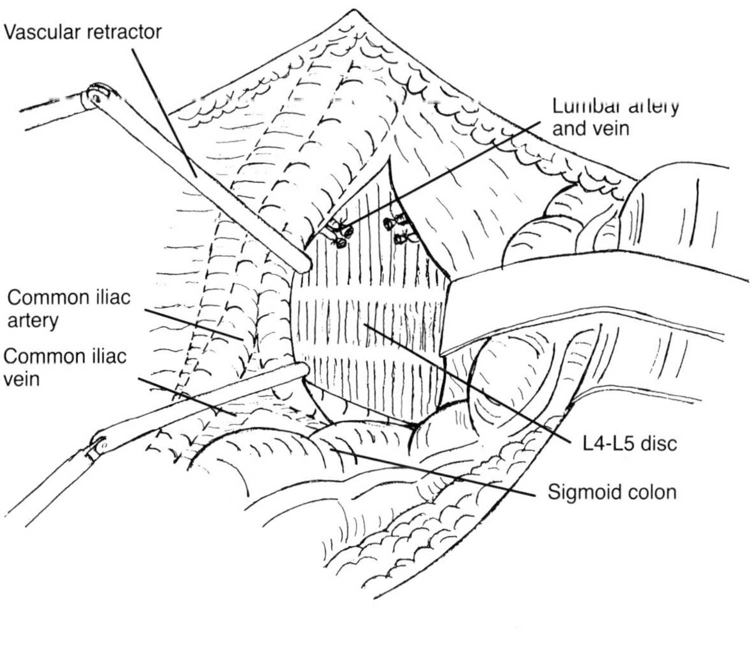

Figure 28 □ Approach to the L4–L5 disc. The large vessels are displaced to the right side.

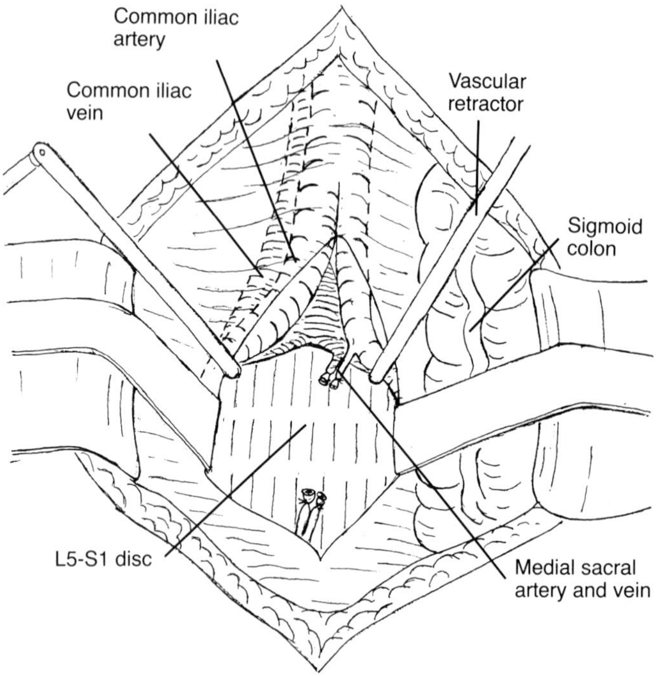

Figure 29 □ Approach to the L5–S1 disc. It can be approached through the space between the common iliac vessels.

inis muscles, and fascia are in one layer, the subcutaneous tissue is in the second, and the skin is in the last.

EXTRAPERITONEAL APPROACH

The preoperative preparation is the same as that for the anterior transperitoneal approach. The patient is given laxatives and enemas prior to the surgery.

The patient is placed in the supine or right lateral position. A left lateral oblique skin incision is made along the midline between the ribs and the iliac crest, to the lateral border of the rectus sheath (Fig. 31). The level of the skin incision is changed, according to the level of the lumbar spine approached. The abdominis obliquus muscles are cut in line with the skin incision by using an electric cautery knife or heat scalpel. Hemostasis should be confirmed as the dissection progresses. The transversus muscle should be cut carefully so as not to cut

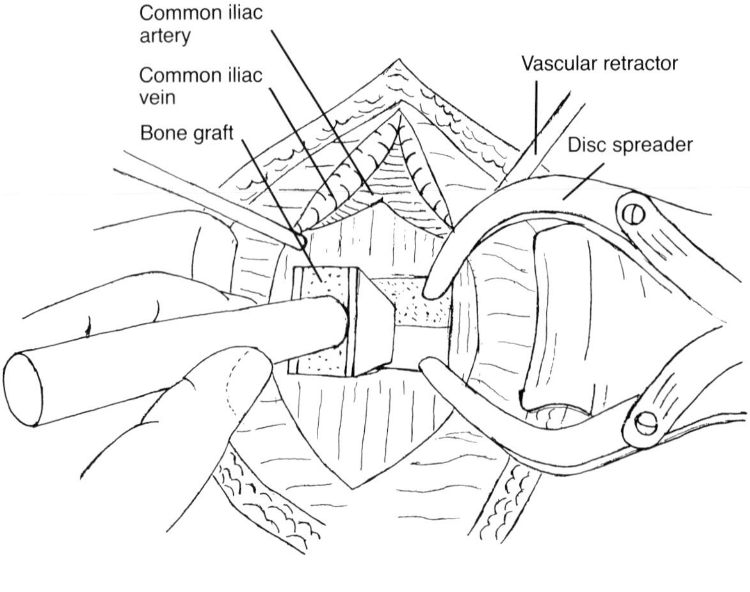

Figure 30 □ The bone grafts are tightly tapped into position by means of the disc spreader.

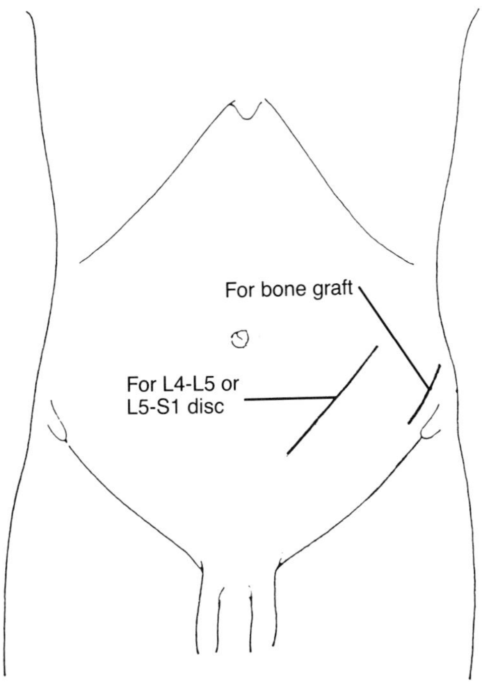

Figure 31 □ The skin incision for the extraperitoneal approach.

the peritoneum. When the opening is made, the peritoneum is carefully separated from the abdominal wall, manually or by using clamp-held compresses. If the peritoneum is injured during the procedure, it should be repaired immediately, because it is sometimes difficult to find the ruptured portion later. The posterior sheath of the rectus muscle is longitudinally cut to the arcuate line to facilitate the retraction of the muscle medially.

Then the intraperitoneal viscera is gradually retracted medially by means of large flexible retractors. When the lateral margin of the psoas muscle is reached, the retraction should be changed anteriorly. Although the ureter, which shows peristaltic movement, is usually retracted with the peritoneum, care must be taken neither to injure nor to ligate it. As the abdominal viscera in the peritoneum are displaced medially, the vertebral column and the pulsating aorta become palpable, and vertebral bodies and discs can be identified. When necessary, an x-ray film should be obtained to confirm the level to be approached. The segmental lumbar vessels may be ligated and cut to mobilize the large vessels (Fig. 32). The truncus sympathicus, which is located at the side of the lumbar spine, should be protected during dissection. After the anterior part of the lumbar spine is fully exposed by this procedure, the discectomy and spine fusion are accomplished by the same procedure described in the anterior transperitoneal approach.

Postoperative Care

Nutrition is supplied by the parenteral route until the patient can clearly pass gas. Elastic stockings should be used after surgery to prevent thrombophlebitis of the lower extremities. Anticoagulant therapy is indicated in patients with a high risk of venous throm-

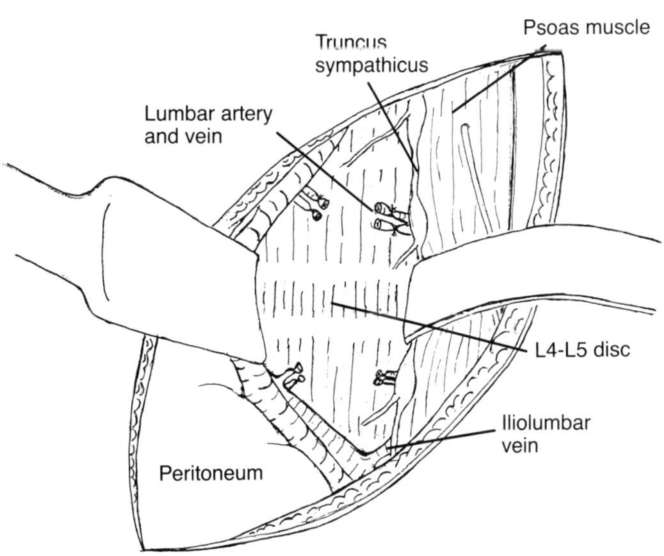

Figure 32 □ The L4–L5 disc space can be approached by displacing the large vessels to the right side, as in the transperitoneal approach. The truncus sympathicus should be protected during dissection.

bosis. The patient is allowed to stand 3 to 4 weeks after the surgery, using a hard corset, which is applied for a 3-month period postoperatively. Thereafter, a soft corset is applied for another 3 months. Vigorous activities are allowed 6 months postoperatively.

PERCUTANEOUS DISCECTOMY

Onik and colleagues[32] have developed a vitrectomy–aspiration type of probe that in 1988 was widely used for percutaneous aspiration of herniated nuclear material. The stimulus for such an approach came from the complications that occurred following the widespread release of chymopapain in the United States. Because of their desire to avoid open discectomy and its attendant scarring, radiologist Onik and neurosurgeon Maroon pioneered the use of the probe (Fig. 33).

It is the author's (J.A.M.) opinion that the limited indications and a higher-than-acceptable recurrence rate will erode the present popularity of this approach. The excitement about this concept is caused by its potential extension to triangulation approaches to the spinal canal, as reported by Schreiber and Suezawa.[35]

SPECIAL SITUATIONS WITH AN HNP

Foraminal HNP

Because of the advent of CT scanning, this syndrome has now gained recognition.[1,7] Most foraminal disc herniations occur in older patients at the L4–L5 interspace and encroach on the fourth lumbar nerve root, causing anterior thigh pain, medial shin numbness, and fourth-root neurologic changes. Figure 34 is a CT scan of a patient with a foraminal disc herniation. The herniation was removed through an approach lateral to the pars interarticularis,[47] as depicted in Figure 35.

HNP with Spondylolisthesis[9]

Patients with a spondylolisthesis may suffer from a disc rupture causing an acute radicular syndrome. Most of these occur at the level above the spondylolisthesis. Figure 36 shows an example of such a patient. A disc herniation into the foramen at the same level of the slip usually occurs, as depicted in Figure 37. For the former situation, a simple disc excision is all that is required; for the latter (disc excision at the slip level), discectomy should be accompanied by a stabilization procedure.

HNP in Spinal Stenosis

Spinal stenosis can occur in the central canal or in the lateral zones. It can be an asymptomatic or a mildly symptomatic condition that can suddenly convert to a significant disability when a disc herniation occurs. Investigation in these patients is somewhat inconclusive if viewed in isolation. Only when the presenting symptoms are analyzed and the dominance of the leg pain in association with significant straight-leg raising reduction does one suspect a small disc herniation in the presence of a stenotic canal or lateral zone. For asymptomatic spinal canal stenosis, simple microsurgical removal of the disc herniation is the proposed method of treatment, unless, based on history, the stenotic component was found to be significantly symptomatic prior to the occurrence of the HNP.

HNP in Instability

Patients with a long history of back pain and significant degenerative disc disease on plain x-ray findings may suffer from a disc herniation at the degenerative level. Whether this instability should be treated at the time of the disc excision is the subject of Posterior Spinal Fusions, later in this chapter, and of Chapter 10.

HNP in the Adolescent Patient

The young patient with a disc herniation is a special problem. As outlined in the series of De Orio and Bianco[6] from the Mayo Clinic, a number of these patients go on to repeat surgical procedures after their initial surgical intervention. Because of the high proteoglycan content of the disc material and the prevalence of disc protrusions, rather than disc extrusions, it is proposed that, in this age group, the optimum treatment is chemonucleolysis rather than surgical intervention.[26]

Text continued on page 419

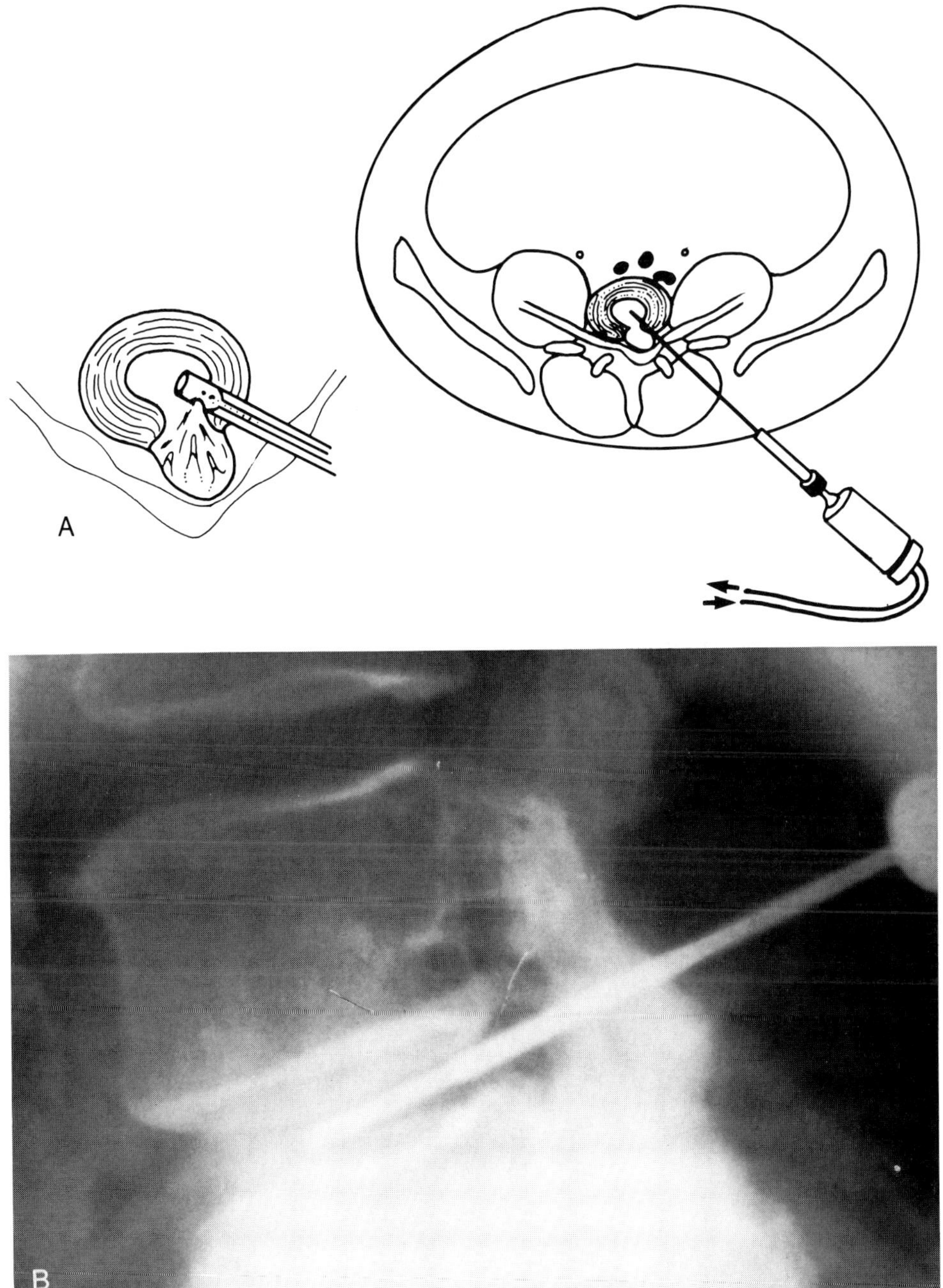

Figure 33 □ *A,* Approach and concept of percutaneous discectomy are shown. *B,* Probe is in the disc space.

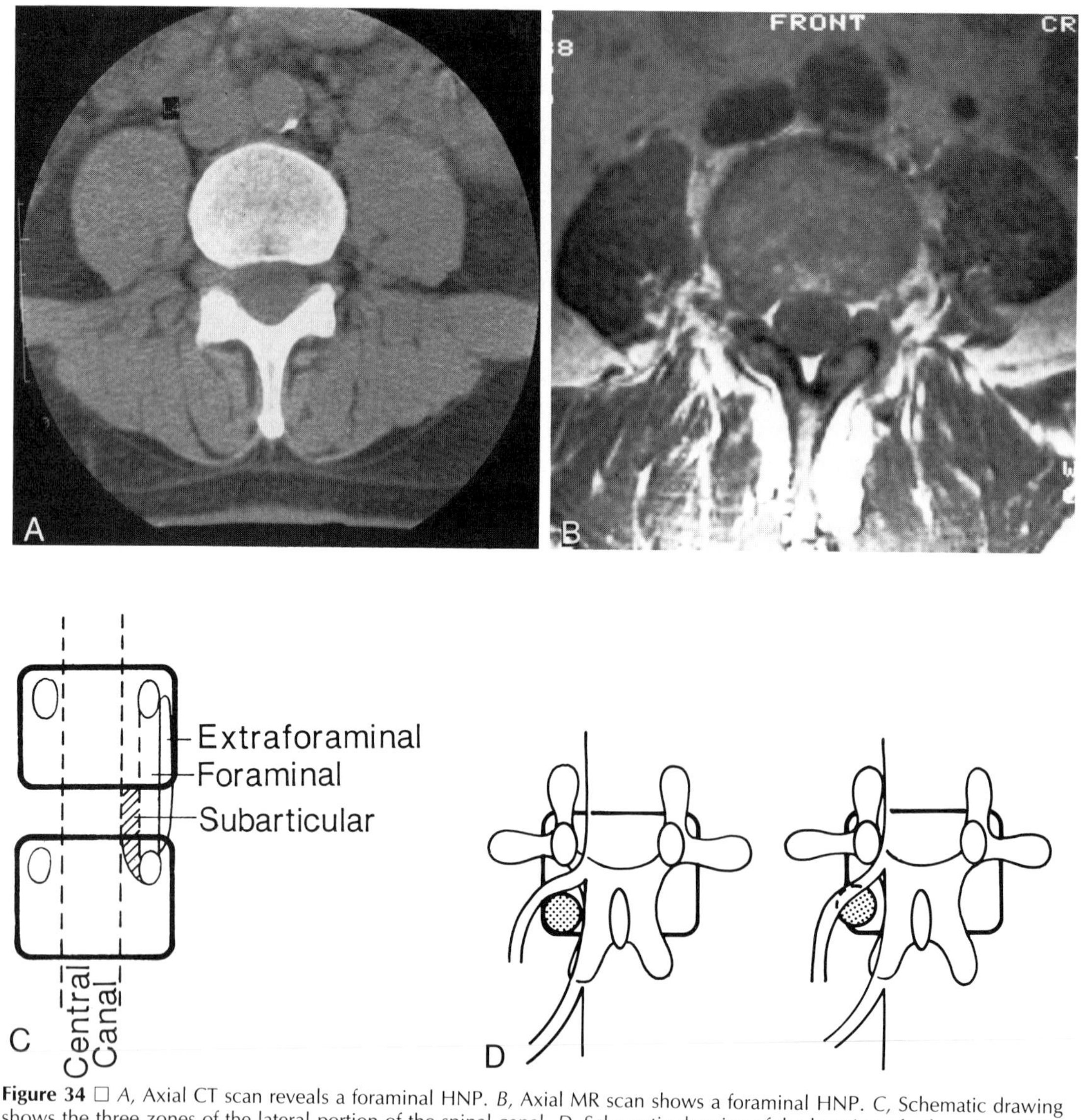

Figure 34 □ *A*, Axial CT scan reveals a foraminal HNP. *B*, Axial MR scan shows a foraminal HNP. *C*, Schematic drawing shows the three zones of the lateral portion of the spinal canal. *D*, Schematic drawing of the location of a foraminal HNP. The more usual location is shown in the drawing on the right.

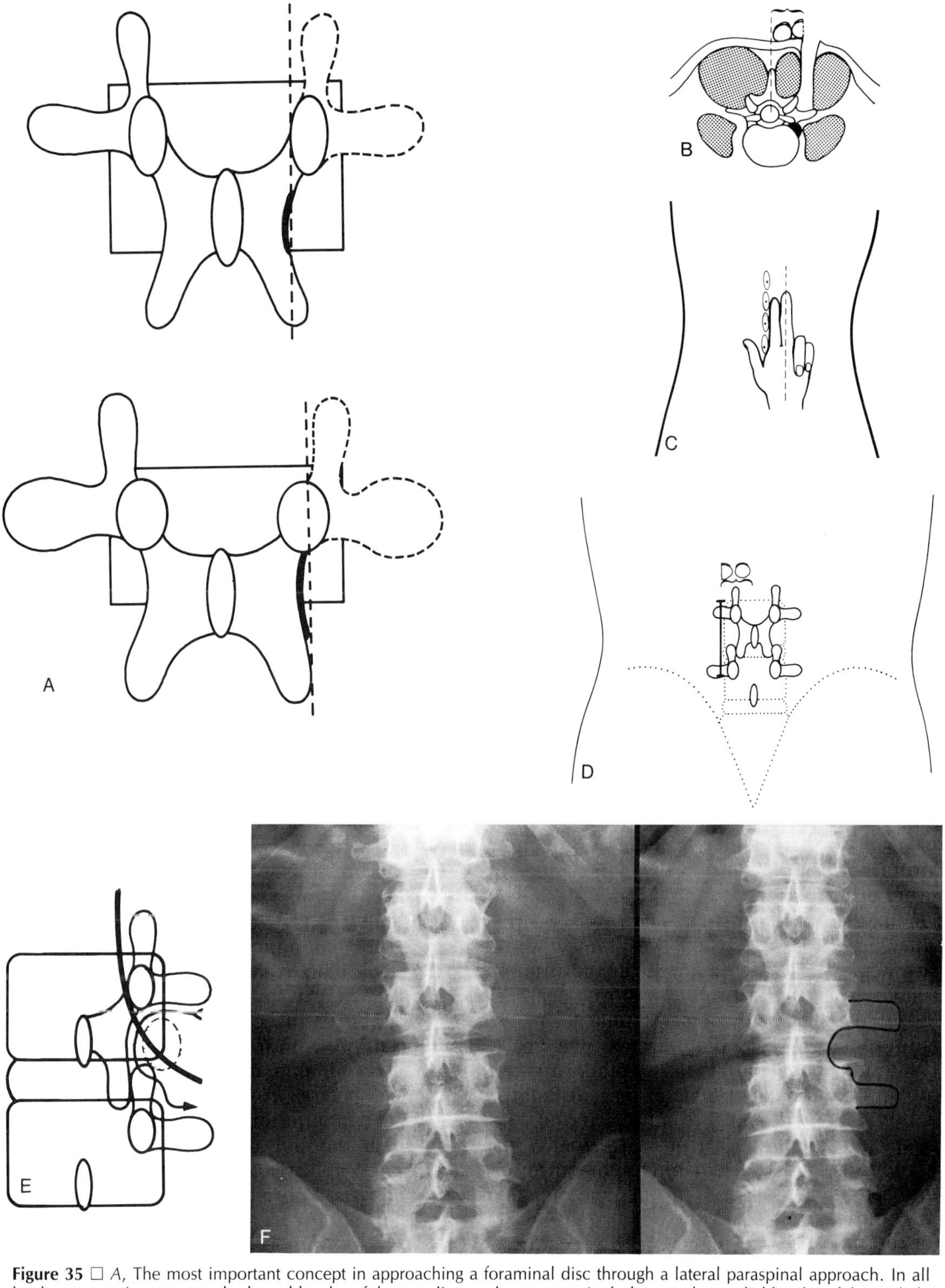

Figure 35 □ *A,* The most important concept in approaching a foraminal disc through a lateral paraspinal approach. In all lumbar anatomic segments the lateral border of the pars lies on the same sagittal plane as the medial border of the pedicle (top). The only exception is L5 (bottom). Retrieving a disc from the foramen by using an interlaminar approach may result in fracturing the pars, sacrificing the inferior facet, and adversely affecting the stability of the segment. *B,* Lateral paraspinal approach to the intertransverse ligament is shown. (Adapted from Wiltse, L.L., Bateman, J. G., Hutchinson, R.H., and Nelson, W.E.: The paraspinal sacrospinalis-splitting approach to the lumbar spine. J. Bone Joint Surg., 50A:919–926, 1968.) *C,* Skin incision is 1½ fingers' breadth from the midline, centered over the pars *(D). E,* To open the intertransverse interval, one starts along the inferior edge of the cephalic transverse process, taking off some of the lateral edge of the pars and removing the tip of the superior facet, as shown. *F,* Postoperative x-ray film showing the exposure, L4–L5, left. Compare this interval to the right side. The right-sided x-ray study shows the exposure outlined. Observe how much of the disc space can be seen from the lateral edge to the pars.

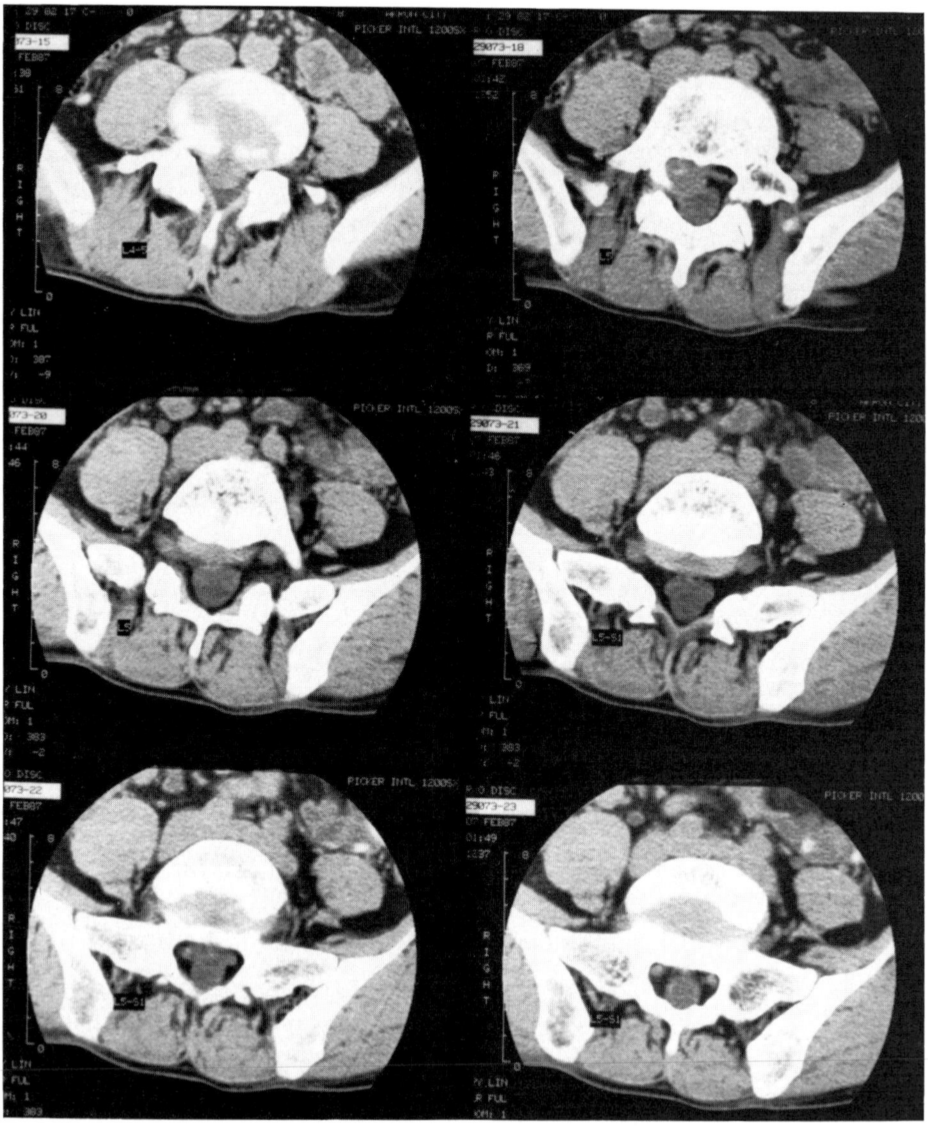

Figure 36 □ Spondylolisthesis, L5 on S1, and a large HNP, L4–L5, are shown in these CT scans.

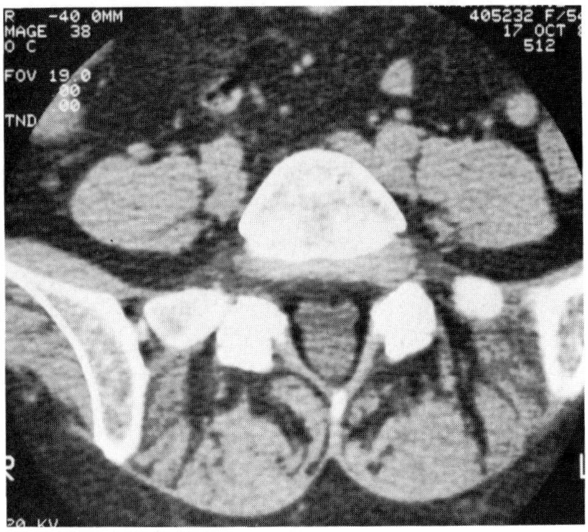

Figure 37 □ Axial CT scan of a foraminal disc, L5, left, that occurred in a slipped segment, L5 on S1.

Recurrent HNP

The prevalence of reherniation of discal material is approximately two to five in 100 cases. The recurrence may occur at any interval after surgery (days to years) and is most often at the same level and same side. If the recurrence is at same level and opposite side or at another level, the principles discussed earlier apply. Unfortunately, most recurrences are at the same level and same side, and scar tissue from the previous surgery introduces a new element in diagnosis and treatment, which can be summarized as follows:

1. Scarring "tacks" down the dura to the back of the disc space so that a smaller amount of herniated nuclear material is capable of producing a significant amount of pain and neurologic deficit.
2. Because of the immobility of the scarred dura, transdural ruptures, although rare, can occur.
3. Determining the anatomic level by clinical assessment can be difficult because
   a. Some neurologic changes are residual from the prior HNP.
   b. The dura may not simply be immobilized; it may be distorted from the scar tissue, leading to root involvement lower than usual for the level of the HNP (e.g., a recurrent L4–L5 HNP may affect a number of sacral roots).
4. Investigation can be difficult to interpret because of the scar tissue. To a large extent, this reduces the reliability of myelography and has led to the use of contrast-enhanced (IV Conray-enhanced) CT (Fig. 38) and IV gadolinium DTPA–enhanced MRI.
5. Not only are the clinical assessment and investigation difficult, the surgery is also difficult and prone to complications such as missed lesions, dural tears, and neurologic damage. A basic principle in repeat surgery is to gain as wide an exposure as possible in order to manage the recurrent pathologic condition. The microsurgeons are flying in the face of this principle, but if preoperative investigation is used to accurately localize the recurrent disease, microsurgical intervention presents some advantages.[11]

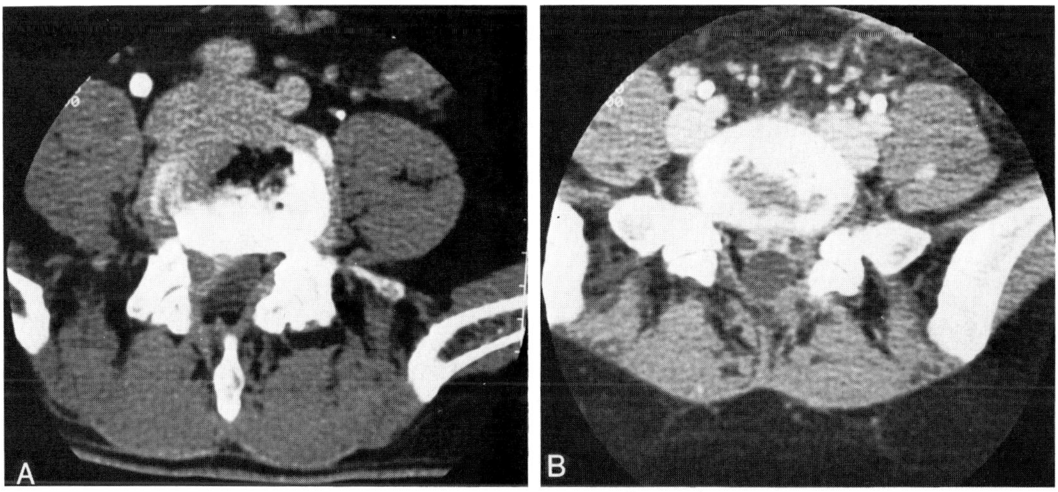

Figure 38 □ *A,* Axial CT scan soon after injection of IV contrast. The scar tissue enhances the image to outline the avascular recurrent HNP. *B,* Axial CT scan with contrast-enhancing scar tissue and no evidence of a recurrent HNP.

Table 14 □ Symptoms and Signs Suggesting a Nonorganic Component to Disability[43]

SYMPTOMS

Pain is multifocal in distribution and nonmechanical (present at rest).

Entire extremity is painful, numb, and/or weak.

Extremity gives way (as a result, the patient carries a cane).

Treatment response: No response; "allergic" to treatment; or not on treatment.

Multiple crises, multiple hospital admissions/ investigations, multiple doctors.

SIGNS

Tenderness is superficial (skin) or nonanatomic (e.g., over body of sacrum).

Simulated movement tests are positive.

Distraction tests are positive.

Entire leg is weak or numb.

CURRENT APPROACH

It is the author's (J.A.M.) current philosophy that a thorough clinical history and physical examination lead to an accurate diagnosis of an acute radicular syndrome resulting from an HNP. The routine clinical assessment should also reveal any nonorganic component to a patient's disability (Table 14). The next step in decision-making is an attempt to establish the anatomic level (Table 15) before reviewing the investigation. Finally, there must be a perfect marriage between the clinical syndrome and the patient's investigation before surgical intervention is undertaken. CT and MRI are facilitating this more accurate definition of the nature and location of the structural lesion. By means of this approach, it will be possible to live up to today's standard for surgical intervention for lumbar disc disease. The standard includes an accurate clinical diagnosis, an accurate surgical procedure without complications, delivery of at least an 85% success rate, and a return-to-work rate of 95%.

Table 15 □ Anatomic Level of HNP

Location of leg pain
- Posterior thigh and calf—L5 or S1, root
- Anterior thigh—L4, L3, or L2, root

Paresthetic discomfort
- Medial shin—L4
- Lateral calf, Dorsum of foot } L5
- Lateral border of foot—S1

Neurologic examination

THE FUTURE

At the time of writing this chapter, there was considerable interest in percutaneous discectomy. It is the author's opinion that this interest will have a limited life span in spinal surgery but will be the beginning of more percutaneous approaches to spinal disorders. For the future, the author envisions triangulation techniques, which are so prevalent in knee and shoulder surgery, being adapted to spinal surgery. Much work is now being undertaken to design an artificial disc. However, it will be long in coming to fruition, and many complications are anticipated before suitable substitute and technique of application are developed.

Probably the greatest development in lumbar disc disease will be in the field of preventing disc degeneration and disc herniation. This is likely to come through better understanding of the biologic, pathologic, and biomechanical factors that lead to disc deterioration and by manipulating those factors.

References

1. Abdullah, A.F., Ditto, E.W., Byrd, E.B., and Williams, S.R.: Extreme lateral lumbar disc herniations: Clinical syndrome and special problems of diagnosis. J. Neurosurg. 41:229–234, 1974.
2. Bell, G.R., and Rothman, R.H.: The conservative treatment of sciatica. Spine 9:54–56, 1984.
3. Caspar, W.: A new surgical procedure for lumbar disc herniation causing less tissue damage through microsurgical approach. Adv. Neurosurg. 4:74–79, 1977.
4. Cotugno, D.: De Ischiade Nervosa, Commentarios. Napoli, Apud Frat, Simonios, 1764.
5. Dandy, W.E.: Loose cartilage from intervertebral disk simulating tumor of the spinal cord. Arch. Surg. (Chicago) 19:660–672, 1929.
6. De Orio, J.K., and Bianco, A.J.: Lumbar disc excision in children and adolescents. J. Bone Joint Surg. 64A:991–996, 1982.
7. Dyck, P.: The femoral nerve traction test in lumbar disc protrusion. Surg. Neurol. 6:163–166, 1976.
8. Fager, C.A., and Freidberg, S.R.: Analysis and failures of poor results of lumbar spine surgery. Spine 5:87–94, 1980.
9. Feldman, R., and McCulloch, J.A.: Acute radicular syndrome in lytic spondylolisthesis. Spine (in press).
10. Feldman, R., and McCulloch, J.A.: Microsurgery for lumbar disc disease (submitted for publication).
11. Goald, H.J.: A new microsurgical reoperation for failed lumbar disc surgery. J. Microsurg. 7:63–66, 1986.

12. Goldthwait, J.: The lumbo-sacral articulation. An explanation of many cases of "lumbago", "sciatica", and paraplegia. Boston Med. Surg. J. 164:365–372, 1911.
13. Hakelius, A.: Prognosis in sciatica: A clinical follow-up of surgical and non-surgical treatment. Acta Orthop. Scand. 129(Suppl.):1–76, 1970.
14. Harmon, P.H.: Anterior excision and vertebral body fusion operation for intervertebral disk syndromes of the lower lumbar spine. Clin. Orthop. 26:107–127, 1963.
15. Helms, C.A., Dorwart, R.H., and Gray, M.: The CT appearance of conjoined nerve roots and differentiation from a herniated nucleus pulposus. Radiology 144:803–807, 1982.
16. Hirabayashi, K.: Anterior lumbar disc lesion. Rinsho Seikei Geka 4:610–623, 1969.
17. Hitselberger, W., and Witten, R.: Abnormal myelograms in asymptomatic patients. J. Neurosurg. 28:204–206, 1968.
18. Hodgson, A.R., and Wong, S.K.: A description of a technic and evaluation of results in anterior spinal fusion for deranged intervertebral disk and spondylolisthesis. Clin. Orthop. 56:133–162, 1968.
19. Hudgins, W.R.: The role of microdiscectomy. Orthop. Clin. North Am. 14:589–603, 1983.
20. Inoue, S., Tateiwa, M., Tsuji, H., et al.: Over ten year follow-up study of anterior lumbar body fusion. Nippon Seikeigeka Gakkai Zasshi 43:749–750, 1969.
21. Inoue, S., Watanabe, T., Hirose, A., et al.: Anterior discectomy and interbody fusion for lumbar disc herniation. Clin. Orthop. 183:22–31, 1984.
22. Kadish, L.J., and Simmons, E.H.: Anomalies of the lumbosacral nerve roots. An anatomical investigation and myelographic study. J. Bone Joint Surg. 66B:411–416, 1984.
23. Lane, J.D., and Moore, E.S.: Transperitoneal approach to the intervertebral disc in the lumbar area. Ann. Surg. 127:537–551, 1948.
24. LaRocca, A., and Macnab, I.: The laminectomy membrane. J. Bone Joint Surg. 56B:545–550, 1974.
25. Lasègue, C.: Considerations sur la Sciatique. Arch. Gen. Med. Serv. 6:558–580, 1864.
26. Lorenz, M., and McCulloch J.: Chemonucleolysis for herniated nucleus pulposus in adolescents. J. Bone Joint Surg. 67A:1402–1404, 1985.
27. Love, J.G.: Removal of protruded intervertebral disc without laminectomy. Proc. Staff Meet. Mayo Clin. 14:800, 1939.
28. Mayfield, F.H.: Complications of laminectomy. Clin. Neurosurg. 23:435–439, 1976.
29. Mixter, W.S., and Barr, I.S.: Rupture of the intervertebral disc without involvement of the spinal cord. N. Engl. J. Med. 211:210–215, 1934.
30. Nakano, N.: Operative result for lumbar disc degeneration. Seikei Geka 23:567–574, 1972.
31. Neidre, A., and Macnab, I.: Anomalies of the lumbosacral nerve roots. Review of 16 cases and classification. Spine 8:294–299, 1983.
32. Onik, G., Helms, C.A., Ginsburg, L., et al.: Percutaneous lumbar discectomy using a new aspiration probe. A.J.N.R. 6:290–293, 1985.
33. Postacchini, F., Urso, S., and Ferro, L.: Lumbosacral root anomalies. J. Bone Joint Surg. 64A:721–729, 1982.
34. Sacks, S.: Anterior interbody fusion of the lumbar spine. J. Bone Joint Surg. 47B:211–223, 1965.
35. Schreiber, A., and Suezawa, Y.: Transdiscoscopic percutaneous nucleotomy in disk herniation. Orthop. Rev. 15:35–38, 1986.
36. Scoville, W.B., and Corkilig, G.: Lumbar disc surgery: Technique of radical removal and early mobilization. J. Neurosurg. 39:265–269, 1973.
37. Spangfort, E.V.: The lumbar disc herniation. A computer-aided analysis of 2,504 operations. Acta Orthop. Scand. 142(Suppl.):1–95, 1972.
38. Spengler, D.M.: Lumbar discectomy: Results with limited disc excision and selective foraminotomy. Spine 7:604–607, 1982.
39. Stauffer, R.N., and Coventry, M.B.: Anterior interbody lumbar spine fusion. J. Bone Joint Surg. 54A:756–768, 1972.
40. Suzuki, J., Ishibashi, B., Sakamaki, K., et al.: Anterior body fusion for lumbar disc herniation. Nippon Seikeigeka Gakkai Zasshi 32:948–950, 1958.
41. Tsuchiya, K.: A long term follow-up study of transperitoneal anterior vertebral body fusion (Suzuki's method) for lumbar disc herniation—especially on the influence of vertebral body fusion upon the lumbar vertebral column. Nippon Seikeigeka Gakkai Zasshi 47:731–767, 1973.
42. Verbiest, H.: Results of surgical treatment of idiopathic developmental stenosis of the lumbar vertebral canal. A review of twenty-seven years' experience. J. Bone Joint Surg. 59B:181–188, 1977.
43. Waddell, G., McCulloch, J.A., Kummel, E.G., and Venner, R.M.: Non-organic physical signs in low back pain. Spine 5:117–125, 1980.
44. Weber, H.: Lumbar disc herniation: A controlled prospective study with 10 years of observation. Spine 8:131–140, 1983.
45. Williams, R.: Microlumbar discectomy. A conservative surgical approach to the virgin herniated lumbar disc. Spine 3:175–182, 1978.
46. Wilson, D., and Harbaugh, R.: Microsurgical and standard removal of protruded lumbar disc. A comparative study. Neurosurgery 8:422–427, 1981.
47. Wiltse, L.L., Bateman, J.G., Hutchinson, R.H., and Nelson, W.E.: The paraspinal sacrospinalis-splitting approach to the lumbar spine. J. Bone Joint Surg. 50A:919–926, 1968.
48. Yasargil, M.G.: Microsurgical operations for herniated lumbar disc. Adv. Neurosurg. 4:81–82, 1977.
49. Yong-Hing, K., Reilly, J., de Korompay, V., and Kirkaldy-Willis, W.H.: Prevention of nerve root adhesions after laminectomy. Spine 5:59–64, 1980.

Facet Syndrome

Vert Mooney

Facet syndrome remains an undefined entity and as such is similar to discogenic pain. The degree to which it is the primary source of pain, rather than a contributing source, for each individual with lumbago and sciatica has not yet been defined. The definition of this clinical entity rests on the validity of findings of pain relief following radiographically controlled, anatomically specific injections. There should be a better means of defining this syndrome. The following discussion is a prologue to a greater future understanding of facet syndrome.

HISTORICAL BACKGROUND

Although the phrase *facet syndrome* was first introduced by Ghormley in 1933,[16] his meaning was different from the one used today. The concept of referred pain had not been developed. Fluoroscopy and the axial view of the spine (computed tomographic [CT] scan) were unknown. The only objective measurement tool for the spine was the standard x-ray film. All that could be seen were narrowed disc spaces with degenerating facet joints. Thus, Ghormley's discussion was about the role of the facet joints in creating nerve pressure and thus providing a potential source of sciatica.

The first clinician to point out the potential role of the apophyseal joints in the production of back pain and leg pain was Goldthwait.[17] Again, using the x-ray study as his only clinical investigative tool, he correlated surgical experience and anatomic dissections with facet joint pathologic conditions. As were many clinicians of that time, Goldthwait was struck by the asymmetry of the facet joints as seen on x-ray studies and believed that it must be a major factor in initiating facet disorders and eventually pain resulting from nerve root pressure. Mechanical pressure on the nerves, he thought, was the source of pain. In fact, it took years and thousands of x-rays before clinicians could lay to rest the concept that facet asymmetry was related to back pain.[27]

The theory of asymmetry and the apparently unbalanced mechanical forces was tantalizing. Several clinicians, in the 1920s, provided anatomic support for the concept.[9, 2, 60] The Italian surgeon, Putti, seems to be the first to have focused specifically on the degenerative process of the articular facets.[43] At first, this degeneration was largely considered to be the cause of sciatica, but Putti hinted at the possibility of nonmechanical sources of nerve irritation and therefore defined the neurologic problem as a neuralgia. He noted the increasing prevalence of facet arthropathy with increasing age. Because he could not specifically pinpoint the disease of the apophyseal joints, he believed that it had to be secondary to the nonsymmetric articulations. Great efforts to measure various angles were made by Putti and by other investigators. On the basis of these measurements, it was noted that even the L4–L5 articulation may not be symmetric, and it was thus entertained that this too could be a source of back pain.

The first clinician who seems to have questioned the idea of facet arthritis as a source of nerve root irritation being an explanation of lumbago and sciatica was Badgley.[3] He noted that fewer than 20% of the patients coming to him with lumbago and sciatica had any neurologic evidence of direct nerve irritation. Also, the great majority were responsive to the conservative care of rest and manipulation; it was difficult to believe that structural abnormalities of a severity sufficient to cause nerve root irritation could be so easily reversible. Apparently, he was the first clinician to consider the radiation of pain down the leg or into the buttock to be based on a referred phenomenon.[4] At that time, however, the concept was so tenuous that it was never published, but only was read at a meeting of the American Academy of Orthopaedic Surgeons (AAOS) in 1936. Badgley did note the understandable phenomenon that with the discovery of the protruding or extruded nucleus pulposus, attention to the facets as major contributors to the back pain problem had greatly diminished. Surgical exposure of the spinal canal to visualize the nucleus pulposus in its relationship to the nerve root in the spinal canal was far more understandable, especially to clinicians who, for the first time, were visualizing the spine at surgery for nonmalignant or traumatic diseases.

Thus, in spite of the emerging surgical enthusiasm for the disc, Badgley made a plea for continuing to focus attention on the facets in order to explain the large numbers of low back clinical problems that were unexplainable by our current understanding of the ruptured disc. His comments in 1941 are probably just as relevant today as they were then:

> The anatomical possibilities of the articular facets to play a more or less active part in the production of low back pain with or without sciatic radiation are obvious, but pathological evidence is not yet sufficient to make this conclusion a fact.[3]

Considering the facet joints to be a source of pain implies, of course, a specific innervation. Pain pathways of the lumbar spine were poorly understood at the time of Badgley's comments. Until the 1940s, it was thought that a portion of the facet joint innervation came from a recurrent branch of the anterior primary division. Dissections of this area by McCotter and Strong were reported by Badgley.[5] They identified a medial branch of the posterior primary ramus as the consistent means of innervation of the capsule and periosteum of the joints. Thus, it was reasonable to propose a concept that irritation of the capsule by the degenerated lumbar facet joints could produce stimuli that, by way of the posterior primary division, could return to the central nervous system and produce referred pain through the distribution of the involved nerves that corresponded to the sciatic radiation. However, his enthusiasm for the facets was essentially unheeded by other clinicians; it was not until the 1970s that additional interest in the facet joints emerged in our literature.

A concept vital to our current understanding of back pain and leg pain related to abnormalities of the lumbar spine is that of referred pain. As mentioned above, the concept was initially tentative. Distribution of abnormal neurologic function according to the distribution of peripheral nerves was mapped out nicely by Foerester.[15] The neuroanatomic distribution of pain and dysesthesia, as well as numbness and motor weakness, fit nicely into the concepts of the ruptured disc defined at the same time in the early 1930s.[35] However, the neurologist Kelgrin noted that stimulation of connective tissue structures could create pain distally in a distribution different from that of the dermatomes. He thus labeled the vague anatomic distributions *sclerotomes*.[24, 25] Referred pain arising from skeletal structures was later identified by Inman and Saunders in 1944.[22]

Various authors recognized that the referred pain phenomenon was far less specific than had originally been proposed. A great overlap of pain patterns was noted in the effort to map specific referral sites.[20, 51] It was recognized that many different anatomic sites could cause pain in the same location. Steindler and Luck, however, did offer direct evidence that referred pain could come from the facet joint.[52] Using percutaneous anatomic landmarks, they injected a local anesthetic into what was presumed to be the facet joint and were able to relieve back pain. They could not, at that time, specifically identify the anatomic structure; nor, of course, could they define whether the location of the material was intracapsular or extracapsular. It also became clear that pain could be created by the irritation of various anatomic structures ranging from the ligaments to the disc as well as to the facet joints. Using hypertonic saline injected with the guidance of x-rays, Hirsch and associates produced pain in living subjects at various anatomic sites. The implication of this work, however, was that most of the pain emerged from the disc.[19]

No specific therapeutic approach to the facet joint emerged until the 1970s. Attention to the facet joint came from a most unusual direction. A general physician by the name of Skirmi Rees, working by himself in a small town in Australia, conceived the notion that one might denervate the posterior structures of the spine and thus relieve back pain.[45] He developed a procedure performed under local anesthesia wherein a special hook blade knife was placed near the facet joint percutaneously. No x-ray studies were included in work-up or treatment. An astounding short-term success was reported. Owing to lack of repeatability and long-term studies, this procedure never entered the mainstream of medicine. Nonetheless, the concept caught the attention of a very imaginative neurosurgeon, Norman Shealy. After visiting Dr. Rees, he attempted to carry out the same procedure but with the neurosurgeon's more specific anatomic knowledge. To his dismay, in an attempt to be thorough in denervating the facet joints by percutaneous incision, significant morbidity resulted because of hemorrhaging from the surrounding tissues. This led Dr. Shealy to use a tool more discrete than the knife—the thermal lesion maker. This tool was currently used for the controllable destruction of neurologic tissue. Initially, Dr. Shealy attempted merely to denervate the capsule, but once the neuroanatomic distribution of facet innervation was understood, he proceeded to approach the articular nerves at specific anatomic sites.[49] He was the first to use fluoroscopic localization of the facet joint in an attempt to specifically treat the anatomic site. I visited Dr. Shealy in 1972 and observed patients in obvious pain and distress being brought to the fluoroscopy unit. Under local anesthesia with the use of the lesion maker, obliteration of innervation of various levels was accomplished. To my astonishment, after this procedure the patients nearly jumped off the table, indicating their significant relief and their great pleasure in the rapid change of events.

It seemed very reasonable to try to duplicate Dr. Shealy's excellent initial results. With the availability of an animal laboratory, it was possible to use the lesion maker and specifically identify the damage done to the articular structures of the facet joint. At that time, the innervation was not clear, and I used the procedure initially advocated by Shealy: destruction of the capsule and thus of the innervation. In a series of procedures involving rabbits, histologic evaluation of the articular structures in our laboratory at Rancho Los Amigos Hospital showed minimal changes in the cartilage. However, the amount of destruction to muscle tissue was notable. The lesion maker had originally been developed for use in the brain or cord, and thus its effect on muscles was not a point of concern. However, muscles were sensitive to thermal injury. On this basis, it seemed inappropriate to create additional structural damage to the back musculature by using this tool. If the pain was arising from arthropathy within the joint, it seemed quite appropriate to approach the joint, as is customary, at other articulations by the injection of steroids. Using the fluoroscopy technique developed by Shealy, we proceeded to inject joints with local anesthesia and steroids. This technique added to our current understanding of the role of facets in relation to back pain.[36] This is discussed in another section.

ANATOMIC ASPECTS

In trying to more clearly understand the facet syndrome, it is important to identify what we know about the structural anatomy of the facet joint. We must recognize at the outset that no radiologic study of the lumbar spine correlates the incidence of lumbago and sciatica with the radiographic features of the degenerating disc and associated arthropathy of the facet joints. Nor does a well-controlled biomechanical study exist, associating variations in lumbar range with symptoms of back pain or sciatica. Diminished range should be associated with facet joint abnormalities. Nonetheless, some individuals, on the occasion of severe back and leg pain, with or without radiographic changes noted in the facet joints, achieve excellent relief of symptoms when only the joint is injected with local anesthesia. Where was the pain coming from? What are the anatomic considerations relative to the facet joint?

A function of the facet joint certainly must be to limit the mechanical range of the disc. The facet joints apparently respond to the aging process.[44] Initially, fetal and infant facet joints are coronally oriented. As the lordotic posture emerges, posterior growth from lateral margins of the facets develops in early childhood so that the eventual orientation is curved and biplanar as the posterior parts approximate a sagittal plane, while the anterior parts of the joint remain in more coronal orientation. As age advances, the anterior aspect of the concaved surface becomes thicker, and cell hypertrophy (i.e., an increased density of cells) is noted in the anterior medial aspect. Vertical fibrillation of the cartilage develops, as do sclerotic changes of the underlying subchondral bone plate (Fig. 1).

On the other hand, the posterior two thirds of the joint have a different deteriorating process. In some specimens, the cartilage appears to split parallel to the cartilage–bone interface. The damaged cartilage remains continuous with the capsular attachment and therefore forms a meniscus-like structure. There is a template-like fit to the underlying cartilage, which indicates that the structure has an articular-cartilage origin

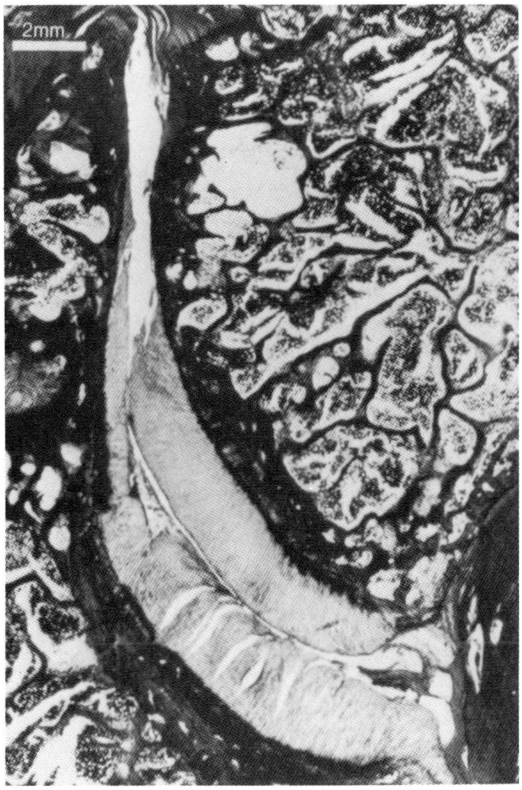

Figure 1 □ In these reproductions of dissections, the two alternative functions of facet joint are noted. The anterior aspect of the joint shows cartilage fibrillation and increased sclerotic changes, suggesting compressive loads. The posterior aspect demonstrates shearing and denuding of cartilage (superior is anterior; inferior is posterior, in this illustration). (From Twomey, L.T., and Taylor, J.R.: Physical Therapy of the Low Back. New York, Churchill Livingstone, 1987.)

and is not from a synovial fold. An interesting anatomic fact is that the multifidus muscle attaches to the capsule and therefore has the potential to move this "meniscus" formed from detached cartilage (Fig. 2). There is a progressive deterioration with age so that moderate to severe fibrillation is noted in patients in their thirties and forties. The changes noted in younger groups continue but with more significant changes. Ultimately, there may be denuding of articular surfaces in the posterior aspect, whereas vertical fibrillation and thickening of the cartilage may continue in the anterior medial aspect. Sclerotic changes continue in the anterior medial aspect, suggesting continued vertical stress loading.

Also associated with the aging process is a reaction phenomenon, that is, the formation of osteophytes. They are often accompanied by enlarged synovial fat pads, which form cushions between the osteophyte and the inferior articular process. The osteophytes develop at the joint margins at the attachment of the ligamentum flavum or the capsule. They are seen most commonly as beaklike extensions from the anterior medial margin of the superior articular process into the ligamentum flavum.

Thus, the deterioration mode of the articular surfaces demonstrates the various functions of the facet joints. The thickening of the anterior medially suggests that this phase of the joint prevents forward translation. The role of the facet joints as the major barrier to excessive lumbar flexion was demonstrated in another study by Twomey and Taylor. They showed that on the occasion of osteotomy of the pedicles (and thus, loss of facet function) excessive and significant lumbar range became available.[58] On the other hand, a posterior sagittal component of the lumbar facet joint demonstrates relatively thin subchondral bone and, thus, apparently limited compressive loading. Shearing forces, as demonstrated by detached articular cartilage attached to the capsular segments parallel to the subchondral bone, are more manifest.

This leads to the subject of the facet joint meniscus, its potential for entrapment, and its possible role in causing the "locked back." Structures located on the dorsal and ventral margins of the joint have been described,[13] but these are very rudimentary and are perhaps more accurately described as capsular invagination. They do not have a cartilaginous core. In the sections of Bogduk and Engel,[6] dense fibrous tissue was not found at the poles. Fibroadipose meniscoids were found to varying degrees; however, they demonstrated only loose connective tissue and synovium connecting the apex to the capsule. The tissue appeared to be too flimsy to form the substantial fibrous connection that would be required if capsular traction were to move it. Thus, there seems to be no demonstration of a primary meniscus that would offer an explanation for the locked back syndrome. Therefore, if a meniscus-like structure develops, it is apparently related to the degenerative process and really is a portion of the original articular cartilage, which has maintained continuity with the capsule.

An alternative description of the patho-

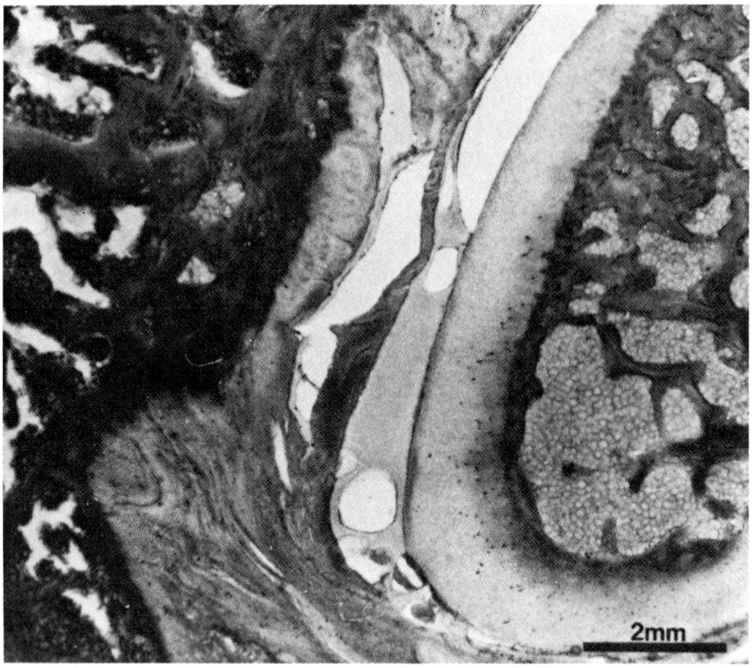

Figure 2 □ The potential for a meniscus-like structure is illustrated from this cartilaginous "flap" attached to the capsule. This again identifies the shearing function of this phase of the joint. (From Twomey, L.T., and Taylor, J.R.: Physical Therapy of the Low Back. New York, Churchill Livingstone, 1987.)

logic changes associated with symptomatic facet joints was presented by Eisenstein and Parry.[12] In this study of 12 patients who had a specific clinical problem (syndrome), which was defined as pain at rest, relieved by motion, and restricted and painful extension associated with normal x-rays, biopsy of the facet joints was achieved on the occasion of fusion surgery. In all these patients, full-thickness cartilage loss or partial necrosis was noted. There was no osteophyte formation. And according to this study, no specific part of the facet joint seemed to be consistently involved. To my knowledge, this is the only study in which symptomatic "facet syndrome" patients were biopsied. These authors drew a parallel between the findings described above and the findings typical of chondromalacia of the patella with its characteristic basal degeneration. The chondromalacia-like changes are different from the degenerative changes noted in the aging cadavers by other authors. On the basis of the relative paucity of pathologic changes (reflected by the lack of radiographic changes) associated with significant pain complaints, the parallel to chondromalacia seems worth considering. On the basis of these findings, the authors propose that the facet syndrome should be called "chondromalacia facetae." This clinical entity should be differentiated from mechanical instability, which is relieved by rest and is aggravated by motion. Of interest in this group of biopsies, the articular ulcer was the major finding. There were no meniscus-like findings or synovial intrusions.

The facet joint obviously takes significant loads during functional activity. Several studies have attempted to evaluate these loads.[18, 56] It must be noted that studies using cadavers probably are not as reliable a representation of true mechanical events as pathologic changes noted in various dissections, as described above. The absence of living musculature and the difference in the compliance of tissues appropriately hydrated in the living organism are large variables in the analysis of loads on cadaver spines. Nonetheless, some principles can be developed. Adams and Hutton, by means of cadaver studies at various angles of loading, determined that the facet joints picked up between 16% and 20% of the load of the entire motion segment.[1] On the other hand, Lorenz and colleagues,[32] using pressure-sensitive film, demonstrated that with increasing loads, less pressure was measured at the joint interface. This is probably due to the translation of the nearly vertically oriented joints and appropriate synovial interfaces. To a certain extent, this hypothesis was confirmed by the study by Yang and King,[61] who noted that excessive facet loads caused the inferior facet to "bottom out" on the pars and then to begin to pivot about the pars to stretch the joint capsule. Thus, the facet joint does not itself take the increasing loads, but rather the capsule and the skeletal structures of the pars take them.

One of the large questions related to the biomechanics of the spine is the participation of the facet joints with the discs in tolerating the stresses of function. In a study of 86 cadavers, Lewin found that intersegmental arthritis of the facet joints occurred occasionally independent of disc degeneration.[28] Indeed, in our own laboratory, Videman and colleagues noted that in 20% of cadaver discograms, which were normal by discography and direct observation, degenerative changes were noted in the facet joints from narrowing of the disc space.[59] Another corollary to this is a study by computed tomographic (CT) examination, in which, of patients complaining of back pain but no neurologic deficit, only 20% had a suggestion of a pathologic disc disorder, whereas 40% showed facet joint changes.[8]

In summary, all that we know about the biomechanical problems of the facet joint suggests that they certainly participate in loads to the lumbar spine. Obviously, their role is to restrain excessive mobility and to distribute axial loading over as broad an area as possible. To a certain extent, the measured mechanical forces do not correlate with those observed in histologic studies. Indeed, various mechanical forces may create varying abnormalities within the facet joint, ranging from sheer overload to peak pressure overload. Necrotic cartilage has been observed in symptomatic joints. Finally, stress to the facet joints may be completely independent of structural overload to the lumbar disc.

From a mechanical standpoint, we are left with the problem of trying to identify the role of the unstable or traumatized facet joint compared with other potential sources of pain. In multiple dissections of the facet joints, Paris has noted that the facet joint capsule is a significant structure.[41] The capacity can be quite variable. There also may be a ridge of synovial lining that may project into the crevice between the articular surfaces. Occasionally, it may take the form of a fat pad. Adhesions have been noted between the capsule and the joint itself. They can be directly observed as a source of limited range of the facet joint.

The facet joint capacity is also quite variable in the living patient. Greater degeneration results in lower capacity, but in individuals without complaint and without radiographic abnormality, arthrography of the facet joint can accept up to 3 cc of fluid before bursting.[11] There is one other aspect of facet disease that may be related to the phenomenon of facet syndrome and appears to be its later disease process: degenerative arthritis. Certainly the facet joint capsule, especially the ligamentum flavum, is close to the nerve root itself. This is beautifully illustrated by the studies of Rauschning, in which the nerve root resides, hugging the pedicle, just superior to the capsule (Fig. 3).[44] The next lower nerve root would be found medial and inferior to the ligamentum flavum. This relationship may explain why it is possible occasionally for individuals with back pain and leg pain of equal inten-

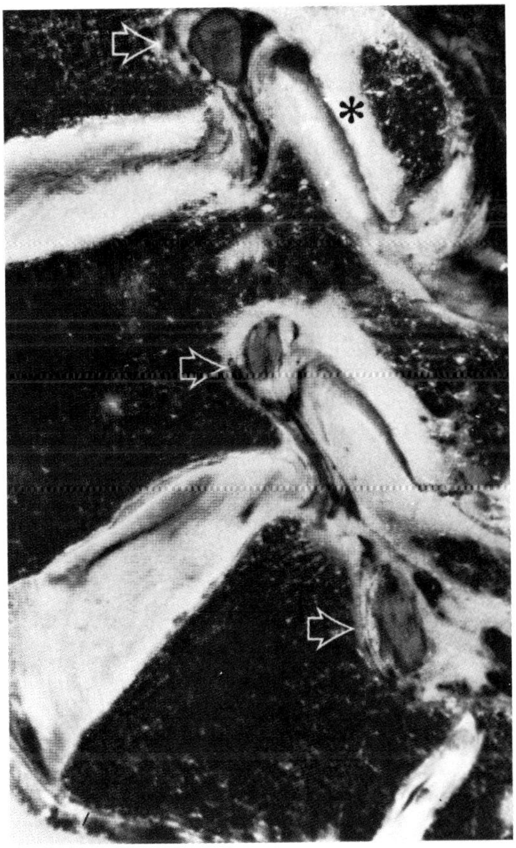

Figure 3 □ Arrows point to the nerve root hugging the inferior pedicle, but, in close association to the superior capsule of the facet joint, the asterisk identifies the inferior facets. (From Rauschning, W.: Computed tomography and cryomicrometry of lumbar spine specimens [a new technique of multi-planar anatomic correlation]. Spine 8:170–180, 1983.)

sity to be significantly relieved by a facet injection. Can we assume capsular reaction is irritating the nerve? Indeed, the degenerative process may be so severe that a synovial cyst emerging from the degenerative joint can create extradural compression.[42] At this point, however, no one has yet to find to what degree mechanical irritation of the nerve root is a source of pain vs. chemically induced noxious stimuli arising from the inflammatory reaction of the overstressed connective tissue structures related to the joint.

The mention of noxious stimuli of course again brings into focus the pathways of innervation of the facet joint itself. The gross anatomic distribution has been described by various dissectors, more recently in a comprehensive description by Paris.[41] The results of his dissection are displayed in Figure 4*A*,*B*. The features of innervation that are pertinent to the discussion of facet syndrome are (1) the profuse innervation of the posterior articular structures and (2) the close association of the nerve root and the spinal ganglion to the facet joint and its capsule. The portion of the capsule in closest relationship to the nerve root is the ligamentum flavum, which has been demonstrated to have significant innervation. The profuse overlapping innervation is pertinent because it explains poor localization of noxious stimuli. If three different neural segmental levels can receive noxious stimuli from one skeletal site, it is not surprising that pain perception at the cerebral level is very blurred. However, the same profuse innervation makes denervation of the facet joint difficult to achieve. It is noted that at all lumbar levels, L1–L5, an ascending branch leaves the medial branch of the posterior primary ramus just before passing through the foramen bounded laterally by the intertransverse ligament. This ascending branch is well clear of the transverse process as it ascends to the facet above. Thus, standard maneuvers to denervate the joint related to specific skeletal sites will miss this tiny nerve. It is

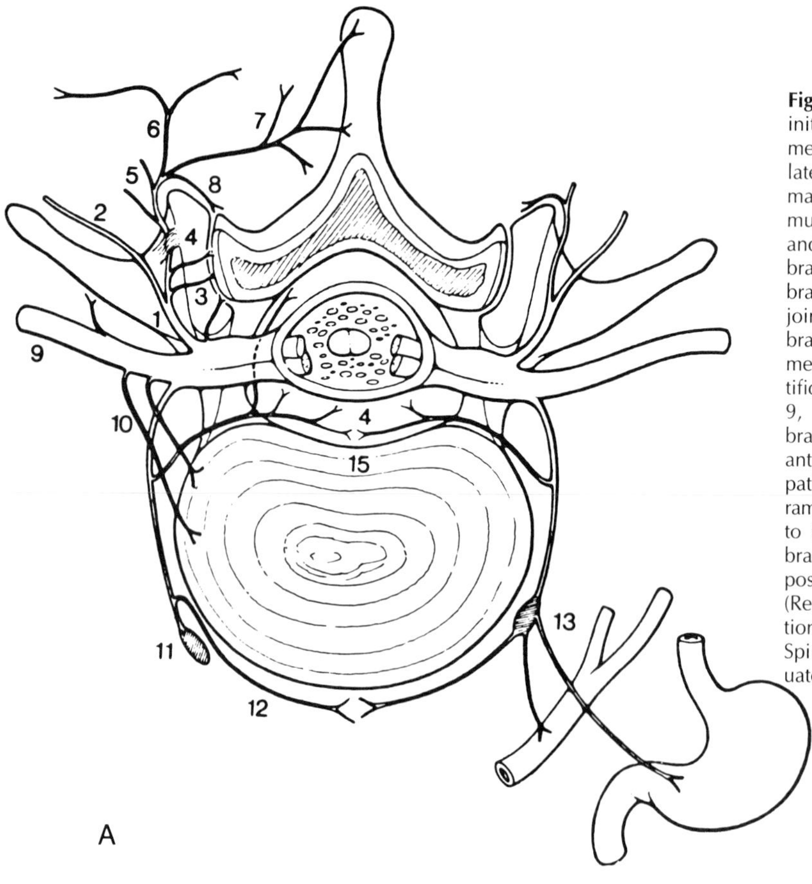

Figure 4 □ *A,* Neuroanatomic definition of the lumbar motion segment. 1, Posterior primary rami; 2, lateral branch of the posterior primary rami to skin and muscles; 3, muscular branches to multifidus and to facet capsule; 4, medial branch posterior primary rami; 5, branch to the posterior sacroiliac joint; 6, muscular and cutaneous branches; 7, muscular and ligamentous branches—large to multifidus; 8, local branch to facet; 9, anterior primary rami; 10, branches to the disc from the anterior primary rami; 11, sympathetic chain; 12, recurrent gray rami communicantes; 13, branches to blood vessels and viscera; 14, branches to dura; 15, branches to posterior longitudinal ligament. (Redrawn, from Paris, S.B.: Functional Anatomy of the Lumbar Spine. Ph.D. Thesis. Union Graduate School, Atlanta, 1983.)

also apparent from this dissection that complete denervation of one segment will require three levels of destroying of innervation. The same overlapping innervation has been confirmed in other primates.[53]

Finally, to confound the innervation even more, it has been well documented that not only do branches of the gray rami communicantes from the sympathetic system supply the lateral aspect of the disc and the anterior longitudinal ligament, but nerve filaments go directly into the ventral ramus before it divides into anterior and posterior branches. Thus, on a neuroanatomic basis, it is possible for an autonomic supply to travel with the segmental innervation of the facet joints.[7]

In summary, it is quite possible for the facet joints to be sufficiently innervated to create noxious stimuli and ultimately to be a source of symptomatic distress. Certainly the facet joints participate in the degenerative process. But typical of degenerative processes elsewhere, the mechanical reflection of excessive stress (i.e., degenerative changes seen on x-ray studies) does not necessarily identify which sites are symptomatic.

DIAGNOSTIC CRITERIA FOR FACET JOINT EVALUATION AND TREATMENT

As mentioned earlier, the availability of fluoroscopy for direct localization of injection into the facet joints made possible various studies in our laboratory to clarify which individuals might benefit from facet injections.[36] In a group of 15 individuals with back and leg pain and five with no complaints, a series of provocative injections was performed. First, under fluoroscopy, the needle was inserted into the facet joint and a few drops of contrast medium were injected to outline the joint. Conray-60, which is nearly isotonic, was used, and no pain was produced. Through the same needle, 1 to 3 cc of 5% hypertonic saline was then injected within the confines of the joint. In all individuals, a pain reaction was noted after a few seconds. At first it was deep, dull, and located near the injection site. However, after several more seconds (up to 20 seconds), the pain seemed to spread into the buttock and posterior thigh. Often the greater trochanter area was painful as well. The pain never radiated cephalad of the

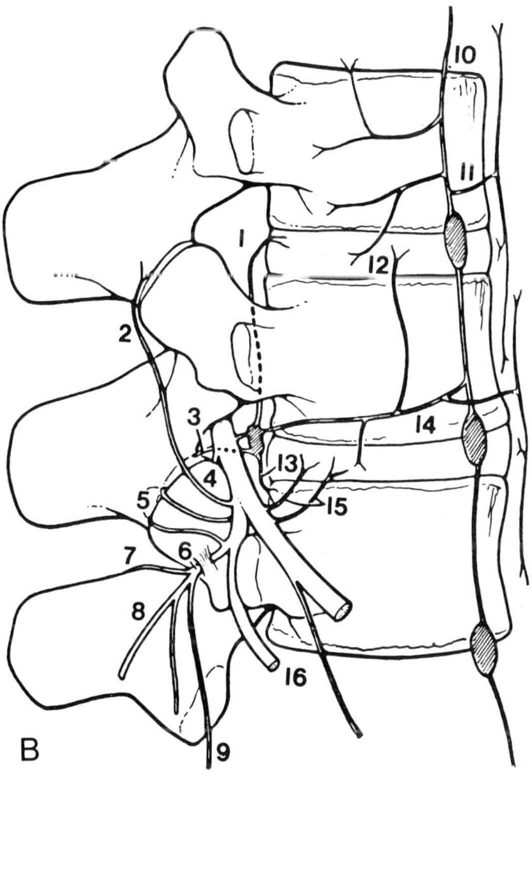

Figure 4 □ *Continued B,* Neuroanatomic definition of the lumbar motion segment. 1, Ascending branch of sinuvertebral nerve; 2, ascending facet branch; 3, sinuvertebral to facet; 4, direct branch to facet; 5, branches to multifidus; 6, medial branch of posterior primary ramus; 7, local facet branch; 8, descending facet branch; 9, branch to sacroiliac; 10, sympathetic chain; 11, branch under anterior longitudinal ligament; 12, branches from gray ramus to disc; 13, sinuvertebral to disc; 14, gray ramus communicans; 15, branches from anterior primary ramus to disc; 16, lateral branch of posterior primary ramus. (Redrawn, from Oudenhoven, R.C.: The role of laminectomy, facet rhizotomy and epidural steroids. Spine 4:145–147, 1979.)

injection site and in only two patients did it radiate across the midline. In three individuals, radiation extended below the knee to the calf. To a certain extent, the volume of injection seemed to correlate with the extent of pain distribution. There was never any evidence of a change of sensation on the skin; no numbness was ever noted, and no consistent pain pattern occurred, regardless of whether the injection was at L4–L5 or L5–S1. The L3–L4 facet injection did tend to produce pain slightly lateral on the thigh compared with the L4–L5 injection. Once the extent of distribution of pain had been determined, the pain could always be obliterated by the injection of a local anesthetic agent.

In two subjects, wire electrodes were placed into the hamstring muscle before the saline was injected into the facet joint. In these individuals with previously normal straight-leg raising test results, approximately 15 seconds following injection of hypertonic saline, myoelectric activity was noted in the hamstring muscles and straight-leg raising was diminished to 70 degrees. This continued for several minutes. The myoelectric activity and the straight-leg raising test returned to normal with the injection of 2 cc of local anesthetic agent into the facet joint. In six patients who demonstrated positive straight-leg raising at about 70 degrees before the injection, all had normal straight-leg raising within 5 minutes after the facet injection with local anesthetic.

Another observation related to the significance of painful stimuli to the nervous system. Three of the experimental patients had depressed achilles reflexes prior to the arthrogram and injection. Following the local anesthetic injection, the reflexes were again tested and they were found to return to normal. We assume the basis for this finding was that the physiologic inhibition of anterior horn cell firing due to noxious stimuli arising from the symptomatic facet joint was obliterated by the instillation of a local anesthetic.

Clinically, it is apparent that pain in the back, buttock, and leg is a nonspecific finding. Certainly, if there is radiculopathy suggesting anterior primary ramus involvement, the anatomic site for this abnormality probably is not the facet joint. However, based on the studies described above, the facet joint could be the source of pain in a wide array of clinical settings. Pain perceived to be in the buttock, posterior or lateral thigh, or even the calf could originate from the facet joint. Diminished straight-leg raising could result from a hamstring spasm secondary to facet initiation. Even minor neurologic abnormalities such as reflex changes may be the result of pathologic disorders of the facet. Thus, in individuals with back and leg pain and no radiculopathy, one is justified in making the clinical diagnosis of facet arthropathy. On the basis of our work, there seems to be no specific pain pattern that would clearly identify the facet joint over other potential sources of noxious neural stimulation.

In a study from Oswestry, similar findings by provocation studies were noted.[34] The study was accomplished on male volunteers who had no history of back pain. The injection was made at the L1–L2 level and at the L4–L5 level, using small amounts of hypertonic saline (0.4 cc) either into the joint itself (as identified by arthrography) or just adjacent to the joint. Little difference in distribution of pain was found between pericapsular and intracapsular injections. The pain was more intense, however, in the pericapsular injections. The sensation was cramp-like and vague with inexact margins. As in our own study, there was a significant delay before the onset of pain perception, of up to 25 seconds. No cephalad radiation of pain occurred, and pain did not cross the midline. Although the L1–L2 injections were more likely to be in the flanks, there was considerable overlap in location with those at the L4–L5 level. Once again, in these studies there was confirmation that the facets could be sources of noxious stimuli, but the pattern of pain was an unreliable predictor of anatomic location.

In an attempt to find out whether there were other aspects of history or examination, a prospective study was accomplished by the same group.[14] In this study, 26 patients with nonradicular back and leg pain were injected; 14 patients had excellent relief of pain after a radiographically controlled local anesthetic injection was made into the facet joint, and they were identified as responders. The rest were nonresponders. When the clinical pictures of the two groups were compared, it was noted that the straight-leg raising was more deficient in the nonresponders, but the responders had more back and thigh pain, whereas the nonresponders had more back and lower leg pain. The responders more frequently had a history of acute onset relieved by walking and exacerbated by sitting. The nonresponders had a gradual onset of pain, which increased by walking and was relieved by sitting. Tenderness was noted in all patients, and the choice of injection site was based on this tenderness. Duration of relief of the responders was quite varied, but 6 of the 14 responders had permanent relief of their pain.

In another more recent study, attempting to identify the clinical picture that most likely will lead to responders for injection, Lewinnek and Warfield could find no correlation with the various criteria suggested by Fairbanks and coworkers.[27] The factor that confounds all of clinical medicine was operative here; that is, the groups were not quite comparable. In the Fairbanks group, no radiographic differences existed between responders and nonresponders. In the Lewinnek group, however, all the responders with x-rays had degenerative changes in the facet joints. In this group of 15 of 20 responders, a clinical picture of pain with rest emerged. The most predictive criterion was awakening at night with pain. Actually, this seemed somewhat reminiscent of Eisenstein's syndrome of facet disease defined as chondromalacia facetae.

What, then, is the clinical picture of facet syndrome? Because no study even approaches a 100% success rate associated with injection of a local anesthetic, it is obvious that we really do not know how to select the patient with pure facet-initiated pain. Lippitt has proposed a clinical syndrome that, based on primarily intuitive concepts, suggests the facet syndrome.[30] The symptoms are described as hip and buttock pain, cramping leg pain (usually above the knee), low back stiffness (especially in the morning or associated with inactivity), and absence of dysesthesias in the limbs. The signs associated with this are local paralumbar tenderness, pain on extension, hip and buttock pain on straight-leg raising, and absence of neurologic deficits. But even in this crisp group of patients, only 66% responded at all. A more critical analysis emerged from Jackson and associates.[23] In this large study of 390 patients (226 individuals receiving Workman's Compensation), injections were done with the assistance of arthrography. In this group, those more likely to respond were individuals with a prior history of back pain, no complaints of leg pain, normal gait, no muscle spasm or tenderness, and maximum pain while extending from the flexed position. Duration or severity, positional aggravating factors, radiographic findings, relief on manipulation, or time off work did not correlate with successful treatment. It was the view of this group that effective treatment was so minimal that the value of the procedure is to be questioned.

The question arises, therefore: Why should we pursue an interest in this phenomenon? One of the justifications is to prove or disprove intuitively developed concepts of the origin of low back pain and sciatica. A paper by Kraft and Levinthal is a good example of anecdotal concepts that are part of our medical heritage and certainly part of the chiropractic and osteopathic view of back pain.[26] These authors, in the 1950s, described what they referred to as a new concept in the etiology of lumbar vertebral derangement. They described a common clinical event. The typical history is the sudden onset of low back pain associated with a twist or bend of the back without radiculopathy. The patient often refers to himself or herself as having a "catch" in the back. Physical examination may even reveal a list of the lumbar spine. The sudden onset seems to suggest some sudden mechanical event. Although the authors produce no specific dissections of their own, they do produce a slide that identifies capsular synovial tissue removed from between facet joints, showing marked fibrosis. It is, therefore, their proposal that pieces of this fibrosis can be caught within the joint itself and explain the clinical events. On this basis, they suggest various manipulative maneuvers that, indeed, were apparently associated with relief sufficient to justify their continued application. As is typical of the literature of that era, no prospective controlled study was undertaken. In fact, there is not even a report of the author's own experience. The proposal seemed so logical that, apparently, none was thought to be needed.

The technical tools currently at our command would seem to make possible some justifiable explanation. At the present, only one paper (Eisenstein's) reports a surgical dissection in patients who are prospectively identified as having a facet syndrome. Most cases of this type are so benign that they do not seem to warrant surgical care and thus the potential for biopsy. Alternatively, perhaps the surgeons have not been as diligent as necessary to achieve biopsy material when fusions are done. Nonetheless, the continued enthusiasm for anecdotal medicine in the care of the back does offer justification for a continued attempt to clarify the anatomic sources of pain in symptomatic individuals.

CURRENT TREATMENT OPTIONS

As noted above, there seems to be little unanimity about what constitutes the facet syndrome. Neuroanatomic, biomechanical, and pathologic changes suggest that any incidence of pain in the back and leg without radiculopathy can be emerging from a deranged facet joint. There seem to be only two alternative sources of pain without radiculopathy: the muscle or ligament attachments to the spine and the disc itself. How can we separate these three categories?

Myofascial pain is described as pain associated with tenderness in various areas of the low back. This is certainly a frequent clinical presentation. Could the associated areas of tenderness described by advocates of facet syndrome really be myofascial abnormalities? Although there have been numerous descriptions of the clinical picture, no pathologic definition of myofasciitis has ever appeared. It is difficult to conceive of an entity lasting for weeks that essentially resulted from an unhealing overload of muscular and fascial tissue. Thus, if we restrict our discussion to subacute and chronic lumbago and sciatica, the presumed disorder, described as myofasciitis, seems unexplainable.

An alternative explanation for this back pain seemed to be pain arising from the disc itself. Again, although hypothetic explanations are available, no specific definition of this pain is available. Many descriptions of successful manipulative care for back complaints are available. None of these has a specific anatomic definition, but many assume abnormalities of structure that are correctable by manipulative treatment and a reduction in symptoms. In the living individual, however, there seems to be no opportunity to identify a specific anatomic source.[54]

Thus, for this particular clinical entity, the opportunity for specific anatomic definition seems available only by the analysis of an anatomically specific approach. Only a radiographically controlled injection can assure a specific anatomic site as the location of injection with local anesthetic or with anti-inflammatory medication. It is impossible for any mechanical therapy to manifest its action on only one specific location, without affecting other structures. Any manipulative maneuver aimed at affecting the disc, myofascial adhesions, or even the relationships of the nerves to other structures, must also affect the facet joint. Only a radiographically controlled injection into the facet without the association of mechanical events can offer some clue as to the relationship of that anatomic site to other painful sources.

RESULTS OF TREATMENT

The major role of injection for a facet syndrome is as a diagnostic procedure, because once an understanding of the location of pain is available, a more rational treatment may be initiated. It is certainly also reasonable to look to the effects of injection as a form of treatment. Because the only definition of efficacy of injection is the patient's stated pain response, assuring an effective treatment is obviously difficult.

The treatment of facet disease can take two forms: (1) One can assume that the joint is a continuing source of noxious stimuli and therefore that denervation of the joint would be appropriate. (2) One can assume that an arthropathy within the joint is causing a reactive inflammation. Anti-inflammatory medication should be beneficial. We will look first to the discussion of results of treatment in the form of denervation. Historically, this is the older procedure.

Results of Denervation

In 1973, Shealy and colleagues made their initial presentation of a large series of facet denervations.[49] At that time, Shealy reported good to excellent results in 80% of patients who had no previous surgery. In those who had previous surgery, only a 40% success rate was reported. He continued to report very favorable results for the next several years.[48] Other neurosurgeons began to utilize this technique and reported high levels of its success. In the report of Lora and Long,[31] the patients were preselected by successful relief of their pain by percutaneous radiographically controlled injection of a local anesthetic into the facet joints. In this series, 234 consecutive cases were reported on. In that group, which included patients with cervical, thoracic, and lumbar pain, about one third failed to respond to facet injections. Patients selected for this procedure were those with chronic pain who had failed investigative procedures to identify spinal canal disease. This was a very chronically affected group of patients, and only 82 had no previous surgery. In this group, 79% claimed benefit from the procedure and 61% indicated 50% or more reduction in pain. Again, because this was such a chronically affected group, the authors noted other findings. In addition to the more effective treatment in those without surgery, no patient who had a serious drug addiction was benefited, nor was any patient who had arachnoiditis. Patients with compression fractures secondary to traumatic reasons were benefited, although compression fractures associated with cancer were not. Unsettled Workman's Compensation claims were poor predictors of success, as well. Multiple surgeries, also, were not associated with pain relief. This point underlined the contention that the treatment was more than a placebo. If it were simply a placebo, some of those who had undergone surgery would have benefited, whereas an overall 61% success was noted in those who had no surgery. Furthermore, in a small group of patients, saline blocks were given. On no occasion did they relieve pain, although a local anesthetic injected into the facet joints relieved pain in two thirds of the patients. In contrast to other observers, these investigators found that the ideal candidate for this procedure was one who was relieved by rest and aggravated by activity. Based on this experience, the authors believed that they could recommend the procedure, not as an end in itself but as part of a total program including various aspects of conservative care. They thought it quite necessary that diagnostic local anesthetic blocks be performed initially. They also recognized that the procedure was in its infancy and were not sure of the long-term results.

In a group of less chronic patients, Oudenhoven reported on 801 facet rhizotomies.[39] The results were initially good, and the report of successful results was 80% at 6-month follow-up. (Postsurgical backs did less well.) With extended follow-up, however, the success rate deteriorated, and some patients had to proceed to surgical care. The success rate fell to 68% in unoperated backs.[40] This was a carefully performed study. The author reported it as a technically successful procedure when fibrillation potentials could be identified in the paraspinal musculature by electromyogram (EMG). This should be appropriate because the medial branch of the posterior primary ramus innervates the multifidus muscles and other paraspinal musculature.

The destruction of the nerve by rhizotomy should therefore lead to a display of fibrillation potentials on the EMG. This raises the question of the role of the muscles in back pain. If their functional loss occasioned by the rhizotomy seems not to be associated with pain, what role would they have if they were healthy? One problem in assessing results is the subjective nature of pain. If the surgeon is asking the patient whether the costly and painful procedure was beneficial, it seems likely that the patient respond favorably to avoid displeasing the surgeon or chastise himself or herself for the waste of time. In these early studies, improvement in function was seldom used as a criterion. Authors who chose improved function, a harsher definition of success, had lower levels of success. When the criterion of success was a doubling of the level of function, only 41% were considered to be successfully treated.[21]

Interestingly, in spite of these remarkable levels of success reported in the 1970s, no recent rhizotomy series has been produced. A review of pertinent spine journals over the past 8 years has failed to produce a single article relative to the use of facet rhizotomies. Personal communication with the originator, Norman Shealy, has indicated that he has given up this procedure.

Because tissue destruction is inevitable with the use of the temperature probe of the lesion maker, alternative means of denervating the articular nerve have been suggested. Injecting the nerve with a destructive agent such as phenol, under radiographic control, has been advocated. This may create less destruction to the surrounding tissue. The procedure has been used in individuals already treated by facet joint injection with steroids. An initial 70% success rate was noted at 6-month follow-up. However, success gradually deteriorated for most of the patients.[37] The procedure has since been given up by the authors.

Another maneuver focused on denervation of the facet uses freezing, rather than heating, as a method of achieving neural destruction. It was anticipated that this method might cause less destruction than the radiofrequency probe, and thus that a return of pain secondary to scarring of structural tissues would be less likely to occur. Short-term results reported with this method were good.[46] None of these studies has reported the patient's condition to be made worse. No subsequent reports with this procedure have emerged. There are still areas in which the procedure is being used because of its relative safety, but no prospective study of comparison has been undertaken.

Results from Steroid Injection

If one assumes that the underlying abnormality of the facet joint is an arthropathy that has created reactive inflammation, the alternative approach to pain control would be to reduce reactive inflammation. In other settings, instillation of steroids into joints has been noted to be beneficial. This would seem to be likely here, as well, unless there is something unique about the arthropathy of the facet joint. My initial report of this procedure was poorly controlled.[36] As with other studies, the only justification for the procedure was the absence of neurologic signs and persistent low back, buttock, and leg pain. We reviewed a group of 100 patients. One third of the patients had previous surgery, and 45% had previous myelograms. All had pain lasting for at least 6 months. The average age was 45 years. Thus, this was a group of individuals with greater chronicity than is typical of its current application. In this group, 62% had initial pain relief, but only 20% had complete pain relief at the end of 6 months. An additional 12% had reported partial pain relief at 6 months. Initially, we had used the injection procedure as an anticipated prologue to denervation by Shealy's method. We had added 1 cc of steroid into each injection. Initially, therefore, it was a diagnostic procedure, but when the remission of symptoms lasted longer than expected, it became apparent that this was also a therapeutic maneuver that had an anatomic basis. It was our impression, at the time, that we were treating something not necessarily defined as a degenerative condition. There was no correlation with radiographic findings of those who responded and those who did not respond. No patients were biopsied, and so we really do not understand the notable abnormalities within the facet joint.

More precise studies have been reported. A French study took the view that interarticular injections of steroids should be accomplished without a local anesthetic, so that the anti-inflammatory effect would be the only potential therapeutic event. They also pointed out that the flow of local anesthesia through the surrounding soft tissues may confound the perception of results, if it is injected at the time of the steroids.[55] Using this method, about 80% improved for at least 3 days. The individuals most likely to improve were those with leg pain rather than back pain. Because this is largely a radiographic study, the authors approached this method chiefly as a diagnostic study to evaluate other methods of care.

Actually, the status of this procedure as a diagnostic study raises the question of who would best perform it. Several radiologists have reported on their experiences.[8, 10] Their results were similar to those reported elsewhere. For instance, Destouet and colleagues reported a 54% success rate initially with an 18% continued success rate. Once again, the choice of patients was vague. In their setting, it was the patients who did not have radiographic findings suggesting a ruptured disc or skeletal sources of pain and who did not have radiculopathy. With a greater availability of tools, however, the radiologists have developed greater skills in approaching the facet joint by the CT scan. Greater success rate in the use of the CT scan has been reported.[38] In this series, with about 50% success rate of pain relief greater than 3 months, more patients were successfully treated with CT scan injection control rather than fluoroscopy.

It seems likely that greater precision of instilling the medication into the joint will offer a more specific method of comparing the structural sources of pain versus placebo or pain arising from nonjointed structures.

Other studies have emerged in the literature. The Lewinnek and Warfield study has already been mentioned.[29] In this group of 21 patients who were widely diverse in age but all of whom had degenerative changes, 75% were successfully treated. In the Lippitt report, again the study of a wide array of patients, 99 individuals were injected with a 54% rate of success;[30] 17% had excellent long-term results. Again there was a diversity between workmen's compensation cases, patients with previous surgery, and varying age groups with varying radiographic findings in the back. A recent study by Lynch and Taylor reported on a series of 50 patients.[33] In this group with selection based on over 6 months complaint and paraspinal tenderness with worsening on extension, 28% had total relief for over 6 months. Initially, 78% had some relief. The Jackson study,[23] when analyzed for patients who might be considered to be better candidates (i.e., those with normal psychologic status [as identified by pain drawings] and private pay status), the initial rate of pain relief was 67%. About 20% had long-term benefit. In another study presented by Shroeder[50] an overall success rate of 56% was reported, but 26% had continued improvement. Selby reported a straightforward series of 100 consecutive office patients who had no response to conservative care, a negative neurologic evaluation, and a negative straight-leg raising test result;[47] 45% had no response, whereas 26% had an excellent response with permanent relief, and 29% had short-term relief.

These are reports by varied groups of clinicians ranging from radiologists to orthopedists and neurosurgeons. Each had varying selection criteria for facet injection and varied criteria for success. The summary of all these studies suggests that a long-term excellent result can be expected in perhaps 20% of the patients and at least some short-term benefit might be expected in around 50% of the patients. The reports are all unsatisfying because no precise criteria for selection have been identified. Facet syndrome exists primarily as a diagnosis of exclusion. No precise criteria for comparison have been identified. Widely ranging age groups and postsurgical status are included in most series. The significance of tenderness or pain on extension is variable among various groups, and the duration since onset is quite variable. The use of various other types of therapeutic methods, before and after the treatment, is seldom defined. We can conclude little from these series other than to state that in some patients the facet joints seem to play a major role in initiating pain in the back with referral to the leg.

AUTHOR'S CURRENT APPROACH

What is the role of facet joint injections in my own current clinical practice? From my standpoint, facet injections serve two significant functions: as a diagnostic tool and as a mechanism to buy time. The more significant role is as a diagnostic tool.

The technique for the facet injection is quite simple, but it does require the use of radiologic equipment for needle localization. It is not possible for us to presume the location of the needle based purely on its "feel" in relation to the bony part of the spine. One is never secure exactly where the medication might be injected without radiographic localization. After 15 years of experience performing facet injections, I find that I am inaccurate as to the presumed level of needle localization in 25% of the cases. I find that I am totally accurate in my initial needle positioning in 5% of the cases. Thus, I believe it is essential that radiographic assistance be available if the procedure is to have diagnostic value.

My technique is as follows. Patients are considered to be appropriate candidates for facet injections if they have had persistent pain complaints in the back, buttock, and posterior thigh. They should not have radiculopathy. Patients fall into two categories: those who have radiographic abnormalities of the facet joints and those who do not. In both cases, injections are made on the side of major pain complaint. Thus, an individual with more pain in the left buttock and down the left thigh will receive facet injections at the L4–L5 and L5–S1 levels on the left. Owing to the overlapping innervation and to the well-known distribution of abnormalities primarily related to the lower two lumbar segments, this seems to be an appropriate semidiagnostic and certainly a potentially therapeutic approach. In patients with radiographic abnormalities, if these radiographic abnormalities correlate with the clinical findings that bring the patient in for a medical review, these facets will be injected.

Frequently, a broad array of radiographic problems are seen. A working man will have degenerative changes noted throughout the lumbar spine; yet, he will have anterior left thigh pain. On this basis the most appropriate approach would be to inject the L3–L4 level and perhaps the L4–L5 level on the left. Personally, I have not found value in tenderness or hyperextension pain as predictors of facet syndrome. At this point I have discovered no particular predictor other than radiographic findings. The individuals who have striking single-level radiographic findings as evidence of progressive degenerative changes located at one level are likely to have significant responses from radiographically controlled facet injections. Aside from this, no reliable predictor has ever emerged. In patients without radiographic findings, the lower two levels on the painful side are injected. The efficacy of facet injections seems to be more reliable in the older age groups. Young people usually have poorer responses to facet injections, and I believe that most of their problems are not related to the facet joint. In the older group, while the disc also is involved with the degenerative process, so are the facet joints. These individuals tend to be more effectively treated with the facet injection.

The patient is brought to the radiology suite without any premedication and is asked to lie prone on the fluoroscopy table with a small pillow under the abdomen. The pillow is found to be useful in that, as the patient is rotated either to the left or right oblique, it maintains the lumbar spine in a more neutral position.

Once the patient has been placed comfortably on the fluoroscopy table, the decision as to which side or whether both sides should be injected is made on the basis of a confirmation of the patient's complaint. Without additional radiographic information, one generally plans to inject both the L4–L5 and the L5–S1 levels. On the other hand, if significant radiographic findings are elsewhere, the patient will be injected at the most appropriate location (Fig. 5). A local anesthetic is injected into the subcutaneous area on the appropriate side. This is accomplished 2 to 3 cm from the midline, anticipating that this overlies the facet joints. In our experience, pain from the facet joint does not cross the midline, and, therefore, unilateral pain is to be treated only on the side to be injected.

Because in its first context, this is a diagnostic procedure, we are hopeful that the smallest feasible number of segments can be injected. Frequently there are no clues for the clinician to help identify the specific area of pain. As has been noted earlier, the referral of pain from a stimulated facet joint is very nonspecific.

To inject the facet joint, disposable 20-gauge spinal needles are inserted perpendicular to the skin at a site 2 cm from the midline, overlying the presumed level of the facet, which is generally at the level of the palpable spinous process. Once the injection has been accomplished, the patient is rotated into the oblique position with the involved side superior. This oblique position brings the joint parallel to the radiographic beam. Often it is necessary to roll the patient further, either toward the lateral or toward the prone position, to orient the facet joints into an alignment that is most parallel to the radiographic beam. Frequently, the various levels are not in the same orientation, and what appears to be an excellent position for visualization of the L5–S1 facet demonstrates the L4–L5 level to be a blur. Additional rotation must be accomplished if the L4–L5 is to be injected too. In the patient who is totally cooperative, one can rotate the pelvis easily; movement under direct visualization may be necessary to identify which is the best position for injection of the facet joint.

The needle is passed through the skin and soft tissues until its further progress is prevented by the presence of bone. Usually, this is not uncomfortable. The skin has been anesthetized, and motion of the needle through the skin is not noted by the patient. In our experience, the patient's response upon striking of the facet joint has not been a good predictor as to the efficacy in an injection. At this point, the position was reviewed with fluoroscopy and was adjusted. Figure 6 demonstrates the usefulness of the vertical approach contrasted with the oblique approach. Often the oblique approach obliterates the facet joints by the presence of the metallic overlay of the needle. If one tries to change needle position, it is usually necessary to withdraw the needle to the subcutaneous space and to reorient it. The 20-gauge needles are too flexible to try to permit reorientation after they have passed through the musculature. The needle positioning vertical to the skin

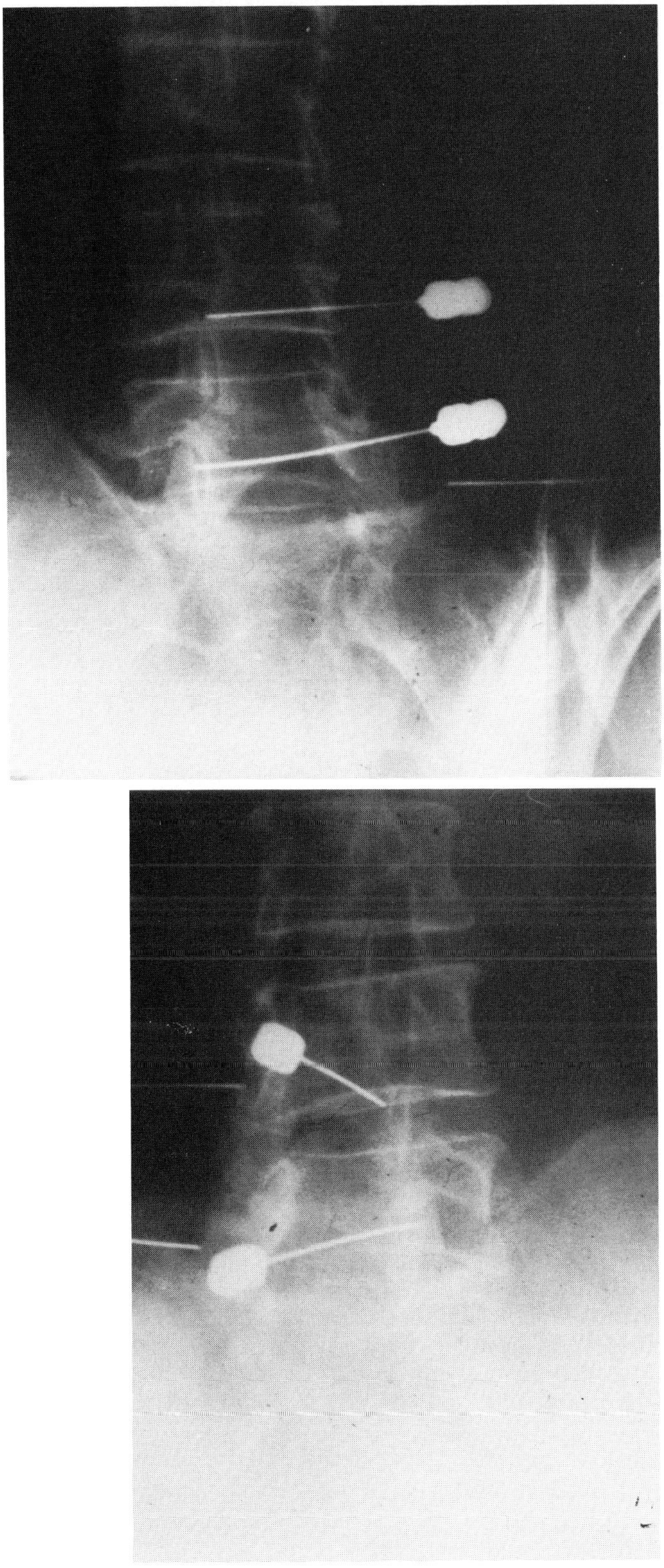

Figure 5 □ This is an example of a bilateral injection for an individual with pain equal on the left versus the right. Minor degenerative changes were noted at L5–S1. The facet injection localization at L4–L5 on the right is not ideal. An effort should have been made to place it more appropriately. The view on the right shows some very minor early degenerative changes at the L4–L5 level. These were not considered symptomatic, and, thus, this level was not injected.

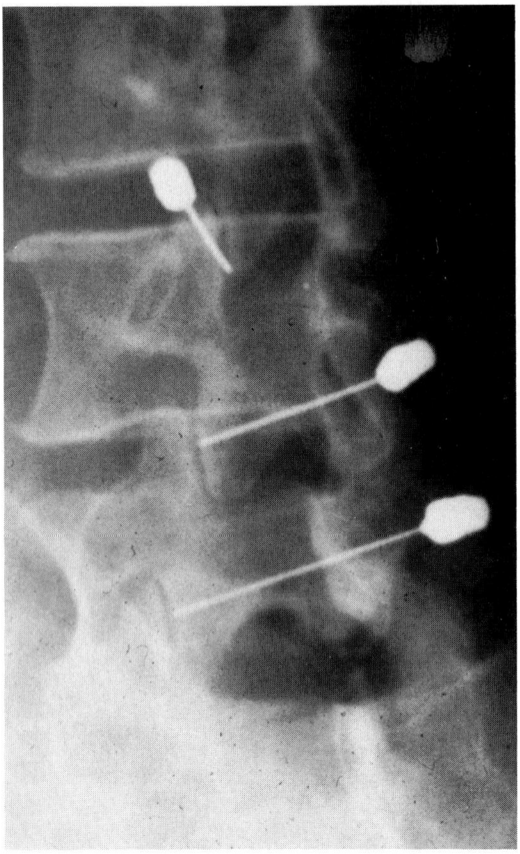

Figure 6 □ Contrast the needle orientation as either vertical to the skin or oblique to the skin. When the injection is accomplished obliquely, there is potential for obliteration of the joints by the metallic needle overlay. A longer needle may also be required.

is also useful in the obese patients, in that the shortest distance from the skin to the facet joint is at a site perpendicular to the facet joint. If an oblique orientation, parallel to the oblique orientation of the facet joint, is undertaken, the distance from skin to facet may be so great in the obese patient that standard needles cannot be used.

Usually, when the needle is passed through the skin and subcutaneous muscles, one strikes the skeletal structures at the expected depth. Confirmation easily notes the variation from medial to lateral at which the needle strikes the joint. Reorientation of the needle into the site of the joint is often easily accomplished. Often one can feel perforation of the capsule with entry into the joint. This is most notable in younger individuals who have no significant degenerative changes. In aged individuals, there may be occasions in which the overgrowth of the degenerative process obliterates the facet joint and it is not possible to enter the joint on the view of fluoroscopy.

The number of levels injected is variable. Unless there is some specific justification for injecting only one level on the basis of findings and radiographic abnormalities, two levels are usually injected. This is done purely on the basis of statistics, but there seems to be no alternative, given the overlapping innervation of the facet joints. Generally, therefore, the L4–L5 and L5–S1 levels are injected, unless there is some reason to choose the L3–L4 level. Where there are single-level degenerative changes, fewer numbers of injections can be performed. Certainly, degenerative changes of the lumbar spine are frequent and often are not associated with back pain. On the other hand, an individual with back pain may certainly have a symptomatic level and this must be clarified by the specific injection. The ideal application of radiographically controlled facet injections is in a setting in which there are significant radiographic changes throughout the spine and in which the contemplation of a further therapeutic approach is necessary. One can very clearly identify the symptomatic level of degenerative disease and perhaps look forward to additional care at that level. Occasionally, this leads to surgical care with fusion.

Unhappily, even in spite of great pains taken to localize the injection, the pain is frequently unresolved over the long term. This should not be surprising because we are treating a chronic process for which the potential for structural change is no greater than for resolving gray hair or lines in the face. Once it is identified that a specific level is the symptomatic source, a rational treatment plan can be initiated. For instance, if a facet joint that has no radiographic clues of abnormality is injected and persistent relief occurs following the injection, one may assume that arthropathy yet too premature to offer radiographic reflection has occurred. At our current level of knowledge, the only rational treatment for abnormalities within the joints is exercise programs that offer stabilization of the range by muscle activity and improved nutrition of the joint by mechanical activity. Thus, the major role of the facet injection in therapeutics is to provide an opportunity for pain relief of duration sufficient that a progressive guided exercise program can be accomplished. It is well recognized that the injection cannot be a definitive approach. However, it can offer short-term relief to allow the patient to progress into an appropriate conservative program. Ultimately, if nothing resolves the pain and it can be localized at specific levels of abnormality, our current surgical solution is a spinal fusion. This can be advocated after frequent injections show recognizable benefit.

WHAT IS THE FUTURE OF THIS LINE OF INVESTIGATION?

Future studies will need to be better controlled. To fully understand the pathophysiology of primary facet arthropathy, one must identify groups of patients early in the disease process. Future investigations should be in the form of comparative studies. Unfortunately, clinical research is extremely difficult in the environment of private medicine. Every effort is focused on improving the patient's condition in the most efficient manner. Therefore, for benign back pain, it is extremely difficult to undertake only one therapeutic maneuver. Ideally, similar groups of patients should be treated in one random group with facet injection, and in an alternative random group with merely localization of the needle into the facet joint. Instillation of local anesthetic might create a reversal of pain of a duration sufficient to allow improvement in exercise tolerance of a degree sufficient to regain control of the motion segment. What agency would pay for the localization of a needle into a joint under x-ray control?

An alternative might be a microsurgical approach to the facet joint on the patients whose pain was significantly relieved upon injection. A biopsy of the joint could also be accomplished by this method, but who would pay for the potential destruction of a normal joint on the occasion of biopsy under direct visualization?

It seems the only maneuver available to us in current clinical practice is the retrospective review of the characterization of responders and nonresponders. Quite a few such controlled studies have been reported, and at this time no clear understanding of a clinical syndrome that would predict the response rate of over 80% is available.

We really await the chemical characterization of the arthropathy. Certainly, the arthropathy is a response to mechanical overload. Why, though, does it sometimes progress to a nonpainful degenerative process, whereas sometimes it becomes an apparent, painful, local, mechanically induced inflammation? It must be the same phenomenon that occurs in knees, hips and other joints, although the mechanism remains undefined.

The role of the facet joint in the disease entities of lumbago and sciatica will only become clearer as a result of closer follow-up on more specifically characterized patients. Ideally, cooperative studies between various groups would be useful so that numbers of statistical significance could be achieved. Restraint from alternative therapeutic approaches would be necessary. Who will volunteer?

References

1. Adams, M.A., and Hutton, W.C.: The effect of posture on the role of the apophyseal joints in resisting intervertebral compressive force. J. Bone Joint Surg. 62B:358–362, 1980.
2. Ayers, C.E.: Lumbo-sacral backache. Boston Med. Surg. J. 196:9–16, 1927.
3. Badgley, C.E.: The articular facets in relationship to low back pain and sciatic radiation. J. Bone Joint Surg. 23A:481–496, 1941.
4. Badgley, C.E.: Clinical and roentgenological study of low back pain with sciatic radiation. A. Clinical aspects. A.J.R. XXXVII:454, 1937.
5. Badgley, C.E.: I. The Importance of the Lumbo-Sacral Joint in Low-Back Pain with Sciatic Radiation. II. A New Theory to Explain Radiation of Pain. Read before the Annual Meeting of the American Academy of Orthopaedic Surgeons. St. Louis, Missouri, Jan. 14, 1936.
6. Bogduk, N., and Engel, R.: The menisci of the lumbar zygoapophyseal joints—a review of their anatomy and clinical significance. Spine 9:454–460, 1984.
7. Bogduk, N., Tynan, W., and Wilson, A.S.: The nerve supply to the human lumbar intervertebral disc. J. Anat. 132:39, 1981.
8. Carrera, G.F.: Lumbar facet joint injection in low back pain and sciatica: Preliminary results. Radiology 137:665–667, 1980.
9. Danforth, M.S., and Wilson, P.D.: The anatomy of the lumbosacral region in relation to sciatic pain. J. Bone Joint Surg. E11:109, 1925.
10. Destouet, J.M., Gilula, L.A., Murphy, W.A., and Monsees, B.: Lumbar facet joint injection: Indication, technique, clinical correlation and preliminary results. Radiology 145:321–325, 1982.
11. Dory, M.A.: Arthrography of the lumbar facet joints. Radiology 140:23–27, 1981.
12. Eisenstein, S.M., and Parry, C.R.: The lumbar facet arthrosis syndrome—clinical presentation and articular surface changes. J. Bone Joint Surg. 69B:3–7, 1987.

13. Engel, R., and Bogduk, N.: The menisci of the lumbar zygoapophyseal joints. J. Anat. 135:795–809, 1982.
14. Fairbank, J.C.T., Park, W.M., McCall, I.W., and O'Brien, J.P.: Apophyseal injection of local anesthetic as a diagnostic aid in primary low back syndromes. Spine 6:598–605, 1981.
15. Foerester: The dermatomes in man. Brain 56:1–39, 1933.
16. Ghormley, R.K.: Low back pain with special reference to the articular facets, with presentation of an operative procedure. J.A.M.A. 101:1773–1777, 1933.
17. Goldthwait, J.E.: The lumbosacral articulation. An explanation of many cases of "lumbago, sciatica, and paraplegia." Boston Med. Surg. J. 164:356–372, 1911.
18. Gotfried, Y., Bradford, D.S., and Oegema, T.R.: Facet joint changes after chemonucleolysis induced disc and space narrowing. Spine 11:944–954, 1986.
19. Hirsch, C., Ingelmark, V.E., and Miller, N.: The anatomic basis for low back pain: Studies on the presence of sensory endings in ligamentous capsular and intervertebral disc structures in the human lumbar spine. Acta Orthop. Scand. 33:1–17, 1963.
20. Hockaday, J.M., and Whitty, C.W.N.: Patterns of referred pain in the normal subject. Brain 90:481–496, 1967.
21. Igneizi, R.J., and Cummings, T.W.: A statistical analysis of percutaneous radiofrequency lesions in the treatment of chronic low back pain and sciatica. Pain 8:181–187, 1980.
22. Inman, V.T., and Saunders, J.B.: Referred pain from skeletal structures. J. Nerv. Ment. Dis. 99:660–667, 1944.
23. Jackson, R.P., Montesano, P.X., and Jacobs, R.R.: Facet Joint Injections in Mechanical Low Back Pain Patients: A Perspective Statistical Study: Abstracts, International Society for the Study of the Lumbar Spine, Dallas, May, 1986.
24. Kelgren, J.H.: Observation on referred pain arising from muscle. Clin. Sci. Molec. Med. 3:175–190, 1938.
25. Kelgren, J.H.: On the distribution of pain arising from deep sematic structures with charts of segmental pain areas. Clin. Sci. Molec. Med. 4:35–46, 1939.
26. Kraft, G.L., and Levinthal, D.H.: Facet synovial impingement—a new concept in etiology of lumbar vertebral derangement. Surg. Gynecol. Obstet. 93: 439–443, 1951.
27. LaRocca, H., and MacNab, I.: Value of pre-employment radiographic assessment of the lumbar spine. Can. Med. Assoc. J. 101:383, 1969.
28. Lewin, T.: Osteoarthritis of the lumbar synovial joints: A morphologic study. Acta Orthop. Scand. (Suppl.)73:6–112, 1964.
29. Lewinnek, G.E., and Warfield, C.A.: Facet joint degeneration as a cause of low back pain. Clin. Orthop. Rel. Res. 213:216–222, 1986.
30. Lippitt, A.B.: The facet joint and its role in spinal pain: Management with facet joint injections. Spine 9:746–750, 1984.
31. Lora, J., and Long, D.: So-called facet denervation in the management of intractable back pain. Spine 1:121–128, 1976.
32. Lorenz, M., Patawardhan, A., and VanDerby, R.: Load-bearing characteristics of lumbar facets in normal and surgically altered spinal segments. Spine 8:122–130, 1983.
33. Lynch, M.C., and Taylor, J.F.: Facet joint injection for low back pain. J. Bone Joint Surg. 68B:138–141, 1986.
34. McCall, E.W., Park, W.M., and O'Brien, J.P.: Induced pain referral from posterior lumbar elements in normal subjects. Spine 4:441–446, 1979.
35. Mixter, W.J., and Barr, J.S.: Rupture of the intervertebral disc with involvement of the spinal canal. N. Engl. J. Med. 211:210, 1934.
36. Mooney, V., and Robertson, J.: The facet syndrome. Clin. Orthop. 115:149–156, 1976.
37. Mooney, V., and Selby, D.: Phenyl Injection into the Facet Articular Nerve. Abstracts of International Society for the Study of the Lumbar Spine. Gothenburg, 1981.
38. Murtagh, F.R.: CT-guided anesthesia and steroid injection in the facet syndrome. Post, M.J.D. (ed.): Computed Tomography of the Spine. Baltimore, Williams & Wilkins, 1984.
39. Oudenhoven, R.C.: Results of Facet Denervation. Presented at the International Society for the Study of the Lumbar Spine. Paris, 1981.
40. Oudenhoven, R.C.: The role of laminectomy, facet rhizotomy and epidural steroids. Spine 4:145–147, 1979.
41. Paris, S.B.: Functional anatomy of the lumbar spine. Ph.D. Thesis. Union Graduate School, Atlanta, 1983.
42. Polivy, K.D., Hanelin, J., and Boyd, R.J.: Synovial facet joint cyst causing extradural compression. Spine 12:412–414, 1987.
43. Putti, V.: New conceptions in the pathogenesis of sciatic pain. Lancet 2:53–60, 1927.
44. Rauschning, W.: Computed tomography and cryomicrometry of lumbar spine specimens (a new technique of multi-planar anatomic correlation). Spine 8:170–180, 1983.
45. Rees, W.E.S.: Multiple bilateral subcutaneous rhizolysis of segmental nerves in the treatment of the intervertebral disc syndrome. Ann. Gen. Pract. 26:126–127, 1971.
46. Schuster, G.D.: The use of cryonalgesia in the painful facet syndrome. J. Neurol. Orthop. Surg. 3:271–274, 1982.
47. Selby, D.K., and Paris, S.V.: Anatomy of facet joints and its correlation with low back pain. Contemp. Orthop. 312:1097–1103, 1981.
48. Shealy, C.N.: Percutaneous radiofrequency denervation of spinal facets and treatment for chronic back pain and sciatica. J. Neurosurg. 43:448–451, 1975.
49. Shealy, C.N., Prieto, A., Burton, C.V., and Long, D.N.: Articular Nerve of Luschka Rhizotomy for the Relief of Back and Leg Pain. Presented at the Annual Meeting of the American Association of Neurologic Surgeons. Los Angeles, 1973.
50. Shroeder, W.F.: The facet syndrome: Diagnosis and treatment. Exhibit presented at the American Academy of the Orthopaedic Surgeon. Atlanta, 1984.
51. Sinclaire, D.C., Feindel, W.H., Waddell, G., and Falconer, M.A.: The intervertebral ligaments as a source of segmental pain. J. Bone Joint Surg. 30B:515–521, 1948.
52. Steindler, A., and Luck, J.V.: Differential diagnosis of pain in the low back: Allocation of the source of pain by procaine hydrochloride method. J.A.M.A. 110:106–113, 1938.

53. Stillwell, D.L.: Nerve supply of vertebral column. Anat. Rec. 125:139–142, 1956.
54. Taylor, J.R., and Twomey, L.T.: Age changes in lumbar zygoapophyseal joints—observations on structure and function. Spine 11:739–745, 1986.
55. Theron, J., Blais, M., Casaco, A., et al.: Lumbar Spine: Therapeutic radiology. J. Neuroradiol. 10:223–230, 1983.
56. Tobias, D., Ziv, I., and Maroudas, A.: Measurement of Facet Cartilage Hydration in Relation to Applied Load. Abstracts, International Society for the Study of the Lumbar Spine. Rome, 1987, p.23.
57. Twomey, L.T., and Taylor, J.R.: Physical Therapy of the Low Back. Melbourne, Churchill Livingstone, 1987.
58. Twomey, L.T., and Taylor, J.R.: Sagittal movements of the human lumbar vertebral column: A quantitative study of the role of the posterior vertebral elements. Arch. Phys. Med. Rehabil. 64:322–325, 1983.
59. Videman, T., Malmivaara, A., and Mooney, V.: The value of axial view in assessing diskograms. An experimental study with cadavers. Spine 12:299–304, 1987.
60. Von Lackum, H.L.: The lumbosacral region: An anatomic study and some clinical observations. J.A.M.A. LXXXII:1109, 1924.
61. Yang, K.H., King, A.I.: Mechanism of facet load transmission as a hypothesis for low back pain. Spine 9:557–565, 1984.

□ Chemonucleolysis

Mark D. Brown
Bradford L. Currier

The concept of enzymatic dissolution of a herniated disc ("chemonucleolysis") was conceived by Lyman Smith. His report in 1963 on the use of chymopapain for the treatment of herniated discs in dogs[63] sparked an explosion of investigation and controversy concerning this subject that has continued for more than 25 years. Over 110,000 patients were injected with the enzyme from 1982 to 1986, but enthusiasm for the procedure has dropped precipitously over the past several years in response to reports of its adverse effects.

The convoluted history of chemonucleolysis has centered around the process of approval of chymopapain and collagenase by the Food and Drug Administration (FDA). Smith became interested in chymopapain in 1959 and experimented with the drug in animals. He sold the patent to the Baxter-Travenol Pharmaceutical firm for $1.00 and formed a research team to conduct further animal studies on the drug. Phase I clinical trials in humans began in 1963. Smith and Brown presented data on the first 75 patients in 1967 and reported successful results in 86% of patients who had had no previous spinal surgery.[64] One patient in that series injected at the C6–C7 level, without a preoperative myelogram, developed a Brown-Séquard syndrome. He was later found to have a malignant hemangioendothelioma, and his neurologic deficit progressed to quadriplegia following laminectomy.[9] As a result of that case, the FDA restricted the use of the drug to the lumbar region. The first reported case of paraplegia following chymopapain injection was also described in that series and led to the routine use of the lateral approach to avoid intrathecal injection. Phase I clinical studies culminated in a symposium published in 1969.[40] Combined data on approximately 600 patients revealed good results in 73%. Interestingly, the drug by-passed Phase II investigations because the original investigators argued that a controlled study was impossible and unethical.[9]

In Phase III, open clinical trials, chymopapain was tested in more than 16,000 patients between 1969 and 1975. A workshop sponsored by the American Academy of Orthopaedic Surgeons reported that 72% of 6,752 patients experienced satisfactory symptomatic relief following chymopapain (Discase) injections.[56] In 1974, 1,600 physicians were trained in the use of the technique in preparation for general release of the drug. At the same time, however, Baxter-Travenol initiated a Phase II double-blind, multicenter controlled study. In July of 1975 the FDA imposed a moratorium on the use of the enzyme except by investigators in the study. In 1976 Schwetschenau and others reported on the preliminary Walter Reed experience in their group of 66 patients injected with either Discase or its diluent cysteine-ethylenediaminetetra-acetic acid (EDTA) iothalamate.[62] They showed no statistically significant difference with chymopapain as compared to placebo in the treatment of proven lumbar disc displacement, leading Baxter-Travenol to withdraw its new drug application for Discase. This sequence of events created tremendous controversy both medically and legally.

In 1975 the Canadian Health Protection Branch, the Canadian counterpart to the FDA, approved chymopapain for general use.[8] This led to the referral of a large number of patients from the United States to Canada for chymopapain injection and allowed one surgeon, John McCulloch, to develop a series of over 7,000 patients.[30, 43]

The validity of the Schwetschenau double-blind study was challenged because of design flaws.[10, 57] A second randomized double-blind study was begun by Javid and associates in 1980.[32] Using Chymodiactin, a second brand of chymopapain from the newly founded Smith Laboratory, they demonstrated a 73% success rate with the drug, compared with 42% in controls by code-break criteria. Based on this study, the FDA released Chymodiactin for Phase IV clinical use in November of 1982.

At about the same time, two additional randomized double-blind studies were being performed using Discase, the original brand of chymopapain. A group of investigators in Australia performed a study comparing intradiscal injection of 8 mg of Discase to saline. Fraser reported that at 2 years, 77% of the 30 patients injected with Discase showed improvement, compared with 47% of the control group.[27] A multicenter randomized triple-blind study, which was carried out in North America by Dabezies and others, compared the efficacy of Discase with that of cysteine-EDTA (the control in the first double-blind study) and saline.[15] This study was designed to correct some of the deficiencies noted in the first study.[10] The dosage of Discase was doubled to 2 cc, versus 1 cc in the original study, and code break was discouraged until 6 weeks after the injection (when it was safe to do so). Travenol Laboratories summarized the early results of this study in a new drug application to the FDA. Approval for Discase was obtained in 1983. The final results of this study were recently reported by Dabezies and coworkers.[15] They demonstrated satisfactory results in 71% of the group injected with Discase, compared with 45% in the cysteine-EDTA control group.

An alternative enzyme to chymopapain, collagenase, was also being investigated during this period. Following animal research[6] and Phase I clinical studies,[67] Bromley and others performed a double-blind trial comparing collagenase to saline in a group of 30 patients.[7] Eight weeks following injection, 80% of the enzyme group and 33% of the control group were believed to have had successful results. Based on this small study, collagenase was approved for Phase III clinical trials in January of 1982.[9]

Collagenase has been shown to have less neurotoxicity, compared with chymopapain.[60, 77] However, intrathecal injection is toxic[51] and it is suggested that collagenase increases postinjection pain[12] and is associated with an increased incidence of transient neurologic deficits.[11] The enzyme is currently undergoing another randomized double-blind study in Europe to assess its efficacy and adverse effects.[66]

Numerous clinical studies have shown that satisfactory results can be expected in approximately 60% to 80% of patients injected with chymopapain.[9] Long-term studies have demonstrated that results do not deteriorate significantly with time. A recent symposium was devoted to this subject and compilation of the data from 14 studies with average follow-up of 8 to 11 years showed that 77% achieved satisfactory results.[49]

Several studies have described the findings at surgery in patients who failed to improve with chemonucleolysis.[3, 13, 18, 20, 37, 38, 44, 55, 65] In these studies the postchemonucleolysis operation rate averaged 20%. Discogenic pathologic conditions were found in 24%[3] to 100%[20] with sequestered fragments identified in 6%[65] to 50%.[20, 44] Spinal stenosis was reported in 0%[20] to 50%.[55] In 0%[20] to 30%[38] of the patients, the explorations were negative. The surgical experience in 82 patients following failed chemonucleolysis with collagenase was similar to that following chymopapain injection.[24] Satisfactory long-term outcomes following laminectomy for failed chemonucleolysis have been reported in 70%[18] and 77%[36] of those given chymopapain and in 87% of those receiving collagenase.[24] Only one study has reported that chymopapain injection compromised the success rate of subsequent surgery.[14] Crawshaw and others found good results in only 36% of their patients undergoing laminectomy following failed chemonucleolysis.[14] This led to the recommendation that patients who do not respond to enzyme injection in the first month should be considered for early surgery to prevent chronic scarring. This is based in part on the observation that surgical treatment is less successful if delayed more than 3 months from the onset of symptoms.[73]

The findings at surgery in cases of failed chemonucleolysis demonstrate the need for careful patient selection. If a sequestered disc is suspected preoperatively, open discectomy should be performed because intradiscal injection of enzyme cannot be expected to reach the fragment. Myelography, computed tomography (CT), and magnetic resonance imaging (MRI) are helpful in differentiating sequestered fragments from protruded or extruded discs and are becoming more reliable.[39] Spinal stenosis is obviously not amenable to treatment by chemonucleolysis and may be exacerbated by disc space narrowing. The finding of stenosis in about 40% of chemonucleolysis failures demonstrates the difficulty in preoperative diagnosis of this condition as well. Improvements in imaging studies have decreased, but not eliminated, this problem. Other conditions thought to be contraindications to the procedure include previous chymopapain injection, history of allergy to papaya or derivatives, previous lumbar spinal surgery, herniation of more than two discs, rapidly progressive neurologic deficit, neurogenic bladder and/or bowel dysfunction, spinal tumor, spondylolisthesis, diabetic neuropathy, and pregnancy.[4, 45]

Several recent studies have suggested additional criteria for patient selection to improve results of chemonucleolysis. Pos tacchini and others demonstrated that chemonucleolysis was slightly better than surgery with small disc herniations, and definitely inferior to surgery with large herniations or when the clinical pattern suggested severe root impingement.[54] Ford, however, has treated some patients who showed a complete block on a myelogram and found that the results with chymopapain injection were as good as in patients with small to moderate lateral disc herniations.[26] Troisier and Cypel found that discography was helpful in predicting outcome.[68] Good results were obtained in 76% of patients who demonstrated a large, well-filled protruded area on discography. In the group of patients who also experienced lateralized pain at the time of discography, 97.5% had good results. Edwards and colleagues analyzed the prognostic value of CT discography in patients undergoing chemonucleolysis.[19] They found that when the herniated disc fragment demonstrated an uptake of contrast material, the success rate was 95%. When no contrast material was taken up by the herniated fragment, the success rate was only 16%.

The treatment options for a patient with a herniated disc have been reviewed earlier in this book. The place of chemonucleolysis can be determined only by comparing its efficacy and adverse effects with the natural history of the disease and other treatment modalities. Weber's classic study comparing the results of surgery with conservative treatment has been extremely valuable in defining the indications for a laminectomy.[73] He is currently comparing the results of chymopapain injection with the natural history of disc herniation. The study is nearing completion and allegedly shows minimal differences.[46] Studies comparing chemonucleolysis with surgical discectomy have not shown a consistent advantage of one technique over the other. Nordby[47] and Leavitt and others[34] have shown an advantage of chemonucleolysis. Onofrio[52] and Weinstein and colleagues[74] have reported that the results are similar to those of surgery, and several groups of investigators have claimed that standard discectomy[14, 20, 72] and, more recently, microdiscectomy[70, 76] are superior. Studies reporting the results of laminectomy alone generally reveal 75% to 95% successful results. Combining the data, it appears that results with chemonucleolysis approach those of standard laminectomy or microsurgical discectomy in carefully selected patients.

The popularity of chemonucleolysis in the United States has dropped dramatically in recent years in response to reports of its adverse effects. The mortality and morbidity rates associated with chemonucleolysis compare favorably with those of surgery.[25] The mortality rates of each are reported to be 0.02%,[25, 58] and the overall incidence of complications is lower with chemonucleolysis.[25] The primary reason that chemonucleolysis has fallen into disfavor is related to the potential for life-threatening anaphylactic reactions and severe and unpredictable neurologic complications. Similar types of complications have been described with both Discase and Chymodiactin,[2, 8, 25, 71] the two commercially available forms of chymopapain. The differences in incidence of the reported adverse effects is probably a result of refinements in patient selection, preoperative planning, and injection technique, rather than to actual differences in the enzymes. Postmarketing surveillance data on the first 110,000 patients injected with Chymodiactin showed that anaphylaxis occurred in 0.5%, neurologic complications in 0.06%, discitis in 0.05%, and mortality in 0.02%.[25]

In Watts' early series on complications of chemonucleolysis, the incidence of anaphylaxis was 1%.[71] More recent reports of 0.35%[30] and 0.5%[25] do not represent the true incidence of anaphylaxis; rather, they reflect improvements in preoperative screening for chymopapain allergy and the use of local, instead of general, anesthesia.

Anaphylaxis is a severe allergic reaction associated with significant hypotension or respiratory distress. In Europe, the reported incidence of anaphylaxis following chymopapain injection is only 0.09%.[5] It is speculated that the difference is related to a greater exposure to papain derivatives in the United States.[46] The reaction occurs more commonly in females than in males and is seen more frequently in Afro-Americans and Hispanics than in Caucasians.[25] Other less severe manifestations of sensitivity to chymopapain are nausea, itching, and urticaria. The clinical manifestations of a chymopapain allergy start with sensitization through previous injection[41, 42, 61] or exposure to papain derivatives in meat tenderizers, beer, toothpaste and fruit juices.[9] Immunoglobulin E antibodies are induced and become attached to the surface of mast cells or basophils. With injection of chymopapain in a sensitized individual, an antigen-antibody reaction occurs and leads to the release of chemically active mediators such as histamine, slow-reacting substance of anaphylaxis, serotonin, and bradykinin. These substances act on target organs to cause increased capillary permeability, increased arterial constriction, and bronchiolar and smooth-muscle contraction.[9, 35]

Anaphylactic reactions can be prevented in several ways. It is clear that patients who have been previously treated with chymopapain should not be reinjected.[61] Patients with a history of allergy to papaya or its derivatives should also not be considered for injection. Tests to detect IgE antibodies are available to screen patients for sensitivity to chymopapain. The radioallergosorbent test (RAST; Pharmacia of New Jersey) is commonly used to test patients for allergies. It is of limited value in screening candidates for chemonucleolysis, however, owing to its lack of sensitivity and specificity.[35] The fluorescent allergosorbent test (ChymoFAST; Allergenetics Reference Laboratory, Division of Axonics), a solid-phase fluorescent enzyme immunoassay for the determination of chymopapain-specific IgE antibodies, has been developed. Postmarketing surveillance data on this test indicate that it is a reasonably reliable screening test.[69] The test is considered to be positive when the IgE concentration is greater than or equal to 0.06 IU/ml. Of patients who had a positive test but still chose to have the injection, 62% experienced an adverse reaction.

Unfortunately, 9 out of 4,763 (0.2%) patients with negative tests who underwent injection also experienced adverse reactions. If the test is considered to be positive when any trace of IgE antibody to chymopapain is detected, the false-negative rate drops to 0.05%, but this excludes 13% of the population from injection.[69]

Skin testing to detect a chymopapain allergy has been described.[29, 41, 42] These preliminary reports suggest that it is rapid, simple, reliable, and safe. Mayer and colleagues performed chymopapain injection on more than 350 patients who had had negative skin tests, and none experienced an anaphylactic reaction.[41] Grammer and coworkers reported a similar experience with 287 patients.[29] Patients with positive skin tests were not injected in these series, but McCulloch found that five of six patients who had a positive test and were injected had reactions.[42] The selectivity of the test is supported by the observation in the series by Mayer and coworkers[41] that the incidence of positive tests increased from around 3% to a maximum of 73%, following chymopapain injection. Interestingly, the skin reactions were found to be time dependent with an increase in the frequency of positive responses between the second and twelfth week followed by a decrease beyond 13 weeks. This suggests that chymopapain allergy may be temporary in some individuals and raises the possibility of repeat injections in patients with negative skin tests. They also demonstrated differences in sensitivity to Discase and Chymodiactin, suggesting that it may be possible to perform selective injections when sensitivity to only one agent is found. More data are needed before a firm conclusion can be drawn for this screening technique.

Preinjection administration of H_1 and H_2 histamine antagonists has been advocated by many. The incidence of reactions is not decreased by histamine receptor blockade, but it has been shown that attenuating the reduction of systemic vascular resistance caused by histamine may diminish the severity of an anaphylactic reaction in animals.[53] The current recommendations are 50 mg diphenhydramine four times daily and 300 mg cimetidine four times daily by mouth, beginning 24 hours prior to injection.[4, 33]

A test dose of chymopapain at the time of intradiscal injection is recommended by the manufacturers to help identify patients who are most sensitive to the enzyme.[4] They recommend injecting a test dose of 0.2 ml of Chymodiactin and observing the patient for 10 to 15 minutes before injecting the full therapeutic dose. Patients exhibiting signs or symptoms of anaphylaxis following the test dose should not receive the remainder of the therapeutic dose. However, there have been reports of patients who did not react to the test dose but developed anaphylaxis following the therapeutic dose. It is not clear whether this represents dose-related sensitivity to chymopapain or a delayed reaction to the test dose. Until further information is available, a test dose is advisable.

The incidence of anaphylaxis has been found to be lower when local anesthesia is employed.[2] In addition, patients are able to report prodromal symptoms of anaphylaxis, thereby allowing earlier treatment.[30] In the Hall and McCulloch series of 4,282 patients treated by chymopapain injection, only 15 (0.35%) sustained an anaphylactic reaction. Twelve of the 15 reported subjective early warning signs before the development of hypotension.[30]

The treatment of anaphylaxis requires rapid and aggressive management. It is essential to have all preparations for this complication complete before the enzyme injection is administered. The keys to successful management include prompt diagnosis; maintenance of the airway; rapid administration of crystalloid, intravenous epinephrine, diphenhydramine, and corticosteroids; and close monitoring of the patient's hemodynamic status.[30, 35] There were no fatalities or long-term sequelae in the Hall and McCulloch series, in which this protocol was used.[30]

The most alarming and dreaded complications associated with chemonucleolysis are neurologic reactions. Agre has carefully reviewed postmarketing surveillance data on approximately 80,000 patients injected with Chymodiactin.[1] As of February, 1985, 51 serious neurologic complications had been reported to the manufacturers, and by January, 1987, the number of neurologic complications had risen to 66.[25] They have included paraplegia and paraparesis, cerebral hemorrhage, seizure disorders, subarachnoid hemorrhage, Guillain-Barré syndrome, and quadriplegia.

Of the 28 patients who developed paraplegia or paresis, 11 patients were thought to have had intrathecal injections of chymopapain and contrast agents. All of these patients had similar clinical courses with rapid irreversible neurologic loss within hours of the injection. The cerebrospinal fluid in each patient was grossly bloody. The pathophysiology of chymopapain-induced paraplegia and paresis has been studied extensively. Chymopapain has been shown to be toxic when it comes in direct contact with nervous tissue.[59, 77] On intrathecal injection, microvascular damage leads to subarachnoid hemorrhage followed by a rapid rise in cerebrospinal fluid (CSF) pressure.[8, 9, 46] Studies on intrathecal injection in baboons have shown that the combination of chymopapain and contrast agents is far more toxic than either agent alone.[1] In addition, discography may decrease the chance of improvement of a neurologic deficit once it occurs.[1]

Acute transverse myelitis (ATM) occurred in at least five of the patients reviewed by Agre.[1] The patients generally left the hospital clinically improved and ambulating. Within 2 to 5 weeks they suddenly developed back and leg pain, and over the next 24 hours they developed irreversible paraplegia.[1, 21] One of these patients had had known violation of the dura from transdural discography 2 days prior to injection. The incidence of ATM following chymopapain is significantly higher than that found in the general population. The etiology is unknown, but theories include a delayed hypersensitivity[33] or immune complex disease and thrombosis of the arterial supply of the cord.[1]

Cerebral hemorrhages were reported in 15 of the patients reviewed by Agre.[1] Eight of these patients died, and autopsies were performed on seven of them. Four patients died of ruptured aneurysms or vascular malformations, and the deaths were believed to be unrelated to the enzyme injection. An intrathecal injection of chymopapain could be directly implicated in one of the other three patients. One patient who developed a cerebral hemorrhage has remained in a comatose state.[16] Discography films, in this case, documented the presence of contrast material in the CSF. Chymopapain injection was performed through the same needle and was thereby implicated in this complication.

Of the four patients who developed seizures, two were thought to be related to contrast material sensitivity and two were believed to be the initial episodes of epilepsy. All the patients recovered completely.

One patient developed Guillain-Barré syndrome following enzyme injection. The patient recovered completely.

There has been one reported case of quadriplegia following lumbar injection of chymopapain. Discography was carried out at the same time as enzyme injection and may have been partially responsible for the hemorrhagic myelitis that led to the quadriplegia.

In addition to discography at the time of chemonucleolysis, other factors that were implicated as increasing the risk of neurologic complications include chymopapain injection at multiple levels and the use of general, instead of local, anesthesia.[1] In 1984 the FDA advised against each of these practices.[23]

The incidence of discitis following chemonucleolysis is 0.08%.[2] There have been two reported fatalities secondary to discitis; one patient died of staphylococcal septicemia, and the other died of staphylococcal meningitis.[1] A strict aseptic technique is the most important factor in preventing discitis. A two-needle technique has been described by McCulloch in order to decrease the risk of disc space infection. This technique is designed to assure that the needle entering the disc has not been contaminated by the skin.[43] Fraser has shown that as few as seven *Staphylococcus epidermidis* bacteria can cause discitis when injected intradiscally.[28]

The most common side effects following chymopapain injection are back pain (50%) and spasms (30%).[4]

The complication rate of chemonucleolysis can be decreased in several ways.[33] First, careful patient selection will prevent injection of a patient who is likely to improve spontaneously or who would be better treated by an open procedure. Patients who have multiple medical problems or are debilitated are also poor candidates for chemonucleolysis. Sensitivity reactions can be avoided by preinjection screening with the ChymoFAST assay[69] and perhaps, in the near future, by skin testing.[29, 41, 42] Chemonucleolysis is contraindicated in patients who have been previously injected or patients with a known sensitivity to papain derivatives.[61] H_1 and H_2 histamine blockers are used 24 hours prior to injection to improve the outcome, in the event of an anaphylactic reaction.[4, 33, 53] Careful preinjection preparation and performance of the procedure in association with a skilled anesthesiologist are mandatory if the anaphylactic reaction is to be treated successfully. The use of local anesthesia will decrease the incidence of anaphylaxis[1, 4] and will permit the patient to report prodromal symptoms, thereby allowing early treatment.[30] It has also been shown to be associated with fewer neurologic complications,[1] perhaps because the patient is able to report pain indicative of needle penetration of nervous tissue.[30, 33] Correct positioning of the patient, optimum fluoroscopic control, and the availability of previous radiographic studies are critical for proper needle placement. The two-needle technique is used to prevent discitis, and the lateral approach is used to avoid intrathecal injection.[33] A test dose is recommended to identify patients who are most sensitive to the enzyme.[4] In order to prevent neurologic complications, one should avoid both discography at the time of chemonucleolysis and multiple-level injections.[1, 23] Finally, if intrathecal injection is recognized at the time of chemonucleolysis, one should be prepared to perform a C1–C2 puncture for venting and irrigation of the dura.[33]

Current research efforts are directed toward finding alternative enzymes that are less toxic than chymopapain or collagenase. Chondroitinase ABC is currently undergoing animal studies. In a rabbit study, all discs injected with Chondroitinase ABC had radiographic evidence of disc space narrowing.[22] Histologic evaluation of the discs indicated a loss of proteoglycans from the nucleus pulposus and annulus fibrosis. The end plates of the adjacent vertebral bodies appeared to be unaffected. Olmarker and coworkers have compared the acute and long-term effects of Chondroitinase ABC with chymopapain and a saline control.[50] In hamsters they demonstrated that Chondroitinase ABC and sterile water both induced a transient reduction in blood flow. A therapeutic concentration of chymopapain immediately stopped the microcirculation in the injected area and caused numerous microhemorrhages at the border zone. Long-term effects of the enzymes and saline were studied in rabbits. Chondroitinase ABC and saline did not cause any effects macroscopically or microangiographically. Light microscopy revealed moderate inflammatory reactions with both substances. Chymopapain induced subcutaneous hemorrhages and necrosis of the overlying skin. Microangiography revealed a vessel-free zone at the injection site. The concentration of Chondroitinase ABC used in this study was four to eight times that likely to be used clinically, suggesting a wide margin of safety for this agent.

In conclusion, chemonucleolysis appears to be a successful treatment for herniated discs in approximately 70% to 80% of patients, and these results are sustained during long-term follow-up. The results approach those obtained by open or microsurgical discectomy in carefully selected patients. The indications for the procedure are more limited than those for standard laminectomy and discectomy. It should be avoided in cases of coexisting spinal stenosis, a suspected sequestered fragment, disc herniations at multiple levels, previous laminectomy, rapidly progressive neurologic deficits, severe allergy or prior sensitization to papain, tumors or spondylolisthesis, and diabetes or pregnancy. Evidence suggests that it should be performed only with small or medium herniations that do not have severe root impingement. Complications can be decreased by careful patient selection, awareness of immunologic factors, and avoidance of technical errors.

In the author's experience, many of the patients fulfilling the selection criteria described above will improve spontaneously. In those who continue to be disabled by pain after 6 weeks of conservative therapy, the options of continued conservative care, open discectomy, and chemonucleolysis are offered. With the present backlash of public opinion about chymopapain, very few patients choose chemonucleolysis. Enthusiasm for the technique of chemonucleolysis will most likely continue to fade unless a safer enzyme becomes available.

References

1. Agre, K.: Serious neurological adverse events associated with administration of Chymodiactin. *In* Brown, J.E., Nordby, E.J., and Smith, L. (eds.): Chemonucleolysis. Thorofare, New Jersey, Slack, 1985.
2. Agre, K., Wilson, R.R., Brim, M., and McDermott, D.J.: Chymodiactin postmarketing surveillance: Demographic and adverse experience data in 29,075 patients. Spine 9:479–485, 1984.
3. Benoist, M., Deburge, A., Heripret, G., et al.: Treatment of lumbar disc herniation by chymopapain chemonucleolysis. A report on 120 patients. Spine 7:613–617, 1982.
4. Boots-Flint Inc.: Package insert for Chymodiactin. Nov., 1987.
5. Bouillet, R.: Complications of discal hernia therapy: Comparative study regarding surgical therapy and nucleolysis by chymopapain. Acta Orthop. Belg. 49(Suppl.)1:48–77, 1983.
6. Bromley, J.W., Hirst, J.W., Osman, M., et al.: Collagenase: An experimental study of intervertebral disc dissolution. Spine 5:126–132, 1980.
7. Bromley, J.W., Varma, A.O., Santoro, A.J., et al.: Double-blind evaluation of collagenase injections for herniated lumbar discs. Spine 9:486–488, 1984.
8. Brown, J.E., Nordby, E.J., and Smith, L.: Chemonucleolysis. Thorofare, New Jersey, Slack, 1985.
9. Brown, M.D.: Intradiscal Therapy: Chymopapain or Collagenase. Chicago, Year Book Medical Publishers, 1983.
10. Brown, M.D., and Daroff, R.B.: The double blind study comparing discase (chymopapain) to placebo. An editorial comment. Spine 2:233–236, 1977.
11. Brown, M.D., and Tompkins, J.: Chemonucleolysis (discolysis) with collagenase. Spine 11:123–130, 1986.
12. Brown, M.D., Tompkins, J., and Mann, H.: Pain response post-chemonucleolysis and laminectomy. Spine 14:321–326, 1989.
13. Cauchoix, J., and Deburge, A.: Operative observations and results of surgery after failure of chemonucleolysis. Acta Orthop. Belg. 49(Suppl.)1:78–89, 1983.

14. Crawshaw, C., Frazer, A.M., and Merriam, W.F.: A comparison of surgery and chemonucleolysis in the treatment of sciatica: A prospective randomized trial. Spine 9:195–198, 1984.
15. Dabezies, E.J., Langford K., and Morris J.: Safety and efficacy of chymopapain (Discase) in the treatment of sciatica due to a herniated nucleus pulposus: Results of a randomized, double-blind study. Spine 13:561–565, 1988.
16. Davis, R.J., North, R.B., Campbell, J.N., and Suss, R.A.: Multiple cerebral hemorrhages following chymopapain chemonucleolysis: A case report. J. Neurosurg. 61:169–171, 1984.
17. Deburge, A., Benoist, M., and Boyer, D.: The diagnosis of disc sequestration. Spine 9:496–499, 1984.
18. Deburge, A., Rocolle, J., and Benoist, M.: Surgical findings and results of surgery after failure of chemonucleolysis. Spine 10:812–815, 1985.
19. Edwards, W.C., Orme, T.J., and Orr-Edwards, G.: CT discography: Prognostic value in the detection of patients for chemonucleolysis. Spine 12:792–795, 1987.
20. Ejeskar, A., Nachemson, A., Herberts, P., et al.: Surgery versus chemonucleolysis for herniated lumbar discs: A prospective study with random assignment. Clin. Orthop. 174:236–242, 1983.
21. Eguro, H.: Transverse myelitis following chemonucleolysis. J. Bone Joint Surg. 65A:1328, 1983.
22. Eurell, J.A., Brown, M.D., and Ramos, M.: The effects of chondroitinase ABC on the rabbit intervertebral disc. A radiologic and histologic study. Accepted for publication in Clin. Orthop. 1989.
23. FDA Drug Bulletin. 14:14–15, 1984.
24. Fisher, R.G., Bromley, J.W., Becker, G.L., et al.: Surgical experience following intervertebral discolysis with collagenase. J. Neurosurg. 64:613–616, 1986.
25. Flint Laboratories, Inc., Spinal Therapies Group: Chemonucleolysis update: Patient selection for chemonucleolysis. Northbrook, Illinois, Flint Laboratories, Inc. Jan., 1987.
26. Ford, L.: Personal communication. Data presented at Low Back and Sciatica Pain Meeting, St. Louis, Missouri, December, 1983.
27. Fraser, R.D.: Chymopapain for the treatment of intervertebral disc herniation: The final report of a double-blind study. Spine 9:815–818, 1984.
28. Fraser, R.D., Osti, O.L., and Vernon-Roberts, B.: Discitis following chemonucleolysis: An experimental study. Spine 11:679–687, 1986.
29. Grammer, L.C., Schafer, M., Bernstein, D., et al.: Prevention of chymopapain anaphylaxis by screening chemonucleolysis candidates with cutaneous chymopapain testing: A preliminary report. Clin. Orthop. 221:202–206, 1987.
30. Hall, B.B., and McCulloch, J.A.: Anaphylactic reactions following the intradiscal injection of chymopapain under local anesthesia. J. Bone J. Surg. 65A:1,215–1,219, 1983.
31. Hirsch, C.: Studies on the pathology of low back pain. J. Bone Joint Surg. 41B:237–243, 1959.
32. Javid, M.J., Nordby, E.J., Ford, L.T., et al.: Safety and efficacy of chymopapain (Chymodiactin) in herniated nucleus pulposus with sciatica: Results of a randomized double-blind study. J.A.M.A. 249:2,489–2,494, 1983.
33. Kitchel, S.H., and Brown, M.D.: Complications of chemonucleolysis. *In* Garfin, S.R. (ed.): Complications of Spine Surgery. London, Williams & Wilkins (in press).
34. Leavitt, F., Garron, D.C., Whister, W.W., and D'Angelo, C.M.: A comparison of surgery and chemonucleolysis in the treatment of sciatica. A prospective randomized trial. Spine 9:195–198, 1980.
35. Levy, J.H., Roizen, M.F., and Morris, J.M.: Anaphylactic and anaphylactoid reactions. A review. Spine 11:282–291, 1986.
36. Maciunas, R.J., and Onofrio, B.M.: The long-term results of chymopapain: Ten-year follow-up of 268 patients after chemonucleolysis. Clin. Orthop. 206:37–41, 1986.
37. Maroon, J.C., Holst, R.A., and Osgood, C.P.: Chymopapain in the treatment of ruptured lumbar discs. J. Neurol. Neurosurg. Psychiatry 39:508–513, 1976.
38. Martins, A.N., Ramirez, A., Johnston, J., and Schwetschenau, P.R.: Double-blind evaluation of chemonucleolysis for herniated lumbar discs. J. Neurosurg. 49:816–827, 1978.
39. Masaryk, T.J., Ross, J.S., and Modic, M.T.: High resolution MR imaging of sequestered lumbar intervertebral disks. Am. J. Neuroradiol. 9:351–358, 1988.
40. Massie, W.K.: Chemonucleolysis. Editorial comment. Clin. Orthop. 67:2–5, 1969.
41. Mayer, H., Wehr, M., Brock, M., and Kaden, B.: Skin testing for chymopapain allergy in chemonucleolysis. Surg. Neurol. 25:283–289, 1986.
42. McCullough, J.A., Canham, W.D., and Dolovich, J.: Skin tests for chymopapain allergy. Ann. Allergy 55:609, 1985.
43. McCulloch, J.A.: Chemonucleolysis experience with 2,000 cases. Clin. Orthop. 146:128–135, 1980.
44. McCulloch, J.A.: Chemonucleolysis. J. Bone Joint Surg. 59B:45–52, 1977.
45. McDermott, D.J., Agre, K., Brim, M., et al.: Chymodiactin in patients with herniated lumbar intervertebral disc(s): An open-label, multicenter study. Spine 10:242–249, 1985.
46. Nachemson, A.L., and Rydevik, B.: Chemonucleolysis for sciatica. A critical review. Acta Orthop. Scand. 59:56–62, 1988.
47. Nordby, E.J.: A comparison of discectomy and chemonucleolysis. Clin. Orthop. 200:279–283, 1985.
48. Nordby, E.J.: Current concepts review: Chymopapain in intradiscal therapy. J. Bone J. Surg. 65A:1,350–1,353, 1983.
49. Nordby, E.J.: Editorial comment. Long-term results in chemonucleolysis. Clin. Orthop. 206:2–3, 1986.
50. Olmarker, K., Danielsen, N., Nannmark, U., et al.: Microvascular effects of Chondroitinase ABC. Accepted for publication in Clin. Orthop. 1989.
51. Olmarker, K., Rydevik, B., Dahlin, L.B., et al.: Effects of epidural and intrathecal application of collagenase in the lumbar spine. An experimental study in rabbits. Spine 12:477–482, 1987.
52. Onofrio, B.M.: Injection of chymopapain into intervertebral disc: Preliminary report on 72 patients with symptoms of disk disease. J. Neurol. Surg. 42:384, 1975.
53. Philbin, D.M., Moss, J., Akins, C.W., et al.: The use of H_1 and H_2 histamine antagonists with morphine anesthesia: A double-blind study. Anesthesiology 55:292–296, 1981.
54. Postacchini, F., Lami, R., and Massobrio, M.: Chemonucleolysis versus surgery in lumbar disc her-

niations: Correlation of the results to preoperative clinical pattern and size of the herniation. Spine 12:87–96, 1987.
55. Ravichandran, G., and Mulholland, R.C.: Chymopapain chemonucleolysis: A preliminary report. Spine 5:380–384, 1980.
56. Report of the Committee on Chymopapain (Discase). Chicago, American Academy of Orthopedic Surgeons, 1975.
57. Reynolds, F.C.: Report on Evaluation of Double-Blind Study of Chymopapain. Chicago, American Academy of Orthopedic Surgeons, 1975.
58. Roberts, M.P.: Mortality Rate of Lumbar Laminectomy for Herniated Intervertebral Disc. Report of 15,378 Cases. Proceedings of the 1984 Annual Meeting of American Association of Neurological Surgeons. San Francisco, Apr. 8–12, 1984, p. 132.
59. Rydevik, B., Branemark, P.I., Nordborg, C., et al.: Effects of chymopapain in nerve tissue. An experimental study on the structure and function of peripheral nerve tissue in rabbits after local application of chymopapain. Spine 1:137–148, 1976.
60. Rydevik, B., Brown, M.D., Ehira, T., and Nordborg, C.: Effects of collagenase on nerve tissue: An experimental study on acute and long-term effects in rabbits. Spine 10:562–566, 1985.
61. Schweigel, J.F., and Berezowsky, J.: Repeat chymopapain injection: Results and complications. Spine 12:800–802, 1987.
62. Schwetschenau, P.R., Ramirez, A., Johnston, J., et al.: Double-blind evaluation of intradiscal chymopapain for herniated lumbar discs. J. Neurosurg. 45:622–627, 1976.
63. Smith, L., Garvin, P.J., Gessler, R.M., and Jennings, R.B.: Enzyme dissolution of the nucleus pulposus. Nature 198:1,311–1,312, 1963.
64. Smith, L., and Brown, J.E.: Treatment of lumbar intervertebral disc lesions by direct injection of chymopapain. J. Bone Joint Surg. 49B:502–519, 1967.
65. Stephens, M.M., and McManus, F.: Chemonucleolysis. Irish J. Med. Sci. 153:174–177, 1984.
66. Stern, H.: Advance Biofacture Corp., 1988.
67. Sussman, B.J., Bromley, J.W., and Gomez, J.G.: Injection of collagenase in the treatment of herniated lumbar disc. J.A.M.A. 245:730–732, 1981.
68. Troisier, O., and Cypel, D.: Discography, an element of decision: Surgery versus chemonucleolysis. Clin. Orthop. 206:70–78, 1986.
69. Tsay, Y., Jonas, R., Calenoff, E., et al.: A preoperative chymopapain sensitivity test for chemonucleolysis candidates. Spine 9:764–768, 1984.
70. Watters, W.C., Mirkovic, S., and Boss, J.: Treatment of the isolated lumbar intervertebral disc herniation: Microdiscectomy versus chemonucleolysis. Spine 13:360–362, 1988.
71. Watts, C.: Complications of chemonucleolysis for lumbar disc disease. Neurosurgery 1:2–5, 1977.
72. Watts, C., Hutchison, G., Stern, J., and Clark, K.: Comparison of intervertebral disc disease treatment by chymopapain injection and open surgery. J. Neurosurg. 42:397–400, 1975.
73. Weber, H.: Lumbar disc herniation. A controlled, prospective study with ten years of observation. Spine 8:131–140, 1983.
74. Weinstein, J., Spratt, K.F., Lehmann, T., et al.: Lumbar disc herniation: A comparison of the results of chemonucleolysis and open discectomy after ten years. J. Bone Joint Surg. 68A:43–54, 1986.
75. Wiltse, L.L., Widell, E.H., and Yuan, H.A.: Chymopapain chemonucleolysis in lumbar disc disease. J.A.M.A. 231:474–479, 1975.
76. Zeigler, H.E.: Comparison of chemonucleolysis and microsurgical discectomy for the treatment of herniated lumbar disc. Spine 12:796–799, 1987.
77. Zook, B.C., and Kobrino, A.I.: Effects of collagenase and chymopapain on spinal nerves and intervertebral discs of Cynomolgus monkeys. J. Neurosurg. 64:474–483, 1986.

□ Pelvic Visceral Dysfunction—Cauda Equina Syndrome

Thomas W. McNeill

The neural elements associated with the lumbosacral spine in adults consist of the termination of the spinal cord (conus medullaris), the lumbar portion of the sympathetic nervous system, the sacral portion of the parasympathetic nervous system, and the lumbosacral nerve roots. Injuries to these neural elements may be associated with concomitant injuries to the bony elements of the lumbosacral spine, may be caused by diseases of the lumbosacral spine, or may arise as a complication of surgical treatment of diseases or injuries of this region of the spine. Whatever the cause of the injury to the neural elements, the potential for significant impairment and subsequent disability is great; this is because, in addition to loss of function of the lower extremities, there may be loss of bowel, bladder, and sexual function. This chapter discusses lumbosacral neural injuries with emphasis on the visceral components of these injuries and the so-called cauda equina syndrome.

ANATOMY AND PHYSIOLOGY

In the adult the conus medullaris, or termination of the spinal cord, occupies the most proximal region of the lumbar spinal canal. The conus medullaris usually overlies the body of L1. It is about 2.5 cm in length, is narrower than the remainder of the spinal cord, and tapers to an ending in the filum terminale. The lumbar nerves and the lumbar sympathetic nerves originate in the lumbar enlargement of the spinal cord immediately proximal to the conus medullaris. The sacral parasympathetic nerves and the sacral sensory paths originate in the conus medullaris.[14, 15] The individual lumbar nerves join the sacral nerves to form the cauda equina, or "horse's tail." The conus medullaris may lie distal to the body of L1 in the adult when the normal ascent with growth is altered by cord tethering, which may occur in a variety of conditions such as myelomeningocele, diastematomyelia, and sacral lipomata.

The lumbar and sacral nerves arise from the lumbar spinal cord as separate dorsal (sensory) and ventral (motor) roots, which join together to form the individual lumbar or sacral nerves. Each pair of nerves exits at its respective level, beginning with the L1 nerves exiting between the L1 and L2 vertebrae. Nerve fibers of the visceral nerves are initially associated with the somatic afferent and efferent nerves. The motor component of the visceral nerves forms the autonomic nervous system. The sensory (afferent) component from the viscera is, technically, not a part of the autonomic nervous system. However, these afferents are an essential part of the reflex arcs by which many of the autonomic functions take place. The autonomic nervous system is, by definition, a motor system that has two components: the sympathetic (thoracolumbar) and parasympathetic (craniosacral) nerves to the viscera. These two components often have contrasting effects, in a general sense. Nevertheless, contributions from both components are required for the normal functioning of the pelvic viscera, which includes defecation, micturition, and sexual responsiveness.

The somatic efferent nerves of the lumbosacral plexus control the striated muscle of the lower extremities, pelvic floor, and external sphincters (i.e., "voluntary" motor functions). The visceral efferent nerves supply the smooth muscle of the colon, rectum, bladder, blood vessels, and sexual organs (i.e., "involuntary" motor functions).

The sympathetic portion of the nervous system originates in preganglionic cells in the thoracic spinal cord and in the first two lumbar segments. The axon from the preganglionic neuron exits the spinal cord and traverses the ventral root, where it creates a synapse with the postganglionic neuron in either the paraspinal sympathetic chain or one of the accessory ganglia (e.g., celiac or superior mesenteric ganglia). Activity in these sympathetic fibers to the lower urinary system results in bladder relaxation, internal sphincter contraction, and urethral smooth muscle sphincter contraction. Sympathetic activity to the rectum and colon results in inhibition of peristalsis. Much of the motor component of orgasm and ejaculation is mediated by the sympathetic fibers, yet penile and clitoral erections are inhibited by sympathetic activity.

The preganglionic cells of the parasympathetic portion of the autonomic system reside in the conus medullaris. These fibers exit along with the sacral roots, form the presacral plexus, and descend to the colon, rectum, bladder, and genital organs. The postganglionic fiber is short and most often begins within the organ that is innervated. Parasympathetic activity results in contraction of the smooth muscle of the bladder and relaxation of the sphincter. In the colon and rectum, parasympathetic activity results in an acceleration of peristalsis and a relaxation of the internal sphincter. Penile erection and clitoral erection and retraction are mediated by parasympathetic outflow, as are vaginal lubrication and engorgement of the labia and vaginal wall.

The sensory portion of the reflex arc from the viscera and sexual organs is necessary for normal function in micturition, defecation, and active sexual function. (Conception does not depend upon these reflexes, and it may occur in paraplegic women.) Furthermore, somatic motor nerves play a major role in the control of micturition and defecation by controlling the striated muscle sphincters and contraction of striated muscle in ejaculation and orgasm.[16, 17]

Defecation and Urination

After infancy, urination (micturition) and defecation are subject to voluntary control.

They are integrated spinal reflexes that require the interactions of higher (cerebral) centers, voluntary (striated muscle) control, parasympathetic motor function, sympathetic motor function, and a complete sensory component of the reflex arc. Urination and defecation are nearly identical insofar as the description of the components of neurologic control are concerned. As the bladder or rectum is distended, a point is reached in which the sensation of fullness is transmitted to centers in the spinal cord, pontine reticular formation, and cerebral cortex. The impulse originates in stretch receptors in the bladder wall or rectal wall, which fire when a certain volume is reached; in the case of the bladder, this volume is approximately 400 cc.[17] These afferent fibers are associated with the parasympathetic efferents and enter the spinal cord via the lower three sacral segments (S3 to S5). Awareness of the need to urinate or defecate is a cortical function that is integrated with the spinal cord, providing control over the motor components of the reflex arc. Proper and complete functioning of the bladder or rectum is not possible without this central control component. During the period in which the bladder or rectum is filling, sympathetic activity inhibits pelvic ganglia, inhibits peristalsis, causes detrusor relaxation, and causes internal smooth muscle sphincter contraction. When inhibition is released, a complex reflex begins. In the case of micturition, the parasympathetic fibers stimulate detrusor muscle contraction (i.e., contraction of the smooth muscle of the bladder wall), sympathetic contraction of the internal sphincter ceases, and voluntary relaxation of the skeletal muscle external sphincter is accompanied by a voluntary increase in the intra-abdominal pressure. For defecation the process is nearly the same, except that in this case sympathetic inhibition of peristalsis ceases and parasympathetic stimulation of peristalsis is facilitated. The internal and external sphincter control in micturition is the same as in defecation, as is the nature of the central control (Table 1).

Sexual Function

Here again, a complex reflex involving cortical functions, spinal cord centers, somatic sensory afferents, somatic motor efferents, sympathetic efferents, and parasympathetic efferents is required for complete function. In both sexes the basic response and its neural control are the same. The obvious differences are those that directly relate to conception. In the male the entire reflex arc from the cord down must function in order for ejaculation to occur, whereas in the female conception can occur without any of the distal neurologic function being present.

In both sexes hormonal stimulation of the sexual organs is an almost essential foundation for the remainder of the response. The next step in the initiation of the sexual autonomic reflexes is some combination of central and peripheral afferent stimulation leading to the excitement phase. This phase requires parasympathetic innervation, which produces genital vasodilation resulting in penile and clitoral erection, penile lubrication, vaginal lubrication, and distention of the labia and vaginal wall. The plateau phase is the same as the excitement phase but has an increase in the same parasympathetic-mediated vascular effects to the

Table 1 □ Pelvic Visceral Neurologic Function

LEVEL	MICTURITION/DEFECATION	SEXUAL: Response	SEXUAL: Orgasm
Cortical, pons	Control by inhibition of reflex	Initiation of excitement phase	
Cord	Integration of reflex	Integration of reflex	
Sensory	Stretch receptor detection of bladder or rectal filling	Initially varied sensory input	Continued genital stimulation required
Motor, sympathetic	Internal sphincter Inhibits detrusor Inhibits peristalsis	Inhibition prior to orgasm	Rhythmic, smooth muscle contraction: male—emission
Motor, parasympathetic	Detrusor contraction Peristalsis	Penile, clitoral, labial engorgement/lubrication	Contraction of vaginal, urethral, uterine muscle: male—ejaculation
Motor, somatic	Inhibition of external sphincter	Pelvic floor contraction	

extent that orgasm occurs if adequate stimulation continues. Orgasm requires both sympathetic and somatic motor efferent discharge. In both sexes orgasm is accompanied by rhythmic contraction of both smooth and striated muscle of the urethra, rectum, and pelvic floor. In the female the vagina and uterus contract also. In the male the sympathetic efferents produce smooth muscle contraction of the prostate, seminal vesicles, vas deferens, and internal sphincter, leading to emission. This is followed by parasympathetic-mediated contraction of striated muscles of the ischiocavernosus, bulbocavernosus, and urethral muscles, leading to ejaculation. In both sexes orgasm is usually followed by resolution of the vasodilation and lubrication. Sympathetic stimulation prior to orgasm results in inhibition of the response, and the sympathetic discharge at the time of orgasm leads to resolution phase of the sexual response (see Table 1).[16]

Effects of Sympathectomy

Lumbar sympathectomy, if unilateral, does not disturb ejaculation but may result in subjective disturbance of sexual function; however, if both sides are removed and if the L1 ganglia are included, then most patients will experience a significant disturbance of sexual function.

Bilateral sympathectomy, which includes the L1 ganglion, results in failure of the emission component of the male sexual response but not ejaculation per se. There is an interference with the smooth muscle function of the vas deferens, prostate, and seminal vesicles, resulting in less fluid being sent into the urethra. Furthermore, because the internal sphincter is relaxed, what fluid is present is expelled into the bladder. The sperm that are present are nonmotile, owing to lack of motility of the vas deferens. Bilateral sympathectomy may also lead to failure of erection, but the mechanism leading to this effect is poorly understood. It may be due to postdenervaton sensitization to circulating catecholamines or to diversion of blood to the denervated lower extremities. Sexual functioning following sympathectomy appears not to be as severely affected in the female as in the male; yet there seems to be no reason why the same mechanisms that lead to failure of erection in the male should not lead to the analogous failure in the female.[18]

Bladder Decentralization

With conus medullaris injury or sacral nerve root injury, one initially sees urinary retention with a flaccid bladder. There may be overflow incontinence, but this is accompanied by poor bladder emptying, increasing residual volumes, and loss of bladder sensation. A cystometrogram will show a flat filling curve. After a variable period of time, uncontrolled spontaneous parasympathetic ganglion activity in the bladder wall causes persistent detrusor activity, which results in a small hypertrophic bladder. In this instance, the voluntary (somatomotor) external skeletal muscle sphincter function is also lost, while the smooth muscle (sympathetically innervated) internal sphincter may remain functional. This results in the need for experienced urologic care, because when urethral resistance exceeds 40 cm of water, ureteral dilation can be expected. If the urethral smooth muscle (sympathetically innervated) sphincter is also paralyzed, severe incontinence results.[18]

Conus Medullaris Syndrome

The sacral parasympathetic motor nerves from S3 to S5, the somatic motor nerves from S3 to S5, and the coccygeal nerve originate in the conus medullaris. The sacral sensory input from S3 to S5 enters the central nervous system here also. Injury or disease of the conus medullaris may result in partial or complete loss of these neural elements. Isolated injury or disease of this small segment of the spinal cord is, fortunately, rare. However, mixed lesions of the cauda equina and conus medullaris are not rare. If an isolated conus medullaris lesion occurs alone, one should expect to see the following: complete loss of sexual function, bladder paralysis, and paralysis of both external sphincters all on a permanent basis. More often, however, clinical findings are either mixed lesions that involve more of the cord to include upper sacral and lumbar segments of the spinal cord or lesions of the nerve roots of the cauda equina distal to the conus medullaris.[15]

CAUDA EQUINA SYNDROME

The cauda equina consists of all of the nerve roots from L1 downward. Paralysis of all of these roots results in the loss of all motor and sensory function of the pelvic viscera, pelvic floor, and both lower extremities. This version of cauda equina syndrome seldom occurs to this extent or degree of severity. A more general definition of cauda equina syndrome will be used in the following discussion: any lesion of the cauda equina (but not the conus medullaris) that results in bladder dysfunction.

Cauda equina syndrome is caused by compression of all or a portion of the nerves of the cauda equina. For bladder involvement to occur, the sacral nerves below S2 must be involved; furthermore, it seems logical that some degree of bilateral involvement is necessary in most instances because it is known that surgical hemisacrectomy for tumor often does not result in significant bladder paralysis. Logic does not always prevail. Clinically, unilateral lesions are seen with some frequency.[6]

Cauda equina syndrome may be caused by any lesion that might produce compression of the cauda equina. These lesions may include fracture, tumor, infection, disc herniation, and spinal stenosis. Disc herniation and spinal stenosis are the most common causes. Most of the disc hernias that produce the cauda equina syndrome occur at L4–L5 and L5–S1 because the overwhelming majority of disc herniations occur at these levels.[7] However, when upper lumbar or intrathecal disc herniations do occur they are individually more likely to result in clinical cauda equina syndrome than are the lower disc lesions.[1, 2, 6, 11]

Typically, the clinical description of cauda equina syndrome includes severe lower back pain, accompanied by severe bilateral sciatica, lower extremity weakness, lower extremity numbness (especially in the soles of the feet), perineal numbness, urinary retention (or incontinence), and fecal incontinence. This description, however, represents only one of several well-recognized variations on this theme.[2–5] There are two large general groups of patients with cauda equina syndrome; they are the acute and chronic varieties. In the acute group the syndrome develops rather suddenly within a week, whereas in the chronic group it evolves slowly over many months, or even years.

Acute cauda equina syndrome may arise suddenly without warning and without previous lumbar spine problems. This is the Group I described by Tandon and Sankaran.[12] In Group II there is a previous history of lower back pains and sciatica on one or several occasions before the acute onset of pelvic visceral paralysis (i.e., typically urinary retention). Group III patients present with lower back pain and either unilateral or bilateral sciatica. Later, they develop bladder paralysis before the acute episode of lower back pain and sciatica is resolved. The acute cauda equina syndrome is most often the result of an acute discal herniation. The herniation may be either a very large extrusion of nuclear material in a normal spinal canal or a moderate protrusion in a stenotic canal. The size of the protrusion or extrusion is not as important as how much of the available space in the canal has suddenly been occupied by the discal hernia. This concept has important implications for treatment.

Group I patients with acute cauda equina syndrome may complain of severe perirectal pain, although the sciatic symptoms may be less severe. Urinary retention and severe lower back pain are nearly constant features. The sciatic pain and paresthesias affect the buttocks, posterior thigh, posterior leg, and sole of the foot. Patients in Group II have these symptoms but differ in that they have had similar episodes in the past, although they were less severe and did not include urinary retention. Those in Group III present initially with lower back pain and sciatica, and gradually they develop urinary retention. This group causes the greatest difficulty for the treating physician. Inability to void is a common complaint, especially among males, who are given narcotic medication and placed at bed rest. Therefore, the beginning bladder paralysis is not appreciated immediately.[2, 8, 12]

Patients with chronic cauda equina syndrome present with symptoms suggestive of spinal stenosis such as pseudoclaudication, back pain, or radicular symptoms of long duration and the additional complaints of perineal pain and difficulties with urination and defecation. The discovery of the urinary complaints may require diligent inquiry on the part of the physician as they may be assumed, by the patient, to be attributable to other causes, even to normal aging. The patients in the chronic group are most often over 50 years of age, whereas those in the acute group are, on the average, at least a decade younger. Compression of multiple lumbosacral nerve roots develops slowly in the patients with chronic cauda equina syndrome, owing to the gradual nature of the change in the volume of the spinal canal. This gradual loss of volume of the spinal canal may be due to spondylosis per se, degenerative spondylolisthesis, or spondylosis superimposed upon a developmentally narrow canal. When chronic cauda equina syndrome develops in a younger patient, it is more likely the result of the gradual development of a central disc protrusion in a developmentally narrow canal.

Iatrogenic cauda equina syndrome may be caused by overly vigorous manipulation of the spine, postoperative bleeding, postoperative infection, and postoperative neural swelling. Typically, the patient who is at risk is the one with the developmentally very narrow canal who is operated upon for discal hernia with an intralaminar approach. Postoperative bleeding may occur days or even weeks after surgery.

The physical findings in patients with cauda equina syndrome may include widespread numbness of the buttocks and perineum, including perianal, penile, scrotal, vulvar, and clitoral numbness. Often, a considerable portion of the thighs and legs is affected. Numbness of the soles of the feet (indicating an S2 lesion) should alert the physician to the possibility of the development of cauda equina syndrome. There will be loss of the anal "wink" reflex, the cremasteric reflex, and the bulbocavernosus reflex in the complete lesions. However, partial lesions may result in significant pelvic visceral dysfunction. Lesions that are more cephalad than S1 will include additional findings of lumbar root involvement. In elderly patients with chronic pelvic visceral neurogenic injury, lower extremity findings are often absent, except by provocative testing. In the acute patients the bladder will be enlarged.

STUDIES

In the acute patient myelography should be performed as soon as is possible and medically appropriate. It is not inappropriate to consider obtaining basic urodynamic studies immediately prior to surgical decompression of the cauda equina. This would provide an invaluable measure of future recovery. In the chronic patient a slow, deliberate, and complete work-up should be performed. This should include an intravenous pyelogram (IVP), kidney function studies, urodynamic studies, sphincter function assessment, myelogram, and computed tomographic (CT) studies, if available.

TREATMENT

For both the acute and chronic varieties of the cauda equina syndrome the treatment is complete decompression of all of the involved neural elements. This has been successfully accomplished by one-sided laminectomy in instances of massive unilateral discal hernia.[1] In most instances, a bilateral laminectomy is probably a more prudent approach, especially when there may be any degree of spinal stenosis. The surgical decompression should be performed promptly. In the acute patient every effort should be made to complete the surgical decompression on the same day that the lesion is detected. This standard has seldom been achieved in the reported cases, and no evidence is available to indicate that a delay of 48 hours results in any deterioration of the final result.

PROGNOSIS

Recovery of normal bladder function is unusual and probably never occurs in patients who present with a complete lesion. Patients with unilateral symptoms, and presumably partial autonomic paralysis, may show significant recovery. Recovery can only be demonstrated by cystometry,[1] as patients may be taught (or may learn on their own) to nearly completely empty the bladder without using a catheter, by increasing intra-abdominal pressure.[9] If saddle anesthesia persists, bladder recovery will not occur, and when saddle anesthesia occurs, it seldom recovers. Genital function is often less severely affected and sexual complaints are often mild or absent. Anal dysfunction may be severe, but symptoms are less often noted and adequate studies are not available. No evidence is available to indicate that there may be an improved prognosis in the acute patients with very early surgical treatment. Aho suggests that there may be some improvement if the surgery takes place within 3 days of the onset of symptoms, but this was by no means conclusively demonstrated in his or in any other material. The commonly made assertion that surgery must be performed within a specified period of time in order for recovery to occur has no basis in fact. Nonetheless, some authors,[6] despite a complete lack of correlation between the duration of preoperative symptoms and eventual recovery, urge early surgery.[10] This attitude seems prudent until evidence to the contrary is presented. Some such evidence may exist in Onkey's unpublished material, suggesting that a short delay (48 hours) may actually be advantageous.

SUMMARY

In the most restrictive sense, cauda equina syndrome is any pelvic visceral dysfunction caused by compression of a part or all of the cauda equina. This compression may be sudden or gradual and may have many causes. However, the most common cause of the sudden onset of cauda equina syndrome is herniation of a lumbar intervertebral disc; for gradual onset, the usual cause is spinal stenosis. It is often the case that combinations of herniation and stenosis are present in an individual patient. The pelvic visceral dysfunction is most often first noticed as difficulty with urination. Eventually, difficulties with defecation and sexual responsiveness are also evident. Associated with the symptoms of pelvic visceral dysfunction are symptoms of back pain and sciatica, in varying degrees. Numbness and paralysis in the lower extremities, perineum, and genitalia are present to some extent. Assessment of the patient must include myelography. The only available treatment is surgical decompression of the cauda equina.

References

Clinical Studies

1. Aho, A.J., Auranen, A., and Pesonen, K.: Analysis of cauda equina symptoms in patients with lumbar disc prolapse. Acta Chir. Scand. 135:413–420, 1969.
2. Anderson, J.T., and Bradley, W.E.: Neurogenic bladder dysfunction in protruded lumbar disk and after laminectomy. Urology 8:94–96, 1976.
3. Choudhury, A., and Taylor, J.C.: Cauda equina syndrome in lumbar disc disease. Acta Orthop. Scand. 51:493–499, 1980.
4. Floman, Y., Wiesel, S.W., and Rothman, R.H.: Cauda equina syndrome presenting as a herniated lumbar disc. Clin Orthop. 147:234–237, 1980.
5. Jennett, B.W.: A study of 25 cases of compression of the cauda equina by prolapsed intervertebral disc. J. Neurol. Neurosurg. Psychiatr. 19:109–116, 1956.
6. Kostuik, J.P., Harrington, I., Alexander, D., et al.: Cauda equina syndrome and lumbar disc herniation. J. Bone Joint Surg. 68A:386–391, 1986.
7. Peyser, E., and Harari, A.: Intradural rupture of lumbar intervertebral disk. Surg. Neurol. 8:95–98, 1977.
8. Raaf, J.: Some observations regarding 905 patients operated upon for protruded lumbar intervertebral disc. Am. J. Surg. 97:388–399, 1959.
9. Scott, P.J.: Bladder paralysis in cauda equina lesions from disc prolapse. J. Bone Joint Surg. 47B:224–235, 1965.
10. Shephard, R.H.: Diagnosis and prognosis of cauda equina syndrome produced by protrusion of lumbar disc. Br. Med. J. 2:1434–1439, 1959.
11. Sprangfort, E.V.: The lumbar disc herniation; a computer-aided analysis of 2,504 operations. Acta Orthop. Scand. (Suppl.)142, 1972.
12. Tandon, P.N., and Sankaran, B.: Cauda equina syndrome due to lumbar disc prolapse. Indian J. Orthop. 1:112–119, 1967.
13. Tay, E.C.K., and Chacha, P.B.: Midline prolapse of a lumbar intervertebral disc with compression of the cauda equina. J. Bone Joint Surg. 41B:43–46, 1979.

Neurology and Physiology

14. Walton, J. (ed.): Brain's Diseases of the Nervous System. Oxford, Oxford University Press, 1985, pp. 593–603.
15. Countee, R.W., Vijayanathan, T., Martin, B.F., et al.: The conus medularis: physiological, anatomical and clinical considerations. *In* Camino, M., and O'Leary, P. (eds.): The Lumbar Spine. New York, Raven Press, 1987, pp. 171–182.
16. Lindsey, D.F., and Holms, J.E.: Basic human neurophysiology. New York, Elsevier Science Publishing Co., Inc., 1984, pp. 269–307.
17. McGuire, E.J.: Neuromuscular dysfunction of the lower urinary tract. *In* Walsh, P.C., Gittes, R.F., Perlmutter, A.D., et al. (eds.): Campbell's Urology. Philadelphia, W.B. Saunders, 1986.
18. Whitelaw, G.P., and Smithwick, R.H.: Some secondary effects of sympathectomy, with particular reference to disturbance of sexual function. N. Engl. J. Med. 245:121–130, 1951.

☐ Posterior Spinal Fusion*

David K. Selby

A posterior spinal fusion is any fusion of the spine that is posterior to the midpoint of the pedicles. This is in contradistinction to an anterior fusion, which is done in the column of the vertebral bodies. Posterior interbody fusion,[5, 6, 27] which is really an anterior fusion performed from the posterior approach, is a separate entity, and no attempt will be made to describe this difficult procedure, with all of its implications, in this chapter.

The following methods of posterior fusion are available to the spine surgeon:

1. **Posterior laminar fusion.** This is a fusion done by laying bone on top of the lamina after roughing up the laminae to make them a suitable site for the bone grafting. This is a technically easy fusion and was the standard of the early spine surgeons. However, it has the following disadvantages:
   a. Continued growth of the bony mass can cause central canal stenosis.
   b. It is not available following laminectomy.
   c. The fusion mass is placed as far away from the axis of rotation of the spine as is possible. This decreases the potential for healing as it is at the end of the motion arm. It also offers the least restraint to motion in the area of the nerve roots and disc.
2. **Facet fusion.** Fusion of the facets tends to have the same disadvantages as described above with no additional advantages that can be seen. Obtaining a facet fusion can be very difficult unless some form of fixation is used.
3. **Transverse process fusion.** An informal poll of the members of the International Society for the Study of the Lumbar Spine would indicate that this is the paragon of fusions, the standard against which other fusions must be measured. Because of this, the content of this chapter concentrates on this fusion, and the technique of fusion is described. It has the following advantages:
   a. Because of its lateral location, it has minimal opportunity to interfere with neural tissues.
   b. It can be used following laminectomy and is available for iatrogenic instability.
   c. It can be used with virtually all types of internal fixation.
   d. It has a high fusion rate, owing to its midposition in regard to the motion segment.
   e. Because of its midposition, it offers better stability to the entire motion segment.

HISTORY

The history of spinal fusion is taken from a monograph by Dr. Lee Wiltse. Portions of the following history are actual quotations from Dr. Wiltse.

The documented history of spinal fusion goes back to 1891 when Bethold Hadra[17] of Galveston wired together the spinous processes. However, none of us would be surprised if a prehistory skeleton was unearthed with evidence of iatrogenic tampering.

From a practical standpoint, spinal fusions started in New York with both Albee and Hibbs publishing the results of their spinal fusions in 1911. Albee's[1] method of fusions consisted of obtaining a strip of autogenous tibia, splitting the spinous process and laying the strip of tibia between the two halves of the spinous process. He then sutured the soft tissue together very securely.

Hibbs'[18] fusion was a more truly classical laminar fusion. He denuded the lamina and feathered the bone, overlapping the bony strips. In his initial description, he did not graft bone per se, but only jointed the feathered strips. Later, he placed graft over the lamina, and this became the standard fusion.

Ghormley[16] in 1933 published a paper in which the use of the iliac crest for graft was advocated; henceforth, that became the procedure of choice for most surgeries in which autologous bone graft was needed.

Campbell[3] of Memphis described the first transverse process fusion per se in the mid-1920s. In this operation, he tamped bone to the tips of the transverse process at L5. He also used the principle of taking strips of iliac crest for graft. Later, it was natural to push bone out on the transverse processes from L4 to S1 in doing lumbar spinal fusion.

In 1948, Cleveland and Bosworth[4] recommended repairing pseudarthrosis by passing through the midline, exposing the transverse processes on one side only and putting autologous iliac strips over this area.

It took 35 years after Campbell described the placing of bone graft out to the tips of L5 before transverse process fusion became commonly used. Many of the older surgeons never stopped using the simple posterior fusion as described by Hibbs, perhaps with some iliac crest graft added. They continued to do this, even though including the transverse process remarkably improved the fusion rates.

INDICATIONS

To be effective, spinal fusion of any type must be performed only when well-defined instabilities can be identified. The practice of doing any fusion automatically in combination with disc removal is a protocol to be condemned.[15, 20, 21, 26, 33, 38–40, 44] Transverse process fusion can offer stability for rotational, translational, and iatrogenic instabilities (see Chapter 10). Transverse process fusion is not helpful for a painful motion segment in the anterior column, and some type of interbody fusion is required for that problem.[33]

What clinical presentation is most likely to need fusion? Certainly, the patient who presents with a sudden onset of leg pain and little or no back pain is experiencing a root compression syndrome, and usually an instability cannot be identified. The patient with instability is having pain mediated through the posterior primary ramus. The pain is in the back with radiation into the hips or midthighs, seldom below the knees. The pain is frequently in a somatic distribution and not dermatomal. These are patients who present for work-up, as described in Chapter 10.

PREOPERATIVE CARE

Any spinal fusion is only one part of a coordinated rehabilitation program to restore the patient to full function. Many surgeons lose sight of this and believe that the operation is curative. This may be the case for an intelligent, well-motivated, self-employed patient. However, even that patient can benefit from a carefully planned preoperative and postoperative program of guidance and information.

Information □ The patient must be fully informed concerning the surgery and all of its ramifications. He must also be aware of the goals, and the surgeon should be sure that he and the patient have the same expectations. The use of videotapes in the office is an easy way to ensure that all of the information is fully provided to the patient.

It is also important that the patient understand the proper use of narcotics and the rationale behind it. A program on endorphins and their depletion by narcotics is helpful in this regard.

Smoking □ There is ample evidence in the literature that smoking influences the outcome of fusion. Most patients are willing to discontinue smoking for 6 months or so. Our minimum goal for the heavy smoker is one half of a pack per day for 6 months. Preferably, they stop completely.

Metabolic Work-up □ The metabolic evaluation of the patient with evidence of bone resorption, such as failed fusion, is directed toward the exclusion of diseases or conditions known to increase bone resorption. The common causes of bone resorption are as follows:

- Estrogen deficient bone loss (involutional osteoporosis, Type I)
- Calcium deficient bone loss (involutional osteoporosis, Type II)
- Hyperparathyroidism
- Hyperthyroidism
- Hypothyroidism
- Diabetes
- Paget's disease
- Cushing's disease or syndrome
- Hepatic insufficiency
- Renal insufficiency
- Gastrointestinal tract disease or surgery
- Drug usage such as loop diuretics, antacids, H_2 blockers, antiepileptics, corticosteroids

The most common cause of bone resorption, involutional osteoporosis, has no characteristic laboratory findings other than normalcy, and it is a questionable cause of fusion failure. The medical history may, in some cases, point to specific causes of bone loss, but the physician is often forced to undertake a general work-up to exclude disorders that may exist, possibly causing significant bone loss while producing only subtle clinical symptoms. The general laboratory evaluation should include the following: complete blood count (CBC); serum calcium; serum phosphorus; glucose; serum albumin; serum protein electrophoresis; 24-hour urine for calcium and creatinine; fasting 2-hour timed urine collection for calcium and creatinine, alkaline phosphatase, blood urea nitrogen (BUN), creatinine, T_4, and liver function tests (LFTs).

The CBC, particularly the hemoglobin, hematocrit, and red blood cell indices, can provide clues to the presence of myeloma, intestinal tract disease producing folate, or B_{12} deficiencies that may be associated with decreased absorption of calcium, alcoholism, or renal disease. A normal fasting glucose test excludes diabetes. The serum calcium and phosphorus are obviously necessary to rule out hyperparathyroidism. The serum calcium should be corrected for the serum albumin level because the normal laboratory ranges for serum calcium assume an albumin level of 4.0.

The serum albumin is an excellent indicator of liver function in addition to the other LFTs such as the serum glutamic-oxaloacetic transaminase (SGOT), serum glutamic-pyruvic transaminase (SGPT), and gamma-glutamyl transpeptidase (GGTP). Failing liver function may be associated with declining 25 vitamin D levels, which would lead to a failure of adequate calcium absorption.

Renal function indicators are the serum creatinine, BUN, and creatinine clearance, which is calculated from the 24-hour urine collection. Declining renal function may be associated with falling 1,25 vitamin D levels, which would also render calcium absorption inadequate. In situations of liver or renal impairment, the 25 and 1,25 vitamin D levels should be measured directly.

Hypercalciuria found on the 24-hour urine collection may be due to renal hypercalciuria or to absorptive hypercalciuria. The fasting 2-hour timed urine collection can help to differentiate between these two entities by measuring the fractional calcium excretion (FC_aE). This is calculated using the following formula:

$$FCA = ([Ca]^{mg/dl} \div [Cr]u^{mg/dl}) \times [Cr]s^{mg/dl}$$

Normal is less than 0.11 mg Ca/100 cc glomerular filtrate. High FCaEs can also be found in patients with 24-hour urine collections that are normal for calcium, usually because of a low dietary intake of calcium. This still implies renal calcium wastage. The test should therefore be performed, even in the presence of a normal 24-hour urine value. Absorptive hypercalciuria is not generally accepted as being a cause of increased bone resorption, even though the 24-urine calcium is high.

The T_4 level excludes most cases of hyperthyroidism and hypothyroidism, but if abnormalities are found they should be confirmed with a thyroid-stimulating hormone (TSH), T_3, and thyroxine-binding globulin (TBG) level. An abnormally high alkaline phosphatase should raise suspicion of Paget disease.

If abnormalities in the serum calcium and phosphorus determinations suggest hyperparathyroidism, a parathyroid hormone (PTH) level and urinary cyclic adenosine monophosphate (cAMP) determination may help to confirm the diagnosis.

A normal serum protein electrophoresis excludes multiple myeloma in about 90% of the cases. If it is abnormal, or if suspicion is high, serum and urine immunophoresis should be carried out. In about 3% of the elderly population, a benign monoclonal gammopathy that is not associated with any pathologic condition will be found.

In the elderly patient or in any patient with a significant gastrointestinal disease or surgery, the vitamin D levels should be measured. In any man with significant osteopenia, the serum testosterone level should be measured to exclude primary or secondary hypogonadism, which might cause bone loss. A low level must then be followed with the measurement of gonadotropins and prolactin.

A medication history should be taken to determine the use of medications that might affect the bone metabolism, such as antacids or H_2 blockers like cimetidine (Tagamet), which could interfere with calcium carbonate absorption; loop diuretics like furosemide (Lasix), which can cause increased renal wastage of calcium; phenytoin (Dilantin), which can interfere with vitamin D metabolism; and corticosteroids, which can have a myriad of adverse effects on bone metabolism.

Finally, it is all too easy to forget a nutritional assessment to rule out dietary calcium deficiency, which is found in 80% of adult Americans today, in men as well as women.

Autologous Blood[20] □ It is advantageous for the patient to supply 2 units 40 days in advance to avoid contagious disease or blood reaction. Patients will participate in this type of program with enthusiasm.

OPERATIVE TECHNIQUE

Exposure and hemostasis are the key elements to a technically competent spinal surgery. Concern as to the length of the incision seems petty when one considers that the patient may have years of pain if the job is not properly accomplished. The incision should be made long enough to comfortably insert the retractors and provide all the necessary exposure. If one is struggling to do a portion of the operation, more exposure is probably needed. A headlight and loupes are helpful in decompression and careful working around neural tissues. The headlight is particularly helpful in the denuding of the transverse processes in the lateral trough, as it is difficult to direct overhead operative lights into that field.

Some type of fixation is highly recommended.[7, 10, 11, 22–25, 28, 29, 35, 39] It has dual advantages. The immobilization greatly increases the fusion rate; it is logical that the bone will heal more rapidly if motion is reduced. Patients can also be started on a much more aggressive program of activity with the extra assurance of internal fixation. They have a feeling of increased stability and their pain decreases, which heightens their enthusiasm. Internal fixation may be in the form of distraction or compression hooks, Luque segmental fixation, pedicle screws, or facet screws (see Chapter 21).

Hemostasis is the second great principle of spinal fusion. Accurate location and manipulation of tissue cannot be accomplished when working under a pool of blood. The following items can influence blood loss:

1. **Patient position.** Any of the many frames used to allow freedom of the abdominal contents will reduce epidural vessel pressure. This directly influences blood loss in a fusion, as some type of decompression is most commonly accomplished at the same time. We use a Wilson frame, which provides a stable base for surgery and prevents the hyperextension common with most methods of the knee–chest position.
2. **Hypotensive anesthesia.**[30] With some exceptions, it is reasonable for the surgeon to insist that the anesthesiologist provide hypotensive anesthesia at the level of 80 to 90 mmHg systolic. The decrease in blood loss is significant enough that continuation of normotensive anesthesia is to be avoided, if possible.
3. **Vessel anatomy.** Most important to hemostasis is the surgeon's knowledge of the anatomy of the blood supply of the spine. The arterial supply is amazingly constant and coagulation of arteries before they become bleeders can greatly reduce blood loss (Fig. 1). With apologies to Dr. Harry Crock,[9] whose book is the classic regarding the blood supply to the spine, the names of the arteries in the accompanying illustrations have been referred to by their anatomic location to help the surgeon better identify them.
   a. *Transverse process artery.* This artery, sometimes called the artery of Macnab,[31] because of his excellent description of it, appears at the upper aspect of the junction of the transverse process and pedicle. In cleaning the soft tissue off the transverse process, it is advisable to first locate and coagulate this vessel. Frequently, the use of curved bayonet forceps facilitates coagulation of this artery.
   b. *Pars artery.* This is lateral to and always closely adjacent to the pars interarticularis. It most commonly comes into play during the initial exposure of the spine. Owing to its juxtaposition with the pars, it is most easily coagulated with bayonet forceps over the bleeder, but touching the bone of the pars. At the sacrum, this vessel emerges from a recess just below an accumulation of fat caudal to the inferior articular facet of L5. Coagulation requires the insertion of the forceps into the recess of bone.
   c. *Sacral arteries.* These protrude from the sacral foramen and can be difficult to control, unless the forceps again are

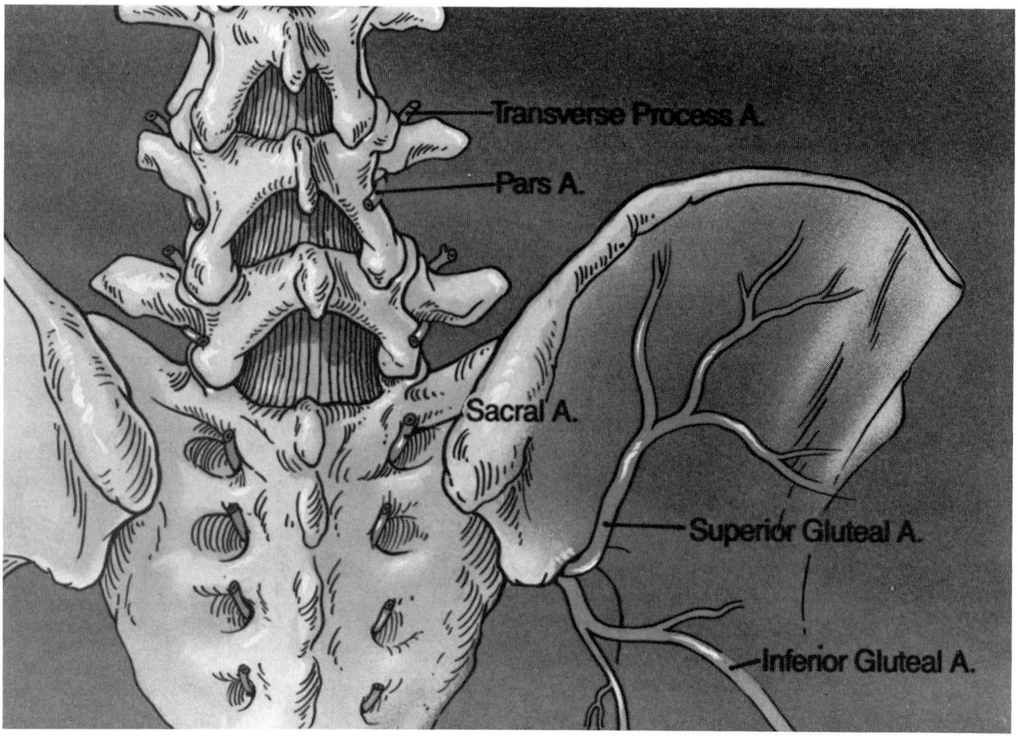

Figure 1 □ The arterial supply of the lumbar spine available for easy hemostasis.

inserted into the bony recess for coagulation.

d. *Superior gluteal artery*. It should be peeled back from the iliac crest during the taking of the bone graft so that it is with the muscle and protected from harm. If interrupted, it can be very difficult to control and the use of vascular clips is advised.

Technique[10, 19, 32, 35, 39, 41]

The incision is made in the midline over the spinous process (Fig. 2). The surgeon is best advised to carry the incision two segments above the fusion level. The lower limit should include most of the sacrum. This allows exposure that includes direct visualization of the transverse processes.

Commonly, a periosteal stripping technique is used to expose the bony structures. A more hemostatic technique (Fig. 3) is to put the tissue on stretch with an elevator and cut with an electric knife set on the coagulation mode. The dissection should follow the spinous processes down to the laminae and then clean the laminae laterally. The muscle should be retracted away from the bone and the coagulative cutting blade should be on the bone for the entire time. After the laminae have been cleared, then the soft tissue between the laminae can be cut and separated. It is here that one frequently encounters the pars artery. It is advantageous to clear off all bony structures with particular attention to the pars (Fig. 4). The pars is the anatomic guide to the pedicle and transverse process of the vertebrae (Fig. 5). Moving cephalad, the pars runs into its pedicle. By continuing cephalad and laterally, one exposes the mammary process of the transverse process and, just a bit above that, the main body of the transverse process. It is relatively easy to become confused about which transverse process may be identified with a level of fusion. By careful dissection of the anatomic structures and use of the pars as a landmark, it becomes easier to identify the specific transverse process of a motion segment. Decortication of the transverse process must be accomplished under direct visualization (Fig. 6). A Hibbs retractor toed in by the assistant, or a Wiltse retractor on the end of the transverse process, will provide excellent exposure. The cortex can then be removed by an instrument

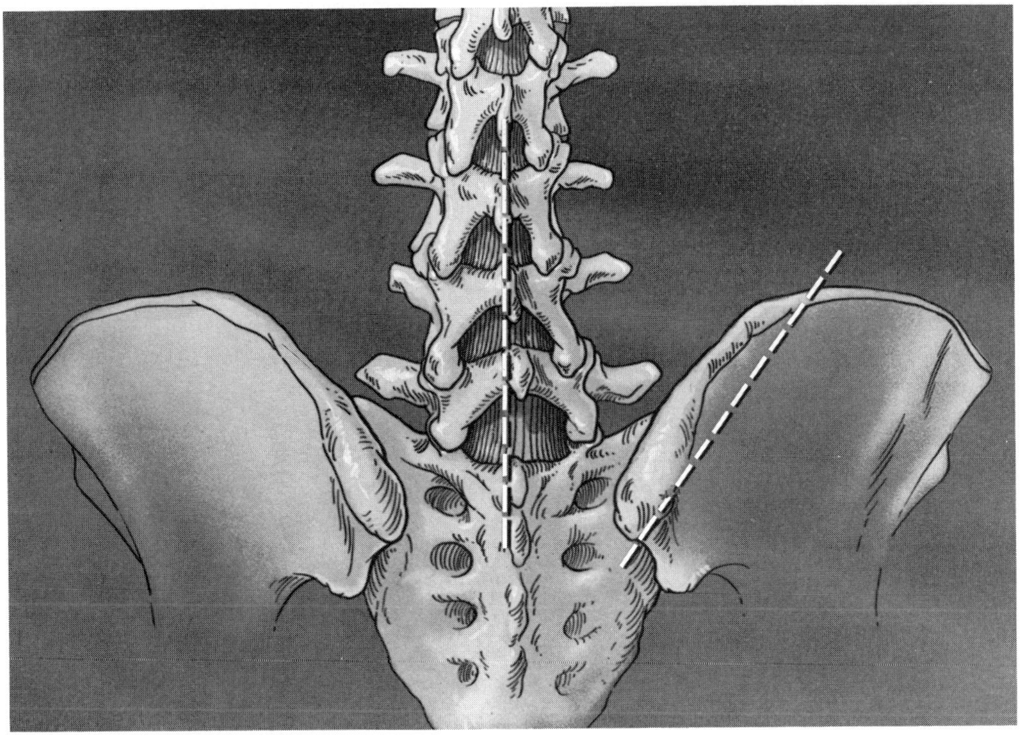

Figure 2 □ The incisions.

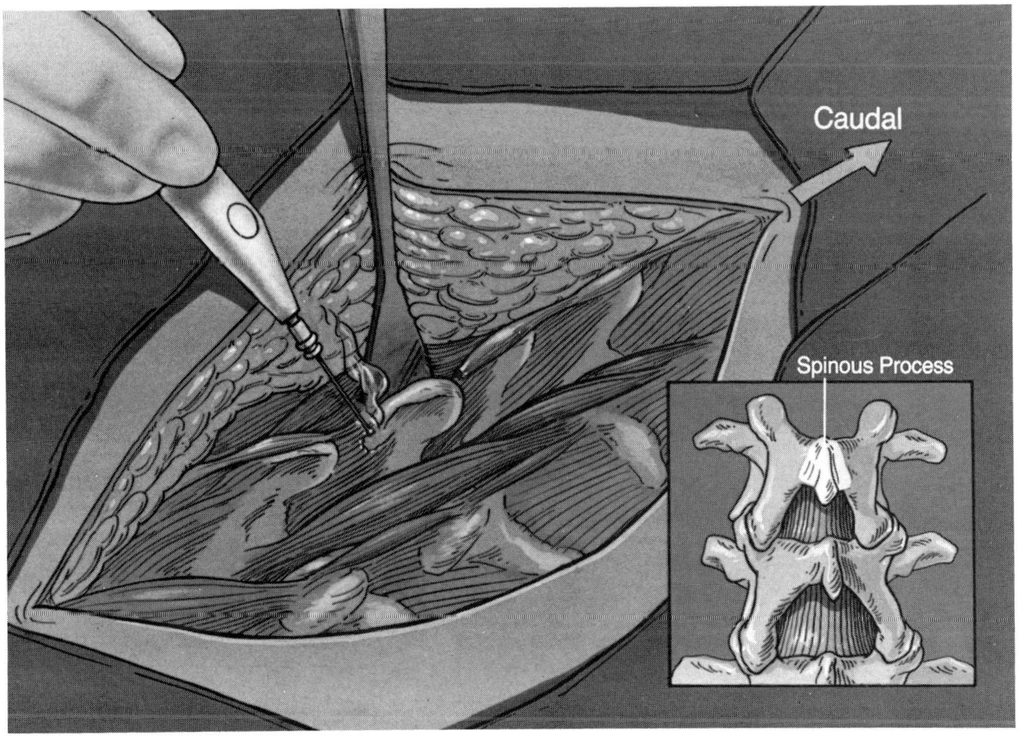

Figure 3 □ Technique of bony exposure. Note that the cautery is on the bone itself and that the dissection is carried down the spinous process and across the lamina.

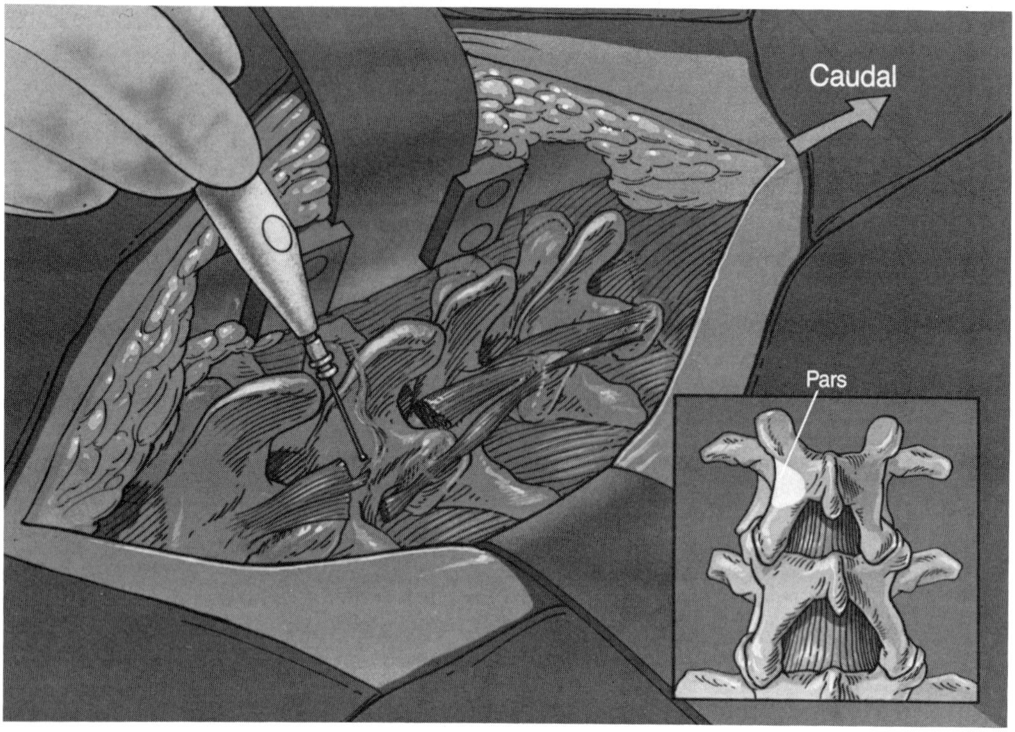

Figure 4 □ Cleaning of the pars.

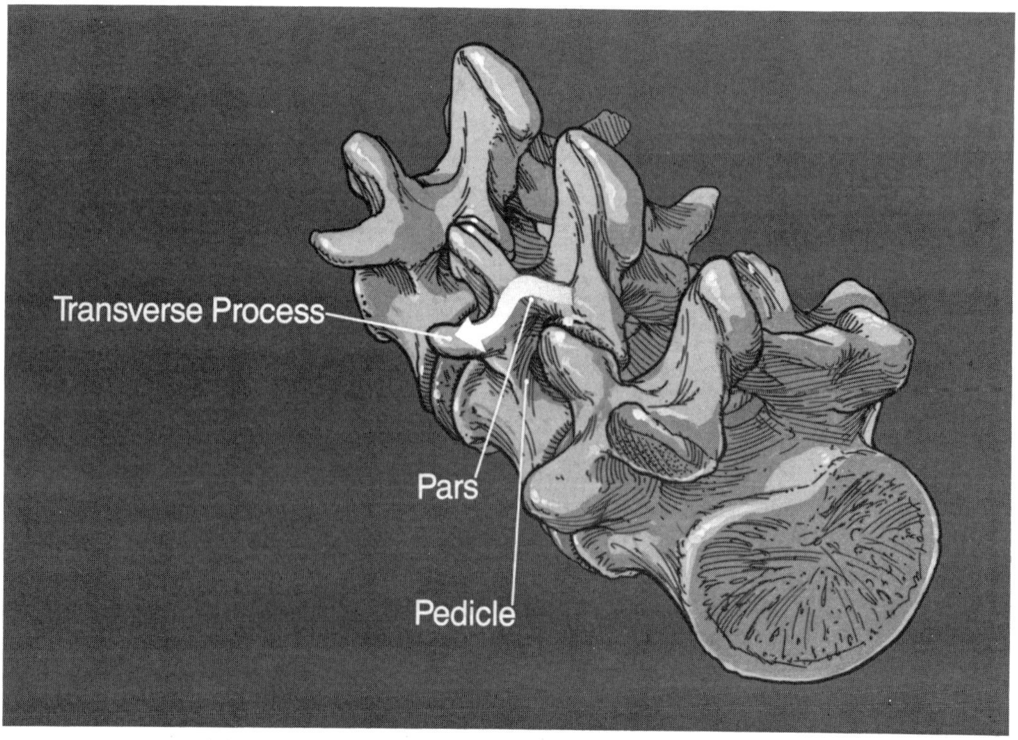

Figure 5 □ The pars is followed to the pedicle and transverse process.

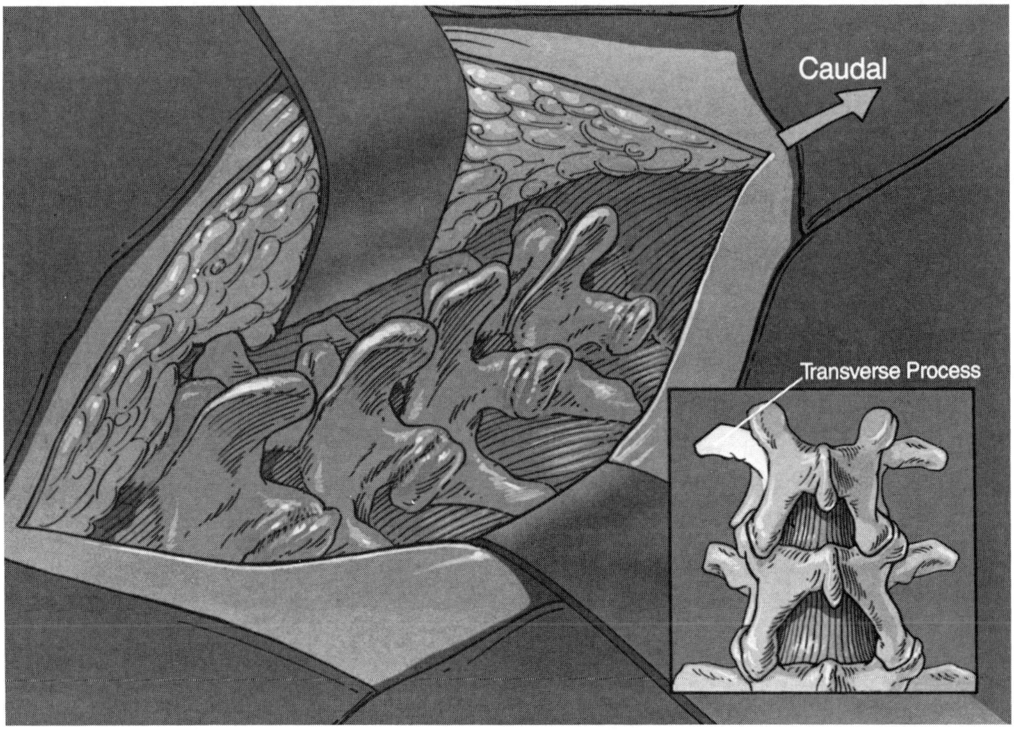

Figure 6 □ Exposure of the transverse process.

of choice. Again, the use of a headlight at this juncture is invaluable. If using the Wiltse retractor, one must be careful of pressure against the transverse process because it will have a tendency to break after a portion of the cortex is removed. It is also important to take the soft tissue off the intertransverse ligament so that one has a trough of bone and ligament without interference by fibrous tissue (Figs. 7 and 8). The ala is transversely cleared of soft tissue, and bites can be made across it with a rongeur. After the soft tissue is cleared from under the alar protuberance, the jaws of a rongeur can be inserted under it; closing the rongeur provides instant exposure of cancellous bone.

The most important part of any grafting procedure is the graft bed, and the most meticulous attention should be paid to its preparation. Figure 9 demonstrates that decortication is carried out not only on the transverse process—the area of the graft bed can be doubled by carrying decortication up the lateral aspect of the pedicle. This can be accomplished without interfering with the facet joint. This is very important at the top level, as iatrogenic invasion of the functioning facet joint above a fusion is a technical error that can lead to an early breakdown of the motion segment.

Bone Graft

Autogenous bone, which is still the most advantageous of graft materials,[40] is then removed from the iliac crest in the following manner (see Fig. 2). A separate incision is made over the iliac crest. The initial midline incision may be carried laterally by a hockey-stick technique, but that tends to increase the incidence of seromas and causes some problems of wound breakdown. After exposure of the iliac crest (Fig. 10), the muscle mass is removed from the lateral aspect of the iliac crest. The cautery technique is recommended for the top 2 cm of muscle removal. The muscle is then stripped with a periosteal elevator (Fig. 11). The cortex is removed with an osteotome to be made into match sticks. The bone is removed with a portion of cortex thin enough to expose the cancellous bone (Fig. 11). The cancellous bone is then removed in thin strips for placement in the graft site (Fig. 12). Care should be taken to stay on the bone and lateral to

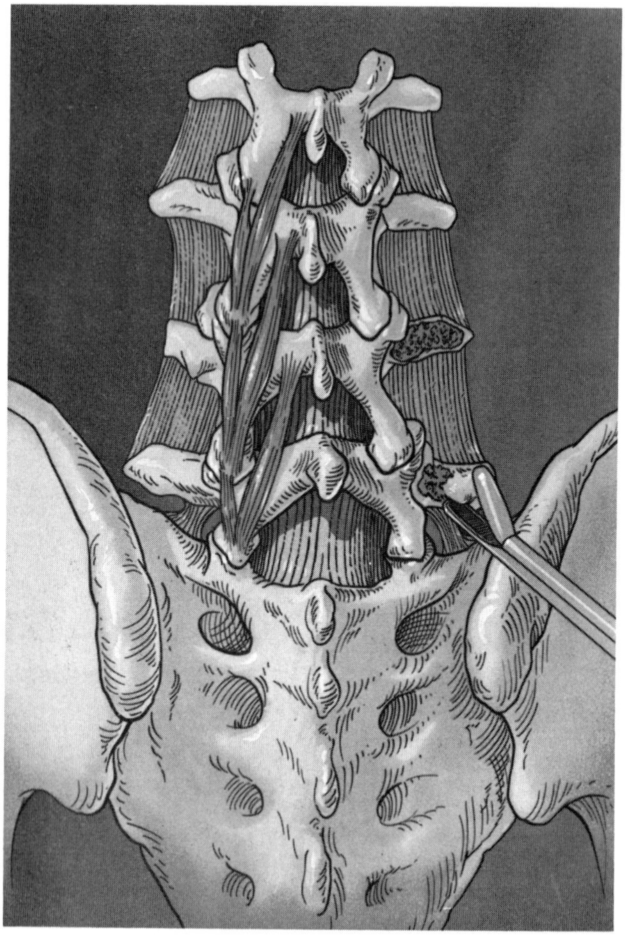

Figure 7 □ Cleaning of the transverse process under direct vision.

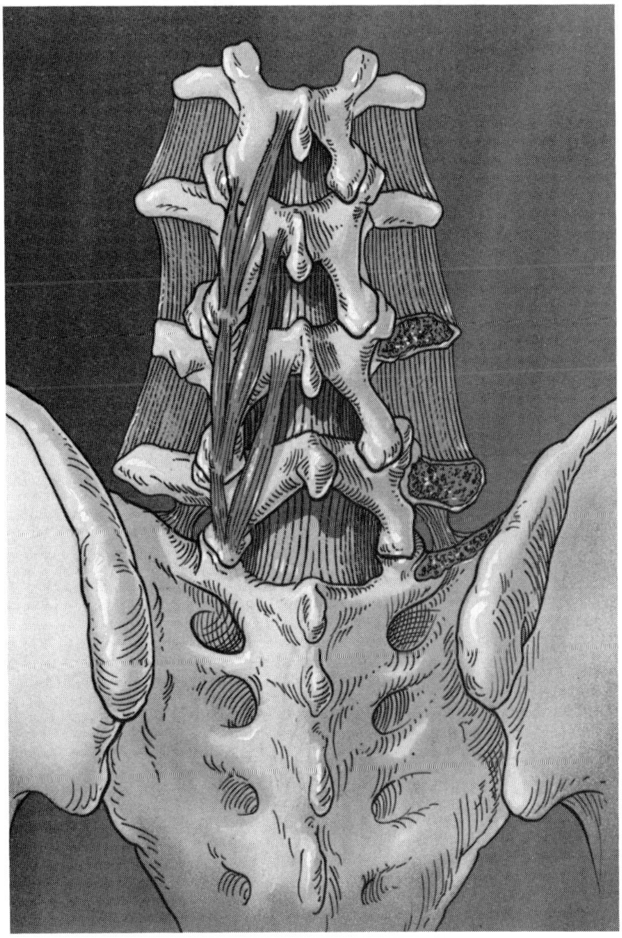

Figure 8 □ Removal of the posterior cortices of the transverse processes.

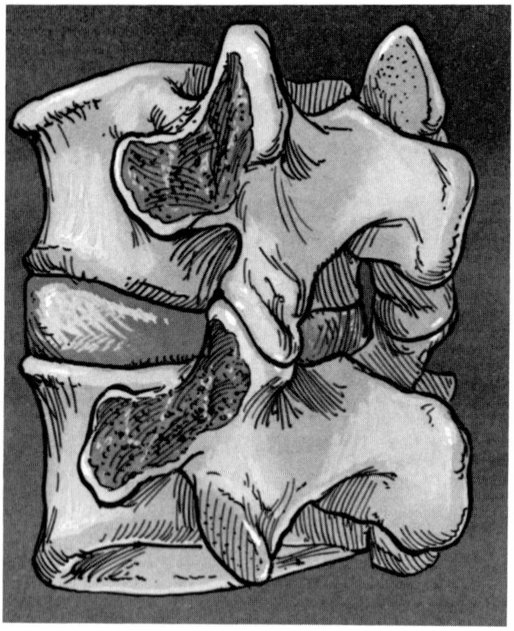

Figure 9 □ The fusion bed. Note that the area of the fusion bed can be greatly extended by going up the side of the pedicle and using the lateral aspect of the facets without invasion of the facet joint.

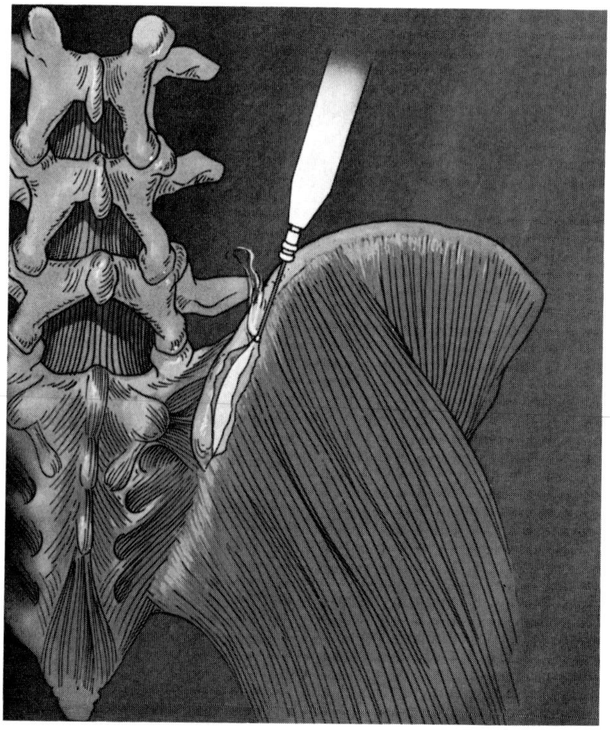

Figure 10 □ Incision into the iliac crest

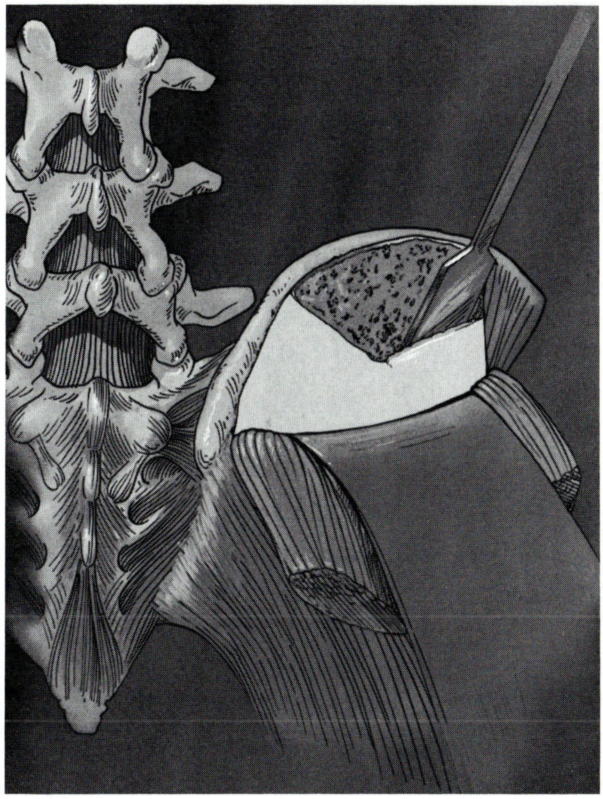

Figure 11 □ Removal of cortical bone for bone graft.

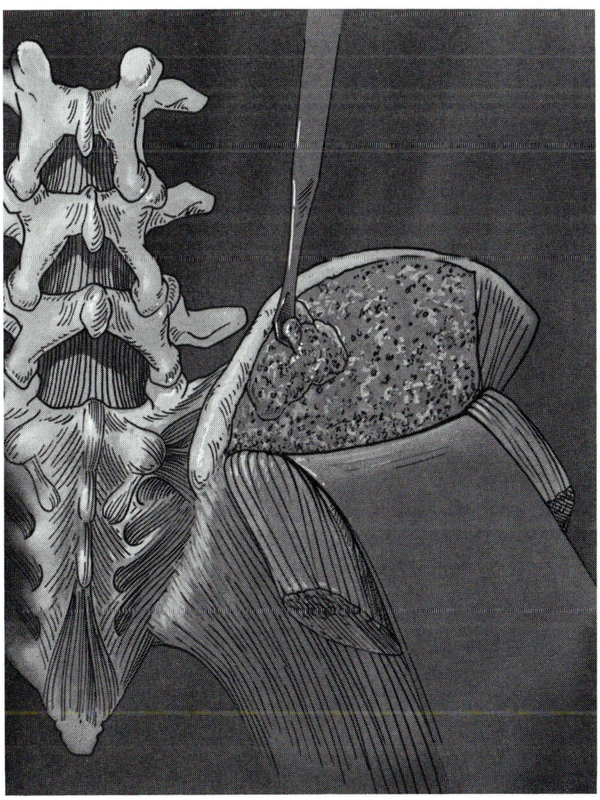

Figure 12 □ R [illegible] bone graft.

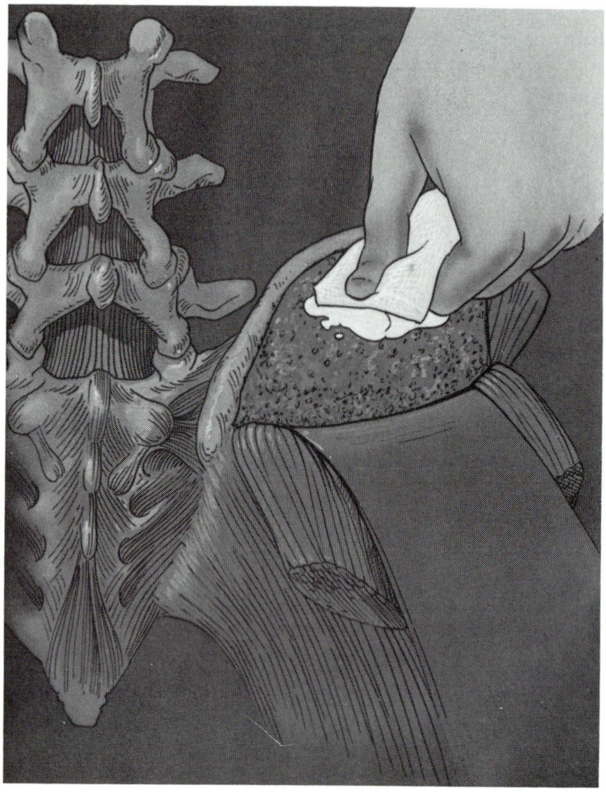

Figure 13 □ Hemostasis with bone wax and Gelfoam.

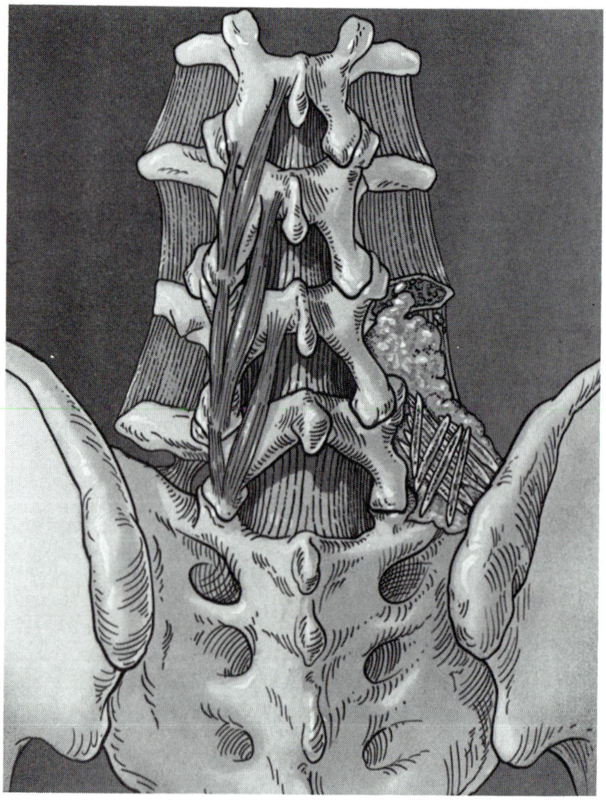

Fig

it, in the anterior portion of the iliac crest. This avoids injury to the cluneal nerve and artery.

The use of bone wax and Gelfoam on the site of the raw bone helps reduce bleeding (Fig. 13). Closure should be performed over drains for both wounds.

The obtained graft material is then packed in the transverse process, with the cancellous bone forming the bed for the cortical strips (Fig. 14). Again, closure should occur over a drain.

POSTOPERATIVE CARE

Catheters are not routinely used, although some patients may need intermittent catheterization for the first several days. The emphasis should be on activity, and patients are encouraged to ambulate the day of surgery if they are sufficiently recovered from the effects of the anesthesia. This walking program is extended to a minimum of 2 miles a day at a 2-month period. It is further explained to the patients that bone responds to the stresses placed across it. The patient can influence the rate and quality of bone fusion by engaging in activities that place some stresses across the back. Thus, no restrictions are imposed on lifting activities and other aspects of activities of daily living. However, the patients are encouraged to control pain with activities and are discouraged from the use of narcotic medication. The average patient can easily control his or her pain with aspirin or acetaminophen (Tylenol) and with the judicious use of activities and rest, given the proper education and motivation. The use of in-hospital back school is invaluable in this regard.

In-hospital back school is conducted on the third and fourth postoperative days to all the patients. This consists of a videotape presentation that can be taken home by the patients, if they wish, and also a personal presentation by the physical therapist that includes the following topics:

- Wound care
- Graduated exercise program with the emphasis on walking
- Body mechanics
- Sex information
- Use of drugs
- Further answering of patient's questions regarding the surgery.

LONG-TERM FOLLOW-UP

It is expected to see early fusion at 4 months, and most self-employed people return to almost any kind of job at 3 to 4 months. Sedentary workers frequently return to their activities as early as 2 months. Mature fusion appears on x-rays at a 6- to 9-month period. If, at 1 year, there is a paucity of bone on the x-ray, the patient probably has nonunion.

SUMMARY

Transverse process fusion is a reliable and technically easy fusion that, with internal fixation, should yield results of fusion rates above 90%.[34, 36, 39] It is adaptable to central canal procedures and most kinds of internal fixation. Exposure and hemostasis are critical to the correct completion of the procedure. The surgeon must place the fusion process within a general frame of rehabilitation. Strong postoperative programs, including in-hospital back school and other educational devices, are highly recommended.

Acknowledgment

The author would like to thank Dr. Sydney Bonnik for her assistance in the metabolic portion of this chapter.

References

1. Albee, F.H.: Transplantation of a portion of the tibia into the spine for Pott's disease. J.A.M.A. 57:885, 1911.
2. Boucher, H.H.: A method of spinal fusion. J. Bone Joint Surg. 41B:248, 1959.
3. Campbell, W.C.: An operation for extra articular arthrodesis of the sacroiliac joint. Surg. Gynecol. Obstet. 45:218, 1927.
4. Cleveland, M., Bosworth, D., and Thompson, F.: Pseudarthrosis of the lumbosacral spine. J. Bone Joint Surg. 30A:302, 1948.
5. Cloward, R.B.: History of Posterior Lumbar Interbody Fusion. Springfield, Charles C Thomas, p. 58, 1982.
6. Cloward, R.B.: The treatment of ruptured intervertebral discs by vertebral body fusion. Ann. Surg. 136:987, 1952.
7. Cotrel, Dubausset: The Use of Pedicle Screws with Universal Instrumentation for Spinal Fixation. Paper presented at the A.O. Trauma Course. Davos, Switzerland, Dec., 1985.
8. Crock, H.V.: Practice of Spinal Surgery. New York, Springer-Verlag.
9. Crock, H.V., and Yoshizawa, H.: The Blood Supply of the Vertebral Column and Spinal Cord in Man. New York, Springer-Verlag, 1977.

10. Dyck, W.: Fixator Interne. Report given at A.O. Trauma Course. Davos, Switzerland, Dec., 1985.
11. Edwards, W.C.: The Sacral Fixation Device: A New Alternative for Lumbosacral Fixation. Paper read at the meeting of the North American Spine Society, Laguna Niguel, Jul., 1985.
12. Eie, N.: Comparison of the results in patients operated upon for ruptured disc with and without spinal fusion. Acta Neurochir. 41:107, 1978.
13. Epstein, J.A., Epstein, B.S., and Lavine, L.S.: The role of spinal fusion. Spine 6:281, 1981.
14. Farfan, H.F., and Kirkaldy-Willis, W.H.: The present status of spinal fusion in the treatment of lumbar intervertebral joint disorders. Clin. Orthop. Rel. Res. 158:198, 1981.
15. Frymoyer, J.W., Matteri, R.E., Hanley, E.N., et al.: Failed lumbar disc surgery requiring second operation—a long term follow-up study. Spine 3:7, 1978.
16. Ghormley, R.K.: Low back pain with special reference to the articular facets with present attention of an operative procedure. J.A.M.A. 101:1773, 1933.
17. Hadra, B.E.: Wiring of the spinous processes in Pott's disease. Trans. Orthop. Assoc. 4:206, 1891.
18. Hibbs, R.H.: An operation for progressive spinal deformities. N. Y. J. Med. 93:1013, 1911.
19. Hoover, N.W.: Methods of lumbar fusion. J. Bone Joint Surg. 50A:194–209, 1968.
20. Howarth, B.: Low back pain and sciatica: Results of surgical treatment, Part I, spine fusion only. J. Bone Joint Surg. 46A:1485–1499, 1964.
21. Howarth, B.: Low back pain and sciatica: Results of surgical treatment, Part II, spine fusion only. J. Bone Joint Surg. 46A:1500–1515, 1964.
22. King, D.: Internal fixation for lumbosacral fusion. Am. J. Surg. Arch. Surg. 66:357, 1944.
23. Kraag, M.H., et al.: An internal fixator for posterior application to short segments of the thoracic, lumbar or lumbosacral spine: Design and testing. Clin. Orthop. Rel. Res. 203:75–99, 1986.
24. Knodt, T.H., and Larrick, R.: Distraction fusion of the lumbar spine. Ohio State Med. J. 62:140, 1964.
25. Kornblatt, M.D., Casey, M.P., and Jacobs, R.R.: Internal fixation in lumbosacral spine fusion: A biomechanical and clinical study. Clin. Orthop. Rel. Res. 203:141–150, 1986.
26. LaMont, R.L., Morawa, L.G., and Pederson, H.E.: Comparison of disc excision with combined disc excision and spinal fusion for lumbar disc ruptures. Clin. Orthop. Rel. Res. 121:212, 1876.
27. Lin, P.M.: Posterior interbody fusion. Springfield, Charles C Thomas, 1982.
28. Louis, R.: Fusion of the Lumbar and Sacral Spines by Internal Fixation with Screw Plates. Clin. Orthop. Rel. Res. 203:18–34, 1986.
29. Luque, E.: The Anatomic Basis and Development of Segmental Spinal Instrumentation. Spine 7, 1982.
30. Mandel, R.J., Brown, M.D., McCollough, N.C., et al.: Hypotensive anesthesia and autotransfusion in spinal surgery. Clin. Orthop. Rel. Res. 154:27, 1981.
31. Macnab, I., and Dall, D.: The blood supply of the lumbar spine and its application to the technique of intertransverse lumbar fusion. J. Bone Joint Surg. 53B:628–638, 1971.
32. McElroy, K.D.: Lumbosacral fusion with bilateral lateral techniques. J. Bone Joint Surg. 43A:918, 1961.
33. O'Brian, J.P.: The role of fusion for chronic low back pain. Orthop. Clin. North Am. 14:639, 1983.
34. Overton, L.W.: Arthrodesis of the lumbosacral spine: A study of end results. Clin. Orthop. Rel. Res. 5:97–102, 1955.
35. Pennal, G.F., McDonald, G.A., and Dale, G.G.: A method of spinal fusion using internal fixation. Clin. Orthop. Rel. Res. 35:86, 1964.
36. Rolander, S.D.: Motion of the lumbar spine with spinal posterior fusion: An experimental study of autopsy specimens. Acta Orthop. Scand. (Suppl.)90, 1966.
37. Rothman, R., and Booth, R.: Failure of spinal fusion. Orthop. Clin. North Am. 6:299, 1975.
38. Schmidt, A.C., Flatley, T.J., and Place, J.S.: Lumbar fusion using facet inlay grafts. South Med. J. 68:209–216, 1975.
39. Selby, D.K.: Internal fixation with Knodt's rods. Clin. Orthop. 203:179–185, 1986.
40. Urist, M.R., and Dawson, E.: Intertransverse process fusion with the aid of chemosterilized autolyzed antigen-extracted allogenic (AAA) bone. Clin. Orthop. Rel. Res. 154:97, 1981.
41. Watkin, R.E.: Posterolateral fusion of the lumbar and lumbosacral spine. J. Bone Joint Surg. 35A: 1014, 1953.
42. White, A.H., Wynne, G., and Taylor, L.W.: Knodt rod distraction lumbar fusion. Spine 8:1983.
43. Wilson, P.D.: Lumbosacral fusion with metallic plate fixation. A.A.O.S. Instruct. Course Lect., Vol. 9, 1952.
44. Young, H., and Love, J.: End results of removal of protruded intervertebral discs with and without fusion. A.A.O.S. Instruct. Course Lect. 16:216–313, 1959.

8 □ Lumbar and Lumbosacral Spondylolisthesis

Leon L. Wiltse
Stephen L.G. Rothman
Kazimiera Milanowska
Edward N. Hanley, Jr.
David S. Bradford

■ CLASSIFICATION, DIAGNOSIS, AND NATURAL HISTORY

Leon L. Wiltse
Stephen L.G. Rothman

Few conditions have fascinated the orthopedic surgeon as has spondylolisthesis. Thousands of articles have been written on the subject, and scarcely a week goes by without a new one appearing in the world literature. In 1782, Herbinaux,[20] a Belgian obstetrician, noted that there were times when a bony prominence was present in front of the sacrum and was thought, perhaps, to cause problems in delivery. He is generally credited with having first described spondylolisthesis, probably the complete type, in which the body of L5 is actually lying in front of the sacrum (i.e., *spondyloptosis*).

Spondylolisthesis is the slippage of all or part of one vertebra onto another. The term, coined by Kilian[27] in 1854, is derived from the Greek *spondylos*, meaning "vertebra," and *olisthesis*, meaning "to slip or slide down a slippery incline." Kilian did not recognize the defect in the pars interarticularis but believed the lesion to be caused by a slow subluxation of the lumbosacral facets. One year later, Robert[49] of Koblenz established the location of the fundamental lesion of the isthmic type in the pars interarticularis, but he did not recognize the nature of the defect. In 1885, Lambl[28a] demonstrated the lesion in the pars. Neugebauer,[34] in 1881, made an extensive study of anatomic specimens throughout Europe and was the first to recognize that slippage can occur by an elongation of the pars without its coming apart. He did, however, confuse the degenerative type with the isthmic type of the disorder.

Newman[35, 36] in "The Etiology of Spondylolisthesis," a paper published in 1963, coined the phrase *degenerative spondylolisthesis*. He was also the first to publish a satisfactory classification of the condition. He separated congenital forms, or "dysplastic" forms (as he called them), from isthmic forms. The names of Macnab,[31] Rosenberg,[50, 51] Gill,[16, 17] Taillard,[64] Wynn-Davies

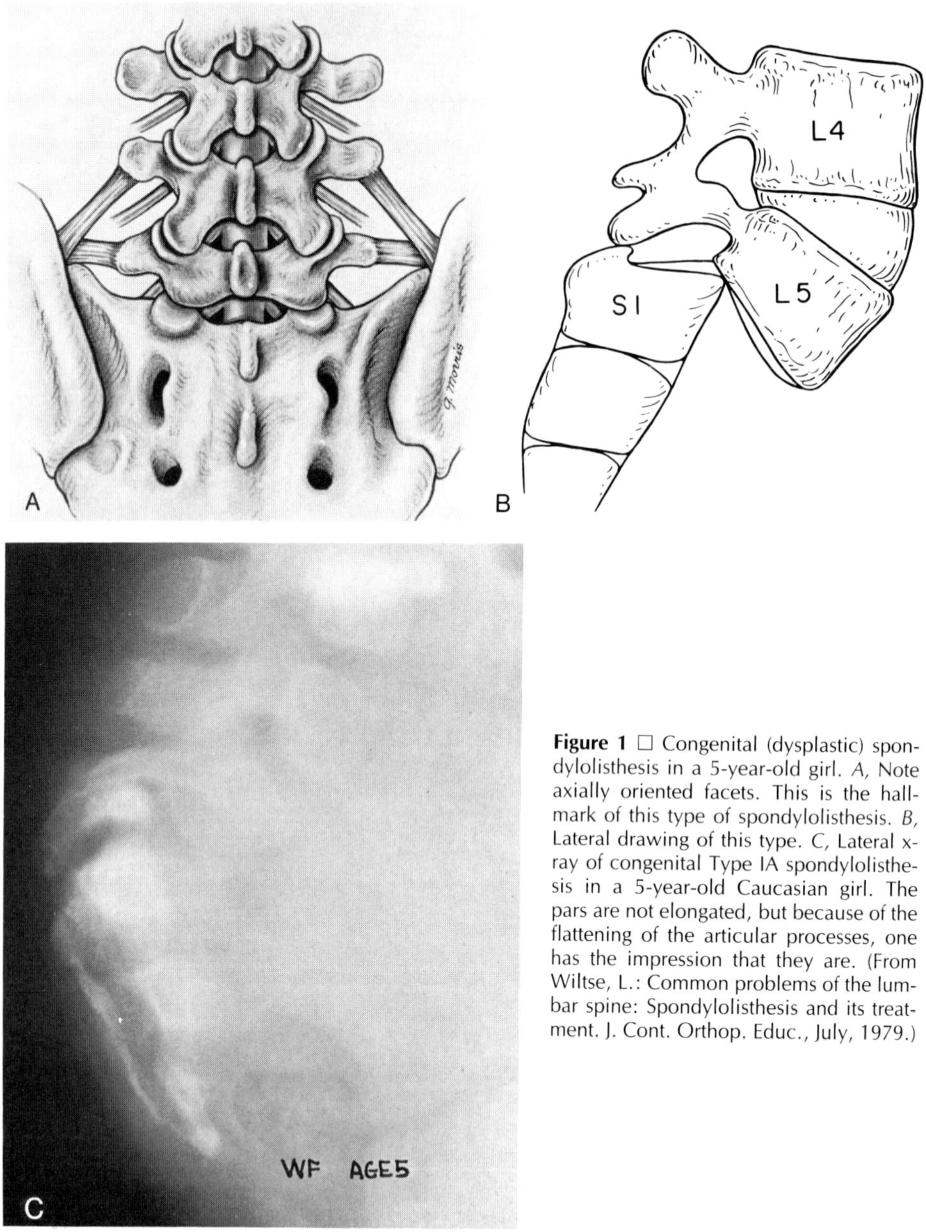

Figure 1 □ Congenital (dysplastic) spondylolisthesis in a 5-year-old girl. *A,* Note axially oriented facets. This is the hallmark of this type of spondylolisthesis. *B,* Lateral drawing of this type. *C,* Lateral x-ray of congenital Type IA spondylolisthesis in a 5-year-old Caucasian girl. The pars are not elongated, but because of the flattening of the articular processes, one has the impression that they are. (From Wiltse, L.: Common problems of the lumbar spine: Spondylolisthesis and its treatment. J. Cont. Orthop. Educ., July, 1979.)

and Scott,[76] and Saraste,[54–58] to name a few, are prominent in the development of our present knowledge of spondylolisthesis.

The types of the condition are as varied as its causes. The type of most clinical importance in persons under the age of 40 years is the one in which the lesion is in the isthmus or the pars interarticularis. However, dysplasia and changes in facet orientation are prominent in its etiology, and several other conditions permit the forward slip of one vertebra on another. This discussion is limited to the lumbar spine, except to point out that the disease does occur in the cervical spine and that a few reports of pars defects in the thoracic spine have been published. Lesions in the thoracic spine are so rare as to be of little importance. The classification of spondylolisthesis that is presented here is based on both anatomic and etiologic criteria and diagnosis.

CLASSIFICATION AND DIAGNOSIS OF SPONDYLOLISTHESIS

Classification

The following classification of spondylolisthesis and spondylolysis has been derived from classifications previously published by various authors.[73] We stress that it is an anatomic one and that the basic congenital condition acting as the etiologic agent may be the same in several types or subtypes.[37]

I. Congenital
   A. This type has dysplastic articular processes at the level of olisthesis; they are axially oriented and are frequently combined with spina bifida. This unstable condition permits the slip to occur (Fig. 1 *A–C*).
   B. This type has a sagittal orientation of the articular processes. As a result, the junction between L5 and S1 is unstable.
   C. Other congenital anomalies of the lumbar spine permit spondylolisthesis to occur. Congenital kyphosis is the principal one.

II. Isthmic—The lesion is in the pars interarticularis. Two types can be recognized.
   A. Lytic—In this type there is a stress fracture of the pars (Fig. 2).[70]
   B. Elongated but intact pars secondary to healed stress fractures (Fig. 3).

III. Degenerative—Due to long-standing intersegmental instability.

IV. Post-traumatic—This results from acute fractures in areas of the bony hook other than the pars (Fig. 4).

V. Pathologic—This type results from generalized or localized bone disease. Destruction of the posterior elements allows the cephalic vertebra to slip forward on the one below.

VI. Postsurgical—This is due to partial or complete loss of posterior bony and/or discogenic support or to stress fractures of the inferior articular processes secondary to surgery.

Types of Spondylolisthesis

Type I. Congenital

TYPE IA

In this subtype, the anomalies of the lumbosacral area are frequently associated with spina bifida occulta of the S1 or L5 segments (Fig. 5). There is also dysplasia (underdevelopment) of the articular processes.[36] These dysplastic articular processes have an axial

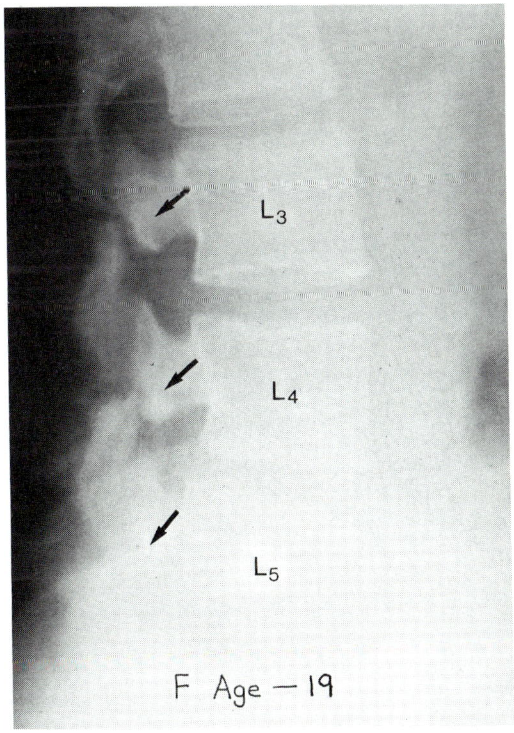

Figure 2 □ Typical stress fractures of the pars in a female equestrian, age 19 years, competing for the Olympic games. The L3 lesion is older than the L4; L5 is intact.

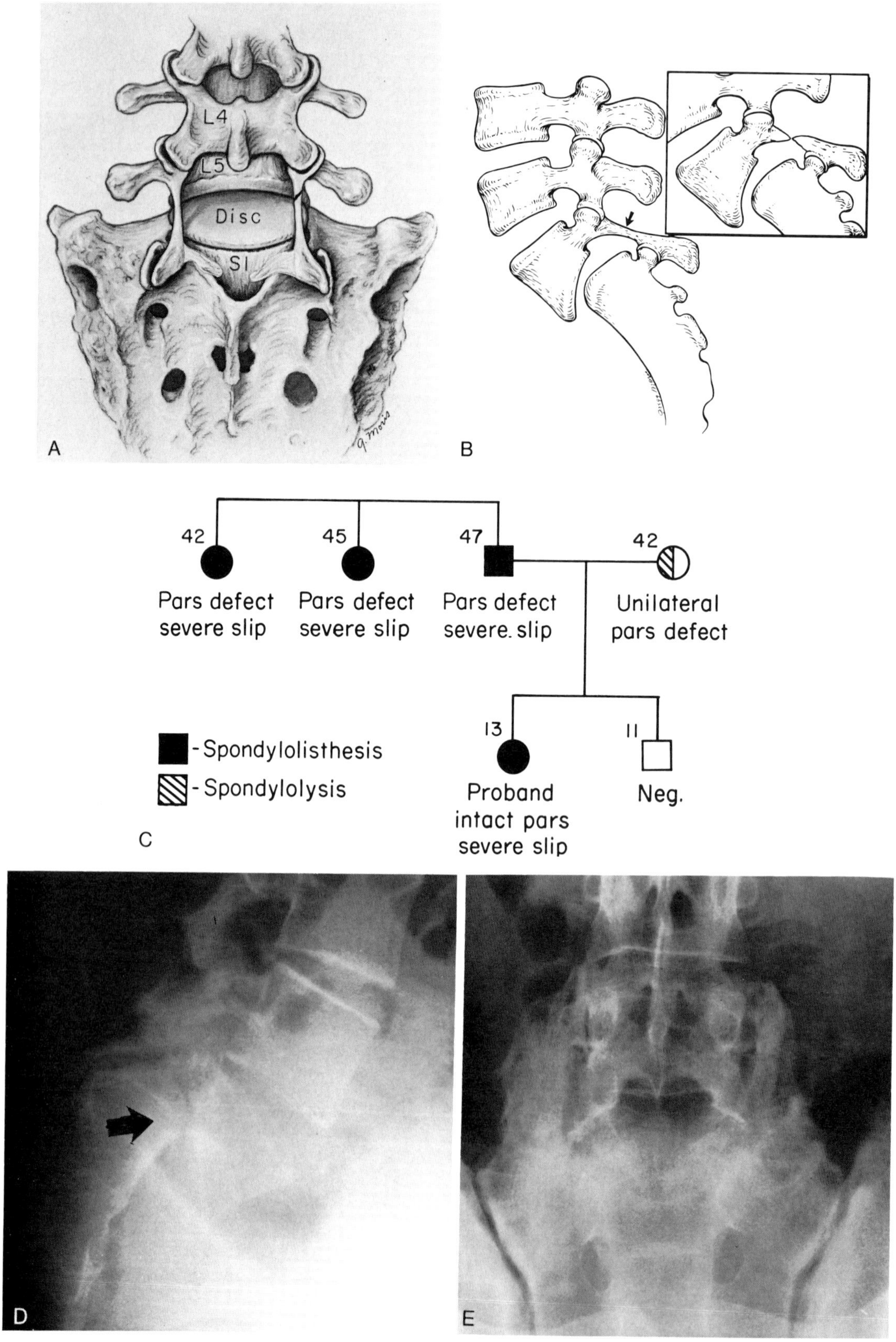

Figure 3 *See legend on opposite page*

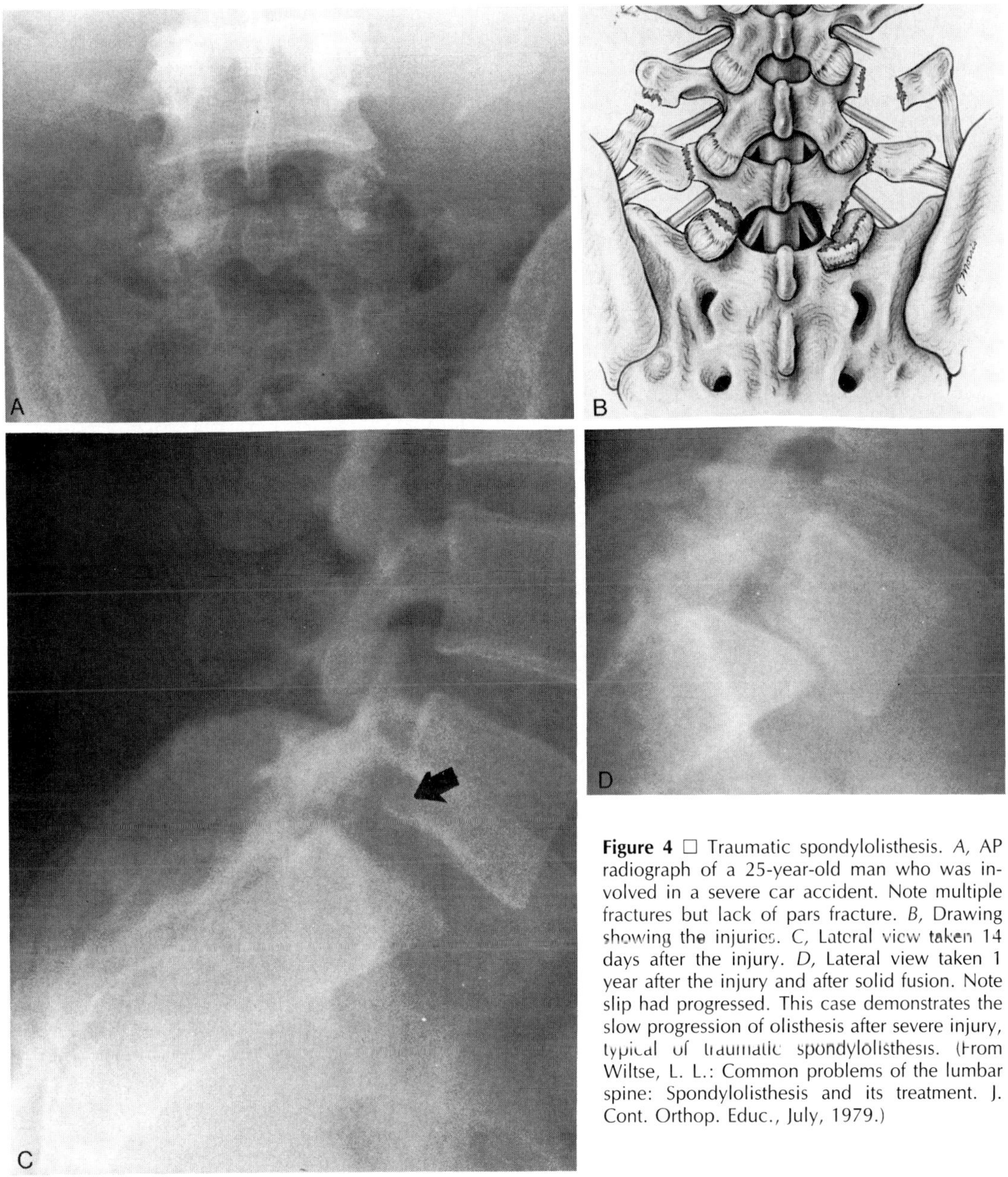

Figure 4 □ Traumatic spondylolisthesis. *A,* AP radiograph of a 25-year-old man who was involved in a severe car accident. Note multiple fractures but lack of pars fracture. *B,* Drawing showing the injuries. *C,* Lateral view taken 14 days after the injury. *D,* Lateral view taken 1 year after the injury and after solid fusion. Note slip had progressed. This case demonstrates the slow progression of olisthesis after severe injury, typical of traumatic spondylolisthesis. (From Wiltse, L. L.: Common problems of the lumbar spine: Spondylolisthesis and its treatment. J. Cont. Orthop. Educ., July, 1979.)

Figure 3 □ Elongated but intact parts (IIB classification). *A,* Drawing made at surgery of elongated but intact pars. On the right, the right pars has cracked through, and the left has elongated but remained intact. It might have healed even if the fusion had not been performed. *B,* Lateral drawing of Type IIB. The pars may stretch for years and then crack and come apart. (From Ruge, D., and Wiltse, L.L.: Spondylolisthesis and its treatment: Conservative treatment, fusion with and without reduction. *In* Spinal Disorders—Diagnosis and Treatment. Philadelphia, Lea & Febiger, 1977.) *C,* Family of one of the author's patients with elongated but intact pars. Only the proband had elongated, but intact, pars. All others had typical Type IIA lesions in the pars. *D,* Preoperative lateral view of same patient as in *A.* Patient is a 16-year-old Caucasian woman. *E,* Anteroposterior (AP) radiograph, after fusion, of patient in *A.* (*C, E,* from Wiltse, L. L., Newman, P. M., Macnab, I: Classification of spondylolysis and spondylolisthesis. Clin. Orthop. 116:25, 1976.)

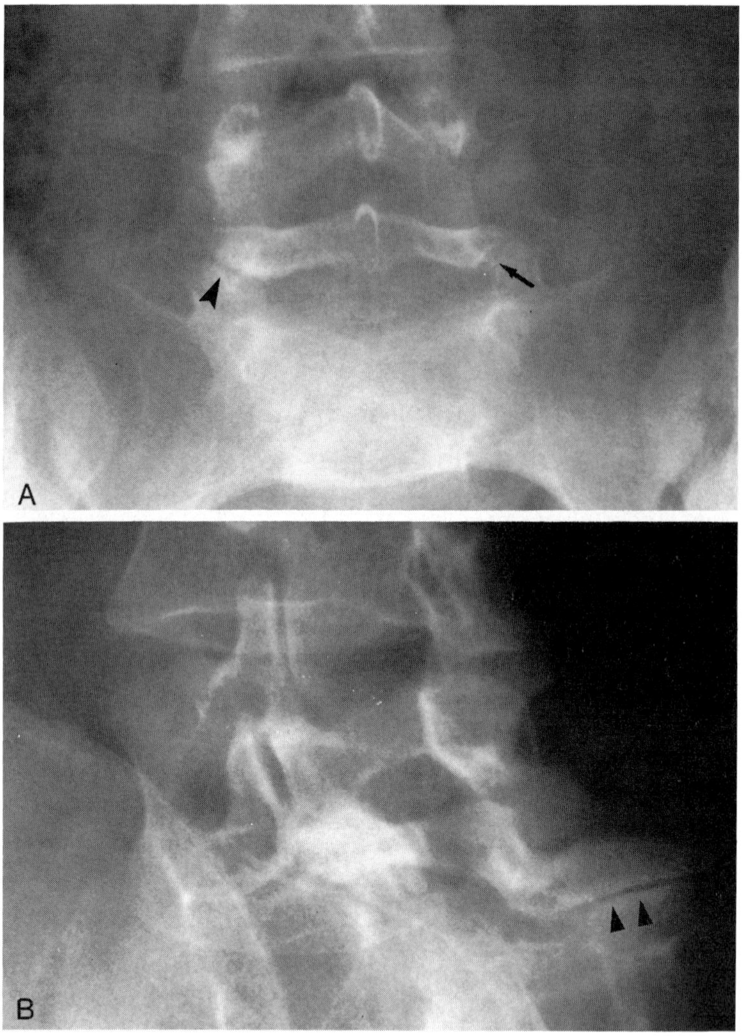

Figure 5 □ *A,* AP view of congenital Type IA spondylolisthesis. This patient had 30% olisthesis. Note axial orientation of facets and tropism of facets. S1 spinous process is bifid, but L5 is not. *B,* Oblique view shows the markedly axial (horizontal) orientation of the left L5–S1 facet in the same case of congenital Type IA. This is the same case as shown in *A.*

orientation, usually more on one side than on the other. The combination of dysplastic articular process, the axial (horizontal) orientation of the facets, and spina bifida makes the area unable to support the superincumbent weight, and spondylolisthesis results. The pars interarticularis may remain unchanged. If it remains completely unchanged and the ring is intact, the slip cannot exceed more than about 35% or there will be too much pressure on the cauda equina. Severe tightness of the hamstrings is likely to result. At least one case is on record in which a cauda equina compression syndrome resulted. Usually, however, the pars interarticularis either elongates or comes apart. If it elongates, healing as it does, it is very difficult to distinguish roentgenographically from Type IIB, in which the pars cracks and heals—elongating as it does so. If it separates, it may be nearly impossible to distinguish from Type IIA. If exposed at operation, the abnormal relationship and subluxation of the facets may still be very difficult to identify. Careful study with computed tomography (CT) usually makes it possible to categorize this type accurately.

Occasionally, a wide-open sacrum exists and the L5 vertebra also shows wide spina bifida. The upper end of the superior surface of the body of S1 is often dysplastic (Fig. 6). In a study by Wynne-Davies and Scott,[76] 11 of 12 patients with a dysplastic lesion had spina bifida occulta in the lumbosacral area. No large series indicate the male-to-female ratio for the congenital type, but in the Wynne-Davies and Scott series there were seven males and five females (ratio 1.4) in the dysplastic group. For the isthmic type with the stress fracture, the male-to-female ratio was 25 to 10, the males being more commonly affected.

There is a strong genetic element to both the dysplastic and isthmic types of spondylolisthesis. In the study by Wynne-Davies and Scott, a radiographic survey was carried out of the 147 first-degree relatives of 47 patients treated in Edinburgh for spondylolisthesis of L5; 12 patients had the congenital type, and 35 had an isthmic defect. The survey identified 19% of relatives with the opposite type, suggesting a close relationship between the causes of the congenital and isthmic types. Index patients with the congenital form had a higher proportion of affected relatives (33%) than had the isthmic type.

Spina bifida occulta at L5 or S1, or both, was more common among all individuals with spondylolysis than among unaffected relatives (congenital form, 94%; isthmic type, 32%; and unaffected relatives, 7%). However, there was no single instance of a neural tube defect (i.e., anencephaly, spina bifida with or without meningocele, other generalized vertebral anomalies, or spinal dysraphism) among 826 first-, second-, or third-degree relatives. Wynne-Davies and

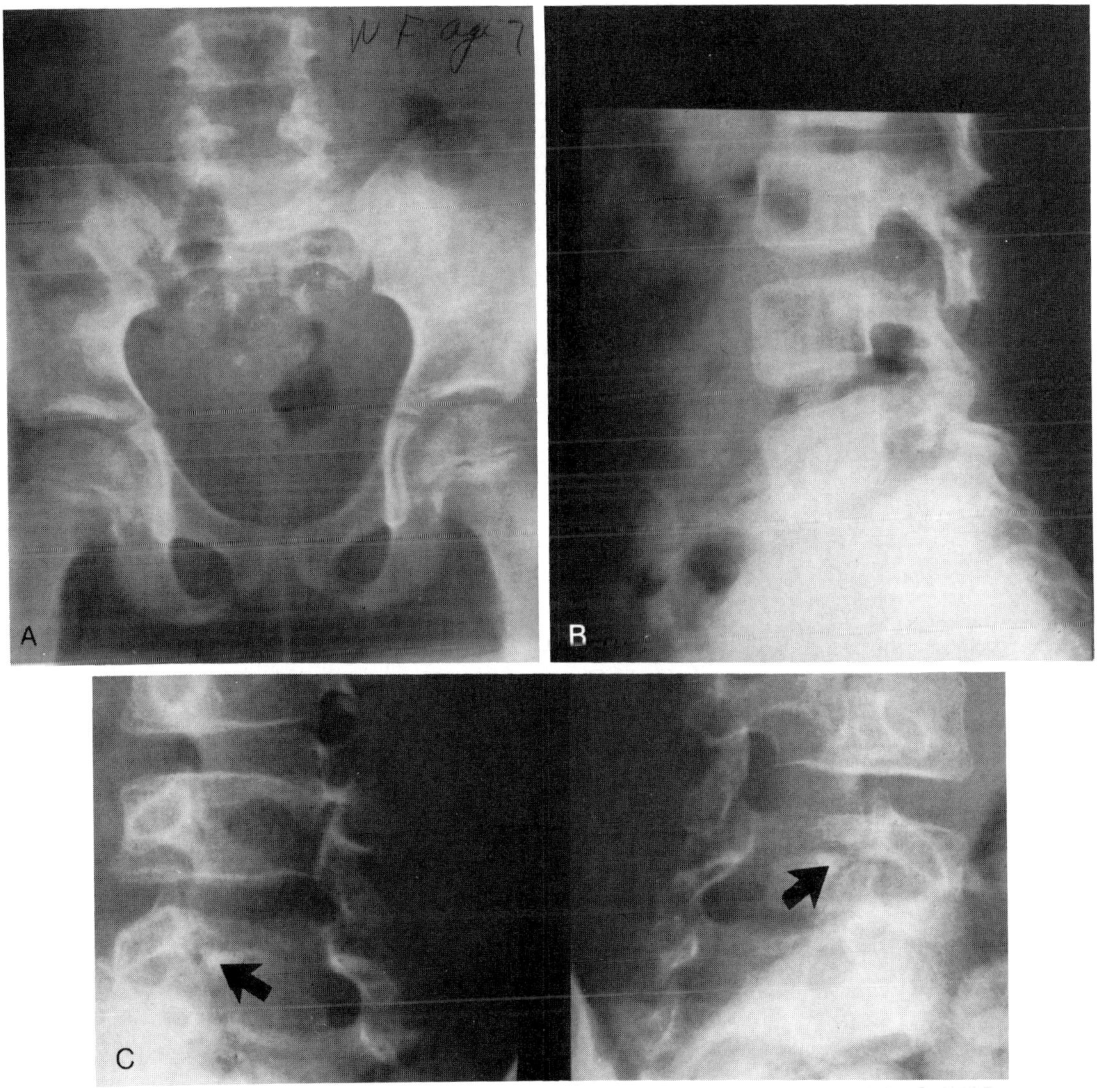

Figure 6 □ *A, B,* AP and lateral views of child with spina bifida of L5 and a wide-open sacrum. Note that in the lateral view the pars is also fractured. *C,* Oblique views of same patient, showing pars fractures.

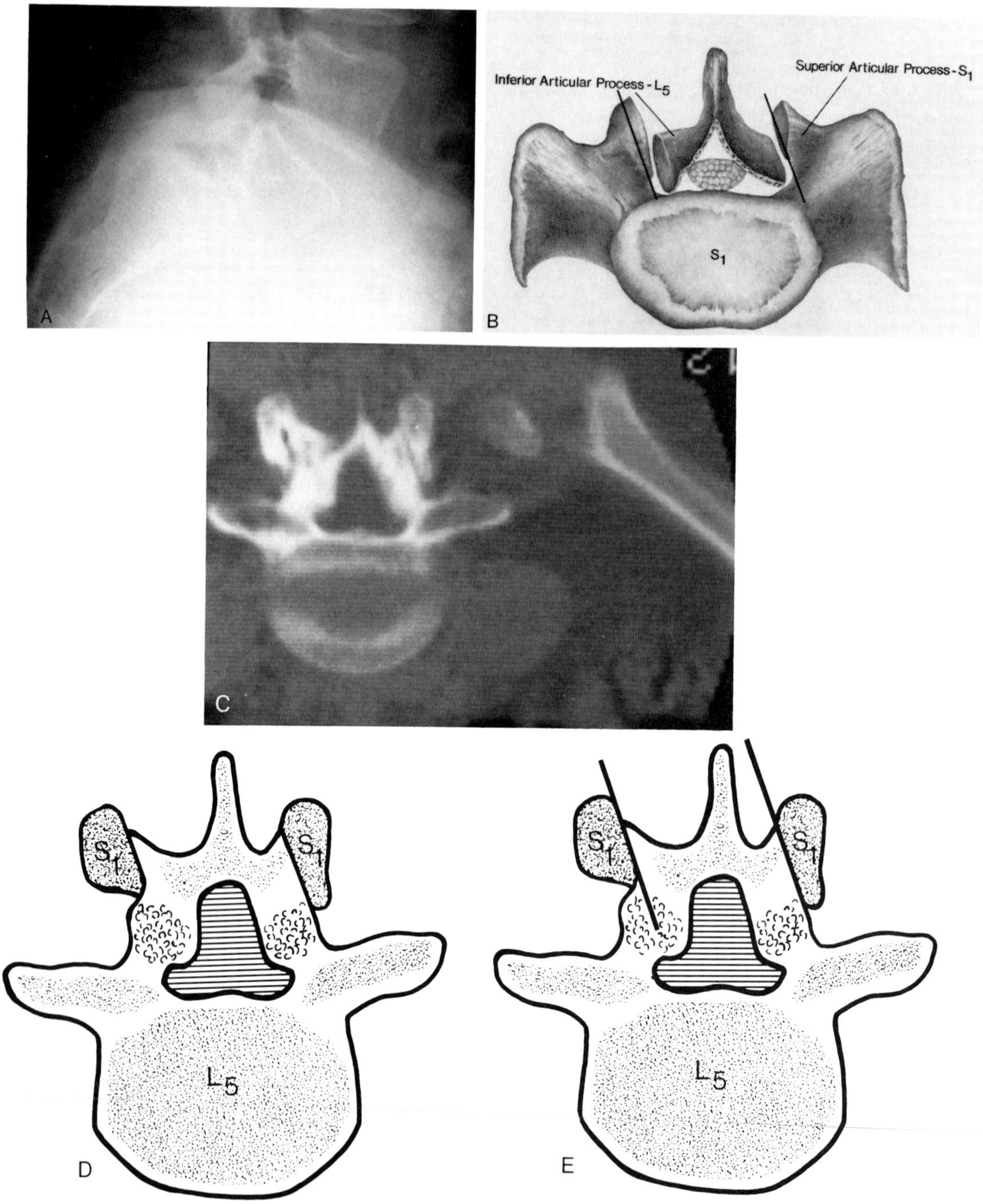

Figure 7 □ *A,* Lateral view of Type IB. Note intact pars and relatively low degree of slip. The pars appears elongated, but what we are actually seeing is the side of the neural ring. *B,* Drawing of the cephalic end of the sacrum in Type IB. This shows the sagittal orientation of the facets. Note that, on the left, the facet is rotated in the direction opposite that of the facet on the right. This peculiar rotation effectively removes the stability normally supplied by the facets. *C,* Axial computed tomographic (CT) section through lower one fourth of the body of L5. Note the sagittal orientation of the facets. Also note how the facets on the right are rotated so that the posterior tip of the facet is more medial than the anterior tip. This peculiar rotation effectively removes the stability normally supplied by the facets. *D,* Drawing of axial CT section shown in C. Facets are sagittally oriented and are also in a state of tropism; the third peculiarity is that the posterior tips of the facets are more medial than the anterior tips. *E,* The lines show the direction of the facets in the axial plane. When both facets are in nearly the same plane, much of the stability normally supplied by the facets is lost.

Scott concluded that the developmental defects of the vertebrae associated with spondylolysis are not etiologically related to neural tube defects.

Congenital spondylolisthesis of Type IA can occur in newborn infants. Zembo and coworkers[78] reported a small series of this type in infants, two of whom had the condition at birth. The representatives of this type appearing at birth usually have the lesion in the lower lumbar spine. Horizontal articular processes and a high grade of slip are present. This type is different from congenital kyphosis, which usually appears in the thoracolumbar area.

TYPE IB

In this type of spondylolisthesis, there is congenital sagittal malorientation of the articular processes. As in Type IA, the posterior elements are often poorly developed (Fig. 7). The slip probably occurs because of the unstable orientation of the facets and the fact that the articular processes at the olisthetic level are, besides being sagittally oriented, rotated so that the posterior tip is more medial than the anterior tip on one side. This type seldom progresses to an extremely high degree of olisthesis because the neural ring is intact.

TYPE IC. OTHER ABNORMALITIES OF THE LUMBAR SPINE

Other, often severe, congenital anomalies of the spine permit spondylolisthesis and spondyloptosis to occur. These are of relatively little importance and are included only because they have been reported.

Congenital kyphosis is probably the principal representative of this type. Winter,[75] in summarizing his previous publications, recognized congenital failure of vertebral body formation, congenital failure of segmentation, and a mixed type of the disorder. Congenital failure of vertebral body formation is, by far, the most significant as a cause of spondyloptosis. This usually occurs at the thoracolumbar junction, rather than down at L4 or L5.

Armstrong and Ye[4] described a congenital condition in which there is forward angulation of the upper sacrum, permitting olisthesis to occur. They described three types based on the angles made by intersecting vertical lines; the first line is through the upper two sacral segments perpendicular to the end plate, and the second through the remainder of the segments.

Type II. Isthmic

This type always has a fracture in the pars interarticularis. Secondary changes (e.g., alteration in the shape of the body of L5) may occur, but these are not fundamental to its cause.

TYPE IIA. LYTIC

Lytic spondylolisthesis is due to separation or dissolution of the pars following a stress fracture (Fig. 8). Statistically, it is seldom seen in patients below the age of 5 years, but it does occasionally occur.[39] The authors' youngest patient having, unquestionably, a lesion of the pars was only age 8 months when the lesion was first discovered.[69] This child's father also had the same lesion.[67] Borkow and Kleiger[6] reported a patient in whom the lesion in the pars was first discovered when the child was only 4 months of age.

If a group of 100 children of 5 years of age were to be studied roentgenographically, probably none would have a pars defect.[53] However, if the same children were exam-

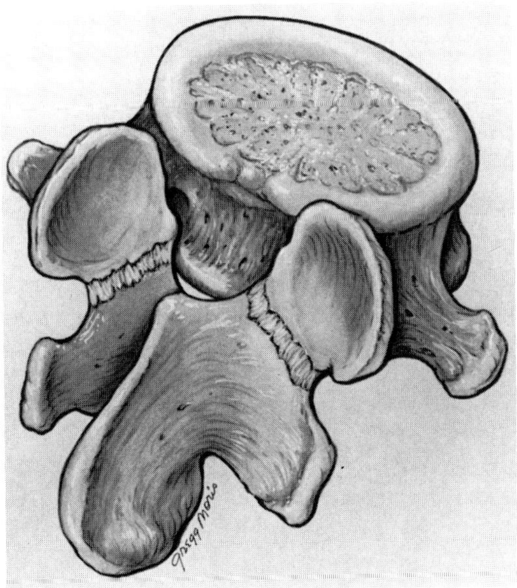

Figure 8 □ Drawing showing the defect in isthmic spondylolysis, classification IIA. (From Ruge, D., and Wiltse, L.L.: Spondylolisthesis and its treatment: Conservative treatment, fusion with and without reduction. *In* Spinal Disorders—Diagnosis and Treatment. Philadelphia, Lea & Febiger, 1977.)

ined toward the end of the first grade (approaching 7 years of age), the incidence would be around 4.4%, which is just slightly below the national average.[40] Baker and McHolick[5] performed a study such as this. They were also able to examine, roentgenographically, the same group when they were approaching adulthood. They found that the incidence had increased 1.4% by the time the group reached 18 years.[15] Most of this increase occurred between ages 11 and 16 years, the time of life when boys and girls are engaging in the very strenuous athletics that produce fatigue fractures.

Just why the period of 5.5 to 7 years of age is the one during which the lesion appears so frequently is not well known. One might postulate either that it is because these children already have the anatomic set-up for pars fractures, and this is the age when children start school and begin to push each other and tumble about, or that for the first time they sit for long periods with a lordotic posture. It is not known whether fracture in the pars is caused by flexion or extension stresses.[59] Probably, it results from both, plus torsional stresses.[11, 65, 66] There is considerable controversy concerning this point. It is known that the fracture never occurs in animals phylogenetically below humans, and only humans have true lordosis.[60] There is, also, a strong hereditary component to the cause of this type.[69] Table 1 shows the proportions of first-degree relatives with spondylolysis or spondylolisthesis.

TYPE IIB

In this type of the disorder, there is elongation of the pars, without separation. This disease is the same as Type IIA. It is secondary to repeated microfractures, which allow the pars to heal in a somewhat elongated position as the body of L5 slides forward.

The senior author has obtained x-ray studies of all available members of five families in whom the probands had elongated but intact pars, whereas several other members of each of their immediate families had typical spondylolysis or spondylolisthesis with the classic pars defect, which is seen in Type IIA. (As noted above, Wynne-Davies and Scott found that index patients of both the isthmic and congenital types had relatives with the opposite type.)

The pars may remain in continuity as it elongates, or it may thin out and finally separate, leaving stumps with a combined length much greater than that of a normal pars (Fig. 9). When this separation occurs, the lesion is reclassified as Type IIA, since it cannot be differentiated from that subtype. The fundamental disease is the same.

In summary, it is likely that there is a common congenital component to the cause of all variations of both the congenital and isthmic types of spondylolisthesis. For this reason the authors have formulated the following hypothesis of etiology.[1, 44]

A Theory Supporting a Common Mechanism of Etiology for Both the Congenital and Isthmic Types

It has been consistently observed that both congenital and isthmic types of spondylolisthesis are often associated with spina bifida of the L5 or S1 segments. The spina bifida defect is much more common at S1 than at L5, but lesions at one or the other, or both, occur considerably more often than in the normal population.[24, 42] Since the advent of the CT scan, our ability to detect associated congenital anomalies has been immeasurably enhanced.[52]

CT scans demonstrate hypoplasia of the superior articular process of S1 in most patients with either type of spondylolisthesis.

We suggest that, except in the young athlete, the congenital propensity for fracture at the pars and also for the slip in the

Table 1 □ Affected First-Degree Relatives of Patients with Spondylolysis or Spondylolisthesis*

PATIENTS	PARENTS	SIBLINGS	CHILDREN	TOTAL
Dysplastic type (congenital)	6 of 18	2 of 12	3 of 3	11 of 33 (33.0%)
Isthmic type	5 of 32	7 of 51	5 of 31	17 of 114 (14.9%)
Total	11 of 50 (22.0%)	9 of 63 (14.3%)	8 of 34 (23.5%)	28 of 147 (19.0%)

*From Wynne-Davies, R., and Scott, J. H. S.: Inheritance and spondylolisthesis: A radiographic family survey. J. Bone Joint Surg. (Br.) 61B:301–305, 1979.

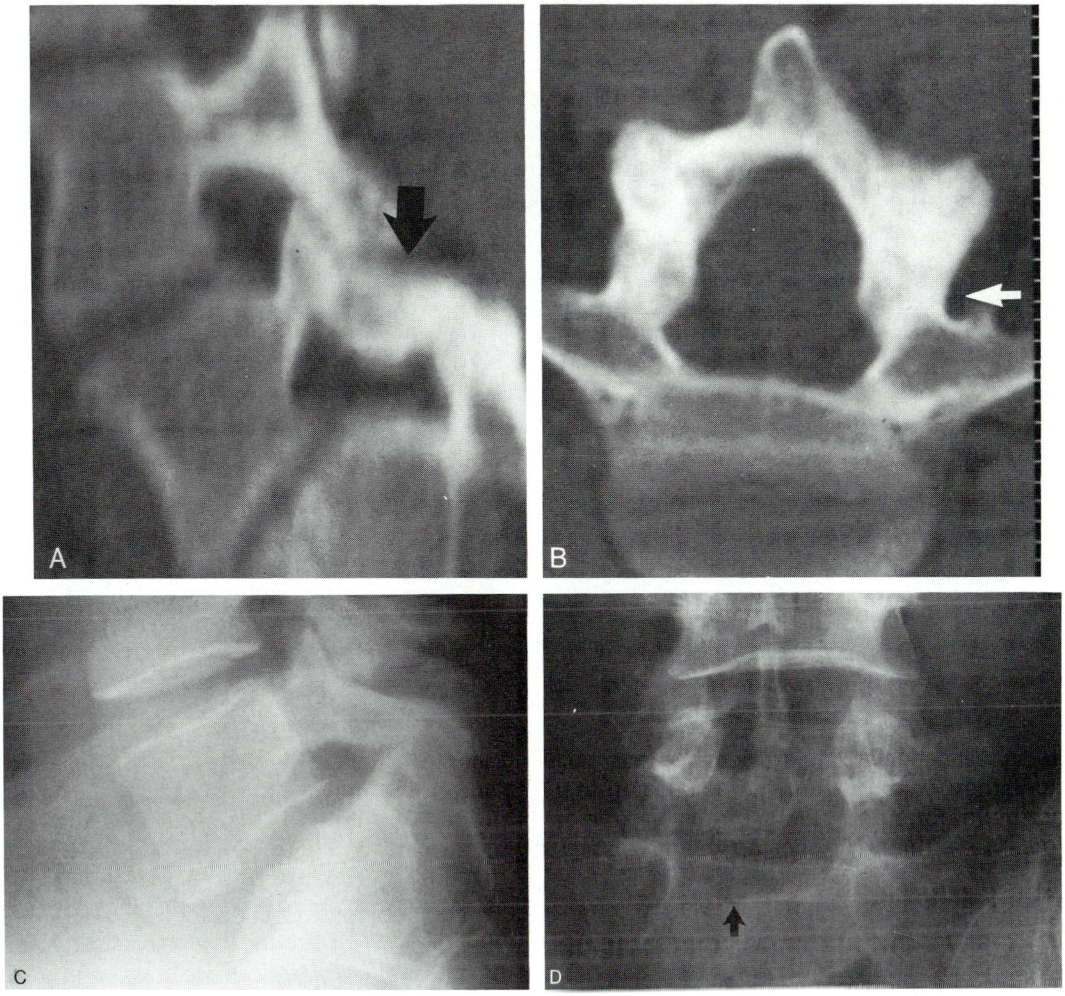

Figure 9 □ *A,* Reconstructed parasagittal view of a healed but elongated pars (Type IIB classification). *B,* Axial view of healed bilateral pars fractures in the same patient as in Figure 9*A*. Arrow points to healed area. Note elongated but healed pars. The radiologist reported, based on the CT scan, "minor spina bifida occulta and hypoplasia of the lumbosacral facets." *C,* AP radiograph of the same patient as in 9*A*. Arrow points to a dysplastic area at the top of the body of S1. *D,* Lateral view of patient in 9*A*. Note dysplastic areas in cranial border of the body of S1. This patient had never been an athlete and stated that he was rather sedentary. Therefore, these fractures are not quite the same as those we see in the teenage superathlete, who seldom has signs of dysplasia. This patient may have developed pars defects because he had abnormal growth of the upper sacrum and facets.

dysplastic type is caused by hypoplasia of the posterior arches of L5 or S1, or both, usually combined with an unstable orientation of the facets.

In the presence of hypoplasia of the facets, because the area of contact is small, the L5 pars is predisposed to stress fracture, because the fulcrum, which should be through the center of the pars, is caudally displaced. The increased length of the lever arm exerts greater stress on the pars, thus predisposing it to fracture.[23]

More severe dysplasia of the L5–S1 joint area with abnormal orientation of the articular processes leads to congenital spondylolisthesis with higher grades of slip. The facets may be sagittally or axially oriented, but never coronally oriented. If they were coronally oriented, olisthesis would be impeded by direct bony contact of the facets. When facets are sagittally or axially oriented, especially when the facet on one side is more medial at its posterior tip than on its anterior tip, only the ligamentous structures check forward gliding. Because the spine is unstable at the articular processes, especially if there is a bifid spinous process, subluxation or luxation occurs.

Because, as is suggested here, the underlying processes are the same, both mechanisms may coexist. Therefore, we find patients with both dysplastic facets and elongated pars. In the isthmic type, as the pars elongates or breaks, the laminae, including the spinous process and inferior articular processes, remain posterior as the anterior parts of the vertebrae slip forward; thus, the cauda equina is not compressed. This accounts for the cases, which we so often see, of an extremely high-grade slip with no neurologic changes and little dysfunction of any kind.

In some patients, after a certain amount of elongation, the pars finally fractures and does not heal. In others, the pars neither elongates nor fractures, but the superior facets glide forward on the inferior facets so that the entire neural ring subluxates forward, causing profound cauda equina compression, even with relatively low degrees of olisthesis. These probably account for the cases in which the severity of pain and hamstring spasm are out of proportion to the relatively low degree of slip. The rare case of cauda equina crisis is, likely, of this type. In the type in which an intact ring glides forward, the spinal nerves caudal to the L5 nerve are compressed, whereas in the type in which the posterior elements remain in normal position, the L5 nerve is compressed by the stumps of pars and the lateral masses of L5.[75]

Inheritance Factor in Types I and II

As of this writing, the pattern of inheritance for Types I and II is not known for certain. Haukipuro and colleagues[19] believe that the pattern definitely results from a dominant gene, as do Amuso and Mankin.[2] Wynne-Davies and Scott[76] believe that it lies between autosomal dominant inheritance with reduced penetrance and multifactorial inheritance.[77]

Based on our own studies carried out in the 1950s,[69] we believed that the pattern of inheritance was attributable to a recessive gene with incomplete penetrance, but in some families the involved gene showed incomplete dominance, in that some affected individuals are carriers (heterozygous) for the gene.

It is very possible that the confusion in deciding upon the inheritance pattern arises from the fact that we are confronted with at least two distinct anatomic types, congenital and isthmic, both having two subtypes and each showing anatomic differences, but having a common congenital cause. Much of the early work on the hereditary aspects was done before these subtypes were recognized and, of course, before the advent of the CT scan. CT has made it possible to see a great deal of bony detail, which had earlier been impossible.

Stress Fracture of the Pars in the Young Athlete

This type is commonly seen in the young athlete engaged in strenuous training.[70] To our knowledge, no genetic surveys have been conducted to determine whether there is an increased incidence among first-degree relatives of this group. In a study from our office of 100 young female gymnasts,[24] 11 had pars defects. This is nearly four times the average for females. Of the 11, 9 had spina bifida of either the L5 or S1 arch, or both. This is higher than average. One problem with studies of spina bifida in children is that the posterior arch does not close until fairly late in adolescence or early adulthood, so the incidence is abnormally high, even in children without pars defects.[32]

In a much more recent study of six young athletes with fresh pars fractures, conducted by one of the authors (S.L.G.R.), all had normal bony anatomy. This leads us to surmise that for this one type of unquestionable stress fracture developing later (i.e., in adolescence) the cause is primarily the extreme stress placed on the pars, which is the most vulnerable point. Young athletes who have spina bifida may be slightly more prone to develop pars defects than those with totally normal bony architecture. This explains the increased incidence of spina bifida in the young athlete with fresh pars fractures.

Type III. Degenerative

The degenerative lesion is attributable to long-standing intersegmental instability.[14] Remodeling of the articular processes occurs at the level of involvement (Fig. 10). Farfan[11]

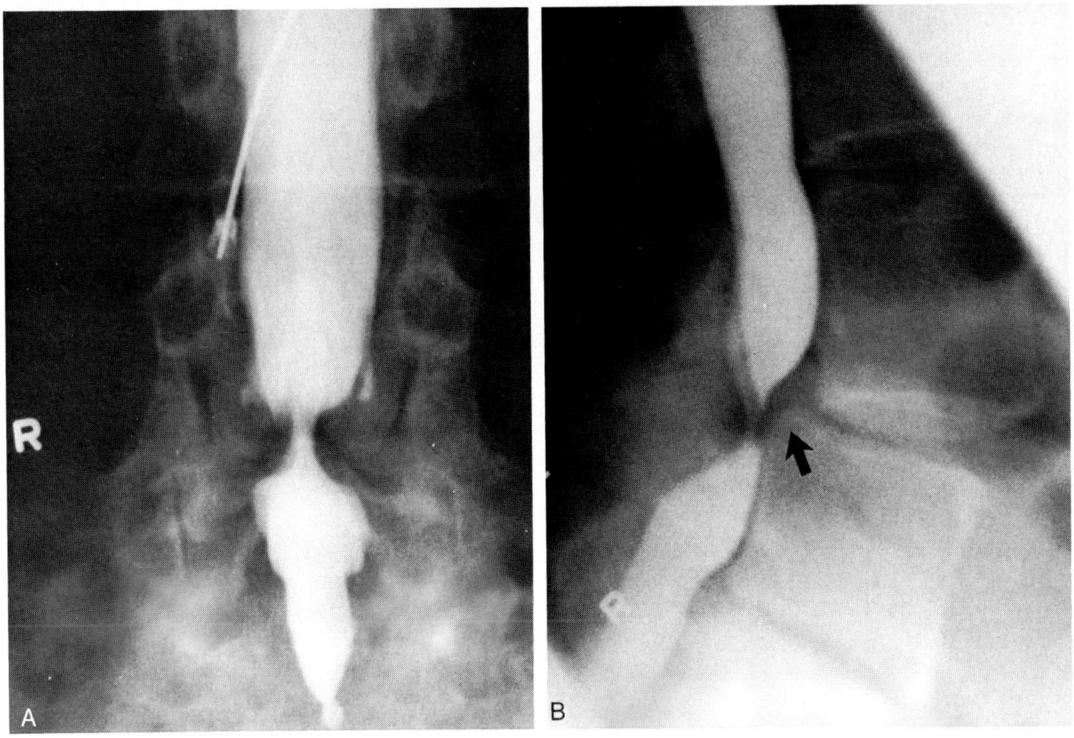

Figure 10 □ Typical AP (*A*) and lateral (*B*) myelograms of a patient with degenerative spondylolisthesis.

believes that there are multiple small compression fractures of the inferior articular processes of the vertebra that slip forward. Because of this, the bone of the articular processes has a peculiar granular appearance on radiographs. As the slip progresses, the articular processes change direction and become more horizontal.[50, 51]

Tropism of the facets is very common. When tropism is present, one side virtually always slips more than the other, and rotation of the vertebra at the level of olisthesis is an integral characteristic. The facets are sagittally oriented. The subluxation is more severe on the side of the more sagittally oriented facet. We cannot be sure, at the moment, whether the more sagittal orientation is the result of the fact that one side has slipped further or whether the increased sagittal orientation is the cause of the increased slip on that side. However, there can be little doubt that rotatory instability is part of degenerative spondylolisthesis.

Degenerative spondylolisthesis occurs six times as frequently in females as in males, six to nine times more frequently at the L4 interspace than at adjoining levels, and four times more frequently when the L5 is sacralized than when it is not.[50, 51] When the lesion is at L4, the L5 vertebra is more stable and less lordotic than average. A horizontal line drawn between the cephalic borders of the iliac crests (intercristal line)[39] passes, on the average, through a more caudal level in the spine in patients who develop degenerative spondylolisthesis than in others. This arrangement increases stress on the joint between L4 and L5, leading to decompensation at the articular processes and multiple microfractures of the inferior articular processes of L4, thereby allowing forward slipping. Farfan[12] says that, when demonstrable degenerative spondylolisthesis is present, the olisthetic joint has lost 50% of its torsion and shear strength.

In previous years, the senior author had not seen this lesion in any patient under 40 years of age, but since we have begun routinely taking standing x-rays on all patients, we have seen slip in patients as young as in their late thirties. We also take Knuttsen[28] flexion and extension views and are seeing instability, a frequent precursor of degenerative spondylolisthesis, at even earlier ages.

Interestingly, the slip in degenerative spondylolisthesis seldom exceeds 33% slip, unless there has been surgical intervention.

Type IV. Post-Traumatic

The post-traumatic type is secondary to an acute injury that fractures parts of the supporting bone other than the pars and allows the forward slip of the upper vertebra on the one below as a secondary phenomenon. Fracture of the pedicle may also be present.

This type of spondylolisthesis is always the result of severe trauma; the slip must occur gradually, over a period of weeks or longer. It is not an acute fracture/dislocation, although the pathologic findings may be virtually the same. Separating this into a distinct type may seem somewhat artificial, but is probably warranted. It is fairly rare. The senior author sees about two new cases a year.

Type V. Pathologic

In pathologic spondylolisthesis, local or generalized bone disease causes the bony mechanism (consisting of the pedicle, the pars, and the superior and inferior articular processes) to fail to hold the forward thrust of the superincumbent body weight. Forward slipping of the vertebra on the one below occurs. It is a fairly rare type.[46]

TYPE VA. GENERALIZED

In this type there are widespread generalized bony changes, as in the following examples:

Albers-Schönberg Disease (Osteopetrosis). □ In this condition fractures of the pars are frequent. These sometimes heal and refracture. Spondylolysis occurs, and often spondylolisthesis (Fig. 11).[63]

Arthrogryposis. □ In a type of arthrogryposis called Kuskokwim disease, several pedicles (L5 in particular) may be elongated, producing spondylolisthesis of L5 on S1.

Syphilitic Disease. □ Spondylolisthesis in the lumbar spine secondary to syphilitic gummas of the articular processes has been reported by Karaharjii and Hunnuksela.[26]

TYPE VB. LOCALIZED

A localized bone infection or a tumor may destroy the supporting structures sufficiently that the cranial vertebra may slip forward on the one that is more caudal.

Type VI. Postsurgical

This is a fairly frequent type of spondylolisthesis.[29, 68] The incidence varies in different reported series but was about 3% to 5% in the series reported by White and Wiltse.[68] The slip occurs because too much of the supporting structure has been removed in an effort to decompress adequately. This group should not include patients developing further olisthesis after decompression of degenerative spondylolisthesis or olisthesis following the removal of the loose element in isthmic spondylolisthesis; but again, the etiologic findings are very similar. This group includes the patients seen after extensive decompression for spinal stenosis, after laminectomy for disc removal, or after any other spine surgery in which it is necessary to destabilize the spine. Several authors have used the term *iatrogenic spondylolisthesis* to describe this type. It is the belief of the senior author that this word is far too harsh, because it implies fault of the surgeon, which is not necessarily so. Often, a minor degree of instability was present before surgery, but could not be detected by ordinary x-ray examination. If a rather wide laminectomy is performed, as is often necessary to adequately decompress, postoperative olisthesis is a common sequel. Also, in the presence of osteoporosis and poor ligamentous support, unanticipated olisthesis may occur. To call this "iatrogenic" is to invite a malpractice suit.

In a study of CT scans made by one of the authors (S.L.G.R.) for patients who had undergone laminectomy, more than 10% were noted to have stress fractures of an inferior articular process at the level of decompression. Mild postsurgical spondylolisthesis is common in these patients. This is somewhat different from instances in which too much bone has been removed. It is suggested that, in these cases, surgical weakening occurs at the base of the articular process, and fracture occurs during normal activity.

NATURAL HISTORY OF SPONDYLOLISTHESIS

The discussion of the natural history will be limited to Types IA, IB, IIA, and IIB. These

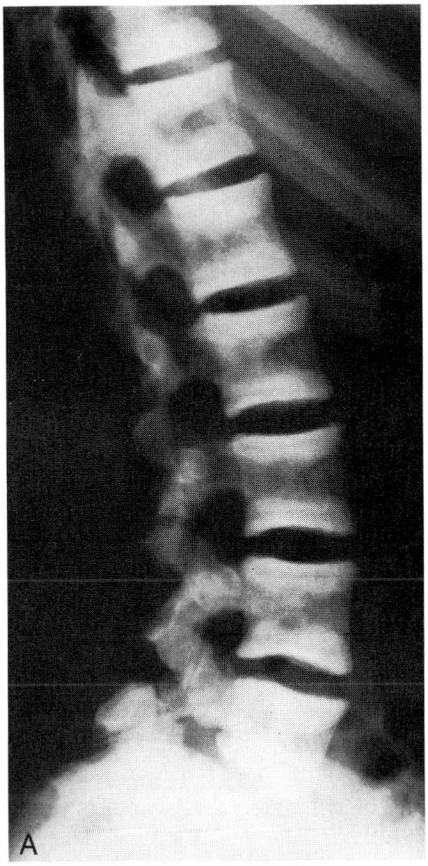

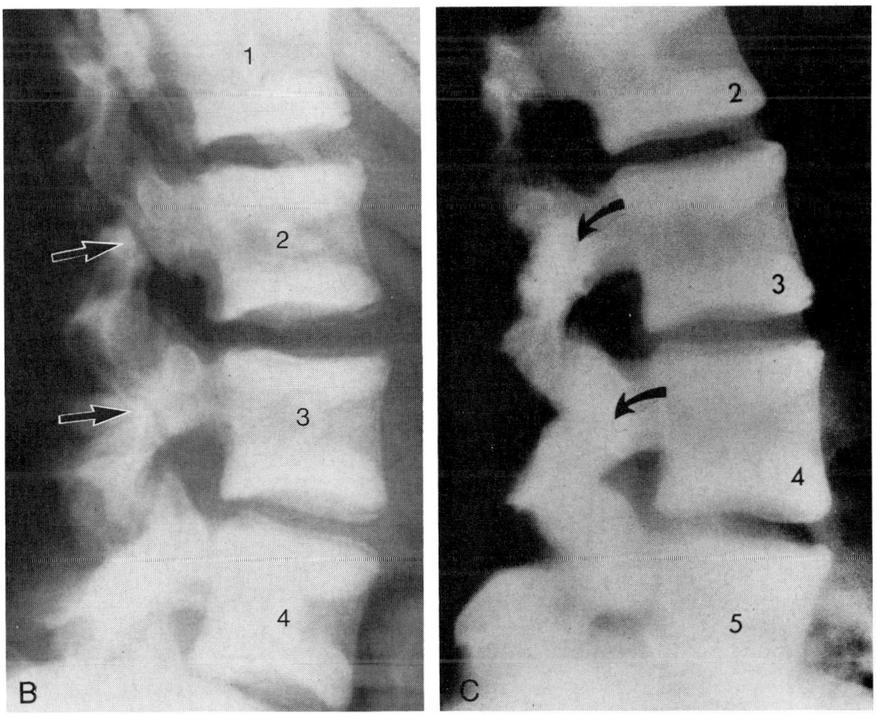

Figure 11 □ Pathologic spondylolisthesis secondary to osteopetrosis, showing cracking and healing of pars. *A,* A 12-year-old girl. Note pars fracture at L5. The partes of L2 and L3 are intact. *B,* Three months later, note spondylolysis of the L2 and the L3 partes. *C,* Seventeen months later the partes of L2 and of L3 have healed. The pars of L5 shows an attempt at healing.

are the congenital and isthmic types. Degenerative spondylolisthesis will also be discussed.

Several studies have been made in an attempt to establish the natural history of Types I and II,[45] but they have been only partially successful. Many problems must be confronted in such studies. It is essential that one be certain of the type of spondylolisthesis being studied. The slip that occurs in the isthmic type in which the loose element remains in its normal position behaves quite differently from the congenital Type IB, in which there are no pars defects and no spina bifida. Most long-range studies also have the problem of poor x-rays or no original x-rays at all available at the time of follow-up study, and one must depend on reports of radiologists who may not have been aware of these subdivisions. Also, the question arises regarding the degree of spondylolisthesis being studied.

High-grade olistheses, especially in the very young patient, with wedging of L5 and rounding of the top of the sacrum, are likely to slip further. Also, especially in children, if standing laterals are taken instead of lying-down x-rays, what would normally be called spondylolysis may slip a little and be called spondylolisthesis. Most patients first come to the doctor because of back pain. This tends to skew the statistics and must be allowed for, because certainly many people have a slip that is just as severe, although they have no back or leg pain.

It appears, based on reviewing several studies,[13, 61, 62] that isthmic spondylolisthesis with olisthesis, up to at least 10%, carries a risk of low back trouble about the same as that for no spondylolisthesis. For a slip of between 10% and 25%, there may be some increase in the incidence of back pain and sciatica.

What about the higher grades (beyond 25%) of slip? Are these patients predisposed to symptoms? We believe that they are, and we have some statistical studies to back up this belief.[22, 58] We do know that, in large studies taken from pre-employment x-rays incidental to pre-employment physical examinations, the incidence of high-grade slip is very low and in many studies nonexistent, suggesting that these people with high-grade slip do not get to the stage of applying for work in the general labor market. Unfortunately, we do not know the incidence of high-grade slip in the general population. Those of us who have large spine practices see few cases of high-grade slip in the elderly as an incidental finding, suggesting that it is not very frequent.

Saraste[58] recently reported a 20-year observation of 255 spondylolysis and spondylolisthesis patients. She noted that progression of slipping was small and not correlated with age at diagnosis or with the initial degree of olisthesis. Disc height reduction at the spondylolytic level occurred earlier and was more severe than in a control group. If the slip was greater than 25%, the patient was at an increased risk of symptoms, compared with the normal population. Wedging of the L5 vertebral body and disc degeneration also increased the likelihood of back pain and sciatica, compared with those without spondylolysis or olisthesis.

Harris and Weinstein[18] compared the long-term clinical results (average of 18 years) of 11 patients with what appeared to be isthmic spondylolisthesis and olisthesis greater than 50% who were treated nonoperatively with another group of 21 who had a slip of a similar percentage treated by posterior in situ fusion. The two groups were compared as to degree of pain, residual neurologic change, bladder or bowel problems, and changes in lifestyle. The two groups fared virtually equally. Only one of each group had significant pain, and all were living normal, active lives. Two in the nonoperated group developed significant slip, so it was concluded that progressive slip was an indication for in situ fusion.

Apel and coworkers[2] reported on a group of 12 patients with first-degree spondylolisthesis and an average follow-up period of 40 years. These patients were treated at Hines Veterans Administration Hospital in Chicago, between 1944 and 1951. In each case, the slip had been classified as Grade 1 and was at the L5–S1 level. Five had been treated conservatively, and seven were treated surgically with a Hibbs posterior fusion from L4 to S1. Of the conservatively managed patients, all functioned well during their working years, although one did have chronic, nondisabling, low back pain. This same patient demonstrated radiographic evidence of progression to a Grade 2 spondylolisthesis. Among those undergoing surgery, the poor results were confined to patients for whom attempts at fusion failed.

The researchers concluded that the management for low-grade spondylolisthesis should be conservative, if possible. When the low back pain is disabling and surgery is resorted to, failure to obtain a fusion portends a poor clinical result. Thus, in this study, conservatively managed patients actually did somewhat better than those who were operated upon.

It can be deduced from these studies that it is best to treat the patient who has either isthmic spondylolisthesis (Types IIA or IIB,) or congenital spondylolisthesis (Types IA or IB) without having to resort to surgery, if that is possible. If pain is severe and persistent to the degree that it alters the patient's lifestyle or if, in a young patient, the slip is increasing then fusion in situ is indicated.[56, 57] There is little danger in continuing conservative treatment indefinitely.

The natural history of the three most important types of spondylolisthesis can be summarized as follows.

Types IA and IB. Congenital

Type IA: If the posterior ring is intact, symptoms will occur with low (35%) slip. If a wide-open spina bifida of L5, S1, or both is present,[55] then:

1. Olisthesis often appears earlier than in others.[36]
2. Slip may be very severe.
3. These patients may have severe hamstring spasm but fare better neurologically than if the posterior elements are intact and still slip forward.
4. These patients probably need fusion more often than others.

Type IB shows altered facet orientation and often an intact posterior ring. The following are associated with the disorder:

1. High-grade slip is uncommon.
2. Leg pain, back spasm, hamstring spasm, and altered gait bring the patient to the doctor.
3. The part of the cauda equina caudal to the L5 nerves is compressed.
4. If fusion in situ without decompression is performed on these patients, they will be slow in getting over their tight hamstrings and altered gait.

Types IIA and IIB. Isthmic

These patients have either a separated fracture in the pars or a pars that has elongated as the vertebral body slips forward, leaving the posterior elements in a more or less normal position.

1. There are few cases before 5 years of age.[53]
2. Most develop during the first year of school.[53]
3. By 7 years of age, 4% of the cases will have appeared.[5]
4. Another 1.4% will appear before adulthood.[5] Most of the 1.4% will appear between the ages of 11 to 15 years and these in the very athletic youngsters.[70]
5. In persons engaged in very strenuous athletics, new cases appear, even into early adulthood.
6. Olisthesis develops any time after the pars fractures occur, but the majority of high grades of slip develop from 10 to 14 years of age (in girls, a year or so earlier than in boys).
7. High-grade slip is four times as likely to occur in girls, compared with boys; yet pars defects are only half as frequent in girls as in boys.[10, 25]
8. Back and leg pain commonly bring the patients to the doctor. Changes in the body contour alone seldom bring children to the doctor.
9. Significant increase in olisthesis after adulthood is sufficiently uncommon that it can be ignored as a significant problem.
10. Olisthesis of up to 10%[32] appears not to increase the likelihood of back problems, even with heavy work. With slip between 10% and 25%, there may be some question, and beyond 25%, it quite clearly does increase the likelihood of a patient's having low back symptoms compared with what would be expected in a population without pars defects.[22, 54, 61]
11. Wedging of the body of L5 also increases the likelihood of symptoms.[54]
12. Increased sagittal rotation causes more change in body contour than that caused by increased olisthesis.
13. Spondylolisthesis, even high-grade, causes no problem with pregnancy.[55]

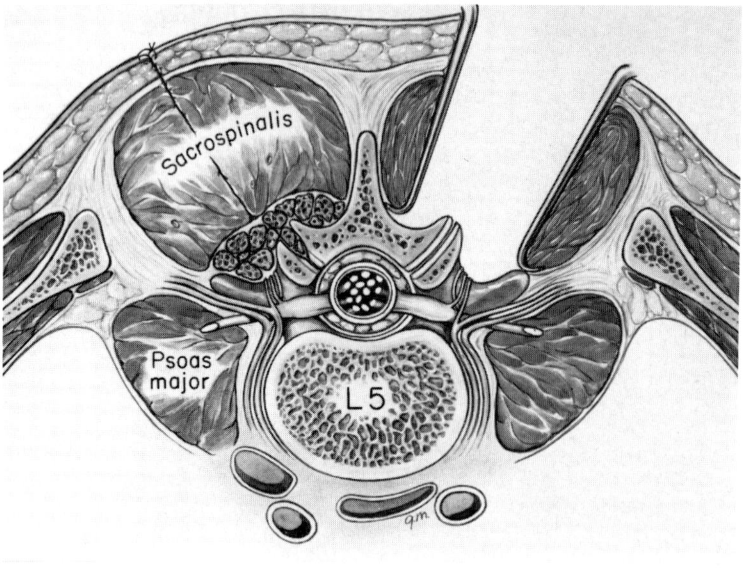

Figure 12 □ We use this paraspinal approach in virtually all cases of spondylolisthesis, Type I and Type II. (From Wiltse, L.L., Bateman, J.G., and Hutchenson, R.H.: The paraspinal sacrospinalis splitting approach to the lumbar spine. J. Bone Joint Surg. 50:A, 1968.)

Natural History of Degenerative Spondylolisthesis

Degenerative spondylolisthesis is characterized by the following:

1. Seldom is seen before age 40 but the incidence increases with age and is common in the very elderly.[14]
2. Women are more commonly affected than men.[50]
3. Pain is of two types: (a) the claudicant, characterized by pain in the calves brought on by walking[47] and (b) the much more common sciatic type, in which pain extends down one leg, resembling the pain from a herniated disc.
4. Slip seldom progresses to more than 33% if no surgery is performed.
5. Severe paralysis is rare, although foot drop—unilateral or rarely bilateral—does occur.
6. Sciatic tension signs are often absent.
7. Most patients can be treated nonoperatively. It has been reported that only one in ten who go to the doctor with slip needs surgery.

SURGERY FOR SPONDYLOLISTHESIS

Type I. Isthmic

Since a complete discussion of the surgery for spondylolisthesis is beyond the scope of this paper, we will limit the discussion to a few areas, especially to areas of controversy.

In children with isthmic spondylolisthesis, we fuse in situ without decompression, no matter how high the degree of slip. This is what we have done for the past 30 years. No child has had less than a good result. Complications have been negligible. We have used a paraspinal approach since 1960 (Fig. 12).[71] Most patients have been allowed to get up in a few days, and normally no corset or brace is used. We know of no failures of fusion (Fig. 13).[48]

In a study of adults with high-grade isthmic spondylolisthesis and sciatica,[43] eight consecutive patients were treated by fusion in situ without decompression. All patients had severe sciatica and neurologic deficits. Anterior displacement ranged from 60% to complete spondyloptosis, the average being 81%. Follow-up ranged from 2.0 to 14.1 years, with an average of 5 years. All eight cases fused solidly with excellent relief of back pain and sciatica. Neurologic deficits resolved with the exception of lost Achilles reflexes in two patients. There have been no serious complications (Fig. 14).

When should the arthrodesis be limited to L5 and S1, and when should L4 be included? Based on the degree of sagittal rotation alone and ignoring, for the moment, such factors as ruptured disc at the L4 level or internal disc disruption[9] at that level, we use the rule of thumb that if the angle of the superior border of L5 to the horizontal (the new sacrohorizontal angle) is less than 55 degrees, we fuse only L5 to S1. If it is greater

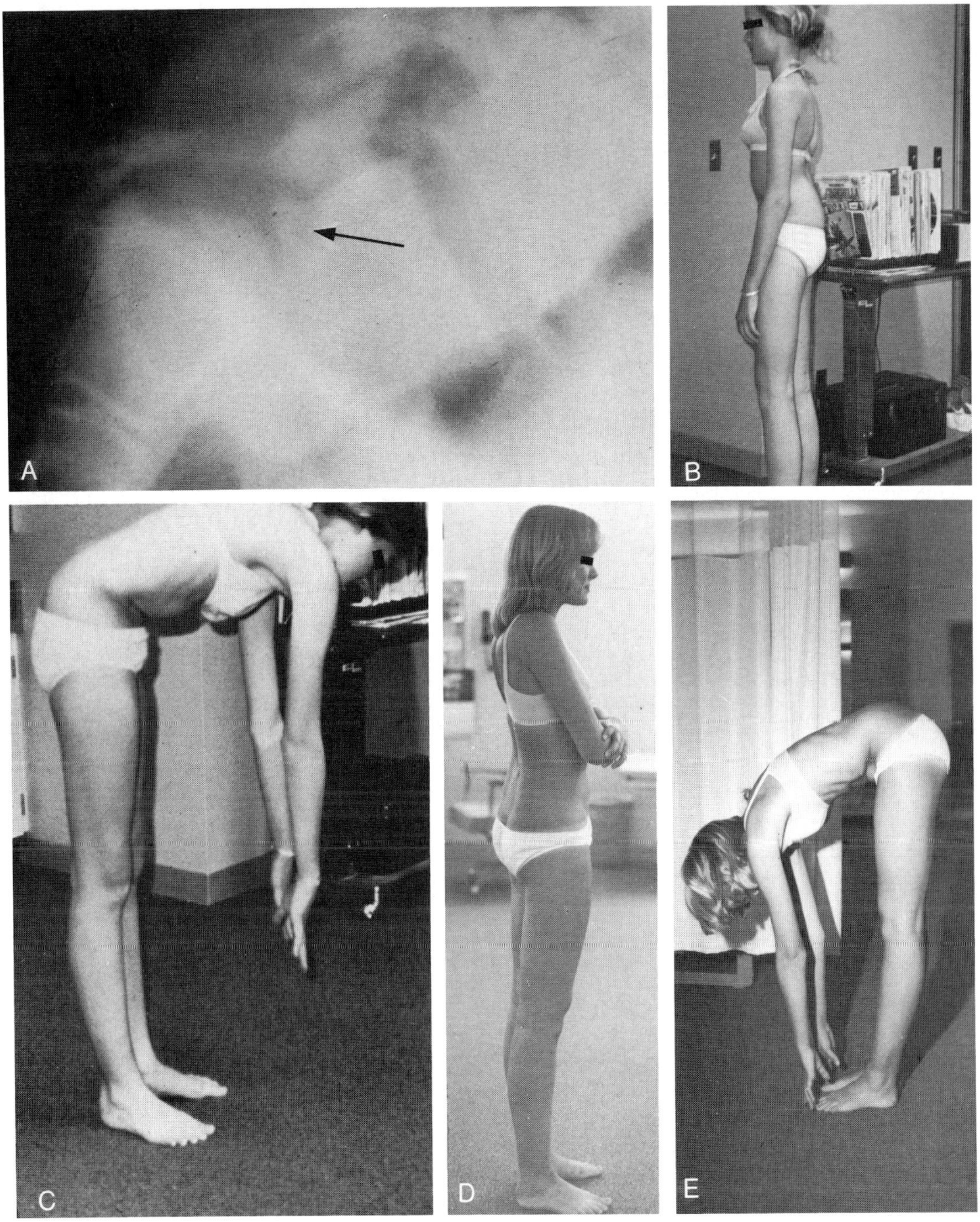

Figure 13 □ *A*, X-ray of a typical 15-year-old female with high-grade slip and marked sagittal rotation of L5. The degree of sagittal rotation is much more important, in regard to the effect on bodily contour, than is the slip. Note that there has been an increase of a few degrees in sagittal rotation and a few degrees of decrease in sacral tilt, but none of olisthesis. This is characteristic. *B*, Note change in body contour. *C*, Note limitation in bending. *D*, One year after fusion. *E*, Bending 1 year after fusion.

Illustration continued on following page

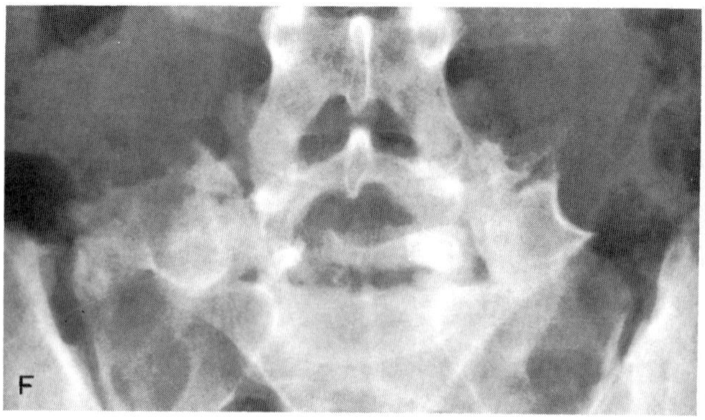

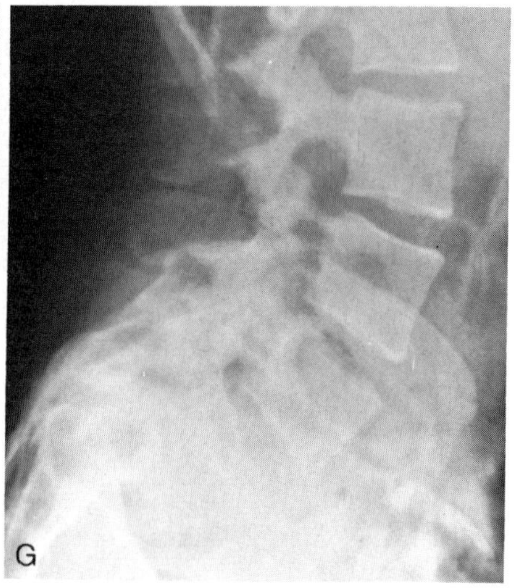

Figure 13 *Continued F,* AP x-ray 11 years after fusion. *G,* Lateral x-ray 11 years after fusion.

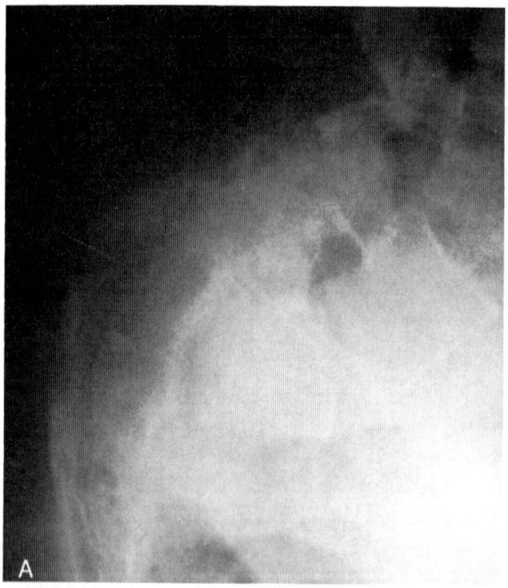

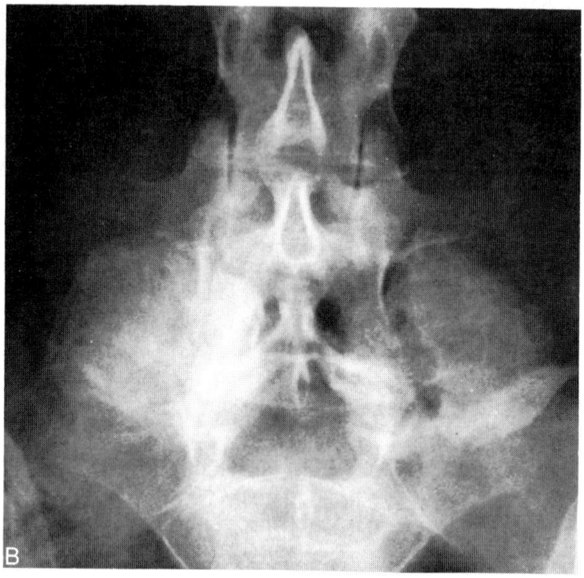

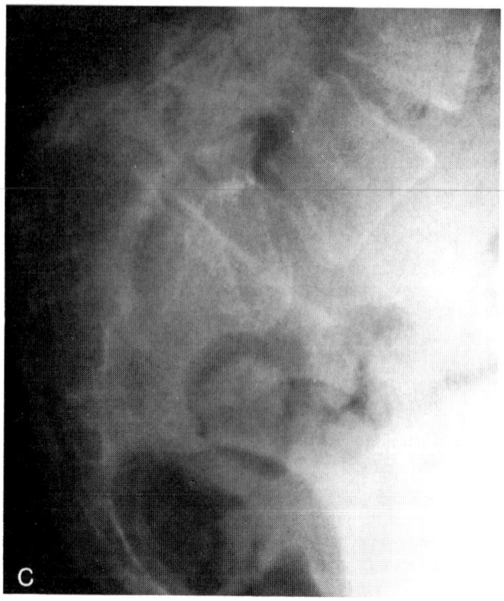

Figure 14 □ *A,* A 34-year-old Caucasian woman with high-grade slip, severe leg pain, and reflex and sensory change in painful leg. *B,* Three and a half years after fusion in situ, no decompression. She was allowed up immediately. No corset or brace was used. *C,* Lateral view. Note that no further olisthesis or sagittal rotation has occurred. She shows an excellent result.

than 55 degrees, we include L4 in the fusion.[74]

Type IA. Congenital

In the congenital Type IA, surgery is identical to that of the isthmic type, but in congenital Type IB, where the posterior arch is intact and there is no defect in the pars, the posterior ring slides forward and compresses the cauda. These cases can have more severe tightness of the hamstrings, and this tightness is slower to resolve after surgery. These cases can be fused in situ, but if the tight hamstrings and peculiar gait persist, a decompression may be necessary and can easily be performed later. We have had to do a late decompression in only one patient out of about four who had intact rings. Once the fusion is solid, there is no danger of further olisthesis, and simple decompression at the L5–S1 level is all that is necessary. It appears that the nerves passing over the posterior superior rim of the body of S1 are compressed in these patients, but one is wise to decompress the L5 nerve as well. It is also important to get out far enough laterally on the L5 nerve to be sure that it is free. Furthermore, a wide fusion should be performed in these patients, so that if decompression is required later, it can be done without compromising the solidity of the fusion. In our experience, the tight hamstrings disappear quite rapidly after decompression. However, if the existing tightness is not too great and not too troublesome, the patient can be left nondecompressed; the gait will return to normal and hamstring tightness will disappear, over a period of a few years. We have noted that in either the isthmic or dysplastic types, pain and hamstring tightness are likely to persist until the fusion is solid. We have had to do a late decompression in only two cases in our entire experience.

When L4 should be included in a fusion performed for an L5–S1 slip is an area of controversy. Many surgeons always include the L4. We believe that short fusions are generally better than long ones, so we do an L5 to S1 fusion, if possible. We have arbitrarily decided that when a line drawn across the top of L5 forms an angle with the horizontal of greater than 55%, only then should the fusion include L4. This will be the "new" sacrohorizontal angle after the fusion becomes solid (Fig. 15).

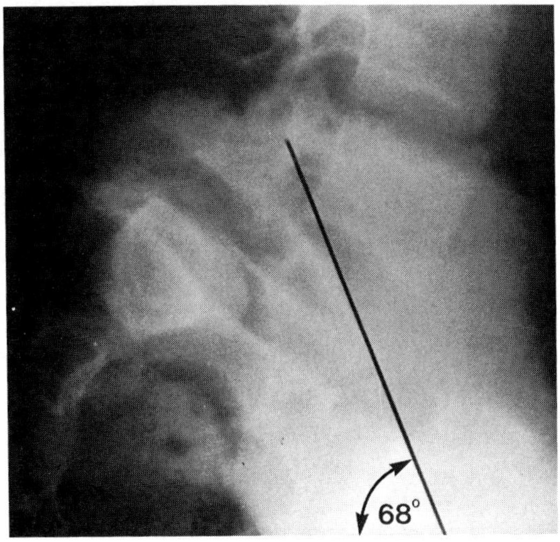

Figure 15 □ Sacrohorizontal angle (x-ray must be taken with the patient standing). When a solid fusion of the lateral masses has been obtained from L5 to S1, it is as though there is a Class IV transitional vertebra with the wings solidly fused to the alae. The top of L5 then becomes the new sacrohorizontal angle. We have arbitrarily chosen 55 degrees as the break-off point for one-level fusions. Beyond 55 degrees we perform a two-level fusion from L4 to S1.

The question of whether discography should be carried out at the first unfused level will not be dealt with here.

Pedicle Screws

We have been using pedicle screws in the adult in whom there has been a failure of previous surgery. We have not made a point of reducing the slip, except in cases of alar transverse process impingement, in which situation we may avoid a decompression by lifting L5 off the sacrum. Pedicle screws have been especially useful in these cases.[72]

By using pedicle screws, the L5 can be jacked cranially and posteriorly, thus lifting the lateral masses off the nerve. Only the one level need be fused. If the vertebrae are very severely separated at surgery, the surgeon may need to add an interbody fusion to take the stress off the screws. We have not added an interbody fusion for any of our patients and no breakage has occurred so far, although our experience is not great. If the surgeon prefers, the nerve can be decompressed by channeling far out laterally; then fixation with rods and pedicle screws with an added fusion can be done (Fig. 16).

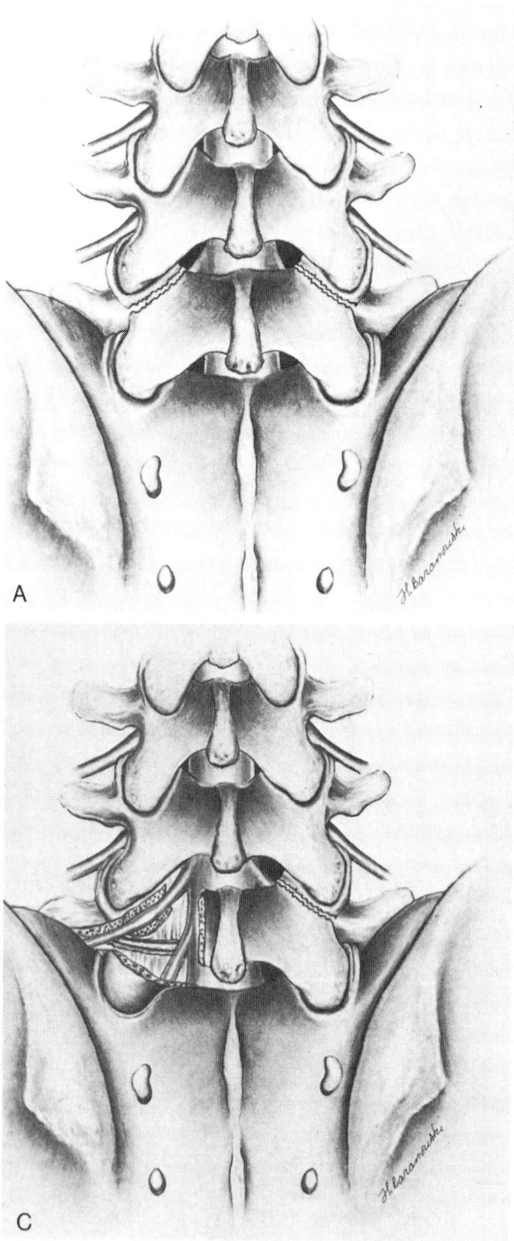

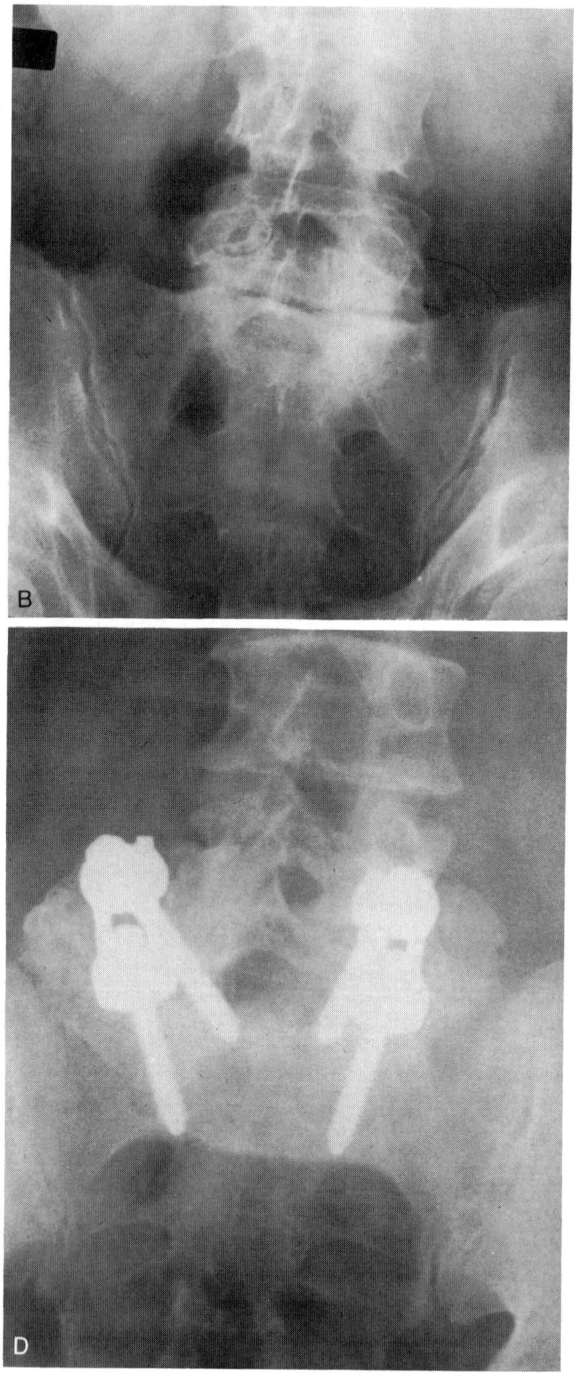

Figure 16 □ *A,* In spondylolisthesis, if the slip is as much as 20%, or perhaps even less, the lateral masses and transverse processes may drop down on the alae and compress the L5 nerve. The drawing attempts to demonstrate this. *B,* In this AP x-ray of a patient with spondylolisthesis and 25% slip, we also see some tilt to the left. In th patient, the lateral mass was jammed down against the ala on the left. He had severe sciatica on the left. *C,* Traditionally, we have decompressed the painful side, as in this drawing, and fused the other side only. In younger people, we would wait about 6 weeks and perform an anterior interbody fusion. *D,* With the use of pedicle screws, we can decompress, as in *C,* and add pedicle screws and rods. An anterior interbody fusion is not necessary. Alternatively, we can spread the left side before tightening down the nuts and thus lift the lateral mass off the L5 nerve, in which case decompression is not necessary.

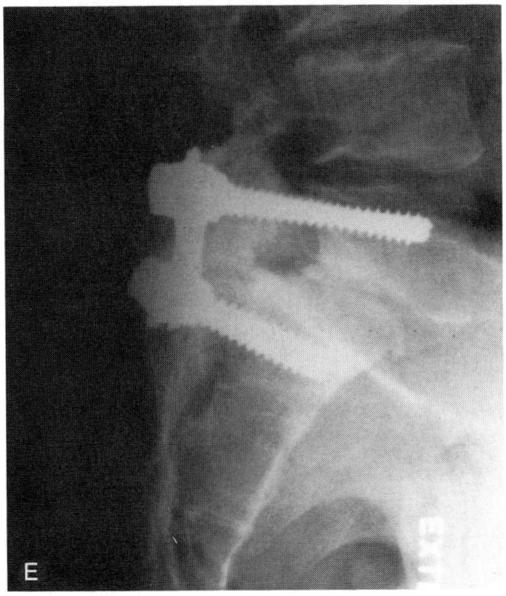

Figure 16 *Continued E,* Lateral view shows solid fusion with pedicle screws and rods in place.

AREAS OF CONTROVERSY/ NEEDS FOR RESEARCH

There is considerable difficulty separating the congenital and isthmic types of spondylolisthesis. Separation is important only in some instances in which one is deciding on a treatment. Both have a hereditary component to their causes, although understanding the patterns of inheritance requires further research. The advent of the CT scan has made this type of study much more exact than it ever was before. Nevertheless, difficulties remain.

It is quite clear that where there is separation at the isthmus and the posterior element remains in the normal position, decompression by removal of the loose element is unnecessary and often harmful because it removes support as well as fusion area. Not so clear is how to determine the circumstances under which decompression is necessary when the arch is intact and olisthesis exists. The CT scan, frontal and lateral re-formations, and physical examination, should make this decision possible.

Burski and coworkers[8] believe that in many cases, because of fibrous attachments between the tips of the broken pars, the loose element follows along as the body slips forward, thus presenting a clinical picture of no pars defect. The authors report that these patients have neurologic change with relatively small degrees of slip. This is an area needing further study by clinicians in collaboration with radiologists. With contrast reformation, it should be possible to confirm or refute the contention that in some patients the loose element moves forward with the anterior elements as olisthesis progresses.

What causes tight hamstrings? At least in some cases, the cause is clearly nerve pressure, but is this always so? Perhaps traction on the nerves plays a part when there is a high-grade slip. We had a patient with congenital spondylolisthesis with about 40% slip. She had been fused from L4 to S1 and had a wide, solid arthrodesis. Her hamstrings before operation were extremely tight so that she had to walk on tiptoe with her feet wide apart and knees flexed. One year after fusion, her hamstring tightness remained unchanged. Her disability was such that she could not even attend school. A myelogram showed no tethering of the filum. Simple decompression of both L5 and S1 nerves was done, saving the wide fusion. The patient was walking normally within 3 weeks (Fig. 17). This represents a case in which the tight hamstrings were caused by compression alone. Once compression was removed, she became normal in a matter of days, after having been virtually unable to walk for over a year.

Marked disagreement still exists concerning when, if ever, reduction should be performed. The results of simple fusion in situ, even in the most severe cases, have been

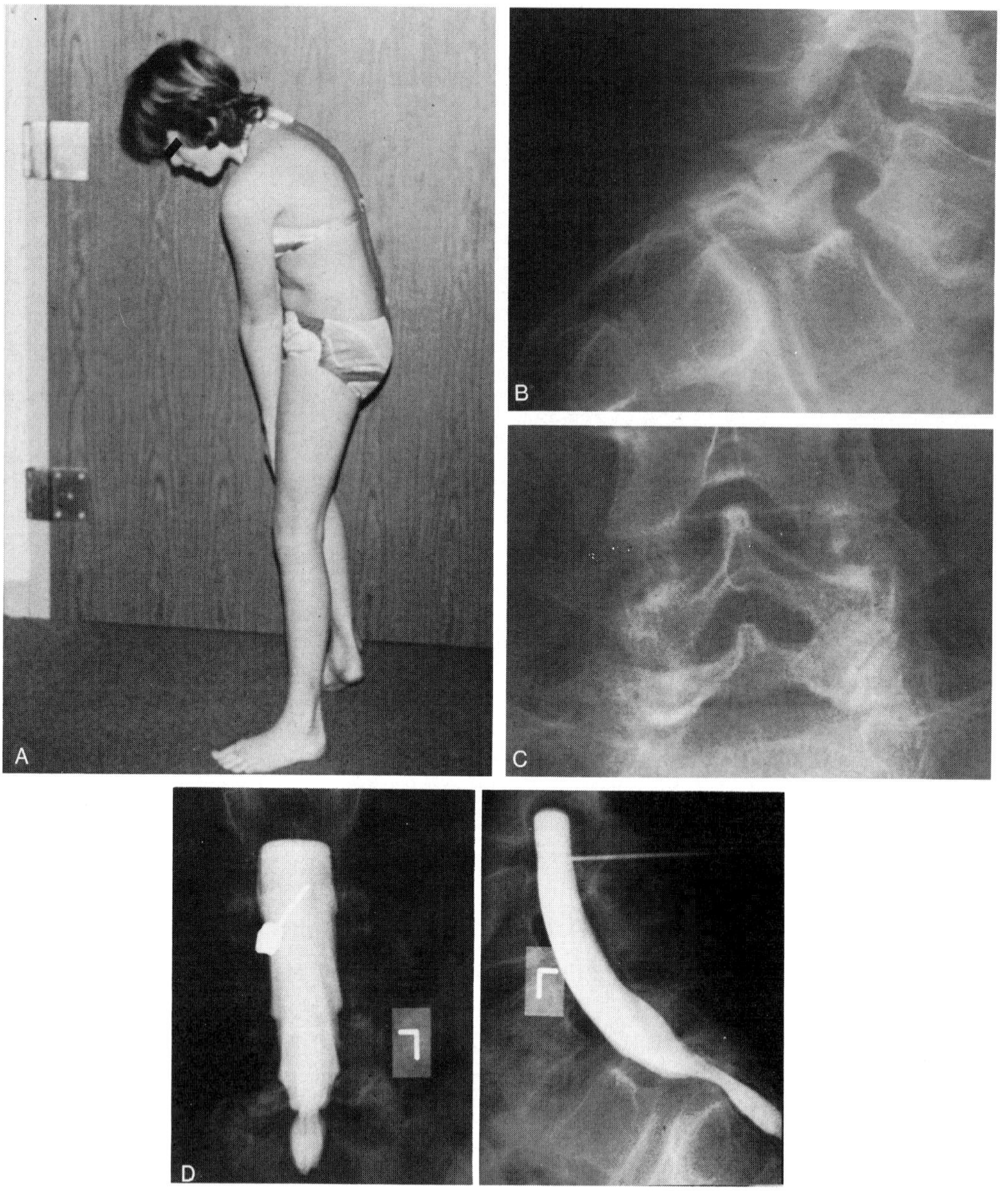

Figure 17 □ *A,* A 12-year-old child with a hamstring spasm so severe that she could not go to school. *B,* Standing lateral view shows a slip of about only 25%, but no pars defect. *C,* AP view shows typical axially oriented facets, and the facets show tropism. Most important, the posterior ring of L5 is intact. *D,* Myelogram shows near-block at L5–S1.

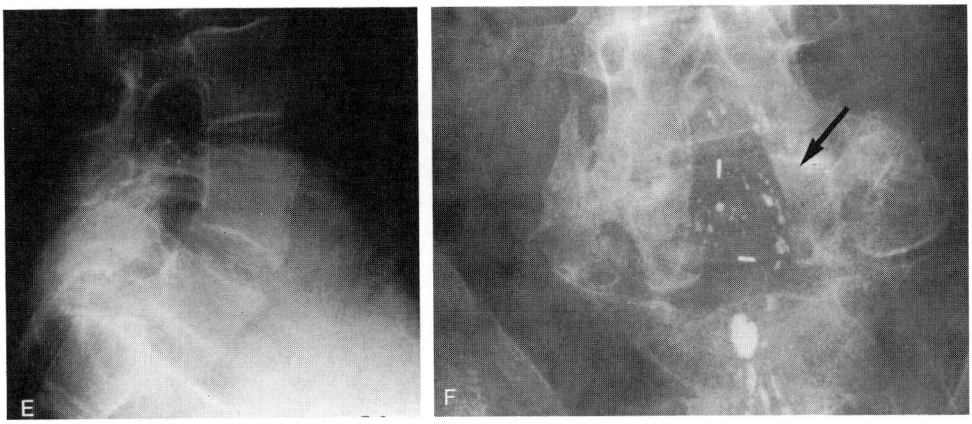

Figure 17 *Continued E,* Lateral view 6 months postoperatively shows solid fusion at L4 to S1 with no further slip. *F,* Because her hamstring spasm was unchanged, a decompression was performed. Within 3 weeks she could walk and bend normally. This case demonstrates that when the posterior arch is intact, a small amount of slip can be devastating. Also, simply removing the pressure cured the patient of all hamstring spasm in a matter of days. This case is important in that the cause of the hamstring spasm in such instances is still a matter of widespread discussion.

good. Although a great deal of discussion has surrounded body contour, the patients themselves seem not to be disturbed about their build.[43] It does seem likely that, as methods of reduction improve, reduction will gain favor in patients with high-grade olistheses.

Will internal fixation be used frequently in the future? It appears that it will. Especially with pedicle screws and the vast array of fixation methods available, it is almost certain that a method will eventually be developed so that the spine can be reduced and internally fixed with relative ease and safety.

Treatment of the stress fracture in the young athlete remains controversial. The young athlete who is training to compete in the Olympics, for example, quite frequently develops stress fractures of the pars or even the pedicles. This produces pain that sends the individual to the doctor, who diagnoses an early stress reaction in the pars and, very rarely, in the pedicle (Fig. 18).[41] If there is an expectation of these healing, and remaining healed, the patient must be taken off athletics and put into a brace or a corset (we use a heavy corset) for at least 8 months. The problem is that the healing rate is rather low (probably because of noncompliance). If the patient is put into a cast from knees to nipples and kept in a horizontal position for at least 4 months, we believe the early fracture will always heal. This appears to be far too severe a treatment, but the question remains: How vigorous should the surgeon be in trying to obtain healing of this relatively benign condition?

At the time of this writing, we are aware of no statistical studies indicating that the

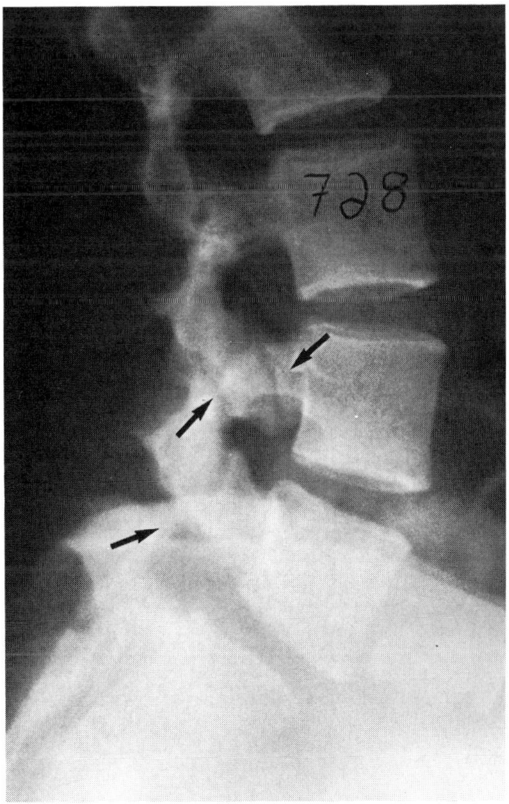

Figure 18 □ The radiograph shows one or two of these cases per year, in which the pars is broken on one side and the pedicle on the other.

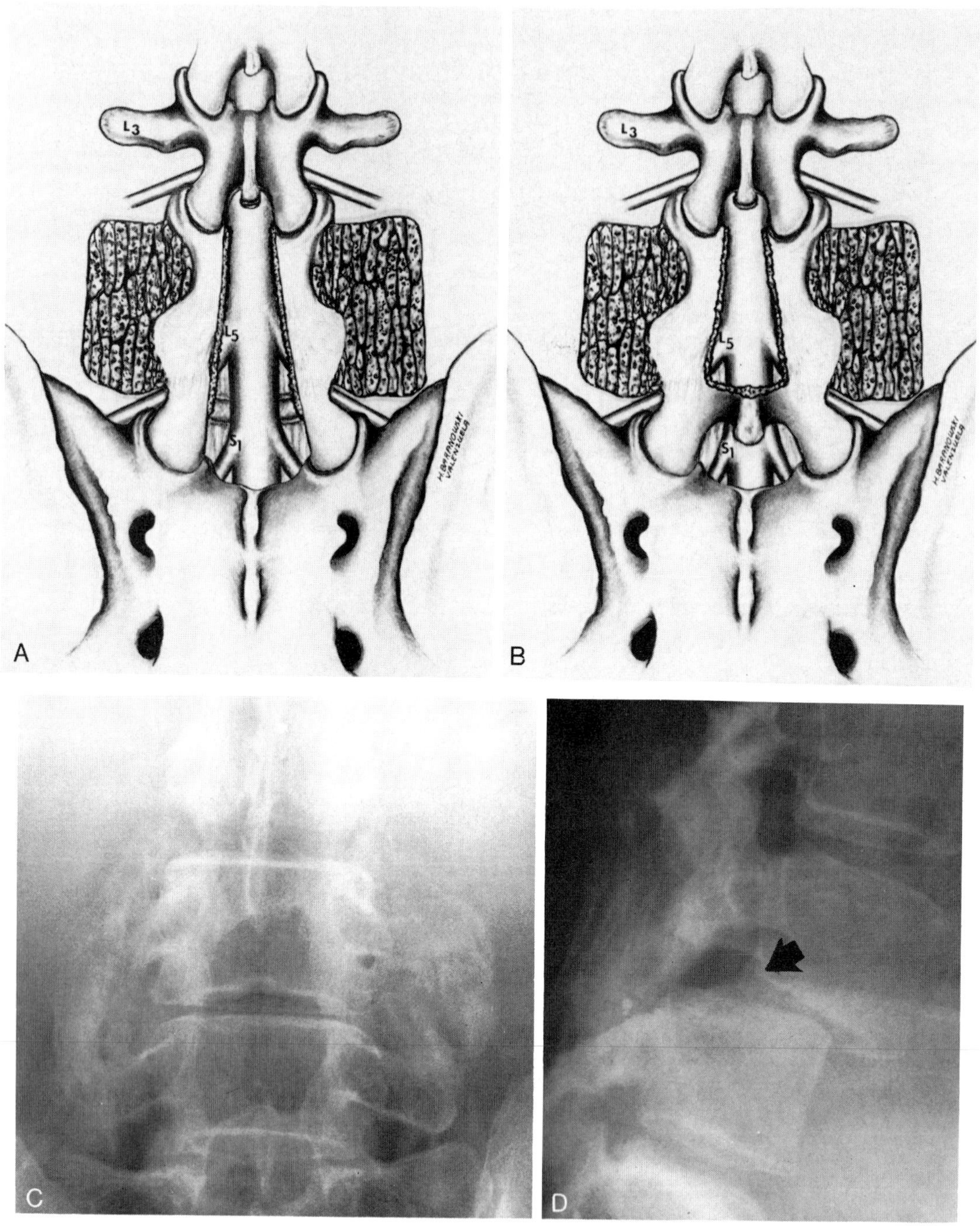

Figure 19 □ *A,* Type of decompression and fusion performed for degenerative spondylolisthesis. *B,* If the L5–S1 level is clearly uninvolved, we do not extend the decompression all the way down to S1. *C,* AP x-ray of a case in which the patient was treated in the above manner. *D,* Lateral x-ray of a case treated in the above manner.

pars fractures that occur in the teenage athlete have a hereditary element. However, some evidence suggests heredity in that the incidence of spina bifida is increased in these children.[24] However, except for the increased incidence of spina bifida, the bony architecture appeared normal on CT scans in the six cases reviewed by us recently.

What is the place of pars interarticularis fusion? At least three methods of fusing the fracture of the pars interarticularis are available.[38] The earliest was described by Buck,[7] who passed a screw down the pars interarticularis, drawing the fragments together and then grafting. Nicol and Scott[37a] advocated a method of passing wires around the base of the transverse processes and tying them around the spinous process. Morscher and colleagues[33] of Switzerland have developed another method using a tiny Harrington-type hook around the loose element and a screw into the lateral mass of L5. All these methods work. All impose a fairly demanding surgical technique. The obvious problem is determining when is it appropriate to perform this rather major operation for a condition from which the child will probably recover and live a nearly pain-free life.

In considering degenerative spondylolisthesis, should every case which is operated on be fused?[29] The authors believe they should. Differences of opinion exist, however, and Herron[21] reports that patients with degenerative spondylolisthesis do just as well with decompression alone, without fusion. What is the best way to fuse? We use an intertransverse process fusion of only the olisthetic vertebra on the one below it. Is internal fixation advisable? Because of the availability of pedicle screws and the ability to fuse very short segments, it may be. The question then arises: Is decompression necessary if one can pull the olisthetic vertebra back into place, spread it apart somewhat, and keep it in the proper degree of lordosis by internal fixation with pedicle screws? Perhaps decompression is not necessary if a reduction can be accomplished. Farfan[11] has for years been an advocate of pulling the olisthetic vertebra backward and not performing decompression.

Should the L5–S1 level also be fused in cases of L4–L5 degenerative spondylolisthesis? It is our belief that in the elderly patient, it is seldom necessary to perform two-level fusion for L4–L5 olisthesis (Fig. 19).

Should retrodisplacement be considered a form of spondylolisthesis and be included in the classification? We believe that it should not. It does not fulfill the requirements of the meaning of the word, because olisthesis means to slip or slide down an incline. In retrodisplacement, the vertebra above slides posteriorly on the one below.

The word "retrolisthesis" is often used to describe this condition, but we prefer *retrodisplacement*. It is primarily a disease of the disc, and the posterior elements may be normal or nearly so.

DISCUSSION

Several articles in the literature state that the division between congenital and isthmic spondylolisthesis is an artificial one and should be abandoned in the classification, because both have hereditary aspects. We have considered this statement but have continued describing the division because the classification presented here is anatomic and only incidentally etiologic. It does seem to us that continuing this separation is indicated, because the case with an intact posterior arc responds differently as olisthesis progresses compared with that having a separate arc, as in the case of pars fractures. Consider the child with an intact posterior ring at L5 and a wide-open sacrum, axially oriented facets between L5 and S1, a 30% slip, and severe hamstring tightness. Should such a child be classified in the same manner as the young athlete with fresh fractures of the pars but otherwise normal anatomy? We believe not.

Another reason for separating the anatomic types is that proper surgical treatment can be quite different.

We left the acute pars fracture resulting from major trauma out of this classification, because it is very rare and virtually never occurs as an isolated lesion, but rather is seen as part of other severe bony injuries to the vertebra. This had been included in a previous classification in which the senior author participated.

SUMMARY

In the classification presented here, we recognize that there is great overlap in the fundamental causes of Types I and II. For example, we find in our consanguinity studies that both have a strong etiologic hereditary component. Both have dysplasia of the facets, and both have an increased incidence of spina bifida. Types IIA and IIB are actually the same disease, except that the pars has healed in Type IIB.

However, important anatomic differences affect prognosis and treatment. For this reason, we have chosen to continue to separate the congenital (dysplastic) from the isthmic and have presented an anatomic classification. We believe that the division will help the physician in his surgical treatment of the patient. We have also chosen to use the word *congenital* instead of "dysplastic" since both types have dysplastic articular processes. Admittedly, we run into some problems with the word congenital, because both types have so many congenital elements within their causes.

The section on surgical treatment presents the methods that the senior author has used for many years with what he believes to be generally good results. In no way is there an attempt to cover the whole field of surgery for spondylolisthesis.

References

1. Albinase, M., and Pizzutillo, P.D.: Family study of spondylolysis and spondylolisthesis. J. Pediatr. Orthop. 2:496–499, 1982.
2. Amuso, S.J., and Mankin, H.J.: Hereditary spondylolisthesis and spina bifida. J. Bone Joint Surg. 49A:507–513, 1967.
3. Apel, D., Lorenz, M., and Zindrick, M.: Symptomatic spondylolisthesis in adults four decades later (awaiting publication, Spine).
4. Armstrong, G.W.D., and Ye, C.B.: Sacral configuration in dysplastic spondylolisthesis (abstr.). J. Bone Joint Surg. 67B:335, 1985.
5. Baker, D.R., and McHolick, W.: Spondylolisthesis and spondylolisthesis in children. J. Bone Joint Surg. 38A:933, 1956.
6. Borkow, S.E., and Kleiger B.: Spondylolisthesis in the newborn, a case report. Clin. Orthop. 81:73–76, 1971.
7. Buck, J.E.: Direct repair of the defect in spondylolysis. J. Bone Joint Surg. 52B:432–437, 1970.
8. Burski, G., McCall, I.W., and O'Brien, J.P.: Myelography in severe lumbosacral spondylolisthesis. J. Bone Joint Surg. 57B:1067–1072, 1984.
9. Crock, H.V.: Observations on management of failed spinal operations. J. Bone Joint Surg. 58B:193, 1976.
10. Dandy, D.J., and Shannon, M.J.: Lumboscral subluxation. J. Bone Joint Surg. 53B:578–592, 1971.
11. Farfan, H.F.: Mechanical Disorders of the Low Back. Philadelphia, Lea & Febiger, 1973.
12. Farfan, H.F.: Personal communication. January, 1988.
13. Ferguson, R.J., McMarter, J.H., and Stanelski, C.L.: Low back pain in college football linemen. Am. J. Sports Med. 2:63–69, 1974.
14. Fitzgerald, J., and Newman P.: Degenerative spondylolisthesis. J. Bone Joint Surg. 58B:184, 1976.
15. Fredrickson, B.E., Baker, D.R., McHolick, W.J., et al.: The natural history of spondylolysis and spondylolisthesis. J. Bone Joint Surg. 66A:699–700, 1984.
16. Gill, G.G.: Long-term follow-up evaluation of a few patients with spondylolisthesis treated by excision of the loose lamina without spinal fusion. Clin. Orthop. 182:215–219, 1984.
17. Gill, G.G., Manning, J.G., and White, H.L.: Surgical treatment of spondylolisthesis without spinal fusion. J. Bone Joint Surg. 33A:493–520, 1955.
18. Harris, I., and Weinstein, S.: Long-term follow-up of spondylolisthesis. J. Bone Joint Surg. 69A:960, 1987.
19. Haukipuro, K., Keranen, N., Koivisto, E., et al.: Familial occurrence of lumbar spondylolysis and spondylolisthesis. Clin. Genet. 13:471–476, 1978.
20. Herbinaux, G.: Traite sur Divers Accouchement Laborieux et sur les Polypes de la Matrice. Bruxelles, De Boubers, 1782.
21. Herron, L., and Trippi, A.: L4–L5 degenerative spondylolisthesis: The results of treatment by decompressive laminectomy without fusion (accepted for publication, Spine, 1988).
22. Hult, L.: The Munkfors investigation. Acta Orthop. Scand. Suppl.:16, 1954.
23. Hutton, W.C., and Cyron, B.M.: Spondylolysis: The role of the posterior elements in resisting the intervertebral compressive force. Acta Orthop. Scand. 49:604–409, 1978.
24. Jackson, D.W., Wiltse, L.L., and Cirincione, R.J.: Spondylolisthesis in the female gymnast. Clin. Orthop. 117:68–73, 1976.
25. Johnson, J.R., and Kerwin, E. O'G.: The long-term results of fusion in situ for severe spondylolisthesis. J. Bone Joint Surg. 65B:43, 1983.
26. Karaharjii, E., and Hunnuksela, M.: Possible syphilitic spondylitis. Acta Orthop. Scand. 44:289, 1973.
27. Kilian, H.F.: Schilderungen neuer Beckenformen and ihres Verhalten im leben Bassermann und Mathy (cit da Brocher). Mannheim, 1854.
28. Knuttsen, F.: Instability associated with disc degeneration. Acta Radiol. 15:593, 1944.

28a. Lambl, W.: Beitrage zur Geburtskunde und Gynäckologie. Von F.W. v. Scanzoni, 1885.

29. Lee, C.K.: Lumbar instability (olisthesis) after extensive posterior spinal decompression. Spine 82:429–433, 1983.
30. Lombardi, J., Wiltse, L.L., Reynolds, J., et al.: Treatment of degenerative spondylolisthesis. Spine 10:821, 1985.
31. Macnab, I.: Spondylolisthesis with an intact neural arch: The so-called pseudospondylolisthesis. J. Bone Joint Surg. 32:325, 1950.
32. McCarroll, J.R., Miller, J.M., and Ritter, M.A.: Lumbar spondylolysis and spondylolisthesis in college football players. Am. J. Sports Med. 14:404–406, 1986.
33. Morscher, E., Gerber, B., and Fasel, J.: Surgical treatment of spondylolysis by bone grafting and direct stabilization of the spondylolysis by means of a hook screw. Arch. Orthop. Trauma Surg. 103:175–178, 1984.
34. Neugebauer, F.I.: Die entschung der spondylolisthesis. Zentrabl. Gynaekol. 5:260–261, 1881.
35. Newman, P.H.: The etiology of spondylolisthesis. J. Bone Joint Surg. 45B:39, 1963.

36. Newman, P.H.: A clinical syndrome associated with severe lumbosacral subluxation. J. Bone Joint Surg. 47B:472–481, 1965.
37. Neuwirth, M.: Dysplastic and isthmic spondylolisthesis. Bull. Hosp. Joint Dis. Orthop. Inst. 41:95–104, 1981.
37a. Nicol, R. O., and Scott, J.: Lytic spondylolysis: Repair by wiring (abstract). J. Bone Joint Surg. 67B:673, 1985.
38. Nicol, R.O., and Seall, J.H.S.: Lytic spondylolysis repair by wiring. Spine 11:127–130, 1987.
39. Oakley, R.H., and Carty, H.: Review of spondylolysis and spondylolisthesis in pediatric practice. Bone Joint Radiol. 57:877–885, 1984.
40. Ohata, H.: Spondylolysis: Familial occurrence and its genetic implication. J. Jpn. Orthop. Assoc. 41: 931–941, 1967.
41. Oland, C., Rineberg, B., Malberg, M., and Fried, S.: Fracture of the pedicle associated with contralateral spondylolysis. J. Bone Joint Surg. 68A:1454–1455, 1986.
42. Patwordhan, A., Lorenz, M., Orenstein, E., et al.: A biomechanical study of spina bifida occulta (awaiting publication, Spine).
43. Peek, R.D., Wiltse, L.L., Reynolds, J.B., et al.: In situ arthrodesis without decompression for Grade III or IV isthmic spondylolisthesis in adults with severe sciatica (accepted for publication, J. Bone Joint Surg.).
44. Pfeil, J., Niethard, F., and Cotta, N.: Pathogenesis of pediatric spondylolisthesis. Z. Orthop. 125:526–533, 1987.
45. Porter, R.W., and Hibbert, C.S.: Symptoms associated with lysis of the pars interarticularis. Spine 9:755–785, 1984.
46. Rask, M.R.: Spondylolisthesis resulting from osteogenesis imperfecta. Clin. Orthop. 139:164–166, 1979.
47. Reynolds, J.R., and Wiltse, L.L.: Degenerative Spondylolisthesis. Paper presented at the meeting of the International Society for the Study of the Lumbar Spine. San Francisco, June, 1978.
48. Reynolds, J.B., and Wiltse, L.L.: The Surgical Treatment of High-Grade Spondylolisthesis in Children by In Situ Fusion. Paper presented at the meeting of the International Society for the Study of the Lumbar Spine. Cambridge, England, spring, 1982.
49. Robert (zu Koblenz): Eine eigentumliche angeborene Lordose, wahrseheinlich bedingt eine Verschiebung des Korpers des letzten Lindenwirbels auf die vordere Flache des ersten Kreuzheinwirbels (Spondylolisthesis Kilian) nebst Bermerlsungen uber due Mechanik dieser Beckenformation. Monatsschr. Geburtskunde Frauenkrank 5:891–894, 1855.
50. Rosenberg, N.J.: Degenerative spondylolisthesis, Predisposing Factors. J. Bone Joint Surg. 57A:467, 1975.
51. Rosenberg, N.J.: Degenerative spondylolisthesis, surgical treatment. Clin. Orthop. 117:112, 1976.
52. Rothman, S.L., and Glenn, W.V.: CT multiplanar reconstruction in 253 cases of lumbar spondylolysis. Am. J. Neuroradiol. 5:81–90, 1984.
53. Rowe, C.G., and Roche, M.B.: The etiology of separate neural arch. J. Bone Joint Surg. 35A:102, 1953.
54. Saraste, H.: Prognostic radiologic aspects of spondylolisthesis. Acta Radiol. 25:427–432, 1984.
55. Saraste, H.: Radiologic assessment of anatomic deviation in lumbar spondylolysis. Acta Radiol. Diagn. (Stockh.) 25:317–323, 1984.
56. Saraste, H.: The etiology of spondylolisthesis. Acta Orthop. Scand. 56:253–255, 1985.
57. Saraste, H.: Spondylolysis and pregnancy—a risk analysis. Acta Obstet. Gynecol. Scand. 65:727–729, 1986.
58. Saraste, H.: A radiological follow up of spondylolysis and spondylolisthesis. J. Pediatr. Orthop. 7:631–638, 1987.
59. Schulitz, K.P., and Lethard, N.: Strain on the interarticular stress distribution. Arch. Orthop. Trauma Surg. 95:197–202, 1980.
60. Schultz, A.H. (Dir. Inst. Anthrop., Zurich, Switzerland): Personal communication, 1962.
61. Semon, R.L., and Spengler, D.: Significance of lumbar spondylolysis in college football players. Spine 6:172, 1981.
62. Splithoff, C.A.: The lumbosacral junction. J. Am. Med. Assoc. 152:1610–1613, 1957.
63. Szappanos, L., Szepesi, K., and Thomazy, V.: Spondylolisthesis in osteopetrosis (awaiting publication, J. Bone Joint Surg. [Br.]).
64. Taillard, W.: Etiology of spondylolisthesis. Clin. Orthop. 117:30–39, 1976.
65. Troup, D.: Paper presented at the meeting of the International Society for the Study of the Lumbar Spine. London, 1975.
66. Troup, J.D.G.: The etiology of spondylolisthesis. Orthop. Clin. North Am. 8:59–64, 1977.
67. West, F.: Personal communication.
68. White, A.H., and Wiltse, L.L.: Spondylolisthesis after extensive lumbar laminectomy. J. Bone Joint Surg. (Proc.) 57A:727, 1975.
69. Wiltse, L.L.: Etiology of spondylolisthesis. J. Bone Joint Surg. 44A:539–560, 1962.
70. Wiltse, L.L.: Fatigue fracture: The basic lesion in isthmic spondylolisthesis. J. Bone Joint Surg. 57A:17–22, 1975.
71. Wiltse, L.L., Bateman, J.G., and Hutchinson, R.H.: The paraspinal sacrospinalis-splitting approach to the lumbar spine. J. Bone Joint Surg. 50A:919, 1968.
72. Wiltse, L.L., Guyer, R.D., Spencer, C.W., et al.: Alar transverse process impingement of the L5 spinal nerve: The far out syndrome. Spine 9:31–41, 1984.
73. Wiltse, L.L., Neuman, P.H., and Macnab, I.: Classification of spondylolisthesis. Clin. Orthop. 117:23–29, 1976.
74. Wiltse, L.L., and Winter, R.B.: Terminology and measurement in spondylolisthesis. J. Bone Joint Surg. 65A:768–772, 1983.
75. Winter, R.B.: Congenital kyphosis. J. Bone Joint Surg. 55A:223–256, 1973.
76. Wynne-Davies, R., and Scott, J.H.S.: Inheritance and spondylolisthesis: A radiographic family survey. J. Bone Joint Surg. (Br.) 61B:301–305, 1979.
77. Yano, T., Meyagi, S., and Ikari, T.: Studies of familial incidence of spondylolisthesis. Singapore Med. J. 8:203, 1967.
78. Zembo, M.M., Roberts, J.M., Burke, S.W., et al.: Congenital spondylolisthesis. Paper presented at Scoliosis Research Society 21st Annual Meeting. Bermuda, September, 1986.

CONSERVATIVE TREATMENT

Kazimiera Milanowska

The aims of therapy for patients with symptomatic spondylolisthesis are as follows:

1. Elimination of pain by relieving compressed nerve roots.
2. Strengthening of trunk muscles by forming a strong "muscle corset" and restoring stability of the spine.
3. Good posture and physical efficiency for functional and work capacity.

None of the treatment methods, independent of the type of spondylolisthesis, effects normal anatomic spine structure and its full physiologic efficacy. Thus, the patient should be informed about the character of changes and the prognosis, and should actively cooperate in his or her treatment. An informative educational type of treatment should be established. The patient should be fully aware that the results of treatment, prevention of changes, progress, and recurrence of pain depend, to a great extent, on the patient's compliance with instructions for systematic rehabilitation treatment, and way of life and work.

The best therapeutic results can be obtained when treatment is based on a full understanding of pathogenesis and pathomechanisms of the changes. In order to reach the three treatment aims mentioned above, therapy cannot be based on one method only—it must be a complex procedure.

In regard to the question of whether therapy should be conservative or surgical, the majority of centers treating patients with spondylolisthesis are of the opinion that Grades I and II, according to the Meyerding classification,[3] as well as degenerative spondylolisthesis are usually treated conservatively.[4] Very often, the decision is made by the patient, who does not agree to surgical treatment and insists on being treated conservatively. Results of conservative rehabilitation treatment in 35 patients with isthmic, dysplastic, and degenerative spondylolisthesis are given later in this chapter.

CHOICE OF CONSERVATIVE REHABILITATION TREATMENT

Based on the available body of knowledge, the treatment of patients with symptomatic spondylolisthesis depends on the clinical presentation and the physical and laboratory findings.

The clinical manifestations of spondylolisthesis are fairly typical of a mechanical disorder.[3] Once the symptoms are initiated, the patient has some constant back discomfort, which is aggravated by such activities as carrying heavy loads and taking long walks and is relieved by rest. Back pain, buttock pain, and radicular pain down to the thigh, leg, or foot are the most frequent findings.[1]

By examining the standing patient, many changes in posture are observed. Shortening of the lumbar part of the trunk, increase of lumbar lordosis (a backward tilt to the pelvis), stiffness of the lumbar spine, hamstring tightness, and a crease in the abdomen occur. On the level of spondylolisthesis there occurs (often palpably) a "step-off" or dimple in the midline at the site of the abnormality.[3]

The patient has typical gait, well-described by Newman[7] and by Phalen and Dickson,[8] with the knees slightly flexed and a tendency to walk on the toes.

Pressure on the nerve roots causes such neurologic symptoms as sensory loss, decreased ankle reflex, and weakness and atrophy of thigh and other leg muscles.

The above-presented clinical picture is a consequence of multidirectional pathologic changes (e.g., those in the intervertebral joints, ligaments, and joint capsules of the spine), which lead to collision of bone elements and nerve roots, and the spinal cord and blood vessels. The damage and flaccidity of spine elastic elements bring about the instability, which itself is the pain-causing factor. Understanding this picture of changes influences the choice of the most effective treatment.

Since 1973, the Rehabilitation Department, Academy of Medicine in Poznań, has elaborated and introduced a complex, systematic rehabilitation training program for patients with back pain, and it has been found to be effective in a large patient population.[6]

Conservative rehabilitation treatment for patients with acute pain syndrome is described below.

First Week

Bed Rest

The most important element of therapy in patients with acute pain syndrome is an adequate period of bed rest. It is expected that the patient remain at complete bed rest, except for having bathroom privileges. For the short period of ambulation necessary to reach the bathroom, I supply the patient with crutches. Crutches provide some relief for the spine and decrease pain during walking. The patient should be placed on a flat bed in the most comfortable and pain-free position. This is usually lying on the back or on the side with the lower extremities flexed in hip and knee joints. This position decreases lumbar lordosis and pelvic anteversion and loosens painful tension in the spine and in the ischiofemoral muscles. Placing a rolled pillow or a composition rubber wad under the knees of the patient (Fig. 1) further increases the comfort of bed rest.

Physical Therapy

Hot paraffin compresses are applied to the lumbar part of the spine, the pelvis, and the lower extremity to which the pain is radiating. The patient is wheeled on the cart in the lying position to the room in which the procedure will be carried out. If the patient does not tolerate hot paraffin compresses (i.e., if a secondary inflammatory reaction occurs), naturally, this procedure is cancelled.

Pain-relieving analgesic electrotherapy, such as diadynamic currents, interferential currents (Nemeca), and anode galvanization are applied. These procedures bring about a marked decrease of pain in the majority of patients.

During this time (i.e., during the first week and bed rest), isometric exercise for the trunk muscles, especially the abdominal muscles, breathing exercises, and active exercises of upper extremities are introduced. These exercises are carried out in a position with good pelvic stabilization and removal of lumbar lordosis; that is, when all factors that may cause or increase pain are eliminated.

Early and properly performed manipulation in Grade 1 and Grade 2 spondylolisthesis, with a slight blockade and good bolting possibilities, brings immediate relief in many patients. It should be taken into consideration, however, that by means of manipulation only functional, reversible spine changes are removed. Thus, manipulation can be included in therapy as one of many procedures present in the complex rehabilitation treatment program for patients with back pain.

Second Week: Pelvic Traction

After the disappearance of acute pain syndrome, pelvic traction in bed with the initial

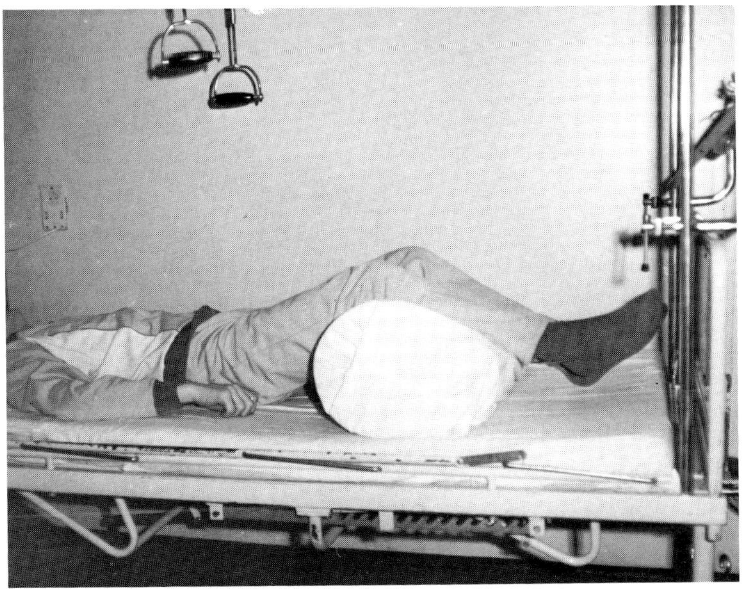

Figure 1 □ Position for bed rest.

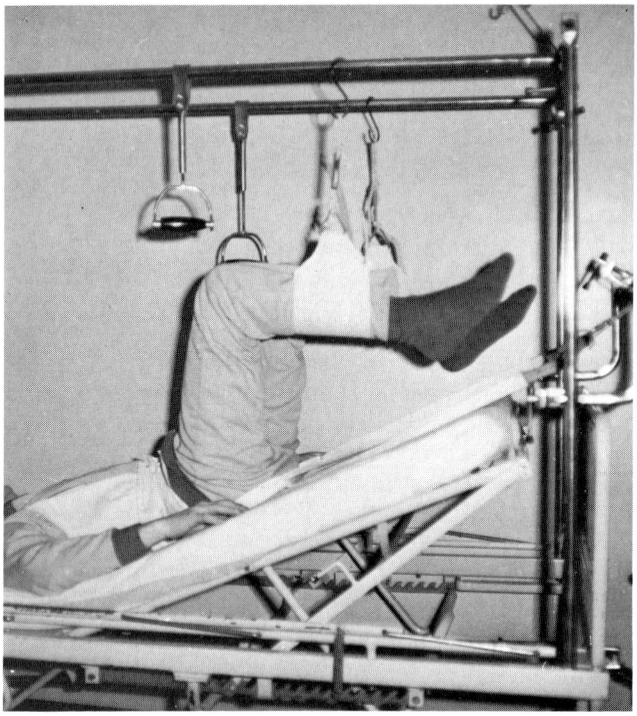

Figure 2 □ Pelvic stable traction on the bed.

load reaching one eighth of the patient's weight (6 to 10 kg) is introduced (Fig. 2). The aims of the traction are as follows:

1. Decompression of intravertebral spaces.
2. Increase of intervertebral foraminal lumen.
3. Widening of spaces between the vertebral corpora.[2]

In cases of pain increase after the traction, which happens in patients who have secondary inflammatory reactions, such a procedure is cancelled.

Isometric exercises of the trunk muscles are continued, and after hot paraffin compresses and electrotherapy, exercises stretching and relaxing the spinal muscles are applied (Figs. 3 to 7). These exercises are particularly advisable in cases of pain-rephlectoric scoliosis and strongly positive Lasègue symptoms. These exercises are carried out in positions with good pelvic stabilization and elimination of lumbar lordosis (i.e., with lower extremities flexed in hip and knee joints).

Autotraction by means of pulling back the pelvis with hands in the outward direction is also recommended (Fig. 3). Besides, the hand pressure on the iliac crest eliminates

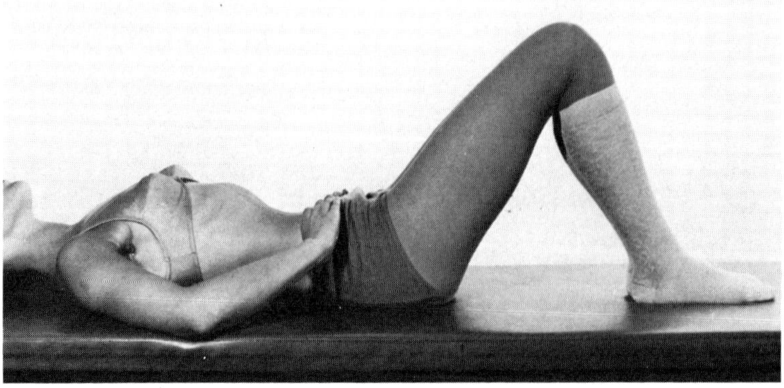

Figure 3 □ Autotraction.

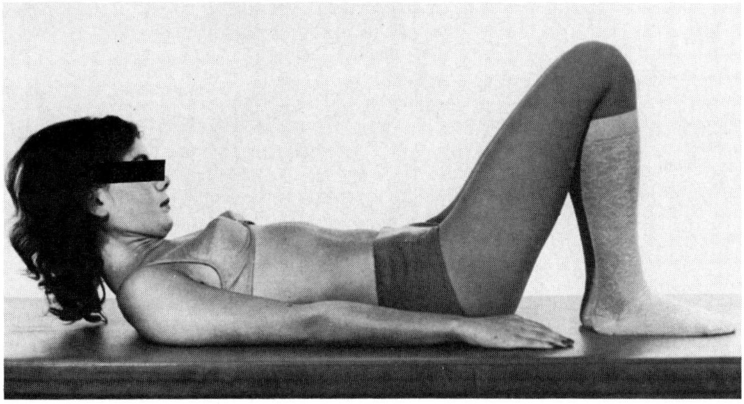

Figure 4 □ Isometric exercises for abdominal muscles.

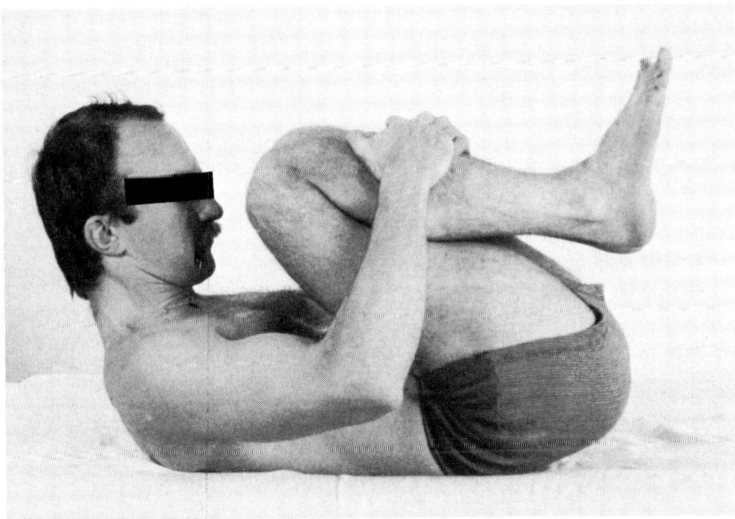

Figure 5 □ Stretching exercises for spinal muscles.

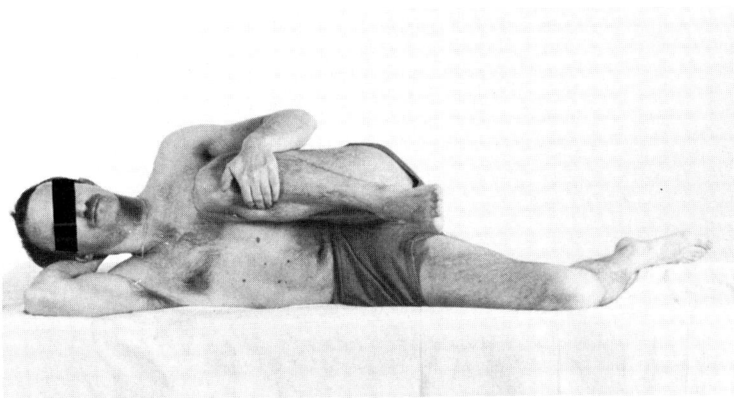

Figure 6 □ Stretching exercises for spinal muscles.

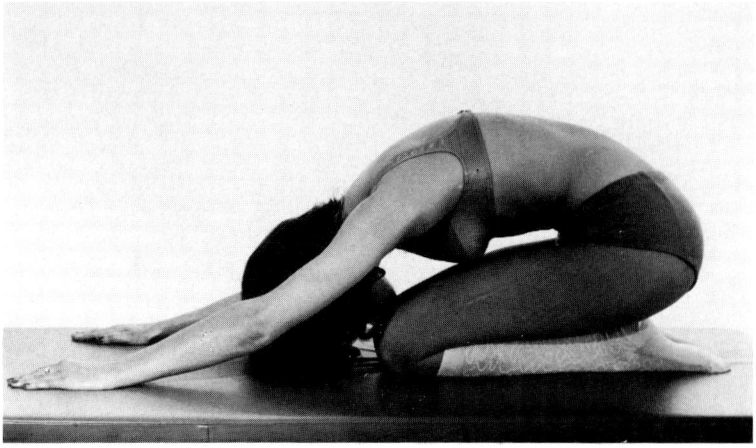

Figure 7 □ Relaxing exercises of the spine.

development of synchronic contractions of abdominal oblique muscles and spinal extensors. Training of rephlectoric mechanisms of abdominal and spinal muscles can reduce by 30% the pressure on the vertebrae in the lower part of the trunk.[5]

Third week: Intermittent Traction

After a few days of traction in bed, intermittent traction on the traction table with a gradual load increase of up to one half of the patient's weight (30 to 40 kg) is introduced (Fig. 8). Intermittent traction is applied after hot paraffin compresses are given over a 12- to 14-day period. Directly after the traction, the patient is lying on his or her back with lower extremities flexed in hip and knee joints for about 1 hour. Still, exercises stretching spinal muscles are continued, and dynamic exercises strengthening trunk muscles are gradually introduced (Figs. 9 to 13). Dynamic exercises are aimed toward achieving spine stabilization.

Fourth Week to Sixth Week: Kinesitherapy

The intensity of exercises is gradually increased, paying attention, first of all, to the strengthening of abdominal, spinal, and gluteal muscles until a strong muscular corset is formed (Figs. 14 to 16). Exercises for the purpose of obtaining proper posture of the body—mainly, lessening of lumbar lordosis and forward tilt of the pelvis—are also applied. During exercises, great attention is paid to the pain factor. The intensification

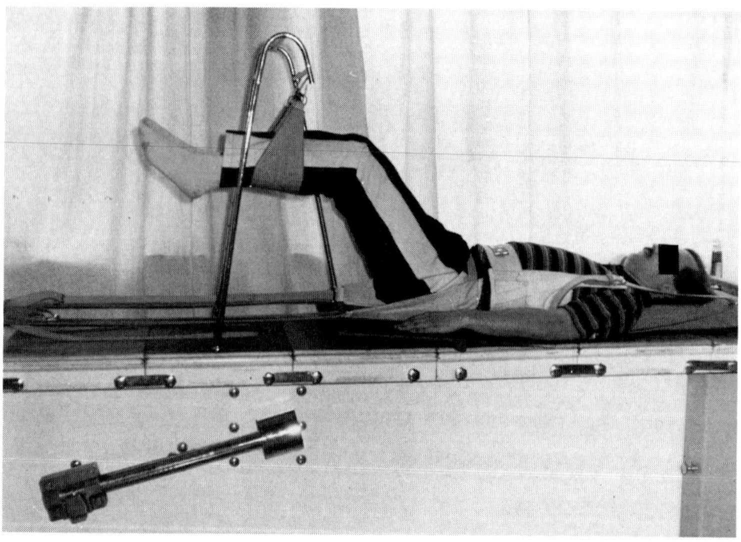

Figure 8 □ Pelvic traction on the traction table.

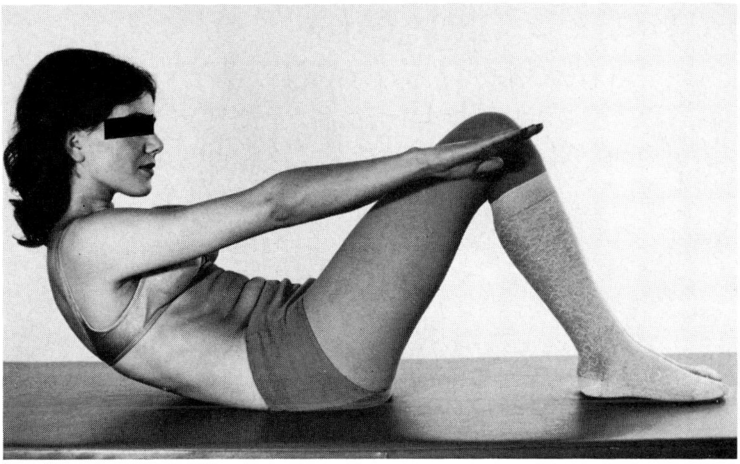

Figure 9 □ Dynamic exercises of abdominal muscles (upper part).

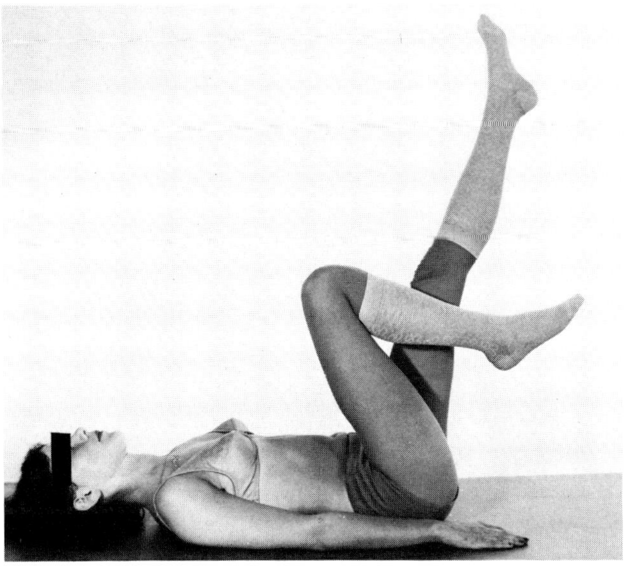

Figure 10 □ Dynamic exercises of abdominal muscles (lower part).

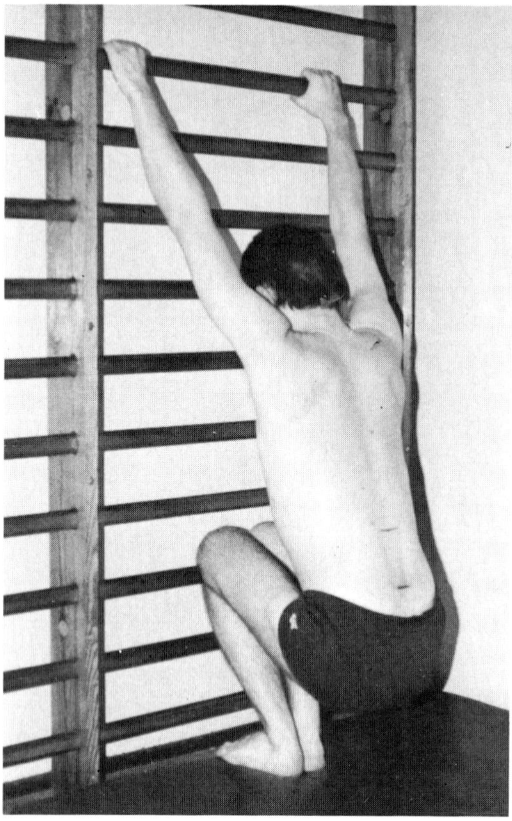

Figure 11 □ Dynamic stretching exercises of the spine.

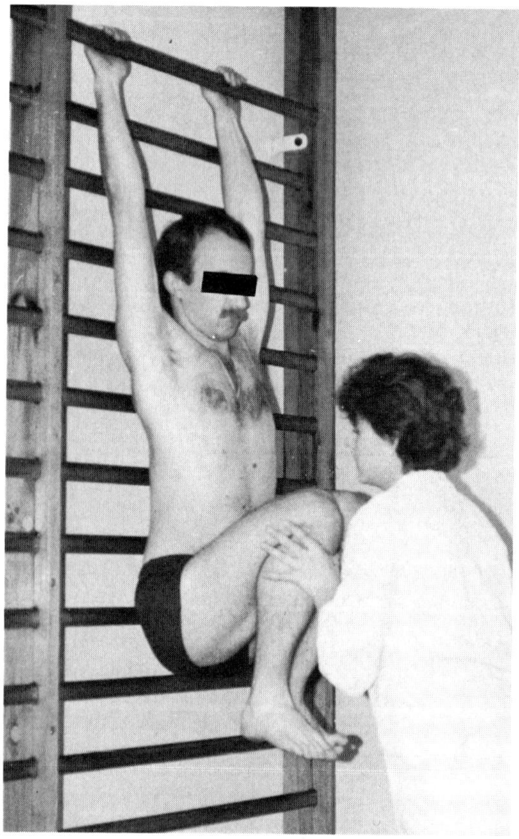

Figure 12 □ Dynamic stretching exercises of abdominal and spinal muscles.

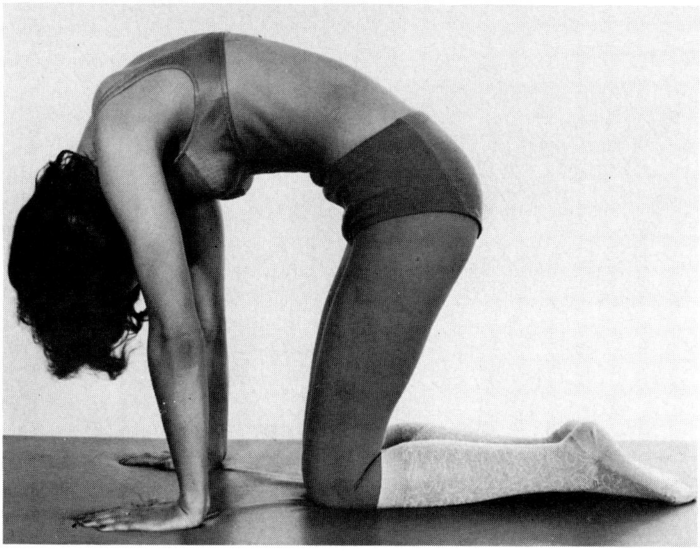

Figure 13 □ Dynamic stretching exercises of the spine ("cat back").

or occurrence of pain during exercise calls for a revision and an analysis of applied exercises, eventual changes in exercise program, or elimination of some exercises. The purpose of the basic re-educational and corrective exercises is restoration of normal spine statokinetics. It is necessary to conduct them systematically, with graduated intensity, starting from exercises performed first in a lying position, then in half-lying, sitting, and standing positions. Classic exercises strengthening trunk muscles, which consist of strenuous flexion and rotation of the trunk that reproduce movements and postures causing back pain, are very harmful.

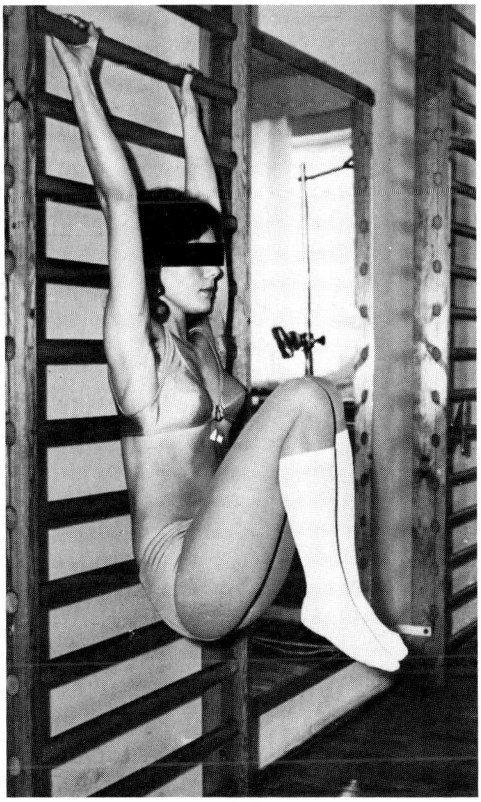

Figure 14 □ Dynamic exercises of abdominal muscles.

After a complete decline in pain, apart from individual exercises, patients take part in group exercises with appropriately chosen movements. They may also exercise in water and swim in a pool with a water temperature of 28° to 30°C.

Patients with low back pain syndrome are being treated, for an average of 6 weeks, in the Rehabilitation Department. After the patient is discharged from the hospital, he or she is advised to exercise systematically for 20 to 30 minutes a day. The aims of these systematic exercises, performed every day, are the formation of a strong muscle corset and good body posture, and the development and maintenance of high physical efficiency. The patient must be clearly informed that only with such treatment may he or she avoid recurrences and regain functional and work capacity.

It is also important to recommend a weight reduction program if the patient is obese. Furthermore, the patient is also instructed about how to live and work with the back problem.

The individual is instructed to sleep on

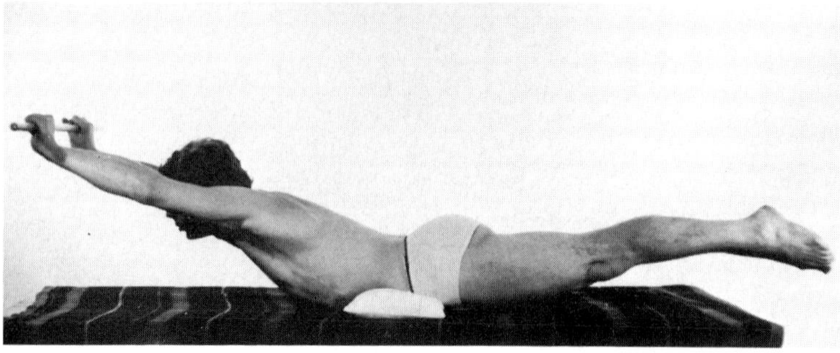

Figure 15 □ Dynamic exercises of spinal and gluteal muscles.

one side or on the back with the knees and hips in a position of flexion. The patient is cautioned against lying in the prone position, which hyperextends the lumbar spine. When sitting in a chair, the individual should sit with the buttocks well forward and the spine in a flexed position. Crossing the legs while seated adds flexion to this position and is also desirable. A rocking chair has been advertised for persons with back problems (Fig. 17).

In everyday activities, especially in housework, when one is performing activities that demand a standing position, one should assume the posture that least overloads the lumbar spine. This is the standing position, with lower extremities slightly flexed in hip and knee joints and the trunk straight. When performing activities demanding longer periods of standing, it is recommended that one support the pelvis or prop up the buttocks against any piece of furniture. In general, long periods of standing and sitting are not recommended.

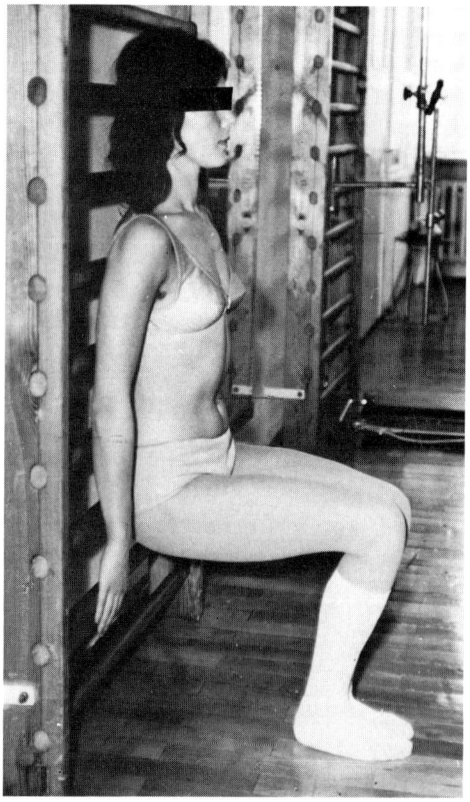

Figure 16 □ Postural exercises.

Carrying and transporting heavy loads are particularly significant in spine overloading. Thus, the patient must be instructed on how to carry and transport heavy loads. While picking up heavy objects from the ground, one should assume the following position: half knee-bending, legs astride and feet parallel, trunk straight, arms close to the trunk, elbows flexed, and chin directed toward the chest. Picking up the load in this position, we keep it close to the trunk. The above positioning of the feet shifts the center of gravity forward and toward the midline, thus increasing body stability and preventing a slip.

The patients, especially those working, are encouraged to rest for 1 hour during the day with the lower extremities flexed in hip and knee joints.

Those patients with less stable spondylolisthesis are provided with a lumbosacral corset, which reduces the forward pelvic tilt, to wear during the day for a period of a few months.

Post-Hospital Treatment

Spa treatment is recommended for patients with spondylolisthesis, especially for those with the degenerative type. Many spas in Europe provide balneophysical treatment for patients with back pain. The most beneficial procedures for patients with back pain are

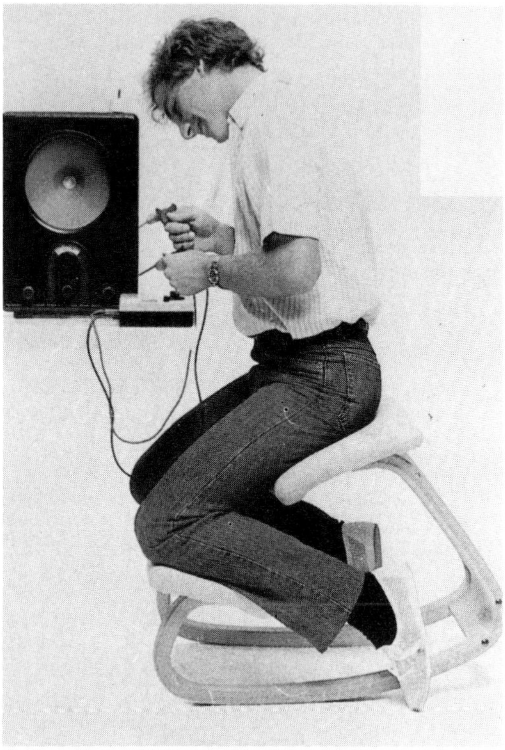

Figure 17 □ Application of the rocking chair at work.

hot peloid-mud compresses or mud baths; pelvic traction in water; underwater massage of the back, buttocks, and lower extremities; and corrective and generally rehabilitating exercises.

My department has 15 beds in Cieplice Sl. Spa, in the south of Poland, where patients are sent for a 24-day post-hospital rehabilitation. The spa physician and therapists are trained in treatment of back pain patients and continue the rehabilitation program devised in the hospital rehabilitation department.

The patients with irreversible spine changes, the category to which persons with spondylolisthesis belong, should be under the constant care of a specialized outpatient department. There is one in the Rehabilitation Department of Academy of Medicine in Poznań. This outpatient department takes care of patients treated in the Rehabilitation Department and those who need only ambulatory observation and treatment. It also carries out systematic checkup examinations (every 6 to 12 weeks, depending on the indications), controls the methods of patients' exercising, and provides instruction regarding how to live and work in order to prevent recurrences and to develop good physical efficiency.

Conclusions

The following conclusions can be drawn in regard to the conservative treatment of patients who have symptomatic spondylolisthesis:

1. Conservative therapy for patients with symptomatic spondylolisthesis should be a form of complex rehabilitation treatment.
2. Kinesitherapy applied in patients with low back pain syndrome requires systematization and gradation; it should not increase pain.
3. The main aims of rehabilitation treatment of patients with spondylolisthesis are as follows:
   a. Strengthening of trunk muscles by forming strong "muscle corset" and restoring stability of the spine,
   b. Formation of good body posture and creation of good physical efficiency for functional and work capacity.
4. The "back school," which teaches the patients how to improve their management of back pain, has been shown to be the most effective way of educating them, preventing recurrences, and lowering the costs for society.

REMOTE RESULTS OF CONSERVATIVE REHABILITATION TREATMENT IN PATIENTS WITH LUMBAR SPONDYLOLISTHESIS

The aim of the following study is evaluation of conservative rehabilitation treatment in patients with isthmic, dysplastic, and degenerative spondylolisthesis.

Material of the Study

Thirty-five patients treated in the Institute of Orthopaedics and Rehabilitation in Poznań in the years 1968 to 1986 were evaluated (Table 1).

Table 1 □ Types of Spondylolisthesis

Isthmic	26
Dysplastic	5
Degenerative	4
	(Total) 35

On the basis of radiologic examinations, L4–L5 spondylolisthesis in 20 patients and L5–S1 in 15 patients were noted.

The observation period lasted from 5 to 18 years; in 15 patients it ranged from 11 to 18 years, and in 20 patients it ranged from 5 to 10 years. Of the studied group, most were between 40 and 49 years of age.

Method of Evaluation

The evaluation of treatment results was based on detailed clinical and radiologic assessments performed at the beginning of treatment and in November 1986. In the clinical examination, lumbar spine mobility and symptoms of neuromuscular disturbances (i.e., pain, the straight leg–raising test, reflexes, sensory disorders, and muscle strength) were evaluated.

In the radiologic examinations, I assessed x-ray studies of the lumbosacral spine in the anteroposterior, lateral, and oblique views, and functional studies in the sagittal plane.

The value of the slip was calculated in millimeters, according to the modified Meschane method (Fig. 18).

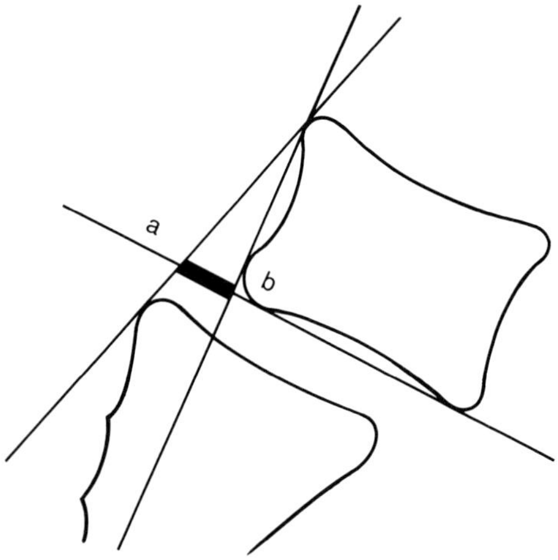

Segment a-b: size of the slip

Figure 18 □ The modified Meschane method.

Treatment

Conservative rehabilitation treatment consisted of the following:

1. In patients with acute back pain we applied absolute bed rest with hips and knees flexed, pelvic stable traction with increasing loads of from 6 to 16 kg, relaxation, and isometric exercises.
2. After pain elimination, systemized exercises were prescribed to strengthen abdominal and gluteal muscles, with particular attention paid to exercises decreasing pelvic tilt. In two children with unstable spondylolisthesis, a plaster corset lengthened to one thigh was applied for 3 months. For the next 3 months they wore Boston orthopedic corsets, and for 1 more year, Hohmann corsets.
3. After hospital treatment the patients were taken care of through the outpatient department, where systematic checkup examinations were performed every 6 to 12 weeks. During the examinations, physiotherapists control the method of doing recommended exercises, instruct patients on how to perform work (how to carry heavy objects), and what shoes to wear. One hour of bed rest during the day with flexed hips and knees is recommended.
4. All patients are provided with lumbosacral corsets, which decrease the pelvic tilt, to wear during the day for several months.

Results

In the checkup assessment in November, 1986, a regression of neurologic symptoms in 26 patients and a marked reduction of ailments in nine patients were found (Table 2).

Radiologic examinations showed a lack of slip progression in 22 patients and slip progressions ranging from 2 to 3 mm in 12 patients. In one patient with a slip progression of up to 6 mm, surgical treatment was applied (Table 3).

Twenty-two patients still work or study, and 13 persons retired or obtained an invalid's pension. Three case histories are described below.

T.K., CASE HISTORY NO. 22.257: 54-YEAR-OLD WOMAN WITH ISTHMIC L4–L5 SPONDYLOLISTHESIS

In 1972, the patient had an unstable slip of 7 mm (Fig. 19). In 1986, a stable slip of 9 mm was found (Fig. 20).

Treatment □ During the first 2 months (in the acute stage), the patient was treated with stable traction with increasing load from 6

Table 2 ☐ Results of Clinical Examinations Before Treatment and in November, 1986

	PAIN RADIATING TO LOWER EXTREMITY	THE STRAIGHT LEG-RAISING TEST			ASYMMETRY OF KNEE AND TARSAL REFLEXES	SENSORY DISTURBANCES	DEFICIENCY OF MUSCLE STRENGTH	SCHOBER'S SYMPTOM	
		30°	60°	Above 60°				Up to 3 cm	Above 3 cm
Before treatment	26	5	15	15	10	8	10	24	11
November, 1986	9	0	6	29	3	3	2	8	27

Table 3 □ Progression of Slip in Comparison with Preliminary Examinations

LEVEL	NUMBER OF PATIENTS FOR EACH INCREMENT OF SLIP				
	0 mm	2 mm	3 mm	6 mm	
L4–L5	10	4	5	1	20
L5–S1	12	2	1	0	15
					(Total) 35

to 20 kg, bed rest, and gradually increasing exercise leading to strengthening the muscle corset. Then a Boston corset was applied for 6 months, and systematic everyday exercise continued until the present.

Preliminary Examination (1972) □ Pain was radiating to the left lower extremity. There was weakness of the quadriceps muscle (4 degrees according to the Lovett scale).

Examinations in 1986 □ Periodic slight pains and normal muscle strength were found. The patient was fully active as a housewife.

M.P., CASE HISTORY NO. 28.607: 14-YEAR-OLD BOY WITH DYSPLASTIC L5–S1 SPONDYLOLISTHESIS

In 1981, an unstable slip of 8 mm was found (Fig. 21), and in 1986, there was a stable slip of 5 mm (Fig. 22).

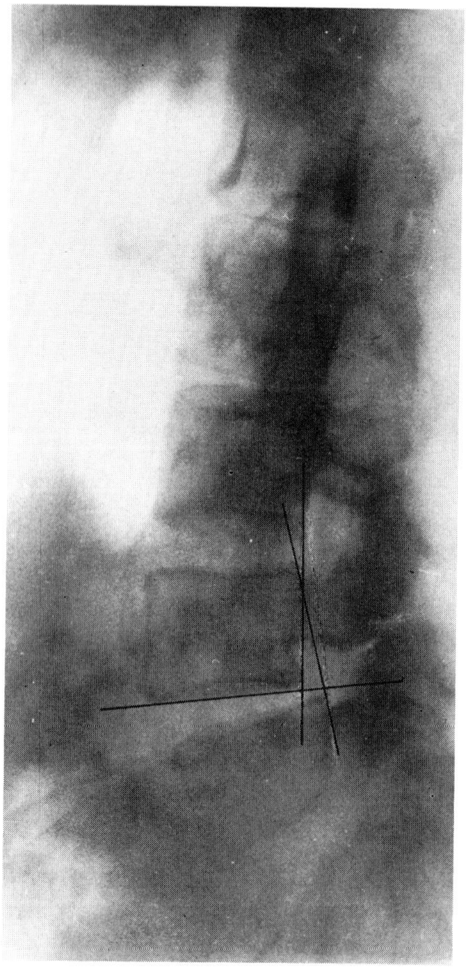

Figure 19 □ X-ray film of L4–L5 isthmic spondylolisthesis, unstable slip of 7 mm (case from 1972).

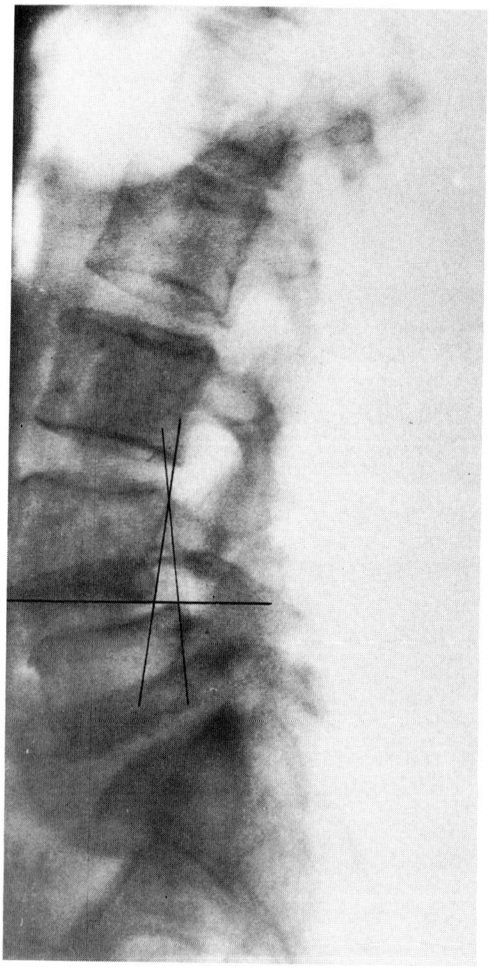

Figure 20 □ X-ray film of L4–L5 isthmic spondylolisthesis, stable slip of 9 mm (case from 1986).

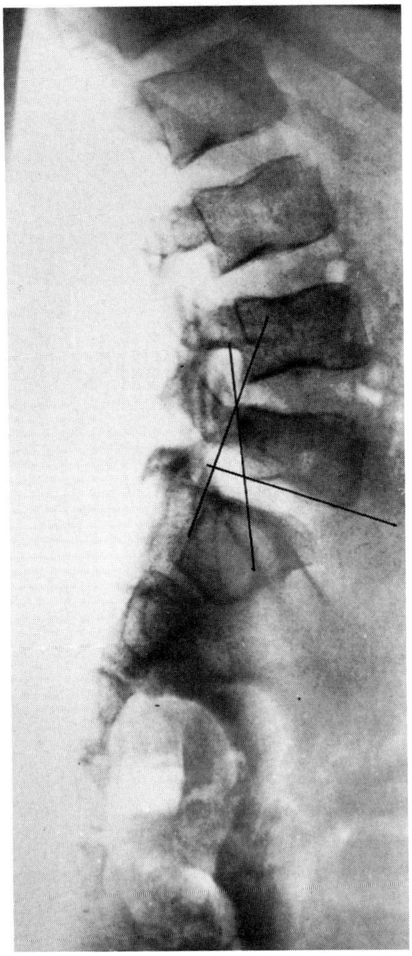

Figure 21 □ X-ray film of L5–S1 dysplastic spondylolisthesis, unstable slip of 8 mm (case from 1981).

Treatment □ For the first 3 months, a plaster corset lengthened to one thigh was applied. For the next 3 months, a Boston orthopedic corset was applied. This was followed by 1 year of wearing a Hohmann corset and introducing gradual exercises, including those strengthening the muscle corset.

Preliminary Examination (1981) □ Lumbosacral pain was radiating to lower extremities. The result of the straight-leg-raising test was 50 degrees. Sensory disturbances and a deficiency of muscle strength were found.

Examination in 1986 (After 5 Years) □ A regression of all symptoms and slight limitation of lumbar spine mobility were found. The boy leads a normal life.

W.N., CASE HISTORY NO. 29.219: 48-YEAR-OLD MAN WITH DEGENERATIVE L4–L5 SPONDYLOLISTHESIS

In 1980, unstable slip of 11 mm was seen (Fig. 23), and in 1986 there was a stable slip of 12 mm (Fig. 24).

Treatment □ During the first 2 months (in the acute stage), the patient was treated with stable traction with increasing loads of from 6 to 20 kg, bed rest, intermittent traction on a traction table with increasing loads of up to 35 kg, and gradually increasing exercise, leading to those strengthening the muscle corset. Physical therapy consisted of hot paraffin compresses on the back and the left lower extremity, interferential currents, and underwater massages. Then the Boston corset was applied, and systematic everyday exercises continued until the present. The

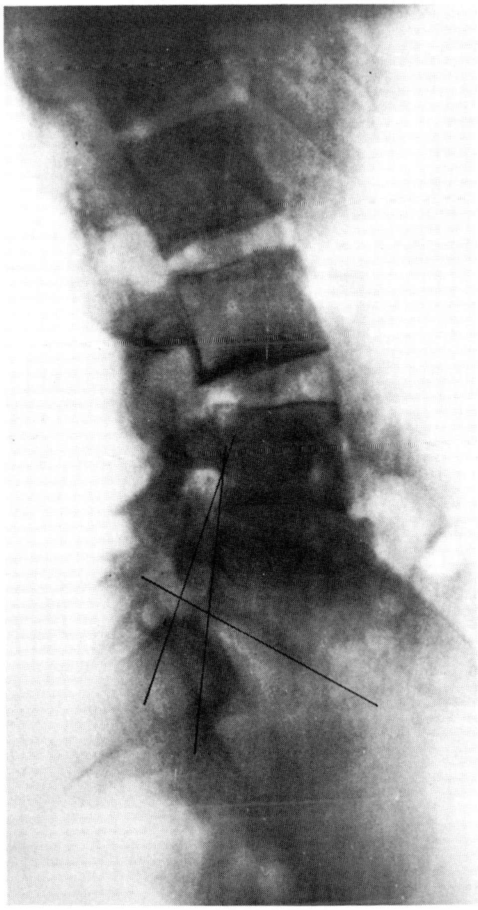

Figure 22 □ X-ray film of L5–S1 dysplastic spondylolisthesis, stable slip of 5 mm (case from 1986).

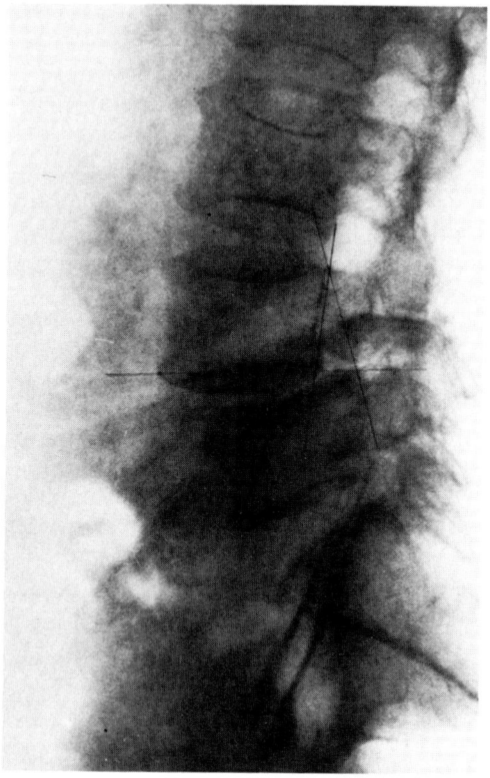

Figure 23 □ X-ray film of L4–L5 degenerative spondylolisthesis, unstable slip of 11 mm (case from 1980).

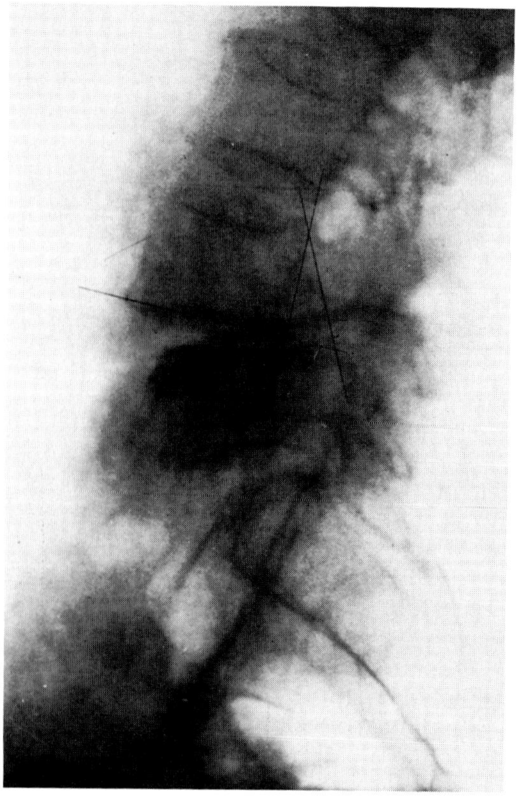

Figure 24 □ X-ray film of L4–L5 degenerative spondylolisthesis, stable slip of 12 mm (case from 1986).

patient attended back school and received spa treatment once a year.

Preliminary Examination (1980) □ Pain was radiating to the left lower extremity, and weakness of muscles in both lower extremities was found. The patient had sensory disturbances.

Examination in 1986 (After 6 years) □ The patient had a regression of all symptoms and full movement range in the lumbar spine. He returned to his previous work as a storekeeper.

References

1. Boxal, D., Bradford, D., Winter, R.B., and Moe, J.H.: Management of severe spondylolisthesis in children and adolescents. J. Bone Joint Surg. 61A:479–495, 1979.
2. Dega, W.: Ortopedia i Rehabilitacja (Orthopaedics and Rehabilitation). P.Z.W.L., Warsaw, 1983.
3. DePalma, A.F., and Rothman, R.H.: The Intervertebral Disc. Philadelphia, W.B. Saunders, 1970.
4. DeSmet, A.A.: Radiology of Spinal Curvature. St. Louis, C.V. Mosby, 1985.
5. Grochmal, St.: Profilaktyka zespolu bolow dolnego odcinka kregoslupa z przeciazenia praca zawodowa (Prophylactics of low back pain overloaded by work). Proc. Symp. Rehab. Comm. Pol. Acad. Sci. Warsaw, 1977.
6. Milanowska, K., Konieczna, D., and Bembnista, A.: Leczenie usprawniajace osob z zespolem bolow dolnego odcinka kregoslupa (Rehabilitating treatment of patients with low back pain). Proc. Symp. Rehab. Comm. Pol. Acad. Sci. Warsaw, 1978.
7. Newman, P.H.: The etiology of spondylolisthesis. J. Bone Joint Surg. 45B:39–59, 1963.
8. Phalen, G.S., and Dickson, J.A.: Spondylolisthesis and tight hamstrings. J. Bone Joint Surg. 43A:505, 1961.
9. Wynne-Davies R., and Scott J.H.S.: Inheritance and spondylolisthesis. J. Bone Joint Surg. 61B:301–305, 1979.

■ OPERATIVE TREATMENT: CHILDREN AND ADOLESCENTS

Edward N. Hanley, Jr.

Spondylolisthesis, the slippage of one vertebra on another, is the result of a loss of the mechanical integrity of the spinal column. Predominantly occurring at the lumbosacral articulation, it is thought to be accentuated by gravitational and postural forces acting on this area as a result of the upright human posture. Although a variety of predisposing factors have been described for spondylolisthesis in children, two types of vertebral slippage predominate in childhood: dysplastic (I) and isthmic (II).[48, 69]

Spondylolisthesis is rarely seen in infancy, but its incidence appears to increase between the ages of 5 and 8 years and stabilizes prior to the third decade of life.[1, 6, 21, 66, 70] Heredity and activity patterns, no doubt, influence its occurrence.[1, 6, 34–36, 38, 39, 57, 60, 65, 66, 69, 70] Progression, when it occurs, appears to predominate in those with the dysplastic type and to be correlated with the adolescence growth spurt.[3, 17, 61] Increasing slippage is infrequently seen thereafter. Symptoms of pain and/or neurologic dysfunction, commonly the presenting symptoms in adults, are less frequently seen in children and adolescents.[8, 17, 28, 35, 41] Although the majority of patients can be satisfactorily managed with nonoperative measures (i.e., rest, immobilization, exercises, and anti-inflammatory medication),[27–29, 48, 50, 60] a subset of individuals remains in whom symptoms or progression of deformity leads to consideration of surgical intervention. Knowledge of the natural history of the disease, risk factors for future problems, and the expected outcome of interventional treatment all play a role in therapeutic decision-making. Similarly, there is no one solution appropriate for all patients, and when operative treatment is elected, one must judiciously select the most appropriate surgical and postsurgical treatment plan for a particular individual. Although in situ arthrodesis remains the standard of operative care, there are instances in which other procedures such as isthmic defect repair or reduction may be indicated. Appropriate selection of the procedure for the patient and meticulous attention to details of the operation serve to minimize problems and complications while maximizing functional return.

RISK FACTORS IN SPONDYLOLISTHESIS

When an individual presents for evaluation or is being followed with a diagnosis of spondylolysis or spondylolisthesis, certain factors should be taken into consideration so that an appropriate treatment or monitoring regimen can be instituted. Clinical and radiographic "risk factors" that may portend a poor result with nonoperative measures should be weighed each time the patient is assessed. Although no exact formula exists for determining when to advise surgery, the following factors should be considered.[29]

Age □ The progression of spondylolisthesis is most likely to occur in individuals under the age of 15 and has been shown to be correlated with the adolescent growth spurt.[3, 17, 61] Significantly increased slippage subsequent to this period is unlikely.[8, 17, 24, 38, 61]

Pain □ Children with symptoms of back pain, particularly those whose painful symptoms are unresponsive to nonoperative measures, are more likely to require surgery. Likewise, if radicular symptoms are present, the likelihood of the need for surgical treatment to control these symptoms is higher. In addition, those with neural symptoms are likely to have a higher grade of slip (>50%), which in itself may be an indication for surgery.[25, 61]

Sex □ Females with spondylolisthesis are more likely to experience progression of displacement.[8, 17, 55, 68] This may be related to the generally more lax nature of their soft tissues.

Ligamentous Laxity □ Generalized laxity of the soft tissues may predispose individuals to progressive slippage. Assessment of joint hyperextension, skin laxity, or a family history of related conditions may be beneficial.

RADIOGRAPHIC RISK FACTORS

Type of Slippage □ In individuals with incomplete and/or abnormal formation of the posterior elements at the lumbosacral articulation, spondylolisthesis of the dysplastic type (Type I) is likely to occur and more likely to progress.[17, 28, 29, 34, 48, 70] Those with the more common isthmic spondylolisthesis tend to acquire their disease later on, and mechanical factors leading to profound progression generally are not present.[48, 70]

Mechanical Insufficiency □ Individuals with anatomic factors leading to mechanical insufficiency at the L5–sacrum level are more likely to exhibit progression. These factors include an eroded, rounded, or dome-shaped sacrum; a trapezoidal shape of the L5 vertebral body; a "teeter-totter" type of alignment of L5 on S1 as described by Hensinger and coworkers;[28, 29] and an abnormally high slip angle (>40 to 50 degrees) indicative of localized kyphosis.[1, 8, 17, 28, 29, 38, 61] The slip angle normally ranges from 0 to 10 degrees and should be measured in all individuals with spondylolisthesis, as this is a very reliable and reproducible sign that correlates well with propensity for further displacement.[8]

Degree of Slippage □ Individuals with spondylolisthesis of greater than 30% have a higher chance of progression, and in those with 50% or greater olisthesis, the likelihood of progression is so great that many authors advocate surgical treatment at this stage, regardless of whether symptoms are present.[1, 8, 28, 45, 61, 66]

Hypermobility □ In individuals in whom the degree of slippage increases when a standing lateral radiograph is compared with a supine view, a tendency to progression exists.[8, 46] Likewise, if on lateral flexion–extension radiographs increased olisthesis or angular hypermobility with opening of the isthmic defect is present, the propensity to slip is increased.[29]

INDICATIONS FOR SURGERY

In children and adolescents, the indications for surgical intervention are different than for adults. Likewise, the results of surgical treatment are generally more favorable in the younger population.[25] Children with spondylolysis or low-grade spondylolisthesis are very likely to respond to nonoperative measures, and often surgery can be avoided

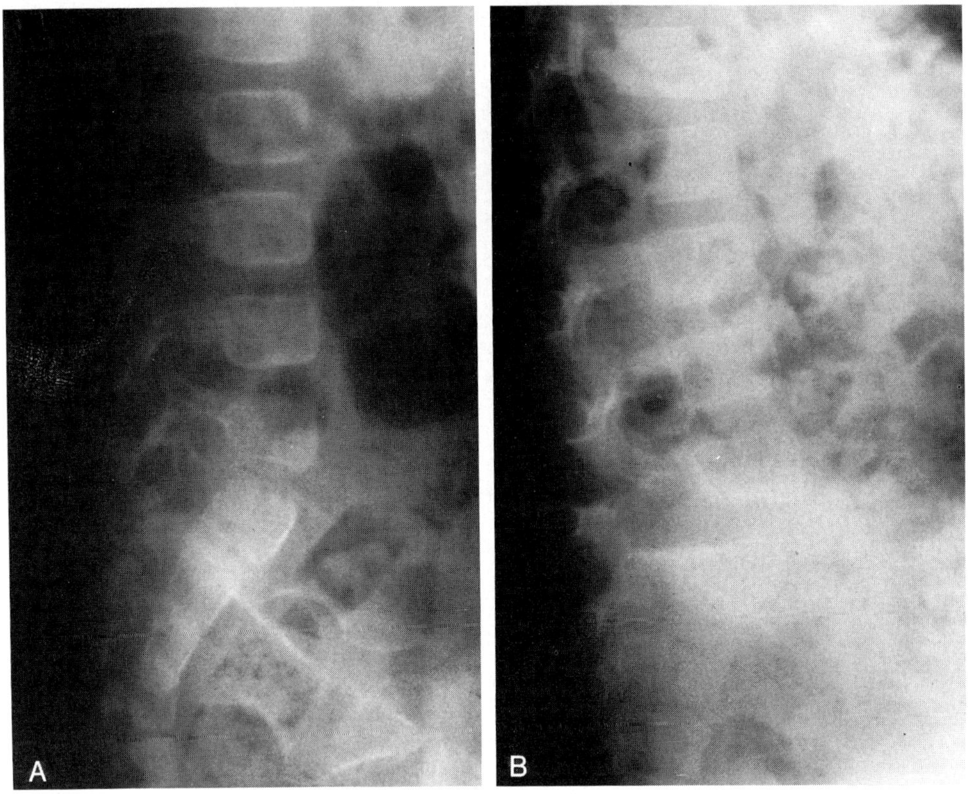

Figure 1 □ *A,* A 2-year-old child with back pain. Sclerosis of the pars interarticularis at L5 is present. *B,* At age 4, the pars defect is apparent and spondylolisthesis of 25% has occurred. Further progression is an indication for surgical stabilization.

in these patients without long-term sequelae.[28, 29, 48, 61, 66, 69, 70] On the other hand, it is generally in childhood that progression of slippage and initial presentation of individuals with higher-grade slips are seen. Some children with significant grades of spondylolisthesis or even spondyloptosis will appear without any symptoms whatsoever.

During evaluation of an individual with spondylolysis or spondylolisthesis, many factors must be taken into consideration, and the indications for surgery may vary between patients. However, based on our knowledge of the natural history of the disease, of risk factors as applied to the individual, and of the outcome of surgical treatment for this condition, broad indications for surgical intervention can be arrived at. They are as follows:

1. Persistence of painful mechanical or neurologic symptoms, despite an appropriate course of nonoperative treatment.[9, 10, 28]
2. Documentation of progresive slippage beyond 25% to 33% (Fig. 1*A*, *B*).[9]
3. Presentation with slippage greater than 50%.[9, 28, 39, 68]
4. Postural deformity and gait abnormality (relative indication) (Fig. 2*A–D*).[28, 29]

OPERATIVE OPTIONS

In Situ Fusion—One Level

In most instances, local one-level arthrodesis of the spine will suffice, providing a stable fusion and symptomatic relief in the majority of patients.[8, 28, 52, 55, 61] This procedure is best performed through a bilateral approach with an intertransverse process or transverse process/sacral ala arthrodesis to stabilize flexion, extension, and rotational forces on the involved segment. For slippage of less than 50% in children and adolescents, this is the procedure of choice. Further slippage postoperatively is less likely if a bilateral muscle splitting, rather than a midline dissection, is utilized.[62]

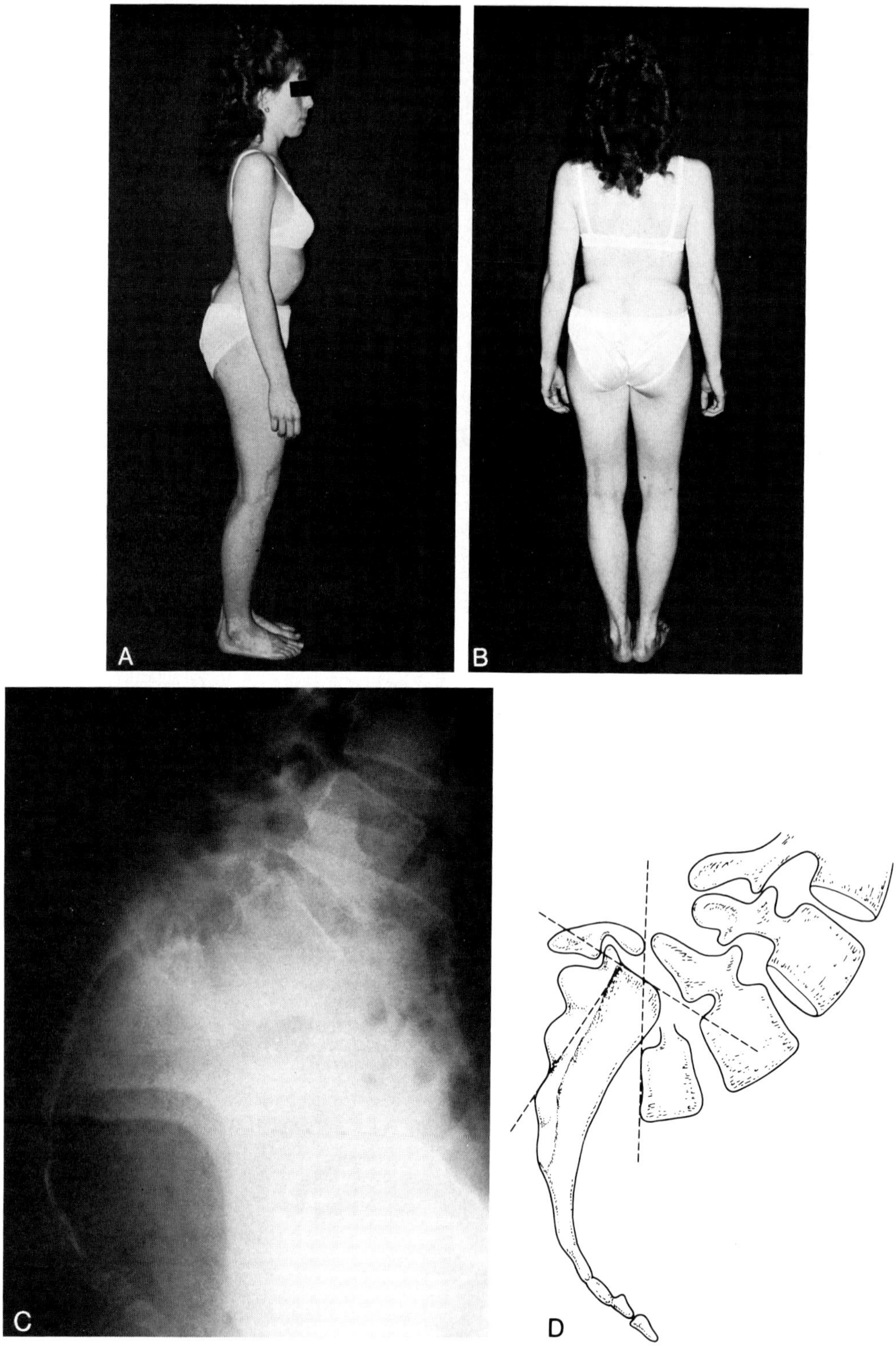

Figure 2 □ *A, B,* Teenage girl with spondyloptosis. Note the characteristic deformity. *C,* Standing lateral radiograph demonstrates complete slippage of the lumbar spine off the pelvis. *D,* Schematic drawing of this patient's radiograph. The slip angle measures 58 degrees and quantifies the localized kyphosis.

In Situ Fusion—Two Levels

When the spondylolisthesis exceeds 50%, the anterior displacement of the vertebral body and, hence, the transverse processes to which the fusion is to be applied makes long-term stabilization less likely with a one-level fusion. In such instances, it is wise to extend the arthrodesis to L4.[9, 12] Despite the immobilization of the additional segment, mobility is remarkably well preserved when pain relief is achieved. The increased incidence of pseudoarthrosis seen in adults with extension of the fusion is not observed in children.[25]

Laminectomy/Laminectomy and Fusion

In adult patients with spondylolisthesis, radicular symptoms are relatively frequently encountered and remain unrelieved unless neural decompressive procedures are performed. In contrast, radiculopathy due to spondylolisthesis is much less frequently seen in childhood. This is likely attributable to the relative lack of hypertrophic tissue about the pars interarticularis lesion, despite the magnitude of the slip. Even in relatively high-grade cases of olisthesis, laminectomy can be avoided, because, with satisfactory arthrodesis and elimination of abnormal motion, nerve-related lower-extremity symptoms will usually resolve.[8, 24, 28, 31] In addition, removal of the posterior ligamentous and osseous elements may add yet another destabilizing factor to an already unstable mechanical situation, thus resulting in predisposition to further slippage, even during the period of arthrodesis consolidation.[37, 68] Owing to these factors, laminectomy alone for spondylolisthesis is never indicated in children and should be combined with fusion only in special circumstances; such situations include laminectomy in conjunction with the reduction of a high-grade spondylolisthesis or spondyloptosis for which the development of neural problems has a significant incidence, or in occasional cases in which the preoperative symptoms are predominantly radicular and in which myelography, computed tomography (CT), and/or magnetic resonance imaging (MRI) show a significant hypertrophic fibrocartilaginous mass encroaching on the nerve roots at the level of the defect.

Anterior Fusion

The indications for anterior arthrodesis in childhood spondylolisthesis appear to be limited. The majority of patients, with the possible exception of high-grade (>75%) slips, achieve satisfactory results with posterior stabilization alone. Although, in experienced hands, anterior lumbosacral interbody fusion is reported to be successful,[22, 54, 62, 64] the technical difficulties presented by the confluence of the great vessels at this level add risk and make this operation more than routine. In addition, the risk of the possible induction of retrograde ejaculation, owing to violation of the presacral plexus, in males should be taken into consideration if this procedure is contemplated.[32] On occasion, however, when deformity is great and a posterior procedure is deemed insufficient, or in instances in which pseudoarthrosis or plastic deformation of the fusion mass has occurred as a result of a high slip angle and/or major translational displacement, a supplementary anterior fusion can be performed.[5, 14, 67] A few surgeons advocate a primary anterior approach with disc excision, thereby facilitating reduction.[40, 56, 58] Good results with interbody fusion through a posterior approach have been reported by Cloward.[16]

Isthmic Defect Repair

First popularized by Buck in 1970,[15] direct repair of the defect can be performed for isolated spondylolysis or low-grade (<25%) spondylolisthesis.[11, 13, 49, 63] The appeal of this technique lies in the preservation of the involved motion segment, thus minimizing abnormal stresses at adjacent levels. It may be performed either by a direct screw technique,[15] or by wiring about the transverse processes and posterior elements, providing a tension band–like effect.[13, 49] It is more easily performed, particularly utilizing the wire technique, at levels above the lumbosacral junction. Bone grafting of the defect to facilitate healing of the pars defect is mandatory. This procedure should not be attempted when the defect distance is substantial (>25% olisthesis) or when an abnormal slip angle is present. Nachemson[47] has suggested direct defect repair in conjunction with lateral arthrodesis. Although seemingly attractive, this technique appears to add little to the success of in situ lateral arthrodesis, because results are satisfactory in most cases, anyway.

Anterior and Posterior Fusion

Combined approaches for spondylolisthesis are advocated by some for higher-grade and more unstable spondylolisthetic patterns.[10, 40, 64] As mentioned previously, this technique is most commonly utilized if a posterior procedure alone might be expected to fail or if a reduction technique is deemed to require a primary anterior release.[14] Possible vascular and neurologic complications should be taken into consideration if one elects this approach.

Reduction of Spondylolisthesis/Spondyloptosis

Despite uncertainty as to the indications for spondylolisthesis/spondyloptosis reduction, a variety of techniques have been described.[2, 10, 18, 19, 23, 26, 30, 33, 36, 40, 42–44, 53, 56, 58] These procedures include preoperative traction and/or cast reduction followed by posterior fusion, (Lance[36] and Scaglietti and coworkers[53]); posterior distraction techniques (DeWald and colleagues,[19] Harrington and Tullos,[26] and Kaneda and coworkers[33]); posterior element wiring with external traction reduction (Balderston and Bradford[2] and Snijder and colleagues[58]); spinal column shortening by L5 vertebrectomy (Gaines and Nichols[23] and Huizenga[30]); combined posterior and anterior procedures (Bradford,[10] Bradford and Gotfried,[14] DeWald and colleagues,[19] and McPhee and O'Brien[42]); and more recently, pedicle screw techniques (Edwards,[20] Louis and Maresca,[40] McQueen and colleagues,[43] Matthiass and Heine,[44] and Sijbrandij[56]).

With all of these methods, a significant incidence (up to 30% in some series) of neural problems has been reported, most commonly involving postoperative dysfunction of the L5 and/or S1 nerve roots. Additionally, loss of reduction is not uncommon, owing to the tremendous mechanical forces that have caused the presenting deformity.[9] Regardless of the technique employed, meticulous attention to the bone grafting arthrodesis technique is necessary; otherwise, deformity and recurrent symptoms ensue. Laminectomy and thorough clearing of the nerve roots at the deformity level are mandatory whenever reduction is undertaken, in order to prevent tethering during the reduction maneuver. Despite this, neural pain or dysfunction is not uncommon after such a procedure. The cause of this is unclear, but it is speculated that it may be related to unrecognized nerve root compression or tension or to vascular factors associated with repositioning of the roots and changes in spinal alignment.

Although pedicle screw techniques seem appealing at this time, the small size of the pedicle in children, particularly in those with dysplastic variations of the disease, sometimes precludes appropriate placement of the screws. This may prevent obtaining an adequate mechanical grasp of the olisthetic vertebra for the reduction maneuver, or the screw itself may impinge on neural structures.

Regardless of the technique employed, postoperative immobilization of the pelvis, either with a cast or brace incorporating one or both thighs, should be considered in order to minimize chances of the loss of reduction.

Pseudoarthrosis Repair

Pseudoarthrosis of an attempted arthrodesis is relatively uncommon in children if appropriate surgical techniques are utilized.[8, 25] As with other arthrodesis procedures, the chances of this occurring are greater with more extensive procedures or when mechanical forces work against bone consolidation. In patients with high-grade slips or those with abnormal slip angles, the arthrodesis may be placed in tension, thus increasing the likelihood of pseudarthrosis. This occurrence can be minimized by using meticulous technique and adequate bone graft material, and by minimizing stress on the fusion site during consolidation. The latter may be accomplished by casting, bracing, or internal fixation.

When failure of fusion occurs, it is generally accompanied by persistent pain, progression of slippage, or recurrence of deformity. Radiographs should be correlated with the clinical symptoms before a secondary procedure is considered. Not infrequently (at least in children), a few months more of immobilization will result in resolution of the problem. When, however, symptoms persist or deformity progresses with clear evidence of failure of fusion, secondary repair with clearing of all fibrous tissue at the defect and fresh bone grafting, should be considered. Usually this will result in a satisfactory outcome. Secondary anterior arthrodesis or addition of instrumentation to the pseudoarthrotic level is usually reserved for older individuals, cases of higher-grade spondylolisthesis, or instances in which two or more posterior operations have failed. Postoperative immobilization for at least 3 months should be utilized in all pseudarthrosis repairs.

POSTOPERATIVE CARE

During childhood and adolescence, excellent fusion success rates in spondylolisthesis have been reported, regardless of the form of immobilization employed. Greater than 90% good results have been reported by Wiltse and Jackson[68] and Rombold[52] utilizing no postoperative immobilization; by Bosworth and coworkers[7] and Nachemsen[47] using a corset; and by Turner and Bianco[61] employing postoperative casting. Bradford has stated that immobilization of the leg is usually not necessary.[9, 11, 12] Despite these reports, there are situations in which immobilization of the lumbar spine and pelvis may play a role.[40] For patients with spondylolisthesis greater than 50% or for those in whom translational or slip angle reduction is attempted, I have employed a cast or brace incorporating the torso and one thigh.[9, 28] Likewise, when instrumentation is utilized for reduction purposes, this type of postoperative restriction may be beneficial in decreasing the incidence of instrument loosening and, hence, of reduction loss. Younger individuals are always able to ambulate, albeit with some loss of speed, in such devices with minimal inconvenience. A reduction of activity by whatever means for a period of 3 months postoperatively is generally sufficient for satisfactory fusion consolidation. The return to relatively normal activity is permitted after 6 months and is unlimited after 1 year if a good result has been achieved. The issue of whether these children should be allowed to return to high-stress endeavors, such as gymnastics or contact sports, following surgery for spondylolisthesis is controversial, and it should be resolved on an individual basis. In patients who have spondylolisthesis with complete resolution of their symptoms, a satisfactory radiographic appearance of the fusion, and normal spinal motion, I generally permit full return to athletic activities without restriction.

SPECIAL CONSIDERATIONS

Spondylolisthesis in Scoliosis

Most scoliosis associated with spondylolisthesis is antalgic and resolves with treatment of the symptomatic slippage. On occasion, however, a patient will be seen with spondylolisthesis in conjunction with a structural scoliosis. Each condition should be treated individually, based on criteria for that condition.[11] Thus, if the spondylolisthesis meets operative criteria and the scoliosis does not, then the spondylolisthesis should be operated upon and the scoliosis treated with whatever nonoperative measures are indicated; the opposite is also true. On rare occasions in which both conditions warrant surgery, it is best to avoid a contiguous fusion to the sacrum. At least a few open lumbar motion segments should be preserved between the two fused portions of the spine. A balanced, mobile spine with some deformity is preferable to a stiff one, regardless of the situation.

Spondylolisthesis Above a Previously Fused Level

In rare instances in children, a spondylolysis or spondylolisthesis will develop above a previously fused segment.[4] This condition should be managed as if it were an isolated problem with whatever nonoperative measures or operative measures are indicated. If surgery is necessary, extension of the fusion should be limited to as few additional segments as possible, preferably to one.

Iatrogenic Spondylolisthesis

Iatrogenic induction of spondylolisthesis in children generally occurs after laminectomy for tumorous conditions. Any child who has undergone such a procedure should be observed closely for the development of deformity, and if this occurs, stabilization should immediately be performed. Patients, especially younger ones, who have had multiple-level laminectomies or in whom the pars interarticularis has been resected, will predictably develop a kyphotic and/or spondylolisthetic deformity, and a prophylactic stabilization procedure is indicated prior to its development.

Operative Treatment of Spondylolisthesis (Author's Preferred Approach)

My approach to surgical treatment for spondylolisthesis varies, depending on the patient's symptoms and mechanical factors influencing the instability pattern. Factors that I believe to influence outcome include the presence or absence of neural symptoms and the slip angle in relationship to the degree of olisthesis. Based on our knowledge of and experience with this disorder, I have adopted relative guidelines to select the indicated procedure for each patient with spondylolisthesis (Table 1).

Patients with spondylolisthesis of less than 25% and no symptoms require observation only. It is most reasonable to follow them on a 6-month basis. If unresponsive symptoms develop or progression to the next grade occurs, then a direct repair or local one-level posterolateral arthrodesis is indicated. Similarly, a one-level in situ stabilization procedure is utilized for patients with Grade 1 or Grade 2 olisthesis whose symptoms have failed to show response. The slip angle is generally not a factor in such patients. Rarely, children and adolescents with slippage of less than 50% will develop neural symptoms as a result of fibrocartilaginous hypertrophy about the pars interarticularis defect. When radiculopathy is encountered in this group of patients, back pain symptoms generally predominate and lower-extremity symptoms will usually resolve with a stabilization procedure and elimination of the abnormal motion causing the nerve root irritation. If, however, radicular symptoms predominate, a situation commonly seen in adults, and appropriate studies reveal profound neural encroachment, then laminectomy and removal of the hypertrophic tissue about the pedicle–pars region may be performed. It is important to do more than just remove the lamina, as failure to clear the roots of compressive tissue will result in the continuation of

Table 1 □ Guidelines for Treatment of Spondylolisthesis Based on Symptoms, Degree of Olisthesis, and Slip Angle

		SLIP ANGLE <45 DEGREES		SLIP ANGLE >45 DEGREES	
	ASYMPTOMATIC	Low Back Pain Only	Back and Neural Symptoms	Low Back Pain Only	Back and Neural Symptoms
I (<25%)	No treatment	One-level fusion*	One-level fusion* Rare neural decompression	One-level fusion*	One-level fusion* Rare neural decompression
II (25–50%)	No treatment versus one-level fusion* if progression is documented	One-level fusion*	One-level fusion* Selective neural decompression	One-level fusion*	One-level fusion* Selective neural decompression
III (50–75%)	Two-level fusion*	Two-level fusion*	Two-level fusion† Neural decompression	Two-level fusion‡ (selective reduction)	Two-level fusion‡ Selective neural decompression (selective reduction)
IV (75–100%)	Two-level fusion†	Two-level fusion† (selective reduction)	Two-level fusion Neural decompression† (selective reduction)	Two-level fusion‡	Two-level fusion‡ Neural decompression (selective reduction)
Spondyloptosis	No treatment versus reduction for functionally cosmetic reasons†	Two-level fusion† (selective reduction)	Two-level fusion Neural decompression† (selective reduction)	Two-level fusion‡ (selective reduction)	Two-level fusion‡ Neural decompression (selective reduction)

*Corset, TLSO, or cast
†TLSO, with thigh extension
‡Preoperative and postoperative extension cast

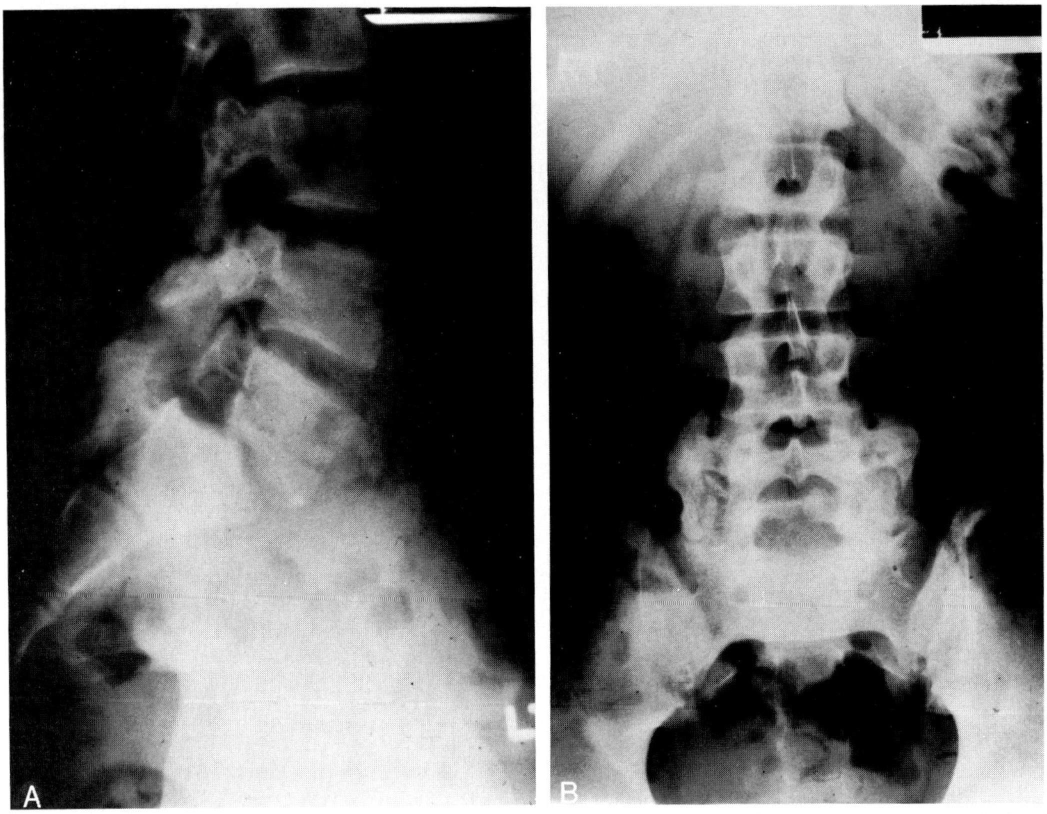

Figure 3 □ *A, B,* Posterolateral in situ arthrodesis for spondylolisthesis in a 14-year-old boy. At 1 year postoperatively, the fusion is consolidated and symptoms are resolved.

symptoms. After such procedures, immobilization in a lumbar corset, thoracolumbosacral orthosis (TLSO), or cast for 3 months facilitates fusion consolidation by generally reducing the patient's activity.

For those patients with olisthesis of from 50% to 75% without abnormal kyphosis, extension of the arthrodesis to another level (e.g., L4 to sacrum for L5–S1 spondylolisthesis) will usually result in a satisfactory outcome (Fig. 3). Extension of the fusion is indicated in such instances, owing to the anterior positioning of the transverse processes, thus permitting a less-than-adequate grasp of the translated vertebra by the fusion that is now placed in tension. By extending the fusion, a more sagittally oriented arthrodesis in relative compression can be achieved. If, however, a laminectomy is deemed necessary for relief of radicular disorders, another element of instability is introduced into the situation. In such instances it has been my practice to immobilize the torso and one thigh postoperatively to limit flexion at the fusion site.

When slippage of greater than 50% is present and the slip angle exceeds 45 degrees, then an attempt to reduce the local kyphotic deformity by extension casting followed by a two-level in situ fusion is employed. Continuation of this immobilization postoperatively facilitates fusion incorporation and limits postoperative progression, particularly in instances in which a midline approach and/or neural decompression has been performed.

In patients with spondylolisthesis of greater than 75% or spondyloptosis, surgical decision-making becomes more difficult. In children and adolescents with a higher-grade spondylolisthesis who are asymptomatic, it is probably best to perform a two-level in situ fusion in order to avoid the potential development of spondyloptosis. Occasionally, a patient will be seen with a completely asymptomatic spondyloptosis. In such instances, in situ stabilization will accomplish nothing and reduction of the deformity is difficult, possibly resulting in the development of neural dysfunction. It is probably best in these situations to do nothing, unless a profound cosmetic abnormality and gait disturbance are present. If reduction is undertaken, the risk-to-benefit ratio must carefully be weighed and discussed with the patient and family prior to such a procedure.

The majority of patients with high-grade spondylolisthesis or spondyloptosis are symptomatic, and the deformity is of the dysplastic type. Almost always, an abnormally high slip angle is present. Not infrequently, radicular symptoms and/or motor or sensory changes are present. In such situations, the minimum surgical intervention is a two-level in situ arthrodesis combined with neural decompression. Extension casting preoperatively and postoperatively is helpful in controlling the slip angle and thus improves spinal balance while retarding pseudarthrosis and/or progression.

The question of whether to attempt reduction of a severe spondylolisthesis remains controversial, owing to the difficulty of accomplishing the reduction and the risk of causing or accentuating neurologic symptoms or deficits. For high-grade spondylolisthesis and spondyloptosis, I have attempted reduction in patients with preoperative neural symptoms and an abnormal slip angle. Previously, I employed a distraction technique utilizing Harrington rods. Although this usually resulted in an initial improvement of the translational abnormality, the slip angle was not decreased, and was often accentuated, by this technique. This resulted not only in instrumentation of an excessive portion of the lumbar spine, but also in gradual loss of reduction with time, despite whether a concomitant anterior fusion was performed. For the past few years, my practice has been to perform a laminectomy and reduction using an isolated posterior approach by employing techniques and instrumentation devised by Charles Edwards of Baltimore (Fig. 4).[20] Although the procedure is technically demanding and time consuming, almost any degree of spondylolisthesis can be reduced by using

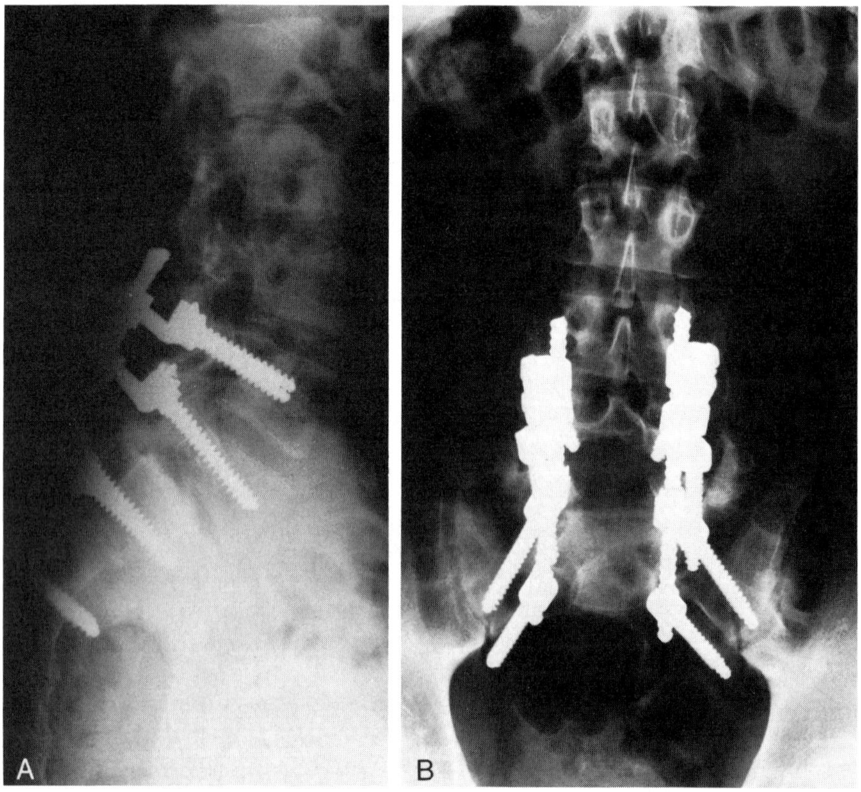

Figure 4 □ *A, B,* Radiographs following reduction and stabilization of spondylolisthesis utilizing a pedicle screw rod technique. After distraction, posteriorly directed forces correct the translational malalignment. Two-level sacral fixation permits correction of the kyphotic deformity during the gradual reduction maneuver. Laminectomy of L5 has been performed.

this technique, with few neurologic sequelae. The procedure is based on the introduction of forces opposite those acting to produce the deformity and on the principle of stress relaxation of soft tissues. This procedure has been performed by several spinal surgeons in the United States, and initial results are encouraging. Meticulous attention to obtaining a good fusion bed and postoperative immobilization of the torso and pelvis are mandatory to avoid instrument or osseous failure and a resultant recurrence of the deformity. This procedure should not be performed without a thorough decompression of the L5 nerve roots prior to the reduction maneuver or by individuals unfamiliar with pedicle screw surgical techniques. In patients under the age of 12 years, the small size of the vertebral elements may preclude adequate screw placement, and other techniques of treatment, such as cast reduction, are advisable.

TECHNICAL CONSIDERATIONS IN THE OPERATIVE TREATMENT OF SPONDYLOLISTHESIS

Posterolateral Spinal Arthrodesis

The procedure is similar for one- or two-level fusions (Fig. 5). When a laminectomy is unnecessary, the spine can be approached by a muscle-splitting technique lateral to the midline, with exposure of the transverse processes, facet joints, and sacral ala. The skin incision can be a single midline one with subcutaneous dissection, or it can be bilateral. The transverse processes are thoroughly denuded and decorticated along with the lateral aspect of the facet joint and pedicle. It is not necessary to destroy the facet joint, and this should be avoided at the superior margin of the fusion so as to minimize damage to the adjacent motion segment. Exposure of the pars interarticularis defect is generally not necessary. At the sacral ala, complete exposure is performed and a large drill hole (5⁄8 inch) placed into it from a superior-to-inferior direction. This establishes a good cancellous fusion bed in the pelvis and permits the fusion mass to assume a more sagittal orientation, thus placing it in relative compression. A large volume of autologous cancellous bone graft is then obtained from the ilium and packed into the fusion bed.

If nerve root decompression is performed in conjunction with arthrodesis, a midline approach is best. The hypermobile posterior elements are removed, either as a unit or piecemeal. At this point it is necessary to proceed superiorly in the epidural space and to identify the ventral area of the pars defect adjacent to the inferolateral aspect of the L4 lamina. Fibrocartilaginous tissue will be noted to proliferate from the pedicle–pars region in a mushroom-like fashion, with the nerve root (L5) coursing under the cap of

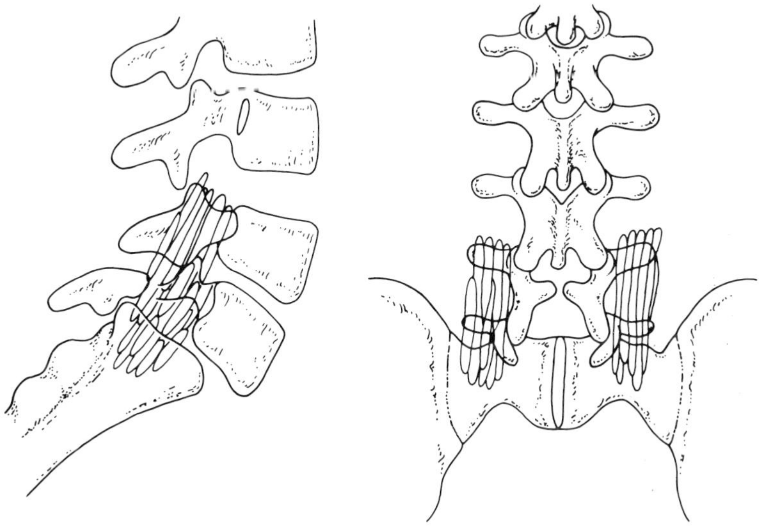

Figure 5 □ Schematic drawing of posterolateral lumbosacral spinal arthrodesis. The bone graft extends into a drill hole placed in the sacral ala.

the mushroom as it exits through the foramen. Removal of this tissue is necessary in order to adequately relieve neural irritation and predictably eliminate symptoms. The inferior roots (S1) at the laminectomy site are rarely the source of neural symptoms, and any irritative forces or stenotic factor will have been relieved by the laminectomy. Following decompression, fusion is performed as noted above. When a laminectomy has been performed, bleeding should be meticulously controlled and a drain inserted prior to closure to avoid the development of a symptomatic epidural hematoma.

Spondylolisthesis Reduction

At this time, my preferred technique for spondylolisthesis reduction is that developed by Edwards.[20] It will be described for treatment of deformity at the L5–sacral level. Through a posterior midline approach, the posterior and lateral elements of L4, L5, S1, and S2 are completely exposed. The loose posterior elements are then removed and the L5 nerve roots dissected free from the superior margin of the pedicle through the entire foramen. They must be completely free so as to permit their unobstructed migration superiorly and dorsally during the reduction maneuver.

Following this, utilizing radiographic control, holes are drilled into the pedicles of L4 and L5 on either side and pedicle screws of an appropriate length (40 to 50 mm) are inserted into these pedicles. At S1 and S2 screws are placed in a lateral orientation to take advantage of the more substantial bone present in this area of the sacrum. All screws are placed in a plane parallel with that of the adjacent vertebral end plate. At the L5 level, this often means an inferiorly directed angle of from 45 to 60 degrees.

After screw placement and confirmation of position, the lateral fusion sites are decorticated. Rods are then inserted, obtaining a stable two-segment base on the sacrum. This permits control of sacral rotation and, hence, correction of the slip angle. Turnbuckle-like pedicle connectors are then applied between the rods and L4 and L5. Moderate distraction force is then instituted in stages, permitting gradual stretching of the soft tissue contractures. If necessary, supplementary distraction may be applied by the Harrington distraction rod (from L1 or L2 to the sacral ala), which can be removed after appropriate distraction has been accomplished. After initial distraction, the translational deformity is gradually corrected by sequentially tightening the threaded pedicle connectors. During this portion of the procedure it is necessary to pause for a while each time translational reduction forces are applied, in order to permit stress relaxation of the soft tissues and to avoid instrument pull-out. Applying a combination of intermittent distraction and translation force permits one to gradually bring the malpositioned spine back into normal alignment. Throughout the procedure the nerve roots need to be observed for tethering and released where necessary. After reduction, all articulations are tightened, and bone graft is applied to the lateral masses. Postoperative immobilization including the torso and one thigh for at least 3 months is mandatory. After this period, gradual resumption of activity is permitted.

SUMMARY

Spondylolysis and spondylolisthesis in childhood and adolescence are relatively common, but the majority of individuals with this condition are asymptomatic or can be effectively managed by nonoperative measures. Surgery may be indicated when symptoms are incapacitating and unresponsive to appropriate nonoperative measures, documented progression of at least one grade has occurred, or olisthesis at presentation is greater than 50%. In situ posterolateral arthrodesis of one or two segments is successful in most instances. Laminectomy in children with spondylolisthesis may predispose them to further deformity and should be avoided when unnecessary. On rare occasion, fusion or a combination of reduction and fusion can be considered for asymptomatic high-grade spondylolisthesis or spondyloptosis with neural symptoms, gait abnormalities, or significant cosmetic deformity. Experience with the techniques necessary to accomplish reduction and a stable arthrodesis and an awareness and acceptance of the possible complications of this maneuver are prerequisites to its performance.

References

1. Baker, D.R., and McHolick, W.: Spondylolysis and spondylolisthesis in children. J. Bone Joint Surg. 38A:933–944, 1956.

2. Balderston, R.A., and Bradford, D.S.: Technique for achievement and maintenance of reduction for severe spondylolisthesis. Spine 10:376–382, 1985.
3. Blackburne, J.S., and Velikas, E.P.: Spondylolisthesis in children and adolescents. J. Bone Joint Surg. 59B:490–494, 1977.
4. Blasier, R.D., and Monson, R.C.: Acquired spondylolysis after posterolateral spinal fusion. J. Pediatr. Orthop. 7:215–217, 1987.
5. Bohlman, H.H., and Cook, S.S.: One-stage decompression and posterolateral and interbody fusion for lumbosacral spondyloptosis through a posterior approach. Report of two cases. J. Bone Joint Surg. 64A:415–418, 1982.
6. Borkow, S.E., and Kleiger, B.: Spondylolisthesis in the newborn. Clin. Orthop. 81:73–76, 1971.
7. Bosworth, D.M., Fielding, W.J., Demarest, L., and Bonaquist, M.: Spondylolisthesis: A critical review of a consecutive series of cases treated by arthrodesis. J. Bone Joint Surg. 37A:767–786, 1955.
8. Boxall, D., Bradford, D.S., Winter, R.B., and Moe, J.H.: Management of severe spondylolisthesis in children and adolescents. J. Bone Joint Surg. 61A:479–495, 1979.
9. Bradford, D.S.: Spondylolysis and spondylolisthesis. *In* Chou, I.S.N., and Seljeskog, E.L. (eds.): Spinal Deformity and Neurological Dysfunction. New York, Raven Press, 1978.
10. Bradford, D.S.: Treatment of severe spondylolisthesis: A combined approach for reduction and stabilization. Spine 4:423–429, 1979.
11. Bradford, D.S.: Management of spondylolysis and spondylolisthesis. Instructional course lectures, A.A.O.S. 32:151–162, 1983.
12. Bradford, D.S.: Spondylolysis and spondylolisthesis in children and adolescents. *In* Bradford, D.S., and Hensinger, R.N. (eds.): Pediatric Spine. New York, Thieme and Stratton, 1985.
13. Bradford, D.S., and Iza, J.: Repair of the defect in spondylolysis or minimal degrees of spondylolisthesis by segmental wire fixation and bone grafting. Spine 10:673–679, 1985.
14. Bradford, D.S., and Gotfried, Y.: Staged salvage reconstruction of Grade IV and V spondylolisthesis. J. Bone Joint Surg. 69A:191–202, 1987.
15. Buck, J.E.: Direct repair of the defect in spondylolisthesis. J. Bone Joint Surg. 52B:432–437, 1970.
16. Cloward, R.B.: Spondylolisthesis: Treatment by laminectomy and posterior interbody fusion. Clin. Orthop. 154:74–82, 1981.
17. Dandy, D.J., and Shannon, M.J.: Lumbosacral subluxation. J. Bone Joint Surg. 53B:578–595, 1971.
18. Del Torto, U.: Surgical reduction and stabilization of spondylolisthesis. Clin. Orthop. 75:281–284, 1971.
19. DeWald, R.L., Faut, M.M., Taddonio, R.F., and Neuwirth, M.G.: Severe lumbosacral spondylolisthesis in adolescents and children: Reduction and staged circumferential fusion. J. Bone Joint Surg. 63A:619–626, 1981.
20. Edwards, C.: Personal communication, 1988.
21. Frederickson, B.E., Baker, D., McHolick, W.J., et al.: The natural history of spondylolysis and spondylolisthesis. J. Bone Joint Surg. 66A:699–707, 1984.
22. Freebody, D., Bendall, R., and Taylor, R.D.: Anterior transperitoneal lumbar fusion. J. Bone Joint Surg. 53B:617–627, 1971.
23. Gaines, R.W., and Nichols, W.K.: Treatment of spondyloptosis by two-stage L5 vertebrectomy and reduction of L4 onto S1. Spine 10:680–686, 1985.
24. Gill, G.G., Manning, J.G., and White, H.L.: Surgical treatment of spondylolisthesis without spine fusion. J. Bone Joint Surg. 37A:493–520, 1955.
25. Hanley, E.N., and Levy, J.A.: Surgical treatment of isthmic lumbosacral spondylolisthesis: Analysis of variables influencing results. Spine 14:48–50, 1989.
26. Harrington, P.R., and Tullos, H.S.: Spondylolisthesis in children; observations and surgical treatment. Clin. Orthop. 79:75–84, 1971.
27. Harris, I.E., and Weinstein, S.L.: Long-term follow-up of patients with Grade III and IV spondylolisthesis. J. Bone Joint Surg. 69A:960–969, 1987.
28. Hensinger, R.N., Lang, J.R., and MacEwen, G.D.: Surgical management of spondylolisthesis in children and adolescents. Spine 1:207–216, 1976.
29. Hensinger, R.N.: Spondylolysis and spondylolisthesis in children. Instructional course lectures, A.A.O.S. 32:132–151, 1983.
30. Huizenga, B.A.: Reduction of spondylolisthesis with two stage vertebrectomy. Orthop. Trans. 7:21, 1983.
31. Johnson, J.R., and Kirwan, E.O.: The long-term results of fusion in situ for severe spondylolisthesis. J. Bone Joint Surg. 65B:43–46, 1983.
32. Johnson, R.M., and McQuire, E.J.: Urogenital complications of anterior approaches to the lumbar spine. Clin. Orthop. 154:114–118, 1981.
33. Kaneda, K., Satoh, S., Nohara, Y., and Tadanori, O.: Distraction rods instrumentation with posterolateral fusion in isthmic spondylolisthesis: 53 cases followed for 18–89 months. Spine 10:383–389, 1985.
34. Kettlekamp, D.B., and Wright, G.D.: Spondylolysis in the Alaskan Eskimo. J. Bone Joint Surg. 53A:563–566, 1971.
35. Lafond, G.: Surgical treatment of spondylolisthesis. Clin. Orthop. 22:175–179, 1962.
36. Lance, E.M.: Treatment of severe spondylolisthesis with neural involvement. J. Bone Joint Surg. 48A:883–891, 1966.
37. Laurent, L.E.: Spondylolisthesis. Acta Orthop. Scand. 35(Suppl.):9–45, 1958.
38. Laurent, L., and Einola, S.: Spondylolisthesis in children and adolescents. Acta Orthop. Scand. 31:45–64, 1961.
39. Laurent, L.E., and Osterman, K.: Operative treatment of spondylolisthesis in young patients. Clin. Orthop. 117:85–91, 1976.
40. Louis, R., and Maresca, C.: Stabilization chirugicale avec reduction des spondylolyses et des spondylolisthesis. Sicot Int. Orthop. 1:215–225, 1977.
41. McKee, B.W., Alexander, W.J., and Dunbar, J.S.: Spondylolysis and spondylolisthesis in children: A review. J. Can. Assoc. Radiol. 22:100–109, 1971.
42. McPhee, I.B., and O'Brien, J.D.: Reduction of severe spondylolisthesis: A preliminary report. Spine 4:430–434, 1979.
43. McQueen, M.M., Court-Brown, C., and Scott, J.H.: Stabilization of spondylolisthesis using Dwyer instrumentation. J. Bone Joint Surg. 68B:185–188, 1986.
44. Matthiass, H.H., and Heine, J.: The surgical reduction of spondylolisthesis. Clin. Orthop. 203:34–44, 1986.
45. Meyerding, H.W.: Spondylolisthesis: Surgical treatment and results. Surg. Gynecol. Obstet. 54:371–377, 1932.
46. Monticelli, G., and Ascani, E.: Spondylolysis and spondylolisthesis. Acta Orthop. Scand. 46:498–506, 1975.

47. Nachemson, A.: Repair of the spondylolisthetic defect and intertransverse fusion for young patients. Clin. Orthop. 117:101–105, 1976.
48. Newman, P.H., and Stone, K.H.: The etiology of spondylolisthesis. J. Bone Joint Surg. 45B:39–59, 1963.
49. Nicol, R.D., and Scott, J.H.: Lytic spondylolysis repair by wiring. Spine 11:1027–1030, 1986.
50. Pederson, A.K., and Hagen, R.: Spondylolysis and spondylolisthesis. Treatment by internal fixation and bone grafting of the defect. J. Bone Joint Surg. 70A:15–24, 1988.
51. Pizzutillo, P.D., Mirenda, W., and MacEwen, G.D.: Posterolateral fusion for spondylolisthesis in adolescence. J. Pediatr. Orthop. 6:311–316, 1986.
52. Rombold, C.: Treatment of spondylolisthesis by postero-lateral fusion. J. Bone Joint Surg. 48A:1282–1300, 1966.
53. Scaglietti, O., Frontino, G., and Bartolozzi, P.: Technique of anatomical reduction of lumbar spondylolisthesis and its surgical stabilization. Clin. Orthop. 117:164–175, 1976.
54. Sevastikoglou, J.A., Spangfort, E., and Aaro, S.: Operative treatment of spondylolisthesis in children and adolescents with tight hamstrings syndrome. Clin. Orthop. 147:192–199, 1980.
55. Sherman, F.C., Rosenthal, R.K., and Hall, J.E.: Spine fusion for spondylolysis and spondylolisthesis in children. Spine 4:59–67, 1979.
56. Sijbrandij, S.: A new technique for the reduction and stabilization of severe spondylolisthesis. A report of nine cases. Int. Orthop. 9:247–253, 1985.
57. Simper, L.B.: Spondylolysis in Eskimo skeletons. Acta Orthop. Scand. 57:78–80, 1986.
58. Snijder, J.G.N., Seroo, J.M., Snijder, C.J., and Schijvens, A.W.M.: Therapy of spondylolisthesis by repositioning and fixation of the olisthetic vertebra. Clin. Orthop. 117:149–155, 1976.
59. Steiner, M.E., and Micheli, L.J.: Treatment of symptomatic spondylolysis and spondylolisthesis with the modified Boston brace. Spine 10:937–943, 1985.
60. Stewart, T.D.: The age incidence of neural arch defects in Alaskan natives considered from the standpoint of etiology. J. Bone Joint Surg. 35A:937–950, 1953.
61. Turner, R.H., and Bianco, A.J., Jr.: Spondylolysis and spondylolisthesis in children and teenagers. J. Bone Joint Surg. 53A:1298–1306, 1971.
62. van Rens, J.G., and van Horn, J.R.: Long-term results in lumbosacral interbody fusion for spondylolisthesis. Acta Orthop. Scand. 53:383–392, 1982.
63. Vender Werf, G.J.I.M., Tonino, A.J., and Zeggers, W.S.: Direct repair of lumbar spondylolisthesis. Acta Orthop. Scand. 56:378–379, 1985.
64. Verbiest, H.: The treatment of lumbar spondyloptosis or impending lumbar spondyloptosis accompanied by neurologic deficit and/or neurogenic intermittent claudication. Spine 4:68–77, 1979.
65. Wertzberger, K.L., and Peterson, H.A.: Acquired spondylolysis and spondylolisthesis in the young child. Spine 5:437–440, 1980.
66. Wiltse, L.L.: Spondylolisthesis in children. Clin. Orthop. 21:156–163, 1961.
67. Wiltse, L.L., and Hutchison, R.: Surgical treatment of spondylolisthesis. Clin. Orthop. 35:116–135, 1964.
68. Wiltse, L.L., and Jackson, D.W.: Treatment of spondylolisthesis and spondylolysis in children. Clin. Orthop. 117:92–100, 1976.
69. Wiltse, L.L., Newman, P.H., and Macnab, I.: Classification of spondylolysis and spondylolisthesis. Clin. Orthop. 117:23–29, 1976.
70. Wiltse, L.L., Widell, E.H., Jr., and Jackson, D.W.: Fatigue fractures: The basic lesion in isthmic spondylolisthesis. J. Bone Joint Surg. 57A:17–22, 1975.

OPERATIVE TREATMENT: ADULTS

David S. Bradford

Spondylolisthesis is defined as a slipping forward of one vertebra on another.[58] Herbiniaux,[37] a Belgian obstetrician, is credited with first describing this condition. Although the entity is not uncommon (i.e., occurs in approximately 5% of the population), symptoms severe enough to require surgical intervention are much less frequent. The cause of these defects in the pars interarticularis, the propensity for a few to lead to progressive deformity, the causes of back or radicular pain, and the optimal conservative or surgical treatment program are but a few of the questions that await a definitive answer.[1, 68]

This chapter reviews the treatment options available for isthmic and dysplastic as well as degenerative spondylolisthesis, primarily focusing on the older adolescent and adult patient. An attempt is made to integrate some of the newer treatment concepts into the more established techniques and to discuss the advantages and disadvantages of each. The classification, diagnosis, and natural history are not discussed, nor is the treatment in the younger child, because these areas are covered in earlier chapters.

DYSPLASTIC AND ISTHMIC SPONDYLOLISTHESIS[87]

Adult and adolescent patients with defects involving the posterior arch may need surgical treatment. The indications for surgery and the type of procedure recommended depend in part on the age of the patient, the type of complaints, and the magnitude of deformity.[10] Adolescent and adult patients seek help primarily because of pain. Their complaints may be one of the following two types: (1) back pain, which may occasionally radiate into the buttocks and which increases with physical activity; (2) radicular pain, usually radiating into the posterior thighs and rarely into the feet. This latter type of pain in the adolescent is usually associated with a high degree of slip. However, in the adult patient with chronic degenerative changes with long-standing spondylolysis, radicular pain from root impingement is not uncommon. The pain magnitude may not always correlate with the magnitude of the slippage. The pain may be associated with the instability from foraminal stenosis, disc degeneration, root entrapment from an uncinate spur or the fibrocartilagenous callus, or finally sacral compression as the sacral plexus passes over the dome of the sacrum.[1] These patients may also complain of significant deformity and a loss of trunk height. More disabling is the loss of sagittal plane alignment that may occur with high degrees of slip (Fig. 1). These patients may be unable to stand fully upright with their knees and hips fully extended because of the severe degree of lumbosacral kyphosis. This abnormal posture places an immense stress across the upper lumbar and thoracic spine as the patients attempt to hyperextend the trunk in order to maintain sagittal plane balance.[36] Patients with high degrees of slip, presenting with this type of problem, which is symptomatic, pose a greater challenge for the treating surgeon in determining the optimal technique to facilitate the return to normal function. The presence or absence of neurologic findings may also affect the treatment decision. It is well known that, in children, surgical stabilization alone usually results in an improvement in neurologic function, and hence decompression has not routinely been advocated in the child.[33, 38, 87] In the older adolescent, and particularly in the adult, it has been the author's experience that in patients presenting with neurologic dysfunction (i.e., motor dysfunction and symptoms of stenosis) maximum clinical improvement may be facilitated by decompression as well as by surgical stabilization procedures.

Another factor that might well affect the indication for surgery would be a full appreciation of the patient's long-term prognosis if he or she is not treated. A definitive answer to this question of surgery may not be stated at this time, but more recent publications have provided the physician with a better "feel" regarding the risk of further progression of the deformity and continued pain, if the individual is not treated. In several series reported to date, it has been noted that skeletally immature patients have a possibility of showing progression of the deformity in 0% to 24% of cases,[28, 60, 80, 81] and this appears to be most likely in the younger female patients with a dysplastic type of lesion that has a high degree of slippage (>50%), or a large slip angle (>45

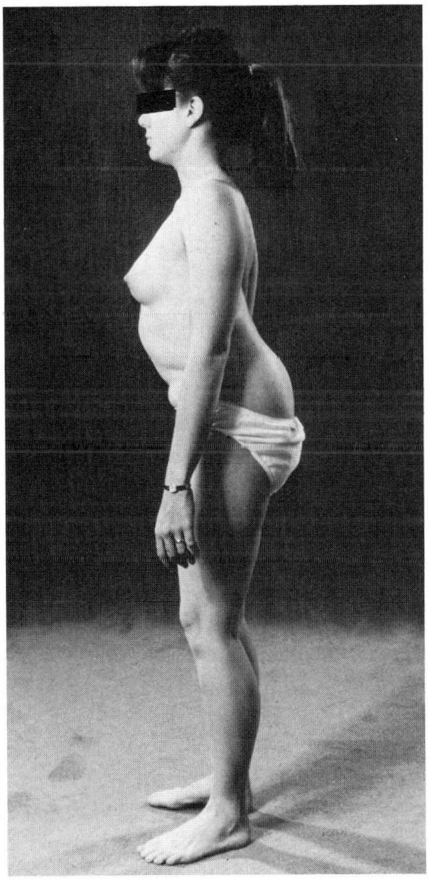

Figure 1 □ This photograph demonstrates the loss of sagittal plane alignment in a patient with a Grade 5 spondylolisthesis. Note the extreme degree of pelvic malrotation, the inability to stand upright with the knees fully extended, and the hyperlumbar lordosis that extends all the way up into the thoracic spine. This posture makes it extremely difficult for the patient to stand and walk for prolonged periods.

degrees) with instability demonstrated on flexion and extension.[6, 11] Untreated patients with slippage of greater than 50% may also show progression after skeletal maturity. Three of the nine patients reported by Harris and Weinstein[35] showed progression. Several patients in our series have also showed continued progression after skeletal maturity, particularly if decompression without stabilization has been carried out. Finally, a poor prognosis would be indicated by a symptomatic L4 spondylolysis or spondylolisthesis that was not managed surgically. These patients would appear to have a high probability of continued pain and disability.[70]

Indications for Surgery

Surgery would be indicated in the adolescent or adult patient with spondylolisthesis of the isthmic or dysplastic type if they presented with continued low back pain that was unresponsive to conservative management, with evidence of progressive slippage of greater than 30% to 50%, with neurologic findings consisting of radicular pain or symptoms of spinal stenosis, and with tension signs with positive straight-leg raising and an inability to stand and walk normally because of loss of sagittal alignment.[9, 11, 50, 62, 78] These patients should obviously be managed initially by nonoperative means consisting of rest and curtailment of activities. As symptoms improve, one could initiate a flexion or extension exercise program with a flexible lumbar back support. Anti-inflammatory medication, likewise, might be useful. Most patients could be significantly relieved with this course of treatment, progressing to full activity once the acute symptoms have subsided. A recurrence of symptoms or symptoms unresponsive to conservative management, of course, would dictate a more aggressive approach.

Surgical Treatment

The mainstay of managing adolescent and adult patients with spondylolisthesis consists of a bilateral lateral fusion in situ with iliac crest bone grafting.[9, 57, 78, 87, 88] We have not recommended instrumentation in the skeletally immature patient because successful arthrodesis by fusion in situ may be expected in greater than 95% of cases. However, once the patient has reached skeletal maturity, I believe that the arthrodesis is enhanced and that there is less likelihood of pseudarthrosis, by using internal fixation. At our center, we would now favor internal fixation for the adult patient, using a transpedicular device coupled with the bilateral lateral fusion. Our recent experience with Steffee instrumentation has provided a fusion rate of 93%[85] compared with Cleveland's reported figures of 17% pseudarthrosis for L4 to sacral fusions.[14] It has been our prejudice that patients return to full activity more expeditiously by augmenting the arthrodesis with rigid fixation. If the slippage is greater than 50%, extension of the fusion to L4 would be recommended.[11]

Decompression

Although the Gill procedure has been advocated in adults as a definitive procedure in spondylolisthesis associated with nerve root entrapment, as an isolated procedure in children it would be contraindicated.[30] Progression of the slippage results in a high percentage following Gill decompression. It has been our experience that, in the adult, the Gill decompression is not an effective procedure to adequately decompress the nerve roots.[86] This has been well noted by Edelson and Nathan,[22] who have demonstrated the residual hooklike projection of the lamina that persists, even after the Gill procedure is performed. To adequately decompress the nerve root underneath the spondylolytic defect, one must remove the residual bone to the base of the pedicle.[1] The indication for doing this would be a presentation with severe tension signs or radicular pain or a cauda equina syndrome.[19] In patients for whom a reduction is planned, a decompression would likewise be necessary.[10]

Operative Procedure

The patient is positioned on a four-poster type of frame, ensuring that the abdomen is completely free. The wound is prepped and draped in a routine fashion, and a midline incision is made from approximately the L3–L4 spinous process to the S1–S2 area. The incision is carried down through the subcutaneous tissue to the deep fascia. If instrumentation and/or a decompression is planned, the incision is continued through the midline, with a subperiosteal dissection off the spinous processes of L5 as well as of L4 if arthrodesis to L4 is planned. The soft tissues are stripped subperiosteally out to the tips of the transverse process and over the lateral aspect of the alar of the sacrum. A decompression, if planned, entails the removal of the loose arch of L5 with a residual hook of bone down the base of the pedicle, completely decompressing the L5 root bilaterally. Transpedicular fixation is then carried out in a customary manner using image control to ensure the proper placement of the pedicular screws. An iliac crest bone graft is taken through the same incision, and copious amounts of bone graft are placed from transverse process to alar of sacrum; spinal plates are placed on top of the screws and locked into position in a routine fashion. The wound is closed with appropriate drains. Approximately 2 days postoperatively the patient is ambulated. A flexible chair back brace may be used for comfort.

If decompression and instrumentation are not carried out, a muscle-splitting incision is made into the deep fascia approximately 2 to 3 inches lateral to the midline, just over the facets, exposing the facet joint and the transverse processes. Decortication and bone grafting are carried out in a routine fashion.

The patient is encouraged to progressively increase his or her activities over the first month postoperatively and, within 6 weeks, to begin a progressive range-of-motion, muscle-strengthening back exercise program to enhance rehabilitation and a return to normal activities.

Operative Management of L1 to L4 Spondylolysis or Spondylolisthesis

Symptomatic spondylolysis and spondylolisthesis above L5 carry a somewhat poorer prognosis for continued low back pain. Saraste has recently noted this association, and that finding has been supported by the clinical experience at our center as well.[69] The options of treatment in this group of patients following a failure of conservative management consist of fusion with or without decompression. Again, it is the author's experience that, if the patient presents with significant radicular pain and evidence of stenosis on computed tomography (CT), decompression along with arthrodesis is the procedure of choice. One may consider performing a free-floating fusion following the decompression; that is, an arthrodesis (for instance) from L4 to L5 in the presence of an L4 defect. This may be supplemented with instrumentation. If there is significant displacement of greater than 25 degrees and reduction is thought to be indicated, a transpedicular device has proven useful, although the implant must be extended to S1. Again, it is the author's impression that a better decompression may be achieved by partial reduction with a transpedicular internal fixation device; however, there are no satisfactory data available at this time to suggest that this may be a preferable alternative to fusion in situ.

A symptomatic defect in the younger adult from L1 to L4 with insignificant displacement may likewise be managed successfully by repairing the pars defect alone.[8] This may be carried out with a single circlage wire passing around the transverse process and secured to the spinous process. Cancellous bone grafts placed from the transverse process to the spinous process underneath the circlage wire following decortication ensure a satisfactory rate of healing. In the patient over 25 or 30 years of age, I would not favor using this technique, especially if there is evidence of facet and disc degeneration. In these cases, a free-floating fusion or arthrodesis and instrumentation to the adjoining vertebra appear to offer the greatest possibility of pain relief.

Alternative Treatments to Posterior Lateral Fusion in Situ

Although reduction of spondylolisthesis was first carried out by Scherb in 1919[74] and first mentioned in the English literature by Jenkins in 1936,[41] little progress was made in furthering this concept until the past few decades. Harris in 1951[36] presented a classic monograph describing the causes of back and radicular pain, the kyphotic relationship of L5 to S1, and the importance of this angulation in producing the severe degree of deformity in high-grade slips. He also described the technique for skeletal traction that could reduce the spondylolisthesis. Subsequent work by Taillard,[80] Newman,[59] Lance,[48] and others[20, 21, 34] further demonstrated techniques for reduction and arthrodesis by the posterior approach. More recent techniques for internal fixation,[23, 53, 56, 79] as well as combined approaches,[10, 12, 29, 39, 89, 90] have been described. Unfortunately, the stated rationale for reduction—that is, restoration of normal biomechanical function, improved likelihood of arthrodesis, reversal of neurologic deficits, and elimination of pain as well as improved cosmesis—has not always been realized by those who advocate reduction techniques.[53] This, coupled with the realization that some patients with high-grade slips function well without reduction, leads some authors to believe that reduction should never be carried out.[35, 57]

It is indeed recognized that the main treatment for spondylolisthesis is surgical arthrodesis. However, it has been known that with high grades of slips, 50% or greater, further slippage may occur, even if the patient remains supine. The incidence of this varies from 10% to 37%[6, 7, 17, 31, 49, 59] and may occur even in the young adult, especially if a posterior decompression concomitant with the fusion is performed. A reduction, or at least a partial reduction, improving the lumbosacral kyphosis would improve the biomechanical orientation of the spine and conceivably facilitate a more certain arthrodesis. Furthermore, reduction would be likely to open the neuroforamina, decompressing the 5th root, and to correct the sagittal plane malalignment, allowing the patient to stand more fully upright with the knees and hips extended. These mechanical principles, coupled with the realization that the natural history of untreated Grade 4 or Grade 5 spondylolisthesis along with fusion in situ may not be quite as favorable as has been suggested, have led many authors to consider undertaking reductions and attempting to redefine their role, although it is an understandably limited one. The data of Harris and Weinstein[35] showed that, of 11 patients with high-grade slips, only 36% were asymptomatic, and 45% had atrophy or positive neurologic findings. Three of the 11 had progressed after maturity. Of 21 patients who had undergone fusion in situ, only 57% were asymptomatic and three of the 21 had progressed. Pregnancy was not a problem, even in the presence of spondyloptosis. This finding has been confirmed by Saraste.[69a]

Cast Reduction Technique

Scaglietti and coworkers[71, 72] noted that by applying a cast in an extension mode across the lumbosacral junction, reduction of the lumbosacral kyphosis was possible (Fig. 2). We have found this technique most useful in the skeletally immature patients with high degrees of slippage and sagittal plane malalignment. However, we have also used it in young adults with flexible deformities in an attempt to correct the kyphosis only. It has not proved effective in correcting translation or the percentage of slippage.[7]

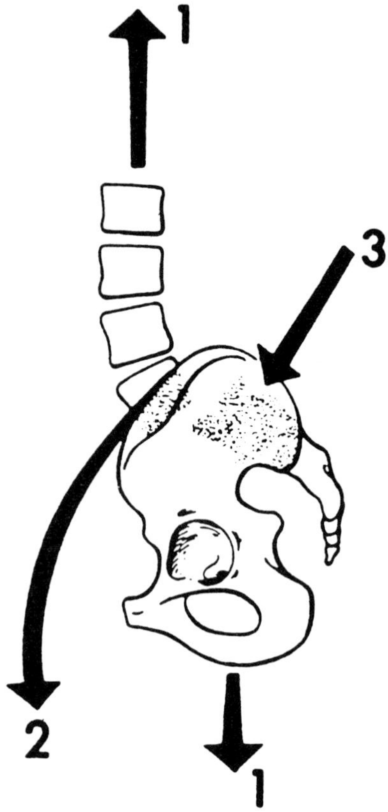

Figure 2 □ The concept of cast reduction for spondylolisthesis is achieved by applying axial traction (1) with pelvic rotation (2, 3); reduction of the lumbosacral kyphosis therefore is possible.

The advantages of this procedure are as follows: (1) The correction of lumbosacral kyphos can be carried out while the patient is awake after a posterior lateral fusion has been performed. (2) A posterior fusion mass is placed under compression, thereby theoretically enhancing the likelihood of healing. (3) At least in the child, the anterior portion of the sacral cortex is decompressed, allowing sacral remodeling to develop. Scaglietti and coworkers[71, 72] have applied this cast 3 or 4 months before the patient has undergone fusion. We found that this is unnecessary and actually carry out the bilateral fusion in situ, applying the cast 1 week after

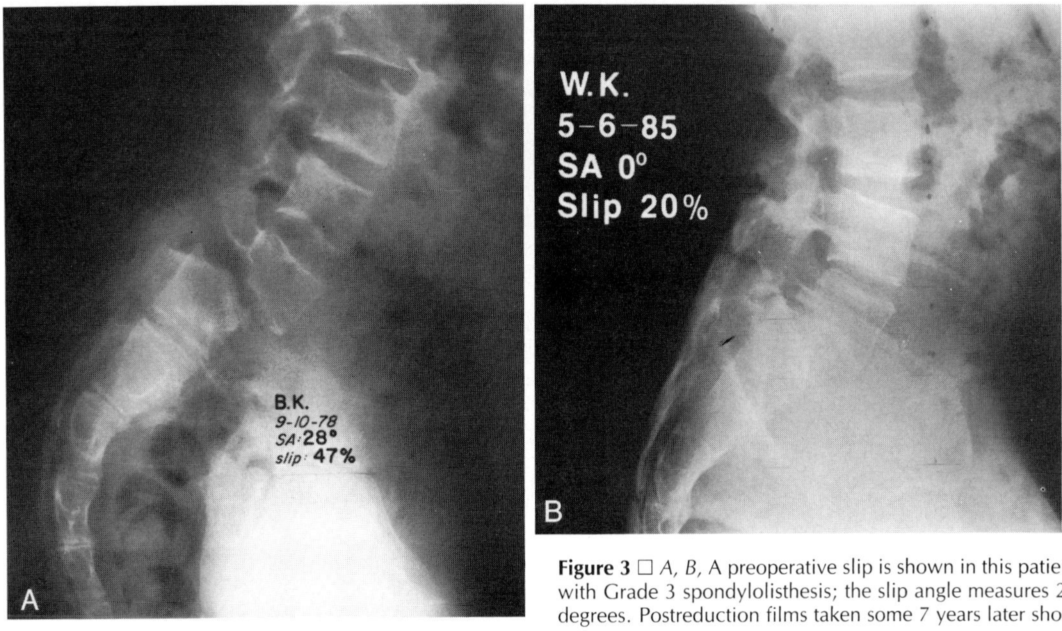

Figure 3 □ *A, B,* A preoperative slip is shown in this patient with Grade 3 spondylolisthesis; the slip angle measures 28 degrees. Postreduction films taken some 7 years later show a 0-degree slip angle and the percentage of slip has actually decreased. Generally speaking, the percentage of slip does not improve so much, and only the angulation of kyphosis improves with this closed reduction technique.

surgery. This procedure is most useful in the child and the young adolescent, as mentioned, because it can be applied to a mature adolescent or younger adult with marked instability in whom instrumentation is not contemplated. If the reduction appears to be reasonably stable and the correction is maintained with the patient upright and in a cast with a single pantaloon, the individual may be ambulated and then converted to an orthosis about 3 to 4 months later.

We have now performed closed reduction techniques in 35 patients (Fig. 3). Results in 22 patients with an average follow-up of 40 months have been reported.[7] The percentage of slip preoperatively averaged 50%; postoperatively, 43%; and at follow-up, 40%. The preoperative slip angle averaged 33 degrees; postreduction, 12 degrees; and at follow-up, 11 degrees. Loss of correction occurred in four patients, and this appeared to be related to a decompression procedure, a high degree of slip, and an inability to correct the relationship of L4 to the sacrum, which we had labeled the "stable zone" (Fig. 4).[11]

Posterior Techniques for Reduction

Distraction techniques for reduction of spondylolisthesis were proposed by Harrington and Tullos in 1971.[34] Others have advocated these techniques as well.[20, 21] It has been our center's experience that the kyphos is poorly corrected by distraction and that, in fact, the deformity above the kyphosis is aggravated by distraction. We have, therefore, favored transpedicular devices such as those reported by Louis,[52] Steffee,[79] and Edwards.[23] These techniques might be considered under the following circumstances:

1. The patient is physiologically mature.
2. The loss of sagittal plane alignment is unacceptable.
3. The bone stock is satisfactory.
4. Decompression is indicated.
5. The patient presents with a high-level slip, greater than 50%, with a significant kyphosis of greater than 45 degrees.

These techniques are highly demanding operative procedures, and great caution should be taken to ensure that the nerve roots are adequately decompressed before, during, and at the completion of the reduction (Fig. 5). If the nerve roots appear tight during any part of the procedure, some residual displacement must be accepted. Nerve conduction studies or a wake-up test during the operation is recommended (Fig. 6).

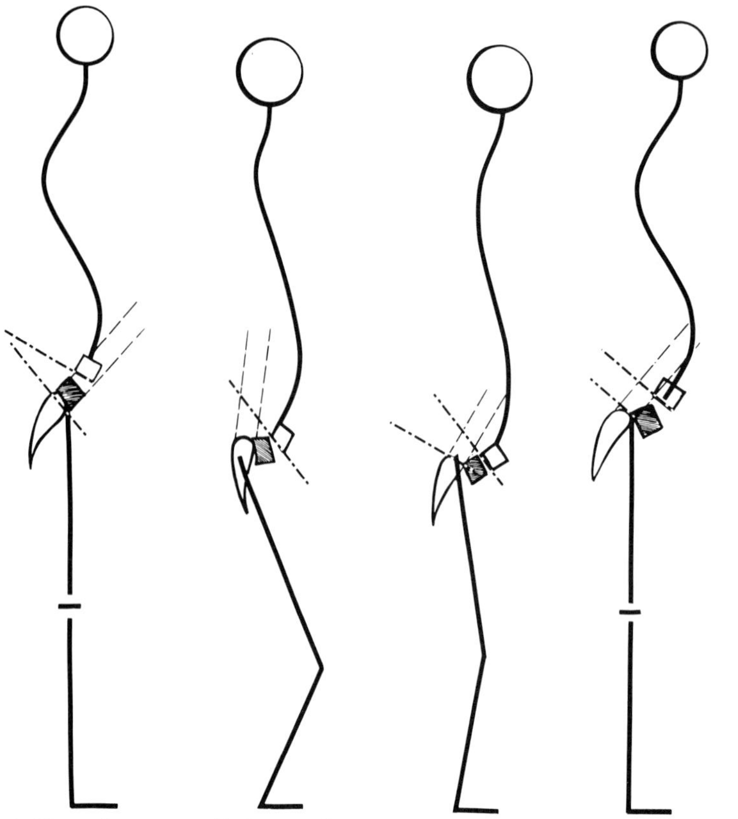

Figure 4 □ *A–D,* Note the anatomic arrangement of a normal spine in relation to the L5–L4 vertebral body and the sacrum in the presence of severe slips and the unsatisfactory reduction in a cast. If L4 is not placed in the so-called stable zone, which is a more cephalic extension of the axis of the sacrum, then the reduction is not maintained and sagittal plane alignment is lost. If, as noted in *D,* L4 is placed into the anatomic zone, a reduction appears to be stable in the author's experience.

Anterior and Combined Approaches to Reduction

Anterior fusion had been recommended by several authors for the treatment of spondylolisthesis because it places the 5th vertebra in a better anatomic relationship and allows positioning of the bone graft under favorable conditions for healing. Several authors[89, 90] had described combined anterior and posterior approaches for reduction.[10, 12, 20, 29, 39, 70, 77] We found these techniques to be most useful when the patient presented with (1) intractable pain (back pain or sciatica), (2) a high-grade slip, (3) a loss of sagittal alignment, and (4) a failure of previous posterior or anterior surgery. In these patients, a single-stage posterior procedure is possible, but it may prove much more difficult, unless a discectomy is done anteriorly or an anterior osteotomy is performed in the presence of a previous anterior interbody fusion. It must be stressed that the indications for these procedures are not common and, in our experience at our center, the need is infrequent.

For combined procedures (Fig. 7*A, B*), the operative technique consists of a first-stage posterior approach with complete decompression and removal of the loose arch of L5. A resection of the dome of the sacrum may be necessary in Grade 4 or Grade 5 slips. Complete decompression of the L5 roots bilaterally is carried out. A bilateral transverse process fusion of L4 to sacrum is then done. If internal fixation has been carried out, transpedicular devices are placed under image control; onc should be certain that the screws are properly seeded in the vertebral body. Slow sustained reduction is

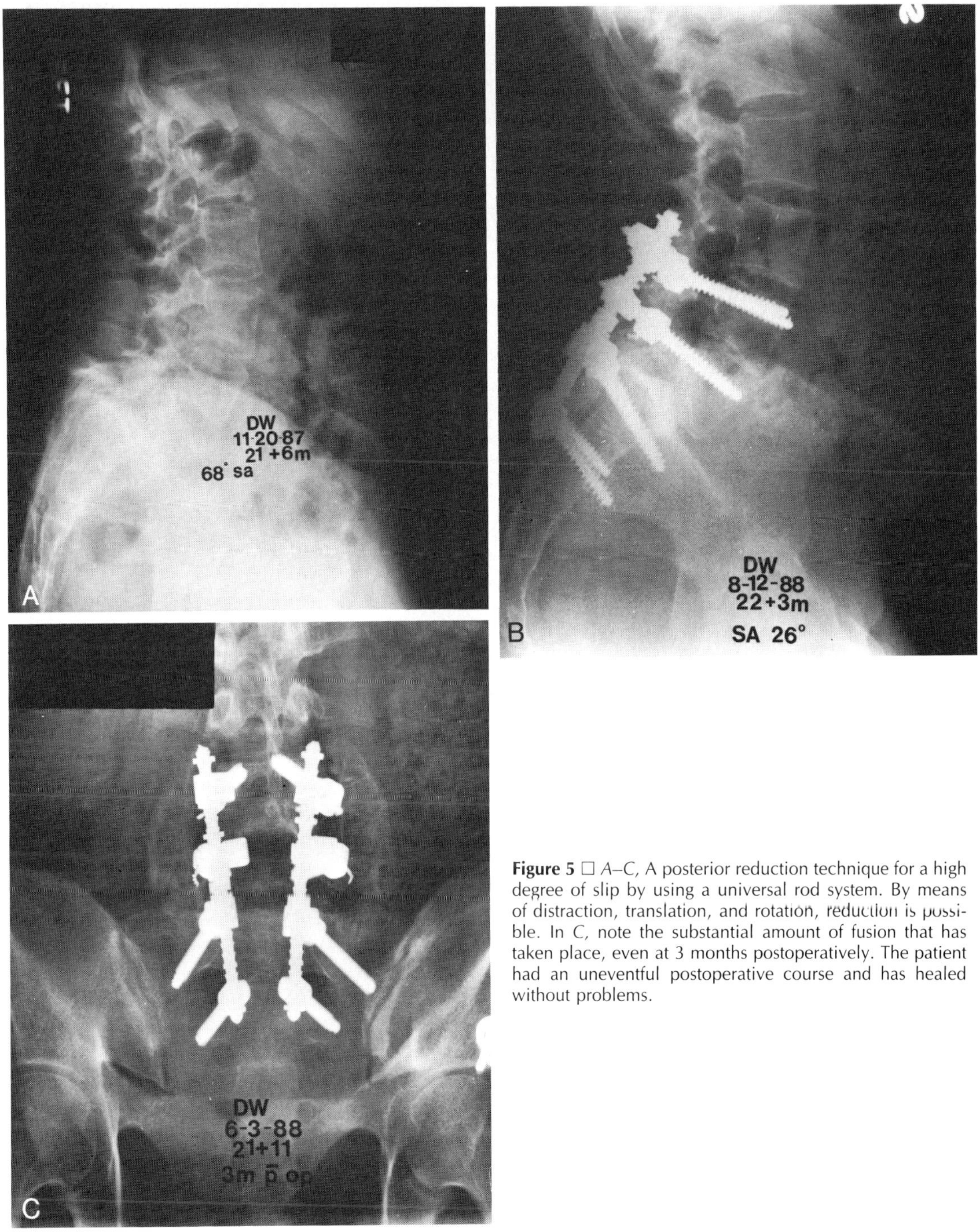

Figure 5 □ *A–C,* A posterior reduction technique for a high degree of slip by using a universal rod system. By means of distraction, translation, and rotation, reduction is possible. In *C,* note the substantial amount of fusion that has taken place, even at 3 months postoperatively. The patient had an uneventful postoperative course and has healed without problems.

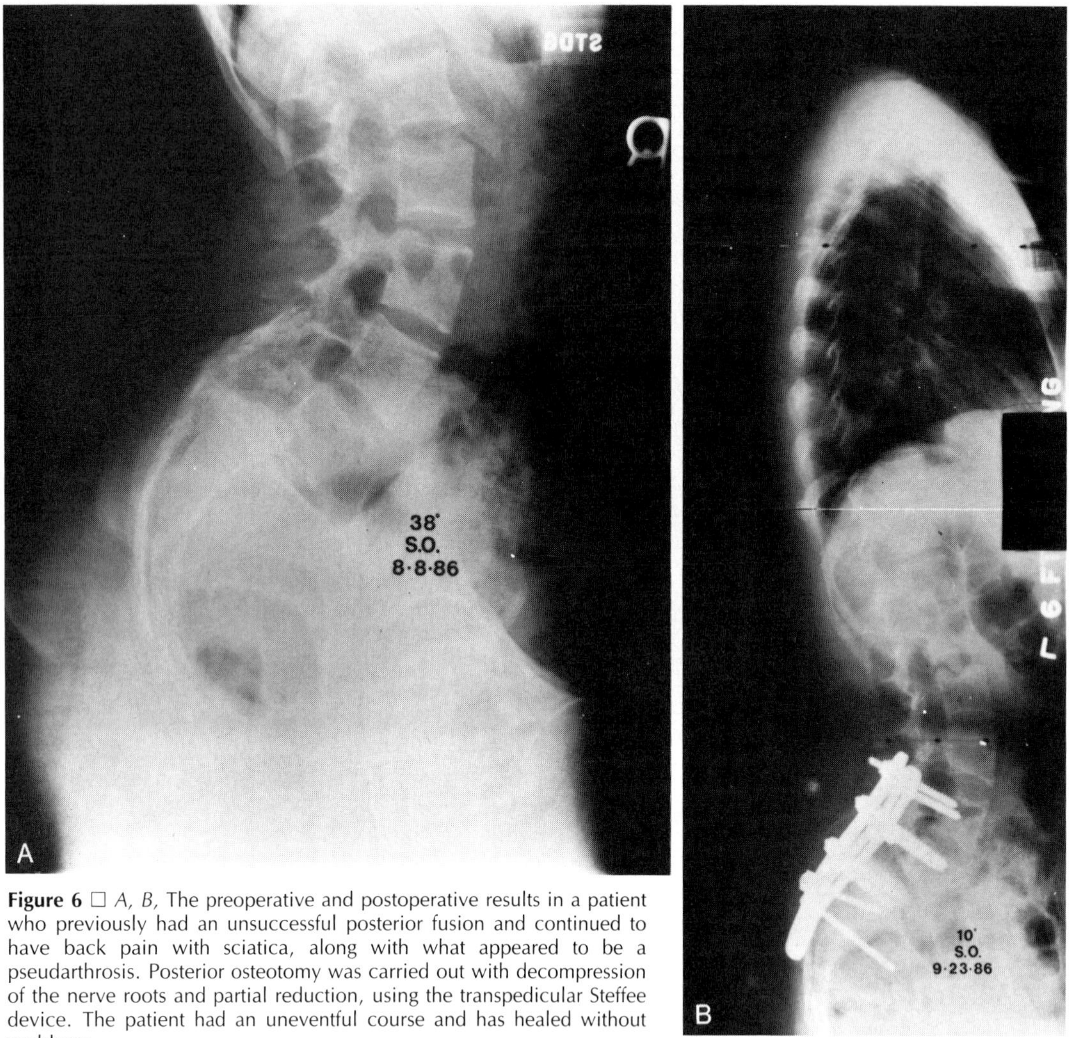

Figure 6 □ *A, B,* The preoperative and postoperative results in a patient who previously had an unsuccessful posterior fusion and continued to have back pain with sciatica, along with what appeared to be a pseudarthrosis. Posterior osteotomy was carried out with decompression of the nerve roots and partial reduction, using the transpedicular Steffee device. The patient had an uneventful course and has healed without problems.

carried out, and multiple wake-up tests are done to assure neurologic integrity.

If a second-stage procedure is being carried out, the patient may be placed in halo, pelvic pin traction between stages, in order to achieve some partial reduction of the kyphosis. One to two weeks later, a retroperitoneal or a transperitoneal approach is performed in the midline with exposure to the L5 vertebral body. Cautery should be used with caution, and the presacral plexus is identified and displaced primarily to the left. The middle sacral artery and vein are ligated, and multiple retractors are placed to facilitate the exposure. The intervertebral disc is excised, and the L5 vertebra is carefully levered up to further correct the kyphosis. The fibula strut graft is obtained and then locked into position underneath the L5 vertebra and into the anterior cortex of S1–S2 level. It must be realized that the sacrum is extremely thin, and great care should be taken to prevent the fibula graft from breaking through the inner cortex of the sacrum.

One week postoperatively an extension cast is applied, incorporating the one leg to the midthigh. The patient remains supine for 2 to 3 months and then ambulates in a cast or brace for an additional 4 to 6 months. Should an L5 vertebral body resection be elected, the anterior approach is done first, followed by a second-stage posterior decompression with repositioning of L4 over the sacrum. Transpedicular fixation is preferred.

Thirty-eight patients up until 1985 were

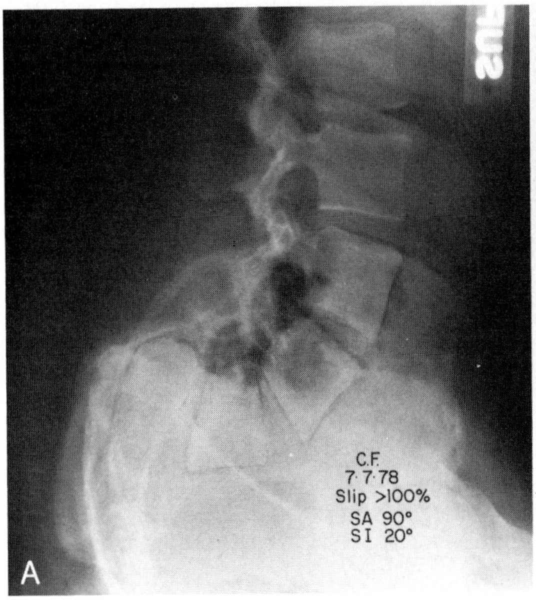

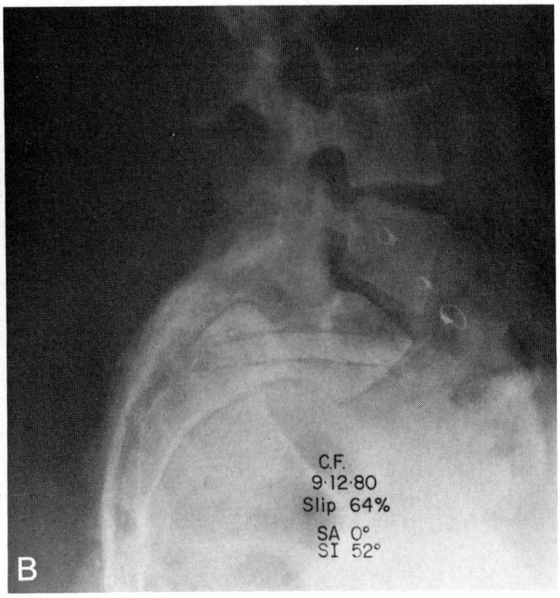

Figure 7 □ *A, B,* The results of a combined approach for reducing a high degree of slip. Although translational displacement has not been substantially corrected, the slip angle has been markedly improved, and the patient is now able to stand upright with the hips and knees fully extended with the normal amount of lumbar lordosis and thoracic kyphus.

operated on at our center using this technique. Sixteen patients have undergone staged reconstruction to salvage a failed result from previous procedures. Twenty-two have not had previous surgery. Five of those were lost to follow-up. Of the 17 patients who have not had previous surgery, the follow-up ranged from 2 to 7.5 years. All have been relieved of their pain. The preoperative slip angle improved from 71 to 32 degrees. The preoperative percentage of slip averaged 100 degrees, and this did not change significantly at follow-up. Pseudarthrosis developed in three patients, and two needed additional surgery to obtain a solid arthrodesis. Three patients developed an L5 neuropathy postoperatively; one recovered, and two were left with mild residual anterior tibial weakness, which was not a functional problem and did not affect ambulation.

The other 16 patients with Grade 4 or 5 spondylolisthesis who had previous surgery obtained similar satisfactory results. All were relieved of their symptoms postoperatively, at an average follow-up of 52 months. The preoperative percentage of slip averaged 100%; postoperatively it averaged 56% and at follow-up, 56%. The slip angle averaged 74 degrees preoperatively, 11 degrees postoperatively, and 11 degrees at follow-up. It is possible that the improved correction in this group was related to the fact that several patients underwent a third-stage posterior spinal fusion with instrumentation. Five patients developed neuropathy, three recovered totally, and two had residual anterior tibial weakness that did not interfere with functional ambulation. All were relieved of their pain (Fig. 8).

Surgical reduction, although an attractive concept, should not be undertaken without careful evaluation. Matthias has reported an incidence of neuropathy of about 5%, which is similar to our finding.[53] The functional disability from this has been negligible, however. One should also remember that neuropathy, or abnormal neurologic findings, may occur in patients without treatment. Saraste reported 18%,[70] Matthiass reported 45%,[53] and Harris reported 45%.[35] Cauda equina compression may also develop without treatment or with bilateral fusion in situ without instrumentation.[70, 75] Even with this in mind, it appears to me that reduction should be undertaken only under the following conditions: (1) a loss of sagittal alignment significantly compromises function, and (2) in the presence of a high-grade slip,

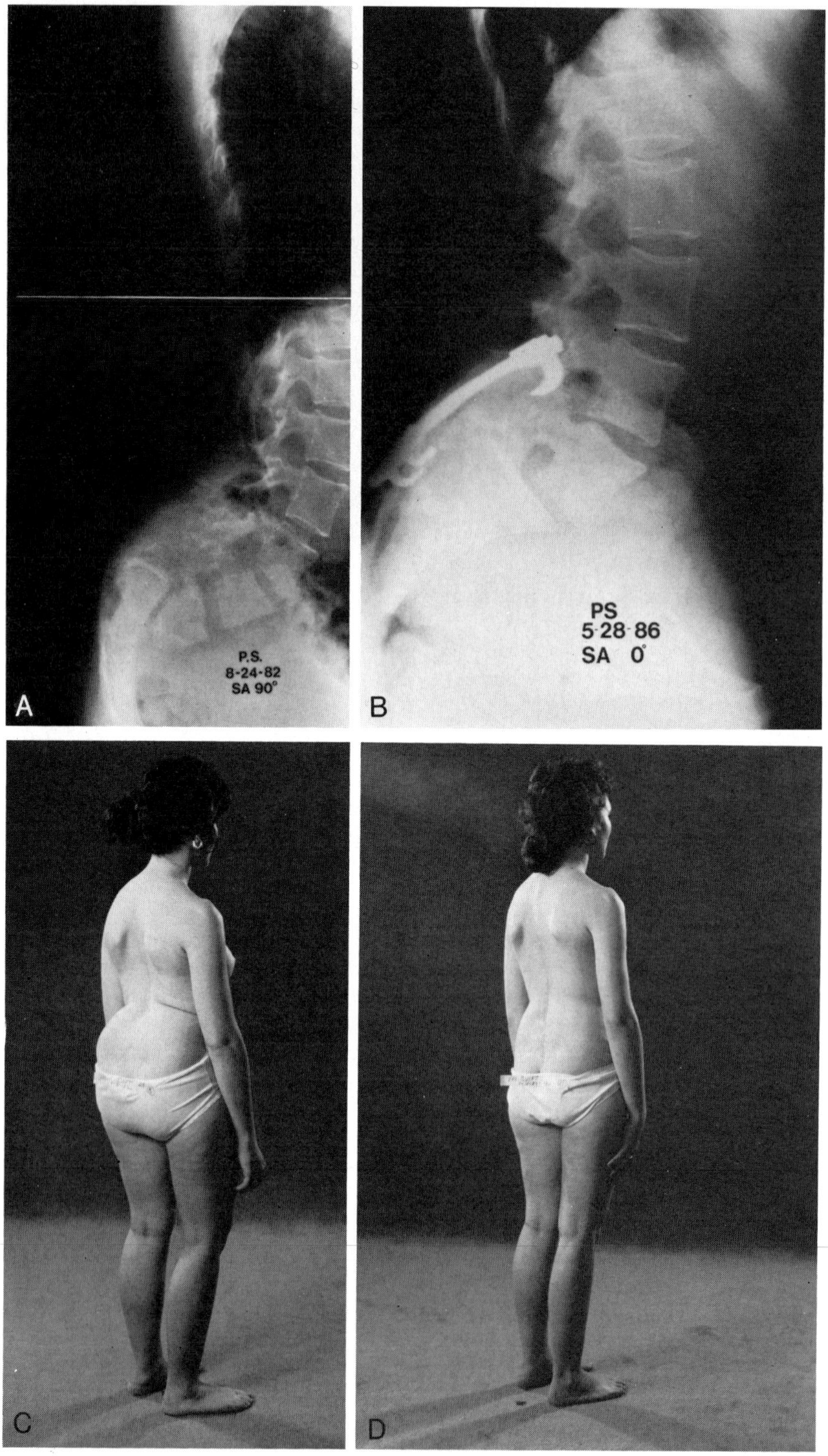

Figure 8 □ A more severe degree of deformity in a patient who had had three previous procedures: two posterior and one anterior. Because of intractable stenotic pain, inability to stand upright, and constant back pain, a staged osteotomy with reconstruction was carried out. The patient had an excellent anatomic correction of her deformity, became able to stand upright with the knees and hips fully extended, and has been relieved of her pain. *A*, A preoperative lateral x-ray. *B*, A 4-year postoperative lateral x-ray. *C*, *D*, Preoperative and postoperative clinical photographs, respectively.

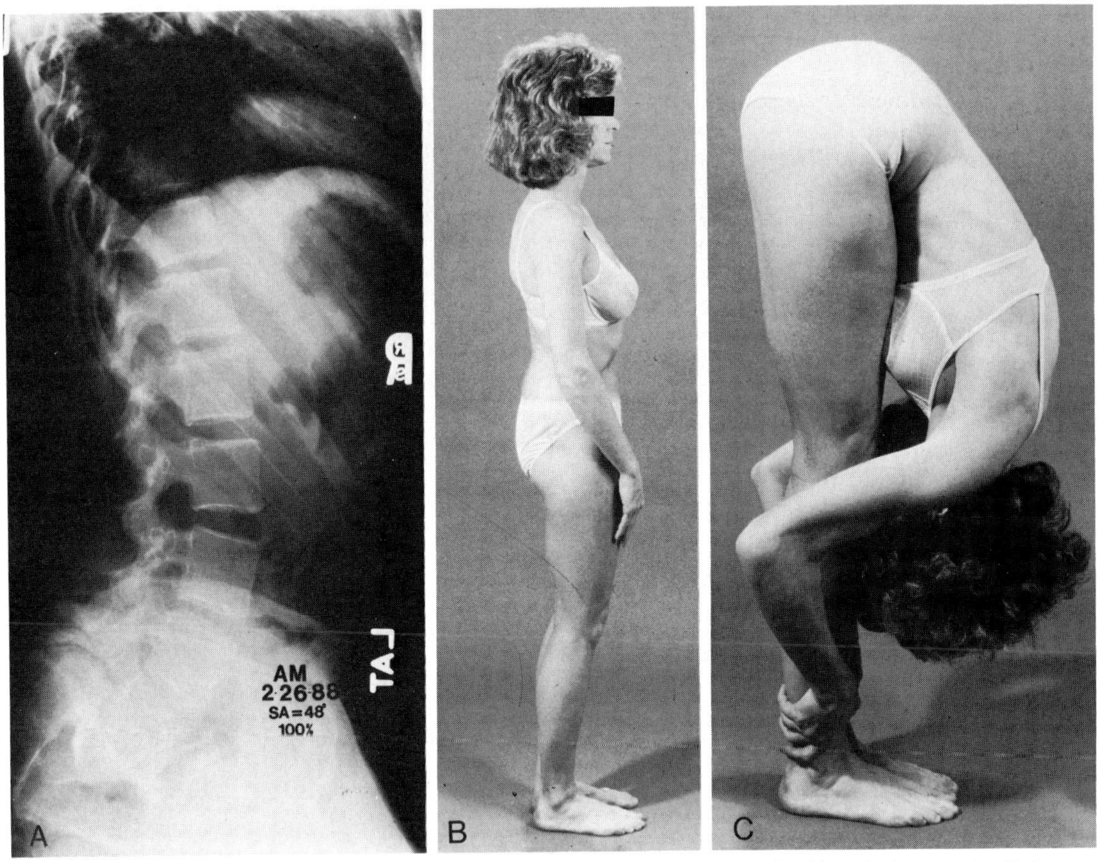

Figure 9 □ The importance of treating the patient and not the x-ray is demonstrated. Although the x-ray itself shows a severe degree of spondyloptosis (*A*), one can see by looking at the patient that she has normal sagittal alignment and excellent flexibility of the lumbar spine as well as of the hips (*B, C*). Surgery was definitely not indicated. Her symptoms were mild, and she was functioning at a high level of performance. She was advised that surgery was not indicated.

decompression is thought necessary and therefore the likelihood of further slippage is increased. It should be remembered that anatomic reduction is not necessary and that neurologic function should be monitored during, as well as after, surgery. We have seen neuropathy develop 2 and 3 days postoperatively, and it appears to be related to root swelling. It is usually reversible. Longer follow-up and greater experience are necessary in order to fully assess the role of surgical reduction and determine whether the increased risk fully justifies the benefits. A fusion in situ is still the most acceptable procedure in the management of spondylolisthesis in the adult as well as the mature adolescent. If pseudarthrosis is probable or develops following an in situ fusion, augmentation is still possible by a posterior interbody fusion, as described by Bohlman,[4, 43] or an anterior strut fusion, as described by Verbiest.[84] We have used both approaches and find they are most helpful in the situations described (Fig. 9).

DEGENERATIVE SPONDYLOLISTHESIS

Degenerative spondylolisthesis, that is, vertebral displacement in the absence of a pars defect, was first described as a pathologic entity by Junghanns in 1930.[44, 45] He identified 11 cases and used the term *pseudospondylolisthesis* to describe the disorder. He noted that it usually occurred at the L4 vertebral level.

In 1950, Macnab[55] reported 22 cases of spondylolisthesis with an intact neural arch, and he coined the phrase "spondylolisthesis with an intact neural arch," objecting to the term pseudospondylolisthesis. He thought that patients presenting with symptoms involving minimal degrees of displacement were well managed with spinal fusion. Those who had more severe symptoms with radiculopathy were best managed by decompression and fusion. Since that time, it is safe to say that the controversy has continued between those who recommend decompression and those who recommend decompression with arthrodesis.

One of the more important studies was that published by Rosenberg in 1975,[65, 66] in which he studied 20 skeletons and reported on 200 patients with degenerative spondylolisthesis. He noted that the slipped vertebra and its adjacent vertebra demonstrated abnormalities in the articular process, particularly with hypertrophy of the superior facet of L5 and encroachment on the spinal canal and spinal stenosis of the lateral recess. He noted that degenerative spondylolisthesis occurs 4 times more frequently in females than in males, 6 to 9 times more frequently at the L4–L5 level than at L5–S1, 3 times more frequently in blacks than in whites, and 4 times more frequently in the presence of a sacralized L5 vertebra. He did not see slippage before the 5th decade. In the absence of decompression, slippage never exceeded 30%. Of particular interest was the finding of Rosenberg that the patients with degenerative spondylolisthesis had reduced lumbar lordosis at the L5–S1 junction, whereas those with isthmic spondylolisthesis showed hyperlordosis at the L5–S1 articulation. The cause of this degenerative process with slippage is not completely known, but it is certain that the degenerative process takes place at the facet joint as well as at the intervertebral disc. Allbrook[2] believed that when the sacrum was relatively high, the L4 vertebra was exposed to greater stresses. Farfan hypothesized that the process was related to a series of forced rotational injuries, usually occurring at the L4–L5 joint.[25, 26] Whether local segmental instability or excessive stresses across that area produce instability cannot conclusively be stated at this time.[47] The fact that there is such a high incidence of sacralization of L5 certainly lends credibility to the concept of abnormal forces and stresses with degenerative changes at that joint.

Clinical Presentation[16, 24, 73, 82]

Patients with degenerative spondylolisthesis usually present with back, buttock, or thigh pain; radicular pain; or neurogenic claudication. Alternatively, they may present with components of all of these symptoms. The pain is described as an aching discomfort in the low back that is aggravated with activity, is relieved by rest, and is often associated with radicular pain not dissimilar to that of disc herniation. A few patients may present with pseudoclaudication type of pain described as weakness and numbness in the legs that begins during walking and is relieved by rest. They may have genital or perineal numbness, or urinary incontinence. Documented neurologic findings may be present in about 40% of the patients and usually involve the L5 nerve root with a diminished sensory perception to pin prick, distal motor weakness, and atrophy.

Radiographic Evaluation

X-ray findings usually demonstrate significant degenerative changes of the posterior facet joints with disc space narrowing at L4–L5 and minimal anterior translation of L4 on L5. A CT scan with or without enhancement will demonstrate significant neural constriction.

Treatment

Treatment may revolve around numerous conservative modalities. All patients should certainly be tried on a conservative regimen before surgery is recommended. These treatments may consist of lumbar exercises, either flexion or extension depending on the patient's tolerance, anti-inflammatory medications, facet joint injections, and occasional epidural blocks. We have sometimes found cutaneous electric stimulation to be of some benefit, although it is rather marginal over a long period of time. Underarm body orthoses may provide significant relief of back pain and even, occasionally, some relief of spinal stenosis–type pain. These braces may not have long-term benefit but certainly they should be tried on all patients before surgical intervention is undertaken (Fig. 10*A*, *B*).

It is the author's impression that the optimal surgical results are obtained with de-

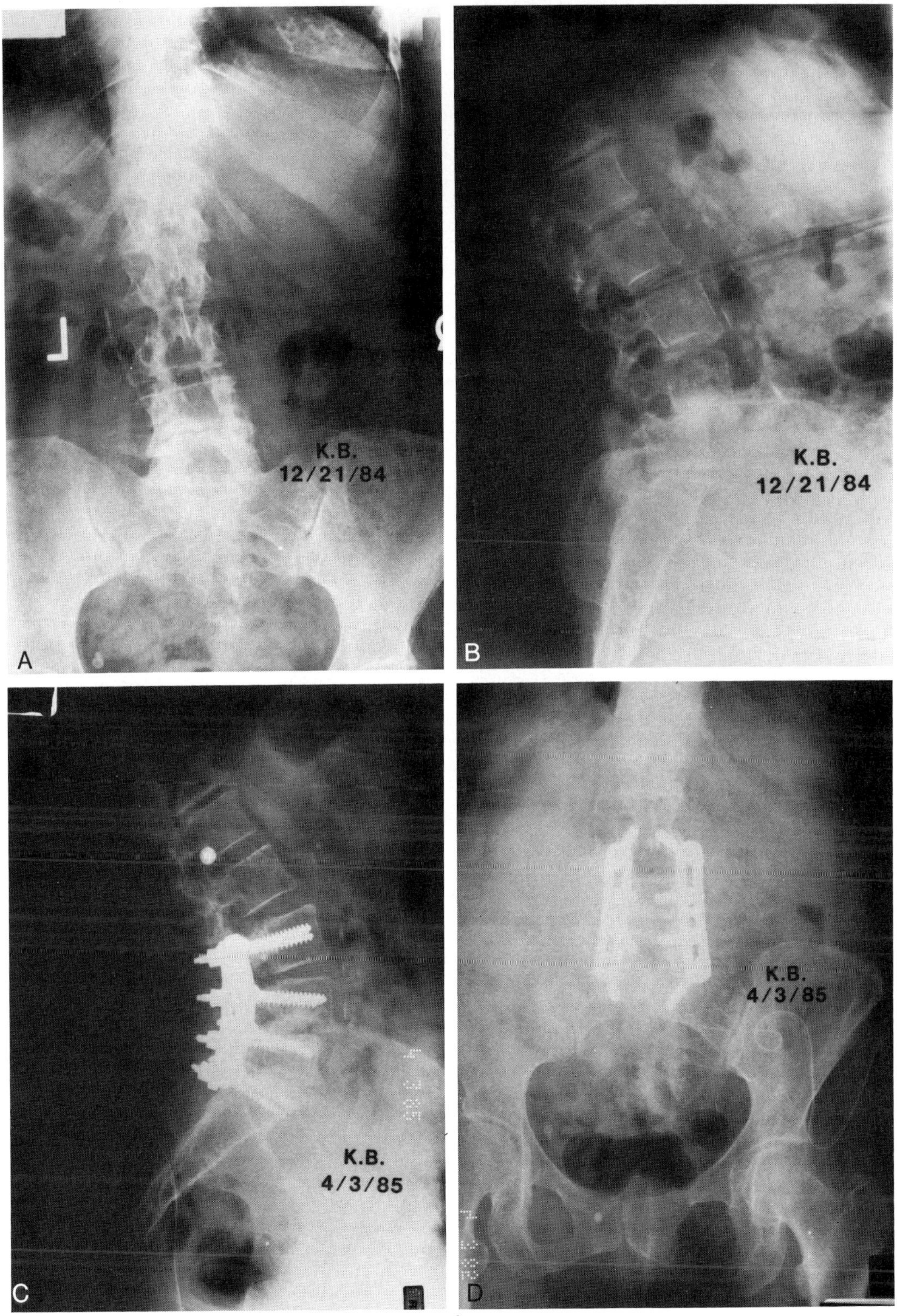

Figure 10 □ The preoperative x-rays, AP and lateral (*A, B*), of a patient with a Grade-3 degenerative spondylolisthesis after laminectomy. Her symptoms have continued; she has recurrence of her radicular pain, and she is incapacitated with back pain. Progressive slippage after this decompression is not uncommon. The patient was subsequently treated with bilateral fusion and transpedicular fixation with partial reduction of the slippage (*C, D*). She has obtained excellent relief from symptoms and has no further radicular or spinal stenotic type of pain.

compression along with arthrodesis. There is considerable controversy, however, as to the need for arthrodesis in all patients[64, 67, 83] Epstein and coworkers published what appeared to be good results with decompression only, but 40 patients were followed for an average of 5.5 months, and the other 20 for 3.5 years.[24] Studies published by Dall,[16] Dandy,[17] Davis,[18, 19] and Laurent and Osterman[49] are among a few that would lead one to think that decompression procedures per se may produce unsatisfactory results in up to 50% of the patients over the long term. In the report of Cedell and Wiberg,[13] none of their patients were symptom free. Furthermore, progressive slippage following decompression has been noted by many authors.[18] Amuso and coworkers[3] reported that 28% of patients in their series developed further progression, and Reynolds and Wiltse[63] noted that it occurred in all of their patients who underwent a more radical facetectomy. Johnsson and colleagues[42] noted a 65% increase in slippage after decompression, and Lee[51] reported postoperative slipping in all of his patients. Nevertheless, it seems certain that the radicality of decompression may affect the results. Greater relief of radicular and stenosis type pain is more likely with more extensive decompression, which also increases the likelihood of slippage.[16] In this regard, it is interesting that more recent studies reported by Kaneda and associates[46] and Hanley,[32] as well as Feffer and coworkers,[27] would lead one to believe that stabilization with the decompression procedure would lead to the optimal long-term result. Anterior fusion without decompression has recently been proposed by Inoue and associates,[40] and their results look most gratifying. It is my experience that single-stage anterior interbody fusion has generally not worked well, and graft collapse with pseudarthrosis is usual.

Author's Preferred Technique

After the patient has been prepared and draped, a midline incision is made and exposure proceeds down the L4–L5 area. The L4 lamina is removed, as is a portion or all of L5 as necessary to totally decompress and expose the canal and the L4–L5 roots. The lateral recesses are completely undercut, and every attempt is made to preserve the facet joints. It is most important to undercut the superior facet to ensure that the 5th root is not impaled and that the L4 root is not compressed as it lies in the recess just superior to the disc space. Once the decompression has been completed, transpedicular fixation is carried out at L4–L5 and S1, resulting in partial, if not complete, correction of the deformity. Care is taken to be sure that no intervertebral disc or osteophyte material is brought back into the canal with reduction of the L4–L5 slippage. A bilateral lateral fusion is performed, using iliac crest bone grafting. A fat graft or absorbable gelatin sponge (Gelfoam) is placed over the dura, and the wound is closed in a routine fashion. It should be appreciated that instrumentation is not necessary to achieve a satisfactory result. I believe, however, that pain relief is greater and early return to activities is more likely with instant stabilization. In the first 61 procedures performed at our center using transpedicular fixation with Steffee plate and screws with a 2-year follow up or more, we have achieved a fusion rate of 92% in patients who had not undergone previous surgery.[85] One patient developed a deep wound infection and the implant had to be removed; four patients developed a pseudarthrosis that subsequently required repair. Two patients developed nerve deficits attributable to screw placement, and both completely recovered over the months following surgery.

One of the disadvantages of using internal fixation is the necessity of usually fusing across the slipped articulation down to the sacrum. Those who advocate decompression and fusion can present convincing evidence that a free-floating fusion at L4–L5 is necessary. If one wished to obtain some reduction, it would be necessary to fuse into the sacrum, in order to have the stable implant base required for an L4–L5 reduction. Furthermore, the bone content of the osteopenic spine is by definition meager, and transpedicular fixation may therefore be jeopardized. That has not been our experience, although it is always a possibility.

In summary, although it is known that decompression should relieve the symptoms of spinal stenosis, for the most part it appears less helpful in relieving back complaints. The emerging general consensus appears to be that the optimal result, in terms of pain relief and improved function, will most likely occur in patients who undergo a decompression procedure along with surgical arthrodesis.

References

1. Adkins, E.W.O.: Spondylolisthesis. J. Bone Joint Surg. 37B:48, 1955.
2. Allbrook, D.: Movements of the lumbar spine column. J. Bone Joint Surg. 39B:339–345, 1957.
3. Amuso, S.J., Neff, R.S., Coulson, D.B., and Laing, P.G.: The surgical treatment of spondylolisthesis by posterior element resection. J. Bone Joint Surg. 52A:529, 1970.
4. Bohlman, H.H., and Cook, S.S.: One-stage decompression and posterolateral and interbody fusion for lumbosacral spondyloptosis through a posterior approach. J. Bone Joint Surg. 64A:415–418, 1982.
5. Bosworth, D.M., Fielding, J.W., Demarest, L., and Bonaquist, M.: Spondylolisthesis: A critical review of a consecutive series of cases treated by arthrodesis. J. Bone Joint Surg. 37A:767, 1955.
6. Boxall, D., Bradford, D.S., Winter, R.B., and Moe, J.H.: Management of severe spondylolisthesis in children and adolescents. J. Bone Joint Surg. 8:12, 1979.
7. Bradford, D.S.: Closed reduction of spondylolisthesis: An experience in 22 patients. Spine 13:580, 1988.
8. Bradford, D.S.: Repair of spondylolysis or minimal degrees of spondylolisthesis by segmental wire fixation and bone grafting. Spine 10:673, 1985.
9. Bradford, D.S.: Spondylolysis and spondylolisthesis in children and adolescents. *In* Bradford, D.S., and Hensinger, R.N. (eds.): Pediatric Spine. New York, Thieme and Stratton, 1985.
10. Bradford, D.S.: Treatment of severe spondylolisthesis: A combined approach for reduction and stabilization. Spine 4:423, 1979.
11. Bradford, D.S.: Spondylolisthesis. *In* Bradford, D.S., et al (eds.): Moe's Textbook of Scoliosis and Other Deformities, 2nd Ed. Philadelphia, W.B. Saunders, 1987.
12. Bradford, D.S., and Gottfried, Y.: Staged salvage reconstruction of grades IV and V spondylolisthesis. J. Bone Joint Surg. 69A:191, 1987.
13. Cedell, C., and Wiberg, G.: Longterm results of laminectomy in spondylolisthesis. Acta Orthop. Scand. 40:773, 1970.
14. Cleveland, M., Bosworth, D.M., and Thompson, F.R.: Pseudarthrosis in the lumbosacral spine. J. Bone Joint Surg. 20A:302, 1948.
15. Cloward, R.B.: Spondylolisthesis: Treatment by laminectomy and posterior interbody fusion. Clin. Orthop. 154:74–82, 1981.
16. Dall, B.E., and Rowe, D.E.: Degenerative spondylolisthesis. Its surgical management. Spine 10:668–672, 1985.
17. Dandy, D.J., and Shannon, M.J.: Lumbosacral subluxation (group I spondylolisthesis). J. Bone Joint Surg. 53B:578, 1971.
18. Davis, I.S., and Bailey, R.W.: Spondylolisthesis. Long-term follow-up study of treatment with total laminectomy. Clin. Orthop. 88:46, 1972.
19. Davis, I.S., and Bailey, R.W.: Spondylolisthesis: Indications for lumbar nerve root decompression and operative technique. Clin. Orthop. 117:129, 1976.
20. DeWald, R.L., Faut, M., Taddonio, R.F., and Neuwirth, M.G.: Severe lumbosacral spondylolisthesis in adolescents and children: Reduction and staged circumferential fusion. J. Bone Joint Surg. 63A:619, 1981.
21. Del Torto, U.: Surgical reduction and stabilization of spondylolisthesis. Clin. Orthop. 75:281, 1971.
22. Edelson, J.G., and Nathan, H.: Nerve root compression in spondylolysis and spondylolisthesis. J. Bone Joint Surg. [Br.] 68:596–599, 1986.
23. Edwards, C.C.: Reduction of spondylolisthesis biomechanics and fixation. Orthop. Trans. 10:543, 1986.
24. Epstein, N.E., Epstein, J.A., Carras, R., and Lavine, L.S.: Degenerative spondylolisthesis with an intact neural arch: A review of 60 cases with an analysis of clinical findings and the development of surgical management. Neurosurgery 13:555–561, 1983.
25. Farfan, H.F., Osteria, V., and Lamy, C.: The mechanical etiology of spondylolysis and spondylolisthesis. Clin. Orthop. 117:40–55, 1976.
26. Farfan, H.F.: A reorientation in the surgical approach to degenerative lumbar intervertebral joint disease. Orthop. Clin. North Am. 8:9, 1977.
27. Feffer, H.L., Wiesel, S., Cuckler, J.M., and Rothman, R.H.: Degenerative spondylolisthesis—to fuse or not to fuse. Spine 10:287–289, 1985.
28. Fredrickson, B.E., Baker, D., McHolick, W.J., et al.: The natural history of spondylolysis and spondylolisthesis. J. Bone Joint Surg. 66A:699, 1984.
29. Gaines, R.W., and Nichols, W.K.: Treatment of spondyloptosis by two stage L5 vertebrectomy and reduction of L4 onto S1. Spine 10:680–687, 1985.
30. Gill, G.G., Manning, J.G., and White, H.L.: Surgical treatment of spondylolisthesis without spine fusion. J. Bone Joint Surg. 37A:493, 1955.
31. Hensinger, R.N., Lang, J.R., and MacEwen, G.D.: Surgical management of spondylolisthesis in children and adolescents. Spine 1:207, 1976.
32. Hanley, E.N.: Decompression and distraction-derotation arthrodesis for degenerative spondylolisthesis. Spine 11:269–276, 1986.
33. Haraldsson, S., and Willner, S.: A comparative study of spondylolisthesis in operations on adolescents and adults. Arch. Orthop. Trauma Surg. 101:101–105, 1983.
34. Harrington, P.R., and Tullos, H.S.: Spondylolisthesis in children. Observation and surgical treatment. Clin. Orthop. 79:75, 1971.
35. Harris, I., and Weinstein, S.L.: Longterm follow-up of spondylolisthesis 50% or greater treated with or without posterior fusion. Orthop. Trans. 8:155, 1984.
36. Harris, R.I.: Spondylolisthesis. Ann. R. Coll. Surg. Engl. 8:259, 1951.
37. Herbiniaux, G.: Traite sur divers accouchements laborieux et sur les polypes de la matrice. Bruxelles, J.L. DeBoubers, 1782.
38. Howorth, B.: Low backache and sciatica: Results of the surgical treatment, Part III. Surgical treatment of spondylolisthesis. J. Bone Joint Surg. 46A:1515, 1964.
39. Huizenga, B.A.: Reduction of spondyloptosis with two-stage vertebrectomy. Orthop. Trans. 7:1, 21, 1983.

40. Inoue, S., Watanabe, T., Goto, S., et al.: Degenerative spondylolisthesis. Pathophysiology and results of anterior interbody fusion. Clin. Orthop. 227:90–98, 1988.
41. Jenkins, J.A.: Spondylolisthesis. Br. J. Surg. 24:80, 1936.
42. Johnsson, K.E., Willner, S., Johnsson, K.: Postoperative instability after decompression for lumbar spinal stenosis. Spine 11:107–110, 1986.
43. Jones, A.A., McAfee, P.C., Robinson, R.A., et al.: Failed arthrodesis of the spine for severe spondylolisthesis. Salvage by interbody arthrodesis. J. Bone Joint Surg. 70:25–30, 1988.
44. Junghanns, H., and Schmorl, G.: The human spine. *In*: Health and Disease. New York, Grune & Stratton, 1959.
45. Junghanns, H.: Spondylolisthesen ohne spalt in zwischengelenkstijck archiv fur orthopadische and unfall-dchirurgie. 29:118–127, 1930.
46. Kaneda, K., Kazama, H., Satoh, S., and Fujiya, M.: Follow-up study of medial facetectomies and posterolateral fusion with instrumentation in unstable degenerative spondylolisthesis. Clin. Orthop. 203: 159–167, 1986.
47. Kirkaldy-Willis, W.H., Wedge, J.H., Yong-Hing, K., and Reilly, J.: Pathology and pathogenesis of lumbar spinal spondylosis and stenosis. Spine 3:319–328, 1978.
48. Lance, E.M.: Treatment of severe spondylolisthesis with natural involvement: A report of two cases. J. Bone Joint Surg. 48A:833, 1966.
49. Laurent, L.E., and Osterman, K.: Spondylolisthesis in children and adolescents: A study of 173 cases. Acta Orthop. Belg. 35:717, 1969.
50. Laurent, L.E.: Spondylolisthesis. Acta Orthop. Scand. 35(Suppl.):1958.
51. Lee, C.K.: Lumbar spinal instability (olisthesis) after extensive posterior spinal decompression. Spine 8:429–433, 1983.
52. Louis, R., and Maresca, C.: Stabilisation chirurgicale avec reduction des spondylolysis et des spondylolisthesis. Int. Orthop. 1:215, 1977.
53. Matthiass, H.H., and Heine, J.: The surgical reduction of spondylolisthesis. Clin. Orthop. 203:34–44, 1986.
54. Macnab, I.: Negative disc exploration and analysis of the causes of nerve root involvement in 68 patients. J. Bone Joint Surg. 99:29–34, 1981.
55. Macnab, I.: Spondylolisthesis with an intact neural arch—the so-called pseudospondylolisthesis. J. Bone Joint Surg. 32B:325–333, 1950.
56. Morscher, E., Gerber, B., and Fasel, J.: Surgical treatment of spondylolisthesis by bone grafting and direct stabilization of spondylolysis by means of a hook screw. Arch. Orthop. Trauma Surg. 103:175–178, 1984.
57. Nachemson, A., and Wiltse, L.L.: Editorial comment: Spondylolisthesis. Clin. Orthop. 117:4, 1976.
58. Neugebauer, F.L.: A new contribution to the history and etiology of spondylolisthesis. New Syndenham Soc. Sel. Monogr. 121:1, 1888.
59. Newman, P.H.: A clinical syndrome associated with severe lumbosacral subluxation. J. Bone Joint Surg. 47B:472, 1965.
60. Newman, P.H.: The etiology of spondylolisthesis. J. Bone Joint Surg. 45B:39–59, 1963.
61. Oakley, R.H., and Carty, H.: Review of spondylolisthesis and spondolysis in paediatric practice. Br. J. Radiol. 57:877, 1984.
62. Osterman, K., Lindholm, T.S., and Laurent, L.E.: Late results of removal of the loose posterior element (Gill's procedure) in the treatment of lytic lumbar spondylolisthesis. Clin. Orthop. 117:121, 1976.
63. Reynolds, J.B., and Wiltse, L.L.: Surgical treatment of degenerative spondylolisthesis. Spine 4:148–149, 1979.
64. Rombold, C.: Treatment of spondylolisthesis by postero-lateral fusion, resection of pars interarticularis and prompt mobilization of the patient. J. Bone Joint Surg. 48A:1282, 1966.
65. Rosenberg, N.J.: Degenerative spondylolisthesis, predisposing factors. J. Bone Joint Surg. 57A:467–475, 1975.
66. Rosenberg, N.J.: Degenerative spondylolisthesis, surgical treatment. Clin. Orthop. 117:112–120, 1975.
67. Rosomoff, H.L.: Neural arch dissection for lumbar spinal stenosis. Clin. Orthop. 154:83–89, 1981.
68. Rowe, G.G., and Roche, M.B.: The etiology of separate neural arch. J. Bone Joint Surg. 35A:102, 1953.
69. Saraste, H.: Long-term clinical and radiological follow-up of spondylolysis and spondylolisthesis. J. Pediatr. Orthop. 7:631–638, 1987.
69a. Saraste, H.: Spondylolysis and pregnancy—a risk analysis. Acta Obstet. Gynecol. Scand. 65:727–729, 1986.
70. Saraste, H.: The etiology of spondylolysis. A retrospective radiographic study. Acta Orthop. Scand. 56:253–255, 1985.
71. Scaglietti, O., Frontino, G., and Bartolozzi, P.: Technique of anatomical reduction of lumbar spondylolisthesis and its surgical stabilization. Clin. Orthop. 117:164, 1976.
72. Scaglietti, O., Frontino, G., and Bartolozzi, P.: Tecnica della redozione de la spondelolistesi lombare esua contenzione definitiva. atti S.I.C.O.T. 292:55, 1970.
73. Schatzker, J., and Pennal, G.F.: Spinal stenosis—a cause of cauda equina compression. J. Bone Joint Surg. 50B:606, 1968.
74. Scherb, R.: Zur indikation and technik der albec de Quervain operation. Schweiz. Med. Wochenschr. 20:763, 1921.
75. Schoenecker, P.L., Cole, H.O., Herring, J.A., and Capelli, A.: Cauda equina syndrome (CES) following in situ fusion of spondylolisthesis of the lumbosacral junction. J. Bone Joint Surg. (in press, 1988).
76. Sijbrandij, S.: Reduction and stabilization of severe spondylolisthesis. J. Bone Joint Surg. 65B:40, 1983.
77. Snijder, J.G.N., Seroo, J.M., Snijder, C.J., and Schijvens, A.W.M.: Therapy of spondylolisthesis by repositioning and fixation of the olisthetic vertebra. Clin. Orthop. 117:149, 1976.
78. Stauffer, R.N., and Coventry, M.B.: Posterolateral lumbar spine fusion. J. Bone Joint Surg. 54A:1195, 1972.
79. Steffee, A.D., and Sitkowski, D.J.: Reduction and stabilization of grade IV spondylolisthesis. Clin. Orthop. 227:82–89, 1988.
80. Taillard, W.: Le spondylolisthesis chez l'enfant et l'adolescent (étude de 50 cas). Acta Orthop. Scand. 25:115, 1954.
81. Turner, R.H., and Bianco, A.J.: Spondylolysis and spondylolisthesis in children and teenagers. J. Bone Joint Surg. 53A:1298, 1971.

82. Verbiest, H.: A radicular syndrome from developmental narrowing of the lumbar vertebral canal. J. Bone Joint Surg. 36B:230–237, 1954.
83. Verbiest, H.: Results of surgical treatment of idiopathic developmental stenosis of the lumbar vertebral canal. A review of 27 years' experience. J. Bone Joint Surg. 59B:181, 1977.
84. Verbiest, H.: The treatment of lumbar spondyloptosis or impending lumbar spondyloptosis accompanied by neurologic deficit and/or neurogenic intermittent claudication. Spine 4:668, 1979.
85. West, J., Bradford, D., and Ogilvie, J.: Steffee instrumentation: 2 year results. Presented at Scoliosis Research Society, 23rd annual meeting. Baltimore, Sept., 1988.
86. Wiltse, L.L., Guyer, R.D., Spencer, C.W., et al.: Alar transverse process impingement of the L5 spinal nerve: The far out syndrome. Spine 9:31–41, 1984.
87. Wiltse, L.L., Newman, P.H., and Macnab, I.: Classification of spondylolysis and spondylolisthesis. Clin. Orthop. 117:23–29, 1976.
88. Wiltse, L.L.: Etiology of spondylolisthesis. Clin. Orthop. 10:48, 1957.
89. Zimmerman, H.: Beitrag zur ventralen interkorporellen spondylodese des lumbosakralbereiches. Z. Orthop. 105:303, 1968.
90. Zimmerman, H.: Die transabdominale reposition und verspagnung fortgeschrittener spondylolisthesis und beginnender spondyloptose. Z. Orthop. 109:467, 1971.

9 □ Lumbar Spinal Stenosis

Henk Verbiest
Richard Porter
Franco Postacchini

MORPHOLOGY, CLASSIFICATION, AND LONG-TERM RESULTS

Henk Verbiest

Because I have already written various chapters about so-called lumbar stenosis, the emphasis here is on existing controversial views of the subject. In addition, a few new diagnostic aids are discussed.

The controversies surrounding concepts of spinal stenosis are interesting because of their very peculiar aspects. A discussion of these aspects will follow "metamedical"* pathways, which may be unusual in a clinical treatise such as this. The following metamedical aspects will be encountered in the discussion of pathomorphology and classification of the spinal stenoses.

1. *The pathology of stenosis is spatial in nature.* Thinking of space in terms of the "macroworld" represents a problem in human thinking, which was well formulated by the eighteenth-century philosophers Leibniz and Kant. Leibniz stated that thinking of space without "things" requires a high degree of abstract thinking. In Kant's view, space was not an independent physical quantity but, as time, was an indispensable condition for the perception of things or events. He considered space to be unrelated to sensation and instead being a concept constructed by the mind. The generic idea of stenosis concerns the pathologic shortage of space, regardless of its cause. Many modern medical diagnostic techniques provide information by means of numbers and symbols, which are the point of departure for reasoning.

Imaging techniques reproducing particularities of morphologic configurations are a basic requirement in the diagnosis of spinal stenosis. The visible "things" causing stenosis occupy subconsciously the position of primacy in reasoning, suppressing the integration of conceptual activities concerning the space involved. Evidence of this statement is provided, for instance, by the way in which computed tomographic (CT) findings of stenotic lumbar vertebral canals are recorded; that is, all attention is given to the visible bony or ligamentous abnormalities causing stenosis, without measuring the residual space inside the vertebral canal. Measurements provide the most concrete data for determining properties of reality; all other interpretations of our sense data are abstractions from reality. However, mismeasurements can be unmasked only by measurements.

In the discussion of the pathomorphology of spinal stenosis, attention will be given first to its definition.

2. *Confusion in terminology and underlying notions do exist.* Charles Burton[20] used the metaphor "The Spinal Column: A Mod-

*Metamedicals is a special branch of the science involved in the study of the inner logic of scientific theories, the relation between experiment and theory, the role of language in scientific communication, and so forth. In metamedicals, the science and practice of medicine is the object of interest and study from the side of the "surrounding" sciences.

ern Tower of Babel," with respect to these problems. The Babylonian confusion of tongues was the Lord's reaction to the people's fatally erroneous concept of space (Gen. 11:3–9). Between the time of my struggle in demonstrating the occurrence of developmental stenosis of the vertebral canal in about 5% to 10% of spinal operations for sciatica and the days when some spinal surgeons told me that about 50% to 80% of their lumbar laminectomies for sciatica concerned cases of lumbar spinal stenosis, about 20 years had elapsed. In contrast to the early years, I found it necessary to reverse my role as a herald of spinal stenosis by contesting its occurrence with such high frequency. This change was the consequence of differences in definitions, semantics of terms and nomenclature, and resulting taxonomy of the stenoses. It was, however, no expression of a Babylonian confusion of tongues but of theories and concepts, which can be discussed by the use of a common language. Important issues related to this subject are (1) whether the words used or the notions given to words are useful tools in describing spinal stenosis and (2) whether the collection of data and the manner of their analysis result in knowledge that may help clarify the nature of the underlying pathologic process, may open paths of research into the unclarified areas, or may help in treatment. This is a pragmatic approach that accepts theories as being true as long as they do not conflict with other well-established theories—as long as they are not falsified.

3. *Classification is another debatable topic*. Every scientific endeavor departs from the axiom that there is order in its field of exploration; otherwise, research would be senseless. The scientist's aim is to detect systems of order, in a field of research, which are shaped by and adapted to his or her mental capacities in the acquisition of new knowledge or understanding is acquired. However, classification has its own rules.

In this chapter, the metamedical principles discussed earlier will be used, when needed, as a touchstone for testing controversies concerning nomenclature, theories, and classification of the spinal stenoses.

HISTORICAL REVIEW

An early description of too-narrow vertebral canals was given by the French anatomist Antoine Portal (1742–1832) in 1803.[88] During autopsic examinations of the vertebral columns of hunchbacks, in those days a frequent deformity that was usually caused by rickets, Portal observed that the abnormal curvatures of the vertebral column had produced a more or less pronounced narrowing of the vertebral canal at the level of one or more vertebrae. In one of his autopsies performed at the Collège de France in 1783, the vertebral canal was found to be reduced to half its normal size. He wrote that his teacher Lieutaud[71] and Morgagni had described similar cases of narrowing of the vertebral canal, but he did not present detailed references. Portal stressed the occurrence of very narrow vertebral canals in the absence of any weakness or atrophy of the legs. In his view, the difference between symptomatic and asymptomatic narrowing of the vertebral canal was attributable to differences in how rapidly compression of the spinal cord evolved.

After 1803, no further reports on narrowed vertebral canals appeared until the early twentieth century. Between 1900 and 1925, a few authors published reports of narrowness of the thoracic vertebral canal caused by thickened laminae.[7,87,96] The patients showed signs of spinal cord compression. The descriptions of the underlying pathologic condition were unclear, although the authors believed that it was inflammatory. Between 1971 and 1982, a few papers on bony hypertrophy or giant articular osteophytes producing stenosis of the thoracic vertebral canal were published.[4,6,58,77] In none of the papers presented up to that point had attention been given to the capacity or diameters of the vertebral canal.

In 1910, Sumita[106] described narrowing of the vertebral canal in achondroplastics. This was a fundamental discovery subsequently verified by many authors.

Another other essential contribution was made by Sarpyener, who in 1945 and 1947 described the occurrence of congenital stricture of the vertebral canal in infants. In most of his patients, it was accompanied by dysraphic anomalies, such as spina bifida, meningomyelocele, or diastematomyelia. In some of his patients, congenital constriction of the vertebral canal was accompanied by other malformations, such as clubfoot and/or dysplasia of the hip joints. Most of the children suffered from disturbances of micturition, spastic paraparesis, or paraplegia.

Of the three clearly different causes of a too-narrow vertebral canal described thus far, two are still valid: inborn errors of skeletal growth and congenital dysraphic conditions. Their frequencies are low. Rickets as a cause of abnormal spinal curvatures has disappeared in modern countries. Abnormal narrowness of vertebral canals may occur in dysplastic and congenitally abnormal spinal curvatures and should be classified accordingly.

In 1949,[113] I published reports of three cases of narrow bony portions of the lumbar vertebral canals in the absence of spinal malformation, abnormal curvature, or other skeletal growth disturbances. In all patients, the laminae were very thick. In two of the patients the dural sac was narrowed and had also to be enlarged during surgical decompression. I used the term *stenosis* to designate this type of narrowness because of the impeded or blocked myelographic passage of the contrast medium through the area of narrowness. From the beginning, I was of the opinion that the diagnosis of stenosis of the vertebral canal should be based on measurements of diameters of the canal and that the measurements should rely on the use of universally applicable reference markers, allowing for comparative studies.

From 1949 until the time of this writing the only diameters that can be rather accurately measured conforming to these criteria are the largest interpedicular distance and the midsagittal diameter. Measurements of the largest interpedicular distances in x-ray films of the area of narrowness of the vertebral canal, corrected by the magnification factor, showed values that were greater than the minimal interpedicular distances found by Elsberg and Dyke[37] in patients with no lesions in these areas and by my comparable measurements of interpedicular distances[113, 114] at each of the five lumbar vertebrae of 100 patients. On the basis of these findings, *it was concluded that in our three patients the narrowness was the result of a reduced midsagittal diameter, thus indicating an isolated growth disturbance of the vertebral arch.* This view was confirmed, in later years, by Larsen and colleagues.[70] Thickening of the laminae and an acute interlaminar angle contributed to the narrowing. Abnormal shortness of the pedicles could not be measured exactly because of their sloping transitions to the vertebral bodies and the partes interarticulares, preventing the use of universally applicable reference markers. A fourth patient presented signs of stenosis in the presence of a slightly bulging disc. It induced me to make a tentative distinction between *absolute stenosis,* capable of producing signs and symptoms in the absence of additional compressive agents, and *relative stenosis,* in which the narrowness was such that only in the absence of slightly bulging intervertebral discs, hard ridges, or infolding ligamenta flava would the patient remain asymptomatic. In 1950 our number of patients had increased to five. A more careful analysis of the profile myelograms revealed that three of the five patients had a posterior impression, partial or complete blocks of the contrast medium, caused by the hypertrophic articular processes. In this paper, neurogenic intermittent claudication was described as a prominent symptom in all five patients.[114]

My next paper,[116] concerning seven cases and written in English, was published after a delay of 2 years because of its frequent rejection by editorial boards of great international journals, who did not believe in the existence of this type of stenosis. When it was published in the British volume of the *Journal of Bone and Joint Surgery,* we had replaced the phrase *stenosis* of the vertebral canal by *narrowing* of the canal. As mentioned above, the term stenosis was applied because of impeded myelographic transport. We changed this name because the pathomechanism of narrowness of the vertebral canal consists of compression of the cauda equina. In order to distinguish the narrowing described in our publications from the earlier described congenital narrowing of the vertebral canal, the adjective *developmental* was introduced, indicating that the narrowness was the consequence of a prenatal and postnatal growth disturbance of the vertebral arch continuing until growth of the vertebral arch was completed. This definition was based upon the fact that the thickness of the bony structures of the vertebral arch found at operation could not be expected to have been present at birth. All patients were more than 20 years old.

Because achondroplastic stenosis of the vertebral canal is also the consequence of disturbed prenatal and postnatal growth, it should also be classified as developmental but resulting from an inborn error of skeletal bone growth. Because the cause of the developmental narrowness I described was unknown and limited to the lumbar vertebral canal without other skeletal growth disturbances (except cervical spinal stenosis in some cases), the term was coined with the additional adjective *idiopathic.*

One of the seven patients suffered from orthostatic lumbago, whereas five of the other six patients presented symptoms of intermittent claudication. Operation revealed thickened laminae in all patients; however, in four patients the medial portions of the hypertrophic articular processes reaching to the midline had to be removed because they encroached upon the vertebral canal. It was stressed that the greatest narrowness of the vertebral canal occurred at the level of the articular processes, if they were hypertrophic.

Before the introduction of the CT body scanners, it was impossible to measure the midsagittal diameters (MSD) of the lumbar vertebral canal in plain-profile x-rays because the projections of the transverse and articular processes overlap the projection of the posterior wall of the vertebral canal. The same structures produce blurring of the posterior wall of the lumbar vertebral canal in sagittal tomograms; this includes the hypercycloidal tomogram, which was applied in later years. In 1949, no literature existed about measurements of MSDs of the lumbar vertebral canal. We requested, therefore, that the anthropologist Dr. Huizinga perform such measurements. A stenosimeter (Fig. 1) was developed for intraoperative measurements of MSDs,[117] so that these findings could be compared with the data collected by Huizinga and coworkers,[65] which were obtained from 51 Dutch skeletal lumbar vertebral columns. Out of six new cases of symptomatic narrowing of the lumbar vertebral canal, only one patient had no additional compressive agents inside the vertebral canal. His smallest lumbar MSD was 10 mm. This finding suggested that an MSD of 10 mm may represent absolute stenosis. This low value was smaller than the lowest value of 11 mm, found by Huizinga and by other authors in later years.[26, 34, 36]

Our other five patients had protruding ridges (hard discs) inside the vertebral canal, the anteroposterior lengths of which varied between 2 and 3 mm. These ridges reduced the original MSDs of the five patients varying between 11 to 12 mm at the corresponding lumbar levels to 8 to 9 mm (diameters measured before and after removal of the ridges). They presented the small variations in MSD found by Huizinga and other authors. These findings supported our early idea of separating a group of those with relative stenosis, because they indicate the risk of people with small but normal (i.e., asymptomatic) variations in the MSD of the lumbar vertebral canal becoming symptomatic when small degenerative protruding agents develop inside the canal and produce absolute stenosis.

The preliminary conclusion was that symptomatic narrowness of the lumbar vertebral canal may occur in the presence of midsagittal diameters of 10 mm or less, regardless of whether this shortness is primary in origin or caused by additional compressive agents.

Because of the low frequency of absolute stenosis and the impossibility to perform intraoperative measurements in a number of patients without damaging caudal nerve roots, many years passed before our experience covered a number of cases sufficient to certify that the upper limit of the midsagittal diameters capable of producing symptomatic narrowness of the lumbar vertebral canal was invariably 10 mm.[120–122]

After our earliest papers in which the word stenosis had been used for the first time in the literature to designate abnormal narrowness of the vertebral canal, a few analogous observations were published in the Netherlands, by French colleagues and former foreign residents. Although these papers appeared after 1954, when I already had replaced the word stenosis by narrowness, some of these authors had used the word stenosis, which may have contributed to stenosis becoming the most frequently used for designating this condition. The first American author to use the name *narrow spinal canal* after the appearance of my English papers was Donald Munro,[83] who mentioned 18 cases of narrow spinal canals out of 166 cases of symptomatic compression of the cauda equina in the absence of disc protrusions or extrusions at L4–L5 and L5–S1. Apart from his comment that the narrow spinal canal is "virtually unrecognizable except at operation," further morphologic characteristics of the narrow spinal canal and references to previous literature were not provided. Epstein in 1960[39] was the first American author to refer to our description of developmental stenosis. In a discussion of his patients he concluded that "congenital narrowing of the canal in the lumbar region, alone or with disc and osteophytic changes, appears to be a definite but inadequately appreciated clinical entity." In his writing, Epstein considered the adjectives *developmental* and *congenital* as synonyms, a view shared by authors in later years until the time of this writing. In 1961, Friedman[50] was the next to describe the occurrence of idiopathic developmental stenosis in North American patients. In 1962, Epstein and coworkers[40] described 29 patients with narrowing of the lumbar vertebral canal accompanied by pathomorphologic findings that were identical to those described in our cases. Special attention was given to the narrowed lateral recesses, in which abnormal notching might occur and produce further narrowing. In the following years, the number of papers on narrowness of the lumbar vertebral canal increased in the United States. In particular, Ehni, Weinstein, and Wilson, in addition to Epstein, promoted the greater knowledge of the narrow lumbar ver-

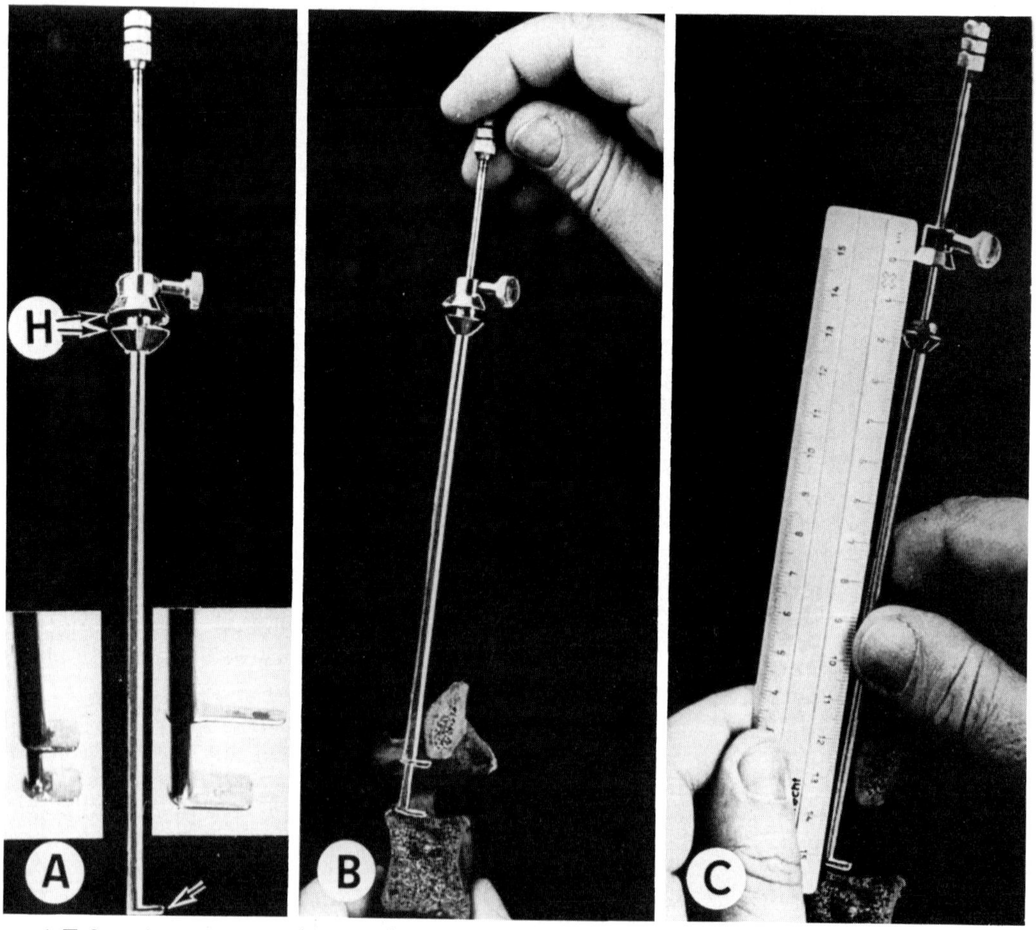

Figure 1 □ Stenosimeter: system of inner caliper. *A,* Hollow cylindric outer bar carries the upper foot (insert) of the measuring device. Arrows at H point to two large metal discs separated by a smaller disc. The lower and the smaller middle discs are fixed to this bar, which surrounds an inner metal rod carrying the lower foot of the caliper. The upper metal disc can move along the inner rod and can be fixed by a screw in any position (see *B* and *C*). *B,* The lower foot is vertically placed on the anterior wall of the vertebral canal, and the upper foot is pressed against the anterior surface of the laminae. The mobile upper disc is placed on the middle disc and fixed by a screw. *C,* Without removing the caliper from the vertebral canal, the outside bar is pressed with its foot against that of the inner rod. The resulting distance between the two large discs corresponds to the midsagittal diameter (MSD) of the portion of the canal measured. The height of the small disc between the two larger metal discs represents the total height of both feet, the smallest MSD that can be measured with this caliper.

tebral canal (see alphabetical references for their numerous contributions).

In 1957, Schlesinger[100] published a report of two cases of compression of spinal nerve roots in the lateral recesses of the lumbar vertebral canal. In 1972, Epstein and coworkers[41] published on 15 cases of nerve root entrapment in lateral recesses but with normal transverse and midsagittal diameters of the vertebral canals. According to their definition, the roof of a lateral recess is formed by the inferior portion of a superior articular facet, which, being oriented in a coronal plane, may, when thickening of investing tissues secondary to trauma or degenerative processes occurs, lead to compression of the underlying portion of the spinal nerve roots. The authors also used the terms *foraminal recess* and *superior facet syndrome* as synonyms so that they considered the lateral recesses to be the parts of the vertebral canal providing access to the lumbar intervertebral foramina.

The years 1975 and 1976 were milestones in the development of clinical knowledge and concepts about the narrow lumbar canal because of the introduction of CT body scanners and the proposition of an "inclusive classification" of the stenoses of the lumbar spine by Arnoldi and 20 well-known coauthors.[3] Because I did not agree entirely with the nomenclature, definitions, and system of classification, I could not—to my regret—accept the invitation to join this group of authors.

Because the classification of Arnoldi and coworkers is the first and still the only "inclusive classification" of the lumbar stenoses ever presented, it will be the touchstone for discussion in the following sections.

NOMENCLATURE AND PRINCIPLES OF CLASSIFICATION OF THE STENOSES OF THE LUMBAR VERTEBRAL CANAL

Basic Principles, Significance, and Limits of Nosologic Classification

In view of the confusion concerning the classification of the spinal stenoses or the too-liberal use of this diagnosis, it seems appropriate to first briefly discuss the basic principles, significance, and limits of nosologic classification.

Classifications aim toward arranging objects or entities on the basis of similarities and differences. Taxonomy has become the proper term for the classification of living things, and its goal is the development of natural systems in which words or symbols express the objective order of the living things in nature. It came into being after the Renaissance. Linnaeus systematized a hierarchy of categories above the level of the species (e.g., genus, family, class) and introduced a binary nomenclature consisting of generic and specific names. In 1730[13] he had already written a *Genera Morborum*, in which he had vainly attempted to classify diseases in the manner of classifications used in zoology and botany. Linnaeus' empirical nosologic taxonomy remained limited to names of diseases and their treatment.

Morgagni's *De Sedibus et Causis Morborum per Anatomum Indagatis* appeared in Venice in 1761, too late for Linnaeus to develop a nosologic taxonomy based upon pathomorphology. The advantage of newer taxonomies based on pathomorphology was that they concern visible nature, which can be reviewed objectively. In later years, with the development of biopsies and imaging methods, the advantages of a morphologic taxonomy also became valid for the taxonomy of pathophysiologic and pathobiochemical characteristics of disease, which are observed during life. The taxonomy required a change in the language of nomenclature adapted to the kind of objective knowledge involved, such as observation terms, observation-dependent, and theory-laden terms.

As in the early period (although for other reasons), modern nosologic taxonomies based on a hierarchic system of categories above the level of the species cannot make use of binary systems because diseases possess a mixture of properties belonging to anatomic, physiologic, biochemical, chronologic, topologic, and other categories. A solution to this taxonomic problem was advanced by Feinstein,[46] who proposed to classify diseases by means of Boolean algebra and Venn diagrams, allowing an overlap of different categoric entities.

The binary classification of Arnoldi and coworkers is incapable of classifying stenotic disease. The old hierarchic binary taxonomy may still be applicable to single categories of properties of stenosis.

The important question concerns the principles of classification of the stenoses that may be of scientific advantage. Nomenclature and classification are interrelated, and their rules are valid for all sorts of sciences, although their methodologic aspects are independent of the scientific field of application. The science of words and their use belongs to linguistics, and the principles of inner logic in systems of classification are subjects of epistemology.

These aspects are rarely recognized by medical nomenclature committees. The participation of medical specialists, preferably those proficient in both medical and nonmedical aspects of nomenclature and classification, is wanting.

It may be useful, here, to quote some of Bronowski's lucid descriptions[19] of important criteria of classification. The first concerns the choice of the kind of order, which cannot be defined on any grounds except its success.

Successful order means that the selection of one set of appearances rather than another gives a better sense of the reality behind the appearances. Any such selection itself implies, and imposes, an interpretation.

A successful order may lead to scientific discoveries as did, for instance, the arrangement of the chemical elements.

Science is a language describing the world, and so the use of language in taxonomy should be concise and explicit. From Bronowski's definition of successful order it follows that there exist no rules of how to develop a successful ordering system, because the success becomes obvious only after the ordering has been achieved. Some objects and some characteristics are ordered in taxonomic systems more successfully than others. On the one hand, Bronowski states

This is the most important step in every science: the construction of a first order which is reasonable in itself and holds to the experimental facts that are known.

On the other hand he writes

Until a science has passed through a long stage of observation and trial, it cannot develop a system of ordering its observations. . . . A science which orders its thoughts too early is stifled.

The classification of Arnoldi and coworkers will be tested with respect to its aims that "it helps the clinician to think of all possible causes of compression in making an accurate diagnosis and in formulating a rational approach to treatment." We have added a third criterion concerning the question of whether this classification provides some means of gaining more insight into the nature of various forms of stenosis.

Definition of Stenosis

The classification of Arnoldi and colleagues reinforces the use of the generic name *stenosis* for designating the too-narrow vertebral canal. The original meaning of the word and its changes during the past ages have been described by me.[122] The word stenosis and its initially more frequently used synonym *stegnosis* were probably first used in the early years AD. Stenosis was derived from the Attic adjective *stenos* originating from the Ionic *steinos*, meaning "being narrow." The Attic suffix-*osis*, used, for example, to indicate pathologic conditions was added. It is useless to study the theory-laden original meaning of stegnosis or stenosis by reading the classics because the words had fallen out of use. The word stegnotic returned, incidentally, in medical writings of the seventeenth century for indicating styptic substances or drugs arresting hemorrhage. The evolution of comparative linguistics in the nineteenth century revived the interest in etymology. The printing of etymologic medical dictionaries may have contributed to the reintroduction of stegnosis and stenosis into the medical nomenclature. The *Oxford Dictionary* mentions the use of the prefix *steno-* in *stenobregmatic* (Pritchard, 1813), for indicating skulls that had an appearance of lateral compression, in *stenocephalic* (Meig, 1866), for indicating a narrow oval form of the skull, in *stenocardia* (Allbutt, 1857) for indicating the feeling of constriction in angina pectoris. *Stenochoria*, a Galenic term, covered all sorts of narrowing of spaces or ducts.

The prefix *steno-* might indicate pathologic conditions, but also anthropologic, zoologic, or botanic morphologic properties defining the species.

The Greek suffix *-osis*, when used in medical terms, always indicates pathologic conditions. Stenosis is mentioned as a synonym of stegnosis in the 2nd and 3rd editions of Kraus' *Kritisch-Etymologisches Lexicon*

(1831, 1844)[68] without further comment, and stegnosis was defined, as in Galen's time, as an obstruction of ducts, by their contents or by their narrowing at certain sites, especially of their orifices. Two other German medical encyclopedias of the middle nineteenth century[90, 94] have listed the word stenosis as a synonym of the German word for narrowing *(Verengerung)*. Stenosis is only one of the many synonyms borrowed from classic Greek, Latin, or Hellenized Latin and designating the excessive narrowness of ducts serving transport, such as *angustatio, angustia, coarctatio, stenochoria, strictura,* and *constriction*. Some of these terms are still used.

Stenosis, according to *Webster's Dictionary*, designates a narrowing or constriction of the diameter of a bodily passage. This definition uses two synonyms, between which the conjunction *or* suggests that they are not absolute, but near, synonyms. *Constriction*, however, is defined in the same dictionary as "being constricted"; *constrict* means "to make narrow." Some nineteenth-century medical dictionaries commented, in addition, that the resulting pathologic organic changes occur at a distance from the site of narrowing.

The French medical literature is known for its early use of the mother language in medical writings. The famous French pathologist Cruveilhier[25] described in his *General Pathology* (1852) the "lésions de canalisation," which he classified as narrowing, obliteration, dilatation, and fistula. This classification was limited to vascular and mucosal channels. The causes of narrowing were divided by Cruveilhier into the following categories: external compression, lesions in the walls of the channels, spasmodic contraction, foreign bodies inside the channels, and congenital deformities. Although in Landais' dictionary (1836)[69] the word stenosis was already listed as a medical term meaning "narrowing or obstruction of ducts," the fifteenth edition of Littré's *Dictionnaire de Médecine* (1884)[73] did not list the term stenosis but rather stegnosis, meaning "constriction of pores and vessels, constipation, and suppression of evacuation." In the nineteenth century, therefore, the word stenosis was used to indicate impeded transport through channels such as arteries, urogenital or gastrointestinal tracts, and airways. Stenosis was not considered to be a disease but only an accompanying symptom of a disease. The use of a number of synonyms for designating this transport disturbance and the use of two or more synonyms for indicating pathologic narrowing of identical types of ducts are an obvious sign of poor motivation in developing one well-defined generic medical term.

Only one other meaning of stenosis was introduced by Virchov[131, 132] in the term *craniostenosis*, used to distinguish some types of abnormally small circumferences of the head, resulting from premature closure of cranial sutures but in the presence of a normally developed brain, from microcephaly consequent to an underdeveloped brain. He classified various types of cranial deformities, with respect to the cranial sutures involved, under the heading *craniostenosis*. As with the use of the prefix *steno-*, Virchov used the word stenosis to indicate the narrowness of the head.

Although Virchov knew that premature closure of cranial sutures is the cause of craniostenosis, it was only through the development of diagnostic radiology, when it became possible to identify premature closure of cranial sutures in the living, that the more informative term *craniosynostosis* was more frequently used. Stenosis is used for no other condition to indicate reduced volume, and in many cases of craniostenosis the synostosis does not reduce the intracranial volume because of compensatory widening of some of its other diameters. Therefore, the word craniosynostosis or the name of the resulting cranial deformity became the more adequate scientific expression, although the word craniostenosis has not, unfortunately, completely disappeared from the medical vocabulary.

The same noncritical use of synonyms exists for indicating forms of compressive stenosis. Compression of the median nerve in the carpal tunnel is called *carpal tunnel syndrome*, indicating the site of compression, whereas stenotic compression of the lateral cutaneous femoral nerve in its pathway through the inguinal ligament is called *meralgia paraesthetica*, designating the consequences of compression. This capricious use of medical terms is the result of a sort of tacit convention that seems to closely resemble that of the vocabulary of common language; in regard to this language, Robins[93] commented that usually the arbitrary and conventional status of the relation between the form and meaning of words prevails, "though the convention is tacit and not explicit." Medical terms resulting from such a tacit convention may block further abstractive processes, becoming "dead-level abstractions." The tacit convention in using the term lumbar stenosis has, however, been canonized by a convention through agreement by a number of medical authorities, despite the ambiguity of the meaning of the dead Greek word stenosis. The alternative term, a *too-narrow vertebral canal,* is clear and can be translated in all languages. In my opinion, factors facilitating this tacit convention regarding the term spinal stenosis are as follows:

1. Medical xenophilic habits in selecting terminology are used.
2. Metaphoric anatomic terminology exists, concerning the vertebral column and its contents. Spinal nerve roots are said to enter or leave the spinal cord; spinal nerves leave the intervertebral foramina. The word canal is used for grooves or closed tubular structures transporting or conveying something. In anatomy, the Latin word *canalis* is often applied to bony tubular structures surrounding other structures that have a conveying function, such as auditory or arterial bony channels.

   The vertebral canal is not a passage for the flow of spinal fluid, because this fluid is intradural and because the constituents of the spinal fluid enter and leave the dural theca at a molecular level through different points of entry and exit.
3. Some diagnostic tests aim at demonstrating possible transport through the vertebral canal. Examples are the propagation of a pressure wave during Queckenstedt's test or the transport of the contrast medium during myelography. It is tempting to introduce these objective abnormal responses to diagnostic tests in the naming of the disease as a specific property, although they do not, per se, represent an essential part of the pathogenetic mechanism of the disease involved.

Problems in the Definition of Lumbar Spinal Stenosis

In the definition of Arnoldi and co-authors, the word stenosis implies any type of narrowing of a hollow tubular structure. The words "any type of narrowing" in their definition would include the frequently encountered narrowing of the vertebral canal at the level of L3 and L4. Huizinga[65] called it a physiologic stenosis, thereby neglecting, as did Arnoldi and associates, that the suffix *-osis* indicates a pathologic condition.

My alternative definition of stenosis is "any type of abnormal narrowing of a hollow tubular structure, an orifice, or a valve." In an editorial comment, two of Arnoldi's coauthors[66] gave an anatomic description of three types of channels for which abnormal narrowing should be listed as spinal stenosis.

Their definitions of two of these channels, namely the spinal canal and the intervertebral foramen, are in agreement with universally accepted notions. The third type of canal, called *nerve root canal,* was defined as follows: "The nerve root canal or tunnel is an essential part of the spinal canal. This canal, an anatomic concept, starts in the spinal canal at the point where the nerve root comes off the dural sac and ends *where the nerve root emerges from the intervertebral foramen.*" Apart from the fact that the spinal nerve, not the nerve root, emerges from the intervertebral foramen, it is obvious that the intervertebral foramen is considered to be a part of the nerve root canal or tunnel. It is not clear why the intervertebral foramen is described as a separate entity.

Next, the statement that the nerve root canal or tunnel is an essential part of the spinal canal is not clear for the following reasons: (1) The essential portions of a canal are its walls and its lumen, but this does not hold for its contents. (2) According to the description of the nerve root canal, a part of its anterior, lateral, and posterior walls are equally parts of the wall of the spinal canal. The intervertebral foramen is not an essential portion of the spinal canal. Part of the medial wall off the nerve root canal is formed, according to the authors, by the lateral wall of the dural sac and the contents of the epidural space. Both belong to the contents but not to the parts of the spinal canal. In reality, there is a continuity between the posterior and anterior extradural space and the so-called nerve root canal. The latter can be considered to be a lateral portion of the extradural space (Fig. 2A). To call the neighboring aspect of the dura the lateral wall of the nerve root canal is to use a metaphor. A wall is a structure that serves to hold back pressure or a structure con-

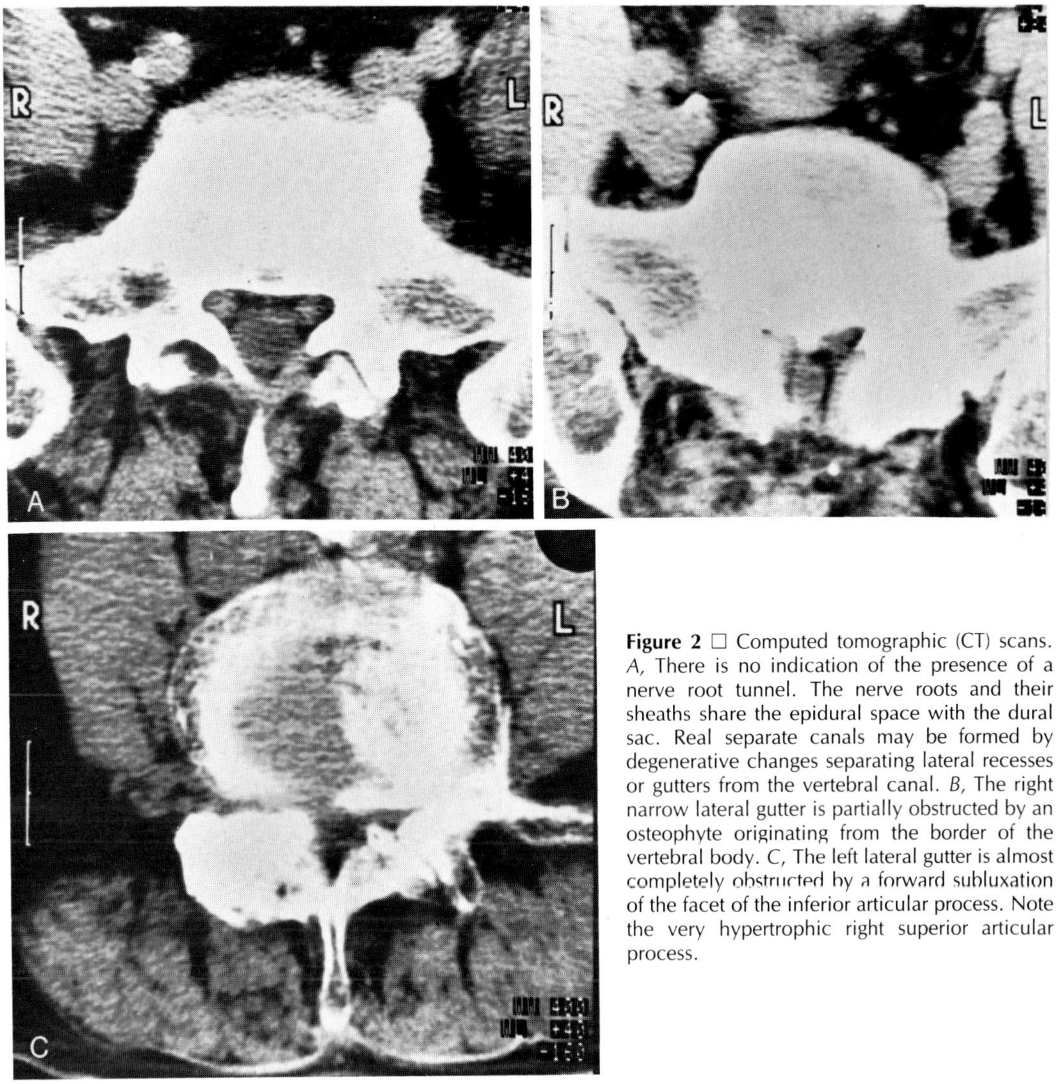

Figure 2 □ Computed tomographic (CT) scans. *A,* There is no indication of the presence of a nerve root tunnel. The nerve roots and their sheaths share the epidural space with the dural sac. Real separate canals may be formed by degenerative changes separating lateral recesses or gutters from the vertebral canal. *B,* The right narrow lateral gutter is partially obstructed by an osteophyte originating from the border of the vertebral body. *C,* The left lateral gutter is almost completely obstructed by a forward subluxation of the facet of the inferior articular process. Note the very hypertrophic right superior articular process.

necting floor and ceiling. The dural theca has no connection with the bony floor and roof of the so-called nerve root canal, and it can easily be displaced. Finally, the authors did not describe the walls between adjacent nerve root canals, and rightly so, because there are no such walls. The authors' statement that the nerve root canal is an anatomic concept does not include correspondence to reality. Just 1 year earlier, one of the subscribers[26] to this classification and nomenclature had produced a quite different definition of the nerve root tunnels when he wrote "the lower lumbar nerve roots gain their sheaths *while still within the spinal canal* and *proximal* to the level of their respective 'nerve root tunnels'." He continued to write that the intervertebral foramen was "a misnomer when applied to the nerve root tunnels, for a foramen is a window or a small opening." It would be, he says, "more appropriate to refer to them as the nerve root tunnels. Each of them has an inlet or inner foramen and an outlet or external foramen." The inner foramina were said to "lead from and *form* an integral part of the lumen of the spinal canal."

Calling a foramen a window means that it is an integral part of a wall but not of an inner space. When the content of this "nerve root tunnel" was discussed, the spinal ganglion occupying the central portion of this tunnel was not mentioned; nor was the spinal nerve, a name given to the nervous continuity between the spinal ganglion and its branching into anterior and posterior primary rami. Because spinal ganglion and spinal nerve occupy more space inside the intervertebral foramen than the nerve roots, the term "nerve root tunnel" is also a misnomer. The inadequate description of the content of the "nerve root canal or tunnel" in both definitions may contribute to the clinician's neglect of the possibility that symptoms resulting from narrowing of these tunnels may be a consequence of compression of the spinal ganglion, rather than compression of the local nerve roots. Apart from the inadequate anatomic description, complete confusion may be created by using the term "nerve root tunnel" to indicate different structures. Furthermore, the word *foramen* also had the meaning of "hole" or "cavity." In anatomy, the word is applied to tunnels that are longer than the lumbar intervertebral foramina, such as the jugular foramen.

On practical grounds, there is good reason to apply the same term to analogous structures at different vertebral levels. At cervical levels, the intervertebral foramina are not tunnel-sized. Besides differences in length, there are differences in the participation of vertebral bodies and articular processes forming the anterior and posterior walls of the intervertebral foramina in the various vertebral regions. It is not possible to indicate all such variations by giving particular names to the various intervertebral foramina. Many words in a language have, apart from their denotative (i.e., explicit or lexical) meaning, a connotative meaning, learned by experience or teaching. Connotative meanings of terms can cover various aspects and only parts of them can be actualized by the context. Nomenclature and binary or ternary taxonomies can function only on the basis of the denotative meaning of one to three words. An all-inclusive definition of intervertebral foramina requires the use of Venn diagrams, but it suggests no adequate nomenclature.

Author's Definition[122, 124, 129]

Because the term *lumbar spinal stenosis* seems to be ineradicable, its definition as a generic term must be applicable to ducts, orifices, or valves involved in the transport of contents and to stenosis consisting of compression of fixed living contents. Consequently, stenosis should be defined as *abnormal narrowness of cavities, tubular organs, orifices or valves, capable of producing disease through its influence upon its contents.* Thus, the concept of stenosis is separated from its causes, because the stenosis is defined by means of the resulting pathologic reduction in space, which can be quantified in terms of cross-sectional surfaces or diameters.

The stenoses can be divided into two subclasses: *transport stenosis* and *compressive stenosis.*[124]

Transport Stenosis of Solid Matter

This is a complicated condition involving many variables. In transport stenosis of fluids and gases, the percentage of reduction of surfaces of cross-sectional areas determines pathologic effects. The transported content is not altered at the site of the stenosis, but the pathologic effects manifest themselves at a distance.

Compressive Stenosis

Compressive stenosis involves not the transport but the compression of fixed living matter. Its biomechanics vary with the anatomic structures involved. In compressive stenosis of the vertebral canal, the pathologic compressive agents are active in transverse planes through the vertebral canal. The degree of stenosis can be expressed in terms of diameters. Abnormal shortness of one of these lengths results in compression of the spinal cord or caudal nerve roots by one pair of opposed aspects of the wall of the vertebral canal.

An abnormal shortness of both lengths results in compression of the cord by two pairs of opposed aspects of this wall, usually resulting in concentric stenosis of the vertebral canal, which is a property of achondroplastic stenosis.

In contrast to transport stenosis, symptomatic compressive stenosis includes damage to the content in the narrowed portion of the canal and distant effects consequent to the local damage. The differences between one-sided compression and stenotic compression of the spinal cord or cauda equina are described below.

One-sided compression results in displacement of the cord and/or caudal nerve roots with the pressure gradient sloping downward in the direction of the displacement. The displacement is accompanied by traction forces along the displaced neural content. Traction is most pronounced in the nerve fibers that are situated at the greatest distance from the compressive agent.

Stenotic compression is a sort of squeezing of the spinal cord or caudal nerve roots between opposed aspects of the wall of the vertebral canal. The squeezing pressure may become greater with increased lumbar lordosis. The limited upward movement of the cord or caudal nerve roots in an axial direction inside the dura, which occurs when one stands up from a sitting position, may be blocked by the stenotic area. This explains the slowly and carefully executed helical movement of the patient's trunk during this change in body posture.

The determinants described so far are essential to defining the differences between transport and compressive stenoses. A number of other determinants of stenotic disease are not active in all types of the transport and compressive disorders, as, for instance, the number of collateral ducts in transport stenosis. Another example is individual differences in the vulnerability of the spinal cord or nerve roots to identical stenotic reductions of diameters of the vertebral canal, and the various influences upon this vulnerability (e.g., constitutional and/or occupational influences and aging processes). These additional influences and morphologic differences do not lend themselves to an inclusive taxonomy. The need for different taxonomies of the stenoses must be bound to their purposes, underlying principles, and results.

TYPES OF CLASSIFICATION OF THE LUMBAR SPINAL STENOSES

Arnoldi and colleagues did not include disc herniations in their classification of the stenoses, except when they occur with other types of stenosis. Depending on their sizes, herniated discs can produce one-sided (anterior) or stenotic compression. No problems in classification are created if a distinction is made between *stenosis of the bony vertebral canal* and *stenosis produced by the ligamentous or cartilagenous portions of the walls of the vertebral canal*. To the latter group belongs stenosis produced by a herniated disc. A herniated disc in patients with stenosis of the bony vertebral canal is an "additional compressive agent."

Arnoldi and colleagues introduced a distinction between stenosis of the central portion and the peripheral portion of the vertebral canal, lateral recesses and nerve root canals (tunnels).

The distinction between stenosis of a central and a peripheral portion of a canal is a paradox, because stenosis always reduces the periphery of an enclosed space. In later years, this linguistic error was partly modified by replacing the word peripheral with the word lateral. The term "stenosis of the central portion of the canal" remains a misnomer. Arnoldi and colleagues defined stenosis as the narrowing of a hollow tubular structure as a whole. Summarizing the various definitions of peripheral portion of canal, lateral recesses, and the ambiguous and imaginary nerve root canal or tunnel, creates complete confusion about names and sites of structures that may, through narrowing, produce signs and symptoms.

The definition, of Epstein and coworkers,[41] of the superior facet syndrome or narrow lateral recess of the vertebral canal is a clear concept that corresponds to anatomic reality.

In the further description of pathomorphology, the term *narrow lateral recess* will be used for the part of the vertebral canal giving access to the intervertebral foramen. If the narrow lateral recess is continuous with a narrowed lateral wing of a trefoil canal, the combination of both will be called the *narrow lateral gutter*[119] of the vertebral canal. We proposed that the inner opening of a lumbar vertebral foramen be called the *ostium*. Figure 2, *B* and *C*, shows that degenerative changes may shut off a lateral recess so that a sort of root canal is formed, which may become stenotic and give rise to signs and symptoms. By CT scanning, such morphologic particularities can be discovered. Because the condition in Figure 2*B* is different from that in Figure 2*C*, the conditions require different treatments. Instead of racking the brain about how to classify such particular acquired variations under a particular name, it seems that a better approach is to integrate the particularities of the findings into the plan for surgical treatment. The same thinking holds for the many variations of intraforaminal compression of the neural contents.

In Arnoldi's inclusive classification, the stenoses are divided into two subclasses: congenital-developmental and acquired stenoses. The words congenital and developmental are apparently considered to be synonymous, because the entities listed under this heading, namely the idiopathic and achondroplastic stenoses, represent types of developmental stenosis. Congenital stenosis has no place in this classification.

The reason to include congenital stenosis as a separate category, distinct from developmental stenosis, is discussed in the next section.

Congenital Stenoses of the Lumbar Vertebral Canal

Congenital spinal stenosis differs from the developmental stenosis in that the stenosis exists at or before birth and is a part of a malformation.

Pathomorphology of Congenital Stenosis

Sarpyener[97, 98] described congenital stenosis observed in children. It was most frequently accompanied by spinal dysraphism and other malformations. I have described the following three types of congenital stenosis:[124, 130]

1. Stenosis as a part of spinal dysraphism. The signs and symptoms in the presence of dysraphism are usually not the consequence of stenosis alone but also of myelodysplasia and eventually are associated with a lipoma. Serious radicular neural deficit occurs frequently in this condition.
2. Stenosis in an area of failure of vertebral segmentation (block vertebrae). It may be associated by hypoplasia of the corresponding apophysial joints and synostosis of the spinous processes. In three cases, observed by the author, stenosis in the area of the block vertebrae was determined by a reduction of the midsagittal diameters of the bony vertebral canal. The signs and symptoms did not differ from those observed in idiopathic developmental stenosis.
3. Intermittent stenosis, the so-called d'Anquin syndrome.[130, 142] The spinous process of S1 is absent, and the laminae of S1 present a large medial cleft. There may be a residual island of bone in the area of the cleft. This malformation is associated with a downward hooklike elongation of the spinous process of L5. During increased lordosis in standing or walking, the tip of the hooklike spinous process of L5 presses directly on the ligamentum bridging the spina bifida occulta of S1 or on the rudimentary bony island in its central portion, reducing the midsagittal diameter of the upper sacral canal. It results in radiating pains in the legs during standing or walking. These disturbances disappear when the patient takes a rest in a flexed sitting position. Removal of the hooked portion of the spinous process of L5 produces permanent relief.

I found that the first symptoms of all three types of congenital stenosis may be manifested in adulthood, so the essential criteria in the classification of congenital stenosis are pathomorphologic.

Classification and Pathomorphology of the Developmental Stenosis of the Bony Lumbar Vertebral Canal (DSBLVC)

DSBLVC is a growth disturbance of vertebral arches that continues until the patient has attained adult age; periosteal apposition of bone continuing into later periods of life is not excluded. The share of prenatal disturbed growth is evident in cases of inborn errors of skeletal growth, but it is unknown in idiopathic DSBLVC.

I have divided the DSBLVC into the following two groups:

1. *Stenosis in the presence of inborn errors of skeletal growth,* in which, besides stenosis of the vertebral canal, other signs of disproportionate skeletal growth are present. The inborn error is hereditary or a consequence of mutation.
2. *Idiopathic stenosis of the lumbar vertebral canal.*

DSBLVC due to Errors of Skeletal Growth

Achondroplasia is the most frequent form. It is a short-limb dwarfism, but the spines of these patients are also abnormally short.[27] The stenosis is concentric.[22, 27] It is the consequence of a premature fusion of the centers of ossification of the vertebral body with those of the vertebral arches and of postnatal excessive apposition of periosteal bone upon the structures of the vertebral arches, resulting in increased stenosis through thickening of the laminae, articular processes, and the short pedicles.[28, 38] The chronology of progressive postnatal narrowing of the vertebral canal characterizes this form of stenosis as belonging to the developmental category.

Bulging discs at multiple levels are additional compressive agents that in older individuals contribute to osteophyte formation at the posterior margins of the vertebral bodies;[1, 28, 38, 60, 133] these together with arthritic hypertrophic apophyseal joints,[27, 49] contribute to a further narrowing of the vertebral canal. Multiple disc herniations above L4 are relatively frequent.[51, 72, 75, 101, 104] Other morphologic properties are multilevel scalloping of the posterior surfaces of the vertebral bodies, most pronounced in the lumbar area. Kyphosis,[1, 6, 28, 75, 133] as a result of wedge deformities of vertebral bodies, and/or narrowing of the foramen magnum and odontoid invagination[80, 146] may contribute to the production of neural deficit.

Morgan and Young[80] divided spinal stenosis in achondroplasia into the following three groups:

1. Upper cervical stenosis accompanied by narrowing of the foramen magnum and odontoid invagination, which is a frequent cause of perinatal death.[146]
2. Symptomatic stenosis at multiple levels.
3. Stenosis at the dorsolumbar and lumbar levels.

Dorsolumbar stenosis is accompanied by symptoms of lower spinal cord compression.[28, 51, 60, 63, 67, 90] A number of symptomatic stenoses may be limited to the lumbar vertebral canal[1, 10, 28, 38, 80] and produce the signs and symptoms observed with idiopathic DSBLVC. Good as well as bad results following surgical decompression of lumbar or dorsolumbar stenosis, whether or not accompanied by disc herniations in this area, have been reported in the literature. Neurogenic intermittent claudication (NICL) is a frequent sign of lumbar stenosis, but it has occurred with stenotic thoracic[87] and stenotic cervical vertebral canals.[118] In NICL due to spinal cord compression, neurologic examination immediately performed after the patient has stopped walking may reveal signs of spinal cord deficit, if this was not present as a permanent phenomenon. Disturbances of bones and joints in achondroplasia may result in walking disturbances, masking the presence of NICL.[6]

In a number of cases of symptomatic dorsolumbar or lumbar stenosis reported in the literature, previous or subsequent operations had to be performed for decompression of other stenotic spinal areas. Although symptomatic achondroplastic stenosis usually develops in patients between 20 and 40 years of age, the first manifestation may occur in 10- to 20-year-old patients.[38, 60, 63, 108] All achondroplastic individuals face an inherent danger of becoming paraplegic. Therefore, the absence of systematic preventive measures in many countries is amazing. I have reviewed this need in detail elsewhere.[130]

A random check of Dutch achondroplastic volunteers[108] revealed a neural deficit that had not been discovered before. Achondroplastic individuals should be regularly checked. An inventory of all vertebral abnormalities should be made soon after birth and followed by yearly checkups. These examinations should include the cervico-occipital transition area, possible presence of kyphotic deformities, and measurements of the diameters of the vertebral canal at all levels.

At the present time, CT is the most important noninvasive aid for measuring these diameters. Regular neurologic examination and orthopedic surveillance are essential. Achondroplastic individuals presenting with signs and symptoms limited to lumbar spinal stenosis should not be subjected to decompressive surgery before an inventory of the condition of the other vertebral regions has been completed. Prophylactic decompression of other severely stenotic but asymptomatic vertebral regions and/or correction of progressive serious kyphosis should, in our opinion, be performed at the same time or soon after decompression of the symptomatic stenotic vertebral region.

Hypochondroplasia (chondrohypoplasia or achondroplasia tarda)[91, 103] is a milder form of disturbed skeletal growth. Spinal stenosis may also occur with this entity.

Morquio disease[81, 82] (in Brailford's terminology, chondro-osteodystrophy[15, 16]) is a much more serious form of dwarfism. The skeletal deformities are more pronounced. Atlanto-occipital instability and odontoid hypoplasia are causes of early death or serious neural deficit. The patients often develop tetraparesis or paraparesis. Spinal stenosis was mentioned to be most pronounced in the lumbar area.[76]

Hereditary multiple exostoses, the transmission of which is autosomal dominant, may produce stenosis of the bony vertebral canal. I have experience[130] with one male patient in whom the exostoses originated from the anterior surface of the fifth and sixth thoracic laminae, producing stenosis. It was associated with acromelic growth disturbances in the form of brachyphalangia. The occurrence of exostoses in the presence of idiopathic DSBLVC is discussed later.

Idiopathic DSBLVC

The term *idiopathic* indicates that the cause is still unknown. No other skeletal growth disturbances are present, with the exception of associated stenoses of the cervical vertebral canal in some patients. The main pathologic features of DSBLVC have already been described. The term developmental was applied, because it is highly improbable that the considerable bony thickening of the elements of the neural arch—pedicles, apophyseal joints, and laminae—were present at birth. We have not encountered this entity in persons under 21 years of age.

Radiodiagnostic Features of Idiopathic DSBLVC

The anteroposterior view is the most informative among the plain radiographic incidences. Increased height of the laminae may completely obliterate the interlaminar spaces, or the interlaminar space may be reduced by a medial extension of hypertrophic articular processes.

Whereas the superior lumbar articular processes have a large base, formed by parts of pedicles, partes interarticulares and lateral cephalic borders of the laminae, the inferior articular processes are downward extensions of the lateral caudal borders of the laminae. The medial borders of the left and right inferior articular processes of normal lumbar vertebrae slope downward in a lateral direction, forming a wide angle between each other at their origin from the laminae. In other cases the origin of the medial borders of the right and left inferior articular processes are separated by a small horizontal lining of the caudal border of the laminae. In idiopathic DSBLVC the medial borders of the inferior articular processes form an acute angle between each other or they may not show any lateral slope in their downward extension. This fact may not be visible in the frontal roentgenograms because of the overlapping projection of the spinous processes (Fig. 3*A*); however, frontal hypocycloidal tomograms through these laminae clearly show this configuration (Fig. 3*B*).[5, 126] CT sections through this area show that the hypertrophic articular processes may reduce the posterior portion of the vertebral canal to a narrow posterior recess, which offers the dura no space (Fig. 3*C*, *D*); consequently, the medial extension of the articular processes results in reduction of the sagittal diameters of the vertebral canal. In all cases of low backache or lumbar radiculopathy, the chronologic order in the use of imaging techniques should begin with plain radiographs of the entire lumbar spine. The anteroposterior view is the most important one for detecting stenotic features discussed above. In case of doubt, frontal hypocycloidal tomograms of this region should be made. Oblique and profile views have no value in the diagnosis of stenosis, although they are needed for the detection of possible other abnormalities such as degenerative spondylolisthesis or other signs of degenerative disease.

Caudography should be performed before CT scanning, because it indicates the number of lumbar levels to be scanned by means of CT and, incidentally, of the lower thoracic levels involved. For economic reasons, routine CT scanning in sciatica is usually limited to the L3–S1 area. Caudography should include the entire lumbar vertebral canal. The contrast medium should be moved into the lower thoracic vertebral canal if there are signs of stenosis of the upper lumbar or of the entire lumbar spinal canal. I have experience with three cases of involvement of the area of T10–T12 in stenosis of the upper or the entire lumbar vertebral canal.[130]

The most typical caudographic findings in stenosis of the lumbar vertebral canal[121, 122, 128] (Figs. 4 and 5*A*) are visualized in the lateral

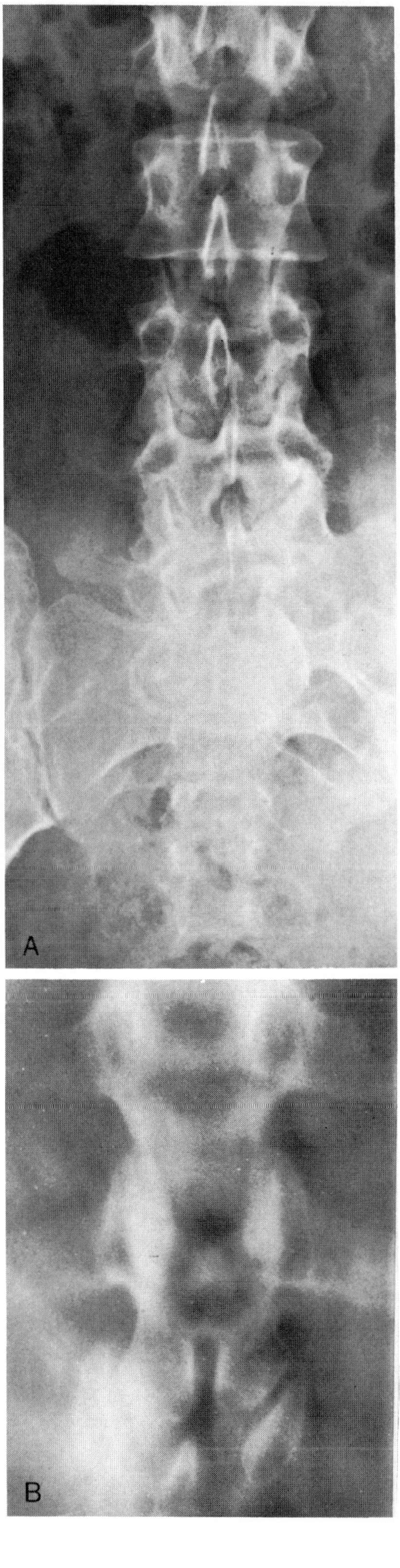

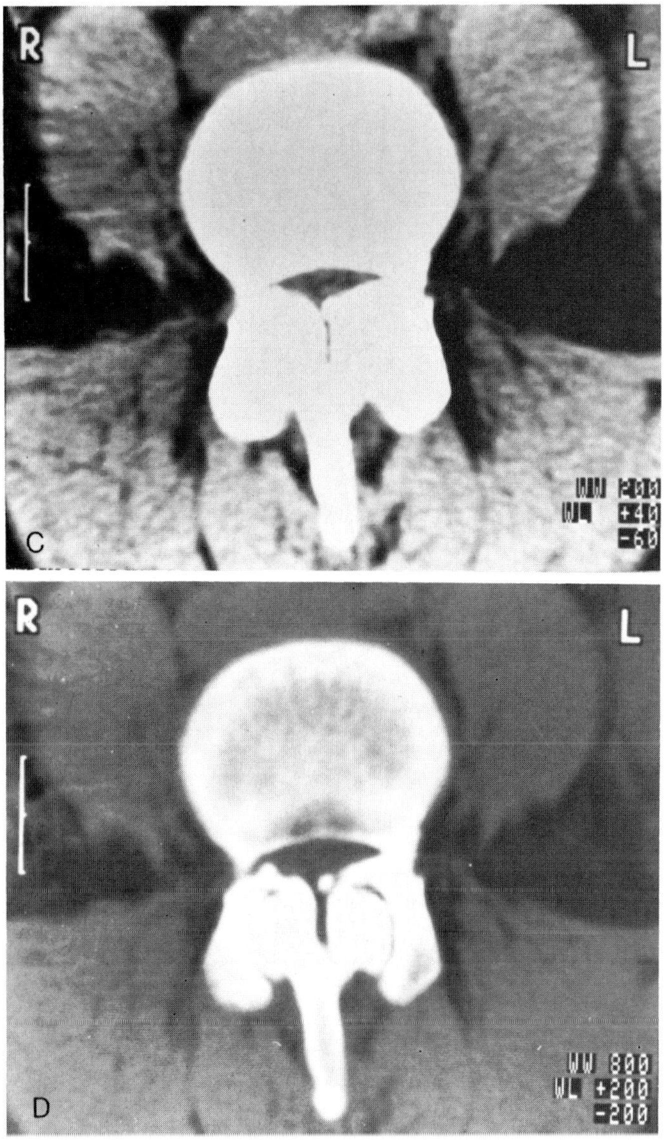

Figure 3 □ *A,* Anteroposterior (AP) plain roentgenogram. The visualization of small angles between the inferior articular processes of L3 and L4 is partly obscured by the overlapping projection of the spinous processes. *B,* Same case. Frontal hypocycloidal tomogram through the laminae and articular processes shows reduction of interlaminar space between the inferior articular processes, a typical sign of the hypertrophic form of idiopathic developmental stenosis of the bony lumbar vertebral canal (DSBLVC). *C, D,* CT scans demonstrate a reduction of the posterior portion of the vertebral canal to a narrow posterior recess as a result of hypertrophy of the articular processes. The vertebral canal has pulled out in an oval shape with an MSD of 6 mm. It demonstrates that hypertrophic articular processes do not invariably produce a trefoil shape of the vertebral canal. CT images of posterior recess of vertebral canal are smaller than actual size, owing to partial volume effect; this more so with the window setting at soft tissue level in *C* than with the window setting at bone level (slice thickness: 3 mm) in *D.*

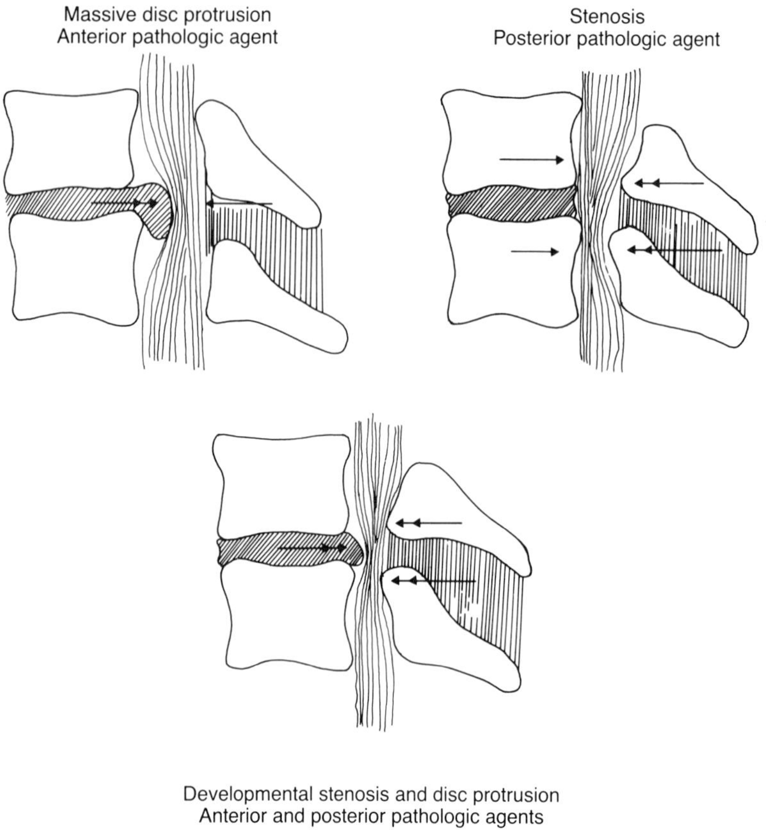

Figure 4 □ Schematic representation of the deformities in the profile myelogram in the presence of stenosis, disc herniations, and a combination of both, if there is no arrest of the contrast medium.

view; these are reduction of the sagittal diameter of the contrast column and posterior impression, and partial or complete block of the contrast medium at the level of the articular processes. The partial and complete blocks of contrast medium often show that their posterior borders are situated more cephalad than their anterior borders if the contrast medium has been introduced above the area of stenosis. This is the result of posterior compression by the hypertrophic articular processes. Because nonionic water-soluble contrast media form sediment rapidly, lateral views with the patient in ventral (more lordotic) decubitus should be made first, once the contrast medium has been injected, for measuring the sagittal diameter[128] of the contrast column. The frontal view may show lateral slanting of the contrast medium (Fig. 5*B*) caused by hypertrophic articular processes.

In stenosis at multiple levels, also involving the portions of the vertebral canal entirely surrounded by bone (at pedicular levels), the caudogram may show a sharp delineation of the caudal nerve roots, which is best seen in the oblique views.[121, 122] Before the introduction of the CT body scanners, the diagnosis of stenosis and its extent was based entirely upon caudography. It is now an indispensable means of determining the area to be examined with CT. Possibly, midsagittal magnetic resonance imaging (MRI) may replace caudography, having the advantages of being noninvasive and avoiding the use of x-rays. Our present experience with the images obtained by means of surface coil MRI is that they are not as accurate as CT images and certainly not more accurate than caudograms, as some other authors contend.[79] MRI may provide information about intradiscal changes (Fig. 6*B*), which cannot be obtained with CT or myelography. However, MRI is much less reliable in measuring MSD (Fig. 6*A*), which is important in the diagnosis of stenosis. Arachnitis may also be missed by MRI.

Because the occurrence of artifacts with MRI is much greater than with CT, great experience is required in the interpretation

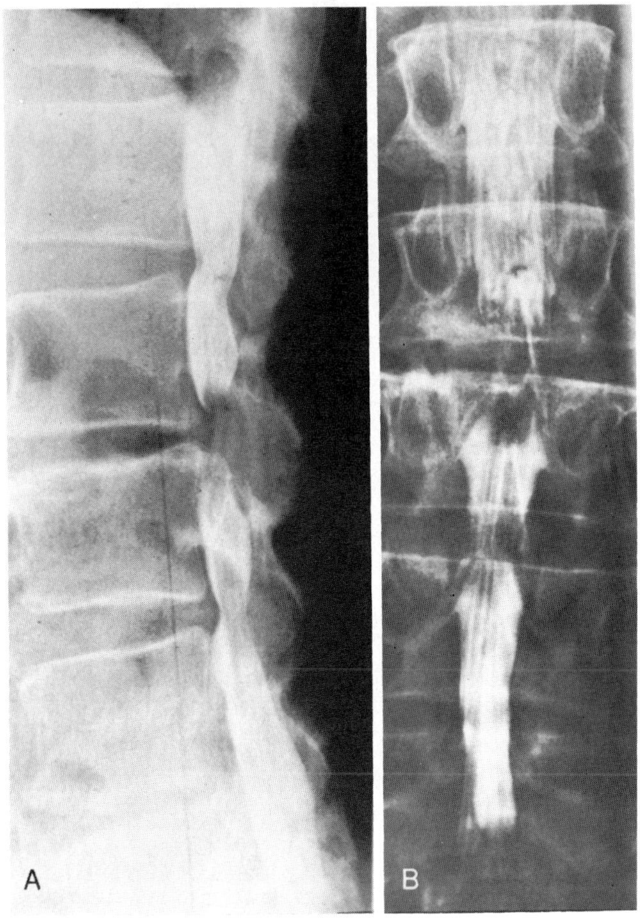

Figure 5 □ Myelograms: idiopathic DSBLVC plus disc herniation. *A,* Profile view shows a flattened disc space at L3–L4. Posterior disc herniation and stenotic canal at that level produce partial arrest and interruption of the contrast column. The hypertrophic articular processes produce a posterior impression of the contrast medium just above the partial arrest at L3–L4. Posterior impressions of the contrast column at L2–L3 and L4–L5 are produced by hypertrophic articular processes. The AP diameters of the contrast column become larger above L2. *B,* The posteroanterior (PA) view shows bilateral slanting of the contrast medium at L4–L5, caused by the hypertrophic articular processes. Interruption of the contrast medium opposite the flattened disc space and disc herniation L3–L4 is shown.

of the MRI findings. At present, CT scanning is always performed when the possibility of stenosis is considered.

Since about 10 years ago we have become familiar with the rearrangement of the data of a series consecutive transaxial CT scans of the spine to provide new slices in other orientations, such as sagittal sections for improved visualization of intervertebral foramina. These so-called multiplanar reformatted (MPR) images remain two dimensional (2-D) and they may show artificial irregularities of configuration resulting from imperfections of the method. Modern 3-D images[74, 112, 147] are less realistic because they produce perceptual depth effects, although the images remain 2-D. Therefore, the 3-D images are referred to as pseudo–3-D or 3-D scenes. Depth perception in these images is obtained by means of i.a. depth encoding: the intensity of surfaces is made inversely proportional to the distance between the observer and those surfaces. In addition, the impression of depth can be created by applying reflective surface shading that is produced by the orientation of a source of virtual light. The use of certain background colors not appearing in the object may produce the impression that the object is in front of the background.

By so-called interaction, the 3-D imaged object can be explored on the screen by changing its position or changing the direction of its illumination.

Hidden structures such as the spinal canal may be visualized by removing parts of surrounding vertebral structures. Figures 7, 8, and 9 show images obtained from 110 consecutive 1.5-mm CT slices taken from the lower end plate of the body of L3 into the inferior border of the sacrum. They represent only a few of the 60 images obtained in various directions or taken after parts of the bony structures have been removed for visualization of the lateral, dorsal, and ventral aspects of the vertebral canal, the surfaces

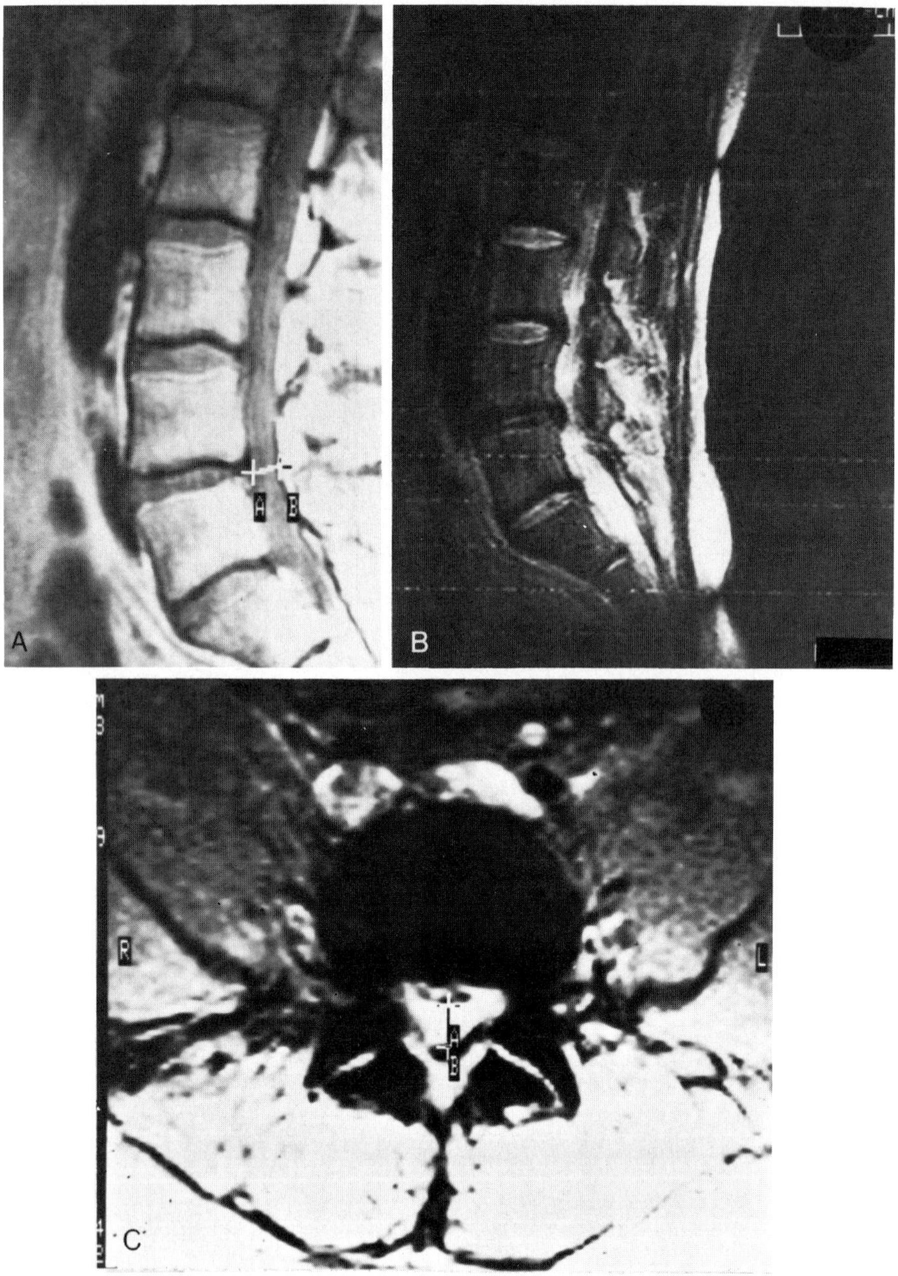

Figure 6 □ Magnetic resonance imaging (MRI) at 1.5 tesla shows profile view of the lumbar spine on a T1-weighted image (SE:TE = 30, TR = 450, not ECG triggered; slice thickness—7 mm; number of measurements—2). This is a case of idiopathic DSBLVC at L3–L5. Disc herniation is at L4–L5. *A,* Patient positioned with increased lordosis results mainly in an increase of the lumbosacral angle. Nonuniform responses of surface coil detector result in high-intensity image of the posterior vertebral structures, which does not allow one to identify the presence of posterior epidural fat, except in the sacral canal around the inferior end of the dural sac. Some fat may be present on the posterior dural aspect at L1 and L2. Longitudinal stripings in the prevertebral abdominal region and in the area of the vertebral canal are artifacts, probably caused by a pulsating aortic blood flow. In the absence of signals from the cortical bony walls of the vertebral canal, approximate MSD measurements can be made from the posterior lining of the vertebral canal to the signal-producing annulus of the intervertebral disc. The MSD opposite the disc L4–L5 is 9 mm, corresponding to an identical value in the CT scan. At L5, L4, and the lower half of L3 the vertebral canal seems to be more shallow than at higher levels, which was confirmed with CT. *B,* In the same patient, the second-echo heavily weighted T2 image produces better visualization of cerebrospinal fluid (CSF) because of a long T2. (SE:TE = 50, TR = 2,000; slice thickness—7 mm; number of measurements—2). This shows degeneration of the L4–L5 disc and bulging of discs at L4–L5 and L3–L4. This estimation of depth of the vertebral canal is impossible. *C,* Transverse section through a degenerated disc at L4–L5 obtained in fast-field sequence with data collection by gradient echos. (Flip angle—12 degrees; TR = 300, TE = 20; slice thickness—6 mm; number of measurements—2). (See text). This technique provides good visualization and a clear demarcation of spinal fluid. Patient is placed in exaggerated lordosis. The homogeneous intensity of the content of the dural theca justifies the presence of a fair amount of CSF. This patient showed a myelographic block above this disc space when standing upright. Midsagittal-diameter of CSF collection is 9 mm, as measured in the T1-weighted image in *A.*

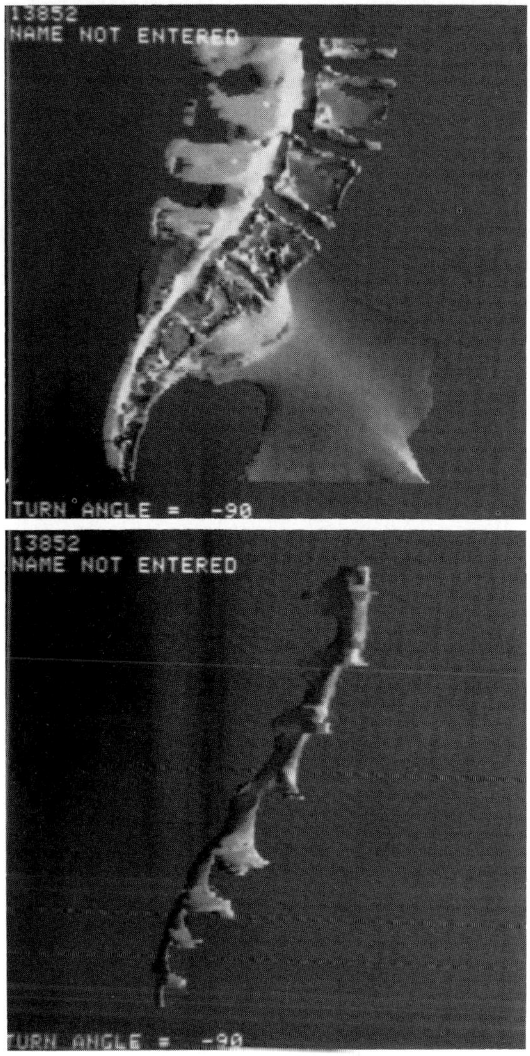

Figure 7 □ 3-D images (see text) of a patient with idiopathic DSBLVC combined with degenerative spondylolisthesis, hemilumbarization of S1, and exostosis. Upper image is of a midsagittal section through 3-D images made from the inferior tip of the sacrum up to the bottom plate of the body of L3, showing degenerative spondylolisthesis of L4. The lumbar vertebral canal is smallest at the levels of L5 and of the partially lumbarized S1. Lower image shows a lateral view of configuration of the vertebral canal defined by interface between surrounding interior surface of the bony canal and adjacent soft tissue and fluid content.

of the sacroiliac joints, and so forth. This procedure required 10 hours. Because the interfaces in this example were determined between bone and air, the patient dose of x-rays per slice was considerably reduced. Obviously such elaborate examination is of interest in particular types of vertebral lesions or diseases, as was the case of the patient in Figures 7, 8, and 9.

The essential and final radiodiagnostic judgment in cases of stenosis of the vertebral canal is based upon CT images, including the qualitative and quantitative aspects. The largest interpedicular distances can be measured in plain frontal x-rays because they concern the distance between the medial surfaces of the pedicles, which are at all lumbar levels tangentially caught by the x-rays and consequently visualized as clear interfaces. In my cases of idiopathic DSBLVC the interpedicular distances measured in the radiographs were corrected by an ample magnification factor (× 1.4).

The smallest value recorded was 20 mm, which is 2 mm more than the lowest value found in skeletal measurements. CT scanning is the most exact method for measuring midsagittal diameter (MSD). It requires that the CT sections are made perpendicular to the anterior wall of the part of the vertebral canal involved. This may be difficult at the level of the lumbosacral angle, where making perpendicular sections depends on the possible angulation of the gantry and degree of obliteration of the lumbosacral angle by positioning the patient. The anthropologic measurements of MSD of skeletal lumbar vertebrae that were reported in the literature were made from the center of the anterior surface of the posterior bony wall of the vertebral foramen to the posterior aspect of the vertebral body. Intraoperative measurements of midsagittal diameters had to be made via interlaminar spaces, if they were not obliterated. It resulted in measurements of MSDs at cephalic and caudal borders of the laminae.

In the absence of stenosis we found that at the caudal border of the laminae the MSD was invariably greater than at their cephalic border. This led to the concept of the ratio of the two MSDs (RMD; the cephalic MSD is the numerator and the caudal MSD is the denominator). Normally the RMD is less than 1.0. This fact has received little attention in anatomic textbooks, although Testut[107] mentioned in 1904 that the laminae do not present a vertical direction but slope slightly in a posteroinferior direction, so that the inferior circumference of the vertebral foramen of each vertebra is larger than its superior circumference (Figs. 10 and 11). The explanation of this fact is that the ligamentum flavum is attached to the front of the lower border of the cephalad laminae and to the back of the superior border of the caudal laminae. Equal lengths of the MSD at the cephalic and caudal borders of laminae would result in a posterior notch inside the vertebral canal, produced by the attachment of the ligamentum flavum to the anterior inferior surface of these laminae.

A caudal MSD smaller than the cephalic MSD would accentuate this notching, which is not seen, however, in the absence of stenosis. *RMDs greater than 1.0 were encountered only with absolute and relative stenosis but not in all cases and, when present, not at all levels of the lumbar vertebral canal involved.* The pathogenesis of reversed RMDs in stenosis has not been explained.

Postacchini and colleagues,[89] in measuring skeletal vertebrae, found that the mean caudal MSDs were equal to the mean cephalic MSDs. Apart from statistical objections that can be made about comparing these means, the main objection to their examination is in the statement of these authors that

> **The caudad MSD was taken as the shortest MSD between the vertebral body and the bony ridge of the attachment of the ligamentum flavum; *when this ridge was located at a lower level with respect to the vertebral body, the caudad MSD was measured at the level of the lower border of the vertebral body.***

The phrase "the bony ridge of attachment of the ligamentum flavum" is a vague one.

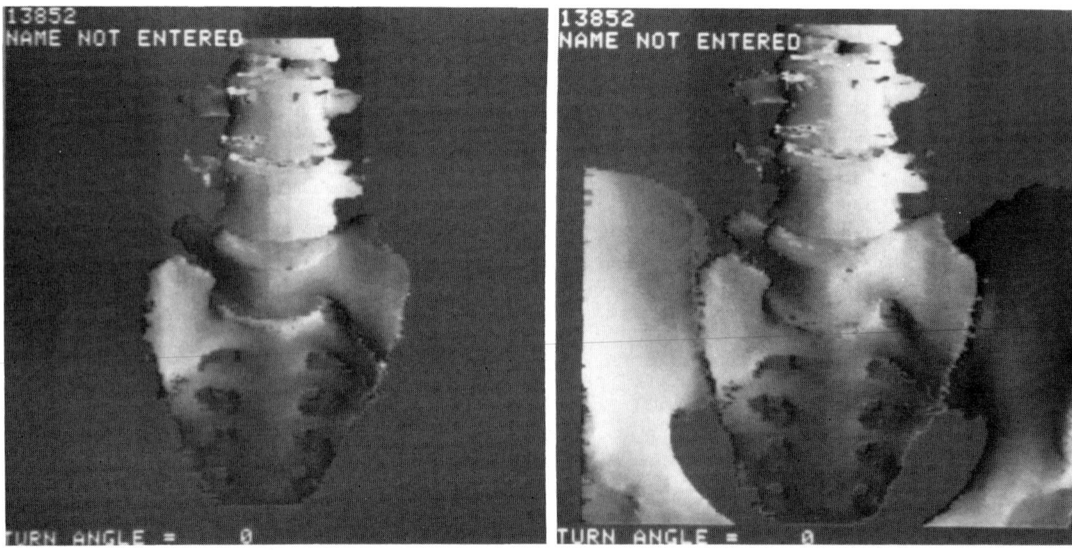

Figure 8 □ Same patient as shown in Figure 7, anterior view of a 3-D image. Right-sided lumbarization of S1 and exostosis at the upper margin of S1 are seen. Left image shows the greatest relief perspective of protruding exostosis through orientation of virtual light with shadow formation and the use of different colors for S1 versus those of the L5 body and of the sacrum below S1. In the right image, the depth effect in the region of the lumbosacral transition area is obtained with virtual light effects alone.

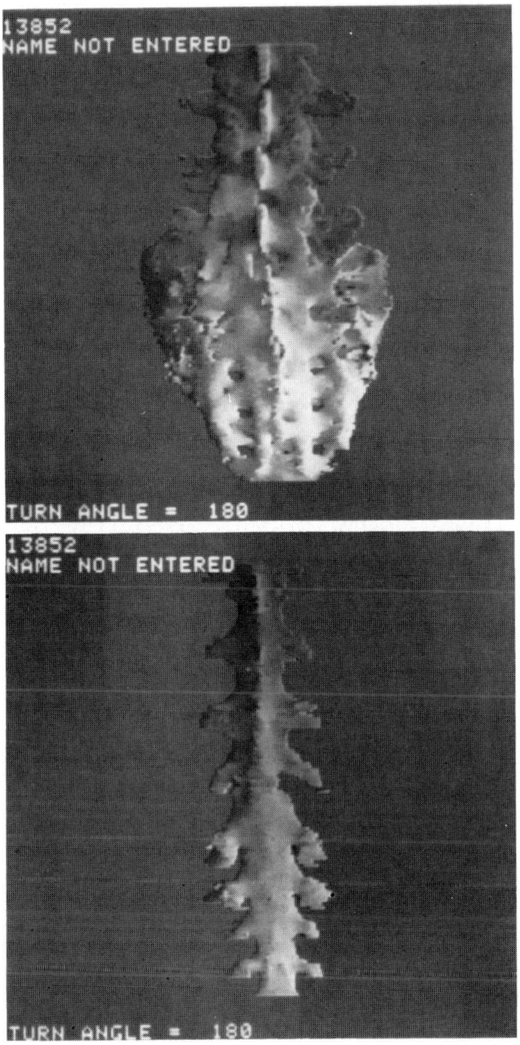

Figure 9 □ Same patient as in Figures 7 and 8. Upper 3-D image shows posterior aspect of the lumbosacral spine. Lower 3-D image shows dorsal interface between the vertebral canal and its wall.

The ligamentum attaches to the lower anterior surfaces of the laminae and not only to their lower borders. Figure 11 shows that the caudal borders of lumbar laminae may (rarely) be situated opposite the vertebral body, but they frequently extend below the level of the body, forming a roof over the intervertebral disc. Because the authors did not give numbers of laminae extending below the vertebral body and did not measure the caudal borders of these laminae, their statistics provide no valid data about the lengths of MSDs at the caudal borders of the laminae.

CT examination of midsagittal diameters.[125] Useful slice thickness is 3 mm. In order to measure MSD at the cephalic border of laminae, the first CT section is made through the centers of the pedicles. Two additional sections in caudal or cephalic direction may be needed to cut the cephalic border of the laminae (Fig. 12*A* and *D*). To measure the MSD at the caudal border of the laminae, the first CT section is made through the center of the disc space and parallel to the inferior end plate of the vertebral body above, followed by a few orienting sections in cephalic and caudal direction, taking care that the sections remain perpendicular to the anterior wall of the vertebral canal. The caudal border of the laminae approximates the shape of an inverted V (Fig. 12*B*). Transarticular sections (Fig. 12*C*) visualize the condition of the articular facets and their influence on the configuration of the vertebral canal. The transdiscal sections may show the presence or absence of disc herniations inside the vertebral canal, in the intervertebral foramina, or in a "far-out" lateral position.

Measurements of the MSD in CT scans are made by means of cursors. Each of the MSDs should be measured at least three times and recorded values should be averaged. Interobserver errors in CT measurements of MSD made by five experienced radiologists were studied by Beers.[9] The greatest difference in average readings was 1.2 mm. No caudal border of the laminae can be measured when they over-roof the superior border of the subjacent laminae, but that condition can already be recognized in plain frontal radiographs. Measurements of MSDs should be routinely performed during CT scanning of the spine. Many radiologists diagnose stenosis of the lumbar vertebral canal merely by sight.

I have tested the measurements made with CT by means of intraoperative measurements. To measure the MSD at the caudal border of the laminae, the attachment of the ligamentum flavum was removed by means of an open-eyed curette. Each MSD was measured three times, and the smallest value found was thought to represent the perpendicular distance. No measurements could be made of over-roofing laminar borders. Some vertebral canals were too narrow to permit the introduction of the stenosimeter without risk of damaging the caudal nerve roots. If under such conditions the interlaminar space could be opened without removing the borders of the laminae, the MSD was measured by introducing a very thin needle through the dura and marking the point of its crossing the anterior border of the laminae. Although the presence of stenosis was obvious in such cases, the quantitative values of MSDs were useful in the study of the pathophysiology of the stenosis and of the accuracy of CT measurements.

Significance of Absolute and Relative Stenoses

In absolute stenosis there is no reserve capacity of the extradural or intradural space to compensate for additional space-occupying agents. In relative stenosis this reserve capacity is very small.

Relative Stenosis

The significance of relative stenosis, as introduced by the author,[113, 117, 122] is not well understood. Postacchini and colleagues[89] wrote that in the "view of Verbiest, MSD less than 12 mm is pathologic," with references to two of my publications. This is an incorrect description of my definition of relative stenosis. Neither in the cited reports[120, 128] nor in my other papers has relative stenosis ever been called "pathologic." On the contrary, I have always stated, beginning with my first paper, that, in the presence of relative stenosis with MSDs of 10 to 13 mm, minimal hard or soft disc bulging that does not exceed 2 mm may already produce symptomatic stenosis. Relative stenosis is no pathologic condition. It is encountered in all vertebrometric statistics, even in 6.3% of 443 lumbar skeletons measured by Eisenstein.[34, 36] Among the lumbar spines studied by Postacchini and colleagues, the minimal MSDs found were in the range of relative stenosis, with the exception of one skeletal lumbar spine for which the smallest MSDs were between 9 and 10 mm. This exceptional spine cannot tell its life story; however, it is proof of the rare chance of encountering absolute stenosis in random

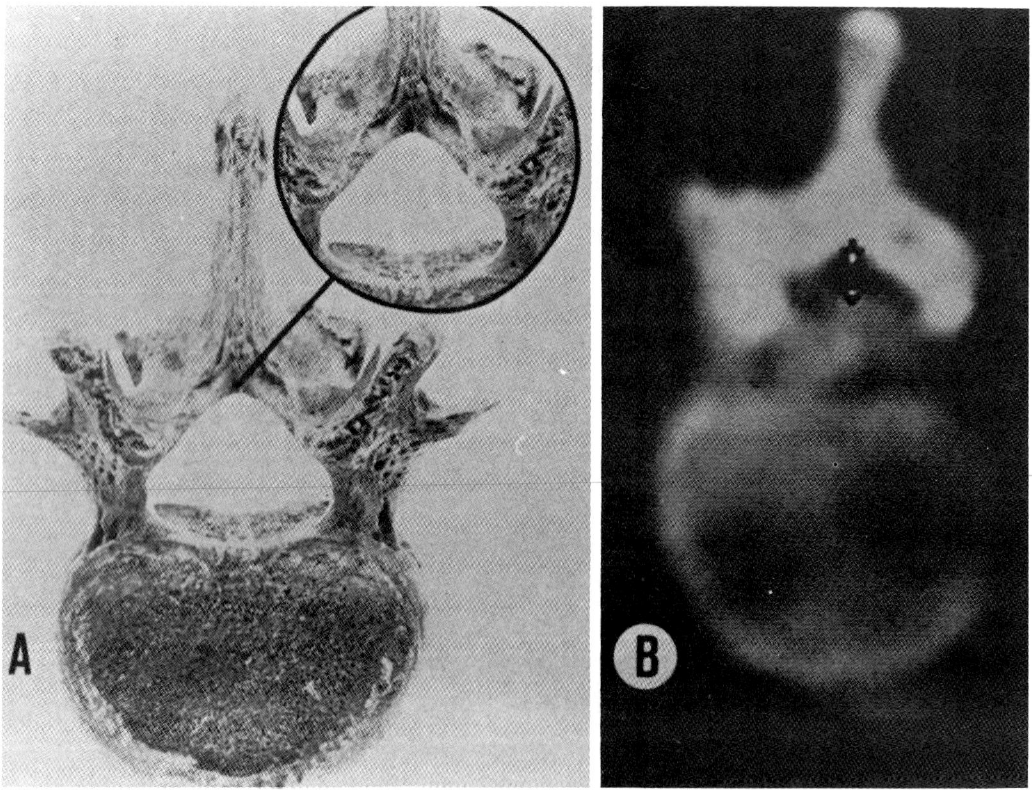

Figure 10 □ *A,* View of lower aspect of lumbar vertebral body shows that the laminae slope posteriorly in a caudal direction, providing room for the portion of ligamentum flavum attached to the caudal anterior surface of the laminae without producing a narrowing of the vertebral canal. *B,* CT scan through caudal border of lumbar laminae. Cursors indicate space occupied by ligamentum flavum, where it attaches to the caudal anterior surface of the laminae.

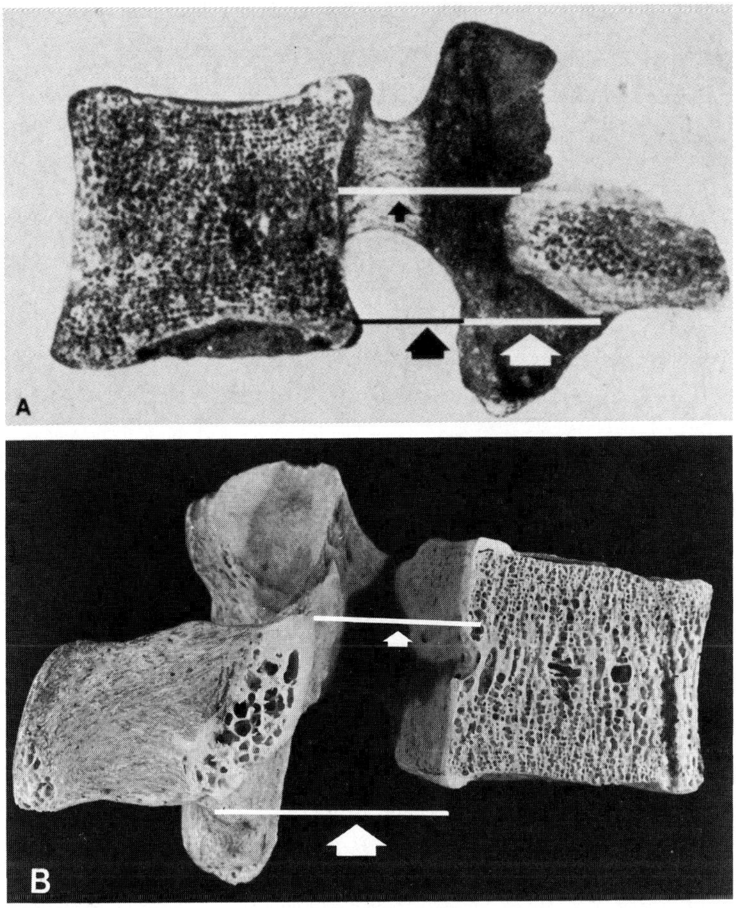

Figure 11 □ Midsagittal sections through two different lumbar vertebrae. *A* shows right half of a lumbar vertebra. The perpendicular (large arrow head) from the center of the caudad border of the laminae arrives at the posterior border of the vertebral body. *B* shows right half of another lumbar vertebra. The perpendicular (large arrow head) from the center of the caudad border of the laminae passes a few mm below the inferior end plate of the vertebral body and through the disc space, if it is not flattened. This type of laminae occurs more frequently than the type shown in A. Bony stenosis at the caudal border of the laminae in A will not directly aggravate the effects of disc protrusions below the body of this vertebra, whereas in B stenosis producing laminae, which roof over a disc protrusion, will aggravate its effects. Therefore measurement of MSD at the caudal border of the laminae of skeletal vertebrae of the type shown in B at a more cephalic level, so that the perpendicular reaches the vertebral body, neglects the real significance of this caudal MSD.

In A and B perpendiculars (small arrow heads) from the cephalad borders of the laminae are clearly smaller than the perpendiculars from their caudad borders of the corresponding laminae.

selections of skeletal vertebrae. In most comparable vertebrometric reports, such small MSDs do not figure at all. Postacchini and colleagues determined lower and upper limits of normal MSDs on the basis of their morphometric findings. The evaluation of these statistical data must be limited to the distribution of the values measured. A distribution curve consisting of values of diameters alone contains no references for separating the normal diameters from the abnormal ones. Normality and abnormality in such statistics can be applied only to the shape of the curves or histograms representing frequencies.

Relations between morphometric properties of the spine and functional disturbances can only be statistically analyzed in comparative studies of patients. Such analyses in our patients have shown that stenosis is one determinant in the production of stenotic disease that may be quantified, but that one or more other indispensable determinants are active in the caudal nerve roots; their nature has not been identified, so their qualification or quantification is not yet possible. Although the inferior limit of MSD of relative stenosis is fixed at 10 mm, representing the upper limit of absolute stenosis, its upper limit, determined by an MSD of 13 mm, may seem to be arbitrary. The reasons are as follows:

1. Reversed RMDs found within this group (Table 2[120, 121, 122]), as in absolute stenosis, were not observed with larger MSDs.
2. Mild hypertrophy of structures of the vertebral arch was incidentally found with MSDs between 10 and 13 mm, but never with larger MSDs.
3. The extension of MSDs between 10 and 13 mm was found to the L2 or L5 vertebrae, where findings of such small MSDs are rare, according to measurements of skeletal vertebrae.
4. An upper limit of MSDs of 14 or 15 mm approaches mean values found with randomized skeletal vertebrometry.

Absolute Stenosis

A number of pathomorphologic features of idiopathic DSBLVC were described earlier. The structures of the vertebral arch are usually very thick, but microscopic examination of the bone involved has not revealed abnormalities, except osteoporosis in some older patients. The hypertrophic joints may show signs of osteoarthritis. Through tacit convention it is usually referred to as hypertrophic osteoarthritis, indicating arthritis as a cause. However, the possibility of primary hypertrophic posterior joints complicated by arthritis cannot be excluded.

The occurrence of trefoil vertebral canals with respect to idiopathic DSNLVC has been discussed by Eisenstein.[35] He observed a tre-

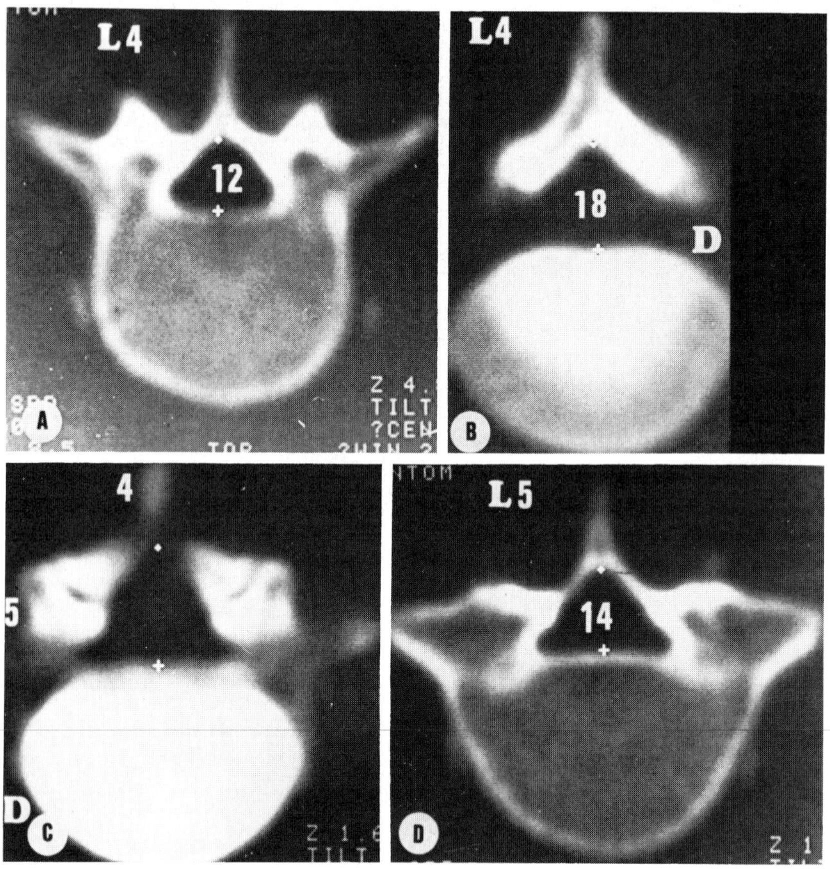

Figure 12 □ Levels of CT sections for measuring MSDs. *A, D,* CT sections taken through the cephalic borders of the laminae of L4 and L5 were used for measuring MSDs at the cephalic borders of the laminae. The sections cut the entirely bony portions of the vertebral canal. *B,* CT section was taken through the caudal border of the laminae of L4 for measuring caudal MSD. It shows the inverted V shape of the laminae. This section passes through the transition between the inferior end plate of the vertebral body of L4 and the disc at L4–L5. *C,* Transarticular CT section is shown (5 indicates superior articular process of L5). The inferior articular processes of L4 are inferior prolongations of the laminae of L4 (4 indicates lower-border posterior tip of spinous process of L4). Numbers printed in the canal are values of the MSDs in millimeters. Note that the MSD at the cephalic border of L4 (*A*) is much smaller than at its caudal border (*B*).

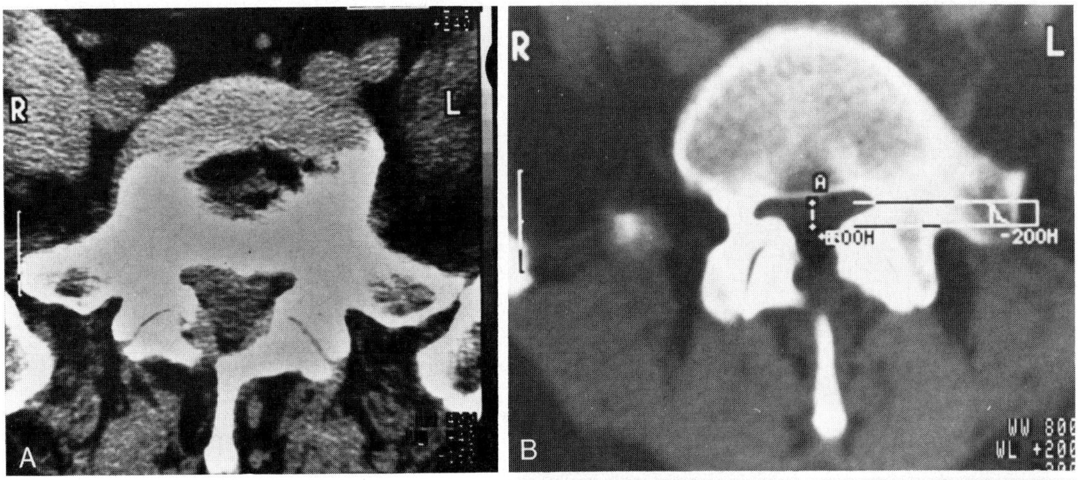

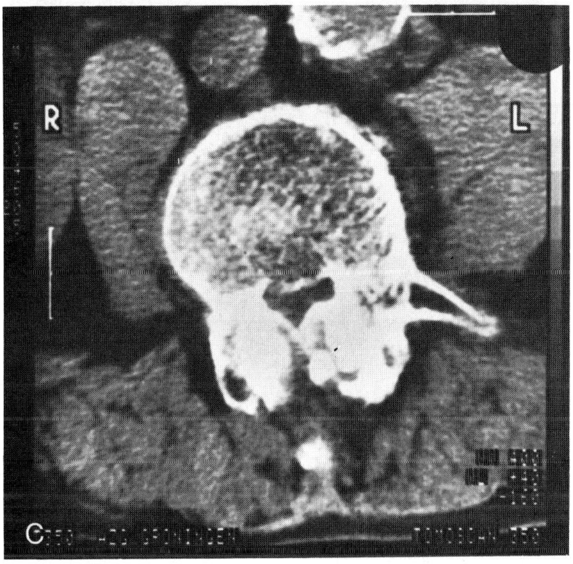

Figure 13 □ CT scans showing lateral recess formation in idiopathic DSBLVC. *A,* CT scan shows an early stage of lateral recess formation as a result of hypertrophy of the superior articular processes; it is most pronounced on the right. *B,* Transitional L5 vertebra. Hypertrophy of right superior articular process produces a very narrow lateral recess. On the left side, the canal is shallow without extralateral recess narrowing. *C,* Asymmetric narrowing of bony portion of the vertebral canal with left-sided lateral recess formation was caused by laminar notching.

foil configuration of the vertebral canal in 14% of 484 skeletons. It was encountered, in descending frequency, at L5, L4, and rarely L3. In his opinion, these findings contradicted my view that facet osteophytes are responsible for the trefoil configuration. My paper[116] was not adequately interpreted because it described only the encroachment of the articular processes upon the vertebral canal; it was then added that "Although spondylosis or arthritis of the vertebral joints was found radiographically in Cases 3, 4, 5, and 6, these changes seemed to have no part in the causation of the narrowing. It may be that it is developmental." The word trefoil was not used in that paper, and no description was provided of the shape of the narrowed vertebral canal. CT made it possible to visualize the effects of the hypertrophic processes or other hypertrophic bony structures on the shape of the vertebral canal. Figure 3, *C* and *D,* show that the hypertrophic articular processes may produce an oval-shaped canal. Alternatively, as shown in Figure 13, *A* to *C,* they may produce asymmetric or approximately symmetric trefoil-shaped canals. Certainly, however, two of the latter three images show the trefoil shape of the transarticular sections of the vertebral canal and not the transpedicular sections, where the occurrence of trefoil shape was examined by Eisenstein and first described by Armstrong.[2] In my experience, idiopathic DSBLVC may produce a trefoil canal at much higher vertebral levels than observed by Eisenstein, as, for instance, in the lower thoracic region.[130] It is an example of the difference between anthropologic and clinical experience.

By making systematic measurements we have found that cases of idiopathic DSBLVC occur in the absence of any bony hypertrophy. When no measurements are made, this condition may pass completely unrecognized during clinical observation and operation.

Determinants of Symptomatic Stenosis of the Lumbar Vertebral Canal: An Analysis of the Share of Morphologic Abnormalities and Reaction of Neural Content in Producing Stenotic Disease

Absolute stenosis, either primary or caused by additional compressive agents, can, in the absence of other compressive agents, produce caudal nerve root disturbances. It means that there is no reserve capacity in the relation between volume of neural content and capacity of the container, (i.e., the vertebral canal). Yet absolute stenosis becomes symptomatic in some patients with MSDs of 10 mm, whereas for other patients it becomes symptomatic with much smaller MSDs. Two explanations of this fact are possible: (1) individual variations in the total cross-sectional surface of the caudal nerve roots in the area of stenosis or (2) individual differences in resistance of the caudal nerve roots to compression. Actually, there is no method of measuring the cross-sectional surface area occupied by the total number of caudal nerve roots in the stenotic canal. There may be variations, some persons having thinner caudal nerve roots than others, that might explain why absolute stenosis becomes symptomatic with smaller MSDs in some patients, compared with other patients.

Findings with a comparative analysis of permanent signs and symptoms versus those of neurogenic intermittent claudication (NICL) in the individual patients indicate that individual differences in resistance of caudal nerve roots to stenotic compression are also determinants in the clinical manifestation of absolute stenosis. We do not know whether absolute stenosis may remain asymptomatic for life. In symptomatic absolute stenosis, regardless of whether it is primary or occurs through additional narrowing of relative stenosis, the signs and symptoms can be divided into permanent radiculopathy and intermittent radicular disturbances during standing and/or NICL. Because orthostatic influences can often be avoided by the patients, this does not hold for walking. Therefore, most systematic information about the occurrence and properties of intermittent radicular disturbances can be obtained from NICL.

The two current theories of the causes of NICL in stenosis are as follows:

1. Increased lordosis during standing and walking produces additional compression of the caudal nerve roots through plication of the dural theca and folding inward the vertebral canal of the ligamenta flava.[29, 143]
2. Increase of blood supply to the nerve roots or spinal ganglia, needed during the exercise of walking or standing, is inhibited through vascular constriction produced by stenosis.[11, 12, 45, 143]

Against the theory of increased compression of the caudal nerve roots producing NICL the point may be advanced that signs and symptoms developing during mechanical compression of a nerve show a certain chronologic order, beginning with paresthesias, which are followed by neural deficits. During recovery after relief of compression, painful paresthesias recur. Paresthesias during NICL were mentioned by only 21 out of 142 patients presenting with NICL.[121, 122]

Recovery from NICL during rest was never accompanied by paresthesias. The occurrence of NICL in the presence of arteriovenous malformations of the cauda equina demonstrates that ischemia of the cauda equina may result in NICL.[121, 122]

Most authors have limited their attention to the presence of permanent radiculopathy as a consequence of the idiopathic DSBLVC, as such, and to temporary signs of radiculopathy during NICL or standing upright, trying to explain the latter by the theories of increased pressure or ischemia, as discussed above. On the basis of these theories, it might be concluded that there are only permanently and temporarily radiculopathic nerves in these cases.

The problem of NICL is more complicated. One of our patients with idiopathic DSBLVC in the area of L3 through L5 whose smallest MSD measured 5 mm, has completely asymptomatic periods interrupted by periods of low backache and NICL. The periods of symptomatic stenosis may be self-limiting while the patient continues work as a waitress, or the patient may recover after a temporary interruption of work. Once recovered, the individual may work for months without any complaints. This simple clinical experience demonstrates that stenosis of the bony vertebral canal is not the only determinant in the production of neural signs and symptoms and that individual variations of the thresholds of vulnerability of the caudal nerve roots to compression are also important determinants in the production of symptomatic stenosis.

The two current criteria for establishing a diagnosis of NICL are as follows:

1. Neural disturbances impede the continuation of walking.
2. Walking can be resumed after 10 to 20 minutes of rest.

For a more selective critical analysis of the signs and symptoms of NICL, we added a third criterion:

3. If the patient presents with permanent neural disturbances, the occurrence of NICL is only accepted if it is caused by disturbances other than the permanent ones. Spread over a larger area of permanent neural disturbances during walking was accepted as a cause of NICL.[121, 122, 127]

On the basis of findings with these three criteria we developed the hypothesis that in DSBLVC three types of caudal nerve roots may be found: normal nerve roots, nerve roots presenting subsymptomatic radiculopathy, and nerve roots presenting manifest permanent radiculopathy.

Gilliatt and Wilson[55, 56] demonstrated the occurrence and properties of subsymptomatic neuropathy in patients presenting partial permanent sensory deficit in the territories of median nerves being compressed in the carpal tunnels. Tourniquet compression of the patients' arms proximal to the carpal tunnel resulted in anesthesia spreading over the entire supply area of the median nerve. In contrast, sensation in the territory of the ulnar nerve, which was equally compressed by the tourniquet, remained normal.

Arguments for the occurrence of subclinical radiculopathy as a cause of NICL in idiopathic DSBLVC are the following:[127]

1. Spread of any type of permanent radicular signs or symptoms during NICL occurred in 79.5% of our 122 patients, representing 41% of the total number of signs and symptoms of permanent radiculopathy in this group.
2. NICL occurred in the absence of permanent neural disturbances. In 20 such patients, the causes of NICL consisted of various combinations of two of the following disturbances: motor deficit, sensory loss, and pains in the legs.
3. NICL may be absent in the presence of permanent neural disturbances.

In 53 of such patients a total of 97 signs of permanent radiculopathy was recorded.[127, 130]

Tables 1 and 2 present comparative data of the laterality of permanent radicular disturbances and those occurring during NICL observed in 195 patients.

The great differences between the laterality of permanent neural disturbances and of

Table 1 □ Comparative Data of the Laterality of Permanent Radicular Disturbances and Those Occurring During NICL, Observed in 195 Patients

RADICULAR DISTURBANCES	PERMANENT	DURING NICL		NO NICL
Bilateral Identical = (BID)*	11.3%	BID	8.7%	2.6%
Bilateral Unequal = (BUD)*	31.7%	BID	12.3%	16.3%
		UD	3.1%	
Unilateral = (UD)*	46.7%	BID	26.2%	8.2%
		BUD	1.0%	
		UD	11.3%	
None (10.3%) = (ND)*	—	BID	8.2%	
		BUD	0.5%	
		UD	1.6%	
Totals	89.7%		72.9%	27.1%

*Abbreviations of terms in left column are used in other columns in Tables 1 and 2.

Table 2 □ Frequencies of Laterality of Radicular Disturbances

	PERMANENT	DURING NICL
BID	11.3%	55.4%
BUD	31.7%	1.5%
UD	46.7%	16.0%

those during NICL (Table 2) as well as the different behavior in laterality of NICL versus the laterality of permanent neural disturbances (Table 1) demonstrate that stenosis affects caudal nerve roots during NICL other than the permanently manifest radiculopathic nerve roots. The conclusion is that NICL is the result of the presence of nerve roots presenting "at-rest" subsymptomatic radiculopathy.

The presence of normal nerve roots in stenotic canals is demonstrated by patients, who, of the three main manifestations of permanent radiculopathy or of NICL (i.e., motor deficit, sensory loss and leg pains) do not show one or two of these disturbances at rest or during NICL. Among these patients are those who present no symptoms at rest and NICL only, and those presenting manifest radiculopathy but no NICL.

The hypothesis that degree of vulnerability of caudal nerve roots is an important determinant in the clinical manifestation of stenosis is founded not only on a comparative analysis of neural signs but also on a morphometric analysis.

In 1976[121, 122] I published reports on the absence of NICL in 13 cases and its presence in 54 cases, with minimal MSDs between 4 and 10 mm and an average MSD of 7.5 mm in both groups.

Twenty-two patients with very small MSDs between 4 and 6 mm suffered from permanent radiculopathy; 18 presented with NICL, whereas 4 patients had no NICL.

Our conclusion is that, in most cases of idiopathic DSBLVC, some caudal nerve root fibers remain normal all the time, some develop subsymptomatic changes, which become symptomatic during standing or walking, and others develop manifest permanent radiculopathy. There is great variety in the quality of permanent radicular disturbances, of radicular disturbances causing NICL, and of permanently absent radicular disturbances. This demonstrates that no general rules have been found concerning which type of caudal nerve fibers are predetermined by some property either to maintain normal function or to develop permanent symptoms or symptoms of NICL in the presence of stenosis. Clinical experience shows that, apart from stenosis, some factor(s) situated in the caudal nerve roots determine the absence or presence of different clinical manifestations of spinal stenosis.

Recording somatosensory evoked potential with patients walking on a traveling band might be interesting for a comparative study of patients with and without NICL.

The occurrence of NICL in spinal stenosis appears to be influenced by two other determinants: the length of the morbid history and the length of the area of stenosis. In an earlier publication I reported the following:[121, 122]

1. NICL occurred in all patients with a morbid history between 4 and 10 years. In patients with morbid histories of between 1 and 4 years, NICL occurred in about 7/10 of the patients, and in those with histories of between 1 and 8 months, in only 1/5 of the patients.
2. NICL was present in almost all cases of stenosis occupying four or five vertebrae, in about 3/4 of stenoses involving three vertebrae, in about 7/10 when involving two vertebrae, and 6/10 when involving one vertebra.

The share of normal, subsymptomatic, and symptomatic nerve roots inside an area of absolute stenosis may be related to influences of constitution, aging, and chronic wear and tear produced by back-and-forth movements of the cauda equina through the stenosed portion of the vertebral canal during flexion or extension movements of the body.

The theory that orthostatic disturbances and NICL are caused by increased lordosis during standing and walking through resulting plication of the dural theca and folding inward of the vertebral canal of the ligamenta flava probably does not represent the whole truth. Because CT and MRI exclude the examination of patients with lumbar stenosis in an upright position, they were placed in dorsal decubitus in the apparatus with a cushion beneath the lumbar region for exaggerating lordosis.

This position did not reproduce intermittent orthostatic disturbances, although the lordosis in dorsal decubitus was much more pronounced than during standing. Figure 6C shows a transverse MR image performed with a fast-field echo technique[140] through an area of absolute stenosis (MSD = 9 mm). There is a clear CSF content in the stenotic area, whereas myelography in this patient had shown a block just above the level of this MRI section.

The patient, who suffered from radiating pains in both legs while standing upright for 5 to 10 minutes, had no such complaints when lying with exaggerated lordosis in dorsal decubitus during 45 minutes of an MRI examination. His permanent backache did increase in this position. Such unexpected findings prove that, apart from degree of narrowness and susceptibility of caudal nerve roots to stenotic compression, the influence of the upright position in the production of NICL must include influences other than dural plication or infolding ligamenta flava in producing NICL or orthostatic radicular disturbances.

Decompressive laminectomy produces relief of NICL. In the few of our patients in whom no relief of NICL was obtained, insufficient decompression of the vertebral canal, of narrowed lateral recesses, or of intervertebral foramina was found.

The theory that NICL is caused by subsymptomatic radiculopathy includes, according to Gilliatt's and Wilson's finding with such nerve fibers, that any additional compression proximal to the stenotic area may produce signs and symptoms. *The view of some surgeons that decompression of absolute stenosis may be limited to the symptomatic area, whatever the definition of such area may be, is erroneous, since, for instance, subsymptomatic caudal nerve roots in the areas of L5 and S1 may also become symptomatic through additional compression at more proximal levels so that all absolutely stenotic levels of the lumbar vertebral canal should be decompressed in all cases.* A discussion of semiology had to be limited in this chapter to aspects of its relationship with the morphologic abnormalities. Other aspects of semiology are left aside.

Extent and Types of Areas of Idiopathic DSBLVC

On the basis of measurements the areas of stenosis could be divided into the following areas:

1. Areas of pure absolute stenosis, all MSDs in the area being 10 mm or smaller.
2. Areas of mixed stenosis with portions presenting MSDs of 10 mm or less and MSDs between 10 and 13 mm.
3. Areas of pure relative stenosis with MSDs between 10 and 13 mm. This distinction is useful because of differences between the three groups in pathogenesis of symptomatic stenosis, methods of treatment, and surgical results.[121–123, 127, 130]

Normal MSDs may occur inside areas of relative stenosis in Groups 2 and 3 but also in the transition between areas of absolute and relative stenosis in Group 2. These normal MSDs are called *discontinuities* (Fig. 14*B*).

Discontinuities may be encountered at only one border of laminae but in one of our patients they occupied one vertebra plus the adjacent laminar border.[128] The surgeon who arrives at a discontinuity during decompression may think that the end of the stenotic area has been reached. This error can be avoided by not terminating previous CT measurements of MSDs before normal MSDs have been found of two vertebrae at the cephalic and of two vertebrae at the caudal (if not sacral) borders of the stenotic area.

Areas of pure absolute and mixed stenosis most frequently involved three vertebrae (61%), followed by involvement of one vertebra only in 24% and of four or five lumbar vertebrae in 15%. Stenosis included S1 in three patients and the area of T10–T12 in three patients.

In pure relative stenosis involvement of only one vertebra was observed in 50% of cases, of two vertebrae in 35%, and of three or four vertebrae in 14%. In all cases involving two or more vertebrae, the lower lumbar vertebrae were more frequently involved than the upper ones. Of all patients, one or more of the L3, L4, and L5 were involved in about 90% of all stenotic vertebral levels. The distribution of values of MSDs, of normal and reversed RMDs, and of the localization, lengths, and extents of discontinuities in areas of stenosis was very irregular. This was illustrated for all cases by means of chains of symbols.[121, 122] This presentation of chaos was criticized by some colleagues who considered the meticulously gathered information about the failure to detect order to be of no practical interest. Such opposi-

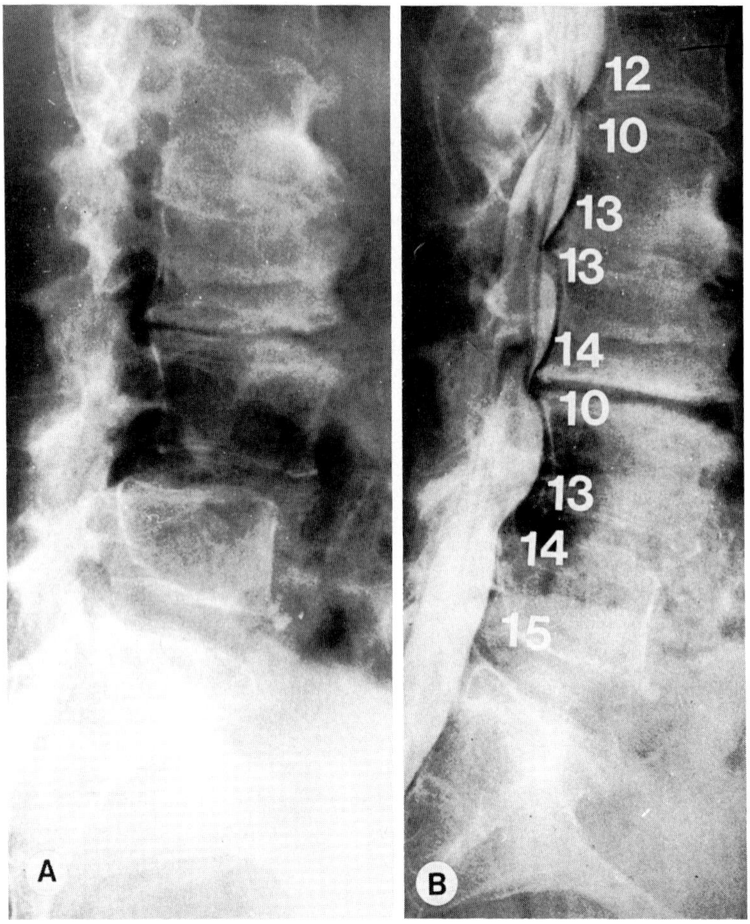

Figure 14 □ Degenerative spondylolisthesis of L4. The numbers printed on vertebral bodies in *B* indicate MSDs at the cephalic and caudal borders of their laminae. *A,* Profile view shows anterior slip of body of L4 and spondylotic changes of vertebral bodies. *B,* Profile myelogram shows pronounced stenosis at L1–L2 and L3–L4 with discontinuities (normal MSDs) between those levels. No stenosis was seen at the level of the degenerative spondylolisthesis.

tion was an interesting psychologic experience.

Additional Compressive Agents in Idiopathic DSBLVC

Remarkable findings were as follows:[127]

1. A more frequent occurrence of herniated discs at two or three levels (25.2% in 99 patients), compared with their occurrence in nonstenotic canals (17.18% of 2,885 of our patients).
2. Frequent localization above L4. Of all herniations in 99 cases, L3–L4 was involved in 25%, L2–L3 in 11%, and L1–L2 in 3%. The corresponding numbers in 2,885 patients with normal vertebral canals were 2.84%, 0.38%, and 0.17%.

In six of our patients a solitary disc herniation was situated outside the area of stenosis, in four above, and in two below. Here there is a risk that existing stenosis is unrecognized.

I described a rare additional compressive agent in a narrow lumbar vertebral canal in 1953[115] as "knotting" of a caudal nerve root. It produced bilateral sciatica without radicular deficit and a complete concave block at myelography. It was rediscovered under the name redundant nerve root in 1968[102] and interpreted as a congenital anomaly. Ehni[32] in 1970 agreed that stenosis of the lumbar vertebral canal was its cause.

Etiology of Idiopathic DSBLVC

Hereditary transmission of idiopathic DSBLVC is rare. We have experience with three brothers in one family being affected, two sisters in another family, and a mother and son in a third family. Mcgret and Marsault[78] reported the occurrence in a brother and a sister.

All our patients operated on between 1948

and 1962 because of pure absolute or mixed stenosis were males, except one. The proportion of females has considerably increased since then. There are no sex differences among patients with pure relative stenosis.[121, 122]

One of our patients with idiopathic DSBLVC was acromegalic.[128] Reports on idiopathic DSBLVC in acromegalic patients are rare.[42, 53] The vertebral changes produced by acromegaly are quite different from those found in idiopathic DSBLVC.

Idiopathic DSBLVC has in common with achondroplastic spinal stenosis the multiplicity of disc herniations, their frequent localization above L4, and postnatal abnormal periosteal bone apposition on structures of the vertebral arch, causing abnormal thickening of these structures. Although the differences between the conditions are greater than the similarities, the similarities are interesting.

Wackenheim[134–137] described a new entity, *cheirolumbar dysostosis,* as a link between acromelic skeletal growth disturbances, such as brachyphalangia, short metacarpal bones or brachypodia, and DSBLVC. In the family described, either acromelic growth disturbances or idiopathic DSBLVC, or a combination of both, were found. Unfortunately, the descriptions of patients were limited to demonstrations of plain radiographs of the spine, hands, and feet and myelograms; CT scans, measurements, clinical data, and surgical reports were not presented. Although the word dysostosis in Wackenheim's terminology is an adequate designation of the defective acromelic skeletal bone growth, this term is not so obviously applicable to the associated developmental stenosis of the bony vertebral canal. Examination of our first six patients by Dr. Huizinga[114] did not reveal any signs of disproportionate skeletal growth.

Remarkable findings in some patients with idiopathic DSBLVC were metaplastic bone formations such as ossifying arachnitis; in scar tissue bridging, hemilaminectomy defects,[121, 122] notching of hypertrophic bony structures of the vertebral arches, and formation of a sort of exostosis (see Figs. 8 and 13C) are also signs of periosteal hyperactivity. No associated cartilage formation was found, as may be seen with multiple exostoses. No signs of paraskeletal bone formation in other regions of the body have been observed in our patients, but no systematic search for occult lesions has been performed.

In some of the cases of idiopathic DSBLVC, the disorder was accompanied by idiopathic developmental absolute or relative stenosis of the cervical vertebral canal. Thickening of the cervical laminae was not observed. This is a remarkable combination because the cervical articular processes do not participate in the formation of the posterior wall of the cervical vertebral canal as they do in the lumbar area. Their medial third forms the posterior border of the cervical intervertebral foramina, whereas the lateral two thirds are fused with the transverse cervical processes. The upper limit of the MSD in cervical absolute stenosis is also about 10 mm. Of our 199 cases of idiopathic DSBLVC, symptomatic cervical relative stenosis occurred in seven patients; it occurred in the presence of absolute lumbar DSBLVC in three patients, and with relative lumbar stenosis in two patients. In two patients, symptomatic absolute cervical stenosis was associated with lumbar absolute stenosis. Epstein and coworkers[44] discussed the surgical aspects of combined lumbar and cervical spinal stenosis.

There are remarkable differences in the occurrence of idiopathic DSBLVC among the populations of various regions, as far as can be estimated from hospital records. I know of clinics in which idiopathic DSBLVC is rarely observed and other clinics in which it is relatively frequently seen. In our department, the yearly operations performed because of idiopathic absolute DSBLVC (pure absolute and mixed stenoses included) varied between 5% and 8% of all laminectomies performed because of sciatica.

Does the Category of "Acquired Stenoses" Have Value in the Classification of the Stenoses?

Although congenital DSBLVC consequent to inborn errors of skeletal growth and idiopathic DSBLVC rightly deserve the generic name stenosis (stenosis being the primary affliction, even though it may be complicated by other pathologic agents), any acquired stenosis is a property of another pathologic condition and may even be an accidental rather than an essential property of that other pathologic condition.

From a pathomorphologic, clinical, or therapeutic point of view, it makes more sense to consider the acquired stenoses as properties of other types of primary abnormalities or diseases. In the taxonomy of such other diseases, stenosis could function as an adjective, indicating a category that belongs to such taxonomies bearing the generic name of the primary other abnormality or disease involved.

Such a conception could fit the statement of Arnoldi and colleagues that a taxonomy makes sense when it is useful in making an accurate diagnosis and formulating a rational approach to treatment. For instance, although spondylolisthesis may produce stenosis, the rational treatment aims at reduction of the vertebral slip and stabilization. Acquired symptomatic stenosis in such a condition would be relieved by this treatment. However, when Arnoldi and coworkers classify degenerative spondylolisthesis as acquired stenosis, the possibility that it has occurred in a region of DSBLVC is neglected. In nine of my patients with symptomatic degenerative spondylolisthesis, the disorder was accompanied by absolute stenosis at other levels.[128, 130] In some of these patients, the diameter of the vertebral canal was even, relatively, largest or normal at the level of the degenerative spondylolisthesis (Fig. 14). Other authors equally described the combination of degenerative spondylolisthesis with stenotic canals extending over larger areas.[43, 143]

The oversimplified classification of the degenerative spondylolisthesis within the category of acquired stenoses is a "booby trap," because degenerative spondyolisthesis can be reduced by means of spinal instrumentation, which would be only part of the cure, when the spinal surgeon neglects the presence of DSBLVC at other vertebral levels.

In the classification of Arnoldi and colleagues, central and peripheral stenoses are considered to be acquired. Earlier, the reasons were given to explain why replacing the terms lateral stenosis and peripheral stenosis by narrow lateral recess and narrow gutter. Even when the terms central stenosis and peripheral stenosis were accepted, the question of why "central" and "lateral" or "peripheral" are invariably classified as acquired would remain. In achondroplastic and idiopathic DSBLVC, the narrowing of the lateral recesses, gutters, or intervertebral foramina may be developmental through abnormal periosteal apposition of bone upon the pedicles and articular processes.

Most mechanisms of foraminal entrapment of nerve roots have been known for many years. The fundamental discoveries of the various foraminal deformities by Gowers,[59] Forestier,[47] Goldthwait,[57] Hadley,[61] and many others are apparently forgotten. Telescoping articular processes, widening of the joint space with relative forward movement of the superior articular process, degenerative vertebral osteophytic lipping, small shifts of vertebral bodies, nerve roots kinked by pedicles, all of which have been treated for many years by experienced spinal surgeons, are actually welcomed into the new family of the peripheral foraminal or subarticular spinal stenoses as if they were new discoveries.

With the exception of the primary stenoses of the intervertebral foramina in achondroplasia or idiopathic DSBLVC, the taxonomy of the stenoses does not provide the key for the treatment of acquired foraminal deformities, because their causes vary greatly, as do the pathobiomechanical mechanisms involved and the surgical techniques applied.

A new term, "far-out lateral spinal stenosis"[21] is being introduced to indicate spinal nerve compression through extraforaminal osteophytes, in contrast to ligamentous extraforaminal spinal nerve compression. It is not clear from the description whether far-out lateral stenosis occurs in a narrowed tunnel-like structure, compressing the spinal nerve on at least two opposed sides; if not, using the word stenosis would make no sense.

The next division of the acquired stenoses in the classification of Arnoldi and colleagues is the *combined,* defined as "any possible combination of congenital/developmental stenosis, degenerative stenosis, and herniations of the nucleus pulposus."

In my opinion, any combination of congenital or developmental stenosis with additional degenerative changes or disc herniations cannot be included under the heading of acquired stenosis, because the developmental or congenital stenosis is already there; the other deformities are no more than additional compressive agents. According to such a classification, many cases of achondroplastic stenosis would be listed under the heading of combined forms of acquired stenosis because of its very frequent complication by herniated discs.

Spondylolisthesis is another category of the acquired stenosis according to Arnoldi and colleagues. Stenosis in spondylolisthesis is only a possible, not always a present, property. Spondylolisthesis should be the generic name of a classification based upon principles leading to greater understanding of its pathomechanism and optimal methods of treatment. With the exception of degenerative spondylolisthesis (for reasons discussed above), the onset of symptomatic stenosis in this condition is only an accidental surgical indication.

Fluorosis and Paget disease are also listed under the acquired stenoses. In these diseases, there is no answer to the question, regardless of whether the onset of stenosis in these conditions depends on previous diameters of the vertebral canal. In any case, stenosis is just one of the accidental properties of fluorosis or Paget disease.

Post-traumatic late changes are equally classified by Arnoldi and colleagues as acquired stenosis. The term *late changes* is vague. Post-traumatic stenosis is an exceptional condition.[17, 99] In my four cases,[124] absolute stenosis was also found beyond the level of the traumatic vertebral deformity.

The last entity classified as acquired stenosis by Arnoldi and colleagues was called *iatrogenic*. It is a medical custom to apply the term iatrogenic to untoward effects induced by a doctor as a result of erroneous or inadvertent treatment.[109] Therefore a difference should be made between iatrogenic results and surgical complications referring to factors that, independent of the method of treatment, modify the course of the disease and for which the individual occurrence cannot be predicted. The formation of a postlaminectomy membrane producing recurrent stenosis is one such complication. Postfusion stenosis was listed as iatrogenic and has been reported by other authors.[18, 23] I have seen cases of large posterior fusion masses in the presence of large vertebral canals.[128, 130] Postfusion iatrogenic stenosis may occur when bone chips have been placed on an exposed dura or when no measures had been taken to avoid displacement of bone chips to that site. Brodsky[18] reported severe stenosis just above the level of posterior fusion being caused by hypertrophic articular processes, disc herniation, thickening of the ligamentum flavum, and ventral projection of the fusion mass into the vertebral canal. In the region of the posterior fusion itself Brodsky observed no narrowing of the vertebral canal, except some at each level of the articular processes. He did not mention which technique of posterior fusion was performed. The fact that the bony mass could project ventrally into the vertebral canal demonstrates, however, that the fusing bone mass reached beyond the laminae at that site.

Iatrogenic stenosis is a highly improbable condition. Iatrogenic aggravation, as Ehni[31, 33] stressed, is caused by the infliction of surgical damage to caudal nerve roots or is a consequence of insufficient decompression of the stenotic area.

STENOSIS OF THE LUMBAR VERTEBRAL CANAL BY THE LIGAMENTOUS PORTIONS OF ITS WALL

This entity is rare and it is mentioned in this chapter only to complete the pathomorphologic taxonomy of the lumbar stenoses. The condition of hypertrophy and ossification of the posterior longitudinal ligament has long been considered to be a Japanese disease,[85] but there are recent reports of its occurrence in Caucasians.[48, 84] It is most frequently localized in the cervical vertebral canal and less frequently in the thoracic canal, but the lumbar region may be involved as well.[48, 64] The disease may produce symptomatic stenosis of the vertebral canal at all levels involved. In the cervical area, anterior decompressive surgery, which presents no problems at this localization, seems to be followed by better results than does decompressive laminectomy.[48] No such experience is available concerning treatment of the lumbar localization.

At one time, hypertrophy of the ligamentum flavum was thought to be capable of producing symptomatic narrowing of a normal lumbar vertebral canal. Van Gelderen[52] described NICL as being caused by hypertrophic ligamenta flava. This author was of the opinion that, in the erect position, resulting lordosis was accompanied by an inward folding of the hypertrophic ligamenta flava, thus producing compression of the dura. This author did not take into account the diameter of the vertebral canal involved. At the time of the publication of his paper, stenosis of the lumbar vertebral canal had not yet been described. Other authors stressed the influence of hypertrophic ligamenta flava in causing caudal nerve root compression.[105, 111] Spurling and coworkers,[105] who once had supported that theory, modified their opinion in later years when they stated that in the absence of disc herniations the ligamenta flava would not produce signs or symptoms.[14] In our cases of idiopathic DSBLVC, the ligamenta flava were thickened in proportion to the thickened laminae. Because, in most cases, the interlaminar spaces were narrowed as a result of the great height of the laminae or by hypertrophic articular processes, there was little possibility of inward folding of these ligamenta during increased lordosis.

Cystic degeneration of the ligamenta flava was observed in only two cases of idiopathic DSBLVC. These cysts plus irregular thickening of the ligaments produced additional narrowing of the vertebral canal.[121, 122]

In three of our cases of pure relative stenosis, hypertrophic ligamenta flava were discovered during operation, although there were no myelographic features to make possible a diagnosis before the operation. Although the ligamentum flavum may fold into the vertebral canal during lordosis, no data are available about the relation between minimal height of the posterior portion of the ligamentum flavum and the depth of the vertebral canal that result in an intensity of dural compression sufficient to produce signs and symptoms.

AUTHOR'S TAXONOMY OF THE SPINAL STENOSES

It is impossible to develop an all-inclusive binary or ternary taxonomy of the stenoses of the vertebral canal.

The taxonomy of the stenoses of the vertebral canal is based upon the following definitions of nomenclature and principles:

- Stenosis means abnormal narrowing of tubular organs, orifices, or valves.
- Stenosis of the vertebral canal is a form of compressive stenosis involving the entire fixed living content of the vertebral canal. The stenosis is only one of the determinants of stenotic disease; the other determinants reside in the compressed neural content.
- A difference is made between absolute stenosis and relative stenosis. The differential diagnosis is made on the basis of measurements of diameters of the vertebral canal in a transverse plane. In absolute stenosis, there is no reserve capacity inside the vertebral canal. It is a pathologic condition. In relative stenosis, the reserve capacity of the vertebral canal is too small, but in itself does not constitute a pathologic condition.
- Acquired other space-occupying changes into these stenotic vertebral canals or intervertebral foramina are called additional compressive agents.
- Reversal of RMDs occurs with absolute and relative stenoses.
- A distinction is made between areas of pure absolute, mixed, and pure relative stenoses. Discontinuities may occur in the areas of relative stenosis in the latter two groups. I have distinguished relative stenosis as a separate entity, which cannot be ordered in the taxonomy presented above. Relative stenosis is not a pathologic condition, although it may share with pure absolute stenosis a few properties, such as reversed RMDs, the occurrence of discontinuities, the extension to lumbar vertebrae other than L3 and L4 (where the minimal values of MSDs occur much less frequently in collections of skeletal vertebrae than with L3 and L4), and, rarely, the presence of hypertrophy of structures of the vertebral arch. Patients with relative stenosis are called symptomatic stenosis–prone, for reasons explained earlier.
- A distinction can be made between uncomplicated stenosis of the bony vertebral canal and stenosis of the bony vertebral canal complicated by the presence of additional compressive agents arising from the nonbony portions of the vertebral canal.

The basic taxonomy of the types of stenoses of the vertebral canal includes stenoses caused by the bony portions of the vertebral canal and those caused by its ligamentous–cartilaginous portions. My pathomorphologic taxonomy of the stenosis of the lumbar vertebral canal is limited to morphologic changes of the walls of the vertebral canal, for which the essential pathologic mechanism consists of stenotic disease caused by compression of the neural content at two or more pairs of opposed sides. The resulting taxonomy is not nosologic in the proper sense, but a taxonomy of one of the two main determinants of stenotic disease, the taxonomy of the stenosis of the bony portions of the vertebral canal, is as follows:

A. Congenital
B. Developmental
   1. Through inborn errors of skeletal bone growth
   2. Idiopathic developmental stenosis
      a. In the presence of bony hypertrophy of structures of the vertebral arch
      b. In the absence of bony hypertrophy of structures of the vertebral arch (rare)

Each of these taxonomies of spinal stenosis is important, but is so with respect to different purposes. Is it impossible to unite all the taxonomic systems in an all-inclusive taxonomy, and there is no need for that. The various taxonomies of the spinal stenosis have no hierarchic relation to one another. Each patient with spinal stenosis is screened in our practice, as to his or her position within the various taxonomies. This guarantees optimal chances of making the much more inclusive inventorial diagnosis that is more important to avoiding therapeutic errors or to researching aspects of spinal stenosis than an all-inclusive lexical listing of conditions that are sometimes accompanied by stenosis.

ACQUIRED STENOSES HAVE NO PLACE IN A TAXONOMY OF VERTEBRAL STENOTIC DISEASES

Acquired stenosis denotes that the vertebral canal previously had normal diameters. Acquired stenosis is one of the properties of diseases for which the primary mechanisms do other than produce stenotic disease. For those conditions, stenosis should not be used as a generic term in related nosologic taxonomies; instead, the name of the underlying disease should be used. The term acquired stenosis may function as an adjective indicating a species in such taxonomies.

Long-Term Results

The results published in the literature are difficult to evaluate because most authors do not make or report having made measurements. Differing opinions about the definition of stenosis contribute to the incommensurability of results reported. Some authors related the results to the findings at operation,[86, 95, 110] whereas others limited the description of functional results to judgments ranging from "excellent" to "bad." For a statistical evaluation of surgical results, a great number of variables would have to be included, such as preoperative duration of signs and symptoms; types of signs and symptoms (NICL as an only complaint is cured in almost all cases); concomitant vertebral abnormalities, such as protruded discs, osteoporosis, and abnormal curvatures; age of the patient; occupation; differences in surgical techniques applied in avoiding damage to the caudal nerve roots in the narrow canal, decompression made on the basis of measurements or of myelographic findings only, complete decompression of the areas of absolute stenosis or decompression limited to so-called symptomatic areas, differences in methods of associated complete or partial foraminal decompression, and associated spinal fusion and type of fusion. In addition, some spinal surgeons modified details of the surgical procedure in the course of time. Statistical processing of data concerning the many variables involved would require the cooperative study of a large number of cases treated according to standardized indications and surgical procedures. The lack of uniformity in documentation and treatment explains the large differences between the frequencies of good or satisfying surgical results reported in the literature, which vary between 60% and 90%.

Before my later results are mentioned, some information about our decompressive surgical techniques is given. Figures 15 and 16 show details of surgical decompression of absolute stenosis by means of the chisel alone, which I have utilized since the early 1950s because I considered this technique to be the safest in avoiding the production of neural damage. My method of ventral foraminal decompression (see Fig. 15) can now more safely be replaced by a paraspinal approach,[21, 92] first developed by Watkins[138, 139] and then modified by Wiltse

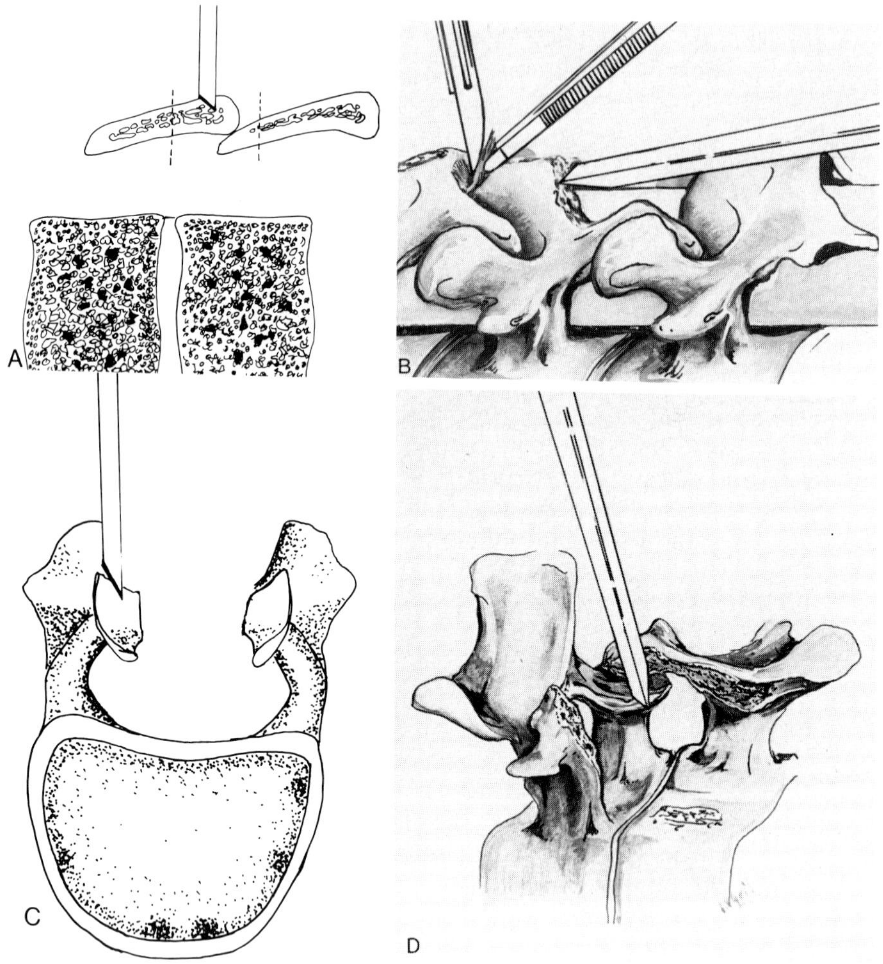

Figure 15 □ The author's decompressive techniques in the surgical treatment of the stenoses by means of chiseling. *A,* Drawing shows, after removal of spinous processes, the position of the beveled surface of the chisel when one is removing portions of laminae over-roofing adjacent laminae. The bevel is reversed for cutting off the underlying portion of the adjacent laminae. *B,* Peeling of layers of hypertrophic laminae is performed with the chisel in a quasiparallel position with the bevel turned downward. With the opposite position of bevel, it may inadvertently penetrate the vertebral canal. *C,* Position of bevel when peeling off medial portions of hypertrophic articular processes. *D,* Removal of the tip of a superior articular process is performed after removal of the medial portion of the overlying inferior articular facet. Next, the tip of the superior facet can be sectioned by careful use of small osteotome or beveled chisel.

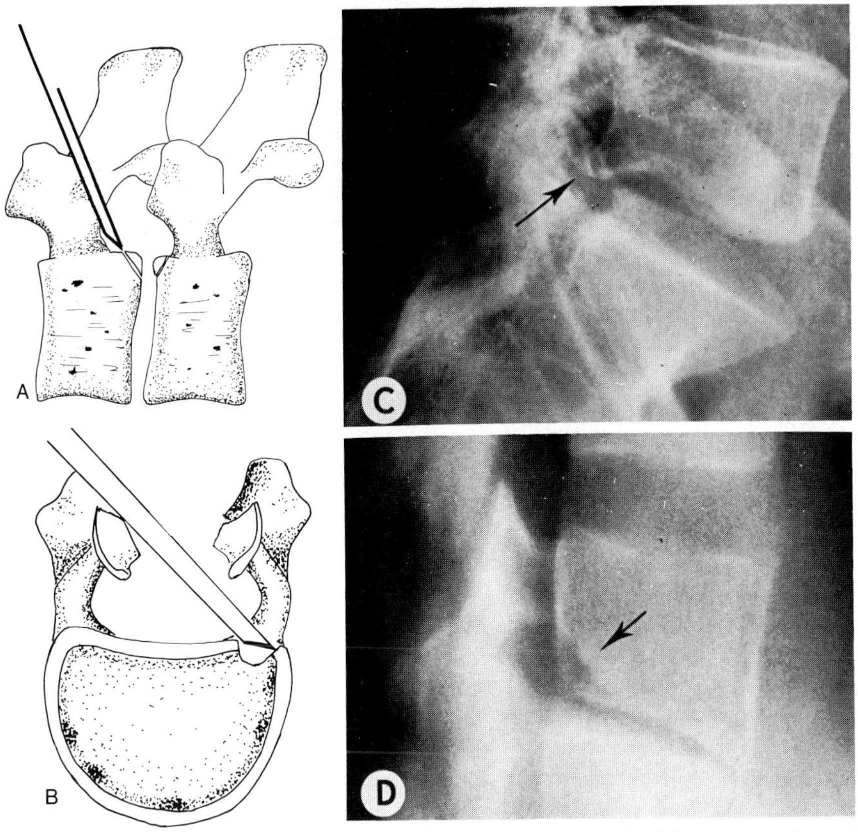

Figure 16 □ In some instances, ventral decompression of a narrowed intervertebral foramen can be achieved by the technique shown in *A* and *B*. *C*, Preoperative profile roentgenograms show posteroinferior rim of the L5 body protruding into the intervertebral foramen at L5 S1. *D*, Postoperative lateral hypocycloidal tomogram shows that this protruding rim has been removed.

Figure 17 □ In symptomatic relative stenosis, the removal of the inferior portion of the laminae, over-roofing the additional compressive agent at disc level, results in sufficient decompression. Arrow points to plane of resection of caudal portion of the laminae.

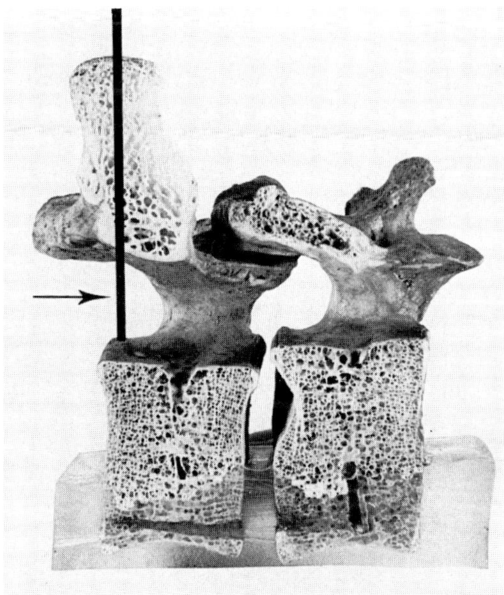

and coworkers.[144, 145] It allows foraminal decompression by means of partial removal of the facets or pedicles, or removal of far-out disc herniations, osteophytes, or protruding rims of vertebral bodies. Knowledge of the many blood vessels in this area is necessary,[24] specifically concerning feeders of the spinal cord or caudal nerve roots.

In the years following laminectomy, limited regrowth of the laminae may be observed. In only one of our patients, operated on in 1948, the laminae had been entirely remodeled, as was seen 30 years later in x-ray studies because the patient complained of backaches.

I have mentioned the reasons why areas of absolute stenosis were completely decompressed, whereas in relative stenosis only the caudal halves of the laminae in the symptomatic area were removed (Fig. 17). During decompression of areas of mixed or of pure relative stenosis I do not prophylactically decompress regions of relative stenosis that are not complicated by any protrusion. I have had experience with only two patients in whom such areas became symptomatic in later years because of ridge formation. Details of other postoperative complications have been reported elsewhere, and they fall outside the scope of a description of late postoperative results. Of 147 patients operated on between 1948 and 1976,[123] the area of stenosis had not been measured or measurement was incomplete in 31 patients because of the risk of damaging caudal nerve roots. The preoperative distribution of signs and symptoms of the 116 patients whose area of stenosis could be completely measured are presented in Table 3 for each of the three types of stenosis. Table 3 shows that NICL as a single symptom occurred only in patients with pure absolute and mixed (absolute plus relative) stenoses and not in those with symptomatic pure relative stenosis.

For those with relative stenosis, the frequency of NICL accompanied by other neural disturbances was also lower than in the other two groups, whereas lumbago and sciatic neuralgia were more frequent with the symptomatic pure relative stenosis.

Of the 116 patients, 25 had disappeared from sight; however, the condition of 92 of the patients could be checked in 1976. Sixty-two percent were free from signs and symptoms of stenosis with postoperative periods of 1 to 2 years in 10 patients, 3 to 7 years in 24 patients, and 7 to 20 years in 28 patients.

Based on the distinction in types of areas of stenosis established earlier, complete recovery was noted in 75% of patients with pure absolute stenosis, in 66% of those with mixed stenosis, and in 50% of those with pure relative stenosis. The difference in results among the three groups is in accordance with the fact that relative stenosis becomes symptomatic stenosis by the evolution of a secondary disease, usually consisting of degenerative spinal disease. Four of 62 cured patients had to be operated on for cervical myelopathy, and one patient for vascular intermittent claudication. Five patients had developed other diseases: mental disturbances (three), Parkinson disease (one) and lung cancer (one).

Of the 30 patients who did not recover or who only partially recovered after surgical decompression, the oldest patient operated on at the age of 85 years, died 4 years later from general asthenia and arteriosclerosis. Two patients developed other diseases: Huntington chorea (one) and amyotrophic lateral sclerosis (one).

Table 4 shows that lumbago is the most frequent residual complaint, by ascending order of types of stenoses from pure absolute

Table 3 □ Preoperative Distribution of Signs and Symptoms

PREOPERATIVE DISTURBANCES	TYPES OF STENOSIS (116 CASES)		
	Pure Absolute (49 cases)	Mixed (35 cases)	Pure Relative (32 cases)
NICL Only	12%	11%	—
NICL and Other Symptoms	67%	74%	56%
Lumbago	67%	69%	78%
Sciatica	10%	11%	47%
Sciatica and Radicular Motor Deficit	57%	49%	47%
Painless Radicular Motor Deficit	20%	29%	—

Table 4 □ Frequencies of Residual Disturbances by Type of Stenosis

RESIDUAL DISTURBANCES	TYPES OF STENOSIS (92 CASES) Pure Absolute (39 cases)	Mixed (27 cases)	Pure Relative (26 cases)
Lumbago	13% (64%)	22% (70%)	27% (77%)
Motor deficit	10% (72%)	19% (78%)	8% (46%)
NICL	3% (87%)	4% (100%)	8% (38%)
Sciatic neuralgia	— (10%)	— (22%)	4% (46%)
Postoperative motor deficit	1 case	1 case	—

In parentheses are percentages of the particular signs and symptoms before operation.

to mixed to pure relative, as an expression of degenerative spinal disease contributing to the manifestation of symptomatic relative stenosis. Poorer results, when degenerative spinal disease had been one of the determinants in producing symptomatic stenosis, was also reported by Getty.[54] The few residual complaints of NICL were all the consequence of insufficient decompression of intervertebral foramina.

Residual motor deficit in the group of the pure relative stenosis was related in all patients to preoperative acute and complete paralysis of the feet, caused by acute massive extrusion of sequestered disc material. Iatrogenic motor deficit was observed in one case of pure absolute and in one case of mixed stenosis.

Acknowledgments

The author is very much obliged to Frans W. Zonneveld, Ph.D., member of the scientific staff of the Department of Diagnostic Radiology, Utrecht University Hospital, and Senior Scientist in CT Applications, Philips Medical Systems, for his skillful 3-D reconstructions from CT images of the stenotic spinal canal, illustrated in Figures 7, 8, and 9.

References

1. Alexander, E.: Significance of the small lumbar canal: Cauda equina compression syndromes due to spondylosis. Part 5: Achondroplasia. J. Neurosurg. 31:513–519, 1969.
2. Armstrong, H.R.: Lumbar Disc Lesions. London, Churchill Livingstone, 1952, p. 18.
3. Arnoldi, C.C., Brodsky, A.E., Cauchoix, J., et al.: Lumbar spinal stenosis and nerve root entrapment syndromes: Definition and classification. Clin. Orthop. Rel. Res. 115:4–5, 1976.
4. Assmann, H., Besel, R.: Aussergewohnlicher Verlauf bei einer Knochernen Stenose des thorakalen Spinalkanals. Zentralbl. Chir. 107:867–872, 1982.
5. Babin, E.: Radiology of the narrow lumbar canal. *In* Wackenheim, A., and Babin, E.: The Narrow Lumbar Canal. New York, Springer-Verlag, 1980.
6. Bailey, J.A.: Orthopaedic aspects of achondroplasia. J. Bone Joint Surg. 52A:1295–1301, 1970.
7. Bailey, P., and Casamajor, L.: Osteoarthritis of the spine as a cause of compression of the spinal cord and its roots. J. Nerv. Ment. Dis. 38:588–609, 1911.
8. Barnett, G.H., Hardy, R.W., Little, J.R., et al.: Thoracic spinal stenosis. J. Neurosurg. 66:338–344, 1987.
9. Beers, G.J., Carter, A.P., Leiter, B.E., et al.: Interobserver discrepancies in distance measurements from lumbar spine CT scans. A.J.R. 144:395–398, 1985.
10. Bergstrom, K., Laurent, U., and Lundberg, P.O.: Neurological symptoms in achondroplasia. Acta Neurol. Scand. 47:59–70, 1971.
11. Blau, J.N., and Logue, V.: Intermittent claudication of the cauda equina. An unusual syndrome resulting from central protrusion of a lumbar intervertebral disc. Lancet 1:1082–1086, 1961.
12. Blau, J.N., and Rushworth, G.: Observations on the blood vessels of the spinal cord and their responses to motor activity. Brain 81:354–363, 1958.
13. Boerman, C.J.: Carolus Linnaeus. Thesis, Utrecht University. Utrecht, Pressa Trajectina, 1953.
14. Bradford, F.K., and Spurling, R.G.: The Intervertebral Disc, 2nd Ed. Springfield, Charles C Thomas, 1945, pp.83–84.
15. Brailsford, J.F.: Chondro-osteo-dystrophy. Am. J. Surg. N.S. 7:404–410, 1929.
16. Brailsford, J.F.: Chondro-osteo-dystrophy. J. Bone Joint Surg. 34B:53–63, 1952.
17. Brish, A., Lerner, M.A., and Braham, J.: Intermittent claudication from compression of the cauda equina by a narrowed spinal canal. J. Neurosurg. 21:207–214, 1964.
18. Brodsky, A.E.: Post-laminectomy and post-fusion stenosis of the lumbar spine. Clin. Orthop. Rel. Res. 115:130–139, 1976.
19. Bronowski, J.: The Common Sense of Science. New York, Vintage Books of Random House, 1978.
20. Burton, Ch.V.: The spinal column: A modern tower of Babel. *In* Watkins, R.G., and Collis, J.S. (eds.): Lumbar Discectomy and Laminectomy. Rockville, Maryland, Aspen Publishers, 1987, pp. 189–193.
21. Burton, Ch. V.: On the diagnosis and surgical treatment of lumbar subarticular and "far out" lateral spinal stenosis. *In* Watkins, R.G., and Collis, J.S.: Lumbar Discectomy and Laminectomy. Rockville, Maryland, Aspen Publishers, 1987, pp. 195–202.

22. Caffey, J.: Achondroplasia of pelvis and lumbosacral spine. Some roentgenographic features. A.J.R. 80:449–457, 1958.
23. Cauchoix, J., Taussig, G., and Nordin, J.Y.: Sciatique et syndrome de la queue de cheval par retrecissement du canal rachidien apres arthrodese lombo-sacree posterieure. Semaine Hopit. Paris 45:2023–2025, 1969.
24. Crock, H.V., and Yoshizawa, H.: The blood supply of the vertebral column and spinal cord in man. New York, Springer-Verlag, 1977.
25. Cruveilhier, J.: Traite d'Anatomie Pathologique Generale, Vol. 2. Paris, Bailliere, 1852, pp. 209–884.
26. Domisse, G.F.: Morphological aspects of the lumbar spine and lumbo-sacral region. Orthop. Clin. North Am. 6:163–175, 1975.
27. Donath, J., and Vogl, A.: Untersuchungen uber den chondrodystropischen Zwergwuchs. Das Verhalten der Wirbelsaule beim achondroplastischen Zwerg. Wiener Arch. Inn. Med. 10:1–44, 1925.
28. Duvoisin, R.C., and Yahr, M.D.: Compressive spinal cord and root syndromes in achondroplastic dwarfs. Neurology 12:202–207, 1962.
29. Ehni, G.: Spondylotic cauda equina radiculopathy. Texas J. Med. 61:746–752, 1965.
30. Ehni, G.: Significance of the small lumbar spinal canal. Cauda equina compression syndromes due to spondylosis. J. Neurosurg. 31:490–494, 1969.
31. Ehni, G.: Significance of the small lumbar spinal canal: Cauda equina compression syndromes due to spondylosis. Acute compression artificially induced during operation. J. Neurosurg. 31:507–512, 1969.
32. Ehni, G.: The redundant or knotted nerve root. A clue to spondylotic cauda equina radiculopathy. J. Neurosurg. 32:252–254, 1970.
33. Ehni, G.: Surgical treatment of spondylotic caudal radiculopathy. *In* Weinstein, Ph.R., Ehni, G., and Wilson, Ch. B. (eds.): Lumbar Spondylosis. Chicago, Year Book Medical Publishers, 1977, pp. 146–183.
34. Eisenstein, S.M.: The morphometry and pathological anatomy of the lumbar spine in South African Negroes and Caucasoids with special reference to spinal stenosis. J. Bone Joint Surg. 59B:173–180, 1977.
35. Eisenstein, S.M.: The trefoil configuration of the lumbar vertebral canal. J. Bone Joint Surg. 62B:73–77, 1980.
36. Eisenstein, S.M.: Lumbar vertebral canal morphometry for computerized tomography in spinal stenosis. Spine 8:187–191, 1983.
37. Elsberg, C.A., and Dyke, C.G.: The diagnosis and localization of tumors of the spinal cord by means of measurements made in x-ray films of the vertebrae, and the correlation of the clinical and x-ray findings. Bull. Neurol. Inst. New York 3:359–394, 1934.
38. Epstein, J.A., and Malis, L.I.: Compression of spinal cord and cauda equina in achondroplastic dwarfs. Neurology 5:875–881, 1955.
39. Epstein, J.A.: Diagnosis and treatment of neurological disorders caused by spondylosis of the lumbar spine. J. Neurosurg. 17:991–1001, 1960.
40. Epstein, J.A., Epstein, B.S., and Lavine, L.S.: Nerve root compression associated with narrowing of the lumbar spinal canal. J. Neurol. Neurosurg. Psychiatr. 25:165–176, 1962.
41. Epstein, J.A., Epstein, B.S., Rosenthal, R.C., and Lavine, S.L.: Sciatica caused by nerve root entrapment in the lateral recess: The superior facet syndrome. J. Neurosurg. 36:584–589, 1972.
42. Epstein, N., Whelan, M., and Benjamin, V.: Acromegaly and spinal stenosis. J. Neurosurg. 56:145–147, 1982.
43. Epstein, N.E., Epstein, J.A., Carras, R. and Lavine, L.S.: Degenerative spondylolisthesis with an intact neural arch: A review of 60 cases with an analysis of clinical findings and the development of surgical management. Neurosurgery 13:555–561, 1983.
44. Epstein, N.E., Epstein, J.A., Carras, R., et al.: Coexisting cervical and lumbar spinal stenosis: Diagnosis and management. Neurosurgery 15:489–495, 1984.
45. Evans, J.G.: Neurogenic intermittent claudication. Br. Med. J. 2:985–987, 1964.
46. Feinstein, A.R.: Clinical Judgment. Baltimore, Williams & Wilkins, 1967.
47. Forestier, J.: Le Trou de Conjugaison Vertebral et l'Espace Epidural. Paris, Jouve et Cie, 1922.
48. Firooznia, H., Benjamin, V.M., Pinto, R.S., et al.: Calcification and ossification of posterior longitudinal ligament of spine: Its role in secondary narrowing of spinal canal and cord compression. New York State J. Med. 82:1193–1198, 1982.
49. Freund, E.: Spastic paraplegia in achondroplasia. Arch. Surg. 27:859–867, 1933.
50. Friedman, E.: Narrowing of the spinal canal due to thickening of the laminae, a cause of low back pain and sciatica. Clin. Ortho. Rel. Res. 21:190–197, 1961.
51. Garde, A., and Mansuy, L.: Compression de la queue de cheval par hernie discale au cours d'une achondroplasie. Rev. Neurol. 97:371–375, 1957.
52. Gelderen, Chr., van: Ein orthotisches (lordotisches) Kaudasyndrom. Acta Psychiatr. (Kbh.) 23:57–68, 1948.
53. Gelman, M.I.: Cauda equina compression in acromegaly. Radiology 112:357–360, 1974.
54. Getty, C.J.M.: Lumbar spinal stenosis. The clinical spectrum and results of operation. J. Bone Joint Surg. 62B:481–485, 1980.
55. Gilliatt, R.W., and Wilson, T.G.: A pneumatic tourniquet test in the carpal tunnel syndrome. Lancet 2:595–597, 1953.
56. Gilliatt, R.W., and Wilson, T.G.: Ischemic sensory loss in patients with peripheral nerve lesions. J. Neurol. Neurosurg. Psychiatr. 17:104–114, 1954.
57. Goldthwait, J.E.: The lumbo-sacral articulation. An explanation of many cases of "Lumbago," "Sciatica" and Paraplegia. Boston Med. Surg. J. 164:365–372, 1911.
58. Govoni, A.F.: Developmental stenosis of thoracic vertebra resulting in narrowing of the spinal canal. A. J. R. 112:401–404, 1971.
59. Gowers, W.R.: A Manual of Diseases of the Nervous System, 2nd Ed., Vol. I. Diseases of the Spinal Cord and Nerves. London, Churchill, 1893, pp. 263–264.
60. Grossiord, A., Guiot, G., Held, J.P., et al.: Lesions medullaires dans l'achondroplasie; role des anomalies vertebrales. Rev. Neurol. 94:329–334, 1956.
61. Hadley, M.D.: Anatomico-Roentgenographic Studies of the Spine. Springfield, Charles C Thomas, 1964, pp. 422–477.
62. Hanai, K., Inouye, Y., Kawai, K., et al.: Anterior

decompression for myelopathy resulting from ossification of the posterior longitudinal ligament. J. Bone Joint Surg. 64B:561–564, 1982.
63. Hancock, D.O., and Phillips, D.G.: Spinal compression in achondroplasia. Paraplegia 3:23–33, 1965.
64. Hasue, M., Kikuchi, S., Sakuyama, Y., and Ito, T.: Anatomic study of the interrelation between lumbosacral nerve roots and their surrounding tissues. Spine 8:50–58, 1983.
65. Huizinga, J., Heiden, J.A., van der, Vinken, P.J.J.G.: The human vertebral canal: A biometric study. Proc. R. Neth. Acad. Sci. C55:22–33, 1952.
66. Kirkaldy-Willis, W.H., and McIvor, G.W.D.: Lumbar spinal stenosis (editorial). Clin. Orthop. Rel. Res. 115:2–3, 1976.
67. Kissel, P., Harteman, P., Barrucaud, D., and Montant, J.: Compression medullaire et achondroplasie. Rev. Neurol. 109:489–498, 1963.
68. Kraus, L.A.: Kritisch-etymologisches medicinisches Lexicon. Gottingen, Deuerlich und Dietrich, 1844.
69. Landais, N.: Dictionnaire general et grammatical des dictionnaires français. Paris, 1834.
70. Larsen, J.L., and Smith, D.: Vertebral body size in lumbar spinal canal stenosis. Acta Radiol. (Diagn.) 21:785–788, 1980.
71. Lieutaud, J.: Anatomie Historique et Pratique. Nouvelle Edition Augmentee de Diverses Remarques Historiques et Critiques et de Nouvelles Planches par M. Portal. Paris, Didot Jeune, 1776–1777.
72. Lindemann, K., and Kuhlendahl, H.: Die Erkrankungen der Wirbelsaule, Stuttgart, Enke, 1953, p. 115.
73. Littré, E.: Dictionnaire de Medecine. Paris, Bailliere, et Fils, 1884.
74. Lobrecht, S., and Kleine Schaars, H.W.G.: Three dimensional imaging and manipulation of CT data. Part I: General principles. Med. Mundi 32:92–98, 1987.
75. Lutter, L.D., and Langer, I.O.: Neurological symptoms in achondroplastic dwarfs. Surgical treatment. J. Bone Joint Surg. 59A:87–92, 1977.
76. Maroteaux, P.: Maladies Osseuses de l'Enfant. Paris, Flammarion, 1974.
77. Marzluff, J.M., Hungerford, G.D., Kempe, L.G., et al.: Thoracic myelopathy caused by osteophytes of the articular processes. Thoracic spondylosis. J. Neurosurg. 50:779–783, 1979.
78. Megret, M., and Marsault, C.: Gas myelography in Verbiest's developmental spinal canal stenosis. *In* Wackenheim, A., and Babin, A. (eds.): The Narrow Lumbar Canal. New York, Springer-Verlag, 1980.
79. Modic, M.T., Masaryk, Th., Boumphrey, F., et al.: Lumbar herniated disc disease and canal stenosis. Prospective evaluation by surface coil MR, CT, and myelography. A.J.R. 147:757–766, 1986.
80. Morgan, D.F., and Young, R.F.: Spinal neurological complications of achondroplasia. Results of surgical treatment. J. Neurosurg. 52:463–472, 1980.
81. Morquio, L.: Sur une forme de dystrophie osseuse familiale. Arch. Med. Infant. 32:129–140, 1929.
82. Morquio, L.: Sur une forme de dystrophie osseuse familiale. Arch. Med. Infant. 38:5–24, 1935.
83. Munro, D.: Lumbar and sacral compression radiculitis (herniated disk syndrome). N. Engl. J. Med. 254:243–252, 1956.
84. Nater, B., Regli, F., Schnyder, P., and De Tribolet, N.: Myelopathie cervicale par ossification du ligament longitudinal posterieur. Rev. Neurol. 142:771–776, 1986.
85. Ono, K., Ota, H., Tada, K., et al.: Ossified posterior longitudinal ligament. A clinical pathological study. Spine 2:126–138, 1977.
86. Paine, K.W.A.: Results of decompression for lumbar stenosis. Clin. Orthop. Rel. Res. 115:96–100, 1976.
87. Parker, H.L., Adson, A.W.: Compression of the spinal cord and its roots by hypertrophic arthritis. Surg. Gynecol. Obstet. 41:1–14, 1925.
88. Portal, A.: Cours d'Anatomie Medicale ou Elemens de l'Anatomie de l'Homme, Vol. I. Paris, Baudoin, 1803, p. 299.
89. Postacchini, F., Ripani, M., and Carpano, S.: Morphometry of the lumbar vertebrae. Clin. Orthop. Rel. Res. 172:296–303, 1983.
90. Prosch, H., and Ploss, H.: Medicinische-chirurgische encyclopedie fur praktische aertze. Leipzig, Brockhaus, 1856.
91. Ravenna, F.: Achondroplasie et chondrohypoplasie. Contribution clinique. Nouv. Icon. Salpetriere 26:157–184, 1913.
92. Ray, Ch.D.: The paralateral approach to decompressions for lateral stenosis and far lateral lesions of the lumbar spine. *In* Watkins, R.G., and Collis, J.S.: Lumbar Discectomy and Laminectomy. Rockville, Maryland, Aspen Publishers, 1987, pp. 217–227.
93. Robins, R.H.: A Short History of Linguistics, 3rd Ed. London, Longman, 1976.
94. Rush, D.W.H., Dieffenbach, J.F., Hecker, J.F.C., et al.: Encyclopadisches Worterbuch der medicinischen Wissenschaften. Berlin, Verlag von Veil et Comp, 1846.
95. Russin, L.A., and Sheldon, J.: Spinal stenosis. Clin. Orthop. Rel. Res. 115:101–103, 1976.
96. Sachs, B., and Fraenkel, J.: Progressive ankylotic rigidity of the spine (spondylose rhizomelique). J. Nerv. Ment. Dis. 27:1–15, 1900.
97. Sarpyener, M.A.: Congenital stricture of the spinal canal. J. Bone Joint Surg. 27:70–79, 1945.
98. Sarpyener, M.A.: Spina bifida aperta and congenital stricture of the spinal canal. J. Bone Joint Surg. 29:817–821, 1947.
99. Schatzker, J., and Pennal, F.: Spinal stenosis, a cause of cauda equina compression. J. Bone Joint Surg. 50B:606–618, 1968.
100. Schlesinger, P.T.: Incarceration of the first sacral nerve in a lateral bony recess of the spinal canal. J. Bone Joint Surg. 37A:115–124, 1955.
101. Schreiber, F., and Rosenthal, H.: Paraplegia from ruptured discs in achondroplastic dwarfs. J. Neurosurg. 9:648–651, 1952.
102. Schut, L., and Groff, R.A.: Redundant nerve roots as a cause of complete myelographic block. J. Neurosurg. 28:394–395, 1968.
103. Silverman, F.N., and Brunner, S.: Errors in the diagnosis of achondroplasia. Acta Radiol. (Diagn.) 6:305–321, 1967.
104. Spillane, J.D.: Three cases of achondroplasia with neurological complications. J. Neurol. Neurosurg. Psychiatr. 15:246–252, 1952.
105. Spurling, R.G., Mayfield, F.H., and Rogers, J.B.: Hypertrophy of the ligamenta flava as a cause of low back pain. J.A.M.A. 109:928–933, 1937.
106. Sumita, M.: Beitrage zur Lehre von der Chondro-

dystrophia foetalis (Kaufmann) und Osteogenesis imperfecta (Vrolik) mit besonderer Berucksichtigung der anatomischen und klinischen Differential Diagnose. Deutsche Z. Chir. 107:1–110, 1910.
107. Testut, L.: Traite d'Anatomie Humaine, 5th Ed., Vol. 1. Paris, Doin, 1904, pp. 62–63.
108. Thomeer, R.T.W.M.: Achondroplasia, Management of Neurological Complications. Thesis, Leiden. Oegstgeest, De Kempenaer, 1982.
109. Thomson, W.A.R.: A Dictionary of Medical Ethics and Practice. Bristol, John Wright, 1977.
110. Tile, M., McNeil, S.R., Zarins, R.K., et al.: Spinal stenosis. Results of treatment. Clin. Orthop. Rel. Res. 115:104–108, 1976.
111. Towne, E.B., and Reichert, F.L.: Compression of the lumbosacral roots of the spinal cord by thickened ligamenta flava. Ann. Surg. 94:327–336, 1931.
112. Udupa, J.K.: Display of 3D information in discrete 3D scenes production by computerized tomography. Proc. I.E.E.E. 71:420–431, 1983.
113. Verbiest, H.: Sur certaines formes rares de compression de la queue de cheval. I. Les sténoses osseuses du canal vertébral. *In* Hommage à Clovis Vincent. Paris, Maloine, 1949.
114. Verbiest, H.: Primaire stenose van het lumbale wervelkanaal bij volwassenen. Een nieuw ziektebeeld. Nederlands Tijdschrift voor Geneeskunde. 94:2415–2433, 1950.
115. Verbiest, H.: Unusual Compression of the Cauda Equina. Report of Two Cases of Lumbosacral Extradural Cysts and of One Case of "Knotting" of Caudal Nerve Root. Valencia. Libro de communicaciones of the combined meeting of the Luso-Spanish Neurosurgical Society and the British Society of Neurological Surgeons. Madrid, April 26, 1951. 1953, pp. 5–14.
116. Verbiest, H.: A radicular syndrome from developmental narrowing of the lumbar vertebral canal. J. Bone Joint Surg. 36B:230–237, 1954.
117. Verbiest, H.: Further experiences on the pathological influence of a developmental narrowness of the bony lumbar vertebral canal. J. Bone Joint Surg. 37B:576–583, 1955.
118. Verbiest, H.: La chirurgie anterieure et laterale du rachis cervical. Neurochirurgie 16 (Suppl.) 2:1–212, 1970.
119. Verbiest, H.: Neurogenic intermittent claudication in cases with absolute and relative stenosis of the lumbar vertebral canal, (ASLC and RSLC), in cases with narrow lumbar intervertebral foramina and in cases with both entities. Clin. Neurosurg. 20:204–214, 1973.
120. Verbiest, H.: Pathomorphologic aspects of developmental lumbar stenosis. Orthop. Clin. North Am. 6:177–196, 1975.
121. Verbiest, H.: Neurogenic intermittent claudication. Lesions of the spinal cord and cauda equina, stenosis of the vertebral canal, narrowing of intervertebral foramina and entrapment of peripheral nerves. *In* Vinken, P.J., and Bruyn, G.W. (eds.): Handbook of Clinical Neurology, 20, Part II. New York, North Holland/American Elsevier, 1976, pp. 611–807.
122. Verbiest, H.: Neurogenic intermittent claudication. With special reference to stenosis of the lumbar vertebral canal. New York, North Holland/American Elsevier, 1976.
123. Verbiest, H.: Results of surgical treatment of idiopathic developmental stenosis of the lumbar vertebral canal. A review of twenty-seven years' experience. J. Bone Joint Surg. 59B:181–188, 1977.
124. Verbiest, H.: Fallacies of the present definition, nomenclature and classification of the stenoses of the lumbar vertebral canal. Spine 1:217–225, 1976.
125. Verbiest, H.: The significance and principles of computerized axial tomography in idiopathic developmental stenosis of the bony lumbar vertebral canal. Spine 4:369–378, 1979.
126. Verbiest, H.: The value of CT of the spine to the neurosurgeon. *In* Post, M.J.D. (ed.): Radiographic Evaluation of the Spine. New York, Masson, 1980.
127. Verbiest, H.: Stenosis of the lumbar vertebral canal and sciatica. Neurosurg. Rev. 3:75–89, 1980.
128. Verbiest, H.: Stenosis of the bony lumbar vertebral canal. *In* Wackenheim, A., and Babin, E. (eds.): The Narrow Lumbar Canal. New York, Springer-Verlag, 1980, pp. 231–270.
129. Verbiest, H.: Introduction. In Hopp (ed.): Spinal Stenosis: State of the Art Review, Vol. 1. Philadelphia, Hanley and Belfus, 1987, pp. 361–367.
130. Verbiest, H.: Lumbar spine stenosis. *In* Youmans, J.R. (ed.): Neurological Surgery, Vol. 6. Philadelphia, W.B. Saunders (in press).
131. Virchov, R.: Gesammelte Abhandelungen. Frankfurt, Meidinger und Sohn, 1856.
132. Virchov, R.: Knochenwachstum und Schaldelformen mit besonderer Rucksicht auf Cretinismus. Virch. Arch. 13:323–357, 1858.
133. Vogl, A., and Osborne, R.I.: Lesions of the spinal cord (transverse myelopathy) in achondroplasia. Arch. Neurol. Psychiatr. 61:644–662, 1949.
134. Wackenheim, A.: Cheirolumbar dysostosis: Developmental brachycheiry and narrowness of the lumbar canal. *In* Wackenheim, A., and Babin, E.: The Narrow Lumbar Canal. New York, Springer-Verlag, 1980, pp. 147–155.
135. Wackenheim, A.: Cheirolumbar Dysostosis. New York, Springer-Verlag, 1980.
136. Wackenheim, A.: A transitional form of cheirolumbar dysostosis. J. Belge Radiol. 64:179–188, 1981.
137. Wackenheim, A.: Cheirolumbar dysostosis. Eur. J. Radiol. 1:189–194, 1981.
138. Watkins, M.B.: Posterolateral fusion of the lumbar and lumbosacral spine. J. Bone Joint Surg. 35A:1014–1018, 1953.
139. Watkins, M.B.: Posterolateral fusion of pseudarthrosis and posterior elements defects of the lumbosacral spine. Clin. Orthop. Rel. Res. 35:80–85, 1964.
140. Wehrli, F.W.: Fast-scan imaging: Principles and contrast phenomenology. *In* Higgins, C.B., and Hricak, H. (eds.): Magnetic Resonance Imaging of the Body. New York, Raven Press, 1987, pp. 23–31.
141. Weinstein, P.R., Ehni, G., and Wilson, Ch.B.: Lumbar Spondylosis: Diagnosis, Management and Treatment. Chicago, Year Book Medical Publishers, 1977.
142. Williams, P.C.: The Lumbosacral Spine. New York, McGraw-Hill, Blakiston division, 1965, pp. 153–157.
143. Wilson, C.B., Ehni, G., and Grollmus, J.: Neuro-

genic intermittent claudication. Clin. Neurosurg. 18:62–82, 1971.
144. Wiltse, L.L., Bateman, J.G., Hutchingson, R.H., and Nelson, W.E.: Paraspinal muscle approach to the lumbar spine. J. Bone Joint Surg. 50A:919–926, 1968.
145. Wiltse, L.L.: The intervertebral foramen. *In* Watkins, R.G., and Collis, J.S.: Lumbar Discectomy and Laminectomy. Rockville, Maryland, Aspen Publishers, 1987, pp. 203–216.
146. Yamada, H., Nakamura, S., Tajami, M., and Kageyama, N.: Neurological manifestations of pediatric achondroplasia. J. Neurosurg. 54:49–57, 1981.
147. Zonneveld, F.W., Meulen, J.C., van der, Akkerveeken, P.F., van, et al.: Three-dimensional imaging and manipulation of CT data. Part II: Clinical applications in orthopaedic and craniofacial surgery. Med. Mundi. 32:99–110, 1987.

DEVELOPMENT OF THE VERTEBRAL CANAL

Richard Porter

CLINICAL RELEVANCE OF THE VERTEBRAL CANAL

There is no doubt about the clinical relevance of a shallow vertebral canal. Following the early papers of Sarpyener,[1] Verbiest,[2] and Van Gelderen,[3] others confirmed that a variety of back pain syndromes are related to spinal pathologic conditions in the presence of an already-small canal.[4–9] Edward and La Rocca[10] showed that 71% of patients with back pain and degenerative change have sagittal diameters below the mean. Kornberg and Rechtine[11] demonstrated an inverse relationship between the vertebral canal size and the morbidity of disc protrusion. Forsberg and Walloe[12] reported that patients who made a poor recovery from disc surgery had canals that were narrower than those of patients who recovered uneventfully.

The size and shape of the vertebral canal have long been neglected factors of back pain, but we now know that a disc prolapse into a restricted space can produce more troublesome symptoms than a protrusion into a wider canal. The trefoil shape is particularly troublesome in the presence of a posterolateral disc protrusion. A far-lateral disc protruding into the root canal, of course, quickly involves the root, irrespective of the size and shape of the central canal (Fig. 1).

In the presence of segmental instability, an adequate canal may ensure that the neural contents are not compromised, but stenotic symptoms can arise with segmental deformation if the canal is small.[13] The vertebral canal is undoubtedly a risk factor in many back pain syndromes.

MULTIFACTORIAL ASPECTS OF BACK PAIN SYNDROMES

There is no single cause of back pain, but each of the syndromes has a multifactorial set of causes. The vertebral canal cannot be described as a cause of back pain, although it is a risk factor and often one of a constellation of factors responsible for the development of symptoms. For example, in symptomatic disc protrusion, we tend to concentrate our attention on the protrusion or sequestration, because this is generally the acute episode that precipitates symptoms. However, in the pathogenesis of the condition we consider the strength of the annulus, which is influenced by familial and occupational factors. Age, sex, and diurnal changes have significance, along with the effects of fatigue and occupational insult, resulting in annular damage. The relative strength of the bone and disc determines whether it is the end plate or the annulus that fails. The integrity of the musculoligamentous complex, muscular strength, and efficient reflex activity also play a part. Biochemical factors and individual differences in the pain mechanism may be important. Constitutional variation occurs in the nerve roots, with variable tethering by dural ligaments[14] and the anomalous roots,[15] which are more readily affected by disc protrusion than is a freely mobile root.

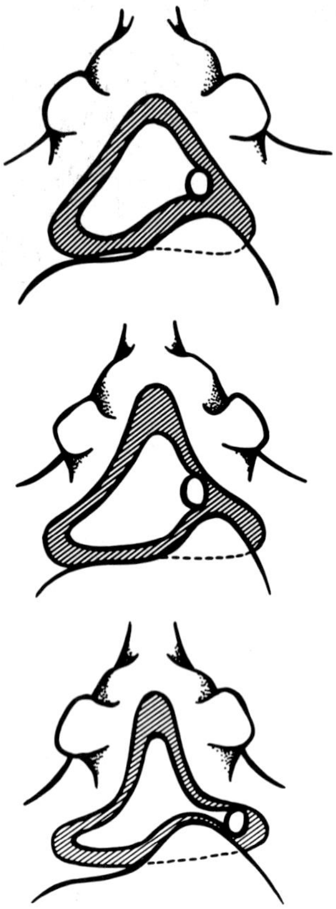

Figure 1 □ Diagram shows that a disc protrusion into a triangular shaped canal merely displaces a mobile root, whereas an equal-size protrusion onto a trefoil-shaped canal can quickly compromise the root.

The space within the bony canal available to the nerve root when compromised by a disc is also an important factor—but, of course, it is only a risk factor. The balance of these factors produces the syndrome.

RELATIVE IMPORTANCE OF THE BONY AND SOFT TISSUE COMPONENT OF THE VERTEBRAL CANAL

The intersegmental region of the vertebral canal is the most important area in which pathologic changes affect the cauda equina and nerve roots. The anterior boundary of the canal indents the dura at disc level in the older patient. The chronically affected disc tends to bulge into the canal, sandwiched between two prominent vertebral bars of the vertebrae above and below. Posteriorly, the attachment of the ligamentum flavum to the cranial end of the lamina also indents the canal. In addition, the thickened capsule around the apophyseal joint can compromise the contents of the canal at the same level. Thus, the soft tissue constitutes the important boundaries of the canal at the intersegmental level. However, that is not to diminish the importance of the bony boundaries of the canal. An individual who has a stenotic bony canal also has limited space at the intersegmental level, even though much of this is composed of soft tissue, whereas large bony diameters ensure more adequate space for the soft tissue contents. In addition, the cranial end of the lamina forms an important bony constriction in central canal stenosis, as do the superior apophyseal joints in both central and root canal stenoses. The fact that soft tissues are important does not negate the relevance of a small bony canal.

WHEN DOES THE BONY CANAL REACH MATURITY?

We examined 155 juvenile vertebrae and compared them with 839 adult vertebrae, observing changes in the size and shape of the vertebral canal with advancing age. It is difficult to obtain archaeologic spines from individuals under 4 years of age, but the vertebrae of that age that we examined had mean midsagittal diameters 10% wider than the mean adult midsagittal diameter at each of the lumbar levels. The reduction in size of the midsagittal diameter throughout childhood is the result of the changing shape of the posterior border of the vertebral body. The mean interpedicular diameter at 4 years of age is approximately 85% of the adult size, and it gradually widens (Fig. 2) with the increasing breadth of the vertebral bodies and the widening pedicles. The upper lumbar vertebrae matured before those in the lower lumbar spine. The trefoil shape was not seen, in our specimens, under 12 years of age and became apparent in about 15% of spines by maturity.[16]

DEVELOPMENT OF THE VERTEBRAL CANAL

Anthropometric measurements provide a clue to the development of the vertebral canal. We examined the vertebral canal in archaeologic specimens and compared it with the length of other bones in the skele-

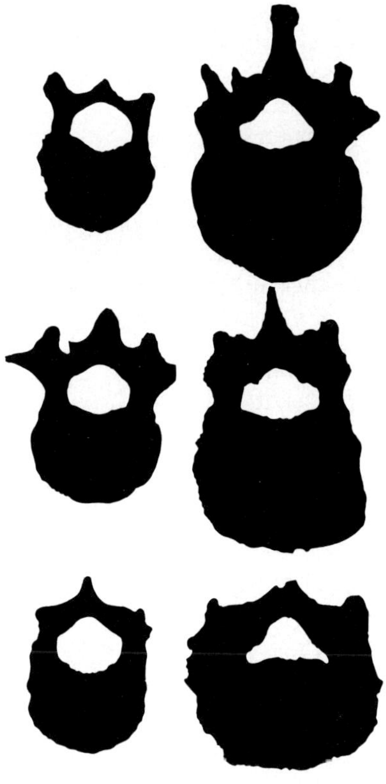

Figure 2 □ Silhouette photographs of vertebrae from children of 4 years of age compared with adult vertebrae. The sagittal diameters are greater in the children's spines than in the adults', although the interpedicular diameters are about 85% of adult size.

ton. There was a useful correlation between the length of the femur and the interpedicular diameter: a tall subject will have a large transverse diameter of the vertebral body and widely spaced pedicles.[16] We did not find many useful correlations between the midsagittal diameter of the canal and other bony measurements. There was a weak correlation between the anteroposterior (AP) and lateral diameters of the skull and the midsagittal diameter of the canal, but this clinically important canal diameter is largely independent of other skeletal growth.

Clark and coworkers[17] suggested that the size of the lumbar vertebral canal may be affected by factors that impair childhood development. They examined two archaeologic populations and found that a malnourished population tended to have shallow vertebral canals. We examined the adult spines of two other archaeologic populations, comparing the canal size with four physiologic stress indicators (cribra orbitalia, porotic hyperostosis, dental hypoplasia, and Harris lines).[18] Dental hypoplasia correlated with a small interpedicular diameter at L1–L2 and L3; Harris lines correlated with a small midsagittal diameter at L1–L3 and L5, a small area at L5, and a more trefoil canal at L4 and L5. We found supportive evidence that an adverse environment in early life is associated with a shallow canal. No doubt, genetic factors influence the canal, but an adverse environment is probably important to impairing its growth.

The differential growth of the canal in the midsagittal and interpedicular diameters makes possible a hypothesis about trefoil development. Impaired early neuro-osseous development can result in an infant's having a small midsagittal diameter. In the absence of catch-up growth, the patient will be left with a shallow canal. However, an improved environment can provide for adequate growth in stature. A tall individual will have long limbs, broad vertebral bodies, and wide pedicles; the catch-up growth still available for the interpedicular diameter will produce a shallow canal that has broadened out into the trefoil shape.

RELATIVE SIZE OF THE VERTEBRAL CANAL AND ITS CONTENTS

One might expect that an individual with a small canal is at no greater disadvantage than another with larger dimensions, because of the relative size of the canal contents resulting in a smaller canal housing a small cauda equina. In utero, however, when the conus is in the sacral canal, the epigenetic influence of the spinal cord on the surrounding bony structures causes the size of the cord and the canal to be related. Impaired neuro-osseous development will result in a small spinal canal being associated with small contents. In infancy, as the conus rises to L2, improved nutrition may be too late to benefit the sagittal diameter of the canal, but with improving stature, longer limbs, good muscles, and large peripheral nerves, the cauda equina will be relatively large within a shallow canal, producing a clinically dangerous situation if that canal is pathologically compromised. Unless there is a disparity between canal size and contents, it is difficult to explain the body of literature on the clinical relevance of the canal.

SPINA BIFIDA AND SPONDYLOLYSIS

The neural tube develops in a craniocaudal manner and is usually complete at the 26th day after gestation. The failure of closure of the neural tube results in spina bifida overta, and failure of closure of the neural arch, in spina bifida occulta. Some evidence suggests that spina bifida occulta is not a single segmental lesion but that its presence is related to changes in the more proximal vertebrae. We have examined the size of the vertebral canal proximal to the spina bifida occulta in affected skeletons and have found a significant increase in the midsagittal diameter at the two more proximal levels ($p < 0.01$).[19] A delay in closure of the neural arch influences at least the two more proximal vertebrae, leaving them wider than those of other skeletons without dysraphism. Spina bifida occulta and spina bifida overta appear to be related conditions. The parents of children with the open spina bifida are four times more likely to have the occult lesion than other members of the population.[20] Neural tube defects are probably related to periconceptional vitamin deficiency,[21] particularly folic acid deficiency.[22] If vitamin deficiency is related to the development of spina bifida occulta, leaving a canal a little larger proximal to the lesion, and if, in another situation, impaired development can result in spinal stenosis, then there are two confounding factors the interaction of which must be complex.

Vertebral displacement in isthmic spondylolisthesis widens the sagittal diameter of the central vertebral canal as the floating lamina is left behind, articulating with the next caudal segment (Fig. 3). Usually the pars is elongated and the canal is dome-shaped. The trefoil configuration is unusual in the presence of spondylolisthesis. For this reason it is unusual to find an isthmic spondylolisthesis in patients with a symptomatic disc lesion or neurogenic claudication.[23] The large vertebral canal protects the cauda equina. Vertebrae with unilateral spondylolysis are asymmetric in shape, and the asymmetry of the canal provides some understanding of the changes observed in bilateral spondylolysis. Elongation of the pars, horizontal orientation of the lamina, and asymmetry of the inferior apophyseal joints and the posterior elements are found. The combination of these effects produces a rotation of the spinous process away from the side of the lesion, and the inferior apophyseal joint on the side of the defect is placed more dorsally than the superior. This produces a

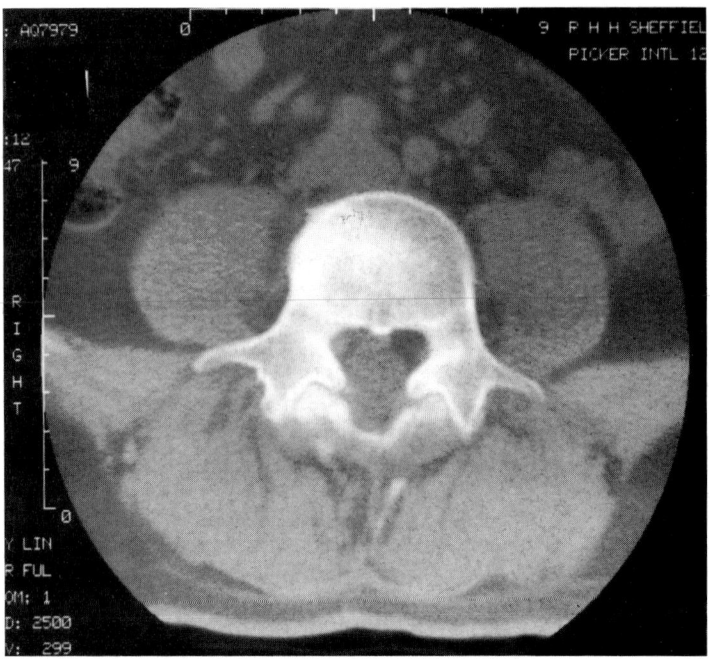

Figure 3 □ Computed tomographic (CT) scan of a patient with isthmic spondylolisthesis at L5 shows a large midsagittal diameter.

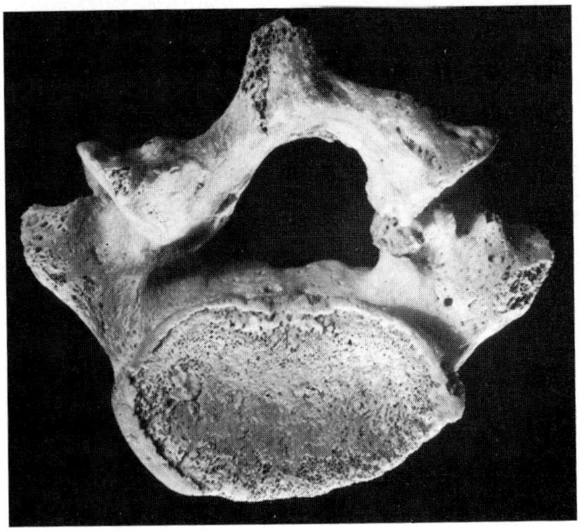

Figure 4 □ Photograph shows a fifth lumbar vertebra, with unilateral right-sided spondylolysis, and asymmetric increase in the canal.

unilaterally capacious vertebral canal (Fig. 4).

NEURO-OSSEOUS DEVELOPMENT AND THE IMMUNE SYSTEM

Clark[24] suggested that infantile malnutrition not only might impair the development of the vertebral canal but also may similarly affect the developing immune and central nervous systems. If the hypothesis is correct, one might expect the small adult vertebral canal, being a marker of deficient early development, also to be associated with poor function of the adult immune and central nervous systems. The growth curves of the thymus and of the central nervous system are similar to that of the spinal neuro-osseous development, and they are likely to be simultaneously affected by an adverse environment.

A relationship exists between the size of the vertebral canal and the thymus hormone, thymosin α_1.[25] This is supported by the observation that adults with spinal stenosis attend their doctors with infections in childhood and in later adulthood more frequently than do subjects with wider canals.[26]

There is also evidence that the academic performance of children with wider vertebral canals at 16 years of age is better than that of their peers with smaller canals; this may, of course, be a reflection of their socioeconomic status rather than of their early neurologic development.

Evidence is growing, suggesting that subjects with spinal stenosis are disadvantaged, not only in relation to back pain, but also in their general health and academic status. A search for factors that affect spinal growth is likely to have wider significance than the investigation of back pain. Our search should probably concentrate on the most rapid phase of growth, from the 8th to 16th weeks in utero, when the crown–rump length of the fetus increases from about 5 to 15 cm.[27] Specific insults to the sensitive enzyme systems at this stage are likely to be more significant than maternal malnutrition, to which the fetus is remarkably resistant.[28] A study of the relation of such factors to the subsequent canal size could be rewarding, and their recognition may have considerable medical, social, and economic significance.

References

1. Sarpyener, M.A.: Congenital stricture of the spinal canal. J. Bone Joint Surg. 27:70–79, 1945.
2. Verbiest, H.: A radicular syndrome from developmental narrowing of the lumbar vertebral canal. J. Bone Joint Surg. 36B:230–237, 1954
3. Van Gelderen, V.: Ein orthotisches (lordotisches) kauda syndrom. Acta Psychiatr. Neurol. Scand. 23:57–68, 1958.
4. Epstein, J.A., Epstein, B.S., and Levine, I.: Nerve root compression associated with narrowing of the lumbar spinal canal. J. Neurol. Neurosurg. Psychiatr. 25:165–176, 1962.
5. Salibi, B.S.: Neurogenic claudication and stenosis of the lumbar spinal canal. Surg. Neurol. 5:269–272, 1976.
6. Porter, R.W., Wicks, M., and Hibbert, C.: The size of the lumbar spinal canal in the symptomatology of disc lesion. J. Bone Joint Surg. 60B:485–487, 1978.
7. Porter, R.W., Hibbert, C., and Wellman, F.: Backache and the lumbar spinal canal. Spine 8:99–105, 1980.
8. Winston, K., Rumbaugh, C., and Colucci, V.: The vertebral canals in lumbar disc disease. Spine 9:414–417, 1984.
9. Heliovaara, M., Vanharanta, H., Korpi, J., and Troup, J.D.G.: Herniated lumbar disc syndrome and vertebral canals. Spine 11:433–435, 1986.
10. Edward, W.C., and La Rocca, S.H.: The developmental segmental sagittal diameter in combined cervical and lumbar spondylosis. Spine 10:42–49, 1985.
11. Kornberg, M., and Rechtine, G.R.: Quantitative assessment of the fifth lumbar spinal canal by computed tomography in symptomatic L4/L5 disc disease. Spine 10:328–330, 1985.
12. Forsberg, L., and Walloe, A.: Ultrasound in sciatica. Acta Orthop. Scand. 53:393–395, 1982.
13. Farfan, H.F., and Gracovetsky, S.: The nature of instability. Spine 9:714–719, 1984.
14. Spencer, D.L., Irwin, G.S., and Miller, J.A.A.: Anat-

omy and significance of fixation of the lumbosacral nerve roots in sciatica. Spine 8:672–679, 1983.
15. Kadish, L.J., and Simmons, E.H.: Anomalies of the lumbosacral nerve roots: An anatomical investigation and myelographic study. J. Bone Joint Surg. 66B:411–416, 1984.
16. Porter, R.W., and Hibbert, C.: Relationship between the spinal canal and other skeletal measurements in a Romano-British population. Ann. R. Coll. Surg. Engl. 63:437, 1981.
17. Clark, G.A., Panjabi, M.M., and Wetzel, F.T.: Can infant malnutrition cause adult vertebral stenosis? Spine 10:165–170, 1985.
18. Porter, R.W., and Pavitt, D.: The vertebral canal, Part 1. Nutrition and development: An archaeological study. Spine 12:901–906, 1987.
19. Porter, R.W., Mills, C., and Powers, R.: Is Spina Bifida a Bonus? Presented to the International Society for the Study of the Lumbar Spine. Miami, 1988.
20. Lorber, J., and Levic, K.K.: Spina bifida cystica. Incidence of spina bifida occulta in parents and controls. Arch. Dis. Child. 42:171–173, 1967.
21. Smithells, R.W., Sheppard, S., and Schorah, C.J.: Apparent prevention of neural tube defects by periconceptional vitamin supplementation. Arch. Dis. Child. 56:911–918, 1981.
22. Laurence, K.M., James, N., Miller, M.H., et al: Double-blind randomised controlled trial of folate treatment before conception to prevent recurrence of neural tube defects. Br. Med. J. 282:1509–1511, 1981.
23. Porter, R.W., and Hibbert, C.S.: Symptoms associated with lysis of the pars interarticularis. Spine 9:755–758, 1984.
24. Clark, G.A.: Heterochrony, allometry, and canalization in the human vertebral column: Examples from prehistoric Amerindian populations. Thesis, Graduate School of the University of Massachusetts, 1985, pp. 375–381.
25. Clark, G.A., Hall, N.R., Aldwin, C.M., et al.: Measures of poor early growth are correlated with lower adult levels of Thymosin α_1 (in press, J. Human Biol.).
26. Porter, R.W., Drinkall, J.N., Porter, D.E., and Thorp, L.: The vertebral canal, Part 2. Health and academic status. Spine 12:907–911, 1987.
27. Thompson D.W.: Maximum velocity of growth at 4th month intrauterine life. *In* Growth and Form, 2nd Ed. London, Cambridge University Press, 1942.
28. Ounstead, M.C.: On fetal growth rate. Clin. Dev. Med. 46:9, 1973.

CLASSIFICATION AND TREATMENT

Franco Postacchini

DEFINITION

The possibility of visualizing the spinal canal in transverse section by means of tomographic transaxial studies has contributed considerably to our knowledge of the pathologic anatomy of the various forms of lumbar stenosis.[6, 7, 16] However, controversy still exists regarding the definition, and thus the concept, of lumbar stenosis and the classification of the different forms of stenosis. The lack of a uniform interpretation of lesions and the frequently inappropriate use of the term *stenosis* produce confusion in the taxonomy of lumboradicular diseases and do not allow a reliable comparison of different clinical series. Attempts to rigorously define the concept of lumbar spinal stenosis arise from the need for this term to be universally employed to indicate a well-determined group of pathologic conditions. This is necessary not only because of the need for precision and uniformity in terminology, but also to prevent an erroneous interpretation of the concept of lumbar stenosis leading to diagnosis and treatment of other pathologic conditions as if they were stenosis.

Lumbar stenosis should be defined, in my opinion, as an *abnormal narrowing of the osteoligamentous vertebral canal and/or the intervertebral foramina, which is responsible for compression of the dural sac and/or the caudal nerve roots. Narrowing of the vertebral canal may involve one or more levels and, at a single level, may affect the entire canal or part of the canal.*[13]

Based on this definition, abnormal narrowing of the spinal canal may be regarded as stenosis if the following criteria are fulfilled: (1) narrowing involves the osteoligamentous spinal canal, and (2) it causes a compression of the nervous structures contained in the canal.

The first criterion implies a sharp distinction between disc disease and stenosis. This distinction may appear to be arbitrary both because of the fact that the intervertebral disc contributes to the delimitation of the spinal canal and because, in stenosis, compression of the nervous structures is often caused by a coexisting disc disease in the form of a more or less marked annular bulging or disc protrusion. However, if the concept of stenosis is not limited to the osteoligamentous vertebral canal, even disc disease becomes a stenotic condition. In fact, in the strictest sense a disc prolapse causes stenosis, that is, a pathologic narrowing of the whole or part of the spinal canal. Because the two conditions—disc herniation and stenosis—differ considerably in the pathogenesis and anatomoclinical characteristics, they cannot be considered as a single pathologic entity. The alternative is to specify, in each instance, whether stenosis has a discal, an osteoligamentous, or some other origin; one hopes that this is not the case because, instead of order and clarity, it would lead to uncertainty in the taxonomy of lumboradicular syndromes. Furthermore, disc changes represent a marginal element in the pathologic anatomy of stenosis. The peculiarity of the latter lies in the compression of the dural sac and the spinal nerve roots by the osteoligamentous components of the canal. Anterior compression by the disc, as well as posterior impingement by thickened ligamenta flava, may increase the narrowing of the spinal canal and contribute to the determination of clinical symptoms and signs, but neither represents an essential factor in the genesis of stenosis. The distinction between disc herniation and stenosis remains valid, even when the two conditions are associated at the same level or at different levels, that is, when disc herniation occurs in a narrow spinal canal. On the other hand, bulging of the annulus fibrosus at multiple levels cannot be regarded as a stenotic condition in the absence of an abnormal narrowing of the osteoligamentous spinal canal.

The second criterion emphasizes the concept of compression of the dural sac and nerve roots, which is implicit in the term stenosis. This term, in fact, indicates a dimensional disproportion of the caliber of the container compared with the volume of the content. If the content is a fluid, as in blood vessels, flow is reduced throughout the stenotic area; conversely, if the content is a solid or semifluid, as in the vertebral canal, the dimensional disproportion results in compression of the content by the walls of the container.[19] The disproportion, however, is not strictly related to the anteroposterior dimensions of the vertebral canal. Severe compression of the nervous structures may occur, even if the sagittal dimensions of the canal are within normal limits. On the other hand, a midsagittal diameter of 10 mm or less does not necessarily lead to compression of the cauda equina. This is probably attributable to the fact that, in normal conditions, the nervous structures contained in the spinal canal develop in harmony with the dimensions of the canal. When this does not occur, the reserve space available for the dural sac and/or the caudal nerve roots is variably reduced and, therefore, acquired constrictive conditions of even minor degree are sufficient to cause stenosis. If the narrowing is not severe enough to cause compression of the nervous structures, the spinal canal is to be considered narrow but not stenotic. This interpretation is supported by two series of observations: (1) of the two skeletal populations (Italian and Asiatic Indian) in which Postacchini and coworkers[14] measured the midsagittal diameter of the vertebral foramen, the Indian showed a lower limit of normal of 11.5 mm, a value generally considered pathologic; (2) The midsagittal diameters of the foramen measured, at one or more vertebral levels, 10.1 to 10.8 mm in 5% of the Italian skeletons and 9 to 10.5 mm in 10% of the Indian skeletons—percentages sufficiently high in comparison with the incidence of lumbar stenosis syndromes to exclude the possibility that during life these narrow canals, or at least most of them, might have been responsible for a cauda equina compression.

The clinical importance of these findings is that diagnosis of stenosis cannot be made on the basis of measurements of the vertebral canal, such as those obtained by computed tomography (CT), or the finding on the lateral myelogram of a uniform narrowing of the contrast medium column throughout the whole, or almost whole, length of the lumbar spinal canal. Diagnosis of stenosis should be based only on the demonstration of compression (which may be clinically symptomatic or asymptomatic) by an abnormally narrow osteoligamentous spinal canal.

As in the spinal canal, the nerve root canal should be considered stenotic when compression of the nerve root is only, or mainly, the result of changes in the osteoligamentous components of the canal. The term stenosis, therefore, is appropriately used when compression of the nerve root is related (as frequently occurs) to a bulging of the annulus fibrosus, unable itself to produce a radicular syndrome in a normal-sized nerve root canal; the term is not appropriate when the radicular syndrome is caused by a disc herniation protruding in a more or less narrow nerve root canal.

Pseudostenosis

This term should be reserved for a few pathologic conditions—isthmic spondylolisthesis, vertebral tumors, and so-called fibrous stenosis—which, although showing several anatomoclinical similarities to typically stenotic conditions, cannot be considered as true forms of stenosis.

In isthmic spondylolisthesis, compression of the nervous structures is attributable to kinking of the dural sac on the vertebra below that presenting olisthesis and to the fibrocartilaginous tissue filling the isthmic defect. In this form of spondylolisthesis, in other words, the osteoligamentous spinal canal is deformed but not narrowed. Indeed, at the level of the olisthetic vertebra, the spinal canal is wider than normal in the sagittal plane, because the dorsal portion of the vertebral arch does not follow the vertebral body in the anterior slipping.

Tumors have such peculiar biologic, pathologic, and clinical characteristics that they cannot be associated with the pathologic conditions responsible for the true forms of stenosis.

So-called fibrous stenosis (postlaminectomy stenosis[2]) is produced by the fibrous or osteofibrous membrane replacing the vertebral arch at the site of a previous laminectomy. The most appropriate term for this condition, as indeed for any form of compression of the nervous structures by epidural scar tissue, is *constrictive epidural fibrosis*.

CLASSIFICATION

Lumbar spinal stenosis may be distinguished, on the grounds of anatomopathologic features, as one of the following: stenosis of the spinal canal, isolated stenosis of the nerve root canal, and stenosis of the intervertebral foramen (Table 1).

In stenosis of the spinal canal, only the central portion may be constricted or, as usually occurs, both the central portion and the nerve root canal, on either one side or both sides.

In isolated stenosis of the nerve root canal, only this canal is narrowed, whereas the central spinal canal is normal in width or has such shape and size as not to cause any compression of the nervous structures. Stenosis may be classified as stenosis of the spinal canal or isolated stenosis of the nerve root canal, depending on the severity of the narrowing of the central spinal canal.

Stenosis of the intervertebral foramen may be isolated or associated with one of the other two forms of lumbar stenosis.

Stenosis of the Spinal Canal

This includes primary, secondary, combined, and mixed forms.

Primary Stenosis

In primary stenosis the lumbar spinal canal may be constricted because of congenital

Table 1 □ Classification of Lumbar Spinal Stenosis

STENOSIS OF THE SPINAL CANAL
Primary
Congenital
Developmental: in achondroplasia or other forms of dwarfism
idiopathic
Secondary
Degenerative (with or without spondylolisthesis)
Late sequelae of fractures
Late sequelae of infections
In systemic bone diseases
Combined
Association of primary and secondary stenosis at the same level
Mixed
Primary and secondary (and/or combined) stenosis at different levels
ISOLATED STENOSIS OF THE NERVE ROOT CANAL
Primary
Secondary
Combined
STENOSIS OF THE INTERVERTEBRAL FORAMEN
Primary
Secondary
Combined

malformations or a disorder in postnatal development of the lumbar vertebrae. In this case, compression of the caudal nerve roots is exclusively or essentially due to the abnormal primary narrowing. Two types of primary stenosis may be identified: congenital and developmental.

Congenital stenosis, which is very rare, is due to congenital malformations of the vertebral body and/or the posterior arch (Fig. 1). The term congenital does not indicate that stenosis is present at birth, but that it is caused exclusively or essentially by a malformative condition. A stenotic condition present at birth has, in fact, never been reported. Compression of the nervous structures usually becomes apparent in adulthood, when primary narrowing of the spinal canal is critically accentuated by osteoligamentous or disc changes, which in a normal-sized spinal canal and because of their mildness would not produce any pathologic effect.

Developmental stenosis may have a known cause or may be idiopathic.

In the former instance, narrowing of the spinal canal is due to known pathologic conditions, such as achondroplasia or Morquio disease, which are related to genetic abnormalities with a hereditary transmission. In the achondroplastic forms, which are the most common, the midsagittal and/or interpedicular diameters of the spinal canal are abnormally short and the nerve root canals show a marked narrowing attributable to shortness of the pedicles (Fig. 2).

In idiopathic developmental stenosis[18, 19] or more simply, idiopathic stenosis, the cause of the defective vertebral development is unknown. In my experience, two types of developmental abnormality may be identified: (1) the abnormality may consist only of a small midsagittal diameter of the spinal canal, or (2) other abnormalities may also be present, particularly an exceedingly sagittal orientation and/or shortness of the laminae.

In stenotic conditions of the first type, in which the spinal canal is narrow in the sagittal plane only, compression of the vertebral nervous structures may occur only in the presence of marked degenerative changes of the spine; for this reason, it may be difficult to differentiate these forms from combined stenoses.

In the forms of the second type, which are the most typical, the spinal canal is abnormally narrow in the interarticular diameter as well, thus tending to assume, in the subpedicular and discal portions, an elongated shape in the sagittal direction. In these forms, the vertebral canal may be only slightly narrower in the sagittal diameter; nevertheless, the disproportion between the volume and shape of the content and the capacity and shape of the container may be such that mild spondylotic changes (such as those normally occurring with aging) are sufficient to cause marked compression of the vertebral nervous structures.

Secondary Stenosis

In secondary stenosis the sagittal dimensions of the spinal canal are normal, even if often at the lower limits, and compression of the caudal nerve roots is exclusively the result of one or more acquired conditions. These are generally represented by spondylotic changes of the vertebral body and/or the facet joints, which may or may not be associated with *degenerative spondylolisthesis* (Fig. 3). In order for compression of the vertebral nervous structures to occur, a general rule is as follows: the wider the dimensions of the canal, the more severe the spondylotic changes have to be, because the reserve capacity of a large spinal canal is greater than that of a narrow canal. It should be pointed out, however, that it is extremely rare for a very wide canal (i.e., with dimensions at the upper limits of normal) to become stenotic; if this occurs, compression of the nervous structures is generally mild and, for this reason, often asymptomatic.

Late fractures or infectious diseases of the spine rarely cause stenosis, either alone or in association with spondylotic changes. Stenosis secondary to *systemic bone diseases,* responsible for an increase in volume and/or deformation of one or more vertebral components, is equally rare.

Some authors[1] also include, among the forms of secondary stenosis, so-called postfusion stenosis (i.e., stenosis presenting in patients who have previously undergone posterior vertebral arthrodesis). This form has not been included in the present classification because it has not yet been established whether, in patients with a posterior lumbar fusion, stenosis results from hyperostosis of articular processes and laminae resulting from arthrodesis, or whether—as I

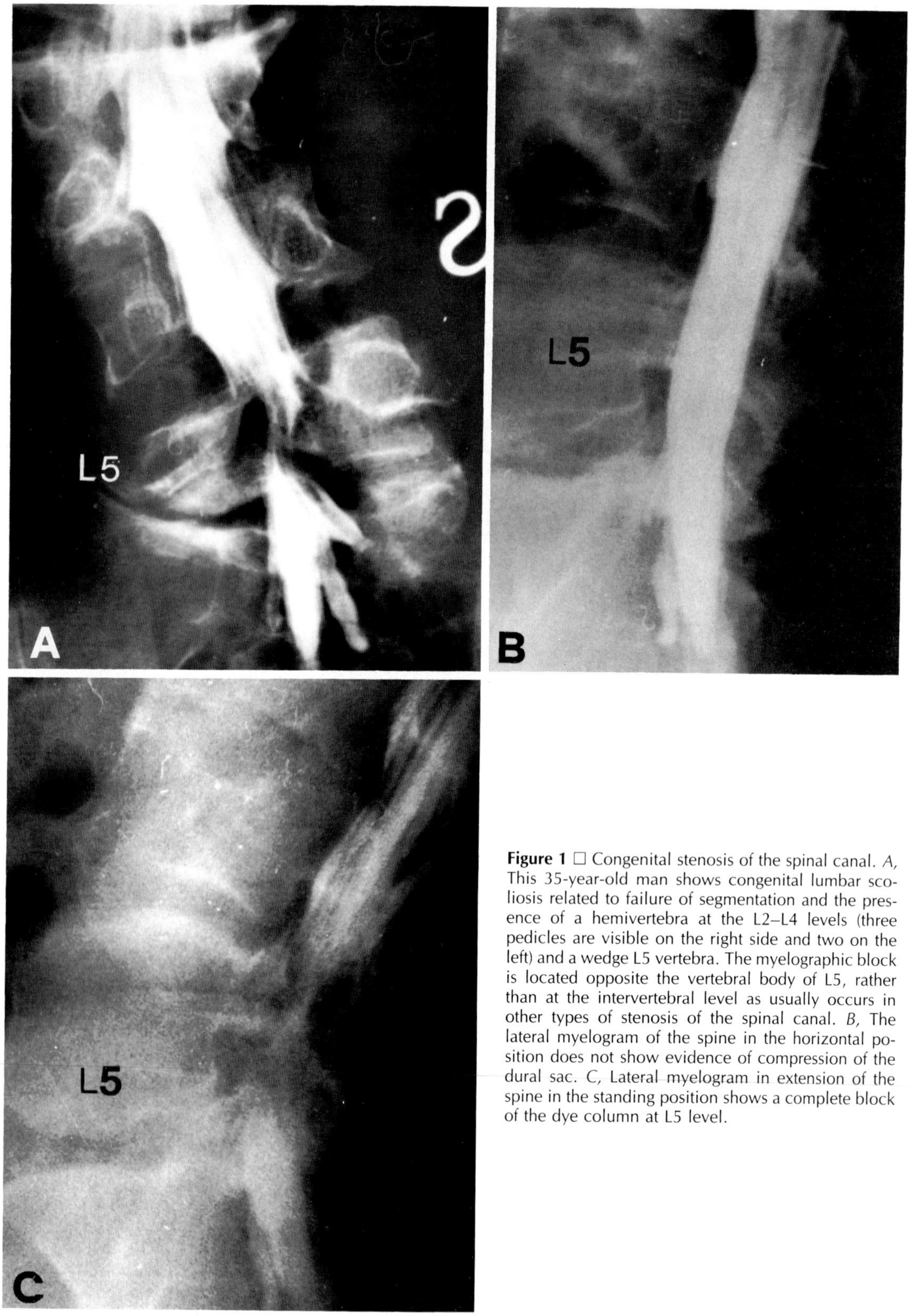

Figure 1 □ Congenital stenosis of the spinal canal. *A,* This 35-year-old man shows congenital lumbar scoliosis related to failure of segmentation and the presence of a hemivertebra at the L2–L4 levels (three pedicles are visible on the right side and two on the left) and a wedge L5 vertebra. The myelographic block is located opposite the vertebral body of L5, rather than at the intervertebral level as usually occurs in other types of stenosis of the spinal canal. *B,* The lateral myelogram of the spine in the horizontal position does not show evidence of compression of the dural sac. *C,* Lateral myelogram in extension of the spine in the standing position shows a complete block of the dye column at L5 level.

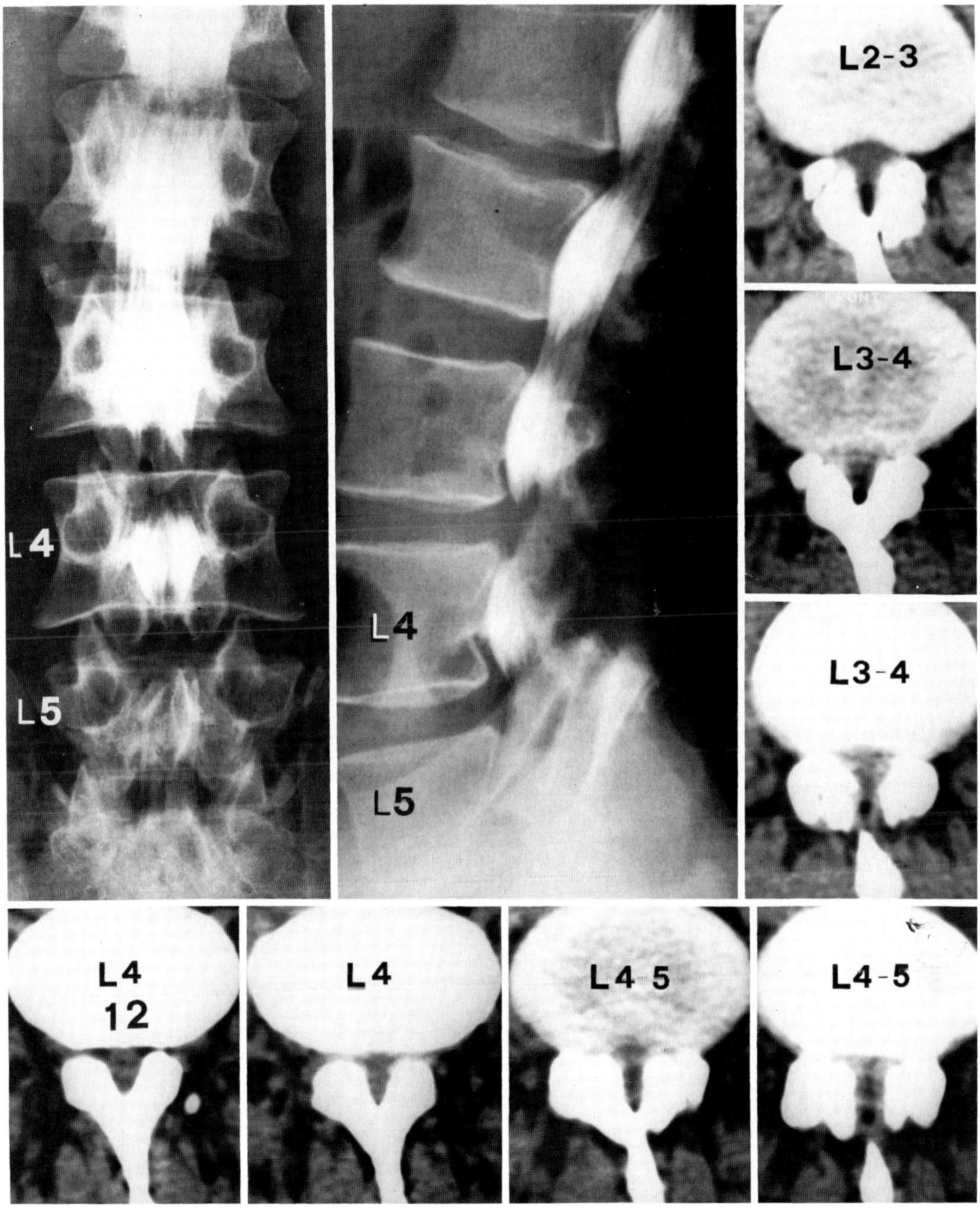

Figure 2 □ Achondroplastic stenosis of the spinal canal. Myelograms show a complete block of the dye column at L3–L4 and L4–L5 and a mild compression of the dural sac at the upper intervertebral levels. Computed tomographic (CT) scans show a moderately short midsagittal diameter of the spinal canal, which measures 12 mm at L4. The interpedicular diameter is markedly narrow at all lumbar levels, and the pedicles are abnormally short. The articular processes encroach on the central spinal canal, particularly at the L4–L5 level.

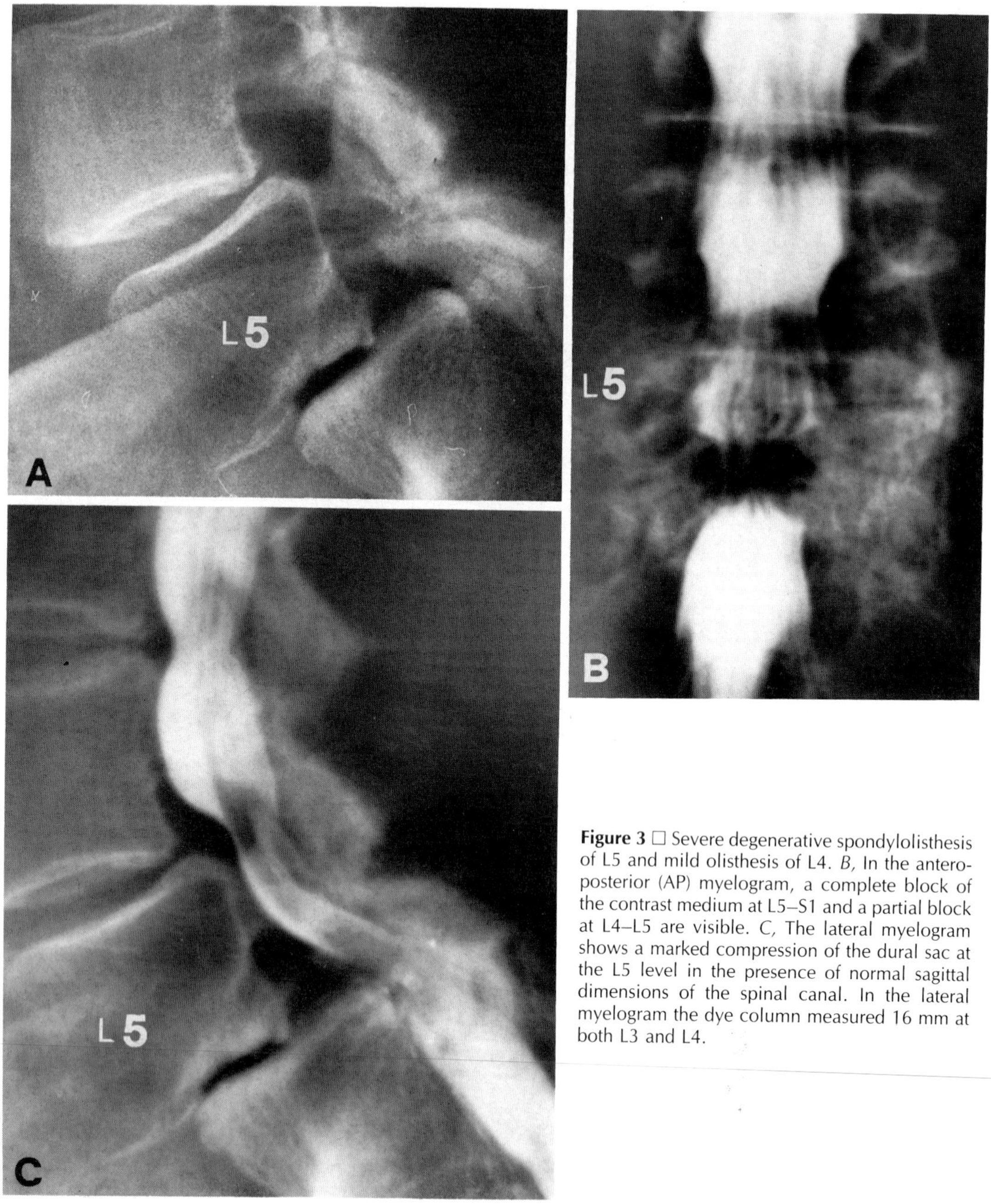

Figure 3 □ Severe degenerative spondylolisthesis of L5 and mild olisthesis of L4. *B,* In the anteroposterior (AP) myelogram, a complete block of the contrast medium at L5–S1 and a partial block at L4–L5 are visible. *C,* The lateral myelogram shows a marked compression of the dural sac at the L5 level in the presence of normal sagittal dimensions of the spinal canal. In the lateral myelogram the dye column measured 16 mm at both L3 and L4.

believe—this is a degenerative or combined form of stenosis that is not dependent on posterior fusion.

Combined Stenosis

Primary narrowing of the spinal canal is associated, at the same vertebral level, with a secondary narrowing, which is generally spondylotic in nature (Figs. 4 and 5). Combined stenosis can be differentiated from primary stenosis by the fact that, in the former, developmental narrowing is usually relatively mild and the degenerative changes are more marked than in the primary forms. The distinction between the various forms of secondary stenosis and combined stenosis is clear-cut for the degenerative forms, but not for the other secondary forms. In fact, in degenerative stenosis the axial tomographic finding of a normal midsagittal diameter of the vertebral canal excludes the possibility that stenosis is combined in nature. In contrast, in the other secondary forms, in which the midsagittal diameter is generally also short, it may be difficult to exclude a primary narrowing.

Mixed Stenosis

Mixed stenosis is characterized by primary stenosis at one or more vertebral levels and secondary or combined stenosis at other levels. This form of stenosis, however, is identified for taxonomic rather than anatomoclinical criteria, because it may be difficult or even impossible to differentiate between mixed stenosis and primary or combined stenosis in vivo.

Nerve Root Canal Stenosis

Stenosis of the nerve root canal may result from (1) disturbances of vertebral development, particularly abnormal shortness of the pedicles, even more so if associated with a trefoil configuration of the spinal canal or anomalous orientation and/or shape of the superior articular process;[4] (2) acquired factors, such as hypertrophy and/or osteophy-

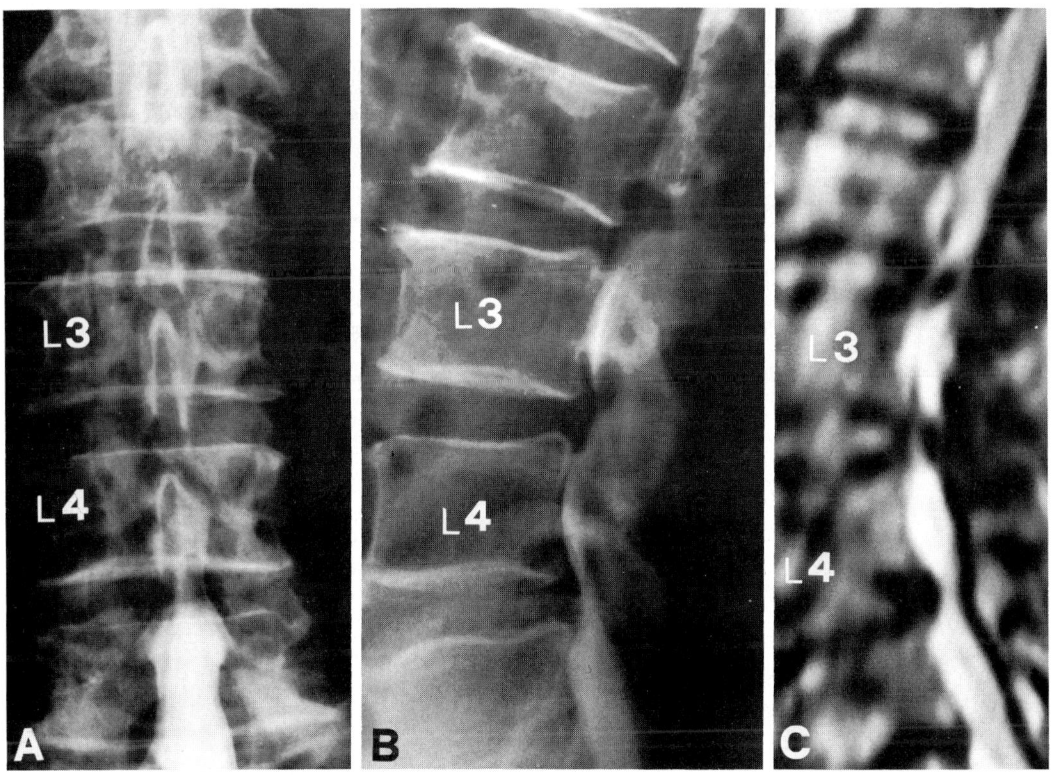

Figure 4 □ Combined stenosis of the spinal canal in a 68-year-old man. Myelograms (*A, B*) show multiple blocks of the contrast medium column from L2 to L5. Magnetic resonance imaging (MRI) (*C*) shows an abnormally short sagittal diameter of the dural sac, measuring 9 mm at L2 to 12 mm at L5, as well as multiple compressions of the nervous structures from L2–L3 to L4–L5.

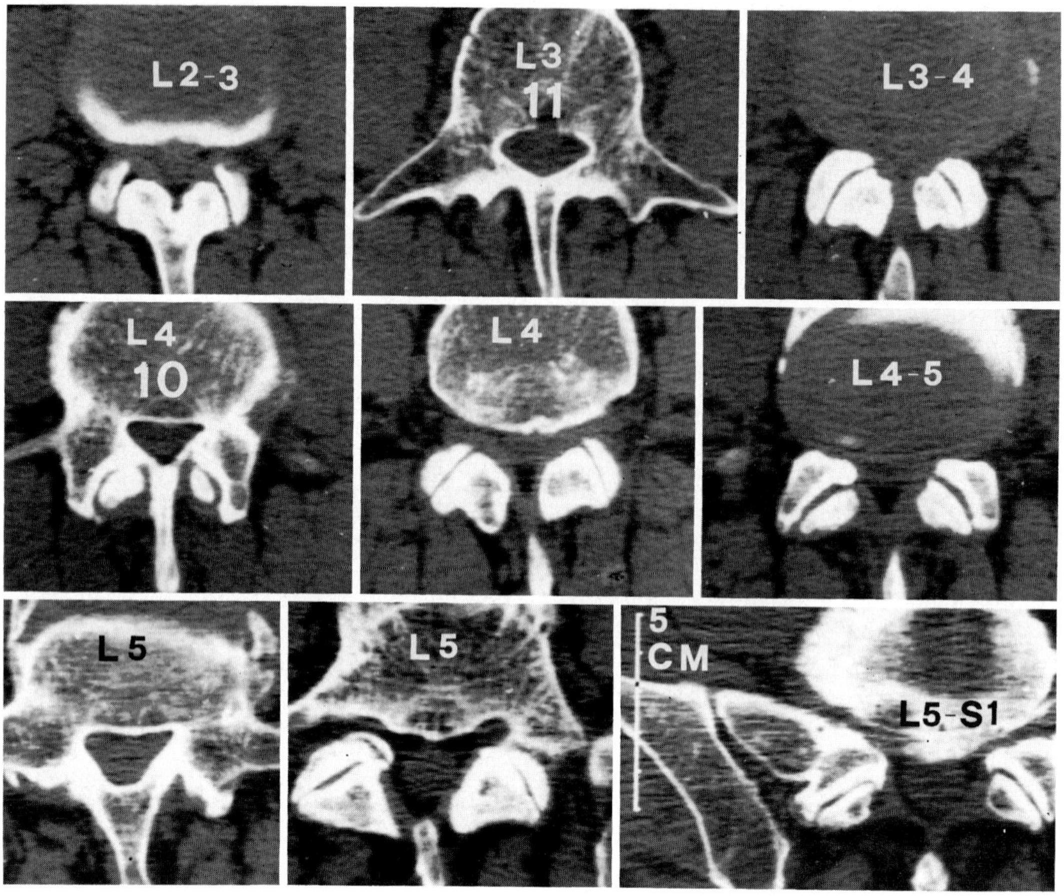

Figure 5 □ Same patient as shown in Figure 4. CT scans show an abnormally short midsagittal diameter of the spinal canal at L3 (11 mm) and L4 (10 mm) and osteoarthritic changes of the articular processes, which encroach on the spinal canal, particularly at the L3–L4 level.

tosis of the superior articular process, osteophytosis of the posterolateral border of the vertebral body, retrolisthesis of the upper adjacent vertebra, and late post-traumatic changes; (3) association (the most frequent occurrence) of primary and secondary pathologic conditions. Therefore, even for stenosis of the nerve root canal, primary, secondary, and combined forms may be identified. The distinctions among the various forms, however, are often difficult to make for individual patients, and are in any event much less clear-cut than for patients with stenosis of the spinal canal.

The nerve root canal may be stenotic at the level of the proximal portion, corresponding to the intervertebral disc, or of the caudal portion, represented by the lateral recess.

The most frequent site of stenosis, or at least of symptomatic stenosis, is the portion corresponding to the intervertebral disc, because at this level the narrowing caused by the bony component of the canal may easily be increased, to a critical extent for the root, by a bulge of varying size of the annulus fibrosus. The second portion, corresponding to the lateral recess, is more rarely stenotic, because the walls of the nerve root canal in this portion are entirely formed by bony structures. Nerve root compression at this level is usually caused by posterior osteophytes of the superior vertebral end plate and/or degenerative changes of the superior articular process at the level of its basal portion, facing the vertebral body. However, stenosis of this second portion of the canal is generally associated with stenosis of the first portion, at least when narrowing is caused by abnormalities of the superior articular process, which usually involve the entire height of the process.

Stenosis of the Intervertebral Foramen

Stenosis of the neuroforamen is often associated with stenosis of the spinal canal, particularly in degenerative forms.[5] On the contrary, it is fairly rare to observe isolated stenosis of the intervertebral foramen. In fact, although one does not infrequently observe abnormal narrowing of the neuroforamen due to excessive shortness of the pedicles, a decrease in height of the intervertebral disc, or osteoarthritic changes of the vertebral body and/or the articular processes, compression of the spinal nerve root is rarely caused by such narrowing. This is because of the fact that the intervertebral foramen has a fairly large reserve capacity. Therefore, the association of two or more pathologic conditions is usually necessary in order for such narrowing to cause nerve root compression.

TREATMENT

Conservative Treatment

The role of nonsurgical treatment in lumbar spinal stenosis differs considerably from that of conservative management in disc herniations. In the latter condition, clinical symptoms and signs show a tendency to improve with time, even to disappear, probably because of the tendency of the herniated nucleus pulposus to show a progressive decrease in volume as a result of tissue dehydration. In stenosis, on the other hand, radicular symptoms tend to become progressively more severe as time passes, on account of the increase in severity of the degenerative changes related to the aging process. In the lumbar stenosis syndrome, therefore, conservative treatment is usually considered to be a second choice or a "wait-and-see" approach, to be employed when surgical treatment is contraindicated owing to a poor general condition of the patient or is not justified on account of mildness of radicular symptoms and signs.

Conservative treatment consists of drug therapy, physiotherapy, and bracing.

Drug Therapy

Low back pain may be lessened by anti-inflammatory noncorticosteroid drugs. For radicular symptoms the use of corticosteroids at low or medium dosage is indicated, if the general condition of the patient allows, for a maximum of 2 weeks.

During the last 20 years, calcitonin and/or mithramycin has been employed in patients with vertebral Paget disease, presenting with clinical and radiographic evidence of compression of the caudal nerve roots, and, in many cases, mild improvement to complete resolution of the radicular symptoms has been reported.[8, 10] A possible explanation for the clinical effects of calcitonin in these cases may be that the highly vascularized pagetic bone exerts a sort of vascular theft, reducing blood flow to the vertebral nervous structures. Because calcitonin reduces the blood flow in the pagetic bone, vascularization of the nervous structures would be improved.

On the grounds of these observations, Porter and Hibbert[12] administered salmon calcitonin (100 units, four times a week) to patients who had lumboradicular intermittent claudication and no evidence of Paget disease and found, in about one fourth of them, a significant improvement in walking capacity after only 4 weeks of treatment. These therapeutic effects of calcitonin, which need to be confirmed, are probably related to a reduction in the skeletal arterial blood flow induced by the hormone[20] and a subsequent increase in the arterial flow in the cauda equina. Alternatively, the hormone might improve the venous blood flow, thus producing a decrease in volume of the venous epidural plexus, with a subsequent increase in the oxygen supply to the cauda equina.

Physiotherapy

Physiotherapy is mainly employed to relieve pain in the low back. It has little or no effect upon radicular symptoms but may be effective, in the form of stimulant electrotherapy and active kinesiotherapy, in the treatment of motor deficits in the lower limbs.

Bracing

The use of a corset may reduce low back pain and, sometimes, radicular symptoms. Lessening of the radiated symptoms, which is usually mild, is likely attributable to the fact that bracing reduces the dynamic stretching and compression of the caudal nerve roots, which may be produced by the articular processes and intervertebral discs during spinal movements. This interpretation is consistent with the observation that bracing leads to the greatest reduction of low back and radicular symptoms in patients showing evidence of vertebral instability, particularly in those with degenerative spondylolisthesis.

Surgical Treatment

Indications and Contraindications

Indications for surgical treatment are based on the results of diagnostic investigations demonstrating compression of the conus medullaris and/or cauda equina and on the presence of cord or nerve root symptoms and signs that correspond, as far as level and side are concerned, to the site of compression of the spinal nervous structures.

In particular, surgical treatment is indicated under the following circumstances:

1. In the presence of sphincteric disturbances due to compression of the conus medullaris, regardless of the severity of radicular symptoms and signs.
2. In patients with severe radicular symptoms (pain, paresthesias, asthenia) and monoradicular or multiradicular motor deficits.
3. In the presence of severe motor deficits and mild or discontinuous radicular symptoms, if stenosis is marked and the patient is not very elderly. In these cases, the indication for surgical treatment is based on the consideration that, as time passes, symptoms usually show a progressive increase in severity; this is not unlike the changes in motor deficits, in which the longer the duration and the greater the entity, the greater is the likelihood that they will be irreversible.
4. In patients with radicular symptoms and no neurologic signs, if the symptoms have been present more than 6 months and show no response to an adequate trial of conservative management. In these cases, investigations should demonstrate a marked compression of the nervous structures, or, in the presence of mild compression, the symptoms should have a precise radicular distribution with involvement of one or more dermatomes at all levels.
5. In patients with severe low back pain and mild radicular symptoms, in whom investigations show evidence of marked compression of the nervous structures.

Conversely, surgery is not generally indicated in the following situations:

1. In patients complaining of vague and imprecise radicular symptoms, when investigations demonstrate only posterior compression of the dural sac.
2. If the clinical picture is characterized by radicular motor deficits only, which, being long-standing, are likely to be irreversible. This is specifically true for subjects of advanced age.
3. In patients complaining of low back pain of varying severity as the main disorder and of mild or discontinuous radicular symptoms, in whom investigations show mild compression of the neurologic structures. The only exceptions are patients with degenerative spondylolisthesis, for whom the aim of treatment may be vertebral stabilization as well as decompression of the caudal nerve roots.

Surgical treatment is contraindicated for the following patients:

1. Those who have a narrow but not stenotic spinal canal.
2. Those for whom investigations carried out to assess an extralumbar condition show a clinically asymptomatic stenosis.

Planning of Surgery

Surgical treatment consists of decompression of the spinal nervous structures by means of bilateral laminectomy or laminotomy at one or more vertebral levels.

It is crucial to accurately plan the extent of decompression before surgery because during the operation it may be difficult to determine with certainty whether, at a certain level, the spinal or nerve root canal is stenotic, particularly if the stenosis is not severe. Lack of sufficient care in planning the operation may give rise to one of the following risks: (1) inadequate decompression, which would leave areas of stenosis, or (2) a too-wide decompression, which could directly or indirectly determine iatrogenic pathologic conditions.

STENOSIS OF THE SPINAL CANAL

Surgical treatment is aimed at decompressing the nervous structures in the areas in which they are compressed. In the narrow but nonstenotic areas of the spinal canal, opening the spinal canal is not generally necessary or useful.[15]

In planning the operative treatment it is necessary to determine the following: the levels that need to be decompressed, the type of procedure (unilateral or bilateral), and the usefulness of performing a vertebral fusion.

NUMBER OF LEVELS TO DECOMPRESS

The stenotic levels may be distinguished, as far as concerns operative treatment, as follows:

1. Levels at which the need for decompression is absolute. At these levels compression of the conus medullaris or cauda equina is marked or, regardless of the severity, is responsible for clinical symptoms and signs. From one to three levels may be involved.
2. Levels at which the need for decompression is relative. At these levels compression of the spinal nervous structures is mild and asymptomatic. In most instances, one or two levels contiguous to the area of "absolute" stenosis are involved. At these levels, myelography usually reveals the following: a posterior indentation on the dural sac, which may be visible only on functional myelograms; lateral indentation or a mild hourglass deformation of the dural sac on the frontal view; or medial deviation and/or partial filling of the nerve root emerging from the dural sac.

The usefulness of carrying out prophylactic decompression at the levels of "relative" stenosis stems from the evaluation of several factors, such as the following:

1. Patient age. In patients of advanced age (i.e., those over 70 years old) the need for a prophylactic decompression is less than is middle-aged or early-old-age patients, because in the latter the chances of stenosis becoming symptomatic as a result of degenerative changes related to the aging process are higher.
2. Site of stenosis. Posterior compression of the dural sac is less likely to become symptomatic than is compression of the nerve roots in the radicular canal.
3. Presence of disc abnormalities. Marked bulging of the annulus fibrosus, which with passing time may become symptomatic, represents an indication for prophylactic decompression. The same is true for posterior somatic osteophytosis, responsible for compression of the dural sac.
4. Electrodiagnostic findings. Evidence of a clinically asymptomatic compression of a nerve root tends to suggest that, over time, compression may become symptomatic.
5. Vertebral stability. In the presence of instability or potential instability of the stenotic motion segment, it is usually advisable to limit the decompression as much as possible. Conversely, the presence of intersomatic osteophytes producing spontaneous vertebral arthrodesis represents a guarantee against postsurgical instability. Similar observations may be made for marked narrowing of the disc space in the absence of other pathologic conditions; loss of disc height, in fact, implies reduced intervertebral motion—thus, vertebral instability is highly unlikely.

In conclusion, it is not generally necessary in very elderly patients to extend laminectomy to areas of mild compression of the nervous structures in the absence of clinical disturbances and electromyographic abnormalities. On the other hand, in middle-aged or early-old-age patients, decompression should be extended to include areas of "relative" stenosis, particularly if there is no specific risk of postoperative instability (e.g., scoliosis, spondylolisthesis, late sequelae of vertebral fractures), and more particularly if vertebral stability is increased, owing to intersomatic osteophytosis or marked resorption of the intervertebral disc.

UNILATERAL OR BILATERAL DECOMPRESSION

For the levels at which the need for decompression is absolute and stenosis is bilateral, the decompression should be performed bilaterally. This is true both for patients with bilateral symptoms and/or signs, and for those with unilateral symptoms. When, at a given level, stenosis is severe and symptomatic on one side and mild and asymptomatic on the other, unilateral decompression may be considered, if discectomy is to be performed for an associated disc disease playing a significant role in the etiology of nerve root compression. In fact, disc excision performed on one side may be sufficient to decompress the nervous structures on the opposite side. However, even in these cases, bilateral decompression is generally recommended.

For levels at which the need for decompression is relative, the choice between unilateral and bilateral decompression should be made, taking into consideration the severity of the stenosis on the two sides, as well as the factors (i.e., patient age, electrodiagnostic findings, vertebral stability) previously taken into account in determining the number of levels to decompress. As a general rule, if bilateral laminectomy is planned at the level of "absolute" stenosis, it is advisable to extend it also to the level of "relative" stenosis. On the other hand, when laminotomy is planned for the area of absolute stenosis, it is often sufficient to limit the decompression for the area of relative stenosis to the side of the more marked compression of the nervous structures.

TYPE OF DECOMPRESSION

The choice of the type of decompression has to be made when the spinal canal is to be opened bilaterally. In these cases, bilateral laminotomy or laminectomy may be carried out. Laminotomy, despite the advantage of almost completely preserving vertebral stability, may be difficult to perform if the interlaminar space is narrow or almost absent because of ossification of the ligamentum flavum. Furthermore, when laminotomy is carried out on the same side, at two adjacent levels, the narrow portion of lamina that should separate the two laminotomies is also often removed; in effect a unilateral laminectomy is thus performed.

The excision of spinous processes and interspinous ligaments that bilateral laminectomy entails undoubtedly reduces vertebral stability, although not to a significant degree and not to an extent such as to make unstable a motion segment that is stable in itself.

Laminectomy, on the other hand, has the advantage of requiring a shorter operative time than laminotomy. In my opinion, bilateral laminectomy is usually preferable when bilateral decompression at two or more vertebral levels is to be performed, particularly if discectomy is not foreseen. Conversely, laminotomy is to be preferred in patients who have stenosis at one or two levels in whom discectomy for a coexisting disc disease will probably be necessary, or in patients in whom the vertebral level to be submitted to decompression is already unstable and for whom spinal fusion is not planned.

LONGITUDINAL AND TRANSVERSE EXTENT OF DECOMPRESSION

Compression of the dural sac and spinal nerve roots usually occurs at the intervertebral level. To be adequate, therefore, decompression of the nervous structures should involve the whole area facing the intervertebral disc. That is, when laminectomy is performed at more than one vertebral level, decompression at the upper limit of the stenotic area should be extended as far as the distal portion of the vertebral body supra-adjacent to the most cephalic of the discs included in the stenotic area and, at the lower limit of the stenotic area, as far as the proximal portion of the vertebral body subadjacent to the most caudal of the discs included in the area of stenosis. A frequent mistake is to decompress to the interlaminar space and (1) not to proceed, at the level of the proximal disc, with removal of the distal portion of the inferior articular processes of the vertebra above and (2) not to proceed, at the level of the distal disc, with removal of the ligamenta flava and the basal portion of the superior articular processes of the vertebra below. As a result, areas of narrowing of the spinal canal may persist; this may be responsible for partial relief only or the recurrence of radicular symptoms and signs.

In a transverse direction, laminectomy or laminotomy should be extensive enough to adequately decompress the dural sac and the spinal nerve roots in the radicular canal. The optimal facetectomy is that in which the medial half, or preferably two thirds, of the superior and inferior articular processes is removed. As time passes, the borders of the residual portion of the articular facets tend to undergo remodeling, which leads to a partial reforming of the facets. When facetectomy is too limited, remodeling of the borders of the articular processes may lead to a recurrence of stenosis in the radicular or spinal canal. However, total facetectomy must be avoided, not only because the far-lateral portion of the articular processes is not usually responsible for compression of the nervous structures but more particularly because total arthrectomy may lead to the risk of postoperative vertebral instability.

VERTEBRAL FUSION

Effects of Laminectomy on Vertebral Stability □ Performing bilateral laminectomy at several levels carries a risk of vertebral instability. Such a risk has often been overestimated, however, to the extent that vertebral fusion has almost consistently been performed in patients undergoing bilateral laminectomy for lumbar stenosis.[11] In my experience, the chances of producing iatrogenic instability are strictly related to the degree of vertebral stability prior to surgery.

When a motion segment is stable before the operation, bilateral laminectomy does not lead to instability if the lateral half or third of the articular processes is preserved and no discectomy is carried out; that is, instability will not occur if the functional integrity of the three columns—the intervertebral disc (and vertebral body) and the two zygapophyseal joints—that are responsible for vertebral stability is preserved.

Similarly, no instability usually occurs when, at an individual level, the lateral half or third of the articular processes on one side is preserved and no discectomy is carried out. Functional integrity of two of the three vertebral columns is, in fact, generally sufficient to guarantee vertebral stability. Furthermore, when facetectomy is subtotal, remodeling of the residual portion of the articular process may restore a sort of joint that contributes, even if to a lesser extent than would a normal joint, to the maintenance of vertebral stability (Fig. 6).

Last, when a motion segment is stable prior to surgery, instability rarely occurs, even when, at an individual intervertebral level, bilateral total facetectomy and unilateral discectomy are carried out. In these cases, vertebral stability is maintained by the anterolateral and residual posterior portions of the annulus fibrosus, if the latter is structurally and functionally intact. On the other hand, the chance of causing instability of a motion segment is great when bilateral facetectomy and discectomy are performed, particularly if the continuity of the posterior longitudinal ligament is interrupted along the midsagittal plane.

If a motion segment is preoperatively unstable, a bilateral laminectomy that extends too far laterally or even a bilateral laminotomy may increase the instability. This is particularly true when a discectomy, especially a bilateral one, is performed.

Indications for Fusion □ Regardless of degenerative spondylolisthesis, vertebral fusion should be planned, in addition to decompression, if the area to decompress is unstable or if bilateral laminectomy and discectomy are to be performed. Spinal fusion is generally indicated in the following patients: (1) in those who are under 70 years of age with stenosis at an unstable level and are to undergo bilateral laminectomy; (2) in young or middle-aged patients with stenosis at one level only for whom bilateral laminectomy has been planned, in whom discectomy will probably be necessary and in whom it may be impossible to adequately preserve the articular processes. This may occur, in particular, for upper lumbar levels, in which the intrinsic shortness of the laminae (which is even more marked in individuals with a narrow spinal canal) may make it difficult to decompress the nervous structures without sacrificing the zygapophyseal joints.

In both cases, the higher (i.e., the more structurally intact) the intervertebral disc, the greater is the need for fusion.

DEGENERATIVE SPONDYLOLISTHESIS

Degenerative spondylolisthesis may be considered a condition of relative vertebral instability. In fact, olisthesis, which is a sign of instability, may or may not be associated with abnormal mobility of the slipped vertebra in flexion–extension movements of the lumbar spine. In the first instance, the olisthetic vertebra is definitely unstable, whereas in the second the instability may be considered only potential.

Planning surgery for patients with degenerative spondylolisthesis depends (1) on the presence (or absence) of hypermobility of the slipped vertebra on functional radiographs and (2) on the degree of slipping and patient age.

When the olisthetic vertebra is only potentially unstable, planning the operation depends on the severity of vertebral slipping and the patient's age. If slipping is mild, surgery should be planned, regardless of whether olisthesis is present and regardless of the patient's age. In these cases, in fact, bilateral laminectomy adequately preserving the articular processes does not lead to postoperative instability. In patients with moderate spondylolisthesis, the treatment of choice is laminotomy (Fig. 7), particularly

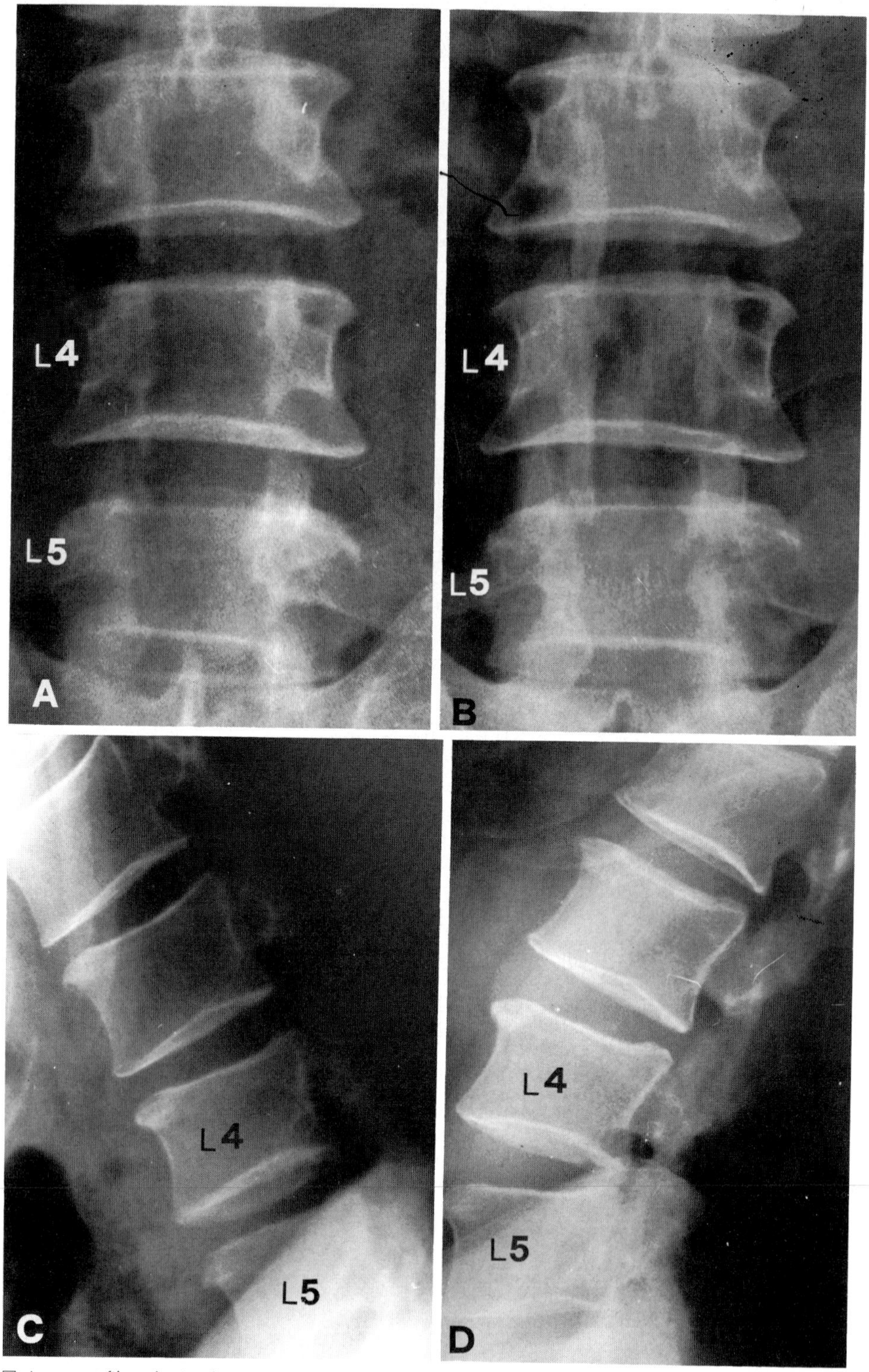

Figure 6 □ An x-ray film obtained 2 months after a wide bilateral laminectomy from L2 to S1. At L3–L4 and L4–L5 a foraminectomy had been performed on the left. No disc had been excised. In an x-ray taken 6 years after surgery, partial reformation of the articular processes on the right side was visible. *C, D,* Flexion–extension x-rays showed, 6 years after surgery, that the spine was stable. The patient had no complaint of low back pain.

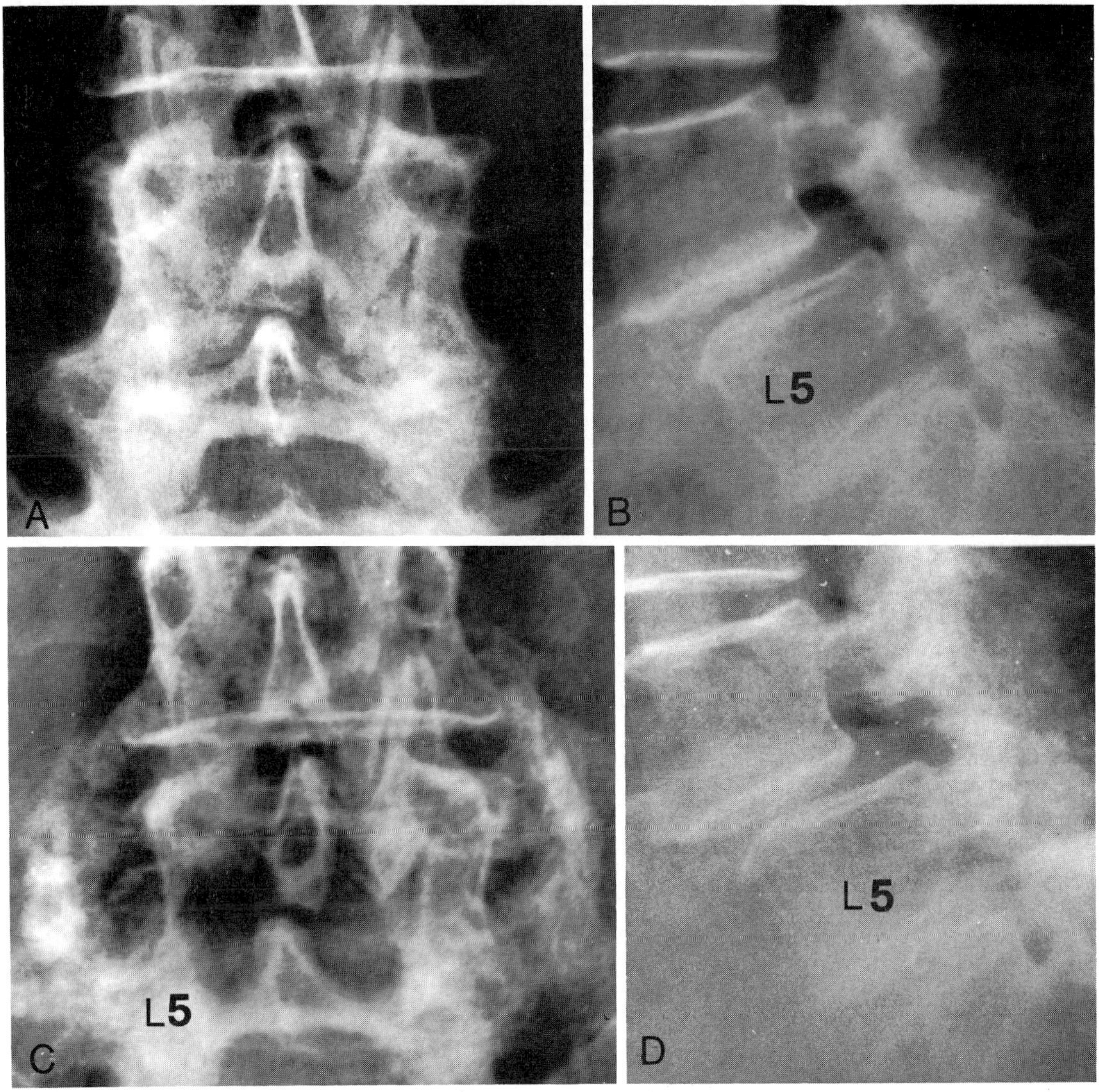

Figure 7 □ Degenerative spondylolisthesis of L4 in a 52-year-old woman who showed a partial myelographic block at L4–L5. *A, B,* Preoperative x-rays show that the fourth lumbar disc has slightly decreased in height. *C,* Operation consisted of bilateral laminotomy and posterolateral fusion at L4–L5. *D,* Despite the fusion, slipping of L4 has slightly increased after surgery.

in the absence of a complete myelographic block, or bilateral laminectomy preserving the lateral half of the articular processes.[17] In both instances, if the patient is under 60 years of age, bilateral posterolateral fusion should be carried out, especially when the normal (or almost normal) height of the disc below the olisthetic vertebra increases the chances of a subsequent vertebral slipping (Fig. 7). If spondylolisthesis is severe, vertebral fusion should be performed in addition to decompression, at least in patients under 70 years of age.

If the olisthetic vertebra is unstable, bilateral posterolateral fusion should always be carried out in addition to decompression. The only exceptions are very elderly patients or patients in poor general condition.

ISOLATED STENOSIS OF THE NERVE ROOT CANAL

Generally, for isolated stenosis of the nerve root canal in which only one vertebral level is usually involved, laminotomy extending distally to a point that varies depending on the site of nerve root compression should be performed.

In the presence, at a single level, of a symptomatic nerve root compression on both sides, bilateral decompression should be carried out. This should be done even if on one of the two sides radicular symptoms are mild and no neurologic abnormality is present (Fig. 8). When, at any one level, myelography and/or CT scans show bilateral nerve root compression in the presence of radicular symptoms and signs on one side only, bilateral decompression should generally be planned, especially if electrodiagnostic investigations show evidence of compression of the clinically asymptomatic nerve root, and if the absence of a significant discogenic component in the nerve root compression tends to suggest that disc excision on one side may not result in adequate decompression of the nerve root on the opposite side. Similar observations apply to patients with unilateral stenosis at two contiguous intervertebral levels. In these patients, unilateral laminectomy or, preferably, two contiguous laminotomies may be performed. Bilateral laminectomy is indicated only in the presence of bilateral stenosis at two or more contiguous levels, when decompression of all the involved roots must be performed, but it is necessary to reduce to a minimum the operative time, which is generally shorter for a bilateral laminectomy than for multiple laminotomies.

Discectomy should generally be planned for patients in whom preoperative investigations show evidence of a bulging intervertebral disc at the stenotic level. Preopera-

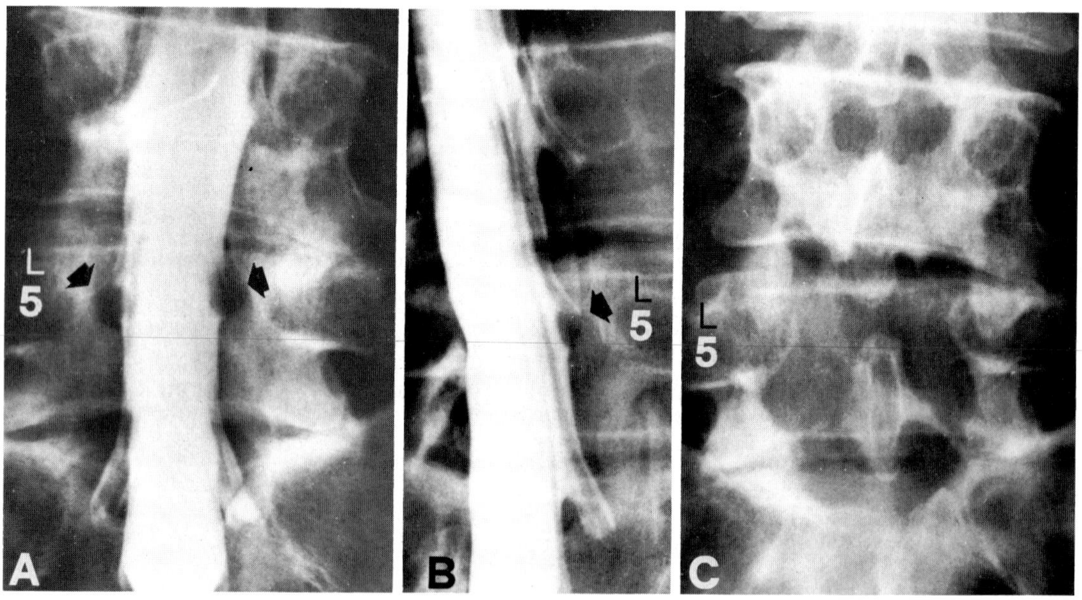

Figure 8 □ Isolated stenosis of the L5 nerve root canal on both sides, in a patient with symptoms and signs of compression of L5 nerve root on the left and only mild radicular discomfort on the right. *A, B,* Myelograms show a filling defect of L5 nerve roots at the level of the pedicles of the fifth lumbar vertebra. *C,* A wide bilateral laminotomy was performed and the L5 nerve roots were decompressed as far as the entrance of the neuroforamen.

tively, however, it is often difficult to determine the precise role played by the intervertebral disc in the etiology of nerve root compression. In these cases, the decision about whether to carry out disc excision must be made during surgery, on the basis of the operative findings.

Spinal fusion is rarely needed in patients who have isolated stenosis of the nerve root canal. Arthrodesis is indicated when bilateral decompression is carried out at a preoperatively unstable level, particularly if a unilateral or bilateral disc excision is performed. Fusion may also be indicated in patients complaining of long-standing low back pain caused by disc degeneration at the stenotic level or levels.

References

1. Arnoldi, C.C., Brodsky, A.E., Cauchoix, J., et al.: Lumbar spinal stenosis and nerve root entrapment syndromes. Definition and classification. Clin. Orthop. Rel. Res. 115:4, 1976.
2. Brodsky, A.E.: Post-laminectomy and post-fusion stenosis of the lumbar spine. Clin. Orthop. Rel. Res. 115:130, 1976.
3. Crock, H.V.: Practice of Spinal Surgery. New York, Springer-Verlag, 1983.
4. Epstein, J.A., Epstein, B.S., Rosenthal, R.C., and Lavine, S.L.: Sciatica caused by nerve root entrapment in the lateral recess: The superior facet syndrome. J. Neurosurg. 36:584, 1972.
5. Epstein, J.A., Epstein, B.S., Lavine, L.S., et al.: Lumbar nerve root compression of the intervertebral foramina caused by arthritis of the posterior facets. J. Neurosurg. 39:362, 1973.
6. Gargano, F.P., Jacobson, R.E., and Rosomoff, H.L.: Transverse axial tomography of the spine. Neuroradiology 6:254, 1974.
7. Glenn, W.V., Jr., Rhodes, M.L., Altschuler, E.M., et al.: Multiplanar display computerized body tomography applications in the lumbar spine. Spine 4:282, 1979.
8. Hadijpavlov, A.B., Tsoukas, G.M., Siller, T.N., et al.: Combination drug therapy in treatment of Paget's disease of bone. J. Bone Joint Surg. 59A:1045, 1977.
9. Hanley, E.N., Jr.: Decompression and distraction–detorsion arthrodesis for degenerative spondylolisthesis. Spine 11:269, 1986.
10. Herzberg, L., and Bayliss, E.: Spinal-cord syndrome due to non-compressive Paget's disease of bone: A spinal artery steal phenomenon reversible with calcitonin. Lancet 2:13, 1980.
11. Kostuik, J.P.: Posterior instrumentation for multiple level instability. Presented at the 7th AOA International Symposium, Chicago, 1986.
12. Porter, R.W., and Hibbert, C.: Calcitonin treatment for neurogenic claudication. Spine 8:585, 1983.
13. Postacchini, F.: Stenosi e pseudostenosi lombari. Definizione e classificazione della patologia stenotica lombare. G. Ital. Ortop. Traumatol. 9:355, 1983.
14. Postacchini, F., Ripani, M., and Carpano, S.: Morphometry of the lumbar vertebrae. An anatomic study in two Caucasoid ethnic groups. Clin. Orthop. Rel. Res. 172:296, 1983.
15. Postacchini, F.: Lumbar Spinal Stenosis. Springer-Verlag, New York, 1989.
16. Postacchini, F., Pezzeri, G., Montanaro, A., and Natali, G.: Computerized tomography in lumbar stenosis. A preliminary report. J. Bone Joint Surg. 62B:78, 1980.
17. Reinolds, J.B., and Wiltse, L.L.: Surgical treatment of degenerative spondylolisthesis. Spine 4:148–149, 1979.
18. Verbiest, H.: A radicular syndrome from developmental narrowing of the lumbar vertebral canal. J. Bone Joint Surg. 36B:230, 1954.
19. Verbiest, H.: Fallacies of the present definition, nomenclature and classification of the stenoses of the lumbar vertebral canal. Spine 1:217, 1976.
20. Wootton, R., Reeve, J., Spellacy, E., and Tellez-Yodilevich, M.: Skeletal blood flow in Paget's disease of bone and its response to calcitonin treatment. Clin. Sci. Mol. Med. 54:69, 1978.

10 □ Segmental Instability

John W. Frymoyer
Malcolm H. Pope
David G. Wilder

A certain amount of care or pain or trouble is necessary for every man at all times. A ship without ballast is unstable and will not go straight.

SCHOPENHAUER

Unstable as water, thou shalt not excel.

GENESIS

In the Presidential Symposium on Instability of the Lumbar Spine, Kirkaldy-Willis posed the following challenges: (1) Define precisely what is meant by the term *instability;* (2) determine how a diagnosis of this phase of the degenerative process can be made; and (3) determine how treatment can be formulated, on a rational basis.[29] Later in that symposium, Nachemson concluded, "We certainly all agree that motion segment instability exists as a clinical problem, hitherto poorly defined." He thereby underscored the conflicting opinions about this topic.[43] In this chapter, the current knowledge about degenerative segmental instability is examined from a clinical and biomechanical perspective.

WHAT IS THE PATHOLOGIC NATURE OF SEGMENTAL INSTABILITY?

Kirkaldy-Willis has conceptualized three stages of the degenerative process: dysfunction, instability, and restabilization.[3] Based on his anatomic review, he has concluded that the unstable phase is characterized by a reduction in disc height and of the disc contents; laxity of the ligaments and facet capsules; and degeneration of the facet joints, which results in an "increased and abnormal range of movement." Although this pathologic description serves as a useful reference point, the clinical correlations have not been proved. However, it has been shown that stability of motion segments is reduced as a function of age and degeneration.[26, 27]

WHAT IS THE BIOMECHANICAL NATURE OF SEGMENTAL INSTABILITY?

Instability is best defined as a lack of stability, although this definition is not particularly useful. The common features in biomechanical descriptions of instability include increased mobility, abnormal spinal motions, and decreased stiffness of the functional spinal unit. The American Academy of Orthopaedic Surgeons defined segmental instability as an abnormal response to applied loads, characterized by activity in the motion segment beyond normal constraints. Pope and Panjabi attempted to illustrate the overall concept of instability by using diagrams (Fig. 1*A–D*).[52] Implicit in them is the crucial importance of the restraining muscles and ligaments to spinal stability, as illustrated in Figure 1*D*. This concept has been substantiated by the experimental observation of spinal buckling, which occurs under imposed axial compressive loads of 4 kg, but is less certain for single functional spinal units. Their working definition of instability is a loss of stiffness, as illustrated

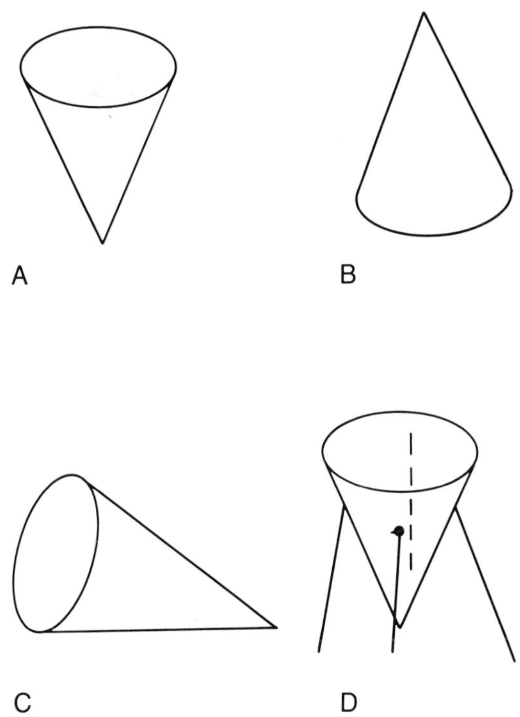

Figure 1 □ Illustration of stable and unstable equilibrium conditions. *A,* If slightly displaced, cone A will move into a new position of equilibrium (unstable equilibrium). *B,* Cone B will return to the same position (stable = equilibrium). *C,* Cone C will stay in the displaced position (neutral equilibrium). *D,* The unstable cone has been made stable by the addition of guy wires to hold it in position. (From Pope, M.H., and Panjabi, M.: Biomechanical definitions of spinal instability. Spine 10:255–256, 1985.)

in Figure 2; however, their conclusion is provocative: "Stability or instability is a mechanical entity, and should be treated as such. Definitions should not be based on suspected injury mechanism or clinical history." From their perspective, clinical measures to quantify instability would be the imposition of standardized external loads or motions, followed by the observation of internal motions or displacements by radiographic techniques.

This general concept of instability as a loss of stiffness has also been implicit in the experiments of Posner and coworkers,[53] who have sequentially sectioned posterior structures of the functional spinal unit and then measured the resultant displacements and coupled motions in six degrees of freedom (see Chapter 4). Based on these experiments, they have created a clinical scoring method for instability that has particular application to spinal trauma yet has proved useful in spinal degeneration.

Another approach has been to study the effects of various injuries that might be important not only to instability but to etiology of the degenerative process (see Chapter 4). A summary of the results of static loading suggests that instability is produced only when acute force applications are carried to failure; thus the relevance of their experiments to our understanding of acute traumatic injuries, or of instability produced by surgical interventions, is greater than to degenerative instability.[42]

Cyclic loading experiments, however, have produced changes that more closely approximate some of the attributes of motion segment degeneration. Brown and colleagues produced a tear throughout the annulus as a result of 1,000 cycles of a compression load of 63.6 N and five degrees of forward flexion at a frequency of 1,100 cycles/min.[6] Adams and Hutton simulated a day of heavy labor involving flexion and torsion at a rate of 40 times/min and produced visible distortions of the lamellae of the annulus fibrosus.[1] Liu and coworkers observed facet or vertebral body failures, or facet capsular ligament tears as a result of a cyclic torque of 0.5 Hz with a 445 N axial preload.[36] Generally, failures occurred in segments subjected to more than 1.5 degrees of axial rotation. Wilder and colleagues further examined the effects of load application at "the balance point."[69, 70] Tencer had pre-

Figure 2 □ A typical load deflection curve of a stable material (S) and an unstable material (U), manifested by loss of stiffness. The stiffness of material U is L/d_2. (From Pope, M.H., and Panjabi, M.: Biomechanical definitions of spinal instability. Spine 10:255–256, 1985.)

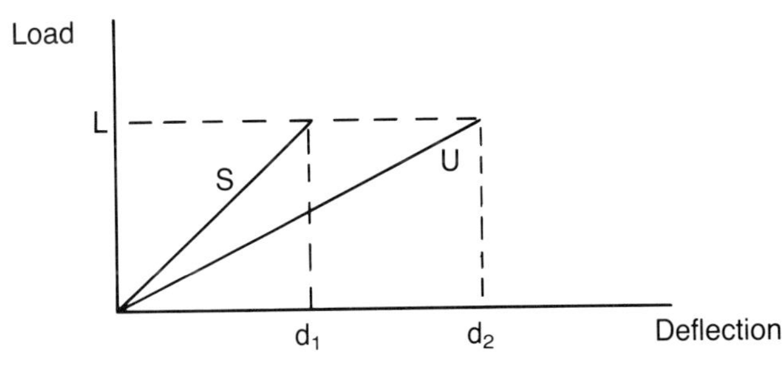

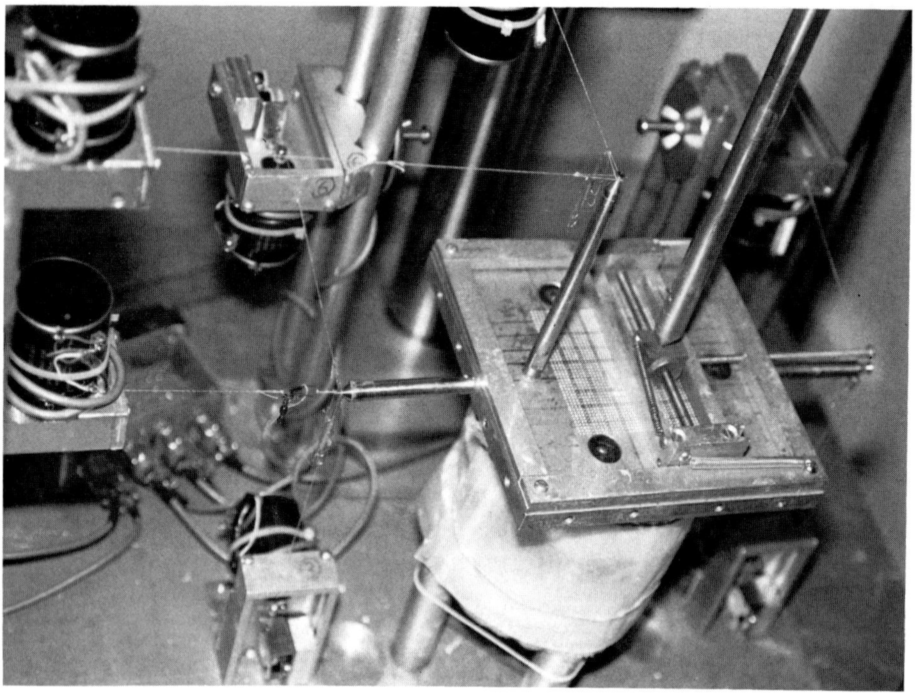

Figure 3 □ Motion sensor in place on materials testing apparatus. Note notches in ends of posts. Kevlar loops fit in notches and are connected to displacement potentiometers. Also, note two-dimensional adjustability of load application point (at end of load application link) for determining balance point location.

viously described this as the point or line at which compressive load application minimized the coupled flexion–extension rotation, but he dismissed its utility because of an inability to reproducibly identify its location.[64] Wilder likened the motion segment to a raft floating in water on which a person is standing. As the person changes position, the raft tends to tip or rotate, but there is a unique point at which no movement other than symmetric depression of the raft in water occurs, which is termed the balance point. He devised an experimental apparatus (Fig. 3) that permitted discrete compressive loads to be applied incrementally over the surface of the disc.[69, 70]

Wilder and colleagues found that the response at the vertical balance point was reproducible for specific loads (Fig. 4) and could be defined within fairly narrow limits (Fig. 5). Specimens were then vibration loaded at 5 Hz to simulate sitting or driving, from a minimum of 330 N to a maximum of 410 N, with a maximum exposure of 18,000 load cycles, and the new location of the balance point was then redetermined when also loaded at the location of the original balance point. Typically, a stable response was observed with minimal displacements, as shown in Figure 6. However, some specimens demonstrated an unstable (nonlinear, buckling) response, which was defined as motions exceeding 1.0 mm of translation or 1.0 degrees of rotation. These specimens also demonstrated loss of stiffness and frequently demonstrated rather dramatic, rapid rotations and displacements, as shown in Figure 7. For example, during a simulated overload event following 1 hour of simulated sitting (either at a desk or during driving), 40% of the segments buckled, often in a combination of flexion and lateral bending and apparently faster than the rate at which the muscles can respond. This motion would place the posterolateral region of the disc at risk of mechanical derangement. Wilder postulated that in the unstable spine minor perturbations may result in displacements sufficient to cause activation of mechanonociceptors, particularly if there was loss of fine neuromuscular control mechanisms. Implicit in this analysis is the concept of short segment buckling, in which the important constraints are the short muscles, such as the rotators, intertransversalis, and multifidi; this is in contrast to the long segment buck-

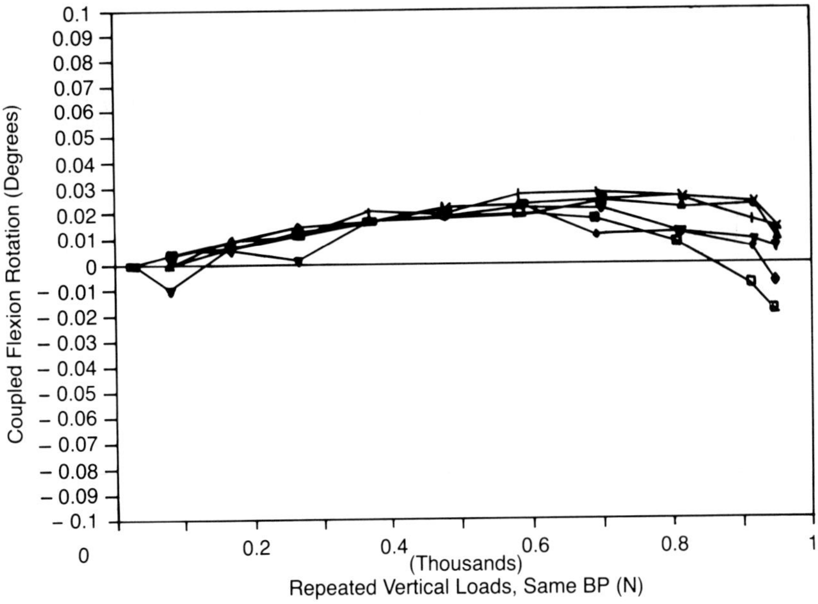

Figure 4 □ Coupled flexion rotation response resulting from a vertical load applied at the balance point. The load was applied six times. Note the consistency and small magnitude of the response.

Figure 5 □ This diagram shows the region in which the projections of the balance points were located in the midtransverse plane. Most of the balance points found were located in a rectangular region of the disc. The region is very thin (6% of the lateral diameter of the endplate) but relatively long (20% of the anteroposterior (AP) diameter of the end plate). It is bilaterally symmetric but is located posterior to the geometric center shown.

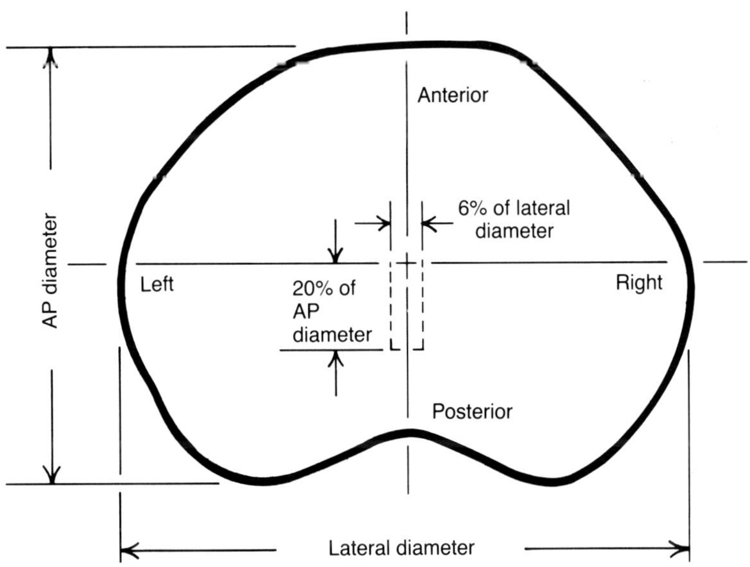

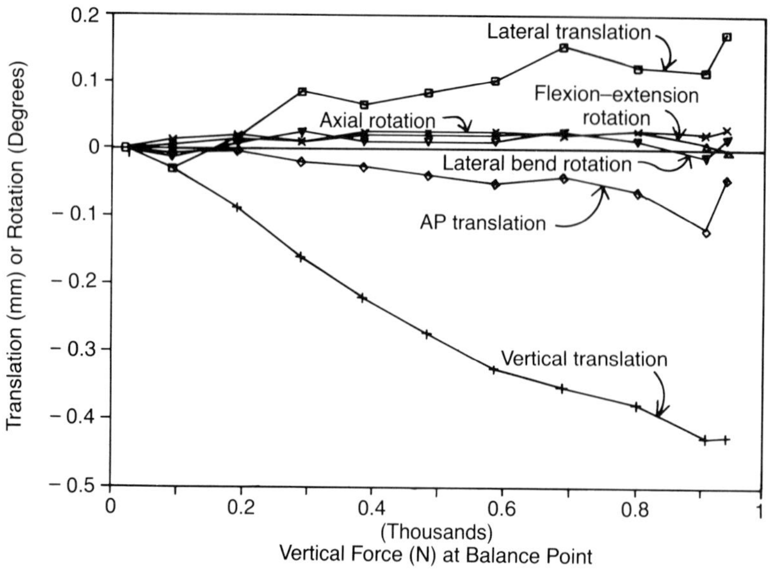

Figure 6 □ Segment response to load—main and coupled effects. Graph shows typical translation and rotation responses of a motion segment (L2–L3) to a compressive load applied at the original balance point. Note the virtually negligible rotations resulting from vertical load applied at the balance point.

ling that is under control of the larger paraspinal muscles.

Yet another experimental approach has been to create animal models that might simulate segmental instability. Earlier animal experiments were primarily directed toward the production of degenerative disc lesions as embodied in the "rat tail model" of Knutsson,[30] the bipedal rat model, and the immobilization models of degeneration produced by either anterior or posterior fusion. Sullivan and colleagues specifically created a model to replicate torsional instability by removing contralateral facets above and below the rabbit functional spinal unit.[62] Based on spinal radiographs, they concluded that this unstable condition resulted in a degenerative lesion of the intervertebral disc. Cauchoix replicated the experiment, using histochemical techniques as his outcome measure of degeneration. Stokes and coworkers similarly replicated the experiment, but they added a second model in which the facets were bilaterally removed.[61] Mechanical stability was assessed in experimental, sham-operated, and control (not op-

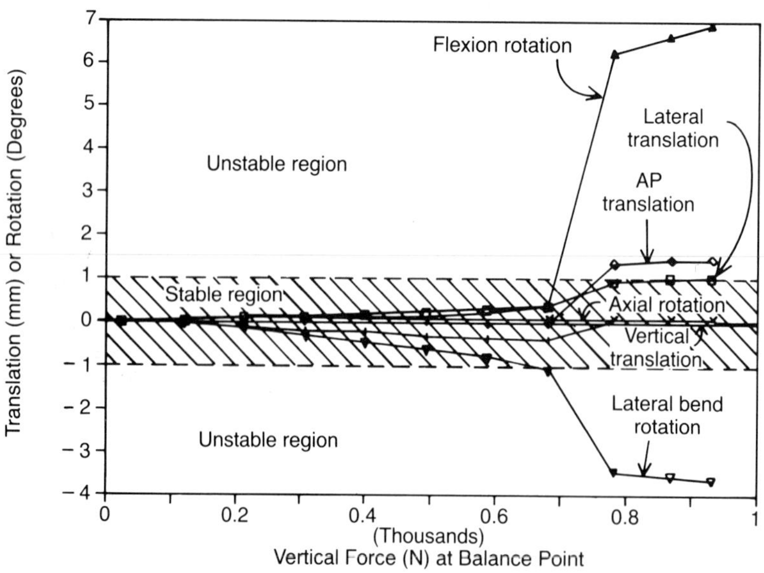

Figure 7 □ This graph shows the stable and unstable translation-load and rotation-load responses of an L2–L3 motion segment tested by using a 100-second load ramp. Note the sudden unstable or buckling response. This response occurred after a 1-hour intervention of vibration loading, loaded at the original balance point.

erated on) rabbits for time intervals of up to 1 year, using a stereophotogrammetric technique.

Degenerative changes were measured by both biochemical and histologic techniques. Although loss of stiffness and increased mobility were demonstrated by both models (Fig. 8), the affected segment tended to restabilize over time. This restabilization proceeded more rapidly in animals subjected to a high activity level than in low-activity-level animals. It was concluded that there was a healing tendency, possibly related to scar formation at the operative site, because osteophyte formation was not observed. These findings are also provocative in light of Rosenberg's observation of a fourfold increase in degenerative spondylolisthesis among diabetics.[57] Insofar as diabetes is associated with abnormalities in collagen cross-linking, soft tissue abnormalities may play a greater role than previously thought in the causation and healing capacity of some forms of degenerative instability.

In summary, the biomechanical data suggest that segmental instability, which most closely approximates the degenerative condition, may be produced by a variety of cyclic or vibrational loading conditions, rather than by acute static loads; the unstable functional spinal unit is characterized by a decrease in stiffness and a resultant increase in motion under load; both the quantity and quality of spinal motions are altered; the buckling motion appears to occur faster than the muscles can respond; the functional spinal segment may behave unstably with relatively minor perturbations, and there is a balance among factors that promote ongoing instability versus healing.

WHAT IS THE CLINICAL DEFINITION OF SEGMENTAL INSTABILITY?

The earliest description of segmental instability seems to be that of Hippocrates who stated, "When a gibbosity seizes a person, it occasions a crisis of the then existing disease." Whether he was referring to spinal tuberculosis or a late effect of trauma is uncertain, but the concept of instability as a crisis has persisted in some definitions.

The simplest of the definitions is that of Kirkaldy-Willis and Farfan, which states that segmental instability exists when minor perturbations produce acute pain.[28] However, Dupuis and coworkers stated, "Little is known about the true clinical presentation of motion segment laxity," and observed that they were unable to correlate specific symptoms with a specific type of instability.[9] They hypothesized that patients might present with a variety of symptoms, including ill-defined central low back pain without leg pain, lateral low back pain with "proximal" sciatica, dynamic nerve root entrapments, or a "catching sensation," which they concluded "is far from being a reliable and

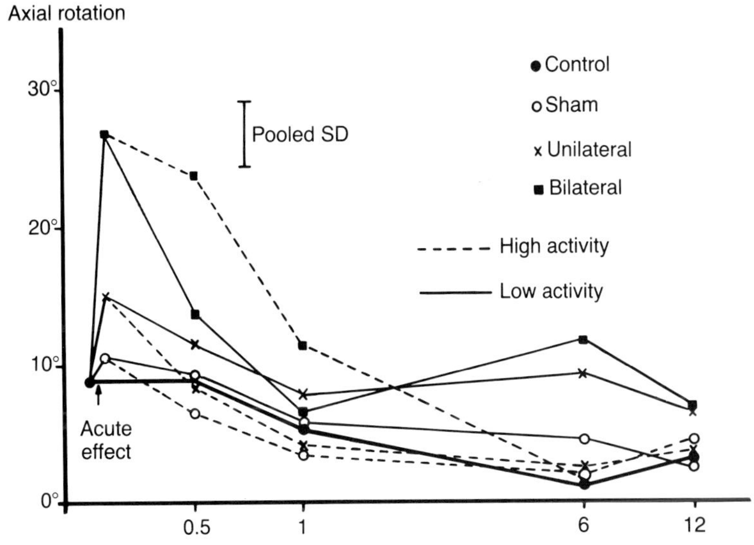

Figure 8 □ The degrees of axial rotation in the four experimental conditions (i.e., control, sham, unilateral facetectomy, and bilateral facetectomy) are illustrated as a function of time. Note that the initial instability in the facetectomized animals tends to become restored and to approach sham and control at 1, 6, and 12 months. (From Stokes, I.A.F., Counts, D.C., and Frymoyer, J.W.: Experimental instability in the rabbit lumbar spine [in press, Spine].)

consistent finding." Nachemson also commented on the well-known "instability catch" observed in patients with pathologic entities such as spondylolisthesis.[43] Paris is more explicit: "A complaint of 'giving away' or 'slipping out' and being able to 'twist it back into position' are definitely due to instability."[51] These later symptoms are reminiscent of the complaints that are frequently reported to represent the "manipulatable back."[22]

Equally elusive are the clinical signs of instability. Frequently noted signs include postural disturbances, such as rotoscoliosis, and intermittent neurologic symptoms and signs. Other observed signs are the presence of a step deformity that is reduced as the patient moves from the standing to the recumbent position, a hypertrophied band of muscle at the affected level that disappears on recumbency, and the palpation of abnormal and excessive motion during spinal flexion and extension. These latter observations, although reported to be reproducible in one study, were not replicated by others.[45]

In summary, much has been speculated about the clinical signs and symptoms of instability, but only minimal reliable and reproducible clinical information is available. There is some consensus that instability is to be suspected when minor activities and movements produce sudden back pain and when neurologic signs and symptoms are variable and often transitory and, furthermore, that a "catch" during spinal flexion and extension represent a clinical manifestation.

WHAT IS THE RADIOLOGIC NATURE OF SEGMENTAL INSTABILITY?

Numerous approaches have been used in the assessment of instability, ranging from plane radiographic findings to single-plane dynamic radiography and to more sophisticated techniques, such as biplanar radiography and the determination of instant centers of motion.

Plane Radiography of Segmental Instability

A variety of plane radiographic findings are reported to be suggestive of segmental instability.

Disc Space Narrowing

There is no question that a narrow lumbar intervertebral disc is degenerate, but the correlation between this finding and clinical symptoms and signs is poor. Torgerson[65] reported that L4–L5 narrowing was more likely to be associated with low back pain, an observation confirmed by Frymoyer and colleagues in their analysis of males of ages 18 to 55 years.[17] Not only was the L4–L5 narrowing more likely to be associated with present and previous complaints of low back pain, but it was also highly correlated with neurologic symptoms such as numbness, weakness, and sciatica. They speculated that such L4–L5 narrowing might represent an unstable motion segment, although they did not perform motion radiography. Others have noted the importance of asymmetric disc space collapse as yet another indicator of an unstable segment.

Osteophytes

Macnab first drew attention to the *traction spur* as an indicator of instability (Fig. 9). He concluded that the traction spur was produced by abnormal stresses on the outermost attachments of the annulus fibrosus, whereas the claw spur was simply a physiologic response to compressive loads and served to stabilize the spine.[40] This latter point has been emphasized by Nathan in his analyses of pathologic specimens and has also been confirmed in epidemiologic studies that correlate claw spurs with a history of heavier labor.[44] Farfan[10] has questioned the existence of the traction spur and suggested it is simply a radiographic aberration produced by rotation.

Spinal Malalignment

There is little doubt that observed spinal malalignments have been most heavily used in the definition of segmental instabilities. Although Junghanns had recognized forward displacement of L4 on L5, a condition he termed *pseudospondylolisthesis,*[25] Macnab's classic article in 1950 focused attention on the clinical signs and symptoms that accompanied the deformity.[39] Others had noted retrolisthetic deformities and concluded that they were causative of low back symptoms and neurologic complaints. Attention has also been directed to other deformities, par-

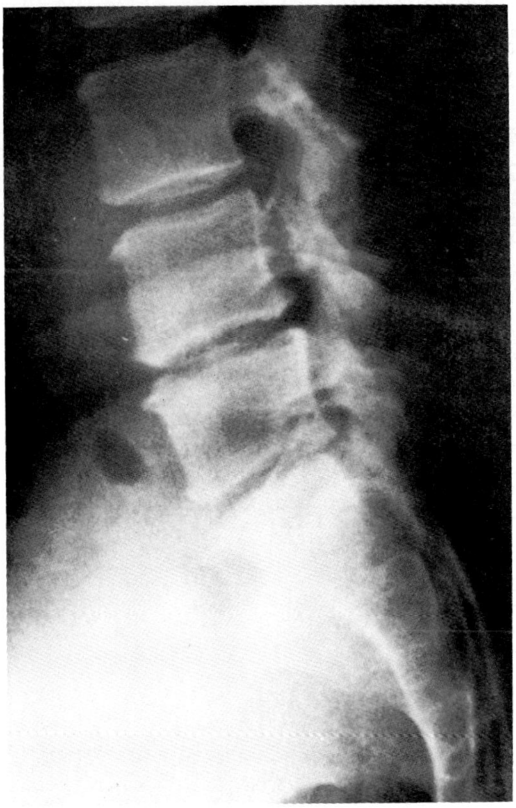

Figure 9 □ Lateral radiograph demonstrating traction spurs at L3–L4 and L4–L5 levels. Note that the spurs are separated from the vertebral end plate by greater than 3 mm, thus fulfilling Macnab's criterion. (From Frymoyer, J.W., Newberg, A., Pope, M.H., et al.: Spine radiographs in patients with low-back pain. J. Bone Joint Surg. 66A:1048–1055, 1984.)

ticularly those that suggest an abnormality in axial rotation. Plane radiographic findings of significance have included rotational deformities of the pedicles and disruption of the normal alignment of the spinous processes, as visualized on the anteroposterior view (Fig. 10).[18] However, the evidence of instability on plane spinal radiographs is presumptive, unless the deformity progresses over time. Newman and Stone noted that degenerative spondylolisthesis progresses at an average of 2 mm every 4 years.[46] Wiltse and Winter have shown "at-risk" signs of progressive deformity and slip (Fig. 11*A–E*) in spondylolisthesis.[72] However, many deformities that might be presumed to be unstable are unassociated with symptoms. For example, the epidemiologic studies of Valkenburg and Haanen have shown that degenerative spondylolisthesis is a common finding, yet many of the individuals they studied had no history of low back pain (Table 1).[66]

Vertebral Body Position

The position of the vertebral bodies relative to the pelvis has been reported as significant, particularly in the etiology of degenerative spondylolisthesis. In his original description of pseudospondylolisthesis, Junghanns[25] noted the condition to be most common at the fourth lumbar level, which was later confirmed by Macnab,[39] and Newman and Stone.[46] Rosenberg's analysis of pathologic and patient material led him to conclude the deformity occurred above a stabilized lumbar segment conferred by either transitional vertebrae or a long transverse process of L5.[57] These anatomic features, therefore, were proposed to place greater stresses on the adjacent L4–L5 level. Fitzgerald's[14] clinical analysis also showed the supracristal line to be lower than in nonaffected patients, a contention supported by Allbrook's studies.[2] These same biomechanical considerations led MacGibbon and Farfan[38] to analyze degenerative patterns as a function of the length of the L5 transverse processes and the relative position of L4 to the intercristal line (Fig. 12). They concluded that an elongated L5 transverse process and a deep-seated L5 vertebra conferred stability on the lumbosacral joint, and thus exposed the L4–L5 intervertebral joint to greater torsional stress and axial rotational deformity. Based on these analyses and the examination of pathologic specimens, Farfan concluded that the major deformity in degenerative spondylolisthesis is rotational.[11] Recently, the analysis by Leong and coworkers of the iliolumbar ligament has reinforced the general concept of these structures protecting the L5 vertebral level, thus placing greater mechanical stresses upon the L4–L5 interspace.[34] This same general hypothesis was tested by Frymoyer and colleagues, who could not demonstrate a predictable relationship between intercristal line position or transverse process length as they affected degeneration at the L4–L5 levels in males of ages 18 to 55 years.[17]

A variant of the mechanical conditions proposed to be important to the cause of L4–L5 degenerative spondylolisthesis also appears to be important in patients who have undergone previous spinal fusion. Long-

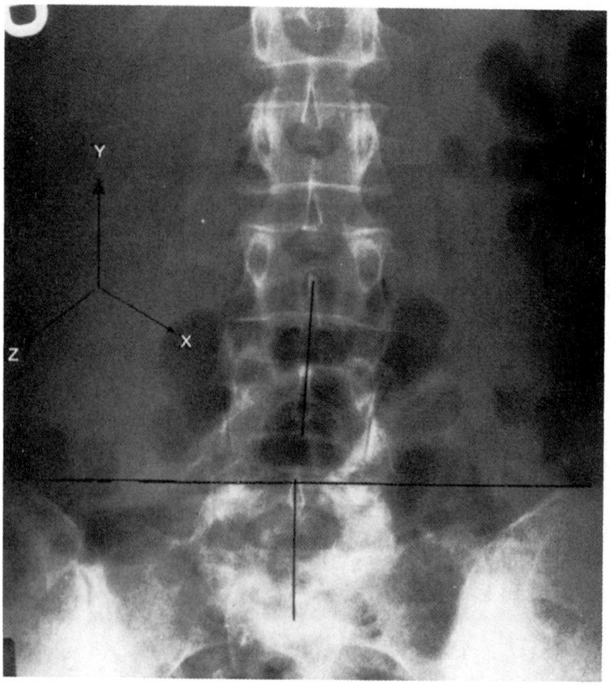

Figure 10 □ AP radiograph demonstrates discontinuity of the L4–L5 spinous process line, one possible sign of a rotational instability. (From Frymoyer, J.W., and Selby, D.K.: Segmental instability. Rationale for treatment. Spine 10:280–286, 1985.)

term follow-up studies have shown that 20% to 45% of patients demonstrate instability (defined in this instance as forward translations of at least 3 mm on flexion–extension films) above a prior L4–sacrum fusion.[16, 33] Moreover, analyses of spinal motion above fusions have indicated that increased shear stresses are produced—as measured by biplanar radiographs—in postoperative patients,[59] in laboratory studies of simulated spinal fusions,[56] and by mathematic modeling.[54]

Motion Radiography in Segmental Instability

The biomechanical concept of segmental instability explicitly proposes that increased motions and displacements are important descriptors for that condition. The idea that increased motion alone is of unique importance is simplistic, in view of the wide variations in normal spinal motion as a function of age, sex, athletic training, and body habitus.[53, 63] Thus, greater importance has

Figure 11 □ Radiographic signs of stability and instability in spondylolisthesis. *A*, The extent of anterior displacement, or slip, is expressed as a percentage obtained by dividing A, the amount of displacement (determined by the relationship of the posterior part of the cortex of the fifth lumbar vertebra to the posterior part of the cortex of the first sacral vertebra), by A^1, the maximum AP diameter of the first sacral vertebra, and multiplying by 100. The smaller drawing shows how to determine the posteroinferior tip of the body of the fifth lumbar vertebra, which is often indistinct because of either hypoplasia or spur formation in this area (x on this drawing). Line a is drawn parallel to the front of the body of the fifth lumbar vertebra. Line b is drawn perpendicular to line a, to the posterosuperior tip of the body of the fifth lumbar vertebra (a point that, usually, is easily located). Line c is drawn parallel to line b and is exactly the same length as line b. The point at which line c intersects the inferior border of the body of the fifth lumbar vertebra is point x. Point x is the relative constant used in measuring the percentage of slip. *B*, Sacral inclination (g) is determined by drawing a line along the posterior border of the first sacral vertebra and measuring the angle created by this line intersecting a true vertical line. *C*, Sagittal rotation is the term used to express the angular relationship between the fifth lumbar vertebra and first sacral vertebra. It is determined by extending a line along the anterior border of the body of the fifth lumbar vertebra until it intersects a line drawn along the posterior border of the body of the first sacral vertebra. The drawing on the right shows an alternative method of measuring sagittal rotation, to be used when the degree of olisthesis is small and lines a and b do not intersect. A third line (c) is added, perpendicular to line a. Lines c and b intersect to form the angle of sagittal rotation.

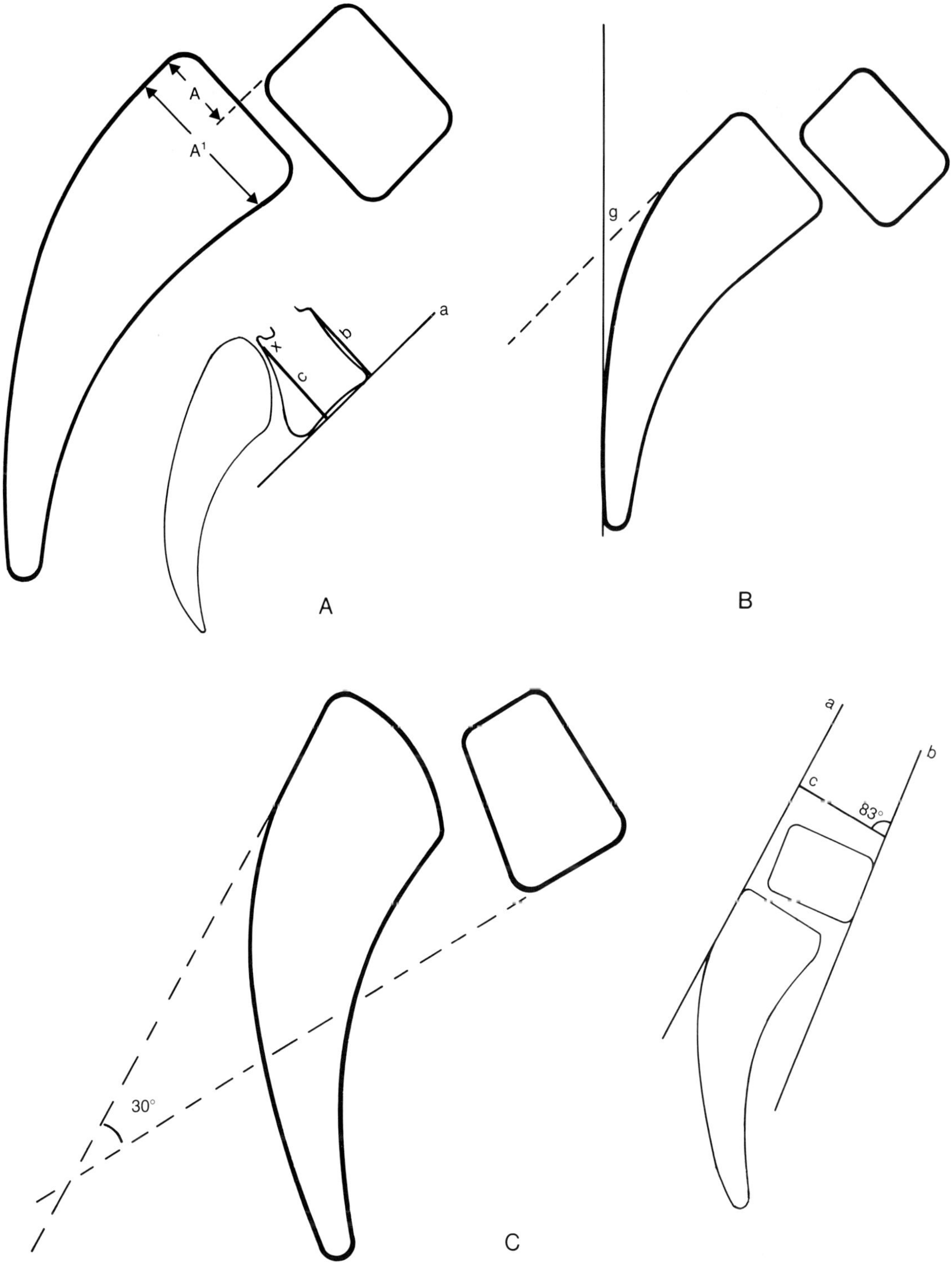

Figure 11 *See legend on opposite page*

Illustration continued on following page

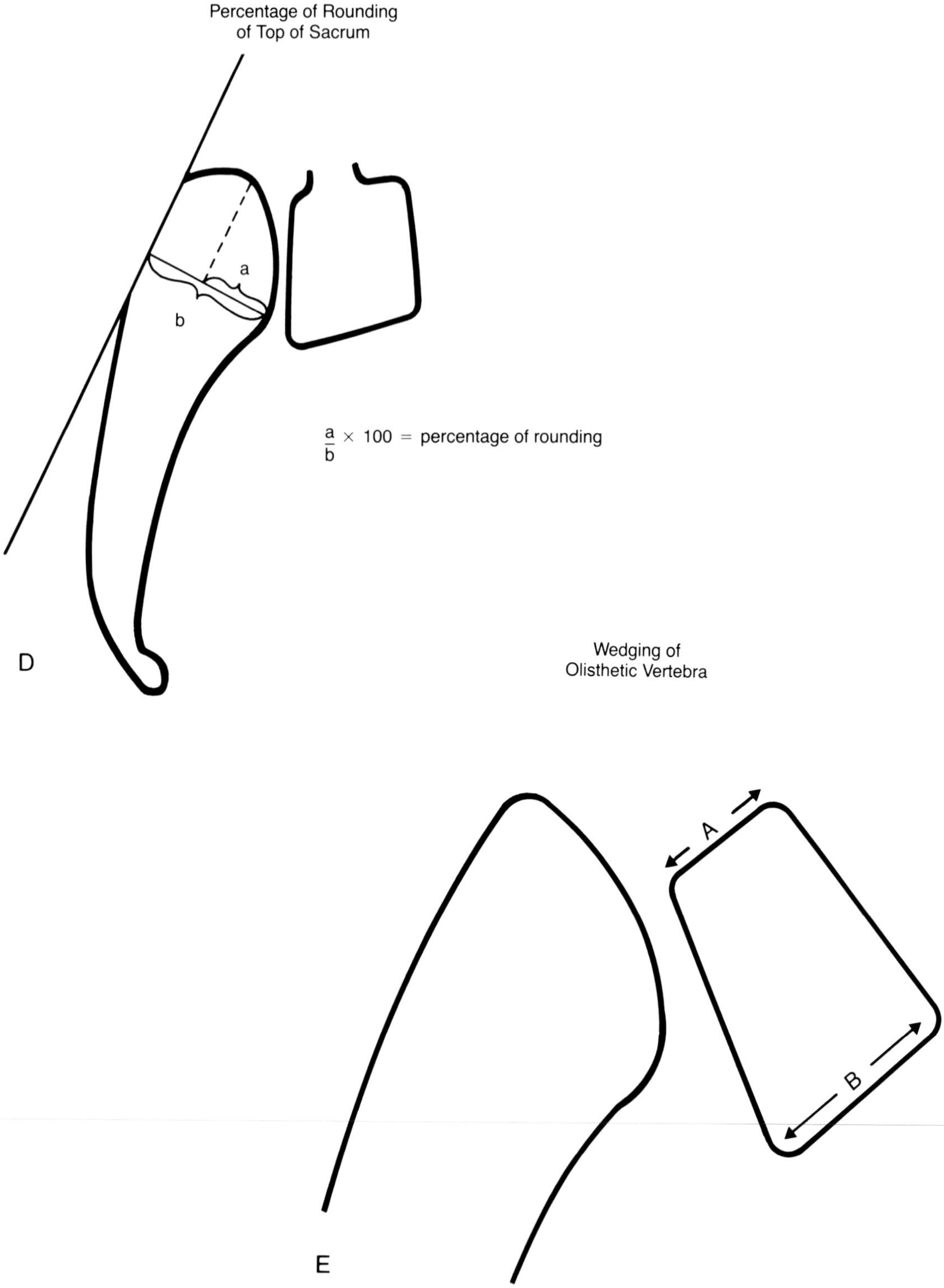

Figure 11 *Continued D,* Rounding of the top of the centrum of the first sacral vertebra is expressed as the relationship between lines a and b, drawn as shown. The result, when multiplied by 100, yields the percentage of rounding of the first sacral vertebra. *E,* Wedging of the olisthetic vertebra is expressed as a percentage determined by dividing line A by line B, drawn as shown, and multiplying by 100. (From Wiltse, L.L., and Winter, R.B.: Terminology and measurement of spondylolisthesis. J. Bone Joint Surg. 65A:768–772, 1983.)

Table 1 □ Age and Sex-Specific Distribution of Radiologic Abnormalities in Men and Women as a Function of Age*

	PERCENTAGES ACCORDING TO AGE GROUP					TOTAL PERCENTAGE
	35	45	55	65	75	
Men						
Lumbar disc degeneration						
Grade 2	32.5	26.9	31.9	31.8	32.6	29.9
Grade ¾	6.4	16.1	27.2	37.9	38.3	21.7
Total grade 2+	38.9	43.0	59.1	69.7	70.9	51.6
(Pseudo)spondylolisthesis						
Grade 2	1.3	2.7	7.0	5.5	7.0	4.1
Grade ¾	0.9	1.5	1.8	3.0	2.3	1.7
Total grade 2+	2.2	4.2	8.8	8.5	9.3	5.8
Immobile lumbar segment						
One	—	14.7	19.4	21.4	14.0	17.0
Two	—	5.2	7.8	11.4	9.3	7.1
Three or four	—	2.2	3.0	6.0	20.9	4.2
Total	—	22.1	30.2	38.8	44.2	28.3
Women						
Lumbar disc degeneration						
Grade 2	32.0	33.9	32.5	31.5	29.4	32.4
Grade ¾	13.5	19.3	25.1	32.1	30.4	23.2
Total grade 2+	45.5	53.2	57.6	63.6	59.8	55.6
(Pseudo)spondylolisthesis						
Grade 2	1.2	2.2	10.6	11.5	17.5	7.1
Grade ¾	0.8	0.9	1.2	2.9	7.8	2.0
Total grade 2+	2.0	3.1	11.8	14.4	25.3	9.1
Immobile lumbar segments						
One	—	19.9	24.1	25.3	19.6	22.0
Two	—	5.9	7.2	8.2	10.3	7.2
Three or four	—	3.7	3.4	7.9	20.6	6.4
Total	—	29.5	34.7	41.4	50.5	35.8

*Reproduced by permission from Valkenburg, Hans A., and Haanen, Huub C. M.: The epidemiology of low back pain. *In* American Academy of Orthopaedic Surgeons: Symposium on Idiopathic Low Back Pain. St. Louis, 1982, The C. V. Mosby Co.

been attached to abnormalities in the plane of motion, because each motion segment can move in six degrees of freedom, along or about three mutually perpendicular axes.[67]

In numerous studies these abnormal motions have been analyzed by flexion–extension, lateral bending, biplanar radiography, or sophisticated analyses of the instant center of rotation.

Knutsson is credited with demonstrating abnormal translations during spinal flexion and extension.[30] During forward flexion, anterior displacements along the z axis greater than 3 mm were postulated to be the earliest sign of intervertebral disc degeneration. Many techniques have been used to quantify these displacements, such as those described by Frymoyer and coworkers,[16] Arkin,[4] Lindahl,[35] and more recently Dupuis and colleagues,[9] whose method is shown in Figure 13*A*, *B*. Knutsson's sign[30] has also been demonstrated in patients with and without low back pain and in those who have undergone lumbar disc excision and lumbar spinal fusions.[16, 32] Similarly, abnormal motions and translations have been observed in the negative z axis (i.e., retrospondylolisthesis), where Lehmann has reported that 30% of patients with low back pain have this finding.[33] During lateral bend, discontinuities in spinous process patterns have been reported,[9] and dynamic computed tomographic (CT) scans are reported to show abnormal and increased rotations about the y axis.[28]

Others have attempted to measure abnormal motion by sophisticated radiographic techniques. For example, Gertzbein and associates have developed a measurement of abnormal motion based upon computations of the instant center of movement.[20] Figure 14*A* illustrates a normal locus found in a nondegenerate segment, whereas Figure 14*B* illustrates a pattern of abnormal motion observed in a degenerating segment. To date, these investigators have not demonstrated

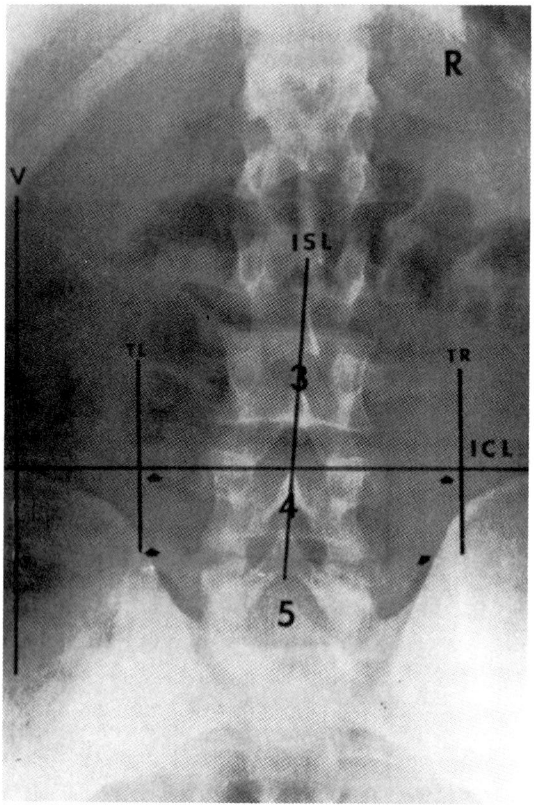

Figure 12 □ AP radiograph demonstrating the construction of the intercristal line (ICL). The interaction of this line with the disc and vertebral body defines greater or less stability of the spine. For example, when the ICL interacts with the body of L5, the L4–L5 level is unprotected and is subject to greater torsional loads. The length of the transverse processes is also considered to be a factor in stability. (From Frymoyer, J.W., Newberg, A., Pope, M.H., et al.: Spine radiographs in patients with low-back pain. J. Bone Joint Surg. 66A(7):1048–1055, 1984.)

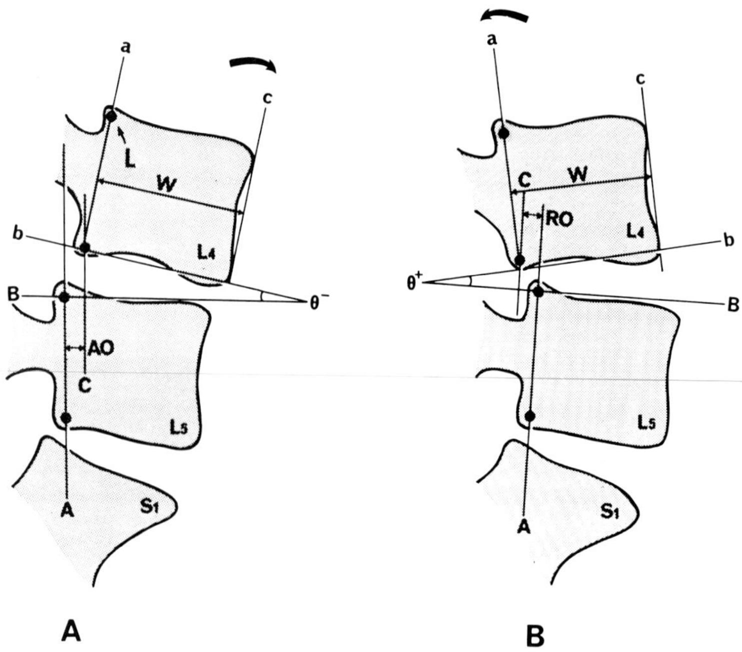

Figure 13 □ *A, B,* Radiographic method of Dupuis and coworkers for the calculation of horizontal and angular displacement in flexion–extension views. (From Dupuis, P.R., Yong-Hing, K., Cassidy, J.D., and Kirkaldy-Willis, W.H.: Radiologic diagnosis of degenerative lumbar spinal instability. Spine 10:262–276, 1985.)

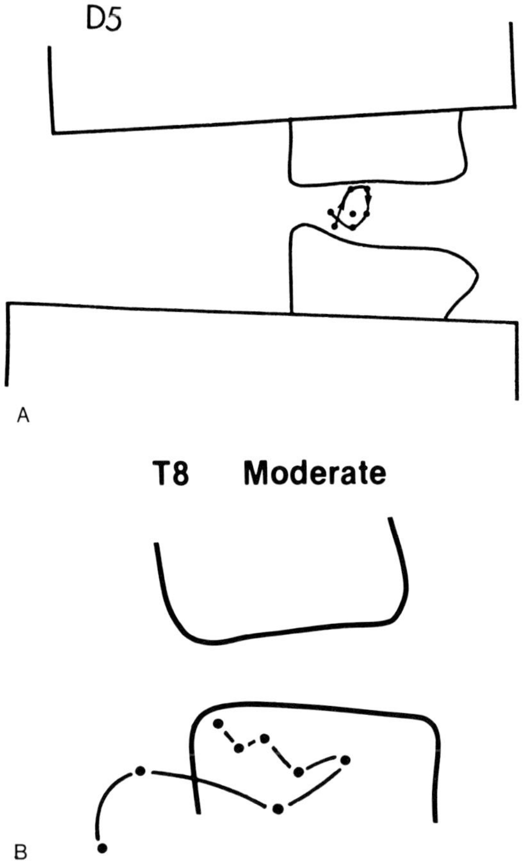

Figure 14 □ *A, B,* The movement of centrodes of motion in mildly and moderately degenerate discs under conditions of flexion and extension is plotted. Note the more erratic and longer course of the centrode in the more severely degenerate condition. (From Gertzbein, S.D., Seligman, J., Holtby, R., et al: Centrode patterns and segmental instability in degenerative disc disease. Spine 10:257–261, 1985.)

the applicability of their method for the clinical setting.

Because spine motion is three-dimensional, other investigators have developed systems for measurement, using biplanar radiographic techniques. Some of these methods have relied on the identification of bony landmarks as reference points,[7, 59] and have developed optimization techniques to minimize the inherent errors that are introduced in the localization of such landmarks.

Others[48–50] have increased the accuracy of the method by implanting discrete metallic markers, which permit accuracy within the range of 0.1 to 0.2 mm, a resolution far greater than that possible using bony landmarks.

The summation of results obtained from these experiments is as follows: (1) Abnormal stresses can be identified, which are principally shear along the forward z axis, particularly in patients who have previously undergone spinal fusion at L4–sacrum.[59] (2) Abnormal coupling of spinal motion can be shown in patients with and without low back pain, but the patterns observed are often paradoxic and bear little relationship to clinical symptoms.[71] (3) Instability is not demonstrated in a predictable fashion in patients with isthmic spondylolisthesis. (4) Patients with spinal fusions have continued movements of at least two degrees, despite apparent relief of symptoms and radiographically solid arthrodesis. (5) Patients who fulfill the clinical criterion of degenerative segmental instability do not have predictable patterns of abnormal motion. In this last study, Stokes and colleagues[60] selected patients who fulfilled the clinical criterion reported to be suggestive of segmental instability, namely, low back pain with recurrent bouts of increasing severity brought on by minimal mechanical stresses. This patient group represented less than 1% of those entering a low back clinic. Each patient was subjected to a detailed protocol of flexion–extension radiography, CT scan, facet blocks at the suspected levels of lesions, and biplanar motion radiography. Although good correlations were demonstrated between flexion–extension mobility measured on plane films and that measured on biplanar radiographs (Table 2), increased shear stresses could be identified (Fig. 15) and no clinically correlated patterns of instability could be demonstrated. The most intriguing possible explanation of their results is that instability cannot be accurately identified in terminal radiographs, either because the instability catch occurs in the middle ranges of spinal motion or, as pointed out by Dupuis,[9] because muscle splinting protects motion in the painful patient. The first of these considerations led Gertzbein and associates[20] to develop their analytic method to determine the instant centers of rotation in cadaveric specimens with varying degrees of intervertebral disc degeneration. The illustration and interpretation of their results have been described previously. Currently, others are experimenting with sophisticated biplanar cineradiography in an attempt to overcome the possible limitations of more

Table 2 □ Sagittal Plane Range of Motion—All Patients

	FLEXION (DEGREE) (STANDING FILMS) (n = 50)	FLEXION (SITTING BIPLANAR) (n = 78)		AP SHEAR (mm) (BIPLANAR FILMS) (n = 78)
		Degrees	Percentage of Total	
L1–L2	9.4 (3–17)	8.8 (2.3–15.6)	24.5 (7.6–57)	1.67 (−1.8–7.3)
L2–L3	9.2 (3–16)	10.0 (3.4–20.2)	28.7 (16–26)	1.69 (−1.9–7.2)
L3–L4	10.3 (2–26)	10.1 (1.2–21.4)	27.2 (6.5–63)	1.35 (−1.9–4.6)
L4–L5	9.5 (−1–22)	8.5 (−3.3–18.8)	19.6 (−99–46)	0.86 (−3.3–7.0)
L5–S1	9.5 (−3–20)	4.6 (1–19)	—	—
All levels	9.6	8.4		1.38

The mean value and the range in parentheses are given in each case.
Percentages are based on the motion in the four lumbar interspaces L1–L2 through L4–L5.

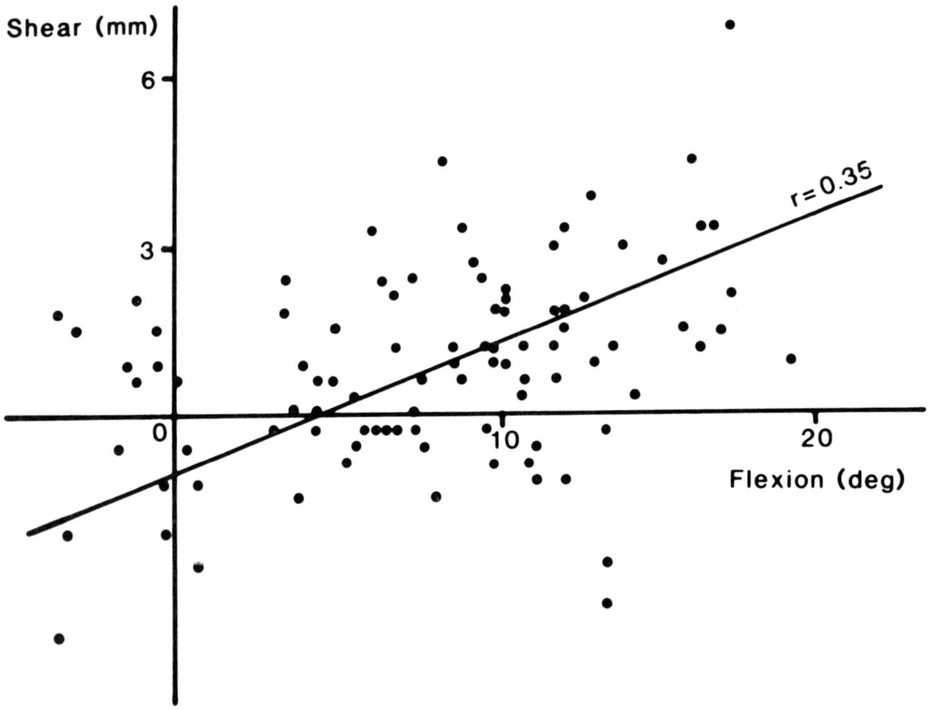

Figure 15 □ The relationship between shear at vertebral levels and range of motion at these levels. Note increased motion is associated with increased shear. (From Stokes, I.A.F., and Frymoyer, J.W.: Segmental motion and instability. Spine 12:688–691, 1987.)

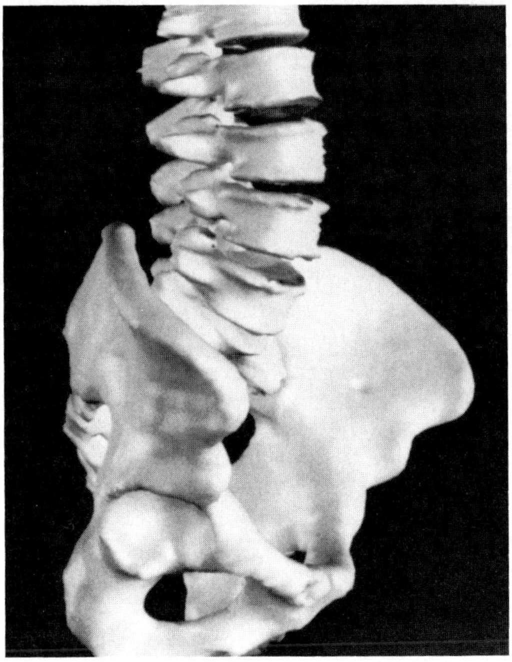

Figure 16 □ Computer-generated model of the spine taken from biplanar motion radiography. Using such models, the 3-D motion of the spine can be precisely quantified. (Courtesy of Robert P. Hubbard, Department of Biomechanics, College of Osteopathic Medicine, Michigan State University.)

conventional biplanar radiography (Fig. 16).[23]

WHAT OTHER METHODS IDENTIFY SEGMENTAL INSTABILITY?

As proposed by Pope and Panjabi,[52] one method of identifying instability is the application of a standardized external load. Historically this technique was proposed as useful in the identification of unstable isthmic and degenerative spondylolisthesis,[37] by comparing radiographs of patients in standing and recumbent positions. Of these patients, 26% showed increased displacements during standing. Evidence of this was cited as important to the diagnosis of an unstable lesion. Recently this technique was used in suspected degenerative instabilities by applying traction, followed by a standard axial load, and measuring displacements before and after the load application. Twenty-four of 45 patients with spondylolisthesis of L5, seven of seven patients with degenerative spondylolisthesis, and 37 of 65 patients with retrospondylolisthesis demonstrated increased displacements.[15]

An alternative method has been to measure the response of patients to immobilization. Historically, the positive response to spinal bracing has been used as an indication for spinal fusion, but it is now well known that braces produce uncertain immobilization, and indeed, may cause increased motions and stresses in the lower lumbar spine (see Chapter 4). Fidler has shown that a one and one half hip spica can produce immobility, at least as determined in the flexion–extension axis.[13] A more dramatic method of testing response to immobilization has been offered by Olerud and coworkers,[47] who have tested pain responses to temporary placement of external fixation devices across the intervertebral level suspected to be causative of symptoms. Their early results are graphically shown in Figure 17. Obviously, such an invasive method re-

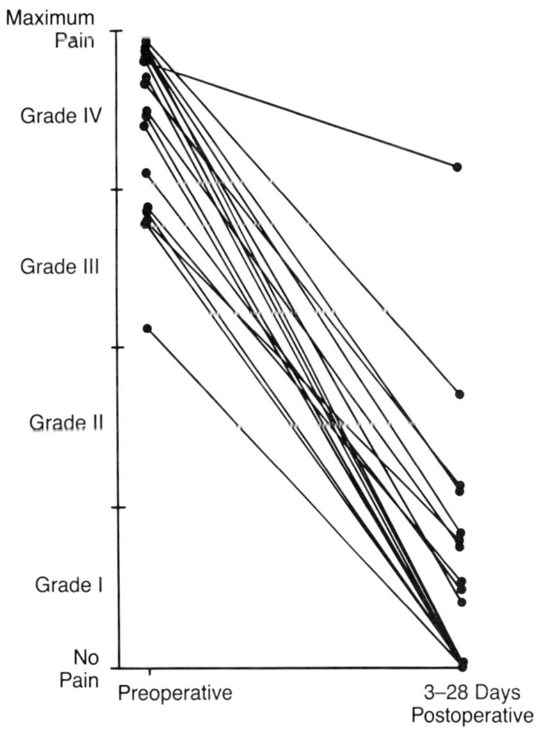

Figure 17 □ Graphic representation of the subjective pain responses of patients before and after the application of external fixation to provide rigid immobilization. (From Olerud, S., Sjostrom, L., Karlstrom, G., and Hamberg, M.: Spontaneous effect of increased stability of the lower spine in cases of severe chronic back pain—the answer of an external transpeduncular fixation test. Clin. Orthop. Rel. Res. 203:67–74, 1986.)

quires far more clinical research before its use can be advocated.

SUMMARY OF EXISTING KNOWLEDGE OF SEGMENTAL INSTABILITY

There seems to be little doubt that in the lumbar spine unstable conditions exist that are best understood in acute spinal trauma, infections, and tumors. They are partially understood in isthmic and congenital spondylolisthesis and only incompletely understood in spinal degeneration. The accumulated biomechanical knowledge indicates that a working hypothesis of instability is loss of normal stiffness and increased and abnormal motions that may be provoked by minimal perturbations of the system. It also suggests that neuromuscular control mechanisms and even soft tissue materials properties are important to etiology. However, clinical symptoms and signs along with plane and motion radiographic confirmation are not sufficiently sensitive or specific to allow clinical syndromes to be described with complete accuracy. Although segmental instability is often used as a synonym of degenerative spondylolisthesis, it is quite clear that numerous other conditions are potentially unstable. The challenge, therefore, is to develop sufficiently sensitive and specific diagnostic tests to more clearly define these syndromes.

AUTHORS' CURRENT CLINICAL APPROACH TO INSTABILITY

Earlier, we defined segmental instability as a loss of motion segment stiffness such that force application to that motion segment produces greater displacement(s) than would be seen in a normal structure.[18, 19] To that earlier definition should be added the following qualifying criteria: the condition causes pain, has the potential to result in progressive deformity, and places neurologic structures at risk. We have previously speculated that, in degenerative segmental instability, "the pattern of deformity should reflect the original directions of instability; hence, the analysis of fixed deformities is one possible method of classifying the preexistent instability state."[18] However, biplanar radiography was not sufficiently accurate to permit us to establish this diagnostic classification before a deformity was evident. We still believe the previously published classification is a useful starting point, but there are no clinical symptoms or physical and radiographic signs sensitive or specific enough to make an accurate diagnosis possible until the later phase of instability. Moreover, we have expanded our original classification to include other degenerative conditions. Important general principles of low back pain diagnosis and treatment are essential in using such a classification scheme.

First, the successful outcome of treatment directly correlates with the precision of the preoperative diagnosis. At one extreme, we can predict successful outcomes of greater than 90% in the treatment of lumbar disc herniation when the symptoms, signs, and radiographic images are highly correlated. At the other extreme, spinal fusion for the diagnosis of low back pain has failure rates that may exceed 70%. By applying this principle to segmental instability, one can see that the likelihood of successful treatment is enhanced when the following conditions are present:

1. A deformity exists (i.e., the patient is already near the end stage of the Kirkaldy-Willis instability phase). The deformity should be visible on plane AP and lateral radiographs. The progression of this deformity over time, as measured by serial radiographs, and its accompanying pain are the most certain evidence of instability. Less certain but presumptive evidence exists when the deformity increases under applied physiologic forces such as spinal motions in the plane of deformity or when increased by axial compressive loads.

We are very cautious in our interpretation of CT and magnetic resonance imaging (MRI). Although disc bulging is proposed by Kirkaldy-Willis[29] as evidence of the unstable phase, this finding is nonspecifically observed in many individuals with and without low back pain.[68] A similar and perhaps greater concern exists for MRI, which is highly sensitive to degenerative changes in the intervertebral disc but is most likely a nonspecific finding in many patients.

2. The clinical signs and symptoms correlate with the patient's level(s) of sus-

pected instability. Among these signs and symptoms, we believe there is the following hierarchy of diminishing importance: neurologic complaints with findings are the most reliable; referred pain, which conforms to sclerotomes consistent with the level of suspected instability, is the next most reliable; the history of repeated episodes of pain brought on by decreasing mechanical overload is the least reliable; and the complaint of low back pain only is unreliable. Rotoscoliosis and instability catches are suggestive but uncertain symptoms.

3. The more focal the lesion, the greater the probability of successful treatment. With the exception of scoliotic and postsurgical multilevel deformities, most instabilities involve a single functional spinal unit segment.
4. Implicit in the diagnosis of segmental instability is that future treatment may require stabilization. Because we do not have the clinical tools necessary to diagnose instability in its earlier phases, stabilization by surgical arthrodesis should be approached cautiously, and general muscular rehabilitation seems to be a rational approach. Moreover, the decision to perform a stabilization procedure should be governed by considerations such as patient age and the presence or absence of neurologic symptoms, as well as by radiographic signs that the patient is advancing into the stabilization phase, such as the presence of marked disc space narrowing and osteophyte formation.

AUTHORS' CURRENT CLASSIFICATION OF SEGMENTAL INSTABILITY

Table 3 provides the overall classification of segmental instability that we currently utilize in our clinic, whereas Table 4 delineates a more complete classification of the conditions that we believe constitute degenerative segmental instabilities.

Primary Instabilities

Type I: Axial Rotational Instability

It is uncertain whether Type I represents a specific subset of instability or is identical with the Type II translational instability There is no doubt that rotational deformities have been identified in pathologic specimens of degenerative spondylolisthesis. The radiographic evidence suggestive of rotation includes malalignments of the spinous processes on anteroposterior radiographs and a rotational deformity of the pedicles on lateral radiographs. Additional criteria thought to place a patient at risk are either a segmentation abnormality or an elongation of the L5 transverse process. In most instances, the deformity affects the L4–L5 intervertebral level and clinical signs, therefore, it may

Table 3 □ Lumbar Segmental Instabilities

I. Fractures and fracture dislocation

II. Infections involving anterior columns with
   A. Progressive loss of vertebral body height and deformity despite antibiotic treatment.
   B. Progressing neurologic symptoms, despite appropriate antibiotic treatment, if accompanied by criterion IIA.

III. Primary and metastatic neoplasms with
   A. Progressive loss of vertebral body height and deformity.
   B. Progressing neurologic symptoms, if symptoms are not the result of direct tumor involvement of the spinal cord, cauda equina, or nerve roots, but result from the conditions of IIIA.
   C. Postsurgical, following resection of neoplasms.

IV. Spondylolisthesis
   A. Isthmic spondylolisthesis
      1. L5–S1 progressive deformity in a child, particularly when accompanied by the radiographic risk signs of Wiltse. Rarely an unstable lesion in the adult.
      2. L4–L5 probably an unstable lesion in the adult.

V. Degenerative

VI. Scoliosis—any progressive deformity in a child further subclassified, per the Scoliosis Research Society.

Table 4 □ Degenerative Segmental Instabilities

A. Primary instabilities
   1. Axial rotational instability.
   2. Translational instability.
   3. Retrolisthetic instability.
   4. Progressing degenerative scoliosis.
   5. (?) Disc disruption syndrome.

B. Secondary instabilities
   1. Post–disc excision—subclassified according to the pattern of instability as described under primary instabilities.
   2. Post–decompressive laminectomy
      a. Accentuation of pre-existent deformity
      b. New deformity, i.e., no deformity existed at the time of original decompression. Further subclassified as for primary instabilities.
   3. Post–spinal fusion
      a. Above or below a spinal fusion, subclassified as for primary instabilities.
      b. Pseudoarthrosis.

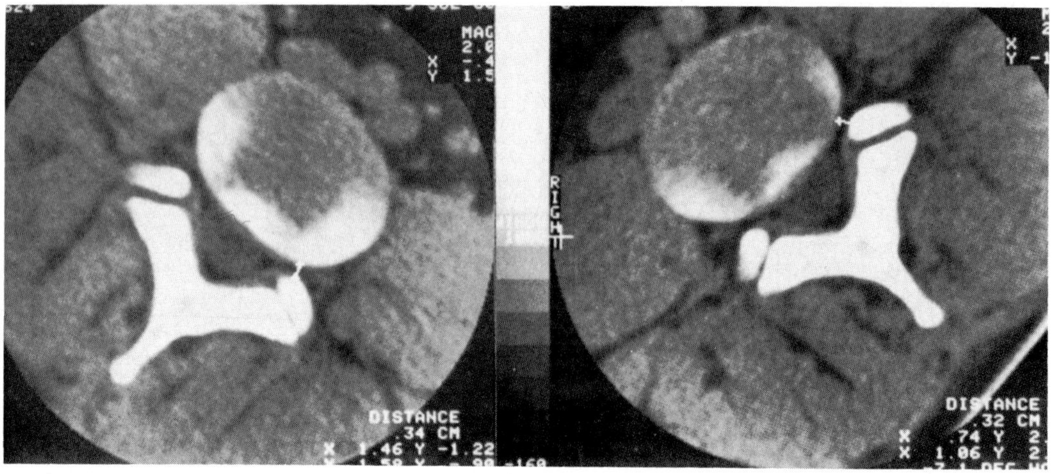

Figure 18 □ CT scans of spine taken with rotational stresses. According to the authors, increased movement and gapping of the facet joints should be observed. (From Kirkaldy-Willis, W.H., and Farfan, H.F.: Instability of the lumbar spine. Clin. Orthop. Rel. Res. 165:110, 1982.)

include L4 or L5 nerve root dysfunction, sclerotome pain in the region of the greater trochanter, and historic or clinical evidence of rotoscoliosis. Nonspecific radiographic findings include annular bulging and asymmetric narrowing of the facet joints. We have not attempted dynamic CT scans, which Kirkaldy-Willis and Farfan[28] suggest are useful in the diagnosis of the rotational deformity (Fig. 18). They also suggest that a pedicle-to-pedicle defect on myelography is an important finding in rotational deformities (Fig. 19). Presently, there is no reliable diagnostic test to identify rotational instability in its earlier phases, although the production of pain on axial rotation is highly suggestive. Our use of facet blocks as an additional diagnostic test has not proven reliable.

If a rotational component can be identified, it would have important implications for selecting the stabilization procedure, because derotation alone may decompress the nerve root(s). Farfan has proposed a derotation facet fusion, which we have performed in over 40 patients, usually supplemented by transverse process fusion.[10] The role of instrumentation is not defined at this time.

Type II: Translational Instability

This is the classic instability of degenerative spondylolisthesis, which may be identical with Type I. In the earlier phases, the Knutsson sign[30] is thought to be diagnostic, although we now believe that 3 mm of displacement is within the range of error in everyday clinical measurement. Additional radiographic signs are disc space narrowing and traction spurs. Females are affected four times more often than males, and diabetics, particularly, are at risk.[57] Proposed fusion

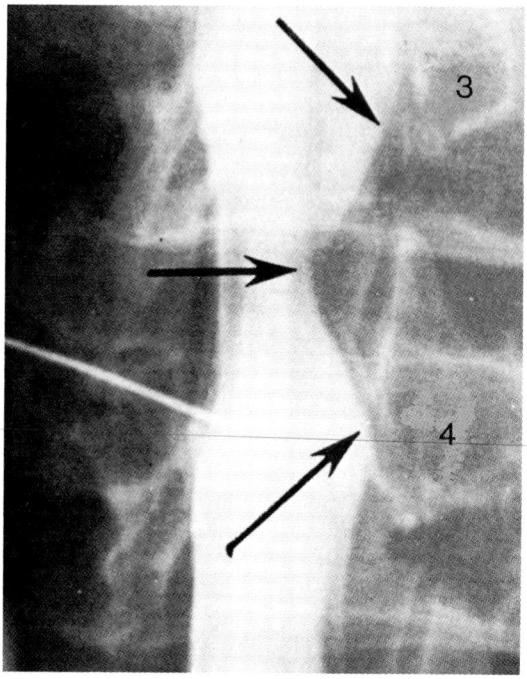

Figure 19 □ A pedicle-to-pedicle defect seen in myelography in a patient with rotational deformity. (From Frymoyer, J.W., and Selby, D.K.: Segmental instability. Rationale for treatment. Spine 10:280–286, 1985.)

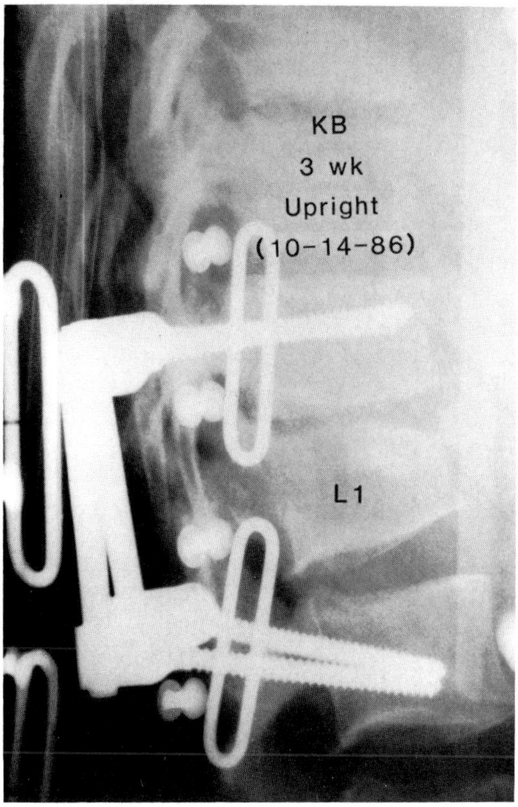

Figure 20 □ Lateral radiograph of the Vermont Spinal Fixateur used for stabilization.

techniques include anterior interbody fusion, if there are no neurologic symptoms,[21] and intertransverse process fusion,[12] which may be supplemented by various forms of internal fixation.[16] Although the evidence is incomplete, fusion seems to yield more favorable results than decompression alone when nerve root symptoms and signs are dominant problems.[12] We currently use our pedicle fixation device (Fig. 20) or, simply, floating transverse process fusion, except in patients in whom the L5–S1 disc space is not well protected by the spinal anatomy (i.e., high-riding vertebrae, short transverse processes).

Type III: Retrolisthetic Instability

The evidence suggests that this lesion is most common at L5–S1 and is frequently associated with symptoms of lateral spinal canal stenosis affecting the S1 nerve root. Flexion in fusion is the most logical approach to this lesion. Historically it has been performed with facet fusion and distraction rods (Knodt)[58] and is currently accomplished by pedicle fixation devices.

Type IV: Progressing Degenerative Scoliosis

Scoliotic deformities may involve single segments, usually accompanied by an axial rotational deformity at multiple levels. Nerve root involvement in the latter cases may involve multiple levels, and the level(s) of decompression and fusion required may be difficult to determine. Fusion supplemented by internal fixation is most appropriate. The best-suited devices are the Cotrell-Dubosais or Zilke apparatus.

Type V: Internal Disc Disruption

We question whether disc disruption is an unstable lesion and isolated disc resorption represents its physiologically stabilized end point. This hypothesis can be tested by measurements of displacement before and after the application of axial compressive loads. Stabilization by anterior interbody fusion currently is the treatment of choice for patients with this condition.

Secondary Instabilities

Type I: Post–disc Excision

We have reported that 20% of the patients who had disc excision 10 or more years previously had a positive Knuttson sign, most commonly in females at the L4–L5 level, but that radiographic findings often did not correlate with symptoms.[16] Three per cent of patients did require stabilization as a secondary procedure for symptoms of low back pain. Diagnostic considerations and treatment are similar to those already described for Types I and II primary instabilities.[16] Some experts believe that these patients can be identified at the time of primary disc excision by flexion–extension radiographs and that primary fusion is a means of preventing the later symptomatic instability.

The frequency with which other patterns of instability follow disc excision is unknown. Retrolisthetic deformities with increasing lateral spinal canal compression of the S1 root are probably the second most common problem identified.

Type II: Post–Decompressive Laminectomy

Accentuation of Pre-existing Deformity □ The most common problem is increasing deformity after decompression of degenerative spondylolisthesis. The likelihood of this increasing deformity is commonly thought to relate to the preoperative extent of the deformity, the patient's age, and the presence or absence of stabilizing osteophytes, whether or not the disc is excised, and the amount of the facets which are removed. Reynolds and Wiltse[55] and Johnsson[24] observed all their patients had increased deformity after radical facetectomies for degenerative spondylolisthesis, often unassociated

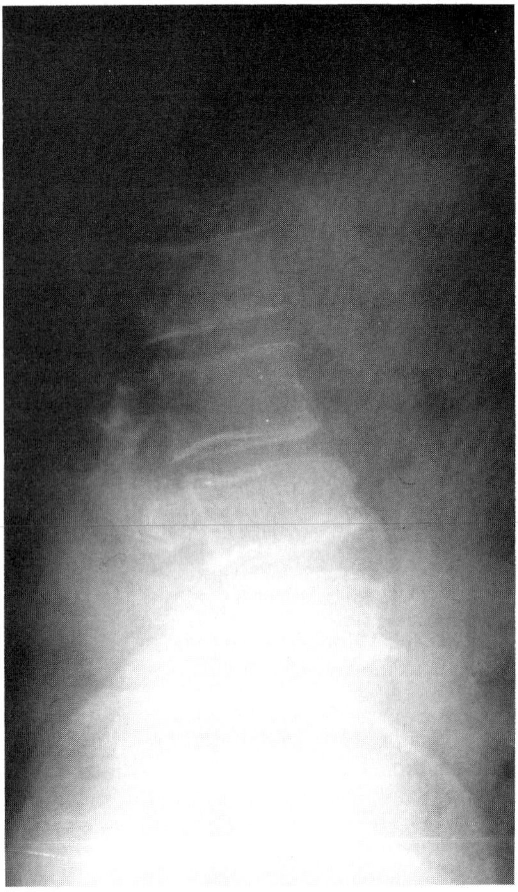

Figure 21 □ This 55-year-old man had multilevel decompressions for severe congenital spinal stenosis with superimposed degeneration. More than one third of the facets were sacrificed. Note the vertebral displacements that have occurred. The patient has nondisabling, with impairing, low back pain.

with new symptoms, an observation also made by Feffer and colleagues.[12] However, Johnsson noted that progression with acquired spinal stenosis had a generally poor result.[24] As a prevention of this occurrence, many experts now recommend fusion,[12] although some reserve that operation for patients under the age of 65.[55]

New Deformity □ This problem is seen in younger patients after extensive decompression for spinal stenosis, and may involve single or multiple levels, often with coexisting, different instability patterns (Fig. 21). The occurrence of this progression was 3.7% in Lee's small series,[31] and it was considerably greater among Johnsson's patients. The prevailing opinion is that the likelihood increases as a function of the magnitude of facet decompression, although Lee's study did not prove that point. For this complex patient group, pedicle fixation devices have proven invaluable.

Type III: Post–Spinal Fusion

Above or Below a Fusion □ There are convincing biomechanical and clinical data that spinal fusion increases the shear stresses in the next adjacent mobile functional spinal unit. Twenty per cent of our patients and 45% of Lehmann's[33] patients who had undergone spinal fusion, 10 or more years previously, demonstrated a positive Knuttson sign, but only 4% had required a fusion for progressing pain and deformity at the L3–L4 level (Fig. 22). In the small group of patients who had previously undergone L5–sacrum fusions, 20% required later stabilization of the L4–L5 level for continuing symptoms, which may have represented instability.[16] Brodsky[5] has emphasized that

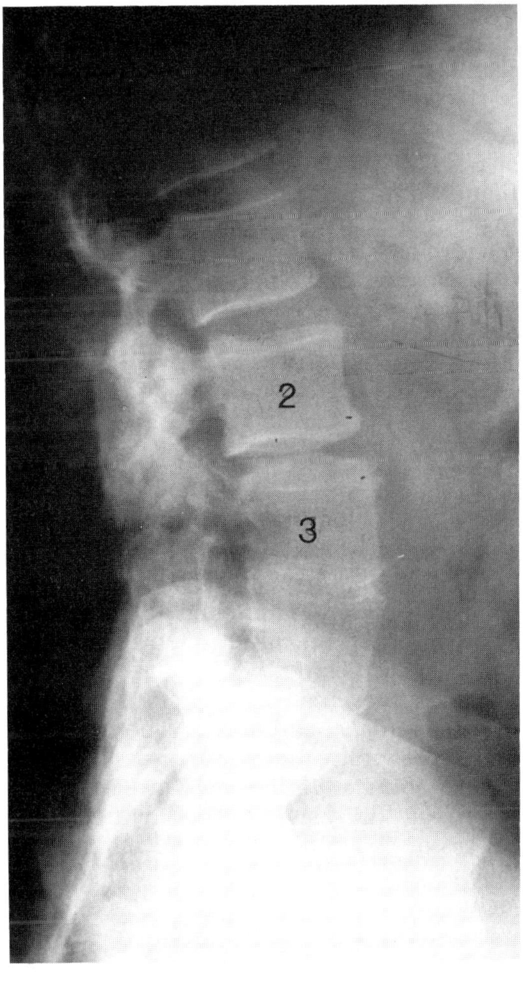

Figure 22 □ This 50-year-old man had previously undergone L4–sacrum fusion. He has developed symptoms of spinal stenosis with an accompanying disc herniation at L3–L4. Note the spondylolisthetic deformity that has occurred.

61. Stokes, I. A. F., and Frymoyer, J. W.: Segmental motion and instability. Spine 12:688–691, 1987.
62. Sullivan, J. D., Farfan, H. F., and Kahn, D. S.: Pathologic changes with intervertebral joint rotational instability in the rabbit. Can. J. Surg. 14:71–79, 1971.
63. Taylor, J., and Twomey, L.: Sagittal and horizontal plane movement of the human lumbar vertebral column in cadavers and in the living. Rheumatol. Rehab. 19:223–232, 1980.
64. Tencer, A. F., and Ahmed, A. M.: The role of secondary variables in the measurement of the mechanical properties of the lumbar intervertebral joint. A.S.M.E. J. Biomech. Engineer. 103:129–137, 1981.
65. Torgerson, W. R., and Dotter, W. E.: Comparative roentgenographic study of the asymptomatic and symptomatic lumbar spine. J. Bone Joint Surg. 58A:850–853, 1976.
66. Valkenburg, H. A., and Haanen, H. C. M.: The epidemiology of low back pain. *In* White, A. A., III, and Gordon, S. L. (eds.): American Academy of Orthopaedic Surgeons Symposium on Idiopathic Low Back Pain. St. Louis, C. V. Mosby, 1982.
67. White, A. A., III, and Panjabi, M. M.: Kinematics of the Spine. *In* White, A. A., III, and Panjabi, M. M. (eds.): Clinical Biomechanics of the Spine. Philadelphia, J. B. Lippincott, 1978.
68. Wiesel, S. W., Tsourmas, N., Feffer, H. I., et al.: A study of computer-assisted tomography. I. The incidence of positive CAT scans in an asymptomatic group of patients. Spine 9:549–551, 1984.
69. Wilder, D. G., Pope, M. H., and Frymoyer, J. W.: The biomechanics of lumbar disc herniation and the effect of overload and instability. (Winner of 1987 American Back Society's Annual Competition.) Presented at the Spring Symposium on Back Pain, American Back Society, Anaheim, California, May, 1987. Am. Back Soc. News. 3:10–11, 1987. (In press, J. Spin. Dis., 1988.)
70. Wilder, D. G.: On Loading of the Human Lumbar Intervertebral Motion Segment. Ph.D. Dissertation, University of Vermont, October 1985. Abstract: Dissertation Abstracts International 46:4328B, 1986. Manuscript #DA8529728: University Microfilms International, Ann Arbor, 1986.
71. Wilder, D. G., Seligson, D., Frymoyer, J. W., and Pope, M. H.: Objective measurement of L4–5 instability: A case report. Spine 5:56, 1980.
72. Wiltse, L. L., and Winter, R. B.: Terminology and measurement of spondylolisthesis. J. Bone Joint Surg. 65A:768–772, 1983.

11 □ Inflammatory Disorders

Michel Benoist
Malcolm I. V. Jayson

INFLAMMATORY SPONDYLOARTHROPATHIES

Michel Benoist

DEFINITION AND HISTORICAL REVIEW

The term *inflammatory spondyloarthropathies* (IS) refers to a group of diseases originally considered to be variants of rheumatoid arthritis (RA). It is now well established that this group is a separate entity, clearly distinct from RA. These disorders include ankylosing spondylitis (AS) and its variants, which are enteropathic arthritis (ulcerative colitis and Crohn disease), psoriatic arthritis, and reactive arthritis (postenteric and postvenereal). The IS group is characterized by varying inflammatory involvement of the axial skeleton (sacroiliac and spinal joints); peripheral synovial and cartilaginous joints; and the entheses, bursae, and tendon sheaths. These disorders share the absence of γ M immunoglobulin (IgM)-agglutinating rheumatoid factor and a familial aggregation, suggesting a genetic susceptibility. The crucial discovery that HLA-B27 was strongly associated with IS and the frequent overlapping of these various inflammatory disorders have justified their identification in a unified group. Moreover, extra-articular symptoms (ocular, mucocutaneous, and genital) are often encountered in the course of the spondyloarthropathies. The triggering role of infectious agents in some cases of "B27–related arthritis" has strongly stimulated the research for both immunogenetics and environmental factors.

Historically, AS was described first. Three eminent neurologists, Von Strümpel, Bechterew, and Pierre Marie, accomplished the pioneer work at the beginning of this century. Later, major contributions were made by Forestier[31] and by Scandinavian authors, especially Romanus and Yden.[53]

Primary AS remains the major and central part of the IS group. AS secondary to enteropathic, psoriatic, and reactive arthritis was subsequently linked to primary AS because of interrelated clinical and radiologic features and because of a common immunogenetic background.

ANKYLOSING SPONDYLITIS

Primary AS is a chronic inflammatory disease of the axial skeleton, often associated with a varying involvement of the peripheral joints and entheses.

Pathology

The main pathologic feature of AS is its tendency to affect the insertion of joint capsules and ligaments into bone (i.e., entheses). In these sites, the inflammation is usually mild and leads to fibrotic and osseous proliferation. Involvement of peripheral joints, bursae, and tendon sheaths is characterized by inflammation of the synovium, usually milder than the one observed in RA. These pathologic changes explain the major features of AS: syndesmophytes, bony ankylosis, and reactive proliferative changes.[14]

Anatomically, the sacroiliac joints are initially involved. Sacroiliitis is the hallmark of the disease, which subsequently spreads to the spinal joints.

Diagnostic Criteria

The diagnosis of AS is based upon the association of characteristic clinical and radiologic features. Episodes of low back pain radiating into the buttocks and the sciatic territory are predominant in the second part of the night. Morning stiffness that subsides with exercise is also highly suggestive. The pain usually starts insidiously in young individuals and progressively spreads to the thoracic and cervical spine. The physical examination may show a decrease of spinal mobility in both anterior and lateral planes, which can be measured by the Schober test. However, the restriction of spinal mobility as well as the loss of lumbar lordosis can be absent in early or mild cases. In this classic form, the diagnosis is usually confirmed by the radiologic demonstration of sacroiliitis and syndesmophytes. Nevertheless, the diagnosis can be difficult early in the course of the disease, when the sacroiliac changes are minimal and doubtful. Criteria for diagnosis of AS have been formulated at conferences in Rome in 1961 and revised in New York in 1966. They are shown in Tables 1 and 2.

Positive results of HLA-B27 testing are helpful in difficult diagnoses; however, these should not be considered to be a diagnostic test. The B27 antigen, although found in the great majority of the white AS patients, can be absent, especially in noncaucasian individuals. On the other hand, a certain number of HLA–positive patients will never have the disease.

Table 1 □ Rome Clinical Criteria for Ankylosing Spondylitis

Low back pain and stiffness for more than 3 months
Pain and stiffness in the thoracic region
Limited motion in the lumbar spine
Limited chest expansion
History or evidence of iritis or its sequelae
Ankylosing spondylitis present if bilateral sacroilitis is associated with any one of the above clinical criteria

Table 2 □ New York Clinical Criteria for Ankylosing Spondylitis

Limitation of motion of the lumbar spine in all three planes (anterior flexion, lateral flexion, and extension)
A history of pain or the presence of pain at the dorsolumbar junction or in the lumbar spine
Limitation of chest expansion to 1 inch (2–5 cm) or less, measured at the level of the fourth intercostal space
Definite ankylosing spondylitis present if:
Grades 3–4 bilateral sacroiliitis associated with at least one clinical criterion
Grades 3–4 unilateral or Grade 2 bilateral sacroiliitis associated with Clinical Criterion 1 or with both Clinical Criteria 2 and 3
Probable ankylosing spondylitis present if:
Grades 3–4 bilateral sacroiliitis exist without any clinical criteria

Other laboratory findings are not specific. The erythrocyte sedimentation rate is usually, but not constantly, elevated. High elevations are found especially in the active forms of the disease with involvement of the peripheral joints. Anorexia with loss of weight and fever can be observed in these patients, as well as in the nontreated initial acute episodes. The synovial fluid in the involved peripheral joints is inflammatory with a predominance of lymphocytes. Histologic examination of the synovium reveals the following nonspecific inflammatory changes similar to those observed in RA: hyperplasia of the synovial lining cells, plasma cells, and lymphocyte infiltrates, with occasional lymphoid follicle formation. However, in most cases the synovial inflammation remains mild.[14]

Radiology

Radiology of AS has recently been reviewed.[34] The diagnosis of AS relies upon suggestive history and clinical symptoms but is mainly based upon the radiographic findings involving the sacroiliac joints and the spine.

The most important diagnostic criterion of AS is a bilateral sacroiliitis affecting the superior and posterior part of the sacroiliac joint. In advanced cases, the radiologic diagnosis is obvious when symmetric bilateral changes are observed, including erosion and widening of the joint space with a reactive, poorly limited band of subchondral bony sclerosis, sometimes progressing to a partial or total bony ankylosis. However, the early changes can be minimal and doubtful. Sacroiliitis may be unilateral at the beginning of the disease and restricted to mild periarticular osteoporosis with minimal erosions. In difficult cases, computed tomographic (CT) examination may reveal erosions and subchondral sclerosis that are not apparent on standard radiographs of the sacroiliac joint. CT examination appears to be the best diagnostic imaging tool in detecting early subtle sacroiliac abnormalities.[37] It should be performed in cases in which history and clinical findings are suggestive of AS. On the other hand, quantitative bone scintigraphy has proven to be less reliable in patients with normal or doubtful radiographs. Numerous causes of errors have been detected, depending upon the effects of age, gender, and laterality.[25]

Radiologic demonstration of sacroiliitis is the major diagnostic criterion of AS. Table 3 summarizes the five grades of sacroiliac changes introduced in the New York diagnostic criteria. AS with a persisting absence of sacroiliitis is extremely rare. In these exceptional cases, the diagnosis relies upon characteristic clinical symptoms, association with uveitis and peripheral arthritis, typical syndesmophytes, and apophyseal joint involvement.

Radiologic abnormalities of the spine are well explained by basic pathology. As mentioned, AS predominantly affects the insertion of ligaments and capsules into bone. Chronic inflammation with bone resorption takes place at the discovertebral junction, where the outer part of the annulus fibrosus inserts into the vertebral body. At this site, bone resorption progresses to erosion and sclerosis. Osseous proliferation, which is the hallmark of the reparative process, leads to ossification of the outer fibers of the annulus fibrosus (syndesmophytes). According to this pathologic process, the initial radiographic finding is erosion with subsequent bony formation at the discovertebral junction, usually occurring at the central part or at the corners of the vertebral body. Syndesmophytes are vertically oriented and follow the outer part of the annulus fibrosus. They are easy to distinguish from osteophytes and from the hyperostotic formations seen in Forestier disease (diffuse idiopathic skeletal hyperostosis). Syndesmophytes are usually bilateral and originally detected at the thoracolumbar region. In advanced stages the ossification can bridge the intervertebral space, creating the classic "bamboo spine," related to an extensive syndesmophytosis. Central and/or lateral discovertebral erosion and destruction with bony sclerosis similar to an infectious spondylodiscitis can occasionally be seen. Inflammation and/or localized fracture with pseudarthrosis are the speculative explanations of this rare radiologic feature.

Involvement of the apophyseal joints with erosions and subchondral sclerosis may progress to bony ankylosis of the facets. This is a frequent finding in the cervical spine. Additional radiologic features include discal calcification and ballooning, and calcification of supraspinous and interspinous ligaments. Involvement of the atlantoaxial joint is not a common feature in AS but is occasionally observed. Axial cartilaginous joints, including symphysis pubis and the manubriosternal joints, are commonly involved. Bony erosions, adjacent sclerosis, and proliferation often lead to complete disappearance of the joints and ankylosis.

Table 3 □ Sacroiliac Changes According to the New York Criteria

Grade	Changes
Grade 0	Normal
Grade 1	Doubtful
Grade 2	Minimal sacroiliitis (discreet blurring—minimal erosions)
Grade 3	Moderate sacroiliitis (definite blurring—erosions and sclerosis)
Grade 4	Ankylosis

Peripheral Joint Involvement

Peripheral joint disease occurs in approximately 25% of the patients. The proximal joints (shoulders and hips) are most frequently involved. Erosions, joint space narrowing, osteophytosis, and sometimes bony ankylosis are the main radiologic features. In the shoulder disease, disruption of the rotator cuff is often associated with articular abnormalities. Other joints (knee, temporomandibular) may also be involved, sometimes late in the evolution of the disease when the axial inflammation has disappeared.[34]

Enthesopathies

The main pathologic feature of AS is inflammation of the enthesis. This is manifested radiologically by osseous erosion, bony sclerosis, and proliferation at the site of insertion of the involved tendons or ligaments. Enthesopathies may be seen in axial sites such as the ischial tuberosity and iliac crest. The most common peripheral insertional lesions include plantar fasciitis, Achilles tendinitis, and dactylitis. Involvement of the calcaneus is a frequent finding.

Systemic Aspects

Extraspinal and extra-articular manifestations may occur during the course of the disease, clearly indicating that AS is a systemic disorder. For references, see a recent review by Bourgeois.[12]

Uveitis

Nongranulomatous anterior uveitis is observed in approximately 25% of AS. It can be an early manifestation of the disease and sometimes precedes the spinal and articular symptoms. Iritis may also develop years after the onset of AS when the spinal disease is inactive. Uveitis is usually mild but can be severe and relapsing. It requires a prompt and adequate treatment, including general and/or local steroid therapy. Uveitis is predominantly seen in B27-positive AS patients with peripheral joint involvement.

Cardiovascular Involvement

Cardiovascular symptoms occur in 1% to 10% of the AS patients. They occur most often in the severe evolutive and relapsing forms of the disease, especially those associated with uveitis and peripheral joint disease.

Aortic incompetence is the most frequent and severe cardiovascular manifestation. Pericarditis is usually latent. Defects in cardiac conduction are frequent and observed in 5% to 8% of the patients. They often consist of incomplete first-degree block, discovered on an electrocardiogram (ECG). However, complete atrioventricular blocks with Adams-Stokes syndrome and cardiac insufficiency may develop. Inflammation and subsequent fibrosis and scar tissue formation primarily affect the aortic valve cusps and the root of the aorta. The lesions progress toward the septum and the main mitral valve with a direct inflammatory involvement of the conduction tissue.

Pulmonary Disease

Involvement of the lung is observed in approximately 1.3% of long-standing cases of AS. Lymphocytic inflammatory infiltrates and progressive interalveolar fibrosis are responsible for the radiographic changes seen mainly in the upper lobe of the lungs but sometimes progressing to the other lobes. The radiographs reveal extensive fibrosis with cyst formation and tissue destruction resembling tuberculosis. The lung involvement is often latent but is occasionally revealed by cough, dyspnea, and hemoptysis. Subsequent *Aspergillus* invasion is a major complication.

Neurologic Manifestation

Cauda equina syndrome is a rare complication of AS but may occur in a long-standing form of the disease when the spinal inflammation has become inactive. Following an insidious onset, the syndrome is revealed by low back and leg pain with reflex, sensory, and sphincter impairment. The motor symptoms usually remain discrete. The myelographic examination reveals enlargement of the dural sac and lumbar diverticula without signs of nerve root compression. Anatomic lesions consist of thickening and fibrotic proliferation of the epidural space and the meningeal envelopes. Surgical treatment may be required, but is difficult and not always rewarding.

A few cases of vertebral cord compression at the thoracic level have been reported, accompanied by similar histologic lesions probably secondary to arachnoiditis.

Amyloidosis

This is a rare but serious complication of AS. It occurs in the severe form of the disease after a long period of evolution; there are numerous relapsing acute episodes, including involvement of the peripheral joints. Very often the disease starts in childhood or adolescence. Amyloid is found in the liver, spleen, and kidneys. Renal involvement may be a cause of death.

The prevalence of amyloidosis in AS is still under discussion. It varies from 4% to 8%. In another study, 3 of 35 patients had amyloid on rectal biopsy.

The Kidney

The glomerular renal function is not impaired in AS. However, vascular abnormalities were found in 11 of 14 renal biopsies. In another study, three cases of renal papillary necrosis were found associated with AS. Cases of γ A immunoglobulin (IgA) nephropathy have also been reported.

Epidemiology

The increased frequency of AS in families of AS patients compared with the general population is now well established. In 1961, de Blecourt and coworkers,[11] studying a series of 7,405 patients, found that the disease was detected 22.6 times more frequently in families of AS patients than in controls. In another study, 16% of the first-degree relatives of 76 AS patients had sacroiliitis.[21]

In 1973, Brewerton and coworkers[13] and Schlosstein and associates[55] independently described the high frequency of HLA-B27 in AS patients and their families. The fact that half of the first-degree relatives of AS patients were HLA-B27 positive explained this familial aggregation. HLA-B27 is genetically transmitted with an autosomal codominant characteristic. The link between HLA-B27 and spondyloarthropathies is discussed later.

Prevalence and Sex Distribution

Primary AS commonly begins in young individuals around 25 years of age, and sometimes before. Classically, there is a striking predominance in males with a male-to-female ratio of 10:1. However, recent studies[17] have shown that AS is much more frequent in women than was thought before, with a female prevalence approaching the frequency in males.

The prevalence of AS in the general population is still under discussion. It is generally estimated to be between 0.5 and 4.0 per 1,000 individuals.[40]

AS develops much more frequently in caucasians than in other populations. The disease is exceptional in black Africans and the Japanese. The rarity of HLA-B27 in these two populations provides a reasonable explanation.[16]

Etiology

The cause of primary AS is unknown. The association with HLA-B27 is well established, but its link with clinical manifestations remains speculative. Involvement of infective agents is still under study. A high fecal carriage of *Klebsiella pneumoniae* in patients with active disease led to speculation that this agent was involved in the pathogenesis.[20] However, other conflicting data, including the absence of lymphocyte transformation to *Klebsiella pneumoniae*,[35] have kept the debate open.

Prognosis

Severity of evolution is hard to predict on the individual level. However, in Western countries extensive spinal disease with peripheral joint and systemic involvement is rare. Proper management usually enables most patients to enjoy normal lives. However, severe forms of disease with total ankylosis and major extraspinal involvement are sometimes encountered. A higher frequency of severe AS with juvenile onset is noted in some regions, such as North Africa.[7] Comparison of AS patients in various populations with similar genetic backgrounds suggests a modulation of the severity of the disease according to the age of exposure to an infectious agent in predisposed individuals.

Treatment

Patient and family education concerning the course of the disease, the prognosis, and the aims and possibilities of therapy are most important. Each patient should be properly informed that there is no definitive cure for the disease, but that relief of pain and maintenance of good posture and activity can be expected with proper management.

Nonsteroidal, anti-inflammatory drug therapy usually relieves inflammation and pain. Phenylbutazone is classically the most effective agent and indeed is sometimes the only efficacious one. However, its potential long-term toxicity or intolerance limits its use. Indomethacin and the newer nonsteroidal anti-inflammatory drugs (NSAID) are often effective. Whatever drug is used, the dosage regimen should be adapted according to the severity of the disease. A high dosage should be used to decrease inflammation during the severe flare-ups of the disease and then carefully tapered off during the nonevolutive periods. If the disease becomes nonactive, continuous therapy does not seem to be necessary. Aspirin and corticoids have a small place in the treatment of AS. Neither gold nor penicillamine has demonstrated efficacy. Whether sulphasalazine is efficacious remains to be determined.

The other major aim of therapy is to avoid ankylosis and curvature. Maintaining good posture and function by extension exercises, swimming, physiotherapy, and adequate attention to day and night position is an important part of the therapeutic regimen.

Vertebral wedge osteotomy may be needed in patients with severe deformities. Spinal fractures or neurologic manifestations need a careful neurosurgical evaluation. Hip arthroplasty, when necessary, contributes to maintaining proper posture and activity.

REACTIVE ARTHRITIS

The term *reactive arthritis* has been proposed to designate aseptic arthritides, which develop after an infection elsewhere in the body, without the microorganism entering in the joint.[4]

Historically, Reiter syndrome, which, in its complete form, associates arthritis with intestinal or genitourinary symptoms, was the first example of reactive arthritis to be described. *Shigella* was the first suspected agent associated with Reiter disease.[23] Subsequently, other postenteric or postvenereal infectious triggering agents have been identified. Table 4 illustrates the frequency of the bacteria identified in 352 cases of reactive arthritis, disclosed in a recent survey of the French Society of Rheumatology.[8] Epidemiology of these agents may vary according to the endemic areas. Complete Reiter syndrome, including arthritis, conjunctivitis, and urethritis, may develop either after an enteric infection or after a sexually transmitted infection. In both cases there is a striking association with the HLA-B27.[16, 32]

Table 4 □ Bacteria Identified in 352 Cases of Reactive Arthritis (National Survey by the French Society of Rheumatology)

BACTERIA	IDENTIFICATION	
	Serology	Culture
Chlamydia trachomatis	61	25
Yersinia enterocolitica	46	3
Yersinia pseudotuberculosis	24	0
Shigella flexneri	29	2
Klebsiella pneumoniae		2
Neisseria gonorrhoeae		6
Ureaplasma urealyticum		7
No bacteria identified in 50% of the cases		

On the other hand, incomplete Reiter syndrome (i.e., reactive arthritis without extra-articular manifestations) following a triggering infection has also been found to be closely associated with HLA-B27. Moreover, a group of HLA-B27–positive patients suffer from a disease exactly resembling reactive arthritis, but they show no evidence of a recent infection.[45]

In the postvenereal form of B27-associated reactive arthritis, *Chlamydia trachomatis* is considered the main etiologic agent.[6, 36] However, in one study *C. trachomatis* was isolated in only 24 cases of 140 posturethritis reactive arthritis.[7]

In the postenteric form, *Shigella, Salmonella, Yersinia,* and *Campylobacter jejuni* infections have been found to be the main triggering agents. However, in some cases these pathogens cannot be identified, and it is likely that other still-unknown etiologic enterobacteria can also be implicated.[2, 3]

Postenteric reactive arthritis affects only a fraction of the HLA-B27 population, although the pathogens found in arthritic and nonarthritic patients do not differ. This clearly indicates the importance of the host response. However, the capacity of the enterobacteria to trigger arthritis appears to differ in some microbial strains. For example, *Shigella flexneri* is arthritogenic and *Shigella sonnei* is not. *Yersinia enterolitica,* Type 03 and Type 09, found in Scandinavia, is associated with reactive arthritis. In contrast, *Y. enterolitica* Type 08 is not arthritogenic.[3, 7]

Rheumatic fever following pharyngeal streptococcal infection is another example of reactive arthritis with no link to the HLA-B27 antigen. Its incidence has dramatically decreased in Western countries. Reactive arthritis can also follow meningococcal, gonococcal, or brucellar infections.

Clinical Picture

The present description addresses only the postenteric and postvenereal HLA B27–associated reactive arthritis, which now represents by far the vast majority of this group.

The onset of the articular symptoms usually begins 1 week to 3 weeks after the infection. Lower extremities are first and almost always affected. Involvement of the upper limbs is not constant. Synovial inflammation appears in the involved joints in rapid succession; there is a predilection for large joints, although feet and hand joints may also be involved. Acute asymmetric oligoarthritis is the typical clinical picture. In approximately one third of the patients, an inflammatory type of back pain and peripheral enthesopathy are observed. These manifestations link the reactive arthritis to the other forms of IS.

Postvenereal arthritis is predominantly observed in young men. It has been suggested that some of the self-limiting seronegative oligoarthritis of unknown cause observed in women may be misdiagnosed episodes of reactive arthritis. Nongonococcal venereal infection is frequently asymptomatic in women. Postenteric arthritis can be observed at all ages with no difference in the sex distribution.

Extra-Articular Symptoms

Urethritis is the triggering infection in the postvenereal form and is probably reactive and less frequent in the postdysenteric form.

Ocular lesions, including conjunctivitis and less frequently uveitis, are part of the complete Reiter syndrome and a common extra-articular feature.[3]

Keratoderma blennorrhagicum is usually seen in patients with a definite diagnosis of Reiter syndrome, appearing on the soles and palms—sometimes with a circinate balanitis. Clinically and histologically, keratoderma is indistinguishable from pustular psoriasis. These skin lesions provide a strong link between B27 reactive arthritis and psoriatic arthritis. Moreover, epidemiologic studies have shown a high prevalence of psoriasis in the relatives of male patients with reactive arthritis.[41] On the other hand, clinical observations have demonstrated that Reiter syndrome could be followed by typical psoriatic arthritis.[59]

Cardiovascular manifestations including valvulitis are rare and, with the exception of myocarditis, usually asymptomatic.[31]

Fatigue and fever are common at the onset of joint inflammation, especially in the postenteric form.

Evolution

Reactive arthritis usually subsides in a few weeks or months. The self-limiting course of the acute attack can be followed by recurrences, especially in the postvenereal form, because of new genital infections or because of the spontaneous recurrence of the nongonococcal urethritis.[32] In some cases chronic deformities with erosive arthritis and cutaneous lesions follow the acute recurrences. In chronic Reiter disease sacroiliitis is a common finding. The sacroiliac changes are often unilateral or asymmetric. Spondylitis can occur in chronic Reiter syndrome but is less frequent than in psoriasis. The paravertebral ossifications are nonmarginal, identical to those described in psoriatic spondylitis, and clearly different from the classic syndesmophytes of primary AS. They randomly affect the lower thoracic and upper lumbar vertebrae.[34]

Long-term follow-up studies also indicate that AS with bilateral sacroiliitis may develop in patients with reactive arthritis, especially in those with postvenereal Reiter syndrome and those with *Shigella* infection.[54]

Diagnosis

The diagnosis of reactive arthritis is based upon the clinical history and physical findings and on identification of the triggering agent. As shown in Table 4, demonstration of the enteric bacteria from the stools is rare. The usual absence of direct bacteriologic evidence is attributable to the fact that cultures are often started too late after the beginning of symptoms, when identification of the bacteria from the stools is no longer possible.

Levels of antibodies for the suspected infectious agent are the second laboratory criterion. The antibody titer has usually reached its peak at the time of the first blood examination and can be expected to show a progressive reduction in the subsequent weeks or months.

The search for *Chlamydia* in posturethritis–reactive arthritis is not always successful. On the other hand, *Chlamydia* can be identified in asymptomatic patients, especially in females. Gamma G immunoglobulin (IgG) *Chlamydia* antibodies are also found in control subjects for a long time after an infection. It is sometimes difficult, therefore, to appreciate the significance of the laboratory findings at the individual level.[7]

Furthermore, as shown in Table 4, in half of the patients with arthritis that closely resembles reactive arthritis, no evidence of recent infection can be demonstrated.[8]

Treatment

Even if the triggering infectious agent has been identified, the treatment of the infection seems to have no influence on the duration of the joint symptoms or on preventing recurrences.[3, 32] However, because of the chronic nature of chlamydial infections, it is appropriate to treat the patient and his or her sexual partner. Patients with postenteric arthritis should be treated only at the beginning of the infection, in instances of persistant diarrhea, fever, and positive stool cultures.

NSAIDs and local injections of corticosteroids are usually efficacious and can control the disease during the course of its self-limiting evolution.

PSORIATIC SPONDYLOARTHROPATHY

An association between psoriasis and seronegative spondyloarthropathies has been demonstrated by family and epidemiologic studies.[57] The studies have also shown that psoriasis and psoriatic spondyloarthropathy are more frequent in the families of patients with psoriatic arthritis. Although a strong genetic factor has been established, its expression is not yet clearly known. No etiologic or environmental factor has been recognized.

Clinical Picture

The skin and nail symptoms usually precede or accompany the arthritis. However, in about 10% of the patients the skin disease appears later than the joints manifestations.[10]

Numerous classifications of psoriatic arthritis have been proposed. They illustrate the heterogeneity of the disease and the various clinical patterns of peripheral and axial joint involvement. The classification by Moll and Wright provides a satisfactory clinical framework. The five categories suggested by these authors are shown in order of frequency in Table 5.[49]

Table 5 □ Classification of Psoriatic Arthritis (After Moll and Wright)

Pauci, asymmetric arthritis	70%
Symmetric polyarthritis	15%
Arthritis mutilans	5%
Asymmetric and exclusive involvement of DIP joints	5%
Ankylosing spondylitis	5%

Sacroiliac and Spinal Involvement

The association of psoriasis and AS with or without peripheral seronegative arthritis is well established. The clinical and radiologic symptoms may be identical to those of primary AS. However, some features often differentiate psoriatic spondylitis from definite AS.

Sacroiliitis develops in approximately 30% to 40% of the patients with psoriatic arthritis.[27] Moreover, about 20% of patients with severe psoriasis have abnormal sacroiliac joints. The radiologic features include erosion, widening of the joint space, and sclerosis. Sclerotic and erosive lesions predominate. Ankylosis is rare. Asymmetric or unilateral involvement may be encountered. Psoriatic sacroiliitis is often asymptomatic and found isolated without spondylitis.[34]

Two types of spondylitis associated with psoriasis have been distinguished. One is clinically and radiologically similar to primary AS. It is considered a chance association of the two diseases. The second group appears to be different, on both clinical and radiologic grounds.[39] The vertebral symptoms appear at an older age and are usually milder than in primary AS. Typical syndesmophytes may be observed but are often replaced by nonmarginal syndesmophytes developing in paravertebral tissues. These ossifications are distant from the vertebral margins and the disc, are more voluminous, and may be unilateral with an asymmetric distribution. Lower thoracic and upper lumbar segments are usually affected, but involvement of the cervical spine may be predominant and is sometimes exclusive. Cervical spinal abnormalities, including paravertebral ossifications and arthritis of the facets, are usually seen in the lower cervical region, but involvement of the atlantoaxial joint may also be observed. These paravertebral ossifications due to calcification of the spinal ligaments are very similar to those observed in Reiter spondylitis. However, nonmarginal spondylitis is usually less extensive in Reiter syndrome than in psoriasis.[34] In general, the clinical spinal symptoms, including pain and stiffness, are less marked in psoriatic spondylitis than in primary AS.[39]

Peripheral Involvement

The peripheral clinical patterns are characterized by an inflammatory arthritis including pain, morning stiffness, articular swelling, and deformities. Radiologically, bone resorption and proliferation are the two important hallmarks of psoriatic arthritis.[39]

Bone resorption often begins at the joint margins, progressing centrally. Destruction of the subchondral bone sometimes leads to the classic "pencil-in-cup" deformity. Interphalangeal joints, metacarpophalangeal and metatarsophalangeal joints of the hands and feet are the usual targets. Severe acro-osteolysis of the phalanges, metatarsi, or metacarpi is characteristic of arthritis mutilans. Bony proliferation often accompanies osseous subchondral destruction, producing a spiculated appearance. Periostitis of the epiphysis and metaphysis of hands and feet bones are frequent, sometimes preceding the joint destruction. Bony proliferation can also produce the so-called ivory appearance of the phalanx and may lead to fusion of distal interphalangeal (DIP) and proximal interphalangeal (PIP) joints. Finally, enthesopathies with calcification at the site of insertion of tendons and ligaments may be seen in the same areas as in primary AS, including ischial tuberosity, calcaneus, and trochanters on the iliac side.[34]

Extra-Articular Involvement

The most severe cases of peripheral arthritis and spondylitis are usually seen in patients with widespread skin disease. However, the psoriatic lesions may be discrete and unnoticed by the patient. They should be carefully looked for, especially in the scalp and in the perineum. In patients with a typical picture of seronegative spondyloarthropathy and an absence of skin lesions, the discovery of nail changes is an important diagnostic aid.

Anterior uveitis occurs in approximately 15% of patients with spinal and sacroiliac involvement but with a much lower frequency in patients with pure peripheral arthritis.[39]

Laboratory Findings

No specific laboratory abnormalities occur in psoriatic seronegative spondyloarthropathy. Psoriasis is associated with HLA-B13 and HLA-B17, but not with HLA-B27. Psoriatic peripheral arthritis is usually seen in the absence of HLA-B27, but 45.5% of the patients are B38 positive.[22] In contrast, HLA-B27 is found in approximately 70% of the patients with sacroiliitis, with or without peripheral involvement. The prevalence of HLA-B27 is higher, approximately 80% in patients with both sacroiliitis and spondylitis.[19]

Prognosis and Therapy

As already mentioned, the axial disease is less severe in psoriatic spondylitis than in primary AS. The loss of motion and pain is less marked and usually controlled by proper management. However, severe psoriatic spondylitis is occasionally seen with pulmonary complications and a fatal outcome.[52]

Severe evolution of the peripheral arthropathy with joint destruction and functional incapacity is observed in about 15% of patients, especially in those with arthritis mutilans.[39]

The treatment of psoriatic spondyloarthropathy must be adapted to the clinical pattern of the disease and to its severity. The management of psoriatic spondylitis is the same as for primary AS, including NSAIDs, exercises, and physiotherapy. NSAIDs with local injections of corticosteroids usually relieve inflammation and pain in the asymmetric oligoarticular arthritis of mild severity. In the serious polyarticular forms, with or without arthritis mutilans, the management can be difficult. NSAIDs and local forms of treatment are not sufficient to control the disease activity and prevent deformations and erosions. In those cases, D penicillamine and gold salts are sometimes beneficial.[18] In more advanced cases, cytotoxic drugs such as azathioprine and methotrexate are often effective. The latter drug acts on both the psoriasis and the arthritis.[38]

INFLAMMATORY BOWEL DISEASE

Inflammatory bowel diseases, including ulcerative colitis, Crohn disease, and Whipple disease, can be associated with peripheral arthritis and axial involvement. Many studies have confirmed the prevalence of seronegative inflammatory spondyloarthropathies in this group of disorders. The same studies have demonstrated that these arthropathies are clearly different from and not coincidental with RA.[1, 9, 15, 26, 47]

Ulcerative Colitis

Peripheral arthritis occurs in approximately 10% of patients with ulcerative colitis.[47] The acute synovial inflammation usually starts in one joint, primarily affecting the large joints of the lower limbs. However, hands and feet are sometimes involved. The synovitis often remains monoarticular or oligoarticular and disappears spontaneously in a few weeks or months. No radiologic changes are usually seen. The arthropathy is primarily observed in patients with widespread and chronic bowel involvement. The synovitis is often associated with exacerbations of the intestinal disease. Moreover, the peripheral arthropathy is particularly frequent in colitic patients with local or general complications. Surgical removal of the colon has a dramatic beneficial effect on the articular symptoms.[60]

AS may also be associated with ulcerative colitis. It sometimes precedes the appearance of the bowel symptoms. Later, there is no relationship between the course of the intestinal disease and the evolution of the spondylitis, which is not affected by colectomy. The sacroiliitis and the spinal changes are exactly the same as those seen in primary AS.[44, 61]

Family studies have shown a strong genetic influence in the development of ulcerative colitis. These studies have also demonstrated an increased prevalance of AS in first-degree relatives of colitic patients, especially those with spondylitis.[42] Histocompatibility studies have shown the presence of the B27 antigen in approximately 65% of patients with ulcerative colitis and AS.[43]

Crohn Disease

The peripheral arthritis associated with Crohn disease closely resembles the arthropathy already described in ulcerative colitis. The seronegative oligoarthritis, affecting primarily the lower limbs, may antedate the bowel symptoms by many years. The temporal relationship between the articular and the intestinal exacerbations is not as striking as in ulcerative colitis.[29]

The spinal disease comprises sacroiliitis with or without spondylitis. The clinical and radiologic features of the axial involvement are similar to those encountered in primary AS.[29, 47] There is no correlation between Crohn disease flare-ups and the evolution of spondylitis, which is not affected by intestinal surgery.

Family studies have demonstrated a strong genetic factor in Crohn disease.[28] They have also shown a genetic association between ulcerative colitis and Crohn disease. Antigen-B27 is found in about 53% of patients with Crohn-associated spondylitis.[30]

Whipple Disease

Whipple disease is a rare form of inflammatory bowel disease produced by an interplay of an infectious agent with host factors. The exact nature of the enterogenic organism is not well established. However, the infectious origin of the disease has been demonstrated by the efficacy of antibiotic therapy.

Peripheral arthritis and spondylitis identical to those found in ulcerative colitis and Crohn disease are seen in a substantial proportion of cases of this rare disease.[33, 51]

ETIOLOGY AND PATHOGENESIS

A close interrelationship between the seronegative spondyloarthropathies is suggested by the numerous overlapping syndromes. Association of AS occurs with psoriatic arthritis and inflammatory bowel disease. As already mentioned, definite AS may follow chronic Reiter syndrome.[54] Other clinical overlaps strongly support the concept of a separate entity. They include an association between psoriatic arthritis and Reiter syndrome, inflammatory bowel disease and psoriasis, and ulcerative colitis and Reiter syndrome.[47, 59]

Moreover, a significantly increased frequency of one or more types of IS is found in families of patients. Such clustering has been found in psoriatic arthritis, in Reiter syndrome, and in the inflammatory bowel disease group. For instance, there is an increased prevalence of spondylitis and of inflammatory bowel disease in families of patients with psoriatic arthritis.[56]

Finally, similar extra-articular involvement, including eye and skin lesions, can be found in any IS. The mucocutaneous lesions of Reiter syndrome can easily be confused with pustular psoriasis.[58] Anterior uveitis is a frequent manifestation of the entire IS group. The overlap of symptoms in the same patient and the evidence of familial associations strongly suggest a common genetic background. Genetic factors have indeed been recognized in each of the spondarthritides by family studies and HLA-antigen investigations.[50] A close relationship between HLA-B27 and axial involvement has been demonstrated.[56] However, the frequency of HLA-B27 is not identical in each disease. HLA-B27 is present in 90% of the patients with AS, 70% to 80% of the patients with psoriasis and spondylitis, 50% to 60% of the patients with inflammatory bowel disease and spondylitis, and 60% to 80% of the patients with urogenital or *Yersinia*-reactive arthritis.[13, 16, 19, 30, 32, 43, 55]

The absence of HLA-B27 in about 10% of primary AS caucasian patients and in a greater proportion in the other seronegative spondyloarthropathies strongly suggests the effect of other genes with polygenic inheritance. However, the strong association of primary AS with HLA-B27 makes it likely that this antigen is the major gene for AS.[56] It remains a hypothetic issue, whether the B27 gene itself has a direct effect on pathogenesis or whether another gene in strong linkage disequilibrium with B27 is the actual disease-susceptibility gene.[5] On the other hand, subtypes of B27 have been recognized, clearly establishing the heterogeneity of the B27 gene.[31] However, the relationship of this heterogeneity to disease remains under intense study.

In addition to genetic predisposition, the importance of environmental factors is now well recognized. The triggering effect of gram-negative enteric bacteria and of genitourinary tract infections has been demonstrated in reactive arthritis.[7] The mechanism of the microbial triggering effect is still under discussion. However, the concept of "molecular mimicry" between antigen HLA-B27 and the microbial antigens is presently the most attractive model. Other hypotheses have been formulated, such as an association of B27 with immune response genes or a modification of the B27 gene by a viral antigen.[7, 48]

No infective agent has been demonstrated in primary AS. The triggering role of *K. pneumoniae* is still a matter of debate. Interestingly, gut inflammatory lesions have been found by ileocoloscopies in 75% of a series of patients with primary AS, suggesting the role of an enterogenic infection.[46] As in inflammatory bowel disease, gut microorganisms could, in genetically predisposed patients, produce immune reactions leading to bowel lesions and extraintestinal symptoms, including peripheral and axial arthropathy.[47]

CONCLUSIONS

Recent clinical and epidemiologic studies and the investigation of HLA associations have shown that the seronegative types of IS can be classified as a distinct group of diseases. Genetic predisposition and especially the role of HLA-B27 have been demonstrated.

However, many questions remain unresolved concerning the exact nature of the genetic constitution, the host's response, and the interaction between genetic factors and the suspected infectious agents.

One hopes that genetic studies, as well as the precise identification of the responsible infective agents, will improve the possibilities of therapy by methods other than symptomatic treatments.

References

1. Acheson, E. D.: An association between ulcerative colitis, regional enteritis and ankylosing spondylitis. Q. J. Med. 29:489, 1960.
2. Aho, K., Ahvonen, P., and Lassus, A.: Yersinia arthritis and related diseases. *In* Dumond, D. C. P. (ed.): Infection and Immunology in the Rheumatic Diseases. Oxford, Blackwell, 1976.
3. Aho, K., Leirisalo-Repo, M., and Repo, H.: Reactive arthritis. Clin. Rheum. Dis. 11:25, 1985.
4. Ahvonen, P., Sievers, K., and Aho, K.: Arthritis

associated with *Yersinia enterolitica* infection. Acta Rheum. Scand. 15:232, 1969.
5. Albert, E., Scholz, S.: Immunogenetics and rheumatic disease. Clin. Exp. Rheumatol. 5/S1:29, 1987.
6. Amor, B.: Chlamydia and Reiter's syndrome. *In* Ziff, M., and Cohen, S. B. (eds.): Advances in Inflammation Research. The Spondyloarthropathies. New York, Raven Press, p. 203, 1985.
7. Amor, B.: Suspected infectious agent and host environment interactions in spondyloarthropathies. Clin. Exp. Rheumatol. 5/S1:19, 1987.
8. Amor, B., Bouchet, H., and Delrieu, F.: Enquête nationale sur les arthrites réactionnelles de la Société Française de Rhumatologie. Rev. Rhum. Mal. Osteoartic. 50:733, 1983.
9. Ansell, B. M., and Wigley, R. A. D.: Arthritic manifestations in regional enteritis. Ann. Rheum. Dis. 23:64, 1964.
10. Baker, H.: Epidemiological aspects of psoriasis and arthritis. Br. J. Dermatol. 78:249, 1966.
11. de Blecourt, J. J., Polman, A., and de Blecourt-Meindersma, T.: Hereditary factors in rheumatoid arthritis and ankylosing spondylitis. Ann. Rheum. Dis. 20:215, 1961.
12. Bourgeois, P.: Aspects systémiques de la spondylarthrite ankylosante. *In* Kahn, M. F., and Peltier, A. P. (eds).: Maladies Dites Systémiques. Paris, Flammarion, 1982.
13. Brewerton, D. A., Caffrey, M., Hart, F. D., et al.: Ankylosing spondylitis and HLA 27. Lancet 1:904, 1973.
14. Bywaters, E. G. L.: Pathology of the spondyloarthropathies. *In* Calin, A. (ed.): Spondyloarthropathies. Orlando, Grune & Stratton, 1984.
15. Bywaters, E. G. L., and Ansell, B. M.: Arthritis associated with ulcerative colitis. Ann. Rheum. Dis. 17:169, 1958.
16. Calin, A.: Spondyloarthropathy in Caucasians and non-Caucasians. J. Rheumatol. 10 (Suppl):16, 1983.
17. Calin, A., and Fries, J. F.: The striking prevalence of ankylosing spondylitis in healthy W27 positive males and females. A controlled study. N. Engl. J. Med. 293:835, 1975.
18. Dowart, B. B., Gall, E. P., Schumaker, H. R., and Krauser, R. E.: Chrysotherapy in psoriatic arthritis. Arthritis Rheum. 21:513, 1978.
19. Eastmond, C. J., and Woodrow, J. C.: The HLA system and the arthropathies associated with psoriasis. Ann. Rheum. Dis. 36:112, 1977.
20. Ebringer, R. W., Cawdell, D. R., Cowling, P., and Ebringer, A.: Sequential studies in ankylosing spondylitis. Association of *Klebsiella pneumoniae* with active disease. Ann. Rheum. Dis. 37:146, 1978.
21. Emery, A. E., and Lawrence, J. S.: Genetics of ankylosing spondylitis. J. Med. Genet. 4:239, 1967.
22. Espinoza, L. R., Vasey, F. B., Wilkinson, O. R., and Osterland, C. K.: Association between BW 38 and peripheral psoriatic arthritis. Arthritis Rheum. 21:72, 1978.
23. Fiessinger, N., and Leroy, E.: Contribution à l'étude d'une épidémie de dysenterie dans la Somme. Bull. Soc. Med. Hôp. Paris 40:20, 1916.
24. Forestier, J., Jacqueline, F., Rotes-Querol, J.: La spondylarthrite ankylosante. Paris, Masson, 1951.
25. Goldberg, R. P., Genant, H. K., Shimshak, R., and Shames, D.: Applications and limitations of quantitative sacroiliac joint scintigraphy. Radiology 128:683, 1978.
26. Hammer, B., Ashurst, P., and Naish, J.: Diseases associated with ulcerative colitis and Crohn's disease. Gut 9:17, 1968.
27. Harvie, J. N., Lester, R. S., and Little, A. H.: Sacroiliitis in severe psoriasis. A. J. R. 127:579, 1976.
28. Haslock, I.: Arthritis and Crohn's disease. A family study. Ann. Rheum. Dis. 32:479, 1973.
29. Haslock, I., and Wright, V.: The musculo-skeletal complications of Crohn's disease. Medicine 52:217, 1973.
30. Huaux, J. P., Fiasse, R., le Bruyere, M., and Nagant de Deuxchaisnes: HLA B27 in regional enteritis with and without ankylosing spondylitis or sacroiliitis. J. Rheum. 3(Suppl. 4):60, 1977.
31. Khan, M. A.: Immunogenetics of ankylosing spondylitis: clinically oriented aspects. Clin. Exp. Rheumatol. 5/S1:49, 1987.
32. Keat, A.: Reiter's syndrome and reactive arthritis in perspective. N. Engl. J. Med. 309:1606, 1983.
33. Kelley, J. J., Weisiger, B. B.: The arthritis of Whipple's disease. Arth. Rheum. 6:615, 1963.
34. Kerr, R., and Resnick, D.: Radiology of the seronegative spondyloarthropathies. Clin. Rheum. Dis. 11:113, 1985.
35. Kinsella, T. D., Lanteigne, C., Fritzler, M. J., et al.: Absence of impaired lymphocyte transformation to *Klebsiella* in ankylosing spondylitis. Ann. Rheum. Dis. 43:590, 1984.
36. Kousa, M., Saikku, P., Richmond, S., and Lassus, A.: Frequent association of chlamydial infection with Reiter's syndrome. Sex. Transm. Dis. 5:57, 1978.
37. Kozin, F., Carrera, G. F., Ryan, L. M., et al.: Computed tomography in the diagnosis of sacroiliitis. Arth. Rheum. 24:1479, 1981.
38. Kragballe, K., Zachariae, E., and Zachariae, H.: Methotrexate in psoriatic arthritis. A retrospective study. Acta Dermatovener. 63:165, 1982.
39. Laurent, R.: Psoriatic arthritis. Clin. Rheum. Dis. 11:61, 1985.
40. Lawrence, J. S.: The prevalence of arthritis. Br. J. Clin. Pract. 17:699, 1963.
41. Lawrence, J. S.: Family survey of Reiter's disease. Br. J. Vener. Dis. 50:140, 1974.
42. MaCrae, I., and Wright, V.: A family study of ulcerative colitis with special reference to ankylosing spondylitis and sacroiliitis. Ann. Rheum. Dis. 32:16, 1973.
43. Mallas, E. G., MacKintosh, P., Asquith, P., and Cooke, W. T.: Histocompatibility antigens in inflammatory bowel disease. Their clinical significance and their association with arthropathy with special reference to HLA-B27. Gut 17:906, 1976.
44. McEwen, C., di Tata, D., Lingg, C.: A comparative study of ankylosing spondylitis and spondylitis accompanying ulcerative colitis, regional enteritis, psoriasis and Reiter's disease. Arthritis Rheum. 14:291, 1971.
45. Meyer, O., Vignalli, M., and Ryckewaert, A.: Rhumatismes inflammatoires inclassables avec HLA B27. Rev. Rhum. Mal. Osteoartic. 49:11, 1982.
46. Mielants, H., Veys, E. M., Cuvelier, C., et al.: Significance of gut inflammation in the seronegative spondylarthropathies. Clin. Exp. Rheumatol. 5/S1:81, 1987.
47. Moll, J. M. H.: Inflammatory bowel disease. Clin. Rheum. Dis. 11:87, 1985.
48. Moll, J. M. H.: Pathogenic mechanism of B27 related

seronegative polyarthritis: Interplay between genetic and environmental factors. Clin. Exp. 5/S1:7, 1987.
49. Moll, J. M. H., Wright, V.: Psoriatic arthritis. Semin. Arth. Rheum. 3:55, 1973.
50. Moller, P.: Genetics of ankylosing spondylitis, psoriatic arthritis and Reiter's syndrome. Clin. Exp. Rheumatol. 5/S1:35, 1987.
51. Puite, R. H., and Tesluk, H.: Whipple's disease. Am. J. Med. 19:383, 1955.
52. Roberts, M. E. T., Wright, V., Hill, A. G. S., and Mehra, A. C.: Psoriatic arthritis. Follow-up study. Ann. Rheum. Dis. 35:206, 1976.
53. Romanus, R., and Yden, S.: Pelvo-spondylitis ossificans. Rheumatoid or ankylosing spondylitis. Copenhagen, Munskgaard, 1955.
54. Sairanen, E., Paronen, I., and Mahonen, H.: Reiter's syndrome. A follow-up study. Acta Med. Scand. 185:57, 1969.
55. Schlosstein, L., Teresaki, P. I., and Bluestone, R. T.: High associations of an HLA antigen W 27, with ankylosing spondylitis. N. Engl. J. Med. 288:704, 1973.
56. Woodrow, J. C.: Genetic aspects of the spondyloarthropathies. Clin. Rheum. Dis. 11:1, 1985.
57. Wright, V.: Psoriatic arthritis. Ann. Rheum. Dis. 20:123, 1961.
58. Wright, V.: Skin and arthritis. Clin. Exp. Rheumatol. 5/S1:75, 1987.
59. Wright, V., and Reed, W. B.: The link between Reiter's syndrome and psoriatic arthritis. Ann. Rheum. Dis. 23:12, 1964.
60. Wright, V., and Watkinson, G.: The arthritis of ulcerative colitis. Br. Med. J. II:670, 1965.
61. Wright, V., and Watkinson, G.: Sacroiliitis and ulcerative colitis. Br. Med. J. II:675, 1965.

FIBROSIS, CHRONIC INFLAMMATION, AND VASCULAR DAMAGE IN BACK PAIN SYNDROMES

Malcolm I. V. Jayson

Back pain is common, and mechanical evidence of degenerative change such as spondylosis or disc disorders is also remarkably frequent. However, the correlation between objective evidence of spinal damage and the development of back pain is poor. For example, in population surveys[1] comparing the prevalence of back pain with radiographic changes in the lumbar spine there is a poor correlation between symptoms and radiographic changes. Those with the worst x-rays showing the most degenerative changes do have a somewhat greater prevalence of back pain than those with normal or nearly normal radiographs. The striking finding is that the difference between the two was remarkably small, and the difference in prevalence between those with the best and the poorest radiographic findings was only 12%. It is therefore difficult to implicate mechanical damage of the spine alone as the source of symptoms.

Simple observation confirms this view. Lumbar spondylosis, once developed, is permanently present and can only slowly deteriorate. However, the symptoms of back pain commonly fluctuate, and many patients have long pain-free periods interspersed with acute episodes of pain and disability. This suggests that there are other poorly recognized factors playing important roles in the pathogenesis of back pain.

Following a prolapse, the disc rupture will lead to local pain in the back and referred pain in the lower limbs. Mechanical pressure alone can produce pain. However, there is good evidence that secondary vascular, fibrosing, and inflammatory changes play an important role in the development of symptoms. For example, studies on nerve roots exposed at the time of operation show that those damaged by a prolapse react abnormally to mechanical stimulation with production of pain, whereas stimulation of nondamaged roots in the same patient and in nonsciatic patients does not elicit pain.[2] This suggests that increased sensitivity in the nerve root damaged by sciatica is increased and is compatible with the suggestion of secondary changes developing after the original mechanical insult. At operation, vascular granulation tissue may be found,[3] particularly so when the disc rupture is complete to the outer border of the annulus fibrosus.[4] Careful histologic examination of damaged nerves shows a high frequency of changes with hyperplasia of the perineurium and chronic inflammatory cell infiltration.[5] Such changes have also been described in nerve roots compressed by spinal stenosis.[6] In the nucleus of prolapsed discs there is an increase in lactate levels with a reduction of pH,[7] and the low pH does correlate both with pain and with evidence of inflammatory reactions and scarring around nerve roots.[8] In disc prolapse in animals, an inflammatory action with granulation tissue has similarly been found, later becoming much more fibrous and with appearances very similar to those found in humans.[9]

Evidence of altered immunity has been found in patients with disc prolapse and degeneration.[10–12] There is inhibition of the migration of lymphocytes by disc homogenate in disc prolapse, and elevated levels of sera IgM are found in individuals with back pain. These changes in immunity are probably secondary to the damage in the disc and surrounding structures, but they may play some role in the chronic scarring and inflammatory changes that are found.

Many patients who have mechanical back problems and in whom the classic inflammatory types of back problem, such as ankylosing spondylitis, have been excluded provide a history of aching and stiffness that are exacerbated by rest. They report marked stiffness early in the morning and after sitting in a chair, and this symptom is ameliorated by exercise and anti-inflammatory drugs. Such a history does suggest a significant inflammatory component to the problem.

ARACHNOIDITIS AND PERIDURAL FIBROSIS

The most florid evidence of chronic inflammation and scarring occurs in patients with arachnoiditis. Thickening and scarring of the arachnoid and dural membranes are a recognized cause of severe back and nerve root problems. Early descriptions of this syndrome were presented as sequels to meningitis attributable to viral or a wide variety of bacterial infections.[13] The use of spinal anesthetics has been suggested.[14] However, it is most commonly recognized in patients who have undergone myelography using oil-based media[15] and in subjects who have undergone previous spinal surgery.[16]

Arachnoiditis has been classified by Burton[17] as follows:

1. *Radiculitis:* inflammation of the pia-arachnoid with associated hyperemia and swelling of the nerve roots of the cauda equina. This stage is characterized by a minimal fibroblast proliferation and the beginning of deposition of strands of collagen between nerve roots and pia-arachnoid.
2. *Arachnoiditis:* progression of fibroblast proliferation and collagen deposition. Nerve root swelling has decreased, and nerve roots are now adherent to each other and to the pia and pia-arachnoid.
3. *Adhesive arachnoiditis:* the end stage of the inflammatory process. Marked pia-arachnoid proliferation with dense collagen deposition has produced complete encapsulation of the nerve roots, which are now hypoemic and have undergone extensive atrophy. This process can involve the nerve root sleeves alone or extend to involve the subarachnoid space.

Of particular interest is the finding in the early stages of a fibrinous exudate with only a small cellular component. The changes in adhesive arachnoiditis are similar to adhesions elsewhere. Fibrin-covered nerve roots and the arachnoid membranes stick together with bands of fibrinous adhesions, forming bridges in which proliferating fibrocytes lay down collagen.[18]

In many biopsy specimens we can show the presence of extensive proliferated collagenous tissue with only a small inflammatory cell infiltration. In places, masses of fibrin blend intimately with the excessive collagen that is deposited (Fig. 1). In postlaminectomy specimens we have found birefringent crystalline material (Fig. 2). In places, this is phagocytosed by macrophages (Fig. 3*A*,*B*) and the sparse chronic inflammatory cell reaction does seem concentrated around these birefringent deposits. By careful histochemical stains and use of enzymes we have shown this material to be identical to fragmented cotton debris presumably from

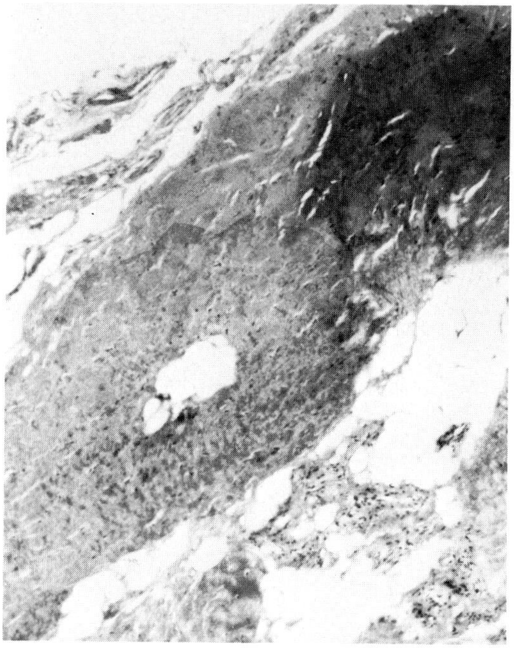

Figure 1 □ Scar tissue from the dural membrane shows collagen proliferation and fibrin deposition. (With thanks to Dr. A.J. Freemont and Dr. J. Hoyland.)

the swabs and patties used during the surgical procedures (Table 1).[19] It seems likely that retained debris from surgical swabs and patties liberated at surgery was responsible for the subsequent development of arachnoiditis. In other specimens we have found retained lipid droplets that are radiopaque and are presumably the retained oily myelographic medium. Of a total of 26 biopsy specimens, we found the birefringent debris in 14 and the lipid material in two more, indicating that foreign material was present in about two thirds of the subjects. Of course this could result from a sampling problem, as we looked only at small specimens and the true frequency of foreign material may actually be much higher. This suggests that retained foreign material, in particular debris from surgical swabs and patties, may be responsible for many cases of postlaminectomy arachnoiditis. In turn, this suggests the need to carefully examine surgical procedures, particularly the linting characteristics of surgical swabs and patties, and to use only materials that are free from this problem.

PATHOLOGIC STUDIES IN LUMBAR SPONDYLOSIS

Recognition of arachnoiditis and nerve root sheath fibrosis can be difficult. It commonly requires specialized imaging techniques, such as radiculography or computed tomography (CT). Without such studies it can be difficult to recognize the disorder.

It has been stated that the conventional spectrum of arachnoiditis is probably only "the tip of the iceberg."[20] Many patients with lumbar spondylosis may have degrees of arachnoiditis or peridural fibrosis that are of clinical significance yet not recognized by conventional examination. The secondary development of scar tissue formation could account for the variable development of back and nerve root pain and especially for the poor association with radiologic evidence of degenerative disease of the spine.

These observations have led us to undertake detailed pathologic studies of cadaveric specimens to identify periradicular changes in specimens with and without evidence of degenerative disease.[21]

Forty-three lumbar spines were examined

Table 1 □ Staining Reactions of Cellulose, Fragmented Surgical Swab and Pattie, and Foreign Material in the Specimens

	CELLULOSE	SURGICAL SWAB AND PATTIE	FOREIGN MATERIAL
Physical			
Polarizing microscopy	Birefringent	Birefringent	Birefringent
Histochemical			
PAS	+ + +	+	+
Congo red	+ + +	+	+
Grocott's Gomori	+ + +	+ +	+ +
Schweizer reagent	Dissolves	Dissolves	Dissolves
Iodine/H_2SO_4	Brown to blue	Brown to blue	Brown to blue
Enzymatic			
Cellulase	+ + +	+ + +	+ + +

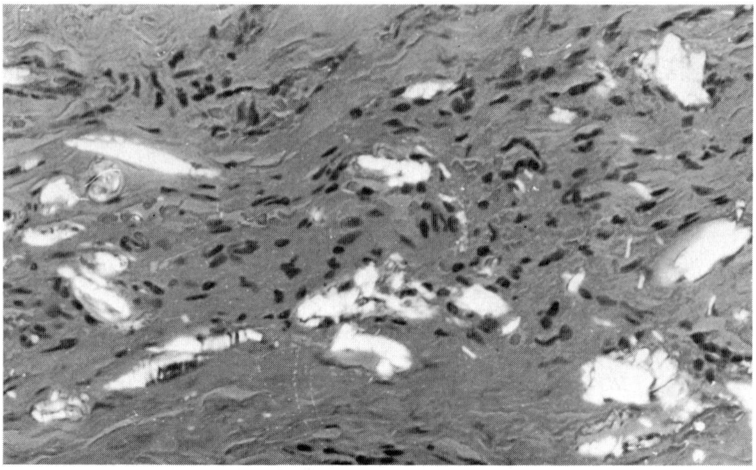

Figure 2 □ Postlaminectomy arachnoiditis. Birefringent material scattered in collagen proliferation with surrounding chronic inflammatory cells. (With thanks to Dr. A.J. Freemont and Dr. J. Hoyland.)

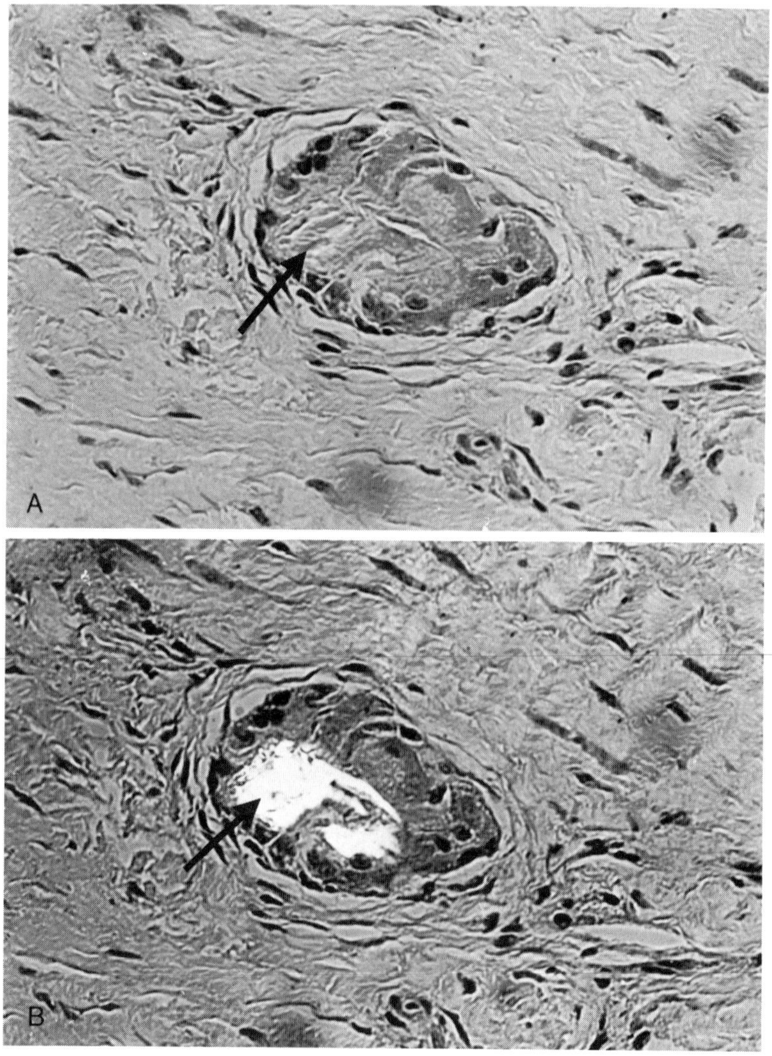

Figure 3 □ Macrophage in postlaminectomy arachnoiditis showing phagocytosed birefringent material (*arrow*). This is shown under normal light (*A*) and under polarized light (*B*). (With thanks to Dr. A.J. Freemont and Dr. J. Hoyland.)

and we studied a total of 160 intervertebral foramina. Serial sections across these foramina were obtained, and disc protrusions were graded according to the proportion of the diameter occupied by the protrusion. This, in turn, was related to compression of the nerve roots and of blood vessels within the intervertebral foramina and connective tissue proliferation.

We found that disc prolapses and osteophytic outgrowths rarely impinge directly on nerve roots (Fig. 4). However, they are commonly associated with fibrous connective tissue proliferation (Fig. 5), and we frequently see evidence of direct venous compression by the disc prolapse and of venous dilatation in the large venous plexus within the intervertebral foramina (Fig. 6). Despite the absence of direct nerve root compression, we do find severe perineural and intraneural changes (see Fig. 5), which are associated with compression and dilatation of the foraminal veins. The changes found within the nerve roots include edema of the nerve roots, fibrosis within the nerve root, and a tendency toward division into several small fasciculi. There is also proliferation of the arachnoid and dilatation of subarachnoid pockets. Blood vessel changes found within the perineural connective tissue sheaths include basement membrane thickening, damage to endothelial cells, and in some cases intravascular fibrin deposition and thromboses. These changes are typical of those associated with endothelial cell injury. We were able to relate the extent of vascular compression to the degree of disc prolapse (Table 2) and the extent of fibrous tissue proliferation to venous compression and dilatation (Fig. 7).

These pathologic changes are very similar to those in other conditions such as venous lipodermatosclerosis, in which venous occlusion leads to vascular injury and fibrosis

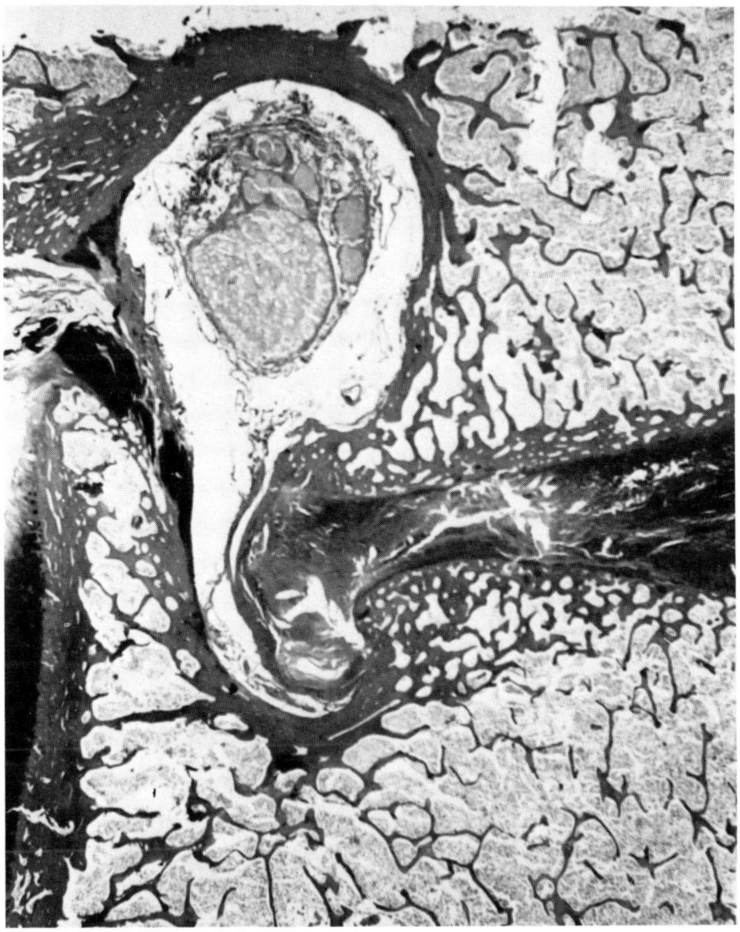

Figure 4 □ Section across the intervertebral foramen showing a disc prolapse. This does not compress the nerve root. There is distortion of the venous plexus by the prolapsed material. (With thanks to Dr. A.J. Freemont and Dr. J. Hoyland.)

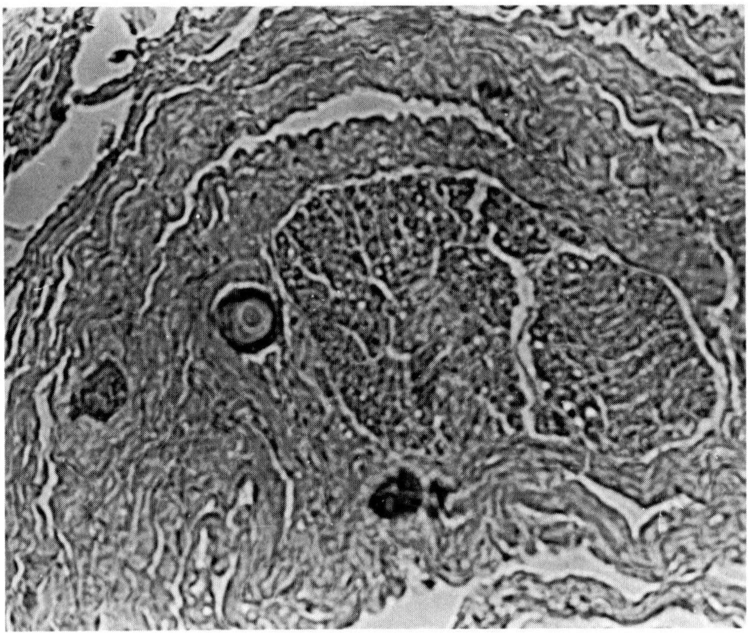

Figure 5 □ Nerve root shows extensive peridural and intraneural fibrosis. (With thanks to Dr. A.J. Freemont and Dr. J. Hoyland.)

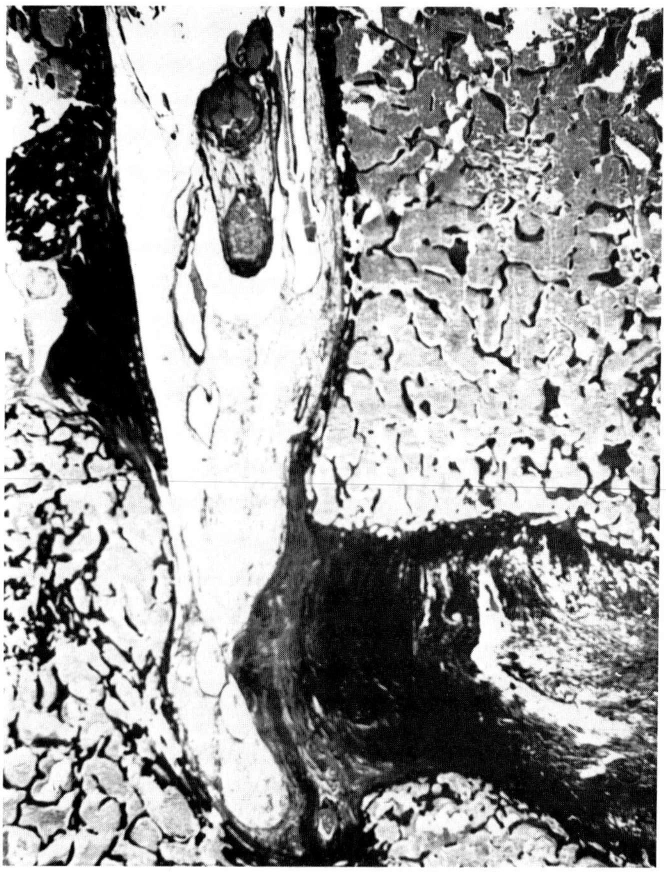

Figure 6 □ There are compression and dilatation of the intraforaminal venous plexus and associated extensive perineural fibrosis. (With thanks to Dr. A.J. Freemont and Dr. J. Hoyland.)

Table 2 □ Association Between Disc Protrusion, Apophyseal Joint Osteophytes, and Vascular and Nerve Root Compression

DISC PROLAPSE (PROPORTION OF IVF)	TOTAL NUMBER	VASCULAR COMPRESSION	NERVE ROOT COMPRESSION
0%	9	0	0
1–10%	59	11	0
11–20%	39	21	0
21–30%	30	20	4
>30%	23	18	3
Apophyseal joint osteophytes	17	5	1

with fibrin deposition in the tissues. It is believed that a defect in the fibrinolytic enzyme system associated with fibrin deposition plays a secondary pathogenic role in the chronicity of the problem. These observations have led to the use of fibrinolytic enhancement therapy, which is effective in correcting the fibrinolytic defect in the blood, reducing the fibrin in the damaged tissues, and improving the clinical problem. It has stimulated us to examine the fibrinolytic system in our chronic back pain patients.

FIBRIN AND THE FIBRINOLYTIC SYSTEM

The deposition of fibrin forms a normal part of the healing process following injury. The fibrin is usually cleared within a few weeks by the fibrinolytic enzyme system.[22] The persistence of fibrin in itself can provoke further tissue damage. The first experimental model of arthritis in animals[23] was produced by intra-articular injection of fibrin in sensitized rabbits. Persistence of fibrin in vessel walls can interfere with diffusion of oxygen

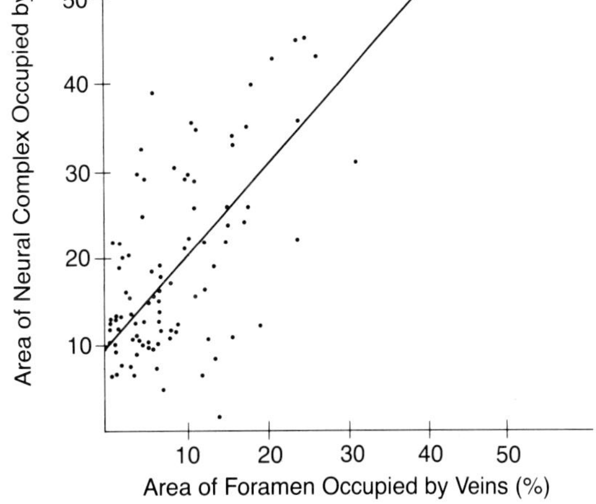

Figure 7 □ Graph shows the correlation between venous compression and dilatation and perineural fibrous tissue proliferation. (With thanks to Dr. J. Hoyland.)

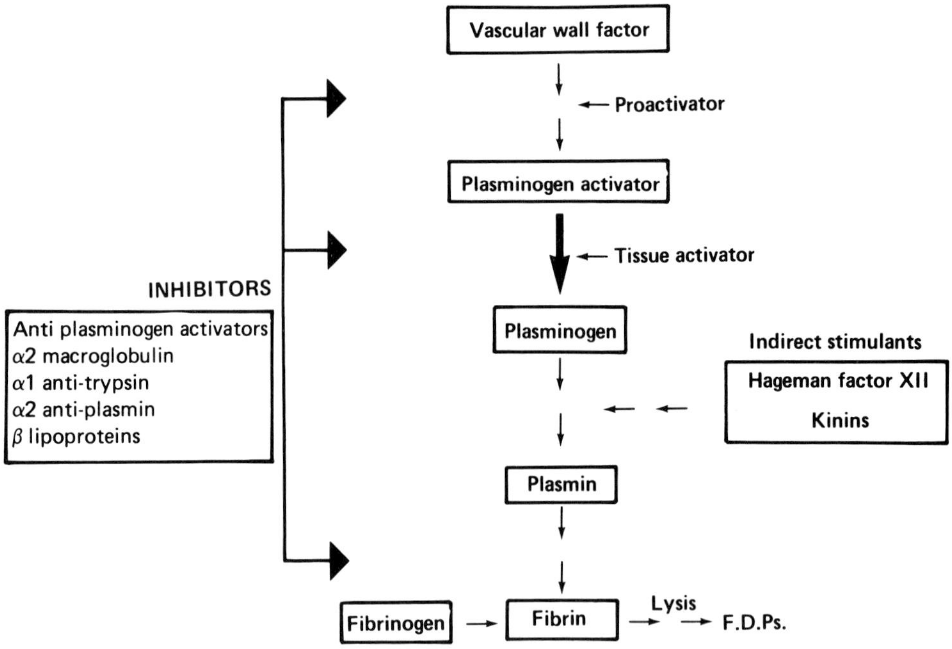

Figure 8 □ The fibrinolytic system is depicted.

and nutrients into tissues and, if deposited around capillaries, may block the diffusion of oxygen through the tissues.[24] These problems could be responsible for the development of chronic tissue damage.

The fibrinolytic system is a complex cascade of reactions by which fibrin is cleaved to various degradation products (Fig. 8). Plasmin is responsible for cleaving fibrin. It is formed from plasminogen activated by plasminogen activator. There are various inhibitors of plasminogen activator, and their increase can lead to defective fibrinolytic activity.

Our present studies of the fibrinolytic system are performed under careful standard basal conditions at the same time in the morning with the subjects rested and not having eaten or smoked for at least ten hours. We measure the fibrin plate lysis area[25] and the euglobulin lysis time,[26] which are direct overall measures of fibrinolytic activity. In addition we measure the levels of fibrinogen[27] and plasminogen, and the inhibitors α-2 antiplasmin and α-2 macroglobulin, using chromogenic substrate assays and immunodiffusion techniques.

FIBRINOLYTIC STUDIES IN PATIENTS WITH CHRONIC BACK PAIN

In a group of patients with chronic back pain of various causes we demonstrated a marked defect in fibrinolytic activity, compared with matched controls.[28] These observations have been extended to a much larger series of patients with separately defined problems such as proven arachnoiditis, possible arachnoiditis, chronic prolapsed intervertebral disc, lumbar spondylosis, and spinal stenosis. Similar defects in fibrinolytic activity were found in all groups, although the most marked changes were found in those with the most severe back problems, namely, proven arachnoiditis. Some of the groups were quite small, so not all the changes were significant compared with controls. Nevertheless, it does appear that this is a common change in chronic mechanical back pains of various causes (Fig. 9).[29]

This has led us to re-examine the correlation between back pain and radiographic change. We have assessed fibrinolytic activity in a group of subjects with chronic back

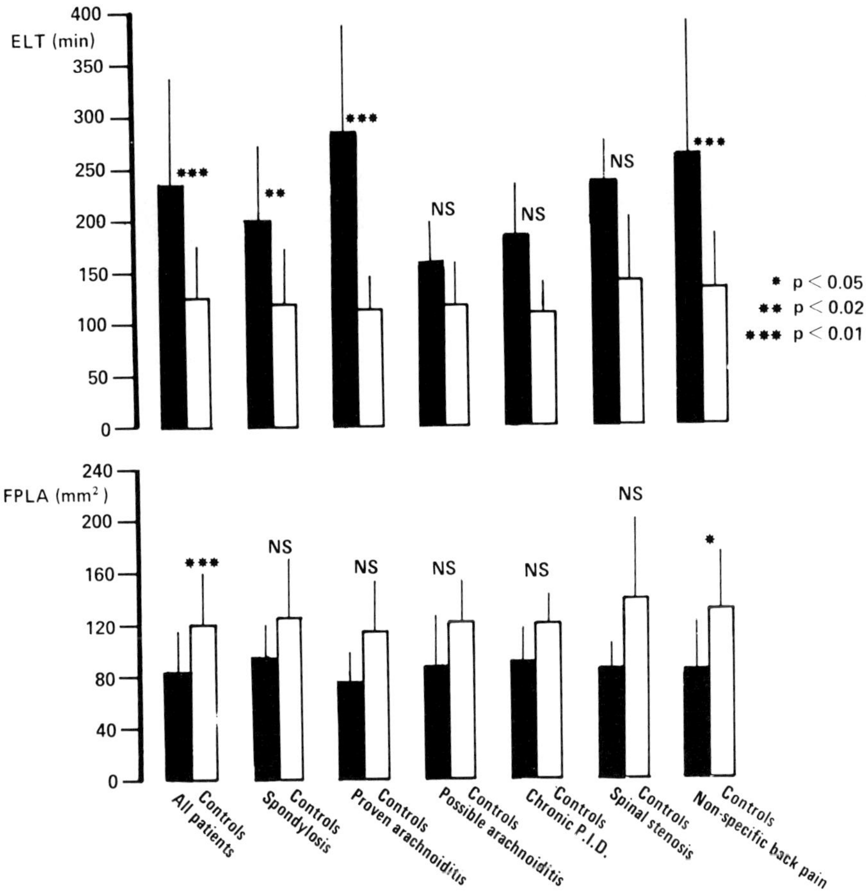

Figure 9 □ Fibrinolytic activity measures the ELT (euglobulin lysis time) and FPLA (fibrin plate lysis areas) in patients with defined chronic back pain syndromes. (From Pountain, G.D., Keegan, A.L., and Jayson, M.I.V.: Impaired fibrinolytic activity in defined chronic back pain syndromes. Spine 12:83–86, 1987.)

pain and Grade III or Grade IV lumbar spondylosis and compared the findings with healthy symptom-free subjects who were shown to have similar degrees of radiographic change. Again, we have found a defect in the fibrinolytic system with prolongation of the euglobulin clot lysis time (ELT) and reduction in the fibrin plate lysis area (FPLA) correlating with the development of back pain (Table 3).

These observations do suggest that the fibrinolytic defect is common in many patients with chronic back pain and does seem to correlate more closely with symptoms than the presence of radiographic changes. We believe that these enzyme changes are markers of vascular and tissue damage, and it is possible that they play a pathogenic role.

In order to analyze the development of

Table 3 □ Fibrinolytic Activity in Symptomatic and Symptomless Lumbar Spondylosis

	ELT (Min)	FPLA (mm^2)	MEAN RADIOLOGIC GRADE OF SPONDYLOSIS
Symptomatic spondylosis n = 15	286 ±124	83 ±36	2.7
Asymptomatic spondylosis n = 8	176 ±54	115 ±42	2.7
p value	p ≤ 0.01	NS	

this defect, we have sequentially studied patients presenting with their first episodes of acute back pain and sciatica and compared them with matched control individuals (Fig. 10*A*,*B*). [30] We have performed serial measurements of fibrinolytic activity throughout a year and compared them with the severity of pain measured on a visual analogue scale. We can see the development of the fibrinolytic defect at presentation or shortly thereafter. At the end of the year we were able to divide the studied individuals into two groups: one recovered; the other had persistent symptoms that failed to resolve. We were able to correlate the changes in the fibrinolytic defect with the symptoms. The patients who normalized their fibrinolytic activity recovered, whereas in those who had a persistent fibrinolytic defect the symptoms failed to diminish.

These observations indicate that the changes in fibrinolytic activity can be related to the severity of symptoms. We believe that they act as a marker of the vascular and soft tissue damage. In addition, by analogy with other conditions such as venous lipodermatosclerosis, we believe that the changes may act as a secondary pathogenic mechanism and that failure to clear fibrin is one important factor contributing to the chronicity of symptoms.

This may explain the association of smoking with back pain that has been found in epidemiologic surveys.[31] Smoking can produce a fibrinolytic defect[32] and so, perhaps, predisposes individuals to back pain by this mechanism.

FIBRINOLYTIC ENHANCEMENT THERAPY

The management of chronic back pain is unsatisfactory. Treatment usually revolves around analgesic and anti-inflammatory drugs and various forms of physiotherapy. In patients with arachnoiditis, surgical removal of the scar tissue leads to short-term improvement, although the recurrence rate is extremely high; recurrence is usually within a few weeks of the operation.

If the fibrinolytic defect is contributing to the chronicity of back pain problems, fibrinolytic enhancement therapy may be of therapeutic value. In venous lipodermatosclerosis, in which similar pathologic and biochemical changes occur, fibrinolytic enhancement has been found to be effective, not only in correcting the biochemical defect in the blood and reducing the fibrin in the tissues but also in reducing the area of liposclerosis and improving symptoms. Similar improvements have been found in rheumatoid arthritis[33] and in cutaneous vasculitis.[34] In systemic sclerosis we have found that fibrinolytic enhancement significantly improves peripheral blood flow with a trend toward reduction of abnormal fibrosis.[35]

Based upon these observations, we are currently undertaking studies of fibrinolytic enhancement therapy in patients with severe chronic back pain problems. The agent used, stanozolol, is a nonvirilizing anabolic steroid. However, it can produce mild androgenic side effects, which does limit its application in some patients, particularly in young females. In addition it may occasionally disturb liver function, and it is important to check the liver function tests from time to time. Other problems include fluid retention and calf cramps.

Our experience to date does suggest that this treatment may be effective in producing significant relief of symptoms (Fig. 11). We avoid patients whose symptoms have a major nonorganic component, using the Waddell screening tests.[36] Treatment is restricted to those with a severe fibrinolytic defect, and the benefit seems most marked in patients with a lot of general aching and stiffness, particularly morning stiffness, which would be characteristic of a significant inflammatory component. It may take some months, even a year or longer, before the value of treatment can be established in an individual. Double-blind controlled trials are in progress to explore properly the value of this approach to therapy.

SUMMARY

It appears that the ways in which mechanical damage can arise in the spine vary widely. Normally, any acute mechanical event would produce a transient episode of back pain from which the patient will recover. The actual incident may produce some localized vascular and tissue damage that will be reflected in a transient abnormality in fibrinolytic activity.

It seems likely that the vascular and tissue damage is associated with fibrin deposition at the time of the fibrinolytic defect in the

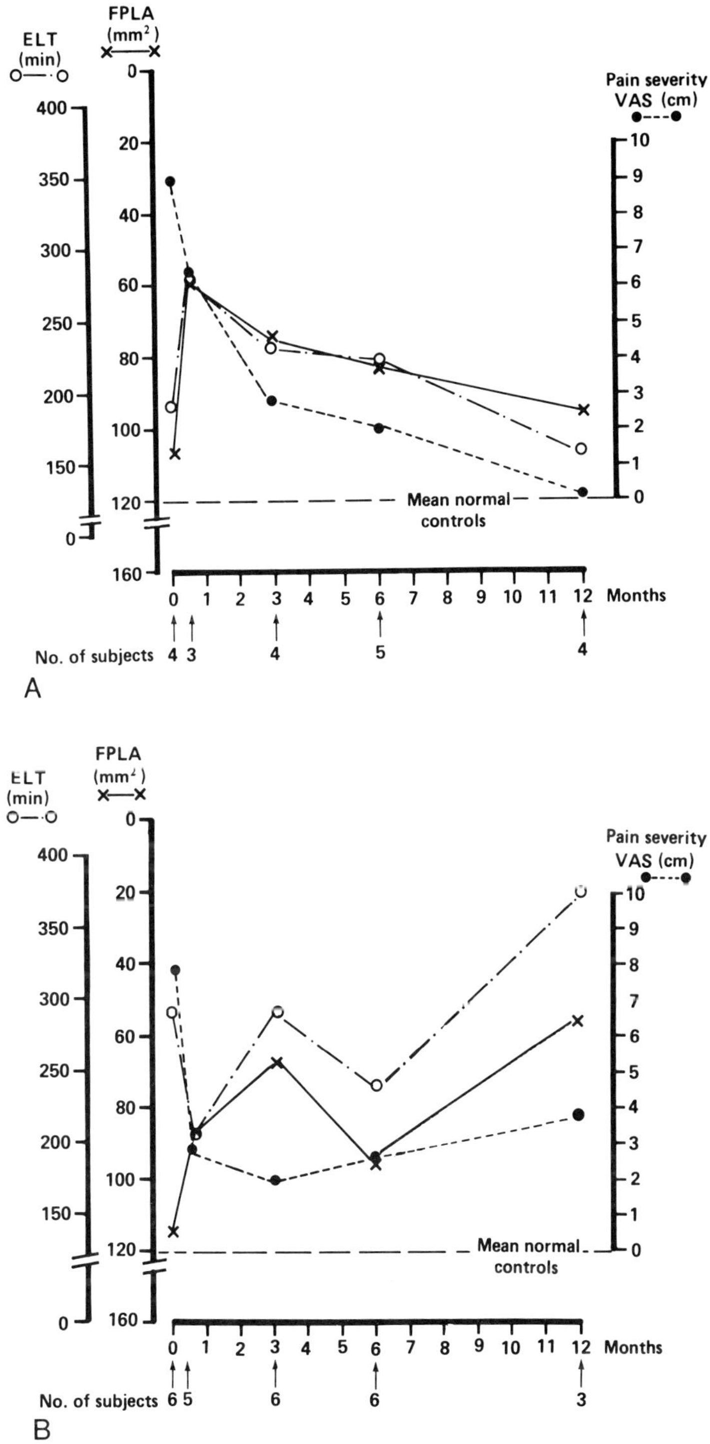

Figure 10 □ Sequential measurements of fibrinolytic activity in patients whose back pain resolved (*A*) and in those whose pain persisted (*B*). The relative pain is measured on a visual analog score and shows correlation of outcome with change in the fibrinolytic foramina. (From Klimiuk, P.S., Pountain, G.D., Keegan, A.L., and Jayson, M.I.V.: Serial measurements of fibrinolytic activity in acute low back pain and sciatica. Spine 12:925–928, 1987.)

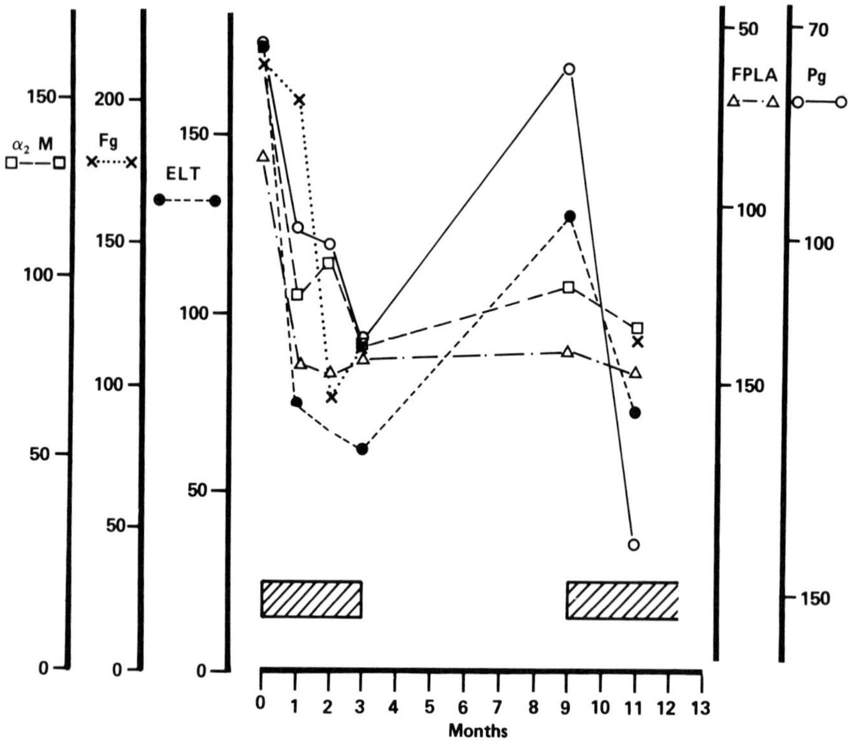

Figure 11 □ Sequential measurements of fibrinolytic activity in a patient with chronic back pain. The patient responded well to treatment. After 3 months, treatment was stopped because of androgenic adverse effects. Over the succeeding 6 months, symptoms gradually relapsed. Treatment was resumed, again with improvement in fibrinolytic parameters.

blood. Normalization of fibrinolytic activity is associated with clearance of fibrin and restoration of damaged tissues toward normal. In some cases, however, there is persistent tissue damage. Blood vessels may be compressed with endothelial damage, fibrin deposition, and thrombosis; this is associated with fibrous proliferation around the nerve roots and in turn may lead to changes within the nerve roots themselves. A persistent fibrinolytic defect is present in the peripheral blood, and this may contribute toward the persistence of the tissue damage. These secondary changes play an important role in the chronicity of the back pain in some individuals.

These abnormalities are most marked in postlaminectomy arachnoiditis, in which there is commonly foreign material that may act as the irritant leading to tissue damage. In particular, cotton debris from swabs and patties seems to be of great importance. Attention must be directed toward further analyzing the problem and preventing fragmentation of swabs and patties in order to avoid this complication.

It appears that a vicious circle may occur, in which chronic vascular and tissue damage develop in association with a defect in the fibrinolytic activity. The tissue damage leads to the fibrinolytic defect, and this in turn leads to failure to clear fibrin and to persistence of the tissue damage (Fig. 12). If this idea is correct, stimulation of the fibrinolytic

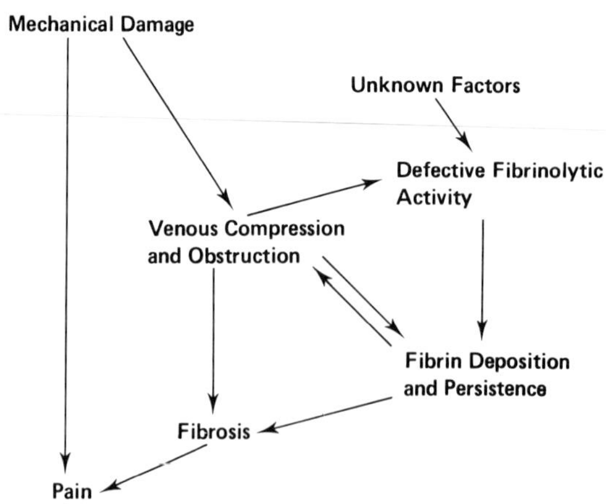

Figure 12 □ A hypothesis of chronic back pain is diagrammed.

system may be helpful in appropriate cases. Preliminary studies of this approach to treatment are encouraging, but further studies are needed.

Acknowledgments

My thanks are due to Dr. A. J. Freemont, Dr. J. Hoyland, Ms. K. Illingworth, Dr. P. Klimiuk, Dr. W. Mitchell, and Dr. W. Morris, all of whom have made major contributions to this research program.

References

1. Lawrence, J. S.: Rheumatism in Populations. London, Heinemann, 1977, pp. 68–97.
2. Lindahl, O.: Hyperalgesia of the lumbar nerve roots in sciatica. Acta Orthop. Scand. 37:367–374, 1966.
3. Goldie, I.: Granulation tissue in the ruptured intervertebral disc. Acta Pathol. Scand. 42:302–304, 1958.
4. Hirsch, C.: Studies on the pathology of low back pain. J. Bone Joint Surg. 41B:237–243, 1959.
5. Lindhal, O., and Rexed, B.: Histological changes in spinal nerve roots of operated cases of sciatica. Acta Orthop. Scand. 20:215–225, 1951.
6. Watanabe, A., and Parke, W. W.: Vascular and neural pathology of lumbosacral spinal stenosis. J. Neurosurg. 64:64–70, 1986.
7. Diamant, B., Karlsson, J., and Nachemson, A.: Correlation between lactate levels and pH of discs of patients with lumbar rhizopathies. Experientia 24:1195–1196, 1968.
8. Nachemson, A.: Intradiscal measurements of pH in patients with lumbar rhizopathies. Acta Orthop. Scand. 40:23–42, 1969.
9. Hansen, H. -J.: A pathologic-anatomical study on disc degeneration in dog. Acta Orthop. Scand. 11(Suppl.):1–117, 1952.
10. Elvis, M. W., Buchnill, T., and Sullivan, M. F.: In-vitro inhibition of leucocyte migration in patients with intervertebral disc lesions. Orthop. Clin. North Am. 6:59–65, 1975.
11. Gertzbein, S. D., Tile, M., Gross, A., and Falk, R.: Auto-immunity in degenerative disc disease of the lumbar spine. Orthop. Clin. North Am. 6:67–73, 1975.
12. Bisca, R. S., Marchisello, T. J., Lockshin, M. D., et al.: Auto-immunological basis of disc degeneration. Clin. Orthop. Rel. Res. 121:205–211, 1976.
13. Elkington, J. St. C.: Meningitis serosa circumscripta spinalis (spinal arachnoiditis. Brain 59:181–203, 1936.
14. Arner, O.: Complications Following Spinal Anaesthesia. Acta Chir. Scand. (Suppl.):167, 1952.
15. Hansen, E. B., Fahrenkrug, A., and Priestholm, J.: Late meningial effects of myelographic contrast media with special reference to metrizamide. Br. J. Radiol. 51:321–327, 1958.
16. de la Porte, C., and Siegfried, J.: Lumbo-sacral spinal fibrosis (Spinal Arachnoiditis). Spine 8:593–603, 1983.
17. Burton, C. V.: Lumbo-sacral arachnoiditis. Spine 3:24–30, 1978.
18. Quiles, M., Marchisello, P. J., and Tsairis, P.: Lumbar adhesive arachnoiditis. Etiologic and pathologic aspects. Spine 3:45–50, 1978.
19. Hoyland, J. A., Freemont, A. J., Denton, J., et al.: Retained surgical swab debris in post-laminectomy arachnoiditis and peridural fibrosis J. Bone Joint Surg. 70B:659–662, 1988.
20. Hoffman, G. S.: Spinal arachnoiditis: What is the clinical spectrum? Spine 8:538–540, 1983.
21. Hoyland, J. A., Freemont, A. J., and Jayson, M. I. V.: Age-related changes in the structures within and bordering the intervertebral foramina: Associations with low back pain. *In* Hukins, D. W., and Nelson, M. A. (eds.): The Ageing Spine. Manchester University Press, 1987, pp. 94–110.
22. Innes, D., and Sevitt, S.: Coagulation and fibrinolysis in injured patients. J. Clin. Pathol. 17:1–13, 1964.
23. Dumonde, D. C., and Glynn, L. E.: The production of arthritis in rabbits by an immunological reaction to fibrin. Br. J. Exp. Pathol. 43:373–383, 1962.
24. Browse, N. L.: Venous ulceration. Br. Med. J. 286:1920–1922, 1983.
25. Haverkate, F., and Brakman, P.: Fibrin Plate Assay. *In* Davidson, J. F., Samama, M. M., and Desmoyers, P. C. (eds.): Progress in Chemical Fibrinolysis and Thrombolysis. New York, Raven Press, pp. 1, 151–159, 1979.
26. Cash, J. D., and Leask, E.: Automatic determination of euglobulin lysis time. J. Clin. Pathol. 18:821–823, 1965.
27. Clauss, A.: Rapid physiological coagulation method in determination of fibrinogen. Acta Haematol. 17:237–246, 1957.
28. Jayson, M. I. V., Keegan, A., Million, R., and Tomlinson, I.: A fibrinolytic defect in chronic back pain syndromes. Lancet 2:1186–1187, 1984.
29. Pountain, G. D., Keegan, A. L., and Jayson, M. I. V.: Impaired fibrinolytic activity in defined chronic back pain syndromes. Spine 12:83–86, 1987.
30. Klimiuk, P. S., Pountain, G. D., Keegan, A. L., and Jayson, M. I. V.: Serial measurements of fibrinolytic activity in acute low back pain and sciatica. Spine 12:925–928, 1987.
31. Frymoyer, J. W., Pope, M. H., Clements, J. H., et al.: Risk factors in low back pain: An epidemiological study. J. Bone Joint Surg. 65A:213–218, 1983.
32. Meade, T. W., Chakrabarti, R., Haines, A. P., et al.: Characteristics affecting fibrinolytic activity and plasma fibrinogen concentrations. Br. Med. J. 1:153–156, 1979.
33. Belch, J. J. F., Madhok, R., McArdle, B., et al.: The effect of increasing fibrinolysis in patients with rheumatoid arthritis: A double blind controlled trial. Q. J. Med. 58:19–27, 1986.
34. Cunliffe, W. J., Dodman, B., Roberts, B. E., and Tebbs, E. M.: Clinical and laboratory double blind investigation of fibrinolytic therapy of cutaneous vasculitis. *In* Davidson, J. F., Samama, M. M., and Desmoyes, P. C. (eds.): Progress in Chemical Fibrinolysis and Thrombolysis. New York, Raven Press, 1975, pp. 325–332.
35. Jayson, M. I. V., Holland, C. D., Keegan, A., et al.: Controlled studies of stanozolol in primary Raynaud's phenomenon (PRP) and in systemic sclerosis (SS). Br. J. Rheumatol. 26(Suppl. 2):24, 1987.
36. Waddell, G.: Understanding the patient with back pain. *In* Jayson, M. I. V. (ed.): The Lumbar Spine and Back Pain. London, Churchill-Livingstone, pp. 419–434, 1987.

12 □ Trauma of the Lumbar Spine: Classification and Treatment

Stanley D. Gertzbein
Frank J. Eismont

Interest has been renewed in the surgical management of lumbar fractures because of the development of new spinal fixation devices. This chapter reviews the relevant anatomy and biomechanics, the concept of spinal instability, the mechanisms of injury, and the classification of lumbar injuries. It addresses the clinical evaluation of patients with these injuries, the diagnostic techniques available, and details of management techniques. The chapter concludes with an algorithm for decision-making.

ANATOMY AND BIOMECHANICS

The vertebral bodies increase in strength from L1 to L5; this is directly related to size rather than mineral content.[70] However, the ability of the vertebrae to resist loads decreases with age.[6] Cancellous bone transmits 55% of the axial load in individuals under the age of 40 years but only 35% over the age of 40 years.[64] Vertebrae fail under compressive loading in different modes that fall into three groups.[46] In the first group, there is decreasing strength in the load deformation curve after loading to failure, which explains progressive collapse when lumbar fractures are axially loaded. In the second group, vertebral strength is constant after failure. In the third group, vertebral strength actually increases; this is most often seen in females under the age of 40 years.

A leash of blood vessels enters the posterior cortex of the vertebral body at the junction of the upper and middle thirds. This is a site of weakness and acts as a stress riser, which results in a typical fracture of the posterior vertebral body commonly seen with burst injuries. This has clearly been demonstrated by Fredrickson and colleagues in experimental studies in the laboratory (Fig. 1).[31]

Considerable importance has been attached to the integrity of the anterior longitudinal ligament[3] and the posterior longitudinal ligament.[5] They are uniaxial structures that resist tensile forces. The site of failure depends on the rate of loading, with bone failing at a slower rate of loading than ligaments.[58]

Most lumbar spinal fractures fail in axial loading or flexion, rather than in rotation. Because of their orientation, the lumbar facet joints limit axial rotation. The intervertebral disc transfers compressive loads from one vertebra to the other through the nucleus pulposus and annulus fibrosus.[72] Increasing axial load may cause the nucleus pulposus to rupture through the end-plates into the adjacent vertebra,[9] resulting in the typical burst fracture.

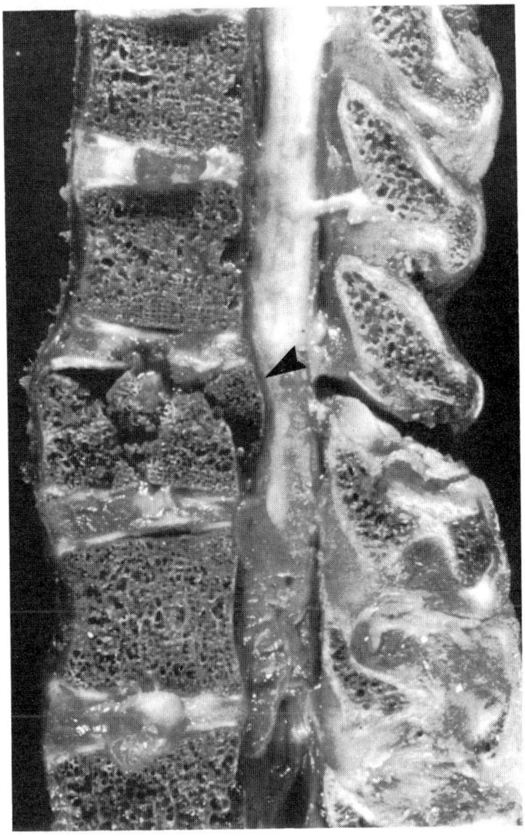

Figure 1 □ Cadaver specimen demonstrates a burst fracture with a fragment of bone penetrating the spinal canal at the junction of the upper and middle thirds of the posterior cortex (*arrow*), a point of entry of a leash of blood vessels that acts as a stress riser. (Courtesy of Dr. B. Fredrickson.)

Because the spinal cord usually ends at the L1–L2 disc, injuries to the first lumbar vertebra commonly involve the conus medullaris and the lumbar nerve rootlets, which arise from the more proximal spinal cord. Below this level the nerve rootlets are involved, and the lesion produced is purely of the lower motor neuron type.

SPINAL INSTABILITY

The concept of instability of the spinal column has been developed over the last 3 or 4 decades by a number of investigators. Nicoll in 1949[56] suggested that the integrity of the interspinous ligaments was the major factor in maintaining stability. Holdsworth[41] described instability as occurring when the entire posterior ligamentous complex was disrupted along with the anterior portion of the spinal column. Bedbrook[2] disagreed with this concept and pointed out that disruption of the posterior ligamentous complex was frequently carried out surgically without resulting instability. Rather, he believed that the integrity of the disc and anterior longitudinal ligament were more important factors in maintaining stability.

The work of Holdsworth was useful in providing an early understanding of the mechanisms of injury, but he did not recognize the significance of instability in flexion–distraction injuries or burst fractures. The use of computed tomography (CT) has helped demonstrate that many spinal fractures are more extensive than formerly realized, leading to a more sophisticated concept of spinal instability.

Denis[18] undertook a retrospective survey of 412 thoracolumbar fractures and introduced the concept of the three-column spine. He also classified spinal fractures according to the mechanisms of injury and their resulting fracture pattern. The three-column concept is a major advance in our understanding of spinal stability, particularly with reference to burst fractures.

Complete disruption of the posterior ligamentous complex is not sufficient to create instability;[3, 59, 62] therefore, the concept of the three-column spine was introduced to explain empirical observations of vertebral collapse and malalignment. When trauma to

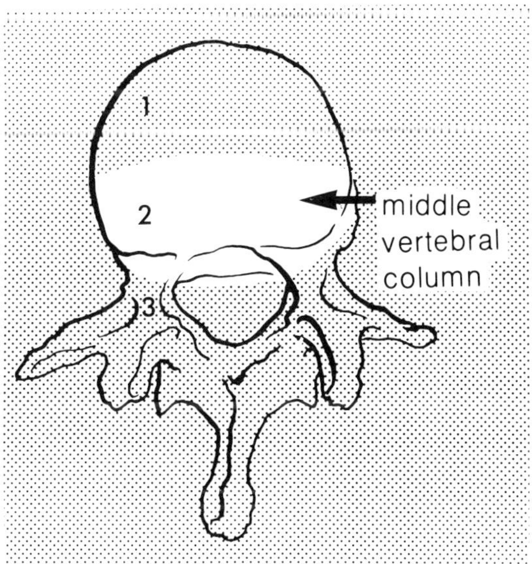

Figure 2 □ Axial cut of a typical lumbar vertebra demonstrates the anterior (1), middle (2), and posterior columns. (Modified from Floman, Y. [ed.]: The Lumbar Spine—Current Concepts. Freund Publishing House Ltd. [in press])

Table 1 □ Modes of Failure of the Three Columns for the Four Major Spinal Injuries*

TYPE	COLUMN		
	Anterior	**Middle**	**Posterior**
Compression	Compression	None	None or distraction (severe)
Burst	Compression	Compression	None or splaying of pedicles
Flexion–distraction	None or distraction	Distraction	Distraction
Fracture/dislocation	Compression Rotation Shear	Distraction Rotation Shear	Distraction Rotation Shear

*From Denis, F., Armstrong, E. W., Searls, K., et al: Acute thoracolumbar burst fractures in the absence of neurological deficit: A comparison between operative and non-operative treatment. Clin. Orthop. 189:142–149, 1984.

the posterior longitudinal ligament and posterior annulus fibrosus occurs, instability in flexion results. The posterior column consists of all structures posterior to the posterior longitudinal ligament, whereas the middle column includes the posterior longitudinal ligament, the posterior annulus fibrosus and the posterior wall of the vertebral body (Fig. 2). The anterior column is formed by the anterior longitudinal ligament, the anterior annulus fibrosus, and the anterior part of the vertebral body. Instability is present when two or three columns are disrupted.

Denis categorized fracture types into four major spinal injuries and four minor injuries. None of the latter types is unstable (Table 1).

MECHANISMS OF INJURY AND CLASSIFICATION

The spine may fail in the following directions: flexion–extension, rotation, side bending, anteroposterior or lateral shear; compression–distraction, or a combination of these; well-recognized patterns of injury result. The forces and vectors applied to the spine have been described by Denis,[18] as related to the fracture patterns (see Table 1). We believe that this classification is the most practical to date, although a number of other recent classifications have been proposed.[27, 48, 50]

COMPRESSION FRACTURES

Compression fractures occur with eccentric axial loading. This load may be applied anterior or lateral to the axis of rotation (Fig. 3), resulting in the common anterior wedge fracture or the less common lateral compression fracture.[18]

On lateral radiographs, anterior compression fractures are characterized by a loss of height in the anterior column. There is usually no damage to the middle or posterior columns, although in younger patients who have had violent injuries the posterior elements may be disrupted (Fig. 4).

The anterior compression fracture has four subtypes. In Type A both end-plates are damaged, whereas in the more common Type B the superior end-plate is fractured. The inferior end-plate alone is fractured in Type C, and in Type D end-plates are intact but the anterior vertebral cortex is compressed.

BURST FRACTURES

These injuries are caused by axial loading (Fig. 5). The end-plates are damaged first, commonly during falls or traffic accidents, although other mechanisms, such as rapid ejection from an aircraft, also result in this type of fracture.[72] The three types of end-plate fracture are (1) those involving the central portion of the end-plate, (2) those occurring at the periphery of the end-plate, and (3) those producing transverse cracks across the end-plate.

The load-bearing capacity of the lumbar vertebra varies with changes in a number of factors, such as the magnitude of the applied axial load, the time over which the load is applied, the spatial orientation of the vertebral column, and the age of the bone.[6] Axially loaded vertebrae in individuals over 60 years of age fail at approximately 4,200 newtons (N), whereas under the age of 40 years the average load to failure is 7,600 N.[60] Increased loading causes a crack in the end-plate to propagate in different directions. This is followed by displacement of the disc into the vertebral body, at which stage the

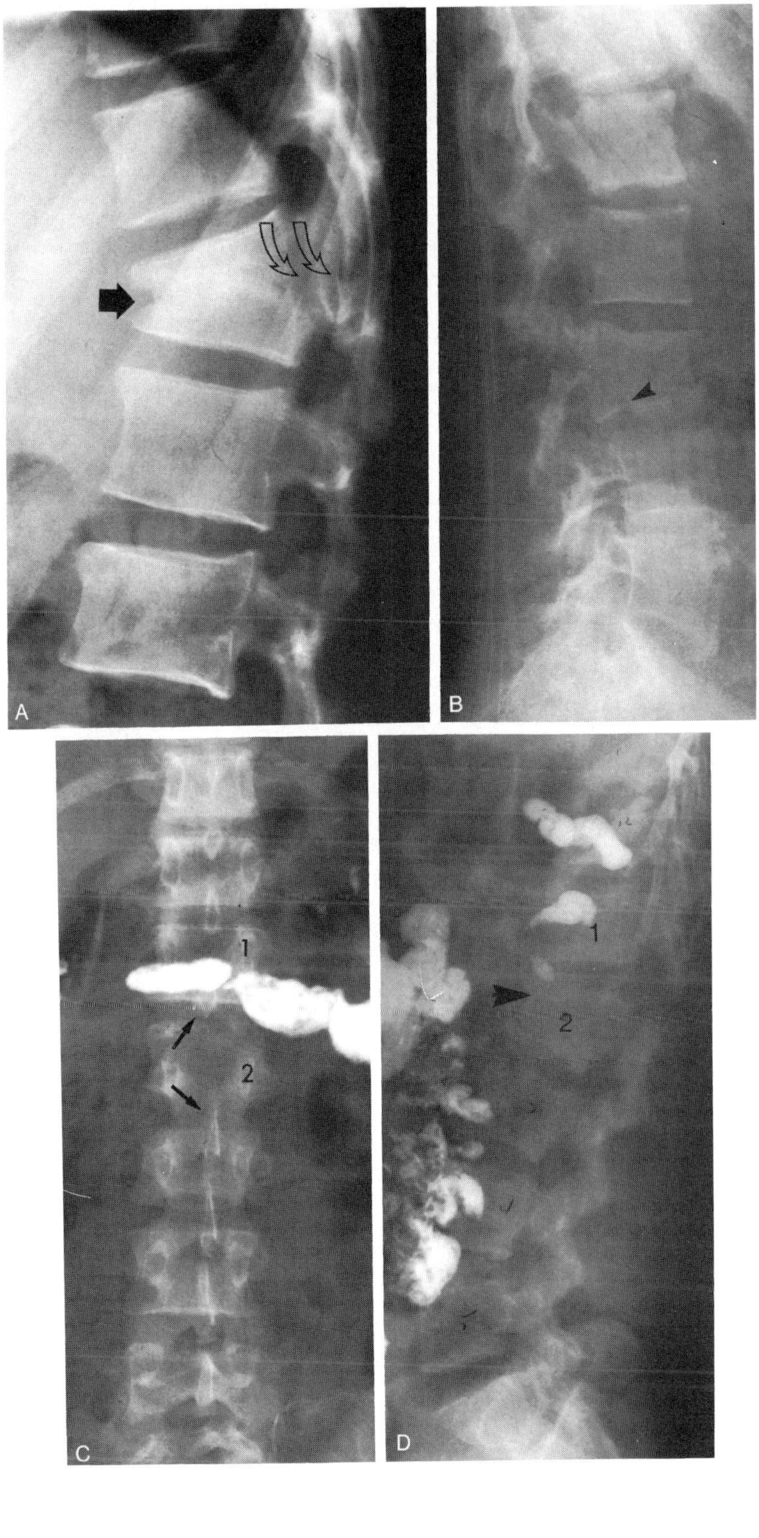

Figure 7 □ Flexion–distraction injuries. *A,* This injury extends through the posterior arch (*open arrows*) and through the vertebral body to the anterior cortex (*arrow*) and is classified as a Type IB injury. *B,* A second example is this flexion–distraction type of injury, which passes between the spinous processes and extends from the midportion of the posterior cortex of the body, inferiorly to the disc space and anteriorly through the disc (*arrow*). *C, D,* A third variant demonstrates a widening of the interspinous spaces (*arrows*), on the AP radiograph between L1 and L2, with a wedge compression component noted on the lateral radiograph (*arrow*). (Modified from Floman, Y. [ed.]: The Lumbar Spine—Current Concepts. Freund Publishing House Ltd. [in press])

that considerable axial loading in the spine occurs early during deceleration. The magnitude of the axial load depends on the G forces encountered during deceleration. In addition, an increase in the axial load occurs late in a deceleration phase, as a result of the body being lifted off the seat and then returning to the sitting position. The most common Chance fracture in this study was Type C(2) (Fig. 6).

An anteroposterior radiograph shows an apparent gap between the posterior elements of the adjacent vertebra caused by the distraction component of the fracture (Fig. 7). There may be an associated anterior compression or burst fracture (Fig. 7). CT scanning may be helpful if an associated burst fracture is suspected.

EXTENSION FRACTURES

This type of injury is rare in the lumbar spine. It may occur with violent extension forces causing loads in tension anteriorly (Fig. 8).

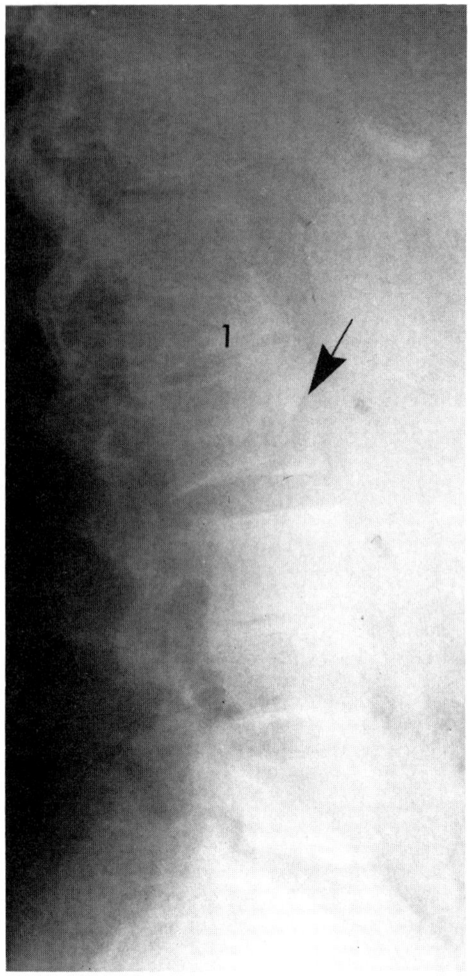

Figure 8 □ Extension fracture: This patient, with an old wedge compression fracture of L1, suffered an extension injury with a teardrop fracture noted at the anteroinferior corner (*arrow*).

FRACTURES/DISLOCATIONS

Fracture/dislocation of the lumbar spine occurs when there is failure of all three columns of the spine under compression, tension, rotation, or shear, or a combination of these forces. The essential feature of this injury is that the magnitude of the applied loads is sufficient to disrupt the intrinsically stable anatomy. Disruption of the facet joints leads to subluxation or dislocation. Occasionally, a fracture/dislocation may be spontaneously reduced, and the true nature of the lesion may be missed on conventional radiographs. CT scans often show the extent of bony injury. Fracture/dislocation injuries can be divided into three types related to the direction of loads applied.[18]

Flexion–Rotation Injuries

This injury occurs when the posterior and middle columns fail under tension and rotation and the anterior column fails under compression and rotation. This leads to anterior wedging of the vertebral body and stripping of the anterior longitudinal ligament from the vertebra below (Fig. 9).

Shear Injuries

All three columns are disrupted by this injury, including the anterior longitudinal ligament. The shear force is usually applied in the lateral direction (Fig. 10) but may also occur in the anteroposterior direction (Fig. 11).[20]

Flexion–Distraction Burst Injuries

This is a variant of the seat belt injury produced by a combination of flexion and distraction.[15] Failure occurs through the ligaments and/or bone in the posterior and middle columns and the disc and/or bone in the anterior column. The anterior longitu-

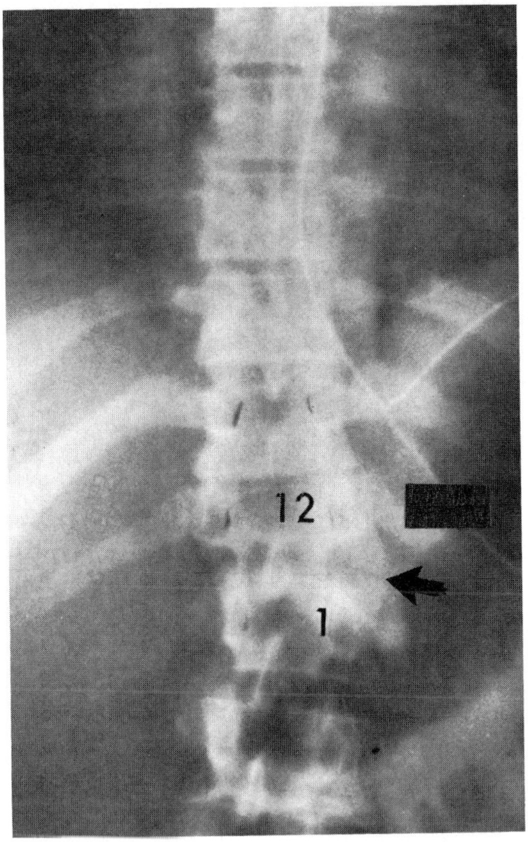

Figure 9 □ Fracture/dislocation of T12–L1 with significant lateral translation (*arrow*) as a result of rotational forces. (Modified from Floman, Y. [ed.]: The Lumbar Spine—Current Concepts. Freund Publishing House Ltd. [in press])

dinal ligament is stripped from the vertebra below (Fig. 12).

POSTERIOR ARCH FRACTURES

Fractures of the posterior vertebral column are stable. They are commonly seen as fractures of the articular processes, the transverse processes, the spinous process, or the pars interarticularis (Fig. 13). Two mechanisms of injury are likely: flexion and axial rotation, and extension. Sometimes these injuries are difficult to diagnose on plain radiographs, and tomography or CT scanning may be required for an accurate diagnosis. Transverse process fractures often result from direct blunt trauma to the spine or avulsion of the tip secondary to violent contraction of the attached muscle. It should be remembered that fractures of the L5 transverse process may be associated with severe pelvic fractures[69] and may provide a clue to the instability of the pelvis. They may also be the direct result of violent lateral flexion. Transverse process fractures of the upper lumbar vertebrae may be associated with hematoma, causing neuropraxia of the femoral nerve as the roots pass through the psoas muscle, although femoral nerve neuropraxia may occur with rupture of the psoas muscle alone.[33]

Posterior element fractures commonly occur in association with more major spinal fractures; an incidence as high as 39% has been noted with Chance fractures.[15]

CLINICAL EVALUATION OF PATIENTS WITH LUMBAR SPINAL FRACTURES

Evaluation begins with obtaining a history of the injury. This often allows the examiner to determine the mechanism and energy of injury. Questioning the patient about neurologic symptoms, even transient extremity weakness or paresthesias, often helps the physician to evaluate the extent of instability and neural compression. Associated injuries can often be detected from a carefully taken history.

A cramping pain in the legs should specifically be questioned because it often indicates neural compression, just as it does with severe spinal stenosis or an impending cauda equina syndrome. Its presence should indicate to the clinician that the extent of neural compression is significant, even if the patient is neurologically normal.

Examination should include an assessment of vital signs; gross examination of the head, trunk, and extremities; and palpation of the spine from the first cervical vertebra to the sacrum. Abdominal abrasions, if present, may indicate a seat belt injury with a flexion–distraction injury of the spine. The clinician should rule out associated intra-abdominal injuries. The back should be inspected to be certain there are no significant abrasions that may influence the decision to perform surgery.

The physical examination should include a sensory and motor examination with careful documentation of the findings. A perineal examination is most important and should include a rectal examination for baseline tone, voluntary sphincter contraction, and perineal sensation, which should indicate the ability to distinguish sharpness from

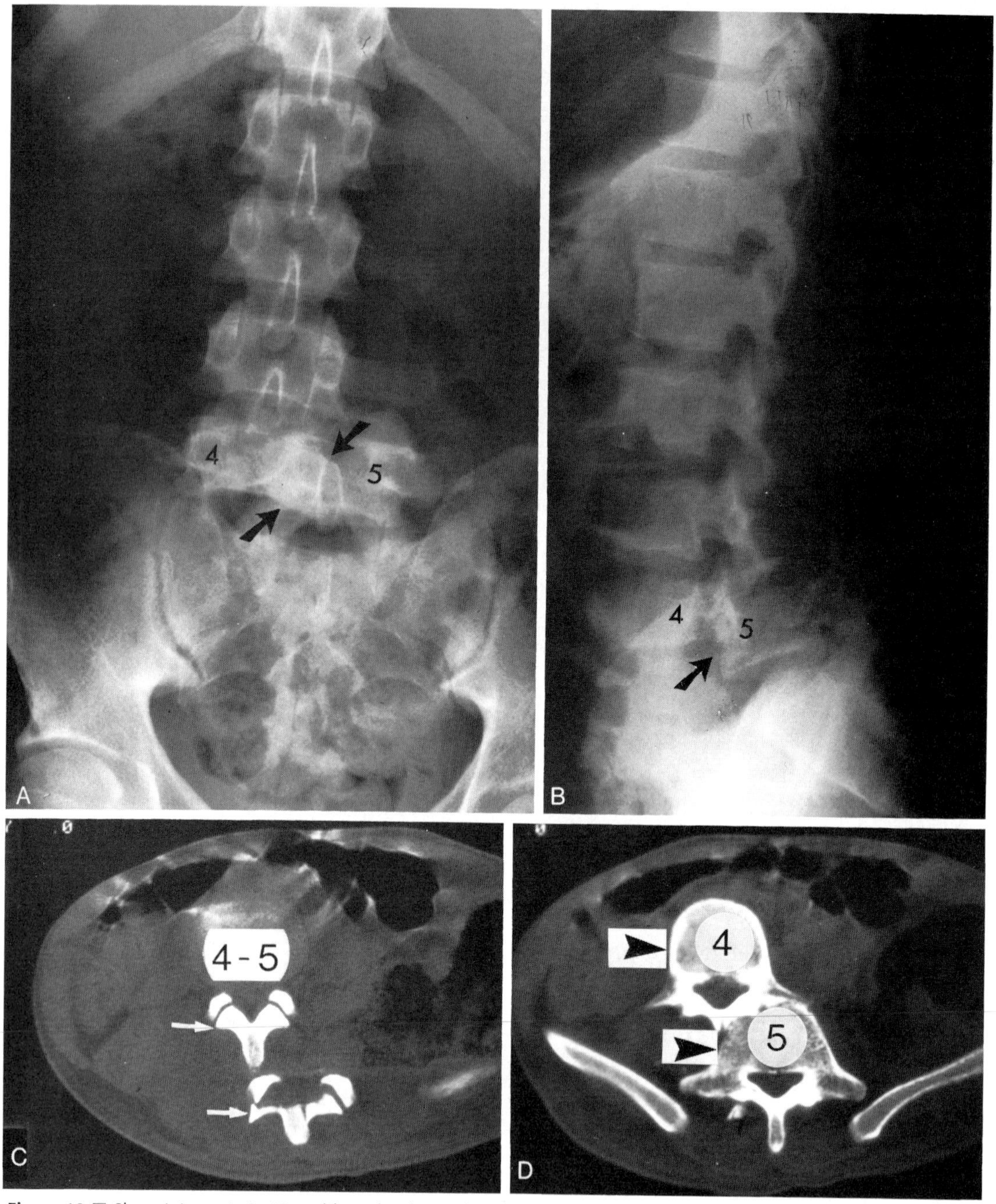

Figure 10 □ Shear injury. *A, B,* AP and lateral radiographs demonstrate displacement of the vertebral column to the right and anteriorly (*arrows*). *C, D,* CT scan of the posterior elements (*white arrows*) and vertebral bodies (*arrowheads*), respectively, seen in the same axial cuts. (Modified from Floman, Y. [ed.]: The Lumbar Spine—Current Concepts. Freund Publishing House Ltd. [in press])

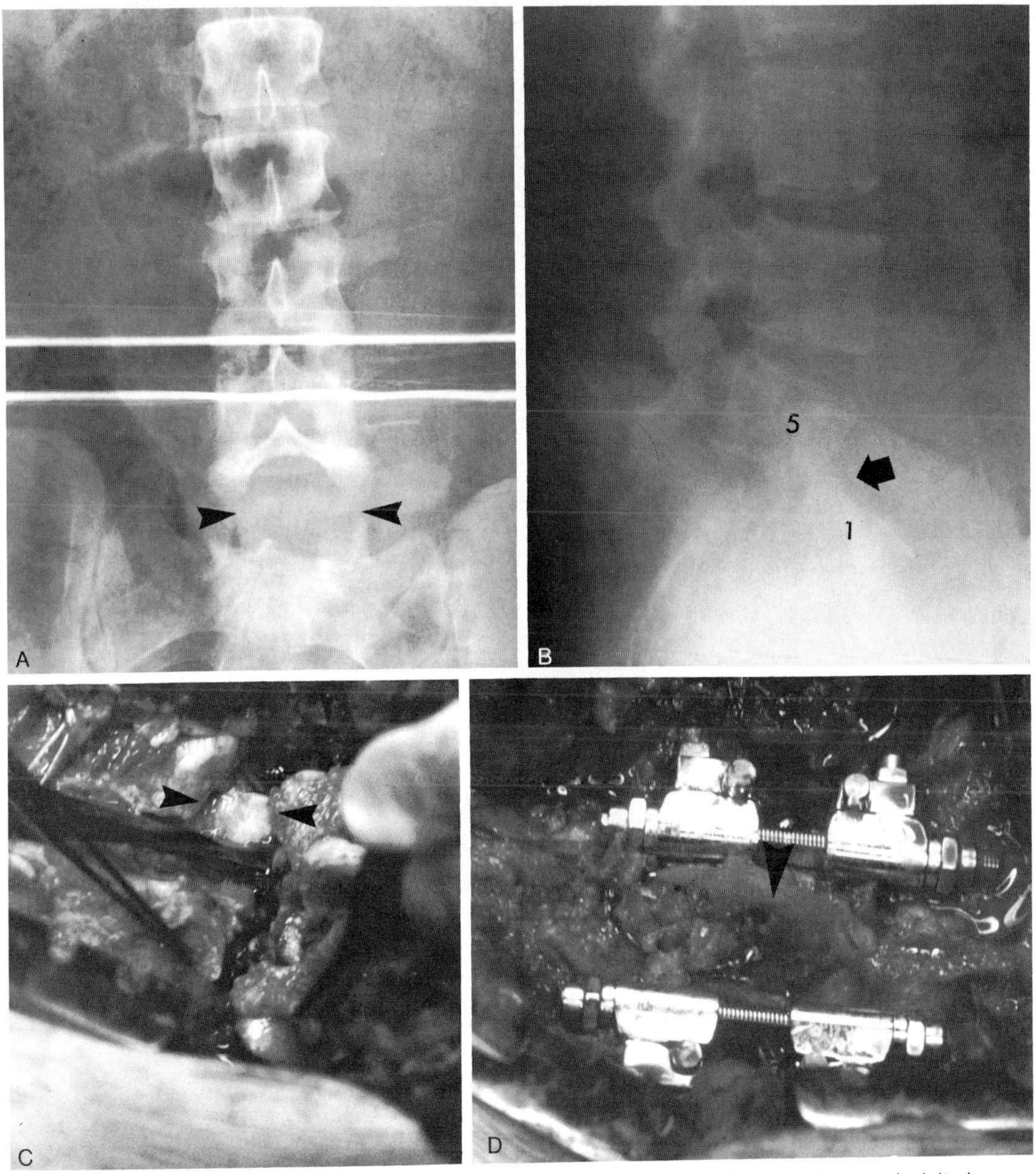

Figure 11 □ Posterior shear injury. *A, B,* AP and lateral radiographs of the lumbosacral junction show marked displacement of the L5 vertebra posteriorly on the sacrum and widening of the L5–S1 interspinous distance (*arrows*). *C,* Severe posterior shear forces have disrupted the soft tissues as seen intraoperatively (*arrows*). *D,* The gap is closed with an interspinous wire, transfacetal screws, and pedicle fixation, using an AO internal fixator (*arrow*).

Illustration continued on following page

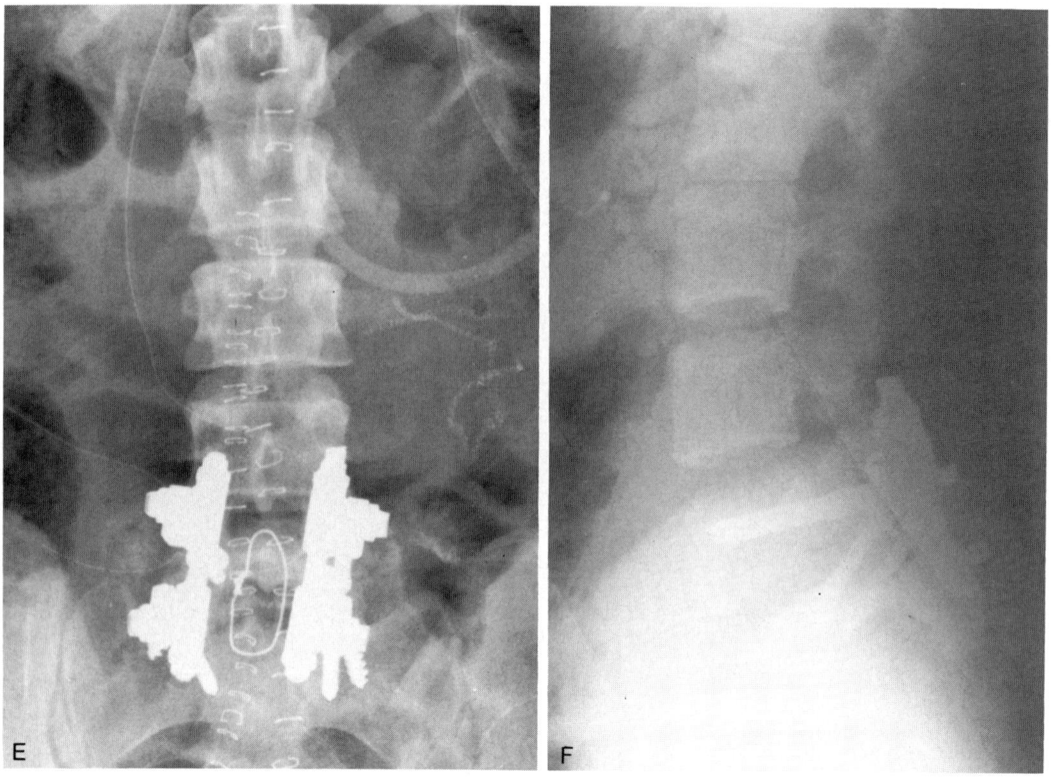

Figure 11 *Continued E, F,* AP and lateral postoperative radiographs demonstrate completed reduction.

dullness during testing with a safety pin. The examination is not complete until a postvoid residual urine volume is assessed, with 50 cc being the upper limit of normal. The importance of this perineal and bladder assessment cannot be overemphasized, because injuries to the conus medullaris or S2–S4 nerve rootlets may be seen in isolation while the remainder of the neurologic examination is entirely normal.

DIAGNOSTIC EVALUATION OF PATIENTS WITH LUMBAR SPINAL FRACTURES

When there is a suspected spinal injury, the patient should remain immobilized on a spine board until the clinical and radiologic assessment has been completed. Plain anteroposterior and lateral radiographs of the affected area of the spine should first be obtained. If there is an associated paralysis, the entire spine should be studied, because there is a 5% or greater incidence of multiple levels of spinal injuries in this group of patients.[11]

CT scans are routinely performed for further evaluation of lumbar spinal fractures, including scans at least one level above and one level below the injured vertebra. These studies are most useful for assessing intrusion of bone fragments into the spinal canal and for evaluation of posterior element fractures, including the lamina fractures often seen in conjunction with burst injuries.[12, 50, 51, 54] They are most limited for the detection of transverse fractures, and significant Chance fractures can often be undetected unless sagittal reconstruction is performed. Disc herniation should be visible on a plain CT scan; however, if there is an associated vertebral subluxation, the disc herniation will often be misinterpreted as an averaging of the signal due to subluxation. Another weakness is that the neural tissues are poorly visualized by CT, unless performed after a myelogram is obtained. When indicated, this can be safely done with the patient remaining immobilized and supine on the spine

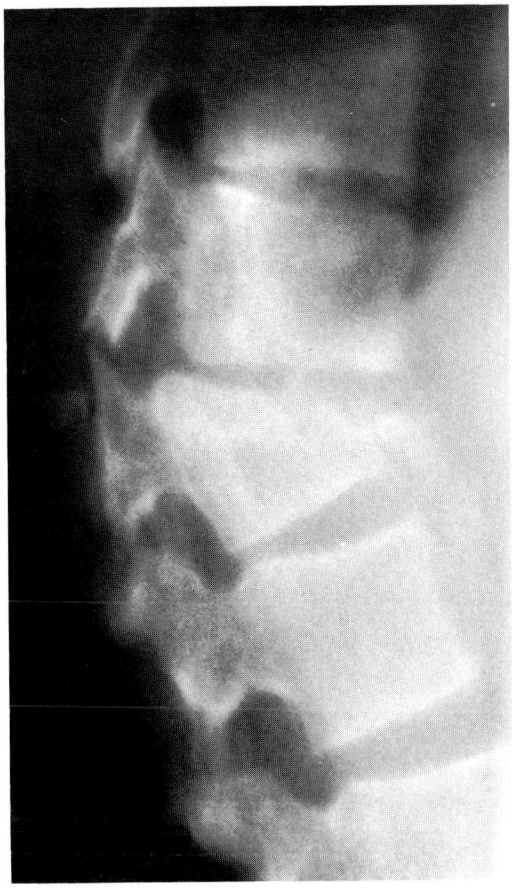

Figure 12 □ Flexion–distraction burst injury. This lateral tomogram demonstrates the combination of flexion–distraction as well as burst injury, representing a complex combination of forces.

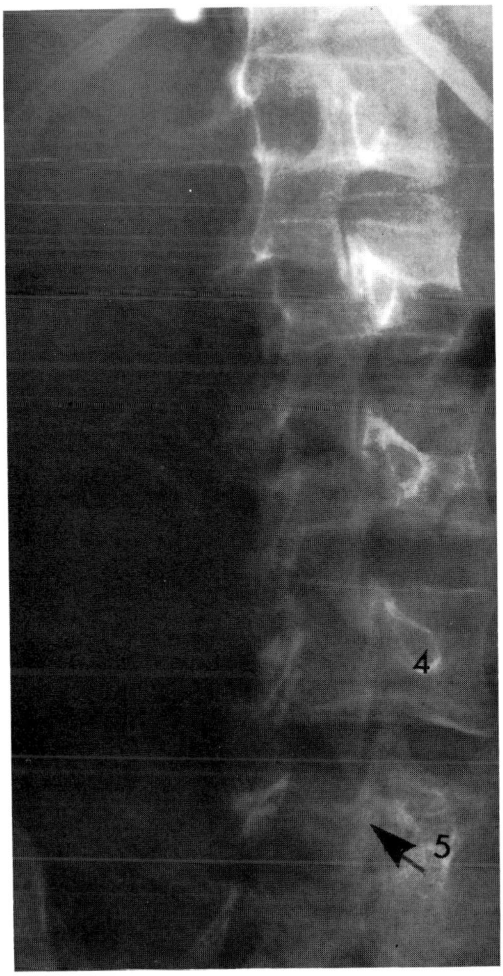

Figure 13 □ Posterior arch injuries. Fracture of the pars interarticularis (*arrow*) has resulted from hyperextension forces. (Modified from Flomen, Y. [ed.]: Spine—Current Concepts. Freund Publishing House Ltd. [in press])

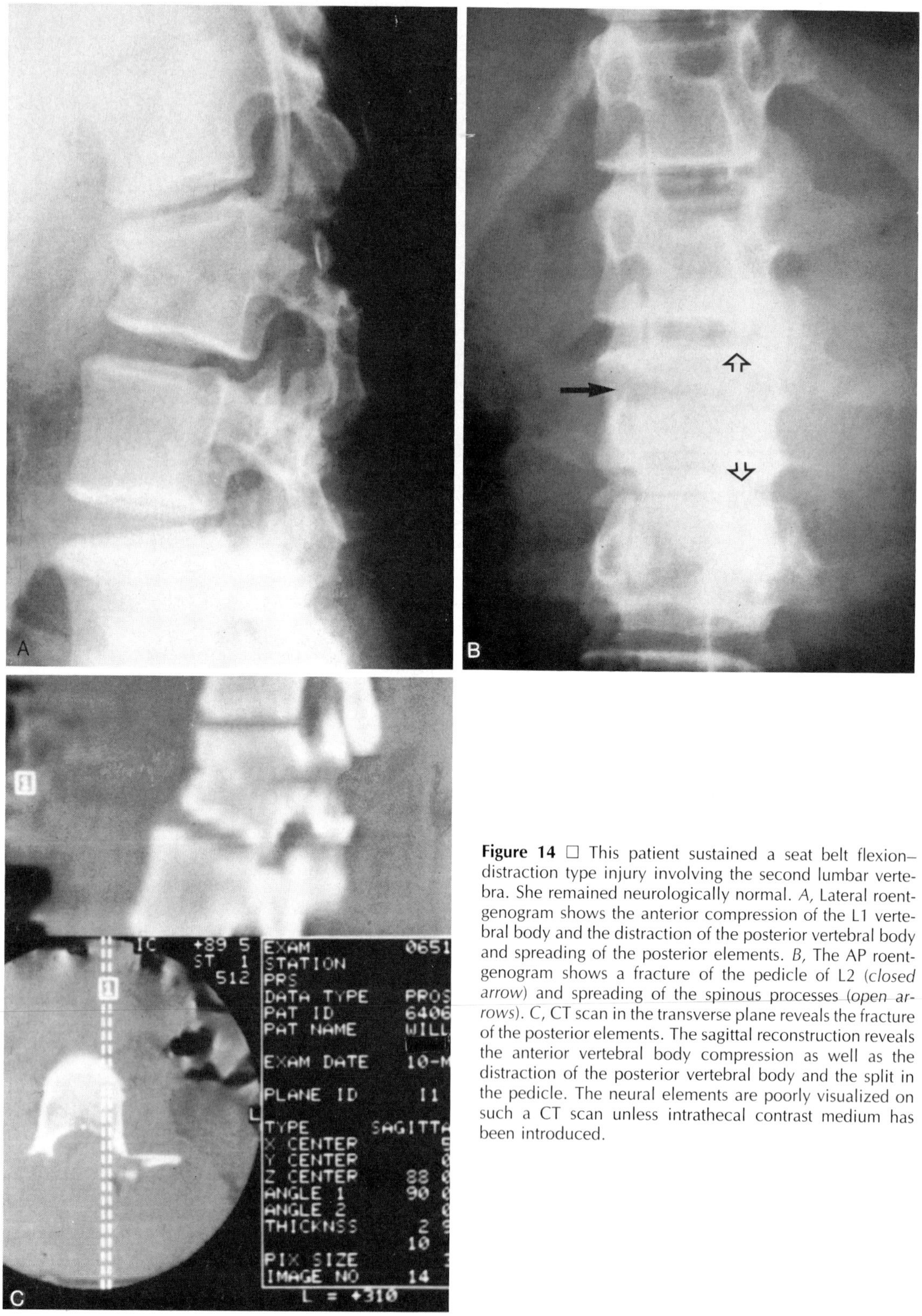

Figure 14 □ This patient sustained a seat belt flexion–distraction type injury involving the second lumbar vertebra. She remained neurologically normal. *A,* Lateral roentgenogram shows the anterior compression of the L1 vertebral body and the distraction of the posterior vertebral body and spreading of the posterior elements. *B,* The AP roentgenogram shows a fracture of the pedicle of L2 (*closed arrow*) and spreading of the spinous processes (*open arrows*). *C,* CT scan in the transverse plane reveals the fracture of the posterior elements. The sagittal reconstruction reveals the anterior vertebral body compression as well as the distraction of the posterior vertebral body and the split in the pedicle. The neural elements are poorly visualized on such a CT scan unless intrathecal contrast medium has been introduced.

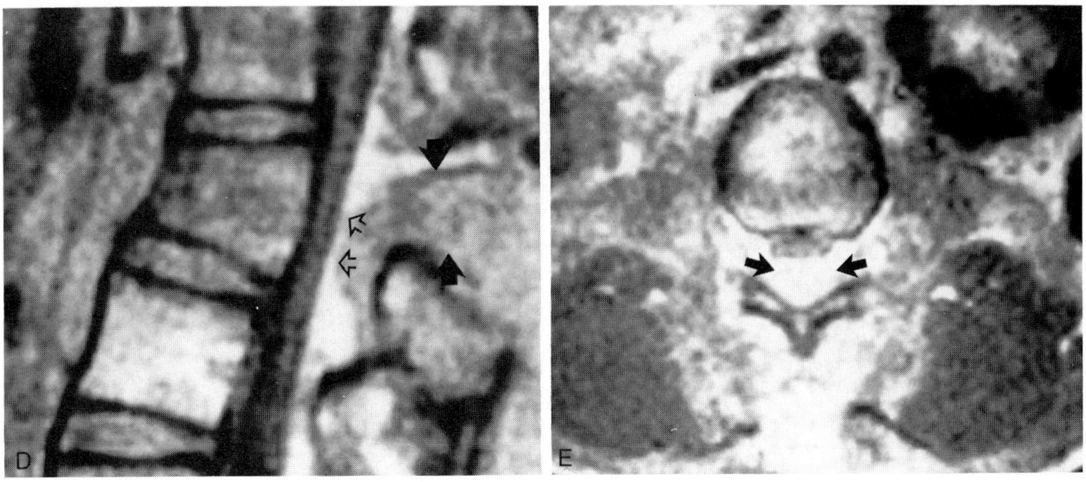

Figure 14 *Continued D,* A midsagittal magnetic resonance (MR) scan shows the bony pathologic condition poorly. The soft tissue visualization, however, is much better, and a hematoma extending from the posterior paraspinal region into the spinal canal (*arrows*) can be seen with the compression of the thecal sac (*open arrows*). *E,* The transverse MR scan again clearly shows the neural compression secondary to hematoma extending to the spinal canal. (Hematoma is marked by arrows.)

board; a lateral C1–C2 needle puncture is performed for introduction of the contrast material.[37] This postmyelogram CT scan is usually reserved for infrequent cases in which the clinical assessment of the patient does not correlate with the radiographic findings and further neural tissue visualization is needed.

Magnetic resonance imaging (MRI) is gradually replacing myelography in the evaluation of patients with spine injuries (Fig. 14). Its major advantages are that it provides much clearer soft tissue visualization than other available tests, and the spinal cord and cauda equina can be assessed for extrinsic compression as well as intrinsic changes. Some preliminary evidence suggests that MRI may be helpful in predicting which spinal cord injuries will be complete and which will be incomplete and potentially reversible.[14] There have also been reports of MRI being used to assess the continuity of the anterior and posterior longitudinal ligaments, which can be helpful information before surgery.[8] Further prospective studies are necessary to better delineate the role of MRI in acute lumbar spine injuries.

Ultrasonography of the spine has been used in the past to transcutaneously assess spinal canal size.[61] The artifacts resulting from the intervening soft tissues and the blockage of the ultrasound signal by the lamina limit its usefulness as a diagnostic test for preoperatively evaluating lumbar spine injuries. It can, however, be used intraoperatively to assess the patency of the spinal canal (Fig. 15).[25, 26, 63]

Any real-time ultrasonography machine that can be set at 7.5 MHz can be used. The tip of the ultrasound probe is covered with a surgical lubricant gel and then covered with a sterile barrier, such as a plastic arthroscopy barrier, while care is taken to eliminate any air bubbles in the gel between the probe tip and the sterile barrier. The surgical wound is then filled with isotonic irrigating solution, and the probe is submerged below the surface to totally eliminate any air interface between the spine and the probe (Fig. 15*B*). A small laminotomy (1.5 cm × 1.0 cm)[26] at the site of injury allows excellent visualization of the thecal sac and its contents. Any anterior neural compression by bone or disc fragments can be clearly documented via the posterior approach to the spine. By simply rotating the probe 90 degrees, the surgeon can obtain either a sagittal or a transverse view of the spinal canal. This is an extremely useful method to check for spinal canal patency, and it can be utilized during and after posterolateral decompression. Because it provides direct visualization of the conus medullaris and/or cauda equina, the information is more detailed than that obtained with an intraoperative myelogram.

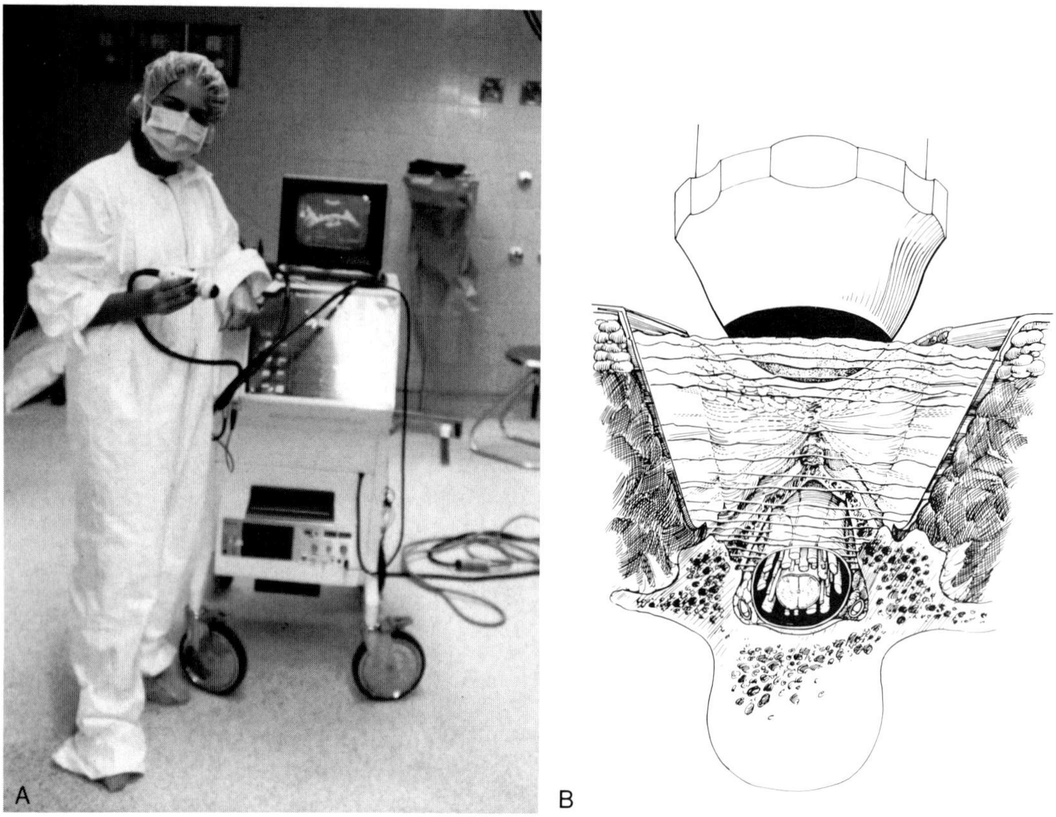

Figure 15 □ *A,* The ultrasonography equipment is shown in the operating room to demonstrate that it is portable and to show the relative size of the probe that is held in the doctor's hand. *B,* This schematic illustration shows the posterior surgical incision with the patient in the prone position and the wound being filled with saline. The probe tip, which has been covered with lubricating gel in a sterile barrier, is then submerged below the surface of the irrigation fluid. Turning the probe 90 degrees allows the surgeon to view the spinal canal in either the transverse plane or the sagittal plane.

MANAGEMENT OF LUMBAR SPINAL INJURIES

Aims of Treatment

The primary aims of treating lumbar spinal injuries are (1) restoration of alignment and stabilization of the spinal column, (2) improvement in neurologic status, and (3) early mobilization and rehabilitation of the patient. Although both nonoperative and operative means are capable of achieving these aims, there has been considerable debate regarding the merits of surgical and nonsurgical treatment for unstable fractures.[71] Interest has increased regarding burst fractures of the lumbar spine and their management by internal fixation, either posteriorly or anteriorly.[19] The nonoperative approach has been recommended by a number of authors,[17, 44, 45] who suggest that most fractures are well-treated by postural reduction and a period of bed rest. Bedbrook has stated that mobilization out of bed has little to recommend it since, in well-disciplined units, mobilization and physical restoration can be practiced equally well while the patient is in bed. It has also been demonstrated that fragments within the spinal canal may resorb with time if treated nonoperatively.[44, 45] Despite the relative success of the multidisciplinary team approach advocated by these authors, the type of unit required is expensive in terms of both man-hours and financial resources, and the late outcome has not been as favorable as one might expect.[19, 43] Many countries have found it to be an untenable concept. Careful documentation of spinal deformity has not been forthcoming in patients treated nonoperatively, so that

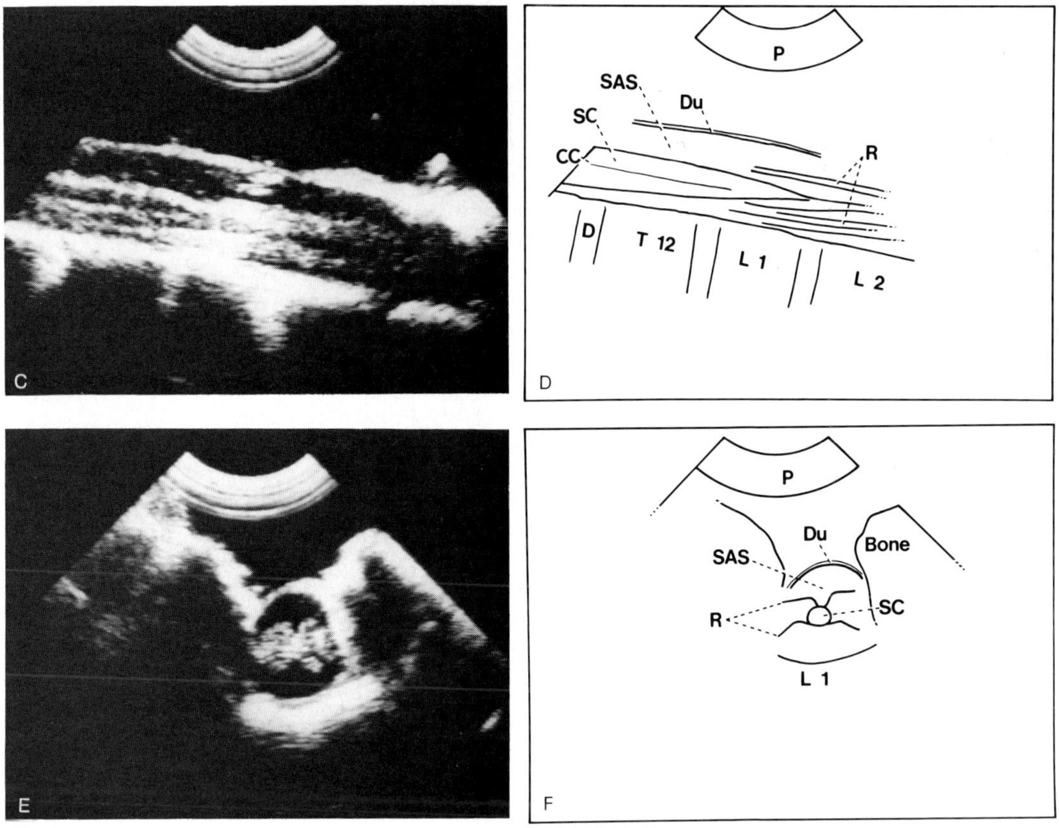

Figure 15 *Continued C,* In this sonogram, the patient has undergone a laminectomy over several levels at the thoracolumbar junction. Ultrasonography allows visualization of the spinal cord, conus medullaris, and the posterior aspect of the vertebral body. *D,* This artist's drawing illustrates the structures visualized in C. (CC = central canal within the spinal cord; D = intervertebral disc; Du = dura; L1 = L1 vertebral body; L2 = L2 vertebral body; P = ultrasound probe tip; R = nerve rootlets; SAS = subarachnoid space; SC = spinal cord; T12 = T12 vertebral body.) *E,* This ultrasonography at the L1 vertebral body level clearly shows the conus medullaris with lumbar and sacral nerve rootlets. The subarachnoid space is clearly visualized. *F,* This artist's drawing depicts what is shown in the ultrasonography in Figure 15F. *A–F,* Eismont, F. J., et al.: The role of intraoperative ultrasonography in the treatment of thoracic and lumbar spine fractures. Spine 9:783–784, 1984.)

late deformity and the sequelae of late pain are uncertain when nonoperative techniques are used. Fewer than 5% of patients treated nonoperatively for unstable injuries require operative intervention[4, 30] because of an inability to maintain an adequate reduction according to the proponents of the conservative approach.

The neurologic improvement in patients with incomplete neurologic deficits treated nonoperatively is not as great as with operative treatment. In patients treated nonoperatively, recovery by at least one Frankel grade is about 60% to 70%,[30, 39, 74] although Davies and colleagues reported an improvement rate of 95%.[17] In patients reviewed in the literature undergoing posterior surgery, the recovery rate is somewhat higher, in the order of 80% to 85%.[20, 22, 24, 51, 53, 65, 66] In patients undergoing anterior decompression surgery, the improvement rates of at least one Frankel grade in those with incomplete neurologic deficit are approximately the same.[23, 49, 53] Reduction of the intraspinal fragment by posterior distraction techniques has been shown to increase the diameter of the spinal canal from a preoperative value of 40% to a postoperative diameter of 75%,[1, 34, 73] if it is performed early. It is not possible to determine whether the neurologic improvement differs statistically because of inadequate measures for comparison. It appears, however, that there is a slight trend toward greater improvement by the surgical approach, compared with the nonoperative approach.

MANAGEMENT OF SPECIFIC LUMBAR SPINAL FRACTURES

Wedge Compression Fractures

Although this injury is considered to be relatively stable, involving the anterior column alone, in some instances there is significant disruption of the soft tissue structures posteriorly to render this a more unstable injury with a distinct potential for progressive collapse and further deformity. An angular deformity of more than 20 to 25 degrees of kyphosis (usually associated with posterior element disruption) may be an indication for a realignment procedure, in spite of the stability of the injury.

In order to re-establish alignment and ensure stability, a posterior approach using a dual rod technique is advocated. Bracing is recommended because a loss of bone substance anteriorly may leave a gap after reduction that could displace over time if external support is lacking (Fig. 16).

Burst Fractures

Most burst fractures of L1–L4 should be stabilized by means of posterior instrumentation. For fractures of L1 and L2, dual rods, extending to the L3 or L4, respectively, will provide sufficient fixation for stability and maintenance of the reduction (Fig. 17).

For all lumbar fractures, pedicle screw fixation devices that are capable of distraction may be used. Our choice is the AO internal fixator,[1, 21] which is recommended because it can provide adequate fixation over one or two motion segments (Fig. 18). We found this device to be particularly valuable in a recent review of 35 patients.[36] Burst fractures of L5 may be difficult to instrument without this type of device and can adequately be treated nonoperatively if the malalignment is not excessive.[16, 31] For injuries at the lumbosacral junction, this device has proven to be very effective, particularly when supplemented with transfacet screw fixation (see Fig. 11).

For patients with lumbar fractures with neurologic deterioration, we recommend immediate neural decompression and spine stabilization. One of the authors (S.D.G.) recommends an anterior decompression followed by anterior instrumentation, if available, or posterior fixation either at the same procedure or shortly thereafter (Fig. 19), because decompression without instrumentation leads to progressive deformity.[17] The other author (F.J.E.) recommends a posterior approach, intraoperative ultrasonography to localize the neural compression, a posterolateral decompression with removal of the medial portion of the pedicle, and stabilization with posterior distraction instrumentation. Postoperative CT scanning should be performed, and anterior decompression and fusion should be performed for significant residual neural compression.

In patients with incomplete neurologic deficit who are improving within the first 48 to 72 hours, posterior instrumentation using distraction techniques, either with dual rods or pedicle screw fixation with the AO internal fixator, is recommended in order to reduce any fragments within the spinal canal. A laminotomy at the level of injury and intraoperative ultrasonography can enable the surgeon to assess anterior neural compression and perform a posterolateral decompression, if needed. If this technique proves to be ineffective, anterior decompression should follow. We do not advocate anterior decompression for burst fractures where there is no neurologic deficit. However, if there is a substantial anterior crush of greater than 50%, one author (S.D.G.) recommends anterior fusion and instrumentation as a stabilizing technique with or without anterior decompression as a supplementary procedure; the other author (F.J.E.) recommends a posterior reduction and fusion using dual distraction rods.

Flexion–Distraction Injuries

Most flexion–distraction or seat belt injuries should be treated with posterior instrumentation, using a compression system such as the 3/16-inch Harrington compression rods (Figs. 20 and 21). In a review of 26 such fractures, 19 patients underwent this treatment.[32] Harrington compression rods were used for two patients with associated burst injuries; an anterior decompression was carried out in one, and distraction techniques to reduce the fragment were carried out in a

Text continued on page 689

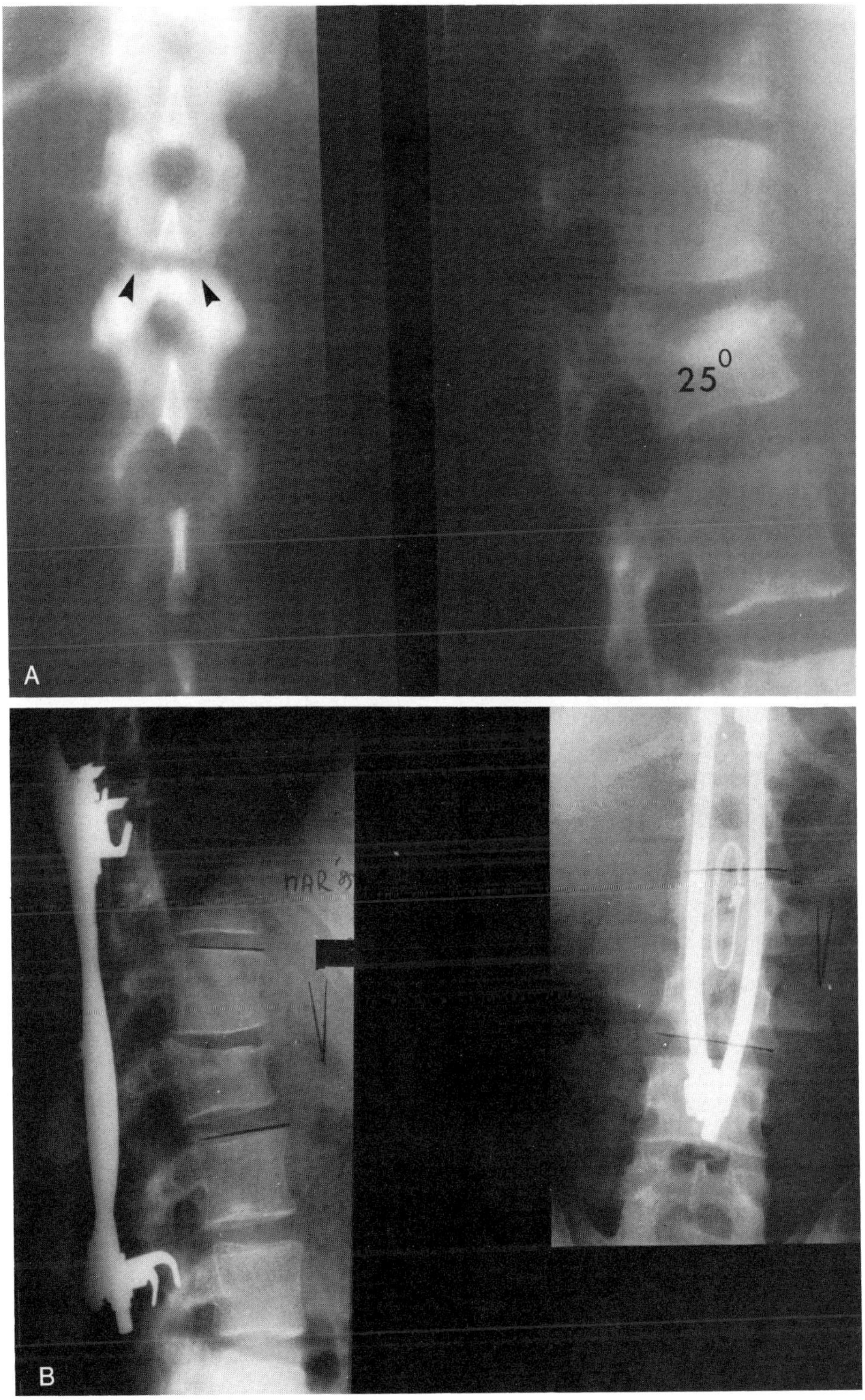

Figure 16 □ Wedge compression fracture with significant deformity. *A*, AP and lateral tomograms demonstrate significant deformity of 25 degrees with disruption of the posterior soft tissue elements (*arrows*). *B*, Deformity corrected by the use of dual locking hook spinal rods.

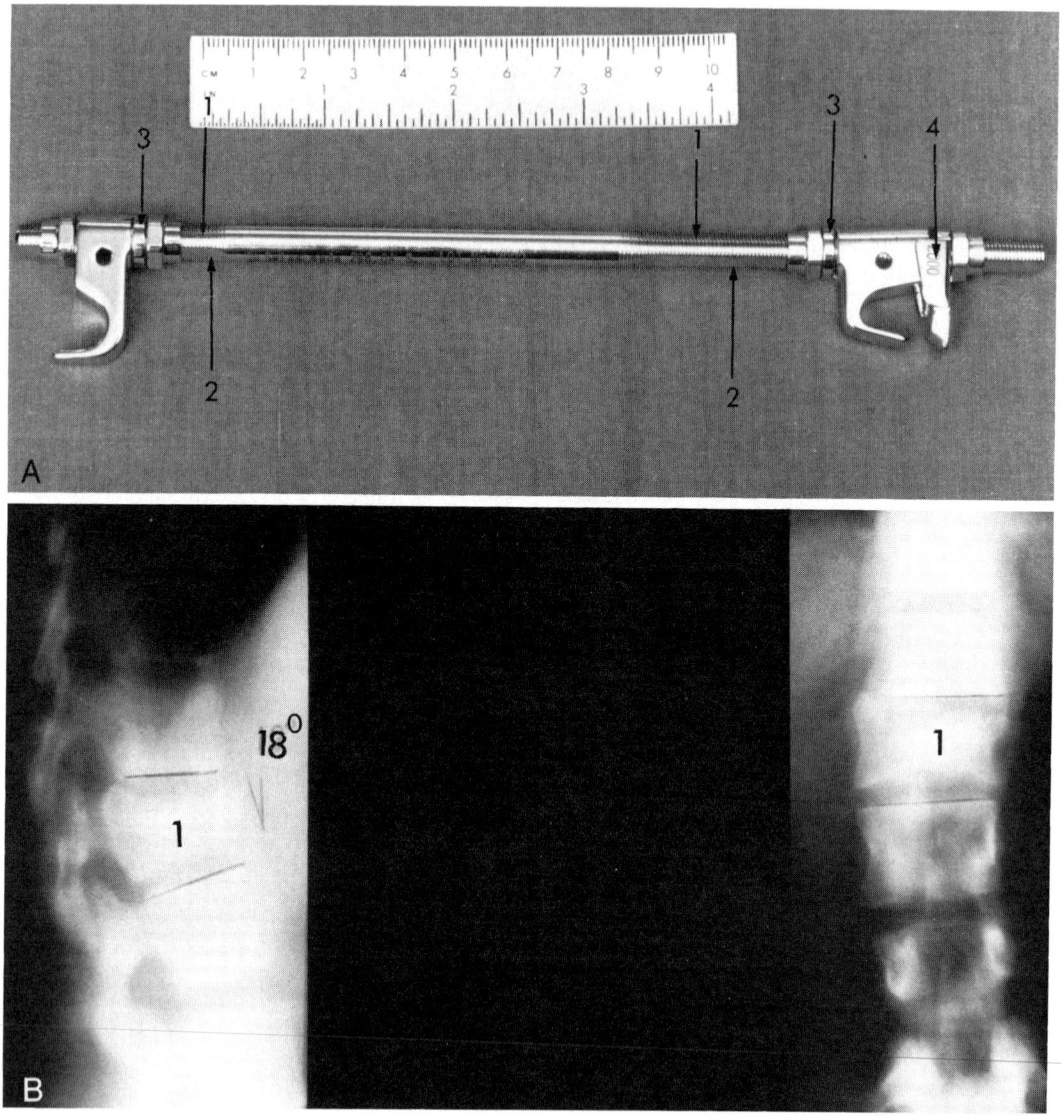

Figure 17 □ Locking hook spinal rod in the treatment of burst fractures. *A,* This rod is 7 mm in diameter, with proximal and distal threaded portions (1) and a flat surface at the threaded portion (2) for the application of a locking washer (3) to each hook. Note the sliding cap (4) at the top hook, which engages the superior lamina and provides good fixation at the upper end of the instrumentation. *B,* AP and lateral radiographs show a burst fracture of L1, with angulation and loss of vertebral height.

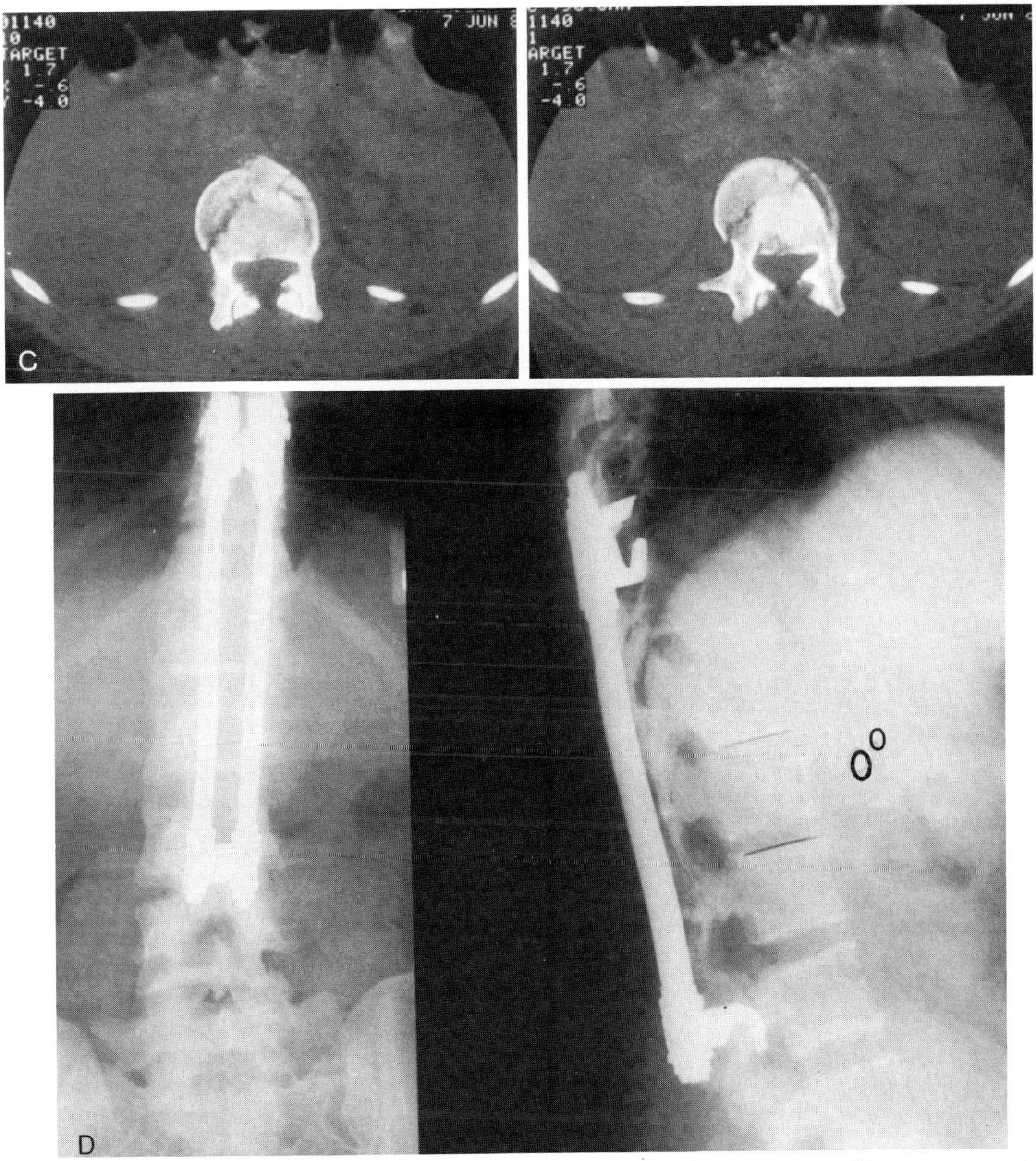

Figure 17 *Continued C,* CT scan demonstrates minor obstruction of the spinal canal. *D,* AP and lateral postoperative radiographs show satisfactory realignment of the spine with the use of the locking hook spinal rod inserted two levels below and three levels above the injury.

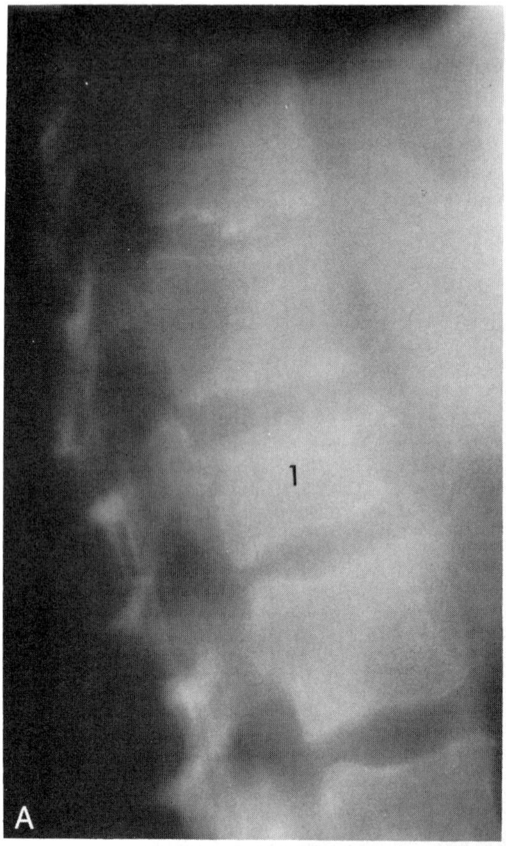

Figure 18 □ Burst fracture treated with AO internal fixator. *A*, Lateral tomogram of burst fracture at L1. *B*, CT scan with significant encroachment by a fragment in the spinal canal. *C*, Reduction of fracture using pedicle fixation (i.e., AO internal fixator).

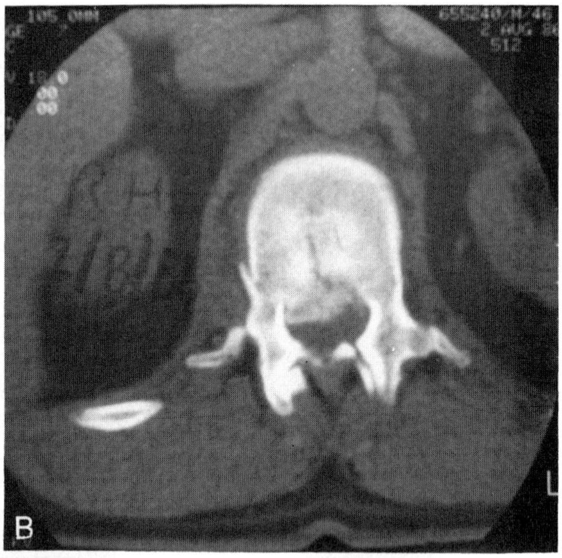

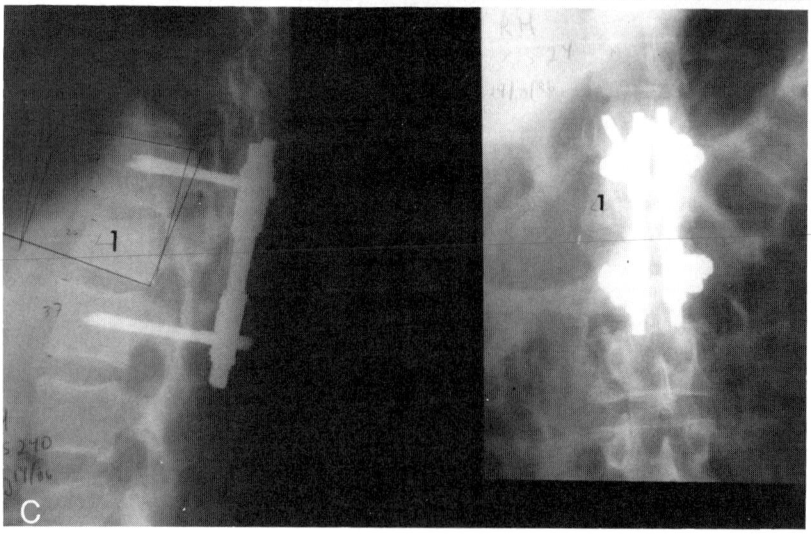

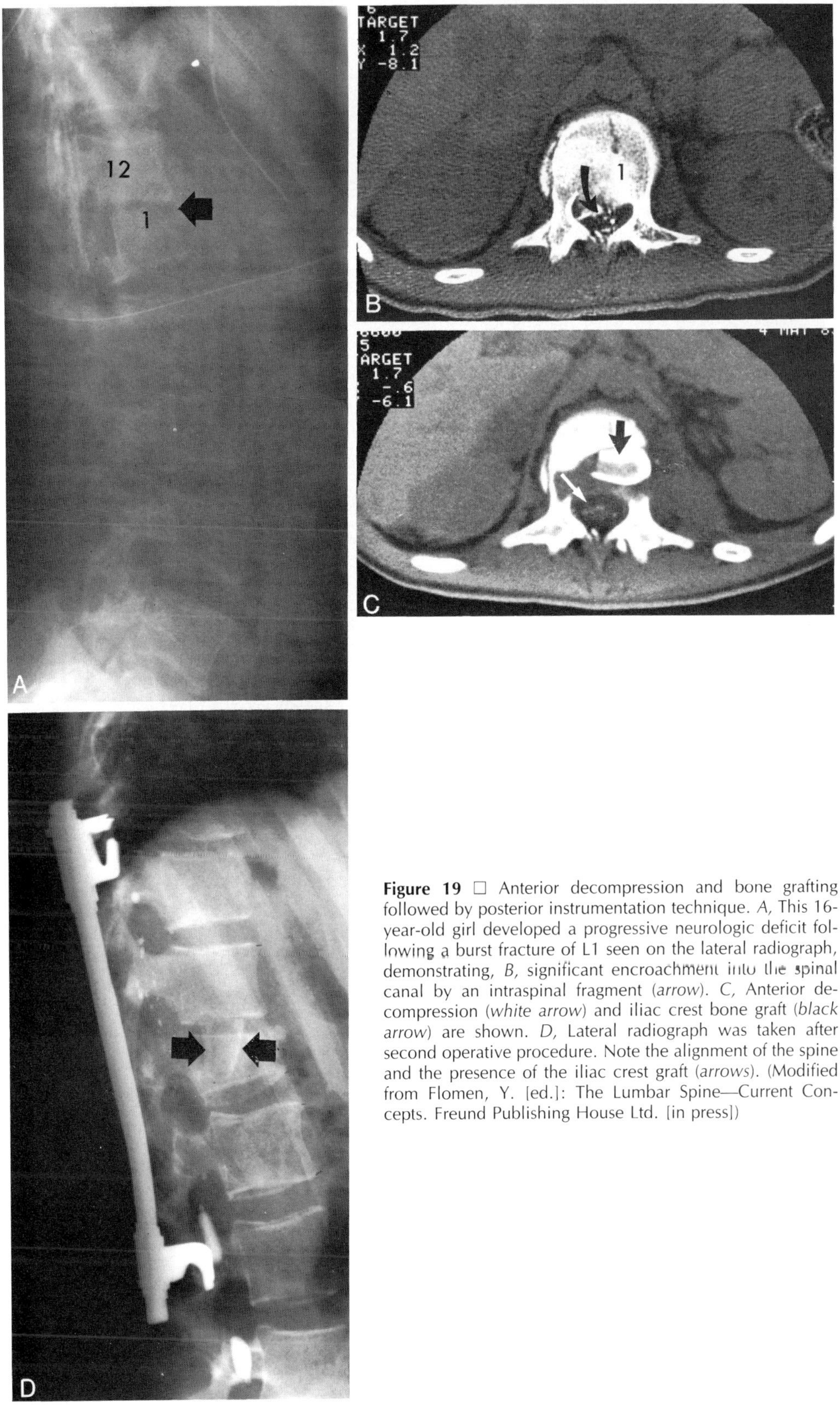

Figure 19 □ Anterior decompression and bone grafting followed by posterior instrumentation technique. *A,* This 16-year-old girl developed a progressive neurologic deficit following a burst fracture of L1 seen on the lateral radiograph, demonstrating, *B,* significant encroachment into the spinal canal by an intraspinal fragment (*arrow*). *C,* Anterior decompression (*white arrow*) and iliac crest bone graft (*black arrow*) are shown. *D,* Lateral radiograph was taken after second operative procedure. Note the alignment of the spine and the presence of the iliac crest graft (*arrows*). (Modified from Flomen, Y. [ed.]: The Lumbar Spine—Current Concepts. Freund Publishing House Ltd. [in press])

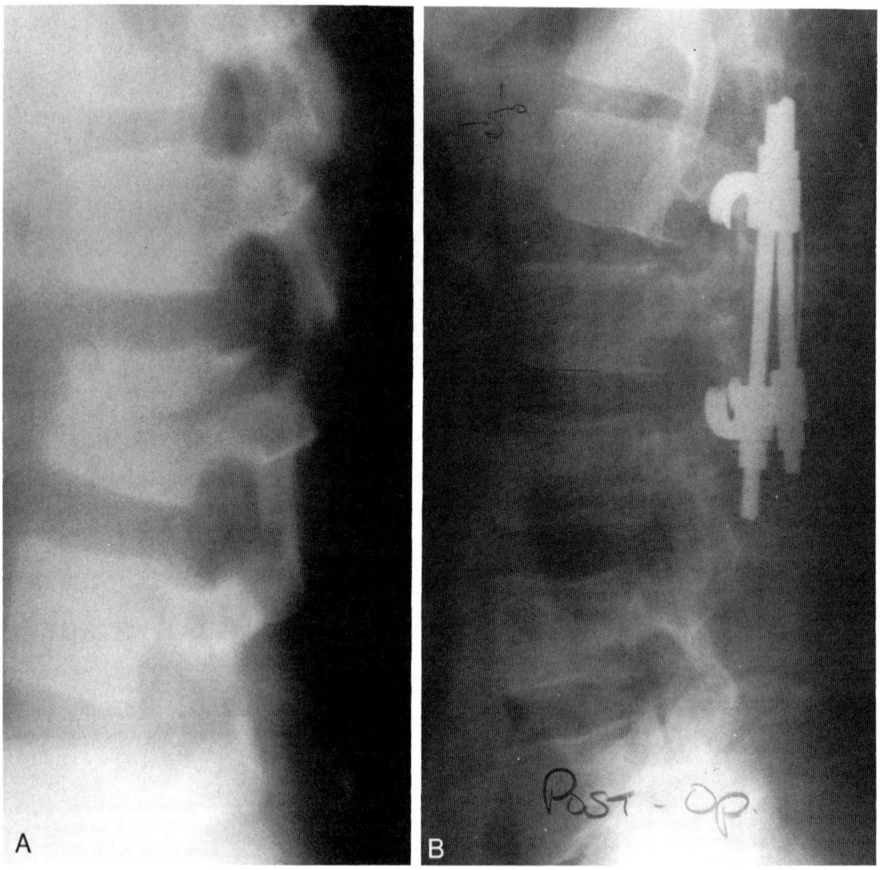

Figure 20 □ Flexion–distraction injury. *A*, This L1–L2 seat belt injury with extension into the L1–L2 disc space was treated by means of two heavy Harrington compression rods (*B*) over a single motion segment; excellent alignment was achieved.

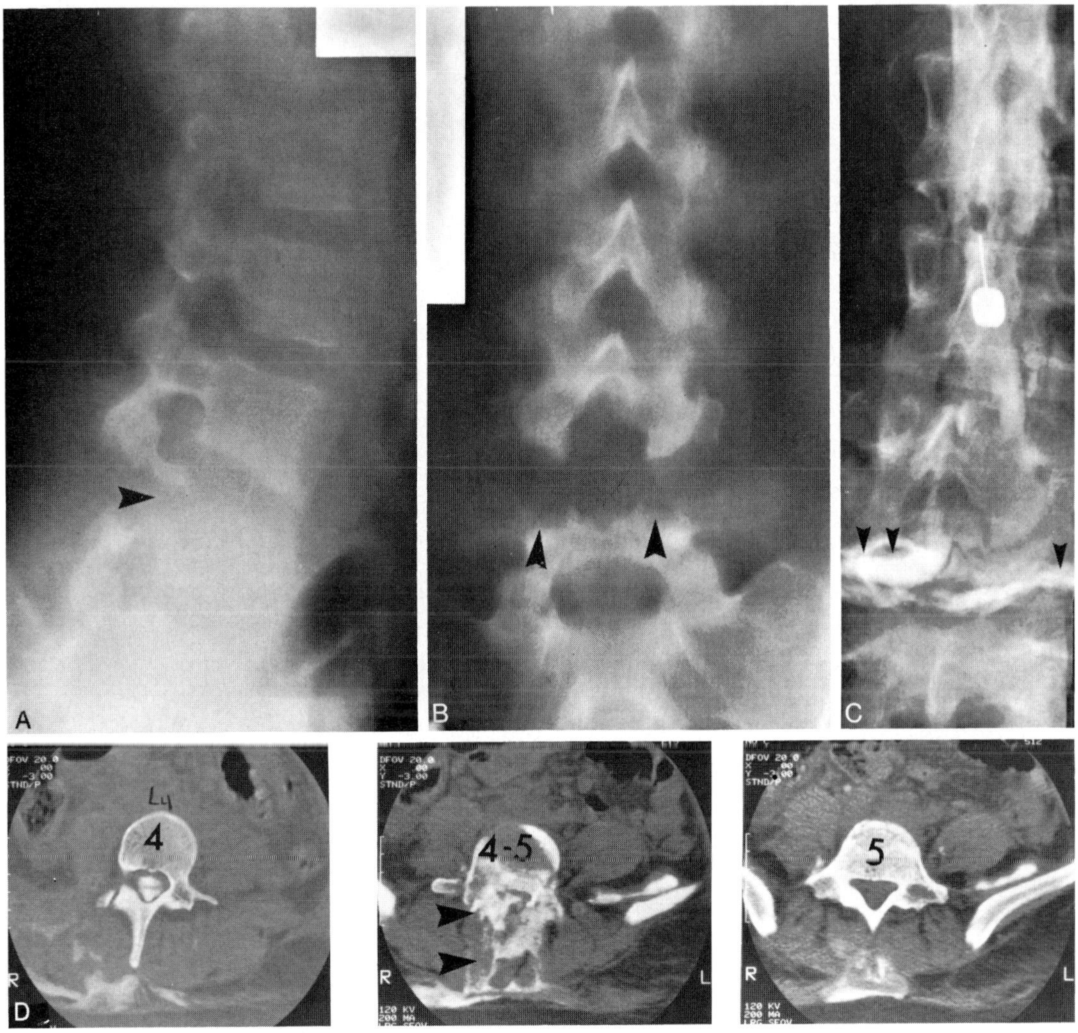

Figure 21 □ Severe flexion–distraction injury. *A, B,* Disruption of the spine through the L4–L5 interspinous space and the corresponding disc (*arrows*). *C, D,* Contrast material is leaking out of the dural space on the routine and CT myelograms.

Illustration continued on following page

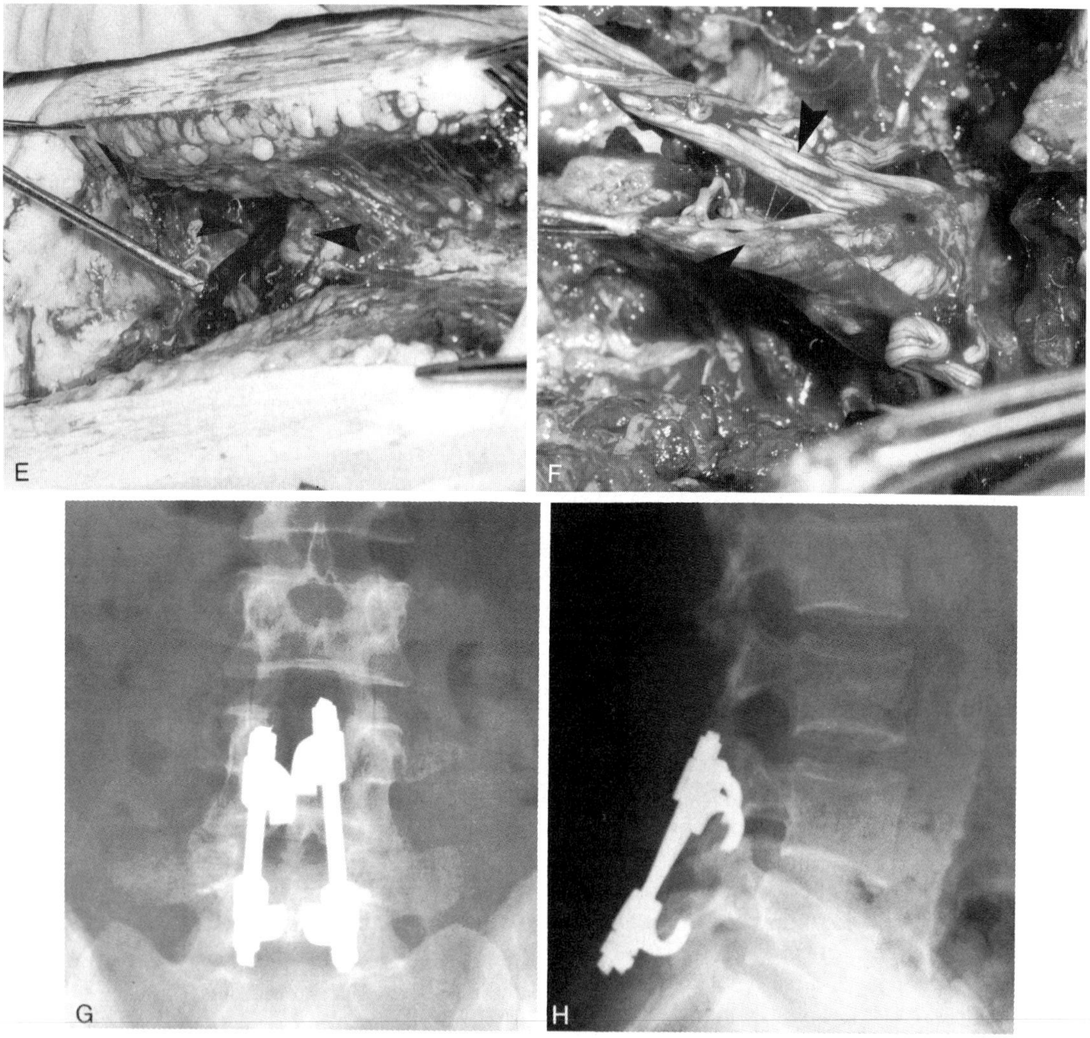

Figure 21 *Continued E,* Intraoperative demonstration shows avulsed ends of the cauda equina (*arrows*) on incising the subcutaneous tissues, and, *F,* on close-up with the distal cauda held by forceps (*arrows*). *G, H,* Postoperative reduction was performed with two Harrington compression rods.

second. The remaining five patients were treated nonoperatively because most of the trauma occurred through the bony elements. These latter patients were kept in bed for several weeks and then mobilized in an extension brace. Of the 26 patients, 25 had minimal or no pain, and their alignment was satisfactorily maintained. The same principles for the management of the neurologic condition apply to this injury, in which there is a burst component to the fracture.

Fracture/Dislocation Injuries

These are the most unstable fractures and include the flexion–rotation injuries, as well as shear fractures and some combined dislocation–burst fractures. The same operative techniques apply, namely, posterior stabilization using dual rods or pedicle screw fixation (Fig. 22). However, these extremely unstable injuries may require additional anterior stabilization, should the primary operative technique be insufficient.

Extension Injuries

These rare fractures tend to be stable in flexion and usually require a period of bed rest, followed by the use of a flexion-type brace (see Fig. 8).

TECHNIQUES OF SURGICAL DECOMPRESSION

The surgical approaches to the lumbar spine have been well-described in the literature.[7, 10, 68] For anterior exposure of L1, either a transthoracic approach[10] or a retroperitoneal approach[68] can be utilized; the diaphragm and part of the crus must be detached from the spine with either approach. The L2–L4 vertebrae are best visualized anteriorly via a retroperitoneal approach.[68] The transperitoneal surgical approach is best for anterior exposure of L5. A midline posterior approach with a posterolateral decompression can be performed for any of the lumbar vertebrae (Fig. 23).

When any decompression is performed, care must be taken to decompress the spinal canal across its entire width from pedicle to pedicle. For posterolateral approaches, the surgeon can utilize intraoperative ultrasonography to be certain that the decompression is adequate.[25, 26, 63] For anterior approaches, the surgeon must rely more on anatomic landmarks; the tendency is to inadequately decompress the spinal canal on the side opposite from that on which the exposure is made.

The technique of posterolateral transpedicular decompression is illustrated in Figure 24. The patient is prone, and the spine is exposed through a midline incision. At the level of injury, a laminotomy is performed to expose the dura for a width of 1.5 cm and a length of 1.0 cm.[26] For most lumbar spine injuries, this means removing the torn or attenuated ligaments and a thin rim of adjacent bone. Only the most medial portion of the facet joint is removed. Intraoperative ultrasonography is then used to visualize the anterior neural compression,[25] which most typically is bone retropulsed into the spinal canal at the level of the pedicle. In the case of an acute lumbar injury, instrumentation should be inserted initially to attempt neural decompression by fracture reduction; this can be visualized by ultrasonography. If the neural compression is not reduced with the instrumentation or if the fracture is not an acute injury, then a posterolateral transpedicular decompression would be performed. The superior portion of the lamina is resected to expose the cephalic two thirds of the pedicle. A power bur is then used to remove the central portion of the pedicle, and this tunnel is extended into the posterior portion of the vertebral body. A fine rongeur is used to remove the remaining medial cortex of the pedicle. Care is taken to protect the nerve root exiting the spinal canal below the level of the partially removed pedicle. Reverse-angle curettes and a mallet are used to pack the bone fragments back into the vertebral body, away from the neural elements. Intraoperative ultrasonography is then used to assess the adequacy of decompression. Posterolateral transpedicular decompression is safest at the level of the cauda equina, but it can be performed at more cephalic levels with the help of ultrasonography and somatosensory evoked responses.

Intraoperative myelography may be used to assess the canal patency if any concern is raised regarding the decompression, should ultrasound be unavailable.

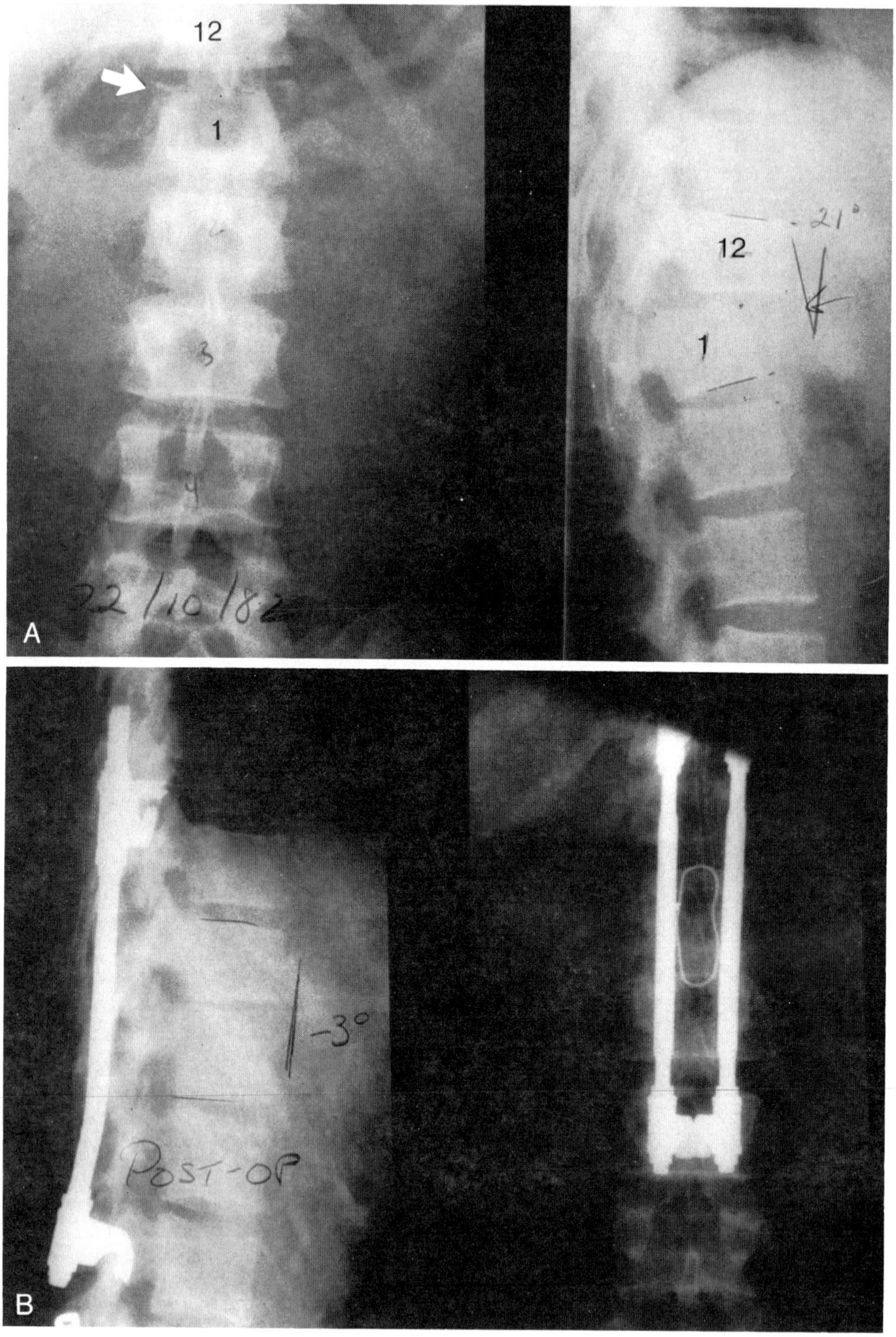

Figure 22 □ Fracture/dislocation. *A,* This unstable fracture/dislocation at T12–L1 required stabilization. *B,* Dual-locking hook spinal rods were required to realign the spinal column and stabilize the injury by fixation, three levels above and two levels below the fracture.

SPINAL ORTHOSES

Basic research has been carried out on spinal orthoses, but these studies have tested only small numbers of volunteers and most often with large variations among volunteers.[28, 47, 55, 57] Some of the difficulties with research in this area have included exposure of volunteers to radiation.[28, 55] and the requirement of invasive procedures such as placing Steinman pins in the spinous processes of the volunteers.[47, 57] There has been no prospective clinical study of spinal orthoses in patients with spinal fractures that includes such information as the amount of motion allowed by the orthoses in different positions. The available reviews show that braces can be effective in three different ways. First, they can physically restrain different spinal motions.[28, 29, 47, 57] Second, they can remind the patient to limit the spinal range of motion by causing discomfort over pressure points.[57] Third, braces can be effective by simply increasing the intra-abdominal pressure, which tends to support the spine and divert weight-bearing forces away from the spine.[52, 55] Different braces apply different principles. A good general review has been published by the American Academy of Orthopaedic Surgeons.[29] Two disadvantages of all types of braces, over which the physician has very little control, are patient obesity and patient compliance.

Three groups of patients with spinal fractures are commonly encountered. The first is the group with stable injuries, for whom a brace is prescribed for comfort only. The second group, of greater clinical concern, consists of those who have minimal to moderate degrees of instability after a spinal injury, who can ambulate in a brace in order to minimize both the expense and the inconvenience of prolonged bed rest. The third group comprises those with moderate to severe degrees of spine instability who have undergone stabilization procedures and require a brace for protected mobilization. These three groups are now considered in relation to lumbar spinal injuries, including both the upper and lower lumbar spine.

Patients with Stable Spinal Fractures

In this group of patients, braces may be prescribed to enhance comfort. For most, a wraparound type of lumbosacral orthosis would be adequate to increase the patient's intra-abdominal pressure and hence make the patient more comfortable.[55] It must be understood that this type of brace would not provide a significant degree of physical restraint. It may or may not provide pressure points to remind the patient to limit his or her range of motion.

Patients with Minimal to Moderate Degrees of Lumbar Spinal Instability

This group of patients is of prime concern to the clinician. In addition to providing comfort for the patient, the goal is to prevent increasing spinal deformity and especially subsequent neurologic deterioration. Hence, this group of patients should be treated with braces that physically restrain the spine. For this purpose, a thoracolumbosacral orthosis (TLSO) must be utilized. The clinician should determine the mechanism of injury from the patient's history, radiographs, and clinical examination, and the brace should be designed to prevent further deformity in those directions. If a patient has a simple flexion injury, such as a compression fracture with no rotational instability, then a TLSO flexion control brace such as a Jewett brace would be adequate. Many types of orthoses primarily utilize cloth with rigid stays; however, these usually fail to provide adequate restraint.[29, 47, 57] The only brace that provides control of flexion, extension, lateral movement, and rotary movement is a TLSO made of a rigid material such as Orthoplast and having total contact over the rib cage, the lumbar spine posteriorly, and the pelvis inferiorly.[29] This can provide adequate support down to L4. Studies have indicated that, in order to adequately immobilize the lumbosacral junction (and this should include significant L5 vertebral fractures), a thigh extension must be included to lock the hip in a neutral position.[28] Reviews have shown that if braces do not immobilize the hip joint, there may actually be compensatory increased movement at the lumbosacral junction with attempts at flexion and extension.[57] Disadvantages of the total-contact individually fitted TLSO are that it must be custom made (and therefore is more expensive) and usually requires several days for fabrication. Compared with the TLSO flexion control brace, it is also more difficult to remove and reapply, and the patient may

Text continued on page 696

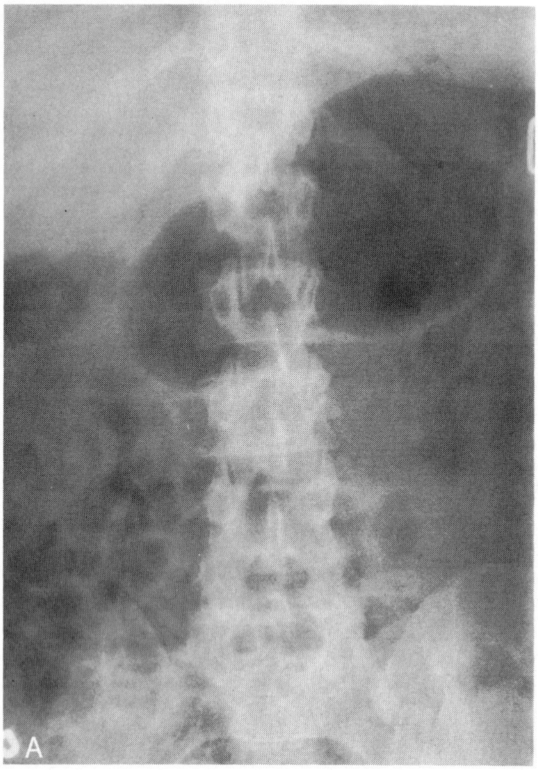

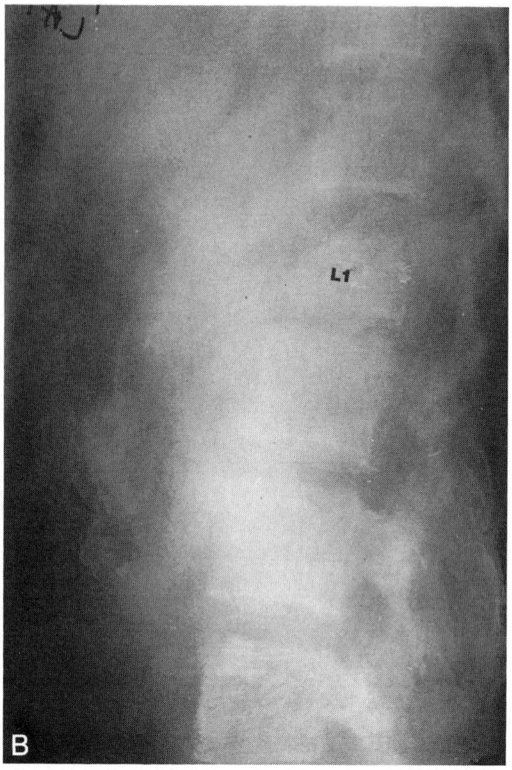

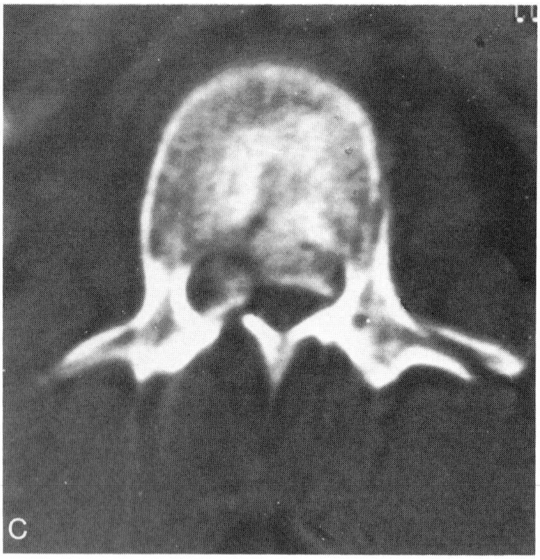

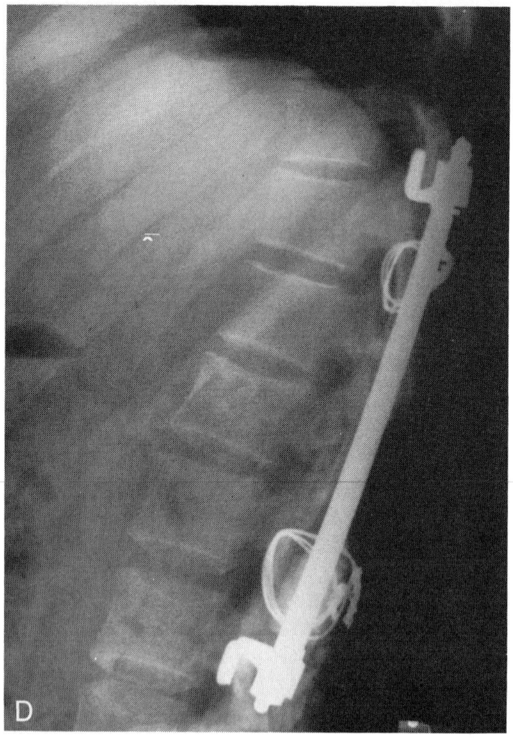

Figure 23 □ This male was injured in a fall from a height. He sustained an L1 burst injury and was transferred to our facility, 2 weeks after injury, with bowel and bladder incontinence and with only minimal motor function in his legs. *A*, This AP roentgenogram appears abnormal, but the L1 fracture cannot be visualized well. *B*, The lateral roentgenogram reveals comminution and significant compression of the L1 vertebral body, especially anteriorly. The extent of bone protruding into the spinal canal is not clearly seen. *C*, The CT scan at the level of injury reveals the disruption of the middle column and protrusion of bone into the spinal canal. It also shows the laminar fractures that are present. The spinal canal is narrowed to 20% of its normal volume. *D*, The patient was treated surgically by means of ultrasonography, an L1 laminectomy in order to extricate extruded nerve roots from between the posterior laminar fractures, and a posterolateral decompression of the spinal canal. Harrington rods with Edward's sleeves were then inserted for stabilization.

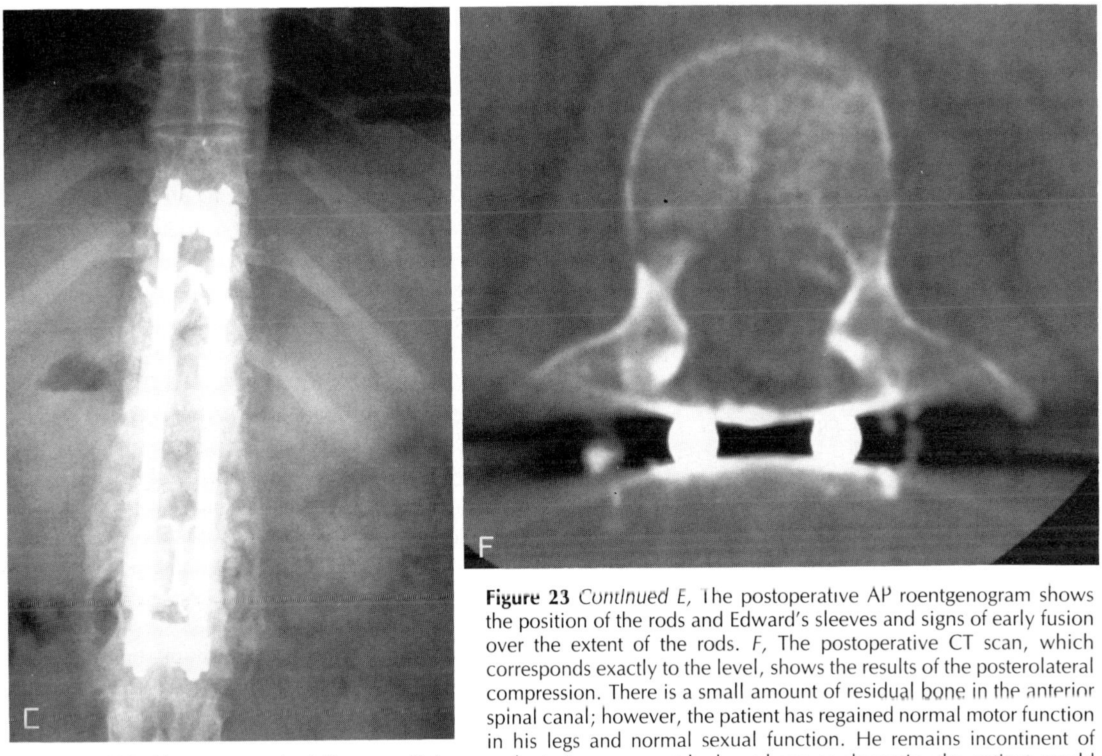

Figure 23 *Continued E,* The postoperative AP roentgenogram shows the position of the rods and Edward's sleeves and signs of early fusion over the extent of the rods. *F,* The postoperative CT scan, which corresponds exactly to the level, shows the results of the posterolateral compression. There is a small amount of residual bone in the anterior spinal canal; however, the patient has regained normal motor function in his legs and normal sexual function. He remains incontinent of bowel and bladder at 6 months follow-up. If the neurologic improvement had not been so dramatic, the patient would have been re-evaluated for consideration for an anterior spinal canal decompression to remove the residual bone from the spinal canal.

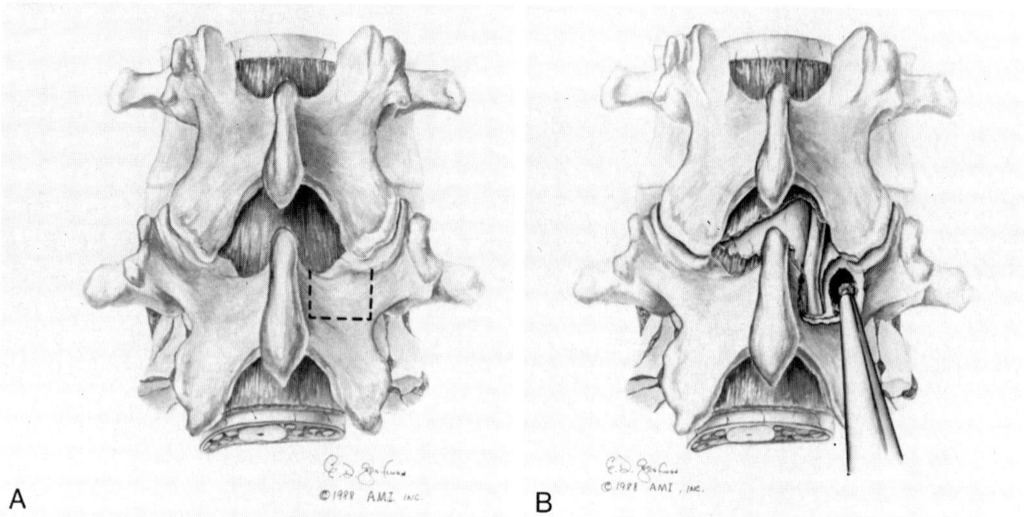

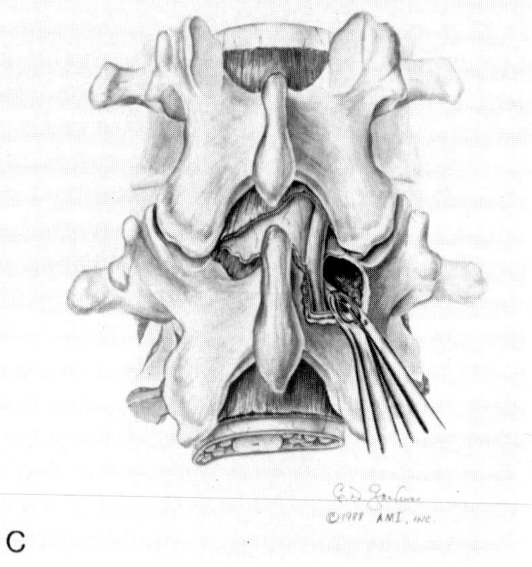

Figure 24 □ This illustrates the technique for posterolateral decompression that would be utilized for treating an L1 burst fracture. (From Levine, A., Garfin, S., and Eismont, F.: Spine Trauma. Philadelphia, W.B. Saunders [in press, 1991].) *A,* Posterior elements of T12 and L1 are illustrated. The dotted lines indicate the bone that would be removed for a posterolateral decompression. (From Levine, A., Garfin, S., and Eismont, F.: Spine Trauma. Philadelphia, W.B. Saunders [in press, 1991].) *B,* This illustrates the central laminotomy that has been performed to facilitate the use of intraoperative ultrasonography. The laminotomy has been extended into the L1 lamina on the side at which the decompression will be performed. Following this laminotomy, a power bur is utilized to drill out the central portion of the pedicle, leaving a thin wall medially and a thicker wall laterally, in order to maintain continuity of the transverse process with the vertebral body. The drill hole is continued down into the vertebral body anteriorly. Care is taken to protect the nerve root exiting at the level of the pedicle. (From Levine, A., Garfin, S., and Eismont, F.: Spine Trauma. Philadelphia, W.B. Saunders [in press, 1991].) *C,* A fine rongeur is utilized to remove the remaining thin medial wall of the pedicle. Again, care is taken to identify and protect the nerve root exiting under that pedicle. (From Levine, A., Garfin, S., and Eismont, F.: Spine Trauma. Philadelphia, W.B. Saunders [in press, 1991].)

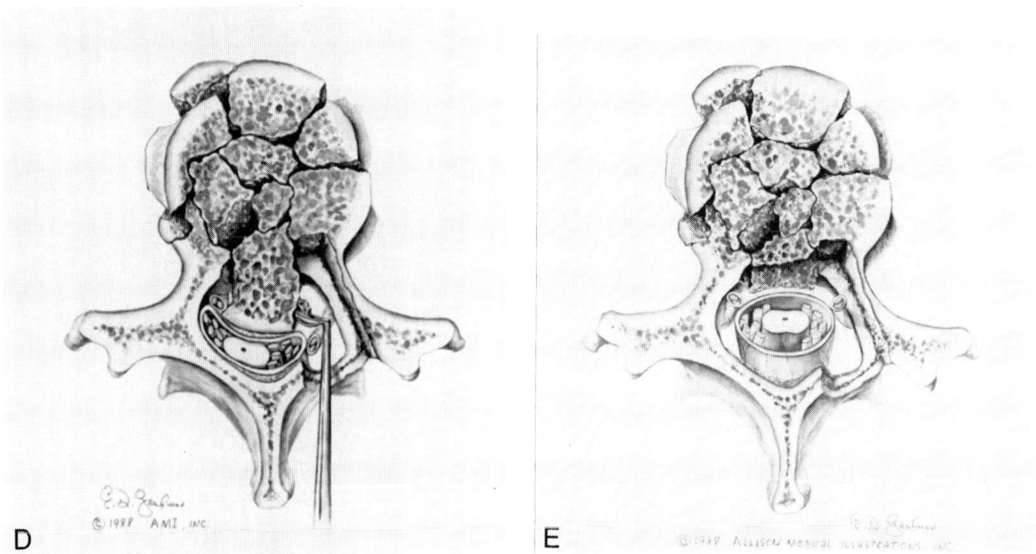

Figure 24 *Continued D,* A reverse-angle curette is introduced into the spinal canal lateral to the dural sac and exiting nerve root. It is used to impact the bone fragments away from the neural elements. Intraoperative ultrasonography is very useful for demonstrating whether residual bone fragments are remaining within the spinal canal and also to document whether the neural elements are being deformed by the bone fragments. (From Levine, A., Garfin, S., and Eismont, F.: Spine Trauma. Philadelphia, W.B. Saunders [in press, 1991].) *E,* This illustrates the ideal final result, showing removal of all bone fragments from the spinal canal. The transverse process maintains continuity with the fractured vertebral body, which will aid in achieving stability with a lateral fusion. (From Levine, A., Garfin, S., and Eismont, F.: Spine Trauma. Philadelphia, W.B. Saunders [in press, 1991].)

need assistance. In the past, emphasis has been placed on adequate relief at all bony prominences in patients with insensate skin. We have not found this to be a problem, even in those with complete paralysis in the lumbar spine, because the skin sensation over the torso remains normal in these patients.

Moderate to Severe Instability in Patients Treated Operatively

The considerations that were discussed for the last group of patients also apply here. If the surgeon is pleased with the degree of stability achieved intraoperatively, then the brace may be prescribed for comfort only, in which case simply increasing the intra-abdominal pressure may be adequate. Various degrees of physical restraint may also be required, in which case a TLSO flexion control brace, a total-contact TLSO, or even a total-contact TLSO with locked thigh extension may be required.

ALGORITHM FOR THE MANAGEMENT OF SPINAL INJURIES

Stable injuries, such as wedge compression fractures of less than 20 degrees and posterior element fractures, are best treated by means of early mobilization and bracing. For upper lumbar fractures a Jewett-type brace is effective; fractures from L3 to the sacrum can be managed by means of a lumbosacral orthosis.

Unstable fractures or stable injuries with a kyphotic deformity of greater than 20 to 30 degrees can usually be treated posteriorly by means of dual rods for the upper lumbar spine or pedicle screw fixation, utilizing a device capable of distraction, compression, or neutralization for either the entire lumbar spine or the lower levels. Compression instrumentation is most suitable for flexion–distraction injuries.

For a progressing neurologic deficit, one author (S.D.G.) recommends an immediate anterior decompression, followed by anterior or posterior instrumentation at the same time or shortly thereafter. The other author (F.J.E.) recommends an immediate surgical treatment with a posterior approach, reduction utilizing posterior instrumentation, evaluation with intraoperative ultrasonography, and posterolateral decompression if indicated.

In the face of a stable neurologic deficit, we recommend posterior instrumentation in an attempt to reduce any intraspinal fragments. Failing sufficient reduction, an anterior procedure should be undertaken using an anterior iliac crest strut graft and anterior instrumentation (if available) for stabilization. The authors disagree on the timing of surgery for this group of patients. One author (S.D.G.) recommends first observing the patient for 2 to 3 days for any neurologic improvement, and the other (F.J.E.) recommends proceeding with surgery as soon as the patient is medically stable.

References

1. Aebi, M., Etter, C., Kehl, T., and Thalgott, J.: Stabilization of the lower thoracic and lumbar spine with internal spinal skeletal fixation system. Indication, techniques and first results of treatment. Spine 12:544–551, 1987.
2. Armstrong, G.: Personal communication.
3. Bedbrook, G. M.: Stability of spinal fractures and fracture dislocations. Paraplegia 9:23–32, 1970.
4. Bedbrook, G. M.: Treatment of thoracolumbar dislocation and fractures with paraplegia. Clin. Orthop. 112:27–43, 1975.
5. Begeman, P. C., King, A. L., and Prasad, P.: Spinal injuries resulting from -Gx acceleration. *In*: Proceedings, 17th S.T.A.F.F. Car Crash Conference. New York, Society of Automotive Engineers Incorporated, pp. 343–360, 1973.
6. Bell, G. H., Dunbar, O., Beck, J. S., and Gibb, A.: Variation in strength of vertebrae with change and their relation to osteoporosis. Calc. Tissue Res. 1:75–86, 1967.
7. Bohlman, H. H., and Eismont, F. J.: Surgical techniques of anterior decompression and fusion for spinal cord injuries. Clin. Orthop. 154:57–67, 1981.
8. Brightman, R. P., Miller, C. A., and Hunt, W. E.: MRI of spinal trauma: Imaging of the anterior and posterior longitudinal ligaments. 14th Annual Scientific Meeting, American Spinal Injury Association, May 2–4, 1988. Abstract Digest, p. 28.
9. Brown, T., Hanson, R., and Yorra, A.: Some mechanical tests on the lumbosacral spine with particular reference to the intervertebral disc. J. Bone Joint Surg. 39A:1135–1164, 1957.
10. Burrington, J. D., Brown, C., Wayne, E. R., and Odom, J.: Anterior approach to the thoracolumbar spine. Arch. Surg. 11:456, 1976.
11. Calenoff, L., Chessare, J. W., Rogers, L. F., et al.: Multiple level spinal injuries: Importance of early recognition. A.J.R. 130:665–669, 1978.
12. Cammisa, F. P., Eismont, F. J., and Green, B. A.: Thoracolumbar burst fractures associated with lamina fractures and dural lacerations. J. Bone Joint Surg. 71A (in press, 1989).
13. Chance, G. Q.: Note on a type of flexion fracture of the spine. Br. J. Radiol. 21:452–453, 1948.
14. Cotler, H. B.: Magnetic resonance imaging in acute spinal cord injury, Presented to Amer. 14th Annual Scientific Meeting, Spinal Injury Association, May 2–4, 1988. Abstract Digest, p. 25.

15. Court-Brown, C. M., Gertzbein, S. D.: Flexion/distraction injuries of the lumbar spine. Clin. Orthop. Rel. Res. 227:52–60, 1988.
16. Court-Brown, C. M., Gertzbein, S. D.: Burst fractures of the fifth lumbar vertebra. Spine 12:305–312, 1987.
17. Davies, W. E., Morris, J. H., and Hill, V.: An analysis of conservative (non-surgical) management of thoracolumbar fractures and fracture/dislocations with neurological damage. J. Bone Joint Surg. 62A:1324–1328, 1980.
18. Denis, F.: Three column spine and its significance in the classification of acute thoracolumbar spinal injuries. Spine 8:8, 817–831, 1983.
19. Denis, F., Armstrong, G. W., Searls, K., et al.: Acute thoracolumbar burst fractures in the absence of neurological deficit. A comparison between operative and non-operative treatment. Clin. Orthop. 189:142–149, 1984.
20. de Oliviera, J. C.: A new type of fracture/dislocation of the thoracolumbar spine. J. Bone Joint Surg. 68:481–488, 1978.
21. Dick, W.: The "Fixateur Interne" as a versatile implant for spine surgery. Spine 9:882–900, 1987.
22. Dickson, J. H., Harrington, T. R., and Erwin, W. D.: Results of reduction and stabilization of the severely fractured thoracic and lumbar spine. J. Bone Joint Surg. 60:799–805, 1978.
23. Dunn, H. K.: Anterior spine stabilization and decompression for thoracolumbar injuries. Orthop. Clin. North Am. 17:113–119, 1986.
24. Edwards, C.C., and Levine, A. M.: Early rod sleeve stabilization of the injured thoracic and lumbar spine. Orthop. Clin. North Am. 17:121–145, 1986.
25. Eismont, F. J., Green, B. A., Berkowitz, B. M., et al.: The role of intraoperative ultrasonography in the treatment of thoracic and lumbar spine fractures. Spine 9:782–787, 1984.
26. Eismont, F. J., Morse, B., Post, J. D., et al.: Intraoperative ultrasonography of the lumbar spine. Annual Meeting I.S.S.L.S., Jun. 3–7, 1984. Abstracts Digest.
27. Ferguson, R. L., and Allen, D. L.: A mechanistic classification of thoracolumbar spine fractures. Clin. Orthop. 189:77–88, 1984.
28. Fidler, M. W., and Plasmans, C. M. T.: The effect of four types of support on the segmental mobility of the lumbosacral spine. J. Bone Joint Surg., 65A:943, 1983.
29. Fishman, S., Berger, N., Edelstein, J. E., and Springer, W. P.: Spinal Orthoses, A.A.O.S. Atlas of Orthotics, 2nd Ed. St. Louis, C.V. Mosby, 1985, 238–256.
30. Frankel, H. L., Hancock, D. O., Hyslop, G., et al.: The value of postural reduction in the initial management of closed injuries of the spine with paraplegia and tetraplegia. Paraplegia 7:179–192, 1969.
31. Fredrickson, B. E., Yuan, H. A., and Miller, H.: Burst fractures of the fifth lumbar vertebra. A report of four cases. J. Bone Joint Surg. 64A:1088–1094, 1982.
32. Gertzbein, S. D., and Court-Brown, C. M.: Rationale for the management of flexion/distraction injuries of the thoracolumbar spine based on a new classification (submitted for publication).
33. Gertzbein, S. D., and Evans, D. C.: Femoral nerve neuropathy complicating iliopsoas hemorrhage in patients without hemophilia. J. Bone Joint Surg. 54B:149–151, 1972.
34. Gertzbein, S. D., Court-Brown, C. M., Jacobs, R. R., et al.: Neurological outcome following surgery for fractures of the thoracic and lumbar spine. (Spine 1988).
35. Gertzbein, S. D., et al.: Decompression and circumferential stabilization of unstable spinal fractures. Spine 13:892–895, 1988.
36. Gertzbein, S. D., Robbins, S., Chow, D., et al.: Preliminary Results of the AO Internal Fixator for Spinal Fractures.
37. Green, B. A., and Callahan, R. A.: A radiological approach to acute spinal cord injury. *In* Post, J. D. (ed.): Radiographic Evaluation of the Spine: Current Advances with Emphasis on Computed Tomography. New York, Masson, 1980.
38. Gumley, G., Taylor, T. K. F., and Ryan, M. D.: Distraction fractures of the lumbar spine. J. Bone Joint Surg. 64B:520–525, 1982.
39. Guttman, L.: Spinal Injuries. Folia, Traumatologica Geigy, 1972.
40. Hall, H. E., Robertson, W. W.: Another Chance: A non–seat belt related fracture of the lumbar spine. J. Trauma 25:1163–1166, 1985.
41. Holdsworth, F. W.: Fractures, dislocations and fracture/dislocations of the spine. J. Bone Joint Surg. 45B:6–20, 1962.
42. Howland, W. J., Curry, J. L., and Buffington, C. B.: Fulcrum fractures of the lumbar spine. J.A.M.A. 193:140–141, 1965.
43. Jacobs, R. R., Asher, M. A., and Snider, R. K.: Thoracolumbar spinal injuries. A comparison study of recumbent and operative treatment in 100 patients. Spine 5:463–477, 1980.
44. Krompinger, W. J., Fredrickson, B. E., Mino, D. E., and Yuan, H. A.: Conservative treatment of fractures of the thoracic and lumbar spine. Orthop. Clin. North Am. 17:161–170, 1986.
45. Krompinger, W. J., Yuan, H. A., Frederickson, B. E., et al.: Non-surgical management of thoracic and lumbar fractures in neurologically intact patients: CT evidence of reabsorption of bony canal compromise. Transactions of the 12th Annual Meeting I.S.S.L.S. 1985, p. 75.
46. Lindahl, O.: Mechanical properties of dried, defatted, spongy bone. Acta Orthop. Scand. 47:11, 1976.
47. Lumsden, R. M., and Morris, J. M.: An in vivo study of axial rotation and immobilization at the lumbosacral joint. J. Bone Joint Surg. 50A:1591, 1968.
48. Magerl, F., and Harms, D.: Classification of thoracic and lumbar fractures. Presented at the Spine Trauma Section, S.I.C.O.T., Munich, Germany, Aug. 1987.
49. McAfee, P. C., Bohlman, H. H., and Yuan, H. A.: Anterior decompression of traumatic thoracolumbar fractures with incomplete neurological deficit using a retroperitoneal approach. J. Bone Joint Surg. 67A:89–104, 1985.
50. McAfee, P. C., Yuan, H. A., Fredrickson, B. E., et al.: The value of computer tomography in thoracolumbar fractures. An analysis of 100 consecutive cases and a new classification. J. Bone Joint Surg. 65:461–473, 1983.
51. McAfee, P. C., Yuan, H. A., and Lasda, N. A.: The unstable burst fracture. Spine 4:365–373, 1982.
52. McCollough, N. C., III: Biomechanical analysis of the spine. *In* A.A.O.S.: Atlas of Orthotics, Biomechanical Principles and Application. Ch. 18, edited by the Committee on Prosthetics and Orthotics, A.A.O.S. St. Louis, C. V. Mosby, 1975.

53. McEvoy, R. D., and Bradford, D. S.: The management of burst fractures of the thoracic and lumbar spine: Experience in 53 patients. Spine 10:631–637, 1985.
54. Miller, C. A., Dewey, R. C., and Hunt, W. E.: Impaction fracture of the lumbar vertebrae with dural tear. J. Neurosurg. 53:765–771, 1980.
55. Morris, J. M., Lucas, D. B., and Bresler, B.: Role of the trunk in stability of the spine. J. Bone Joint Surg. 43A:327, 1961.
56. Nicoll, E. A.: Fractures of the dorsolumbar spine. J. Bone Joint Surg. 31B:376–394, 1949.
57. Norton, P. L., and Brown, T.: The immobilizing efficiency of back braces: Their effect on the posture and motion of the lumbosacral spine. J. Bone Joint Surg. 39A:111, 1957.
58. Noyes, F. R., Torvin, P. J., Hyde, W. B., and LeLucas, J. L.: Biomechanics of ligament failure: An analysis of immobilization, exercise and reconditioning effects in primates. J. Bone Joint Surg. 56A:1406–1418, 1974.
59. Panjabi, M. M., White, A. A., and Johnson, R. M.: Cervical spine mechanics as a function of transection of components. J. Biomech. 8:327–336, 1975.
60. Perey, O.: Fractures of the vertebral end plate in the lumbar spine. Acta Orthop. Scand. 25 (Suppl.):237–238, 1957.
61. Porter, R. A., Hibbert, C. S., and Wicks, M.: The spinal canal in symptomatic lumbar disc lesions. J. Bone Joint Surg. 60B:485–487, 1978.
62. Purcell, G. A., Markolf, K. L., and Dawson, E. G.: Twelfth thoracic first lumbar vertebral mechanical instability of fractures after Harrington rod instrumentation. J. Bone Joint Surg. 53A:71–78, 1981.
63. Quencer, R. M., Montalvo, B. M., Eismont, F. J., and Green, B. A.: Intraoperative spinal sonography in thoracic and lumbar fractures: Evaluation of Harrington rod instrumentation, A.J.N.R. 6:353–359, 1985.
64. Rockoff, S. D., Sweet, E., and Bleustein, J.: The relative contribution of trabecular and cortical bone to the strength of human and lumbar vertebrae. Calc. Tissue Res. 3:163–175, 1969.
65. Roy-Camille, R., Saillant, G., and Mazel, C.: Plating of thoracic, thoracolumbar and lumbar injuries with pedicle screw plates. Orthop. Clin. North Am. 17:147–159, 1986.
66. Ryan, M. D., and Taylor, T. K. F.: The early management of thoracolumbar fractures by ORIF. Aust. N.Z. J. Surg. 52:236–244, 1982.
67. Smith, W. S., and Kaufer, H.: Patterns and mechanisms of lumbar injuries associated with lap seat belts. J. Bone Joint Surg. 51A:239–259, 1969.
68. Southwick, W. O., and Robinson, R. A.: Surgical approaches to the vertebral bodies in the cervical and lumbar regions. J. Bone Joint Surg. 39A:631, 1957.
69. Tile, M.: Fractures of the Pelvis and Acetabulum. Baltimore, Williams & Wilkins, 1984.
70. Weaver, J. K., and Chalmers, J.: Bone: Its strength and changes with aging and an evaluation of some methods for measuring its mineral content. J. Bone Joint Surg. 41A:935–941, 1961.
71. Weinstein, J., Collalto, P., and Lehmann, T.: Thoracolumbar burst fractures treated conservatively: A long-term followup. Spine 13:33–38, 1988.
72. White, A. A., and Panjabi, M. M.: Clinical biomechanics of the spine. Philadelphia, J. B. Lippincott, 1978.
73. Willen, J., Lindahl, S., Irstram, L., and Nordwall, A.: Unstable thoracolumbar fractures. A study by CT and conventional roentgenology. The reduction effective Harrington instrumentation. Spine 9:214–219, 1984.
74. Young, J. S., and Dexter, W. R.: Neurological recovery distal to the zone of injury in 172 cases of closed traumatic spinal cord injury. Paraplegia 16:39–49, 1978.

13 □ Spinal Infections

John C.Y. Leong
Robert D. Fraser

PYOGENIC AND TUBERCULOUS INFECTIONS

John C.Y. Leong

The following discussion deals mainly with tuberculosis and pyogenic infections of the spine. Other rare or unusual infections occur, but only a short description of them is given here.

Infection of the spine is not an uncommon disease. The frequency of tuberculosis relative to pyogenic infection varies among countries. Poor social conditions, poor environmental hygiene, and a dense population tend to favor the development of tuberculosis. Pyogenic infection, on the other hand, is less influenced by such factors. Therefore, in so-called advanced countries tuberculosis is seen less often, but it does exist. Its relative rarity has unfortunately decreased the awareness of the condition and led to a marked delay in its diagnosis.[50] The disease has recently been raising its head again because of immigration from third-world countries, chronically debilitating conditions such as alcoholism, and immunocompromised patients such as those with acquired immunodeficiency syndrome (AIDS). Pyogenic infections may present in otherwise healthy individuals, patients with a septic focus elsewhere in the body, and not uncommonly in drug addicts.

The main controversies surrounding spinal infection are about conservative and surgical treatment; if surgical treatment is indicated, they are also about the extent of excision of the diseased focus and the use of bone grafts to achieve a solid fusion.

TUBERCULOSIS OF THE SPINE

Tuberculosis of the spine is a secondary infection. The primary lesion may be in the lung (Ghon focus), the alimentary tract, or the tonsil. The primary focus is small but evokes a marked regional lymph node response; together these features are called the primary complex. This may occur in childhood with reactivation in adulthood, or it may occur in adulthood de novo.

Over 1,000 cases of tuberculosis of the spine were studied from 1955 to 1960 by the University of Hong Kong. The distribution according to level of involvement is seen in Figure 1. Although the frequency per year has dropped to about 40, the pattern continues. The most common site is therefore the thoracolumbar region. The three main patterns of clinical presentation are as follows:

1. Typical presentation—the classic clinical features include back pain and a gibbus. Other features may be present, such as an abscess in the loin, groin, trochanteric area, or the buttock; paraplegia or paraparesis may occur, with or without bladder and bowel involvement. It is also pertinent to mention that in young children with high thoracic involvement a paraspinal abscess may lead to bronchial compression and irritation, and a symptom known as *asthma Millari* (simulating asthmatic bronchitis) occurs when the patient lies down at night.

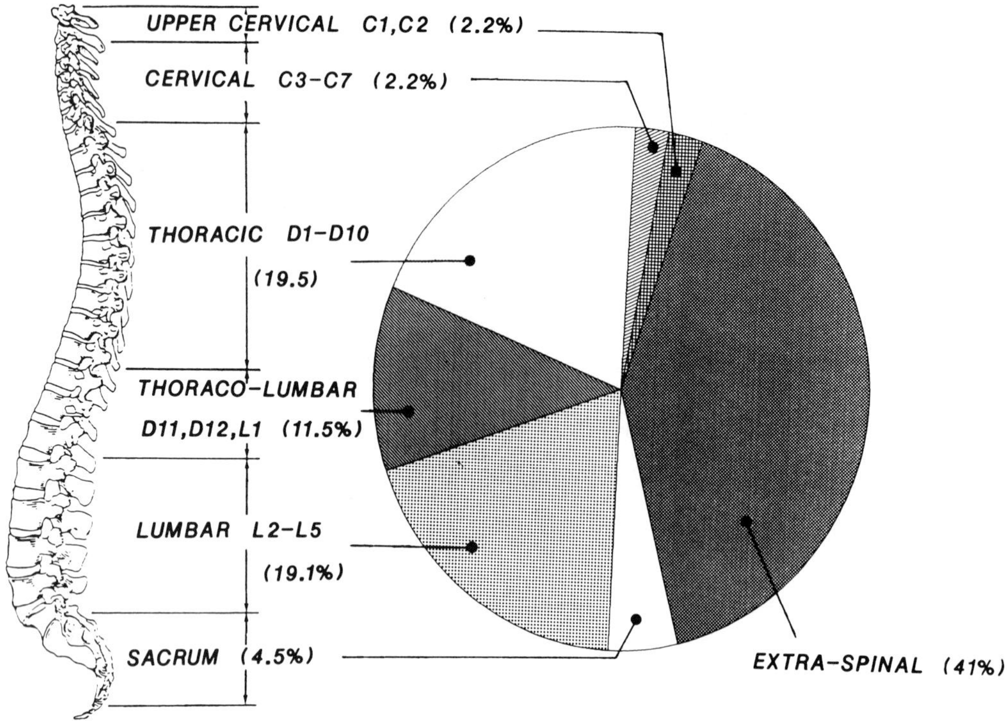

Figure 1 □ Distribution of spinal and extraspinal bone and joint tuberculosis by site in 2000 cases studied from 1955 to 1960.

2. Atypical presentation—involvement of the neural arch alone, an epidural abscess, or extensive external pachymeningitis, without significant anterior vertebral involvement, is rare. The clinical features are significantly different. Paraparesis or paraplegia occur much more commonly, and may be highly spastic, simulating a spinal cord tumor. External pachymeningitis with resulting arachnoiditis may produce a picture of fluctuating neurologic deficit.
3. Presentation with a difficult clinical problem.
   a. Kyphosis—severe angular kyphosis with marked pulmonary function restriction. It may be associated with paraplegia of spontaneous onset.
   b. Reactivation in old age[25]—another difficult situation is one in which extensive spinal tuberculosis has occurred during early adulthood, a full course of antituberculous chemotherapy has been administered for conservative treatment, and the disease is deemed to be cured. Significant kyphosis has resulted because of the extent of the disease. Some 30 to 40 years later the disease is reactivated, and there may or may not be cord compression. Patients in this age group have very osteoporotic bone, and after surgical excision of the diseased tissue the stable seating of bone grafts is extremely difficult to achieve.
   c. Disease affecting the lumbosacral junction[42]—surgical access is difficult to obtain in this area. On the other hand, conservative treatment is usually followed by a kyphotic deformity. Besides being unsightly, this leads to compensatory hyperlordosis above the junction, which is frequently associated with significant low back pain.

Pott's Paraplegia

Sorrel and Sorrel-Dejerine[48] classified paraplegia or paraparesis due to tuberculosis of the spine into the following groups: (1) paraplegia of early onset, and (2) paraplegia of late onset. Hodgson and Yau[19] proposed a classification based on the in vivo pathologic process. From direct observation of the pathologic process during anterior radical resection and spinal fusion, they classified patients as follows: (1) those with paraplegia of active disease, and (2) those with paraplegia of healed disease.

In paraplegia of active disease, there is direct cord compression by the tuberculous abscess, caseous material, necrotic bone, and sometimes sequestered disc. Subluxation and concertina collapse of the vertebral body may also cause pressure. Spinal artery thrombosis may also cause paraplegia (*unrelated* to pressure). When there is external pachymeningitis, direct involvement of the dura and even of the spinal cord will lead to a very severe and spastic form of paraplegia.[16] This may sometimes be mistaken for a spinal cord tumor.

Paraplegia of healed disease has a different pathogenesis. In patients with significant destruction of the vertebral body, especially if more than one or two levels are affected, the spine tends to become markedly kyphotic. Even if healing occurs, either spontaneously or as a result of conservative treatment with chemotherapy, the newly formed bone at the diseased site is soft, and the effect of gravity will tend to exaggerate the kyphosis. There may also be repeated microfatigue fracturing of the newly formed bone. Gradually the latter becomes consolidated, but in the process it is being slowly retropulsed posteriorly, forming an internal ridge. This causes pressure on the anterior aspect of the spinal cord.

Hsu and coworkers[21] have recently confirmed the pathologic process of active disease causing paraplegia of early onset. They have also shown that in paraplegia of late onset, a combination of active and healed disease, or healed disease alone, may be present. Hodgson and coworkers[20] found that anterior decompression and spinal fusion for Pott's paraplegia due to active disease led to rapid recovery of the paraplegia in the majority of patients. Hsu and colleagues[21] have shown that in paraplegia of late onset, the prognosis is significantly worse in patients with healed disease, compared with those who have active disease. Surgical decompression of healed disease is technically difficult, and the outcome is also markedly less favorable.

Radiographic Appearances

The disease may affect the following main sites in the vertebrae:[18] (1) the paradiscal region, (2) the center of the vertebral body, and (3) the anterior aspect of the vertebral body. Involvement of the paradiscal region is most common. Paradiscal disease is usually present on either side of the intervertebral disc, leading to early narrowing of the disc (Fig. 2*A*, *B*). When the center of the vertebral body is involved, a concertina collapse occurs, commonly associated with paraplegia. This type of change is more common in children (Fig. 3). Involvement of the anterior aspect of the vertebral body is due to extension of a paravertebral abscess, which strips up the periosteum and ligaments from the spine with the peripheral periosteal blood supply. The disease then attacks this devitalized bone and leads to anterior scalloping. This is sometimes referred to as an *aneurysmal syndrome*. It is most common in the thoracic spine and in children (Fig 4).

Tuberculous infection rarely involves the transverse processes, the pedicles, the laminae, or the spinal processes. When it does, it falls into the group of patients with atypical presentation.

Malalignment of the spine may result from the disease, including scoliosis (sometimes mistaken for a hemivertebra (Fig. 5), bayonet deformity (Fig. 6*A*, *B*), subluxation and dislocation (Fig. 7), and in the lower lumbar region a reversed spondylolisthesis (Fig. 8). Subluxation or dislocation occurs when there is destruction of two or three vertebrae. In the dorsolumbar region, the anterior surface of the lowest thoracic vertebra or disc attached to it comes to lie on the upper surface of the first remaining lumbar vertebra or the disc. Reversed spondylolisthesis occurs because narrowing of the intervertebral disc causes the vertebral bodies to become closer together. The inclination of the facet joints dictates that the upper body moves backward on the lower ones.

In the lumbar spine another radiographic feature may be present. This is a bony bridging across the sides of two adjacent vertebrae. Masmonteil and Beclere[28] named it *becs de perroquet*. It is probably a true ossification of the paravertebral ligaments, possibly occurring as a response to infection.

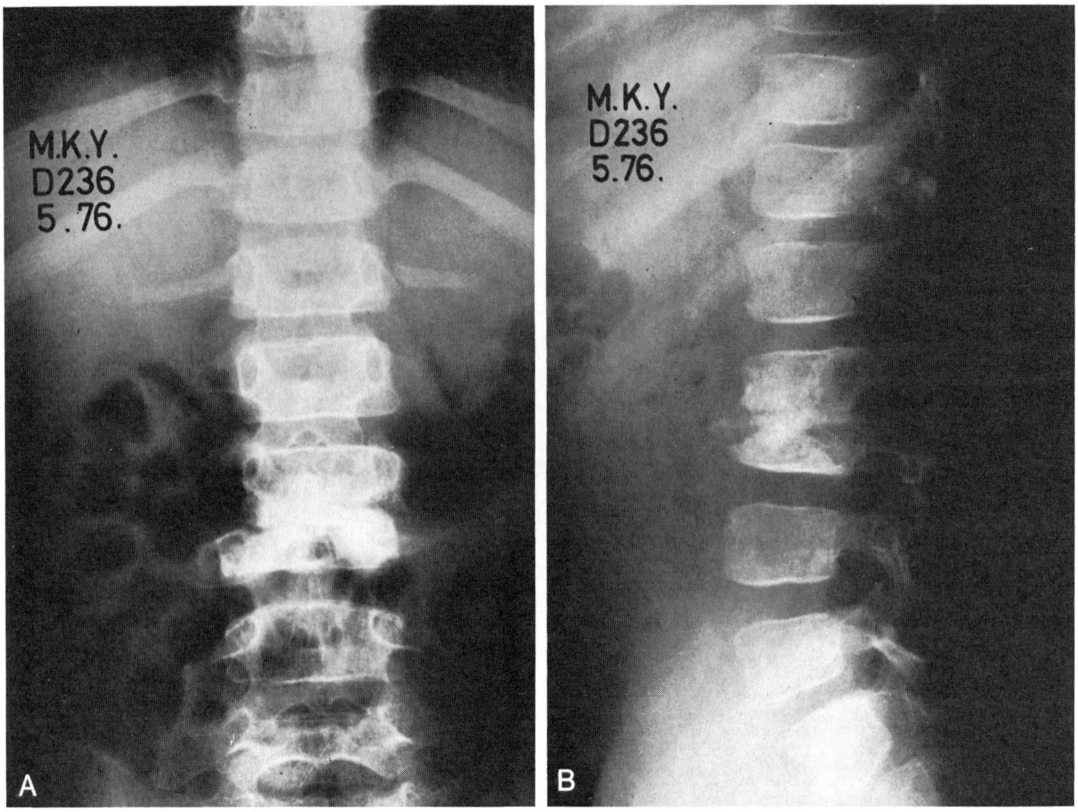

Figure 2 □ *A,* AP x-ray showing early disc narrowing in tuberculosis of the spine. *B,* Lateral x-ray showing early disc space narrowing.

A paravertebral abscess is commonly seen in the cervical, cervicodorsal, and thoracic regions. In the lumbar spine, however, because of the multiple origins of the psoas muscle arising from the vertebral bodies and intervertebral discs, the pus passes through a small opening to form an abscess in the psoas muscle. The psoas abscess does not show up well on plain x-rays. If the disease affects the L5 vertebra or the sacrum, a presacral abscess forms, which again is difficult to detect by plain x-rays, unless calcification has occurred.

Conservative Treatment for Tuberculosis of the Spine

The mainstay of treatment is antituberculous chemotherapy.[3] These drugs vary in (1) their bactericidal action, which is their ability to kill large numbers of actively metabolizing bacilli rapidly, (2) their sterilizing action, which is their capacity to kill slowly or intermittently metabolizing semidormant bacilli, and (3) their ability to prevent emergence of acquired resistance by suppressing drug-resistant mutants. Isoniazid (INH) is the most potent bactericidal drug, and rifampicin is also an important one. On the other hand, rifampicin and pyrazinamide are the most important sterilizing drugs. INH, rifampicin, streptomycin, and ethambutol are effective in preventing the emergence of acquired resistance.

Short-course chemotherapy[3] is now widely accepted as the treatment of choice for tuberculosis. The recommended regimen for newly diagnosed patients is 2 months of pyrazinamide, INH, and rifampicin given daily, followed by 4 months of INH and rifampicin given daily. The dosage for INH is 5 mg/kg of body weight, for rifampicin it is 10 mg/kg, and for pyrazinamide 35 mg/kg. An alternative (and less potent) regimen is INH and rifampicin given daily for 9 months, with or without the addition of streptomycin or ethambutol daily for the first 2 months. (The dosage for streptomycin is 15 to 20 mg/kg of body weight.) The number of viable bacilli contained in bone and joint tubercu-

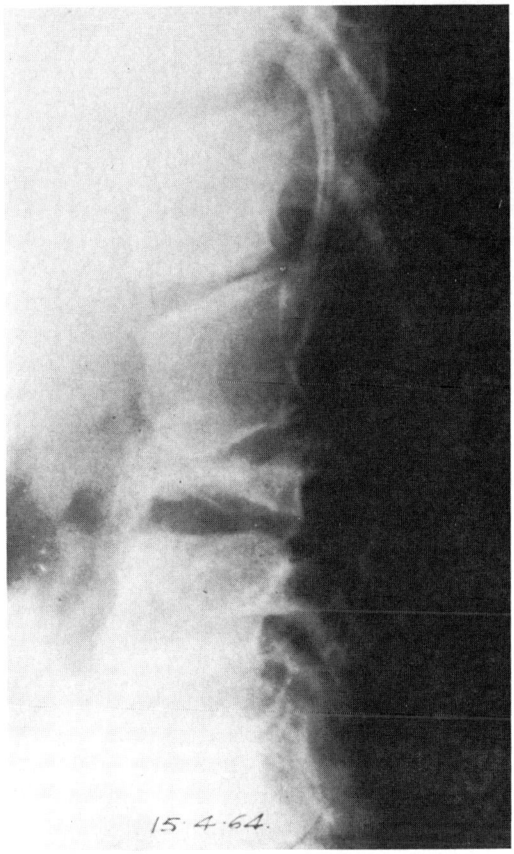

Figure 3 □ Concertina collapse of L3 vertebra in tuberculosis of the spine.

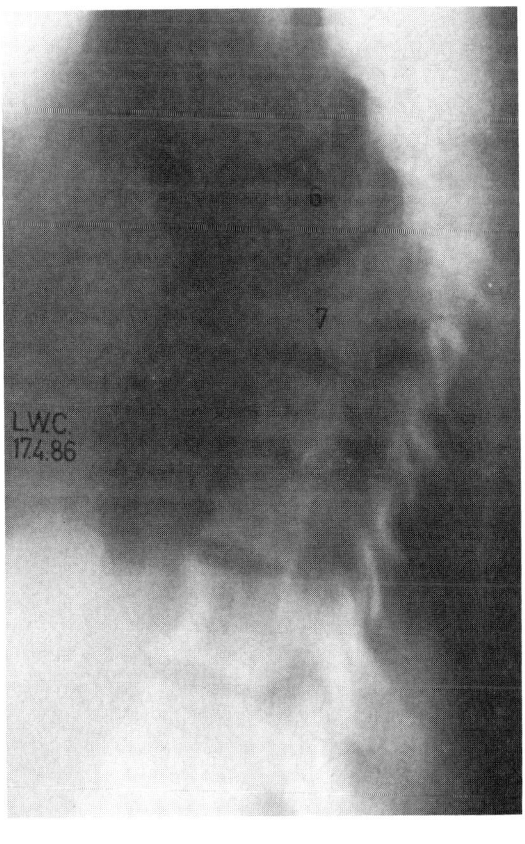

Figure 4 □ Aneurysmal syndrome affecting D6-11 in tuberculosis of the spine.

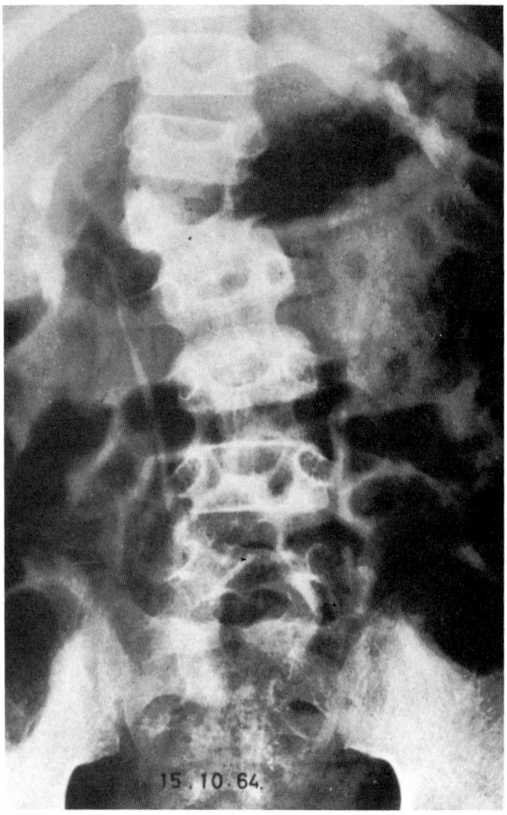

Figure 5 □ Tuberculosis of the spine mimicking a hemivertebra.

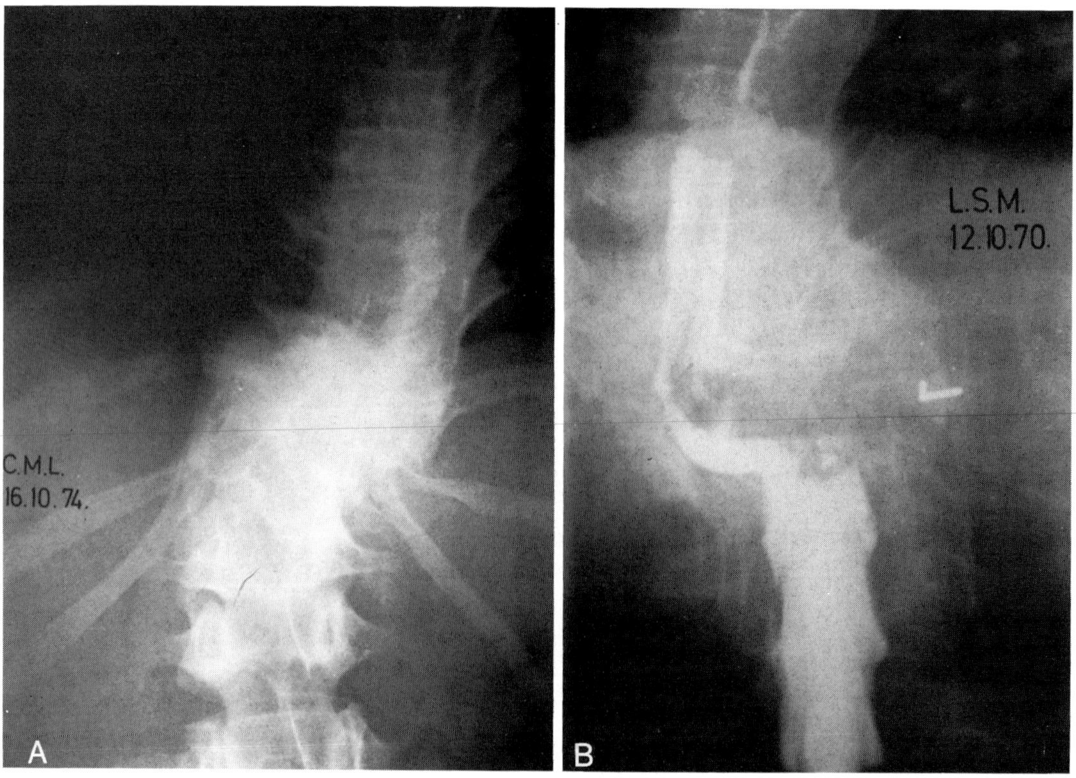

Figure 6 □ *A,* Bayonet deformity in tuberculosis of the spine. *B,* Myelogram of a different patient showing the same deformity.

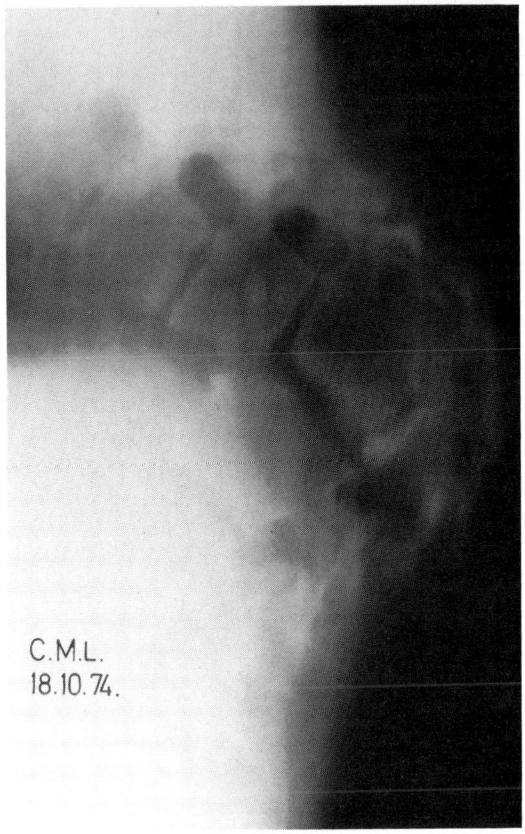

Figure 7 □ Dorsolumbar subluxation in tuberculosis of the spine.

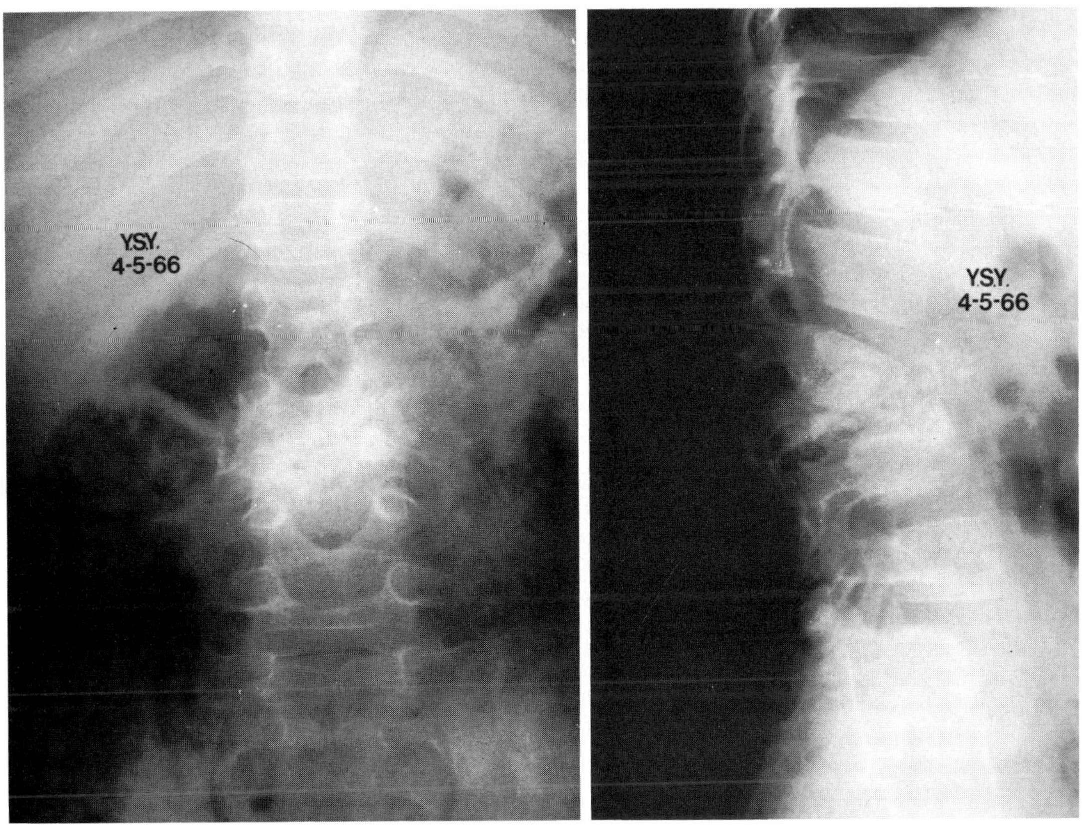

Figure 8 □ Reversed spondylolisthesis of L3 on L4 in tuberculosis of the spine.

losis is small compared with the number in pulmonary lesions. A two-drug regimen, for example, 9 months of INH and rifampicin, is theoretically effective provided it is known that the level of initial resistance to INH in the population is low.

The Medical Research Council (MRC) of Britain has conducted clinical trials comparing the effectiveness of ambulant chemotherapy alone, or in combination with (1) bed rest for 6 months, (2) plaster jacket immobilization for 9 months, (3) surgical débridement (without fusion), and (4) anterior radical excision of disease focus and anterior spinal fusion. These are multicenter trials, some mainly studying children, and others mainly studying adults. The locations of centers include South Korea, Bulawayo, Hong Kong, and Madras.

They have compared the efficacy of different treatment regimens based on the percentages of patients achieving *favorable status* after 3, 5, and 10 years.[30–36] Favorable status is defined as full physical activity with clinically and radiographically quiescent disease, no sinuses or clinically evident abscesses, no myelopathy with functional impairment, and no modification of the allocated regimen. The first series, which was started in 1965, used a chemotherapy regimen consisting of 18 months of daily INH plus para-aminosalicylic acid (PAS), with or without streptomycin for the first 3 months. The percentage of patients with favorable status at 3 years was approximately 85% in all the groups. These results have been maintained at 5 and 10 years. If the remaining patients who attained a favorable status after additional chemotherapy and/or operation were included, the proportion in all groups would rise to between 95% and 100%.

However, it must be emphasized that favorable status does *not* take into account symptomatic relief, fusion rate, or angle of kyphosis.

A second series of studies was begun a few years ago, using short-course regimens of 6 or 9 months of INH and rifampicin with or without streptomycin. The 3-year[37] results showed that favorable status was achieved in a slightly higher percentage in patients treated with the radical operation (plus chemotherapy) compared with ambulant chemotherapy alone, except in Madras.

Anterior Radical Resection and Anterior Spinal Fusion for Tuberculosis of the Spine

The rationale for surgical treatment is based on the following findings:

1. The patient's general condition improves dramatically immediately after evacuation of the abscess.
2. Avascular material can be removed, and the insertion of an anterior strut graft under compression will lead to early fusion.
3. Late recurrence is uncommon (after radical excision of the disease focus and solid fusion has been achieved).
4. Diseased material may be obtained for a definitive diagnosis.
5. Increasing deformity can be prevented.
6. Paraplegia can be prevented, or when established, anterior decompression with bone grafting leads to rapid recovery.

Tuberculosis of the spine mimicks other conditions. Although diagnosis does not usually pose a problem in developing countries in which the disease is rife, it can be difficult in more affluent countries in which the condition is uncommon.

In the first 100 cases reported from our center in 1960,[17] followed for an average of 3 years, the fusion rate was 94%. Our first 300 cases,[15] published in 1964, had an overall radiologic fusion rate of 80%. However, among those without radiologic union, 4.7% had died during the follow up period, and 3% did not have bone grafts inserted because of technical reasons. The average time for fusion was 22.2 months, the shortest was 7 months, and the longest was 42 months. These contained cases of very extensive disease, including involvement of up to eight vertebral bodies.

In the same series of 300 cases, with 80% followed for over 5 years, there was a recurrence rate of 3.3%. Another series[4] of 100 consecutive children from 18 months to 10 years old, after an average follow-up period of 8 years and 2 months (range from 1 to 15 years), again showed a low recurrence rate of 2%. Although the true incidence of reactivation after healing as a result of conservative treatment is unknown, there is evi-

Table 1 □ Changes in the Angle of Kyphosis at 5 Years of Follow-up

	PATIENTS ASSESSED	DECREASE 11° OR MORE	MEAN INCREASE	INCREASE		
				11°–30°	31°–50°	51°–70°
Hong Kong operation	60	12	0	9	0	0
Debridement (Bulawayo)	38	0	12	11	3	0
Conservative treatment (Korea)	271	26	12	88	31	12

dence from the MRC trials that a large proportion (50%) of children undergoing conservative treatment do not show evidence of bony fusion at up to 5 years[33] of follow-up; even at 10 years[36] 27% still have *not* fused. This compares with 90% fused with the radical procedure at the 5-year follow-up,[34] and 97% at 10 years.[35]

The changes in the angle of kyphosis were compared at a 5-year follow-up among patients treated by the radical operation in Hong Kong, débridement in Bulawayo, and conservative measures in South Korea. The initial mean angles of kyphosis for the three groups were similar. Sixty patients in Hong Kong, 38 in Bulawayo, and 271 in Korea were assessed. The radically treated group had no change in the mean angle, whereas both those treated with débridement and those conservatively treated had a mean *increase* of 12 degrees in their kyphosis. More detailed analysis (Table 1) showed that 5% of patients in the conservative treatment group had an *increase* in their angle of kyphosis of 51 to 70 degrees. At 10 years of follow-up, although the number of patients assessed was smaller, those treated by the radical operation showed a mean *decrease* in kyphosis of 1.4 degrees in the thoracic and thoracolumbar regions, and 0.5 degrees in the lumbar region, compared with an *increase* in the débridement group of 9.8 and 7.6 degrees, respectively, and in the conservative treatment group an *increase* of 17.8 and 5.2 degrees, respectively. Of 160 patients assessed for the conservative treatment, 52 patients *increased* their kyphosis between 11 and 30 degrees, 27 between 31 and 50 degrees, and 9 between 51 and 70 degrees. This poses a severe problem for the future (Table 2).

Preferred Method of Treatment

The form of treatment offered should provide rapid relief from symptoms, especially pain and paraparesis or paraplegia. The end result should be firm evidence of eradication of the disease, as shown by a solid bony fusion with little or no deformity. This can be achieved predictably and in the majority of patients only by anterior radical resection of the diseased focus and anterior spinal fusion. This requires good surgical expertise, good general anesthesia, and a high standard of postoperative care.

In the cervical spine, there is no place for conservative treatment alone. In the thoracic spine and the thoracolumbar junction, when there is early and limited disease without a large abscess causing pain, ambulant chemotherapy is justifiable. More extensive disease, significant pain, paraparesis, and presence of a kyphosis are strong indications for

Table 2 □ Changes in the Angle of Kyphosis at 10 Years of Follow-up

		PATIENTS ASSESSED	MEAN INCREASE*	INCREASE		
				11°–30°	31°–50°	51°–70°
Hong Kong	T†&TL‡	27	−1.4	4	0	0
	Lumbar	4	−0.5			
Debridement	T&TL	21	9.8	9	3	0
	Lumbar	12	7.6			
Conservative	T&TL	125	17.8	52	27	9
	Lumbar	35	5.2			

*Mean increase. Negative values indicate a *decrease* in kyphosis.
†T = thoracic spine.
‡TL = thoracolumbar spine.

surgical treatment. It must be remembered that at 10 years of follow-up in the MRC trials, the average increase of kyphosis in the conservatively treated group amounted to 17.8 degrees. This is completely unacceptable in the thoracolumbar junction.

In the lumbar spine, the average increase in kyphosis for the conservatively treated group averaged only 5.2 degrees. Technically, radical resection and anterior spinal fusion become more difficult with more caudal involvement. This is because the common iliac and segmental vessels may be involved in the abscess itself; sometimes their walls become very friable because of the inflammatory process, increasing the risk of damage that can lead to massive bleeding. The indication for ambulant chemotherapy is therefore stronger, unless there is extensive disease or significant deformity. At times, when surgical approach to the spine becomes too difficult, one can compromise by simply draining the abscess. Ideally, anterior radical resection and spinal fusion still give the best end result (Fig. 9*A*, *B*).

Tuberculosis affecting the lumbosacral junction[42] is uncommon. Experience with 37 patients, 26 of whom had adequate records and follow-up (average 20.2 years, range 6 to 34.5 years) revealed that conservative and surgical treatment both resulted in firm fusion. However, only 25% of the group treated by anterior spinal fusion had kyphosis (averaging 10.5 degrees) compared with 100% of the group treated conservatively resulting in kyphosis (averaging 60.4 degrees). Significant low back pain and a narrowed pelvic outlet necessitating caesarean section for pregnancy were correlated with the spinal deformity. The lumbosacral junction is technically highly demanding to operate on, but if the expertise is available the outcome will be superior (Fig. 10*A*, *B*, *C*). Conservative treatment cures the disease but results in significant deformity (Fig. 11*A*, *B*).

PYOGENIC INFECTIONS OF THE SPINE

Pyogenic infections have significant differences in clinical presentation, diagnostic criteria, treatment modalities, and outcome, as well as in causative organisms[5, 7, 43] compared with tuberculosis of the spine. Three different groups of clinical entities have been described, although the relative frequency of occurrence of these groups vary from one another. They are as follows:

1. Pyogenic spondylitis—the infection lies in the vertebral body and usually starts in the region of the end plates. Involvement of the neural arch is rare.
2. Intervertebral discitis.
3. Spinal epidural abscess.

Pyogenic Spondylitis

Pyogenic infections[43] of the spine constitute only about 1% of cases of osteomyelitis. The presentation may be acute or chronic. In the acute form, pain is the most constant symptom, whereas pyrexia, local tenderness, muscle spasm, constitutional upset, and neurologic involvement may or may not be present. The pain may radiate to the abdomen or legs. The presence of abdominal pain may confuse the diagnosis. The incidence of paraplegia or paraparesis varies from 3% to 15% in different series. Radiculopathy may also occur. It appears that increased age, a more cephalad level of infection, and associated diseases of diabetes mellitus and rheumatoid arthritis predispose one to paraplegia.

In about half the cases, *Staphylococcus* is the causative organism, with *Streptococcus*, *Proteus*, and *Escherichia coli* involved in most of the remainder. Other organisms occasionally involved include *Pseudomonas*, *Klebsiella*, *Salmonella typhi*, *Brucella*, and *pneumococci*.

The evidence is that the infection is hematogenous, with the urinary tract being the most common primary focus. Spinal infection has arisen after cardiac or urinary catheterization. Drug addicts and diabetics are also vulnerable.

Investigations

Erythrocyte sedimentation rate elevation is the most consistently positive investigation. Elevation of the white cell count and a positive blood culture occur less consistently. Rising antibody titers, in response to specific organisms or antigens, when present, are valuable diagnostic aids.[8] These include anti–alpha and anti–gamma staphylococcal hemolysin, antistreptolysin-O, brucellin antibody, Widal tests for *Salmonella typhi*, and gonococcal complement tests.

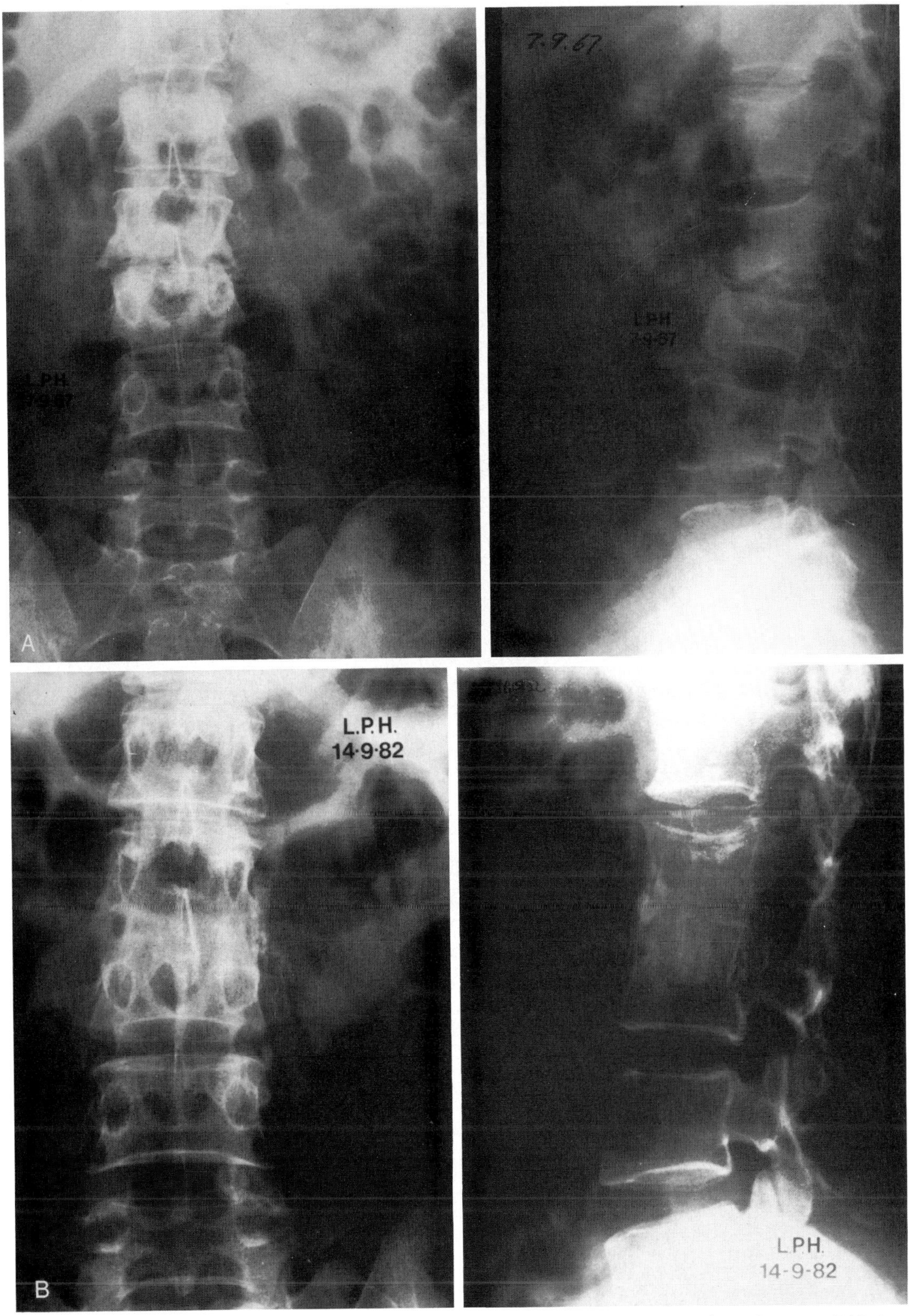

Figure 9 □ *A*, Tuberculosis affecting L2 and L3. *B*, 15 years after anterior excision and strut grafting, showing solid fusion.

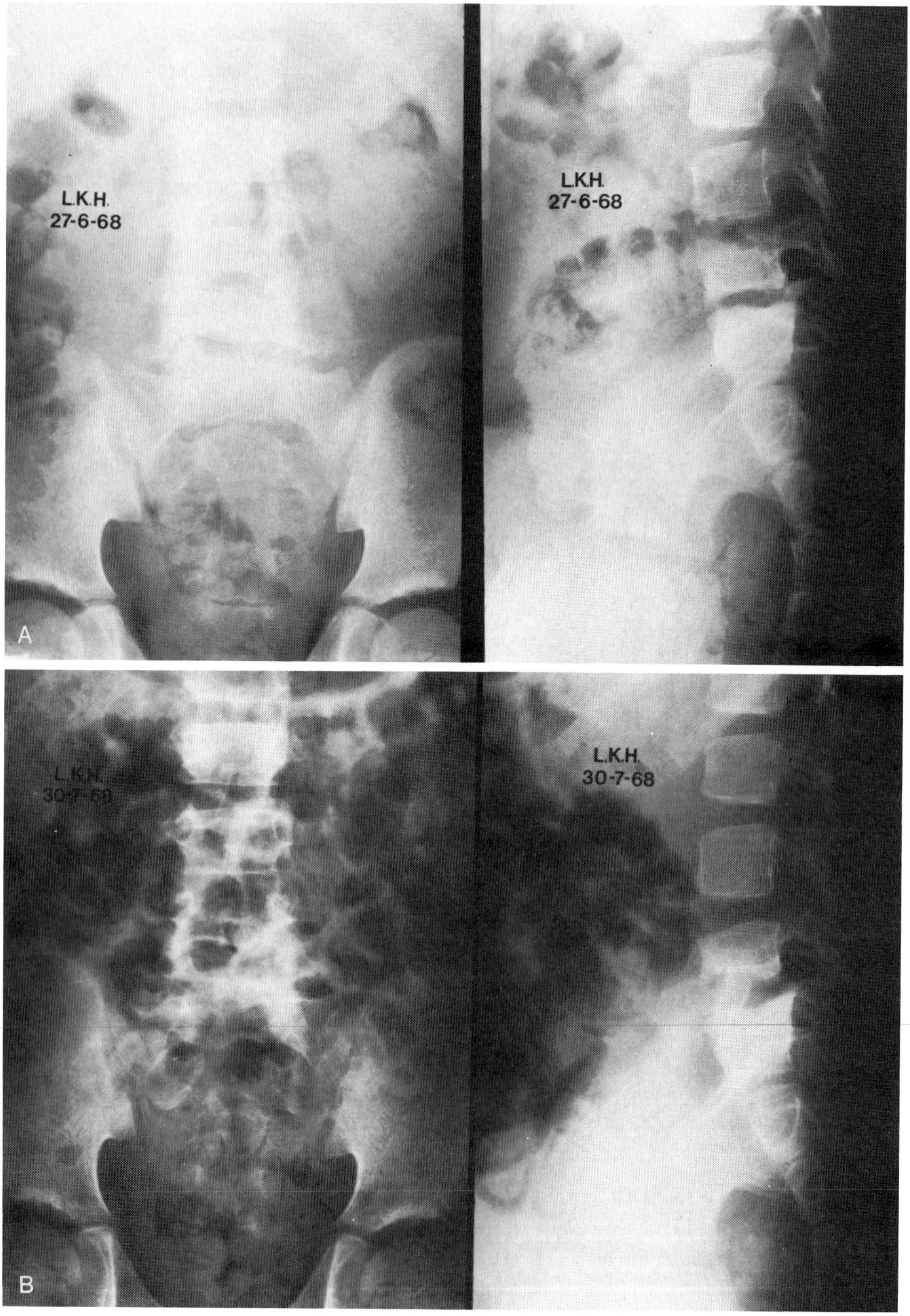

Figure 10 □ *A,* Tuberculosis affecting lumbosacral junction. *B,* After anterior excision and strut grafting.

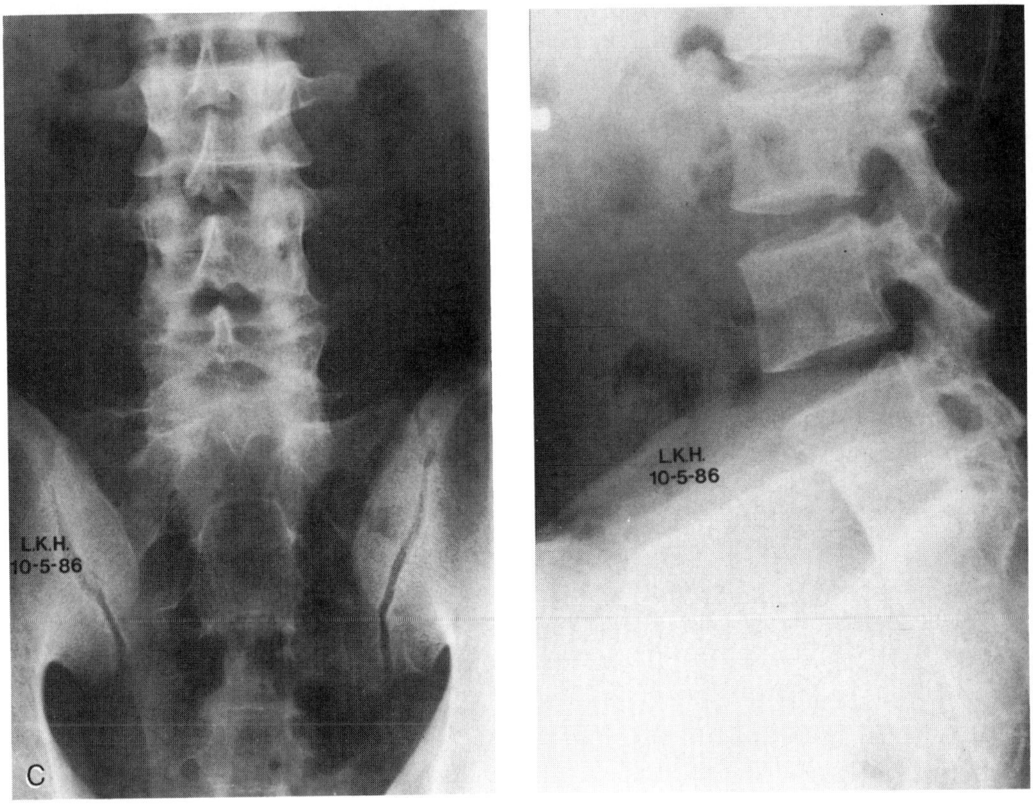

Figure 10 *Continued C,* 18 years later showing solid anterior fusion.

Needle biopsy is a useful procedure in obtaining material for both culture and pathologic study. However, the success rate of the procedure for diagnosis varies from 20% to 100%.

Radiographic Appearances

Plain X-ray Films

No radiologic pattern is completely reliable in distinguishing a pyogenic infection from a tuberculous one. One or more of the following features may be present:[12]

1. Symmetric destruction of the adjacent surfaces of two vertebrae—this is not a specific feature (Fig. 12).
2. Loss of disc space—this may be variable in amount and is not a specific feature (Fig. 13).
3. New bone formation—this is much more common in pyogenic infections compared with tuberculous ones. In a prospective study of 45 patients[2] with spinal infection proven by bacteriologic and/or histologic findings, new bone formation occurred in 50% of white patients with pyogenic infection, but none occurred in tuberculous infection. However, in black patients, new bone formation occurred in 20% with tuberculous infection (Fig. 14).
4. Sclerosis of bone, with or without marked destruction—this is more common in pyogenic infections (Fig. 14).
5. Paravertebral abscess—this is uncommon, and even when present it is less prominent.
6. Kyphosis and subluxation—this is not a specific feature, and it tends to be less severe than in tuberculosis, because the number of vertebrae involved is usually smaller (Fig. 15).

Computed Tomography

There are certain advantages of this type of radiologic investigation.[6] These are as follows:

1. Multiplanar depictions of disturbances of bone integrity are possible by means of image reformation.

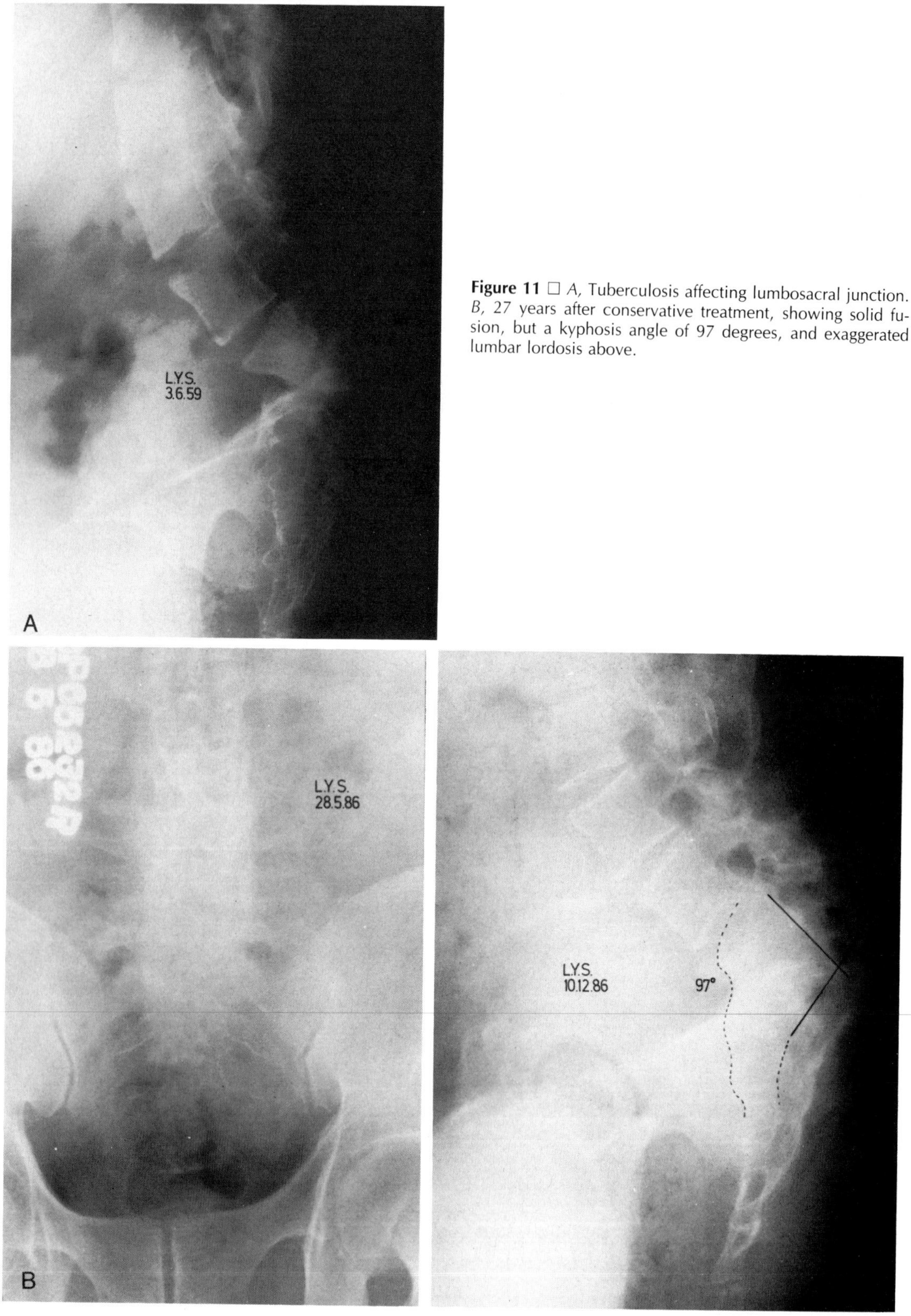

Figure 11 □ *A,* Tuberculosis affecting lumbosacral junction. *B,* 27 years after conservative treatment, showing solid fusion, but a kyphosis angle of 97 degrees, and exaggerated lumbar lordosis above.

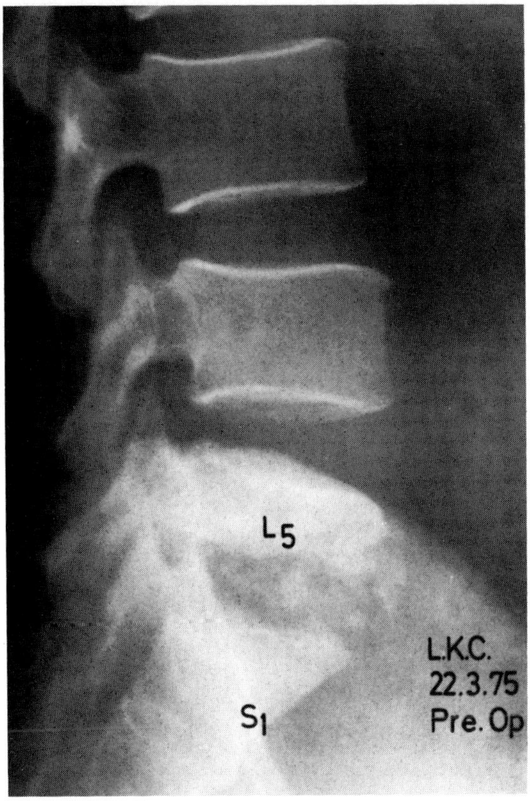

Figure 12 □ Pyogenic spondylitis showing symmetric destruction of the adjacent surfaces of L5 and S1.

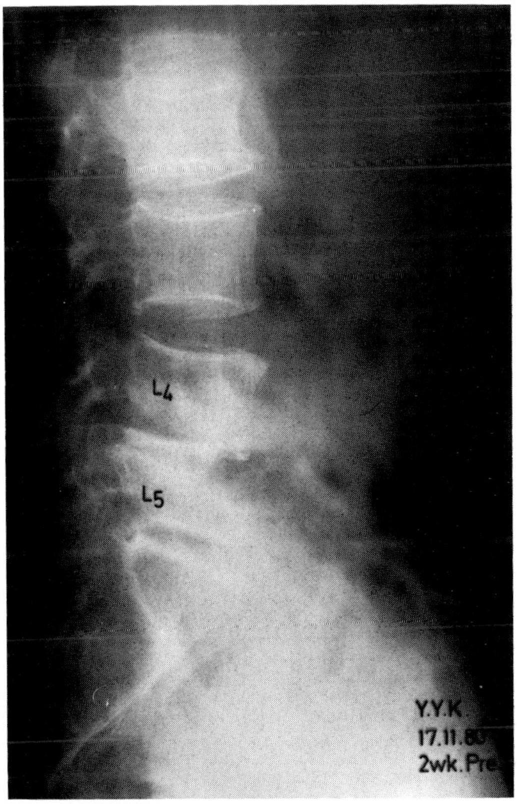

Figure 13 □ Pyogenic spondylitis showing early loss of joint space between L4 and L5.

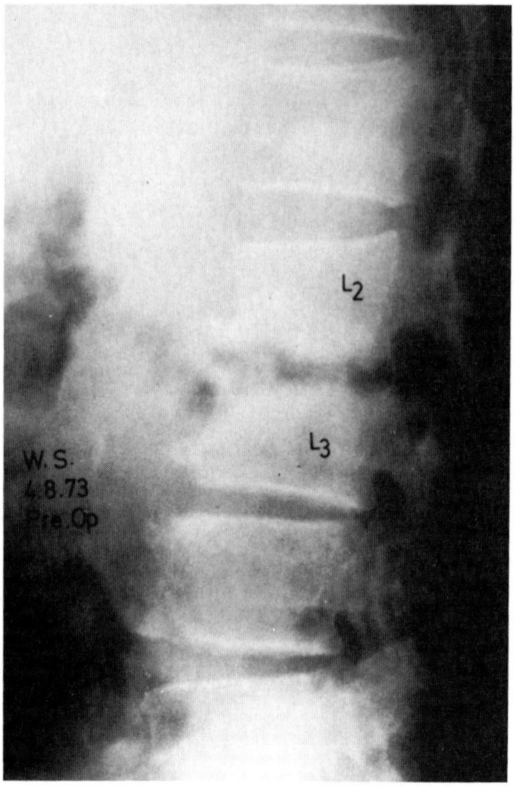

Figure 14 □ Pyogenic spondylitis showing subchondral and adjacent bone sclerosis and new bone formation anteriorly.

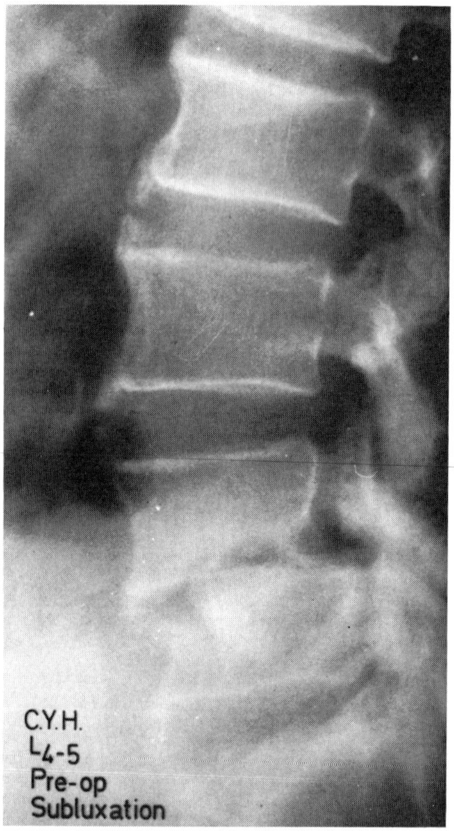

Figure 15 □ Lumbar pyogenic spondylitis showing mild anterior subluxation.

2. Precise definition of paraspinal soft tissue is possible. This is most useful in detecting paravertebral abscess formation, as well as extension of the disease process into the spinal canal. The combination of computed tomography (CT) and small-volume, low concentration metrizamide administration in the subarachnoid space will also increase accuracy.
3. CT can also be used to guide percutaneous needle biopsy.

There is no evidence to show, however, that CT is more sensitive than conventional radiography in the earliest stages of spinal infection.

Other Radiologic Investigations

Radionuclide Bone Imaging[1, 12]

Technetium-99m–labeled methylene diphosphonate (^{99m}Tc MDP) is the most sensitive screening test. An abnormal bone image increases the probability of the disease, even if findings of conventional x-ray films and CT scans are normal. A normal bone image virtually rules out suspected acute or chronic active osteomyelitis. The sensitivity of the three-phase bone scan varies from 89% in osteomyelitis to 100% in vertebral osteomyelitis.

Total-body gallium-67 (^{67}Ga) is usually used sequentially after ^{99m}Tc MDP. An abnormal ^{67}Ga image following an abnormal ^{99m}Tc bone image increases the specificity of the diagnosis. Normal technetium and gallium bone images of the vertebra virtually exclude the diagnosis of pyogenic spondylitis.

In patients with paravertebral abscesses, abnormalities on both technetium and gallium scans may extend into the paravertebral region. The pattern of this uptake has been termed the *butterfly sign*.

Magnetic Resonance Imaging

This is more useful in evaluating intervertebral discitis (see below).

Septic Intervertebral Discitis

This condition is believed to be a pyogenic infection arising primarily in the intervertebral disc. In children,[46] as a rule, the disease is relatively benign with rapid resolution of symptoms. Many patients respond well with bed rest or immobilization alone. Because of that, there is doubt as to whether it is a true bacterial infection. In late adolescence and adulthood, intervertebral discitis is a more ominous disease.

A significant percentage of adult patients with intervertebral discitis present with prodromal infection, suggesting that, like pyogenic spondylitis, the bacteria reach the spine by a hematogenous route. There is controversy as to whether it is due to venous or arterial spread. Doyle[9] postulated that infections occurred via the vertebral venous plexus of Batson. However, Wiley and Trueta[49] demonstrated by vascular studies that it was extremely unlikely that the venous plexus was responsible for the spread of infection to the spine. They believed that arterial spread was the more likely route. Although it is generally stated that the intervertebral disc becomes avascular in adult life, Wiley and Trueta,[49] Mineiro,[38] and Hassler[13] showed that although the blood supply to the intervertebral disc diminished with age, the main decrease was in the number of vessels that enter the nucleus pulposus from the adjacent vertebrae via the end plates, but that an adequate circumferential supply was maintained from the periphery, with vessels penetrating as far as the junction between the annulus fibrosus and the nucleus pulposus.

The clinical picture may include features of a prodromal infection before spinal involvement. Locally, there are back pain with or without referred pain of femoral or sciatic distribution, point tenderness, paravertebral muscle spasm, and limitation of movement. Paraparesis or paraplegia occurs in as many as 40% of patients. The level of involvement varies from one series to another, but is mainly thoracic and lumbar, with infrequent involvement of the neck, except in children.

Blood Investigations

Investigations similar to those used in pyogenic spondylitis may be helpful, although a normal value will not rule out the diagnosis.

Radiographic Appearances

The following features are observed in the plain films.[23] They tend to occur in sequence,

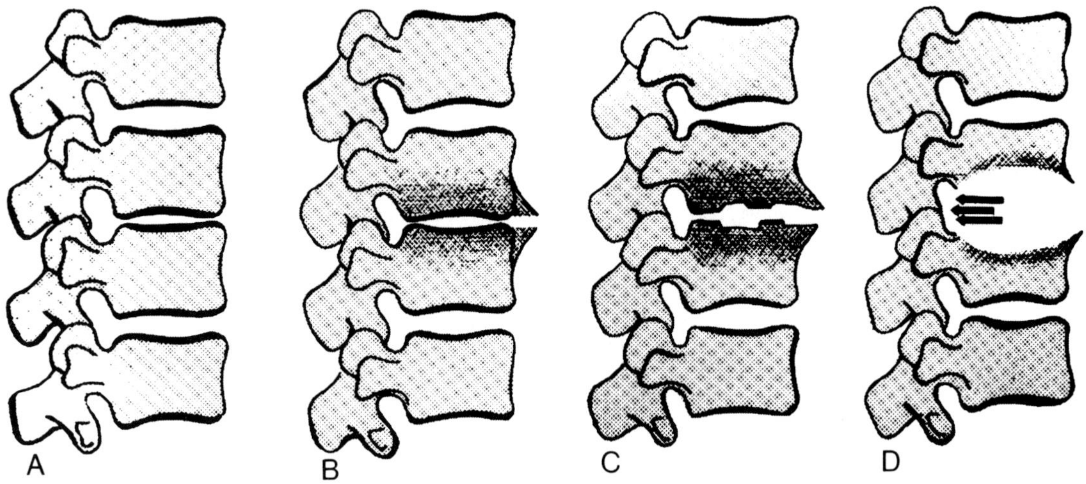

Figure 16 □ *A* to *D,* Septic intervertebral discitis showing different stages of radiographic presentation. (From Kemp, H. B. S., Jackson, J. W., Jeremiah, J. D., and Hall, A. J.: Pyogenic infections occurring primarily in intervertebral discs. J. Bone Joint Surg. 55:701, 1973.)

although in individual cases it depends on the stage at which the patient presents (Fig. 16*A*, *B*, *C*, *D*).

1. Decrease in the vertical height of the affected intervertebral disc space—this feature is most constant and occurs during the first 3 months of the disease. The degree of narrowing is variable but does not relate to the subsequent progress of the disease (Fig. 16*A*).
2. Progressive sclerosis of the subchondral bone together with increase in radiodensity of the adjacent area of the vertebral bodies on either side of the affected disc. It usually follows disc space narrowing by 2 to 3 months. The density results from deposition of new bone on existing trabeculae, as well as associated subperiosteal new bone formation (Fig. 16*B*).
3. Progressive irregularity of the adjacent vertebral end plates—Kemp and coworkers[23] demonstrated that these changes were a local extension of the inflammatory process, which in turn evoked sclerosis of the margins of the vertebral body (Fig. 16*C*).
4. In 50% of the cases, the narrowing of disc space and adjacent sclerosis would increase further. In the rest, there may be "ballooning" of the disc space as a result of erosion of the vertebral body (Fig. 16*D*).
5. Circumferential formation of bone around the annulus. This is attempted repair of the disease. Radiologically, it appears as a bony bridge.

In both tuberculous and pyogenic spondylitis, narrowing and subsequent loss of disc space is an early and relatively common feature. In tuberculous spondylitis, there is early destruction of bone, leading to loss of definition and collapse of the affected vertebral body. In pyogenic spondylitis, spontaneous intervertebral fusion occurs, which is not seen in septic discitis. Abscess formation is also extremely rare in septic discitis, although involvement of the spinal cord leading to paraplegia can occur by either pressure from inflammatory granulomatous tissue or septic thrombosis of spinal blood vessels.

Other Radiologic Investigations

Radionuclide Uptake Scanning

Both ^{99m}Tc MDP and ^{67}Ga have been shown to be very useful in the early diagnosis of this condition.

Magnetic Resonance Imaging

There is evidence that MRI is at least as sensitive, and more specific, than radionuclide uptake scanning in disc space infection. In adults,[39] using a relatively long echo time (120-msec TE) and repetition time (3-sec TR) shows a markedly increased signal intensity of the entire disc as well as the adjacent end plates. A 60-msec TE/1-sec TR pulse sequence will only produce an isointense signal of the body and disc space. In children[14] an increase in signal intensity is not obtained, but an affected disc will still show up as being different from the adjacent normal structures.

Compared with radionuclide bone scanning, MRI specifically localizes the diseased process to the disc space and has the added advantage of being completely noninvasive. It is known that technetium scans have been found to be abnormal within 7 days of onset of symptoms in cases of intervertebral septic discitis. This is much earlier than x-ray findings, in which usually 2 to 6 weeks must pass before changes are apparent. Whether MRI changes occur even earlier is not clear at this stage.

Spinal Epidural Abscesses

This condition is relatively uncommon,[22, 24] and patients are more frequently referred to neurosurgeons than to orthopedic surgeons.

Clinical Features

Back pain is invariably present. Pyrexia may or may not be present. Root pain commonly follows. The incidence of paraparesis or paraplegia is high, ranging from 75% to 100%.

The presentation may be acute or chronic. The thoracic and lumbar spine are most commonly involved, and the disease is rarely seen in children under 12 years old.

Investigations

Erythrocyte sedimentation rate is usually raised, and leukocytosis may or may not be present. The useful investigations include the following:

1. Lumbar puncture with analysis of the cerebrospinal fluid—the CSF is commonly turbid or xanthochromic, but it can be clear. The protein concentration is usually increased and may be marked in patients with complete spinal block. A glucose content below 40 mg% may be found when there is coexistent bacterial meningitis.
2. Plain x-rays of the spine—these may be completely normal. If a spinal epidural abscess is secondary to a disc space infection or spondylitis, there may be corresponding x-ray changes.
3. Myelography with water-soluble contrast media—this is the most useful investigation. However, occasionally false negatives occur, such as when lesions are too thin to displace the dural sheath; myelography may also fail to show up multiple lesions.
4. The value of CT and magnetic resonance imaging has not been thoroughly investigated in this condition as yet.

Conservative Treatment

Pyogenic Spondylitis

A patient presenting with clinical features suggestive of this disease should be investigated with a blood culture or urine culture and plain x-rays of the spine. The outcome will lead to the following alternatives and the logical plan of management:[47]

1. Radiologic evidence and a positive blood culture—this group of patients should be treated by the appropriate antibiotics intravenously for 6 weeks, then orally for a minimum of another 6 weeks. Bed rest is essential during the acute stage. When severe pain and muscle spasm have been alleviated, usually after 2 to 3 weeks of antibiotic administration, the patients can be mobilized with an external light spinal brace.
2. Positive radiologic evidence but negative blood and urine cultures—if there is a known prodromal infection, then the organism is assumed to be the same. The appropriate antibiotic can then be selected. Specific antibodies to the more common infections, such as *Staphylococcus* and *Streptococcus*, can be helpful if present. If the antibodies are absent and the disease is not responding to the chosen antibiotic, then a needle biopsy is indicated to obtain material for culture.
3. No radiologic evidence—a radionuclide bone scan (^{m99}Tc MDP) is indicated to identify a lesion in the spine and the level of involvement. If it is followed by a ^{67}Ga scan the specificity is increased. A positive bone scan, together with a positive blood culture, puts the patient into the same plan of treatment as in the first group. If the bone scan is positive, but the blood culture is negative, the plan of treatment is the same as in the second group. Occasionally, a repeat needle bi-

it occurred at one level of a two-level fusion in the cervical spine. Two patients had an abnormally long fusion time. One patient had a disappearing graft in the initial few months after surgery, but this gradually reappeared on the subsequent radiographs, and radiologic fusion was seen at 28 months.

Two patients had recurrence. One had a chronic sinus and an acute abscess in the subcutaneous region of the scar 3 years after the surgery. This was treated by drainage of the abscess and excision of the sinus. The sinus was deep but did not involve the spine. The other patient had an adjacent (L1–L2) vertebral involvement by chronic spondylitis 2 years after the primary (D12–L1) surgery. This was treated similarly with excision and anterior spinal fusion. A few months later, involvement of the L4–L5 vertebrae was noticed. This was treated by débridement without formal fusion. Chronic osteomyelitis was confirmed each time by histologic examination. At 14 years of follow-up, fusion was present in all the surgically treated levels. However, there was late onset of lower limb weakness (some years after the third surgery), and a myelogram showed chronic adhesive arachnoiditis.

Thirteen patients had neurologic involvement. Eight had radiculopathy, and five had myelopathy. All those with radiculopathy improved after the operation. Of those with myelopathy, three were Frankel Grade C, and two Grade D, preoperatively. Postoperatively, four recovered fully (Grade E), and one improved from Grade C to D. On the long term follow-up, one of the patients who improved from Grade D preoperatively to Grade E postoperatively subsequently had late deterioration to Grade C (this is the patient with the multiple-level recurrence, referred to above).

Twenty-six patients returned to the same work that they had before surgery, whereas three had to change their jobs (one owing to weakness, another owing to concomitant systemic lupus erythematosus, and the third because his job involved heavy manual labor). Of the 26 patients who returned to their original work, six had occasional pain, one had a distinct limp, one had residual weakness, and four had mild deformity of the spine that did not bother them.

These results show that with adequate excision of the disease focus and the appropriate antibiotic given for an adequate period, bone-graft survival is not a problem in pyogenic spondylitis. Indeed the fusion rate is over 93%. Neurologic involvement is generally well alleviated, which is the experience of other authors as well.

Eismont and coworkers[10] reported a series of 31 patients affected by pyogenic spondylitis with paraparesis. Twenty-two were followed for more than 2 years. They showed that laminectomy for decompression did not achieve good results. Anterior débridement with or without grafting produced superior results. They thought that if only minimum decompression with limited bone grafting were needed, the costotransversectomy approach would be preferred. If extensive resection of necrotic bone with strut grafting were needed, then the transthoracic or extraperitoneal approach would be preferable. We have found that the costotransversectomy approach offers very limited exposure and is useful only when a severe kyphosis is present, which rarely occurs in pyogenic spondylitis.

Septic Intervertebral Discitis

The absolute indication for surgical intervention is paraparesis or paraplegia. As noted before, the incidence is higher than in pyogenic spondylitis, by as much as 40%. Also, the onset is rapid and more frequently irreversible. Kemp and coworkers,[23] from operative findings, showed that paraplegia in this condition is mainly the result of direct extension of the inflammatory granulations posteriorly to involve the meninges and (occasionally) the cord. Septic thrombosis of spinal vessels may also be a cause.

Kemp and coworkers[23] advocated surgical clearance of diseased tissue in this condition, even in the absence of cord compression. His reasons included preventing recurrence of the condition in some patients who had been treated conservatively, promoting rapid relief of symptoms, and obtaining material for culture of the infecting organism.

Spinal Epidural Abscess

The treatment of this condition constitutes an emergency, as permanent paraplegia or quadriplegia may otherwise result.[22, 24] The extent of the infection may span the length of many vertebrae and is most common at the thoracic and lumbar regions. Ventrally, the epidural space is practically nonexistent, but dorsally there is a larger amount of areolar tissue and a rich vascular plexus, where infection easily lodges. Therefore, a logical treatment is laminectomy over the entire extent of the infection, evacuation of abscess, and application of local as well as systemic antibiotics. Postoperative drains are recommended.

The results are worse if the patient has an acute presentation and if the infection has a subdural or intramedullary component. Mortality rate is still significant and varies from 3% to 30%. Morbidity in the form of residual weakness or sensory disturbance is also common (from 11% to 30%).

There is some suggestion that hyperbaric oxygen treatment may improve the outcome.[44] One center recommended one session per day, lasting 40 to 60 minutes at 1.7 to 2 units of atmospheric pressure. Ten to twenty sessions were needed.

Other Uncommon Infections

These infections may be bacterial or fungal. Most are insidious in onset, and a long interval may exist between onset of symptoms and diagnosis. Changes on x-ray films are slow to appear and are often nonspecific. Not infrequently, multiple levels of involvement may be present. The diagnosis is made possible only by awareness of such conditions, by the application of specific serologic tests, and by histologic examination of biopsy material.

Brucellosis Vertebral Osteomyelitis[26]

Brucellae are small non-motile gram-negative capnophilic coccobacilli. There are three main species: *Brucella melitensis*, *Brucella abortus*, and *Brucella suis*. Brucellosis is an occupational disease found mainly in farmers, people working in meat-packing plants, veterinary surgeons, and livestock producers. Serologic studies include a brucelloslide test which, if positive, is followed by a *Brucella* antibody tube dilution titer. The diagnosis depends on (1) a minimum *Brucella* antibody titer of 1:80, (2) radiographic evidence of spinal involvement, and (3) a clinical response to treatment. The lumbar spine, especially the lumbosacral region, is more commonly involved than other parts. The lesions may be single or multiple. Treatment consists of a combination of tetracycline and streptomycin, cotrimoxazole alone, or a combination of cotrimoxazole and rifampicin. Treatment should be for at least 3 months. Surgical decompression is required if there is neurologic involvement.

Actinobacillus Actinomycetemcomitans *Vertebral Osteomyelitis*[40]

This is an extremely rare condition. The organism is part of the indigenous flora of the mouth. It is a gram-negative microaerophilic coccobacillus with fastidious growth requirements. There is no specific serologic test. Diagnosis depends on histologic findings and culture of the organism. Radiologically, the lesion may be osteoblastic. The bacteria are usually sensitive to streptomycin, tetracycline, and chloramphenicol.

Nocardial Vertebral Osteomyelitis[51]

Again this is a very rare infection. *Nocardia* organisms are true bacteria, gram-positive and partially acid fast. The most frequent primary site of involvement by the disease is the pulmonary system. The x-ray findings in the spine are nonspecific, but multiple involvement sites are not uncommon. No specific serologic test is available. The mainstays of treatment are the sulfonamides. Minocycline is also effective.

Cryptococcal Vertebral Osteomyelitis[27]

This again is a rare condition. *Cryptococcus* infection is a true fungal infection. Diagnosis can be made by demonstrating rising serum cryptococcal titer (latex agglutination). Antifungal therapy, such as amphotericin B, may be useful.

References

1. Adatepe, M. H., Powell, O. M., Isaacs, G. H., et al.: Hematogenous pyogenic vertebral osteomyelitis: Diagnostic value of radionuclide bone imaging. J. Nucl. Med. 27:1680–1685, 1986.
2. Allen, E. H., Cosgrove, D., and Millard, F. J. C.: The radiological changes in infections of the spine and their diagnostic value. Clin. Radiol. 29:31–40, 1978.
3. Antituberculosis Regimens of Chemotherapy: Bull. Int. Union Tuber. Lung Dis. 63:60–64, 1988.
4. Bailey, H. L., Gabriel, M., Hodgson, A. R., and Shin, J. S.: Tuberculosis of the spine in children. J. Bone Joint Surg. 54:1633, 1972.

5. Bonfiglio, M., Lange, T. A., and Kim, Y. M.: Pyogenic vertebral osteomyelitis. Clin. Orthop. Rel. Res. 96:234–247, 1973.
6. Brant-Zawadzki, M., Burke, V. D., and Jeffrey, R. B.: CT in the evaluation of spine infection. Spine 8:358–364, 1983.
7. Collert, S.: Osteomyelitis of the Spine. Acta Orthop. Scand. 48:283–290, 1977.
8. Digby, J. M., and Kersley, J. B.: Pyogenic nontuberculous spinal infection. J. Bone Joint Surg. 61:47–55, 1979.
9. Doyle, J. R.: Narrowing of the intervertebral-disc space in children. J. Bone Joint Surg. 42:1191, 1960.
10. Eismont, F. J., Bohlman, H. H., Soni, P. L., et al.: Pyogenic and fungal vertebral osteomyelitis with paralysis. J. Bone Joint Surg. 65:19–29, 1983.
11. Fang, D., Remedios, I., and Leong, J. C. Y.: Pyogenic spondylitis: Results of anterior excision and anterior spinal fusion (submitted, J. Bone Joint Surg. [Br.]).
12. Fernandez-Ulloa, M., Vasavada, P. J., Hanslits, M. L., et al.: Diagnosis of vertebral osteomyelitis: Clinical, radiological and scintigraphic features. Orthopedics 8:1144–1150, 1985.
13. Hassler, O.: The human intervertebral disc. Acta Orthop. Scand. 40:765, 1970.
14. Heller, R. M., Szalay, E. A., Green, N. E., et al.: Disc space infection in children: Magnetic resonance imaging. Radiol. Clin. North Am. 26:207–209, 1988.
15. Hodgson, A. R.: Report on the findings and results in 300 cases of Pott's disease treated by anterior fusion of the spine. J. West. Pacific Orthop. Assoc. 1:3–7, 1964.
16. Hodgson, A. R., Skinsnes, O. K., and Leong, J. C. Y.: The Pathogenesis of Pott's Paraplegia. J. Bone Joint Surg. 49:1147, 1967.
17. Hodgson, A. R., and Stock, F. E.: Anterior spine fusion for the treatment of tuberculosis of the spine. J. Bone Joint Surg. 42:295–310, 1960.
18. Hodgson, A. R., Wong, W., and Yau, A.: X-ray appearances of tuberculosis of the spine. Springfield, Charles C Thomas, 1969.
19. Hodgson, A. R., and Yau, A.: Pott's paraplegia: A classification based upon the living pathology. Paraplegia 5:1–16, 1967.
20. Hodgson, A. R., Yau, A., Kwon, J. S., and Kim, D.: A clinical study of 100 consecutive cases of Pott's paraplegia. Clin. Orthop. 36:128–149, 1964.
21. Hsu, L. C. S., Cheng, C. L., and Leong, J. C. Y.: Pott's paraplegia of late onset. J. Bone Joint Surg. 70:534–538, 1988.
22. Kaufman, D. M., Kaplan, J. G., and Litman, N.: Infectious agents in spinal epidural abscesses. Neurology 30:844–850, 1980.
23. Kemp, H. B. S., Jackson, J. W., Jeremiah, J. D., and Hall, A. J.: Pyogenic infections occurring primarily in intervertebral discs. J. Bone Joint Surg. 55:698–714, 1973.
24. Kumar, S., and Gulati, D. R.: Spinal abscesses. Neurol. India 26:193–195, 1978.
25. Leong, J. C. Y., and Hodgson, A. R.: Surgical treatment of tuberculosis of the spine. *In* Leach, R. E., Hoaglund, F. T., and Riseborough E. J. (eds.): Controversies in Orthopaedic Surgery. Philadelphia, W. B. Saunders, 1982, pp. 472–486.
26. Lifeso, R. M., Harder, E., and McCorkell, S. J.: Spinal brucellosis. J. Bone Joint Surg. 67:345–351, 1985.
27. Litvinoff, J., and Nelson, M.: Extradural lumbar cryptococcosis. J. Neurosurg. 49:921–923, 1978.
28. Masmonteil, F., and Beclere, H.: Diagnostic radiographique des tuberculoses osteo-articulaires. J. Radiol. Electr. 7:259–266, 1923.
29. McCain, G. A., Harth, M., Bell, D. A., et al.: Septic discitis. J. Rheumatol. 8:100–109, 1981.
30. Medical Research Council Working Party on Tuberculosis of the Spine (First Report): A controlled trial of ambulant out-patient treatment and in-patient rest in bed in the management of tuberculosis of the spine in young Korean patients on standard chemotherapy. A study in Masan, Korea. J. Bone Joint Surg. 55:678–697, 1973.
31. Medical Research Council Working Party on Tuberculosis of the Spine (Third Report): A controlled trial of débridement and ambulatory treatment in the management of tuberculosis of the spine in patients on standard chemotherapy. A study in Bulawayo, Rhodesia. J. Trop. Med. Hyg. 77:72–92, 1974.
32. Medical Research Council Working Party on Tuberculosis of the Spine (Fourth Report): A controlled trial of anterior spinal fusion and débridement in the surgical management of tuberculosis of the spine in patients on standard chemotherapy. A study in Hong Kong. Br. J. Surg. 61:853–866, 1974.
33. Medical Research Council Working Party on Tuberculosis of the Spine (Fifth Report): A five-year assessment of controlled trials of in-patient and out-patient treatment and of plaster-of-Paris jackets for tuberculosis of the spine in children on standard chemotherapy. Studies in Masan and Pusan, Korea. J. Bone Joint Surg. 58:399–411, 1976.
34. Medical Research Council Working Party on Tuberculosis of the Spine (Sixth Report): A five-year assessments of controlled trials of ambulatory treatment, débridement and anterior spinal fusion in the management of tuberculosis of the spine. J. Bone Joint Surg. 60:163–177, 1978.
35. Medical Research Council Working Party on Tuberculosis of the Spine (Eighth Report): A 10-year assessment of a controlled trial comparing débridement and anterior spinal fusion in the management of tuberculosis of the spine in patients on standard chemotherapy in Hong Kong. J. Bone Joint Surg. 64:393–398, 1982.
36. Medical Research Council Working Party on Tuberculosis of the Spine (Ninth Report): A 10-Year assessment of controlled trials of inpatient and outpatient treatment and of plaster-of-Paris jackets for tuberculosis of the spine in children on standard chemotherapy. J. Bone Joint Surg. 67:103–110, 1985.
37. Medical Research Council Working Party on Tuberculosis of the Spine (Tenth Report): A controlled trial of 6-month and 9-month regimens of chemotherapy in patients undergoing radical surgery for tuberculosis of the spine in Hong Kong. Tubercle 67:243–259, 1986.
38. Mineiro, J. D.: Coluna vertebral humana: Alguns aspectos da sua estrutura e vascularizacao. University, Lisbon. Ph.D. dissertation, 1965.
39. Modic, M. T., Pavlicek, W., Weinstein, M. A., et al.: Magnetic resonance imaging of intervertebral disk disease. Radiology 152:103–111, 1984.
40. Muhle, I., Rau, J., and Ruskin, J.: Vertebral osteomyelitis due to *Actinobacilius actinomycetemcomitans*. J.A.M.A. 241:1824–1825, 1979.
41. Onofrio, B. M.: Intervetebral discitis: Incidence, diagnosis, and management. Clin. Neurosurg. 27:481–516, 1980.

42. Pun, W. K., Chow, S. P., Luk, K. D. K., et al.: Long-term follow-up on tuberculosis affecting the lumbosacral junction (accepted for publication. J. Bone Joint Surg. [Br.] July, 1990).
43. Pyogenic infections of the spine. Lancet 1:619–620, 1985.
44. Ravicovitch, M. A., and Spallone, A.: Spinal epidural abscesses. Eur. Neurol. 21:347–357, 1982.
45. Ryan, M. D., and Taylor, T. K. F.: The bacteriological diagnosis and antibiotic treatment of haematogenous vertebral osteomyelitis in adults. Aust. N. Z. J. Surg. 48:81–83, 1978.
46. Scoles, P. V., and Quinn, T. P.: Intervertebral discitis in children and adolescents. Clin. Orthop. Rel. Res. 162:31–36, 1982.
47. Silverthorn, K. G., and Gillespie, W. J.: Pyogenic spinal osteomyelitis: A review of 61 cases. N. Z. Med. J. 99:62–65, 1986.
48. Sorrel, E., and Sorrel-Dejerine, Y.: Recherches sur la transit du lipoidal par voie sousarachnoidienne dans les différentes formes de paraplégie pottigue. Rev. Neurol. 2:88, 1924.
49. Wiley, A. M., and Trueta, J.: The vascular anatomy of the spine and its relationship to pyogenic vertebral osteomyelitis. J. Bone Joint Surg. 41:796, 1959.
50. Wolfgang, G. L.: Tuberculosis joint infection. Clin. Orthop. 136:257–263, 1978.
51. Yanoff, D. B., and Church, McG. L.: Nocardial vertebral osteomyelitis. Clin. Orthop. Rel. Res. 175:223–226, 1983.

IATROGENIC DISCITIS

Robert D. Fraser

Discitis is a potential complication of any procedure that involves entering the intervertebral disc. In addition to contamination during surgical removal of the nucleus pulposus, discitis may result from the use of a contaminated needle during such procedures as discography, chemonucleolysis, lumbar puncture, myelography, and chemical sympathectomy.

Very few reports have described possible local complications of intradiscal injection. Discitis following discography with contrast material has been considered a rare complication,[2, 3, 15, 21–23, 26, 31, 35] some investigators attributing it to a chemical or aseptic reaction.[3, 4, 22, 35] In recent times it was suggested that discitis following discography was more common than previously recognized and was likely to occur as often as once in 30 cases.[4, 8, 10]

The term discitis has been more commonly associated with chemonucleolysis because of the exacerbation of back pain that frequently follows this procedure. Radiographic evidence of discitis following chemonucleolysis has been reported in as many as 2%[24] of patients and was generally attributed to a chemical or an aseptic process. More recent studies described infective discitis following chemonucleolysis, but this seems to have been regarded as a separate entity.[1] In a review of 29,075 patients in the United States treated with chymopapain, Agre and colleagues[1] reported that 22 patients had developed discitis. The patients had developed severe back pain and spasm from a few days to many weeks following injection. In nine of them bacterial infection had been confirmed by culture. A number of the remaining patients were considered to have aseptic discitis on the basis of negative cultures, and some had been treated with steroid therapy. The authors did not state the time intervals between discography and needle biopsy. McCulloch and Macnab[25] reported no cases of infective discitis following chemonucleolysis in over 6,000 patients. They believed that the incidence of "chemical" discitis was probably less than 1%, and they explained the apparently low incidence of infective discitis on the bactericidal effect of chymopapain.

The evidence used to support the idea of a noninfective cause of discitis following discography and after chemonucleolysis was the following: the failure to isolate bacteria from biopsy material in most cases; the associated raised erythrocyte sedimentation rate (ESR) in the presence of a normal white cell count; the histopathologic findings of a chronic inflammatory process with lymphoid cell infiltration; and the tendency toward natural resolution. The same reasons have been advanced to support the idea of a noninfective cause for some cases of discitis after discectomy, although most authors consider discitis following open procedures to be infective.[7, 19, 20, 28] In a review of the literature concerning postlaminectomy disc space infection, Fernand and Lee[7] stated that the route of infection was still not clear, as both hematogenous spread and local contamination may occur in a surgically traumatized area that has a poor blood supply.[19, 20, 34]

Until recently, discitis following discography was considered to be a rare occurrence with a reported incidence of about 0.1%.[2, 3, 15, 21, 26, 31] More recent studies have reported a higher incidence of discitis following both discography and treatment with chymopapain.[4, 5, 10, 24] However, because many individuals present with less severe symptoms, and the disorder apparently resolves without treatment, the actual incidence of discitis following both discectomy and intradiscal injections is likely to be higher than the reported rates. The reported incidence of discitis following a standard discectomy varies from 0% to 2.8%,[7, 14] whereas the use of the operating microscope has been associated with a higher rate of discitis.[18, 24]

ETIOLOGY

There is conclusive evidence that all cases of discitis with accompanying end-plate changes which occur as a result of an intradiscal procedure are due to bacterial contamination and are not due to a chemical, allergic, or some other aseptic process. The evidence for this is based on clinical and experimental studies:

1. In a clinical study[10] the case records and radiographs of 432 patients who had undergone lumbar discography were reviewed. When an 18-gauge needle without a stilette had been used, discitis was diagnosed in 2.7% of 222 patients, but stiletted needles in a two-needle technique at each level reduced the incidence to 0.7%. Seven patients with discitis after discography required anterior discectomy and fusion; their histopathologic findings were those of a chronic inflammatory response. Bacteria were isolated only from the discs of three of the four patients who had open biopsy less than 6 weeks from the time of discography. These findings suggest that bacteria were initiators rather than promoters of the response.

2. In an experimental study[10] multiple-level lumbar discography was carried out in 11 mature sheep by injecting contrast material with or without various concentrations of bacteria. Radiographs were taken, and the discs and end plates were examined histologically and cultured for bacteria at intervals after injection. None of the controls showed any evidence of discitis, but all sheep injected with bacteria had typical radiographic and pathologic changes of discitis by 6 weeks although cultures were almost all negative. The process did not seem to be dose related, and only a few bacteria were required to produce discitis. At 1 and 2 weeks after injection, bacteria could be isolated, but usually this could not be done after 3 weeks.

3. Despite the known bactericidal effect of chymopapain, similar results were obtained in a further experimental study.[9] Multiple-level lumbar intradiscal injections of chymopapain were carried out in eight mature sheep. Sixteen discs in four sheep were injected with a mixture of reconstituted chymopapain and a *Staphylococcus epidermidis* suspension, and 16 discs in another four sheep were injected with reconstituted chymopapain only. All sheep were sacrificed at 6 weeks. The discs and end plates were examined by means of radiologic and histopathologic procedures, and nuclear material was cultured for bacteria. None of the controls showed evidence of discitis, whereas all sheep injected with bacteria showed typical radiographic and pathologic changes of discitis, which occurred after the injection of very few bacteria. However, for most cases in which end-plate lesions were well established, there was no evidence of bacteria at sacrifice.

4. The intradiscal use of cephazolin (Kefzol) in discography has resulted in the incidence of discitis falling from 4.9% of 61 patients for one radiology practice[10] in a 12-month period to 0% of more than 100 patients during the first 12-month period when prophylactic antibiotics were employed. The role of prophylactic antibiotics in the prevention of discitis following discography and chemonucleolysis was tested in another experimental study.[12] In 16 adult sheep lumbar intradiscal injections of bacteria were carried out at five adjacent levels. Half the animals were treated with intradiscal cephazolin, and the other half were treated with a single intravenous injection of cephazolin. At the time of sacrifice at 6 weeks, all sheep showed no evidence of discitis at any level,

and all cultures of disc material were negative. The results of this study indicated that either intradiscal or intravenous cephazolin was likely to substantially reduce the incidence of iatrogenic discitis resulting from intradiscal procedures.

PATHOLOGY

The histopathologic findings after discography of seven patients with discitis who required anterior discectomy and fusion are summarized in Table 1. Bacteria were recovered from three of four patients who had open biopsies carried out within 6 weeks of discography, but they were not isolated from any of the three patients who had open biopsies carried out more than 6 weeks after discography. The observation of disc vascularization, mature granulation tissue formation in both discs and vertebral bodies, the association of the more marked histologic changes with vertical disc protrusions, and the occasional presence of acute inflammatory cells in addition to chronic inflammation were features also common to the pathologic changes observed in experimental studies of discitis in sheep.[9, 10] In these studies the histologic findings suggested that the earliest change was the disorganization of the end-plate region associated with granulation tissue and herniation of the nucleus pulposus. Although lesions were not visible at 1 week after injection, at 2 weeks macroscopic examination of the affected discs showed small herniations of nuclear material with an inflammatory reaction confined to the zone close to the end plate. Microscopically, the bony end plates and hyaline laminae had been breached in several places by granulation tissue (Fig. 1) and by the herniation of nuclear material. At 3 weeks there was much more extensive loss of the end plates and hyaline laminae associated with larger protrusions of nuclear material into the vertebral bodies. The extruded nuclear material showed marked "capping" by neutrophil polymorphs in some places (Fig. 2), but the granulation tissue generally showed a paucity of acute inflammatory cells. A striking feature was the extensive replacement of vertebral bone by granulation tissue, even in regions where the end plate and nucleus were normal (Fig. 3). By 6 weeks extruded and residual nuclear material had been extensively replaced by relatively avascular fibrous tissue and with evidence of new bone forming at the periphery

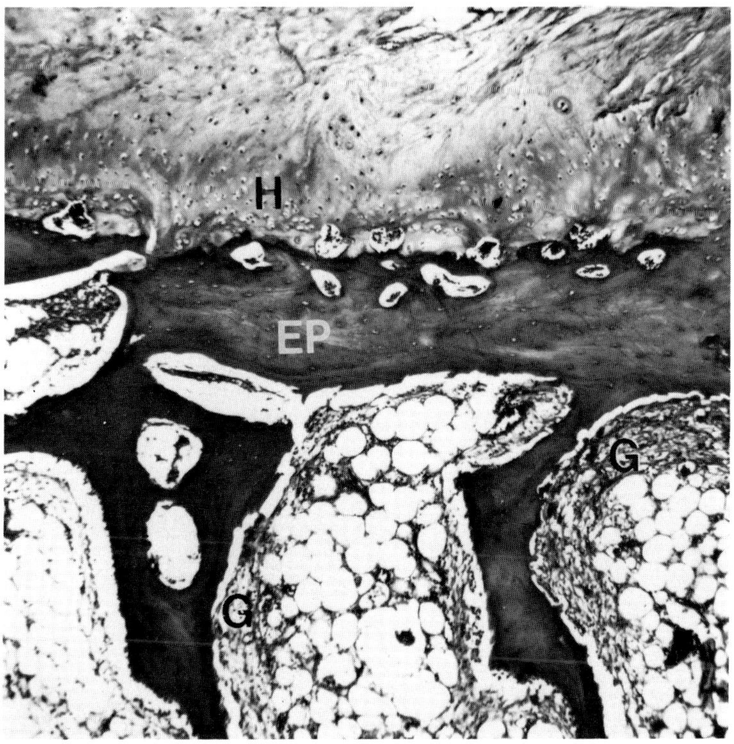

Figure 1 □ Low-power micrography of L1–L2 disc in a sheep 2 weeks after injection of meglumine iothalamate 60% (Conray) and *Staphylococcus epidermidis*. It shows intact regions of the end plate (EP) and prominent vascular channels extending into the hyaline lamina (H). The marrow spaces in the adjoining bone show young granulation tissue (G) extending along the trabecular surfaces, which are undergoing resorption. (Hematoxylin and eosin, × 50.) (From Fraser, R. D., Osti, O. L., and Vernon-Roberts, B.: Discitis after discography. J. Bone Joint Surg. 69B:26–35, 1987.)

Table 1 □ Summary and Grading of Histopathologic Features

		DISC FEATURES					VERTEBRAL BODY FEATURES					
		Vascular-ization	Granulation Tissue	Mature Fibrous Tissue	Inflammatory Cells		End Plate Defects	Nuclear Herniation	Granulation Tissue	Mature Fibrous Tissue	Inflammatory Cells	
CASE	DISC				ACUTE	CHRONIC					ACUTE	CHRONIC
1	L5/S1	++	+	—	—	—	++	—	++	++	+	++
2	L4/L5	+++	+++	++++	—	+	+++	++	++	+++	—	+
3	L4/L5	+++	+++	+++	—	+	++++	++	+	++	—	++
4	L5/S1	++	—	—	++	—	+	—	++	++	++	++
5	L4/L5	++	++++	++++	++	+++	++++	++	+++	++	++	+++
6	L4/L5	++	+	—	+	+	+	—	+	—	+	—
7	L4/L5	+++	+++	+++	—	+	+++	++	+++	++	—	+

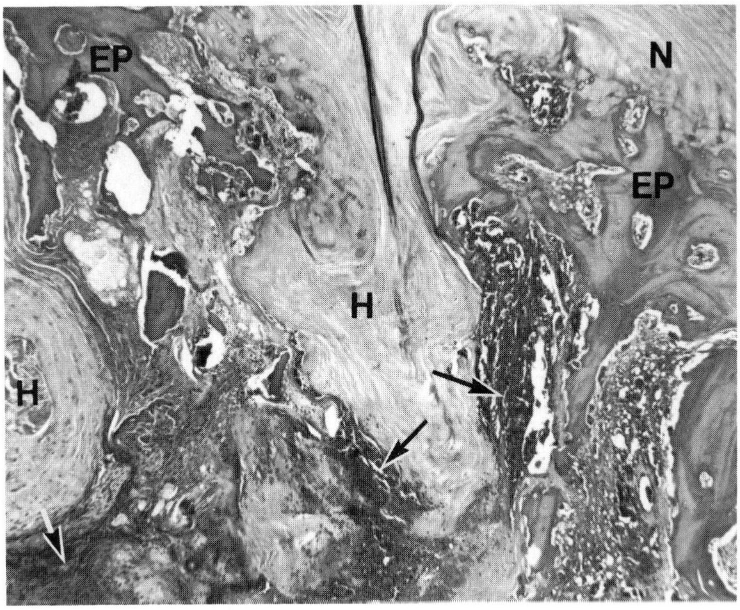

Figure 2 □ Low-power micrograph of L2–L3 disc in a sheep 3 weeks after injection of Conray and *S. epidermidis*. It shows herniations (H) of material from the nucleus pulposus (N) through the end plate (EP). The dark areas (*arrows*) capping the herniations represent an acute inflammatory reaction with numerous neutrophil polymorphs. (Hematoxylin and eosin, × 50.)

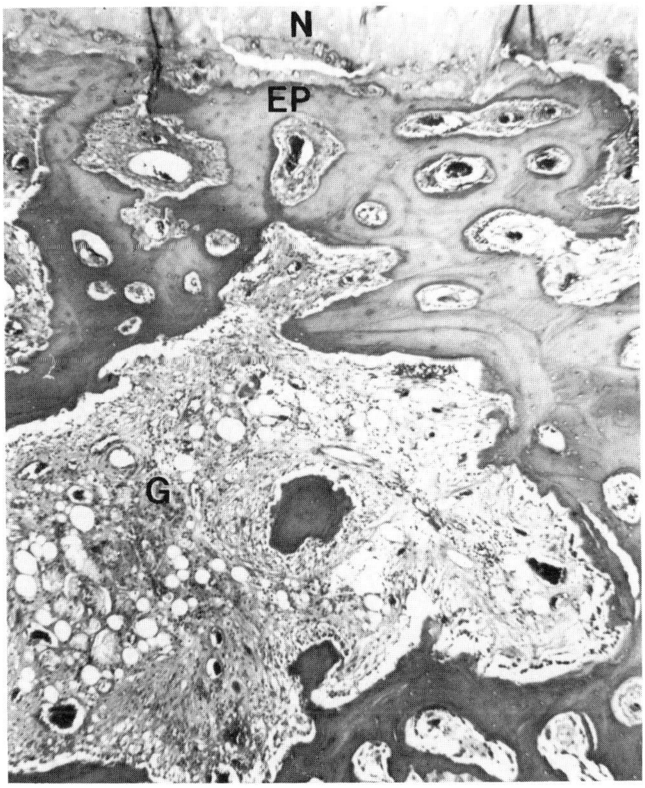

Figure 3 □ Low-power micrograph of L2–L3 disc in a sheep 3 weeks after injection of Conray and *S. epidermidis*. It shows extensive replacement of vertebral cancellous bone by granulation tissue (G) adjoining the intact end plate (EP) and normal nucleus. (N = nucleus pulposis.) (Hematoxylin and eosin, × 50.) (From Fraser, R. D., Osti, O. L., and Vernon-Roberts, B.: Discitis after discography. J. Bone Joint Surg. 69B:26–35, 1987.)

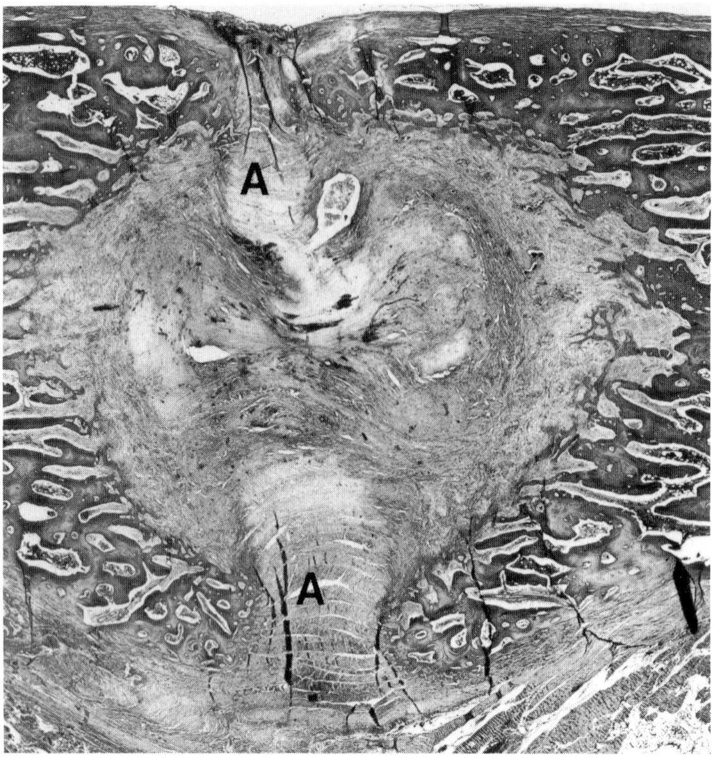

Figure 4 □ Low-power micrograph of L3–L4 disc in a sheep 6 weeks after injection of Conray and *S. epidermidis*. It shows the disorganization of the nucleus with preservation of the outer annulus (A), disappearance of end plates and adjoining vertebral cancellous bone, herniation of nuclear material into both vertebral bodies, granulation tissue and fibrous tissue extending into the central region of the disc with (dark) intradiscal hemorrhages, and new bone forming at the junction of fibrous tissues with the residual cancellous bone of the vertebral bodies. (Hematoxylin and eosin, × 8.) (From Fraser, R. D., Osti, O. L., and Vernon-Roberts, B.: Discitis after discography. J. Bone Joint Surg. 69B:26–35, 1987.)

of the lesions in the vertebral bodies (Fig. 4). In most of the lesions the granulation tissue contained moderate to few inflammatory cells, and these were mainly lymphocytes and plasma cells forming small aggregates. However, one or two microabscesses were found in the granulation tissue in a few discs (Fig. 5).

As has been seen in human specimens, the site of the lesion in experimental discitis corresponds to the needle-tip position (Fig. 6).

The following stages in the development of discitis after intradiscal procedures have been determined (Fig. 7):

1. Bacteria are introduced on the tip of a needle.
2. At 1 week the bacteria have multiplied, but there are no other abnormalities.
3. At 2 weeks the end plate is thin but may still be intact. Immature granulation tissue has formed on the vertebral side of the end plate, and this is surrounded by a vascular response.
4. Three weeks after inoculation the end plates have been ruptured with the herniation of nuclear material into the vertebral bodies. Granulation tissue lies against the herniated nucleus, and a more marked vascular response is present. At this stage the bacteria are usually destroyed.
5. By 6 weeks the lesion is approaching maturity with appositional new bone formation, and the nuclear material has been largely replaced by granulation tissue. In most cases the bacteria have been eradicated. In a few instances the lesion takes longer to reach maturity, and bacteria may persist leading to osteomyelitis.

The pathologic response in postdiscectomy discitis is altered by the extent of the disc space clearance. As with postinjection discitis at a level with gross degenerative changes, the end-plate lesion produced in postdiscectomy discitis tends to be more diffuse, as distinct from the classic discrete lesions of discitis following discography at a normal level.

PRESENTATION AND CLINICAL COURSE

Although the severity of symptoms of discitis vary widely, the clinical features are

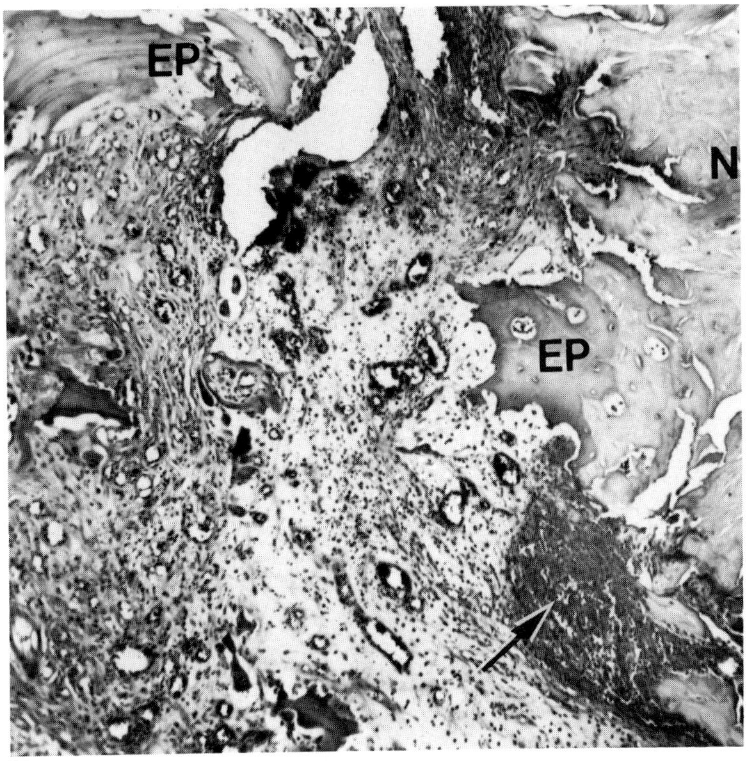

Figure 5 □ Low-power micrograph of L2–L3 in a sheep 6 weeks after injection of Conray and *S. epidermidis*. It shows that the end-plate (EP) has been breached by granulation tissue extending into the nucleus (N), and the presence of a microabscess (*arrow*). (Hematoxylin and eosin, × 50.)

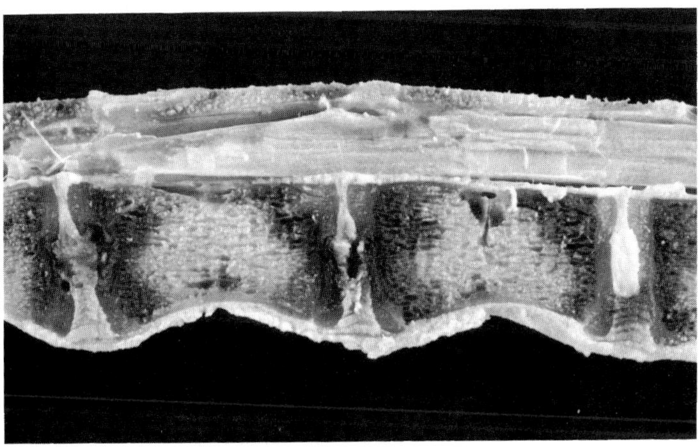

Figure 6 □ Macroscopic view of portion of spine in a sheep following injection of chymopapain and bacteria at all three levels illustrated. L3–L4 disc (*left*) shows largely central discitis; L2–L3 disc (*center*) shows combination of central and anterior discitis; and L1–L2 disk (*right*) shows anterior discitis alone. (From Fraser, R. D., Osti, O. L., and Vernon-Roberts, B.: Discitis following chemonucleolysis: An experimental study. Spine 11:34–43, 1986.)

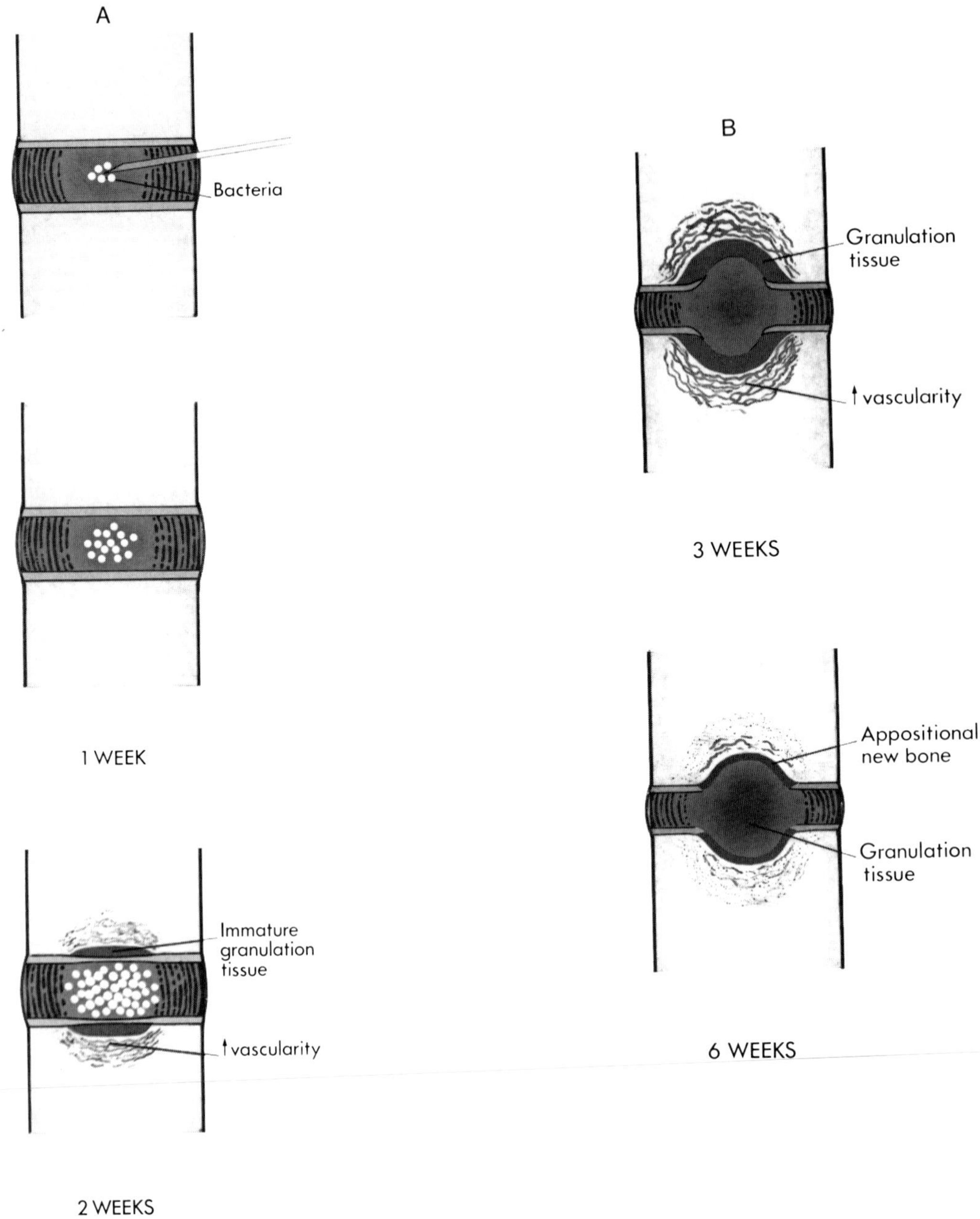

Figure 7 □ *A, B,* The stages in the development of discitis after discography are shown.

similar, irrespective of the cause. The clinical hallmark of discitis is back pain. Postoperative or postinjection pain may persist and then gradually increase in severity. In some individuals the pain is excruciating, not relieved by rest, and poorly relieved by narcotic analgesics. The pain is aggravated by any attempt at movement and is accompanied by severe muscle spasm. Often the spine is held rigidly in extension in a manner similar to that seen in childhood discitis. Not only does the patient resist moving the back, but straight-leg raising is grossly limited on both sides by back pain. In this more severe form of postinjection discitis, fever may be present for 1 or 2 days, but in most cases the patient remains afebrile. An elevated temperature is more commonly associated with discitis after open procedures.[7, 20] The severity of symptoms from discitis varies considerably, and some patients have increased back pain, which develops insidiously following the procedure and may slowly subside over a period of several weeks or months.

The diagnosis of iatrogenic discitis may be overlooked because of the marked variability in clinical expression of the disease and because the physical, laboratory, and radiologic findings may be masked by the recent intervention. Some patients are likely to be regarded as hyper-reacting to operative or postinjection pain or may be dismissed as "functional" problems. Many patients experience an exacerbation of back pain following intradiscal injections, possibly owing to a mechanical or chemical effect, but this invariably resolves spontaneously within 1 to 2 weeks.

Although the clinical course of postinjection discitis varies considerably, there is a tendency for spontaneous resolution over a period of several weeks to 6 months or so, in which the patient's symptoms usually gradually subside. Sometimes, however, disabling back symptoms persist. Although the infective process is usually self limiting, individuals occasionally progress to a vertebral osteomyelitis and the possible extension of an abscess to the epidural space.[5]

In a review of 33 patients with discitis following open discectomy, Lindholm and Pylkkanen[20] found the average duration of the disease was 7.4 months (R = 1.5 months to 2 years). At an average follow-up of 7.5 years they found most patients had disabling back symptoms, and more than 60% had still not returned to work. Radiographic assessment revealed that bone-bridging or spontaneous fusion had occurred in 42% of cases. They advised prophylaxis and early appropriate treatment to prevent a chronic disorder and protracted disability.

INVESTIGATIONS

The ESR is usually increased, but in postoperative cases this is likely to be partly attributable to the surgical procedure itself. Following contamination by an intradiscal needle, the ESR may not become elevated for 10 to 14 days, even in patients who have increased back pain with associated muscle spasms within a few days of the procedure. There is variation in the effect on the ESR, which has ranged from normal to 90 mm/hr in our experience.

The white cell count nearly always remains normal, although it may be near the upper limit of normal, and an associated neutrophilia is not uncommon. A leukocytosis is more commonly associated with postdiscectomy discitis and is partly attributable to the procedure itself. Blood cultures are usually negative, unless obtained early in the disease process. This is similar to the findings in childhood discitis; in one large series[33] blood cultures were positive only within the first 6 weeks of the onset of symptoms.

The earliest radiographic change is narrowing of the height of the disc space, which may occur as early as 2 to 3 weeks after the procedure but in some cases may take some months to develop. As time passes, there is usually loss of definition of the bony end plate as seen on radiographs, and vertebral erosions may be seen. These changes are better demonstrated by lateral tomography (Fig. 8), or by computed tomography (CT), although generally 2 or 3 weeks must pass before they appear. This sequence of radiographic changes in the human is very similar in timing and extent to that seen in experimental discitis in the sheep (Fig. 9).

A technetium bone scan often confirms the diagnosis of discitis following an intradiscal injection, but it is less useful in diagnosis following open surgery because of the increased tracer around the surgically treated vertebral segment. Sometimes the identification of the level or levels involved

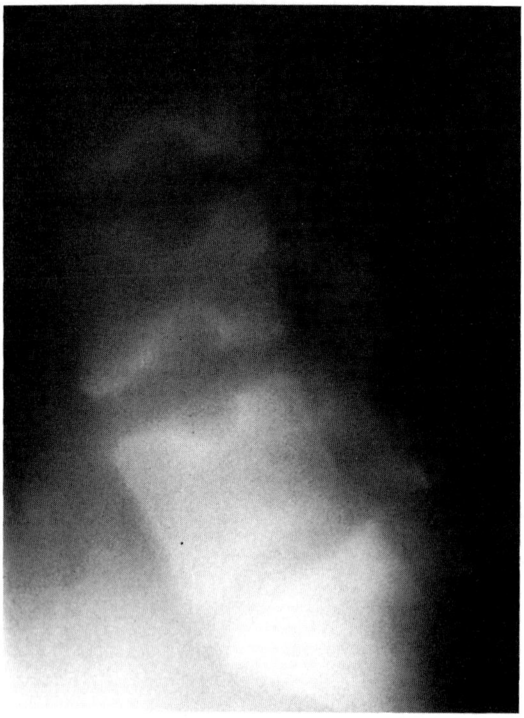

Figure 8 □ Lateral tomogram of lumbar spine 3 months after two-level discography shows the erosions of the end plates at both levels, a classic characteristic of postdiscogram discitis. The sclerotic margins of the erosions are typical of late lesions.

when multiple-level discography has been carried out can be difficult because a technetium bone scan is not always positive. It is probable that magnetic resonance imaging (MRI) would confirm the diagnosis early in the disease process by an alteration of the signal in the end-plate region.[27]

ILLUSTRATIVE CASES

From 1982 to 1984, seven patients with discitis after discography required anterior discectomy and fusion at the affected level. At operation the disc and adjacent end plates were removed en bloc using dowel-cutting instruments.[4] Swabs were taken from the disc space and sent for microbiologic examination. The case histories of these patients are summarized in Table 2 and the histopathologic findings in Table 1. Two illustrative cases are reported in detail.

Case 1

A 28-year-old soldier presented with an 8-month history of increasing low back pain following repeated falls at work, where he was an army physical instructor. Examination revealed bilateral restriction of straight-leg raising to 45 degrees by back pain, and there were no abnormal neurologic signs in the lower limbs. Discography at the L4–L5 level demonstrated a normal disc with no pain reproduction (Fig. 10). At the L5–S1 level the injection was directed into a false cavity in the annulus and was reported to reproduce the patient's typical symptoms. Immediately following discography the pain was more severe. Six weeks later the patient's ESR was 24 mm/hr. Under general anesthesia discography was repeated, and a major extravasation of contrast material was observed through the upper and lower end plates of the L4–L5 level (Fig. 11). At the L5–S1 level a more limited end-plate lesion was demonstrated posteriorly, corresponding to the position of the false cavity injection. The patient underwent anterior disc clearance and interbody fusion at L4–L5 and L5–S1, using a muscle-splitting retroperitoneal approach. Histologic examination of

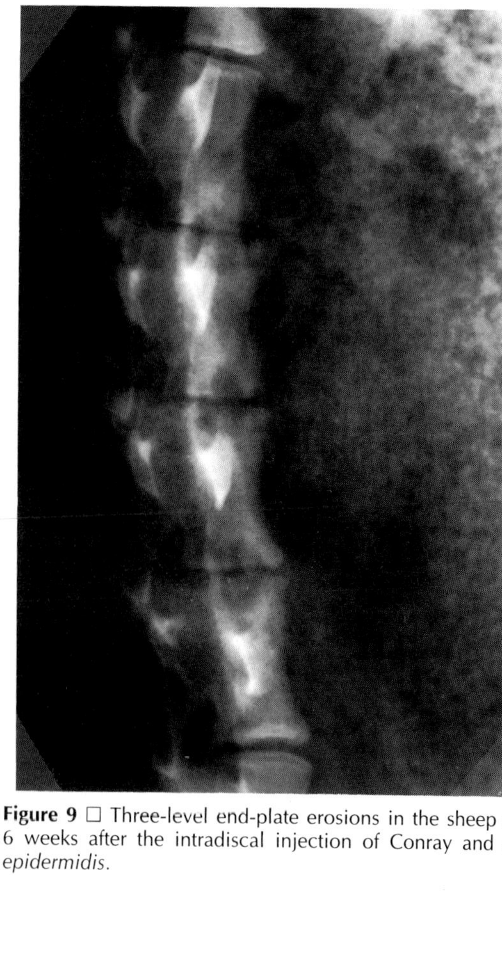

Figure 9 □ Three-level end-plate erosions in the sheep at 6 weeks after the intradiscal injection of Conray and *S. epidermidis*.

Table 2 □ Details of Seven Patients Having an Open Biopsy After Discography

CASE	AGE IN YEARS	ORIGINAL DIAGNOSIS	ESR* BETWEEN DISCOGRAPHY AND SURGERY (mm/hr)	RADIOGRAPHS	BONE SCAN	INTERVAL BETWEEN DISCOGRAPHY AND BIOPSY	HISTOLOGIC EVIDENCE OF DISCITIS	BACTERIAL CULTURE
1	28	L5–S1 internal disc disruption	24	Large end plate erosion	—	5 weeks	Yes	*Pseudomonas aeruginosa* (light growth)
2	21	Grade I isthmic spondylolisthesis L5–S1	2	Large end plate erosion L4–L5	—	3 months	Yes	No growth
3	47	Discogenic back pain L5–S1	50	End plate erosion L4–L5	Patchy nonspecific uptake	6 months	Yes	No growth
4	38	Back pain after compression fracture of L4	30	End plate erosion L5–S1	Positive L5–S1	4 weeks	Yes	*Staphylococcus epidermidis*
5	40	Grade II traumatic spondylolisthesis	99	—	Positive L4–L5	3 weeks	Yes	No growth
6	18	Grade II isthmic spondylolisthesis	—	—	—	4 weeks	No	*Klebsiella pneumoniae*
7	46	Grade II degenerative spondylolisthesis	105	End plate erosion L4–L5	Positive L4–L5	3 months	Yes	No growth

*ESR = erythrocyte sedimentation rate.

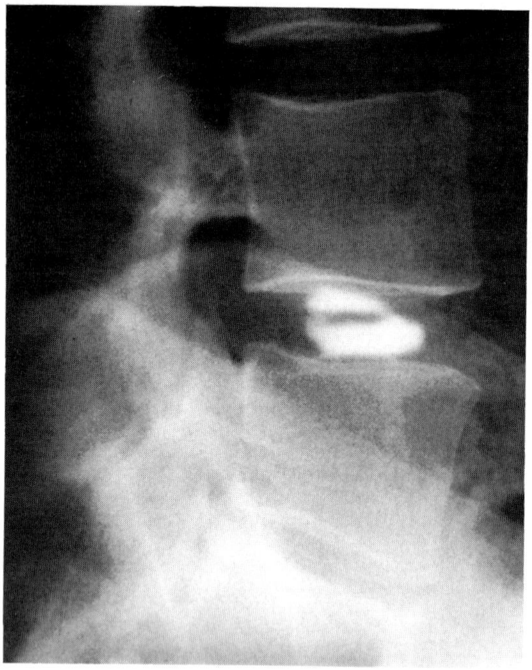

Figure 10 □ Normal L4–L5 discogram (Case 1) is shown. (From Fraser, R. D., Osti, O. L., and Vernon-Roberts, B.: Discitis after discography. J. Bone Joint Surg. 69B:26–35, 1987.)

L5–S1 disc material showed heavily inflamed granulation tissue in both the hyaline laminae and the bone of the region of the end plate; acute inflammatory cells and chronic inflammation in disc material were observed (Fig. 12). A culture of this material demonstrated a light growth of *Pseudomonas aeruginosa*. The postoperative course was uneventful, and 9 months after the procedure the patient was assessed as being pain free. X-ray studies demonstrated consolidation at both levels.

Case 2

A 21-year-old naval rating presented with a 12-month history of disabling low back pain after lifting heavy drums along a gangway. He was unable to work, and his condition failed to respond to conservative treatment. Plain x-ray findings demonstrated a Grade 1 spondylolisthesis. He was investigated by lumbar discography, which demonstrated minimal nuclear degeneration at the L4–L5 level and a degenerate disc at L5–S1 with reproduction of his typical back pain (Fig. 13). His symptoms became progressively more severe following discography, and arrangements were made to carry out an anterior interbody fusion at the L5–S1 level. A diagnosis of discitis was considered at the time but was thought to have been excluded by an ESR of only 22 mm/hour and a plain lateral x-ray study 1 month after discography, which showed no evidence of disc space narrowing or erosion. Two weeks after anterior interbody fusion at L5–S1 (Fig. 14) he was still complaining of severe pain and needed a parenteral narcotic. He continued to require large amounts of analgesics, and 3 months after his interbody fusion plain x-ray films demonstrated that the disc space narrowing had occurred at the L4–L5 level together with a massive erosion in the L5

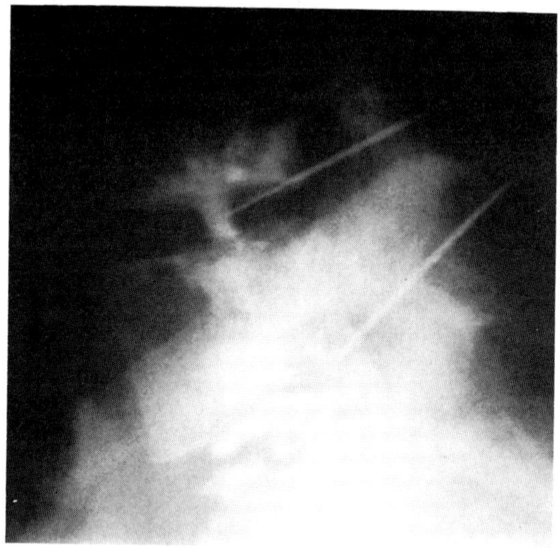

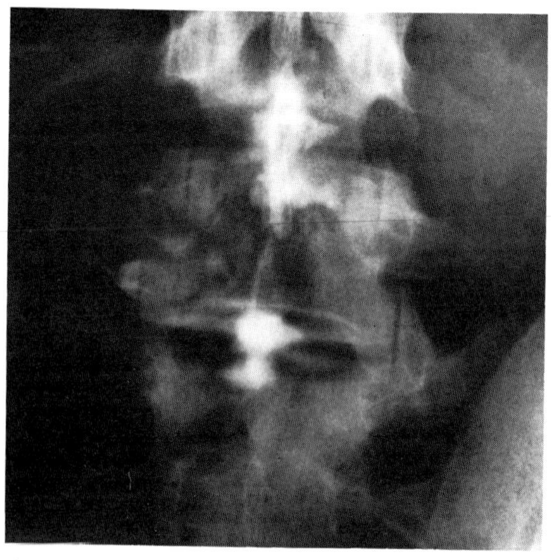

Figure 11 □ Lateral and AP discograms 5 weeks later show end-plate disruption at L4–L5 and L5–S1 (Case 1).

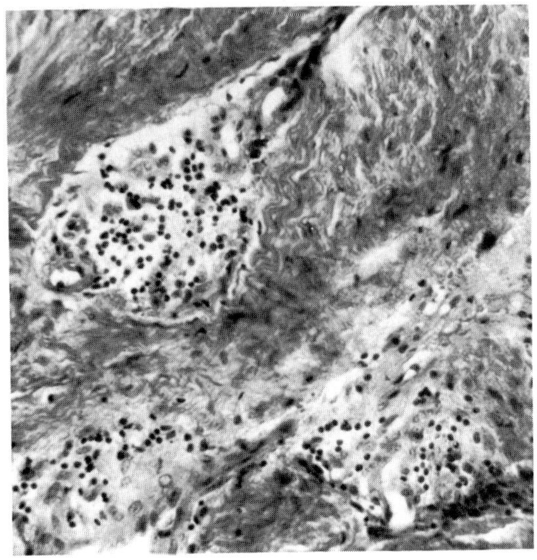

Figure 12 □ Chronic inflammation in the mature fibrous scar tissue within the disc shows clusters of lymphocytes grouped around small blood vessels (Case 1). (Hematoxylin and eosin, × 100.) (From Fraser, R. D., Osti, O. L., and Vernon-Roberts, B.: Discitis after discography. J. Bone Joint Surg. 69B:26–35, 1987.)

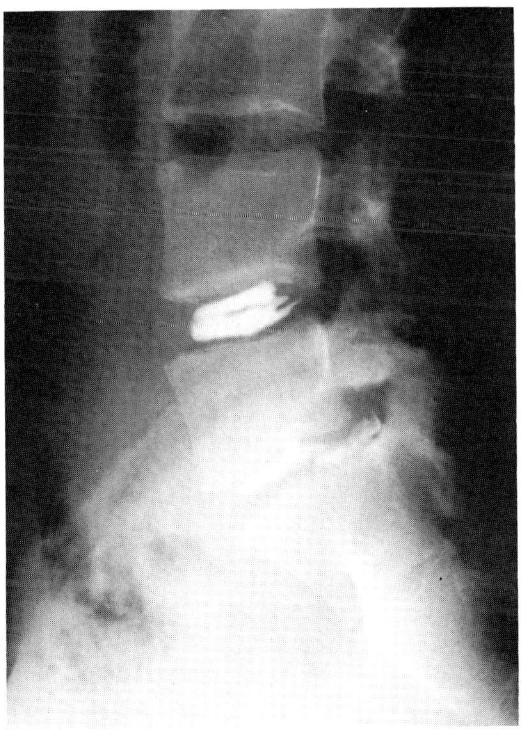

Figure 13 □ Lateral discograms demonstrate minimal nuclear degeneration at L4–L5 and a degenerate disc at L5–S1 (Case 2). (From Fraser, R. D., Osti, O. L., and Vernon-Roberts, B.: Discitis after discography. J. Bone Joint Surg. 69B:26–35, 1987.)

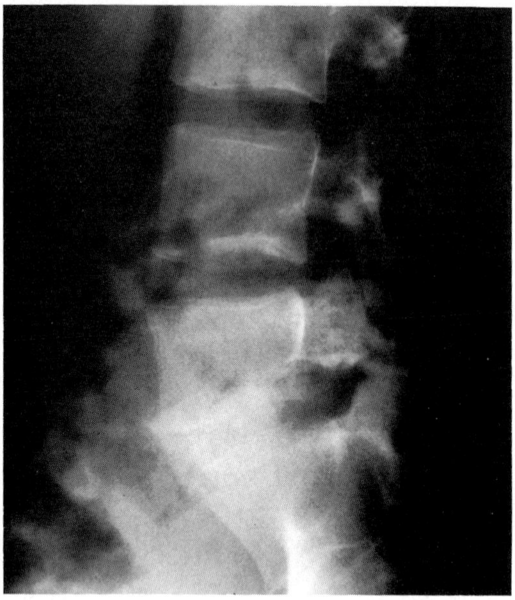

Figure 14 □ Lateral radiograph was taken 6 weeks after discography and 2 weeks after anterior interbody fusion at L5–S1 (Case 2).

vertebral body (Fig. 15). Under general anesthesia, aspiration biopsy of the L4–L5 disc space was carried out, but a culture of this failed to reveal an organism. Contrast material was injected to outline the defect (Fig. 16), and he was treated with an intradiscal

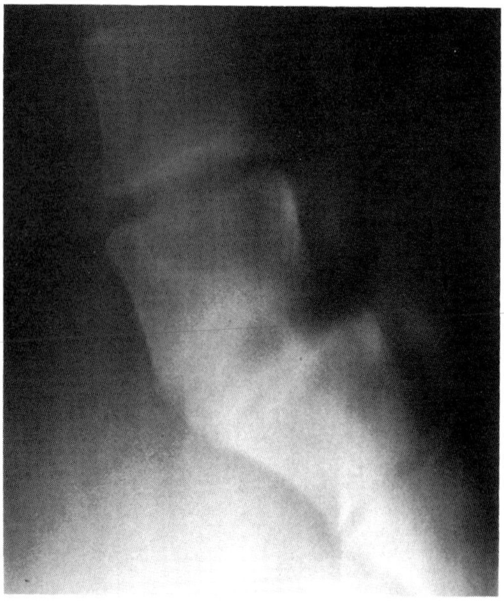

Figure 15 □ Lateral radiograph 3 months after interbody fusion demonstrates disc space narrowing at L4–L5 and a massive erosion of L5 vertebral body (Case 2).

corticosteroid. This failed to result in the relief of his symptoms, and he had not improved after 6 weeks immobilization in a brace. Seven months after the initial discogram had been carried out he underwent anterior disc clearance and interbody fusion at the L4–L5 level, and this was followed by dramatic pain relief that has been sustained. Histologic examination of the L4–L5 intervertebral disc and adjacent end plates showed extensive destruction of the endplate region (Fig. 17). There was abundant anterior granulation and fibrous tissue extending into the nucleus, but chronic inflammatory cells were few.

TREATMENT

Treatment should be mainly directed toward prevention. A strict aseptic technique is required for any intradiscal procedure. The skin should be prepared over a wide area, and the drapes firmly fixed. The patient should be sedated to minimize movement for procedures carried out under local anesthesia. Care must be taken to avoid contamination of the drapes by x-ray equipment. Only stiletted needles should be used for intradiscal injection procedures, and a two-needle technique for each level is recommended. The operator should avoid touching the needle shaft, particularly near the tip, and a separate needle should be used for each skin puncture. Similar principles should be observed during percutaneous discectomy. Because of the increased incidence of discitis accompanying the use of the operative microscope, one should take great care when using this equipment to avoid contaminating the gloves and the operative field.

Clinical and experimental evidence now supports the prophylactic use of a suitable antibiotic such as cephazolin administered either intradiscally or intravenously. For intradiscal injection procedures we recommend that cephazolin be added to the contrast agent, when this is used, to a concentration of 1 mg/ml. For other intradiscal procedures we recommend the intravenous administration of 1 to 2 grams of cephazolin just before the commencement of the procedure.

Some doubt remains about the role of antibiotics in the treatment of established discitis. Although in most cases the bacterial

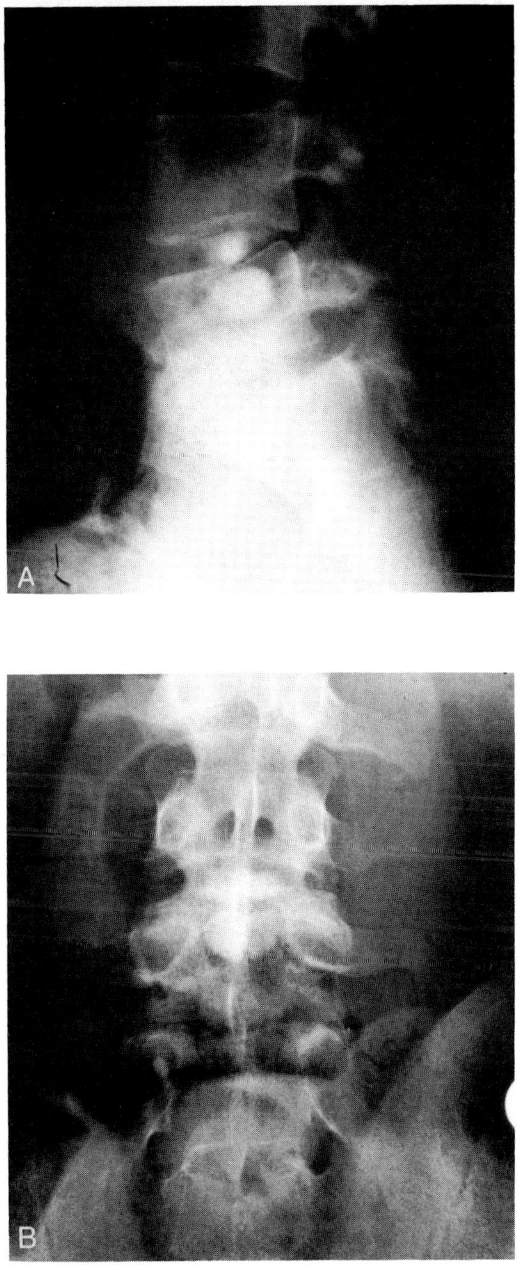

Figure 16 □ *A,* Lateral discogram demonstrates end plate disruption 4 months after discography and 3 months after anterior interbody fusion at L5–S1 (Case 2). *B,* Anteroposterior (AP) discogram demonstrates end-plate disruption (Case 2). (From Fraser, R. D., Osti, O. L., and Vernon-Roberts, B.: Discitis after discography. J. Bone Joint Surg. 69B:26–35, 1987.)

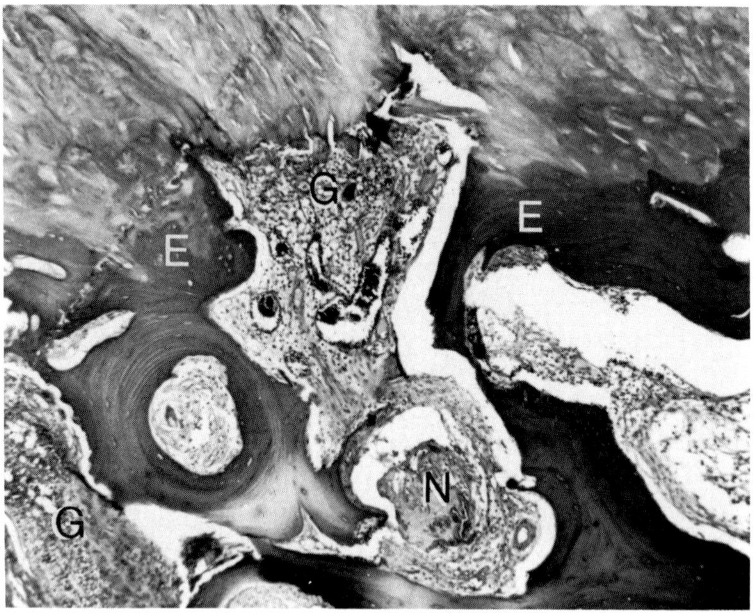

Figure 17 □ Low-power view shows a breach in the end plate (E) with herniation of nuclear material (N) and granulation tissue (G) extending into the disc and marrow spaces (Case 2). (Hematoxylin and eosin, × 50.) (From Fraser, R. D., Osti, O. L., and Vernon-Roberts, B.: Discitis after discography. J. Bone Joint Surg. 69B:26–35, 1987.)

response is self limited, appropriate antibiotics may hasten recovery, however, this has yet to be proved. Pilgaard[28] found that antibiotics made no difference in the outcome of disc space infection following laminectomy. However, most authors have advocated the use of antibiotics when a bacteriologic diagnosis has been made.[7, 19, 20] Gibson and coworkers[13] were unable to assay antibiotics from disc material in humans after the intravenous injection of high doses of various preparations. Other studies have since demonstrated by indirect means that antibiotics do cross the end plate[6, 12] and that in sufficient amounts they eradicate up to 2,000 bacteria.[11] Recent research has failed to demonstrate any therapeutic effect of antibiotics in the control of established discitis.[11] Antibiotics may, however, have a definite role in the few cases in which iatrogenic discitis proceeds to a vertebral osteomyelitis. Because of this small but important group of patients, a case can be made for an early attempt to isolate the bacteria by a needle biopsy of the affected disc followed by the intravenous administration of an appropriate antibiotic.

Some patients gain worthwhile symptomatic relief from the use of a brace or spinal jacket, which may need to be worn for 3 to 6 months. Successful treatment of postinjection discitis has been reported with both intradiscal[4] and systemic[11] steroids. In the light of recent work,[9, 10] steroids should be considered only in the late phase when the radiographic lesion is quiescent with a smooth sclerotic margin demonstrated by lateral tomography.

When a patient with disabling back symptoms develops discitis following preoperative discography at either the intended or adjacent level of the spinal fusion, it seems appropriate to treat the patient by means of anterior disc clearance and interbody fusion once the diagnosis has been confirmed, rather than wait for spontaneous resolution of the discitis, which would at best return the patient to the preinjection level of symptoms. In patients who have already undergone surgery prior to the development of postdiscographic discitis at an adjacent level, conservative measures as detailed above seem more appropriate in the first instance. In cases of postinjection discitis in which the patient has persistent severe pain that does not respond to appropriate vigorous conservative measures, anterior disc clearance and interbody fusion should be considered. In the experience of 33 patients with postoperative discitis following discography reported by Lindholm and Pylkkanen,[20] the average duration of the disease was 7.4 months, most patients complaining of disabling back symptoms at an average follow-up of 7.5 years. In the light of these poor results of conservative measures, anterior disc clearance and interbody fusion should be considered if the patient shows few signs of responding to early appropriate treatment.

NOMENCLATURE

The term discitis is logically reserved for a primary infection of the intervertebral disc. Spontaneously occurring "discitis" in the adult is undoubtedly an osteomyelitis of the vertebral body with secondary involvement of the intervertebral disc space and as such should be referred to as a *vertebral osteomyelitis*. The pathology of this condition and its treatment is in most cases quite different from that of iatrogenic discitis. In most cases of iatrogenic discitis the bacteria are removed once the vertebral end plate is reached. However, in a few cases a secondary vertebral osteomyelitis develops.

Apart from iatrogenic discitis, primary disc space infection may only occur in childhood. Some authorities consider discitis of childhood to be always secondary to osteomyelitis.[29, 33] Schmorl and Junghanns[30] described the sequence of the development of a small abscess in the end-plate region of the vertebral body with subsequent eruption into the adjacent disc rather than destruction of the vertebral bone. Childhood discitis is typified by radiographic disc space narrowing, and both end plates are usually involved. The observation that one end-plate lesion is larger than the other has been used as evidence to support the contention that discitis in childhood is a vertebral osteomyelitis with secondary involvement of the disc.[33] However, asymmetric adjacent end-plate lesions have commonly been encountered with iatrogenic discitis, and in some cases an end plate lesion on one side only (usually the lower end plate) occurs.[11]

In fact the clinical picture and clinical course of childhood discitis closely parallel those of iatrogenic discitis; both conditions are dissimilar to spontaneously occurring discitis in the adult, except for the development of spontaneous interbody fusion that rarely occurs in the child. Frank purulence and paravertebral abscesses are extremely rare complications of childhood discitis[17, 29] and only occur in iatrogenic discitis in association with a secondary vertebral osteomyelitis. The sheep studies have demonstrated that very few bacteria are required to produce iatrogenic discitis, and it seems quite possible that a few bacteria could find their way into the inner annulus of a child's intervertebral disc from a vascular outer annulus. In further support of this contention, we have been unable to produce vertebral osteomyelitis in the sheep by the placement of several hundred thousand staphylococci directly into the vertebral end plate, whereas we have never failed to produce discitis by the injection of an estimated 10 bacteria into the intervertebral disc itself.[9–11]

CONCLUSION

All iatrogenic discitis with accompanying end-plate changes resulting from an intradiscal procedure is attributable to bacterial contamination. In most cases the bacterial infection resolves spontaneously, even though the patient may continue to have disabling back symptoms. It is likely that the incidence of discitis is higher than that reported in most series. The increased popularity of percutaneous disc excision[16] is likely to be associated with a significant incidence of discitis unless appropriate preventive measures are taken, including the prophylactic use of a suitable antibiotic.

References

1. Agre, K., Wilson, R. R., Brim, M., and McDermot, D. J.: Chymodiactin: Post marketing surveillance: Domographic and adverse experience data in 29,075 patients. Spine 9:479–485, 1984.
2. Brodsky, A. E., and Binder, W. F.: Lumbar discography—its value in diagnosis and treatment of lumbar disc lesions. Spine 4:110–120, 1979.
3. Collis, J. S., and Gardner, W. J.: Lumbar discography: An analysis of one thousand cases. J. Neurosurg. 19:452–461, 1962.
4. Crock, H. V.: Practice of Spinal Surgery. Wien, Springer-Verlag, 1983.
5. Crock, H. V.: Unpublished data, 1986.
6. Eismont, F. J., Wiesel, S. W., Brighton, C. T., and Rothman, R. H.: Antibiotic penetration into rabbit nucleus pulposus. Spine 12:254–256, 1987.
7. Fernand, R., and Lee, C. K.: Post laminectomy disc space infection: A review of the literature and a report of three cases. Clin. Orthop. Rel. Res. 209:215–218, 1986.
8. Fraser, R. D.: Chymopapain for the treatment of intervertebral disc herniation: The final report of a double-blind study. Spine 9:815–818, 1984.

9. Fraser, R. D., Osti, O. L., and Vernon-Roberts, B.: Discitis following chemonucleolysis: An experimental study. Spine 11:34–43, 1986.
10. Fraser, R. D., Osti, O. L., and Vernon-Roberts, B.: Discitis after discography. J. Bone Joint Surg. 69B:26–35, 1987.
11. Fraser, R. D., Osti, O. L., and Vernon-Roberts, B.: Unpublished data, 1988.
12. Fraser, R. D., Zhang, Y. -F., and Vernon-Roberts, B.: The Role of Prophylactic Antibiotics in the Prevention of Discitis Following Chemonucleolysis: An Experimental Study. Presented to the Annual Meeting of The I.S.S.L.S. Rome, 1986.
13. Gibson, M. J., Karpinsky, M. R. K., Slack, R. C. B., et al.: The penetration of antibiotics into the normal intervertebral disc. J. Bone Joint Surg. 69B:784–786, 1987.
14. Graf, R., Reinhardt, H., and Gratzl, O.: Prolapses in adolescents of lumbar intervertebral discs: I—Clinical observations. Neurochir. 27:12–15, 1984.
15. Gresham, J. L., and Miller, R.: Evaluation of the lumbar spine by discography and its use in selection of proper treatment of the herniated disc syndrome. Clin. Orthop. Rel. Res. 67:29–41, 1969.
16. Kambin, P., and Sampson, S.: Posterolateral percutaneous suction-excision of herniated lumbar intervertebral discs: Report of interim results. Clin. Orthop. Rel. Res. 207:37–43, 1986.
17. Kemp, H. B. S., Jackson, J. W., Jeremiah, J. D., and Hall, A. J.: Pyogenic infections occurring primarily in intervertebral discs. J. Bone Joint Surg. 55B:698–714, 1973.
18. Kho, H. C. H., and Steudel, W. I.: Comparison between lumbar microdiscectomy and standard discectomy in lumbar disc herniations: A retrospective analysis of 267 cases. Neurochir. 29:181–185, 1986.
19. Kirkaldy-Willis, W. H.: Complications of disc surgery—discitis. Orthop. Trans. No. 7:110, 1983.
20. Lindholm, T. S., and Pylkkanen, P.: Discitis following removal of intervertebral disc. Spine 7:618–622, 1982.
21. Massie, W. K., and Stevens, D. B.: A critical evaluation of discography. J. Bone Joint Surg. 49A:1243–1244, 1967.
22. McCulloch, J. A.: Chemonucleolysis. J. Bone Joint Surg. 59B:45–52, 1977.
23. McCulloch, J. A.: Chemonucleolysis: Experience with 2,000 cases. Clin. Orthop. Rel. Res. 146:128–135, 1980.
24. McCulloch, J. A.: Unpublished data, 1985.
25. McCulloch, J. A., and MacNab, I.: Sciatica and chymopapain. Baltimore, Williams & Wilkins 203, 1983.
26. McCulloch, J. A., and Waddell, G.: Lateral lumbar discography. Br. J. Radiol. 51:498–502, 1978.
27. Mulholland, R., Gibson, M., Buckley, J., and Worthington, B.: The Changes in the Intervertebral Disc After Chemonucleolysis Shown by MRI. Presented at the Annual Meeting of the I.S.S.L.S. Dallas, May 28–June 2, 1986.
28. Pilgaard, S.: Discitis (closed space infection) following removal of intervertebral disc. J. Bone Joint Surg. 51A:713–716, 1969.
29. Ryan, M. D., and Taylor, T. K. F.: Septic discitis—a misnomer. Med. J. Aust. 147:415, 1987.
30. Schmorl, G., and Junghanns, H.: The Human Spine in Health and Disease, 2nd Ed. (Am.) Besemann, E. F. (trans.). New York, Grune & Stratton, 1971.
31. Simmon, E. H., and Segil, C. M.: An evaluation of discography in the localization of symptomatic levels in discogenic disease of the spine. Clin. Orthop. Rel. Res. 108:57–69, 1975.
32. Smith, R. F., and Taylor, T. K. F.: Inflammatory lesions of intervertebral discs in children. J. Bone Joint Surg. 49A:1508–1520, 1967.
33. Wenger, D. R., Bobechko, W. P., and Gilday, D. L.: The spectrum of intervertebal disc–space infection in children. J. Bone Joint Surg. 60A:100–108, 1978.
34. Wiley, A. M., and Trueta, J.: The vascular anatomy of the spine and its relationships to pyogenic vertebral osteomyelitis. J. Bone Joint Surg. 41B:796–809, 1959.
35. Wiltse, L. L., Widell, E. H., and Yuan, H. L.: Chymopapain chemonucleolysis in lumbar disc disease. J. Am. Med. Assoc. 231:474–479, 1975.

14 □ Spinal Tumors

James N. Weinstein

Primary tumors of *bone* are rare, accounting for approximately 0.4% of all tumors. Primary tumors of the *spine* account for less than 10% of all bone tumors.[6] Primary tumors are far less common than metastatic spinal lesions, particularly in adults.[28] Other non-neoplastic conditions producing spinal symptoms are much more common. Nevertheless, primary tumors of the spine represent a diagnostic and therapeutic challenge to the spinal surgeon.[6, 7, 11, 30, 33, 35, 39] One must have a high index of suspicion if one is to accurately diagnose and successfully treat these lesions, because the most common early complaint is back pain—an almost universal complaint among humans. These lesions are often found in compromising locations, specifically, around the spinal cord, nerve roots, major organs, and blood vessels; nevertheless, the results of treatment can positively affect survival and quality of life.

PRIMARY TUMORS

Clinical Observations

The clinical presentation can vary considerably from patient to patient, but the primary complaint of most is back pain (Tables 1 and 2).[45] Symptoms of back pain at night, pain at rest, or a neurologic deficit should prompt consideration of a spinal tumor. In one series, 84% of patients presented with some complaint of pain, either localized back pain (60%) or radicular pain (24%). There was no symptomatic distinction made between benign and malignant tumors.[45] In such cases the pain is not usually relieved by rest or recumbency. It is usually of an insidious onset and is usually progressive over time.

Despite these complaints, diagnosis is often delayed.[25, 45] The delays are usually in terms of years. Unfortunately, delays affect adequate (optimal) treatment and survival. Patients often relate their pain to a fall or some other mishap, thus providing the unsuspecting physician with a likely but incorrect explanation of their pain. At the time of the initial neurologic examination, an objective deficit may be identified in 50% of patients.[33, 35, 39, 42, 45] This is directly related to the location and nature of the tumor mass. Herniated discs and various types of spinal stenoses have been confused with primary tumors.[35] A palpable detectable mass is uncommon.[45]

The interval from onset of symptoms to diagnosis is often prolonged, particularly in individuals with benign lesions.

Judicious use of roentgenographic investigations is essential. Plain radiographs are satisfactory in a majority of spinal tumors, with thoracic spinal lesions being the most difficult to see.[11, 12, 28, 30, 35, 45] Treatment plans, however, must be supplemented with appropriate use of bone scans, computed tomographic (CT) scans, magnetic resonance imaging (MRI) tomography, and occasionally myelography and angiography. With these techniques and appropriate preoperative x-

Table 1 □ Patterns of Presenting Symptoms

PRESENTING SYMPTOM	NUMBER OF PATIENTS	PERCENTAGE OF PATIENTS
Back pain	25	30.50
Radicular pain	8	9.75
Weakness	7	8.50
Back pain and weakness	15	18.30
Radicular pain and weakness	8	9.75
Mass	4	4.90
Pain and mass	9	11.00
Pain, weakness, and bowel and bladder dysfunction	4	4.90
No symptoms	2	2.40
Total	82	100

From Weinstein, J. N., and McLain, R.: Primary tumors of the spine. Spine 12:843–851, 1987.

Table 2 □ Incidence of Presenting Symptoms

PRESENTING SYMPTOM	PERCENTAGE OF PATIENTS
Pain: localized or radicular	84.2
Weakness	41.5
Mass	15.9

From Weinstein, J. N., and McLain, R.: Primary tumors of the spine. Spine 12:843–851, 1987.

ray staging, a treatment algorithm can be instituted (Fig. 1). On plain radiographs, cortical disruptions and/or soft tissue masses are common for both benign and malignant spinal tumors. Fluoroscopy using C-arm control or CT scan–guided techniques is useful when closed percutaneous biopsies are indicated (Fig. 2). It is strongly recommended that spinal tumors be biopsied and treated only by surgeons experienced in the approach and management of these most difficult problems.[24, 45]

Bone Scan

The ^{99m}Tc bone scan is the most sensitive diagnostic tool for detecting spinal metastases. However, false-negatives do occur if vascular response has been low because of the tumor. Primary tumors such as multiple myeloma and some sarcomas may be negative on bone scan. Also, the extent of ^{99m}Tc uptake does not necessarily correlate with the extent of tumor involvement.[14]

Computed Tomography (CT)

CT may be the best diagnostic and surgical planning tool. It provides clear visualization of even minimal vertebral destruction and a good look at the surrounding soft tissues, allowing surgical decisions to be made based on a clear visualization of the extent of invasion of the spinal canal.[45] A small amount of water-soluble dye in the subarachnoid space, used to enhance CT, will aid in distinguishing tumor from thecal sac. Myelography by itself is rarely indicated, although it can be useful to define extent of involvement or multiple site involvement.[14, 45] Today, however, MRI has, in my opinion, replaced myelography for use in delineating multiple site involvement and

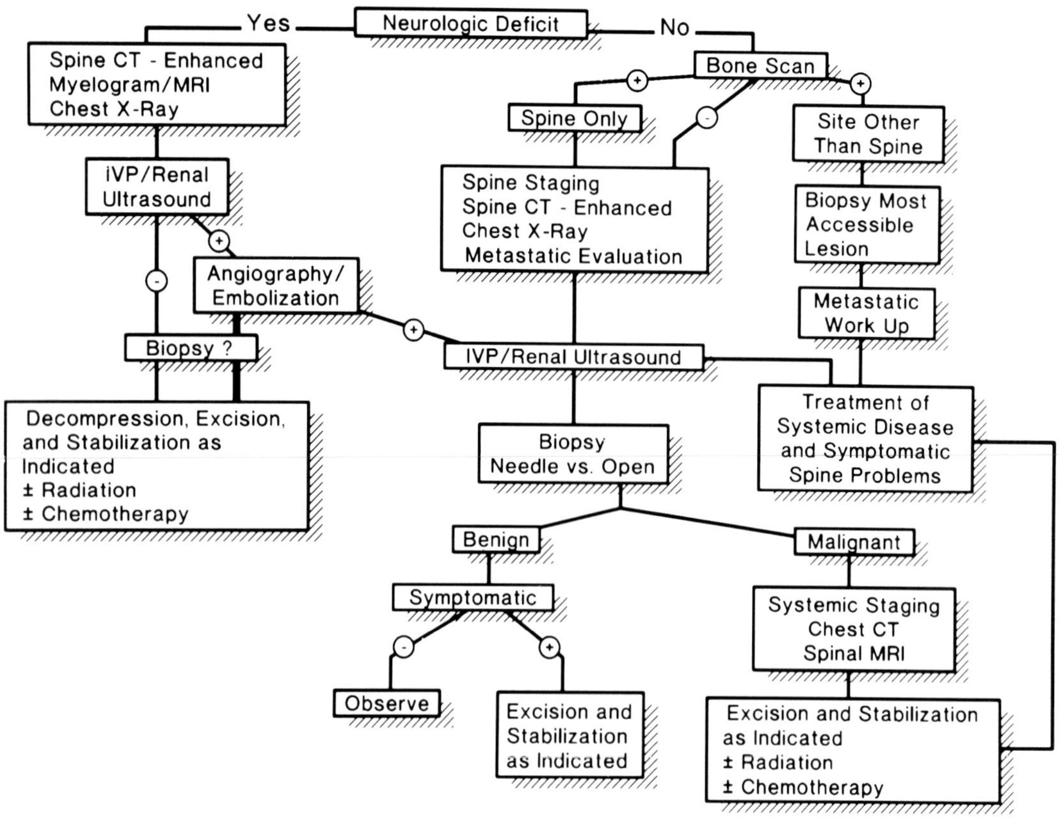

Figure 1 □ Algorithm for an approach to spine tumors.

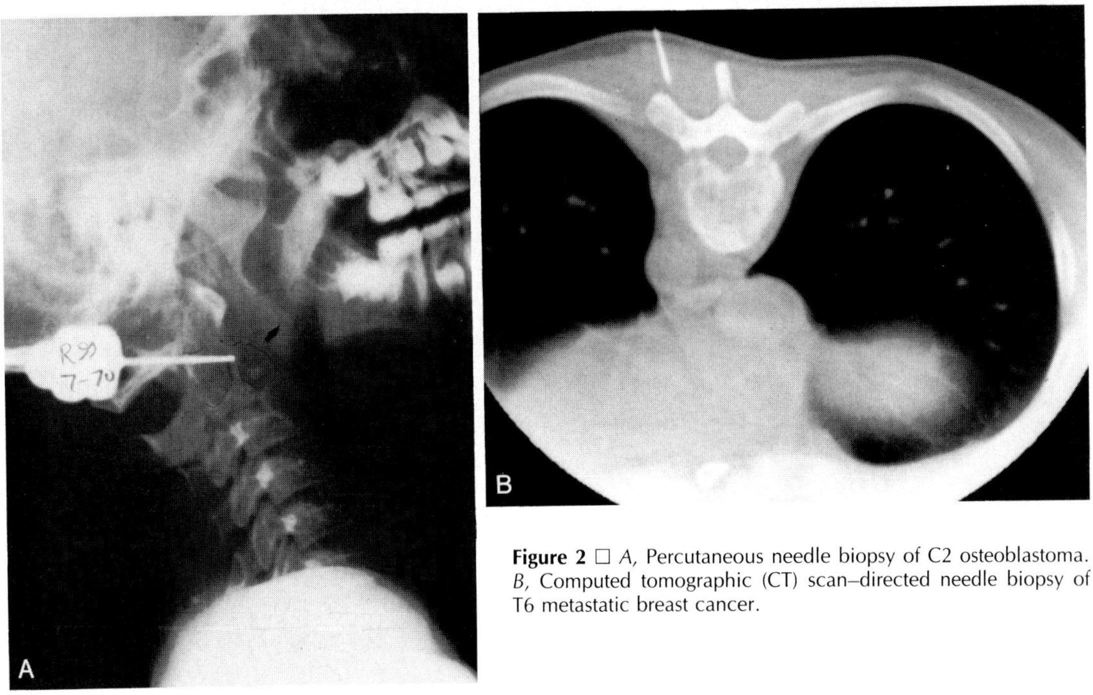

Figure 2 □ *A,* Percutaneous needle biopsy of C2 osteoblastoma. *B,* Computed tomographic (CT) scan–directed needle biopsy of T6 metastatic breast cancer.

extent of disease. Myelographic or MRI blocks do not necessarily correlate with symptoms or outcome.[1] The progressive neurologic compromise, rather than the diagnostic studies, indicates the treatment course to be taken.

Angiography

The effectiveness of spinal surgery is sometimes compromised by excessive bleeding. Metastatic renal cell and thyroid carcinomas can be highly vascular, increasing morbidity and mortality. Aneurysmal bone cyst, hemangiosarcoma, and other primary tumors may also present a vascular challenge to the spinal surgeon. Angiography with selective embolization can be an effective way to manage such lesions. Use of this technique can reduce intraoperative blood loss and perioperative morbidity and mortality. Identification of the origin of the artery of Adamkiewich may also be helpful.[37]

Location

Primary spinal tumors involve all spinal segments. Cervical spinal tumors are, however, less common than thoracic, lumbar, and sacral lesions (Fig. 3).[45] The vertebral body is four times more likely to be involved with primary malignant tumors than are the posterior elements (Fig. 4).[10, 19, 28, 33, 45]

BENIGN TUMORS

Benign tumors of the spine, as those elsewhere in the musculoskeletal system, generally carry a better prognosis than do malignant neoplasms. Surprisingly, with the exception of giant cell tumors, survival does not appear to correlate with treatment.[8, 31, 45] Giant cell tumors of the spine, as those in other locations, tend to have recurrences, and these are extremely difficult to treat.[8, 21, 22, 31, 41] Radiation therapy is almost never indicated in the treatment of benign spinal lesions.

The more common benign spinal lesions are hemangioma (Fig. 5), osteoid osteoma (Fig. 6),[20] and osteoblastoma (Fig. 7).[20] These are followed in frequency by osteochondroma (Fig. 8), giant cell tumor (Fig. 9) and aneurysmal bone cyst (Fig. 10).[39] Eosinophilic granuloma and other lesions such as angiolipoma are less common but must be part of the differential diagnosis. Eosinophilic granuloma (Fig. 11) is part of the

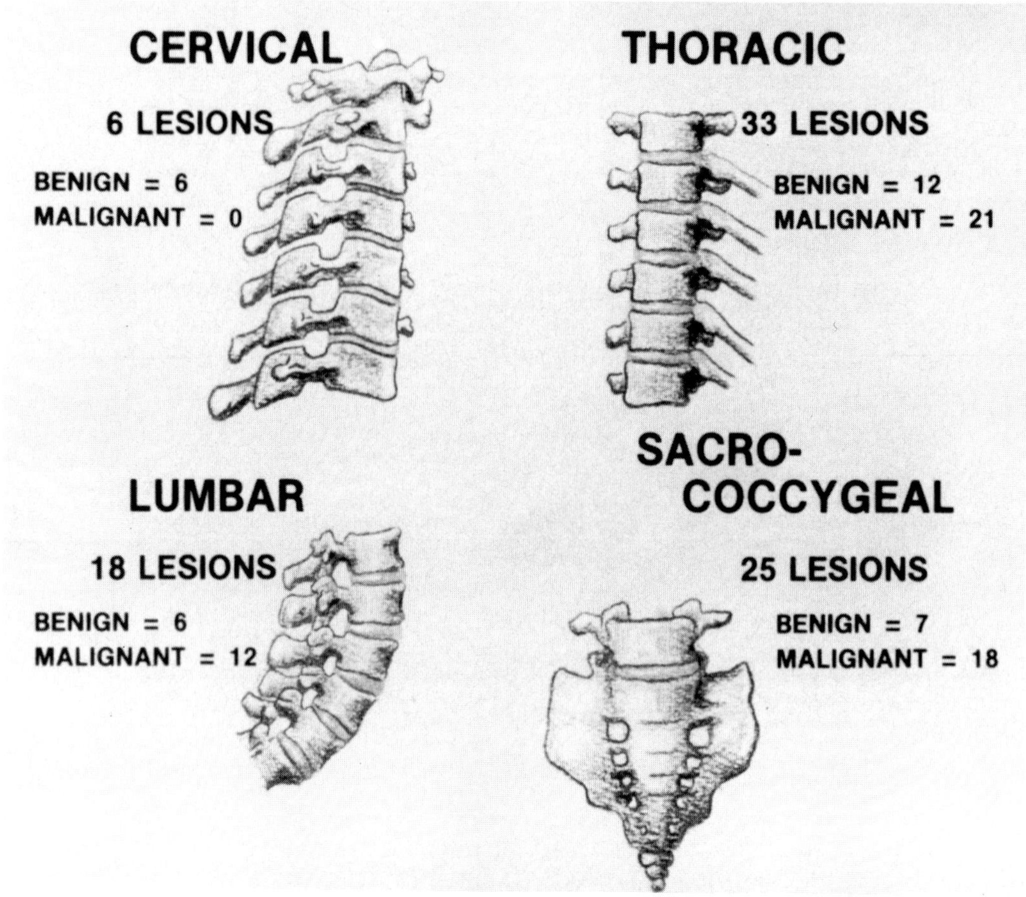

Figure 3 □ Primary spine tumors by location.

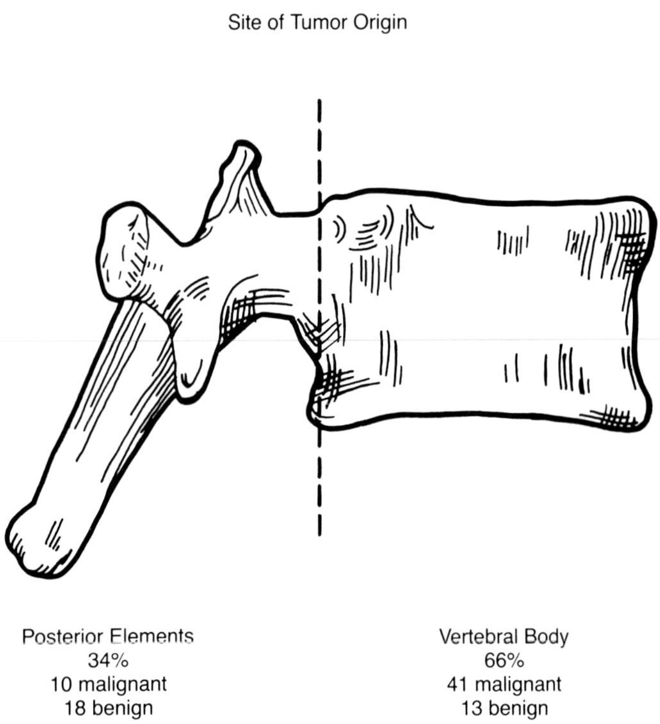

Figure 4 □ Location of tumor origin by tumor grade, benign versus malignant.

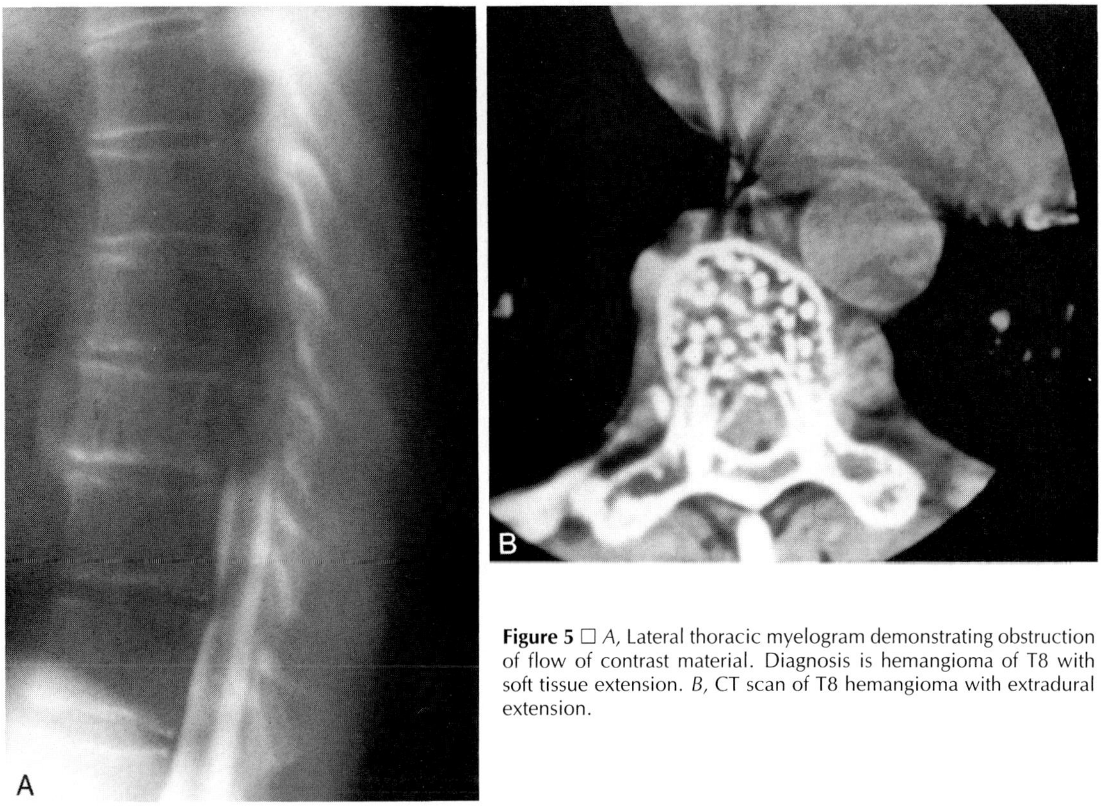

Figure 5 □ *A*, Lateral thoracic myelogram demonstrating obstruction of flow of contrast material. Diagnosis is hemangioma of T8 with soft tissue extension. *B*, CT scan of T8 hemangioma with extradural extension.

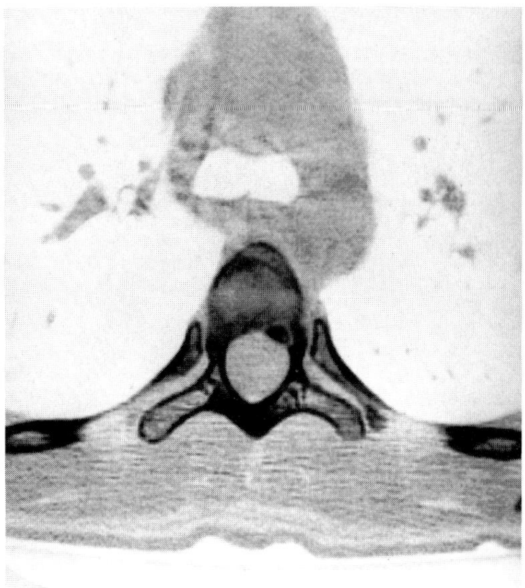

Figure 6 □ CT scan of osteoid osteoma T4. Plain x-ray studies were negative.

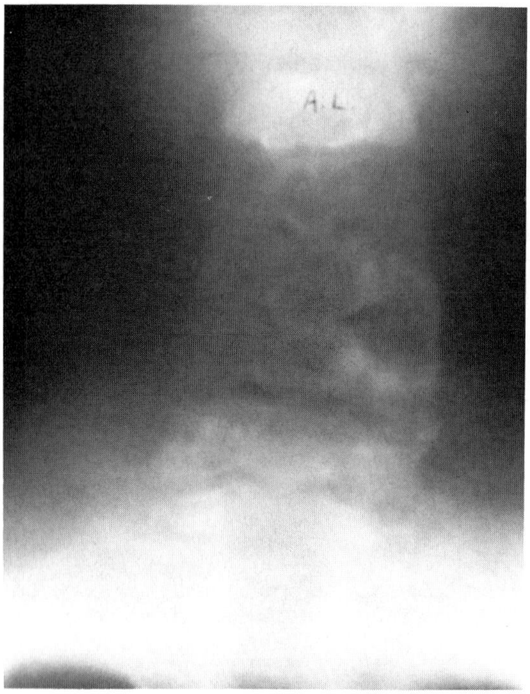

Figure 7. □ Osteoblastoma at C5.

histiocytosis X series, but is benign and can usually be treated by benign observation.[16]

Hemangioma is rarely symptomatic and is found in approximately 10% of all spines. It usually is located between T12 and L4. Women are affected three times more often than men. Usually this lesion is an incidental x-ray finding or is found at autopsy without known clinical symptoms. Hemangiomas have the classic vertical reticular stripelike appearance on x-ray films. Rarely, hemangiomas expand to the adjacent pedicles and lamina or adjoining ribs. Soft tissue extension of hemangiomas causing neurologic deficit has been reported.[42] No treatment is required if the lesion is not symptomatic. However, with soft tissue extension and/or ballooning of the bone, causing symptoms of nerve root or spinal cord impingement, radiation therapy and/or surgical decompression should be considered.[44, 45]

Young patients with acute scoliosis who complain of back pain that is worse at night and during recumbency are suspected of having an osteoid osteoma. Their symptoms are usually relieved by aspirin.[32] Roentgenograms supplemented by CT and/or bone scan may be necessary to demonstrate and appropriately treat these lesions. Treatment in symptomatic cases should be directed at marginal to wide excision of the lesion and appropriate stabilization if necessary (Fig. 12). The scoliosis and pain usually resolve with treatment of the tumor.

MALIGNANT TUMORS

The outcome for patients with malignant tumors of the spine varies with the specific tumor type and the extent of the initial surgical excision.[8, 43, 45]

Malignant neoplasms are much more likely to arise from the vertebral body than are benign lesions.[10, 19, 28, 33, 45] The correlation between age at diagnosis and tumor type is significant.[11, 30, 35, 45] The mean age at diagnosis is significantly higher for patients with malignant tumors than for those with benign tumors (49 versus 21 years). In one series of 51 primary spinal tumors reported in patients over 18 years of age, 80% had malignant neoplasms.[45]

Patients with primary malignant tumors of the spine more commonly have associated neurologic findings, have a propensity for vertebral body involvement, and are older at the time of diagnosis (Table 3).[33, 35, 39, 45]

The most common malignant spinal lesion is plasmacytoma (myeloma). Other, less common, primary malignant tumors of the spine are chordoma, chondrosarcoma, lymphoma, Ewing sarcoma, and osteosarcoma.

Slow-growing, locally aggressive tumors are associated with greater mean, and overall, survival compared to rapidly progressive and early metastasizing lesions. Multimodality therapy has allowed for some long-term survivals in aggressive lesions.[29] Patients with solitary plasmacytoma and

Table 3 □ Clinical Features of Patients with Spinal Neoplasms

	BENIGN	MALIGNANT	p VALUE
Mean age at diagnosis	20.9 yr	48.7 yr	.0001
Age greater than 18 years	32%	80%	.0001
Neurologic deficit	35%	55%	.09
Anterior location	42%	80%	.0005

From Weinstein, J. N., and McLain, R.: Primary tumors of the spine. Spine 12:843–851, 1987.

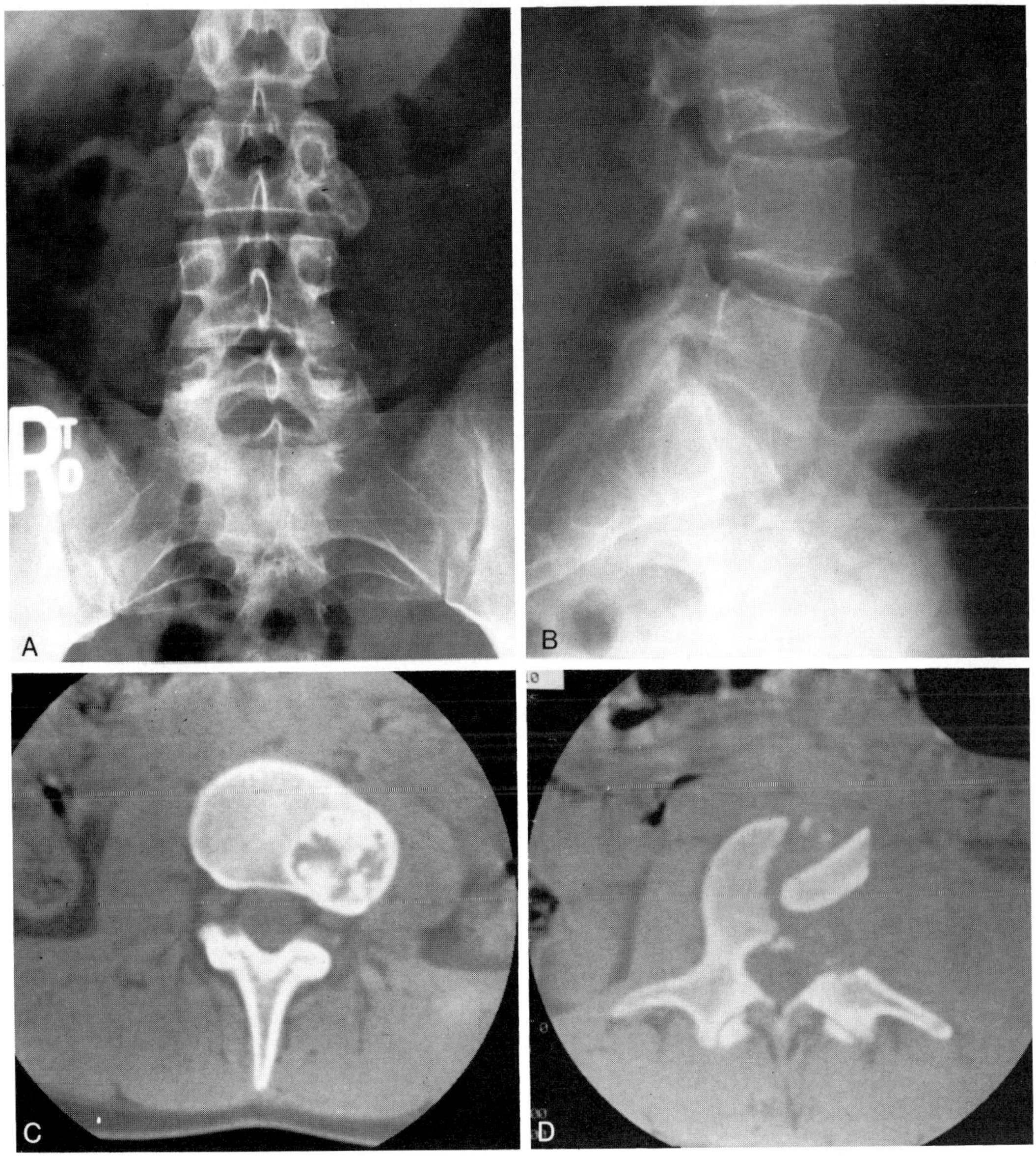

Figure 8 □ *A, B,* Osteochondroma at L3 (anteroposterior [AP] and lateral x-ray films). *C,* Osteochondroma at L3 (CT scan). *D,* Osteochondroma at L3 (CT scan 2 years postoperatively).

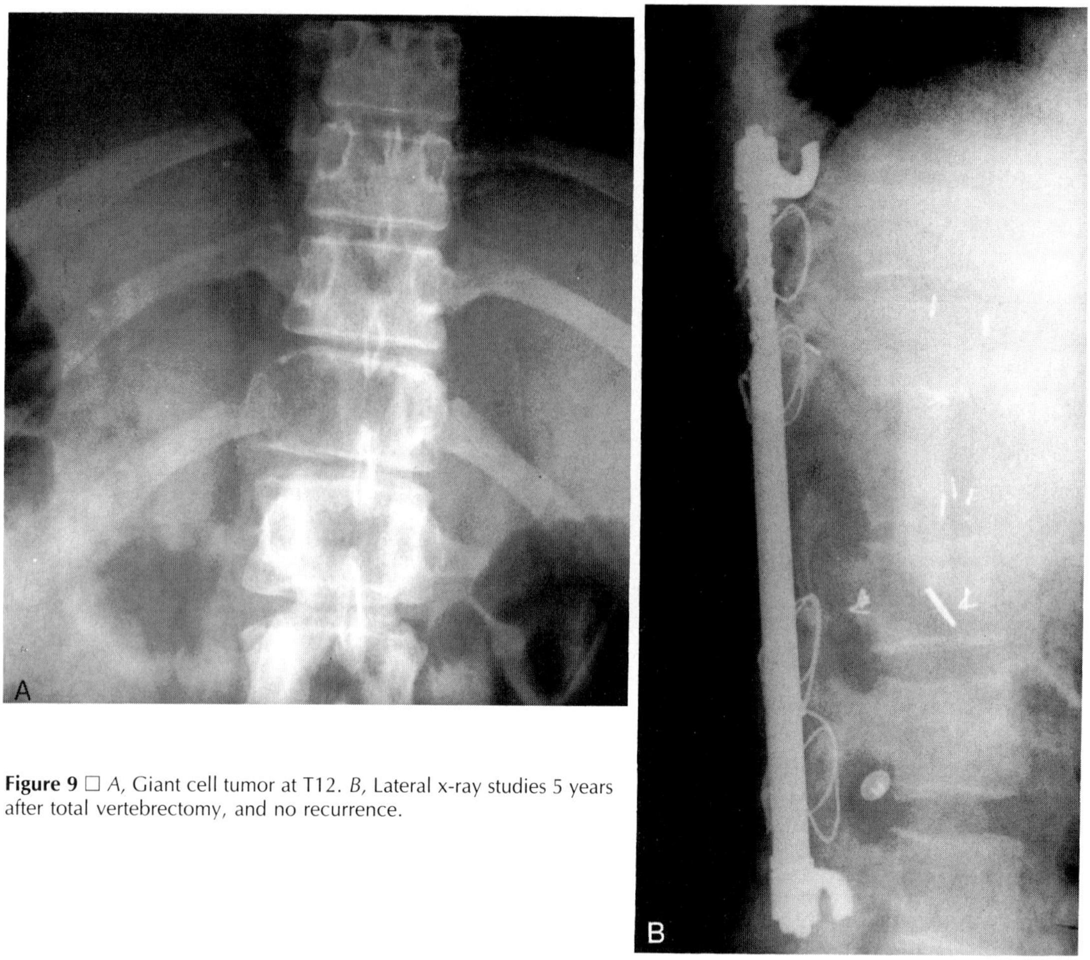

Figure 9 □ *A,* Giant cell tumor at T12. *B,* Lateral x-ray studies 5 years after total vertebrectomy, and no recurrence.

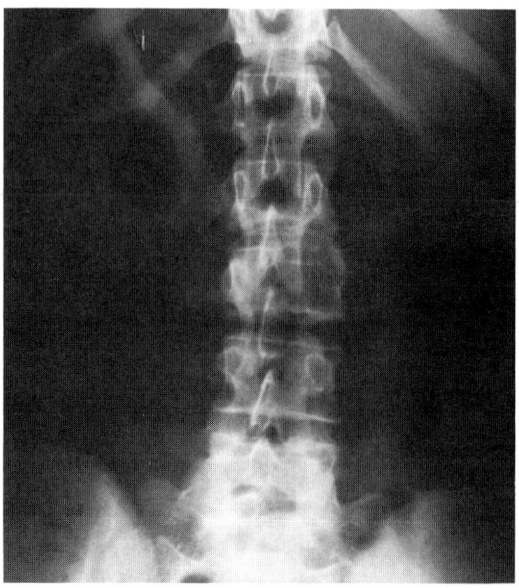

Figure 10 □ Aneurysmal bone cyst at L3.

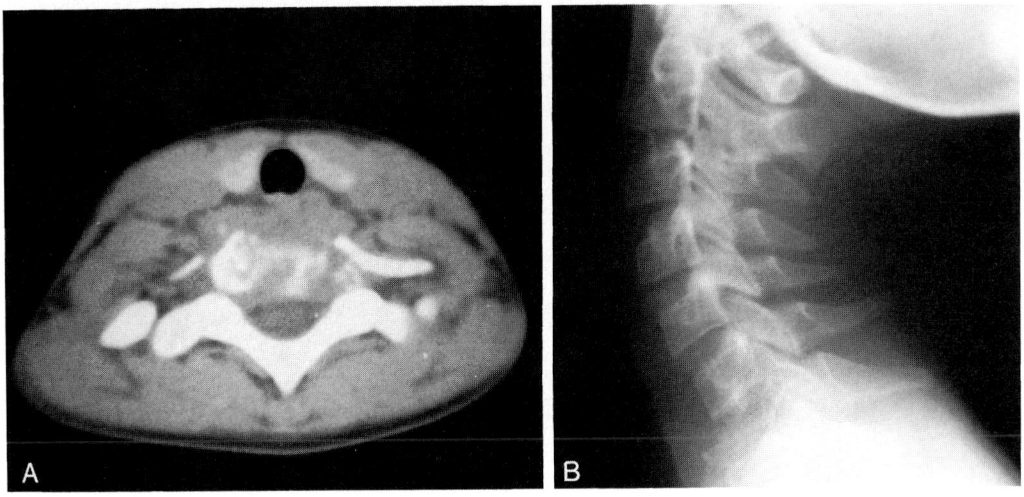

Figure 11 □ *A,* Eosinophilic granuloma at C7. *B,* Lateral x-ray and CT scan of C7 eosinophilic granuloma.

Figure 12 □ Illustration from CT scan of Figure 6, T4 osteoid osteoma, following resection and rib grafting.

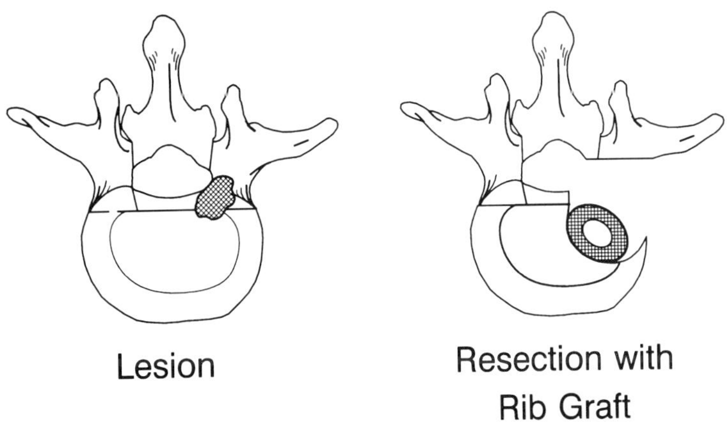

Table 4 □ Survival in Patients with Spinal Malignancy, by Tumor Type

TUMOR TYPE	N	MEAN SURVIVAL (months)*
Solitary plasmacytoma	15	38.27
Chondrosarcoma	4	28.00
Chordoma	11	27.73
Ewing's sarcoma	4	27.50
Osteogenic sarcoma	3	18.33
Lymphoma	5	13.40
Others	4	36.25

*Survival scores truncated to 60 months.
From Weinstein, J. N., and McLain, R.: Primary tumors of the spine. Spine 12:843–851, 1987.

chondrosarcoma have greater overall survival rates than patients with osteosarcoma and lymphoma (Table 4).[45] Solitary plasmacytoma is very sensitive to irradiation, and such treatment positively affects the survival of patients.[23, 27, 42] However, if one eliminates this bias for plasmacytoma in assessment of the long-term survival of malignant spine neoplasms, the relative outcome of surgically treated lesions was only significantly affected by complete surgical excision of the tumor when compared with other less aggressive treatments.[45] Thus, the best treatment results (i.e., survival) are effected by the most radical surgical extirpation of malignant spinal lesions (Table 5).[21, 26, 33, 36–38, 45]

METASTATIC TUMORS

Cancer in general is the second leading cause of death in the United States.[14] There are nearly one million new cases per year. Two thirds of these cases develop metastases, the skeletal system being the third most common site. These metastatic foci are sometimes painful secondary to fracture, marrow disruption, and neural deficits. The most common primary tumors metastatic to bone are breast and prostate (84%), thyroid (50%), lung (44%), and kidney (37%).

Lymphoma and myeloma are also commonly metastatic. The spine is the most common site of skeletal metastasis, irrespective of the primary tumor that is involved. It is followed by the ribs, pelvis, proximal long bones, sternum, and skull. However, vertebral metastases are often asymptomatic and are often discovered only by routine bone scans performed as part of a protocol to follow tumor patients.

In the spine the vertebral body is usually the first anatomic part to be involved, although pedicle destruction is often the first part involved on roentgenographic observation. This is easily explained by the fact that 30% to 50% of the vertebral body must be destroyed before these changes can be recognized on a roentgenogram. However, with only minimal involvement, the pedicle exhibits early roentgenographic cortical changes that can be seen when one looks at the pedicle in cross section on an anteroposterior roentgenogram. Metastases to the posterior elements are seen in about 14% of cases.[17, 40] Thoracic spine metastases are usually from lung and breast, whereas lumbar spinal metastases are more commonly of a prostatic origin. Spinal cord and nerve root compression occur only rarely (5%).[4, 5] Spinal cord compression can occur at multiple levels in the same patient. This possibility, although rare, must be considered prior to treatment. If the symptoms are not consistent with routine roentgenographic studies, MRI or myelogram should be performed to rule out the possibility of multiple-level involvement.

The prognosis for metastatic spinal disease is variable. The rapidity of neurologic deficit is extremely important and generally correlates with the ultimate prognosis. In general, a rapidly declining neurologic picture yields a poor prognosis, whereas individuals with slowly progressive (days to

Table 5 □ Survival in Patients with Spinal Malignancy by Surgical Excision

TYPE OF SURGICAL TREATMENT	N	MEAN SURVIVAL (months)*	PERCENTAGE WITH FIVE-YEAR SURVIVAL
None	5	17.00	15.0
Curettage	4	17.50	0.0
Incomplete resection	17	23.18	18.7
Biopsy only	10	33.50	33.0
Complete resection	10	48.40	75.0

*Survival scores truncated to 60 months.
From Weinstein, J. N., and McLain, R.: Primary tumors of the Spine. Spine 12:843–851, 1987.

weeks) neurologic pictures have much more favorable outcomes.[14]

Treatment for metastatic spinal lesions falls into two general categories: operative and nonoperative.[1, 3–5, 7, 9, 13–15, 17, 18, 34, 40, 45, 46]

Patients with roentgenographic evidence of spinal metastases or a positive bone scan but no bony vertebral collapse or neurologic impairment are candidates for irradiation, if their pain has been unresponsive to chemotherapy or hormonal manipulation. These patients may temporarily respond to epidural narcotics for pain management. Certain tumors (renal cell) with single metastatic foci without vertebral collapse are best treated by extirpation, when possible, and no irradiation, in order to allow the best long-term survival.[38]

In patients without bony collapse or instability but with neurologic deficit and/or pain secondary to soft tissue involvement, the response to irradiation is usually good. However, depending on the tumor type and its particular prognosis, surgical extirpation followed by appropriate spinal stabilization and irradiation may be the procedure of choice.[34] This view is contrary to the work by Gilbert and colleagues, who reported that irradiation alone was as effective as decompressive laminectomy in the treatment of patients with epidural cord compression.[13]

In patients with widespread metastases involving multiple levels, Fitzpatrick and Rider advocated hemibody irradiation of 700 to 1,000 rads. Fifty-three per cent of those who received hemibody irradiation obtained complete or partial relief of their pain, despite disease progression.[9]

Patients who have vertebral collapse and progressive pain, are unlikely to be relieved by irradiation alone. In these patients, the pain is due to a mechanical problem, of the bone, disc, or other structures, and surgery plus or minus irradiation and chemotherapy may be the best course of treatment.

SPINAL STABILITY AND SPINAL TUMORS

Vertebral motion segment stability and the indications for fusion have long been highly controversial topics.[7, 46, 47] To this end, various definitions and classifications of spinal stability have developed.[7, 47] Denis has written about the three-column spine.[7] He states that if the anterior and middle columns are involved, the spine is unstable. Mechanically this may be true, but clinically many tumor patients have both the anterior and middle columns involved and have done very well for many years without surgical intervention. Likewise, kyphosis by itself is not necessarily associated with increased pain and neurologic deficit.[46] However, for patients with progressive kyphosis and increasing pain or neurologic deficit, then appropriate decompression, stabilization, and possibly irradiation may be indicated.[7, 15, 34, 46, 47] Most classifications of spinal stability are based on acute traumatic involvement of the spine and not on primary or secondary tumor involvement.

The scenario for tumors is quite different. To this end, an approach for primary and metastatic tumors of the spine has been developed.[45] The approach appears useful in the management and prognostication of these most difficult spinal lesions. The single most important factor in determining the prognosis of the patient with a primary spinal malignancy is the ability to obtain a complete excision at the initial surgery, particularly with respect to the chordomas and chondrosarcomas.[2, 26, 45] Although some authors have advised that attempts of surgical extripation are fruitless and should not be made,[3] it is clear from others[33, 36–38, 45] that the ability to remove the entire primary tumor, depending on location, plays a significant role in overall patient survival.[36–38, 45]

As in the extremities, certain high-grade tumors necessitate more aggressive surgery when possible.[8] Certain anatomic structures in and around the spine provide for natural planes of dissection. The bony vertebral bod ies, intervertebral discs, anterior and posterior longitudinal ligaments, and the dura are often resected to provide adequate tumor margins.[36–38] Neural, muscular, and vascular structures can also be safely sacrificed in order to achieve adequate surgical margins.[33, 37, 38, 45] Surgical treatment significantly influences outcome in malignant lesions,[33, 36, 45] in terms of both longevity and quality of life. Thus, it appears that surgical extripation allows the best prognosis for local control and cure of the disease.[8, 36–38, 45]

The problems of the spine are obviously different from those of the extremities. Compartments for resection are complicated by the spinal cord and its component parts. Amputations in the form of hemicorporectomy have been described, but its limitations are obvious.

ANATOMIC EXTENT OF SPINAL TUMORS

If spinal tumors are to be surgically treated, it is evident that a logical and consistent approach is needed. To this end, an anatomically based scheme has been developed to aid the surgeon's approach to these most difficult lesions.

Anatomic Extent by Zone (Fig. 13)

Zones I to IV	Site A—intraosseous; site B— extraosseous; site C*—regional or distant metastasis.

*Not shown in figures.

Zones IA to IVA	Intraosseous lesions confined within the cortical boundaries.
Zone IA	Includes spinous processes to the pars interarticularis and inferior articular processes.
Zone IIA	Includes the transverse processes, superior articular processes, and the pedicles to their junction with the vertebral body.
Zone IIIA	Anterior three fourths of the vertebral body.
Zone IVA	Posterior and medial one fourth of the vertebral body.
Zones IB to IVB	Extraosseous extension beyond the cortical boundaries. Lesions having extraosseous extension extend

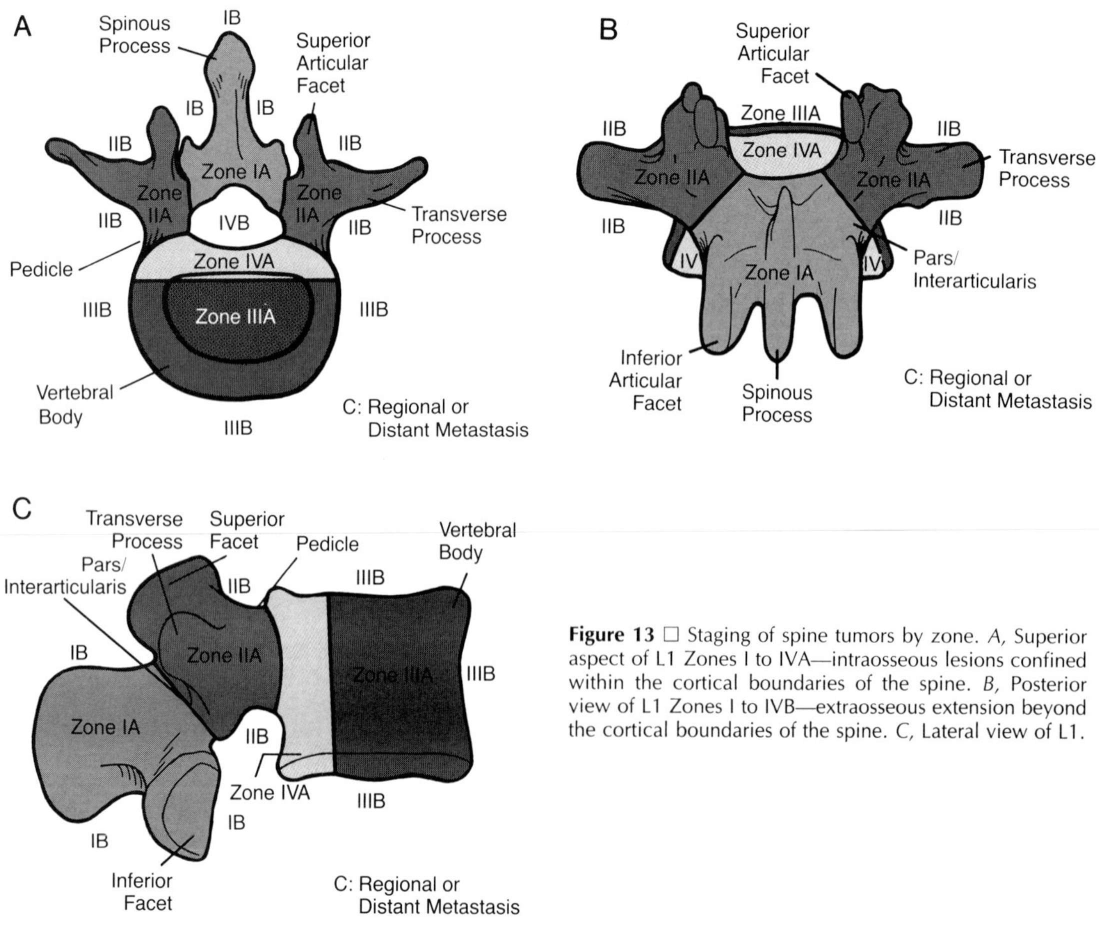

Figure 13 □ Staging of spine tumors by zone. *A,* Superior aspect of L1 Zones I to IVA—intraosseous lesions confined within the cortical boundaries of the spine. *B,* Posterior view of L1 Zones I to IVB—extraosseous extension beyond the cortical boundaries of the spine. *C,* Lateral view of L1.

	beyond the bony margins of their respective zones.
Zones IC to IVC	Intraosseous or extraosseous lesions associated with regional or distant metastases.

These anatomic zones are useful in surgical planning. Surgical outcome is ultimately affected by the zones involved; by whether the lesion is intraosseous (A) extraosseous (B), or metastatic (C); and by the type of tumor and its grade. Likewise, the ability to extirpate these tumors can directly affect prognosis, depending on tumor type, grade, and location.[36, 43, 45]

SURGICAL PROCEDURES

Isolated (A) lesions, in Zones IA through IVA, can be completely resected by a wide excision, whereas extraosseous (B) lesions of the spine are extremely difficult to resect with good margins, especially in the lumbosacral and cervical spine,[36, 45] without neurovascular compromise. Surgery is often marginal at best, and usually intralesional. The decision to perform wide excision must be weighed against the risk. However, using the classification as outlined, wide excision is possible in many cases.[36-38, 45]

SURGICAL APPROACHES BASED ON ANATOMIC EXTENT

(Table 6; see Fig. 13; Fig. 14)

Posterior Approach □ Zone I (A,B,C) lesions are best approached posteriorly. The resulting tensile loads are best minimized by posterior fixation of the surgeon's choice.

Zone II (A,B,C) lesions are also, in general, best approached posteriorly. Zone II lesions may be stabilized by posterior fixation alone.

Table 6 □ Surgical Approach by Zone and Potential Margin of Resection

ZONE	PROCEDURE FOR EXCISION	POTENTIAL MARGIN
IA* (B,C)	Posterior	Wide
IIA* (B,C)	Posterior	Wide/marginal
IIIA* (B,C)	Anterior	Wide/marginal
IVA*(B,C)	Anterior/posterior	Wide/intralesional

*The extent of extraosseous soft tissue (nerve, vessel, muscle) involvement may limit the potential margin of excision for Zones I to IV, B and C lesions.

From Weinstein, J. N., and McLain, R.: Primary tumors of the spine. Spine 12:843–851, 1987.

Anterior Approach □ Zone III lesions should be approached anteriorly. Adequate resection and reconstruction with or without internal fixation can usually be performed in this zone throughout the spine.

Combined Approach □ Zone IV lesions present the most difficult area to approach and reconstruct. One must traverse Zone I, Zone II, and/or Zone III to reach Zone IV lesions. For some Zone IV lesions (e.g., in the lumbar spine), resection demands anterior and posterior stabilization following extirpation of the lesion (Fig. 15).

This scheme, anatomic approach by zone, is an attempt to unify the approach to these difficult problems. It must be critically analyzed and retrospectively reviewed to determine its efficacy.

This type of classification scheme is relevant to both surgical planning and reporting end results of treatment for spine tumors. Depending on the location and extent of the lesion as determined by complete preoperative work-ups, the following types of procedures may be performed: (1) wide excision, (2) marginal excision, or (3) intralesional excision. Appropriate reconstruction can and must be accomplished.[36–38, 45] Once the tumor has been removed and the spinal cord and nerve roots decompressed, if indicated, stabilization of the spine is performed (Fig. 16).[45] For Zone III lesions, some spinal surgeons use corticocancellous anterior interbody graft keyed into the vertebral end plates. The patient is then immobilized in an orthosis until the graft is incorporated (see Fig. 13). If a patient is chronically debilitated and/or is facing further treatment such as chemotherapy or irradiation, this may be an unsatisfactory management plan; internal fixation with grafting may be a more effective approach. Depending on location, age, and tumor type, stabilization augmented with methyl methacrylate cement may be the procedure of choice (Fig. 17).

SUMMARY

The goals of treatment of spinal tumors should focus on (1) obtaining a definitive diagnosis through an appropriate biopsy or primary excision, (2) instituting appropriate surgical or nonsurgical treatment as indicated by tumor type at the time of the initial procedure, (3) preserving or restoring normal

Text continued on page 758

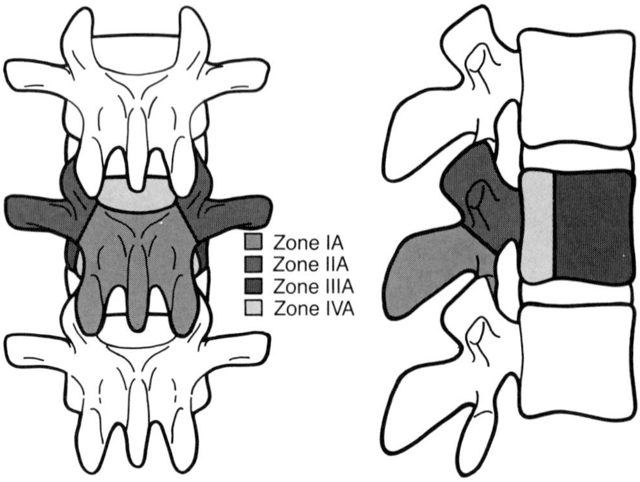

Figure 14 □ Posterior and lateral views L1 to L3.

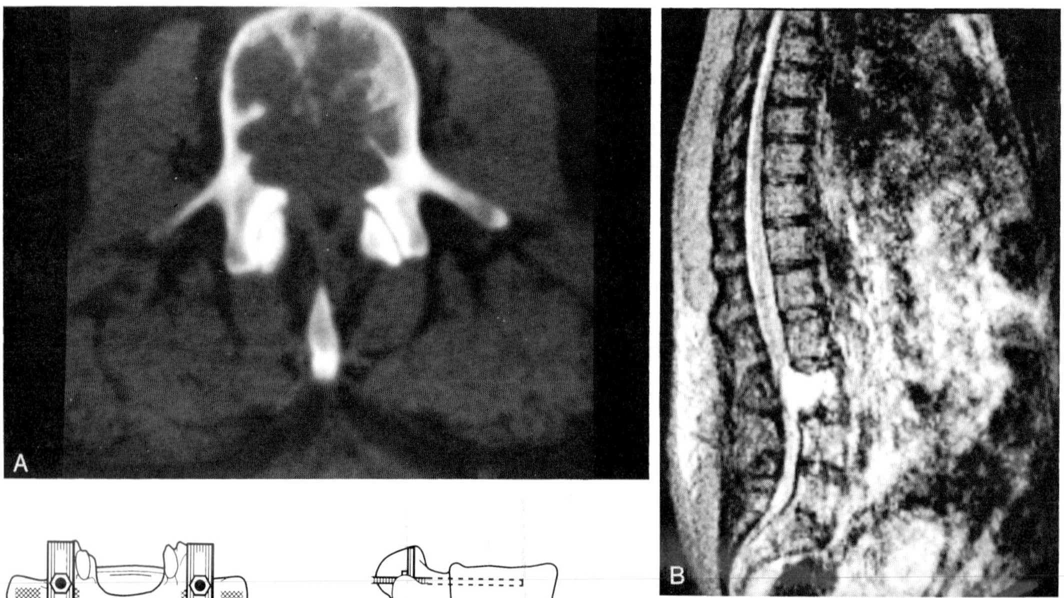

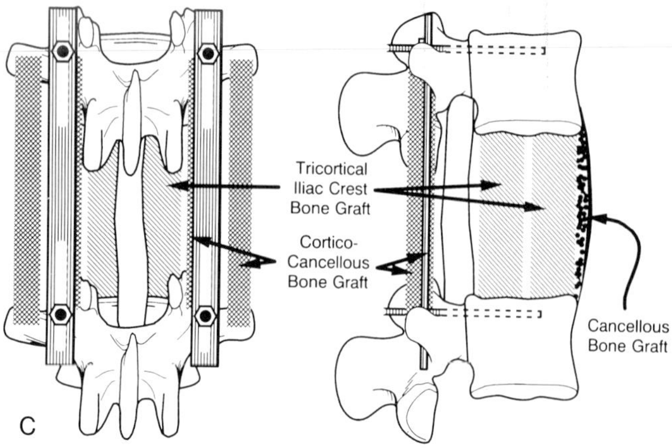

Figure 15 □ *A,* CT scan of an L3 chordoma involving Zones IIA and B, IIIA, and IVA and B. *B,* Magnetic resonance (MR) scan of same patient, T2 image. *C,* Illustration of reconstruction performed.

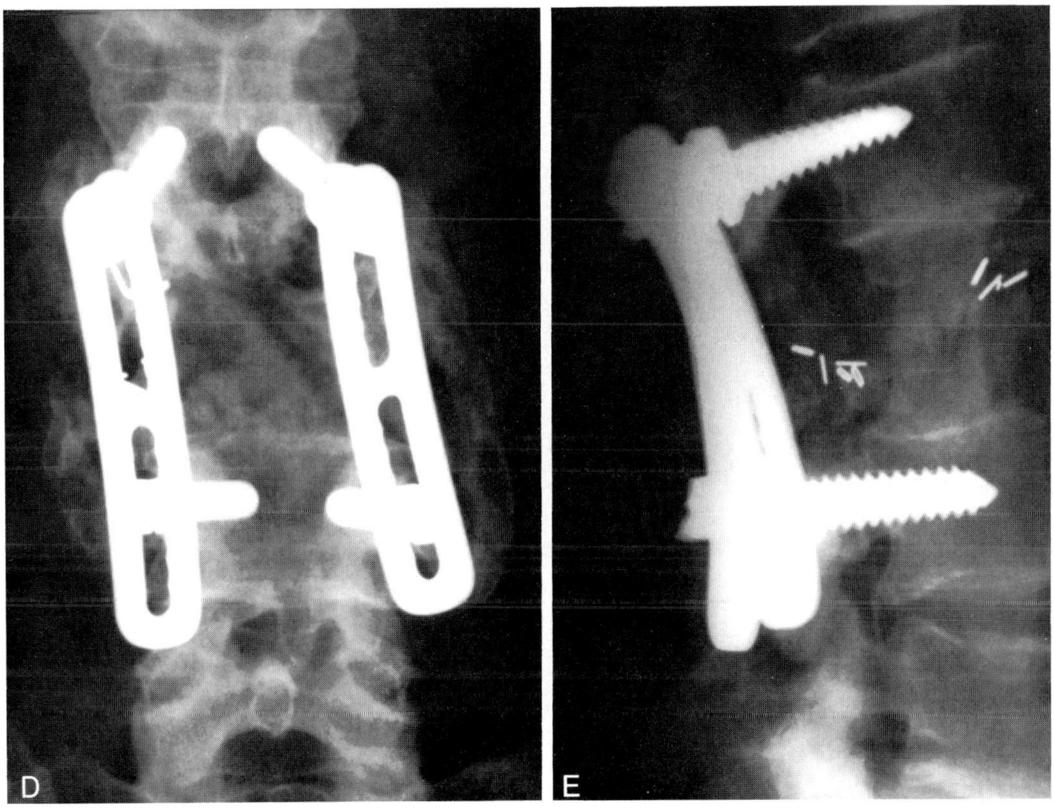

Figure 15 *Continued D, E,* AP and lateral x-rays taken 3 years postoperatively. No signs of recurrence to date.

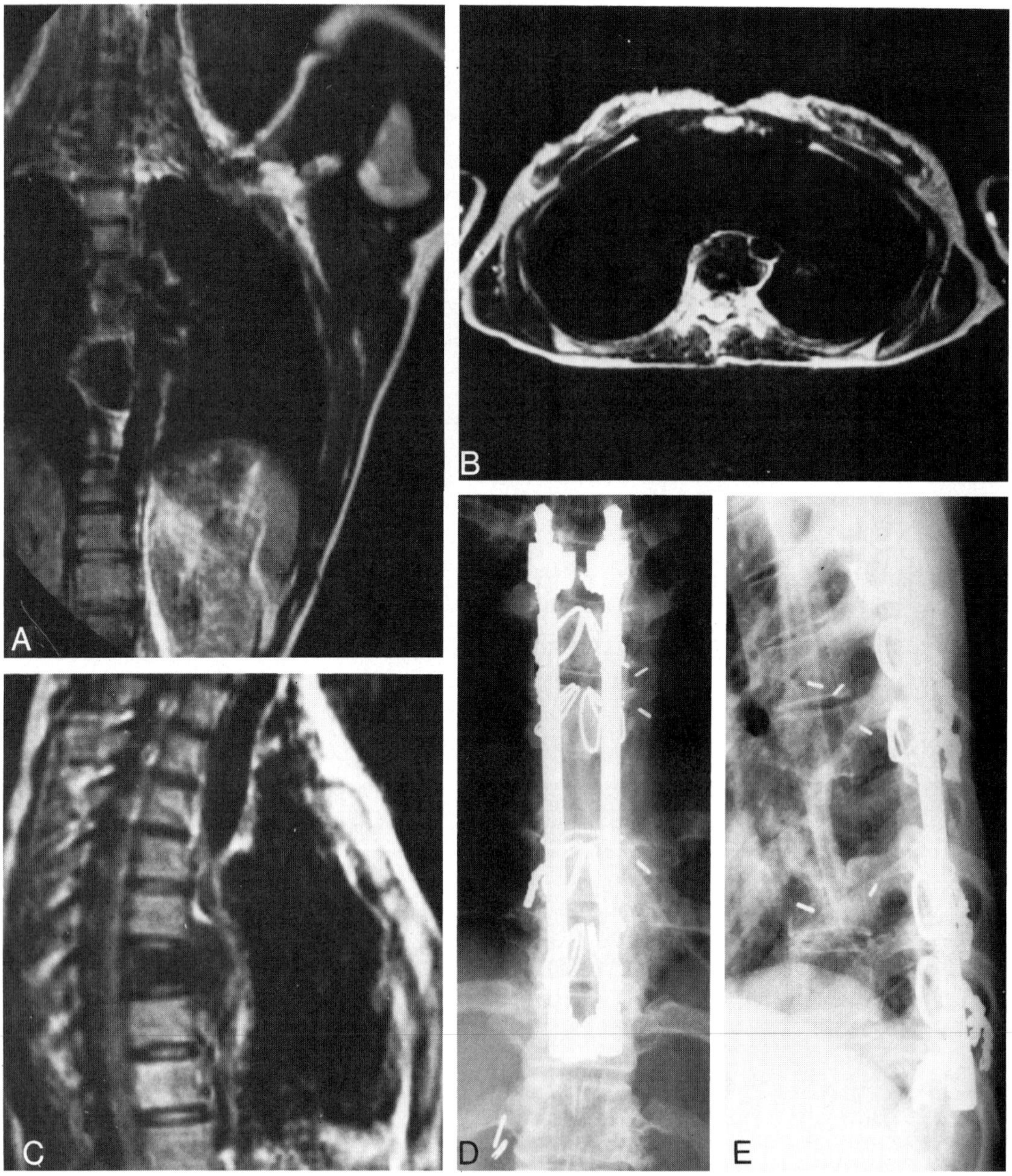

Figure 16 □ *A–C,* MR scans (AP, axial, and sagittal, respectively) of T7 metastatic clear cell sarcoma, adherent to the descending aorta. *D,* AP and *E,* lateral x-ray studies 3 years following tumor resection. A vascular rib graft was used anteriorly.

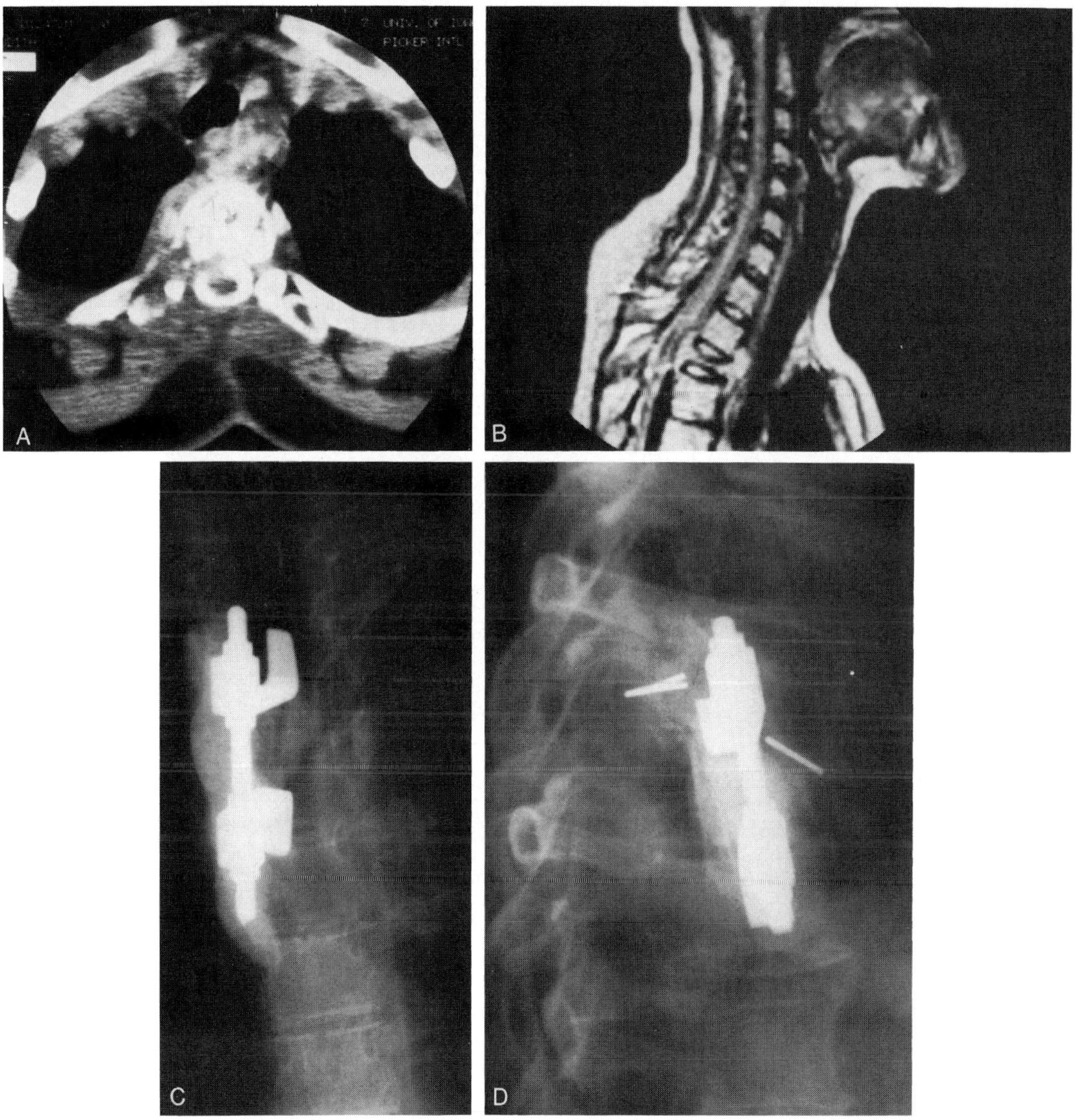

Figure 17 □ *A*, CT and *B*, MR scans of a 36-year-old woman with polyostotic metastatic breast cancer and spinal cord compression of T2, with paraparesis. *C*, AP and *D*, lateral x-ray film following surgery—paraparesis is resolved.

neurologic function, and (4) maintaining spinal stability.

Acknowledgments

The author wishes to extend his appreciation to Dr. Bertil Stener, Gothenburg, Sweden, for his comments and suggestions. This work was supported in part by NIHAR34344 and OREF 87-6-Co.

References

1. Bernat, J. L., Greenberg, E. R., and Barrett, J.: Suspected epidural compression of the spinal cord and cauda equina by metastatic carcinoma. Clin. Diagn. Surviv. Cancer 51:1953–1957, 1983.
2. Blalock, R. L., and Kempe, L. G.: Chondrosarcoma of the cervical spine. J. Neurosurg. 44:500–503, 1976.
3. Bohlman, H. H., Sachs, B. L., Carter, J. R., et al.: Primary neoplasms of the cervical spine. J. Bone Joint Surg. 68A:483–494, 1986.
4. Boland, P. J., Lane, J. M., and Sundaresan, N.: Metastatic disease of the spine. Clin. Orthop. 169:95–102, 1982.
5. Constans, J. P., DeVitus, E., Donzelli, R., et al.: Spinal metastases with neurological manifestations. Review of 600 cases. J. Neurosurg. 59:111–118, 1983.
6. Dahlin, D. C.: Bone tumors: General aspects and data on 6,221 cases. Springfield, Charles C Thomas, 1986.
7. Denis, F.: Spinal instability as defined by the three-column spine concept in acute spinal trauma. Clin. Orthop. 189:65–76, 1984.
8. Enneking, W. F.: Musculoskeletal Tumor Surgery. New York, Churchill Livingstone, 1983.
9. Fitzpatrick, P. J., and Rider, W. D.: Half body radiotherapy. Int. J. Radiol. Oncol. Biol. Phys. 1:197–207, 1976.
10. Floman, Y., Milgrom, C., Kenan, S., et al.: Spongious and cortical osteoblastoma of the axial skeleton. Orthopaedics 8:1478–1484, 1985.
11. Francis, K. C., and Hutter, R. V. P.: Neoplasms of the spine in the aged. Clin. Orthop. Rel. Res. 26:54–66, 1963.
12. Fraser, R. D., Paterson, D. C., and Simpson, D. A.: Orthopaedic aspects of spinal tumors in children. J. Bone Joint Surg. 59B:143–151, 1977.
13. Gilbert, R. W., Kim, J. H., and Posner, J. B.: Epidural spinal cord compression from metastatic tumor: Diagnosis and treatment. Ann. Neurol. 3:40–51, 1978.
14. Harrington, K. D.: Metastatic disease of the spine, current concepts. J. Bone Joint Surg. 68A7:1110–1115, 1986.
15. Harrington, K. D.: Anterior cord decompression and spinal stabilization for patients with metastatic lesions of the spine. J. Neurosurg. 61:107–117, 1984.
16. Ippolito, E., Farsetti, P., and Tudisco, C.: Vertebral plana. J. Bone Joint Surg. 66A9:1364–1368, 1984.
17. Jaffee, W. L.: Tumors and Tumorous Conditions of the Bones and Joints. Philadelphia, Lea & Febiger, 1958.
18. Johnson, J. R., Leatherman, K. D., and Holt, R. T.: Anterior decompression of the spinal cord for neurological deficit. Spine 8:396–405, 1983.
19. Keim, H. A., and Reina, E. G.: Osteoid osteoma as a cause of scoliosis. J. Bone Joint Surg. 57A:159–163, 1975.
20. Kirwan, E. O., Hutton, P. A. N., Pozo, J. L., and Ransford, A. O.: Osteoid osteoma and benign osteoblastoma of the spine. J. Bone Joint Surg. 66B:21–26, 1984.
21. Larsson, S. E., Lorentzon, R., and Boquist, L.: Giant cell tumors of the spine and sacrum causing neurologic symptoms. Clin. Orthop. Rel. Res. 111:201–211, 1975.
22. Larsson, S. E., Lorentzon, R., and Boquist, L.: Giant cell tumor of bone. J. Bone Joint Surg. 57A:167–173, 1975.
23. Lichtenstein, L.: Bone Tumors. St. Louis, C. V. Mosby, 1965.
24. Mankin, H. J., Lange, T. A., and Spainer, S. S.: The hazards of biopsy in patients with malignant primary bone and soft-tissue tumors. J. Bone Joint Surg. 64A8:1121–1127, 1982.
25. McLain, R., and Weinstein, J. N.: Primary tumors of the spine. Iowa Orthop. J. 7:32–38, 1987.
26. Mindell, E. R.: Chordoma: Current concepts review. J. Bone Joint Surg. 63A:501–505, 1981.
27. Raven, R. W., and Willis, R. A.: Solitary plasmacytoma of the spine. J. Bone Joint Surg. 31B:369–375, 1949.
28. Rothman, R. H., and Simeone, F. A.: The Spine, 2nd Ed. Philadelphia, W. B. Saunders, 1982.
29. Russin, L. A., Robinson, M. J., Engle, H. A., and Sonni, A.: Ewing's sarcoma of the lumbar spine. Clin. Orthop. Rel. Res. 164:126–129, 1982.
30. Sachs, B. L., Makley, J. T., Carter, J. R., et al.: Primary osseous neoplasms of the thoracic and lumbar spine. Orthop. Trans. 8:422–423, 1984.
31. Schajowicz, F.: Solitary plasmacytomas. *In*: Tumors and Tumor-Like Lesions of the Bone and Joints. New York, Springer-Verlag, 1981, pp. 296–298.
32. Sherman, M. S., and McFarland, G., Jr.: Mechanism of pain in osteoid osteoma. South. Med. J. 58:163–166, 1965.
33. Shives, T. C., Dahlin, D. C., Sim, F. H., et al.: Osteosarcoma of the spine. J. Bone Joint Surg. 68A:660–668, 1986.
34. Siegal, T., Tiqva, P., and Siegal, T.: Vertebral body resection for epidural compression by malignant tumors. J. Bone Joint Surg. 67A3:375–382, 1985.
35. Sim, F. H., Dahlin, D. C., Stauffer, R. N., and Laws, E. R., Jr.: Primary bone tumors simulating lumbar disc syndrome. Spine 2:65–74, 1977.
36. Stener, B.: Total spondylectomy in chondrosarcoma arising from the seventh thoracic vertebra. J. Bone Joint Surg. 53B:288–295, 1971.
37. Stener, B.: Total spondylectomy for removal of a giant-cell tumor in the eleventh thoracic vertebra. Spine 2:197–201, 1977.
38. Stener, B., Henriksson, C., Johansson, S., et al.: Surgical removal of bone and muscle metastases of renal cancer. Acta Orthop. Scand. 55:491–500, 1984.
39. Thommesen, P., and Poulsen, J. O.: Primary tumors in the spine and pelvis in adolescents: Clinical and

radiological features. Acta Orthop. Scand. 47:170–174, 1976.

40. Thompson, J. E., and Keiller, V. H.: Multiple skeletal metastases from cancer of the breast. Surg. Gynecol. Obstet. 38:367–375, 1924.
41. Tillman, B. P., Dahlin, D. C., Lipscomb, P. R., and Stewart, J. R.: Aneurysmal bone cyst: An analysis of 95 cases. Mayo Clin. Proc. 43:478–495, 1968.
42. Valderama, J. A. F., and Bullough, P. G.: Solitary myeloma of the spine. J. Bone Joint Surg. 50B:82–90, 1968.
43. Verbiest, H.: Giant cell tumors and aneurysmal bone cysts of the spine. J. Bone Joint Surg. 47B:699–713, 1965.
44. Virinder, M., Gupta, S. K., Tuli, S. M., and Sanyal, B.: Symptomatic vertebral hemangiomas. Clin. Radiol. 31:575–579, 1980.
45. Weinstein, J. N., and McLain, R.: Primary tumors of the spine. Spine 12:843–851, 1987.
46. Weinstein, J. N., Collalto, P., and Lehmann, T. R.: Long-term follow-up of nonoperatively treated thoracolumbar spine fractures. J. Orthop. Trauma 3(1):152–159, 1988.
47. White, A. A., III, and Panjabi, M. M.: Clinical Biomechanics of the Spine, Philadelphia, J. B. Lippincott, 1978, pp. 394, 424–425.

15 □ Osteoporosis

Neil Kahanovitz

Bone loss is a normal phenomenon that occurs during the aging process. As do all aspects of aging, the rate and severity of the bone loss vary widely. This variability has made osteoporosis one of the most difficult clinical entities to diagnose, quantify, treat, and, most importantly, prevent.

Although researchers recognized osteoporosis by the fragile and brittle appearance of the bones early in the last century, not until the clinical use of roentgenograms became widespread shortly after the turn of the century did serious clinical and scientific work begin to be reported.[34, 50] In the late 1930s, Fuller Albright reported on the clinical aspects of postmenopausal osteoporosis.[1] This study appears to be the first in a continuing search for insight into the clinical manifestations of osteoporosis.

However, it was not only the availability of roentgenograms that improved the diagnosis and treatment of osteoporosis. As medical care in general advanced early in this century, people continued to live longer. In the past, the cumulative effects of progressive bone loss did not become clinically apparent because people did not live long enough to become symptomatic. As the life expectancy of the adult population continues to increase, the clinical manifestations of osteoporosis are now clearly recognized in an ever-increasing population of senior citizens. It is estimated that osteoporosis is casually related to approximately 1.2 million fractures annually in the United States.[23] Overall, the cost of osteoporosis-related fractures and disability is roughtly $6.1 billion a year in the United States.[20]

Millions of dollars have been spent in the last decade by large pharmaceutical companies to inform the elderly and postmenopausal populations of the risks of osteoporosis, in hopes of selling calcium supplements and other nonprescription medications for the prevention and treatment of the illness. Unfortunately, a great deal of this advertising has led to many misconceptions about the proper treatment and natural history of osteoporosis. It is of the utmost importance that the knowledge of the natural history and treatment of osteoporosis be put into the proper prospective. In this way appropriate counseling, guidance, and treatment of the postmenopausal and elderly patient may begin to alleviate many of the anxieties related to this commercially exploited illness.

Despite efforts to define the exact physiologic alterations, there persists much confusion about the proper terminology for describing osteoporosis and other related metabolic bone diseases. In order to discuss the various diagnostic categories, as well as specific treatment modalities, one must understand the most often confused terms that refer to the various metabolic bone diseases.

Osteopenia is often inappropriately used interchangeably with osteoporosis. However, osteopenia simply means that there is less bone tissue than normal.[13] The term osteopenia is most often used by radiologists to describe a radiograph in which the bone tissue appears less mineralized than expected. The abnormal bone tissue may be osteomalacic or osteoporotic, but as long as the amount of bone tissue is less than normal the bone may be described as osteopenic.

The exact definition of osteoporosis is not clear and varies among authors. As more is known about the pathophysiology of the illness, its definition is increasingly refined. Most authors agree that osteoporosis is a decrease in the normal volume or amount of bone.[14, 36] Controversy beyond this basic definition remains, as there can be relative differences in the loss of cortical and trabecular bone. Differentiation is often dependent on the cause of the osteoporosis. However, the absolute decrease in apparently normal bone tissue is generally agreed to be the hallmark of osteoporosis and is used to differentiate this metabolic bone disease from the others.

The vast majority of patients with osteoporosis have the idiopathic variety; that is, no discrete identifiable metabolic deficit is responsible for the bone loss. However, it is important not to confuse patients with idiopathic osteoporosis and those with a more appropriately termed involutional osteoporosis. Obviously, patients with idiopathic osteoporosis may also be included in the involutional group, but some younger idiopathic osteoporotic patients would not appropriately be included in the involutional group. Therefore, to further clarify this often confusing classification system, it is more applicable to use the term involutional osteoporosis, instead of idiopathic osteoporosis, to describe age-related bone loss.

To further define involutional osteoporosis, there are now two distinct groups recognized within this large group of patients.[37] Type I, or postmenopausal, osteoporosis is found in women within 15 to 20 years after menopause. The cause is not clearly understood, but it appears to be related to hormonal and physiologic changes brought about by menopause.[36]

Type II, or senile, osteoporosis occurs in an older population, usually around age 70 years. It is found much more commonly in men than is Type I osteoporosis, but it predominates in females with a ratio of 2:1. As for Type I, the cause is not entirely clear, but appears to be related to the physiologic events that accompany the aging process.

Before describing the physiologic and clinical vagaries that distinguish these two most common types of osteoporosis, it is important to briefly examine the normal physiology of bone growth and aging.

Bone tissue is of two distinct types. The first is the solid cortical or compact bone, and the other is trabecular or cancellous bone. Cortical bone constitutes 80% of the total bone volume, but because of the broad surface area of the cancellous bone it constitutes only 30% of the total surface area.[41] The vertebrae consist of both cortical and cancellous bone. The posterior elements—lamina, spinous process, transverse processes, pars, facets, and pedicles—consist principally of cortical bone. On the other hand, the vertebral body is composed of an outer shell of cortical bone, but primarily is composed of cancellous or trabecular bone. Although the cortex of the vertebral body is relatively thin (0.5 to 1.0 mm), it accounts for half of the compressive strength of the vertebra.[40] The vertebral end-plate, which is in contact with the cortical bone, is actually composed of layers of trabecular bone densely and compactly arranged. These horizontally arranged layers of trabeculae may be several millimeters wide and are usually thickest in the central portion of the body where the cortical bone is found to be thinnest.[3]

The cellular components of normal bone consist of osteoblasts, osteocytes, and osteoclasts. Osteoblasts are mature cells unable to proliferate or divide and are usually found on the bony surfaces in a single layer. Osteoblasts develop from precursor cells in the marrow and vascular channels of the bone. The chief role of the osteoblast is to synthesize the matrix and ground substance and to control the mineralization necessary for new bone growth.

As new bone is formed by the osteoblast, new layers of bone are deposited. The osteoblasts are then encased in new bone formation and thereby become osteocytes. Osteocytes appear to be enclosed by a space or lacuna surrounded by bone tissue. It is not clear what exact function the osteocyte plays in normal bone metabolism, but it appears to have a role in local tissue repair, mineral homeostasis, and local perilacunar resorption.[31, 32]

Normal bone resorption is primarily carried out by the osteoclast. Osteoclasts are typically found on bony surfaces and are usually multinucleate giant cells. Blood-borne osteoclasts as well as those in the bone marrow develop from precursor cells.[32]

Along with the cellular components of bone, the matrix is equally responsible for the unique physiologic and mechanical properties of bone tissue. Normal bone tissue contains 20% tissue water, 10% crystal-bound water, 30% organic material, and 40% mineral.[33] As the normal aging of bone tissue occurs, the crystal-bound water decreases as the mineral increases. The backbone of the matrix consists of collagen. In fact, collagen accounts for 90% of the weight of the matrix. The collagen is oriented horizontally in three helical polypeptide chains.

The ground substance is composed of proteoglycans and glycoproteins. The proteoglycans consist of mucopolysaccharides, and chondroitin sulfate is the principal mucopolysaccharide found in bone.

The glycoproteins are somewhat smaller and are more diverse in structure than the proteoglycans. The major mineral components of bone tissue are calcium, phosphorus, and carbonate.[33] These minerals are found in either crystalline form or amorphous form. As time passes, the amorphous form of the mineral slowly becomes more crystalline, resulting in the typical lattice configuration.

The primary microstructural bone unit is the haversian system. This unit consists of concentric layers, or lamellae, in which there are scattered lacunae containing osteocytes. A central canal in the haversian system contains the neurovascular structures supplying each individual unit. Canaliculi allow communication between the adjacent osteocytes. Transverse Volksmann canals carry vessels communicating between adjacent haversian systems.

Before discussing the metabolic, physiologic, and mechanical alterations produced by osteoporosis it is important to review the normal metabolic pathways of calcium, phosphorus, and the various hormones controlling their fate. Calcium is absorbed mainly in the small intestine and excreted in the urine and stool. The amount of calcium absorption is related to bodily needs and is increased in the metabolic states in which there is an increased need for calcium (e.g., pregnancy) or a relative deficit (e.g., dietary deficiency). The average recommended intake of calcium remains controversial. However, a daily adult intake of 800 to 1,000 mg appears to be adequate.[48] It is generally agreed that the daily minimal calcium requirements are greater in perimenopausal women. During the perimenopausal and postmenopausal years, the calcium intake should increase to 1,600 mg daily.[19] Phosphorus is also absorbed through the intestinal tract, principally in the distal portions of the small intestine. The predominant method of excretion is by the kidney. The daily requirement for phosphorus ranges from 1,000 mg to 1,200 mg.

1,25-Dihydroxycholecalciferol is the active form of vitamin D. Vitamin D_3 is hydroxylated first in the liver[25] and then in the kidney[1] to become the metabolically active form. Vitamin D plays an active role in the metabolism of calcium in the intestinal tract, kidney, and bone. Intestinal absorption of calcium is increased by an active transport mechanism stimulated by vitamin D. Vitamin D also affects both calcium and phosphate resorption in the kidney. Osteoclastic activity and resorption of bone are enhanced by vitamin D. In combination with parathyroid hormone (PTH), vitamin D increases calcium release from bone. There is also evidence that a lack of vitamin D may have an adverse effect on matrix synthesis and mineralization by depressing the normal activity of the osteoblast.[12]

PTH is secreted by the four parathyroid glands. Secretion of PTH is regulated by alterations in the plasma ionized calcium concentration. A decrease in calcium concentration causes an increase in PTH secretion, and an increase in calcium concentration results in decreased PTH secretion. In addition to this direct effect on the parathyroid glands, other metabolic changes, particularly those affecting calcium metabolism, may alter the secretion of PTH. The direct effects of PTH on bone are not entirely clear, but there is a direct relationship between increased PTH secretion and a subsequent increase in serum calcium. This probably results from a combined action on the osteoblast and osteoclast of bone as well as the renal tubular function.

In contrast to PTH, which raises serum calcium, calcitonin is a hormone that is responsible for lowering serum calcium. Calcitonin is produced in the thyroid gland by the C cells or parafollicular cells. Contrary to the action of calcium on PTH secretion, increased serum calcium causes an increase in the secretion of calcitonin, whereas a decrease in serum calcium causes a decrease in calcitonin secretion. Calcitonin slows bone resorption by inhibiting the osteoclastic activity and increases renal excretion of calcium, thereby opposing the normal actions of PTH.

Although vitamin D, PTH, and calcitonin have the most prominent metabolic effects on calcium and normal bone metabolism, there are many more physiologic and metabolic activities affecting bone metabolism that cannot be discussed in a short review such as this. However, the activities of these metabolites were briefly discussed in this section to improve understanding of the pathogenesis and, more importantly, of the treatment and prevention of osteoporosis.

Normal bone mass continues to increase until late into the third decade. After age 30 years, there is a gradual trend toward bone loss as the ratio of osteoblastic remodeling and replacement to osteoclastic resorption changes. Most studies suggest that trabecular bone density begins to decrease between ages 30 and 35 years.[28] As bone loss continues into later life, as much as 50% of trabecular bone may be lost in females and one third less in males.[28]

Following the peak bone mass reached around age 30 years, there appear to be two distinct types of bone loss that may affect the trabecular bone of the vertebral body. After the third decade, there appears to be a slow consistent loss of bone. This slow phase results from an alteration in the normal osteoblastic remodeling and osteoclastic resorption. After peak bone mass is attained, the osteoblasts are no longer able to keep up with the resorptive activity of the osteoclast, leaving areas of resorption that are not remodeled by the osteoblasts.

Following menopause or surgical oophorectomy, there appears to be a second type of bone loss that is much more rapid than the constant but slower age-related phase.[11, 15, 36] An exact physiologic hormonal link has not been established for this accelerated phase of bone loss, but the decrease in estrogen appears to have a significant effect on increasing osteoclast activity and accelerating bone resorption.

Because osteoporosis is a relative decrease in the normal bone density at any given age, it is important to note that osteoporosis may occur in two ways. Once peak bone mass is attained, the normal phases of bone loss occur as described above. An abnormal increase or acceleration of this normal physiologic bone loss will result in an osteoporotic state. In contrast, a normal and expected amount of postmenopausal and age-related bone loss may result in osteoporosis if the peak bone mass attained by the third decade is below the normal predicted value. Therefore, osteoporosis may result not only from increased bone loss over the expected physiologic loss but also by normal physiologic bone loss occurring in an individual with an abnormally low peak bone mass. Both pathways may ultimately lead to the same clinically and radiographically indistinguishable manifestations of osteoporosis.

Based on a study of plain radiographs, 29% of women and 18% of men will have radiographic osteoporosis between the ages of 45 and 79 years.[27] However, in a study utilizing absorptiometry, it was found that 50% of women over the age of 65 years had a bone density below the predicted fracture threshold.[39] Approximately 350,000 fractures a year are directly related to an abnormally low bone density in women over age 45 years. However, the types of fracture are not evenly distributed among the common fracture sites as one grows older. Vertebral compression fractures and Colles fractures are much more common in the postmenopausal years. Type I, or postmenopausal, osteoporosis affects trabecular loss much more than cortical; therefore, many more vertebral fractures than hip fractures are found in this younger age group.[36] Between ages 51 and 75 years, there is a female-to-male predominance of this fracture pattern in a ratio of as high as 6:1.

Over age 70 years there is combined cortical and trabecular bone loss with a concomitant rise in the number of hip fractures. With Type II, or senile, osteoporosis, a female predominance continues but it is much less marked, with a ratio of 2:1 over age 70 years.[36] Although the number of vertebral fractures rises dramatically in the postmenopausal years, there continues to be a slow, steady increase in the number of vertebral fractures as the years pass, and Type II osteoporosis becomes more common.

Not all postmenopausal women or elderly males are equally predisposed to develop osteoporosis. Any condition that hastens the onset of menopause increases the chances of developing Type I osteoporosis and vertebral compression fractures.[29] Surgical oophorectomy, ovarian dysfunction, and premature menopause are associated with an increased risk and incidence of Type I postmenopausal osteoporosis.[6, 22] In addition, a relatively low total bone mass by the third decade also is a risk factor predisposing individuals to develop earlier and more severe osteoporosis.

A variety of alterations in the normal physiologic and metabolic processes may also increase one's chance of developing osteoporosis. Malnutrition, particularly a diet with poor calcium intake, is commonly observed in older individuals and frequently results in osteoporosis. Inadequate exposure to sunlight results in decreased vitamin D synthesis and osteoporosis. Diabetes mellitus, hyperthyroidism, Cushing syndrome, acromegaly, and homocystinuria may all result in decreased bone density and osteoporosis. Long-standing use of corticosteroids and antacids, and prolonged heavy coffee intake may also result in an increased risk of osteoporosis.[18, 30] Excessive smoking and alcohol intake have also been implicated in the development of osteoporosis.[45]

The racial distribution of osteoporosis is similarly not uniform. Black individuals appear much less prone to develop osteoporosis than a similar group of white individuals.[17] Body habitus also seems to alter the predisposition to developing osteoporosis. Overweight femals are less prone than thin women to develop osteoporosis. In addition to the mechanical stresses on bone brought about by the added weight, the additional body fat allows for greater stores of estrogen.[10]

Vertebral compression fractures or wedge fractures are estimated to occur in 5% to 40% of white postmenopausal women.[9] Most fractures occur in the middle and lower thoracic or lumbar vertebrae (Fig. 1). Acute localized nonradicular pain is the typical presentation of these patients. Osteoporosis alone does not cause pain unless there are structural changes within the vertebrae, even though these changes may be microscopic and not visible on routine radiographic studies. In fact, it is postulated that many of the early symptoms are due to microfractures occurring within the osteoporotic vertebrae. These fractures are often associated with miminal or no trauma. The microfractures occur when small but significant loading of the vertebra is able to overcome the decreased fracture threshold of these osteoporotic vertebrae, resulting in microscopic but symptomatic fractures undetectable on plain radiographs. Radiographically evident compression fractures occur when larger loads are applied to the vertebrae and the fracture threshold is exceeded to a far greater degree. Similarly, cumulative microfractures resulting from smaller but repetitive loading may also result in structurally apparent compression fractures.

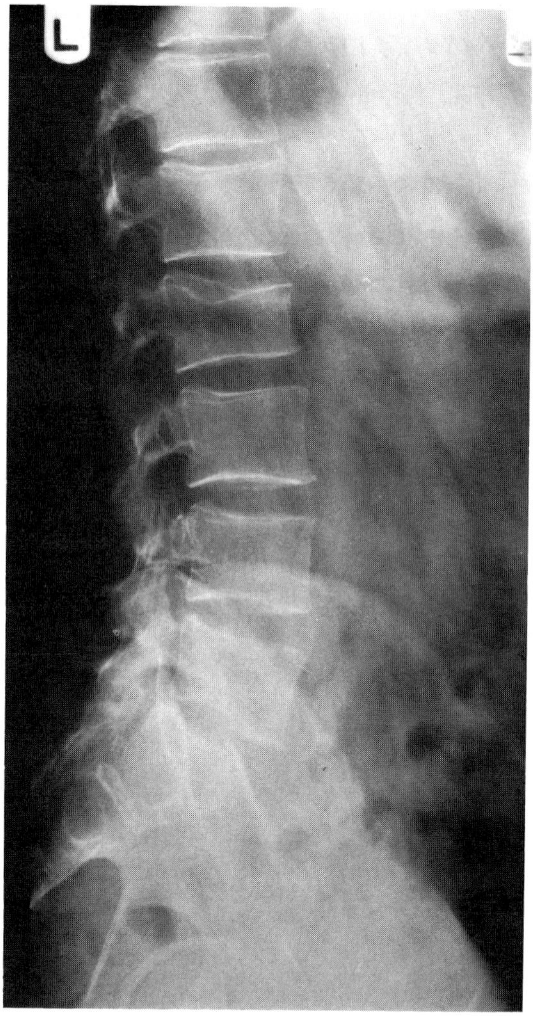

Figure 1 □ Mild compression fracture following minor trauma in a 30-year-old woman undergoing long-term corticosteroid treatment for chronic asthma.

These compression fractures usually heal within 2 to 3 months. By this time the back pain most often slowly resolves. Persistent back pain after fracture healing is usually attributable to alterations in the normal mechanics of the articulations of the affected vertebrae. Single osteoporotic compression fractures as well as compression fractures of purely traumatic causes usually heal uneventfully if the resultant anterior compression deformity is less than 30% to 35% of the vertebral body height. As the severity of the deformity increases, alterations in the normal vertebral motion segment function may occur. With increasing anterior collapse, abnormal stress and ultimately subluxation of the posterior facet joints and ligamentous structures occur. These mechanical alterations are usually responsible for the chronic back pain remaining after bony healing of the more severe compression fractures.

Unless the compression fracture is quite severe or there are several fractured vertebrae, it is unusual for a significant gibbous or sharply kyphotic deformity to occur. It is much more common to have multiple compressed vertebrae leading to an abnormal increase in the thoracic kyphosis or flattening or reversal of the normal lumbar lordosis (Fig. 2). Localized back pain and locally referred pain often accompany the structural kyphotic deformity. In addition to the mechanical pain, fatigue pain of the trunk extensor muscles is also common. These muscles are abnormally stretched over the increased kyphosis and are fatigued easily, resulting in localized pain.

Although kyphotic deformities are the most common of the vertebral deformities associated with osteoporosis, there is also an unusually high incidence of scoliosis found in osteoporotic patients.[16] However, it is not clear what etiologic role the scoliosis or the osteoporosis plays in this higher-than-expected association.

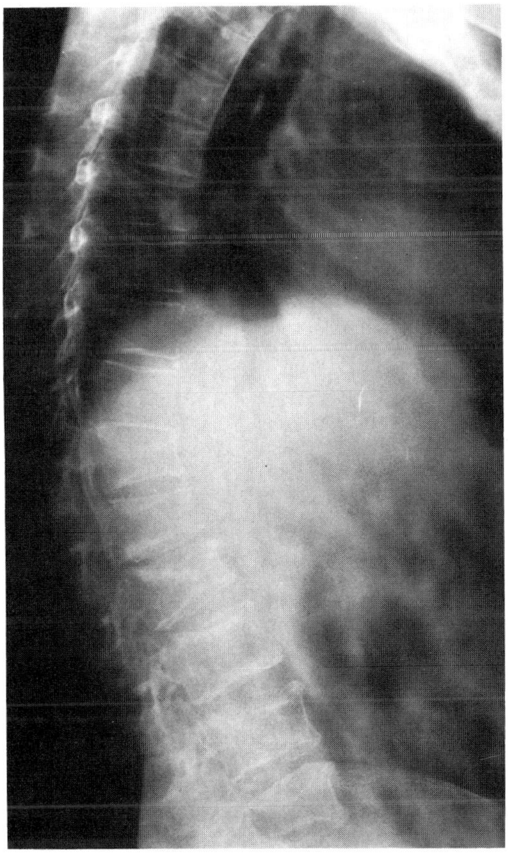

Figure 2 □ Multiple compression fracture in a 74-year-old female. Note the loss of normal lumbar lordosis.

It is uncommon for osteoporotic compression fractures to present with neurologic involvement. There is usually no structural interruption of the posterior wall or middle column of the vertebral body following a compression fracture. Maintenance of the integrity of the posterior cortex of the vertebral body allows for protection of the neural elements. Infrequently, an osteoporotic burst fracture may occur with concomitant neurologic involvement. This occurs much less often than the more common osteoporotic compression fracture. The burst fracture is usually the result of excessive loading and force applied to the vertebra in a somewhat different pattern. This may result in a potentially neurologically unstable type of fracture.

Although quite uncommon, symptomatic spinal cord or cauda equina compression may result from the mechanical compression of a severe kyphotic or gibbous deformity. The osteoporosis is usually quite severe in these cases and is more frequently found in older patients with severely involved vertebrae. The neurologic involvement may range from acute onset of paraplegia to long-standing but minimal lower extremity spasticity. Even though neurologic involvement is unusual in the typical osteoporotic fracture, it is essential to perform a thorough neurologic examination in all patients suspected of having a fracture, in order to detect any early or subtle neurologic changes.

Even though osteoporotic compression fractures may be highly suspected by their clinical presentation, the actual diagnosis must be made radiographically and, on occasion, by utilizing additional diagnostic studies. On plain spinal radiographs it is often difficult to definitively diagnose osteoporosis until it is rather advanced and the characteristic fractures and deformities are present. Unfortunately, at least 30% of the bone mass must be lost before detectable radiolucent changes are seen on plain radiographs.[26] Although osteoporosis is the most common cause of vertebral osteopenia in the postmenopausal and elderly groups, it is virtually impossible to distinguish it from many other less common disease states causing radiographic vertebral osteopenia.[43]

After the osteoporosis has progressed and resulted in vertebral fracture and deformity, there are several characteristic radiographic findings. Once the fracture threshold has been exceeded, most osteoporotic fractures are found to be wedged anteriorly. In postmenopausal women sustaining a vertebral fracture, there is a 98% incidence of coexistent osteoporosis, regardless of the primary cause of the fracture.[4] However, there is usually no involvement of the posterior elements. Involvement of the posterior elements as well as fractures above the T6 level should generally be considered not to be secondary to osteoporosis but to be another pathologic condition, most often metastatic disease or infection.[22] Unless there is the pathognomonic appearance of an osteoporotic wedge compression fracture, it is often quite difficult to assess the cause of the bone loss and fracture on plain radiographs.

Radionuclide bone scanning is helpful in determining whether a vertebral fracture has recently occurred. Acute fractures are typically seen as locally increased uptake at the site of the fracture. The uptake gradually declines over time, and by 24 months it may be only slightly elevated or normal.[43] On occasion, in patients with osteoporosis, there may be a generalized poor uptake of radionuclide throughout the affected bone. However, this is not diagnostic of osteoporosis and may be seen in many other conditions resulting in osteopenia. Unfortunately, radionuclide bone scanning is not helpful in the definitive diagnosis of osteoporosis. Its role in the diagnosis and treatment of osteoporosis lies mainly in its ability to differentiate acute and long-standing healed vertebral fractures. It is not helpful in determining the exact pathologic process causing the increased uptake seen with a recent vertebral fracture or whether osteoporosis and another pathologic process are present concurrently in the fractured vertebra.

Since the advent of dual-photon absorptiometry and the adoption of CT scanning, relative bone density can now be measured with much greater accuracy than in the past. Improvements in the single-photon absorptiometer have enabled the use of two photons of different energies to be used in the development of the dual-photon absorptiometer. The asborption of two different photons allows for less soft tissue interference and more accurate recording of bone density with a relatively low radiation exposure of 5 to 15 mR.[43] The precision of dual-photon absorptiometry has been reported to be 2% to 3% on measurements of spinal bone density.[47] Calculation of the bone mineral content of the spine has also led to the development of guidelines for relative risk of vertebral compression fractures. Statistical analysis of patients with nontraumatic compression fractures has provided comparative data to predict the relative fracture risk for the lumbar vertebrae.[47]

It is obvious that dual-photon absorptiometry has been a tremendous benefit in the diagnosis and treatment of osteoporosis, but there are some drawbacks to its use. Dual-photon absorptiometry measures mineral mass in a two-dimensional area but is unable to accurately distinguish between cortical and trabecular bone. In addition, large-osteophyte formation and compression fractures may affect the true calculation of bone density with the dual-photon absorptiometer.

Quantitative computed tomography (CT) is able to differentiate cortical from trabecular bone when used to calculate bone mineral content. However, unlike dual-photon absorptiometry, its measurement of trabecular bone may be affected by the amount of fat in the bone marrow. Despite the apparent advantages of CT scanning over dual-photon absorptiometry by examining only the trabecular bone of the vertebra, one method appears to have no significant advantage over the other in predicting the probability of fracture.[24] Nevertheless, they are currently the two best methods for quantifying bone mineral content in both the diagnosis and treatment of osteoporosis.

There are several other methods of quantifying the bone mineral content of the skeleton, but these are primarily research techniques. Neutron activation analysis and Compton scattering utilize different radiation sources to quantify bone density.[43] Ultrasonic measurement of bone density uses no ionizing radiation to measure bone density and is used solely as a research technique.

Despite these rapid advances in the radiographic diagnosis and the ability to quantify the extent of bone mineral loss, there are still many cases in which the diagnosis of osteoporosis cannot definitively be made radiographically. In the elderly patient it is common to find radiographic evidence of vertebral osteopenia secondary to a variety of metabolic bone diseases other than osteoporosis. The most distressing diagnostic dilemma is the differentiation of vertebral osteoporosis and primary or metastatic disease affecting the vertebra. These can often be impossible to differentiate radiographically, although radionuclide and CT scanning are frequently helpful.

For patients for whom a definitive diagnosis cannot be made radiographically, it is essential that the diagnosis be made histologically to avoid improper and delayed treatment. Vertebral body involvement of the lumbar spine may be easily biopsied utilizing a lateral approach with a Craig needle. However, as with any needle biopsy, a significant number of false-negative results are encountered in using this technique. Therefore, if a needle biopsy is unsuccessful in providing a definitive diagnosis, open biopsy is recommended. Open biopsy in the lumbar or thoracic spine may be accomplished through an anterolateral approach or costotransversectomy in the thoracic spine. In order to avoid a life-threatening misdiagnosis and inappropriate treatment, only a definitive histologic diagnosis is considered to be acceptable when there is confusion about the exact cause of the radiographic abnormalities.

Once a definitive diagnosis of vertebral osteoporosis is established, treatment becomes the next consideration. The first line of treatment, and the easiest, is prevention. As previously discussed, a number of factors have been found to increase the risk of osteoporosis. Many elderly people do not have a sufficient dietary calcium intake. A careful dietary history should be taken to ensure that the daily intake of calcium as well as of the other necessary vitamins and minerals is adequate. The recommended daily intake of calcium for postmenopausal and elderly patients is approximately 1,600 mg/day.[19]

In addition to dietary calcium deficiency, excessive and prolonged consumption of alcohol, tobbacco, coffee, antacids, corticosteroids, and foods high in phosphorus should be discontinued. Unfortunately, outside of these relatively easily preventive factors, there is no real consensus about the appropriate treatment for osteoporosis. In fact, a survey conducted to determine the preferred treatment for osteoporosis showed a dramatic lack of consistency among the 116 physicians surveyed with respect to the various treatment modalities.[44]

Exercise has long been known to have a beneficial effect on bone metabolism and bone mineral content. In contrast, bed rest of even short duration results in accelerated and rapid decrease in vertebral bone mineral content.[25] Despite the recognition that exercise is beneficial in the prevention and treatment of osteoporosis, it is not clear how much exercise is needed. A controlled prospective study showed a 3.5% increase in lumbar spinal bone mineral content with 1 hour of supervised exercise twice a week for 8 months.[24] Similiar recommendations of exercise three times a week for 30 to 60 minutes also appeared to have a beneficial effect on bone mineral content.[2]

The role of estrogen in the prevention and treatment of osteoporosis is also not clear. However, it is clear that the use of estrogens retards normal postmenopausal bone loss and in fact may increase bone density in some individuals.[10] Outside of the general consensus that estrogens are effective in slowly advancing postmenopausal bone loss, there is virtually no agreement on the appropriate timing of treatment, length of treatment, or dose of estrogen.

The most feared risks of estrogen therapy are those of endometrial and breast cancer. Unfortunately, the exact risk is unknown, as contradictory reports of both a higher risk and a normal risk of cancer are available in the literature.[8, 21, 46] However, whatever the effect estrogen may have in increasing the incidence of endometrial cancer in postmenopausal women, the concomitant use of progestogens may reduce this risk. The combined use of estrogens and progestons or progestogens may also lower the incidence of thromboembolic complication, which increases with the use of estrogens alone.[10]

The appropriate timing for the start of estrogen treatment is also unclear. It has been shown that whenever treatment is begun there is a beneficial effect on bone loss. It appears that the best results for preventing postmenopausal osteoporotic bone loss is when treatment is begun within 4 years after menopause.[5, 10] Regardless of when estrogen treatment is begun, once it is stopped there appears to be a rebound phenonemon in which bone loss is accelerated.

Regardless of the controversy surrounding the use of estrogens, its use in the treatment of osteoporosis is becoming more commonplace. It is now widely recognized that women who are at high risk of developing osteoporosis, or who have already developed it, should be considered candidates for estrogen replacement. The recommended regimen is 0.65 mg/day of conjugated estrogen for the first 25 days of the month and the addition of a progestational agent.[10] This regimen is best started shortly after menopause in high-risk women and may be continued indefinitely, although the length of treatment remains controversial. As long as treatment continues, routine periodic examinations for endometrial and breast cancer are imperative.

In addition to calcium supplementation, other therapeutic agents are being used and investigated in hopes of preventing bone loss by possibly affecting calcium and bone metabolism. Supplemental fluoride appears to stimulate osteoblastic activity. Its use in conjunction with both calcium supplements and calcium and estrogen replacement has a beneficial effect, lowering the incidence of vertebral fractures in postmenopausal women.[38] Despite its apparent clinical benefits, a large number of patients cannot tolerate the drug because of a high incidence of side effects, including gastric irritation and lower extremity pain.

The use of vitamin D would initially appear to have a beneficial effect on the absorption of calcium. However, the use of vitamin D in the treatment of osteoporosis is not indicated unless a deficiency of vitamin D can be identified. Although vitamin D does improve calcium absorption, it has a much less beneficial effect on bone loss, particularly in the postmenopausal patient; in large doses it may actually result in hypercalcemia, osteomalacia, and possibly renal failure.[27, 36] Other compounds, such as calcitonin, low-dose PTH, diphosphonates, and anabolic steroids, have been used in studies attempting to prevent or decrease osteoporotic bone loss.[36] The results of these studies are all of a preliminary nature, and none of these treatment modalities is currently being used outside of an experimental setting.

As overall medical care improves, the world population continues to live longer; consequently, osteoporosis is becoming more prevalent. As clinical awareness increases and diagnostic abilities improve, osteoporosis continues to be more readily diagnosed. The cornerstone of treatment is early recognition and prevention. Avoiding and discontinuing harmful practices that increase risks as well as maintaining an active exercise program constitute the simplest form of prevention. Supplemental calcium and estrogen replacement when indicated are the mainstays of pharmalogic treatment and should be started early in the evaluation and treatment of osteoporosis.

For the unfortunate patient with a symptomatic vertebral compression fracture, treatment should be supportive and directed toward returning the patient to an active and productive life. Fortunately, very few of these patients need treatment other than symptomatic relief, and only a small minority require surgical intervention.

References

1. Albright, F., Smith, P. H., and Richardson, A. M.: Postmenopausal osteoporosis. Its clinical features. J.A.M.A. 116:2465, 1941.
2. Aloia, J. F., Cohn, S. H., Ostuni, J. A., et al.: Prevention of involutional bone loss by exercise. Ann. Intern. Med. 89:356–358, 1978.
3. Amstutz, H. C., and Sissons, H. A.: The structure of the vertebral spongiosa. J. Bone Joint Surg. 51B:540, 1969.
4. Avioli, L. V.: Osteoporosis problem. Curr. Concepts Nutr. 5:99–103, 1977.
5. Boyle, L. T.: Treatments for postmenopausal osteoporosis. Lancet 1:376, 1981.
6. Brown, D. M., Jowsey, J., and Bradford, D. S.: Osteoporosis in ovarian dysgenesis. J. Pediatr. 84:816–820, 1974.
7. Burch, J. C., Byrd, B. F., and Vaughn, W. K.: The effect of long term estrogen replacement therapy. I. Metabolic effects. Am. J. Obstet. Gynecol. 133:525–526, 1979.
8. Chu, J., Schweid, A. I., and Weiss, N. S.: Survival among women with endometrial cancer: A comparison of estrogen users and non-users. Am. J. Obstet. Gynecol. 143:569–573, 1982.
9. Cummings, S. R.: Epidemiology of osteoporotic fractures: Selected topics. *In:* Roche, A. F. (ed.): Osteoporosis: Current Concepts, 1987, pp. 3–7.
10. Diddle, A. W., and Smith, I. Q.: Postmenopausal osteoporosis: The role of estrogens. South. Med. J. 77:868–874, 1984.
11. Eriksen, E. F., Mosekilde, L., and Melson, F.: Trabecular bone resorption depth decreases with age: Differences between males and females. Bone 6:141–146, 1985.
12. Frame, B., and Parfitt, A. M.: Osteomalacia: Current concepts. Ann. Intern. Med. 89:966–982, 1978.
13. Frost, H. M.: The pathemechanics of osteoporosis. Clin. Orthop. 200:198, 1985.
14. Frost, H. M.: Bone Remodeling and Its Relationship

to Metabolic Bone Disease. Springfield, Charles C Thomas, 1973.
15. Genant, H. K., Cann, C. E., Ettinger, B., and Gordon, G. S.: Quantitative computed tomography of vertebral spongiosa: A sensitive method for detecting early bone loss after oophorectomy. Ann. Intern. Med. 97:699–705, 1982.
16. Healey, J. H., and Lane, J. M.: Structural scoliosis in osteoporotic women. Clin. Orthop. 195:216–223, 1985.
17. Heaney, R. P.: Prevention of age-related osteoporosis in women. *In:* Avioli, L. V. (ed.): The Osteoporotic Syndrome. New York, Grune & Stratton, 1983, pp. 123–124.
18. Heaney, R. P., and Recker, R. R.: Effects of nitrogen, phosphorus and caffeine on calcium balance in women. J. Lab. Clin. Med. 99:46–55, 1982.
19. Heaney, R. P., Recker, R. R., and Saville, P. D.: Calcium balance and calcium requirements in middle-aged women. Am. J. Clin. Nutr. 30:1603–1611, 1977.
20. Holbrook, T. L., Grazier, K., Kelsey, J. L., and Strauffer, R. N.: The Frequency of Occurrence, Impact and Cost of Selected Musculoskeletal Conditions in the United States. Chicago, American Academy of Orthopaedic Surgeons, 1984.
21. Hormone Replacement Therapy and Endometrial Cancer (editorial). Lancet 1:577–578, 1977.
22. Johansson, B. W., Kaij, L., and Kullander, S.: On some late effects of bilateral oophorectomy in the age range 15–30 years. Acta Obstet. Gynecol. Scand. 54:449–461, 1975.
23. Kelsey, J. F.: Osteoporosis: Prevalence and incidence. *In:* Proceedings of the NIH Consensus Development Conference. Apr. 2–4, 1984, pp. 25–28.
24. Krolner, B., Toft, B., Nielsen, S. P., and Tondevold, E.: Physical exercise as prophylaxis against involutional vertebral bone loss: A controlled trial. Clin. Sci. 64:541–546, 1983.
25. Krolner, B., and Toft, B.: Vertebral bone loss: An unheeded side effect of therapeutic bed rest. Clin. Sci. 64:537–540, 1983.
26. Lachman, E.: Osteoporosis: The potentialities and limitations of its roentgenographic diagnosis. A.J.R. 74:712–715, 1955.
27. Lukert, B. P.: Osteoporosis—a review and update. Arch. Phys. Med. Rehab. 63:480–487, 1982.
28. Mazess, R. B.: On aging bone loss. Clin. Orthop. 165:239–252, 1982.
29. Meema, H. E., Bunker, M. L., and Meema, S.: Loss of compact bone due to menopause. Obstet. Gynecol. 26:333–343, 1965.
30. Pagninini-Hill, A., Ross, R. K., and Gerkins, V. R.: Menopausal estrogen therapy and hip fractures. Ann. Intern. Med. 95:28–31, 1981.
31. Parfitt, A. M.: The actions of parathyroid hormone on bone. Relation to bone remodeling and turnover, calcium homeostasis and metabolic bone disease. Metabolism 25:809, 1976.
32. Parfitt, A. M.: The physiologic and clinical significance of bone histomorphometric data. *In:* Recker, R. (ed.): Bone histomorphometry: Techniques and Interpretations. Boca Raton, C.R.C. Press, Inc., 1983.
33. Parfitt, A. M., and Kleerekoper, M.: The Divalention Homeostatic System: Physiology and Metabolism of Calcium, Phosphorus, Magnesium and Bone. *In:* Maxwell, M. H., and Kleeman, C. R. (eds.): Clinical Disorders of Fluid and Electrolyte Metabolism. New York, McGraw-Hill, 1979, pp. 269–398.
34. Pommer, G.: Untersuchungen uber Osteomalacie und Rachitis Neb Beitragen Zur Kenntnis der Krochen Resporation Und Apposition in Verschiedenen Altersperioden Und Der Durchborende Gefasse. Leipzig.
35. Raymakers, J. A., Hoekstra, O., Van Putten, J., et al.: Fracture prevalence and bone mineral mass in osteoporosis measured with computed tomography and dual energy photon absorptiometry. Skeletal Radiol. 15:191–197, 1986.
36. Riggs, B. L., and Melton, L. J.: Involutional Osteoporosis. N. Engl. J. Med. 314:1676, 1986.
37. Riggs, B. L., and Melton, L. J.: Evidence for two distinct syndromes of involutional osteoporosis. Am. J. Med. 75:899, 1983.
38. Riggs, B. L., Seeman, E., Hodgson, S. F., et al.: Effects of the fluoride/calcium regimen on vertebral fracture occurrence in postmenopausal osteoporosis. N. Engl. J. Med. 306:446–450, 1982.
39. Riggs, B. L., Wahner, H. W., Dunn, W. L., et al.: Differential changes in bone mineral density of appendicular and axial skeleton with aging. J. Clin. Invest. 67:328–335, 1981.
40. Rockoff, S. D., Sweet, E., and Bleustein, J.: The relative contribution of trabecular and cortical bone to the strength of human lumbar vertebrae. Calc. Tissue Res. 3:163, 1969.
41. Rothman, R. H., and Simeon, E. A.: The Spine. Philadelphia, W. B. Saunders, 1982.
42. Salmi, T.: Risk factors in endometrial carcinoma with special reference to the use of estrogens. Acta Obstet. Gynecol. Scand. 86(Suppl.):1–119, 1979.
43. Schneider, R.: Radiologic methods of evaluating generalized osteopenia. Orthop. Clin. North Am. 15:631–650, 1984.
44. Schwartz, M., Anwah, I., and Levy, R. N.: Variations in treatment of postmenopausal osteoporosis. Clin. Orthop. 192:180–184, 1985.
45. Seeman, E., Melton, L. J., III, O'Fallon, W. M., and Riggs, B. L.: Risk factors for spinal osteoporosis in Men. Am. J. Med. 75:977–983, 1983.
46. Teter, J.: International congress on the menopause. Am. Geriatr. Soc. Grande Matte, France, August 1976. Cited by Patton, G. D.: The Estrogen Controversy. Female Patient 7:47–49, 1982.
47. Wahner, H. W., Dunn, W. L., and Riggs, L. B.: Assessment of bone mineral. Part 2. J. Nucl. Med. 25:1241–1253, 1984.
48. Walker, A. R. P.: The human requirement of calcium. Should low intakes be supplemented? Am. J. Clin. Nutr. 25:518–520, 1972.
49. Whitehead, M. I., Campbell, S. C., King, R. J. B., et al.: Estrogen Treatment and Endometrial Carcinoma (letter). Br. Med. J. 2:453–454, 1977.
50. Wolff, J.: Das Gesetz Der Transformation der Knochen. Berlin, A. Hirchwald, 1892.

16 □ Rehabilitation

Arthur H. White
Robin McKenzie
Stanley V. Paris
Daniel Stein
Yizhar Floman
Tom G. Mayer

BACK SCHOOL: STATE OF THE ART

Arthur H. White

Education, exercise, and body positioning have been used as a treatment for low back pain for hundreds of years.[3] Not until the middle of the twentieth century, however, did modern medicine begin to formulate structured educational and exercise programs for a large number of patients.[59, 60]

By 1960 some physicians, such as Fahrni,[23, 24, 25] had subspecialized, researched, and formulated conservative care programs for their patients. In the 1960s Sweden was one of the most active areas of spinal research in the world. Back education was provided at the Volvo factory outside of Goteborg and was referred to as *back school*. Later, one of the most significant articles in the literature was written from that experience.[11] In the early 1970s other physicians, as a result of their growing interest in spinal problems, developed back schools in their areas of the world.[39, 40, 56, 69, 70, 107, 108, 117–119] By 1980, there were hundreds of back schools throughout the world, and now there are thousands.[87]

There is no single formula by which all back schools operate. The specific needs of therapists, trainers, and physicians have led to a wide variety of back schools.[7–9, 13, 22, 41, 50, 62, 65, 83, 87, 89, 93, 99, 108–115, 120] The only common denominator among all of these schools seems to be education. Some provide education only and no exercise training. Others are primarily exercise programs, some providing large and expensive exercise machines and little or no education, except for perhaps a booklet or videotape on proper back health care.

In the scientific literature there is little agreement as to what should be taught in back schools. So many studies on low back pain have been performed that one can validate almost any personal point of view and thus validate the philosophy of any back school.[1, 16, 19, 64, 92] However, some agreement and a common approach to education and exercises exist in most back schools.[57]

EDUCATION

Education has been the strongest tool that the medical profession has had available. We have fought every disease with education, from the bubonic plague of centuries ago to the current plague of acquired immunodeficiency syndrome (AIDS). Currently, medicine is verifying the value of education for such diseases as diabetes and hemophilia.[46, 53, 67, 74, 91] Education has also proven to be effective in decreasing the incidence of low back pain and the amount of lost time and number of dollars spent in industrial low back injuries.[11, 70]

As the subspecialty of the diagnosis and treatment of low back pain developed over the last 50 years, it was only a matter of time before specialists began to use the tools of education and to perfect the means of delivery. Currently back school education is found in virtually every spine center and is available through most physical therapists. Formal back schools, although once unique physical structures, now blend imperceptibly into most spine centers, rehabilitation programs, and physical therapy offices. One does not need to take a special course or build a specific structure within which to establish a back school. Back school can be offered on the examining table, in a classroom, or by cassettes and videotapes.[109]

EXERCISE

It is well known that smoking, vibration, weakness, and labor that overutilizes the spine are detrimental factors that contribute to low back pain.[5, 33, 34, 47, 48, 54, 83, 116] General exercise, strengthening abdominal and trunk muscles, and stretching to attain flexibility are useful for back health care.[6, 9, 14, 15, 22, 30–32, 49, 50, 59, 60, 82, 83, 95] Stretching the hamstrings, in particular, is taught to enable facile body positioning without overusing the spine.[31, 49, 50, 59] Similarly, strength of the lower extremities is thought to give the pelvis and spine a stronger base from which to function and position.[66, 85] The intradiscal pressure studies have led to some of the teaching about body positioning and the avoidance of certain postures, especially sitting.[2, 4, 5, 10, 18, 78, 79, 81] There has recently been a surge in the popularity of trunk-strengthening machines that use computerized methods of testing.[64, 68, 72, 86, 98, 101] For various theoretical reasons, the abdominal musculature and extensor trunk musculature are strengthened.[45, 71, 80, 88, 96, 97, 102, 103] Such simple exercises as partial sit-ups or prone back extension exercises are used in some clinics, whereas others use pieces of computerized exercise equipment that cost tens of thousands of dollars.

The "proper" methods of human bending, lifting, and locomotion have been developed in order to position the pelvis under the spine and to allow for the most efficient use of spinal musculature and ligaments.[23, 25, 59, 60, 110] Lifting techniques have been standardized for keeping the load close to the body and the spine straight, and for bending the knees.[111] Much of this has come from biomechanical studies.[76, 77, 90, 106]

Any or all of these principles can be applied to any area of daily living. One can theorize and, using these principles, teach such things as how to make a bed most safely, get into and out of a car, and perform other activities related to housework, athletics, and labor.[111]

When one superimposes on this basic knowledge the pathophysiologic or pathoanatomic findings of a particular patient, more specific back education and training develop. If, for example, a patient is known to have severe spinal stenosis that creates leg pain, numbness, and tingling with spinal extension, the patient is taught to avoid extension, develop strength, and apply body mechanics that allow the performance of normal activities with the pelvis and the lumbar spine aligned in a more flexed posture. The opposite posturing of spinal extension may be used for a patient with a disc problem that has typically created pain with lumbar flexion and has been relieved by repeated extension; the McKenzie exercises are an example.[73] As practitioners have worked with a great variety of patients over the years, innumerable exercises, body mechanics concepts, and mobilization and manipulation programs have developed and have been incorporated into back schools.

Some of the more common principles and programs will now be described. None of the following information is intended to be offered as absolutely scientifically validated; it is information that I find most commonly provided in back schools, generally in a form that patients understand, and that has been shown to reduce the incidence of low back pain in various patient populations.[11, 57, 63, 70, 99]

Severe back pain is usually a sign that the back has been abused, and the conditions surrounding the incident should be investigated. Although muscles may occasionally be the primary source of severe low back pain, they frequently go into protective muscle spasm in response to a more significant pathoanatomic lesion.[26–29, 35, 37, 78–83, 87] Disregarding a single incident of acute low back pain is probably not in the best interest of a patient. Evaluating the conditions surrounding the low back incident need not be very time consuming or expensive.[57, 98, 110] Simple measures can be instituted to make changes in a patient's weaknesses, inflexibilities, body mechanics, understanding, and the ergonomics during work and recreation.[11, 70, 99, 107, 111]

Resting an acutely painful back is a principle common to most back schools.[9, 17, 23, 25] More than a few days of bed rest, however, is generally believed to be harmful, from weakness and stiffness, rather than helpful.[17, 42–44, 61, 105] Pain control measures, such as locally applied ice, are taught to the patient. If certain postures and exercises have been found to be helpful in evaluating patients, they are taught and used on a regular basis while the individuals are observed for improvement.[111] Restful positions are then taught to the patients while they are on their feet. There is a perfect alignment position for each pathoanatomic entity, in which there is less pain and less spasm. This type of positioning for improving the body mechanics of the activities of daily living is taught to and practiced by each patient.[75, 104, 111]

After the acute phase has subsided, more generalized strengthening, flexibility, and body mechanics principles are taught and practiced.[1, 111] A nurse, for example, who has recurrent injuries from lifting patients in bed would develop the strength, flexibility, and a better understanding of the body mechanics necessary to perform that task and practice it repeatedly in an attempt to form new and improved habits. As tasks become more complex and uncontrollable, the back school training, also, can become quite complex.[110] Similarly, as the underlying pathoanatomic lesion becomes more severe, the changes in strength and intensity of body mechanics become more difficult. For these reasons the specific type of back school training called *stabilization* has developed.[12, 21, 38, 51, 52, 58, 75, 100, 104, 106]

STABILIZATION TRAINING

One definition of stabilization training is placing the diseased spinal segment in its most anatomic, pain-free, and balanced position and holding it there with muscular forces while accomplishing tasks of living. The strength and coordination, trial and error, concentration, and repetition needed by some individuals to accomplish stabilization is phenomenal. When a patient is strongly motivated and the trainer or therapist is well trained and has patience, the activities of almost any low back patient can be improved, and many can return to normal activities.

Some of the techniques and exercises for stabilization training are as follows.

An average patient with a disc problem without significant neurologic loss would begin stabilization training while lying supine. Tightening the abdominal musculature is first practiced by doing partial sit-up exercises, contracting the diaphragm and learning to continue to breathe while doing so. Range of motion from the extreme of maximal lordosis to maximal pelvic tilt is practiced until a comfortable position of spinal alignment is obtained (Fig. 1). The trainer's hand can be placed underneath the area of the patient's lumbar lordosis to assure the neutral position. Some patients find comfort with forceful flattening of the spine. Other patients need maximum lordosis for comfort. Most patients are comfortable between the extremes of lordosis and pelvic tilt. Once the optimum position is achieved, the abdominal musculature is contracted and the diaphragm is stabilized. Motion of the extremities can then begin; one extremity at a time is lifted slowly as the therapist verifies the patient's ability to maintain the stabilized neutral position. The extremities are then raised faster and alternately until the patient is simultaneously doing a bicycling motion with the legs and a waving motion of the arms, from side to side and over the head (Fig. 2). There should be no pain, and the patient should show no evidence of spinal motion. This can be accentuated by balancing a stick horizontally across the patient's abdomen or chest (Fig. 3) or by again placing a hand behind the patient's back with a finger in each interspinous space to feel for motion.

Stabilization training is also performed with the patient lying prone (Fig. 4). This is slightly more difficult than lying supine, for most patients. The prone patient is instructed to, again, alternately raise one extremity (Fig. 5) and then the other; then the two are raised simultaneously, while the painless neutral position is maintained. It is easier to observe the spine for motion in this position (Fig. 6).

The next logical progression from the prone position is to the position of kneeling. A patient kneels, finds the neutral, balanced pain-free position with a cat-like rounding of the back, and then relaxes into lordosis

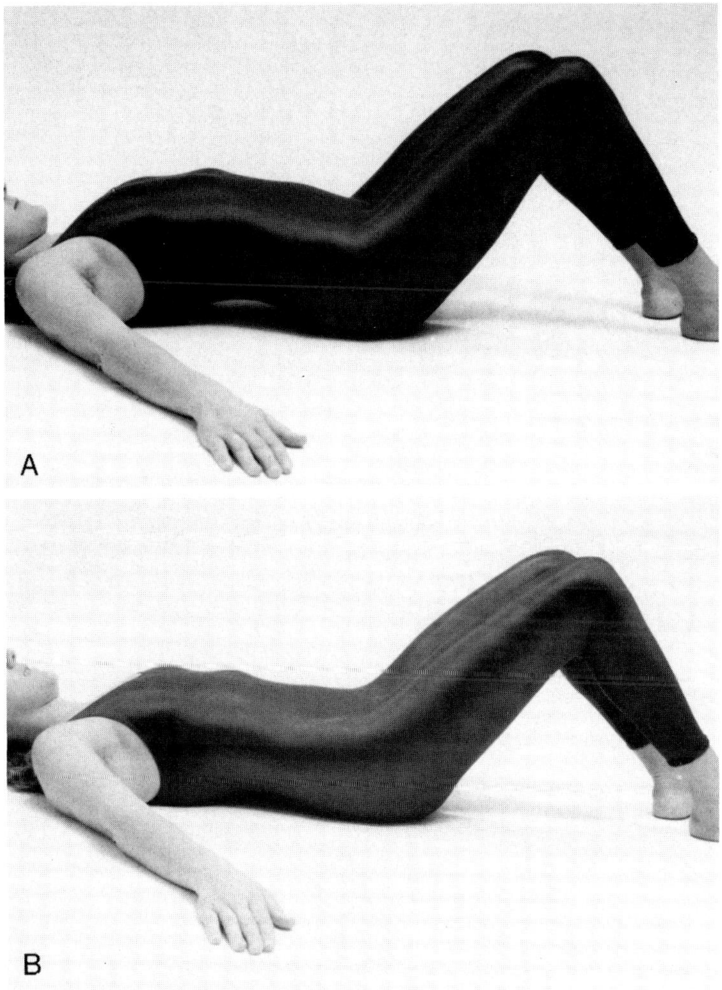

Figure 1 □ *A, B,* Neutral position is found by having the patient test range of motion from maximal lordosis to maximal pelvic tilt. Most patients find that the neutral, pain-free position is between these extremes.

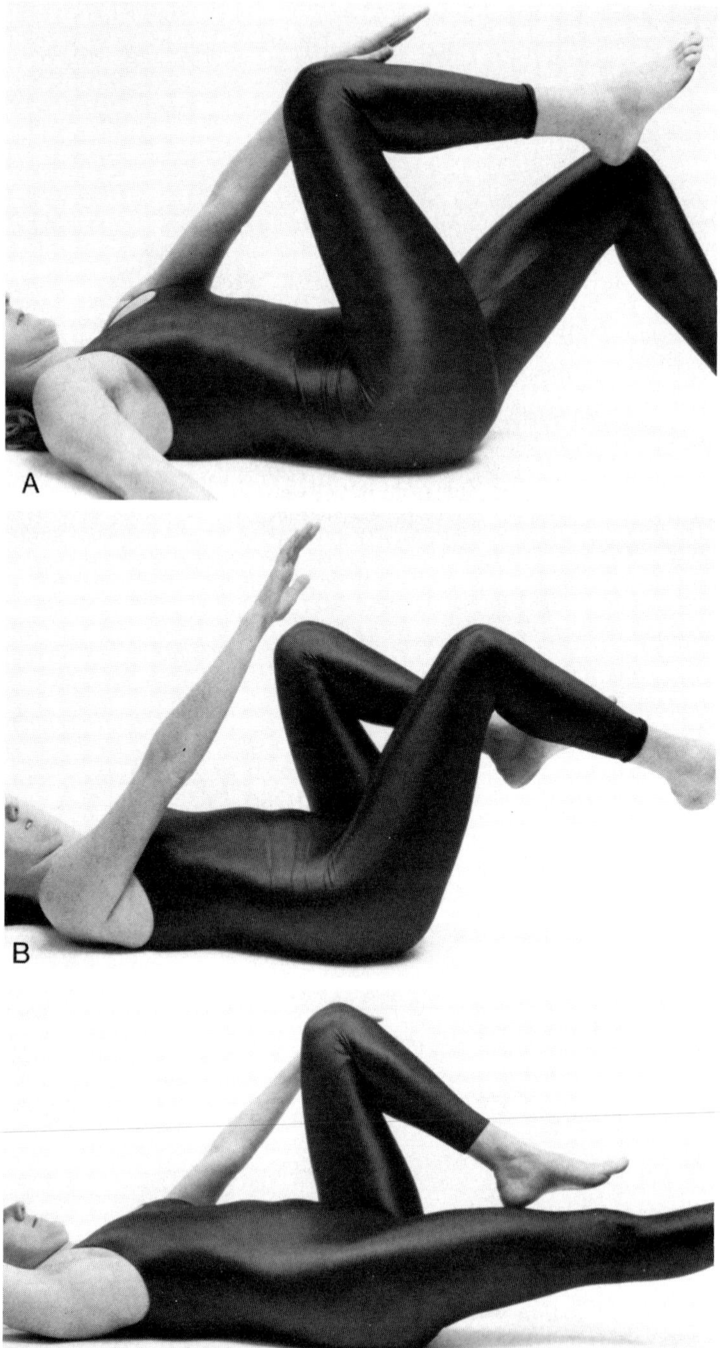

Figure 2 □ *A–C,* Photographs demonstrate maintenance of the neutral position while the extremities are raised, as the patient is taught to move the extremities faster and faster.

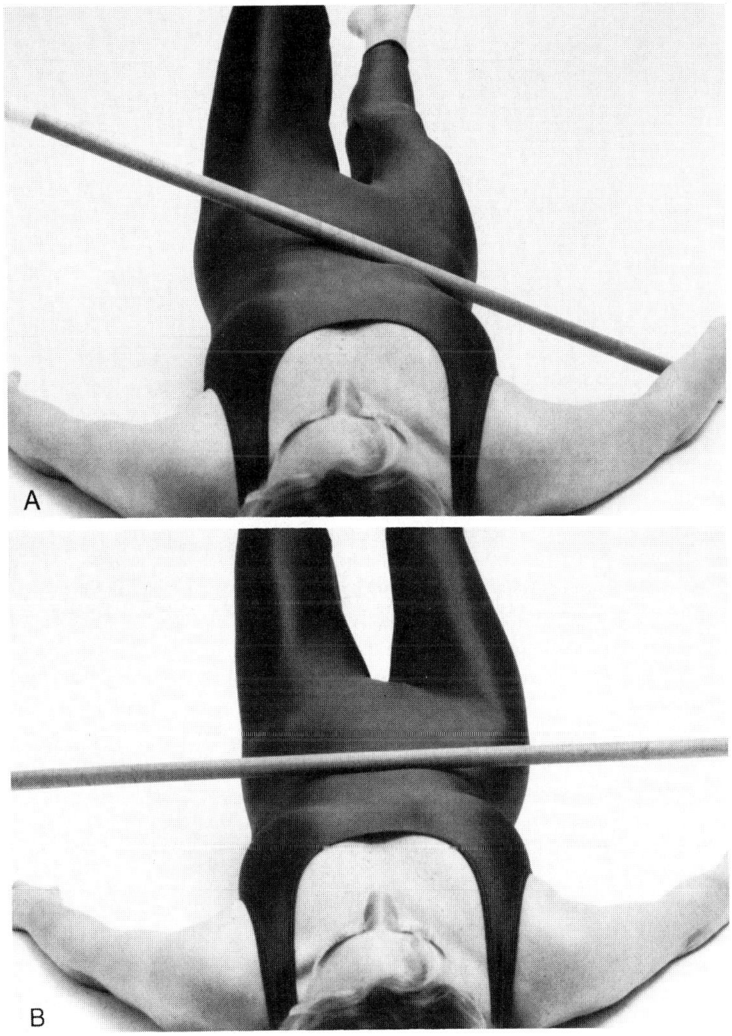

Figure 3 □ *A, B,* Photographs demonstrate the use of a wooden stick across the abdomen to assess stabilization skills or lack thereof.

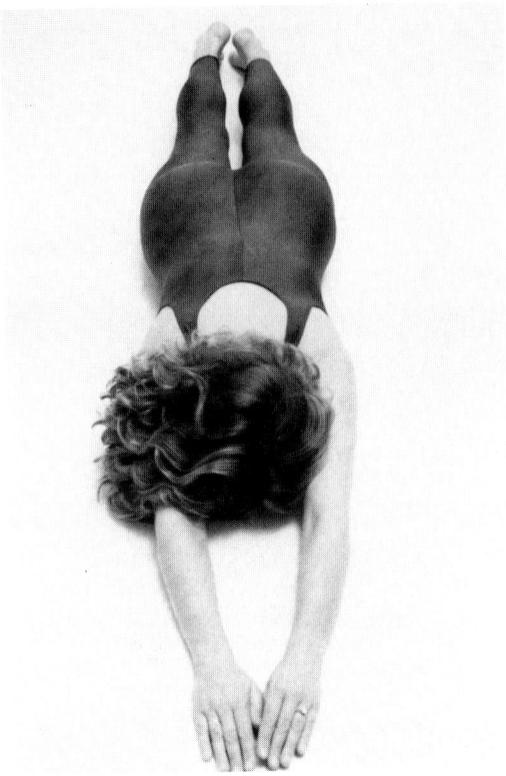

Figure 4 □ Determining neutral position for stabilization in the prone position.

(hump–sag) exercises (Fig. 7). Once the neutral, balanced pain-free kneeling position is found, the patient practices raising one extremity, then another, and eventually two extremities without having pain or any spinal motion. Again, a good test for motion, and a useful example for the patient, is balancing a stick horizontally across the patient's back while he or she watches in the mirror to see that the stick may be wavering, if not falling off the back (Fig. 8).

Stabilization can next be carried into the standing position. An infinite variety of floor exercises can be performed using such objects as Swedish balls, which are large air-filled rubber balls on which the legs are balanced as the patient lies supine in a hip- and knee-flexed position (90/90). The ball creates less stability than the floor and requires greater strength and stabilization control to avoid spinal motion (Fig. 9). Mirrors are extremely valuable in standing stabilization; the patients can watch themselves as they stand and find the neutral position (Fig. 10). They may first back up against a wall to find the neutral stabilized position and then move away from the wall to begin moving one extremity after another, eventually standing on one foot (Fig. 11), perhaps even with a weight in one hand. Increasing degrees of force are then introduced as an attempt to offset the patient's stability. This includes jousting with patient partners. Two patients face each other and grasp a stick or baton, which is mutually held between them. They try to force each other off center, attempting to maintain a neutral position. (This is somewhat akin to Little John fighting on the bridge with his staff.) Instead of striking, however, the opponents slowly exert displacing forces under the direction and supervision of the trainer, who assesses the stabilizing capabilities as the patients joust (Fig. 12).

As a patient's physical demands for such activities of heavy labor and contact sports increase, the stabilization training needs to be similarly aggressive. Until this point in the training, the stabilization has been relatively impractical, although tremendous strength and endurance have been achieved. The exercises described so far are rarely

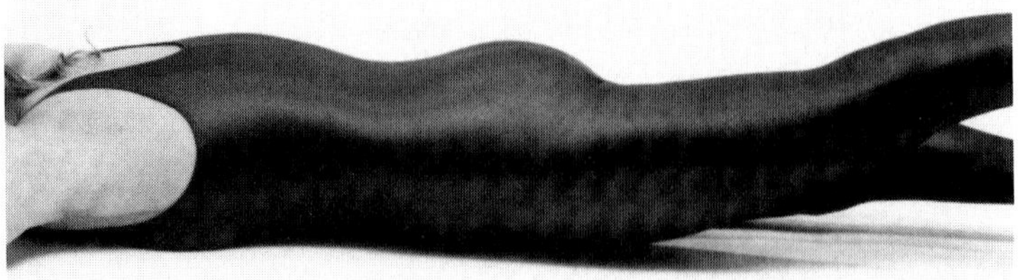

Figure 5 □ Maintaining the neutral position in the prone position and attempting to raise the leg.

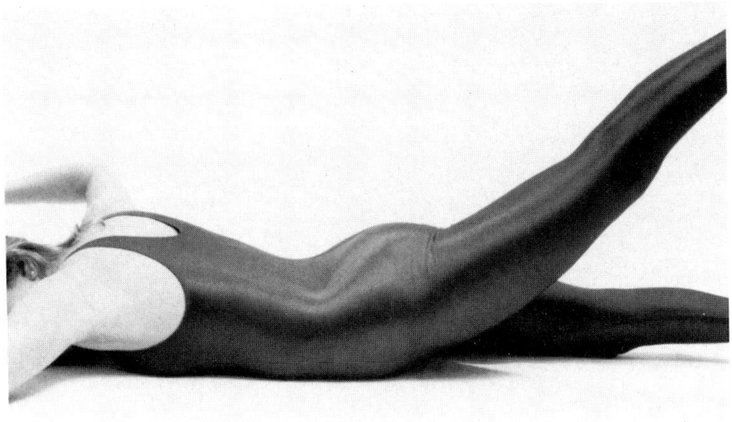

Figure 6 □ Losing the neutral positioning while raising opposite extremities.

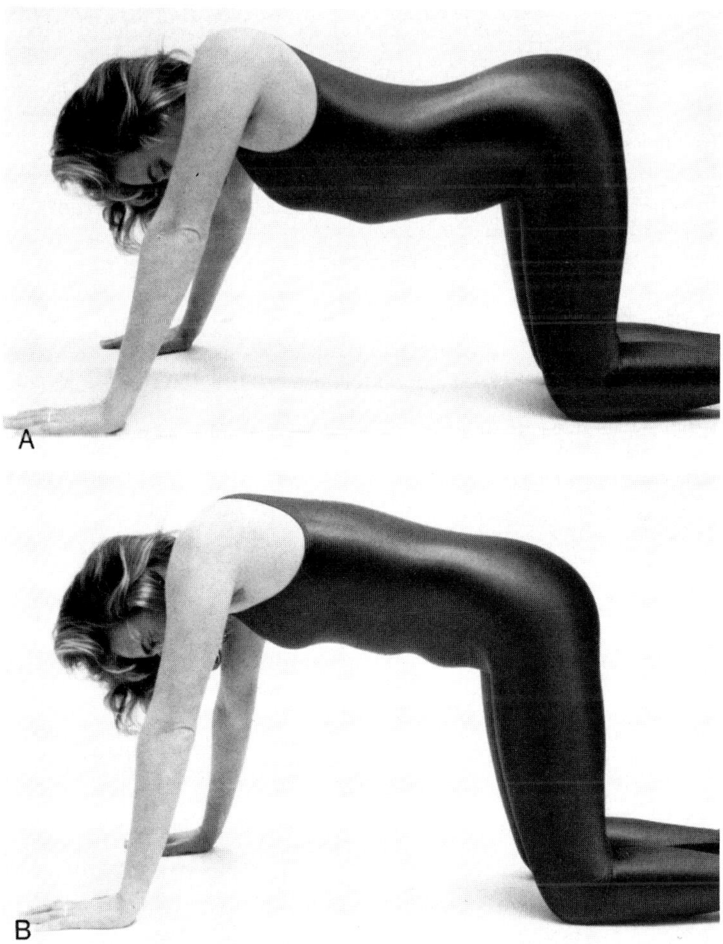

Figure 7 □ *A, B,* Finding and maintaining the neutral position on all fours.

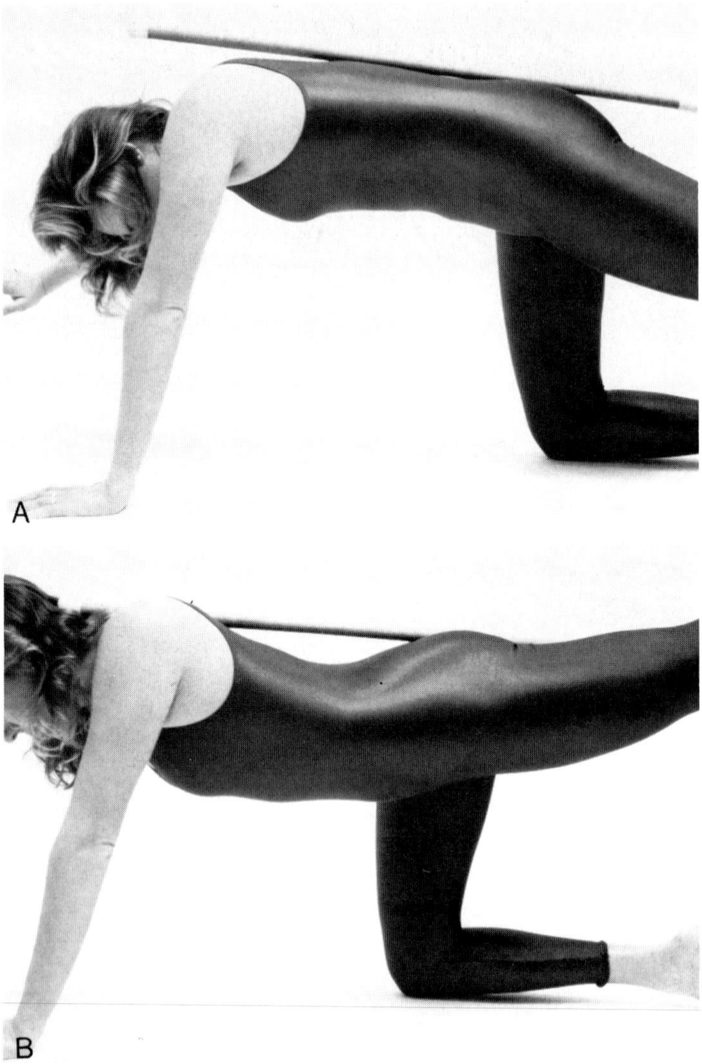

Figure 8 □ *A, B,* Using the wooden stick to monitor stabilization skills or to observe inability to maintain a neutral position while kneeling.

applicable to daily activities. At this point in training, patients need to move about more freely and actively, just as they do in their daily lives, performing such activities as walking rapidly with weights in their hands while maintaining stabilization. A treadmill may first be utilized so that the trainer can easily test and verify satisfactory stabilization techniques. Once these are verified, the patients are allowed to take long walks on their own, remaining pain free and testing their endurance. Low-impact aerobics and dancing programs can be used to teach stabilization techniques under more enjoyable circumstances. Jogging with stabilization can be practiced on a treadmill, then continued daily. This is a new way to jog. It is difficult to breathe while tightening the abdominal musculature. The impact of the foot hitting the ground produces a vibration through the leg and pelvis into the spine. This vibration is cushioned by stabilization of the spine, not only by means of the abdominal musculature, but also by using greater knee flexion and making more use of the quadriceps and hamstring muscles to cushion part of the vibration on the spine.

Contact sports require patients to receive blows by other individuals. This frequently entails unexpected trauma or a very short warning time in which to prepare to receive a blow. Practice, therefore, must lead to rapid stabilization followed by receiving blows of increasing intensity (Fig. 13). We have developed programs for professional athletes of competitive sports by having them train in the martial arts. The martial arts, of course, have dealt with blows, trauma, and human interaction for centuries. Specific techniques have been developed and honed to fine training programs.

No activity simulation program can surpass the activity itself. If the patient is a second-base baseball player, there is no better place to train him than at second base. All the required positions and motions are analyzed for efficiency, stabilization, and energy conservation. The player must be able to stabilize the spine while jumping, falling, rolling, throwing, and catching (Figs. 14 and 15), and the required maneuvers are taught and practiced until they become virtually natural reflexes.

It is amazing, and probably the basis of all low back pain problems, that many physically accomplished individuals and athletes are seemingly nontrainable because of established patterns of movement that lead to injury after injury (perfect body mechanics are not a requirement for superb athletic performance). However, we have known for years that teaching patterns of movement and posture can greatly improve athletic and artistic prowess. Similarly, the martial arts can advance an individual from a brown belt to a black belt as he or she perfects movement, posture, and body mechanics (Fig. 16). There is no end to the training that we can accomplish with posture, strength, and body mechanics—and now with stabilization.

Although some movement patterns may make an individual highly susceptible to back injuries and others virtually immune to them, it is possible to improve the strength, body mechanics, and stabilization capability of any human being, despite the present level of conditioning. A thorough analysis of the individual's needs, strengths, and weaknesses is necessary to devise a useful training program. If we can train patients to protect their backs during times of potential injury, we can possibly eliminate the epidemic of low back pain.

OTHER SPECIFIC BACK SCHOOL SUBDIVISIONS

After basic back school principles have been taught and basic body mechanics have been learned, most mild and moderate back problems will have been controlled. If, however, the underlying condition is more severe, such as that of a frankly herniated lumbar disc, advanced spinal stenosis, nerve root irritation, and instability, it will require more than simply education and deliberate cautious movement (body mechanics).

Hospital Back School

A patient whose back problem is so severe that standing or self care is virtually impossible may require hospitalization. This individual needs to be able to find a pain-free position in bed and simply get into and out of bed without causing further damage or increasing pain. Exercises can be performed in bed; these include isometric abdominal strengthening, quadriceps isometric strengthening, and perhaps upper-extremity strengthening with weights, rings, or pulleys. We do not want patients to be-

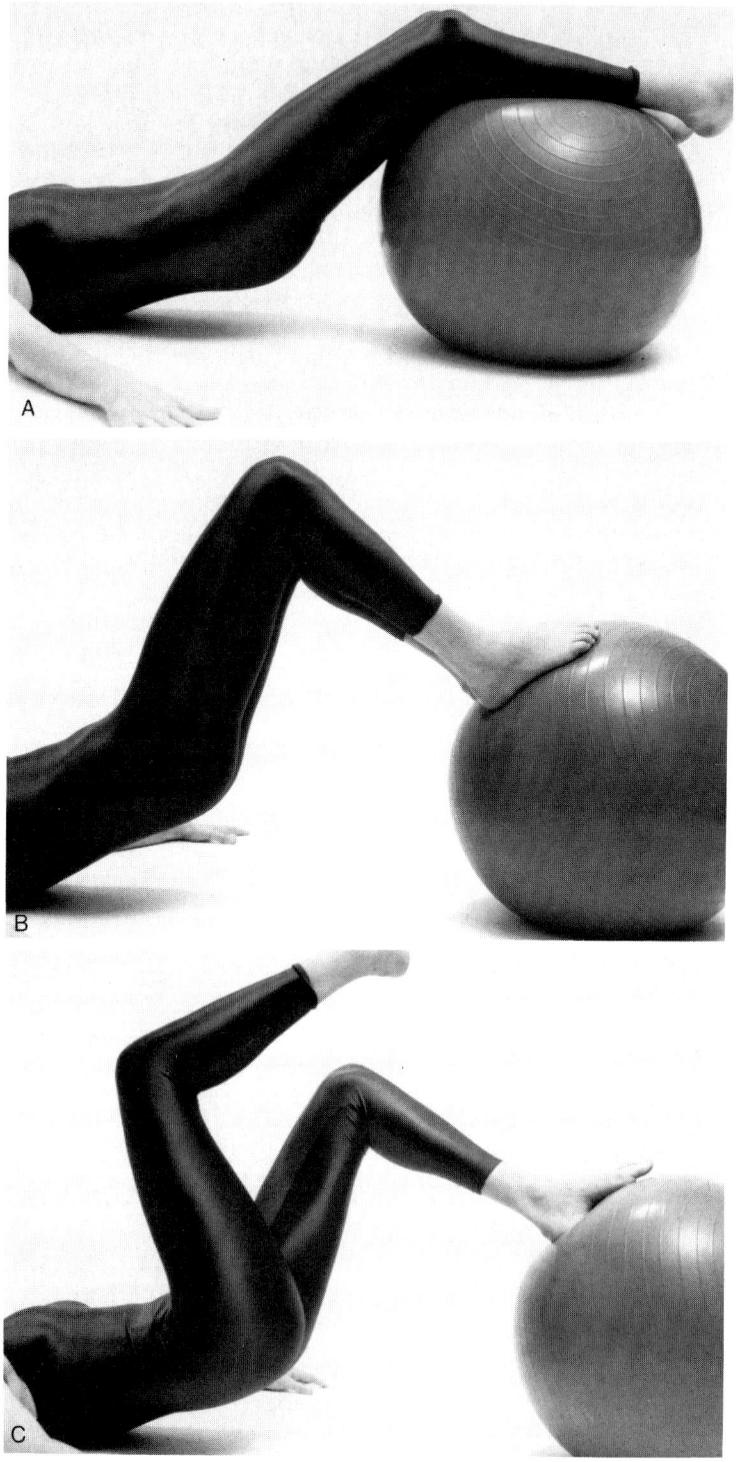

Figure 9 □ *A–E,* Swedish balls are used to assess the patient's stabilization skills before training is carried to the standing position.

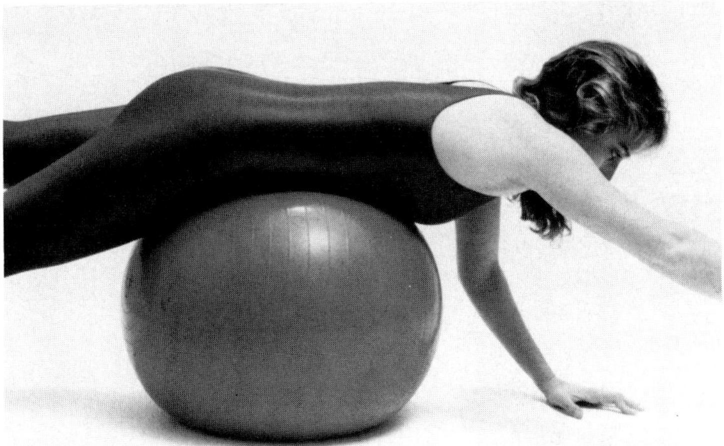

D

Figure 9 *Continued*

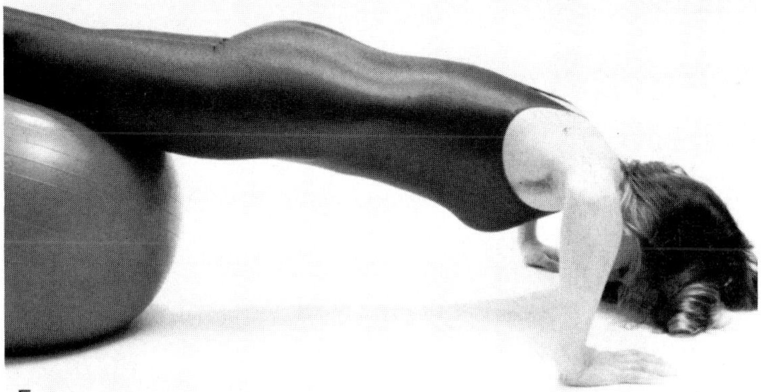

E

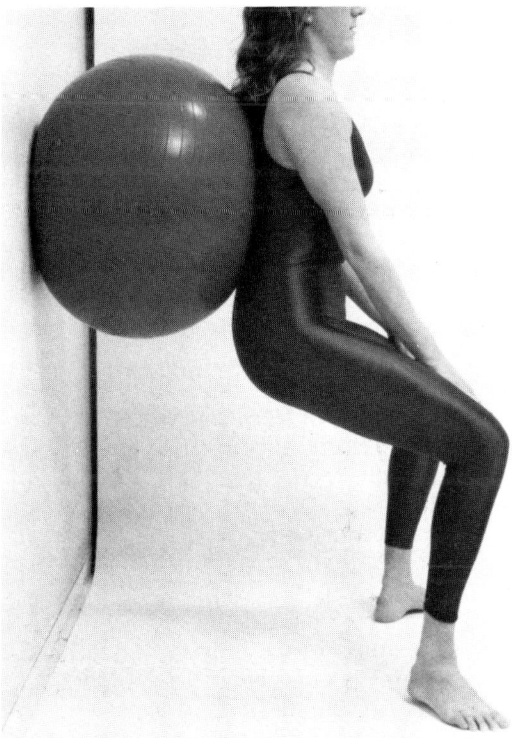

Figure 10 □ Neutral positioning with the Swedish ball behind the back to develop and advance stabilization skills.

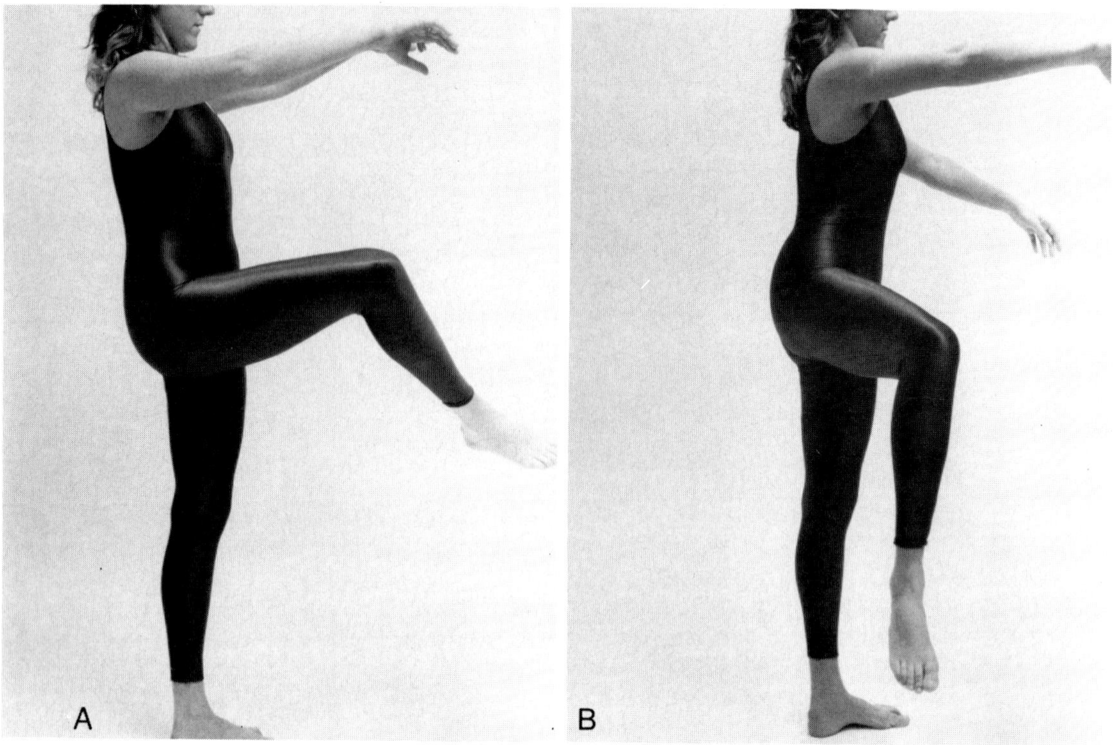

Figure 11 □ *A, B,* Holding a neutral position while standing on one leg.

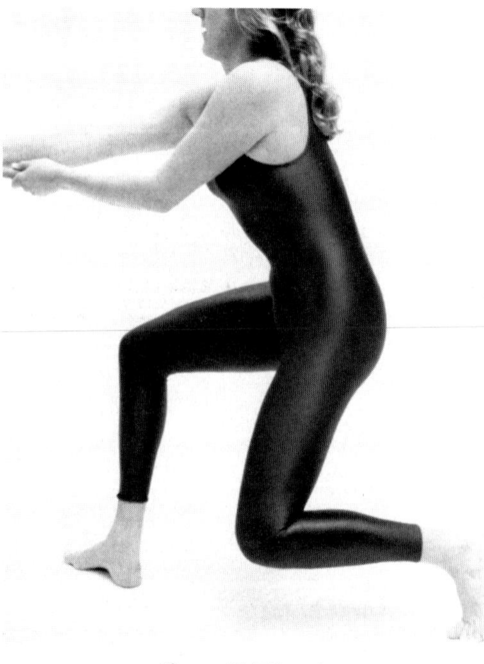

Figure 12 □ Jousting.

come weaker and stiffer while undergoing diagnostic evaluations or while waiting for bed rest to reduce inflammation. Epidural blocks are frequently used in order to reduce vertebral canal inflammation and reduce the need for bed rest. At any rate, the patient needs to achieve a pain-free state and maintain it with training, abdominal bracing, and cautious positioning and movement.

Some spinal conditions can be improved with positions of extension, and others with positions of flexion. A hospital back school therapist, after consultation with the physician, may attempt various positioning techniques to relieve the patient's pain and improve function. If, for example, a patient improves while lying prone rather than supine and then improves further with progressive extension exercises, additional training of the same type is pursued. Other patients improve with flexion. Once the position of maximum benefit is understood, further back school training based on the

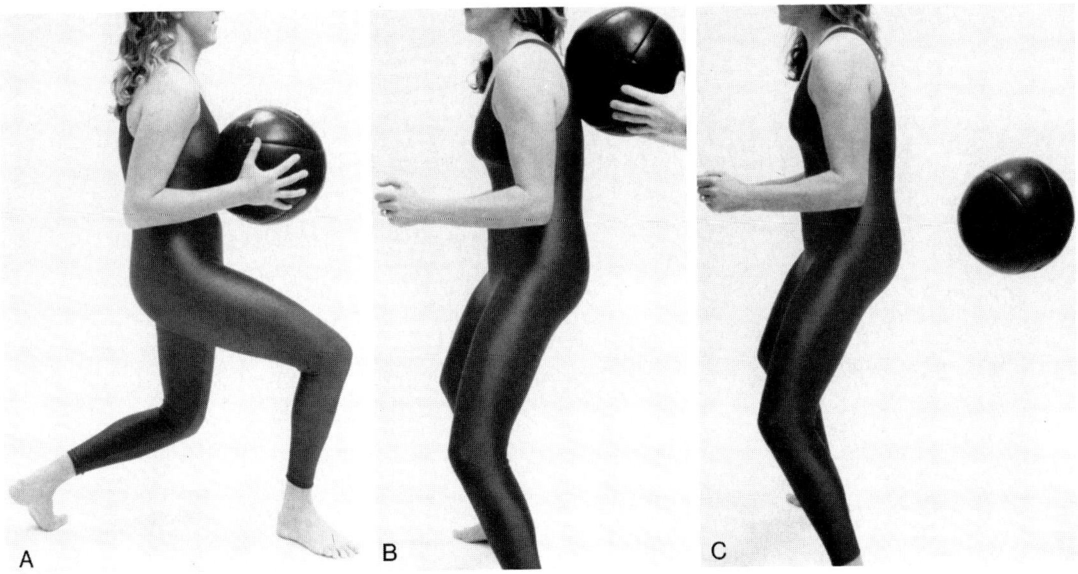

Figure 13 □ *A–C,* Using a medicine ball to initially train the athlete-patient how to receive blows sustained during contact sports.

same principles is offered. Patients who become ambulatory and can be discharged from the hospital by using these techniques are then transferred to an outpatient back school for long-range strengthening, increasing flexibility, and training in body mechanics.

If surgery is necessary, back school in the hospital teaches patients what to expect afterward. They are taught how to log roll, transfer, and get into and out of bed in the least traumatic fashion.

When surgery is required, the patient has been trained and can rapidly and safely become active after surgery. If a fusion has been performed, stabilization in a neutral position is emphasized. If a posterior interbody fusion has been performed, the patient has been trained and will maintain an extension posture. With an anterior interbody fusion, a lumbar flexion posture is adopted. Simple laminectomy and discectomy allow midrange movement, but full flexion and loading are avoided for several months. All surgical patients continue training to achieve maximum flexibility of hamstrings and hip joints. Exercises to strengthen the abdomen, gluteus, and quadriceps are continued throughout all phases of rehabilitation.

Back school trainers also participate in training more disabled patients to use supportive devices such as walkers, crutches, and canes. They are taught to order and fit lumbosacral corsets and body jackets. Gravity traction, inversion traction, autotraction, and other forms of passive and active positioning are available to the well-trained back school specialist.

In the diagnostic phase of hospitalization, back school therapists participate by doing dynamic evaluations when the patient is first admitted to the hospital and then repeating similar evaluations after each diagnostic block and each trial of therapy. The back school therapist participates in team meetings to confirm his or her findings throughout the diagnostic evaluation and make recommendations with regard to strengthening, flexibility, endurance, and body mechanics.

Activity Simulation

As back schools expand to increasingly difficult situations, it has become necessary to improve techniques of training and education. Innumerable audiovisuals, exercise programs, books, and pamphlets have been developed. Specialists in communication have made the information related to back school understandable for all levels of society. The information has also been translated into many languages. There is now nothing to prevent one from communicating this information to any patient.

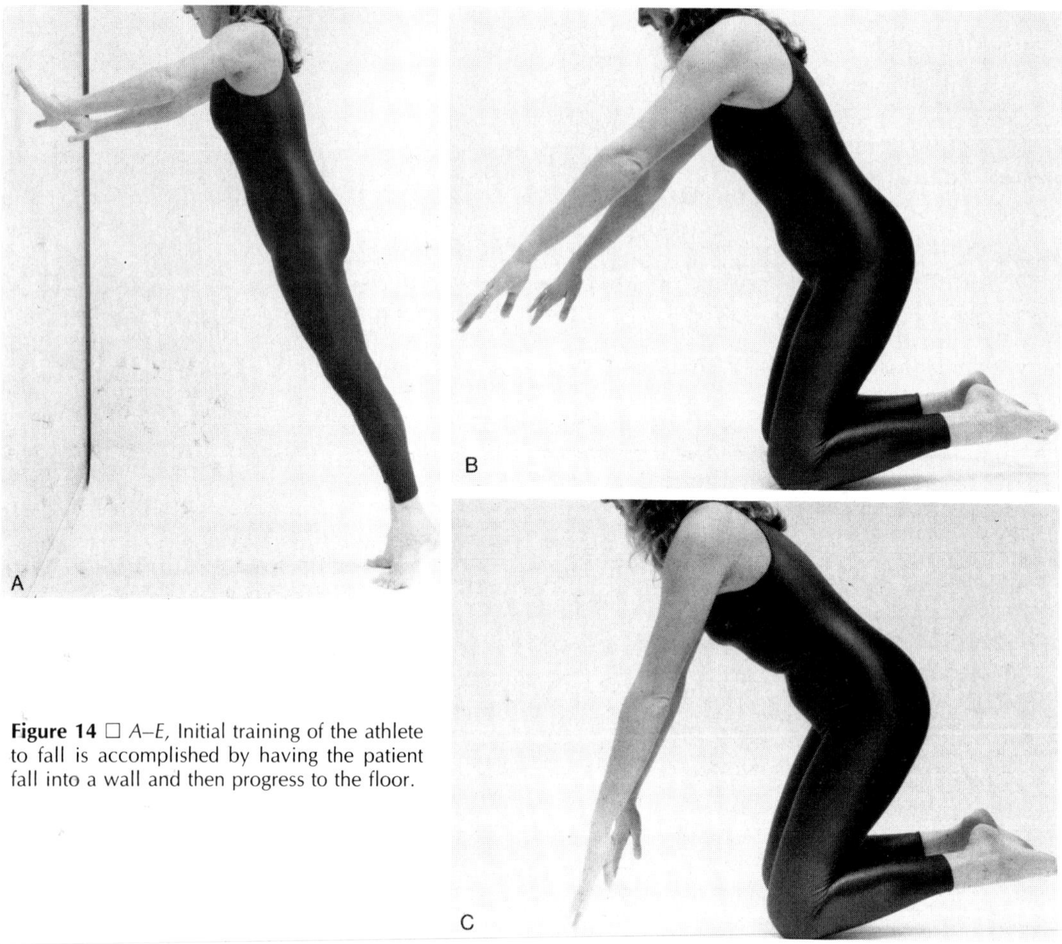

Figure 14 □ *A–E,* Initial training of the athlete to fall is accomplished by having the patient fall into a wall and then progress to the floor.

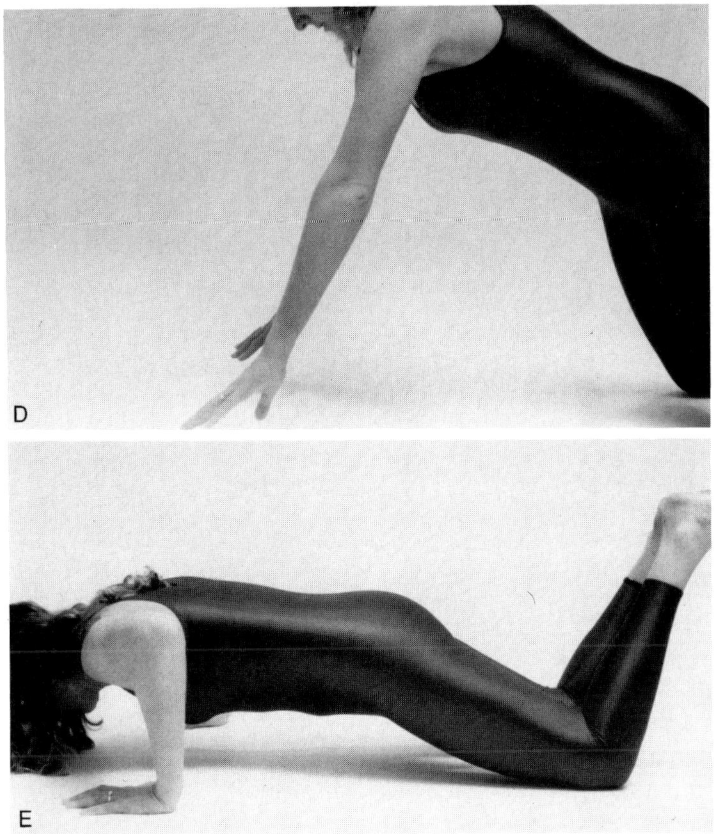

Figure 14 *Continued*

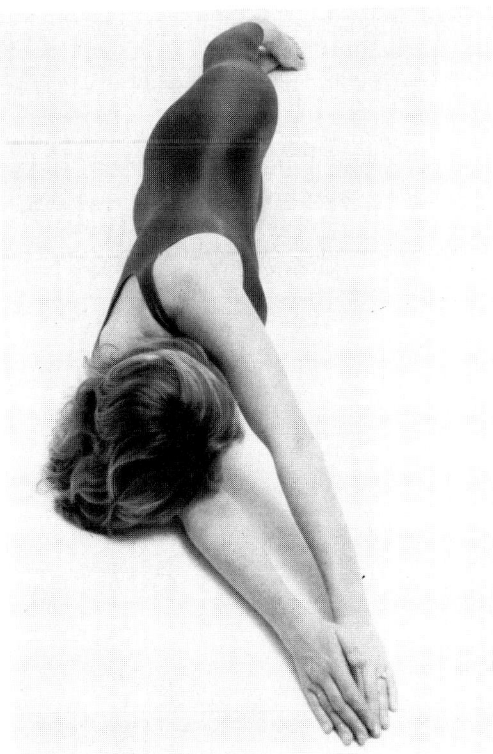

Figure 15 □ As a drill, the athlete-patient learns to maintain neutral positioning while rolling on the floor.

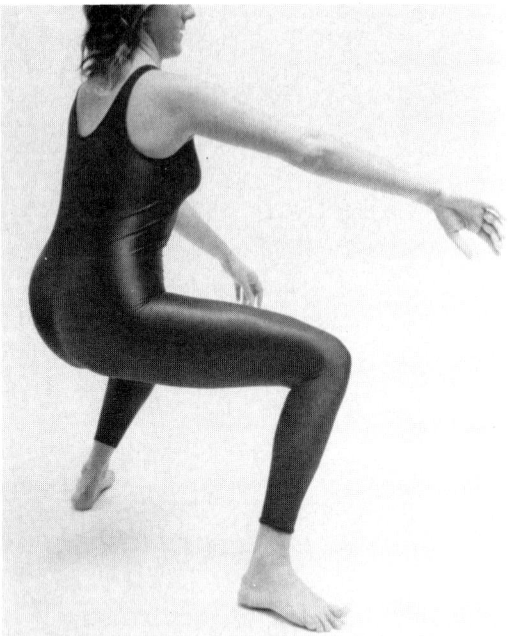

Figure 16 □ Martial arts techniques are useful in teaching stabilization.

Training is another issue, however. As with any other coordination activity, such as juggling, dancing, or pole vaulting, many resistance factors must be overcome. Individuals can learn to do these coordinated activities to varying degrees at different speeds. Some of the factors that determine such capabilities are hereditary coordination, past similar experiences, strength, endurance, concentration, practice, and a trainer. When the combination of these factors is favorable, individuals may learn a new task very rapidly. When they are unfavorable, the job may never be accomplished.

In back school, therefore, it is necessary to analyze an individual's capabilities, the work requirements, and underlying pathologic condition. An equation can be developed, taking into account these various factors, so that the patient, third-party payer, employer, family, and all others concerned understand the underlying problem, resources, goals, and the time frames.

Success in back school needs to be defined. Unfortunately, the gold standard of success in most scientific areas of low back pain has been the return to work—especially work that the patient was previously performing. This is frequently not possible. Once a major spinal pathologic condition is present, it may not be corrected to a level that would permit the return to heavy labor or contact sports. A patient of this sort could be trained for years and never return to a physically demanding occupation. Changing the patient's job might be the most economical and realistic back school accomplishment.

It is difficult to accurately determine the level of work appropriate for a patient with a particular pathologic entity. There are innumerable types of jobs, patient resources, and diagnoses of low back pain.

To simplify matters, we can divide each variable of the "equation" into five levels. Table 1 demonstrates the five levels of each of the three variables. The lightest working situation is basically sedentary, entails no bending or lifting, and allows frequent change in position. Work becomes more difficult until, by the fifth category, it involves the heavy bending and lifting required in labor jobs and/or contact sports. Similarly, a patient's underlying pathologic condition can be graded. The most minimal level, Grade 1, represents such entities as early minimal facet arthritis and early degenerative disc disease (sprain or strain). Grades 2 and 3 are progressively increasing, degenerative segment disease. By Grade 4, patients experience nerve root irritation and significant pathoanatomic changes. Grade 5, which comprises the most severe disease, would represent frank neurologic losses, weakness, and severe pain. The next and last variable of this equation is the most difficult to define, being more subjective and multifaceted. This factor consists of personal resources, environment, psychosocial factors and vocational factors.

Being in back school can be thought of as embarking on a journey. We know our destination, and we know our means of trans-

Table 1 □ Success Rating for Low Back Pain Treatment

GRADE	PHYSICAL CAPACITY	PHYSICAL DEMAND	PSYCHOSOCIAL RESOURCES
Most favorable	1	1	1
Slightly favorable	2	2	2
Moderately favorable	3	3	3
Moderately severe	4	4	4
Least favorable	5	5	5

portation. Now we have to identify all the obstacles along the way, including weather, terrain, nourishment, and fatigue. The journey might be graded as very difficult or "a piece of cake." For the patient in back school, we can grade his or her resources and all the subjective factors of strength, coordination, background, motivation, transportation, pain behavior, and family support from 1 to 5; an assignment of Grade 1 would strongly favor the patient's success, whereas by Grade 5 the obstacles would be overwhelming.

It is now possible to look at these three factors and determine realistic goals of success. For example, consider a patient with a minor pathoanatomic lesion who has both a job with light physical demands and good resources. One can anticipate that this patient will return to his or her previous occupation in a fairly short period of time. One might even decide that success would be considered to be returning to work within 2 weeks. At the other extreme, one might predict that a patient who has a severe anatomic lesion, a job with heavy physical demands, and no resources may never be able to return to a previous job. In this situation, what variable can be changed to obtain the greatest possible success? What would constitute success for this individual? The underlying pathoanatomic condition cannot be altered unless surgery is performed. We can take a critical look at the patient's resources and try to improve them from perhaps a grade of 5 to a grade of 4 or 3. The only variable left to change in the equation then is the patient's job. If we alter it from a heavy labor job with a level of 5 to one with a level of 3, we can now predict the possibility of success for this patient returning to work at a new level.

This is a fairly realistic approach to the treatment of low back pain patients, compared with our current method of placing every patient in the same exercise program or of operating on patients and considering success to be a return to previous work.

In summary, the first factor in our equation might be called physical capacity. This is not determined just on the basis of the pathologic entity that the patient has but includes the individual's ability to cope physically with that underlying condition. For example, an individual may have a very severe underlying pathologic herniated disc but may also have great strength, body mechanics, and stabilization ability and perhaps is working in a job with reasonable physical demands. That individual's physical capacity might be Grade 2. The same pathologic herniated disc in an individual who is weak, obese, and uncoordinated could be devastated by the disease and have a very low physical capacity, considered to be Grade 5.

The second factor then is the level of physical demand. This is essentially determined by the job that the patient is expected to return to or the demands that are placed on the individual, both at home and at work. Heavy labor and heavy contact sports would be Grade 5, whereas the inability to work at all or to engage in any sports would be Grade 1. (Note that the higher numbers are applied to the worst conditions and most difficult situations.)

The third factor pertains to the psychosocial environment. It also includes the availability of vocational retraining. Thus, here we are considering the resources that an individual has personally, psychologically, socially and environmentally. The Grade 5 patient is the one who is addicted, financially devastated, depressed, angry, hysterical, or hypochondriacal or who demonstrates severe pain behavior.

Variations of Back School

There is a "most appropriate" conservative care treatment, which will be different for every patient. The decision as to which appropriate treatment is to be selected will depend upon many factors, including the underlying pathoanatomic condition, the patient's demands at work and at home, and the patient's resources. For example, a minor pathologic condition with minimal demands may require little more than education in order for the patient's treatment to be considered a success and for the patient to function normally and happily. As the pathologic condition becomes more severe, the physical and psychologic resources become less and the physical demands become greater, we need heavier amounts of training and different types of approaches to training. Some back school training will have heavy behavioral modification overtones. If strength and endurance are the only problem, a gym program may be all that is necessary. A spectrum of education and training exists to match the range of disease and resources. Following are the four common types of back school training:

1. Back school education only.
2. Back school education, body mechanics training, and stabilization.
3. Back school, gym training, and functional restoration.
4. Back school education training and behavioral modification.

Prevention programs in industry and schools require education. It is one of our strongest medical tools and is probably the one that will eventually wipe out the epidemic of low back pain. A core of educational material needs to be supplied—not only to every individual for prevention, but for all patients who have back pain interfering with their lives. Every patient should certainly have some concept of the origin of the pain. This can be supplied simply by likening the intervertebral discs to jelly doughnuts or shock absorbers that have been damaged by age or abusive activities. This anatomic and pathoanatomic information can be very specific and intricate for patients who have an interest level and intelligence level sufficient to make use of the information. If we know the exact diagnosis, patients deserve to have that information, if they so desire.

Other basic information includes epidemiologic facts, such as that smoking and vibration are associated with a higher incidence of low back pain.

It is surprising that low back pain patients have such little insight into factors aggravating and relieving pain. Back school education points out that certain positions and activities are abusive to the low back and that patients with low back pain frequently find that the pain is more severe with certain positions of bending, lifting, reaching, and twisting.

The public is not generally aware of alternative ways to sit, stand, move, lift, bend, and exercise. Simply being aware of these factors and thinking about their backs are enough to prevent and control many episodes of low back pain.

Back Education in the Public Schools

If the low back pain epidemic is going to be fought through education, we need to educate the public, just as the dentists have done by showing brushing and flossing across the nation's television screens. This has been started in the public school system in several areas of the United States.[15, 62, 110]

In one public educational program, we devised a prospective study to determine what educational information can be incorporated in a normal public school educational curriculum. We took many of the basic principles that have been taught in back school for years and taught them to teachers of biology, physical education, and health education classes. We then had these teachers include this information in their classes. We tested the students at the beginning and end of each year for 3 years. We will continue to follow the students included in this study for many years to see what information is retained and whether there is any long-range effect upon the incidence of low back pain.

The experience with this public school educational program and the experience of many of the formal back school programs around the world is that teaching the concepts of the source and prevention of low back pain and proper care of the back is relatively simple. The concepts can be easily adjusted to the age and educational level of any individual beginning at about the third grade. The concepts of being physically fit and doing regular exercise are almost common knowledge. The proper, or safe, way to lift has also become fairly common knowledge.[111] Students readily grasp the concept that the spine is supported by trunk musculature and that strong abdominal and leg muscles will allow safer and more efficient positioning of the body for lifting, working, and sports activities. Flexibility is also a concept quickly adopted. Most individuals have already been educated by their parents about posture, slouching, and improper chairs and beds—regardless of whether these concepts have any validity. From an educational standpoint, then, the information is somewhat familiar and is therefore easily absorbed and remembered.

However, teaching about body mechanics and coordination both in the back schools and the public schools is not easy. It is difficult to change habit patterns, postures, and movement patterns by means of lectures, videotapes, pictures, or anything short of one-on-one practice and repetition. Unfortunately, this is not practical in the public school model. It is difficult to convince teachers or students who do not have back pain to move in a different manner or exert more energy in maintaining a particular posture of sitting or standing than is required when the individual is relaxed. There seems to be a natural tendency for humans to preserve energy. Sitting, to most individuals, means relaxing or not expending the energy required for walking or standing. It means, to them, to take the load off the feet and off the muscles, and usually to place it onto the spine with the lumbar segments in full flexion.[2, 10, 18, 78, 79, 81, 82] Although students quickly learn the concept of "sitting supported or sitting straight," they do not use such protective mechanisms on a regular basis.

Our experience in attempting to teach body mechanics and to change habit patterns through public education over the past 20 years indicates that we are fighting a losing battle. Our usual methods of education are not working. It is necessary to penetrate to the essence of society, culture, and human behavior and to appeal to the emotions as do those who sell cigarettes and cosmetics. Good body mechanics need to be made attractive and enjoyable. For example, attractive, athletic modern dancers, doing straight-back bends and exercising with excellent flexibility and strength, might attract the attention of a cigarette-smoking laborer in a high-risk job faster than another sign in the work place stating, "knees bent, back straight, abdomen tight."

Incorporating good spinal body mechanics into athletics, dance classes, and other enjoyable recreational activities at an early age may provide us with some long-range success. We learn how to stand in positions of readiness during racquet sports, and we learn straight-back, coordinated activities on the basketball court, in martial arts, and during other athletic endeavors and other athletic fields.[111]

The world has not recognized widely enough the cost of low back pain. There are very few grants, public television programs, fund-raising organizations or public awareness movements to help solve the problem, even though its solution is ridiculously simple in concept. As for tooth decay, AIDS, and heart disease, the source of the problem is well understood. Preventive measures are available for those who care, and education is the key to success. Perhaps we will someday find a cure through chemistry, immunology, or pharmacology. In the meantime, we need to make much more efficient use of the ubiquitous tool of education in our schools.

References

1. Aberg, J.: Evaluation of an advanced back pain rehabilitation program. Spine 9:317–318, 1984.
2. Anderson, G., Ortengren, R., and Nachemson, A.: The sitting posture: An electromyographic and discometric study. Orthop. Clin. North Am. 6:105–120, 1975.
3. Anderson, R.: Spinal Disease from Prehistory to Present. Conservative Care of Low Back Pain. St. Louis, C. V. Mosby, 1989.
4. Anderson, G. B. J., Ortengren, R., and Herberts, P.: Quanitization electromyographic studies of back muscle activity related to posture and loading. Orthop. Clin. North Am. 8:85–96, 1977.
5. Anderson, G. B. J.: Epidemiologic aspects of back pain in industry. Spine 6:53–57, 1981.
6. Appenzeller, O., Standefer, J., et al.: Neurology of endurance training: Endorphins. Neurology 30:418–419, 1980.
7. Attix, E. A., and Tate, M. A.: Low back school: A conservative method for the treatment of low back pain. J. Miss. State Med. Assoc. 20:4–9, 1979.
8. Back School of Atlanta: Informational pamphlets to patients and insurance carriers. 1981.
9. Bell, G., and Rothman, R.: The conservative treatment of sciatica. Spine 9:54–56, 1984.
10. Bandix, T., Krohn, L., et al.: Trunk posture and trapezius muscle load while working in standing, supported-standing, and sitting positions. Spine 10:433–439, 1985.
11. Berquist-Ullman, M., and Larsson, U.: Acute low back pain in industry. Acta Orthop. Scand. (Suppl.):170, 1977.
12. Brodin, Band, Bechgaard, et al.: Manipulation or Ryggraden. Scandinavian University Books, 1972.
13. Blush, K.: From the Clinic: Back School. Am. Correct. Ther. J. 31:23–25, 1979.
14. Cady, L. D.: Strength and fitness and subsequent back injuries in firefighters. J. Occup. Med. 21:269–272, 1979.
15. Carr, D. B., Bullen, B. A., Skrinar, G. S., et al.: Physical conditioning facilitates the exercise-induced secretion of beta-endorphins and betalipotropin in women. N. Engl. J. Med. 305:560–563, 1981.
16. Chartworks: A review of articles published from April, 1983 through December, 1986. Edited by Chart Hawaii staff. Chart Corporation, Denver, Colorado.
17. Deyo, R. A., Diehl, A. K., and Rosenthal, M.: How many days of bedrest for acute low back pain? A randomized clinical trial. N. Engl. J. Med. 315:1064–1070, 1986.
18. During, J., Goudfrooij, H., Keessen, W., et al.: Towards standards for posture: Postural characteristics of the lower back system in normal and pathologic conditions. Spine 10:83–87, 1985.
19. Dutro, C. L., and Wheeler, L.: Back school and chiropractic practice. J. Manip. Phys. Ther. 9:209–211, 1986.
20. Egbert, L. D., Battit, G. E., Welch, C. E., et al.: Reduction of post operative pain by encourage-

ment and instruction of patients. N. Engl. J. Med. 270:825–827, 1964.
21. Evjenth, O., and Hamberg, J.: Muscle Stretching in Manual Therapy, Vols. I and II. Alfta Rehabilitation, 1984.
22. Facchini, Metal: Comparison of the Results of Various Forms of Conservative Treatment in Low Back Pain. Paper presented at the I.S.S.L.S. Fourteenth Annual Meeting, 1987.
23. Fahrni, W. H.: Backache Relieved. Springfield, Charles C Thomas, 1966.
24. Fahrni, W. H.: Conservative treatment of lumbar disc degeneration: Our primary responsibility. Orthop. Clin. North Am. 6:93–103, 1975.
25. Fahrni, W. H.: Backache: Assessment and Treatment. Vancouver, Musqueam Publishers, 1976.
26. Farfan, H. F.: The effects of torsion on the lumbar vertebral joints: The roles of torsion in the production of disc degeneration. J. Bone Joint Surg. 52A:468–497, 1970.
27. Farfan, H. F.: Mechanical Disorders of the Low Back. Philadelphia, Lea & Febiger, 1979.
28. Farfan, H. F.: Muscular mechanism of the lumbar spine and the position of power and efficiency. Orthop. Clin. North Am. 6:135–144, 1975.
29. Farfan, H. F., and Gracovetsky, S.: The nature of instability. Spine 9:714–719, 1984.
30. Flint, M.: Abdominal muscle involvement during performance of various forms of sit-up exercise: An EMG study. Am. J. Phys. Med. 44:224–234, 1965.
31. Flint, M.: Effect of increasing back and abdominal strength in low back pain. Resident Q. 29:160–171, 1958.
32. Fraioli, F., Moretti, C., Paolucci, D., et al.: Physical exercise stimulates marked concomitant release of beta-endorphin and adrenocorticotropic hormone (ACTH) in peripheral blood in man. Experientia 36:987–989, 1980.
33. Frymoyer, J. W., et al.: Epidemiologic studies of low back pain. Spine 5:419–423, 1980.
34. Frymoyer, J. W., Pope, M. H., Clements, et al.: Risk factors in low back pain. J. Bone Joint Surg. 65A:213–218, 1983.
35. Gracovetsky, S., Farfan, H. F., and Lamy, C.: Mechanism of the lumbar spine. Spine 6:249–262, 1981.
36. Gracovetsky, S., Farfan, H., and Helleur, C.: The abdominal mechanism. Spine 10:317–324, 1985.
37. Gracovetsky, S., and Farfan, H. F.: The optimum spine. Spine 11:543–573, 1986.
38. Grieve, G.: Common Vertebral Joint Problems. New York, Churchill Livingstone, 1981.
39. Hall, H.: The Toronto Back Education Unit—An Approach to the Management of Chronic Mechanical Back Pain. W.C.P.T., Tel Aviv, Israel, 1978.
40. Hall, H.: The Canadian back education units. Physiotherapy 66:115–117, 1980.
41. Hall, H.: Back school (an overview with reference to the Canadian back education units). Clin. Orthop. 179:10–17, 1983.
42. Hansson, T., Roos, B., and Nachemson A.: Development of osteopenia in the fourth lumbar vertebra during prolonged bedrest after operation for scoliosis. Acta Orthop. Scand. 6:621–630, 1975.
43. Hansson, T., Roos, B., and Nachemson, A.: The long-term restitution of bone mineral density after prolonged bedrest (unpublished manuscript).
44. Hansson, T., Sandström, B., Roos, B., et al.: The bone mineral content of the lumbar spine in patients with chronic low back pain. Spine 10:158–159, 1985.
45. Hasue, M., Masatoshi, I., and Kikuchi, S.: A new method of quantitative measurement of abdominal and back muscle strength. Spine 5:143–148, 1980.
46. Healy, K. M.: Does preoperative instruction make a difference? Am. J. Nurs. 68:62, 1968.
47. Heliovaara, M.: Body height, obesity and risk of herniated lumbar intervertebral disc. Spine 12:469–472, 1987.
48. Holm, S., and Nachemson, A.: Nutrition of the Intervertebral Disc: Acute Effects of Cigarette Smoking: An Experimental Animal Study. Presented at the I.S.S.L.S. Eleventh Annual Meeting, 1984.
49. Jackson, C., and Brown, M.: Is there a role for exercise in the treatment of patients with low back pain? Clin. Orthop. 179:39–45, 1983.
50. Jackson, C., and Brown, M.: Analysis of current approaches and a practical guide to prescription of exercise. Clin. Orthop. 179:46–54, 1983.
51. Kaltenborn, F.: Mobilization of the Extremity Joints, 3rd Ed. Sydney, Australia, Norlis Bokhandel, 1980.
52. Kapandji, I. A.: The Physiology of the Joints, Vol. III. New York, Churchill Livingstone, 1977.
53. Kaye, R. L., and Hammond, A. H.: Understanding rheumatoid arthritis: Evaluation of a patient education program. J.A.M.A. 239:2466, 1978.
54. Kelsey, J. L.: An epidemiological study of acute herniated lumbar intervertebral discs. Rheumatol. Rehab. 14:144–159, 1975.
55. Kendell, P., and Jenkins, J.: Exercises for backache: Double blind controlled trial. Phys. Ther. 54:154–157, 1968.
56. Kennedy Mapa, B.: An Australian programme for management of back problems. Physiotherapy 66:108–111, 1980.
57. Klaber Moffett, J. A., Chase, S. M., Portek, I., and Ennis, J. R.: A controlled prospective study to evaluate the effectiveness of a back school in the relief of chronic low back pain. Spine 11:120–122, 1986.
58. Knott, M., and Voss, D.: Proprioceptive Neuromuscular Facilitation, Patterns and Techniques, 2nd Ed. New York, Harper & Row, 1968.
59. Kraus, H.: Prevention of low back pain. J. Assoc. Phys. Ment. Rehab. 6:12–15, 1952.
60. Krause, H.: Diagnosis and treatment of low back pain. Gen. Pract. 5:35–39, 1952.
61. Krolner, B., and Toft, B.: Vertebral bone loss: An unheeded side effect of therapeutic bedrest. Clin. Sci. 64:537–540, 1983.
62. Kunse, P., and White, A. H.: Instruction of Preventive Back Care in the Public School System. Presented at the North American Spine Society Second Annual Meeting, 1987.
63. Kvien, T. K., Nilsen, H., and Vik, P.: Education and self-care of patients with low back pain. Scand. J. Rheumatol. 10:318–320, 1981.
64. Langrana, N. A., Lee, C. K., Alexander, H., et al.: Quantitative assessment of back strength using isokinetic testing. Spine 9:287–290, 1984.
65. Lawlis, G. F., and Hennig, E. G., Jr.: The Spine Education Center: An Evaluation of Individualized Educational Services for the Prevention of Industrial Back Injuries. A Program Evaluation. North Texas State University, 1982.
66. Lichter, R.: Simulated Job Training Using Work

Performance for Worker Rehabilitation and Testing. Paper Presented at the Challenge of the Lumbar Spine Ninth Annual Meeting, 1987.
67. Levine, P. H., and Britten, A. F.: Supervised patient-management of hemophilia: A study of 45 patients with hemophilia A and B. Ann. Intern. Med. 78:195–201, 1973.
68. Marras, W. S., King, A. I., and Joynt, R. L.: Measurements of loads on the lumbar spine under isometric and isokinetic conditions. Spine 9:176–187, 1984.
69. Mattmiller, A. W.: The California back school. Physiotherapy 66:118–121, 1980.
70. Mattmiller, A. W.: Low Back Injury Prevention in Southern Pacific Railroad: A Five-Year Follow-Up Study. Paper Presented at the I.S.S.L.S. Eighth Annual Meeting, 1981.
71. Mayen, L., and Greenberg, B. B.: Measurements of the strength of trunk muscles. J. Bone Joint Surg. 24:812–856, 1942.
72. Mayer, T. G., Smith, S., et al.: Quantification of lumbar function: Part 2: Sagittal plane trunk strength in chronic low back pain patients. Spine 8:765–772, 1985.
73. McKenzie, R. A.: The Lumbar Spine: Mechanical Diagnosis and Therapy. New Zealand, Spinal Publications, 1981.
74. Miller, L. V., and Goldstein, J.: More efficient care of diabetic patients in a country-hospital setting. N. Engl. J. Med. 286:1388–1391, 1972.
75. Moore, M.: Personal Communication, 1985.
76. Morris, J. M.: Biomechanics of the Spine. Arch. Surg. 107:418–423, 1973.
77. Morris, J. M.: Intervertebral disc disease of the lumbosacral spine: Biomechanical observations. *In* American Academy of Orthopaedic Surgeons Symposium on the Lumbar Spine, New Zealand, pp. 3–15, 1979.
78. Nachemson, A.: Lumbar intradiscal pressure. Acta Orthop. Scand. 45(Suppl):1–104, 1960.
79. Nachemson, A.: The load on lumbar discs in different positions of the body. Clin. Orthop. 45:107–122, 1966.
80. Nachemson, A., and Lind, H. M.: Measurement of abdominal and back muscle strength with and without low back pain. Scand. J. Rehab. Med. 1:60–65, 1969.
81. Nachemson, A., and Elfstrom, G.: Intravital dynamic pressure in measurements of lumbar discs. Scand. J. Rehab. Med. 1(Suppl.):1–39, 1970.
82. Nachemson, A.: Towards a better understanding of low back pain: A review of the mechanics of the lumbar disc. Rheumatol. Rehabil. 14:129–143, 1975.
83. Nachemson, A.: The lumbar spine. An orthopedic challenge. Spine 1:59, 1976.
84. Nachemson, A., and Holm, S.: Nutrition of the Intervetebral Disc: Effects Induced by Vibrations. Presented at the I.S.S.L.S. Twelfth Annual Meeting, 1985.
85. Nicholas, J. A., Strizak, A. M., and Veras, G.: A study of thigh muscle weakness in different pathological studies of the lower extremity. Am. J. Sports Med. 4:241–248, 1976.
86. Nordin, M., Kahanovitz, N., Verderane, R., et al.: Normal trunk strength and endurance in women and the effect of exercises and electrical stimulation. Part 1: Normal endurance and trunk muscle strength in 101 women. Spine 112:105–118, 1987.
87. North American Back School Association Files.
88. Ortengren, R., Anderson, G., Nachemson, A.: Studies of relationships between lumbar disc pressure, myoelectric back muscle activity, and intra-abdominal (intragastric) pressure. Spine 6:98–103, 1981.
89. Pawlicki, R. E., Gil, K. M., Jopling, C. A., et al.: The low back school: A new palliative approach to low back pain. W. Va. Med. J. 78:249–251, 1982.
90. Pope, M. H., Wilder, D. G., Stokes, I. A. F., et al.: Biomechanical testing as an aid to decision making in low back pain patient. Spine 7:135–140, 1979.
91. Rosenberg, S. G.: Patient education leads to better care for heart patients. H.S.M.H.A. Health Rep. 86:793, 1971.
92. Selby, D. K.: Conservative care of non-specific low back pain. Orthop. Clin. North Am. 13:427–437, 1982.
93. Sikorski, J. M.: A rationalized approach to physiotherapy for low back pain. Spine 10:571–579, 1985.
94. Simmons, J. W., Dennis, M. D., and Rath, D.: The back school—a total back management problem. Orthopaedics 7:1453–1456, 1984.
95. Sjolund, B. H., and Eriksson, M. B. E.: Endorphins and Analgesia Produced By Peripheral Conditioning Stimulation. New York, Raven Press, 1979.
96. Smidt, G., Herring, T., Amundsen, L., et al.: Assessment of abdominal and back extensor strength. A quantitative approach and results for chronic back pain patients. Spine 8:211–219, 1983.
97. Smidt, G. L., Amundsen, L. R., and Dostal, W. F.: Muscle strength at the trunk. J. Orthop. Sports Phys. Ther. 1:165–170, 1980.
98. Smith, S., Mayer, T. G., et al.: Quantification of lumbar function: Part 1: Isometric and multispeed isokinetic trunk strength measures in sagittal and axial planes in normal subjects. Spine 8:757–764, 1985.
99. Sparrell, C. F., and McKeon, W. F.: Preventing low back pain in industry. Bus. Health May:16–19, 1985.
100. Stoddard, A.: Manual of Osteopathic Technique, 4th Ed. Hutchinson, 1980.
101. Suzuki, N., Endo, S.: A quantitative study of trunk muscle strength and fatigability in the low back pain syndrome. Spine 8:1–2, 1983.
102. Thorstensson, A., and Nilsson, J.: Trunk muscle strength during constant velocity movements. Scand. J. Rehab. Med. 14:61–68, 1982.
103. Troup, J. D. G., and Chapman, A. F.: The strength of the flexor and extensor muscles of the trunk. J. Biomech. 2:49–62, 1969.
104. Vollowitz, E.: Personal communication, 1987.
105. Waddell, G.: A New Clinical Model For Treatment of Low Back Pain. (Volvo Award.) Paper Presented at the I.S.S.L.S. Fourteenth Annual Meeting, 1987.
106. White, A. A., and Panjabi, M.: Clinical Biomechanics of the Spine. Philadelphia, J. B. Lippincott, 1978.
107. White, A. H., and Mattmiller, A. W.: Back school for the conservative care of low back pain. Paper Presented at the American Academy of Orthopaedic Surgeons, 1978.
108. White, A. H.: Evaluation of the Chronic Pain Patient. Symposium on the Lumbar Spine. St. Louis, C. V. Mosby, 1979, pp. 54–66.

109. White, A. H.: Low Back Patient Goes To School. Symposium on the Lumbar Spine. St. Louis, C. V. Mosby, 1979, pp. 236–239.
110. White, A. H., et al.: The Back School: An Audiovisual Team Approach to Low Back Pain. St. Louis, C. V. Mosby, 1981.
111. White, A. H.: Back School and Other Conservative Approaches to Low Back Pain. St. Louis, C. V. Mosby, 1983.
112. White, A. H.: A model for conservative care of low back pain: Back school, epidural blocks, mobilization. Am. Acad. Orthop. Surg. Instruct. Course Lect. 34:78–84, 1985.
113. White, A. H.: Low Back Pain. Am. Acad. Orthop. Surg. Instruct. Course Lect. 34:78–84, 1985.
114. White, A. H.: Conservative Care of Low Back Pain. Spine Update 1987. Radiology, Pain, and Research and Education Foundation, San Francisco, 1987, pp. 283–285.
115. White, A. H.: The Degeneration Trap. Paper presented at the Commonwealth Club of San Francisco, 1987.
116. Wilder, D. G., Woodworth, B. B., Frymoyer, J. W., and Pope, M. H.: Vibration and the Human Spine. Spine 7:243–254, 1982.
117. Zachrisson, M.: The Low Back Pain School. Sound and Slide Program, Danderyd, Sweden, Danderyd Hospital, 1970.
118. Zachrisson-Forsell, M.: The Swedish back school. Physiotherapy 66:112–114, 1980.
119. Zachrisson-Forsell, M.: The back school. Spine 6:104–106, 1981.
120. Zucherman, J. F., and White, A. H.: The "back school" approach to low back pain. J. Musculoskel. Med. 1:13–22, 1984.

MECHANICAL DIAGNOSIS AND THERAPY FOR LOW BACK PAIN: TOWARD A BETTER UNDERSTANDING

Robin McKenzie

In the past little was known about the likely causes of low back pain, and every health-related specialty attempted to obtain for itself the role of responsibility for care of the back by administering the skills of that particular specialty. The situation persists today to a lesser degree; thus, some physicians propose that the answers to most back problems lie in the dispensing of medicines, pills, and embrocations, despite evidence to support the view that most LBP is mechanical and not inflammatory in nature. Surgeons attempt to provide solutions by removing, replacing, or modifying various parts of the spinal column, and osteopaths and chiropractors have for almost 100 years applied spinal manipulative therapy (SMT) to the painful back, albeit for different reasons. Physiotherapists have traditionally used heat, massage, exercises, and electrotherapeutic modalities, which are still used in some clinics today. Only in the past 40 years have physiotherapists adopted manipulative procedures for spinal therapy.

Since Hippocrates over 2,000 years ago first described methods of treatment for low back pain mechanical therapy has played a dominant role in the conservative care of patients suffering from the disorder. In the early stages of the problem, especially, it is unusual for a patient not to receive some form of conservative care from a physiotherapist, a chiropractor, or an osteopath. These professionals dominate the field of health care providers that dispense mechanical therapies; the most common in use today are exercise, traction, massage, mobilization, and spinal manipulation.

The competing professions vie with one another for recognition as providers of the most effective conservative health care for common spinal problems. Society will eventually choose the system that provides cost-effective therapies that have the potential to dispense a long-term benefit. No treatment has yet been found to provide a reliable long-term benefit for people with low back pain.

For the physician wishing to obtain for a patient the very best conservative care, the claims and counterclaims from proponents of mechanical therapies must be bewildering indeed. I am attempting, here, to persuade those interested in the topic that a more organized and rational approach to the mechanical treatment of spinal pain is desirable and, furthermore, that it is available now. Presently, the diversity and complexity of therapeutic approaches confuse most of us when we are first introduced to the therapeutic "scene." It often seems easier to turn away than to become embroiled in the confusion.

Chiropractors have adopted some of the orthodox elements of medicine and have attempted to moderate the extravagant claims that persist from the past.

Chiropractors are now employing modalities commonly seen in physiotherapy clinics. It is almost certain that if you go to a chiropractor you will receive SMT. It is unnecessary and unacceptable to deliver manipulative therapy to every patient with back pain in order to deliver the procedure to the very few who really need it. The chiropractic concept that an alteration of the pathologic state or modulation of the neurophysiology is *best* achieved by the delivery of mechanical forces applied from without remains controversial.

Within medicine, this leaves only the physiotherapists as providers of conservative mechanical treatment. The very nature of physiotherapy and its practice should make physiotherapists and doctors interdependent upon one another. Most doctors have neither the time nor the skills to deliver mechanical therapy in its modern form, and if patients are to receive appropriate modern mechanical therapy they must avail themselves of the services of a modern mechanical therapist. Physiotherapists with new concepts in mechanical pathology can deliver a complete spectrum of mechanical forces (including SMT), which when applied with appropriate guidelines can provide outcome predictors, remove clinical guesswork, and thereby prevent time being wasted by the application of treatment modalities that have dubious value.

Over the next few years, physiotherapists will have an opportunity to be the key professionals within medicine responsible for the delivery of conservative care for mechanical disorders of the spine. They will earn that responsibility only by working within medicine and thereby subjecting themselves to the stringent criticism so necessary for scientific evolution.

In order to better understand the present predicament, it is necessary to review some aspects of pathology, the treatments delivered, and the philosophies of various approaches.

PATHOLOGY

The pathologic processes or the micromechanical disorders that give rise to LBP are still rather obscure, just as they were when Hippocrates first described his methods of treatment for "hyboma," or acute lumbar kyphosis.[22] Hippocrates believed the cause to be a backward dislocation of one vertebra onto another. Although our understanding has improved immensely, especially in the past 20 years, with the exception of the sequestered disc we are still unable to identify with certainty or precision the offending structure causing pain in many particular instances.[35]

Since the search for exact cause of low back pain began, every structure in the lower back was suspect at one time or another. The reasons proposed for onset of pain have been innumerable, but they have ranged from the witch's curse inflaming the nerves to the proverbial chill in the kidneys acquired by sitting in a draft.

Modern medicine has advanced with such rapidity that it can be fairly stated that we have learned more of the precise nature of the causes of spinal pain in the past 20 years than we have in all of previous recorded history, and the search has narrowed to two structures likely to be involved in the production of most mechanical back pain.[35]

The intervertebral disc, with its strong annulus fibrosus retaining the gel-like nucleus, probably attracts the most attention. Since first appearing in 1974, the journal *Spine* has published the results of innumerable studies aimed at the examination of intervertebral disc structure, function, pathology, and treatment. The other mobile structures to capture the attention of those investigating back pain are the zygapophyseal joints. These are also probable sources of pain, but the precise pathologic conditions causing the pain have been difficult to identify.

The pathologic changes occurring between

birth and death are now well described, but disagreement remains about certain fundamental aspects of those changes.[6, 7, 47, 49] Recently, for instance, it has been proposed that the intervertebral disc actually thickens, rather than thins, as the aging process advances.[47] If true, this must inevitably lead to reappraisal of the hypothetic basis of some of our therapies. Indeed, until more sophisticated technology provides an answer, our conceptualization regarding the reasons for treatment effectiveness must continue to remain flexible and open to change.

Although so much about the causes of low back pain remains to be discovered, many health care professionals either remain unaware or choose to ignore certain established findings within orthopedics. Disorders of the sacroiliac joint occur without doubt, but most are inflammatory in origin. That true mechanical lesions occur is also recognized. They are, however, uncommon and usually occur only after pregnancy.[12] Physiotherapists, especially in North America and wherever therapists are receiving instruction from osteopaths, are "discovering" sacroiliac disorders in many of their patients.[41] It is likely that either the proponents are wrong or the literature is in error. The historical obsession of physiotherapists with the musculature as the main source of backache has already been exposed.[9] Although orthopedic opinion does not support the proposal,[46] muscle imbalance and muscle strain are still considered by some physiotherapists to be common causes of persistent back pain and to account for the degree of existing lordosis.

It appears now to be generally accepted within medicine that the origin of most common low back pain is mechanical, probably arising in the intervertebral disc early in life and in the apophyseal joints much later in life.[6, 7, 33, 47, 49] The treatment for these particular problems, therefore, should mainly be mechanical. This fact has been recognized through 2,500 years of recorded history, and most treatments provided today for the alleviation of back pain contain mechanical components.[43]

The problem exists, however, and it is unlikely to change in the forseeable future. Even with the most sophisticated and detailed investigations, the precise pathologic process responsible for the pain remains a mystery. In their attempts to perhaps provide answers to fill this void, some therapists develop a system of "pathology," and a consequent terminology, separate from and contradictory to that existing within medicine as a whole, and orthopedics in particular. Medicine has always been able to exert control over and put pressure on its wayward practitioners in order to protect the public from outrageous claims and methods of treatment. It is time that similar controls were applied to physiotherapy, especially when we see such fringe concepts as cranial suture mobilization, craniosacral techniques and myofascial release techniques being taught to physiotherapists without the slightest scientific evidence to support their consideration as tools for the treatment of spinal pathologic conditions. If we fail to curb the development of unscientific cultism, we deserve to lose what should be our rightful place within the medical team.

DIAGNOSIS

It is frustrating to have to accept that often we lack a complete or even partial diagnosis when commencing our therapies. But as physiotherapists we have one important advantage over our colleagues in the medical profession. By the nature of their training as well as the expectations of the public, physicians and surgeons are predisposed to prescribe drugs for inflamed or painful joints, to surgically immobilize or even remove severely painful joints, and to replace them with metal implants. The surgical procedures must be executed with a high degree of accuracy if success is to follow.

A successful outcome of treatment is dependent, therefore, on positive identification of the site of the lesion. Because physiotherapists are not engaged in delivering invasive patient therapies, the precise identification of the structure affected and location of the offending lesion is less critical.

It has been my belief that prior to commencing mechanical therapy the patient should be screened by the family medical practitioner. Thus, we will receive into our clinics patients who have been appropriately screened, who are judged to have mechanical disorders, and in whom serious pathologic processes have been eliminated. We are then in a position to attempt the definition of the mechanical problem.

MECHANICAL DIAGNOSIS

There are many views regarding the best method of establishing a mechanical diagnosis. There is almost universal agreement that it is necessary to obtain detailed information from the patient by way of a history, but confusion reigns about the relevance of various questions and answers.

Some clinicians attach much more importance to a particular response; others disregard the response as irrelevant. Some clinicians obtain large amounts of detailed information, which is idealistically appropriate but may not be practically useful. We are told that the clinician has a simple choice. If he or she wishes to obtain a large range of detailed information he must realize that much of it will be irrelevant or unreliable.[37] If the clinician is prepared to limit the information, then he or she will increase its reliability and relevance.

Some clinicians decide the nature of the mechanical problem principally by palpation; some even claim to be able to determine by palpation alone the extent of the existing disorders. Although many have found that rather gross losses of movement are detectable by palpation, I am aware of only one study that indicates that palpation is reliable. Unfortunately, it is seriously flawed by having no objective and independent assessors involved in the outcomes.[24] On the contrary, intertherapist reliability, especially regarding palpatory skills, has been shown to be extremely poor.[20, 32, 36] A recent study comparing intertester reliabilities in the examination of sacroiliac dysfunction has also shown extremely poor correlation: in 11 of 13 tests, agreement was 50% or less. Palpatory skills were fundamental to 10 of the 13 cases. All the therapists involved were experienced and trained in orthopedic manual therapy.[41]

Those who base their diagnosis mainly on palpatory findings tend to confuse the issues of whether the information they receive is derived from tactile sources alone—a claim that is frequently made—and whether the information is imparted to them by stressing the offending structure during the process of palpation, thus reproducing the patient's symptoms. Pain produced by localized movement or pressure from palpation itself has been found to be more reliable.[32, 41] It is time, therefore, that those who claim to have developed finely tuned "magic fingers" recognize that their skill requires only the ability to detect the patient's painful response in order to identify affected levels.

Chiropractors rely on a combination of diagnostic criteria, but mainly on information obtained from palpatory and radiographic findings. In addition to palpatory assessment being unreliable, a study showed that radiographs analyzed by a either a chiropractor or a radiologist have little value in detecting the presence or absence of back pain.[18] Thus, both tools are of dubious value.

Physiotherapists in various parts of the world exhibit differing attitudes to the problem of mechanical diagnosis. This has come about because of the influence of three people in particular. (1) Some, especially in Europe and countries influenced by the Norwegian system, have opted to follow the osteopathic concepts and subsequent modifications developed by Freddy Kaltenborn, a Norwegian physiotherapist. (2) Others, mainly in Commonwealth countries, have adopted a more orthopedically oriented approach, probably because of the influence of James Cyriax. (3) In Australia, Geoffrey Maitland, also a physiotherapist, has developed a blend of the orthopedic together with his own system of palpatory examination and treatment.

In the long run, however, and irrespective of the amount of data obtained from the patient's history, examination, and laboratory tests, the final decision as to the mechanical approach to be adopted is determined by the patient's response to the mechanical forces applied. The clinician's conception of the appropriate treatment is frequently and must always be over-ruled by the emergence of an adverse painful reaction in response to the initiation of that treatment.

After excluding serious and unsuitable disorders, it is my contention that the remaining nonspecific back problems (which affect the great majority of our patients) are best evaluated with an organized dynamic mechanical assessment that can determine (usually on the first day) the status of the structures and their potential to react to certain maneuvers.

AFFECTING PAIN PATTERNS BY MECHANICAL THERAPY

Those familiar with my approach to patient selection will realize that serious pathologic processes should already have been eliminated from the patient population by the medical screening. Radiologic assessment eliminates most disorders unsuited to the mechanical approach but is otherwise not helpful in determining patient suitability. Palpatory diagnosis is rejected because of the widespread incidence of tropism[10, 52] and our inability to demonstrate intertester reliability.

I have based my search for diagnostic information on mechanical principles. Increasing mechanical deformation of a structure results in increasing pain. It also causes radiating and referred pain. Reducing mechanical deformation obviously reduces the intensity and radiation of pain. The effects that mechanical forces have on existing pain patterns are therefore likely to be more reliable in determining the nature of the mechanical disorder than any palpatory radiologic or other laboratory investigations. Thus, a dynamic mechanical evaluation using repetitive end range motion as the tool is a basis for my examination and assessment; the consequent expression of pain and whether it peripheralizes or centralizes determine the mechanical diagnosis. No longer is it sufficient to ask the patient during the physical examination if a single movement performed in each direction produces pain. It is of paramount importance to assess the effects of repeating end-range movement in each direction. One movement may well increase peripheral symptoms—but what if repetition of that movement were to abolish those same symptoms? Judgment made on the performance of one movement may well have deprived the patient of a solution to the problem.

Not unusually, information derived from the initial assessment identifies patients with pathologic conditions unsuitable for the mechanical approach. It may not, of course, identify the pathologic process itself, but under certain circumstances may indicate the nature of the problem.

Provocation of and increase of referred symptoms while using all variables *during the course of the initial assessment* is almost certain to expose discogenic disorders unsuited to mechanical treatment at their current stage.

Information emerging from the use of repetitive end-range motion also identifies rapid responders and separates slow responders from nonresponders. The process enables the health provider to determine on the first day the directions in which patients should be moved and those in which they should not be moved. Movements that, when repeated, cause symptoms to diminish progressively or that cause pain to change from the periphery to a more central location are considered desirable and should be encouraged and used as a basis for self treatment. Movements that cause symptoms to become increasingly painful or referred more peripherally are considered undesirable and, once identified, must be avoided. Likewise, positions that produce pain should be avoided and substituted by positions that abolish pain.

My conclusions from this evaluation process are based almost entirely on the effects produced on the patients' symptoms by repeating well-defined movements performed in the standing and recumbent positions (Fig. 1). Special importance is placed on the development of the process of centralization of pain, which I regard as absolutely reliable in predicting successful outcome in the treatment of mechanical disorders of the low back (Fig. 2). This reliability has recently been supported in a study by Donelson and coworkers.[13]

The effects of repetitive end-range motion on the patient's pain pattern identify three main subgroups in the nonspecific spectrum. Each subgroup describes differing pain responses to the application of similar mechanical forces. Individuals in each subgroup describe similar pain responses to the application of similar mechanical forces. Following assessment by repetitive motion, a subdivision of patients within the nonspecific spectrum of back pain is possible, allowing us to classify them into categories I have chosen to call the *postural dysfunction and derangement syndromes*. Patients in the derangement syndrome category are further subdivided into seven clinically identifiable entities. The precise means of identification and the concepts and methods of treatment of these syndromes are described in detail elsewhere.[29] A brief summary only is provided here.

Postural Syndrome

Patients with this syndrome are usually under 30 years of age, have sedentary occupa-

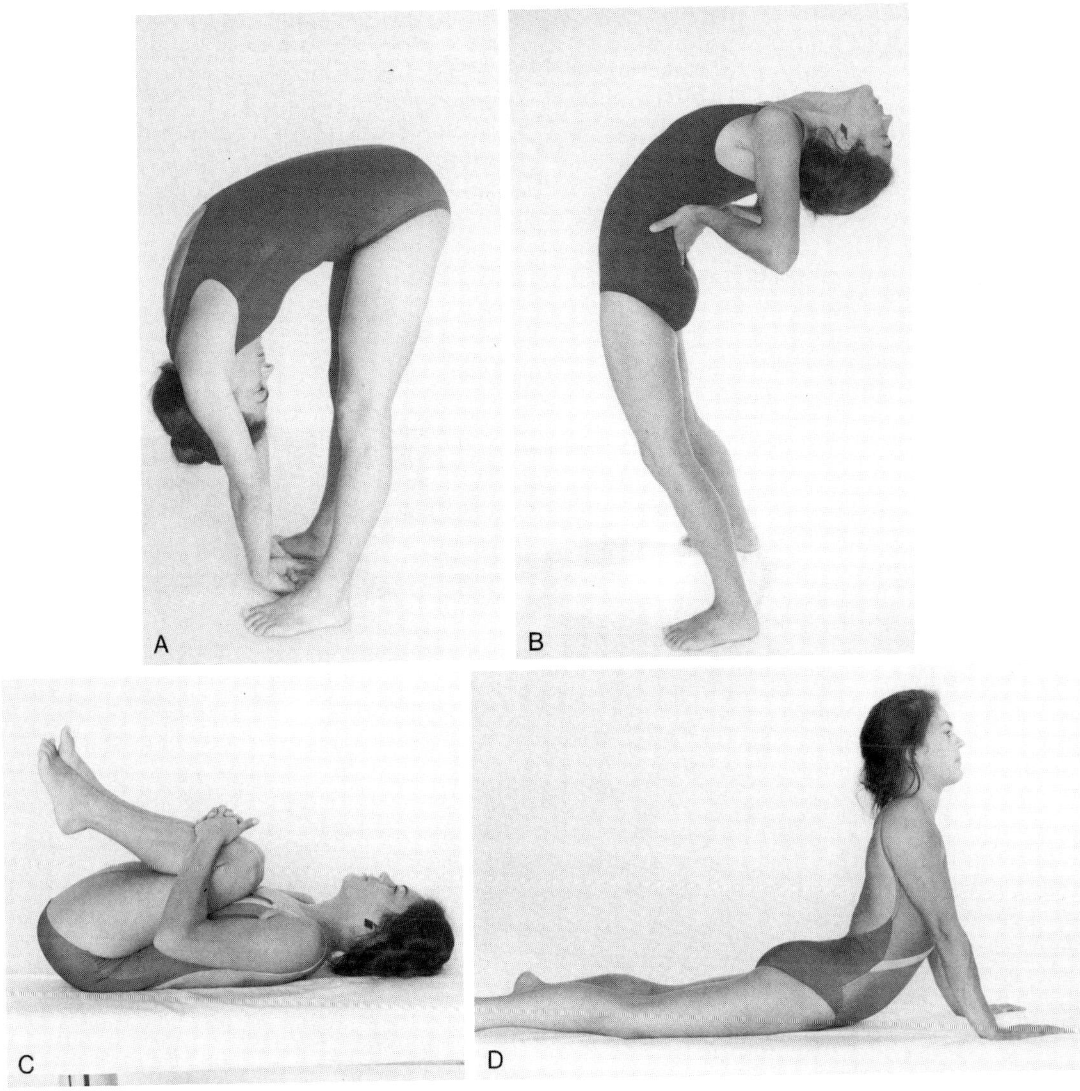

Figure 1 □ *A–D,* Effects of repeating well-defined movements performed in the standing and lying positions are observed.

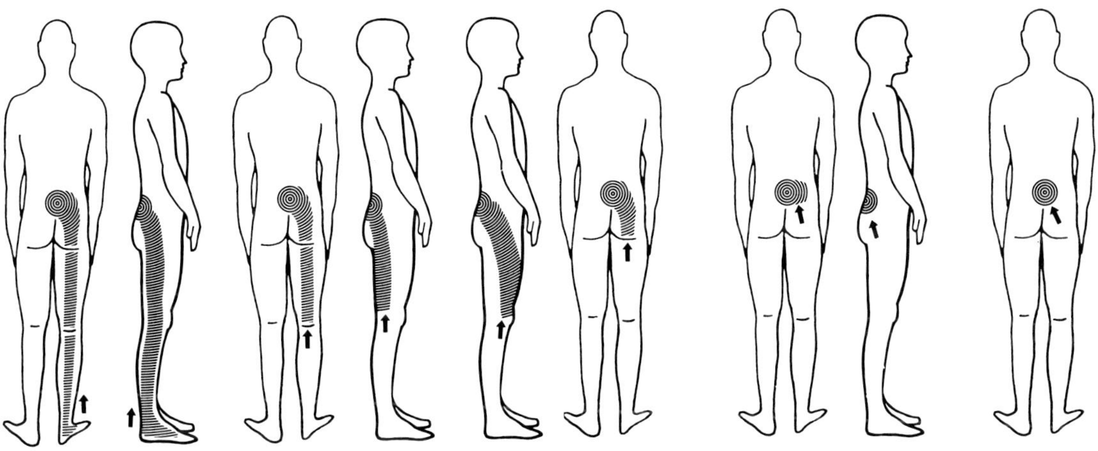

Figure 2 □ Progressive centralization of pain indicates the suitability of the exercise program.

tions, and frequently do not engage in regular exercise. They develop pain that appears locally, usually adjacent to the midline of the spinal column. The pain is provoked by mechanical deformation of soft tissues, which occurs only when spinal segments are subjected to prolonged static loading with joints held at end range. This occurs most commonly when poor sitting or standing postures are adopted and when the individual is required to maintain a prolonged bending or stooping position.

The affected individuals frequently complain of pain felt either separately or simultaneously in the cervical, thoracic, and lumbar areas.

Pain from the postural syndrome is never induced by movement, never referred, and never constant. No pathologic process, no loss of movement, and no signs are found in this syndrome. There is nothing to see.

Movements are normal, and patients with this syndrome are sometimes described as being hypermobile. The only objective information is discovered on examination of posture at the time of onset of pain, when the patient is seen to adopt slouched postures and to "hang" at the end range of ligamentous and capsular tension.

Pain from the postural syndrome can arise from any part of the mobile segment or from the adjacent soft tissues. It is probably ligamentous or periarticular in origin. Described simply, postural pain eventually appears by prolonged overstretching of normal tissue.

Dysfunction Syndrome

Patients with this syndrome are usually over 30 years of age, except for those in whom trauma can be identified as the original cause of their problem. They commonly exhibit poor posture and are frequently under-exercised.

Their pain remains after the initial acute symptoms resolve and may subsequently increase insidiously over a long period. Pain is provoked on attempting full movement by mechanically deforming shortened soft tissues in segments that have reduced elasticity and movement. The pain is always felt at end range, and never during the movement. With the exception of a patient with an adherent nerve root, pain from dysfunction is never referred.

The loss of movement evident in the dysfunction syndrome arises from two common causes. The first and most common cause of reduced spinal mobility is the maintenance of poor postural habits during the first few decades of life. This is likely to occur, especially if the individual does not exercise regularly. Poor postural habits allow adaptive shortening of certain structures. The result is a gradual reduction of mobility with aging. The movements reduced are usually the extension movements essential for the maintenance of the very erect posture. The second cause of reduced spinal mobility is contracture of fibrous scar tissue developed during repair following trauma. Thus, an inextensible scar can form within or adjacent to otherwise healthy structures and will cause reduced mobility. The pain resulting from stretching of this inextensible scar appears *only* on attempting full end-range movement. The pain does not occur during the movement or before the structure is placed under tension. Surrounding healthy structures would be capable of further extensibility but are now restricted by the scar.

It is not possible to identify the structure causing the pain of dysfunction, but any of the soft tissues adjacent to the vertebral column may adaptively shorten or may be damaged. Thus the pain may result from adaptive shortening of or injury to any of the ligamentous structures in the segment, from the intervertebral disc, the zygapophyseal joints, or the superficial or deep muscles or their attachments. The pain may also result from the adherence of the spinal nerve root or dura following severe intervertebral disc bulging or rupture, but this is more easily identified. Described simply, the pain of dysfunction is produced immediately by the overstretching of shortened tissues.

Derangement Syndrome

Patients with the derangement syndrome are usually between 20 and 55 years of age. They invariably have a poor sitting posture.

They develop pain, usually of sudden onset; that is, in a matter of a few hours or over the period of 1 or 2 days they change from completely normal to significantly disabled individuals. Often this syndrome appears for no apparent reason. The symptoms may be felt locally, adjacent to the midline of the spinal column, and may radiate and be referred distally in the form of pain, parasthesia, or numbness. The symptoms are produced, abolished, increased, or reduced by the performance of certain movements or the maintenance of certain positions.

Pain from the derangement syndrome may alter and change in regard to both the site of the pain and the extent of the affected area. Pain from the derangement syndrome may cross the midline and move, for example, from the right of the low back to the left.

My belief is that embryonic discogenic pathologic processes must always be suspected when the patient describes the pain as changing position and radiating when he or she changes position or performs different movements. When referred pain changes its distribution, shape, or location, this may signify the development of nuclear displacement through incomplete annular cracks or tears within the intervertebral disc as the disc changes its shape or position during movement or sustained postures.[2, 26, 49]

Pain from the derangement syndrome frequently is constant. There may be no position in which the patient can find relief. Therefore, the pain may be present regardless of whether movement is performed, is usually described as an ache that at times can be severe. The ache is then made more severe by movement in certain directions and is reduced by movement in other directions.

In patients with the derangement syndrome, especially those with severe cases, gross obstruction of movement may occur; postural deformities, such as kyphosis and scoliosis, are also seen frequently. Sudden obstruction to movement with loss of spinal mobility and the sudden appearance of postural deformity in acute low back and neck pain may be likened to the sudden locking that may occur in the knee joint, in which internal derangement of the meniscus is common.

The mechanism of internal derangement of the intervertebral disc is not fully understood. That the nucleus pulposus can be displaced toward and escape through a damaged annular wall is inarguable.[1, 2] It is highly likely that this is a consequence of sudden or violent movement or a result of postures sustained by younger patients. Older patients have a stiffer, less fluid nucleus, which is less likely to be displaced from within its annular envelope.[1, 2, 15] It is also hypothesized that, prior to a frank annular lesion with nuclear herniation, there are incomplete tears into which nuclear material may be displaced. This alters the joint biomechanics and may be responsible for the temporary postural deformities (e.g., localized scoliosis, kyphosis).

Creep of the fluid nucleus–annulus complex will disturb the normal alignment of adjacent vertebrae and change the resting shape of the disc.[15, 39] This change of shape will also affect the ability of the joint surface to move in its normal pathway, and deviation to the right or left of the sagittal plane will result when flexion or extension is attempted.[39] Laboratory and cadaveric observations carried out by Stahl[45] and Vogel[50] in 1977 and described in a monograph by Kramer[26] exactly duplicated the conceptual model that I presented in 1980,[29] in which I proposed a simple mechanism of displacement that could account for the production of acute low back problems, especially those causing acute lumbar list and acute kyphosis.[26, 29, 31]

Described simply, the pain of derangement occurs as the consequence of a change in disc shape with related malalignment of the mobile segment and its associated abnormal stresses.

Identification of the different syndromes is based on the following: the effects that movements have on the initiation of the pain; the point in the movement pathway at which pain is first perceived; the site of the pain and subsequent change of location of the pain toward peripheralization or centralization; the increasing or decreasing intensity of the pain; and, finally, abolition of the pain. Mechanical pain can arise only from a limited number of events or combination of events causing force to be applied to innervated soft tissues. Those soft tissues may be in a normal state, a shortened state, or in an anatomically altered state with a change in the shape or distribution of the disc and its fluids. Any of these events can be identified by the response of the patient's pain to the deliberate application of certain mechanical forces.

Patients with inflammatory disorders, with spondylolisthesis or other undetected minor fractures and with pathologic conditions unsuited to mechanical therapies will not respond in a predictable fashion. They will be quickly exposed and recognized when tested in the manner I have described.[25]

MECHANICAL TREATMENTS

Spinal Manipulative Therapy

All over the world enthusiastic physiotherapists, frustrated by years of control by medicine or disillusioned by the use of ineffectual methods of physical therapy, are rediscovering mobilization and manipulation and are providing it as the treatment of choice for many patients with spinal pain. No one experienced in the use of such therapy has failed to be excited on the many occasions when a spectacular improvement is obtained. Undoubtedly, many patients benefit from SMT. Several studies support the view that a short-term benefit results from using the therapy.[4, 14, 16, 21, 23, 44]

From within the ranks of the physiotherapists and especially from chiropractors and osteopaths, there emerge claims expounding the advantages of one form of SMT over another. Although one cannot with any hope of resolution enter the arguments for or against the concepts attached to the various systems, it is comparatively simple to demystify the procedures utilized to achieve the same result. As far as I am aware, no study demonstrates that any one form of SMT is superior to another. In one study at least, it has been established that osteopathic manipulation at the end of 4 weeks was no better than a placebo (detuned short-wave diathermy).[19] Schiotz and Cyriax[43] describe these situations well: "It is not the elegance or alleged specificity of some maneuver that matters, it is its therapeutic effectiveness." The effectiveness of repetitive motion is frequently superior to the most elegant SMT technique.

Physiotherapists should not allow history to repeat itself, as there is already a tendency for those schooled in one particular method of mobilization to denigrate other systems. Already we can see Kaltenborn, Maitland, Cyriax, and Paris devotees all enthusiastically supporting their particular "gurus" and failing to recognize that each group is probably dispensing the same mechanical maneuver using a different title, philosophy, and technique.

Once familiar with the various techniques of SMT, it becomes clear that the basic maneuvers in common usage today, by whichever profession, are essentially the same. Although differences may exist in the manner of delivery, these differences have not yet been shown to affect the final outcome. I am sure this statement will be strenuously challenged by the purists. This is the way it should be, of course, and we eagerly await the definitive study that demonstrates the superiority of one form of SMT over another.

In essence, the manipulative treatments are now dispensed by the physiotherapist well trained in modern mechanical concepts. The modern mechanical physiotherapist has the advantage of being able to use the entire spectrum of mechanical concepts and tools. So in considering the form of mechanical therapy most appropriate for the patient, whether it be exercise, traction, mobilization, or manipulation, the well-trained modern mechanical therapist can provide this treatment.

Several problems and concerns arise from the current wave of enthusiasm for SMT and its related techniques. These problems exist because in many parts of the world manipulation by physiotherapists is just now being developed; the initial enthusiasm, although understandable, must be tempered and brought into perspective. Inexperienced physical therapists see manipulation as the answer to the back problem and a panacea for whatever ails the patient.

Those in the profession who have a longer experience of the benefits and limitations of SMT must make that experience available in order to moderate the enthusiasm of those entering the field. Until we have learned to distinguish between a patient's responsiveness to treatment and a natural resolution of symptoms with the passage of time, our credibility is at risk. When our patients improve over a period of 3 to 4 months, can we seriously attribute their recovery to the manipulative or mechanical treatments delivered during this period? Failure to recognize and understand the natural history and the self-limiting characteristics of the low back problem perpetuates an inability to critically review treatment methods and results.

In order to dispense SMT, it has always

been necessary for the therapist to do something to the patient. Thus, irrespective of whether the patient's improvement is a result of the passage of time or to the techniques of therapy, the patient, correctly or incorrectly, attributes the recovery to the treatment. The individual becomes dependent on the therapy and in the event of recurrence hurries back to the therapist. In the mind of the patient and often in the mind of the therapist, the patient must receive more of the same treatment in order to recover.

It has been demonstrated that SMT provides a short-term benefit.[4, 14, 16, 21, 23, 44] There are no known long-term benefits.[34] If physiotherapists within medicine are to become the professionals responsible for the conservative treatment and management of people with mechanical spinal problems, we must provide the treatment that has the potential to provide long-term benefits.

In 1956 I witnessed the first of several observations of patients experiencing rapid and inexplicable improvement from the performance of casual movements or positions. The observations clearly demonstrated a cause-and-effect relationship between these movements or positions and the presence or intensity of symptoms. One patient who had been in pain for 3 weeks lay inadvertently in a certain position on a treatment table. After about 10 minutes he arose, completely relieved of leg pain. He returned the following day almost totally symptom free. Another patient, after a change of position, experienced a complete reversal of his pain from the right to the left side: another patient with a neck problem abolished all symptoms by repeatedly combing his hair with the head laterally flexed to one side. The pain did not return. These and other clinical observations allowed me to develop several rather different avenues of diagnosis and therapy.[29]

The main conclusions arising from these observations were that patients, using self-treatment principles and without manipulation by a therapist, could significantly affect the courses of their own disorders. In the nonspecific spectrum of back pain, I estimate that over 70% of patients can be taught these principles and achieve a good result with greater safety, more rapidly and efficiently, less expensively, and with lasting benefit.[30] *We cannot therefore justify the routine use of SMT for the treatment of low back pain if the same result can be obtained using forces applied by the patient.*

The time to apply special techniques of mobilization and manipulation arrives only after the patient has exhausted all self-treatment options without success. Temporary improvement for only a few hours following self treatment suggests that the applied forces, although appropriate directionally, were inadequate in degree. The introduction of mobilization at this time is indicated. Failing improvement with the use of mobilization, then and only then is manipulation indicated.

I have further proposed that we should postpone or avoid mobilization and manipulation until we have determined that resolution of the problem is impossible utilizing the patient's own movements and positions. Patients unable to apply self-treatment procedures with lasting benefit and those with any lumbar or sciatic list will always require the special skills of the physiotherapist versed in correction of this problem.[31] Others will require techniques in the form of mobilization, and a few of those will additionally require manipulative thrust procedures.[29]

Thus, the gradual development of increasing force to bring about change is a logical and safe method of applying mechanical therapies, assuming that vertebral and vascular pathologic processes are excluded. The ultimate weapon we have is the manipulative thrust technique. Why immediately use that technique when the patient may well be capable of causing the change without the help of the therapist, at the same time learning an important self-management lesson?

I am not proposing that mobilization and manipulation are no longer required. SMT has a particular and important part to play in the treatment of mechanical spinal pain, but is greatly misused. The time has come when we must rationalize the use of such methods. We are now able to determine, usually within the first 24-hour period after assessment, whether manipulative therapy will be needed, and it should no longer be necessary to apply SMT in order to find out retrospectively whether the procedure was indicated. Spinal mobilization and manipulation should not be dispensed to the entire population of patients with back pain in order to ensure that the very few who really need it actually receive it. That philosophy is no longer acceptable. It is conceivable that in the not-too-distant future, apart from the obvious exceptions, mechanical spinal disorders will be so well understood that few problems affecting the spinal segments will require manipulation and most patients themselves will be able to treat mechanical disorders.

Traction

As with studies of the efficacy of SMT,[4] most of the studies investigating clinical efficacy of traction are flawed. However, some evidence remains to suggest that it is premature to discard the treatment as entirely ineffectual. The most recent addition to the various types of traction is the autotraction table, which was devised by Lind but studied by Larsson.[27]

Originally designed for the treatment of frank disc herniation causing sciatic syndromes, autotraction has been recommended by some in the United States as a panacea for back pain in general, and its worth may be misjudged accordingly. No such claims were made by its innovator, and hopefully it will be further investigated by independent assessors, although one recent study indicated that the response to autotraction was no different from the response to manual traction at 2 weeks and 3 months.[28] Another study[3] indicates that during autotraction pressures within the disc increased considerably. No negative pressures were recorded.

Gravity traction and inversion traction are other methods of treatment currently in vogue in the United States. I am aware of no reliable data or objective assessments that indicate its value. As is true of other therapies, improvement with traction must be seen to result from the treatment and not from the passage of 3 or 4 weeks of time as the natural history of the condition runs its course.

It has been my experience that patients other than those I have classified as having derangement six,[29] will benefit more rapidly by using self-treatment procedures than from undergoing traction. The disorders of patients with derangement six (sciatica with list and neurologic deficit), in my experience, appear to resolve with passing time rather than from traction itself, but the advent of autotraction may alter this view.

Massage

Massage is still used for the treatment of low back pain, and it can certainly have a mechanical effect on superficial structures. When it is applied with sufficient pressure, there must also be a mechanical effect on the articulations of the spine. Under certain circumstances, it is likely that firm massage is as beneficial as gentle mobilization.

Exercise

Exercise has been the mainstay of the physiotherapy profession, especially since the development of Swedish Remedial Exercises in the early part of the century.[42] In the treatment of spinal disorders conflict has always existed between those who have advocated flexion exercises based on the rationale proposed by Williams,[51] and those who have advocated extension to treat low back pain.[9, 22, 29] Williams' philosophy is most strongly established in the United States and Canada, where almost anyone with low back pain or sciatica receives the standard flexion procedure.

Extension, on the other hand, having been graphically described by Hippocrates,[22] has been used throughout the rest of the world, it seems, since the earliest records were kept.[43]

Of course, it is not possible to arbitrarily impose one treatment on the entire spectrum of mechanical disorders of the low back, deciding that all patients must flex or all must extend. Several studies indicate that exercises tailored to suit individual needs are of benefit.[13, 25, 30, 38, 40, 48] The majority, but not all, of the patients benefit from extension. Flexion and lateral flexion as indicated by centralizing pain patterns are also necessary. By utilizing repetitive end-range movements[29] and centralizing pain phenomena, it is possible to determine the direction in which any particular patient must be moved in order to bring about resolution of the particular problem.

It is now clear that some patients must flex in a particular way in order to abolish pain; others must extend in a particular way to achieve that state. Still others must first flex and then immediately extend in order to become free of symptoms.

SUMMARY

Pathology

With one exception,[35] we are not yet in a position to positively identify precisely the structures involved in the production of common low back problems. Until recently, treatment has been by trial and error, and no reliable predictors of outcome have been available. Although further research is required, the centralization of pain phenomena appears to offer promise as a reliable prognostic indicator.[13]

Responsibility

Physiotherapists, by virtue of their training, their relationship with the medical profession, and their now-improved public esteem, are without a doubt the professionals most appropriately equipped to assume responsibility to dispense conservative spinal therapy for mechanical disorders.

We must ensure, however, that this opportunity is not lost by allowing some of our less discriminating colleagues to perpetuate the deceptive use of nonvalidated treatments. Ridding ourselves of outmoded therapies is an urgent priority. It is appropriate at this point to quote directly from Nachemson:

> In the therapeutic field today, it is virtually impossible to introduce a new drug without clinical and laboratory tests to prove its effectiveness, and we are increasingly alert to and critical of different types of pharmacological side effects. The same approach should be used for the different forms of treatment of low back pain and we should critically re-assess our present methods.[35]

Mechanical Diagnosis and Treatment

Three clinically identifiable syndromes exist in the nonspecific spectrum of low back pain.[29] Identification of any one of these syndromes is not dependent on the identification of the structures responsible for the presenting symptoms. Soft tissues are affected by mechanical forces that will result in the production of pain only under three particular conditions: (1) normal, (2) shortened, and (3) anatomically disrupted and displaced.

Postural Syndrome

Normal tissues can become painful in daily life by the application of prolonged stresses commonly appearing during static postural loading conditions, such as prolonged sitting, standing, or bending.

Treatment □ Correction of faulty postural habit removes causative stresses. No other treatment is required. SMT mobilization and traction are of no use. In order to remove the cause of pain, the therapist must instruct the patient as to the correct position.

Dysfunction Syndrome

Shortened structures limit movement and simultaneously cause pain when the shortened structure is stretched.

Treatment □ Essentially, it is a remodeling process. Short structures are lengthened by the regular application of stretching exercises. Dysfunction is not rapidly reversible; weeks are required to remodel and lengthen. SMT is of no use. Structures that have adaptively shortened over weeks and months cannot suddenly lengthen by the application of high-velocity thrusts without incurring damage.

Derangement Syndrome

An example of this syndrome would be the presence of frank tears of the annulus fibrosus with nuclear displacement or annular bulging. The patient experiences aching without movement, increased pain with movement in certain directions as displacement increases, and reduced pain in other directions as displacement decreases.

Treatment □ This syndrome is subject to mostly rapid reversal. The derangement is reduced by applying appropriate movements; the reduction is maintained by correcting posture and avoiding wrong positions; function is restored before adaptive changes are established.

Mechanical forces used to treat mechanical disorders of the low back should be applied in a graduated form, first by utilizing the repeated movements of self treatment, then progressing through mobilization, and finally applying manipulative procedures.

With no resolution of symptoms, use of other mechanical devices such as traction should follow. The only patients to receive modalities should be those failing to respond to the mechnical approach. Electrotherapeutic modalities such as transcutaneous electrical nerve stimulator (TENS), interferential therapy, microwave, and others should be used only to modulate pain when mechanical methods have failed. Physiotherapy professionals, however, must ask themselves whether modulating pain by using expensive modalities is of greater benefit to the patient and society than dispensing rather inexpensive medications.

References

1. Adams, M. A., and Hutton, W. C.: Prolapsed intervertebral disc: A hyperflexion injury. Spine 7:3, 1982.
2. Adams, M. A., Hutton, W. C.: Gradual disc prolapse. Spine 10:6, 1985.
3. Andersson, B. J. G., Schulz, A. B., and Nachemson, A.: Intervertebral disc pressures during traction. J. Rehab. Med. 9(Suppl.):88, 1983.
4. Brunarski, D. J.: Clinical trials of spinal manipulation. J. Manip. Physiol. Ther. 7:4, 1984.
5. Carron, H., DeGood, D. E., and Tait, R.: A comparison of low back pain patients in the United States and New Zealand: Psychosocial and economic factors affecting severity of disability. Pain 21:77–89, 1985.
6. Coventry, M. B., Ghormley, R. K., and Kernohan, J. W.: The intervertebral disc: Part II. Changes in the intervertebral disc concomitant with age. J. Bone Joint Surg. 27:233, 1945.
7. Coventry, M. B., Ghormley, R. K., and Kernohan, J. W.: The intervertebral disc: Part III. Pathological changes in the intervertebral disc. J. Bone Joint Surg. 27:460, 1945.
8. Cyriax, J.: Textbook of Orthopaedic Medicine, Vol. 1. London, Bailliere Tindall, 1954.
9. Cyriax, J.: Textbook of Orthopaedic Medicine, 5th Ed., Vol. 1. London, Bailliere Tindall, 1980.
10. Cyron, B. M., Hutton, W. C.: Articular tropism and instability of the lumbar spine. Spine 5:168, 1980.
11. DiMaggio, A., and Mooney, V.: Conservative care for low back pain: What works? J. Musculoskel. Med. 4:27–34, 1987.
12. Dixon, A.: Diagnosis of low back pain. *In* Jayson, M. (ed.): The Lumbar Spine and Back Pain. Tunbridge Wells, Pitman Medical, 1980.
13. Donelson, R., Murphy, K., and Silva, G.: Centralization Phenomenon: Its Usefulness in Evaluating and Treating Sciatica. Annual Meeting of I.S.S.L.S. Dallas, 1986.
14. Doran, M. L., and Newell, D. J.: Manipulation in treatment of low back pain: A multicentre study. Br. Med. J. 2:161, 1975.
15. Farfan, H. F.: Mechanical Disorders of the Low Back. Philadelphia, Lea & Febiger, 1973.
16. Farrell, J. B., and Twomey, L. T.: Acute low back pain. Comparison of two conservative treatment approaches. Proceedings of Manipulative Therapists Association of Australia, Perth, Western Australia, 1983, p. 162.
17. Fredrickson, B., Murphy, K., Donelson, R., and Yuan, H.: McKenzie Treatment of Low Back Pain: A Correlation of Significant Factors in Determining Prognosis. Annual Meeting of I.S.S.L.S. Dallas, 1986.
18. Frymoyer, J. W., Phillips, R. B., Newberg, A. H., and MacPherson, B. V.: A comparative analysis of the interpretations of lumbar spinal radiographs by chiropractors and medical doctors. Spine 11:10, 1986.
19. Gibson, T., Blagrave, P., and Harkness, J.: Low back pain treated by an osteopath. Br. J. Rheumatol. 24:92, 1985.
20. Gonella, C., Paris, S., and Kutner, M.: Reliability in evaluating passive intervertebral motion. Phys. Ther. 62:437, 1982.
21. Hadler, N. M., Curtis, P., Gillings, D. B., and Stinnett, S.: A benefit of spinal manipulation as adjunctive therapy for acute low-back pain: A stratified controlled trial. Spine 12:7, 1987.
22. Hippocrates: Corpus Hippocrateum. Peri Arthron. Chapter 47, 400 BC (cited by Cyriax, 1980).
23. Hoehler, F. K., Tobis, J. S., and Buerger, A. A.: Spinal manipulation for low back pain. J.A.M.A. 245:1835, 1981.
24. Jull, G.: The reliability of manual palpation. Proceedings of the Manipulative Therapists Association of Australia Conference. Brisbane, 1985.
25. Kopp, J. R., Alexander, A. H., and Turocy, R. H.: The use of lumbar extension in the evaluation and treatment of patients with acute herniated nucleus pulposus. Clin. Orthop. Vol. 202, Jan. 1986.
26. Kramer, J.: Intervertebral Disk Diseases, 1st Ed. Chicago, Year Book Medical Publishers, 1981.
27. Larsson, U., Choler, U., and Lidstrom, A.: Auto traction for treatment of lumbago-sciatica. Acta Orthop. Scand. 51:791, 1980.
28. Ljunggren, A. E., Webber, H., and Larson, S.: Auto traction v. manual traction in patients with prolapsed lumbar intervertebral discs. Scand. J. Rehab. Med. 16:17, 1984.
29. McKenzie, R. A.: The Lumbar Spine. New Zealand, Spinal Publications, 1980.
30. McKenzie, R. A.: Prophylaxis in recurrent low back pain. N.Z. Med. J. 89:627, 1979.
31. McKenzie, R. A.: Manual correction of sciatic scolisis. N.Z. Med. J. 76:484, 1972.
32. Matyas, T. A., and Bach, T. M.: The reliability of selected techniques in clinical arthrometrics. Aust. J. Physiother. 1:175, 1985.
33. Mooney, V.: Presidential Address. Spine 12:8, 1987.
34. Moritz, U.: Evaluation of manipulation and other manual therapy. Criteria for measuring the effect of treatment. Scand. J. Rehab. Med. 11:173, 1979.
35. Nachemson, A.: A critical look at conservative treatment of low back pain. *In* Jayson, M. (ed.): The Lumbar Spine and Back Pain. Tunbridge Wells, Pitman Medical, 1980. p. 355.
36. Nachemson, A.: Lumbar spine instability. Spine 10:3, 1985.
37. Nelson, M. A., Allen, P., and Clamp, S.: Reliability

and reproducibility of clinical findings in low-back pain. Spine 4:2, 1979.
38. Nwuga, G., and Nwuga, V.: Relative therapeutic efficacy of the Williams and McKenzie protocols in back pain management. Physiother. Pract. 1:99–106, 1985.
39. Panjabi, M., Krag, M. H., and Chung, T. Q.: Effects of disc injury on mechanical behaviour of the human spine. Spine 9:7, 1984.
40. Ponte, D. J., Jensen, G. J., and Kent, B. E.: A preliminary report on the use of the McKenzie protocol versus Williams protocol in the treatment of low back pain. J. Orthop. Sports Phys. Ther. 6:2, 1984.
41. Potter, N. A., and Rothstein, J. M.: Intertester reliability for selected clinical tests of the sacroiliac joint. Phys. Ther. 65:1671, 1985.
42. Prosser, E.: Manual of massage and movements. London, Faber & Faber, 1945.
43. Schiotz, E. H., and Cyriax, J.: Manipulation, Past and Present. London, Heinmann, 1975.
44. Sims-Williams, H., Jayson, M. I. V., and Young, S. M. S.: Controlled trial of mobilisation and manipulation for patients with low back pain in general practice. Br. Med. J. 2:1338, 1978.
45. Stahl, C.: Experimentelle Untersuchungen zur Biomechanik der Halswirbelsaule Med. Diss., Dusseldorf, 1977.
46. Suzuki, N., and Seiichi, E.: A quantitative study of trunk muscle strength and fatigability in the low back pain syndrome. Spine 8:1, 1983.
47. Twomey, L., and Taylor, J.: Age changes in the lumbar intervertebral discs. Acta Orthop. Scand. 56:6, 496, 1985.
48. Vanharanta, H., Videman, T., and Mooney, V.: A Comparison of McKenzie Exercises, Back Trac and Back School in Lumbar Syndrome; Preliminary Results. Annual Meeting of I.S.S.L.S. Dallas, 1986.
49. Vernon-Roberts, B.: Pathology and interrelation of intervertebral disc lesions. Jayson, M. (ed.): The Lumbar Spine and Back Pain, 2nd Ed. Tunbridge Wells, Pitman Medical, 1980.
50. Vogel, G.: Experimentelle Untersuchungen zur Mobilitat des nucleus pulposus in lumbalen Bandscheiben. Med. Diss., Dusseldorf, 1977.
51. Williams, C. P.: The Lumbosacral Spine. New York, McGraw-Hill, 1965.
52. Willis, T. A.: The lumbo-sacral anomalies. J. Bone Joint Surg. 41A:935, 1959.

MANIPULATION OF THE LUMBAR SPINE

Stanley V. Paris

Spinal manipulation is perhaps the most controversial of conservative spinal management techniques. The controversy is no doubt attributable to the fact that the origin and development of the technique have been outside the sphere of orthodox medical influence. Recent times have given rise to the bone setters of England and Europe and the osteopaths and chiropractors of North America. Although it incurs the healthy skepticism of the medical profession, spinal manipulation enjoys ever-increasing acceptance by physical therapists and, indirectly, by their referring medical colleagues. The methods by which manipulation is practiced differs greatly among the various professional groups, and even within those groups. However, there is a trend toward conformity as some of the more cultish methods give way to those based, at least to some extent, on science.

Until recently, little was known of the mechanism underlying the reported benefits from manipulation of the spine. With the development of information on collagen synthesis and on the mechanisms for the formation of capsular restrictions, a mechanical basis for stretching joints to improve motion has emerged. Again, the neurophysiologic responses of articular mechanoreceptors have been identified[25] as possibly underlying the relief from pain provided by manipulative techniques, especially those that incorporate repeated motions or oscillations.

Both mechanical and neurophysiologic effects can be added to the already recognized psychologic or placebo effect of the intensive manipulation and, of course, the occasional audible crack or snap of the joint, to which many patients and some practitioners attach great importance.

Attempts at clinical investigations into the possible benefits of manipulation have been relatively recent. At present these investigations attempt to compare manipulation with other modalities, such as medication, bed rest, physiotherapy, and placebo. The studies illustrate that manipulation is most effective in acute back pain states. However, there is still no study of manipulation as it is practiced by most practitioners (physical therapists) in North America, who use manipulation not as the sole treatment but along with preparatory modalities, such as heat and massage, and supportive modalities, such as exercises, posture, and back school. Just as back surgery is not practiced without explanation, anesthesia, medication, and supportive care (e.g., physical therapy), neither is manipulation practiced without them. Thus, to assess it as an isolated treatment is meaningless and will have little effect on its acceptance or dismissal.

DEFINITION OF JOINT MANIPULATION

Joint manipulation has been defined as "the skilled, passive movement of a joint (or spinal segment), either within or beyond its active range of motion."[21] The definition contains no mention of the term *thrust* or *force*. It uses the word *skilled*, and it does not distinguish between the words *mobilization* and *manipulation*, which I hold to be synonymous. Therefore, the techniques of manipulation may be gentle oscillations within the existing range, stretches at the end of range, or thrusts either within or at the end of range. One joint sound commonly heard, especially when joints are moved passively, is a "pop," which is probably caused by the release of gas from the joint fluid. This results, no doubt, in an increase in the intra-articular volume and thus produces a temporary increase in range of motion. The pop and its resultant swelling are also thought to have an effect on the muscle tone inhibitors of the Type III mechanoreceptors in the joint capsule and/or the Golgi tendon end organs in the overlying multifidus muscle, which also attaches to the capsule. In either case, a temporary increase in range of motion results, along with a sensation of pain relief. This is the common experience of individuals who crack their own backs. The pain relief could be explained by the gate control mechanisms postulated by Melzack[14] and the muscle relaxation response from the Golgi tendon end organs in the multifidus muscle.

A multitude of techniques are available, each with different objectives and adherents, who are usually divided along professional lines. Furthermore, most practitioners who have taken graduate education in manipulation rarely use it as the sole modality. Preparatory treatment of, for example, heat and massage, followed by a manipulation for either relieving pain (usually gentle oscillations) or increasing the range (usually stretch techniques) are essential to obtaining the best results from treatment. The treatments are followed by rest, exercises, and of course education in the use and care of the back. Unfortunately, most of the research on manipulation fails to take into account these factors and renders on an unprepared individual either a rotary thrust to the lumbar spine or a passive hip flexion, one being considered to be a test of manipulation and the other to be a test of mobilization.[26] This is an outdated approach that may represent the medical practitioner's idea of manipulation, but it is not practiced by most physical therapists and chiropractors who have specialized in manipulative techniques. Manipulation without appropriate preparatory and supportive treatments does not fairly represent the current state of practice.

Thrust techniques are still common in chiropractic but are becoming less so since the gentler techniques of progressive stretch produce similar results that are less likely to aggravate the underlying complaint. When practiced by chiropractors, thrust techniques may either be specific, in which

Table 1 □ Classification of Lumbar Manipulative Techniques

NONTHRUST

- **Oscillations**—principal effect is neurophysiologic; several grades, classification depending on range and force
- **Stretches**—principal effect is mechanical on the capsule and adjacent myofascia
  - Sustained, which are done within comfort
  - Repeated, which are more comfortable
  - Progressive, in which repeated maneuvers go progressively further

THRUST

- **Specific**—usually used to correct a vertebral position (chiropractic) or to a movement restriction (physical therapy)
- **Nonspecific**—usually directed toward a region of the spine and usually involves a torque; commonly the method practiced by physicians who have not had formal training in manipulative techniques

DISTRACTION (a more precise term for traction)—may be intermittent or sustained in combination with positioning for the involved segment and side of the segment, or without positioning.

case the force is directed to a vertebra, or nonspecific, in which case they are applied to an area. Physical therapy thrust techniques, and indeed most techniques, are not directed against vertebrae but rather against the joint in order to increase its range. Far more common in physical therapy is a stretch technique directed primarily toward one facet joint or segment for the purpose of increasing range.

Manipulation is used, therefore, for its mechanical effects to increase range, its neurophysiologic effects to abate pain, and of course the placebo effect, which no doubt is enhanced by the "hands on" nature of both the examination and the treatment.

Table 1 delineates the classification of manipulative techniques for the lumbar spine.

HISTORY

First described by Hippocrates,[24] spinal manipulation has been practiced by distinguished forefathers of orthopedics, including Galen,[18] Sir James Paget,[19] Hugh Owen Thomas (whose father was a bone setter [lay manipulator]),[13] Hood,[9] Mennell[5,16] and Cyriax.[3] In the United States osteopathy, beginning in the 1870s, and chiropractic, beginning in the 1890s, generated more practitioners of manipulation.

By the 1920s, physical therapists in Scandinavia, England, and the United States had taken an interest in manipulation.[6] Since the 1960s the technique has become well established in their practices; articles and texts have been written by myself[20,21,22] and other physical therapists.[5,11]

Most physical therapists use manipulation not as the sole modality but in conjunction with preparatory modalities of heat and massage and supportive modalities of exercises, posture, and back school.

PURPOSE

The principal purpose of manipulation is to increase the range of motion in a spinal segment, which in turn is believed to help improve nutrition, gate pain, increase tolerence to insult, and improve function.

Manipulation has two primary effects: the first is on pain, and the second is on mechanics. In the relief from pain, particularly acute pain, manipulation appears to fare better than all other modalities and procedures. A recent paper presented at The International Society for the Study of the Lumbar Spine in Rome, 1987,[23] showed manipulation in the treatment of acute low back pain with or without leg pain to be superior to drug therapy, physiotherapy, bed rest, and placebo. However, for chronic back and leg pain, manipulation slipped to third place, behind physiotherapy and back school. In fact, this is the combination used by most therapists practicing manipulation (i.e., with physical therapy and back school).

These data point to the effects of manipulation on pain. The effect of the technique seems to resemble that of Codman's exercises on the shoulder;[2] that is, the gentle oscillatory motions appear to control the onward transmission of nociceptive impulses[14,25] and thus close the gate to pain. Not only is the pain relieved, but the involuntary muscle holding is also abated and function is improved. Although oscillations are usually performed manually, some manipulation tables permit patients to oscillate their own lumbar spines (Fig. 1.)

Mechanically, manipulation may stretch tightened capsular adhesions[1] of the facet joints and help restore shortened muscles to normal length (Fig. 2). On occasion, manipulation may correct the alignment of a joint, such as the sacroiliac joint, which owing to hypermobility may have over-ridden its normal restraints and become locked in a faulty position.

Neither manipulation nor the closely related distraction (traction) has been shown to have long-term effect on the intervertebral disc.[12] When relief of pain follows manipulation in patients diagnosed as having disc

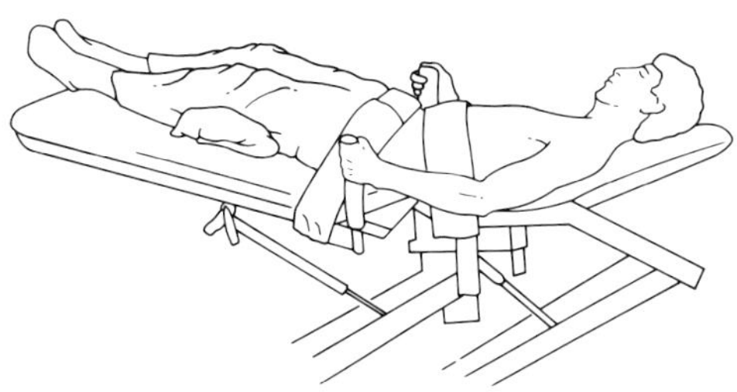

Figure 1 □ Automanipulation is an effective means of introducing motion into the acute spine. The patient controls the movement and can use the low back muscles to assist in motion. The use and effect is akin to that of Codman's exercises for the shoulder. (From Payton, O.D. [ed.]: Manual of Physical Therapy. New York, Churchill Livingstone, 1989.)

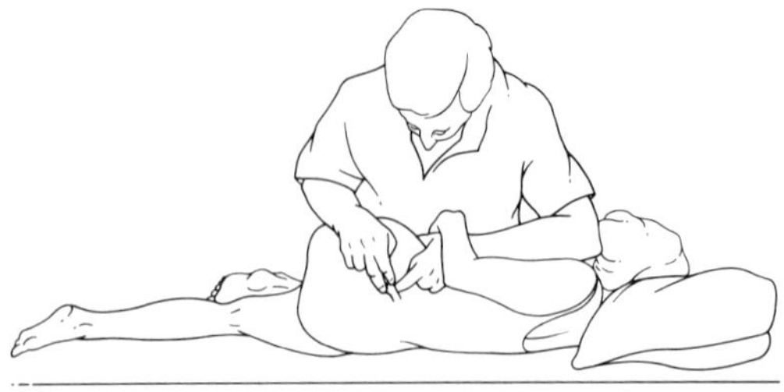

Figure 2 □ Midlumbar rotation stretching the left capsule at L4–L5 is used to regain range of motion or to release a mechanical locking or an incarcerated capsule. The forces are localized by placing the subject in a forward-bending position and then by rotation to the desired level. The position is held by pressure on the shoulder and pelvis and further localized with pressure on the adjacent spinous processes. (From Payton, O.D. [ed.]: Manual of Physical Therapy. New York, Churchill Livingstone, 1989.)

lesions, one can only assume that the disc was not the primary or sole cause of the pain.

Likewise, the use of manipulation to correct (adjust) vertebral misalignments has not been shown to be a valid concept. The principal protagonists of its use for this purpose are chiropractors, and they are currently showing an increasing interest in manipulation for correcting movement dysfunctions rather than vertebral misalignments.

INDICATIONS

The indications for manipulation vary, depending on the stage of the condition. Clinically, low back pain can be divided into immediate, acute, subacute, settled, and chronic stages. The treatment at each of these stages is somewhat different.

Immediate and Acute Stages

In the immediate and acute stages, it is sometimes observed that a patient presents with a combination of forward bending and side bending. In the absence of a current history and neurologic signs, the most likely cause of this posture is either a mechanical lock of the facets or the voluntary adoption of a posture that unburdens the side of the back that is in pain as a result of, perhaps, a painful capsular entrapment.

If the examination of the passive movements detects a locked facet, then the treatment of choice is a facet distraction technique, actually rotation to the segment (Fig. 2). However, if the posture has been maintained for any length of time, backward bending as both a passive and an active exercise may also need to be added once the facet mechanical lock or painful entrapment has been released (Fig. 3). Of course one could argue about whether facets are capable of becoming locked. Given that they—like the knee, wrist, or temporomandibular joint—possess menisci and that these former joints do have a history of spontaneous locking, it seems plausible that the same mechanism may occasionally affect the spine.

If the examination suggests a possible acute facet capsule entrapment as evidenced by a restriction (by pain) of movements that increase the load of the involved facet (i.e., backward bending or side bending to the painful side and by rotation to the opposite side), then an exercise or a manipulation technique that calls on a strong isometric contraction of the multifidus muscle may be successful. The mechanism at work here is the use of the multifidus attachment to the facet capsule to pull out the entrapped capsule; in the clinical picture just described, it is highly effective (Fig. 4). The principle of

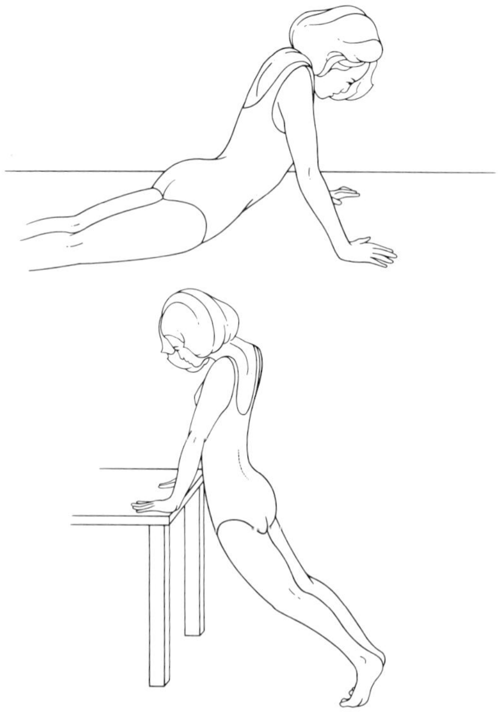

Figure 3 □ *A, B,* Backward bending to provide motion and to gate pain may be accomplished in a number of ways, as depicted in these illustrations. (From Payton, O.D. [ed.]: Manual of Physical Therapy. New York, Churchill Livingstone, 1989.)

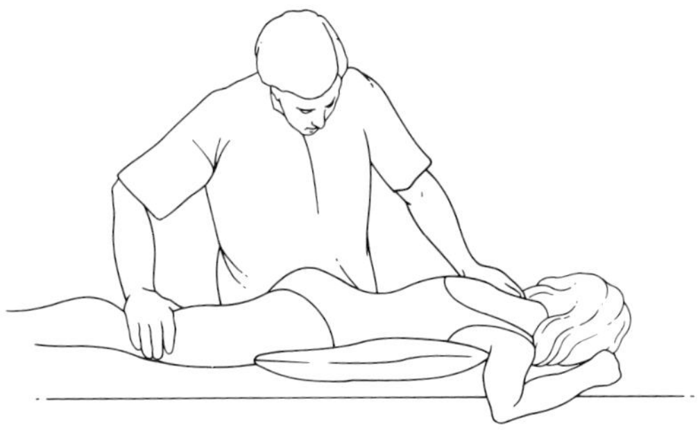

Figure 4 □ Utilizing isometric multifidus contraction to pull on the capsule of a suspected facet capsular impingement. The shoulder on the afflicted side and the pelvis on the opposite side are held firm while a leg raise is requested. Note that the lumbar spine should be supported with one or more firm pillows. (From Payton, O.D. [ed.]: Manual of Physical Therapy. New York, Churchill Livingstone, 1989.)

this procedure is not unlike using the capsular attachment of rectus femoris to avoid painful passive hip flexion. If this is not successful, then the distraction technique illustrated in Figure 2 modified by using more side bending over, for example, a pillow may be effective.

Subacute Stage

In the subacute stage, once any postural malalignment has been corrected, the emphasis is on maintaining range of motion and facilitating healing. Forceful manipulations have no place, but oscillatory and active exercises are quite valuable.

Settled Stage

In the settled stage, usually at around the tenth day after the injury, manipulation, particularly that of a mechanical nature, will be at its most effective. Tired and cramped muscles may be assisted by heat, massage, and manipulative stretching, and any adhesions that may be forming within either the facet joints or the soft tissues surrounding them can also be stretched at this stage, with little risk of causing a regression of symptoms.

Likewise, back school concepts will have already been introduced along with whatever exercises the patient's condition indicates may be of assistance. Furthermore, the therapist will have looked at not only the lumbar spine but also at such factors as a pronated foot, which would functionally shorten the leg and result in lateral curvature. Likewise, a hip restriction or a tight iliopsoas might well influence spinal function and thus be either a factor causing the patient's complaint or one prolonging it.

Chronic Stage

In the chronic stage, which begins about 3 months later, manipulation as the sole treatment does not fare as well as the combined physical therapy, heat massage, and back school. In addition, the emphasis is placed on improving physical fitness, increasing work activity, and, if necessary, using some behavioral techniques.

LIMITATIONS

Manipulation will not be successful in all cases of low back pain, but when combined with education in the form of back school and general physical therapy it offers the best possible approach to low back conditions in patients for whom surgery is not indicated.

There are contraindications to some forms of manipulation. However, even in the presence of nearby fracture or disease, gentle oscillations may provide a significant degree of relief from pain.

Some practitioners have stated that pain below the buttock[10] or pain below the knee[8] is a contraindication to manipulation, no doubt because of the assumption that such pains are discogenic in origin and thus indicate considerable severity. However, Mooney and Robertson[18] showed that such pains can come from facet joints. In addition, the nerves of the lumbar spine also receive nociception from the muscles and ligaments of the lumbar spine as well as from the facets and discs. Furthermore, the sacroiliac joint is likewise innervated by the lumbar nerves, notably the medial branch of the postprimary rami from L4 and L5 and from S1–S3. These nerves would also have the ability of forwarding noxious stimuli, which could be interpreted as back and leg pains. Thus, leg pain does not seem to be a contraindication to manipulation. Nevertheless, most practitioners agree that, when the procedure reproduces the patient's complaint of pain and especially when it increases its radiation, the procedure should be abandoned because it will probably aggravate the condition.

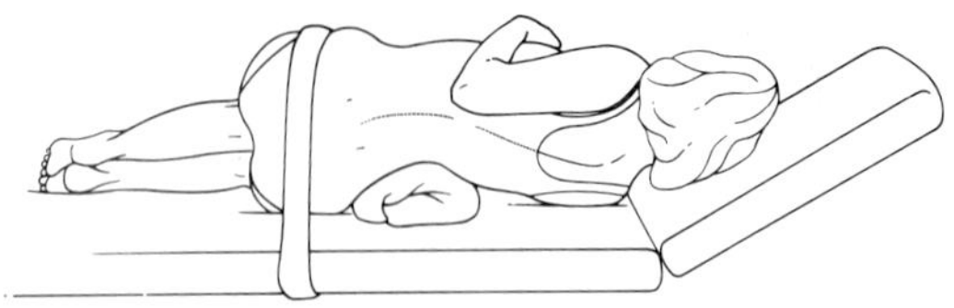

Figure 5 □ When neurologic signs suggest nerve root pressure, this form of distraction (traction), in which the patient is placed over a bolster during side bending and forward bending to the involved level, is effective in gaining a wide opening of the intervertebral foramen. It should not be used with the acute disc, in which case there may be a danger of increasing the disc injury. (From Payton, O.D. [ed.]: Manual of Physical Therapy. New York, Churchill Livingstone, 1989.)

Many practitioners consider that manipulation has little, if any, beneficial effect on intervertebral disc dysfunction. The movement of manipulation may help relieve the patient's discomfort and encourage a return to activity. However, there is very little evidence that a pathologic process in the disc can be reversed by manipulation or, for that matter, by lumbar traction.

Most practitioners are careful to avoid placing a rotary or torque stress on an intervertebral disc when signs of imminent disc disease are present. Instead, a distraction or side-bending technique designed to open up the foramen and flatten the natural disc convexity is preferred. The effect of such maneuvers may be to relieve pressure on a nerve root, thus reducing its sensitivity. These techniques are termed positional distraction, and are illustrated in Figure 5.

When a proven disc herniation is thought to be the cause of the patient's pain, manipulation is probably not indicated[21] and should be replaced by positional distraction techniques during the settled stage. However, in several studies manipulation has been performed in the presence of demonstrated myelographic defects and has resulted in good or excellent pain relief, although no discernible difference was observed in the myelogram.[4] It must be concluded that its use in the presence of a known or suspected disc lesion must be carefully graded and monitored and is at best controversial.

CONCLUSION

In a number of studies spinal manipulation has been shown to be the superior treatment modality for the relief of low back pain in the acute phase. In the chronic stages of low back and leg pain, spinal manipulation as a treatment by itself has not been shown to produce any advantage over other conservative treatment. However, manipulation combined with physical therapy and back school techniques provide the most favorable clinical results. This is the manner in which increasing numbers of physical therapists practice manipulation.

References

1. Akeson, W. H., Amiel, D., and Woo, S.: Immobility effects of synovial joints: The pathomechanics of joint contracture. Biorheology 17:95, 1980.
2. Codman, E. A.: The Shoulder. Boston, Thomas Todd, 1934.
3. Cyriax, J. H.: Textbook of Orthopaedic Medicine, 8th Ed., Vol. I. Diagnosis of Soft Tissue Lesions. London, Bailliere and Tindall, 1982.
4. Doran, P. M. L., and Newall, P. J.: Manipulation in the treatment of low back pain: A multicenter study. Br. J. Med. 2:161, 1975.
5. Edwards, B. C.: Low back pain and pain resulting from lumbar spine conditions: A comparison of treatment results. Aust J. Physiother. 15:104, 1969.
6. Grunewald, L. R.: A study of physiotherapy as a vocation. Physiother. Rev. 8:38–39, 1928.
7. Glover, J. R., Morris, J. G., and Knosla, T.: Back pain: A randomized clinical trial of rotational manipulation of the trunk. Br. J. Indust. Med. 31:39, 1974.
8. Hay, M. C.: Incidence of Low Back Pain in Busselton. Proceedings of Conference on Low Back Pain, West Australia Institute of Technology, Sept. 7–13, 1974.
9. Hood, W.: A Treatise on Bone-Setting. London, 1871.
10. Hooper, J.: Low back pain and manipulation: Paraparesis after treatment of low back pain by physical methods. Med. J. Aust. 1:549, 1973.
11. Maitland, G. D.: Vertebral Manipulation, Stoneham, Butterworths, 1964.
12. Mathews, J. A., and Yates, D. A.: Reduction of lumbar disc prolapse by manipulation. Br. Med. J. 3:696, 1969.
13. McMurray, T. P.: Life of Hugh Owen Thomas. Centenary Lecture, Liverpool Medical Institution, Feb. 7, 1935. Liverpool Med. Chir. J. 43:3, 1935.
14. Melzack, R.: The Puzzle of Pain. London, Penguin, 1973.
15. Mennell, J.: Physical Treatment by Movement, Manipulation and Massage. London, Churchill, 1934.
16. Menell, J.: Back Pain. Boston, Little, Brown & Company, 1960.
17. Mensor, M. C.: Non-operative treatment including manipulation for lumbar intervertebral disc syndrome. J. Bone Joint Surg. 17A:925, 1955.
18. Mooney, V. T., and Robertson, J.: The facet syndrome. Clin. Orthop. Rel. Res. 115:149, 1976.
19. Paget, J.: Cases that Bonesetters Cure. Br. Med. J. 1867, p. 1.
20. Paris, S. V.: The theory and technique of specific spinal manipulation. N. Z. Med. J. 62:320, 1963.

21. Paris, S. V.: Spinal manipulative therapy. Clin. Orthop. Rel. Res. 179:55–61, 1983.
22. Paris, S. V.: The Spinal Lesion. San Diego, Pegasus Press, 1965.
23. Posstacchini, F., Facchini, M., and Palieri, P.: Efficacy of Various Forms of Conservative Treatment in Low Back Pain. A Comparative Study. Paper presented at I.S.S.L.S., Rome, 1987.
24. Withington, E. T.: Hippocrates with an English Translation, Vol. 3. Cambridge, Harvard University Press, 1959, pp. 278–307.
25. Wyke, B. D.: The neurology of low back pain in the lumbar spine. *In* Jayson, I. V. (ed.): Back Pain. London, Pitman Medical, 1980, pp. 265–339.
26. Hadler, N. M., et al.: A benefit of spinal manipulation as adjunctive therapy for acute low-back pain: A stratified controlled trial. Spine 12:703–706, 1987.

PSYCHOLOGIC APPROACHES TO THE MANAGEMENT AND TREATMENT OF CHRONIC LOW BACK PAIN

Daniel Stein
Yizhar Floman

Chronic low back pain (CLBP) is defined as pain in the lumbosacral region that occurs daily for a period of at least 6 months.[111, 122] Some studies, however, have required that the definition specify a longer period, emphasizing the association of the duration of the illness with various dimensions of CLBP.[117] At the time of this writing, CLBP is regarded as one of the most common chronic pain disorders that lead to interference with the patient's lifestyle.[117] Traditional approaches to chronic pain have been characterized by means of a somatosensory model.[130] Pain has been seen as a purely sensory event, and the pain experience has been assumed to be directly proportional to the peripheral damage.[86, 130] Although the model may be appropriate for acute pain,[116] it may be misleading and inadequate in regard to chronic pain.[9, 130] This assumption stems from the many instances of chronic pain that has no discernible peripheral damage,[86] from the fact that emotional conditions can lead to the development of chronic pain,[44] and from the clinical reports on the absence of pain expression despite severe injury.[130] In addition, many studies have demonstrated that various psychosocial variables may be closely related to CLBP[32, 55] and that CLBP may have a significant influence on the patient's psychosocial adaptation.[50, 109] Melzack and Wall[82] have been the first to incorporate such observations into their multidimensional model of chronic pain. Their Gate Control Theory emphasizes the link between neurophysiology and psychology and defines three principal dimensions of pain perception. While the sensory-discriminative dimension provides a "neutral" description of the input, the motivational–affective and cognitive–evaluative dimensions modulate the perception of the input according to the affective state and interpretation of the input. It is thus suggested that complex biopsychosocial models may be applicable for the understanding of CLBP.[9, 43] This highlights the role of the psychiatrist as part of a multidisciplinary team evaluating and treating CLBP patients.[116] This subchapter focuses on the following dimensions: psychologic and social factors associated with CLBP; the risk of the chronification of acute low back pain; the controversial issue of "organic" versus "psychogenic" CLBP; the indications for psychiatric assessment in CLBP; the role of the psychiatrist in a team evaluating and treating CLBP patients; and the most important drug and psychologic treatments of CLBP.

PSYCHOLOGIC AND SOCIAL FACTORS ASSOCIATED WITH CHRONIC LOW BACK PAIN AND DEPRESSION

A close link between the experience of chronic pain and the state of depression has been described in many studies.[9, 50] Several findings strongly support the association between CLBP and depression, although the exact nature of this relationship remains unclear.[22, 38] The findings are as follows:

1. CLBP patients are often depressed.[50, 63] Between 60% and 100% of these patients have demonstrable symptoms of a depressive disorder.[6, 104]
2. CLBP patients often demonstrate neurovegetative symptoms of depression.[1, 122]
3. Many patients with a depressive disorder (between 60% and 100%) report considerable somatic pain.[134, 136]
4. CLBP patients have been shown to have significantly increased rate of affective disorders (particularly unipolar depression) and alcoholism among first-degree relatives.[1, 39] These results are similar to the findings in depression.[95] Interestingly, a significantly higher incidence of major depression has been found in first-degree relatives of depressed CLBP patients, compared with those of nondepressed CLBP patients.[39]
5. In a manner resembling that of depressed patients,[114] individuals with CLBP demonstrate an increased rate of neuroendocrine abnormalities, for example, nonsuppression as shown on the dexamethasone suppression test (DST)[1, 12] or a blunted thyrotropin response to administration of thyrotropin-releasing hormone.[40] They also demonstrate shortened rapid eye movement (REM) latency on the polysomogram.[1, 10] Moreover, CLBP patients with major depression have been differentiated from CLBP patients without depression on the basis on DST nonsuppression.[41]
6. Many patients with chronic pain improve significantly with either antidepressive medications[47, 109, 135] or electroconvulsive therapy.[15, 75]

Various suggestions have been offered to explain the associations between CLBP and depression, reflecting the ambiguity and inconsistencies regarding these relationships. The suggestions are as follows:

1. CLBP leads to the development of depression.[9, 62] Ranga Rama Krishnan and colleagues,[104] for example, have found in a study of 71 CLBP patients that in the majority the depression developed after the onset of pain. Hendler[50] regards depression as a normal reaction in CLBP. Blumer suggests that "the depressive symptomatology of the chronic pain patients tends to be viewed as the consequence of physical suffering from which there appears to be no relief."[9]
2. A depressive disorder may lead to the development of CLBP.[6] This hypothesis stems probably from the well-known finding that depression is often manifested in somatic complaints, including pain.[9, 62] Although Hendler claims that "depression is rarely manifested by chronic pain,"[50] other studies have found that depressive symptoms usually precede the pain[87] and that relief from pain is concomitant with relief from the depression.[15, 89, 136]
3. CLBP is regarded as "masked" depression[71, 122] or as a specific variant of the depressive disease.[11] This suggestion probably reflects the well-known finding that CLBP patients tend to deny or have difficulty in expressing feelings.[43, 72] Thus, when such patients develop depression, it is not expressed directly as an emotional state but rather indirectly as a somatic disorder, including pain.[43, 62]
4. Some authors suggest that chronic pain may be neither primary nor secondary to depression[1, 9] but that similar mechanisms may be involved in developing chronic pain or depression.[62] The aforementioned findings of an increased incidence of depression in first-degree relatives of CLBP patients may be related to a genetic vulnerability to depression in these patients.[39] In addition, similar biologic abnormalities, mainly depletion of serotonin in critical central nervous system (CNS) synapses[48] and the previously mentioned neuroendocrine abnormalities, reported in both cases, may suggest some common underlying biologic basis.

Most depressed CLBP patients apparently do not demonstrate a major (endogenous) depressive disorder, according to standardized psychiatric diagnostic criteria.[2] The rate of major depression in these patients is between 20% and 45%.[6, 38, 72, 104] Thus, it seems that most depressed CLBP patients demonstrate an atypical depressive picture.[119] Some studies,[6, 104] employing standardized diagnostic criteria, have identified subgroups of depressed patients in those with CLBP. These studies emphasized that the depression seen in CLBP represents a continuum, ranging from no depression to major depression. Interestingly, 20% of CLBP patients have no depression at all.[38, 104] Some controversy seems to exist regarding the association between depression and the organicity of the CLBP. Although Magni[74] and Crisson and associates[28] have reported similar rates of depression in CLBP of organic or functional origin, Ranga Rama Krishnan and colleagues[104] have found the incidence of major depression to be twice as high among patients without organic findings.

Chronic Low Back Pain and Other Psychodynamic Factors

Many different psychodynamic factors have been found to be associated with CLBP. The following list seems to point out the most consistent and significant ones:

1. The development and persistence of CLBP as a fulfillment of unmet and unacknowledged passive–dependent wishes[9] as well as wishes to receive affection.[11]
2. Inhibition and repression of aggressive impulses that may lead to muscular activation and increased muscular tonus, and thus to the development of CLBP.[33, 36]
3. A sustained cycle of anxiety and muscle tension causing pain, which causes more anxiety.[86] Although anxiety has primarily been associated with the reaction to acute pain,[52, 117] it is nevertheless often found in CLBP.[105, 117] An association has also been demonstrated between chronic pain and various anxiety disorders.[88]
4. The somatic expression of unresolved psychic pain.[9, 130]
5. Imitation of or identification with a significant person with a crippling disease or chronic pain.[11]
6. The finding, by projective psychologic tests, that CLBP patients derive little pleasure from life, suffer considerable tension,[68] are overly adapted,[107] and demonstrate self-criticism and guilt.[14]

CLPB has often been associated with various forms of the somatoform disorders,[2] known in the past as hysterical neuroses.[86] These include the conversion disorders,[85] somatization disorders,[115] psychogenic pain disorder,[115] and hypochondriasis.[85] These definitions all imply that the painful physical complaints or irrational anxiety and conviction about physical illness exist in the absence of organic findings or known physiologic mechanisms[44] and suggest the existence of some basic underlying repressed psychologic conflict as the cause of the disorder.[9] Some controversy seems to exist, however, regarding the association between CLBP and hysteria. Merskey,[85] summarizing the results of many of his studies, suggests that in many patients with chronic pain, a conversive or hysterical mechanism represents a leading cause, and that these patients often demonstrate a histrionic personality. On the other hand, Blumer[9] claims that suggesting a connection between chronic pain and hysteria is highly inappropriate. Most chronic pain patients lack the colorful and highly dramatic presentation and the "belle indifference" of a classic hysteric, and histrionic personality traits tend to be noticeably absent.

The extensive employment of the Minnesota Multiphasic Personality Inventory (MMPI) in the study of CLBP has also demonstrated an apparent association between chronic pain, somatization, and hypochondriasis. This instrument is a broad-based, self-administered inventory, consisting of 566 true/false questions and yielding data on 10 clinical scales.[45] A frequent finding in CLBP patients is the *conversion* V[43] or *somatization*[120] profile of the MMPI. This constellation is characterized by significant elevations of *hysteria* (Scale 3) and *hypochondriasis* (Scale 5), and to a lesser degree, an elevation of *depression* (Scale 4). Many studies have consistently described this profile in CLBP.[1, 122, 140] A controversy seems to exist, however, regarding the interpretation of these findings. Goldstein[43] suggests the conversion V pattern to reflect a conversion reaction in which the CLBP substitutes for depression. Similarly, Dhanens and Jarrett[30] claim that this pattern is indicative of the defensive style of the psychogenic patient, who exhibits a denial of awareness of psychologic conflict and a subsequent expression of this conflict through somatic concerns. On the other hand, Sternbach and colleagues[122] see this pattern as an example of a psychophysiologic disorder with depression. Keel[62] also suggests that these patients can be characterized as typical psychosomatic patients, that is, demonstrating a physical condition affected by psychologic factors. Interestingly, some researchers argue that the conversion V pattern of the MMPI is representative of a group average that actually disguises important subgroup differences in the psychologic adjustment to CLBP.[1, 73] The introduction of multivariate statistical techniques has yielded strong support for the contention that several distinct subtypes of psychologic response to CLBP can be identified with the use of the MMPI.[1, 73] Several recent studies have by now reported such results,[1, 16, 65, 120] casting considerable doubt regarding the apparent psychologic homogeneity of CLBP patients.[9, 101]

Some attempts have been made to provide support for some of the outlined psychodynamic assumptions. Employing various electromyographic (EMG) techniques, some studies have found EMG changes—reflecting muscular hyperactivity—associated with various psychologic conflicts or stressors.[26, 31] Unfortunately, most of these studies, with the exception of those of Collins and coworkers[26] and Turk and Flor[130] are uncontrolled, and they suffer from various methodologic problems.[130] Other studies have demonstrated a correlation between decreased mobility in CLBP patients and various psychodynamic factors.[36, 91]

Chronic Low Back Pain and Alexithymia—the Psychophysiologic Model

Many studies have consistently reported that CLBP patients tend to have difficulty recognizing and expressing their feelings, particularly those of hostility and anger.[9, 102, 122, 133] Sifneos[118] has coined the term *alexithymia* to refer to this condition; it has been suggested that alexithymia is common not only in chronic pain, but in psychosomatic (or psychophysiologic) disorders in general.[9, 62] In this context pain is viewed as a kind of body language expressing feelings that these patients cannot otherwise show.[9, 62] Approximately 45% of CLBP patients demonstrate significant alexithymia.[4, 83] It has been found that patients who report preoccupation with their symptoms and difficulty expressing emotional distress are more significantly impaired by persistent pain than patients who do not report such responses.[64, 102]

Chronic Low Back Pain and Personality

Many researchers attempted to correlate the development of CLBP with various specific personality types. The most frequent personality disorders associated with CLBP were dependent personality[52] and histrionic (hysterical) personality.[52, 85] Keel[62] suggested that some patients may be more vulnerable and prone to develop chronic pain than others in similar conditions. Engel[33] and Blumer[11] coined the term *pain-prone personality (or disorder)* in agreement with such a hypothesis. In his retrospective studies of a large number of chronic pain patients, Blumer[9] noticed a remarkable psychologic homogeneity. Prior to the development of pain these patients tended to demonstrate excessive work performance, industriousness, overactivity, and a general denial of interpersonal difficulties and hostile aggressive trends. Following a significant loss or disappointment and often with the advent of an injury, these patients tended to develop intractable pain and a complete alteration in lifestyle, changing from responsible, overly active, and industrious individuals to passive-dependent invalids. Blumer suggested that in these patients basic passive-dependent needs are concealed and denied as unacceptable from an early age, only to reappear when pain ensues. However, the multiplicity of personality subtypes found by using the MMPI seem to contradict the tendency to associate chronic pain with only one specific or a few specific personality types.[1, 73, 91]

It is generally agreed that chronic pain as a major complaint is rare among patients with schizophrenia.[86] It is not common among those with major (endogenous) depression,[72, 86] and is often associated with other types of depression[38, 85] and anxiety.[85, 105] Although some authors claim that "chronic pain due to neurotic illness (mainly somatoform disorders or hysteria) and personality disorder is probably the most common variant,"[86] others suggest that the CLBP patient has basically a psychosomatic (psychophysiologic) disorder.[9, 122] The difference between the two definitions is obvious. Whereas hysteria relates to pain in the absence of organic findings, the psychophysiologic model suggests some organic dysfunction attributable to emotional causes. It should be noted that at least some CLBP patients (as many as 20% to 30% in some studies)[1, 6] do not demonstrate evidence of psychopathology.[52, 85]

Another important, and still controversial, issue is whether the psychodynamic and personality factors mentioned precede or result from CLBP. It is obviously difficult to reach a definite conclusion, owing to difficulties in performing prospective studies in this case. Several studies suggest that the patient's emotional condition not only precedes the pain[52] but is actually associated with its development.[77, 86] Pilowsky and Spence[103] have found that the illness behavior of patients with chronic pain (i.e., how they perceive, evaluate and act upon their symptoms)[78] is significantly associated with pre-existing personality factors. Similarly, although patients with clearly physical lesions and good premorbid adjustment do not demonstrate significant emotional and personality changes,[52, 85] those with chronic pain thought to reflect a psychogenic cause tend to report at least some premorbid disturbance.[52, 85] In addition, the pretreatment psychologic condition of CLBP patients as evaluated by the MMPI[73] and other tests[52] has been found to be significantly related to treatment results, including surgery; poor pretreatment adjustment has been consistently linked with a poor response. On the other hand, some authors suggest that CLBP may lead to the development of emotional and even personality changes.[85, 109] For example, Pelz and Merskey[100] have found that chronic pain due to organic causes results in emotional responses and disturbances in the patient's personal and social life (e.g., a significant degree of disturbance of work, sleep, leisure, and social activities and of sexual relationships). Other authors emphasize that CLBP patients develop a variety of psychologic, cognitive, and behavioral coping strategies to adjust and manage their pain.[50, 110] In addition, it has been demonstrated that the relief of chronic pain may result in some amelioration of personality change and psychologic disturbance.[123, 139]

Chronic Low Back Pain and Interpersonal (Environmental) Stressors

In recent years there has been a growing body of research suggesting an association between various environmental (psychosocial) stressors and the development, maintenance, and exacerbation of CLBP.[43, 62, 130] Increased pain has thus been related to increased psychosocial stress.[34, 36] Regarding the role of the family in chronic pain, it has been demonstrated that a number of variables indicating family-related distress (e.g., family conflict or marital dissatisfaction) may be increased in CLBP patients compared with a control group.[34, 90] Factors reflecting familial maladjustment have also been associated with increased pain perception in CLBP patients.[34] In addition, it has been suggested that "pain may run in families," specifically, that relatives of patients with CLBP have been found to demonstrate substantially more complaints of pain than controls.[11] Although attempts have been made to identify specific family models of CLBP patients[69, 138] and to associate them with "psychosomatic families" in general,[130] specific characteristics of families of chronic pain patients have been only rarely delineated.[34] In general, it has been suggested that the patient's pain may fulfill the emotional needs of other family members. Thus, although acute pain appears at random, it may evolve into a chronic pain problem if it fulfills the object-related needs of a family.[69, 138] Similarly, the immediate precipitation of the symptom may be caused, according to these assumptions, by a threat to the family homeostasis.[69] It is important to note that in addition to the contribution of the family to the development and maintenance of CLBP, chronic pain may exert a significant influence on the family.[11, 89] Extrafamilial stressors have also been associated with CLBP. These include mainly factors related to work, such as type of occupation,[85] increased vocational stress,[90] reduced work satisfaction,[126] or decreased peer cohesion at work.[34] Interestingly, patients with CLBP judged to have an organic cause have been found to demonstrate an increased rate of overall psychosocial distress.[46]

CHRONIFICATION OF ACUTE LOW BACK PAIN

Acute low back pain (LBP) is generally defined as pain of a duration not exceeding 6 months.[104, 117] This dichotomy between acute LBP and CLBP is somewhat arbitrary,[122] as changes in pain experience may be gradual,[49] and highly associated with the duration of the illness.[49, 117] In general, it seems that CLBP patients demonstrate significantly more psychopathology than acute patients.[50, 117, 122] Whereas acute LBP may not be associated with significant emotional disturbance (with the exception of anxiety),[133] chronification has been found to lead to increased depression,[52, 122] anxiety,[117] and somatic preoccupation[50, 122] and to decreased coping ability.[50] The development of chronic pain has been also associated with alterations in pain perception and tolerance.[117] Fordyce[37] and Schofferman[116] claim that acute pain tends to persist if it is treated solely as the result of a local lesion, while important psychologic considerations are ignored. Keel[62] has identified the following biopsychosocial factors that may lead to the chronification of LBP: (1) repeated investigations that fail to bring out a clear course or explanation for the illness, and repeated treatment failures; (2) persistent disability and prolonged absence from work; (3) increasing physical inactivity; (4) "secondary" gains presumably associated with the illness, for example, improvement in family relations, the chance of being freed from an unpleasant duty, and financial compensation; (5) the development of medication abuse; (6) negative side effects of surgery or drugs that may increase the patient's suffering and hypochondriasis.

ORGANIC VERSUS PSYCHOGENIC (FUNCTIONAL) CHRONIC LOW BACK PAIN

The concept of psychogeneity has often been applied to the problem of CLBP because many patients report greater suffering and disability than their organic lesions apparently warrant.[46, 79, 112] Many studies have attempted to differentiate between demonstrable organic causation and a nonorganic, presumably psychogenic (functional) disorder. This dichotomy is currently regarded as a most complex and controversial issue.[22, 73, 79] The differentiation would be valid if consistent and replicable findings would appear in various centers using different assessment techniques, and if it would demonstrate predictive validity regarding differences in prognosis or on the effects of various treatment modalities. Some studies claim this is the current state of the art.[52, 76] They have found, for example, that patients with CLBP of organic causes demonstrate a favorable response to conservative,[50, 65] as well as surgical,[52, 96] treatment. Other studies, on the other hand, regard the organic-psychogenic dichotomy as confusing and misleading[19, 43, 44, 73, 128] and as being of limited value in regard to prognosis and treatment decisions.[73, 128] They suggest that an integrated approach, emphasizing complex interactions between biologic, psychologic, and social correlates is more applicable for the understanding of CLBP;[9, 43, 62, 130] they also recommend the formation of valid and reliable subgroups of patients, according to their psychosocial adjustment and ability to cope with CLBP.[73, 128]

The differentiation between organic and psychogenic CLBP is still established according to physical examination, x-ray study, computerized tomography, myelography, electromyography, and nerve conduction, as well as by magnetic resonance imaging. The entire approach emphasizes the definition of psychogenic CLBP as nonorganic; that is, the disorder is presumably functional when there is no evidence of objective organic findings.[128] As do other authors,[6, 22, 54, 115] we suggest that an organic disease and a psychiatric disorder may coexist independently; thus, the definition of functional causation should be based on the existence of positive psychologic findings.

The rate of presumably "psychogenic" patients in various populations suffering from CLBP is found to be between 20% to 50%.[52, 65, 104, 112, 115, 122, 128] Most studies suggest that patients with functional disorders demonstrate a significantly higher level of psychosocial disturbance compared with those who have organic disorders.[56, 62, 88, 104, 112] This relates, for example, to increased premorbid personality disturbance[52] and psychosocial maladjustment,[52, 112] or increased depression[52, 104] and anxiety.[52] Other studies, however, have found either no difference between the groups[105, 122] or increased psychopathology among the organic patients.[46]

Various psychologic assessment procedures have been used to differentiate between organic and functional CLBP. Hackett and Bouckoms[44] have identified some clinical characteristics that correlate with the psychogenicity of pain. The pain is in more than one place or is of more than one variety; the patient seems interested more in convincing others that the pain is genuine than in receiving a cure for it; the presence of emotional problems is denied; the pain is reported to be insensitive to any emotional state; the pain varies according to the interpersonal setting; the patient is convinced about the uniqueness and singularity of the pain; the patient projects to the physician the attitude that "only you can save me"; the pain either does not fluctuate in the course of time or only consistently becomes more severe, and nothing alleviates it.

Some studies found the MMPI to be useful in differentiating organic and psychogenic CLBP.[21, 42, 76] Psychogenic patients were thought to demonstrate the conversion V pattern of the MMPI to a greater degree.[42, 76] In addition, specific scales[21] consisting of selected MMPI items were constructed to distinguish between the two populations. Many studies, however, found a considerable similarity and overlap between the MMPI profiles of functional and organic CLBP patients.[6, 54, 65, 73, 122] Some authors suggested this overlap to be a valid finding.[1, 6, 122] Others claimed that this state actually reflects the inadequacy of the MMPI scale in the assessment of CLBP patients and that other procedures could be more effective in distinguishing organic and functional patients.[54, 65] The following instruments have been used:

Pain Drawing Test[106] □ This test consists of an outline drawing of the human body on which patients map the nature and distribution of their pain. In CLBP of an organic origin, the pain drawings should match the organic diagnosis; in psychogenic CLBP, the pain drawings tend to be bizarre, and the pain spreads to a nonrelated area of the body.[43, 106, 112] Various scoring systems have been developed to standardize the results. Although some studies have found this instrument to discriminate significantly between organic and functional pain,[106, 112] others have failed to replicate these findings.[7]

McGill Pain Questionnaire (MPQ)[80] □ This instrument, developed by Melzack, consists of 20 sets of adjectives from which the patient is asked to choose the words best describing his or her pain. It also includes a pain drawing test, a rating of present pain intensity, and words that describe the temporal quality of the pain. Although some studies have found organic CLBP patients to imply different wordings and descriptions,[88] others have found a considerable overlap.[85] All the words employed in the MPQ imply some physical change in the body.[85] Although the MPQ can identify certain CLBP patients with certain patterns of psychologic disturbance, it is not considered effective in distinguishing organic from functional pain.[62]

Back Pain Classification Scale (BPCS)[66] □ This instrument, developed by Leavitt and associates, consists of various pain-related terms. The patient is instructed to choose the terms best describing his or her pain. By means of discriminant analysis, Leavitt has identified 13 items reliably differentiating organic from functional CLBP.[66] These results, however, were mostly replicated by his own group.[65, 67]

Mensana Clinic Back Pain Test[54] □ This 15-question test, which is essentially a structured medical interview, records the patient's physical and psychologic response to CLBP. It has been found to differentiate between organic and functional pain in some studies.[52, 54] Other specific pain questionnaires have also attempted to tackle this issue,[97, 112] although so far their use has been limited.

In summary, despite the many controversies and inconsistencies associated with the distinction between organic and functional CLBP, treatment is still often recommended (or not recommended) on this basis.[52, 128] This may lead to serious errors in treatment of patients with either disorder.[128] We suggest that in each case, the organic and psychologic conditions have to be carefully scrutinized. Decisions as to the prognosis of treatment should be based simultaneously on the orthopedic evaluation and the patient's ability to benefit from the treatment.

ROLE OF THE PSYCHIATRIST IN A TEAM EVALUATING AND TREATING CHRONIC LOW BACK PAIN

The previous sections have emphasized the highly complex interactions between physical and emotional dimensions in CLBP. Psychologic factors have a great influence on the development of chronicity,[6, 62] and different personality profiles[73] or coping styles[110] are found to be associated with the prognosis and differential responses to treatment. Such a view seems to call for a radical change in the role of the psychiatric consultant as it has been regarded. Traditionally, psychiatrists have been employed when pain has continued for a long time and has become resistant to all sorts of conventional therapies, and when pain behaviors appear inappropriate to the organic condition (i.e., employed to solve issues of organicity versus psychologic overlay.[43, 62, 133]) Thus, the psychiatrist has been called relatively late in the treatment, when patient and doctor are already highly frustrated and equally mistrustful.[44] More recently, it has been suggested that the psychiatric consultant should be brought into the case early.[44] All patients have to be routinely assessed by a psychiatrist if the pain does not improve by conventional treatment within a few weeks, because only such early screening may prevent chronicity.[62] Moreover, the psychiatrist should be an integral part of a multidisciplinary team employing a biopsychosocial approach,[44, 116] and should be introduced to the patients as such.[44] One role of the psychiatrist is to evaluate and identify the psychiatric condition, the emotional adjustment, and the success in coping with pain according to standardized interviews, including those with family members and accepted psychologic batteries.[44] In addition, the psychiatrist should serve as a consultant to the other professions and as a full-fledged member in an integrated team.[44, 116] According to Schofferman, a CLBP management program "that uses a multidisciplinary team approach and a biopsychosocial treatment model, may have the highest likelihood of success."[116] This team includes the following professionals: an orthopedic surgeon, a psychiatrist or psychologist, a physical therapist, an occupational therapist, an anesthesiologist, and occasionally a neurosurgeon.[116]

DRUG TREATMENT IN CHRONIC LOW BACK PAIN

The typical patient with CLBP suffers from backache for more than 6 months. Although the individual usually has a defined disorder in the lumbar spine, the pain is out of proportion to the organic lesion and is not amenable to standard treatment modalities, including surgical intervention. These patients are not working, are increasingly incapacitated, and consume improper medications such as narcotic analgesics and tranquilizers. These drugs usually provide little, if any, help. Pain plays a major role in the lives of these patients and their families.[5]

About 50% of patients admitted to chronic pain programs are routinely using narcotic analgesics, tranquilizers, hypnotic sedatives, and muscle relaxants.[108] These medications not only provide little relief from pain but also possess a strong potential for exacerbating the pain and the related symptoms. Narcotic analgesics lose their effectiveness in reducing chronic back pain because of tolerance.[18] In addition they lead to dependence and depression. The use of benzodiazepines as tranquilizers for treating CLBP patients, diazepam (Valium) for example, is inappropriate and contraindicated. By virtue of the ability of these agents to deplete serotonin levels in the central nervous system, they decrease the pain threshold and induce depression, habituation, and sleep disturbances.[48] Unfortunately, these are the drugs most commonly prescribed by many practitioners managing CLBP.[47] Therefore, the essential first step in any CLBP program is to discontinue the use of these harmful agents. After the medications are successfully discontinued, patients may even notice some alleviation of pain.[146] (For the description of a detoxification program, see the later discussion of Operant Behavioral Treatment Programs.) Sleep disturbances that were present before detoxification or were brought about by the process are managed by the administration of tricyclic antidepressants (TCAs) in increasing dosages.

Sympathetic overactivity is an important feature of acute pain. In chronic pain, on the other hand, the sympathetic activity subsides, and appetite and sleep disturbances, irritability, and somatic preoccupation increase.[109] Therefore, the pharmacologic management of acute pain is completely different from that of chronic pain. For treating acute pain, analgesics are in order. For treating chronic pain, narcotics and tranquilizers may be harmful, and tricyclic antidepressants and phenothiazines are in order. The analgesic efficacy of TCAs in treating chronic pain has been documented in peripheral neuropathies, postherpetic neuralgia, and tic douloureux.[29] Because pain and depression coexist in patients with CLBP, it is reasonable to administer TCAs. Sternbach[121] hypothesized that chronic pain is associated with the depletion of brain serotonin. This depletion accounts for the frequent occurrence of depression in chronic pain. Sternbach and colleagues[124] also speculated that serotonergic TCAs (e.g., amitriptyline or chlorimipramine), by virtue of correcting the serotonin deficit, will successfully ameliorate depression and chronic pain. Indeed, a single dose of 40 mg of fenfluramine, a selective releaser of serotonin, will reduce both pain and depression in some patients with CLBP.[137] Others have hypothesized that TCAs may relieve pain by affecting endogenous opiates[44] or by reducing anxiety or muscle tension.[48] Ward[135] conducted a double-blind study testing the effects of desipramine or doxepin on patients with CLBP and depression. Sixty per cent of the patients had significant pain relief as well as relief of the depression on either drug. Patients who had pain relief following an acute challenge with fenfluramine were significantly more likely to have pain relief on either antidepressant.[135] Neither drug changed cerebrospinal β-endorphin levels, acute pain tolerance, or electromyogram levels. Ward[135] suggested that his data may support the idea of a serotonergic mechanism of action for TCAs in chronic pain. Although desipramine is usually regarded as a noradrenergic antidepressant, and the exact mechanism of action of doxepin is uncertain, both drugs may exert serotonergic uptake blocking effects.[135] Amitriptyline, doxepin, or chlorimipramine may be administered to fight CLBP, anxiety, depression, and insomnia. Because TCAs have anticholinergic side effects on the cardiovascular, gastrointestinal, and genitourinary systems, care should be exercised in elderly patients and in those with cardiac disease, prostatism, and glaucoma. Dose is increased gradually, starting with 25 to 50 mg at bedtime.[47] A daily dose of 100 to 250 mg should be attained. The full effect may not be noticed before 2 to 4 weeks.[47]

The association between the effect of TCAs on amelioration of pain and improvement of depression in chronic pain patients is equivocal. Some studies found simultaneous improvement in both aspects upon the administration of TCAs.[15, 136] They also found that the duration of treatment (about 4 weeks) and the dosage of TCAs (150 to 250 mg daily) are similar for chronic pain and depressive disorders.[59, 136] Others suggest that TCAs may have a differential effect on CLBP and depression.[141] Pain amelioration may be attained in smaller doses[141] and in a shorter duration,[47] as compared with the time and dose required to affect depression. This means that antidepressants should be administered to patients with CLBP, regardless of whether they have concomitant depression. If therapy is successful, it should be maintained for 3 to 6 months. The success rate of TCAs has been documented, by several investigators, to be about 60% to 70%.[11, 70] Anxiety commonly complicates CLBP. The usual antianxiety agents, such as diazepam, are contraindicated in chronic pain syndromes because they deplete brain serotonin. On the other hand, phenothiazine tranquilizers, which are potent anxiolytics,[47] are also quite effective in the management of CLBP.[47, 109] Chlorpromazine, a classic standard of phenothiazines, blocks dopamine postsynaptically, has α-blocking effects, and has a strong atropine-like action. Haloperidol has the fewest effects on acetylcholine and strong dopaminergic and α-blockade effects. In addition, haloperidol has been shown to bind to opiate receptors as an agonist. The combination of TCAs and phenothiazines may be more efficacious than either drug alone.[50, 109]

In summary, the goals of drug therapy in CLBP are (1) withdrawal of inappropriate drugs; (2) management of pain, depression, and anxiety; (3) management of sleep disturbances, and (4) appropriate use of analgesics.[47]

PSYCHOLOGIC TREATMENT OF CHRONIC LOW BACK PAIN PATIENTS

General Principles

Mental health professionals are playing an increasingly important part in the management of CLBP. Although they are still concerned with the various psychosocial aspects of pain,[44] psychologists and psychiatrists are also currently involved in the treatment of chronic pain. In this regard, some important psychologic principles have been established, which are considered by many to be an integral part of the treatment of CLBP patients.

Patients with chronic pain must be treated in a manner very different from that for patients with acute pain.[116] The treatment goal often becomes not eliminating the pain[116] but learning how to live with it.[23, 62, 116] Thus, the continuation or resumption of work and other regular activities becomes a paramount goal in the treatment of CLBP.[9, 116] Characteristically, most psychologic treatments stress the importance of the patient taking an active role in the treatment and the establishment of a cooperative relationship with the therapists.[23, 130] Patients must experience their own actions influencing the pain, thus gaining a sense of control and mastery over their situations.[23, 62] In addition, patients must receive clearly presented information about their illness and its treatment.[62] This orientation should also include the spouse and other family members who may otherwise continue to reinforce pain behaviors, because of the association of such behaviors with conflicts in the family.[9, 62] If the cause of CLBP is presumably mainly psychogenic, the therapists should respond to it as they would to real pain.[9] Patients have to be told that pain of an uncertain origin or resulting from mental stress may exist and can be treated.[9, 62] This must be conveyed to the patient in an empathic and accepting attitude.[62] Although the exact nature of a psychogenic origin (e.g., depression, anxiety) has to be elucidated and treated,[9, 116] invasive somatic investigations must be avoided in these cases, unless they are absolutely indicated.[9, 62]

In the next paragraphs, the currently available psychologic treatments will be reviewed. It should be emphasized, however, that regardless of the treatment, the best results are achieved when the psychologists and psychiatrists are an integral part of a multidisciplinary team, including professionals from several specialties.[116, 130] This has been established in various studies,[13, 129] emphasizing the importance of treating CLBP as a multifunctional problem that requires attention to the physical as well as psychologic and social aspects of pain.[130]

Behavioral Intervention Procedures

Operant Behavioral Treatment Programs

Operant approaches do not deal with the pain experience per se but rather with its behavioral consequences.[62, 130] The goals of operant treatment are the extinction of maladaptive pain behaviors (e.g., verbal pain complaints, taking medications, and avoiding activities associated with pain) and the promotion of "well" behaviors (e.g., exercise and work).[23, 109, 130] To increase the rate of the desired behaviors, they should systematically be followed by effective positive reinforcement. Unwanted pain behaviors are usually reduced by extinction (i.e., by withdrawal of attention and reinforcements for these behaviors).[23, 62, 109, 130] As Reuler and associates[109] have described, "if a CLBP patient lies in bed excessively, one can either withdraw the reinforcers for remaining in bed, such as withdrawing housecleaning services, or give reinforcement to walking as mechanisms to increase up time."

Another goal of operant treatment is to increase physical activity.[62, 109, 130] This is achieved through step-by-step training programs,[62] in which activity is associated with various positive reinforcers, but not with pain.[9, 109, 130] A third goal of such programs is the elimination or reduction of medications.[9, 23, 62, 109, 130] After the establishment of the required dosage, medications are not prescribed as needed, but are provided at regular time intervals. Thus, medication administration and the attention associated with it are no longer contingent upon pain. Because the medication is in liquid form, masked for color and taste, and given in the same volume for each dose, the total amount of medication may be gradually reduced.[9, 62, 109, 130]

Operant programs must usually be conducted on an inpatient basis[9, 109, 130] and are quite costly, time consuming, and complex.[23] Some uncontrolled studies have reported significant increases in activity and employability and significant medication reduction, both after treatment and at follow-up.[3, 19] However, with the exception of the study of Cairns and Paslino,[20] no control group studies have been conducted to test the efficacy of the operant approach in treating CLBP patients.[23, 130] Although they are considered to be promising, operant treatments have several limitations.[130] Reinforcements seem to fail to generalize to activities that are not directly treated, and the results may be not maintained when the reinforcers are removed.[20, 130] Another issue to be considered is the importance of the family involvement and the patient's natural environment in the maintenance of treatment effects.[36]

Respondent Treatment Approaches

The respondent treatment approaches include distraction, relaxation, imagery techniques, and biofeedback. The goal of these treatments is to influence the assumed psychologic basis of CLBP.[130] The theoretical basis of this approach is the assumption of a pain–tension–pain circle. Accordingly, treatment should interrupt this vicious circle by replacing the increased muscular tension with an adequate and tension-incompatible reaction, such as relaxation.[67, 130] These techniques all aim to assist the patients in controlling and regulating the sensory input and thus in experiencing mastery over the pain experience.[62]

DISTRACTION (ATTENTION DIVERSION)

The rationale of this technique is concentration on thoughts to divert the patient's attention from the pain.[130] Attention diversion can be also achieved through a variety of activities, such as walking, talking, or exercising.[62] These activities should require enough attention to make the patient forget the pain. The efficacy of this technique has been demonstrated in patients suffering from CLBP.[62, 116]

RELAXATION

A variety of procedures can be used to induce profound muscular relaxation. The most prevalent method, progressive muscular relaxation,[58] consists of having the patient tense and then relax the major muscle groups of the body in a fixed and systematic order.[17] The rationale is that the patient's negative expectations about pain can increase anxiety; this, in turn, fosters muscle tension, which leads to more pain and consequently more anxiety.[62, 130] This cycle can be interrupted by relaxation.[62, 130] In addition, improvement may be also related to changes in the sympathetic nervous system.[57] Studies evaluating the efficacy of relaxation techniques in CLBP, with concomitant biofeedback[8, 60] or without it,[62, 116, 131] including those with controlled designs,[131] have reported this modality to be quite useful. In addition, relaxation is relatively inexpensive and easy to manage, in both outpatient and group settings.[62, 131]

IMAGERY TECHNIQUES

In these procedures, the patient focuses attention on a comfortable picture that is incompatible with pain or tries to transform the pain perception or the situation (context) in which the pain is perceived. Examples for imaginative pain-perception transformation are reinterpreting the CLBP as mildly disturbing, instead of extremely painful, or imagining comfortable warmth spreading into the painful areas. Changing the context may be accomplished by imagining, for example, the CLBP to be the result of strenuous work, while realizing that one is now resting in a comfortable chair.[62]

BIOFEEDBACK

Biofeedback is the process of providing visual or auditory information-feedback to a subject of the status of some somatic or autonomic function.[53, 109] With biofeedback-measuring devices sensitive to responses in the body beneath the threshold of usual awareness (e.g., visceral responses and muscular tension), it is possible to provide moment-to-moment information about these responses and thus to help the patient control and modify them.[125] Two types of biofeedback application may be distinguished. One is a specific type in which the patient is provided feedback about the actual condition that needs to be controlled. The other, more applicable to CLBP, is the nonspecific type. The patient is taught a more general skill—such as controlling the amplitude of the α component in the electroencephalogram (EEG) or electromyographic (EMG) reduction in various muscles—that has been found to be associated with pain reduction.[53, 125] In EMG biofeedback, for example, the patient may hear a clanging signal, the rate of which increases as the EMG level rises and decreases as the EMG level falls. The patient's task is to learn to relax with the biofeedback's assistance.

Most studies on biofeedback treatment in CLBP are anecdotal or systematic case studies[8, 93] or group outcome or comparison studies.[51, 60, 99] Only a few controlled studies have been performed.[35, 94] In general, the biofeedback studies are difficult to evaluate. According to Turk and Flor,[130] "Different methodological procedures, different patient groups, variation in the number and length of treatment sessions and numerous design studies, including the combination of biofeedback with relaxation training in some studies but not in others, make conclusions tentative." The evaluation of biofeedback effects in CLBP, in general, permits no clear conclusions.[23] When pain reduction is used as the relevant criterion, some studies report significant reductions in pain intensity and/or frequency after treatment,[8, 35, 93, 94] whereas others have not found significant change.[51, 60, 99] When EMG values are used as the criterion, the results are still not clear. Some studies have demonstrated significant post-treatment EMG reductions,[35] whereas others have not shown significant changes.[51, 99] However, the two controlled studies that have assessed the influence of biofeedback alone in CLBP[35, 94] demonstrate strong effects of EMG biofeedback on pain and tension levels. Thus, it is suggested that, although the research on the efficacy of biofeedback in CLBP is preliminary,[35] it appears to be a promising treatment modality for such patients.[53, 130] Some authors[62, 132] emphasize, however, that because biofeedback is a costly and complex procedure, it should be reserved for patients who have no success with other behavioral techniques. In addition, it has been demonstrated that the nonspecific type of biofeedback application often requires continued and frequent practice. This raises such issues as how to transfer the training to the real world from a quiet, clinical setting.[125]

The mechanisms presumed to underly EMG biofeedback effectiveness in CLBP are the reduction of both muscular hyper-reaction and anxiety.[130] Although some studies have demonstrated a significant association between muscle tension and/or anxiety reduction and a decrease in pain,[35] others have not.[51, 94] Thus, the following other mechanisms have been proposed: distraction,[81] suggestion,[81] increase of the patient's sense of control and mastery over the pain,[53, 81] the "mental calm" experienced by patients receiving EMG biofeedback,[142] and the effect of biofeedback on modifying maladaptive cognitive evaluations and responses associated with the experience of pain.[35, 94]

Cognitive Approaches

The cognitive approaches are closely related to the gate control model of pain of Melzack and Wall.[82] As mentioned earlier, this model emphasizes that motivational-affective and cognitive-evaluative dimensions may modulate the perception of the sensory input. The basic assumption underlying the cognitive perception is that the behavior of individuals is determined not only by sensory phenomena (e.g., pain), but also by the way they construe their world and apply meaning to it.[130] The goal of these approaches is to alter maladaptive thoughts, feelings, or behaviors related to pain and thereby to modify the experience of pain.[130] The treatment involves educating the patient about the identification of pain-eliciting and pain-aggravating situations, thoughts, and behaviors, as well as the identification and modification of maladaptive pain-related cognition.[129] The cognitive approach has successfully been employed in various pain syndromes, including CLBP.[131] A significant reduction in pain intensity and general suffering and a concomitant decrease in the use of the health care system have been reported. Cognitive treatment also has the advantage of being applicable in group and outpatient settings.[130, 131]

Hypnosis

When employing hypnosis in the management of chronic pain syndromes, various induction and deepening procedures are typically used and followed by specific analgesia-inducing techniques. These may include the direct suggestion of analgesia (e.g., loss or decrease of sensation in the affected body part), transformation of the pain experience (e.g., moving the pain from one part of the body to another where it is more manageable), and various forms of attention-diversion.[56, 113]

Most studies evaluating the effects of hypnosis in pain control are uncontrolled clinical case studies, in which the subjective report of pain reduction is often the sole criterion of success.[130] Usually these studies report impressive pain reduction.[77, 113] However, the total lack of controlled clinical research precludes confident conclusions about the efficacy of hypnosis in CLBP.[130] Interestingly, some leading authorities in the field of pain have considerable reservations regarding the employment of hypnosis in chronic pain. Hacket and Bouckoms have found that "only about one in four subjects is able to achieve (in hypnosis) a state of concentration of sufficient magnitude for lasting pain control."[44] Merskey emphasizes that relief of pain with hypnotic techniques is "rarely complete where there is an important physical cause of pain, and frequently it is of only modest proportions."[84] In Orne's experience,[98] on the other hand, although hypnotherapy has been found to be efficacious in chronic organic pain, it is frequently ineffective in relieving functional pain. Hendler and Fernandez[53] suggest that, although hypnosis is an effective treatment for acute pain problems, there is only limited evidence of its efficacy in treating patients with chronic pain, with the exception of chronic muscle tension and its resulting pain.

Psychodynamic Psychotherapy

Psychodynamic psychotherapy, when offered as the sole treatment, has been found to have only limited success in alleviating CLBP.[44] Psychotherapy may, however, produce significant benefit if used in conjunction with other treatment modalities, such as behavioral therapy.[44, 116] Its role then is mainly to gain the patient's cooperation in the treatment program and to promote realistic expectations in order to help the individual adjust to the chronic pain and to achieve insight into the psychosocial problems associated with pain. Merskey[84] suggests that psychotherapy may be useful, particularly for pain of assumed psychogenic origin, although it may also assist the patient with organic pain to maintain a more useful and effective adjustment. In his experience, a relatively brief psychotherapy (10 to 12 sessions), is usually sufficient. If it does not work within this sort of time schedule, the chances for any significant change are minimal. When intensive psychotherapy is not appropriate, patients may nevertheless be helped by supportive psychotherapy[84] or counseling.[116] Keel[62] suggests that, because many CLBP patients are alexithymic, methods that help activate feelings or that focus on body awareness seem more suitable than psychodynamic psychotherapy.

Group Treatments and Eclectic Approaches

Group programs have become popular in the treatment of CLBP patients.[116] Various models exist. The main principles of group treatment may be elucidated through one model, the *pain control classes*.[55] These include chronic pain patients in various stages of treatment, and therapists experienced both in group treatment and in the various mechanisms of CLBP. The goals of these classes are to correct misconceptions and reduce fears about illness, to replace self-defeating patterns of thinking with more constructive ones, and to provide a forum for mastery experience. Each meeting consists of the following parts: (1) educating the patients about the nature of their attitudes to pain and how to modify them, (2) conducting group interactions and discussions related to pain, and (3) conducting group experience of various behavioral techniques. The efficacy of the pain control classes has been associated with several factors. The group experience involves exposure to others and thus forces the individual to change the pain-related thinking and behavior.[55] The group may instill hope through processes such as imparting information, encouragement, group support, and constant feedback.[55, 143] During group interaction, patients may explore and vent their pain-related feelings, and perceive the universality of their problem (i.e., others also have CLBP).[55, 143] In addition, good role models are provided by inviting successful graduates of preceding groups to each new group.[55, 120] Employing this model in CLBP, Herman and Baptiste[55] have demonstrated a considerable reduction in depression, pain perception, and analgesic intake, and a significant increase in employment rates following treatment. Other models of group programs, combining several different treatment methods, have also been found to be quite successful.[22, 127] Obvious advantages of group treatment in CLBP are that it is inexpensive and may be employed on an outpatient basis.

Another relatively recent development in the treatment of CLBP includes the eclectic (or comprehensive) approaches.[62, 116, 130] These simultaneously employ a range of techniques that draw from various theoretical perspectives, such as operant behavioral procedures, physical rehabilitation, family participation, group discussions, biofeedback and relaxation, and supportive treatment.[127] Most eclectic studies,[24, 127] although not all of them,[25] provide some evidence for the usefulness of such programs; the combinations are probably more efficient than each treatment alone.[62, 116] They report, for example, a significant reduction in pain and use of medication, an increase in activity, and significant vocational rehabilitation in a large number of patients. However, the lack of control groups and comprehensive pain assessment in these studies, and the uncertainty about the effective components, prevent drawing definite conclusions.[130]

References

1. Adams, K. M., Heilbronn, M., and Blumer, D.: A multimethod evaluation of the MMPI in a chronic pain patient sample. J. Clin. Psychol. 42:878–886, 1986.
2. American Psychiatric Association: Diagnostic and Statistical Manual of Mental Disorders, 3rd Ed., revised. Washington, D.C., 1987.
3. Anderson, T. P., Cole, T. M., Gullickson, G., et al.: Behavior modification of chronic pain: A treatment program by a multidisciplinary team. Clin. Orthop. Rel. Res. 129:96–100, 1977.
4. Antczak-Bouckoms, A., and Bouckoms, A. J.: Affective disturbance and the denial of problems in dental patients with pain. Int. J. Psychosom. 32:9–11, 1985.
5. Aronoff, G. M., and Evans, W. O.: Evaluation and treatment of chronic pain at the Boston Pain Center. J. Clin. Psychiatr. 4(Suppl.):4–9, 1982.
6. Atkinson, J. H., Jr., Ingram, R. E., Kremer, E. F., and Saccuzzo, D. P.: MMPI subgroups and affective disorder in chronic pain patients. J. Nerv. Ment. Dis. 174:408–413, 1986.
7. Bayer, von, C. L.: Invalid use of pain drawings in psychological screening of back pain patients. Pain 16:103–107, 1983.
8. Belar, C. D., and Cohen, T. L.: The use of EMG feedback and progressive muscle relaxation in the treatment of a woman with chronic back pain. Biofeedback Self Regul. 4:349–352, 1979.
9. Blumer, D.: Psychiatric aspects of chronic pain: Nature identification and treatment of the pain-prone disorder. *In* Rothman, R. H., and Simeone, F. A. (eds.): The Spine, 2nd Ed. Philadelphia, W. B. Saunders, 1982, pp. 1090–1117.
10. Blumer, D., Roth, T., and Heilbronn, M.: Biological Markers for Depression in Chronic Pain. Paper presented at the Annual Meeting of the American Psychiatric Association, New Orleans, May, 1981.
11. Blumer, D., and Hilbronn, M.: Chronic pain as a variant of depressive disease. The pain-prone disorder. J. Nerv. Ment. Dis. 170:381–406, 1982.
12. Blumer, D., Zorick, F., and Heilbronn, M.: Biological markers for depression in chronic pain. J. Nerv. Ment. Dis. 170:425–420, 1902.
13. Bonica, J. J.: Basic principles in managing chronic pain. Arch. Surg. 112:783–788, 1977.
14. Bouras, N.: Psychological aspects of patients having multiple operations for low back pain. Br. J. Med. Psychol. 57:147–151, 1984.
15. Bradley, J. J.: Severe localized pain associated with the depressive syndrome. Br. J. Psychiatry 109:741–745, 1963.
16. Bradley, L. A., and Van der Heide, L. H.: Pain-related correlates of MMPI profile subgroups among back pain patients. Health Psychol. 3:157–174, 1984.
17. Brady, J. P.: Behavior therapy. *In* Kaplan, H. I., and Sadock, B. J. (eds.): Comprehensive Textbook of Psychiatry, 4th Ed. Baltimore, Williams & Wilkins, 1985, pp. 1365–1373.
18. Brodner, R. A., and Taub, A.: Chronic pain exacerbated by long term narcotic use in patients with nonmalignant disease: Clinical syndrome and treatment. Mount Sinai J. Med. 45:233–237, 1978.
19. Cairns, D., Thomas, L., Mooney, V., and Pace, J. B.: A comprehensive treatment approach to chronic low back pain. Pain 2:301–308, 1976.
20. Cairns, D., and Pasino, J. A.: Comparison of verbal reinforcement of feedback in the operant treatment of disability due to chronic low back pain. Behav. Ther. 8:621–630, 1977.
21. Calsyn, D. A., Louks, J., and Freeman, C. W.: The use of the MMPI with chronic low back pain patients with mixed diagnosis. J. Clin. Psychol. 32:532–536, 1976.
22. Cameron, A. J. R., and Shepel, L. F.: Psychological assessment. *In* Kirkaldy-Willis, W. H. (ed.): Managing Low Back Pain. New York, Churchill Livingstone, 1983, pp. 63–73.
23. Cameron, A. J. R., Shepel, L. F., and Bowen, R. C.: Psychological treatment of back pain and associated problems. *In* Kirkaldy-Willis, W. H.: Managing Low Back Pain. New York, Churchill Livingstone, 1983, pp. 229–239.
24. Chapman, S. L., Brena, S. F., and Bradford, L. A.: Treatment outcome in a chronic pain rehabilitation program. Pain 11:255–268, 1981.
25. Cohen, M. J., Heinrich, R. L., Collins, G. A., and Bonebakker, A. D.: Group outpatient physical or behavioral therapy for chronic low back pain. Paper presented at the Annual Meeting of the American Pain Society, New York, Sept., 1980.
26. Collins, G. A., Cohen, M. J., Naliboff, B. D., and Schandler, S. L.: Comparative analysis of paraspinal and frontalis EMG, heart rate, and skin conductance in chronic low back pain patients and normals in various postures and stress. Scand. J. Rehabil. Med. 14:39–46, 1982.
27. Crasilneck, H. B.: Hypnosis in the control of chronic low back pain. Am. J. Clin. Hypn. 22:71–78, 1979.
28. Crisson, J., Keele, F. J., Wilkins, R. H., et al.: Self-report of depressive symptoms in low back pain patients. J. Clin. Psychol. 42:425–430, 1986.
29. Davis, J. L., Lewis, S. B., Gerlich, J. E., et al.: Peripheral diabetic neuropathy treated with amitriptyline and fluphenazine. J.A.M.A. 238:2291–2293, 1977.
30. Dhanens, T. P., and Jarrett, S. R.: MMPI assessment index. Predictive and concurrent validity. Int. J. Clin. Neuropsychol. 6:46–49, 1984.
31. Dorpat, T. L., and Holmes, T. H.: Backache and muscle tension origin. *In* Kroger, W. S. (ed.): Psychosomatic Obstetrics, Gynecology, and Endocrinology. Springfield, Charles C Thomas, 1962.
32. Edelstein, E. L.: Experience and mastery of pain. Israel Ann. Psychiatry Re. Disc. 12:216–226, 1974.
33. Engel, G.: "Psychogenic" pain and the pain-prone patient. Am. J. Med. 26:899–918, 1959.
34. Feuerstein, S., Sult, S., and Houle, M.: Environmental stressors and chronic low back pain: Life events, family and work environment. Pain 22:295–307, 1985.
35. Flor, H., Haag, G., Turk, D. C., and Koehler, H.: Efficacy of EMG biofeedback pseudotherapy and

conventional medical treatment for chronic rheumatic back pain. Pain 17:21–31, 1983.
36. Fordyce, W. E.: Behavioral Methods for Chronic Pain and Illness. St. Louis, C. V. Mosby, 1976.
37. Fordyce, W. E.: Learning processes in pain. *In* Sternbach, R. A.: The Psychology of Pain. New York, Raven Press, 1978, pp. 49–72.
38. France, R. D., Houpt, J. L., Skott, A., et al.: Depression as a psychopathological disorder in chronic low back pain patients. J. Psychosom. Res. 30:127–133, 1986.
39. France, R. D., Ranga Rama Krishnan, K., and Trainor, M.: Chronic pain and depression. III. Family history study of depression and alcoholism in chronic low back pain patients. Pain 24:185–190, 1986.
40. France, R. D., Ranga Rama Krishnan, K., Galli, V., et al.: Preliminary study of thyrotropin-releasing hormone stimulation test in chronic low back pain patients. Pain 27:51–55, 1986.
41. France, R. D., Ranga Rama Krishnan, K., Trainor, M., and Pelton, S.: Chronic pain and depression. IV. DST as a discriminator between chronic pain and depression. Pain 28:39–44, 1987.
42. Gentry, W. D., Shows, W. D., and Thomas, M.: Chronic low back pain: A psychological profile. Psychosomatics 15:174–177, 1974.
43. Goldstein, R.: Psychological evaluation of low back pain. *In* White, A. H. (ed.): Failed Back Surgery Syndrome, evaluation and treatment, Vol. 1. Spine: State of the Art Reviews. Philadelphia, Hanley and Belfus, 1986, pp. 103–114.
44. Hackett, T. P., and Bouckoms, A.: The pain patient: Evaluation and treatment. *In* Hackett, T. P., and Cassem, N. M. (eds.): Massachusetts General Hospital Handbook of General Hospital Psychiatry. Littleton, Massachusetts, PSG Publishing Company, Inc., 1987, pp. 42–68.
45. Hathaway, S. R., and McKinley, J. C.: Minnesota Multiphasic Personality Inventory Manual. Revised Edition. New York, Psychological Corporation, 1951.
46. Heaton, R. K., Getto, C. J., and Lehman, R. A. W.: A standardized evaluation of psychosocial factors in chronic pain. Pain 12:165–174, 1982.
47. Hendler, N.: Use of analgesic and psychotropic drugs for chronic pain of benign origin. Contemp. Neurosurg. 1:1–5, 1981.
48. Hendler, N.: The anatomy and psychopharmacology of chronic pain. J. Clin. Psychiatr. 43:15–20, 1982.
49. Hendler, N.: The four stages of pain. *In* Hendler, N., Long, D., and Wise, T. N. (eds.): Diagnosis and treatment of chronic pain. Littleton, Massachusetts, PSG Publishing Company, Inc., 1983.
50. Hendler, N.: Depression caused by chronic pain. J. Clin. Psychiatr. 45:30–36, 1984.
51. Hendler, N., Derogatis, L., Avella, J., and Long, D.: EMG biofeedback in patients with chronic pain. Dis. Nerv. Sys. 38:505–514, 1977.
52. Hendler, N., Viernstein, M., Gucer, P., and Long, D.: A preoperative screening test for chronic back pain patients. Psychosomatics 20:801–808, 1979.
53. Hendler, N., and Fernandez, P.: Alternative treatments for patients with chronic pain. Psychiatr. Ann. 10:25–30, 1980.
54. Hendler, N., Mallett, A., Vierotein, M., et al.: A comparison between the MMPI and the "Mensana Clinic Back Pain Test" for validating the complaint of chronic back pain in women. Pain 23:243–251, 1985.
55. Herman, E., and Baptiste, S.: Pain control: Mastery through experience. Pain 10:79–86, 1981.
56. Hilgard, E. R.: The alleviation of pain by hypnosis. Pain 1:213–231, 1975.
57. Hoffman, J. W., Benson, H., and Arns, P. A.: Reduced sympathetic nervous system responsivity associated with the relaxation response. Science 215:1190, 1982.
58. Jacobson, E.: Progressive Relaxation. Chicago, University of Chicago Press, 1938.
59. Johansson, D., and von-Knorring, L.: A double blind controlled study of a serotonin uptake inhibitor (Zimelidine) versus placebo in chronic pain patients. Pain 7:69–78, 1979.
60. Keefe, F. J., Black, A. F., Williams, R. B., and Surwit, R. S.: Behavioral treatment of chronic back pain. Clinical outcome and individual differences in pain relief. Pain 11:221–231, 1981.
61. Keefe, F. J., Crisson, J. E., Maltbie, A., et al.: Illness behavior as a predictor of pain and overt behavior patterns in chronic low back pain patients. J. Psychosomat. Res. 30:543–551, 1986.
62. Keel, P. J.: Psychological evaluation and management of low back pain. *In* Floman, Y. (ed.): Disorders of the Lumbar Spine. Rockville, MD, Aspen Publishers, Inc., 1989.
63. Kraemlinger, K. G., Swanson, D. W., and Maruta, T.: Are patients with chronic pain depressed? Am. J. Psychiatr. 140:747–749, 1983.
64. Large, R. G., and Mullins, P. R.: Illness behavior profiles in chronic pain: The Auckland Experience. Pain 10:231–239, 1981.
65. Leavitt, F.: Comparison of three measures for detecting psychological disturbance in patients with low back pain. Pain 13:299–305, 1982.
66. Leavitt, F., and Garron, D. C.: The detection of psychological disturbance in patients with low back pain. J. Psychosom. Res. 23:149–154, 1979.
67. Leavitt, F., and Garron, D. C.: Validity of a back pain classification scale among patients with low back pain not associated with demonstrable organic disease. J. Psychosomat. Res. 23:301–306, 1979.
68. Leavitt, F., and Garron, D. C.: Rorschach and pain characteristics of patients with low back pain and "Conversion V" MMPI profiles. J. Pers. Assess. 46:18–25, 1982.
69. Liebman, R., Honig, P., and Berger, H.: An integrated treatment program for psychogenic pain. Fam. Process 15:307–406, 1976.
70. Lindsay, P., and Wyckoff, M.: The depression-pain syndrome and its response to antidepressants. Psychosomatics 22:571–577, 1981.
71. Lopez-Ibor, T. J.: Masked depression. Br. J. Psychiatr. 120:245–258, 1972.
72. Love, A. W.: Depression in chronic low back pain patients. Diagnostic efficiency of three self-report questionnaires. J. Clin. Psychol. 43:85–89, 1987.
73. Love, A. W., and Peck, C. L.: The MMPI and psychological factors in chronic low back pain: A review. Pain 28:1–12, 1987.
74. Magni, G.: Chronic low-back pain and depression: An epidemiological survey. Acta Psychiatr. Scand. 70:614–617, 1984.
75. Mandel, M. R.: Electroconvulsive therapy for chronic pain associated with depression. Am. J. Psychiatry 132:632–636, 1975.

76. McCreary, C. P., Turner, J., and Dawson, E.: Emotional disturbance and chronic low back pain. J. Clin. Psychol. 36:700–715, 1979.
77. McNeill, T. W., Sinkora, G., and Leavitt, F.: Psychologic classification of low-back pain patients: A progressive tool. Spine 11:955–959, 1986.
78. Mechanic, D.: The concept of illness behavior. J. Chronic Dis. 15:189–194, 1962.
79. Mechanic, D., and Angel, R. J.: Some factors associated with the report and evaluation of back pain. J. Health Soc. Behav. 28:131–139, 1987.
80. Melzack, R.: The McGill pain questionnaire: Major properties and scoring methods. Pain 1:277–299, 1975.
81. Melzak, R.: The promise of biofeedback: Don't hold the party yet. Psychol. Today July:18–23, 1975.
82. Melzack, R., and Wall, P. D.: Pain mechanisms: A new theory. Science 150:971–979, 1965.
83. Mendelson, G.: Alexithymia and chronic pain: Prevalence, correlates and treatment results. Psychother. Psychosom. 37:154–164, 1982.
84. Merskey, H.: Psychological aspects, hypnotherapy and psychotropic drugs. *In* Swerdlow, M. (ed.): Relief of intractable pain. Amsterdam, Excerpta Medica, 1974, pp. 90–115.
85. Merskey, H.: Pain and personality. *In* Sternbach, R. A. (ed.): The Psychology of Pain. New York, Raven Press, 1978, pp. 111–127.
86. Merskey, H.: Psychiatry and the treatment of pain. Br. J. Psychiatr. 136:600–602, 1980.
87. Merskey, H., and Spear, F. G.: Pain: Psychological and psychiatric aspects. London, Bailliere-Tindall and Cassell, 1967.
88. Merskey, H., and Boyd, D. B.: Emotional adjustment and chronic pain. Pain 5:173–178, 1978.
89. Mohamed, S. N., Weisz, G. M., and Waring, E. N.: The relationship of chronic pain to depression, marital maladjustment and family dynamics. Pain 5:285–292, 1978.
90. Nagi, S. Z., Riley, L. E., and Newby, L. G.: A social epidemiology of back pain in a general population. J. Chronic Dis. 27:769–779, 1973.
91. Naliboff, B. D., Cohen, M. J., and Yellen, A. N.: Does the MMPI differentiate chronic illness from chronic pain? Pain 13:333–341, 1982.
92. Newman, R. I., Seres, J. L., and Yospe, L. P.: Multidisciplinary treatment of chronic pain: Long-term follow-up of low-back pain patients. Pain 4:283–292, 1978.
93. Nigl, A. J., and Fisher-Williams, M.: Treatment of low back strain with electromyographic biofeedback and relaxation training. Psychosomatics 21:495–499, 1980.
94. Nouwen, A., and Solinger, J. W.: The effectiveness of EMG biofeedback training in low back pain. Biofeedback Self Regulat. 4:103–111, 1979.
95. Nurnberger, F. I., and Gershon, E. S.: Genetics. *In* Raykel, E. S. (ed.): Handbook of Affective Disorders. New York, Guilford Press, 1982, pp. 126–145.
96. O'Brien, J. P.: The role of fusion for chronic low back pain. Orthop. Clin. North Am. 14:639–647, 1983.
97. Oostdam, E. M. M., and Duivenvoorden, H. J.: Description of pain and the degree to which the complaints fit the organic diagnosis of low back pain. Pain 18:71–82, 1984.
98. Orne, M. T.: Pain suppression by hypnosis and related phenomena. Adv. Neurol. 4:563–572, 1974.
99. Peck, C., and Kraft, G.: Electromyographic biofeedback for pain related to muscle tension. Arch. Surg. 112:889–895, 1977.
100. Pelz, M., and Merskey, H.: A description of the psychological effects of chronic painful lesions. Pain 14:293–301, 1982.
101. Pilling, L. F., Bronnick, T. L., and Swenson, W. M.: Psychologic characteristics of psychiatric patients having pain as a presenting symptom. Can. Med. Assoc. J. 97:387–394, 1967.
102. Pilowsky, I., and Spence, N. D.: Pain and illness behavior: A comparative study. J. Psychosomat. Res. 20:131–134, 1976.
103. Pilowsky, I., and Spence, N.: Illness behavior syndromes associated with intractable pain. Pain 2:61–71, 1976.
104. Ranga Rama Krishnan, K., France, R. D., Pelton, S., et al.: Chronic pain and depression. I. Classification of depression in chronic low back pain patients. Pain 22:279–287, 1985.
105. Ranga Rama Krishnan, K., France, R. D., Pelton, S., et al.: Chronic pain and depression. II. Symptoms of anxiety in chronic low back pain patients and their relationship to subtypes of depression. Pain 22:289–294, 1985.
106. Ransford, A. O., Cairns, D., and Mooney, V.: The pain drawing as an aid to the psychologic evaluation of patients with low-back pain. Spine 1:127–134, 1976.
107. Rauchfleisch, U.: Handbruch zum Rosenzweig Picture Frustration Test (PFT). Bern, Huber, 1979.
108. Ready, L. B., Sarkis, E., and Turner, J. A.: Self-reported vs. actual use of medications in chronic pain patients. Pain 12:285–294, 1982.
109. Reuler, J. B., Girard, D. E., and Nardone, D. A.: The chronic pain syndrome: Misconceptions and management. Ann. Intern. Med. 93:588–596, 1980.
110. Rosenstiel, A. K., and Keefe, F. J.: The use of coping strategies in chronic low back pain patients: Relationship to patient characteristics and current adjustment. Pain 17:33–44, 1983.
111. Roy, R.: Measurement of chronic pain in pain-depression literature during the 1980s: A review. Int. J. Psychiatry Med. 16:179–188, 1986–87.
112. Ryden, O., Lindal, E., Uden, A., and Hansson, S. B.: Differentiation of back pain patients using a pain questionnaire. Scand. J. Rehab. Med. 17:155–161, 1985.
113. Sacerdote, P.: Teaching self-hypnosis to patients with chronic pain. J. Hum. Stress 4:18–21, 1978.
114. Sachar, E. F.: Endocrine abnormalities in depression. *In* Paykel, E. S. (ed.): Handbook of Affective Disorders. New York, Guilford Press, 1982, pp. 191–201.
115. Sanders, S. H.: Cross-validation of the back pain classification scale with chronic, intractable pain patients. Pain 22:271–277, 1985.
116. Schofferman, J.: Management of chronic pain. *In* White, A. H. (ed.): Failed Back Surgery Syndrome, Evaluation and Treatment, Vol. 1. Spine: State of the Art Reviews. Philadelphia, Hanley and Belfus, 1986, pp. 115–127.
117. Sedlak, K.: Low-back pain: Perception and tolerance. Spine 10:440–443, 1985.
118. Sifneos, P. E.: Clinical Observations on Some

Patients Suffering from a Variety of Psychosomatic Diseases. Proceedings of the Seventh European Conference on Psychosomatic Research, Basel, Karger, 1967.
119. Skevington, S. M.: Chronic pain and depression: Universal or personal helplessness. Pain 15:309–317, 1983.
120. Sternbach, R. A.: Pain patients, traits, and treatment. New York, Academic Press, 1974.
121. Sternbach, R. A.: The need for an animal model of chronic pain. Pain 2:2–4, 1976.
122. Sternbach, R. A., Wolf, S. R., Murphy, R. W., and Akeson, W. H.: Traits of pain patients: The low-back "loser." Psychosomatics 14:226–229, 1973.
123. Sternbach, R. A., and Timmermans, G.: Personality changes associated with reduction of pain. Pain 1:177–181, 1975.
124. Sternbach, R. A., Janowsky, D. S., Huey, L. Y., and Segal, D. S.: Effects of altering brain serotonin activity on human chronic pain. *In* Bonica, J. J., and Albee-Fessard, D. (ed.): Advances in Pain Research and Therapy, Vol. 1. New York, Raven Press, 1976, pp. 601–606.
125. Stroebel, C. F.: Biofeedback and behavioral medicine. *In* Kaplan, H. I., and Sadock, B. J. (eds.): Comprehensive Textbook of Psychiatry, 4th Ed. Baltimore, Williams & Wilkins, 1985, pp. 1467–1473.
126. Svenson, H. O., and Anderson, G. J.: Low back pain in 40–47 year old men: Work history and work environment factors. Spine 8:272–276, 1983.
127. Swanson, D., Floreen, A., and Swenson, W.: Program for managing chronic pain. II. Short-term results. Mayo Clin. Proc. 51:409–411, 1976.
128. Trief, P. M., Elliott, D. J., Stein, N., and Frederickson, B. E.: Functional vs. organic pain: A meaningful distinction? J. Clin. Psychol. 43:219–226, 1987.
129. Turk, D. C., and Kerns, R. D.: Conceptual issues in the assessment of clinical pain. Int. J. Psychiatr. Med. 113:57–68, 1983.
130. Turk, D. C., and Flor, H.: Etiological theories and treatments for chronic back pain. II. Psychological models and interventions. Pain 19:209–230, 1984.
131. Turner, J. A.: Comparison of group progressive-relaxant training and cognitive-behavioral therapy for chronic low back pain. J. Consult. Clin. Psychol. 50:757–765, 1982.
132. Turner, J. A., and Chapman, C. R.: Psychological interventions for chronic pain: A critical review. I. Relaxation training and biofeedback. Pain 12:1–21, 1982.
133. Villard, H. P., Imbeault, J., and Duguay, M.: Low-back pain: A psychosomatic clinical study. Psychother. Psychosomat. 45:78–83, 1986.
134. Von Knorring, L.: The experience of pain in depressed patients. Neuropsychobiology 1:155–165, 1975.
135. Ward, N. G.: Tricyclic antidepressants for chronic low-back pain. Spine 11:661–665, 1986.
136. Ward, N. G., Bloom, V. L., and Friedel, R. O.: The effectiveness of tricyclic antidepressants in the treatment of coexisting pain and depression. Pain 7:331–341, 1979.
137. Ward, N. G., Bokon, J. A., Ang, J., and Butler, S. H.: Differential effects of fenfluramine and dextroamphetamine on acute and chronic pain. *In* Fields, H. L., Dunber, R., and Cervero, F. (eds.): Advances in Pain Research and Therapy. New York, Raven Press, 1985, pp. 753–760.
138. Waring, E. M.: The role of the family in symptom selection and perception in psychosomatic illness. Psychother. Psychosom. 28:253–259, 1977.
139. Watkins, R. G., O'Brien, J. P., Draugelis, R., and Jones, D.: Comparisons of preoperative and postoperative MMPI data in chronic back patients. Spine 11:385–390, 1986.
140. Watson, D.: Neurotic tendencies among chronic pain patients: An MMPI item analysis. Pain 14:365–385, 1982.
141. Whitlock, F. A.: Hypoalgesia in depressive illness. Br. J. Psychiatr. 140:549–550, 1982.
142. Williams, R., and Rhoads, J.: Biofeedback: An Adjunct for Psychiatric Treatment. Paper presented at the Annual Meeting of the American Psychiatric Association. Anaheim, California, 1975.
143. Yalom, I. D.: The Theory and Practice of Group Psychotherapy, 2nd Ed. New York, Basic Books Inc., 1975.

FUNCTIONAL RESTORATION FOR THE PATIENT WITH CHRONIC LOW BACK PAIN

Tom G. Mayer

FUNCTIONAL RESTORATION PERSPECTIVE

Problems related to the lumbar spine are of great fascination to the array of scientists whose thoughts are contained in this volume (see Chapters 1, 2, and 4 for a description of the scope of the problem). The interests of the general public, it is safe to say, are focused on only two issues: cost and human suffering. The latter category includes two subissues: pain and disability.

The staggering costs have been reported variously, depending on which aspects of cost are included (e.g., weekly benefits, permanent disability payments, Social Security and long-term disability payments, loss of productivity, medical costs, and vocational retraining) at from $20 to $60 billion annually in the United States. Comparable costs relative to population demographics are experienced in other industrialized countries, although costs decline for countries in which life-and-death issues prevail over quality-of-life issues.

The subjectivity of pain and its expression and secondary gain characteristics have also been well covered in the literature.[15, 49, 51] The perception of pain, regardless of whether it is related to structural, functional capacity or psychosocioeconomic issues, remains an unverifiable factor and is therefore the most difficult one to manage. Although several authors have created standardized measures of pain and disability, they are useful for intraindividual comparisons only, because similar lesions may produce highly variable reports among individuals.[17, 28, 38, 41]

The issue of disability has received relatively scant attention in comparison with the other two issues (i.e., cost and pain). Yet, it probably represents the central problem from which all others spring. Lower productivity of individual labor certainly results in major losses for society. It has also been found to produce a loss of self-confidence and self-esteem in most individuals, although a small percentage of patients may enjoy the advantage of an opportunity for "premature retirement." Disability may lead to mental and physical deconditioning, which perpetuates itself and produces a general decline in human performance. Yet, many of our treatments, if devoted solely to relief from pain, fail to ensure the alleviation of disability. As clinicians, we may sometimes even blame the patient for therapeutic failures in the guise of recognizing "secondary gain" concomitant to their failure to become well.

The rate of the rise of low back disability in the United States has been accelerating dramatically over the past 20 years[31] with a staggering 14-fold increase in disability in the United States during the 1970s.[16] This increase can no longer be ignored, particularly in view of the declining work force. The recognition of disability as the central problem related to lumbar dysfunction characterizes the functional restoration approach. The primary goal of functional restoration is the elimination of disability; once this has been accomplished, pain relief and cost control can be anticipated as secondary phenomena.

IDENTIFICATION OF LUMBAR DYSFUNCTION: MEASUREMENT IS THE KEY

Principles of Measurement

Consciously or unconsciously, measurement is a part of all of our activities of daily living. We regularly utilize our senses to determine temperature, distance, size, or texture of objects. Often a fairly qualitative evaluation suffices, usually because no visual or tactile limitation is placed on the frequently repeated assessment of the object in question. Examples of such qualitative evaluation include observing a moving vehicle in traffic or placing food in our mouths. Sometimes, however, greater precision is necessary, usually when the object in question is *not* amenable to regular visual inspection. In these cases the quantitative assessment is usually associated with a range of normal values (obtained by testing, for example, many "normal" patients). A patient's variation from a mean score is then used for evaluating the presence of disease or dysfunction, or the return to an improved state from an abnormal one. The spinal anatomy does not lend itself easily to visual or tactile examination and thus demands indirect, quantitative measurement to describe its performance.

Musculoskeletal clinicians are somewhat spoiled by having visual access to most parts of our organ system. They have not had to develop the discipline of the hematologist and cardiologist, who must rely on indirect measurements (e.g., those of blood components, heart rate, and blood pressure) to diagnose abnormalities. Although quantitative measures of joint motion or muscle strength have been available for many years, all too often a hasty qualitative assessment is substituted for the quantitative one. The novice physician or therapist soon learns that quantitative measurements are time consuming and generally unnecessary for routine clinical practice. Instead, one "eyeballs" the comparison of the motion of both knees and of the size of quadriceps (often without even using a tape measure), reserving the use of a goniometer or isokinetic testing device for special occasions on which an evaluation request specifies quantification.

In the spinal anatomy, the small, inaccessible, three-joint complexes stacked upon each other do not lend themselves to easy inspection. Intersegmental spinal movement is difficult to measure, even with biplanar x-ray devices. Multiple small muscles interdigitate over variable numbers of segments, and ligamentous structures may share surprising amounts of load in certain joint positions. Moreover, bilateral comparisons are impossible to make. Until recently, there were no valid indirect measurement methods to assess available spinal function; this resulted in an ignorance of pathologic processes in the vast majority of patients with spinal dysfunction that did not resolve spontaneously. Currently, however, although an absence of methodology for direct visualization persists, novel technology for assessing spinal function has become part of the clinical routine. Nevertheless, many clinicians demonstrate a persistent lack of familiarity with such technology. In so doing, therapeutic errors are encouraged, outcomes remain unevaluated, and fringe or fad treatments are perpetuated.

The weaker clinical areas must be recognized before it is possible to move forward. In the case of diagnosis of spinal disorders, the lack of recognition of the deconditioning syndrome has adversely affected our therapeutics. Many individuals currently embracing "work hardening" (often as fervently as they previously embraced "pain management") continue to do so with eclectic therapies applied uniformly to all patients, rather than individualized on the basis of functional testing.

Surgical treatment is performed on only 2% to 3% of patients with spinal disorders. Nevertheless, surgeons will search diligently for that small percentage with a wide variety of expensive and sophisticated diagnostic tools (e.g., computed tomography [CT], magnetic resonance imaging [MRI], electromyography, myelography). A structural diagnosis, when made, may lead to the ability to "fix" an anatomic aberration, such as a prolapsed disc. For the remaining 97% of the back-injured population, spontaneous recovery may account for many so-called cures. However, a substantial percentage of patients, perhaps as high as 30% to 40%, show some evidence of disuse and deconditioning, making them candidates for physical retraining once the functional deficits are identified. Without quantification the deficits are simply not recognizable; this results in an inevitable overutilization or underutilization of therapeutic services. This observation has not escaped the attention of health care planners. Medicare requires periodic testing to document progress in other areas of rehabilitation. It is likely that similar rules will ultimately apply to the treatment of spinal problems, once their necessity becomes more generally perceived.

Design of Efficient Measurements of the Spine

The term *deconditioning syndrome* has been applied to the changes of cumulative disuse produced in the chronically disabled patient suffering from spinal dysfunction. It is initially produced by the immobilization and inactivity attendant upon injury. It is supplemented by the disruption of spinal soft tissues and scarring resulting from a surgical approach or repetitive microtrauma. As pain perception is enhanced, learned protective mechanisms lead to a vicious circle of inactivity and disuse. As physical capacity decreases, the likelihood of fresh sprains or strains to unprotected joints, muscles, ligaments, and discs increases. These inevitable alterations of pain and function are perceived by the patient as a recurrence or a reinjury.

In assessing spinal function, we have initially determined the critical elements that are of value in predicting the performance of physiologic functional units of extremities. Such factors as range of motion, strength, neurologic status, endurance combined with whole-body aerobic capacity, and activities of daily living are some of the major factors traditionally assessed. Unfortunately, the evaluation of the neurologic function of extremities (e.g., straight-leg raising, lower-extremity strength, sensation, and reflexes in dermatomal/myotomal patterns) is still viewed by most clinicians as the ideal functional evaluation of the spine. In view of the aforementioned, it is necessary to recognize that the neuro leg tests are simply adjunctive, being used to find the 2% to 3% of patients requiring surgical intervention. As measures of spinal function these tests are irrelevant for several reasons. First, they measure acute change related only to disorders requiring surgery. In patients with chronic disorders the persistence of neurologic changes generally reflects epidural fibrosis or other permanent, noncorrectable anatomic abnormalities. Second, the abnormalities, although emanating from spinal structures, are perceived by the patient as *extremity abnormalities* producing pain, sensory changes, and weakness of the arms and/or legs. Once appropriate surgical decompression has been achieved, rehabilitative treatment of, for example, a foot drop is focused on bracing, mobilizing, and strengthening the foot and ankle, not to retraining the back. In summary, what the clinician currently views as standard objective functional tests may provide no useful information to overcome spinal deconditioning.

Isometric lifting tests have been used to "measure back strength."[7, 24] In fact, although engineering principles require that the force of an isometric test be transmitted through the body from the hands to foot or floor contact, the spine can often be placed into such a position that virtually no spinal muscular strength is required to support the load.[20] This exemplifies the first criterion for any functional evaluation: the test must be *relevant* to the physiologic factor being measured. If one wishes to assess isolated spinal muscular strength, then measures of trunk torques in flexion and extension, rotation, or lateral bend must be sought, not whole-body tasks such as lifting.

A second criterion of measurement is knowing the *validity* and *reproducibility* of the measurement. Validity refers to the accuracy of the test device itself, whereas reproducibility refers to the ability of the test (device *plus* subject) to yield a repeatable and precise measurement of a clinical variable. *A valid test is not necessarily reproducible, and vice versa.* An invalid test is simply useless, but an irreproducible test may reflect clinical reality (such as comparing intersubject body weight or changes in spinal mobility before and after exercise in the same individual). As in the examples, reproducibility problems can often be corrected by restructuring the test protocol.

Once a functional test has been found to be valid, reproducible, and relevant, an *effort factor* must be defined. Without the ability to identify suboptimal effort, invalid low readings may be accepted as true physical deficits. Although a patient's suboptimal effort may reflect a clinical abnormality (such as low motivation or a personality disorder leading to conscious malingering), the clinician must be able to assess whether this is a true physical deficit.

Finally, once the appropriate device and test protocol have been chosen, the difficult work begins. A *normative data base* must be compiled on a large population sample to permit comparisons with a smaller group of patients. The degree of deviation from "normal" may significantly affect treatment protocols. Although much more should be said about measurement criteria, it is most important to select the optimal measurement device in the first place, in order to avoid the tedious task of collecting additional normative data.[23, 24, 31, 33, 34–37, 47]

SPECIFICS OF QUANTITATIVE FUNCTIONAL EVALUATION

Evaluation of Range of Motion

Trunk motion is a compound movement combining intersegmental and hip motion components. Thus, a patient with a completely fused spine can often bend forward to perform toe touches using hip motion alone. Although it is not yet possible to measure intersegmental motion noninvasively, biplanar radiography may confirm inclinometry in selected cases.[43, 44] Inclinometers may be used to separate the hip motion component from the lumbar spinal motion component and derive valuable information.[23, 37] As in all functional capacity measurements, information obtained with range-of-motion techniques must be compared with a normal data base. In addition, an *effort factor* must be available to validate adequate motivation in performing the test. For range of motion, this effort factor is generally the repeatability of sequential measures. However, in the most important spine flexion measure, in which ultimate range of motion is approximately the same in the hips and the six lumbar motion segments, the comparison of the hip motion component with the supine straight-leg raising measurement creates an effective effort factor.[23, 28, 31] In the sagittal plane, the inclinometers, which are available in mechanical or computerized forms from various manufacturers, may be positioned at two points or may be moved from one point to another.[28]

Measurements are taken in both flexion and extension and are validated through the effort factor of straight-leg raising. There are many reasons for a limitation of effort on any single test; thus, the effort factor is not a test for malingering. Effort may be reduced by pain, fear of injury, physiologic perception of excessive load, or psychologic factors of anxiety or depression, or by a conscious effort to mislead the examiner.

In addition to sagittal movement of the spine, coronal motion can be assessed just as easily by simply rotating the inclinometer 90 degrees in the axial plane. This keeps the inclinometer moving within the gravitational field, which is necessary for its proper function. Rotation may also be measured, although the very small range of lumbar torsion makes this a far less reliable test. If performed in a standardized manner with good effort by the patient, the techniques are highly reproducible. However, with suboptimal patient effort, considerable variability is noted on repeat measurements.

Many alternative techniques for spinal mobility measurement have been described.[10] However, many of them are relatively cumbersome to perform or require large and expensive pieces of equipment such as the 3-D digitizer. Probably the most commonly utilized technique is the Schober method,[46] which is essentially useful only for measuring true spinal flexion isolated from the hip component. Unfortunately, there are several problems with this technique, including the variable number of segments measured and the absence of the "dimples of Venus" (a critical anatomic marker) in a significant percentage of subjects. Careful evaluation of all available spinal motion techniques leads to the inescapable conclusion that inclinometry is the only technique combining simplicity, relevance, validity, and reproducibility. As noted above, these are the essential prerequisites for the development of a normative data base using any functional capacity measurement.

Motion measurement techniques can be used for several purposes. To assess function on a one-time basis, the technique can demonstrate the actual range of motion in the T12–S1 segment during sagittal and coronal plane bending (true lumbar motion). Suboptimal effort may lead to more careful scrutiny of other components of the functional capacity test battery and psychosocial barriers to a return to productivity. However, even in the presence of poor effort, the determination of normal or abnormal motion can be made by comparing the motion ratios of the spine and hip. In the normally mobile spine, the sequence of forward bending generally involves spinal flexion considerably more than hip flexion during the initial phases, until the spine seems to be hanging on its ligaments. At that point, hip motion alone increases.[28, 37] If, even in the presence of suboptimal effort, a normal spine-to-hip ratio exists for any given total flexion angle, the clinician can usually conclude that normal spinal mobility *would have been present* if the patient had provided sufficient effort. Conversely, in the presence of an abnormal spine-to-hip ratio, with or without good effort, some actual limitation of spinal mobility can be inferred (postfusion ankylosis or postoperative/disuse stiffness).

Several problems account for the slow acceptance of inclinometry since its advent and use by British rheumatologists and the British Back Pain Association.[26] These problems include a combination of the lack of development of standardized protocols for compound joint motion measurement[37] and the availability of mechanical devices that necessitate cumbersome mental calculations. Subsequently, two computerized devices have become available, including the OrthoRanger (Orthotronics, Daytona Beach, Florida) and the Cybex EDI-320 (Lumex, Ronkonkoma, New York) (Fig. 1). Both inclinometers provide precise measurements. The first device has the advantages of versatility and print-out documentation; the second is inexpensive and compact, with greater convenience and portability. Once mastered, the technique is less time consuming than obtaining a blood pressure. Postural measures may be obtained by associating a lumbosacral angle to a reference surface, such as a wall or table. Nevertheless, it is likely that many physicians will prefer to have these measurements taken by nurses, therapists, or technicians.

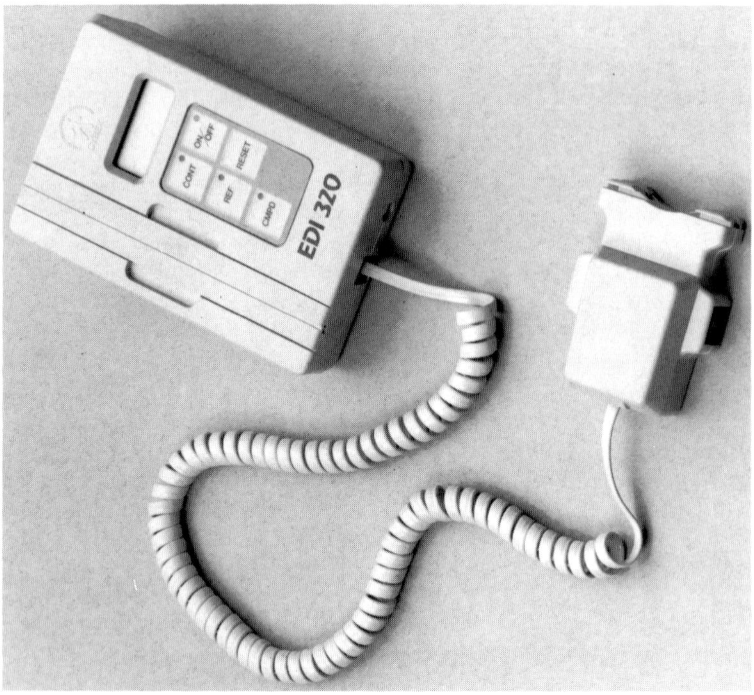

Figure 1 □ Cybex EDI-320 (Lumex; Ronkonkoma, New York), a small, portable, computerized device for measuring joint motion, simple (i.e., in the extremities) and compound (i.e., in the spine and shoulder girdle).

As in all other physiologic measurements, there is some variation in the normal population. Interestingly, our normative data show that the mean true lumbar motions in males and females are almost identical, even though females tend to have higher hip and straight-leg raising mobility components. Patient values are expressed as a percentage of normal as related to mean scores of the asymptomatic subject population. These scores may be normalized for such factors as age, gender, and anthropometric factors (especially body weight), when applicable. The system allows the clinician to judge the significance of small deviations from the anticipated value. More importantly, the clinician may track the progress of the rehabilitation process and patient effort from one examination to the next.

Evaluation of Isolated Trunk Strength

Isolated trunk strength assessment devices measure the torques generated dynamically and isokinetically in the thoracolumbar functional unit of the biomechanical chain. This functional unit is involved in transmitting forces from the hands through the trunk to the ground and is frequently the weak link in the performance of tasks such as lifting, bending, and twisting, once a traumatic incident has occurred. Isokinetic measurements are a form of dynamic evaluation allowing the clinician to preselect a fixed speed of motion and distance moved so as to isolate torque as the only independent variable. Great care is also taken in anatomic stabilization of the hips and lower extremities, so that only torques generated in the thoracolumbar functional unit are measured. This system provides incalculable advantages over static systems (isometrics) and other dynamic systems unable to control multiple independent variables. In particular, the ability of isokinetics to eliminate changes in the preselected fixed variables of velocity, acceleration, distance traveled, and extraneous motion of adjacent functional units (through anatomic stabilization) permits the development of measurements of sensitivity and specificity far greater than those obtained when multiple factors are permitted to vary independently.

At present, several devices are commercially available for assessing isokinetic trunk strength. As discussed above, selection of a device must consider not only such commercial aspects as price, tolerance of abuse, repair record, and resale but also the critical factors of *validity, reproducibility, rele-*

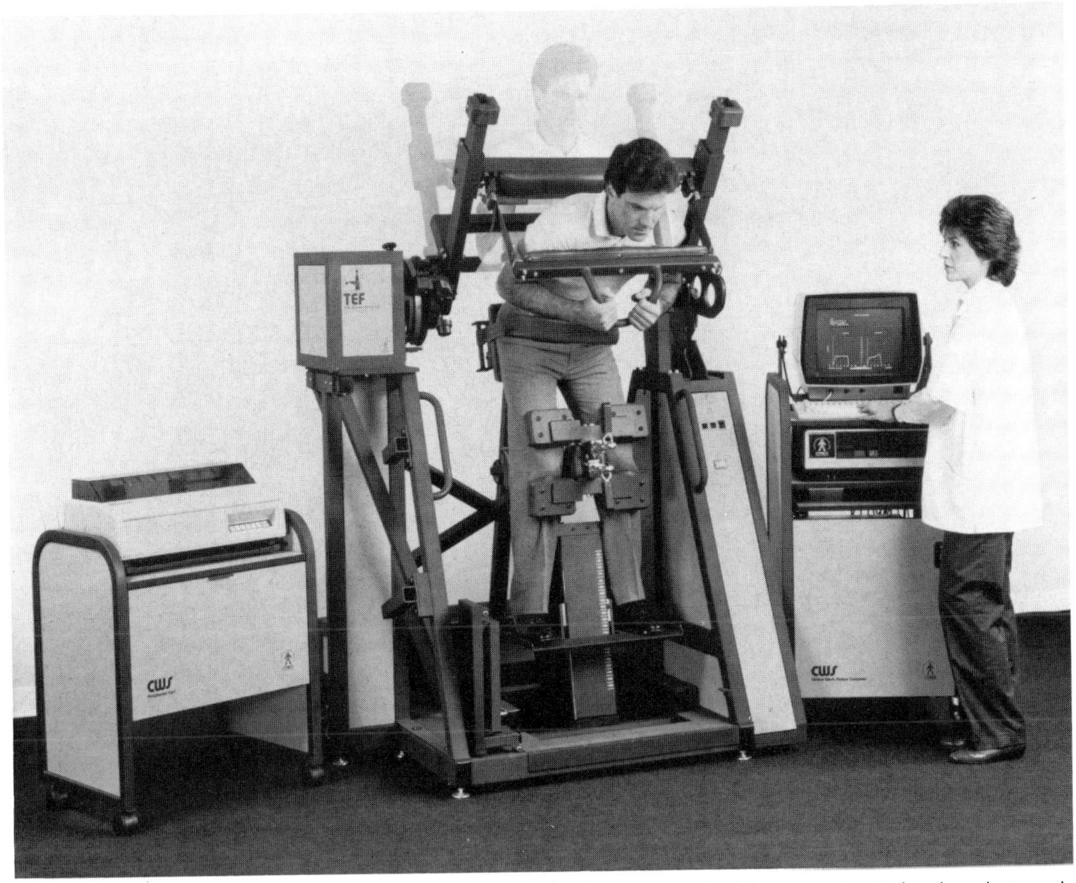

Figure 2 □ Cybex Trunk Extension/Flexion Unit (Lumex; Ronkonkoma, New York) for measuring isolated trunk strength.

vance, *effort factor*, and *simplicity of operation*. At first, the University of Texas Southwestern Medical Center and PRIDE groups had the advantage of working with prototype Cybex (the developers of isokinetics) devices; several other units are now commercially available. They include sitting and standing models, stand-alone devices, or "add-on" units combining extremity and spinal measurement capabilities. The Cybex TEF unit (Lumex, Ronkonkoma, New York) (Fig. 2) is the first sagittal strength testing unit that restricts motion to the sagittal plane only. This manufacturer also has an axial (torsional) measurement device. Biodex, on the other hand, has a reclining unit that adds on to its all-purpose dynamometer (Biodex, Inc., Shirley, New York) (Fig. 3). The dynamometer may be disconnected from the sitting isokinetic sagittal plane unit for use on a variety of alternative fixtures used for isolated extremity joint measures. Lido (Loredan Corp., Davis, California) and Kin-Com (Chatteck Corp., Chattanooga, Tennessee) also manufacture isokinetic trunk strength testing equipment. Lido permits both sitting and standing measurements on a dedicated isokinetic sagittal plane testing unit. Nonisokinetic devices are also available, utilizing isometric, isotonic, or isoinertial systems. Although these devices may have advantages for physical training, particularly when multiplanar motion capability is present, they lack the following advantages of isokinetics that are critical for useful measurement: (1) isolating a single independent variable (torque) rather than allowing changes in multiple independent variables; and (2) dynamic motion with greater safety ensured by *accommodating resistance*.

Major differences between the trunk strength, in both sagittal and axial planes, of a normal individual and of a patient population have been demonstrated.[10, 35, 36, 47, 50] Moreover, through efforts at functional restoration with a sports medicine approach,

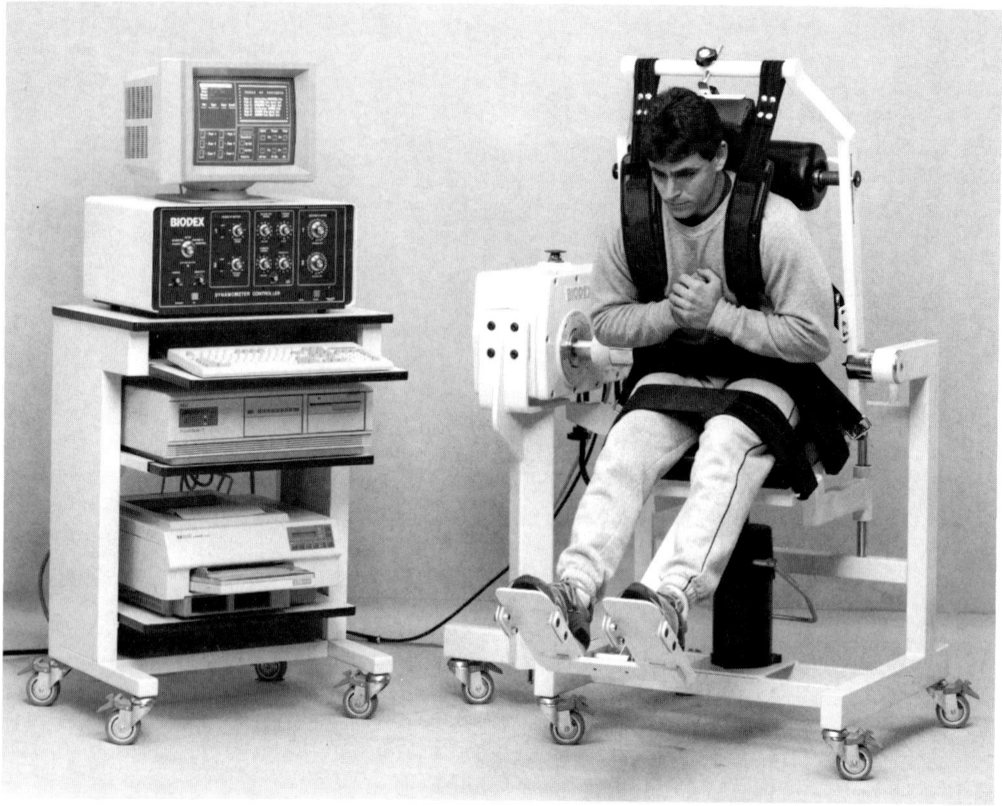

Figure 3 □ Biodex spine strength measurement accessory (Biodex Corp.; Shirley, New York) for assessing trunk strength in the sagittal plane from a semireclining position.

trunk strength in the patient population can be markedly improved.[33] Effort can generally be assessed by the repeatability of curve production, and information on work performance, power consumption, and endurance can be delivered by the computerized assessment devices. It is interesting to note that trunk strength deficits may exist independent of symptoms and may act to produce a risk of recurrent injury.

Evaluation of Cardiovascular Fitness

Inactivity associated with deconditioning may also produce declines in aerobic fitness. Bicycle ergometry that compares the response of heart rate to a predetermined work load can be used to assess cardiovascular fitness with minimal equipment and time commitment. Surprising deficits in aerobic capacity are frequently present in patients with chronic and postoperative low back pain and are somewhat proportional to the duration of disability and the degree of inactivity. Because inactivity may also produce deconditioning of lower-extremity skeletal muscle, the ergometry test may also be terminated by extremity fatigue, rather than by a decline in cardiovascular fitness alone. However, these alternatives can usually be distinguished by noting the heart rate achieved at the point of voluntary test conclusion, as well as by comparing the bicycle ergometry results with those of a treadmill exercise tolerance test. In most deconditioned patients, however, an exaggerated heart rate response to relatively low work loads is usually the limiting factor and is indicative of aerobic capacity deficits. Such testing leads to a determination of the extent to which aerobic capacity and/or lower-extremity strength training needs to be added to the functional restoration program.

Evaluation of Lifting Capacity

The previously described tests of mobility and strength focus primarily on the alterations in the lumbar spine functional unit that are induced by injury or disuse. Measurement of whole-body task performance represents the interaction of multiple functional unit links in the biomechanical chain. Although the body may compensate for deficits in the performance of one body link by substituting the higher performance of another (e.g., substituting squatting for bending after back injury), this is not the optimal biomechanical situation and requires frequent conscious compromises of function that predispose to recurrent injury. Optimum physical capacity involves the highest possible functioning of each functional unit involved in a task and a relearning of tasks in coordination/agility dimensions linking the functional units, to provide optimum safety and efficiency.

Although functional task performance measurements measure what the patient can do in the "real world," a price must be paid for this information. The linking of multiple functional units allows one unit to substitute for another. The lack of anatomic stabilization, and multiplanar motion and postures, interferes with the ability to stabilize anatomic and motion variables. Because of this, tests of whole-body task performance can generally be anticipated to be less precise, sensitive, and specific than isolated trunk mobility or strength measures. Nonetheless, such is the importance of these whole-body tasks that the information is valuable even though certain compromises must be made.

One approach taken at the Productive Rehabilitation Institute of Dallas for Ergonomics (PRIDE) is to perform multiple tests of varying complexity to examine a single task. A case in point is examination of lifting, which has been implicated in 60% to 70% of back injuries. Three separate tests of lifting, all performed along standardized protocols in the sagittal plane, are used. An *isometric* test sequence is performed according to the National Institute of Occupational Safety and Health (NIOSH) guidelines produced by Chaffin and colleagues.[7, 8] *Isokinetic* tests are performed utilizing the Cybex Liftask (Lumex, Ronkonkoma, New York), currently the only available isokinetic lifting device.[24, 31] Finally, a progressive *isoinertial* lifting evaluation (the PILE) is performed to simulate "real-world" lifting while a standardized protocol is used to control vertical distance, weight, and duration of lift in order to produce comparable data.[29, 30] The tests are normalized to age, gender, and a body weight variable.

Positional and activity tolerance is another area of interest in functional task measurement directed toward return to productivity. Following spinal surgery, patients often cannot tolerate the long static positioning (sitting or standing) and often complain of the inability to perform various tasks, such as squatting, kneeling, walking, carrying, or climbing. We have devised an obstacle course requiring the use of multiple positions in an attempt to assess the patient's tolerance of a variety of positions and daily living activities. Observation of the patient through a testing or training session can provide the therapist with an idea of the patient's activity tolerance. Because of the lack of corroborative tests, the latter measures are somewhat less objective than the battery of lifting tests.

Quantification of physical function represents a new and important tool in assessing patients with chronic disabling low back pain. Although the measures are in a relatively early stage of development and standardization, experience with extremity rehabilitation suggests that these tests will, in time, become an important supplement to our sophisticated but expensive imaging devices in determining the full gamut of spinal treatments. Quantification of physical functional capacity requires patient motivation, but because an effort factor can be identified with each functional capacity test, suboptimal effort can be recognized and utilized to validate the actual test scores. In general, the clinician attempts to shorten and simplify the battery of tests in the desire to identify a single number that will be useful in making a decision. Unfortunately, from my point of view, having been involved in research in this area for the past several years, the number of measures is likely to increase rather than decrease in the short run. Tests commonly recognized as being important in the extremities, such as stability, fatigue resistance, and coordination/balance, either are currently unavailable for the spine or are in laboratory development only. Considerably more clinical experience will be necessary before the usefulness of the various tests and their cost/benefit ratios can be assessed.

BARRIERS TO FUNCTIONAL RECOVERY

A multitude of psychosocial and socioeconomic problems may confront the patient recovering from a spinal disorder, particularly if disability from a productive lifestyle is associated with the back pain. The patient's inability to see the proverbial light at the end of the tunnel may involve a severe situational depression often associated with severe anxiety and agitation. The back injury itself may be a sign of emotional conflicts and rebellion against authority associated with job dissatisfaction.[3,4,48] These personality changes may be manifested in anger, hostility, and noncompliance directed at the therapeutic team. Minor head injuries, limited intelligence, or organic brain dysfunction from age, alcohol, or drugs may produce cognitive disorders that make patients difficult to manage and refractory to education. A variety of personality disorders such as sociopathy may also complicate treatment.[17,18,31,33,34]

Many chronic spinal disorders exist within a disability system. Workers' compensation laws were initially devised to protect workers' income and provide timely medical benefits following industrial accidents. Employers ultimately agreed to this because of a compensatory benefit: in return for providing these workers' rights, they were absolved of certain consequences of negligence, generally including cost-capped liability for any injury, no matter how severe, and established by state law. As occurs in any compromise situation, certain disincentives to rational behavior may be produced. One outcome of a guaranteed paycheck while Temporary Total Disability persists is that there may be no clear incentive for an early return to work. A casual approach to surgical decision-making and rehabilitation may lead to further deconditioning, both mental and physical, thus making ultimate recovery more problematic. Complicating matters even further is the observation that *no group* (other than the employer) has a verifiable financial incentive to return patients to productivity as soon as possible. In consequence, an odd assortment of health professionals, attorneys, insurance companies, and vocational rehabilitation specialists may be minimally motivated to combat foot-dragging in regard to the disability issue. Altering the contingencies may correct some of the problems. However, this assumes that the present system has not already evolved to a nearly perfect balance of interests or that legislators will respond to changes in outlook regarding optimal patient care.

FUNCTIONAL RESTORATION PROGRAM

Pain clinics have proliferated over the past 25 to 30 years in response to the recognition that surgical correction of structural deficits could address spinal pain perception in only a small percentage of chronically affected patients and in some cases was associated with a prolongation of disability in the "failed back surgery syndrome." In patients employed in industry poor surgical results associated with psychosocioeconomic disincentives have been documented from several quarters.[1,13,15,22,32] However, successful-outcome studies using objective criteria from the large number of pain clinics actively treating chronically disabled back (and other) pain patients have failed to materialize. Rather, subjective reports by patients of level of pain, use of medication, and levels of stress have appeared as criteria of improvement in the pain literature. The originators of pain management made brilliant diagnostic contributions to the field by recognizing the importance of psychosocial factors, including stress, to the problem of chronic low back pain. The major problems arose not in diagnosis but in treatment. Behavioral modification principles were translated from simple animal models to complex human contingencies. Generally, passive physical therapy approaches and unquantified reactivation programs failed to address the physical deconditioning component of chronic pain. Pain, which is a subjective individual perception that is refractory to external measurement, remained the major focus of both the treatment process and outcome goals. Increased pain all too often resulted in the return to additional passive care, sympathetic attention, inactivity, and avoidance behavior. Disability and its modification were most often ignored.

A conceptual breakthrough was the recognition of the relationship between fitness and back pain. Although Cady's initial study was limited primarily by reliance on cardiovascular fitness measures, engineers and clinicians added substantially to the body of knowledge in this area, leading ultimately to the technology for quantification of function that was discussed previously.[5,19,23–25,35,36,45,47,50] All that remained was the need

Table 1 □ Critical Elements of a Functional Restoration Program

Quantification of physical function and patient self-report
Physical reconditioning of the injured functional unit
Work simulation and whole-body retraining
Cognitive-behavioral multimodal disability management program
Ongoing outcome assessment utilizing objective criteria

to develop truly objective outcome criteria to assess the capability of a treatment program to address *disability*, not merely a subjective *pain* report by the patient. Nachemson summarized the interrelationship between cost and disability and set the stage for the use of objective outcome criteria to assess *cost* and *disability* responses to rehabilitation programs.[42]

In this way, the evolution to the functional restoration program occurred. There are five critical elements of the program, as shown in Table 1. First of all, quantification of function is the key to the entire process (discussed earlier). Patient's self-report of pain, disability, and affective disorders is a necessary part of the process, and standardized self-report tests to permit intraindividual comparisons can be very helpful. These may include, but are not restricted to, the Million Analog, Beck Depression Inventory, Millon Behavioral Health Inventory, Oswestry Rating Scale, Quantified Pain Drawing, Hamilton Depression Scale, and SCL-90.[2, 6, 11, 12, 14, 38, 39, 41] The MMPI, although it is a standard in the field, may provide inadequate information, considering the time involvement and expense of performing the test. It is primarily a stress indicator and as such shows marked improvement in scores with resolution of disability issues. Certain subscales (such as the McAndrews) may be helpful.

The reconditioning and work simulation aspects of the program involve physical and occupational therapists utilizing active, not passive, treatment modalities. This may be difficult to encourage in view of traditional reimbursement schedules used in much of the industrialized world that encourage passive treatments that produce temporary comfort and discourage exercise and education. Quantification is necessary for these aspects of the program because they provide the initial levels of exercise from which a progressive resistive program emerges. The indirect assessments confirm functional deficits and psychosocial barriers to effort, leading to a combination of education and exercise training to resolve the deconditioning syndrome. Initial treatment is directed toward mobilizing and strengthening the weak link in the biomechanical chain, whereas whole-body work simulation integrates the performance of this link with other parts of the body that have been deconditioned simply by inactivity.

The cognitive-behavioral multimodal disability management program initially focuses on the diagnosis of psychosocioeconomic barriers to functional recovery in a given individual by means of the assessment mentioned above, and then on specific treatments for these problems. The initial treatment may be pharmacologic, involving detoxification from habituating opiate and tranquilizer medications, use of antidepressants and anti-inflammatory medications, occasionally including major tranquilizers. Remaining treatments include a cognitively-behaviorally based program of education and counseling, including stress management, that is time limited and aggressively oriented toward sequential goal-setting. Failure to meet mutually prearranged goals may result in dismissal from the program (an event currently occurring in about 5% of comprehensive program admissions). In practice, education and counseling account for approximately one half of the total program time, with the remainder being spent in physical training.

Finally, just as the quantification of physical function and self-report provides feedback about physical performance to the staff and patient, so measures of follow-up outcome provide objective statistical confirmation of the level of success in achieving program goals. The PRIDE comprehensive program performs 1- and 2-year structured follow-up telephone interviews as a routine part of its ongoing program, at no additional cost. During the interview, information is obtained on working status; additional surgical, medical, or chiropractic treatment; resolution of compensation issues (e.g., long-term disability, Social Security disability, permanent partial or total disability); and injury recurrence. At PRIDE we have found that it may be difficult to entice workers to return for 1- and 2-year physical evaluations to obtain quantified physical capacity and pain or disability self-report scores, although it may be possible to obtain this information in a higher percentage of patients in other locations. However, with judicious attempts to maintain patient contact, a high rate of success in performing follow-up interviews may be anticipated. The interviews must be performed within the context of possible barriers to full disclosure by the patient; further investigation may be necessary, for example, contacts with employers, attorneys, family members, or third-party pairs. Combining the follow-up interview information with preprogram demographic data on the same individuals can provide valid statistical comparisons of the ability of a comprehensive functional restoration program to manage disability and cost. Because the patient with chronic low back pain accounts for 80% of the cost of low back pain problems through a combination of medical treatment, lost productivity, indemnity, and government support, program evaluation—including the involvement of other members of the disability system—is a major resource to clinicians, employers, health care planners, and legislators.

Unfortunately, although functional restoration of the patient with chronic low back pain is the area of the highest anticipated benefit per dollar in low back disability, employers and government agencies are often unmotivated to change their policies. Although the Boeing study clearly demonstrates[3, 4, 48] that job dissatisfaction and personnel relations problems may be the most reliable (or only) predictor of ostensible back injury, the use of the medical system to avoid responsibility for good personnel relations has become endemic in some industries. These employers and government agencies may find it easier to ascribe back injury to the "cost of doing business" and pass these expenses on to the consumer or taxpayer. An adversarial relationship filled with rancor often alters the status of the patient from employee to claimant. Instead of too readily labeling the injured worker who seeks redress from the perceived punitive actions of an employer as a faker or a malingerer, it is necessary to consider the many factors in the evolution of the worker's compensation and in the situations involving personal injury.

CONCLUSION

The future lies in finding solutions that involve communication and cooperation among members of the disability system. The injured patient with low back pain must be provided an opportunity for appropriate medical care, re-employment, and compensation for injury as is provided for others with industrial or personal injuries. If objective structural documentation cannot provide the adequate means for assessing impairment, scheduled or functional assessment-based awards must be considered. At this time, judicious combinations of surgical treatment (if appropriate) and functional restoration rehabilitation are available; these should be the first line of defense.

Quantification may also lead to prevention through worker selection and incumbent motivation assessment. Prevention programs should be combined with the analysis and redesign of jobs following risk assessment and with the enlightened education of high-risk workers *and their personnel managers and supervisors.* Multidisciplinary combinations of occupational health professionals who provide optimum early and late care for the entire range of industrial injuries in a cost-effective manner is our ultimate goal. To this end we continue to increase our knowledge by improving the technology for structural and physical capacity measurement.

References

1. Beals, R.: Compensation and recovery from injury. West. J. Med. 104:233–237, 1984.
2. Beck, A.: Depression: Clinical, Experimental, and Theoretical Aspects. New York, Harper & Row, 1967.
3. Bigos, S., Spengler, D., Martin, N., et al.: Back injuries in industry: A retrospective study. II. Injury factors. Spine 11:246–251, 1986.
4. Bigos, S., Spengler, D., Martin, N., et al.: Back injuries in industry: A retrospective study. III. Employee-related factors. Spine 11:252–256, 1986.
5. Cady, L., Bischoff, D., O'Connel, E., et al.: Strength and fitness and subsequent back injuries in firefighters. J. Occup. Med. 21:269–272, 1979.
6. Capra, P., Mayer, T., and Gatchel, R.: Adding psychological scales to assess back pain. J. Musc. Med. 7:41–52, 1985.
7. Chaffin, D.: Pre-employment strength testing: Updated position. J. Occup. Med. 10:105–110, 1978.
8. Chaffin, D., and Andersson, G.: Occupational Biomechanics. New York, Wiley-Intersciences, 1984.
9. Chaffin, D., Herrin, G., and Keyserling, W.: Preemployment strength testing: An updated position. J. Occup. Med. 20:403–408, 1978.
10. Davies, G., and Gould, J.: Trunk testing using a prototype Cybex II isokinetic stabilization system. J. Orthop. Sports Phys. Ther. 3:164–170, 1982.
11. Derogatis, L., Lipman, R., and Covi, L.: The SCL-90: An outpatient psychiatric rating scale. Psychopharm. Bull. 9:13–28, 1973.

12. Derogatis, L. R., Rickels, K., and Rock, A.: SCL-90 and the MMPI: A step in the validation of a new self-report scale. Br. J. Psychiatry 128:280–289, 1976.
13. Dzioba, R., and Doxey, N.: A prospective investigation into the orthopaedic and psychologic predictors of outcome of first lumbar surgery following industrial injury. Spine 9:614–623, 1984.
14. Fairbank, J., Davies, J., Couper, J., and O'Brien, J.: The Oswestry Low Back Pain Disability Questionnaire. Physiotherapy 66:271–273, 1980.
15. Fordyce, W., Roberts, A., and Sternbach, R.: The behavioral management of chronic pain: A response to critics. Pain 22:112–125, 1985.
16. Frymoyer, J., and Mooney, V.: Current concepts review: Occupational orthopedics. J. Bone Joint Surg. 68A:469–474, 1986.
17. Gatchel, R., Mayer, T., Capra, P., et al.: Quantification of lumbar function, Part 6: The use of psychological measures in guiding physical functional restoration. Spine 11:36–42, 1986.
18. Gatchel, R., Mayer, T., Capra, P., et al.: Millon Behavioral Health Inventory: Its utility in predicting physical function in patients with low back pain. Arch. Phys. Med. Rehabil. 67:878–882, 1986.
19. Gould, J., and Davies, G. (eds.): Orthopedic and Sports Physical Therapy. St. Louis, C. V. Mosby, 1985.
20. Gracovetsky, S., and Farfan, H.: The optimum spine. Spine 11:543–573, 1986.
21. Hamilton, M.: A rating scale for depression. J. Neurol. Neuropsychiatr. 12:56–62, 1968.
22. Jackson, R., Boston, D., and Edge, A.: Lateral mass fusion: A prospective study of a consecutive series with long-term follow-up. Spine 10:828–833, 1983.
23. Keeley, J., Mayer, T., Cox, R., et al.: Quantification of lumbar function, Part 5: Reliability of range of motion measures in the sagittal plane and an *in vivo* torso rotation measurement technique. Spine 11:31–35, 1986.
24. Kishino, N., Mayer, T., Gatchel, R., et al.: Quantification of lumbar function, Part 4: Isometric and isokinetic lifting simulation in normal subjects and low back dysfunction patients. Spine 10:921–927, 1985.
25. Langrana, N., and Lee, C.: Isokinetic evaluation of trunk muscles. Spine 9:171–175, 1984.
26. Loebl, W.: Measurements of spinal posture and range in spinal movements. Ann. Phys. Med. 9:103, 1967.
27. Loebl, W.: Regional rotation of the spine. Rheumatol. Rehabil. 12:223, 1973.
28. Mayer, T.: Using physical measurements to assess low back pain. J. Musculoskel. Med. 2:44–59, 1985.
29. Mayer, T., Barnes, D., Nichols, G., et al.: Progressive isoinertial lifting evaluation, Part I: A standardized protocol and normative database. Spine 13:993–997, 1988.
30. Mayer, T., Barnes, D., Nichols, G., et al.: Progressive isoinertial lifting evaluation, Part II: A comparison with isokinetic in a disabled chronic low back pain industrial population. Spine 13:993–997, 1988.
31. Mayer, T., and Gatchel, R.: Functional Restoration for Spinal Disorders: The Sports Medicine Approach to Low Back Pain. Philadelphia, Lea & Febiger, 1988.
32. Mayer, T., Gatchel, R., Kishino, N., et al.: A prospective short-term study of chronic low back pain patients utilizing novel objective functional measurement. Pain 25:53–68, 1986.
33. Mayer, T., Gatchel, R., Kishino, N., et al.: Objective assessment of spine function following industrial injury: A prospective study with comparison group and one-year follow-up (Volvo Award in clinical sciences). Spine 10:482–493, 1985.
34. Mayer, T., Gatchel, R., Mayer, H., et al.: A prospective two-year study of functional restoration in industrial low back injury: An objective assessment procedure. J.A.M.A. 258:1763–1767, 1987.
35. Mayer, T., Smith, S., Keeley, J., and Mooney, V.: Quantification of lumbar function, Part 2: Sagittal plane trunk strength in chronic low back pain patients. Spine 10:765–772, 1985.
36. Mayer, T., Smith, S., Kondraske, G., et al.: Quantification of lumbar function, Part 3: Preliminary data on isokinetic torso rotation testing with myoelectric spectral analysis in normal and low back pain subjects. Spine 10:912–920, 1985.
37. Mayer, T., Tencer, A., Kristoferson, S., and Mooney, V.: Use of noninvasive techniques for quantification of spinal range-of-motion in normal subjects and chronic low-back dysfunction patients. Spine 9:588–595, 1984.
38. Million, R., Haavik, N., Jayson, M., and Balser, R.: Evaluation of low back pain and assessment of lumbar corsets with and without back support. Ann. Rheum. Dis. 40:449–545, 1981.
39. Millon, T., Green, C., and Meagher, R.: Millon Behavioral Health Inventory, 3rd Ed. Minneapolis, Interpretive Scoring System, 1982.
40. Moll, J., and Wright, V.: Measurement of spinal movement in the lumbar spine and the back pain. Jayson, M. (ed.): New York, Grune & Stratton, 1976, pp. 93–112.
41. Mooney, V., and Robertson, J.: The facet syndrome. Clin. Orthop. 115:149–156, 1976.
42. Nachemson, A.: Work for all. Clin. Orthop. Rel. Res. 179:77–82, 1983.
43. Pearcy, M., Portek, I., and Sheperd, J.: The effect of low back pain on lumbar spinal movements measured by three-dimensional x-ray analysis. Spine 10:150–153, 1985.
44. Pearcy, M., and Sheperd, J.: Is there instability in spondylolisthesis? Spine 10:175–177, 1985.
45. Pope, M., Frymoyer, J., and Andersson, G.: Occupational Low Back Pain. New York, Praeger Publications, 1984.
46. Schober, P.: Lendenwirbelsaule Und Kreuzschcmerzen. Munch. Med. Woche. 84:336, 1937.
47. Smith, S., Mayer, T., Gatchel, R., and Becker, T.: Quantification of lumbar function, Part 1: Isometric and multi-speed isokinetic trunk strength measures in sagittal and axial planes in normal subject patients. Spine 10:757–764, 1985.
48. Spengler, D., Bigos, S., Martin, N., et al.: Back injuries in industry: A retrospective study, 1. Overview and cost analysis. Spine 11:241–245, 1986.
49. Sternbach, R.: Pain patients: Traits and treatments. New York, Academic Press, 1983.
50. Thompson, N., Gould, J., Davies, G., et al.: Descriptive measures of isokinetic trunk testing. J. Orthop. Sports Phys. Ther. 7:43–49, 1985.
51. Turk, D., Meichenbaum, D., and Genest, M.: Pain and Behavioral Medicine: A Cognitive-Behavior Perspective. New York, Gilford Press, 1983.
52. Ward, N.: Tricyclic antidepressants for chronic low back pain: Mechanisms of action and predictors of response (1986 Volvo Award in clinical sciences). Spine 11:661–665, 1986.

17 □ Low Back Pain in Pregnancy

Gunnar B. J. Andersson

Pregnant women often develop low back pain, and women with previous or ongoing back pain are often afraid of pregnancy, which they believe will increase their pain or cause it to recur. The association of pregnancy and back pain, therefore, is a topic with which all individuals involved in back care and those involved in maternity care need to be familiar. The epidemiology of the problem is discussed here first; a discussion of diagnostic aspects, treatment, and prevention then follows.

EPIDEMIOLOGIC ASPECTS

Back pain is common during pregnancy. Mantle and associates[11] reported that 48% of a consecutive, retrospective sample of 180 pregnant women experienced backache during pregnancy and that the pain was severe in one third of these women. Fast and colleagues,[2] in a similar retrospective study of 200 women, estimated the 9-month prevalence to be 56% and stated that pain usually developed between the 5th and 7th months.

A prospective Swedish study reported a prevalence during the pregnancy period of 49%.[5] Of the women in that study, 9% had back pain of sufficient severity that they were referred for orthopedic evaluation, and 19% were at some time placed on the sick list because of their problem. In another prospective Swedish study, Ostgaard and Andersson[16] found the 9-month prevalence to be 49% with a point prevalence of between 22% and 28% from the 12th week on, until delivery. Previous back problems increased the risk of back pain, as did young age, multiparity, and several physical and psychologic work factors.

Other studies have shown that women with backache often experience the first episode of low back pain during pregnancy. In a study by Svensson and colleagues[21] the reported first-time incidence was 10%, while Biering-Sorensen[1] reported that 20% of women with back pain related its onset to pregnancy and delivery. Because these studies are retrospective, the recall factor can easily explain the difference between them. Svensson and colleagues,[21] Mantle and colleagues,[11] Frymoyer and associates,[3] and Videman and associates[22] all found that a high number of live births increased the risk of back pain.

Disc herniations, although rare, also occur during pregnancy. Both O'Connell[14] and Kelsey and associates[7, 8] found that previous pregnancies increased the risk of disc herniations. Kelsey's study indicates that the risk is even greater among multipari. Heliovaara,[6] on the other hand, did not find any association between the prevalence of disc herniations and the number of births in a large cross-sectional study of Finnish women.

The risk of developing back pain during pregnancy when such pain has been a previous problem was studied prospectively by Ostgaard and Andersson.[17] Women with a history of back pain experienced back pain twice as often during pregnancy as women who never had such a history. Furthermore, the pain experienced by these women was more intense. The risk of "pregnancy back pain" increased with greater numbers of previous episodes and with longer previous episodes of back pain.

CLINICAL PRESENTATION

Low back pain during pregnancy does not differ significantly in its clinical presentation from other types of low back pain. The only major difference is that a larger proportion of the pregnant women have pain over the sacroiliac joints than is usually the case with back pain. Using pain drawings, Ostgaard and associates[16] were able to differentiate three groups of women with different distributions of pain during pregnancy. The first group, and the smallest, included women with pain in the thoracic region only. A second group consisted of women who had pain in the lumbar region with or without radiation into one or both legs. The third group were women with pain primarily over the sacroiliac joint areas, sometimes radiating into the thighs (Fig. 1). Interestingly, the relative proportion of patients with sacroiliac joint area pain increased as pregnancy progressed, whereas in the group with low back pain the proportion of those with back complaints decreased (Fig. 2). Generally, the point prevalence of back pain remained the same at various times during pregnancy, ranging from 22% to 28%.

Most women have troublesome but not severe pain. However, in a Swedish study about 19% of the women had disability sufficient to result in their placement on the sick list for significant periods during their pregnancies.[5] Women with pain localized to the sacroiliac joint areas in that study seemed to present with the more severe complaints. Thus, almost 50% of these women had difficulties walking with a normal stride length compared with only about 20% of women with pain in the lumbar or thoracic region. Furthermore, these women had difficulty walking on stairs and inclines.

For most pregnant women who have them, back problems increase toward the end of the day. Back pain is usually aggravated by physical fatigue, bending, lifting, and twisting. Some women have greater pain during sitting, but most are more troubled during standing and walking. Mantle and colleagues[11] found that sexual intercourse was an aggravating factor for only a few women. Fast and coworkers[2] noted that as many as 36% of women with pain during pregnancy complained of night pain. This proportion is higher than that usually found with "mechanical" back pain, indicating that the underlying mechanisms may be different.

Unfortunately, back pain occurring during pregnancy does not disappear as a result of delivery. On the contrary, some women actually develop greater pain in the early postpartum period. In a Norwegian study,[9] the prevalence of back pain immediately after delivery was about 20%, and at 3 and 12 months post partum it was 26.5% and 20%, respectively. As during pregnancy, the pain was usually troublesome, but not severe.

Melzack and Schaffelberg[13] recorded pain during labor. They concluded that 33% of

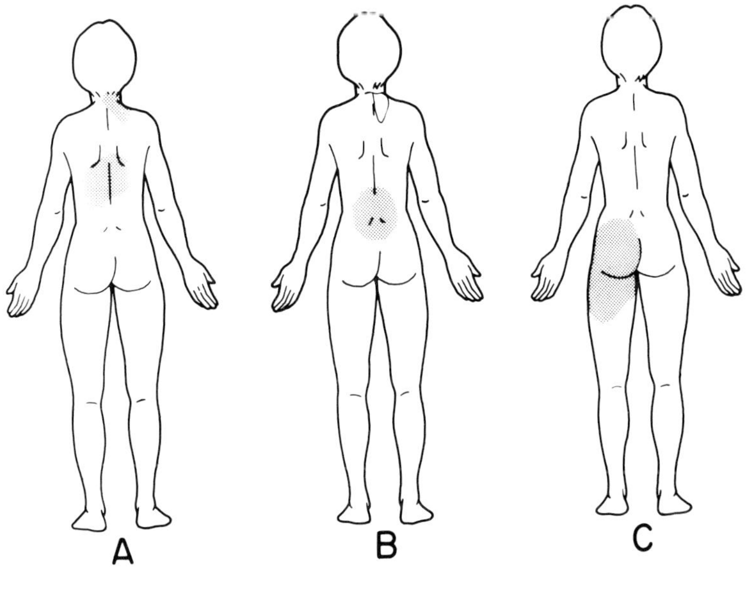

Figure 1 □ Three groups of women with different distribution of pain were identified by Ostgaard and colleagues:[16–18] *A,* women with pain above the lumbar region, *B,* women with pain in the lumbar region (and sometimes down one or both legs), and *C,* women with pain in the sacroiliac joint areas. (Modified from Ostgaard, H.C., Andersson, G.B.J., and Karlsson, K.: Prevalence of back pain in pregnancy [submitted to J. Bone Jt. Surg. (Br.), 1989].)

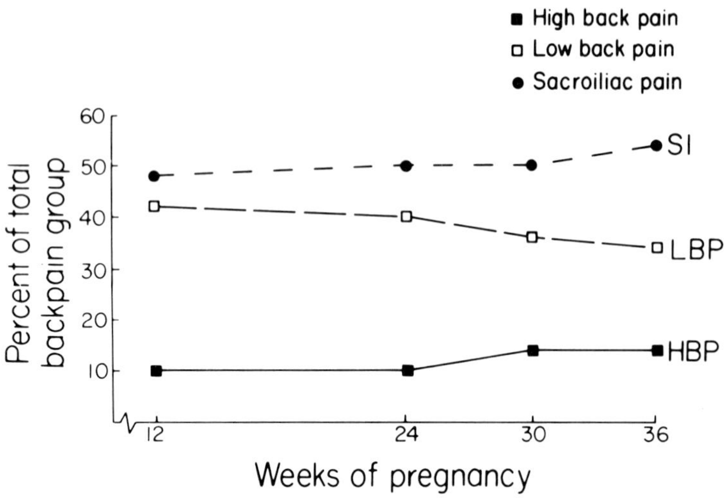

Figure 2 □ The proportion of women with sacroiliac (SI) area pain increased as pregnancy progressed, whereas the proportion of women with lumbar pain (LBP) decreased. The point-prevalence of back pain was similar at each time during the pregnancy. (Modified from Ostgaard, H.C., Andersson, G.B.J., and Karlsson, K.: Prevalence of back pain in pregnancy [submitted to J. Bone Jt. Surg. (Br.), 1989].)

the women had continuous, quite severe low back pain, which was qualitatively different from the pain associated with uterine contractions. It was believed to be attributable to distention and pressure on visceral and neural structures in the peritoneum. No attempt was made to follow the course of pain after labor.

A separate group consists of women with rheumatoid arthritis and associated low back problems. Approximately 75% of women with rheumatoid arthritis have a pregnancy-induced remission. Of those women, however, 75% show improvement during the first trimester, another 20% improve during the second trimester, and about 5% during the third (Fig. 3). About 90% of patients experience a flare-up of their arthritis after delivery, including women who had disease activity that was unchanged during the pregnancy period. Most commonly, this flare-up occurs in the second and third months post partum. It is unrelated to the return of menses and to breast feeding.[15]

PATHOGENESIS

The reason for pregnancy influencing the natural history of back pain is not completely known. However, several hypotheses can be made. Pregnancy causes an increase in the biomechanical load on the spine with an increased forward bending moment that varies somewhat among women and increases as pregnancy progresses. The shape of the spine changes as a consequence of pregnancy. The effects on the anteroposterior curve and on the lumbar tilt are variable.

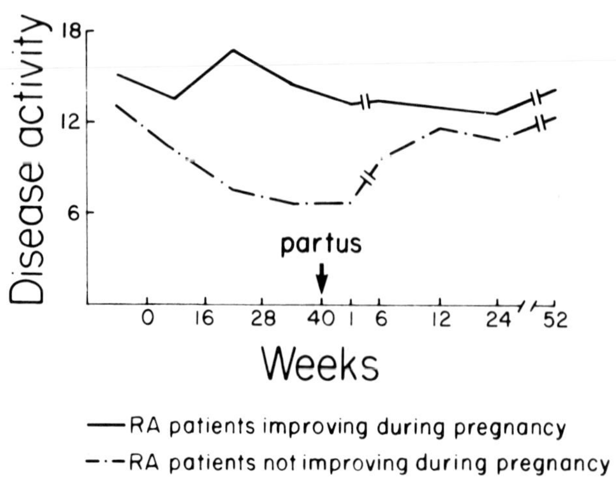

Figure 3 □ Of women with rheumatoid arthritis, 75% have pregnancy-induced remission. After delivery, the disease activity increases to prepregnancy levels. (Modified from Ostenson, M., and Husby, G.: Ensuring a healthy pregnancy for the woman with severe RA. J. Musculoskel. Med. 5(1):13–25, 1988.)

Snijders and colleagues[19] found that the lumbar spine straightened during pregnancy, and they postulated that this was due to equilibrium requirements of moments about the hip joint. This alone does not explain the straightening of the lumbar lordosis, because equilibrium could be accomplished by a backward leaning of the trunk. Mantle and colleagues[11] concluded that weight, obesity, index weight gain, and the baby's weight were not associated with an increased risk of backache during pregnancy. Furthermore, it seems from most of the studies that there is no continuous increase in pain as pregnancy progresses.

An alternative hypothesis is that an increased laxity in collagen tissue occurs during pregnancy; this would make the spine and the pelvic joint less stiff, altering the response to mechanical loading. It is known that the relaxin content in serum increases up to 10-fold during pregnancy.[23] These levels seem to reach a maximum between the 38th and 42nd weeks and decline rapidly after birth. The natural history of back pain during pregnancy does not seem to be directly related to the changes in relaxin levels. The combined effects of increased mechanical load and decreased collagen tissue stiffness can, however, be the cause of back pain in many pregnant women.

In patients with rheumatoid arthritis, changes in steroid hormone levels and pregnancy-associated proteins have been thought to be important. Placenta-eluted γ-globulins have also been suggested as causes of pregnancy-induced remission. Nevertheless, the role of any of these factors remains unclear.

EXAMINATION

In any patient with low back problems, the physical examination is the cornerstone of examinations. Indeed, in the pregnant patient this examination is even more important because the use of structural examinations is limited by the need to avoid irradiation. As mentioned above, a pain drawing is very helpful in outlining the specific distribution of pain, which may provide clues to its origin. The patient history should include questions about previous back problems, the work situation, and any factors associated with relief or aggravation of the pain. In the physical examination, two specific areas need more attention, compared with that given to other low back patients. These are the symphysis and the sacroiliac areas. Symphysiolysis (diastasis of the symphysis pubis) is detected as pain induced by pressure over the symphysis pubis as well as anterior pain induced by compression of the pelvis and by standing on one leg. These women also present with painful restriction of abduction and rotation of both hips. Symphysiolysis generally becomes a problem postpartum.

A multitude of tests are believed to be specific to the sacroiliac region.[4, 10, 20] These include the Patrick test, the knee-shoulder test, the hyperextended hip test, the sacral compression test, the pelvis separation test (ventral gapping), the pelvic compression test (dorsal gapping), the Gaenslen test, and a multitude of other tests. In my opinion, none of these tests is entirely specific. However, increased pain during the performance of any of these tests would seem to be more likely to originate from the sacroiliac joints than from the lumbar spine. Several test results being positive at the same time would strengthen this diagnosis.

Neither radiographs nor a bone scan should be obtained during pregnancy. The effect of magnetic resonance imaging on the fetus is not sufficiently clarified to warrant recommending this method of investigation. Thus, structural examinations are usually out of the question. This is not a great loss because structural examinations usually add little to the treatment decisions. Furthermore, the disease is not so severe as to require these examinations with great urgency.

Laboratory examinations are usually not helpful in evaluating patients with low back pain during pregnancy for subsequent treatment.

TREATMENT

The treatment of back pain in pregnancy is influenced by the fact that pregnancy, in and of itself, precludes the use of some treatment modalities and also the use of some types of medication. Consequently, prevention is the best treatment method.

Information is an indispensable part of treatment. Women should be informed (reassured) that, although the back problem may be annoying, it is not in any way dangerous either to them or to their child and that usually the course is benign. They should also be taught proper body mechanics adapted to pregnancy and appropriate methods of relaxation.

Only patients with significant pain and discomfort should be given medication. They should first be advised about the possible risks, and physicians practicing in the United States should strongly consider having the patients sign a consent form documenting that this information has been transmitted. Drugs with short half-lives are preferred, and of course the smallest possible dosage should be used for the shortest possible period. Simple analgesics such as acetaminophen are not believed to be teratogenic and therefore can be used safely during both pregnancy and lactation. Salicylates have not been shown to have teratogenic effects. However, prolonged gestation and labor as well as maternal and neonatal bleeding and respiratory distress in the neonate have been reported as side effects.[15] For that reason, low doses should be given and treatment should be terminated 6 to 4 weeks before delivery. The same is true for indomethacin, naproxen (Naprosyn), ibuprofen, and diflunisal. These nonsteroidal anti-inflammatory drugs (NSAIDs) should not be given during the third trimester of pregnancy. Further, salicylates and indomethacin should not be given to lactating women because they are excreted in breast milk and have significant side effects on nursing infants.

Corsets may be used during pregnancy, and specific corsets have been designed, called maternity corsets, which allow for the increasing change in abdominal width as pregnancy progresses. These corsets can provide significant support, particularly at the end of the day when fatigue often causes additional pain. Manipulation is not recommended, whereas physical therapy adapted to the maternity situation may prove beneficial. Abdominal muscle and pelvic floor muscle exercises are the ones most commonly employed. Using a small cushion behind the back during sitting and resting in the early afternoon can also be helpful.

Almost all pregnant women with back pain can easily be managed with proper advice, appropriately reduced physical activities, mild analgesics, and perhaps a supporting corset.

Surgery, obviously, should always be avoided in a pregnant woman. Even in patients with muscle weakness due to a disc herniation, the prognosis without surgery is good. Although O'Connell[14] found significant weakness and sometimes paresis in a few patients with disc herniations, the pain was later relieved and strength either recovered or improved without a surgical intervention. The only indication for disc surgery during pregnancy is severe neurologic dysfunction, as in a cauda equina syndrome.

Backache and sciatica during pregnancy are not an indication for abortion.

POSTPARTUM BACK PAIN

Usually, the low back pain that sometimes follows delivery is a continuing pain from the later part of pregnancy. Sometimes, however, back pain occurs during delivery and remains for a period of time. Kogstad,[9] when examining a group of women post partum, found that low back pain in the preceding year, low back pain immediately after delivery, and smoking were negative factors with respect to continuous back pain during the first year after delivery. About one third of the women examined by Kogstad were believed to have a relaxation of the pelvic girdle affecting primarily the sacroiliac joints and the symphysis pubis.

PREVENTION

Prevention of backache in pregnancy can be accomplished by any of three main approaches. The first is to change the lifestyle and work environment to reduce the load on the spine. This is particularly helpful for women who have a history of back pain and who have had many previous pregnancies, some of which have been complicated by back pain. In these women, a modification of heavy physical work can be quite beneficial. The second approach is one of education. This includes prophylactic back education with an emphasis on posture, working positions, lifting technique, and methods of avoiding or alleviating backache. A "pregnancy back school" is preferably combined with some abdominal muscle contraction and pelvic floor contraction exercises to enhance the muscle support. To those can be added instruction both in methods of coping with stress and discomfort and in methods of relaxation. Indeed, the effect of a pregnancy low back school was tested by Mantle and colleagues,[12] and it was found that women who were educated had less troublesome and severe backache than a control group who were not placed in the program.

The third method of prevention is to place pregnant women in a prophylactic corset or brace. Because this has significant negative effects on the trunk muscles and is cumbersome, it cannot be recommended at this time. This is particularly true because there is no study supporting the beneficial effect of such prophylactic efforts.

CONCLUSIONS

Back pain is quite common in pregnancy, and the risk of back pain is greater in people who have had a previous back problem. Usually, however, pain is not severe and unremitting but rather is moderate, although annoying, in nature. A separate group of women tend to have problems that are more localized to the sacroiliac region; for this group the prognosis is not as good as for those with pain in the lower back and upper back. Prophylactic pregnancy back care school programs should, ideally, be provided for all pregnant women. Should back pain occur, information and the judicious use of medication may be necessary. In the more severe cases, it may be necessary to use pregnancy corsets. Unfortunately, the back problem does not seem to immediately disappear after pregnancy, and it may cause a problem for the patient, particularly during the first year post partum. Women need not be fearful of back problems occurring during pregnancy; rather, they need to be informed about the benign nature of these problems and ways of coping with them, should they occur.

References

1. Biering-Sorensen, F.: A prospective study of low back pain in a general population. I. Occurrence, recurrence and aetiology. Scand. J. Rehabil. Med. 15:71–79, 1983.
2. Fast, A., Shapiro, D., Ducommun, E. J., et al.: Low back pain in pregnancy. Spine 12:368–371, 1987.
3. Frymoyer, J. W., Pope, M. H., Costanza, M. C., et al.: Epidemiologic studies of low-back pain. Spine 5:419–423, 1980.
4. Grieve, G. P.: The sacro-iliac joint: Physiotherapy 62:384–400, 1976.
5. Hammar, M., Berg, G., Lillieskold, U., et al.: Low-back pain and pregnancy—incidence, diagnostics and background factors. J. Swedish Med. Assoc. 83:1960–1962, 1983.
6. Heliovaara, M.: Epidemiology of sciatica and herniated lumbar intervertebral disc. Publications of the Social Insurance Institution. Helsinki, Finland, 1988.
7. Kelsey, J. L., White, III, A. A.: Epidemiology and impact of low-back pain. Spine 2:133–142, 1980.
8. Kelsey, J. L., Greenberg, R. A., Hardy, R. J., and Johnson, M. F.: Pregnancy and the syndrome of herniated lumbar intervertebral disc; an epidemiological study. Yale J. Biol. Med. 48:361–368, 1975.
9. Kogstad, O.: Low back pain. Post partum (submitted to Spine, 1988).
10. Lewit, K.: Manuelle Medizin in Rahmen des medizinischen rehabiliteirung. Leipzig, Johan Ambrousius Barth, 1977.
11. Mantle, M. J., Greenwood, R. M., and Currey, H. L. F.: Backache in pregnancy. Rheumatol. Rehabil. 16:95–101, 1977.
12. Mantle, M. J., Holmers, J., and Currey, H. L. F.: Backache in pregnancy. II. Prophylactic influence of back care classes. Rheumatol. Rehabil. 20:227–232, 1981.
13. Melzack, R., and Schaeffelberg, D.: Low back pain during labor. Am. J. Obstet. Gynecol. 156:901–905, 1987.
14. O'Connell, J. E. A.: Lumbar disc protrusion in pregnancy. J. Neurol. Neurosurg. Psychiatry 23:138–141, 1960.
15. Ostenson, M., and Husby, G.: Ensuring a healthy pregnancy for the woman with severe RA. J. Musculoskel. Med. pp. 13–25, 1988.
16. Ostgaard, H. C., and Andersson, G. B. J.: Low back pain in pregnancy. *In* The Abstract Book, The International Society for the Study of the Lumbar Spine, Rome, 1987.
17. Ostgaard, H. C., and Andersson, G. B. J.: Previous back pain and risk of back pain during pregnancy. *In* The Abstract Book, The International Society for the Study of the Lumbar Spine, Miami, 1988 (abstr 42).
18. Ostgaard, H. C., Andersson, G. B. J., and Karlsson, K.: Prevalence of back pain in pregnancy (submitted to J. Bone Jt. Surg. [Br], 1989).
19. Snijders, C. J., Scroo, J. M., Snijder, J. G., and Hoedt, H. T.: Change in form of the spine as a consequence of pregnancy. *In* Digest of the 11th International Conference on Medical and Biological Engineering, Abstract No. 49.4, Ottawa, 1976.
20. Stoddard, A.: Manual of osteopathic technique. London, Hutchinson Medical Publications, 1964.
21. Svensson, H.-O., Andersson, G. B. J., Johansson, S., and Wilhelmsson, V. A.: A retrospective study of low-back pain in 38–64 year old women. Spine 13:548–552, 1988.
22. Videman, T., Nurminen, T., Tola, S., et al.: Low-back pain in nurses and some loading factors of work. Spine 9:400–404, 1984.
23. Zarrow, M., Holmstrom, E. G., and Salhanich, H. A.: The concentration of relaxin in the blood serum and other tissues of women during pregnancy. J. Clin. Endocrinol. 15:22–27, 1955.

18 □ Industrial Low Back Pain

Stanley J. Bigos
Michele Crites Battié
Margareta Nordin
Dan M. Spengler
David P. Guy

RISK FACTORS

Stanley J. Bigos
Michele Crites Battié

Risk factors related to back problems have been a topic of interest in the literature since the 1920s. Congenital abnormalities demonstrated on plain lumbar radiographs were among the first factors recommended for use in identifying individuals at risk for back problems. Although early evidence cast doubt on the effectiveness of this approach, it did not seem to daunt the advocation and adoption of x-ray screening within many industries.

In 1929, Bohart observed no difference in the incidences of low back pain syndrome, comparing patients with and without congenital abnormalities,[18] whereas Cushway and Mailer reported that more than 44 % of 931 asymptomatic individuals evaluated had congenital or developmental abnormalities.[29] In both studies the authors recognized that the abnormalities were not necessarily the cause of back problems, yet they recommended the use of lumbosacral spine radiographs for screening employees who were to work in jobs in which injury to the back was a concern. To date, more than 25,000 sets of radiographs have been evaluated in a controlled fashion, and the findings do not justify the use of pre-employment screening.[32, 39, 46, 60, 75, 87, 88, 103, 106, 110, 118] Pre-employment x-ray screening as well as other types of interventions used in an attempt to reduce the back problem have met with little success.

Back problems remain the most expensive musuloskeletal malady in the industrialized nations of the world, with estimated costs being as high as $30 billion per year in the United States alone.[90] Most of this cost reflects a loss in worker productivity resulting from short-term or long-term disability.

Reportedly, back problems are the most common cause of disability in persons under 45 years of age and thus are an extremely expensive health care problem in the working age group.[49, 66, 69, 114] The costs are assessed not only in dollars but also in the suffering and diminished quality of life for affected individuals and their families. Moreover, back problems exert an impact far beyond the affected individual by increasing costs to society for the production of goods and services or by adding a tax burden for care of the disabled and their families.[112, 114]

Until the 1979 report of Cady and colleagues on firefighters, our knowledge about risk factors related to back pain was limited predominantly to retrospective data and reports.[22] Previously, screening practices had concentrated on congenital abnormalities, medical histories, and physical examinations. However, as Snook pointed out in 1978, in industries employing such practices, their value in reducing incidents of back pain or the associated costs is questionable at best.[111]

Other physical findings, such as strength and flexibility, have been strongly recommended as screening tools but in the absence of adequate scientific testing of their impact on the problem. Physical aspects of the work place and the work task have also been accused of increasing the risk of back problems; these have led to recommendations for ergonomic interventions and training. Yet, it remains unclear whether such factors cause back pain or simply tend to aggravate symptoms once the problem exists. The fact that the industrial back pain problem continues to grow at the expense of society, industry, and individual suffering indicates that other important factors have been overlooked in examining this complex medical puzzle.

BACK PROBLEMS VERSUS BACK INJURY CLAIMS

For insurance purposes, industry has attempted to categorize back problems according to an injury model similar to that used for other more obvious musculoskeletal problems. However, the use of the injury model is complicated by the confusion surrounding the etiology and inciting causes of back symptoms and the effect that environmental and personal factors have on the back injury claims process. Filing of back injury claims seems to involve more than just the presence of back pain, backache, sciatica, sprain, or strain. Current knowledge about the prevalence, incidence, and onset of back symptoms does not easily support the injury model of disease.[47]

ETIOLOGY AND INCITING CAUSES

Epidemiologists tell us that as many as 85% of adults, irrespective of occupation, eventually experience back problems that interfere with work or recreational activity,[55, 59, 60, 93] and up to 25% between the ages of 30 and 50 years report the presence of back symptoms at the time surveyed.[1, 3, 52, 120, 131] The common and usually transitory nature of back pain has led some observers to question whether it can be called a disease, let alone fit into an injury model.[107]

Additional questions about the injury model arise during the study of the onset of back problems. Onset is commonly gradual and not related to an accidental cause.[47, 55, 105, 106, 133] In a recent study of patients with acute, subacute, and chronic back pain at our institution, we found that 77% of a patient population could not relate the onset of symptoms to a time within 24 hours of an accident or unusual activity.[47]

The failure of the injury model to explain industrial back problems has led to the cumulative trauma model, which is now proposed to explain musculoskeletal problems of gradual onset among workers. Unfortunately, the difficulties in monitoring off-work activities make it virtually impossible to control all the factors needed to verify scientifically the cumulative model as an explanation of industrial back problems.

Medical technology allows us to determine a pathoanatomic diagnosis in only 12% to 15% of individuals.[10, 31] Thus, there need be no objective diagnosable condition to explain back symptoms or to file a back injury claim. Commonly used diagnostic terms such as back sprain or strain, myofascitis, disc syndrome, facet syndrome, and subluxations are not verified objectively and for scientific purposes must be considered synonyms for idiopathic back pain. Thus, the basis for studying back problems is less objective than for studying more easily diagnosable problems such as fractures or lacerations.

In summary, both the injury model and the cumulative trauma model are clouded by a number of problems. The documentation of either is difficult, and medical science is unable to provide a specific diagnosis in the majority of cases. More important, both models may distort the perceptions of those attempting to find solutions to industrial back problems as well as the perceptions of those afflicted.

PERCEPTIONS AFFECTING THE CLAIM-FILING PROCESS

Because medical technology usually cannot provide a verifiable diagnosis of back injury,[10, 31] often none is needed for a back injury claim to be filed or accepted. Therefore, the claim-filing process is somewhat subjective, and the perceptions of the employee seem especially significant. Although back symptoms may be the basis of a claim, the employee's perceptions about the *safety* of continuing to work and about the *impact* of a back injury claim on his or her personal situation may determine whether or not a claim is filed. Programs involving the interpretation and presentation of information about symptoms, safety, and personal environment have been proved to affect an individual's perceptions and the back injury claim process, for better or for worse.[40, 41, 104, 140]

Severity of Symptoms

Back problems are so common that there is little reason to question whether an individual has symptoms when a back injury claim is made.[1, 3, 31, 52, 55, 59, 60, 107, 120, 131] The presence of symptoms alone may lead to a back injury claim, especially if they are severe or if the individual believes the problem is unusual, caused by an accident, or is the fault of another person. However, comparing the high incidence (85% of adults) and point prevalence (as high as 30% in the 30- to 50-year age group) of back problems to the actual number of expected injury claims (2% to 5% of workers in the United States per year)[19, 78, 95, 130] indicates that all workers with symptoms do not file a claim.[112] In addition, 10% of individuals who file do not miss work because of their problem.[117]

Perceptions of Safety

Many workers with back symptoms are apparently confident that they can safely perform tasks without jeopardizing their future health. Seemingly, if symptoms are minor, they continue working despite some back discomfort.

The physical requirements of a job can have a major impact on the decision to file a back injury claim.[112] Back symptoms that would lay up a furniture mover or heavy laborer may not interfere with the work of an administrator, foreman, or clerk. If a worker perceives that performing certain tasks will actually cause physical harm, it is unlikely that the person will continue to work, if the industrial environment is insured. Changing only the perceptions about a job can also affect the claim-filing process. Ironically, there is evidence that increasing the employee's awareness of back-related work hazards, in an attempt to improve job safety, increases both the number and cost of back injuries.[104]

Perceptions of Impact

For some individuals with back symptoms, the desire to continue working overcomes difficulties with tasks or the fear of further injury. Common examples are the farmer wearing a footdrop brace in order to harvest crops before taking time for a surgical evaluation; the independent house framer continuing to work in order to avoid leaving the crew unsupervised during the busy season; or the mother with small children and inadequate social support continuing to carry out activities for her family. They illustrate that, in certain situations, concerns about back problems may be overcome by the need to continue activities that are essential to or that positively affect an individual's personal situation.

Indirect evidence also suggests that similar scenarios occur in the industrial setting. Some jobs are stressful to the back but rarely generate back injury claims. In some instances, camaraderie and financial or personal status make the positions very desirable. Surely some of these workers have back discomfort, but perhaps not sufficient to warrant filing a back injury claim and risking transfer to a less desirable position.

Conversely, suppose that the task at hand is not so coveted or is even dreaded. A back injury claim may lead to an escape or time out from the pressures of daily living or an unsatisfactory job or task. A back injury claim may also provide an opportunity to prove a point about a certain task that is perceived as dangerous. Filing a back injury claim could even become a more socially acceptable alternative to quitting a job.[13]

Perceptions about the potential personal impact of a back injury claim commonly raise questions about malingering. However, most employees filing injury claims under the above conditions seem to be reacting to misconceptions about back pain, back injury claims, or safety, which can be fueled by personal problems in the work or off-hours environment. The process rarely seems conscious or deliberate,[58, 113] and we caution against the use of the term *malingering* in regard to these situations. Furthermore, malingering is virtually impossible to document, and such accusations can jeopardize a successful resolution of the individual's medical, insurance, and livelihood problems.

CONTROVERSIES SURROUNDING RETROSPECTIVE DATA

Unfortunately, the interpretation of retrospective data, predominantly from insurance records, has generated controversy and has led, overall, to little progress in curbing the industrial back problem.[1, 112] Reasons for the varied interpretations seem to be related to the data.

As is shown in Table 1, numerous publications have reported on multiple factors in relationship to industrial back problems. Yet much information about these various factors is conflicting. The inconsistencies have several possible explanations. First, Andersson found the data concerning many factors to be misleading; this was because the data

Table 1 □ Summary of Retrospective Study Findings of Risk Factors Related to Industrial Back Pain

	BACK PAIN		HERNIATED DISC	
	Risk	**No Risk**	**Risk**	**No Risk**
INDIVIDUAL FACTORS				
Age	3, 9, 15, 17, 23, 35, 30, 55, 59, 60, 106, 108, 109, 121, 137, 146, 147	—	21, 50, 57, 66, 68, 116, 132	—
Sex	15	—	20, 116	
Height	57, 64, 65, 76	15, 36, 52, 54, 59, 60, 109, 124, 135, 136	—	—
Weight	20, 62	15	—	—
Posture	11	9, 10, 54, 55, 59, 60, 85, 94, 102, 106, 115	—	—
Strength	—	10, 94, 102	—	—
Scoliosis <80	—	28, 73, 91, 97	—	—
Fitness level	—	—	64, 65	—
Spinal mobility	56	123	—	—
Smoking	44, 45, 122			
RADIOGRAPHIC FINDINGS				
Severe multiple disc degeneration	3, 17, 24, 59, 60, 76, 77, 86, 108, 109, 126, 141		—	—
Moderate degeneration	—	2, 52, 55, 59, 60, 61, 86, 118	—	—
Congenital anomalies	55, 60, 75, 79, 99, 118, 125, 142	53, 54, 55, 59, 60, 75, 103, 108, 116	—	—
Spondylolisthesis	39, 55, 60, 143	54, 75, 107, 108, 118	—	—
WORK PLACE FACTORS				
Heavy physical work	4, 9, 25, 26, 30, 51, 59, 60, 62, 72, 76, 80, 81, 96, 100, 106, 121, 137, 138	64, 65, 101	—	—
Sedentary work	34, 64, 65, 74, 82, 100, 135	—	69	—
Frequent bending and twisting	25, 83, 84	—	—	—
Lifting (moderate)	—	25, 60, 62, 64, 65, 69, 82	—	—
Frequent heavy lifting	26, 36, 37, 38, 59, 60, 62, 76, 43, 63	—	—	—
Vibration	43, 63	—	—	—
Driving vehicles	48, 57, 67, 127	—	—	—
PSYCHOLOGIC FACTORS				
Psychologic test results	8, 10, 140, 145	9, 139	—	—
Drug and alcohol abuse	51, 79, 83, 84, 96, 137	—	—	—

The numbers in this table are reference numbers.

had been derived from insurance company reports and absenteeism reports, which were incomplete and categorized for purposes other than back research.[1] Another explanation is inadequate study design. Stover Snook at the 1980 National Institute of Arthritis, Diabetes, and Digestive and Kidney (NIADDK) Diseases Conference in Florida pointed out that "Most studies of low back pain are of small-sample, short-term, and retrospective studies done without control groups."[112] Thus, the retrospective nature, expectant bias, and controversial data available from most studies help explain why solutions to the industrial back problem have been so slow in coming.

PROSPECTIVE STUDIES

At the NIADDK Diseases Conference Snook emphasized,

> The greatest need . . . is for a long-term, controlled longitudinal study that . . . controls the many variables involved in low back pain. . . . Nevertheless we can approach the ideal experiment with a large sample, control groups, good experimental design, adequate statistical treatment, and sufficient funds and time to complete the study.[112]

Owing to the cost and effort required to meet these ideals, only a few prospective studies have been conducted to date.

In 1979, Cady and colleagues reported their study,[22] which examined the back injury experience of 1,654 firefighters over a 3-year period. They analyzed anthropometry, posture, physical fitness, cardiovascular risk information, and several medical tests related to cardiovascular health (Table 2). They found that a high level of fitness emphasizing endurance (according to cardiovascular fitness parameters) but including strength and flexibility provided protection from back problems.[22]

A broader study performed by Biering-Sorensen was reported in 1985.[11] A group of 929 individuals were interviewed and examined, and a history and physical examination were repeated after 1 year (Table 2). Biering-Sorensen's findings indicate that the chance of having back discomfort is increased if (1) the back problems begin early in life, (2) sciatica is present, or (3) there is a history of previous use of medical services for back problems. Those who previously suffered from continuous back problems or recurrent episodes prior to the initial evaluation were found to have weak trunk muscles and reduced flexibility of the back and hamstring muscles.[11,12]

The predictors of the first episode of back trouble following the initial examination were (1) being a man with a lack of back muscle endurance, and (2) being a man with a high degree of back flexibility. Those who had stiffer backs were at less risk for their first episode of back discomfort than were those who were more flexible.[12]

It is important to note that the studies by Cady and Biering-Sorensen differed in population and outcome parameters. The Cady study involved back injury claims of those involved in the very stressful work of firefighting, whereas the Biering-Sorensen study evaluated back troubles, not back injury claims, in a general population.

McDonald and colleagues[89] performed a more limited study, which involved ultrasound measurement of the lumbar canal to compare relative canal size with back problems in mine workers. The population included 204 of 373 miners solicited. Their previous medical and work attendance records were reviewed, and the individuals were followed for 3 years to observe absence from work and change of employment. Those who remained on the job had spinal canal measurements significantly larger than those who retired. However, the evaluation was complicated because of the high retirement rate due to the reduction in the size of the work force for economic reasons; thus, some of the information that led to the final conclusions had to be dealt with retrospectively.[89]

In 1980, Keyserling and Chaffin and coworkers[70, 71] reported two studies examining the correlation between lifting strength, with respect to job requirements, and musculoskeletal injuries. The first study compared medical reports among two groups of employees of a tire and rubber plant. One group was selected for job positions based upon screening tests demonstrating strength to match job task requirements. A second group did not undergo strength testing prior to employment. The authors found a greater tendency toward medical complaints over the following year among employees who were not matched to the job on the basis of meeting strength requirements ($p = .10$).

Table 2 □ Summary of Prospective Studies of Causes of Back Pain

STUDY POPULATION/ SOLICITED FOLLOW-UP DURATION	BIERING-SORENSEN[11, 12] 929 of 1,141 12 months	CADY ET AL[22] 1652 of 1,900 36 months	CHAFFIN & PARK 411 of ? 36 months	TROUP ET AL[128] 2,890 of ? 12 months	BOEING STUDY[5–7] 3,020 of 4,027 48 months
Premorbid data					
Physical					
Antropometry	x	x	x	x	x
Posture	x	x			x
Spinal canal diameter					x
Back examination	x	EX			x
Capacity					
Flexibility	x	x		x	x
Strength	x	x	x	x	x
Endurance	x	x			x
Health					
Past medical history					
Previous back problems	x	EX	x	x	x
Habits (smoking)	x	x		x	x
Physical activity		x			x
Demographics					
Employment history	x				x
Marital status	x				x
Education level	x				x
Social					
Work APGAR					N
Family APGAR					N
Psychologic					
Health locus of control					N
MMPI					N
Job tasks					
Motor vehicle exposure					N
Perception—heavy	x			x	x
Perception—tiring					N
Estimated back load					x
Job demands vs strength			x		
Employment status					
Performance appraisal					N
Job level					N
Prior attendance record					N
Postmorbid Data					
Injury data					
Description	x	x			x
Physical examination	x				x
Work-up		x			x
Treatment					x
Diagnosis if possible	x	x			x
Attendance—postinjury		x			x

x = tested.
EX = exclusion criteria for participation in study.
N = factors not previously studied prospectively.
APGAR = *A*daptability, *P*artnership, *G*rowth, *A*ffection, *R*esolve.
MMPI = Minnesota Multiphasic Personality Inventory.

There were too few musculoskeletal or low back injury reports in the study group to allow for analysis of these subsets of medical complaints.[70]

The second report involved aluminum reduction workers. In this study, the investigators found that workers who were required to lift more than 75% of their maximum capacity, as determined by maximum isometric strength testing, were at an increased risk of medical complaints and musculoskeletal injury reports. This study did not indicate, however, that strength exceeding the job requirements provided any extra protection from back problems. In addition, the relationship between strength inadequate to meet job demands and increased injury reports did not hold true for all strength-testing positions. Employees with strength that matched job requirements in the arm lift position actually had the highest incidence of injury reports. This finding led the investigators to conclude that before using isometric testing as a screening tool "a pilot study should always be performed using incumbent employees."[71] Neither study differentiated between back problems and other musculoskeletal problems. The two previous studies expanded on the work reported by Chaffin and Park indicating a possible association between inadequate strength to meet job demands and a higher incidence of back injury reports.[26]

Troup and coworkers evaluated 2,891 British workers and questioned them 1 year later about back symptoms since their evaluation.[128] They found that perceived physical capacities were actually more important than directly measured capacities, such as isometric lifting strength, for the prediction of back problems, although both were poor predictors. A history of previous back problems was the strongest risk factor of the variables studied, and it enhanced the predictive ability of other variables.

In 1985, Cady and associates reported the results of their cardiovascular fitness intervention program.[23] They found cardiovascular fitness, termed physical work capacity training, improved not only stamina and endurance but also the test results for strength and flexibility. More importantly, workers' compensation costs were reduced by 25% among firefighters. This reduction was associated with a significant improvement in cardiovascular fitness (measured as physical work capacity), without a significant increase in strength or flexibility.

Data have recently been reported from a prospective, multifactorial study concerning risks related to the report of acute industrial back problems. The final goal of this study is to gain a better understanding of risk factors for both acute back problems and the development of chronic back pain disability. Over 3,000 employees from a Boeing aircraft manufacturing plant in the state of Washington volunteered to take part in the study. Premorbid data were collected between July 1982 and September 1983, which included individual physical characteristics and demographic, psychosocial, and work-place factors. Subsequently, back injury reports have been tracked for over 3 years, recorded, and analyzed to identify risk factors related to the incidence of industrial back pain reports.

Among the physical characteristics studied were isometric lifting strength, flexibility, and cardiovascular fitness. Isometric lifting strength testing was limited to 2,178 individuals, owing to the presence of symptoms or other health risks. Standardized arm, leg, and back lift test positions were utilized. The wide variety of activities performed by the workers made specific lifting simulations impractical. No significant difference was found in comparing the strength of injured versus non-injured individuals of similiar age and sex, performing similar tasks. Surprisingly, those with more strength tended to file more back injury claims than did weaker workers.[6]

Flexibility was evaluated in 3,020 subjects, using common clinical measures (modified Schober, sit-and-reach, side bending). No significant difference between premorbid spinal flexibility in flexion or side bending was found between individuals reporting subsequent back problems and those who did not. The Boeing study results demonstrate no clear connection between clinically tested spinal flexibility and the risk of acute industrial back injury. In addition, considering the specturm of "normal" flexibility values found in active working adults, it may be time to reconsider the role that spinal flexibility measures have played in making important decisions based on pre-employment screening or rating impairment and disability.[5]

Cardiovascular fitness was measured by

submaximal treadmill testing. The results did not reveal a correlation between cardiovascular fitness, as measured through predicted VO_{2max}, and subsequent industrial back pain reports. This finding suggests that, for the Boeing study group, higher cardiovascular fitness alone did not provide protection from acute back problems.[7]

Smoking was positively correlated with the subsequent report of acute back pain.[7] This finding is in agreement with several recently published retrospective studies.[44, 45, 122]

A previous history of back problems was a significant risk factor for reporting acute industrial back problems. Although often labeled *re-injuries*, recurrences are expected following an episode of back symptoms, as has been described by many others.[9, 115, 129, 130]

Because the goal of our investigation with aircraft manufacturing employees is to study risk factors not only for the report of back problems but also for disability lasting longer than 3 months, our study is comprehensive, examining both physical and nonphysical factors. This comprehensive approach offers the unique opportunity to study prospectively many psychosocial factors. Although we originally intended to study their potential as risk factors for chronic disability, we also examined psychosocial factors as predictors of acute back injury claims. Of the nearly 150 variables studied, half were physical and half were nonphysical.[16] Evaluation of the p-values from a wide range of significance levels (p = .05 to .0001) revealed that more than 60% of the variable demonstrating a significant relationship with risk of reporting an acute back problem were in the nonphysical category. The two strongest variables for predicting acute industrial back problems came from the Minnesota Multiphasic Personality Inventory (MMPI) and the modified Work APGAR. A previous history of back problems coupled with an expression of distress on the MMPI and low job task enjoyment (Work APGAR) appear to place individuals at greatest risk of reporting acute back problems. This finding indicates that medical and engineering principles alone do

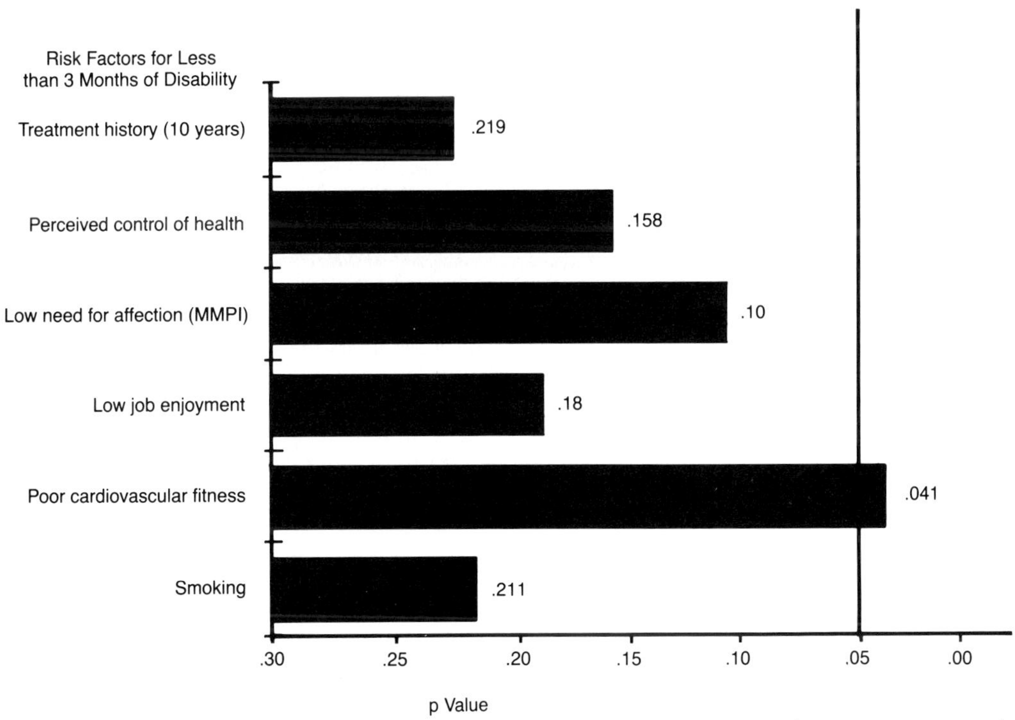

Figure 1 □ This graph displays the trends detected in the first 26 subjects in the Boeing study, experiencing more than 3 months of disability because of back problems, as compared with age- and sex-matched controls. It must be noted that these findings are *preliminary*, owing to the small number of subjects, which have yet to be compared with the general population.

not seem to be the key to solving the back problem in industry.

To our knowledge, this study on hourly aircraft employees is the first longitudinal prospective risk factor study examining industrial back pain disability lasting 3 months or more. These employees with long-term disability account for 10% of employees with industrial back problems, but 80% of the costs.[117] Some interesting trends are emerging from the preliminary data available on these employees (Fig. 1). As in two previous studies of back pain risk factors, low endurance, smoking, and a previous history of back problems appear to be important from preliminary analyses.[11, 22] Only when greater numbers of employees with 3 months or more of disability are available in this longitudinal study will it be possible to develop a clearer perspective of the importance of previously found physical factors, psychosocial factors, and work perceptions.

DISABILITY RELATED TO CHRONIC BACK PAIN

The reduction of disability costs, as accomplished by Cady and colleagues, tends to reflect a reduction in the amount of time off work.[23] The prevention of chronic back pain disability could dramatically reduce costs and the amount of suffering and loss of livelihood experienced by individuals and their families.

Of those who file claims, 90% experience very little individual suffering or loss of livelihood.[29, 78] These individuals return to work rapidly and account for only about 20% of back pain injury claim costs.[78, 117] Epidemiologic studies indicate that recovery from back pain is usually rapid. Fifty percent to 60% of patients with back pain recover from their symptoms within 1 week, and 50% of those with sciatica recover within 1 month.[92, 93, 134, 135]

However, among patients with back pain and those with sciatica, about 10% continue to have problems for 3 months or longer.[92] Because 80% of the disability costs are accounted for by 10% of the back injury claims, one can see that chronic disability because of back pain is the most expensive and devastating component of the industrial back problem.[78, 112, 117]

Our retrospective evaluation of industrial back problems revealed these skewed cost tendencies.[117] The first thought was that the high-cost claims included the most serious injuries. However, only 2 of the 900 back injury claims involved vertebral compression fractures, and neither was associated with long-term disability or became an expensive back injury claim.[14] On the other hand, our data indicated that back injury claims and chronic injury problems were associated with a poor employee appraisal rating. Employee appraisal data were based on evaluation by an immediate supervisor within the 6-month period prior to the back injury claim.[15] This finding raises the concern that the outcome of industrial injury claims can be influenced by nonphysical factors.

Psychosocial and environmental difficulties have been associated with a longer period of disability.[1, 8, 33, 42] Once an individual is off work, perceptions about *symptoms*, about the *safety* of returning to work, and about the *impact* of returning to work on one's personal life can affect recovery even in the most well-meaning worker. Furthermore, a relief from work and personal pressures may become apparent only after a back problem affords a time-out from life stresses.

Return to work may be further complicated by the individual's need to process emotionally the perceived loss of a youthful back. This process can resemble a grief reaction. The claim also may become a solution to other problems, such as the pressures of poor work conditions or the threat of being laid off or fired. Wanted nurturing and support from family and friends, personal support from employers, insurance companies, attorneys, and medical systems may come only when an individual is incapacitated by back pain.

A study by Weber nicely elucidated the relative influence of psychosocial and physical factors upon disability.[133] His 10-year follow-up on patients with disc hernias causing nerve root irritation treated either surgically or nonsurgically found that a small number in both groups were still receiving total disability supplements. However, after 10 years of continued disability these individuals were engaging in strenuous daily physical activities. Factors other than physical impairment seemed to influence their disability. Overall, the same perceptions that may lead to the report of a back injury claim also can affect the period of time for which an individual is disabled.

CONCLUSION

Presently, we unsuccessfully attempt, as we have done in the past, to limit the effects of back problems by the use of back injury, re-injury, and cumulative trauma models. Until our level of knowledge and sophistication about back pain and the complexities of managing the back injury claim system is vastly improved, it seems most prudent to concentrate our efforts on the risk factors related to back pain disability. This approach is especially valid in light of a recent study in Gothenburg, Sweden, conducted by Choler and colleagues, demonstrating that chronic back pain disability can be prevented by emphasizing proven effective treatment methods.[27] This study provides a foundation for us to advance the prevention of back pain disability by realistically using the available risk factor data in conjunction with realistic programs that address industrial back problems for the uninjured work force. Defining a problem through risk factor studies is of little use unless those data can be used to reduce or control the effects of the problem itself. Because only successful intervention can confirm the usefulness of present knowledge about risk factors, we submit the following recommendations:

1. Use the best treatment information available to warn workers about the potential debilitation of excessive bed rest, the dangers of overmedication, and the inadvisability of surgery without strong preoperative indications. At the same time, promote back health and long-term disability prevention by using treatment methods with proven effectiveness, and provide realistic expectations.
2. Utilize the scientific information available to curb the unfounded tendency to label normally occuring back symptoms as industrial injuries. Recurrent symptoms, in particular, are to be expected after a significant back problem and should not be classified as re-injury.
3. Define the psychosocial problems in the work site, in the home, or from previous experiences that may affect perceptions influencing the recovery from symptoms and the return to work.
4. Evaluate means of bolstering the individual's resources, to discourage maladaptive ways of handling life stresses.
5. Use a knowledge of ergonomics to minimize the level of stress on the spine so that a job can be performed safely without exacerbating back symptoms. This would promote continued work or a rapid return to work for those having back discomfort.
6. Continue to use better scientific means for evaluating the industrial back problem, including nonphysical factors, so that the problem can be more clearly defined, and prevention and management strategies can be improved.
7. If data from further studies support our findings to date, we may prepare to help management and labor develop a more meaningful concept of work. The impact of work perceptions and psychosocial factors on the report of acute industrial back problems may encourage industry to explore new ways to enhance worker satisfaction. Alf Nachemson has stated, "A man needs to work like a bird needs to fly." Yet most of us dream of the achievements of flying more than of work. Some studies indicate that the manager who fosters a feeling of worth and achievement among hourly employees would do more to raise productivity and combat disability than would wage increases and standard benefits alone.[27, 40, 41, 148]

References

1. Andersson, B. J.: Epidemiological aspects of low back pain in industry. Spine 6:53–60, 1981.
2. Andersson, G., and Irstam, L.: Radiographic studies in low back pain patients. S.P.R.I. Rapport 22:42–49, 1979.
3. Andersson, G., and Svensson, H. O.: Prevalence of low back pain. S.P.R.I. Rapport 22:11–23, 1979.
4. Anderson, J. A. D., and Duthie, J. J. R.: Rheumatic complaints in dockyard workers. Ann Rheum. Dis. 22:401–409, 1963.
5. Battié, M. C., Bigos, S. J., and Sheehy, A.: The role of clinical measurement of spinal range of motion in back pain assesment. Presented at A.A.O.S. 54th Annual Meeting, San Francisco, Jan., 1987.
6. Battié, M. C., Bigos, S. J., Fisher, L. D., et al. Isometric lifting strength as a predictor of industrial low back pain. Spine, in press.
7. Battié, M. C., Bigos, S. J., Fisher, L. D., et al.: A prospective study of the role of cardiovascular risk factors and fitness in industrial back pain complaints. Spine 14:141–147, 1989).
8. Beals, R. K., and Hickman, N. W.: Industrial injuries of the back and extremities. J. Bone Joint Surg. 54A:1539–1611, 1972.
9. Bergquist-Ullman, M., and Larsson, U.: Acute low back pain in industry. Acta Orthop. Scand. 170(Suppl.):1–117, 1977.
10. Berkson, M. H., Nachemson, A., and Schultz, A. B.: Mechanical properties of human lumbar spine motion segments. Part II. Responses in compres-

sion and shear; influence of gross morphology. J Biomech. Eng. 101:53–57, 1979.
11. Biering-Sorensen, F.: A one-year prospective study of low back trouble in a general population. Laegeforenengens Forlag, 1984. (Accepted for publication in the Danish Medical Bulletin).
12. Biering-Sorensen, F.: Physical measurements as indicators for low-back trouble over a one-year period. Spine 9:106–119, 1984.
13. Bigos, S. J.: Low back pain—potential solution. *In* Fitzgerald, R. H. (ed.): Orthopaedic Knowledge Update II—Home Study Syllabus Video. Chicago, American Academy of Orthopaedic Surgeons, 1987.
14. Bigos, S. J., Spengler, D. M., Martin, N. A., et al.: Back injuries in industry: A retrospective study. II. Injury factors. Spine 11:246–251, 1986.
15. Bigos, S. J., Spengler, D. M., Martin, N. A., et al: Back injuries in industry: A retrospective study. III. Employee-related factors. Spine 11:252–256, 1986.
16. Bigos, S. J., Battié, M. C., Fisher, L. D., et al.: Predictive factors for the report of back problems in industry. The Boeing Study. Paper presented at I.S.S.L.S. Annual Meeting, Miami, 1988.
17. Bistrom, O.: Congenital anomalies of the lumbar spine of persons with painless backs. Ann. Chir. Gynaecol. Fenn. 43:102–115, 1954.
18. Bohart W. H.: Anatomic variations and anomalies of the spine relation to prognosis and length of disability. J.A.M.A. 92:698–701, 1929.
19. Bond, M. B.: Low back injuries in industry. Industr. Med. Surg. 39:28–32, 1970.
20. Brown, J. R.: Manual lifting and handling: An annotated bibliography. Labour Safety Council of Ontario, Ontario Ministry of Labour, 1972.
21. Brown, J. R.: Lifting as an industrial hazard. Am. Ind. Hyg. Assoc. J. 34:292–297, 1973.
22. Cady, L. D., Bischoff, D. P., O'Connell, E. R., et al.: Strength and fitness and subsequent back injuries in firefighters. J. Occup. Med. 21:269–272, 1979.
23. Cady, L. D., Thomas, P. C., and Karwasky, R. J.: Program for increasing health and physical fitness of firefighters. J. Occup. Med. 27:110–114, 1985.
24. Caplan, P. S., Freedman, L. M. J., and Connelly, T. P.: Degenerative joint disease of the lumbar spine in coal miners—a clinical and x-ray study. Arthritis Rheum. 9:693–702, 1966.
25. Chaffin, D. B.: Localized muscle fatigue—definition and measurement. J. Ocup. Med. 15:346–354, 1973.
26. Chaffin, D. B., and Park, K. S.: A longitudinal study of low-back pain as associated with occupational weight lifting factors. Am. Industr. Hyg. Assoc. J. 34:513–525, 1973.
27. Choler, U., Larsson, R. Nachemson, A. L., and Peterson, L. E.: Pain in the Back. S.P.R.I. Rapport 22:188, 1985.
28. Collis, D. K., and Ponseti, I. V.: Long-term followup of ptients with idiopathic scoliosis not treated surgically. J. Bone Joint Surg. 51A:425–455, 1969.
29. Cushway, B. C., and Mailer, R. J.: Routine examination of the spine for industrial employees. J.A.M.A. 92:701–705, 1929.
30. Delin, O., Hedenrud, B., and Horal, J.: Back symptoms in nursing aides in a geriatric hospital. Scand. J. Rehabil. Med. 8:47–53, 1976.
31. Dillane, J. B., Fry, J., and Kalton, G.: Acute back syndrome—a study from general practice. Br. Med. J. 2:82–84, 1966.
32. Dively, R. L., and Oglevie, R. R.: Pre-employment examination of the low back. J.A.M.A. 160:856–858, 1956.
33. Dzioba, R. B., and Doxey, N. C.: A prospective investigation into the orthopaedic and psychologic predictors of outcome of first lumbar surgery following industrial injury. Spine 9:614, 1984.
34. Eklundh, M.: Prevalence of musculoskeletal problems in office work. Socialmed. T. 6:1–9, 1967.
35. Englund, A.: Experiences from the building industry. Forsvarsmedicin 1(Suppl.)23–27, 1974.
36. Ferguson, D. A.: Changing the work process to overcome the back injury hazard. *In* Back Injuries at Work. New Zealand Institute of Industrial Safety, 1970, pp. 42–50.
37. Ferguson, D. A.: Strain injuries in hospital employees. Med. J. Aust. 1:376–379, 1970.
38. Ferguson, D. A.: The work causes of back injury. *In* Back Injuries at Work. New Zealand Institute of Industrial Safety, 1970, pp. 24–40.
39. Fischer, F. J., Friedman, M. M., and Denmark, R. E., van: Roentgenographic abnormalities in soldiers with low back pain: A comparative study. A.J.R 79:673–676, 1958.
40. Fitzler, S. L., and Berger, R. A.: Attitudinal change: The Chelsea back program. Occup. Health Safety 51:24–26, 1982.
41. Fitzler, S. L., and Berger, R. A.: Chelsea back program: One year later. Occup. Health Safety 52:52–54, 1983.
42. Flynn, J. C.: Anterior fusion of the lumbar spine. End-result study with long-term follow-up. J. Bone Joint Surg. 61:1143–1150, 1979.
43. Frymoyer, J. W., Clements, J. Wilder, D., et al.: Epidemiology of low back pain. Part II. Presented at the Seventh Annual Meeting I.S.S.L.S., New Orleans, May 24–28, 1980.
44. Frymoyer, J. W., Pope, M. H., Costanza, M. C., et al.: Epidemiologic studies of low-back pain. Spine 5:419–423, 1980.
45. Frymoyer, J. W., Pope, M. H., Clements, J. H., et al.: Risk factors in low back pain—an epidemiological survey. J. Bone Joint Surg. 65A:213–218, 1983.
46. Fullenlove, T. M., and Williams, A. J.: Comparative roentgen findings in symptomatic and asymptomatic backs. Radiology 68:572–574, 1957.
47. Green, M., Battié, M. C., and Bigos, S. J.: The role of acute back injuries in lower back pain (submitted to J. Spinal Dis., 1989).
48. Gruber, G. J., and Ziperman, H. H.: Relationship between whole-body vibration and morbidity patterns among motor coach operators. Washington, DC, H.E.W. Publication No. (N.I.O.S.H.), 75–104, 1974.
49. Haber, L. D.: Disabling effects of chronic disease and impairment. J. Chronic Dis. 24:469–487, 1971.
50. Hakelius, A.: Prognosis in sciatica. A clinical follow-up of surgical and non-surgical treatment. Acta Orthop. Scand. 129(Suppl.):1–76, 1970.
51. Helander, E.: Back pain and work disability. Socialmed. T. 50:398–404, 1973.
52. Hirsch, C, Jonsson, B., and Lewin, T.: Low back symptoms in a Swedish female population. Clin. Orthop. 63:171–176, 1969.
53. Hodges, F. J., and Peck, W. S.: Clinical and roent-

genological study of low back pain with sciatic radiation. B. Roentgenological aspects. A.J.R. 37:461–466, 1937.
54. Hodgson, S., Shannon, H. S., and Troup, J. D. G.: The prevention of spinal disorders in dock workers. Report to National Dock Labour Board, 1974.
55. Horal, J.: The clinical appearance of low back pain disorders in the city of Gothenburg, Sweden. Acta Orthop. Scand. 118(Suppl.):1–109, 1969.
56. Howell, D. W.: Musculoskeletal profile and incidence of musculoskeletal injuries in lightweight women rowers. Am. J. Sports Med. 12:278–282, 1984.
57. Hrubec, A., and Nashbold, B. S., Jr.: Epidemiology of lumbar disc lesions in the military in World War II. Am. J. Epidemiol. 102:366–376, 1975.
58. Huddleson, J. H.: Accidents, Neuroses and Compensation. Baltimore, Williams & Wilkins Company, 1932.
59. Hult, L.: The Munksfors investigation. Acta Orthop. Scand. 16(Suppl.)1–76, 1954.
60. Hult, L.: Cervical, dorsal, and lumbar spinal syndromes. Acta Orthop. Scand. 17(Suppl.)1–102, 1954.
61. Hussar, A. E., and Guller, E. J.: Correlation of pain and the roentgenographic findings of spondylosis of the cervical and lumbar spine. Am. J. Med. Sci. 232:518–527, 1956.
62. Ikata, T.: Statistical and dynamic studies of lesions due to overloading on the spine. Shikoku Acta Med. 40:262–286, 1965.
63. Junghanns, H.: Die Wirbelsaule in der Arbeitsmedizin. Die Wirbelsaule in Forschung und Praxis 79:1–396, 1979.
64. Kelsey, J. L.: An epidemiological study of acute horniated lumbar intervertebral discs. Rheumatol. Rehabil. 14:144–155, 1975.
65. Kelsey, J. L.: An epidemiological study of the relationship between occupations and acute herniated lumbar intervertebral discs. Int. J. Epidemiol. 4:197–204, 1975.
66. Kelsey, J. L.: Epidemiology of radiculopathies. Adv. Neurol. 19:385–396, 1978.
67. Kelsey, J. L., and Hardy, R. J.: Driving of motor vehicles as a risk factor for acute herniated lumbar intervertebral disc. Am. J. Epidemiol. 102:63–73, 1975.
68. Kelsey, J. L., and Ostfeld, A. M.: Demographic characteristics of persons with acute herniated lumbar intervertebral disc. J. Chronic Dis. 28:37–50, 1975.
69. Kelsey, J. L., and White, A. A. III: Epidemiology and impact of low back pain. Spine 5:133–142, 1980.
70. Keyserling, W. M., Herrin, G. D., and Chaffin, D. B.: Isometric strength testing as a measure of controlling incidents on strenuous jobs. J. Occup. Med. 22:332–336, 1980.
71. Keyserling, W. M., Herrin, G. D., Chaffin, D. B., et al.: Establishing an industrial strength testing program. Am. Industr. Hyg. Assoc. J. 41:730–736, 1980.
72. Kogstad, O., and Gudmundsen, I.: Back Problems in Skien 1971–1972. Presented at the Telemark Sentralsjukehus, Skien, 1973.
73. Kostuick, J., and Bentivoglio, J.: The incidence of low back pain in adult scoliosis. Presented at the Seventh Annual Meeting I.S.S.L.S., New Orleans, May 24–28, 1980.
74. Kroemen, K. H. E., and Robinette, J. C.: Ergonomics in the design of office furniture. Industr. Med. Surg. 38:115–125, 1969.
75. LaRocca, H., and Macnab, I.: Value of pre-employment radiographic assessment of the lumbar spine. Can. Med. Assoc. J. 101:49–54, 1969.
76. Lawrence, J. S.: Rheumatism in coal miners. Part III. Occupational factors. Br. J. Indust. Med. 12:249–261, 1955.
77. Lawrence, J. S.: Disc degeneration. Its frequency and relationship to symptoms. Ann. Rheum. Dis. 28:121–137, 1969.
78. Leavitt, S. S., Johnson, T. L., and Beyer, R. D.: The process of recovery: Patterns in industrial back injury. Part I. Costs and other quantitative measures of effort. Indust. Med. Surg. 40:7–14, 1971.
79. Lokanden, S.: Sick absence in a Swedish company. A sociomedical study. Acta Med. Scand. 377(Suppl):1–172, 1962.
80. Magora, A.: Investigation of the relation between low back pain and occupation. 1. Age, sex, community, education and other factors. Industr. Med. Surg. 39:465–471, 1970.
81. Magora, A.: Investigation of the relation between low back pain and occupation. 2. Work history. Industr. Med. Surg. 39:504–510, 1970.
82. Magora, A.: Investigation of the relation between low back pain and occupation. 3. Physical requirements: Sitting, standing and weight lifting. Industr. Med. Surg. 41:5–9, 1972.
83. Magora, A.: Investigation of the relation between low back pain and occupation. 4. Physical requirements: Bending, rotation, reaching and sudden maximal effort. Scand. J. Rehabil. Med. 5:191–196, 1973.
84. Magora, A.: Investigation of the relation between low back pain and occupation. 5. Psychological aspects. Scand. J. Rehabil. Med. 5:186–190, 1973.
85. Magora, A.: Investigation of the relation between low back pain and occupation. 7. Neurologic and orthopaedic conditions. Scand. J. Rehabil. Med. 7:146–151, 1975.
86. Magora, A., and Schwartz, A.: Relation between the low back pain syndrome and x-ray findings. 1. Degenerative osteoarthritis. Scand. J. Rehabil. Med. 8:115–125, 1976.
87. Magora, A., and Schwartz, A.: Relation between the low back syndrome and x-ray findings. 2. Transitional vertebrae (mainly sacralization). Scand. J. Rehabil. Med. 10:135–145, 1978.
88. Magora, A., and Schwartz, A.: Relation between low back pain and x-ray changes. 4. Lysis and olisthesis. Scand. J. Rehabil. Med. 12:47–52, 1980.
89. McDonald, E. B., Porter, R. Hibbert, C., and Hart, J.: The relationship between spinal canal diameters and back pain in coal miners. Ultrasonic measurement as a screening test? J. Occup. Med. 26:23–28, 1984.
90. Morris, A.: Identifying workers at risk to back injury is not guesswork. Occup. Health Safety 54:16–20, 1985.
91. Nachemson, A. L.: Back problems in childhood and adolescence. Lakartidningen 65:2831–2843, 1968.
92. Nachemson, A. L.: The lumbar spine. An orthopaedic challenge. Spine 1:59–71, 1976.
93. Nachemson, A. L.: The natural history of low back pain. *In* White, A. A., and Gordon, S. L. (eds.): Symposium on Idiopathic Low Back Pain. St. Louis, C. V. Mosby, 1982, p. 46.
94. Nachemson, A. L., and Lindh, M.: Measurement

of abdominal and back muscle strength with and without low back pain. Scand. J. Rehabil. Med. 1:60–65, 1969.

95. National Safety Council: Accident Facts. Chicago, National Safety Council, 1976.
96. Natvig, H.: Sociomedical aspects of low back pain causing prolonged sick leave: A retrospective study. Acta Sociomed. Scand. 2:117, 1970.
97. Nilsonne, U., and Lundgren, K. D.: Long-term prognosis in idiopathic scoliosis. Acta Orthop. Scand. 39:456–465, 1968.
98. Nordgren, B.: Low back pain in elderly military recruits. Forsvarsmedicin 10(Suppl.):17–19, 1974.
99. Paillas, J. E., Winninger, J., and Louis, R.: Role des malformations lombosacrees dans les sciatiques et les lombalgies: Etude de 1,500 dossiers radiocliniques dont 500 hernies discales verifiees. Presse Med. 77:853–855, 1969.
100. Partridge, R. E., and Anderson, J. A.: Back pain in industrial workers. *In* Proceedings of the International Rheumatology Congress. Abstract 284, Prague, 1969.
101. Partridge, R. E., and Duthie, J. J. R.: Rheumatism in dockers and civil servants. A comparison of heavy manual and sedentary workers. Ann. Rheum. Dis. 27:559–568, 1968.
102. Pedersen, O. F., Petersen, R., and Staffeldt, E. S.: Back pain and isometric back muscle strength of workers in a Danish factory. Scand. J. Rehabil. Med. 7:125–128, 1975.
103. Redfield, J. T.: The low back x-rays as a pre-employment screening tool in the forest products industry. J. Occup. Med. 13:219–226, 1971.
104. Robertson, L. S., and Keeve, J. P.: Worker injuries: The effects of workers compensation and O.S.H.A. inspections. J. Health Polit. Policy Law 8:581–597, 1983.
105. Roland, M., and Morris, R.: A study of the natural history of low back pain. Part III: Development of guidelines for trials of treatment in primary care. Spine 8:145–150, 1983.
106. Rowe, M. L.: Low back pain in industry. A position paper. J. Occup. Med. 11:161–169, 1969.
107. Rowe, M. L.: Low back disability in industry: Updated position. J. Occup. Med. 13:476–478, 1971.
108. Rowe, M. L.: Preliminary statistical study of low back pain. J. Occup. Med. 5:336–341, 1963.
109. Rowe, M. L.: Disc surgery and chronic low-back pain. J. Occup. Med. 7:196–202, 1965.
110. Runge, C. F.: Pre-existing structural defects and severity of compensation back injuries. Indust. Med. Surg. 27:249–252, 1958.
111. Snook, S. H., Campanelli, R. A., and Hart, J. W.: A study of three preventive approaches to low back injury. J. Occup. Med. 20:478–481, 1978.
112. Snook, S. H.: Low back pain in industry. *In* White, A. A., and Gordon, S. L. (eds.): Symposium on Idiopathic Low Back Pain. St. Louis, C. V. Mosby, 1982, p. 23.
113. Social Security Commission on Evaluation of Pain. Report to Federal Congress (submitted for publication in 1979).
114. Social Security Statistical Supplement (1977–79), Sup. Doc. No. HE 3.3/3:979, Washington, D. C., Government Printing Office.
115. Sorensen, K. H.: Scheuermann's Juvenile Kyphosis. Thesis. Copenhagen, Munksgaard, 1964.
116. Spangfort, E. V.: The lumbar disc herniation, a computer-aided analysis of 2504 operations. Acta Orthop. Scand. 142(Suppl.):1–93, 1972.
117. Spengler, D. M., Bigos, S. J., Martin, N. A., et al.: Back injuries in industry; A retrospective study. I. Overview and cost analysis. Spine 11:241–245, 1986.
118. Splithoff, C. A.: Lumbosacral junction. Roentgenographic comparison of patients with and without backaches. J.A.M.A. 152:1610–1613, 1953.
119. Sternbach, R. A., Murphy, R. W., Akeson, W. H., and Wolf, S. R.: Chronic low-back pain. the "low-back loser." Postgrad. Med. 53:135–138, 1973.
120. Svensson, H. O., and Andersson, G. B. J.: Low back pain in 40- to 47-year-old men. I. Frequency of occurrence and impact on medical services. Scand. J. Rehabil. Med. 14:47–53, 1982.
121. Svensson, H. O., and Andersson, G. B. J.: Low back pain in 40- to 47-year old men: Work history and work env ronment factors. Spine 8:272–276, 1983.
122. Svensson, H. O., Vedin, A., Wilhelmsson, C., and Andersson, G. B. J.: Low-back pain in relation to other diseases and cardiovascular risk factors. Spine 8:277–284, 1983.
123. Sweetman, B. J., Anderson, J. A. D., and Dalton, E. R.: The relationships between little-finger mobility, lumbar mobility, straight-leg raising, and low-back pain. Rheum. Rehabil. 13:161–166, 1974.
124. Tauber, J.: An unorthodox look at backaches. J. Occup. Med. 12:128–130, 1970.
125. Tilley, P.: Is sacralization a significant factor in lumbar pain? J. Am. Osteopath. Assoc. 70:238–241, 1970.
126. Torgerson, B. R., and Dotter, W. E.: Comparative roentgenographic study of the asymptomatic and symptomatic lumbar spine. J. Bone Joint Surg. 58A:850–853, 1976.
127. Troup, J. D. G.: The spine of the tractor driver. Rural Med. 1:9–12, 1969.
128. Troup, J. D. G., Foreman, T. K., Baxter, C. E., Brown D.: The perception of back pain and the role of psychophysical test of lifting capacity. Spine 12:645–657, 1987.
129. Troup, J. D. G., Martin, J. W., and Lloyd, D. C. E. F.: Back pain in industry: A prospective study. Spine 6:61–69, 1981.
130. Vallfors, B.: Acute, subacute and chronic low back pain. Clinical Symptoms, absenteeism and working environment. Scand. J. Rehabil. Med. Suppl. No. 11, 1985.
131. Valkenburg, H. A., Haanen H. C. N.: The epidemiology of low back pain. *In* White, A. A., and Gordon, S. L. (eds.): Symposium on Idiopathic Low Back Pain. St. Louis, C. V. Mosby, 1982, p. 0.
132. Waris, W.: Lumbar disc herniation. Clinical studies and late results of 374 cases of sciatica. Acta Chir. Scand. 140(Suppl.):1–134, 1948.
133. Weber, H.: Lumbar disc herniation: A controlled, prospective study with ten years of observation. Spine 8:131–140, 1983.
134. Weber, H.: Lumbar disc herniation. Part I. J. Oslo City Hosp. 28:33–64, 1978.
135. Weber, H.: Lumbar disc hernation. Part II. J. Oslo City Hosp. 28:89–120, 1978.
136. Westrin, C. G.: Low back sick-listing. A nosologi-

cal and medical insurance investigation. Scand. J. Soc. Med. 7(Suppl.):1–116, 1973.
137. Westrin, C. G.: Low back sick-listing. A nosological and medical insurance investigation. Acta Sociomed. Scand. 2:127–134, 1970.
138. White, A. W. M.: Low back pain in men receiving workman's compensation. Can. Med. Assoc. J. 95:50–56, 1966.
139. White, A. A., Southwick, W. O., and DePonte, R.: Cervical spine fusions: Psychological and social considerations. Arch. Surg. 106:150–152, 1973.
140. Wiesel, S. W., Feffer, H. L., and Rothman, R. H.: Industrial low-back—a prospective evaluation of a standardized diagnostic and treatment protocol. Spine 9:199–203, 1984.
141. Wiffling, F. J., Klonoff, H., and Kokan, P.: Psychological, demographic and orthopaedic factors associated with prediciton of outcome of spinal fusion. Clin. Orthop. 90:153–160, 1973.
142. Wiikeri, M., Nummi, J., Riihimaki, H., and Wickstrom, G.: Radiologically detectable lumbar disc degeneration in reinforcement workers. Scand. J. Work Environ. Health 1(Suppl.)4:47–53, 1978.
143. Wiltse, L. L.: Lumbosacral Strain and Instability. Proceedings of The A.A.O.S. Symposium on the Spine. 1969, pp. 54–83.
144. Wiltse, L. L., and Hutchinson, R. H.: Surgical treatment of spondylolisthesis. Clin. Orthop. 35:116–135, 1964.
145. Wiltse, L. L., and Rocchio, P. D.: Preoperative tests as predictors of success of chemonucleolysis in the treatment of the low-back syndrome. J. Bone Joint Surg. 57A:478–483, 1975.
146. Wood, P. H. N.: Epidemiology of back pain. *In* Jayson, M. (ed.): The Lumbar Spine and Back Pain. London, Pitman, 1976, pp. 13–27.
147. Wood, P. H. N. and McLeish, C. L.: Statistical appendix. Ann. Rheum. Dis. 33:93–105, 1974.
148. Wood, D. J.: Design and evaluation of a back injury prevention program within a geriatric hospital. Spine 12:77–82, 1987.

TRUNK STRENGTH AND ENDURANCE: MEASUREMENT TECHNIQUES

Margareta Nordin

Six occupational factors have been associated with an increased loss of work time due to low back pain symptoms: physically heavy work, static work postures, frequent bending and twisting, lifting and sudden forceful incidents, repetitive work, and vibrational exposure.[12] In a large retrospective survey, lifting or bending episodes accounted for 33% of all work-related causes of back pain.[11]

Troup and colleagues[59] have identified the combination of lifting with lateral bending or twisting as a frequent cause of back injury in the work place. Magora[35] demonstrated an association between occasional bending, excessive bending, and low back pain. It is not known precisely how these factors are involved in the mechanism of back injury. Several reports in the biomedical literature, however, provide a foundation on which to construct further studies for investigating the nature of this injury mechanism.[1, 15, 18, 60]

Hickey and Hukins[18] have focused on the effect of forward-bending postures on the integrity of the annulus fibrosus and the interspinous ligament. They found that torsion and bending may cause failure of the annulus and thereby lead to protrusion of the nucleus pulposus. Adams and Hutton[1] showed that the interspinous ligament was the first structure to be damaged in hyperflexion, and surgical results corroborated that a prolapsed disc is usually associated with a ruptured or slack interspinous ligament.[53] An in vitro study indicated that when the spine was under compression and hyperflexed only a few degrees, the risk of back injury was significantly increased. The possibility of an injury is increased if lateral bending accompanies forward flexion of the trunk during a lifting task.[2, 60]

Studies have reported that work tasks requiring over 400 repetitive trunk motions a week and those requiring bending, twisting, and lifting over 25 times a day (with a weight of 11.3 kg) were associated with a high risk of a herniated disc and back injury.[26]

This subchapter describes different modes

of measuring muscle performance and their applicability to trunk strength and endurance.

MODES OF MEASURING STRENGTH AND ENDURANCE APPLICABLE TO THE TRUNK

It may be reasonable to start with some basic definitions of terms. Muscle performance for any joint or joint complex can be categorized according to (1) strength, (2) endurance, and (3) coordination. Muscle strength is the capacity to produce torque or work by voluntary contraction.[31] Muscle endurance is the ability to maintain torque or work over a period of time.[31] Coordination, in this context, is defined as adjustment or action of muscles in producing movements and maintaining quality of motor output (torque, velocity, range of motion).

Muscle performance can, with these concepts borne in mind, be measured in either a static or a dynamic manner.

In medical literature, no motion of the joint or joint complex is presumed for the static measurement, whereas for the dynamic measurement the joint or joint complex is presumed to move. This definition found in medical literature is to be compared with the clearly defined concept of statics and dynamics in engineering. In engineering literature, *statics* is defined as "the study of forces acting on a body in equilibrium," and *dynamics* is defined as "the study of forces acting on a body in motion."

In measuring muscle performance, a contraction of the muscle is necessary in order to produce a measurable entity. The active state of muscle contraction occurs when tension is generated through the biophysical bonding of actin and myosin filaments.[13, 47] Depending on the external load, the direction of the action, and the magnitude,[29, 30] contractions can be further classified as shown in Table 1.

When muscles develop tension, exerting a pull on the bony component, movement of the proximal bony lever or the distal bony lever occurs, depending on which is fixed and which is free to move. If the force exerted by the muscle on the free bony lever is greater than the force offered by the external load, then the muscle shortens and produces a concentric contraction.[30, 54] When the internal force developed by the muscle on the bony lever is equal to the external load, no change in joint position is seen, no visible change in muscle length is observed, and an isometric contraction occurs. When the external load is greater than the total force generated by the muscle, then the muscle lengthens and an eccentric contraction occurs.[28–30, 54]

Tension developed in a muscle varies with the type of contraction. Isometric contractions produce more tension than concentric contractions. The tension developed in an eccentric contraction is greater than that which can be developed in a muscle during an isometric or a concentric contraction.[28] This is thought to be due largely to supplemental tension produced in the series of elastic muscle components.[28]

Muscle force production that is constant through a range of motion is called *isotonic*.[54] This commonly used definition does not take into account the leverage effects at the joint. Because of these effects, the force developed by the muscles will actually be changing and should therefore be called *nonisotonic*.[54] During this movement the velocity of the body segment varies with the degree of contraction.[19]

When the rate of shortening or lengthening

Table 1 □ Definitions of Commonly Used Modes of Measuring Muscle Strength

Concentric—a state of contraction occurring when a muscle is shortening under load. The net muscle moment is in the same direction as the change in joint angle,[54] and the mechanical work is positive.[30]

Eccentric—a state of contraction occurring when a muscle is being overcome by an external load, resulting in progressive lengthening of that muscle.[54] The net muscle moment is in the direction opposite to the change in joint angle,[54] and the mechanical work is negative.[30]

Isometric—the state of muscle contraction occurring when no change exists in the distance between its points of attachment and in which, therefore, no change in joint angle occurs.[54] The contractile components of a muscle shorten at the expense of the series elastic structures,[54] and mechanical work is considered to be zero.[30]

Isokinetic muscle action—muscle action in which the rate of shortening or lengthening of the muscle is constant.[54] When measured, it assumes maximal voluntary contraction to be exhibited by the individual or patient.

Isotonic contraction—contraction in which the muscle force is constant through a range of motion.[54]

Isoinertial contraction—movement in which muscles contract against a constant resistance and the limb accelerates or decelerates if the generated torque is greater or smaller than the set resistance.[31]

of the muscle is constant, that muscle action is termed *isokinetic*.[19, 54] Because velocity is held constant, energy cannot be dissipated through acceleration and is converted to a resisting force, which is proportional to the magnitude of the muscular input or muscular force. Force varies in relation to the efficiency of the skeletal leverage.[19] When the resistance is kept constant as it is during isoinertial contraction, the surplus of muscular force produced will display acceleration or deceleration of the measured body segment.[31]

Because muscles usually shorten or lengthen at varying rates and tensions, it is clear that isokinetic and isoinertial movements are somewhat artificial and are usually produced by constraining a subject to a device such as a dynamometer, which helps to control limb segment speed, range of motion, and/or resistance.

In summary, muscles composed of active contractile and passive elastic elements and attached to bony levers are capable of exerting tension. This tension can produce a shortening contraction of the muscle, an isometric contraction, or be subjected to a lengthening contraction, or it can produce any combination of these three types. Movement can be isotonic, with the force remaining constant (more unlikely); it can be isokinetic, with the velocity remaining constant; or it can be isoinertial, with implied resistance remaining constant. These types of movement can be mixed and matched in any fashion necessary for executing a dynamic task.

TRUNK MUSCLE STRENGTH

The lack of trunk muscle strength and endurance has frequently been cited as a factor in the cause of low back pain. Several investigators have suggested that the trunk muscles of asymptomatic individuals are stronger than those of patients with low back pain.[3, 4, 8, 38, 41, 56, 57] A study of inpatients with severe back disorders showed that the back muscle strength of the patients was less than that of the matched asymptomatic individuals.[3] However, outpatients with low back disorders were as strong as asymptomatic individuals. The existence of pain augmented the measured strength in the study of Addison and Schultz.[3] Although their testing methodologies differ from one another in terms of testing methods and positions, the results are similar. Patients with acute low back pain have weaker trunk muscles than individuals in an asymptomatic control group. Patients with chronic low back pain may or may not have weaker trunk muscles than a control group, depending on the testing methods used.[38, 57] However, there is very little consistency among investigators with respect to the methods and types of testing performed. People who are physically fit have a significantly decreased incidence of musculoskeletal impairment, although they do not necessarily have less low back pain. Increasing trunk muscle endurance has been observed to reduce the incidence of first-time low back pain.[8] The objective evaluation of the strength and endurance of trunk musculature may, therefore, be of significant value if adapted to the required job or physical activity performed.

Alston and colleagues[4] and Nachemson and Lindh[40] measured the isometric strength of the trunk flexors and extensors with a cable tensiometer. Since then, researchers have been evaluating various body positions and testing methods to establish the normal strength of trunk muscles. Other investigators evaluated isometric strength in the standing position with a cable tensiometer and isokinetic dynamometers in the side-lying, standing, and sitting positions.[4, 16, 33, 38, 43, 55, 58] Table 2 shows selected studies of trunk muscle strength in populations of adult women.

In isometric testing of the trunk muscles, a supine position (for testing abdominal muscles) and a prone position (for testing back muscles) are frequently used. Nachemson and Lindh[41] suggested that by placing the hips and knees in a flexed position, the iliopsoas muscle is at a mechanical disadvantage. However, Alston[4] compared the two recumbent positions in measuring trunk flexion strength; in one position the hips and knees were straight, and in the other the hips and knees were flexed. According to their findings, these two positions showed no significant difference in strength.

In comparing the isokinetic means and peak values for trunk flexion and extension in two studies,[16, 43] the results in the study of Nordin and coworkers[43] were about 30% lower, even though the test situations were comparable. A possible explanation of this discrepancy is that the axis of rotation in

Table 2 □ Summary of Selected Previous Studies Concerning Trunk Muscle Strength in Normal Adult Women

AUTHORS	NUMBER OF WOMEN	TYPE OF TESTING	TESTING POSITION	TESTING METHOD	TRUNK FLEXION Force (N)	TRUNK FLEXION Moment (N • m)	TRUNK EXTENSION Force (N)	TRUNK EXTENSION Moment (N • m)	RATIO Trunk Flexion–Extension
Addison and Schultz, 1980	30	Isometric	Standing	Harness strain-gauge	257	87	347	117	0.74
Hasue et al., 1930	50	Isometric	Lying	Cybex II		50–105		91–150	0.70–0.55
		Isokinetic				41–98		75–120	0.82–0.55
Langrana et al., 1984b	26	Isometric	Sitting	Cybex II		64		123	0.51
		Isokinetic				60		98	0.61
McNeill et al., 1980	30	Isometric	Standing	Harness strain-gauge	257	87	347	117	0.74
Nachemson and Lindh,	20	Isometric	Standing	Zadig dynamometer	279		453		0.59
1969		Isometric	Lying				469		
Smidt et al., 1983	12	Isometric	Lying	Iowa trunk dynamometer		150		209	0.75
		Isokinetic				90		160	0.56
Nordin et al., 1987	101	Isometric	Lying	Cybex II		19–109		38–160	0.57–0.182
		Isokinetic	Sitting 30 deg/sec	Cybex II		47–183		52–234	
			Sitting 60 deg/sec	Cybex II		17–191		14–208	

the study of Hasue and coworkers[16] was closer to the hip joint than to the lumbrosacral joint. Thorstensson and Nilsson[58] studied the effect of the change of axis of rotation and showed that the contribution of the hip joint muscles varied according to the placement of the axis of rotation. If the axis was below the origin of the hip muscles, a greater contribution of these muscles was shown, and the values for trunk flexion torque increased.

The Natick test, a pull test, was developed by the United States Army.[27] The test procedures are highly standardized, and the values can easily be compared. The mean values for two studies for 38-cm pull were 20%, a discrepancy that can be explained by the fact that subjects from the study of Nordin and associates[43] were older and randomly selected from a general population, whereas the subjects recruited by the Army[27] were preselected and younger.

TRUNK MUSCLE ENDURANCE

It is generally assumed that local muscular fatigue predisposes an individual to injury. Chaffin[10] clearly stated that reduction of precise motor control accompanies muscular fatigue. The industrial engineering and sports medicine literature points to many observations indicating that the skill of the worker is affected by fatigue.[5, 6, 20, 22, 32] However, despite the significance of muscular fatigue and endurance, few prospective long-term studies can be cited from the literature.

Jorgensen[23] found that in order to maintain a stooped position during a work day, the maximum isometric strength of the back muscles must exceed two thirds of the body weight. In the general population with no acute low back pain, it was found that trunk muscles tended to be weaker among those who experienced a recurrence of low back pain during a follow-up year compared with those who had no recurrence. Because persons with first-time low back pain during the follow-up year did not have trunk strength differing from those with recurrent or chronic low back pain, the results of trunk strength measurements seem to be of little value as a predictor of low back pain.[7, 8, 24, 42]

Suzuki and Endo[57] demonstrated that trunk flexors developed fatigue faster than the trunk extensors during isometric contraction. The fatigability of trunk flexors was significantly higher in the patients with low back pain than in the control group; however, this was not observed with respect to trunk extensors.

Dynamic endurance of trunk flexors and extensors in the sitting posture was measured as the time needed for the maximum concentric torque decreased by 25%, using an isokinetic dynamometer at 30 deg/sec.[56] It was demonstrated that trunk extensors were more resistant to fatigue than trunk flexors and that men had less endurance than females. Langrana and Lee[33] using the same protocol, confirmed the results of Smidt and colleagues.[56] It should be noted that at such a slow speed (30 deg/sec) there may be sufficient time for blood to flow into the muscles. In addition, given the dominance of the fatigue-resistant fiber type of the extensor muscles, the protocol was less appropriate for endurance measurement.[21]

Heyward[17] found that the critical occluding strength was to be about 60% of maximal voluntary capacity for low-strength individuals, thus explaining why the endurance time of the low-strength group was significantly greater than that of the high-strength group. Marras and colleagues[36] pointed to the differences in recruitment patterns and functions of trunk muscles among various modes of contraction, thereby explaining the discrepancy between the investigations extensively reviewed by Ortengren and Andersson.[45] An urgent need exists in the ergonomic and medical community to replace the static endurance models of the trunk[24, 37, 42, 48] with more realistic, dynamic ones.

The combination of a 3-D motion monitoring system and a controllable resistance system has evaded researchers until now. The simultaneous measurement of motor output (torque) and movement pattern (angular position and velocity profile) in three dimensions would permit assessment of fatigue as a functional state to which the individual with an intact nervous system could adapt to perform the required task.[48, 49, 51]

Parnianpour and colleagues[48] studied the effects of isoinertial fatiguing of flexion and extension trunk movements on the movement patterns and the motor output of the trunk.

Twenty males with no history of low back pain for the previous 6 months volunteered for the study. A triaxial dynamometer was used; it simultaneously provided measurement of torque, angular position, and velocity of each axis. Resistances were set independently for each axis by an interfaced computer.

The subjects performed trunk flexion and extension movement against a sagittal plane resistance equal to 70% of their maximum isometric extension strength in the upright position. The minimum resistances in the coronal and transverse planes were set up at 7 N • m. The subjects were asked to perform trunk movement as quickly and as accurately as possible, while exerting the maximum efforts until reaching exhaustion.

All the selected parameters (torque, velocity, and range of motion) were significantly ($p < .05$) reduced in the sagittal plane. The individuals displayed significantly less motor control and greater range of motion in the coronal and transverse planes while performing the primary task of flexion and extension (Fig. 1*A–D*).

The reduction in the functional capacity of the primary muscles performing the required task is compensated for by secondary muscle groups, and the spinal structure is loaded in a more injury-prone pattern, as identified by finite element models.[60] In addition, it is suggested that the fatigued muscles would be less able to compensate any perturbation in the load or position of the trunk. The repetitive loading results in a weakening of the viscoelastic passive elements of the spine structure. The loss of ability to protect these weakened passive elements makes the spine more susceptible to injuries.

When similar fatigue studies were performed for lateral bending and axial rotation, the changes resulting from fatigue were significant only in the primary plane of motion. Individuals mainly reduced their torque, velocity, and range of motion in the intended plane and consequently were able to perform the task at a lower intensity level. These studies show different effects due to fatigue when motor ouputs for flexion–extension are compared with those of rotation and lateral bending.[49, 50]

CORRELATIONS AMONG DIFFERENT TESTS OF TRUNK STRENGTH AND ENDURANCE

Some confusion and controversy exist about the inter-relationship of various modes of testing trunk strength and endurance. A study by Parnianpour and colleagues[56] investigated the intercorrelations between isometric, isokinetic strength and isometric endurance of capacity of the back muscles in 131 healthy women. All subjects underwent a comprehensive test battery that consisted of isometric and isokinetic strength testing of abdominal and back muscles using an isokinetic Dynamometer Natick upright pull test,[27] and the Sorensen endurance test.[8] The test trials were randomly ordered, except for the Sorensen test, which was performed last. Isometric back and abdominal muscle

Table 3 □ Correlation Coefficients for Trunk Strength Tests
Significant Coefficients Only Displayed ($p < 0.05$; $n = 131$ Women)

	1	2	3	4	5	6	7	8	9	10	11	12	13
Endurance													
1. Sorensen		.27	.26	NS	.33	.40	.39	.37	.20	.37	.40	.39	.40
Natick													
2. Upright			.52	NS	.28	.31	.36	.30	.20	.32	.34	.34	.29
3. Bent knees				NS	.48	.46	.48	.41	.44	.43	.41	.42	.33
Flexion													
4. Isometric (supine)					NS	NS	NS	NS	NS	NS	NS	NS	NS
5. Isokinetic 30°/s Peak						.84	.87	.69	NS	79	.71	.74	.60
6. Total energy							.81	.81	.34	.73	.82	.68	.66
7. Isokinetic 60°/s Peak								.82	.43	.78	.72	.85	.74
8. Total energy									.25	.63	.70	.73	.83
Extension													
9. Isometric (prone)										.52	.44	.44	.33
10. Isokinetic 30°/s Peak											.91	.86	.73
11. Total energy												.80	.79
12. Isokinetic 60°/s Peak													.74
13. Total energy													

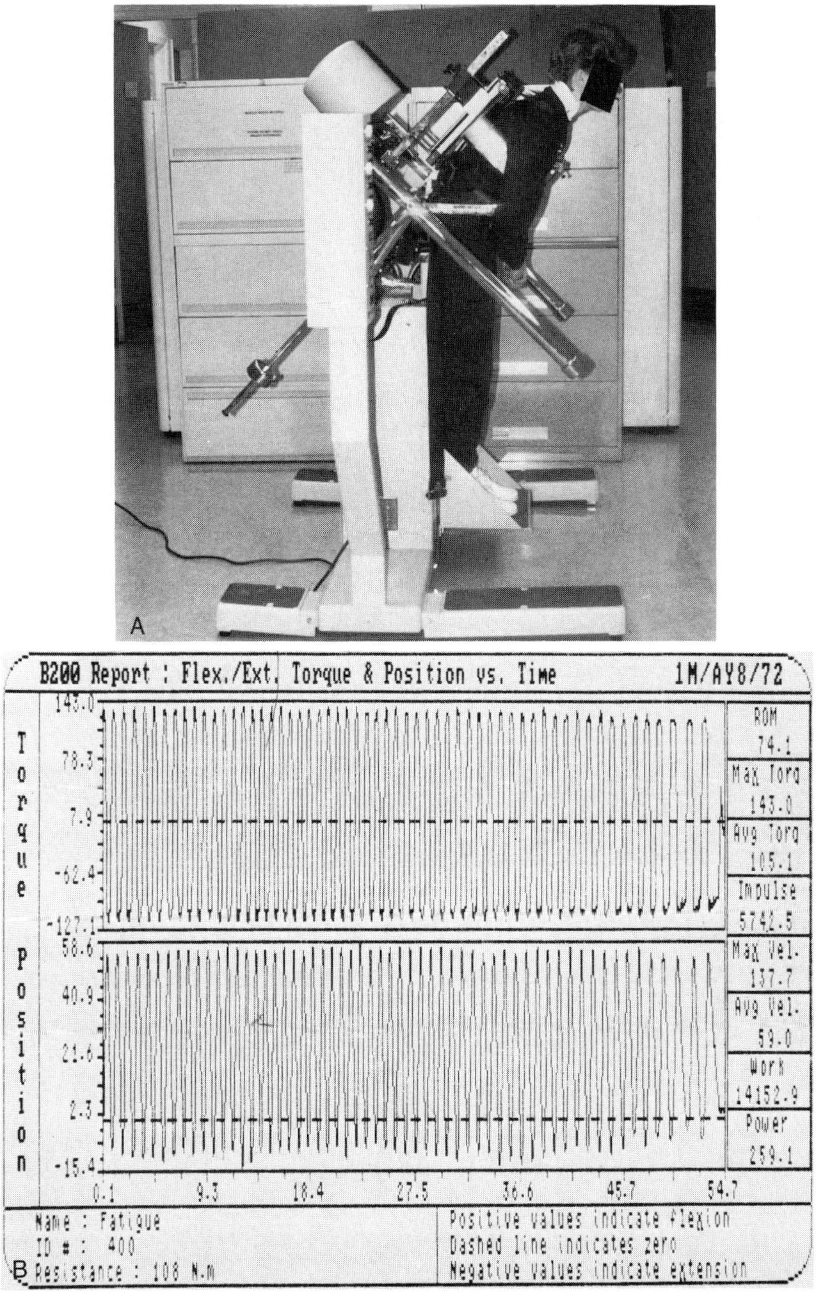

Figure 1 □ *A*, Triaxial dynamometer. *B*, Primary plane motor output, flexion/extension, torque versus angular position curves for one subject.

Illustration continued on following page

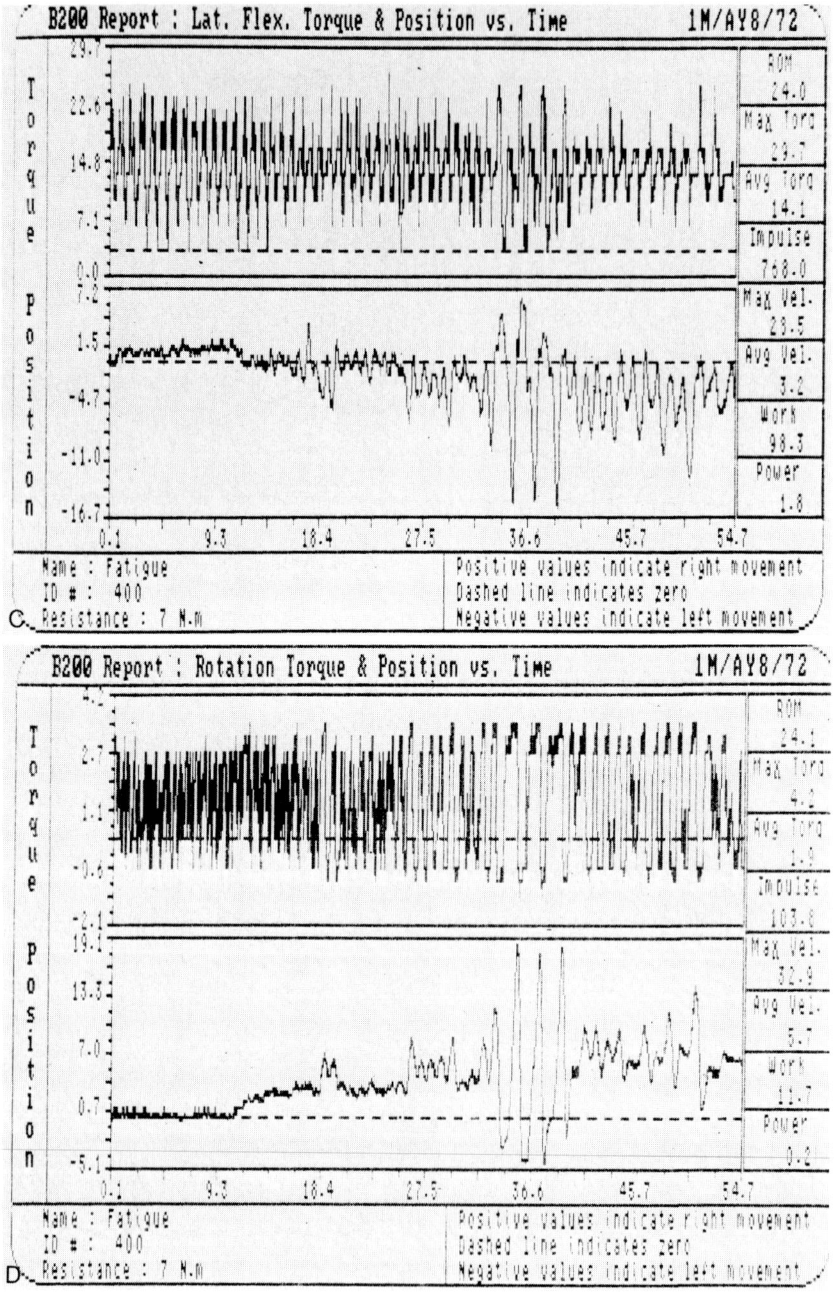

Figure 1 *Continued C*, Accessory plane motor output, lateral flexion, torque versus angular position curves for the same subject. *D*, Accessory plane motor output, axial rotation, torque versus angular position curves for the same subject. (From Parnianpour, M., Nordin, M., Kahanovitz, N., and Frankel, V.H.: The triaxial coupling of torque generation of trunk muscles during isometric exertions and the effect of fatiguing isoinertial movements on the motor output and movement patterns. Spine 13(9):982–992, 1988.)

strength was measured in prone and supine positions. The isokinetic tests were performed in a sitting position at 30 and 60 deg/sec. The Natick upright pull tests were performed in two different postures: (1) upright with the handle at the level of the axilla and with a straight back and knees and (2) upright with the handle 38 cm above the floor and with a straight back and bent knees. The Sorensen test was performed in the prone position. The results are displayed in Table 3. A number of significant correlations exist but are too weak to have any predictive power. The unexpected results were that isometric endurance had a stronger correlation with isokinetic parameters than with isometric strength parameters.

The correlations among the isometric tests were low. The isometric results also showed a weak correlation with isokinetic testing modes. There were no significant correlations between the maximum isometric flexion and any isometric or isokinetic extension parameter. However, there were strong correlations among the isokinetic extension parameters.

These results are in agreement with those of Thorstensson and Nilsson[58] and Ostering and colleagues.[46] Thorstensson and Nilsson[58] showed that the strength is a function of movement velocity, body position, and center of rotation. These data further support the conclusion of Mital and Karwowski,[39] who showed that the use of static strength testing to develop the human performance limit for dynamic tasks is fundamentally incorrect because the inertial forces are ignored. Marras and colleagues[31, 32] showed that muscle recruitment patterns of static and isokinetic movements are drastically different. Another ignored parameter is the time available to complete a lifting task. Hall[14] demonstrated that more rapid lifting significantly increased compressive and shear forces at the L5–S1 level and generated a higher external moment to be balanced by the muscles and other structures of the back. Strength is a complicated quantity that has to be measured through a number of parameters, and based on this study static tests cannot be substituted for dynamic tests. McNeill and colleagues[38] showed isometric trunk muscle strength for back patients and normal individuals to be equal. However, Langrana and coworkers[33, 34] showed significant differences in isokinetic torque curves between patients and normal individuals, thus demonstrating that dynamic strength and endurance assessments are indispensable.

References

1. Adams, M. A., and Hutton, W. C.: The relevance of torsion to the mechanical derangement of the lumbar spine. Spine 6:241–248, 1981.
2. Adams, M. A., and Hutton, W. C.: Prolapsed intervertebral disc. A hyperflexion injury. Spine 7:184–191, 1982.
3. Addison, R. and Schultz, A.: Trunk strength in patients seeking hospitalization for chronic low back disorders. Spine 5:539–544, 1980.
4. Alston, W., Carlson, K. E., Feldman, D. J., et al.: A quantitiative study of muscle factors in chronic low back syndrome. J. Am. Geriatr. Soc. 14:1041–1047, 1966.
5. Asmussen, E.: Muscle fatigue. Med. Sci. Sports 11:313–321, 1979.
6. Bates, B. T., Osternig, L. R., and James, S. L.: Fatigue effects in running. J. Motor Behav. 9:203–207, 1977.
7. Battié, M.: The Reliability of Physical Factors as Predictors of the Occurrence of Back Pain Reporters; A Prospective Study Within Industry. Thesis, Gothenburg University, Gothenburg, Sweden, 1989.
8. Biering-Sorensen, F.: Physical measurements as risk indicators for low back trouble over a one-year period. Spine 9:106–119, 1984.
9. Cady, L. D., Bischoff, D. P., O'Connell, E. R., et al: Strength and fitness and subsequent back injuries in firefighters. J. Occup. Med. 21:269–272, 1979.
10. Chaffin, D. B.: Localized muscle fatigue-definition and measurement. J. Occup. Med. 15:346–354, 1973.
11. Damkot, P. K., Pope, M. H., Lord, J., and Frymoyer, J. W.: The relationship between work history, work environment, and low back pain in men. Spine 9:395–399, 1984.
12. Frymoyer, J. W., Pope, M. H., Clements, J. H., et al.: Risk factors in low back pain. J. Bone Joint Surg. 65:213–218, 1983.
13. Gowitzke, B. A., and Milner, M.: Understanding the Scientific Bases of Human Movement, 2nd Ed. Baltimore, Williams & Wilkins, 1980.
14. Hall, S.: Effect of attempted lifting speed on forces and torque exerted on the lumbar spine. Med. Sci. Sports Exerc. 15:440–444, 1985.
15. Hansson, T., and Roos, B.: The relation between bone mineral content, experimental compression fractures and disc degeneration in lumbar vertebrae. Spine 6:147–150, 1981.
16. Hasue, M., Fujiwara, M., and Kikuchi, S.: A new method of quantitative measurement of abdominal and back muscle strength. Spine 5:143–148, 1980.
17. Heyward, V.: Influence of static strength and intramuscular occlusion on submaximal static muscle endurance. Res. Q. 46:393–402, 1974.
18. Hickey, D. S., and Hukins, D. W. L.: Relation between the structure of the annulus fibrosus and the function and failure of the intervertebral disc. Spine 5:106–116, 1980.
19. Hislop, H. J., and Perrine, J. J.: The isokinetic concept of exercise. Phys. Ther. 47:114–117, 1967.

20. Holding, D. H.: Fatigue. *In* Hockey, R. (ed.): Stress and Fatigue in Human Performance. New York, John Wiley & Sons, 1983, pp. 145–165.
21. Johnson, M. A., Polgar, J., Weightman, D., and Appleton, D.: Data on distribution of fibre types in thirty-six human muscles: an autopsy study. J. Neurosci. 18:111–129, 1973.
22. Jones, L. A., and Hunter, I. W.: Perceived force in fatiguing isometric contraction. Percept. Psychophysics 33:369–374, 1983.
23. Jorgensen, K.: Back muscle strength and body weight as limiting factors for work in the standing slightly-stooped position. Scand. J. Rehabil. Med. 2:149–153, 1970.
24. Jorgensen, K., and Nicolaisen, T.: Trunk extensor endurance: Determination and relation to low-back trouble. Ergonomics 30:259–267, 1987.
25. Kelsey, J. L., White, A. A., Pastides, H., and Bisbee, G. E., Jr.: The impact of musculoskeletal disorders on the population of the United States. J. Bone Joint Surg. 61:959–964, 1979.
26. Kelsey, J. L., Githens, P. B., and White, A. A.: An epidemiologic study of lifting and twisting on the job and risk for acute prolapsed lumbar invertebral disc. J. Orthop. Res. 2:61–66, 1984.
27. Knapik, J. J., Vogel, J. A., and Wright, J. E.: Measurement of isometric strength in an upright pull at 38 cm. Natick, Massachusetts, U.S.A. Medical Research Institute of Environmental Medicine, Report Number T3/81, Apr. 1, 1981.
28. Komi, P. V.: Neuromuscular performance: Factors influencing force and speed production. Scand. J. Sports Sci. 1:2–15, 1979.
29. Komi, P. V.: Physiological and biomechanical correlates of muscle structure and stretch-shortening cycle on force and speed. Exerc. Sports Sci. Rev. 12:81–121, 1984.
30. Komi, P. V.: The stretch-shortening cycle and human power output. *In* Jones, N. L., McCartney, N. and McConas, A. J. (eds.): Human Muscle Power. Champaign, Illinois, Human Kinetics, 1986, pp. 27–39.
31. Kroemer, K. H.: An isoinertial technique to assess individual lifting capability. Hum. Factors 25:493–506, 1983.
32. Lance, B. M., and Chaffin, D. B.: The effect of prior muscle exertions on simple movements. Hum. Factors 13:355–362, 1971.
33. Langrana, N. A., Lee, C. K., Alexander, H. and Mayott, C. W.: Quantitative assessment of back strength using isokinetic testing. Spine 9:287–290, 1984a.
34. Langrana, N., and Lee, C.: Isokinetic evaluation of trunk muscles. Spine 9:171–175, 1984b.
35. Magora, A.: Investigation of the relation between low back pain and occupation 3 physical requirements: Sitting, standing, and weight lifting. Indust. Med. Surg. 41:5–9, 1972.
36. Marras, W. S., King, A. I., and Joynt, R. L.: Measurements of the loads on the lumbar spine under isometric and isokinetic conditions. Spine 9:176–187, 1984.
37. Marras, W. S., Rangarajulu, S. L., and Lavender, S. A.: Trunk loading and expectation. Ergonomics 30:551–562, 1987.
38. McNeill, T., Warwick, D., Andersson, G., and Schultz, A.: Trunk strength in attempted flexion, extension, and lateral bending in healthy subjects and patients with low-back disorders. Spine 5:529–538, 1980.
39. Mital, A., and Karwoski, W.: Use of Simulated Job Dynamic Strength (SJDS) in Screening Workers for Manual Lifting Task. Proceedings of Human Factors Society, 29th annual meeting, p. 513, 1985.
40. Nachemson, A.: The possible importance of the psoas muscle for stabilization of the lumbar spine. Acta Orthop. Scand. 39:47–57, 1968.
41. Nachemson, A., and Lindh M: Measurement of abdominal and back muscle strength with and without pain. Scand. J. Rehabil. Med. 1:60–65, 1969.
42. Nicolaisen, T., and Jorgensen, K.: Trunk strength, back muscle endurance and low-back trouble. Scand. J. Rehabil. Med. 17:121–127, 1985.
43. Nordin, M., Kahanovitz, N., Verderame, R., et al.: Normal trunk muscle strength and endurance in women and the effect of electrical stimulation. Part 1: Normal endurance and trunk muscle strength in 101 women. Spine 12:105–111, 1987.
44. Norkin, C., and Levange, P.: Joint Structure and Function: A Comprehensive Analysis. Philadelphia, F. A. Davis, 1983.
45. Ortengren, R., and Andersson, G.: Electromyographic studies of trunk muscles with special reference to functional anatomy of lumbar spine. Spine 2:44–52, 1977.
46. Ostering, R., Bates, B., and James, S.: Isokinetic and isometric torque relationship. Arch. Phys. Med. Rehabil. 58:254–259, 1977.
47. Ottoson, D.: Physiology of the Nervous System. New York, Oxford University Press, 1983.
48. Parnianpour, M., Nordin, M., Kahanovitz, N., and Frankel, V. H.: The triaxial coupling of torque generation of trunk muscles during isometric exertions and the effect of fatiguing isoinertial movements on the motor output and movement patterns. Spine 13:982–992, 1988.
49. Parnianpour, M., Nordin, M., Brisson, P., et al.: The effects of isoinertial fatiguing trunk axial rotation on the parameters of motor output and movement patterns (unpublished data), 1988.
50. Parnianpour, M., Nordin, M., Brisson, P., et al.: The effects of isoinertial fatiguing trunk lateral bending on the parameters of motor output and movement patterns (abstr.) I.S.S.L.S., Kyoto, Japan, 1989.
51. Parnianpour, M.: The Effect of Fatiguing Isoinertial Flexion and Extension of Trunk on the Motor Output and Movement Patterns. Doctoral dissertation, New York University, New York, 1987.
52. Parnianpour, M., Nordin, M., Moritz, U., and Kahanowitz, N.: Correlation Between Different Tests of Trunk Strength. *In* Buckle, P. (ed.): Musculoskeletal Disorders at Work. New York, Taylor & Francis, 1987.
53. Rissanen, P. M.: The surgical anatomy and pathology of the supraspinous and interspinous ligaments of the lumbar spine with special references to ligament ruptures. Acta Orthop. Scand. 46(Suppl.):1960.
54. Rodgers, M. M., and Cavanagh, P. R.: Glossary of biomechanical terms, concepts and units. Phys. Ther. 64:1886–1902, 1984.
55. Smidt, G. L., Amundsen, L. R., and Dostal, W. F.: Muscle strength at the trunk. The Journal of Occupational and Sports Physical Therapy 1:165–170, 1980.

56. Smidt, G., Herin, T., Amundsen, L., et al.: Assessment of abdominal and back extensor function. Spine 8:211–219, 1983.
57. Suzuki, N., and Endo, S.: A quantitative study of trunk muscle strength and fatigability in the low-back-pain syndrome. Spine 8:69–74, 1983.
58. Thorstensson, A., and Nilsson, J.: Trunk muscle strength during constant velocity movements. Scand. J. Rehabil. Med. 14:61– 68, 1982.
59. Troup, J. D. G., Martin, J. W., and Lloyd, D. C.: Back pain in industry: A prospective survey. Spine 6:61–69, 1981.
60. Wilder, D. G., Pope, M. H., Seroussi, R. E., and Dimnet, J.: Sudden unstable rotation responses to an overload in the lumbar spine. Proceedings of International Society of the Study of the Lumbar Spine, 1987, p. 76.

INDUSTRIAL LOW BACK PAIN: A PRACTICAL APPROACH

Dan M. Spengler
David P. Guy

Complaints of low back pain result in a significant loss of time from productive activity among employees. As a result of the time loss, industry suffers major financial losses. Not only must the company provide compensation and medical costs for the individual employee; in most instances, another worker must be hired to replace the injured worker. In the United States, costs associated with the low back problem have been estimated to exceed $30 billion per annum. Many authors have highlighted the significance of the problem; few, however, have proposed solutions.[1–4, 11–15] Here we provide a rational approach to the management of back-injured employees in industry.

We believe that the best strategy for the management of employees who incur low back injury or, perhaps more accurately stated, develop low back pain, is based on early assessment, diagnosis, and treatment.[9] Deyo has reported that the vast majority of employees who incur low back pain should be able to resume work within 48 hours.[6] The great majority of low back events cannot be classified within a specific diagnostic subset. The term *idiopathic low back pain,* which reflects the lack of an anatomically specific focus, can serve as an appropriate, commonly used, nonspecific diagnosis. Specific diagnoses such as herniated lumbar disc, vertebral compression fracture, and lumbar segmental instability, are easily described and can be quantified through well-established diagnostic criteria. Nonspecific (idiopathic) low back pain problems are the focus of this subchapter. This focus is justified because the majority of financial resources are directed to these nonspecific problems, rather than to specific diagnoses. In a recent review of Tennessee workers' compensation data, we found that 90% of the injuries and 40% of the costs were classified as nonspecific.[7]

The natural history of low back pain has a most favorable prognosis; most employees are able to return to work in a matter of days.[6, 16, 17] Patients with radicular complaints constitute a separate diagnostic subset and will not be considered here. Even when sciatica is present, the majority of patients resume full activity within 30 days.[10]

Treatment of employees who experience a low back event should be directed to promptly return to activity. Appropriate management consists of antiinflammatory medications (e.g., salicylates, nonsteroidal anti-inflammatory drugs [NSAIDs]), short-term rest (2 to 3 days), and early return to work. Trunk flexion and extension exercises may be initiated within the first week. An aerobic activity of choice is also recommended. Appropriate aerobic activities include bicycling, walking, swimming, jogging, and/or running. A return to work can often be facilitated by a transitional job program within the company. Given the widespread success of the above programs, why is low back pain such a significant problem in the industrial setting? The answer to this question is multifaceted. All involved parties contribute to the expanding nature of the back pain problem. These parties include the doctor, employer, employees, ancillary health care personnel (such as the ubiquitous rehabilitation nurse), the insurance carriers, and of course the attorneys who represent the various parties.[8]

Hadler has elucidated the concept of "disability contest," which results when the involved parties become entangled in attempting to resolve a specific claim.[8] The contentious nature of the dispute has more to do with the prolongation of the problem than does the nocioceptive or tissue damage factor as determined by a careful medical assessment. Thus, the problem of low back disability reflects the underlying political, social, legal, and economic climate more than it does a medical disorder. Attempting to resolve the problem through aggressive medical treatment frequently results in overtreatment, with a genuinely adverse impact on recovery. Overtreatment reinforces illness behavior, because the patient becomes convinced of having a serious medical malady as a result of the multiple treatments provided by the health care professionals.

Results of treatment are difficult to extract from the voluminous literature, much of which consists of non–peer-reviewed anecdotal events. Deyo has chided our profession for lacking attention to detail when analyzing clinical results and relating the outcome to the medical intervention utilized.[5] Because the natural history of low back pain is so short-lived, the main objective of treatment should be to avoid inhibiting nature's rapid resolution of the problem.

Our approach to this problem centers on prompt recognition and early intervention. The employee who reports a low back event is immediately directed to a triage area, which is staffed by skilled, trained physical therapists and registered nurses. If objective findings are identified on physical examination, the employee is referred on an urgent or emergent basis to a participating orthopedist. If no objective findings are discovered, the employee is directed back to work, either to full duty or to modified duty contingent upon his or her particular work tasks. Thus, the supervisors who oversee the injured employees must be aware of this approach and the reasons for early work return. Refusing to accept the employee back until he or she is 100% symptom free will result in gradually increasing alienation, with an unlimited potential for the loss of valuable employees as well as an enormous financial loss for both the employer and employee.

Employees who for whatever reason do not resume work within 30 days should be evaluated in a very thorough fashion. Comprehensive assessment in our center includes a careful examination with a review of the initial event. In addition, plain radiographs and a magnetic resonance scan are obtained. A functional capacity assessment is completed, including a multiaxis back testing device. Psychologic testing and evaluation are also performed. Of equal importance is the comprehensive vocational assessment that establishes work-place skills and job capabilities. Based on this early comprehensive assessment, we believe that the vast majority of employees can be appropriately classified and that specific interventions can be recommended to facilitate return to work. Employees who are amplifying symptoms can be identified, and return to work recommended, on a purely objective basis.[15] Employees who have clear-cut disc disorders can also be managed with job modification or other intervention, depending on the specific circumstances.

We are very optimistic about the future of the employee with a low back injury.[10, 15] The natural history reflects a high rate of symptom resolution. We hope that the contentious nature of the resolution of many of these problems will be averted through education directed to the legislative and judicial branches of government, and that huge settlements for nonspecific low back events will become a matter of historical interest. Perhaps low back pain will be viewed in the year 2000 as the common cold is today, a malady that is a nuisance, but one that will surely pass.

References

1. Beals, R. K., and Hickman, N. W.: Industrial injuries to the back and extremities. J. Bone Joint Surg. 54A:1593–1611, 1972.
2. Bigos, S. J., Spengler, D. M., et al.: Back injuries in industry: A retrospective study. II. Injury factors. Spine 11:246–251, 1986.
3. Bigos, S. J., Spengler, D. M., et al.: Back injuries in industry: A retrospective study. III. Employee-related factors. Spine 11:252–256, 1986.
4. Bigos, S. J., Battié, M. C.: Acute care to prevent back disability. Clin. Orthop. 221:121–130, 1987.
5. Deyo, R. A.: Conservative treatment for low back pain. J.A.M.A. 250:1057–1062, 1983.

6. Deyo, R. A., Diehl, A. K., and Rosenthal, M.: How many days bed rest for acute low back pain? A randomized clinical trial. N. Engl. J. Med. 315:1064–1070, 1986.
7. Federspiel, C. F., Guy, D. P., Kane, M. A., and Spengler, D. M.: Expenditures for back injuries in the workplace: A statewide study of worker's compensation (in press).
8. Hadler, N. M.: Legal ramifications of the medical definition of back disease. Ann. Intern. Med. 89:992, 1978.
9. Mayer, T. G., Gatchel, R. J., et al.: A prospective short-term study of chronic low back pain patients utilizing novel objective functional measurement. Pain 25:53–68, 1986.
10. Nachemson, A. L.: Work for all, for those with low back pain as well. Clin. Orthop. 179:77–85, 1983.
11. Snook, S. H., and Webster, B. S.: The cost of disability. Clin. Orthop. 221:77–84, 1987.
12. Spengler, D. M ., Bigos, S. J., et al.: Back injuries in industry: A retrospective study, I. Overview and cost analysis. Spine 11:241–245, 1986.
13. Spengler, D. M.: Chronic low back pain: the team approach. Clin. Orthop. 179:71–76, 1983.
14. Spengler, D. M.: Fundamentals of pain: A review for orthopaedists. Orthop. Surg. (update series) 3:1–7, 1984.
15. Spengler, D. M.: Do the bells toll for idiopathic low back pain? One author's opinion. Iowa Orthop. J. 7:20–21, 1987.
16. Waddell, G.: Clinical assessment of lumbar impairment. Clin. Orthop. 221:110–120, 1987.
17. Waddell, G., Main, C. J., et al.: Chronic low-back pain, psychologic distress, and illness behavior. Spine 9:209–213, 1983.
18. Waddell, G., McCulloch, J. A., et al.: Nonorganic physical signs in low-back pain. Spine 5:117–125, 1980.

19 □ Failed Lumbar Surgery: Principles of Management

Henry La Rocca

In reviewing 2,504 patients in whom lumbar disc excision had been performed by a total of 39 orthopedic surgeons, Spangfort[19] found that complete relief of both sciatica and low back pain was achieved in 60.2% of the total group. Furthermore, the rate of persisting low back pain was 31.5%, a figure in agreement with a number of other reports cited. Weber[23] presented the results of a prospective study of 270 patients undergoing similar surgery performed by neurosurgeons and noted that at the final follow-up examination 4 years after surgery, 58% of the patients were completely free of back pain and 72% were completely relieved of sciatica. Of the entire group, 15% had residual pain described as "considerable." Accepting these figures as universally applicable, one must infer that lumbar disc excision is curative of all pain in 60% of patients undergoing the operation. Therefore, 40% have residual problems, and 15% fall into the unfortunate category known as the *failed back.*

The widely accepted estimate of the number of surgical cases of disc excision in the United States is 200,000 per annum. If 15% of these are failures, then 30,000 people per year enter the group with failed lumbar surgery. The ravages inflicted by this problem include chronic suffering and disability in the individual and heavy burdens upon the family, the employer, the insurance companies, the health care delivery system, and ultimately society itself. This extraordinarily costly problem must be examined closely and in detail if progress is to be made in reducing its magnitude.

It must be stated herewith that these figures are not an indictment against surgery itself, for without it the number of chronically disabled people would be far greater than the 15% figure employed in the calculations. As shown by Dzioba and Doxey, when surgery is indicated and recommended but delayed by the patient, there is only a 20% probability of a satisfactory outcome 1 year later, as opposed to a 65% probability in a group having the surgery.[3] Instead, every effort must be expended to improve the surgical results to the maximum consistent with the disease process.

RESULTS OF INITIAL SURGERY

When one strictly adheres to the indications for disc excision proposed by Hirsch and Nachemson[9] in 1963, results better than those cited above can be produced. These authors showed that if there are root tension signs, neurologic deficits, and a positive corroborating myelogram, then up to 96% of patients will benefit from such surgery. Given those clinical findings, definite herniation of the intervertebral disc will be found at surgery, and addressing it will almost always resolve the sciatica. Hence, the

Table 1 □ Summary of Results of Disc Operation

AUTHOR	PATIENTS WITH RELIEF Sciatica (%)	PATIENTS WITH RELIEF Back Pain (%)
Mixter and Barr[15]	77	52
Falconer et al.[5]	72	65
Spurling and Grantham[20]	79	40
O'Connell[17]	77	60
Jackson[10]	83	53
Weber[23]	72	58

Modified from Nelson, M. A.: Surgery of the spine. *In* Jayson, M. (ed.): The Lumbar Spine and Back Pain. London, Pitman, 1976, pp. 467–509.

operation is an excellent one for relieving sciatic pain. A review of several other major series (Table 1) shows that the operation has a poorer record for the management of back pain. In these series, relief of sciatica was achieved in approximately 80% of the patients, but relief of back pain was accomplished in only about 55% of patients. The inescapable conclusion is that the disc excision operation is not a good treatment for back pain alone. As a corollary, one cannot escape the fact that intervertebral disc herniation is not the cause of most cases of lumbar pain.

In a poignantly honest recent report, Rish[18] described the kind of results he experienced in conducting a private neurosurgical practice. Reviewing 205 of his own cases, he indicated that patients in the following four diagnostic categories presented for surgical management: single-level herniated nucleus pulposus, herniated nucleus pulposus with lumbar spondylosis, spinal stenosis with lumbar spondylosis, and miscellaneous other problems. These patients were treated with four different types of lumbar surgery, including laminotomy with disc excision, disc excision with foraminotomy, posterior lumbar interbody fusion, and decompressive laminectomy. The overall results were satisfactory in 64%. They were poor in 24% and were considered to show failure in an additional 12%. Of the total group, 18% required additional surgery. Failure occurred at the L4–L5 level five times more frequently than at L5–S1.

These data all indicate that lumbar surgery for relief of pain, as currently practiced, is not nearly as effective as surgery for correction of spinal deformity, internal fixation of fracture, or replacement of deranged appendicular joints. In order to attempt to achieve the same high order of excellent results common to these latter three types of surgery, current practice must be analyzed for deficiencies and modified with appropriate proven techniques either currently available or yet to be developed.

REASONS FOR FAILURE

The initial wave of enthusiasm for the disc excision operation began to wane somewhat by the 1950s when the number of unacceptable results began to demand pause for reflection. Armstrong[1] in 1951 published an analysis of the problem, indicating 12 causes of failure (Table 2). The first three are failures resulting from error, on the part of the surgeon, in locating the lesion, and in defining the total problem. The fourth and fifth causes are recurrent herniation at the same level and side of the original lesion, as well as the occurrence of a new herniation at a different location, following an initial period of improvement.

The sixth, seventh, and eighth recognized causes of failure result from nerve root injury. A root may be traumatized as it is being

Table 2 □ Causes of Failure of Disc Excision

1. Failure to locate the lesion
2. Failure to recognize a double lesion
3. Failure to address a bilateral lesion
4. Recurrent herniation
5. New herniation
6. Root damage
7. Root adherence
8. Permanent root changes
9. Damage to articular facets
10. Arthritis of the intervertebral joint
11. Infection
12. Damage to dura, cauda equina

From Armstrong, J. R.: The causes of unsatisfactory results from the operative treatment of lumbar disc lesions. J. Bone Joint Surg. 33B:31–35, 1951.

Table 3 □ Causes of Failure in the Disc Operation

CAUSES	FREQUENCY (N)
Different site of herniation	16
Recurrence at same site	17
Root adhesion	24
Missed herniations	4
Migrated fragments	5
Infection of disc	1

Modified from Greenwood, J., McGuire, T. H., Kimbell, F.: A study of the causes of failure in the herniated intervertebral disc operation. J. Neurosurg. 9:15–20, 1952.

separated from the herniated disc material or if it is retracted too vigorously. Furthermore, failure to protect the root, as completely as possible, from scarring can lead to adherence of the root at the site of disc excision or to the formation of the laminectomy membrane.[12] Additional root damage may result from delay in the performance of surgery when the root is compressed or stretched by disc tissue for too long a period. In all three instances, a permanent radiculopathy may result, giving rise to chronic pain.

The ninth and tenth causes of failure of disc excision are related to damage inflicted to the apophyseal joint during surgery or to activation of arthritic changes in these joints by poorly timed rehabilitative efforts in the early postoperative weeks. The eleventh cause is wound infection that may lead to septic spondylitis or to extensive scarring about the nerve roots. Damage to the dura or the cauda equina from poor surgical technique yielding possibly catastrophic results completes the list.

From the neurosurgical literature, the paper of Greenwood and colleagues[8] addressed the causes of failure in the herniated disc operation. Sixty-seven patients returned for a second lumbar operation, and the causes of failure were found to be herniation at a site different from the original problem in 16 patients, recurrent herniation at the same site as the previous surgery in 17, adhesions or bony encroachment in 24, and missed or migrated fragments in 8 (Table 3). Results of the second operation indicate excellent salvage with recurrent or new herniation, but very poor outcomes in the face of neural adhesion.

In 1971, Macnab[14] analyzed the cause of persisting nerve root involvement following initial surgery in 68 patients (Table 4). His report is invaluable because it points out that there are causes other than disc herniation, which were not addressed at the initial surgery because of failure to recognize them. These include pedicular kinking of the root, facet impingement upon the root, and lateral stenosis. Furthermore, Macnab indicated that a herniation may be located more lateral to the site of previous exploration and that fragments may migrate into a foramen that was left unexplored. Echoing the Greenwood report, he also demonstrated that neural adhesions may cause significant problems that are only poorly relieved by repeat surgery for adhesion lysis.

In a penetrating review analyzing failure of lumbar disc surgery, Fager and Friedberg in 1980 studied 105 cases of failed spinal surgery in which fusion had been performed in only 10.[6] The surgery in question, therefore, is disc excision. Those authors reviewed the preoperative records and clinical studies and determined that in 68% of the patients surgery was not indicated, owing to such factors as the absence of preoperative leg pain and the presence of normal myelograms. The patients had been subjected to disc excision without adequate evidence of disc herniation. Failure could have been

Table 4 □ The Cause of Radiculopathy in Negative Disc Explorations

PATHOLOGY	FREQUENCY (N)	SATISFACTORY RESULTS (%)*
Foraminal migration	9	88
Pedicular kinking	12	91
Facet impingement	19	84
Spinal stenosis	8	87
Lateral herniation	2	100
Root adhesion	6	0
No abnormality detected	12	50

*Percentages are given only for emphasis; the numbers in each group are too small to indicate anything but trends.

From Macnab, I.: Negative disc exploration. An analysis of the causes of nerve-root involvement in 68 patients. J. Bone Joint Surg. 53A:891–903, 1971.

predicted in this group. When surgery was found to have been justifiable, the reasons for failure were found to be a retained disc fragment, surgery at the wrong level, inadequate decompression from limited exposure, and scar formation.

Regardless of the problem of poor patient selection arising from psychosocial disorders, these four reports indicate a number of factors that, if eliminated, would permit an immediate improvement in the results of disc excision. First and foremost should be an awareness that disc excision is not an acceptable treatment for back pain alone. It is highly effective if the clinical problem is sciatic pain that is more severe than back pain and accompanied by root tension signs, neurologic deficit, and positive visualization of the disc herniation with contemporary diagnostic studies. Such studies can allow a definition of the total pathologic process preoperatively so that migrated fragments, lateral stenosis, facet impingement, and other causes of root entrapment will not be missed during the operation. Furthermore, meticulous attention to technique during surgery can reduce the failure rate arising from error. Being certain of the correct level requires an adequate incision so that the sacrum can be unquestionably identified, permitting accurate counting upward. In the absence of this certainty, placement of a needle for radiographic verification of level becomes mandatory, as is also the case when there are segmentation anomalies in the lower lumbar spine. With the level accurately localized, an adequate laminotomy should then be performed to permit an approach to the disc lateral to the emerging nerve root. This will facilitate retrieving the herniated material without undue retraction of the root. More liberal exposure is required when the lesion extends above and beyond the disc herniation. Partial facetectomy, foraminotomy, and decompression by removal of bone from the inferior lamina laterally may be necessary to obtain adequate root clearance. The disc excision itself should be performed through a clean annular incision that leaves behind no tags to which the root might adhere. To guard against recurrent herniation, all degenerate nuclear material should be extracted. Bleeding within the canal should be controlled with bipolar cautery because hematoma generates and guides the formation of an adhering scar.[12] Finally, the laminotomy defect should be covered with an interposition membrane of either free fat grafts or an absorbable gelatin sponge (Gelfoam) (the preferred covering is still a debatable topic). Wound drainage and prophylactic antibiotic coverage help guard against the complication of infection.

RESULTS OF REPEAT SURGERY

Beyond analysis of the causes of failure of intervertebral disc excision, another fruitful source of information for decision-making in the event of failed lumbar surgery is an awareness of the results of repeat surgery. The thesis here is that if one knows the procedures capable of effective salvage, then the application of such procedures at the time of the first surgery might yield more favorable outcomes. Furthermore, when presented with the patient who has already failed, the surgeon is better advised as to how to proceed.

An early report from the Mayo Clinic[11] reviewed the result of treatment of a group of 54 patients who had two prior unsuccessful disc excision operations. Half of these people were treated conservatively with an improvement rate of only 50%. The other half were treated surgically with repeat disc excision and spinal fusion as their third operation. The results of the third operation were acceptable in 13 of 15 patients in whom a frank protrusion of the disc was found. On the other hand, a favorable outcome occurred in only 5 of 12 patients in whom no frank protrusion was identified. This report is important information for it indicates that if there is a correctable pathologic condition, repeat surgery can still be effective. It also suggests that fusion should be part of a repeat procedure.

The study of Greenwood and coworkers[8] referred to above indicated satisfactory outcomes in repeat surgery for removal of a new herniation at another location or removal of a recurrent herniation at the same location. Root decompression is also capable of securing a satisfactory outcome (Table 5). Rhizotomy is mentioned as yielding 66% satisfactory results. The authors pointed out that bony prominences that compromise the nerve root should be leveled by gently hammering them down. They comment that the worst results were obtained in patients with persisting back pain without sciatica. Once

Table 5 □ Results of Repeat Surgery

PROCEDURE	SATISFACTORY RESULT (%)
Root decompression	81
Rhizotomy	66
Removal of new herniation	74
Removal of recurrent herniation	100

From Greenwood, J., McGuire, T. H., and Kimbell, F.: A study of the causes of failure in the herniated intervertebral disc operation. J. Neurosurg. 9:15–20, 1952.

again, the indications are that repeat surgery can be successful in the presence of a definite correctable lesion. Epstein and colleagues[4] echo this experience, demonstrating that surgical results in patients with new or recurrent herniations, treated with disc excision and root decompression at repeat surgery, can compare favorably with the response to the first surgical procedure.

In the orthopedic literature, the report of Barr and colleagues[2] reviewed 120 patients who underwent repeat surgery following prior failure. Their material can be sorted into three groups. In the first, there were 67 patients with either recurrent herniations or unstable segments. They were treated by excision of the recurrent fragment and by fusion. Favorable outcomes occurred in 79%. In the second group, patients were treated for failure of prior fusion with canal exploration and fusion repair. Results in this group were quite poor, with only 47% improving. The finding of poor results from attempted repair of the fusion in its own bed are repeated throughout the past literature to the present. The third group of patients was treated for infection, retained foreign material, or a tumor missed at previous surgery, and their results were poorest, with improvement occurring only in 20%.

A new dimension was added to the orthopedic literature with the realization that certain psychologic factors exerted a negative effect on surgical outcomes and that these factors could be measured preoperatively and used as predictors of such outcomes. This information has obvious bearing on the decision-making process in both initial and repeat surgery. Wiltse and Rocchio[22] evaluated psychologic testing with the Minnesota Multiphasic Personality Inventory (MMPI) and the surgeons' rating of the psychogenic component of the patient's pain prior to administering chemonucleolysis to patients considered to be candidates for disc excision. They found that the best predictors of the symptomatic result were the hypochondriasis and hysteria scales of the MMPI. If the scores were 85 or above, the chances of a good result were only 10%, whereas if they were no higher than 45, the chances of good or excellent recovery rose to 90%. Comparable results were obtained in a smaller group of patients who underwent laminectomy with disc excision. The strength of prediction of outcome could be augmented by the surgeon's preoperative assessment of the degree to which the patient's symptoms were thought to be psychogenic. When the surgeon preoperatively assesses no apparent psychogenic component, results are better then when he or she assesses a predominant or a severe psychogenic component.

Another important finding from the study of Wiltse and Rocchio was that the hypochondriasis and hysteria scores rose proportionately as the number of back operations increased. This finding may mean either that repeat surgery causes the increase in these scales or that persons with initially high scales are more likely to present for repeat surgery.

The reports describing the results of repeat surgery given above are generally somewhat optimistic regarding expected outcomes. A much more pessimistic posture is taken by Waddell and associates who reported on results of repeat surgery performed on 103 patients who were on workers' compensation.[21] This group of patients differs from those in previous studies that reported on the experience of specialized units primarily treating noncompensation patients. Hence, the effect of the issue of compensation could be isolated. All patients were personally evaluated by an independent orthopedic surgeon who was not present at the surgery. In the follow-up assessment, the MMPI was completed by 80 patients, although not by the remainder, owing to language or reading difficulties. Of the group of compensation patients who underwent one lumbar procedure, 15% had a second operation, 6% a third, and 1.4% a fourth. The success rate of the second operation was 50%, whereas 20% of the patients considered themselves to be in worse condition. Following a third operation the success rate was 30%, and 25% of patients considered their conditions to be worse. After the fourth operation success was only 20%, and 45% of patients considered their conditions to be worse. At the time they were evaluated, 97% of these patients had persisting back pain, 77% had reduced lumbar motion, 39% had persistent neurologic deficit, and 6% had root tension signs. Of those tested psychologically, 65% demonstrated findings not previously recognized, including anxiety, depression, hypochondriasis, and conversion. There was a strong correlation between psychologic factors and poor results of repeat surgery. No determination could be made as to whether these psychologic problems were the cause or the effect of the surgical failure.

Fewer than 40% of men and 23% of women undergoing a second operation resumed employment. The figures declined progressively as the number of surgeries increased.

Of 68 patients undergoing a repeat operation during the calendar year 1975 (Table 6), satisfactory results were achieved in three of four patients undergoing excision of a disc at a new level, consistent with earlier reports. Approximately one third of patients undergoing either decompression alone or fusion alone experienced satisfactory results. The combination of decompression and fusion raised the successful outcome rate to 50%. Consistent with the figures of Barr and coworkers,[2] the results of surgery for pseudarthrosis repair were almost uniformly poor.

The causes of failure of surgery in the 103 patients are listed as follows: inadequate indications, technical error, iatrogenic complications, recurrent disc prolapse, and psychologic factors. Regarding repeat surgery, the factors associated with successful outcomes were a pain-free interval of 6 months or more, sciatica more severe than back pain, and definite recurrence of disc herniation.

Table 6 □ Effect of Prodecure of Repeat Operation on Result

PROCEDURE	SUCCESSFUL RESULT/NUMBER OF CASES
Disc excision	3/4
Decompression	10/36
Fusion	3/9
Decompression and fusion	6/12
Pseudarthrosis repair	1/7

From Waddell, G., Kummel, E. G., Lotto, W. N., et al.: Failed lumbar disc surgery and repeat surgery following industrial injuries. J. Bone Joint Surg. 61A:201–207, 1979.

Factors that mitigated against a successful outcome included the following: scarring and neurolysis, previous infection, repair of pseudarthrosis, and adverse psychologic problems.

Waddell and coworkers[21] comment that 11 comparative published studies indicated that any form of treatment of low back pain in compensation patients produced results 30% poorer than in noncompensation patients. However, they indicate that with rigid criteria, successful results are possible, even after two or more previous procedures. They recommend that repeat surgery should be performed only if the reason for failure can be clearly identified and confidently overcome at the next operation. In the event of a new disc herniation at a previously unexplored level, simple disc excision is advised. In the absence of that, decompression of the identified lesion site combined with fusion offers the greatest chance of improvement, and in these cases the bilateral intertransverse fusion is favored. The authors conclude that the most important element required for success in this difficult group of patients is rigorous selection accompanied by strict adherence to proper surgical indications.

Appearing in the same year as the report of Waddell and colleagues was that of Finnegan and associates.[7] They studied 67 patients who had undergone multiple lumbar operative procedures and who were evaluated regarding pain relief for up to 4 years after the most recent operation. These patients had undergone a variety of surgical procedures, including disc excision, decompression, or neurolysis alone, or the same procedures combined with fusion. Surgery was performed for one or more of five diagnostic categories: fibrosis, new disc herniation, pseudarthrosis, instability, and spinal stenosis. The overall results were good in 8, fair in 46, and poor in 13. Over 80% of the patients considered the repeat procedure to have been worthwhile. Better results were achieved with decompression of stenosis, excision of a herniated disc, and fusion of an unstable segment. The poorest results were obtained in surgery for fibrosis or for repair of pseudarthrosis. Whereas all patients had a total disability before the repeat surgery, 19 had no disability at follow-up, and 31 had a partial disability. These results indicate a significant benefit to society.

When there was no compensation or litigation the rate of success of repeat surgery was considerably better (94%) than when there was one (37%).

The data of all these authors showed the following factors to favor a successful outcome: a pain-free interval of 1 year, complete myelographic blocks, operative findings of true herniation of the disc, and positive evidence of instability. On the other hand, factors that mitigated against a successful outcome included the following five: neurolysis as the major objective of surgery; predominant fibrosis at operation; no pain-free interval; more than two previous operations; and psychologic problems, compensation, and litigation.

Lehmann and LaRocca[13] reviewed 36 cases of patients with prior surgery including 10 patients with prior fusion attempts, 8 of which failed. After appropriate assessment, the combined procedure of decompression and posterolateral fusion as later recommended by Waddell was applied to all 36. Before this surgery, the potentially correctable lesion was thought to be compressive radiculopathy in 18 patients, instability in 13, and pseudarthrosis in 5. The results as appraised by an independent orthopedic surgeon required symptomatic improvement, but it did not demand a return to work in an attempt to separate the variable of symptomatic improvement after repeat surgery from the social issue of return to work. As Greenwood and coworkers had noted earlier, many patients are improved but are classified as failures because they have not returned to work.[8]

Lehmann's and LaRocca's results according to the type of surgery were satisfactory in 74% when facetectomy and foraminotomy were carried out; in 61% with excision of a recurrent disc herniation; in 47% with neurolysis; and in only 37% with repair of a pseudarthrosis.

On the issue of pseudarthrosis, of the 21 patients of this series enjoying a satisfactory outcome, 17 had gone on to solid fusion, whereas 4 had not. In the group of 15 patients with unsatisfactory results, only 6 had gone on to solid fusion, and 9 had not. These figures are considered to indicate that with the posterolateral fusion technique, solid fusion is necessary for a satisfactory outcome. The results also point out the problem of attempting to secure solid fusion with repair of a pseudarthrosis in its own bed. All of the series quoted, including the presently discussed one, indicate that pseudarthrosis repair yields poor results. This most likely arises from high fusion repair failure rates and gives rise to the recommendation that some alternative technique to treat those with pseudarthrosis be attempted, instead of grafting the same bed alone. Such options would include anterior interbody fusion or repeat posterolateral grafting supplemented with internal fixation.

The results according to pathologic findings show that patients with definite compressive radiculopathy experienced a 67% satisfactory outcome, those with instability had a 58% satisfactory outcome (related to success of the fusion attempt), and those with pseudarthrosis had only a 20% satisfactory outcome rate. These results support the recommendation of Waddell and colleagues[21] that repeat lumbar surgery should include both decompression and fusion. The overall results are better than those of the Waddell study, even though many of the patients in this series were on compensation. Again, however, a return to work was not required in this series as it was in the other.

A curious finding in a small number of patients was that three of four patients who had four prior lumbar operations demonstrated satisfactory improvement. This supported Waddell's contention that if there is a definite correctable pathologic condition, repeat surgery can be effective.

APPROACH TO THE PATIENT WITH FAILED LUMBAR SURGERY

The preceding discussion pointed out reasons for the failure of initial lumbar surgery. These may be broadly categorized as follows: inadequate diagnostic appraisal before the surgery, technical error and iatrogenic complications, and poor patient selection. The most frequent and serious reason appears to be performing disc excision when the problem is back pain and not confirmed radiculopathy. The discussion of the results of repeat surgery provides a clear warning about the futility of attempting to manage neural adhesions by means of neurolysis, pseudarthroses with repair in the same bed, or any surgery in patients with significant and untreatable psychologic derangement.

On the other hand, it does point out that properly indicated repeat surgery can be successful in the presence of a correctable lesion ideally treated with decompression and fusion. These lessons must be brought to bear in the approach to the patient with failed lumbar surgery if the results are to be improved. Considerable expertise and experience in performing lumbar surgery seem to be a prerequisite for the surgeon who attempts such treatment.

Two determinations are of paramount importance in evaluating the patient with failed lumbar surgery. First, one must determine whether a correctable lesion is present, and second, one must appraise the patient's psychologic status. For the former, the full battery of contemporary diagnostic studies may have to be deployed. For the latter, a basic minimum of a pain drawing must be obtained to determine whether formal psychologic appraisal is necessary.

In the diagnostic studies, a detailed history and physical examination are required, and previous diagnostic studies and operative reports should ideally be part of this information. Radiographic assessment must include dynamic flexion and extension lateral views in order to assess spinal stability. The spinal canal and its subdivisions must be investigated with contrast-enhanced computed tomography (CT) in both the horizontal and sagittal planes. Magnetic resonance imaging (MRI) will have an increasing role in this kind of survey and will also indicate intervertebral disc degeneration and evidence of sepsis. Myelography can be useful, particularly in missed tumors, but in the postoperative patient it is often difficult to interpret because of the scarring phenomenon. Hence, when done it should be supplemented with the scanning procedures. This is especially the case because spinal stenosis may be masquerading as an arachnoiditis.

Full assessment of root function demands studying both the sensory and motor sides of the lumbar and upper sacral roots with somatosensory evoked potentials and electromyography. Nerve conduction velocity studies in the limb may demonstrate evidence of diabetic or other forms of neuropathy. The lower sacral roots must be investigated by visceral studies, including cystometrograms with bladder sphincter electromyography.

Pain-provocative diagnostic radiographic techniques are of the utmost importance for a full definition of the problem in these difficult patients. These would include discography, facet arthrography and blocking, and selective nerve root anesthetization. Each of these studies can identify a source of pain by provoking familiar pain. Furthermore, each can suggest whether permanent relief can be obtained by producing pain relief while the anesthetic agent is active. Such studies help plan the scope and detail of the intended repeat surgery. If the source of the pain can be identified as a correctable lesion, then the repeat surgery is likely to be of definite benefit. If the problem identified is nerve scarring, neurolysis has already been demonstrated to be ineffective, and the patient should instead be considered as a potential candidate for rhizotomy. Alternatively, the scarring may have provoked a reflex sympathetic dystrophy, which can be treated with sympathectomy.

As indicated earlier, the MMPI scores tend to rise with each successive back operation; hence, patients presenting for repeat surgery are likely to show distortions on the MMPI. This does not mean that a correctable lesion should not be operated on in every instance of distorted MMPI scores, but it does mean that special efforts at rehabilitation following repeat surgery may be necessary to restore the patient to a higher level of function. Treatment in a center for chronic pain following suitable surgical recovery time can increase the yield of favorable results in this difficult group of individuals.

If a thorough organic appraisal does not indicate an unequivocal correctable lesion, and if the psychologic appraisal is strongly abnormal, then obviously no repeat surgery would be useful and the patient should promptly be referred to a chronic pain center.

For patients on compensation or in litigation, the decision to proceed with repeat surgery must be made in light of knowing that results will be far less favorable than in patient not so involved. Clearly, this kind of decision should not even be entertained by the occasional spinal surgeon, who should defer any opinion in the matter by referring the patient to a center offering more expertise.

SUMMARY

In summary, the following statements can be made in regard to the management of failed lumbar surgery:

1. Failure to obtain relief of pain after an initial surgical procedure means that either the pathologic condition was not accurately identified or it was not treated appropriately.
2. Inappropriate treatment at the first surgery includes error in selecting the correct procedure for the problem (e.g., removing a disc that is not herniated) or error in the technical performance of the operation (e.g., wrong level, inadequate exposure).
3. Recurrent herniation after a long asymptomatic interval offers the best results in cases of repeat surgery.
4. A new herniation at another location offers results as good as those of a first operation.
5. Anything contributing to chronic radiculopathy may lead to an almost insoluble clinical problem. Such factors include excessive delay in securing root decompression, inadequate surgical decompression, damage to a root during surgery, and fibrosis of the root as a consequence of surgery.
6. In the presence of an identifiable and correctable pathologic condition, repeat surgery can yield acceptable results and can be worthwhile.
7. Psychosocial factors can undermine the effectiveness of the most expertly executed surgical procedure.
8. Repeat surgery yields diminishing returns as the number of procedures increases.
9. The scope of repeat surgery should be definitive; this most often means combining root decompression and spinal stabilization. The only exceptions are in the case of true recurrence of herniation after a long asymptomatic interval and that of the appearance of a new herniation at a different site. In these instances, disc excision alone may provide a satisfactory outcome as after the first operation.
10. Repeat surgery for the lysis of neural adhesions or for the repair of a pseudarthrosis in its own bed yields predictably poor results. In the case of neural fibrosis without residual root compression, neuroablation or augmentation might offer a more acceptable salvage. For pseudarthrosis, repair in a new bed or repair supplemented by internal fixation is recommended.
11. Repeat surgery should be avoided altogether by the occasional lumbar surgeon and by those who have limited training and experience.

References

1. Armstrong, J. R.: The causes of unsatisfactory results from the operative treatment of lumbar disc lesions. J. Bone Joint Surg. 33B:31–35, 1951.
2. Barr, J. S., Riseborough, E. J., and Freeman, P. A.: Failed surgery for low back and sciatic pain. J. Bone Joint Surg. 45A:1553, 1963.
3. Dzioba, R. D., and Doxey, N. C.: A prospective investigation into the orthopaedic and psychological predictors of outcome of first lumbar surgery following industrial injury. Spine 9:614–623, 1984.
4. Epstein, J. A., Lavine, L. S., and Epstein, B. S.: Recurrent herniation of lumbar intervertebral disc. Clin. Orthop. 52:169–178, 1967.
5. Falconer, M. A., McGeorge, M., and Beeg, M. C.: Surgery of lumbar intervertebral disc protrusions. Br. J. Surg. 35:225, 1947.
6. Fager, C. A., Friedberg, S. R.: Analysis of failures and poor results of lumbar spine surgery. Spine 5:87–94, 1980.
7. Finnegan, W. J., Fenlin, J. M., Marvel, J. P., et al: Results of surgical intervention in the symptomatic multiply operated back patient. J. Bone Joint Surg. 61A:1077–1082, 1979.
8. Greenwood, J., McGuire, T. H., and Kimbell, F.: A study of the causes of failure in the herniated intervertebral disc operation. J. Neurosurg. 9:15–20, 1952.
9. Hirsch, C., and Nachemson, A.: The reliability of lumbar disc surgery. Clin. Orthop. 29:189–195, 1963.
10. Jackson, R. K.: The long-term effects of wide laminectomy for lumbar disc excision. J. Bone Joint Surg. 53B:609–616, 1971.
11. Kelley, J. H., Voris, D. C., Svien, H. J., and Ghormley, R. K.: Multiple operations for protruded intervertebral discs. Proc. Staff Meet. Mayo Clin. 29:546–550, 1954.
12. LaRocca, H., and Macnab, I.: The laminectomy membrane: Studies in its evolution, characteristics, effects, and prophylaxis. J. Bone Joint Surg. 563:545–550, 1974.
13. Lehmann, T. R., and LaRocca, H.: Repeat lumbar surgery. A review of patients with failure from previous lumbar surgery treated with spinal canal exploration and lumbar spine fusion. Spine 6:615–619, 1981.
14. Macnab, I.: Negative disc exploration. An analysis of the causes of nerve-root involvement in 68 patients. J. Bone Joint Surg. 53A:891–903, 1971.
15. Mixter, W. J., and Barr, J. S.: Rupture of the intervertebral disc with involvement of the spinal canal. N. Engl. J. Med. 211:210–215, 1934.
16. Nelson, M. A.: Surgery of the spine. *In* Jayson, M. (ed.): The Lumbar Spine and Back Pain. London, Pitman, 1976, pp. 467–509.

17. O'Connell, J. E. A.: Protrusion of lumbar intervertebral discs. J. Bone Joint Surg. 33B:8–30, 1951.
18. Rish, B. L.: A critique of the surgical management of lumbar disc disease in a private neurosurgical practice. Spine 9:500–504, 1984.
19. Spangfort, E. V.: The lumbar disc herniation. Acta Orthop. Scand. (Suppl.):142, 1972.
20. Spurling, R. G., and Grantham, E. G.: The end results of surgery for ruptured lumbar intervertebral discs. J. Neurosurg. 6:57–64, 1949.
21. Waddell, G., Kummel, E. G., Lotto, W. N., et al.: Failed lumbar disc surgery and repeat surgery following industrial injuries. J. Bone Joint Surg. 61A:201–207, 1979.
22. Wiltse, L. L., and Rocchio, P. D.: Preoperative psychological tests as predictors of success of chemonucleolysis in the treatment of the low back syndrome. J. Bone Joint Surg. 57A:478–483, 1975.
23. Weber, H.: Lumbar disc herniation. A prospective study of prognostic factors including a controlled trial. J. Oslo City Hosp. 28:33–61, 91–113, 1978.

20 □ Adult Scoliosis

John P. Kostuik

Adult scoliosis has been defined as the presentation of scoliosis following skeletal maturity. Some definitions have included all scoliotic deformities that patients beyond the age of 20 years present for treatment.

Scoliosis in adults is of two basic types: the first has its onset before skeletal maturity, and the second arises de nouveau in adult life, secondary to osteoporosis, osteomalacia, or iatrogenic factors, such as multiple-level decompressions for spinal stenosis.

Our concern here is primarily the deformities that present in adult life but have an onset prior to skeletal maturity. However, many of the techniques and investigations described are equally applicable to all deformities, primary or secondary.

EPIDEMIOLOGY

Vanderpool and colleagues[34] in 1969 stated that 6% of adults over the age of 50 years showed radiographic evidence of scoliosis. They thought that most of these cases were attributable to compression fractures, osteoporosis, or osteomalacia.

Kostuik and Bentivoglio[9] in 1981, in a review of 5,000 intravenous pyelograms in adults, found an incidence of scoliosis of 3.9%. These were curves of 10 degrees or more; 86% of them were idiopathic. Dewar[3] found a 4% incidence of thoracic curves on routine preadmission chest x-ray studies performed in the 1950s in an adults-only hospital. The 3.9% incidence on the intravenous pyelograms were in lumbar and thoracolumbar areas, yielding an overall incidence of approximately 8%.

In the review of thoracolumbar and lumbar curves as reported by Kostuik and Bentivoglio,[9] the incidence of low back pain was 59%. This is approximately the same as the incidence of back pain in the general population. The group of 189 patients discovered to have scoliosis on intravenous pyelograms were matched for age, sex, and occupation with a similar group of 100 patients without scoliosis, who similarly had an intravenous pyelogram. The incidence of pain was the same in both populations. Of the patients presenting with pain, 44% had mild pain, 49% had moderate pain, and only 7% had severe pain. However, only 4% of the patients had curves of greater than 45 degrees. When one correlates pain with age, the pattern seems to follow a bell curve, and the majority of patients with pain are in the 6th, 7th, and 8th decades of life. Pain appeared to reach its maximum severity between 40 and 60 years of age, which corresponds to the maximum incidence of pain from spondylogenic or discogenic causes in the nonscoliotic population. When one correlates occupation and pain, there appears to be a distinct preference for lighter work by scoliotic patients, although only 21% of patients in this series of patients studied by intravenous pyelograms were aware that they had scoliosis. Drummond and coworkers[4] also have suggested that scoliotics prefer lighter work. The type of occupation was not a factor predisposing individuals to pain in this review, although those with jobs requiring heavier work seemed to be less able to cope and missed more time from work, or were more likely to be incapacitated. Patients with curves greater than 45 degrees had a statistically more significant degree of incapacitating pain than those with curves of less than 45 degrees. The increasing incapacity due to pain with greater curves together with an increasing severity of pain with increasing age tends to suggest that curves of 45 degrees or greater at the end of growth will tend to become more clinically significant with increasing age. For those with lumbar and thoracolumbar curves, pain was more noticeable with the more severe curves. In attempting to correlate pain with plain radiographic changes, all patients with radiographic changes of degenerative processes of the apex of curves also demonstrated similar changes at the lumbosacral junction. Facet sclerosis correlated with a history of pain in 64% of patients. The presence of osteophytes bore little relationship to pain.

A 100% correlation between degenerative changes of the lumbosacral junction and apex of the curve clearly demonstrates the difficulty in assessing the origin of pain in the patient with scoliosis and points out the necessity for the use of discography and facet blocks in helping to assess pain in the disabled scoliotic. Only three patients who had pain provided a history of nerve root entrapment. This correlates with the incidence of nerve root entrapment in an initial review by this author[10] of 227 adult scoliotic treated operatively for pain in which the incidence of root pain was only 2.2% (five patients). In the author's experience, root pain in the scoliotic is uncommon. This is probably because of the slow adaptive changes that occur as a scoliotic curve progresses. Conversely, referred pain above the knee anteriorly must be differentiated from root pain in the distribution of the femoral nerve.

Nachemson[24] found a similar incidence of pain among scoliotics, although the incidence of pain was less than in the population study of Kostuik and Bentivoglio.[9]

Simmons and coworkers[8, 28] in studies of patients requiring operative intervention have shown that radicular symptoms may arise in the compensatory curve below a thoracolumbar curve and that these symptoms may show a marked improvement following correction of the major curve via anterior instrumentation. In the author's experience, this procedure has been less successful.

Collis and Ponsetti,[2] Kostuik and Bentivoglio,[9] Nilsonne and Lundgren,[26] Ponseti,[27] and Stagnara and coworkers,[30–33] among others, have shown that curves in the adult may progress and that frequently these same curves are painful. Recent work by Weinstein and Ponseti[36] has shown etiologic factors that are responsible for continued progression in adult life. Thoracic curves between 50 and 75 degrees at skeletal maturity increased by an average of 30 degrees during a long-term follow-up period. Thoracolumbar curves 50 to 75 degrees at skeletal maturity increased 22.3 degrees over 40 years. In the lumbar spine, curves in which the L5 vertebra was not well seated and apical rotation was greater than 33% progressed the most and had the worst prognosis. The curve with the worst prognosis in adult life is found in the young adult or adolescent who presents with an imbalanced lumbar curve or thoracolumbar curve in which the L5 vertebra is not parallel with the sacrum and the curve emanates from the lumbosacral junction. This curve presents the greatest technicologic difficulty for correction in later adult life, and I believe is often best treated at an earlier age if possible.

Other curves with a poor prognosis include the following: those in which the apex falls at the L2–L3 and L3–L4 area, those with a significant Grade-3 rotation, those that are imbalanced and have a secondary compensatory curve that is sharp and angular at the L4–S1 area. These curves may be treated and rebalanced by focusing on the compensatory curve at one or two levels, if these are the levels of pain, rather than treating for the more proximal curve of five to seven levels.

Cochran and coworkers[1] in a long-term anatomic and functional review of patients with adolescent idiopathic scoliosis treated by Harrington rod fusion have shown a proportionally greater incidence of degenerative changes the more distal the fusion performed in adolescence. There was an incidence of approximately 20% of degenerative changes with pain below fusions ending at L2, approximately 40% at L3, 60% at L4, and 80% at L5. Edgar and Mehta[7] similarly found an increased incidence of degenerative changes associated with pain at levels below a posterior fusion that extended to L3 or L4.

PATIENT EVALUATION

As it is for most patients with spinal problems, history is the primary means of evaluating a scoliotic patient.

A relevant family history of deformity may provide some indication of prognosis. For example, a near relative who has a progressive severe deformity and is older than the patient may supply some insight into the patient's future. The date of onset of the deformity should be considered but is not, in itself, usually important.

A history of curve progression can be determined by the history obtained from the patient or the relatives. For example a change in clothes, increasing rib hump, a loss of height, and a loss of waist line are relevant. Ideally, progression is best obtained by serial x-ray studies, but these are often not available, particularly in the case of thoracolumbar or lumbar curves, in which the deformity may not be noticed until adult life. The psychologic aspects of the patient's deformity should be considered. Many adults are reluctant to discuss their deformity from an aesthetic point of view, unless they are directly asked. Many of them have learned to live with their deformity, and it does not present a problem to them. Conversely, for a number of patients the deformity continues to play a significant psychologic role; this has been found in 10% of the patients in our series.

A pain questionnaire is important to help determine the location of pain. Pain may be apical or below the apex. Often the patient may indicate with the palm of the hand the source of pain. It is important to know the duration of pain and how it affects activities of daily living, social function, occupation, home life, and sexual life. It is important to know what aggravates the pain and what alleviates it. If the pain has a radicular nature that is suggestive of root irritation, it is important to obtain a history of this as well. Radicular pain may be related to the apex of the curve, and if the irritation is in the thoracic or thoracolumbar area, the pain may be costal in nature. Radicular pain may also arise from the compensatory curve in the case of a thoracolumbar curve, as noted by Simmons and coworkers.[8, 28] If the root irritation is in the lumbar area, pain may be referred into the lower extremities. True sciatica extends below the knee; pain above the knee may simply be referred, but it may be of nerve root origin as well.

A history of bowel and bladder function should be obtained. An associated spinal stenosis may initially present with bladder incontinence, particularly in females. Incontinence in the elderly woman is often attributable to spinal stenosis and not, as is commonly assumed, to the effects of childbearing. The history frequently reveals a recent onset of bladder incontinence.

Respiratory malfunction may be the presenting symptom in scoliosis but usually only in the paralytic or severe congenital curves. The patient may describe respiratory problems as shortness of breath in climbing stairs or during other activities, or simply as fatigue. Obtaining a good history of respiratory function is important. A review of 200 consecutive adults with idiopathic scoliosis by the author revealed no cases of severe dysfunction, even in curves of 100 degrees or more. Ventilation was often decreased, by as much as 25% of predicted normal value, but rarely was of functional significance. Arterial blood gases were generally normal. Presentation of severe problems in perfusion or ventilation in the presence of scoliosis indicates congenital scoliosis, unless it is ruled out. There would appear to be a correlation between curve size and pulmonary insufficiency above 60 degrees, but in over 20 years of experience this author has seen no pulmonary deaths associated with idiopathic scoliosis. All deaths were in congenital or in paralytic curves. The only exception to this rule in idiopathic scoliosis is the patient who has a marked thoracic lordosis or whose disorder is of juvenile or infantile onset.

Current theories as to the cause of thoracic curves suggests an anterior tether of the thoracic spine resulting in a lordosis and scoliosis. In patients with a marked thoracic lordosis, pulmonary function may be severely affected.

At the present time, pulmonary function tests are performed only for thoracic curves of greater than 60 degrees or in cases of paralytic or congenital scoliosis.

Physical examination naturally focuses on the spinal deformity. However, a complete examination is necessary, including a full neurologic examination and a cardiopulmonary evaluation. The 3-D nature of the curve should be assessed. A kyphotic or lordotic element should be looked for in the presence of a scoliosis, and its effect on pulmonary function assessed.

The degree of decompensation, the flexibility, and the size of the rib hump should be measured, as should be the patient's height. Signs of subtle neurologic dysfunction should be sought, particularly in left thoracic idiopathic curves, which are often associated with syringomyelia. Mild clawing of the toes may indicate a tethered cord.

Muscle fatigue after exercise in the presence of a history of spinal stenosis associated with scoliosis should be looked for.

Radiology

Following the clinical determination of scoliosis or kyphosis, initial radiographic analysis should include posteroanterior and lateral 3-foot (1-m) x-ray studies. These will indicate the degree of the deformity, local pathologic conditions (if any), and the degree of decompensation. In the presence of pain, localized x-ray films should be taken to look for such findings as enlarged facets, congenital anomalies, disc narrowing, and other specific findings.

In our experience, bending x-rays indicate flexibility of the curve, if one is present, but do not provide any formula as to the degree of correction that might be expected by surgical intervention. In mobile thoracolumbar curves treated by anterior Zielke instrumentation, the amount of correction obtained was twice that obtained by means of bending x-rays.

Traction films are occasionally of value in attempting to show whether distraction will overcome decompensation. A supine posteroanterior film may also help in decision-making about decompensation.

Hyperextension views of a kyphotic area are of value only if the kyphosis is flexible. Flexion views are used for evaluation of excessive lordosis.

Because scoliosis is a rotational deformity, Stagnara views, particularly in cases of kyphoscoliosis, best demonstrate the deformity. They are essentially oblique views. Special studies include bone scanning, myelography, discography, computed tomography (CT), and magnetic resonance imaging (MRI). Bone scans are rarely indicated but are sometimes of value in the young adult with a minor curve in order to rule out a lesion, such as tumor, as a cause of the scoliosis. Myelography is indicated in patients with neuropathologic findings and congenital curves. In any patient undergoing surgical correction for a painful deformity, preoperative myelography is of value in order to rule out cauda equina or cord compression prior to corrective surgery.

CT has not proven to be of value in assessing the contents of the dural canal in scoliosis, and in our experience it is best combined with myelography in which nonionic dyes are used. The scanning is performed from 3 to 4 hours following the myelogram. In low back problems of a degenerative nature, myelography or CT scans often have a 30% false-positive value. The combination of myelography and CT scanning, however, has proven to be accurate in more than 90% of patients. The role of MRI appears to be promising, although it is still somewhat experimental in the study of spinal deformities.

Discography and the use of facet blocks are discussed under Pain Evaluation.

CONSERVATIVE NONOPERATIVE CARE

Nonoperative care is for patients in whom operative indications are not present, or correspondingly for other reasons that preclude operative intervention. Among these reasons are serious cardiac or respiratory disease, or psychologic reasons.

The mainstays of nonoperative treatment are drugs, physical therapeutic modalities, and orthotic devices, as well as a general understanding of the patient's condition and prognosis.

Excluding cosmetic deformity, significant progression, or neurologic problems, the major indication for operative intervention is pain. Prior to operative intervention, in the absence of neurologic problems, nonoperative treatment should be tried.

The use of nonsteroidal anti-inflammatory drugs may be of value and are worth trying. Enteric-coated aspirin is often as valuable as other more expensive nonsteroidal anti-inflammatory drugs and can be used on a long-term basis. Medications such as muscle relaxants or analgesics with high doses of narcotics such as codeine, 30 mg or more, or some of the synthetic narcotic drugs should be avoided, except during very acute phases of severe pain.

Physiotherapy, particularly in the form of exercises, is rarely successful in controlling pain in adult scoliotics. In painful cases, motion usually aggravates the symptom. However, flexibility and stretching exercises may be of value in tiding over a patient for a period of time. Exercises must be tailored to include only motions that avoid pain. Low-thrust aerobics, cycling exercises, and swimming exercises are of value.

No physiotherapeutic modality or exercises will prevent the progression of a curve, but they may maintain, to some degree, the flexibility and make easier subsequent surgical treatment, if it is necessary.

In the elderly scoliotic who is fifty years old or older, the use of an orthosis, particularly in women, may be of great value. These need to be rigid and shaped to the patient's deformity. They should be worn while the patient is ambulatory and may adequately support the patient over for many months or even years. However, in the author's experience, the majority of patients who have worn an orthosis subsequently came to operative intervention. If an orthosis is provided, an attempt should be made to involve the patient in a general exercise program in order to maintain both mobility of the deformity and general muscle tone.

Other aspects of nonoperative treatments that must be considered are a normal regular diet, as well as a general understanding of the cause of scoliosis, and a prognosis for the patient's particular deformity.

Because osteoporosis plays a major role in the progression of deformity in the postmenopausal woman, it is important that women who are discovered to have scoliosis before menopause be sure to exercise. Twenty minutes of general low-impact aerobics four times a week for 10 years before menopause will prevent postmenopausal osteoporosis in most women. In postmenopausal women, the use of exercise combined with hormonal therapy and calcium under the supervision of a physician may help prevent osteoporosis in the first 10 years after menopause.

SURGICAL INDICATIONS: LUMBAR AND THORACOLUMBAR SPINE

The indications for scoliotic surgery in the adult generally are, first, pain; second, progression of deformity; third, neurologic disability; fourth, cosmesis; fifth, progression associated with pain below previous fusions for spinal deformity; and sixth, iatrogenic flat back (kyphosis).

The younger adult who presents before the age of 35 years without pain but who has an obvious documented increasing curvature and whose lumbar or thoracolumbar curve measures approximately 45 degrees is best treated surgically, because inevitably these disorders will progress, and a painful low back will develop. This is particularly true of female patients with a significant lumbar thoracolumbar curve that, because of degenerative changes, may in later adulthood convert from primary scoliosis with retention of lumbar lordosis to kyphoscoli-

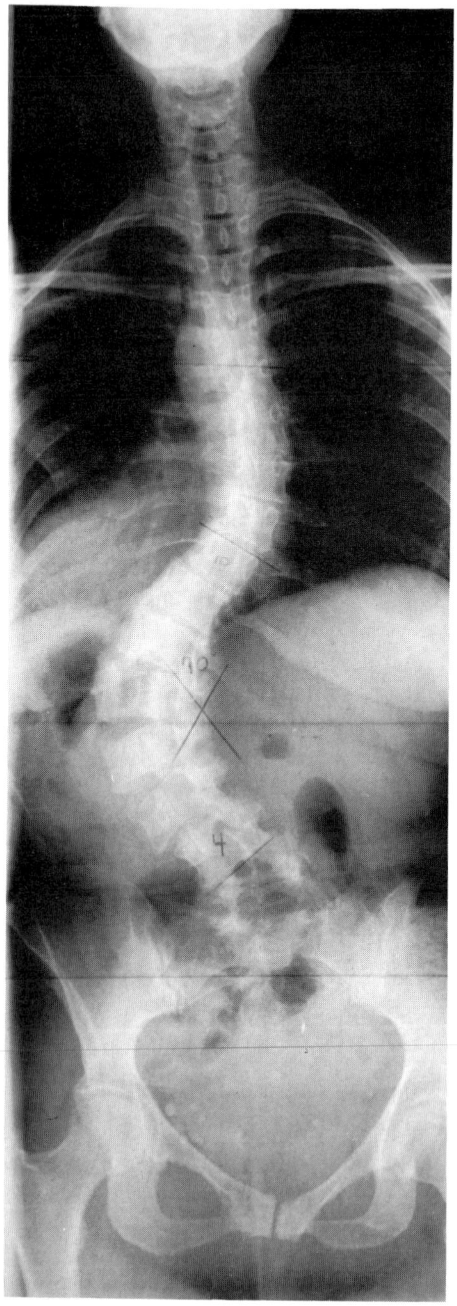

Figure 1 □ Woman, 28 years old, with progressive curvature. Preoperative curve Cobb angle at T10–L4 measured 82 degrees with marked rotation.

osis, which becomes rigid and may require two-stage surgery.

These people can be readily be treated anteriorly with good correction of their deformity using Zielke instrumentation with minimal morbidity (Figs. 1 and 2) The unanswered question is, of course, What happens to the levels below the fusion? Edgar and Mehta[7] and Cochran and coworkers[1] have recently pointed out the problem related to posterior instrumentation that has extended to the L3 or L4 level as an increased incidence of degenerative changes below the fusion associated with pain. Advice to these people who have undergone surgery, as it is to all patients (in particular, the younger patient), is that they must become involved in athletic endeavors in order to maintain a satisfactory level of physical fitness. They must practice good back hygiene and routinely perform low back exercises on a daily basis. The exercises are tailored to the individual's tolerance level. For example, many people with a fusion to L4 or L5 cannot do sit-ups. Furthermore, it is important that patients participate in a general fitness program.

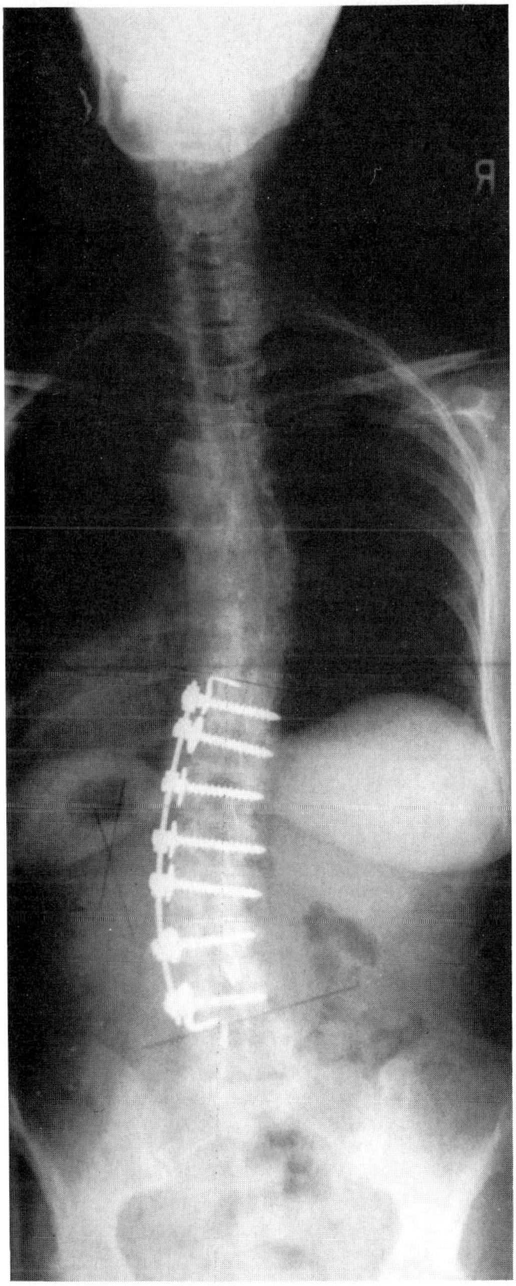

Figure 2 □ Postoperative curve measured 26 degrees at 2 years. Lordosis was maintained. The proximal compensatory thoracic curve remains reduced. (Same patient as in Fig. 1.)

The imbalanced younger patient whose major curve may measure 40 degrees or more and may extend to L3 or L4 but who has a compensatory curve at L4–L5, L5–S1 and who is imbalanced may often have the primary curve significantly reduced by rebalancing through the lower curve. However, this should only be done if the lower curve is painful. These patients may run the risk of progression of the upper curve at a later date, and it should be explained to them that they may later require a more proximal extension of their fusion. To date, however, the technique has worked satisfactorily in a small number of patients (six), and although the follow-up is of short duration, the average degree of correction of the major curve has been more than 50% (Figs. 3 and 4). Pain patterns must be proven preoperatively by discography and facet blocks.

In a series of more than 1,000 adults with scoliosis treated surgically, neurologic deficit has rarely been an indication for surgical intervention. However, in an aging population, greater numbers of patients are seen with an associated spinal stenosis. Surgical decompression via laminectomy is rarely indicated, and in a 1978 review,[10] only 5 of 227 patients treated surgically for a painful scoliosis required associated decompression.

Simmons and colleagues[8, 28] have shown that patients with radicular symptoms present in the compensatory curve may show marked improvement following correction of the major curve via an anterior procedure.

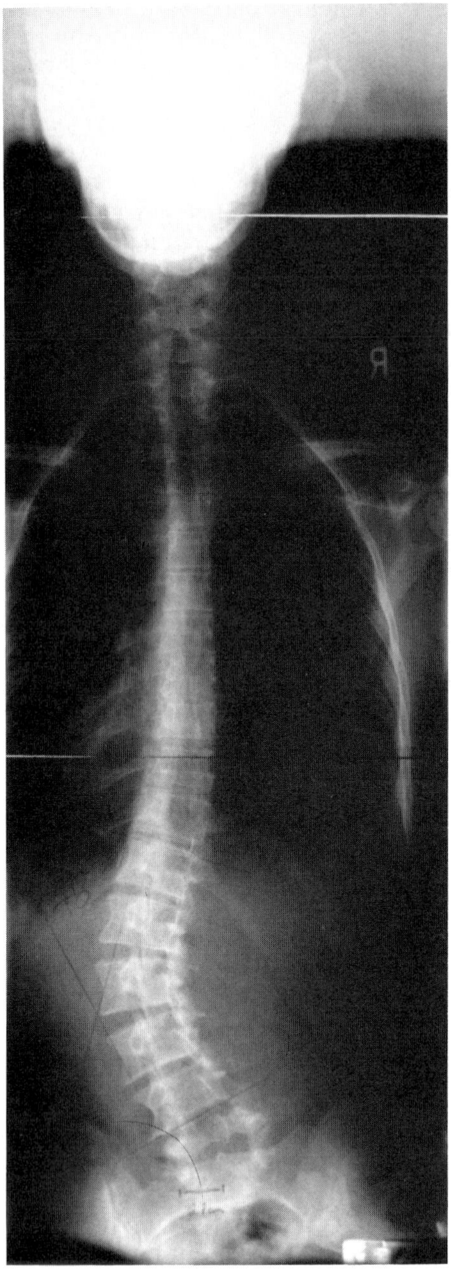

Figure 3 □ Woman, 32 years old. Preoperative curve measures 45 degrees. The patient is imbalanced 4.5 cm to the left. Based on discography and facet blocks, pain was localized to the L4–L5 and L5–S1 levels.

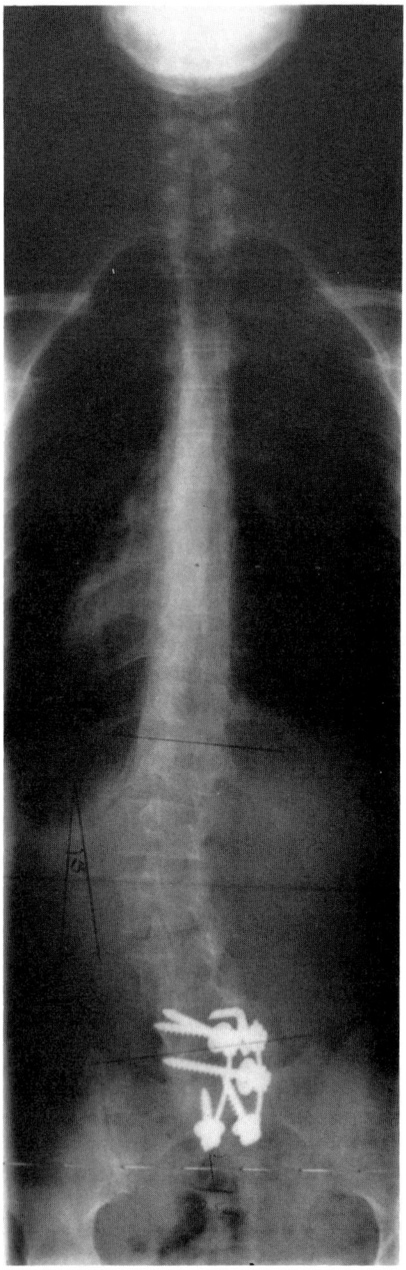

Figure 4 □ At follow-up at 2 years (same patient as in Fig. 3) the curve measures 15 degrees and pain has been alleviated by an anterior two-level Zielke instrumentation and fusion. Partial rebalance has been achieved by closing the disk spaces and removing bone at the L4–L5 level on the compensatory functional L4–S1 right-sided curve.

In my experience this has been less successful.

All patients who complain preoperatively of significant pain should undergo preoperative myelography to rule out other causes of pain such as intradural or extradural tumors. It is believed that adults with significant lumbar and thoracolumbar curves of greater than 45 degrees should undergo preoperative myelography, particularly if they have pain, because the problem of spinal stenosis may be present primarily in patients over the age of sixty years.

PAIN ASSESSMENT

Early attempts made by the author in the late 1960s and 1970s to treat painful lumbar and thoracolumbar curves using Harrington instrumentation and fusion, without preoperative pain assessment by discography and facet blocks, left a significant number of patients complaining of pain. Only 65% to 70% of these patients had pain relief. Subsequent evaluation of pain using discography and facet blocks has demonstrated improved results to between 80% and 90% good pain relief.

The patient may localize the pain to the low back or to the apex of the curvature or to both sites. Frequently, however, the symptoms are vague. Macnab[20] has previously shown that a hypertonic saline injection into the supraspinous ligament at the thoracolumbar junction can reproduce pain at the lumbosacral junction.

With this finding in mind, in the early 1970s this author[10] did a prospective study using discography to help differentiate sources of pain. The current use of discography is limited to an assessment of the lower levels of the lumbar spine, namely, to L3–L4, L4–L5, and the lumbosacral junction. Rarely are discograms now performed at the apex of the curve.

Discography is used to assess whether these levels are degenerative and/or painful. Facet blocks are similarly used. Discography is usually done from a posterolateral approach, although occasionally because of deformity it may be necessary to transgress the dura. Facet blocks are done using bupivacaine hydrochloride (Marcaine) with infiltration of the posterior ramus. It is recognized that levels other than the L5–S1 articulation have multiple innervations, and if the L4–L5 level is to be assessed, then the L3–L4 level must be infiltrated as well.

Our current practice in treatment for painful lumbar and thoracolumbar curves is to perform discography at the lower levels of the lumbar spine and facet blocks at the lowermost level, L5–S1, which has a single innervation, or at L4–L5.

If facet blocks relieve pain and discography reproduces pain at the lumbosacral junction, then fusion will have to be extended to the sacrum. Results before discography, as previously indicated, in which the fusion was not extended to the sacrum, led many patients to continue to complain of pain despite correction of the deformity from either a posterior or an anterior approach. Extension of fusion to the sacrum with preservation of lumbar lordosis and the ability to obtain a solid arthrodesis has resulted in good results in 90% of such cases.

Conversely, if discography does not reproduce the patient's pain and if facet blocks at the lumbosacral junction do not relieve the patient of pain, then it is assumed that the pain arises in the curve itself. If L5 is not part of the curve, the curve alone is dealt with, preferably by an anterior approach.

It is important to have a thorough understanding of the patient's pain, which should be mechanical in nature and not clouded by significant psychologic difficulties.

SURGICAL TECHNIQUES

Today, Harrington posterior instrumentation is rarely indicated in treatment of the adult with a scoliotic deformity of the lumbar or thoracolumbar spine. The reason is that even by using sacroalar hooks, broad sleeves, or contouring of rods or by using square-ended rods with distraction, a loss of lumbar lordosis is inevitable. The majority of lumbar and thoracolumbar curves today are being handled by anterior instrumentation using the Zielke[37] technique, provided there is no associated kyphosis.

However, Zielke instrumentation is of no value if a true kyphosis is present. This can only be evaluated by oblique or Stagnara views. If a significant kyphosis is present, Zielke instrumentation may increase it. In a kyphoscoliosis, which is a common problem encountered in elderly individuals over 50 years of age, in order to restore balance and relieve pain in the lumbar spine it is necessary to restore lumbar lordosis. This can be achieved only if the kyphus is rigid, by a two-stage procedure. Initially, an anterior approach is performed with multiple-level discectomies and fusions followed 2 weeks later by Cotrel-Dubousset instrumentation (Figs. 5 to 8). However, if the kyphoscoliosis is mobile, this may be achieved by single-stage posterior Cotrel-Dubousset instrumentation, which will derotate the spine and restore lordosis.

The advent of Luque instrumentation[20] in

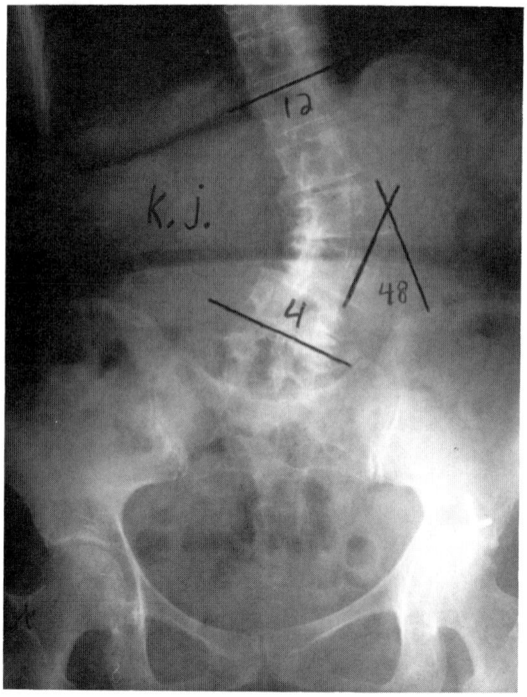

Figure 5 □ Woman, 62 years old, presented with a painful lumbar kyphoscoliosis with progression as evidenced by loss of height. L5–S1 level was not a source of pain on discography and facet blocks. Preoperative curve measures T12–L4, 48 degrees.

1976 has caused the use of segmental fixation posteriorly to gain great popularity. In the lumbar spine Harrington instrumentation with segmental wiring does not suffice for lumbar or thoracolumbar curves. The use of double L rods or rectangular rods may be indicated. Initial fixation to the pelvis with Luque rods contoured by using the Galveston technique showed great promise; however, recent reports indicate that many of these people develop pain related to the sacroiliac joint in the presence of a solid fusion of the lumbar spine.

Today, the use of sublaminar wiring has been abandoned, except in cases of tumor and in some cases of paralytic scoliosis. Cotrel-Dubousset instrumentation has made sublaminar wiring no longer necessary.

Zielke Instrumentation

The primary indication for Zielke instrumentation is a thoracolumbar or lumbar curve that does not require extension of the fusion to the sacrum and is shown to be mobile by bending x-rays, and not kyphotic. For cases associated with pain, if the disorder is accurately assessed preoperatively with discography and facet blocks, as indicated previously, correction of the deformity should be obtained by using Zielke instrumentation. In the mature adult, the entire curve should be incorporated in the instrumentation. In the less mature individual, levels comparable to the level found in adolescence will suffice. From a technical viewpoint, the major problem in many adults has to do with the problem of osteoporosis. This can be overcome by injecting methyl methacrylate into predrilled screw holes in the vertebral bodies. If possible, the screw should be angled toward the contralateral junction of the pedicle with the vertebral body. This necessitates very careful

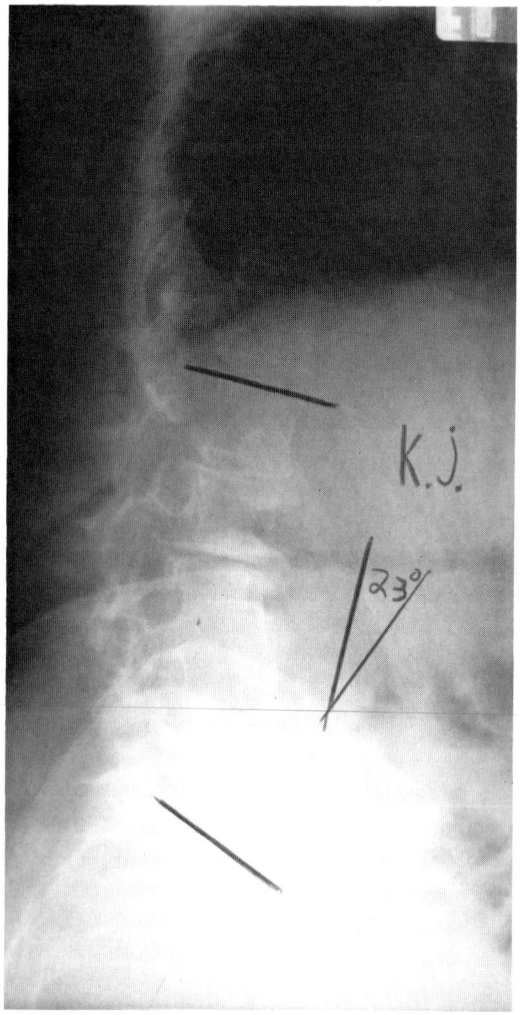

Figure 6 □ Preoperative lateral film taken in the standing position shows a lordosis of minus 23 degrees. (Same patient as in Fig. 5.)

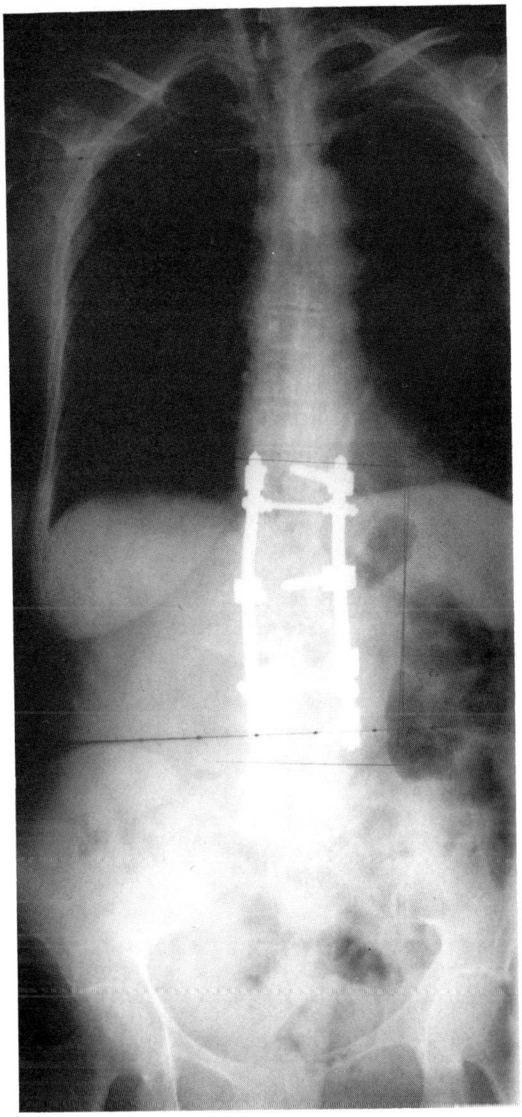

Figure 7 □ Following two-stage surgery consisting of multiple anterior discectomies of T12–L4, with the addition of bone graft, and a second-stage Cotrel-Dubousset derotation, the curve has been completely reduced. (Same patient as in Fig. 5.)

cleaning of the disc space, including the end plates, back to the posterior longitudinal ligament so that an accurate line can be obtained for insertion of the screws. In order to ensure that the opposite cortex is penetrated, a depth gauge is used to measure the line in the interspace that the screw will follow. Following this, 2 mm can be added to the depth of the screw, although frequently if there is lipping of the vertebral body, particularly in cases associated with marked degeneration, this is not necessary.

Cooling the methyl methacrylate or using a low-viscosity methyl methacrylate will allow increased working time for the injection of methyl methacrylate into enlarged screw holes. Frequently, the use of a curet inside the screw hole will enlarge the space within the vertebral body for retention of the cement to enhance fixation of the screws.

The most significant technical difficulty has been a pull-out of the most proximal

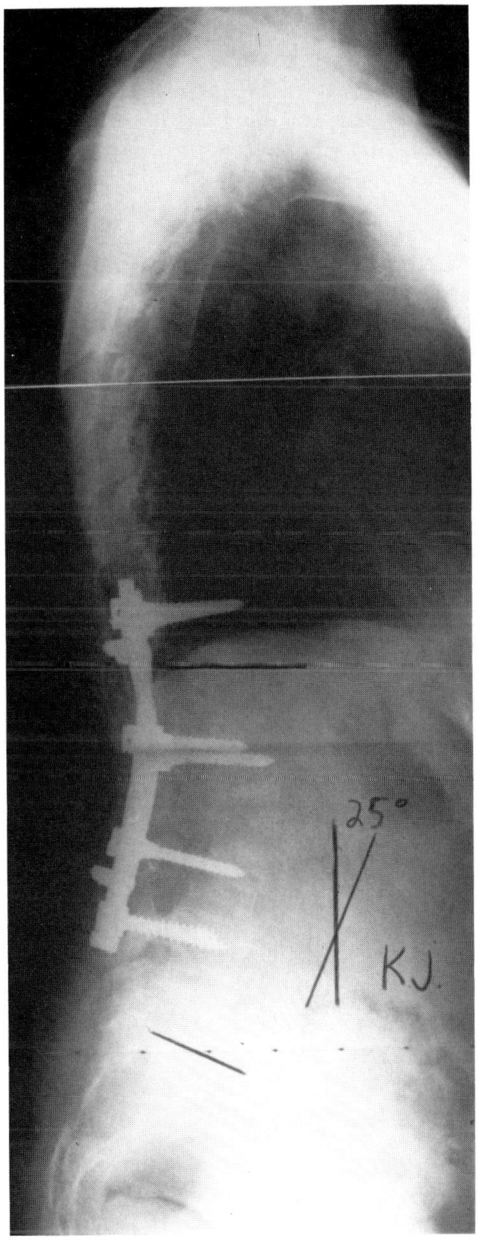

Figure 8 □ Postoperative lordosis measures 25 degrees, a gain of 48 degrees. Pain has been alleviated. (Same patient as in Fig. 5.)

screw. I do not believe that an extra level should be incorporated across a nonfused space in order to prevent this problem. In postmenopausal women bone cement is added routinely to the upper level at the time of screw insertion.

There has been no difficulty in regard to fusions extending proximally from L5. The iliolumbar veins at the L5 level must be ligated in order to allow mobilization of the common iliac system.

Extension to the sacrum using Zielke instrumentation is done only for patients in whom fusion to the sacrum is performed based on preoperative assessment (as indicated previously) and is combined with a posterior fusion. Extension of Zielke instrumentation above T9 or T10 is rarely of value because the disc spaces are so narrow that little correction can be accomplished. The use of the derotator is almost routine in order to reproduce lordosis or reduce kyphosis of the thoracolumbar spine. This has been a marked advantage over the previously used Dwyer instrumentation, which is no longer used and which tended frequently to produce a kyphosis despite accurate screw placement. Autogenous bone graft is used, and this consists of the excised rib cut up into very small fragments.

Bits of block graft or minced graft placed more anteriorly in the disc space helps to maintain or increase lordosis, with the use of Zielke instrumentation. We do not use iliac crest bone. With the use of hypotensive anesthesia and the use of cell savers, the average blood loss has been 1,750 cc. Transfusions using bank blood have been kept to a minimum. Hypotensive anesthesia is not used in people above the age of fifty years.

Zielke instrumentation can be used safely in patients in the 8th decade of life, although it is usually necessary to incorporate methyl methacrylate with the screws (Figs. 9 and 10).

Correction using Zielke instrumentation has been markedly improved over that using Dwyer instrumentation and posterior segmental instrumentation. A long-term review of our first 57 patients treated by Zielke instrumentation revealed that the average correction was 70% versus 45% with the Dwyer[6] instrumentation.

The use of the derotational device improved correction of the curve in both the sagittal plane and the anteroposterior plane, with improved rotation by approximately one grade according to the Nash-Moe method of rotational classification. Intraoperative complications included five fractured vertebral bodies, which were overcome by the use of methyl methacrylate. Postoperative complications included three lateral femoral cutaneous nerve entrapments, one of which required surgical decompression. Two post-thoracotomy syn-

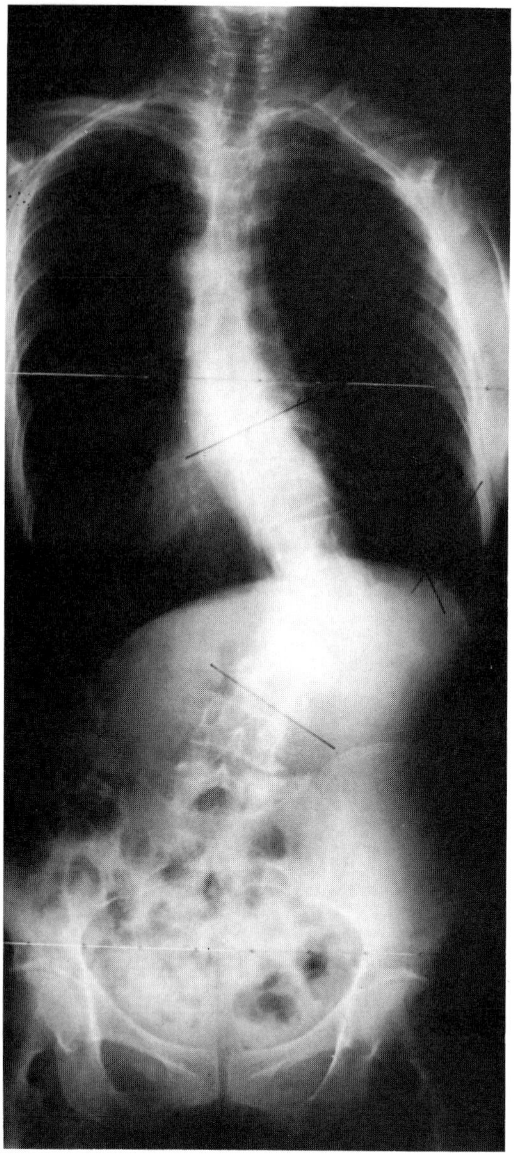

Figure 9 □ Woman, 72 years old. Preoperative thoracolumbar curve T9–L3 measured 75 degrees. Preoperative discography and facet blocks revealed no pathologic condition at L4–L5 or L5–S1 levels. The only surgical intervention was for unremitting pain unresponsive to nonoperative care.

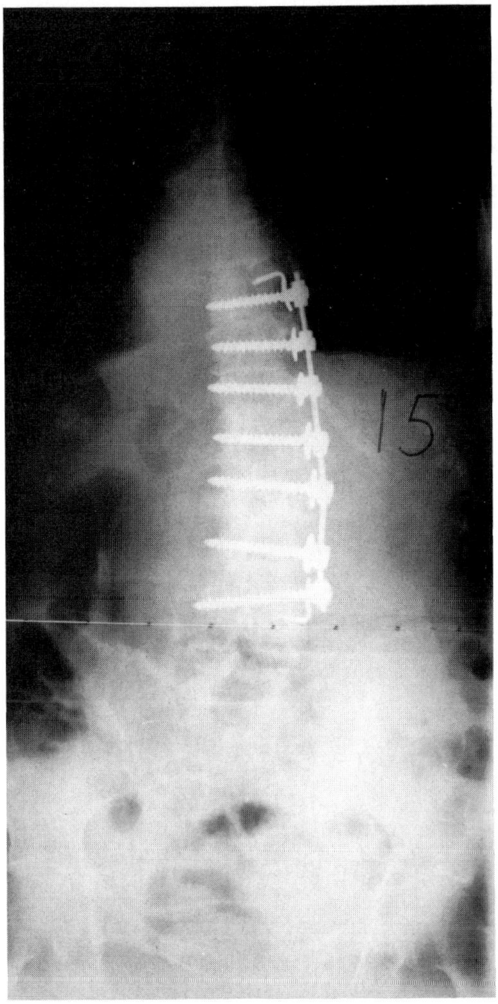

Figure 10 □ Same woman as shown in Figure 9. Postoperatively, her curve measured 15 degrees. At 2 years follow-up she had no pain.

dromes were encountered, and these settled down with time. There were ten cases of atelectasis and pleural effusions that did not require major treatment. In one case the instrumentation failed, requiring subsequent posterior surgery. Proximal staple pull-out occurred at two levels. Nuts backed off the screw head in 10 patients, without any curve deterioration or rod displacement. Rod disengagement from intermediate screw heads was noted in six patients without loss of correction over the immediately postoperative x-ray film. Six cases had partial staple disengagement including the case noted (Figs. 11 to 14). At an average follow-up of 2 years, the average loss of correction was less than 1 degree.

In double idiopathic curves, the average correction was 62%. At 24 months the mean loss was 3.4 degrees (4%). The noninstrumented proximal thoracic curve improved 38% after correction of the distal lumbar curve, without deterioration at follow-up (Figs. 15 and 16). All surgical results revealed an improvement of 50% correction over that anticipated based on preoperative bending anteroposterior radiographs.

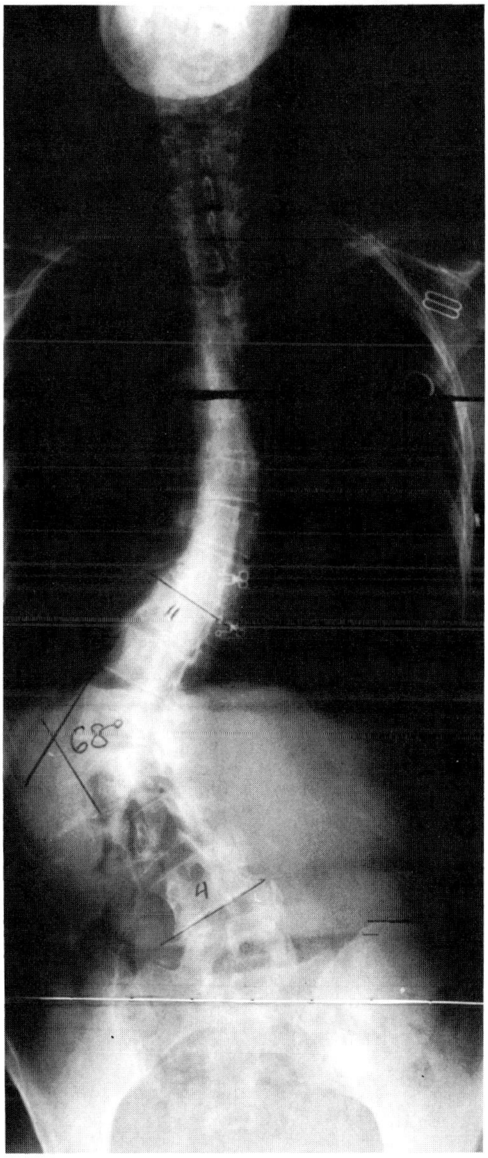

Figure 11 □ Woman physician, 50 years old. Surgical indications were a progressive deformity and pain with an inability to work full time. Preoperative curve measured 68 degrees at T11–L4. Discography and facet blocks at L5–S1 revealed this level not to be a source of pain.

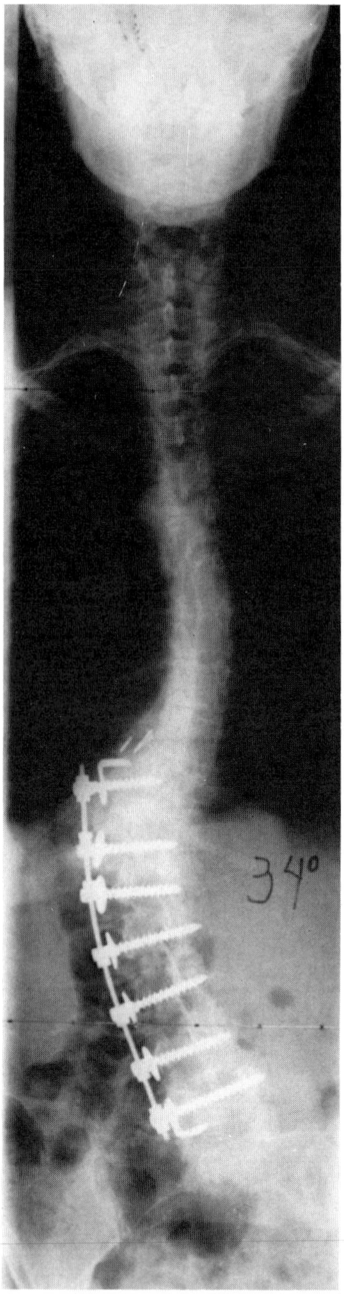

Figure 12 □ Postoperative curve measured 34 degrees. Proximal partial staple pull-out occurred early with no further loss of correction. Pain was relieved, and the patient works full time. (Same patient as in Fig. 11.)

An analysis of Zielke instrumentation used posteriorly in cases of scoliosis with pedicle fixation for degenerative disease has revealed a high incidence of rod breakage. As a result, it is our policy to no longer use Zielke instrumentation posteriorly. This has been surpassed by the use of Cotrel-Dubousset or Kostuik-Harrington instrumentation posteriorly.

Zielke instrumentation has also been used in six patients with imbalance, in the distal convex side of fractional lumbosacral curves (see Figs. 3 and 4). This has resulted in a slightly greater than 50% correction of the proximal major curve. This was done only in patients in whom the distal fractional

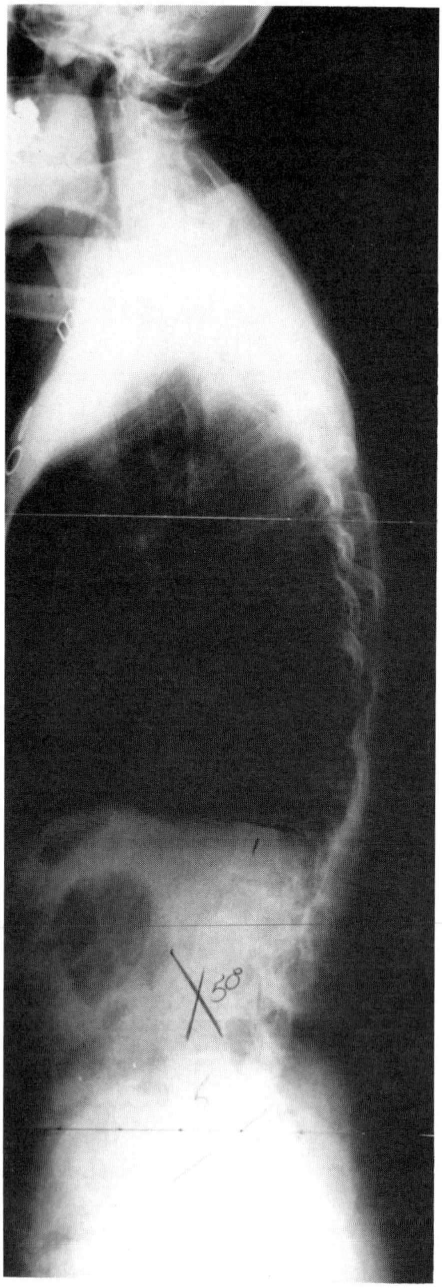

Figure 13 □ Preoperative lordosis measured 50 degrees at L1–S1. (Same patient as in Fig. 11.)

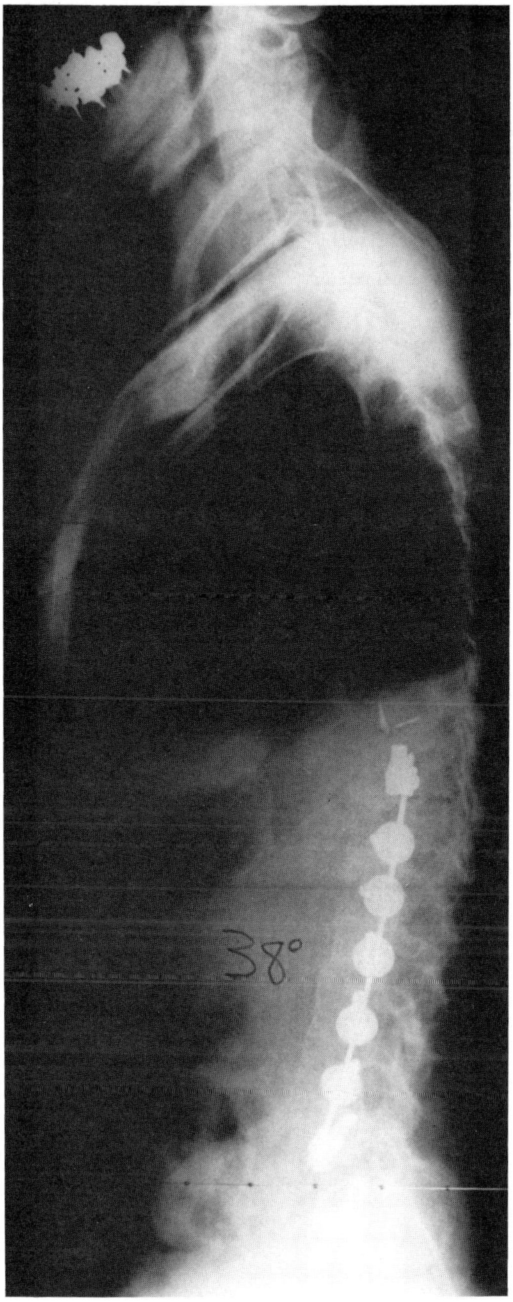

Figure 14 □ Postoperative lordosis measured 38 degrees. The difference was not clinically significant. (Same patient as in Fig. 11.)

curve has been a source of pain and in whom balance has not been shown to be restored on bending x-ray films of the major curve. It is recognized that the follow-up is only 2 years in these patients and that they may well require further treatment of the major curve at a later date. I believe that this technique should be reserved only for fractional curves in the lower lumbar and lumbosacral spine in which this is the source of the pain as shown on discography and facet blocks, and if the patient is imbalanced.

Treatment of Kyphoscoliosis

The use of sublaminar wiring described by Luque has been disbanded in the treatment of scoliosis, except in some cases of paralytic scoliosis. This follows its use in over 200 cases of adult spinal deformity. Reasons for

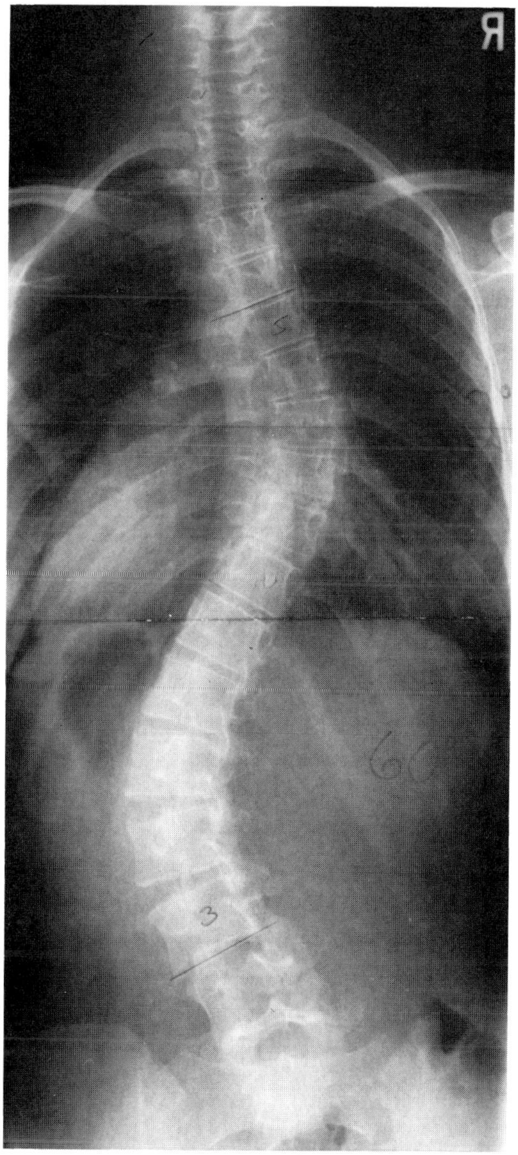

Figure 15 □ Woman, 24 years old. Preoperative curves measured 52 degrees at T5–T11 and 60 degrees at T11–L3.

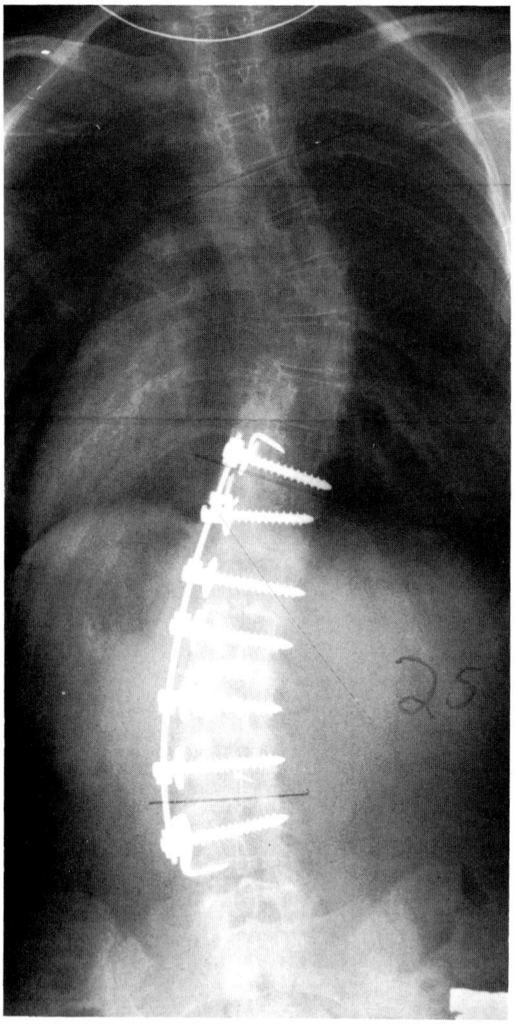

Figure 16 □ At 2 years postoperatively, the curves measured 24 degrees at T5–T11 and 25 degrees at T11–L3. (Same patient as in Fig. 15.)

its abandonment are that with the advent of Cotrel-Dubousset instrumentation and pedicle fixation, more rigid fixation is available, as are true means of correcting deformity, particularly the derotation and restoration of lordosis. In cases of mobile curves in which it is believed that anterior surgery may not be justified (for example, in cases of significant arteriosclerosis with anterior calcification of the aorta) or in cases of marked anterior osteopenia in which the curve is still mobile, Cotrel-Dubousset[5] instrumentation can serve to derotate the spine and restore lordosis.

In cases of significant rigid kyphoscoliosis, Cotrel-Dubousset instrumentation has proved to be invaluable for restoring lordosis and relieving pain following anterior multiple discectomies with the use of minced bone graft in the interbody spaces. The instrumentation is carried out about 2 weeks after anterior surgery is performed and can be used even in the presence of extensive laminectomies for spinal stenosis (Figs. 5 to 8 and 17 to 20). To date experience is limited to a follow-up of only 30 months; however, this procedure has proven to be extremely exciting and offers a means of managing the rigid painful kyphoscoliotic patient, in particular, the elderly person, with excellent

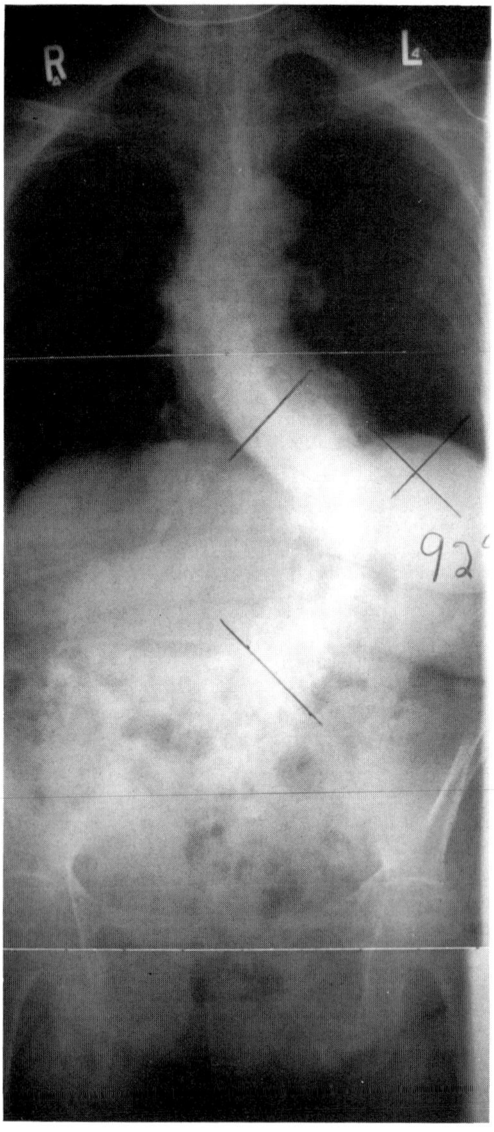

Figure 17 □ Woman, 57 years old. She had noted losing 4 inches of height and an increasing and painful deformity. Preoperative curve measured 92 degrees at T10–L4.

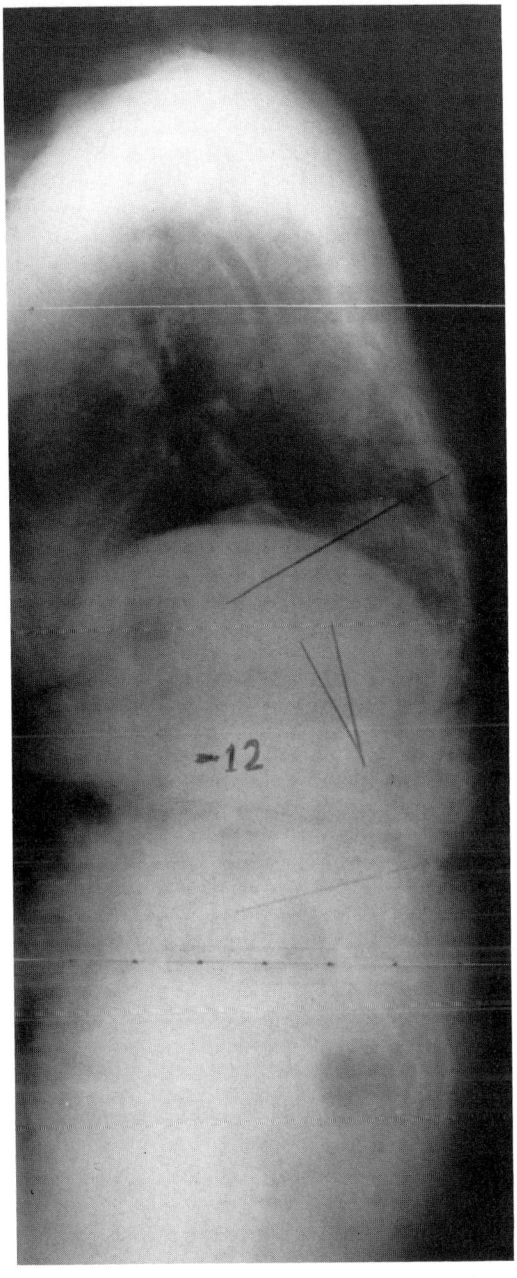

Figure 18 □ Preoperative lordosis at L1–S1 measured −12 degrees. (Same patient as in Fig. 17.)

results to date and no neurologic or vascular complications related to instrumentation.

Fusions to the Sacrum

In a review of fusions to the sacrum by means of Harrington instrumentation, loss of lumbar lordosis was noted by the author[12] in approximately 50% of patients and was clinically significant, requiring revision surgery, in one half of the patients. It was not recognized until the late 1970s that distraction of the thoracolumbar and lumbar spine might result in a loss of lordosis, even with contouring of the Harrington rod and using square-ended Moe rods and sacroalar hooks. The use of Luque L rods across the sacroiliac joint and subsequently the refinement of this with the Galveston technique was believed to result in the improved maintenance of lordosis and an enhanced rate of fusion for posterior instrumentation to the sacrum. The initial incidence of pseudarthrosis to the sacrum using Harrington rods, with either a sacral bar or alar hooks, was 40%. A recent review of Luque instrumentation to the sacrum revealed that the incidence of pseudarthrosis had decreased to 15%. The incidence of flat back in fusions to the sacrum was

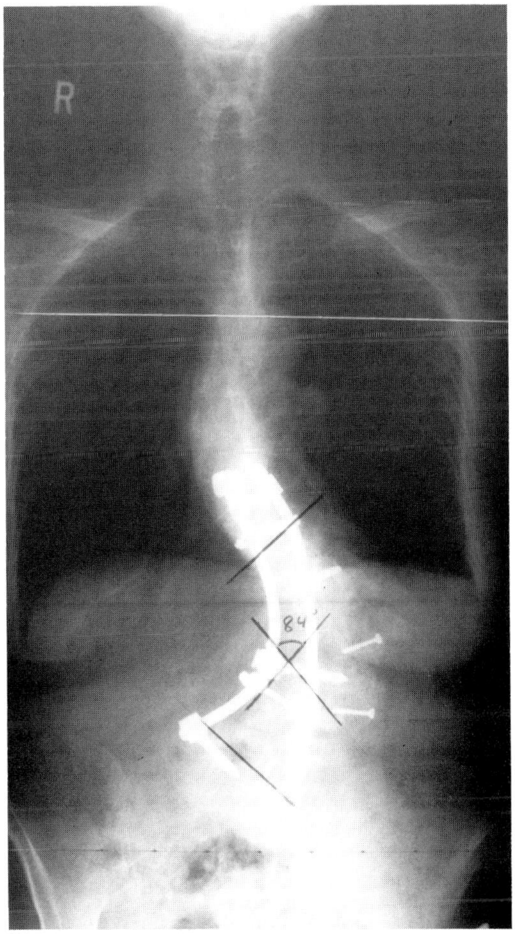

Figure 19 □ The anteroposterior (AP) postoperative radiograph measures 84 degrees. (Same patient as in Fig. 17.)

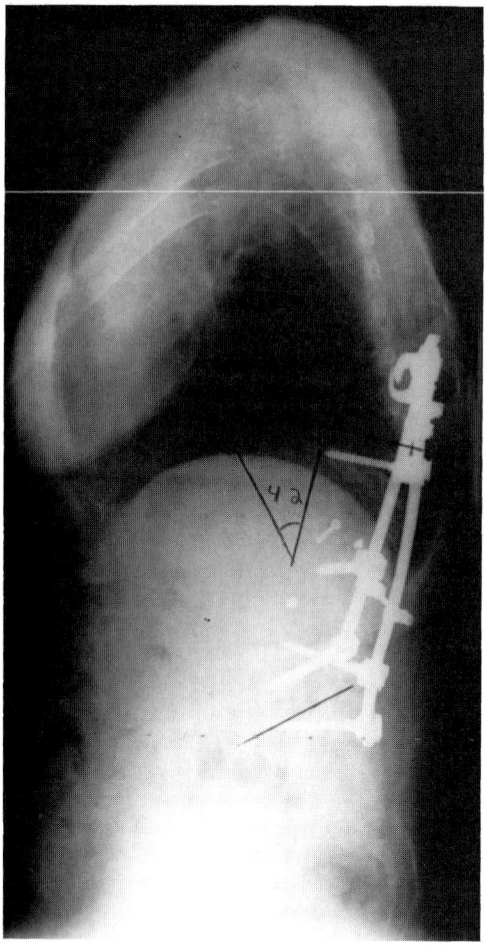

Figure 20 □ Postoperative lordosis has been restored to 42 degrees for a gain of 54 degrees. Pain has been alleviated by the two-stage operation consisting of multiple anterior discectomies and bone grafting followed by second-stage posterior osteotomies and partial derotation using the Cotrel-Dubousset instrumentation. (Same patient as in Fig. 17.)

reduced to only 25%. This occurred despite marked contouring of the L rods into lordosis and was believed to be due to simple loss of mobility; it occurred only in patients who were kyphoscoliotic and was generally not as severe as that encountered when using Harrington instrumentation.[12] To date, the use of Cotrel-Dubousset instrumentation has not had this problem because of the introduction of increased lordosis.

Presently, when fusion to the sacrum is indicated, a two-stage procedure is performed. If the patient is scoliotic with reasonable lordosis and a mobile curve, an initial anterior instrumentation using Zielke instrumentation is done. Although the use of Zielke instrumentation anterior to the sacrum is technically demanding, it has not resulted in any problems related to the common iliac vessels (i.e., either to arteries or to veins). Careful technique avoiding any impingement of screw heads against the vessels has resulted in no vascular complications. The rod can safely pass beneath the common iliac vessels because the rods are small and close to the vertebral body. Occasionally, two rods at the distal two to three levels (see Fig. 4) are used in order to help control rotation at the lumbosacral junction. A second-stage posterior fusion using segmental wiring was initially performed, but this has been replaced by the use of pedicle fixation (Cotrel-Dubousset instrumentation).

If the patient is kyphoscoliotic and requires fusions to the sacrum, the first stage is also anterior, consisting of multiple anterior discectomies with minced bone fusion in the interbody spaces, using either rib or iliac crest. This is followed at about 2 weeks later by posterior Cotrel-Dubousset instrumentation to derotate the spine and restore lordosis (see Figs. 5 to 8 and 17 to 20). If, on the other hand, the curve is mobile and has scoliosis with good preservation of lordosis following the anterior Zielke instrumentation, a posterior instrumentation is performed using either Cotrel-Dubousset instrumentation or posterior Kostuik-Harrington instrumentation. The latter is less expensive and is used over the distal few levels, in order to supplement fixation of the lumbosacral junction.

In over 300 patients with anterior instrumentation in both the thoracic and lumbar spine, the author has not encountered any late vascular problems.

During an anterior instrumentation ligation of the segmental vessels, particularly in a left retroperitoneal approach, the aorta and common iliac vessels fall away from the vertebral bodies and more room is allowed for placement of the internal fixation devices. Because the majority of lumbar and thoracolumbar curves are left-sided, this approach is most commonly used.

Bicortical grafts from the iliac crest in younger people or tricortical in more osteoporotic people are used to maintain disc height at L4–L5 and at L4–S1 and, indeed, to enhance lordosis anteriorly. Internal fixation is used to enhance fixation because iliac crest bone is unable to support loads much greater than body weight alone, without the use of internal fixation. With the use of combined anterior and posterior approaches, no instances of pseudarthrosis have been encountered in the last 20 such cases.

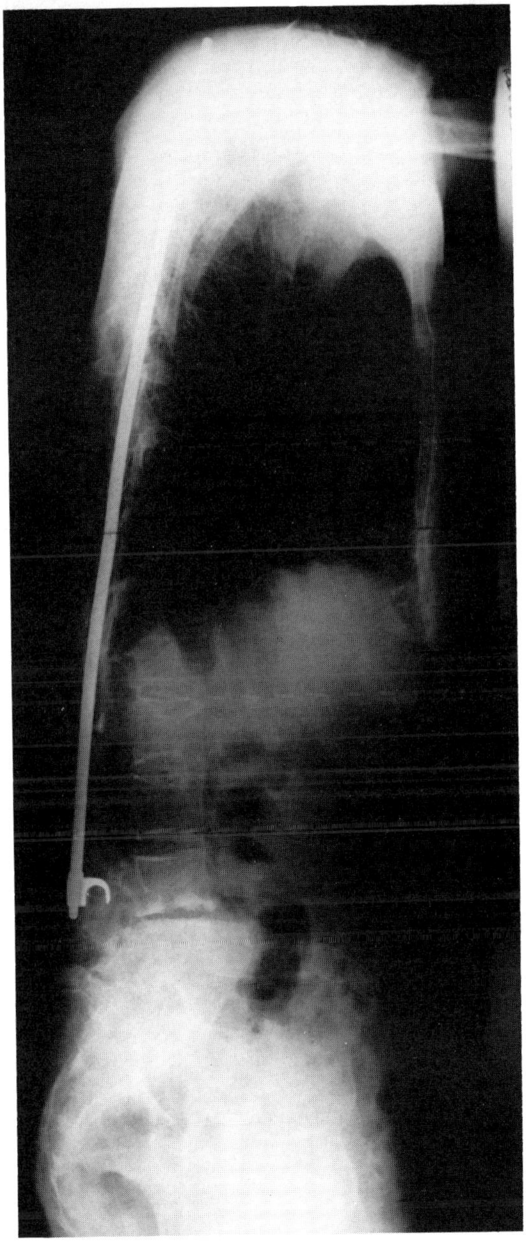

Figure 21 □ Woman, 52 years old. Previous Harrington distraction instrumentation to L4 16 years previously. Note the loss of lordosis attributable to loss of disc height at L4–L5 and L5–S1 secondary to precocious degeneration resulting from increased stress after Harrington distraction at these levels, as well as the use of a stringent distraction rod in the lumbar spine.

Extensions of Fusions in the Lumbar Spine

Recent reports by Edgar and Mehta[7] and Cochran and coworkers[1] and a review of our own statistics show that patients who have had previous fusions to L2, L3, or L4 are at an increased risk of developing degenerative changes below their fusion.

These patients require extension of the fusion if nonoperative means fail to control pain and the problem becomes a progressive one, often associated with some degree of spinal stenosis at the level immediately below the fusion. If, after investigative studies, including myelography, CT scanning, discography, and facet blocks, a fusion does not require extension to the sacrum, then posterior instrumentation or anterior instrumentation alone will suffice. However, if extension of the fusion to the sacrum is required, then a combined approach will be necessary (Figs. 21 to 24) Extension of fusion to the sacrum is usually carried out at a single stage. This is done with posterior pedicle fixation and anterior Zielke instrumentation. In order to improve lordosis, some of the posterior laminae at L4–L5, L3–L4, and L5–S1 can be removed, and compression is applied to the pedicles to increase lordosis. Anteriorly, interbody grafts are performed after the disc space is opened as widely as is possible. Double Zielke rods are used anteriorly. The best results have been obtained by removing posterior bone in order to increase lordosis, rather than simply by fusing the spine in situ with instrumentation posteriorly and then anteriorly with interbody graft and instrumentation. A recent review of 24 cases of extension fusion to the sacrum revealed that of six cases of fusion posteriorly with Harrington rods only, five failed owing to the development of pseudarthrosis and a flat back. Nine were fused anteriorly in situ with interbody grafts and instrumentation used to maintain lordosis; these were supplemented either at the same stage or at a second stage with posterior instrumentation and fusion. With this technique, three pseudarthroses with associated flat back occurred. However, ten fusions done at a single stage with an associated removal of bone posteriorly through the pars interarticularis and an increased opening of an interbody space an-

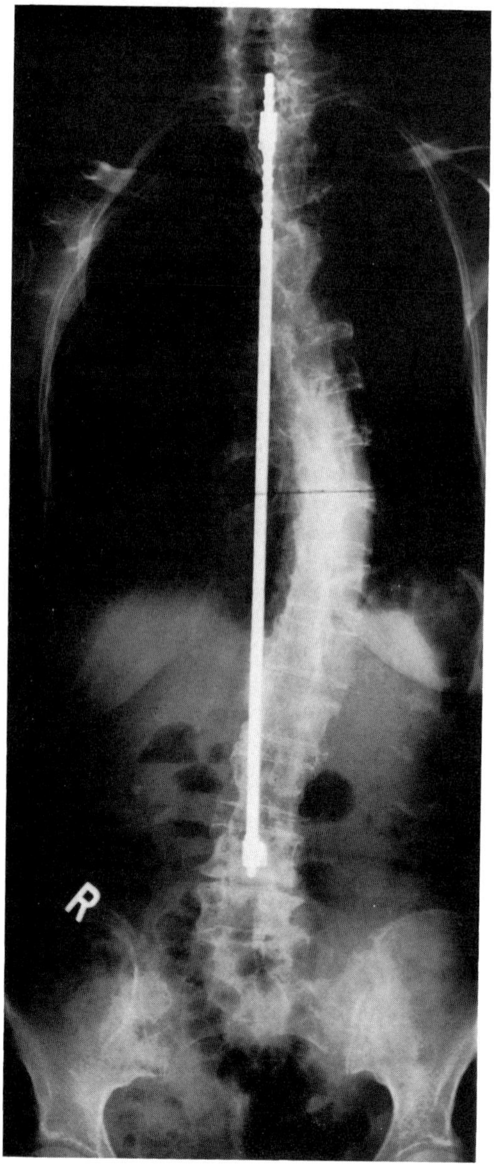

Figure 22 □ AP views of same patient as in Figure 21.

teriorly with bone grafts and instrumentation had satisfactory results, with only one instance of pseudarthrosis.

TREATMENT OF SEVERE RIGID SCOLIOTIC DEFORMITIES

In 1980 the author[10] reported on 85 patients with deformities of 90 degrees or greater, whose curves failed to change as seen on bending x-ray films.

Fifteen of these patients were primarily kyphotic, 42 had idiopathic curves, and 28 had congenital curves. The majority were thoracic and thoracolumbar curves. There were 32 patients who had fusions, as a result of either congenital failures of segmentation (28) or spontaneous fusions (four). Thirty-three patients had been untreated but were shown to be rigid on bending x-rays, although at the time of surgery they were found to have no spontaneous fusion. Twenty patients had previous fusions and presented with a progression of deformity and pain. All patients underwent posterior releases, including (as necessary) osteotomies of previous fusions or congenitally fused spines. Posterior osteotomies were done at multiple levels, usually averaging four in number. These were associated with rib releases over three to four levels on the concavity, and with transverse process osteotomies and rib resections of between five and six ribs on the convexity. Patients had associated anterior osteotomies as well. The age range of the patients was from 20 to 55 years, and the curve magnitude was from 75 to 180 degrees.

Second-stage surgery was performed 2 weeks later. At the time of primary release surgery, traction was applied in one of two forms; in 32 patients halo femoral traction was used, and more recently, halo pelvic distraction was applied. The latter form of traction continues to be used in very severe curves. It has been replaced to some degree by halo-dependent traction either in a circoelectric bed at 30 degrees of dependency or in association with halo wheelchair traction. A second-stage procedure performed 2 weeks later consisted of posterior instrumentation, originally done with Harrington instrumentation and then superseded by sublaminar wiring techniques and more recently by Cotrel-Dubousset instrumentation.

The degree of correction averaged 40% with halo pelvic and 32% with halo femoral distraction. Subsequent Harrington instrumentation added a further 8% to correction. Overall correction in this rigid group of curves was 40%. This was comparable to a previously reported series of mobile curves. The degree of correction of idiopathic curves was an average of 48%, and of congenital curves it was 33%.

Cosmesis

In a review of the first 1,000 patients with scoliosis treated by the author, approxi-

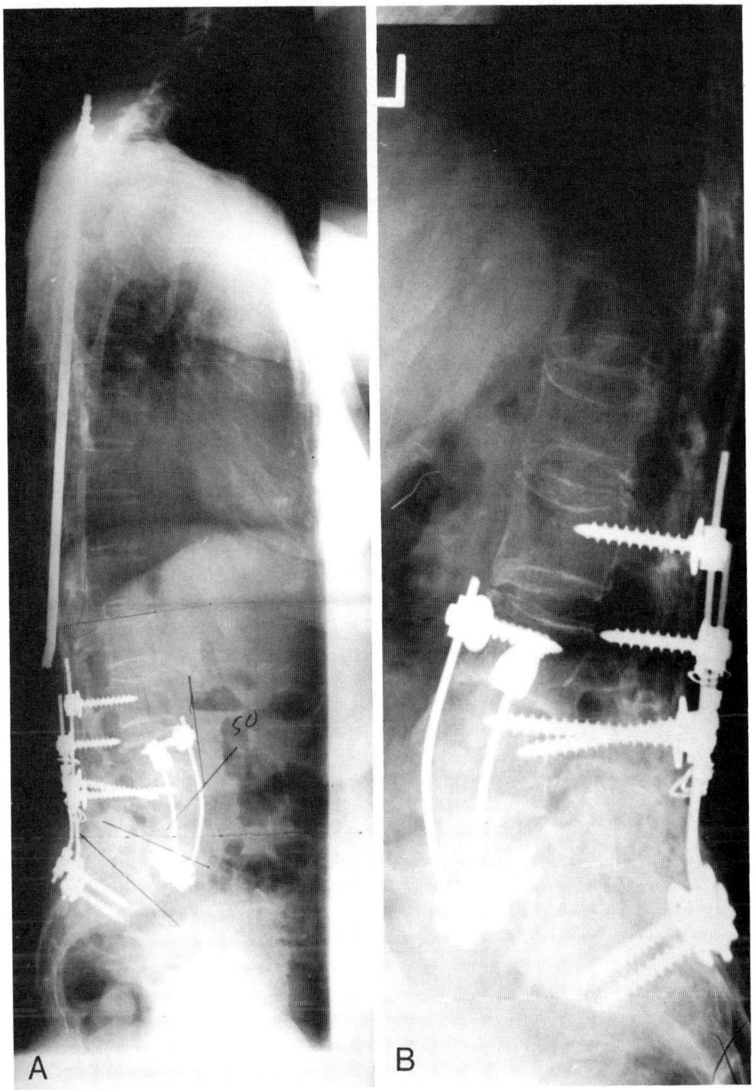

Figure 23 □ *A, B,* Postoperative lateral. The L4–L5 and L5–S1 disc spaces have been opened to restore lordosis with a net gain of 22 degrees at L1–S1. Fixation has been with Zielke instrumentation, anteriorly and posteriorly, at a single stage, in order to assure a solid fusion (see text). (Same patient as in Fig. 21.)

mately 10% were treated for essentially cosmetic reasons. These were primarily thoracic curves with a range of from 45 to 75 degrees. The age range was from 20 to 42 years; 90% were female.

The correction of thoracic deformities for cosmetic reasons in the adult should be given serious consideration. Not all patients were single, and many were happily married but continued to be concerned about their cosmetic deformity.

Following careful assessment of the desire for surgery, together with a careful explanation of the procedure and its postoperative course and complications, such surgery should not be denied the adult, provided that the surgeon is highly experienced and has the full support of the institutional facilities and care.

The past few years have seen a return to excision of the rib hump. This is particularly valuable for rigid curves in the thoracic spine and especially in the sagittal plane where there is hypokyphosis. In more mobile curves, the use of Cotrel-Dubousset instrumentation to derotate the spine helps decrease the rib hump. An associated rib excision can be done at the same time.

In a review of 20 patients who underwent rib excision consisting of five to six ribs on the convexity, patients with very rigid deformities of 90 degrees or greater revealed

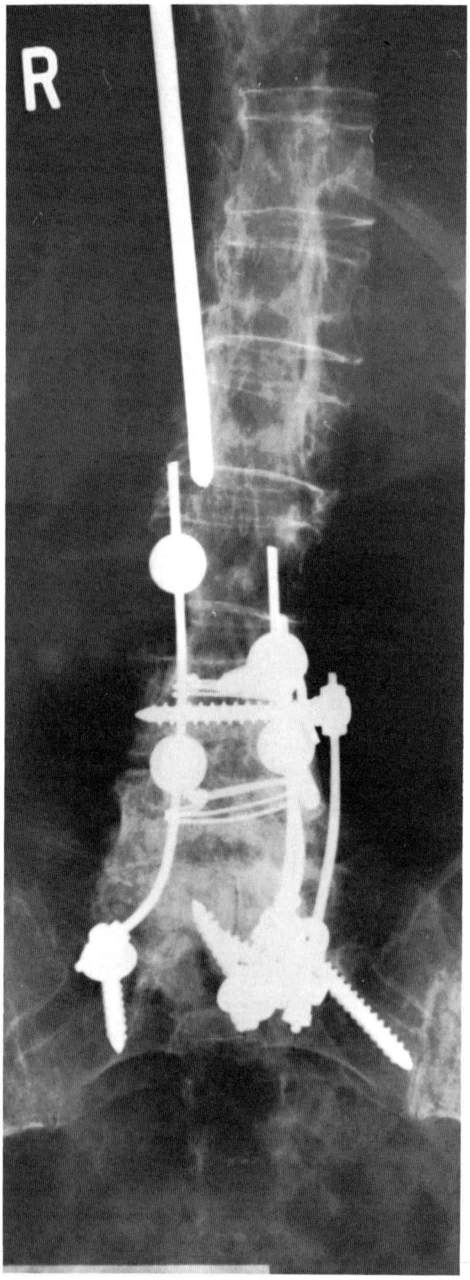

Figure 24 □ Postoperative AP radiograph. Pain has been relieved. (Same patient as in Fig. 21.)

no untoward morbidity. There were no changes in preoperative and postoperative ventilation studies. Rib hump excision in the presence of a severe thoracic scoliosis that is rigid can markedly improve the cosmetic result.

In mobile curves the use of Cotrel-Dubousset instrumentation is preferred. Because of its enhanced stability today, Cotrel-Dubousset instrumentation is also used in patients with rigid curves. No postoperative orthoses are necessary.

At the time of rib excision, the bone may be cut up into small fragments to be used as graft material.

The problem of cosmesis in the lumbar and thoracolumbar spine in adults is a rare one, in the young adult who is unbalanced and in the elderly individual with a kyphoscoliotic lumbar spine. The latter should not be operated on for cosmetic reasons alone.

Treatment of Structural Disabilities

Patients who have a paralytic scoliosis may find sitting at a desk or wheelchair difficult because of marked pelvic obliquity or an associated kyphosis with a collapsing spine or hyperlordosis. The latter is encountered particularly in patients who have had lumbar peritoneal shunts in childhood. Patients with paralytic scoliosis are still best treated by a combined anterior and posterior approach, which eliminates the need for external postoperative immobilization and allows for early ambulation in a wheelchair.

Individuals with certain paralytic curves of a collapsing nature, in whom respiratory function is decreasing, can be significantly helped by correction of their deformity. This results in improved diaphragmatic breathing. A preoperative trial of halo-dependent traction may show an improvement in respiratory function and demonstrate, with little morbidity, the advantages of surgical correction of the deformity to improve respiratory function by lifting the diaphragm out of the abdomen.

The use of Cotrel-Dubousset instrumentation has not yet proven to be sufficient in the treatment of paralytic deformities that extend into the distal lumbar spine, for which we advocate an anterior and posterior approach. Certainly, in children, the use of Luque instrumentation to the pelvis, using L rods or the Galveston modification has proven to be of value in that age group, but in our experience with adults this is insufficient, and a two-stage anterior and posterior procedure is necessary.

Treatment of Spinal Deformities Over 50 Years of Age

The adult over 50 years of age presents with a complex problem. The deformity is often rigid and may be associated with significant imbalance and loss of normal lordosis of the lumbar spine. The bone is frequently osteopenic, and there may be associated neurologic problems related to spinal stenosis. The major indication for presentation is pain. The early experience of the author was such that major spinal deformities in patients over 50 years of age could only be corrected in terms of deformity at great risk to the neurologic structures, because the vast majority of these curves are rigid. As a result, in the early experience, most such deformities were simply stabilized by means of Harrington instrumentation with little attempt made at correction. This often resulted in continuing kyphosis, which in itself was a problem.

Because of the improved techniques of anterior fixation, such as Zielke instrumentation, and posterior fixation techniques, such as Cotrel-Dubousset instrumentation, correction can now be safely achieved. In the presence of a thoracolumbar or lumbar deformity with good preservation of lordosis, an anterior Zielke instrumentation can be safely used. The use of methyl methacrylate has greatly enhanced the holding power of screws in the vertebral bodies. Methyl methacrylate should not be used posteriorly in the pedicles, except in the first sacral pedicle, because the cement may exude out of the osteopenic pedicle in elderly adults and result in canal compromise. In the presence of a rigid kyphoscoliosis or where there is minimal lumbar lordosis, a two-stage procedure is preferable. The first stage consists of a multiple disc excisions and interbody graft by using small bone fragments followed 10 days later by posterior derotation by means of Cotrel-Dubousset instrumentation to correct the curve and restore lumbar lordosis (see Figs. 5 to 8 and 17 to 20). This has proved to be extremely valuable over the last few years.

A recent review of 80 patients over 50 years of age was performed by the author. Fifty had idiopathic curves, and the remainder had a congenital curve, a paralytic curve, or a pure kyphotic deformity. Twelve of the idiopathic curves were thoracic, nine were thoracolumbar, and 17 were lumbar; there were 12 double curves. All patients presented with back pain. Eight patients had a progressive pulmonary dysfunction, usually related to an increasing kyphosis. Fifty-seven percent of cases had documented evidence of progression of greater than 10 degrees in the 3 years preoperatively. Sixteen patients had associated root pain. These 80 underwent 100 procedures. Twenty patients had a second-stage procedure either anterior or posterior for increased stabilization. Twelve patients had concurrent anterior and posterior procedures performed largely for correction of flat back syndrome through a single-stage combined posterior and anterior osteotomy with anterior and posterior fixation. Although 20 patients who underwent a second-stage procedure for stabilization, most had rigid kyphoscoliosis. Fourteen had a second-stage anterior procedure because fusion was carried to the sacrum posteriorly, and in order to ensure a solid fusion, anterior fixation and fusion were carried out (as described under the discussion of fusions to the sacrum). In a review of all cases, excellent to good results were achieved in 69%, of which 56.5% were good and 12.5% excellent. Fair and poor results occurred in 31%, 25% of which were poor. No pain was noted in 27 patients postoperatively (34%); root pain was relieved in all patients.

It is absolutely contraindicated, in the presence of spinal stenosis or other causes of root pain in a scoliosis, to perform a posterior decompression alone, particularly if more than one level is decompressed. An associated stabilization procedure should always be performed. The author has encountered many patients who have undergone posterior decompression for spinal stenosis in the presence of scoliosis, only to have the patient present within months to years with significant collapsing, progressive, painful scoliosis. These patients present marked difficulties in obtaining a subsequently stable fused spine because of the lack of bone stock as a result of the decompression and subsequent scarring, and they generally require an anterior and a posterior procedure to ensure bone union.

In this group of 80 patients over 50 years of age, curve correction was 22% with Harrington instrumentation and 22% with sublaminar wired Harrington rods. Twenty-one percent correction was achieved with Harrington rods combined with L rods, and 33% with double L rods. Curve correction with Dwyer instrumentation was 42%, and with Zielke instrumentation it was 67%. This result compares favorably with the 70% of all adults corrected by Zielke instrumentation over the age of 20 years. The average correction obtained with Cotrel-Dubousset instrumentation was 50%. Thirteen of the patients treated with Harrington instrumentation alone developed flat back syndrome. Posterior distraction in the lumbar spine at any age should be avoided at all cost, except for anterior distraction for kyphotic deformities. Pure kyphotic deformities are best treated by anterior instrumentation as noted in a section on kyphotic deformities. Instrumentation failure in this group of elderly adults occurred in 11 patients (14%), six of whom were Harrington rod fractures, dislodgment of a rod in one case, two cases of L rod migration, one case of anterior screw breakage, and one case of broken posterior Zielke rods. The infection rate was 1%. Pulmonary complications including atelectasis and pneumonia, and adult respiratory distress syndrome occurred in 24%. Intraoperative bone fracture of either laminae or vertebral bodies occurred in seven cases and was overcome with the use of methyl methacrylate associated with internal fixation devices. Thirteen patients developed iatrogenic flat back secondary to Harrington distraction. Four of these subsequently underwent restoration of lordosis by single-stage anterior and posterior osteotomies. One patient became paraparetic as a result of surgery and had partial improvement. Pseudarthrosis was found in 21%, primarily in the Harrington series. To date, there have been no pseudarthroses with the use of Zielke instrumentation or Cotrel-Dubousset instrumentation. Twenty-five percent of pseudarthroses were found in fusions carried to L5, and 24% were found in fusions carried to the sacrum. All pseudarthroses to the sacrum occurred prior to the development of two-stage surgery for fusions to the sacrum as described elsewhere in this subchapter. Nine patients developed a kyphosis secondary to osteopenic factors proximal to their instrumentation with improved diagnostic capabilities and improved postoperative care and the advent of improved fixation, such as posterior pedicle fixation, particularly of the Cotrel-Dubousset type. Anterior Zielke instrumentation morbidity has been reduced by 50% in the last 5 years. The importance of restoration of lordosis cannot be over emphasized, particularly in cases of kyphoscoliosis. The use of multiple-level releases anteriorly followed by posterior derotation with Cotrel-Dubousset instrumentation, and if necessary, posterior osteotomy through the pars interarticularis increases lordosis, which markedly improves the quality of life of these senior patients.

Treatment of Iatrogenic Lumbar Kyphosis

Fusions to the sacrum performed in adults by the author with posterior Harrington distraction instrumentation led to a significant loss of lumbar lordosis in 50% of patients.[12] Half of them required restorative surgery. Although adolescents compensate well, it is not unusual for a patient who has had a fusion to the sacrum in adolescence to begin complaining of fatigue symptoms and pain during the 3rd, 4th, or 5th decades of life. Care must be taken to ascertain that this problem does not arise from the sacroiliac joint.

Loss of lumbar lordosis results in an increasingly forward flexed attitude as the day progresses, and the patients walk with their knees and hips flexed. This is an unsightly deformity (Figs. 25 and 26). Despite a solid fusion, these patients complain of increasing pain and fatigue. Unfortunately, this problem was not recognized until the late 1970s. The author presented a preliminary report of 10 cases in 1980 and a further review of 33 patients in 1984,[13] in which a combined anterior and posterior osteotomy was used for restoration of lordosis. A combined approach offers more than a posterior osteotomy, and in an old fusion mass, greater correction can be obtained and it is not necessary to immobilize the patients in a hip spica postoperatively. Moreover, the use of posterior osteotomy alone has in the author's experience in at least two cases resulted in a late recurrence of deformity. A recent report by Lagronde et al[19] also indicated that the best results can be obtained by anterior and posterior procedures. A combined anteroposterior approach, together with internal fixation and the use of a simple lumbar orthosis postoperatively, allows for early ambulation.

Etiologic factors that may lead to a loss of lumbar lordosis are as follows, in descending order of frequency: distraction instrumentation, the lower end of which is at the

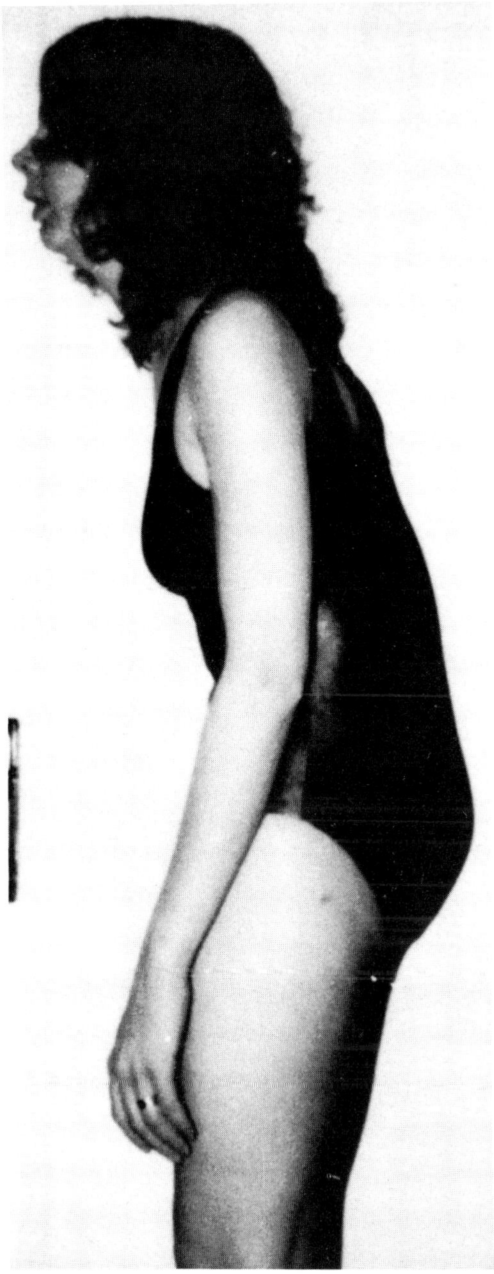

Figure 25 □ Photograph taken following Harrington distraction on the lumbar spine. The lumbar spine, unless kyphotic, should never be distracted posteriorly.

L5 or S1 vertebral level; thoracolumbar junction kyphosis greater than 15 degrees, especially if associated with kypokyphotic thoracic spine; degenerative changes above and/or below a previous fusion, due to loss of disc height that occurs more commonly below a previous fusion ending at L3, L4, or L5.

If loss of lumbar lordosis is also associated with a pseudarthrosis, repair of the pseudarthrosis alone does not suffice to relieve the patient's symptoms.

If the patient is imbalanced in the anteroposterior plane, a quadrilateral-type wedge osteotomy performed anteriorly and posteriorly can be done to restore balance in the

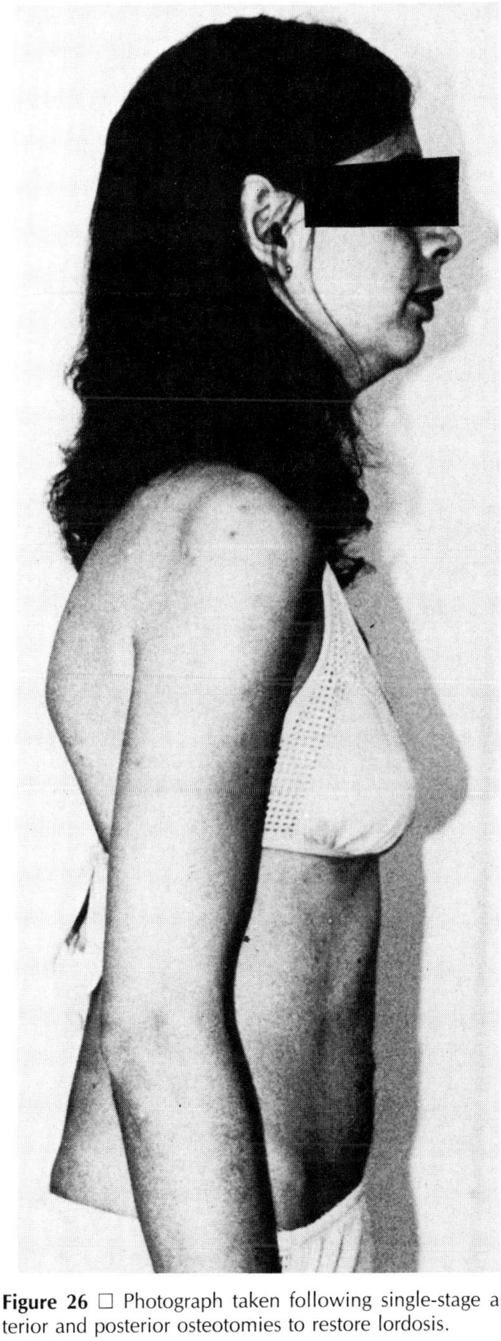

Figure 26 □ Photograph taken following single-stage anterior and posterior osteotomies to restore lordosis.

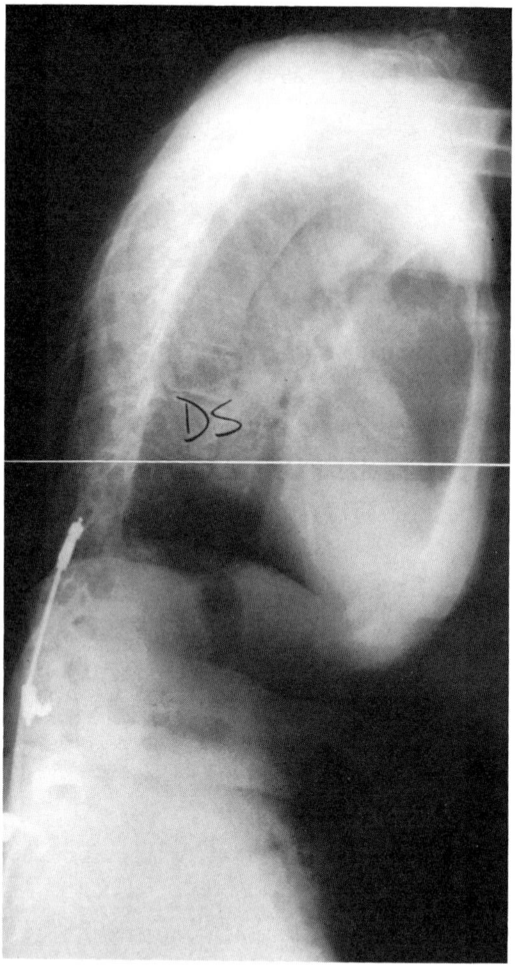

Figure 27 □ Woman, 44 years old. Previous Harrington distraction instrumentation was performed in the lumbar spine with loss of lordosis. The distraction rod was removed. The fusion was solid.

frontal plane as well as to restore lumbar lordosis in the sagittal plane (Figs. 27 to 30). If the fusion is solid, the osteotomy is carried out, usually at the L3–L4 level; otherwise it may be carried out through the posterior pseudarthrosis, which is enlarged. The nerve roots at the level of the posterior osteotomy must be clearly identified, and an osteotomy analogous to that described by Smith Peterson and coworkers[29] is used. Dwyer screws and cables used in the lateral fusion mass posteriorly are ideal for closing the osteotomy site. Eight screws are used. These consist of four screws proximal to and four screws distal to the osteotomy site (Figs. 31 to 34). These are used on either side of the midline, and in the author's opinion it appears to be simpler to use than other forms of fixation. A midline contoured AO plate is used to help control rotation; at least two screws are proximal and distal to the osteotomy site. Concomitant to the posterior approach, an anterior approach is carried out at the L3–L4 level or at the apex of the frontal curve and corresponding to the posterior osteotomy. An opening wedge osteotomy is performed through the disc, or if there has been a previous anterior fusion, through the anterior fusion mass. The opening of the osteotomy anteriorly is carried out simultaneously with Kostuik-Harrington instrumentation (Figs. 33 and 34), while the posterior osteotomy is closed with a Dwyer instrumentation. A tricortical or bicortical iliac crest graft is used anteriorly. A review of 54 patients[14] treated in this fashion revealed excellent results, with pain relief in

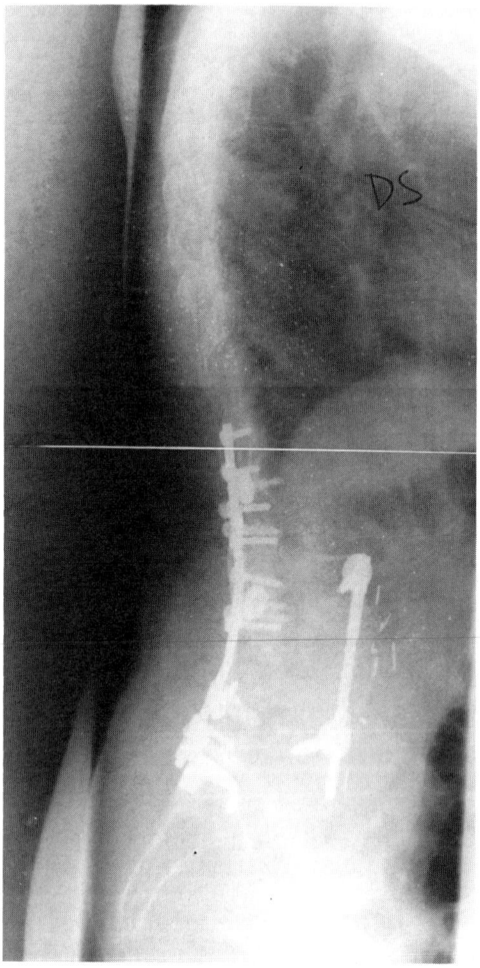

Figure 28 □ Lordosis has been restored by single-stage anterior and posterior osteotomies with fixation (see text) and relief of symptoms.

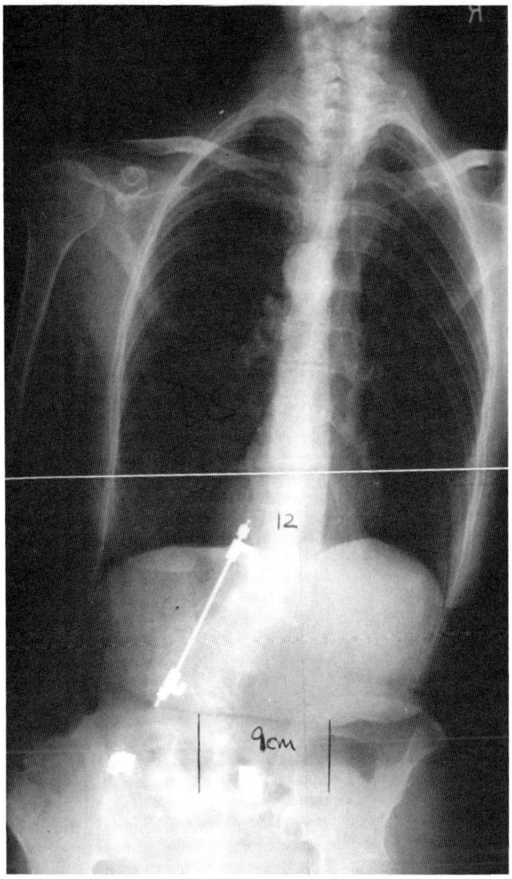

Figure 29 □ Note the marked imbalance on the AP radiograph.

48 (90%). Delayed union occurred in three patients because of anterior graft collapse, one of whom requested a reoperation. Neurologic complications were found in two patients; one had a permanent deficit of weakness of the dorsi and plantar flexors of her feet and inconsistent bladder control.

Follow-up is at 4 years. Average preosteotomy lordosis, L1–S1, was 21.5 degrees and was restored to 49 degrees, which indeed was equal to lordosis before the initial posterior scoliosis surgery. This is an average of 29 degrees of correction with a range of 24 to 63 degrees.

Attention to prevention of this complication is paramount (see discussion of Fusion to the Sacrum).

Treatment of Adult Kyphotic Deformities

The posterior elements of the spine are under tension, and the anterior elements are under compression. Kyphosis may occur when either of these two components are disrupted. An increase in physiologic loads both in magnitude and direction may result in a kyphotic deformity. An increase in angulation results in an increased in the moment arm and as pointed out by White and Panjabi,[35] may result in an increase in load

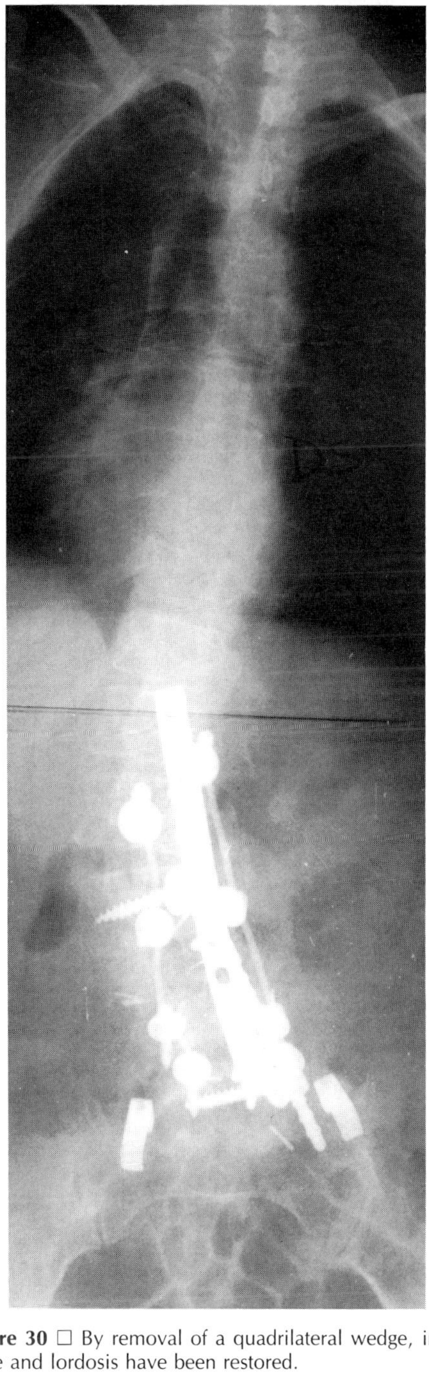

Figure 30 □ By removal of a quadrilateral wedge, imbalance and lordosis have been restored.

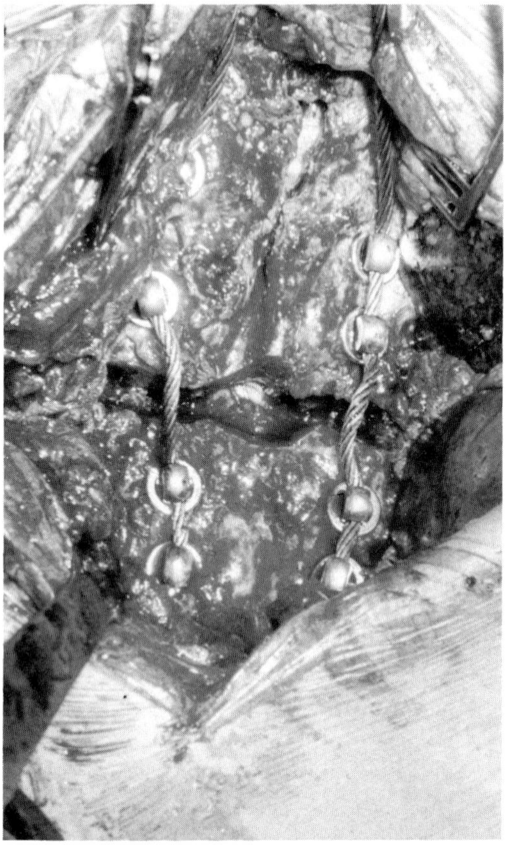

Figure 31 □ An osteotomy has been performed, usually about 1.5 cm in width through the posterior fusion mass. Note placement of the Dwyer screws, once washers are placed in the lateral fusion masses. Also note the dura in the midline.

and increased wedging of the vertebral bodies. Increased wedging increases angulation and results in a vicious circle (Fig. 35).

The treatment of severe kyphosis involves one or more steps, including, if necessary, adequate decompression of the spinal cord and the application of forces to correct the deformity. These corrective forces consist of axial traction and sagittal plane bending moments (transverse loading). These correctional forces reverse the role of the anterior and posterior structures.

Posterior fusions are generally under tension in a kyphosis and are usually thin and susceptible to stress fracture, and they may bend. A posterior fusion is usually considered to be more stable, the greater its length. Nevertheless, pseudarthrosis rates and failure to maintain correction are as high as 40% in the treatment of Scheuermann's disease in adults.[15] Conversely, anterior fusions are under compression and are therefore ideal. In the beginning of 1979, the author started to use Harrington instrumentation anteriorly for the correction of kyphotic deformities. Instrumentation consists of a rachet screw for the rachet end of the round Harrington rods and a collar-ended screw (Fig. 36). The instrumentation was initially developed for the treatment of burst fractures that were decompressed anteriorly. Two rods were used: a rachet-ended rod and a heavy Harrington compression rod. These rods were used in the form of a rectangular parallelogram (they are preferably coupled). This led to the subsequent use of the instrumentation for the correction of other kyphotic deformities, in particular, post-traumatic kyphosis, Scheuermann's kyphosis, a small number of congenital kyphotics, iatrogenic loss of lumbar lordosis, rigid round back, postlaminectomy kyphosis, and kyphosis secondary to tumor and secondary to metabolic osteoporosis with fractures. As of October 1987, 279 cases of anterior instru-

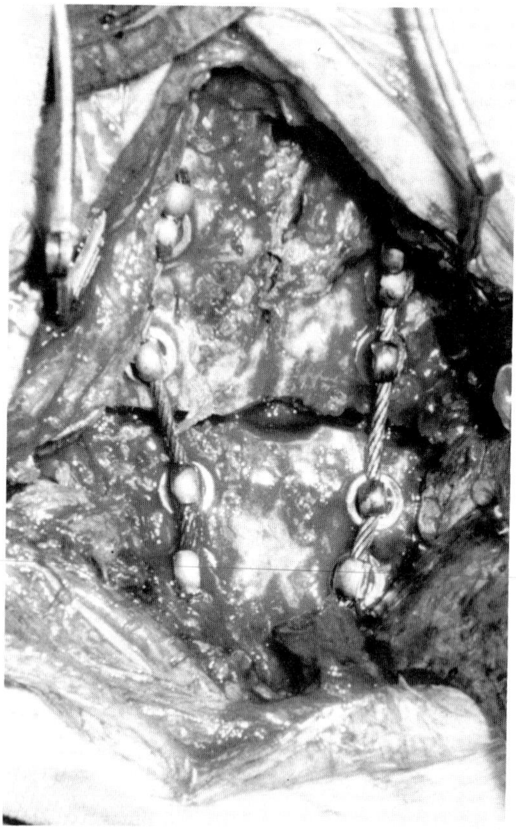

Figure 32 □ The cables have been tightened simultaneously with the opening of the anterior osteotomy. A midline AO plate contoured to the restored lordosis is added posteriorly to control rotation (see Fig. 30).

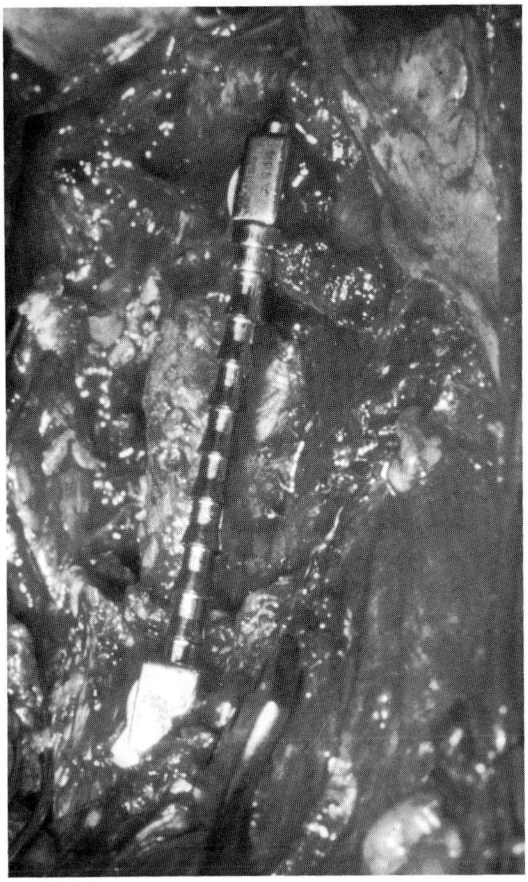

Figure 33 □ The anterior osteotomy is opened with the Kostuik-Harrington instrumentation (see Fig. 28). A tricortical or bicortical iliac crest graft is added.

mentation have been carried out using the system.[18] These consist of 100 burst fractures,[16] 45 post-traumatic kyphotics,[17] 36 Scheuermann's kyphotics, 3 rigid round backs, 4 acute angled rigid kyphotics, 21 postlaminectomy kyphotics, 56 iatrogenic lumbar kyphotics, 10 with kyphosis secondary to tumor, and 4 with secondary to osteoporotic fractures. The instrumentation has also been used posteriorly in 50 cases of pedicle fixation. Complications have consisted of screw breakage in 35, primarily in the earlier models of untapered thin shank screws. Two distraction rods have fractured without any sequelae. Vertebral body fractures occurred in 8, all intraoperatively in osteoporotic bone, and they were salvaged by the use of methyl methacrylate. There have been no early or late vascular or neurologic problems. Of the 45 patients with post-traumatic kyphosis, all of whom presented with pain, excellent to good pain relief occurred in 37. Screw breakage occurred in three cases. Late neurologic improvement occurred in 33% (3 of 10) (Figs. 37 and 38).

Previous studies by the author[15] of the surgical treatment of adults with Scheuermann's kyphosis by posterior instrumentation indicate a progressive loss at long-term follow-up (minimum, 6 years). Loss of correction is a result of the fusion being on the tensile side of the spine with high pseudarthrosis rates (40%)[15] and later is because of late stress fractures resulting from repetitive cyclical loading on the tensile side of the spine. Previously, studies by Morscher[23] and Malcolm and Bradford[22] of anterior interbody fusion performed alone without instrumentation have shown inadequate maintenance and correction of the deformity. The unsuccessful techniques of posterior instrumentation and fusion with high pseudarthrosis rates and subsequent secondary surgical procedures due to loss of correction from the above causes led to the development and use of Kostuik-Harrington instrumentation anteriorly, combined with interbody fusion for the correction of Scheuermann's kyphosis. The use of this

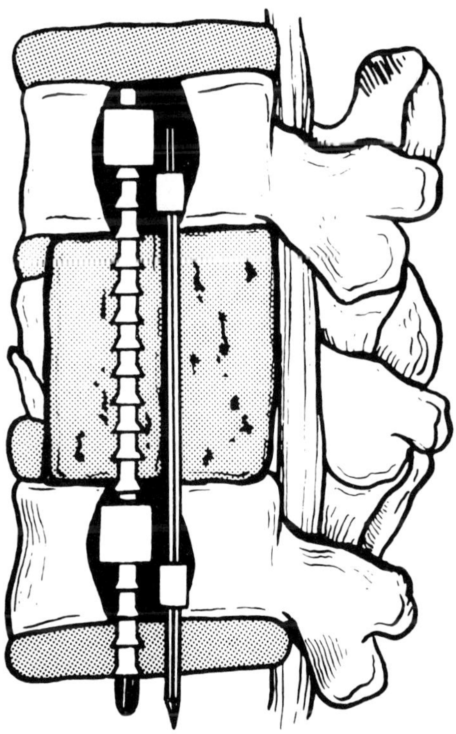

Figure 34 □ A second heavy Harrington compression rod is added for rotational stability.

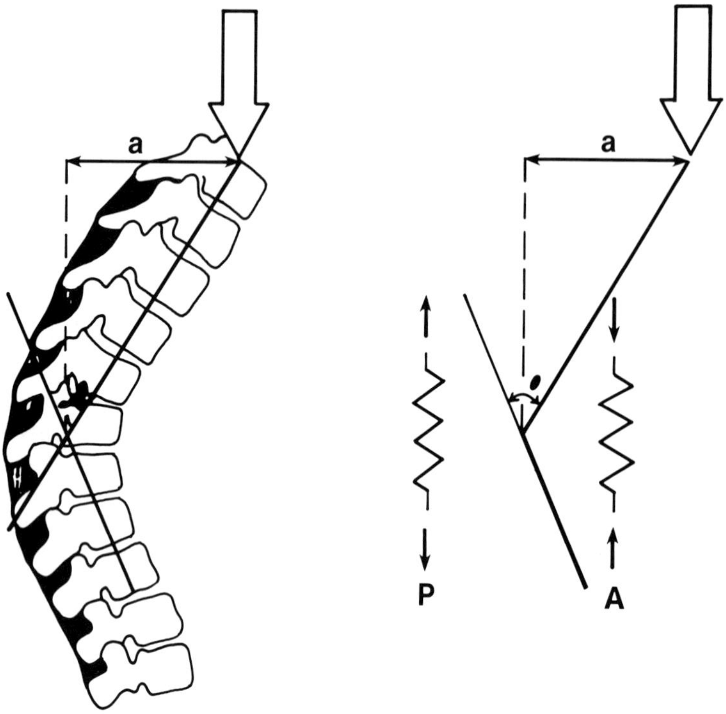

Figure 35 □ The pathomechanics of kyphosis. An increase in load results in increased kyphosis. As well, an increase in angulation results in an increased moment arm (a). A vicious cycle ensues. (A = anterior; P = posterior.)

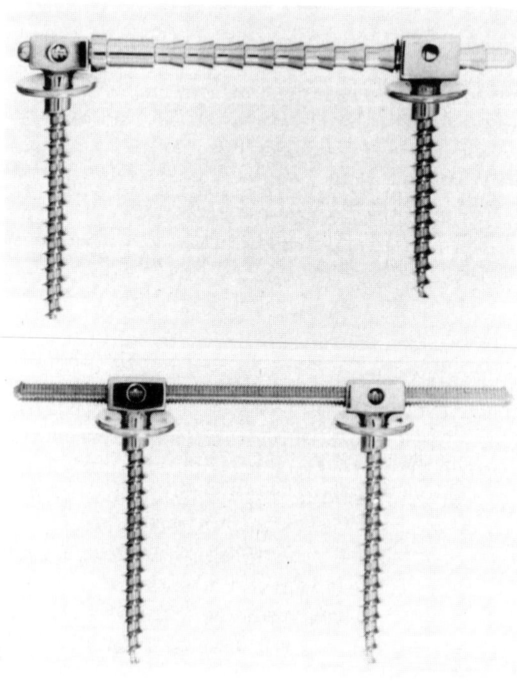

Figure 36 □ Kostuik-Harrington instrumentation. Staples, instead of washers, may be used to increase the couple. The screws consist of a rachet screw for the round-ended Harrington distraction rod and collar-ended screws. The collar-ended screws are usually crimped over the heavy Harrington compression rod, although nuts may be used.

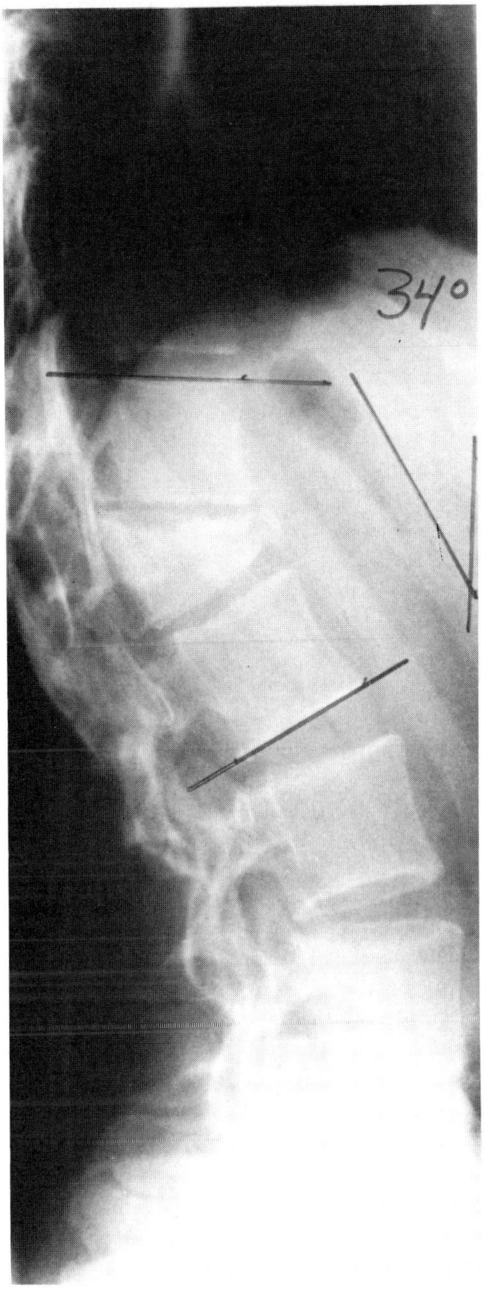

Figure 37 □ Burst fracture at L1, which occurred 4 years previously. One year postinjury a posterior fusion was performed without relief of pain. Re-exploration revealed a solid fusion. Late neurologic signs and symptoms developed. Kyphosis measured 34 degrees.

technique correlates with the ideals in the correction of kyphotic deformities by providing axial distraction in reducing bending moments and by producing a fusion mass that is under tension and that is long and far from the neutral axis and interbody.

Although space does not permit a description of the technique here, it should be pointed out that screws must pierce the cortices of both bodies. (Figs. 39 and 40). Osteopenic bone can be enhanced by the use of methyl methacrylate. The indications for the correction of Scheuermann's kyphosis in adults are for deformities of 75 degrees or greater, particularly in women, and in those who have a documented progression of the kyphosis.

Between 1982 and 1987, 36 patients at an average age of 27.5 years were treated; the mean preoperative curve was 75 degrees, and the postoperative curve was reduced to 56 degrees. (Figs. 41 to 43) At follow-up at 2 years, the average curve was 60 degrees. One pseudarthrosis occurred. Four screw fractures occurred with some loss of correction. Postoperatively, a plastic orthosis was

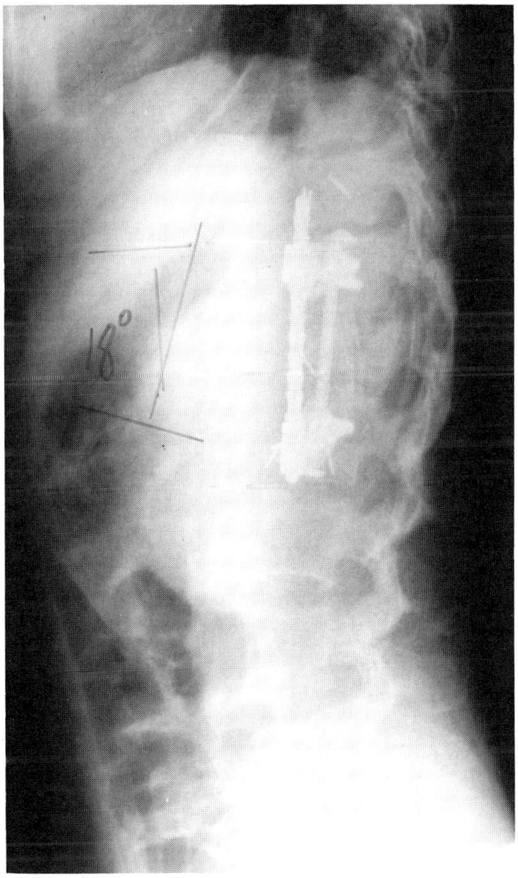

Figure 38 □ The angulation has been reduced to 18 degrees with Kostuik-Harrington anterior instrumentation without osteotomy of the solid fusion mass. Anterior decompression relieved the patient's signs and symptoms. An iliac crest graft (bicortical) was added.

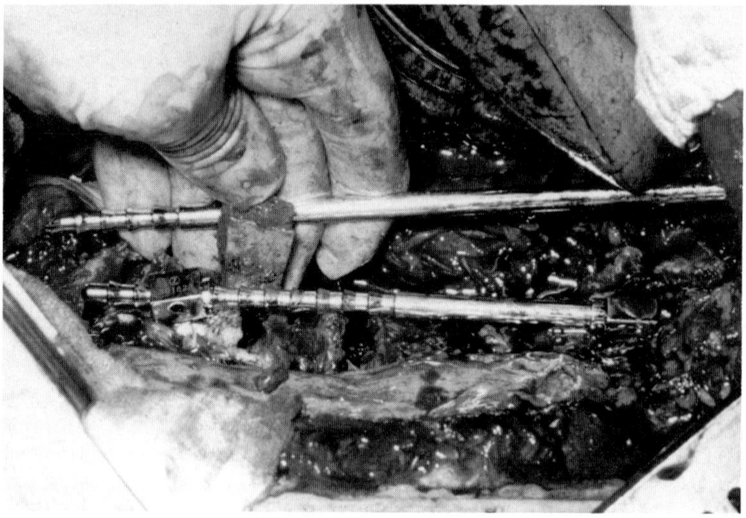

Figure 39 □ Scheuermann's kyphosis: anterior approach. Note the two distraction rods and multiple discectomies. Bicortical iliac crest grafts are used as interbody grafts.

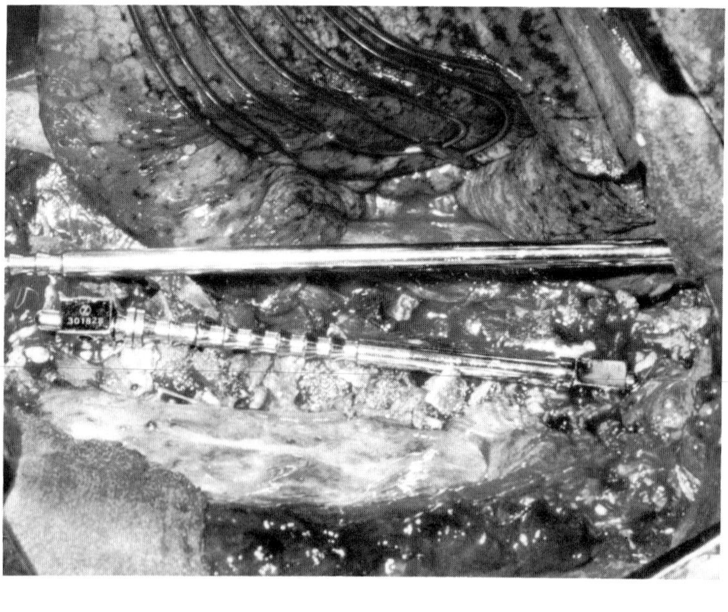

Figure 40 □ Immediately postoperative views with all grafts in place.

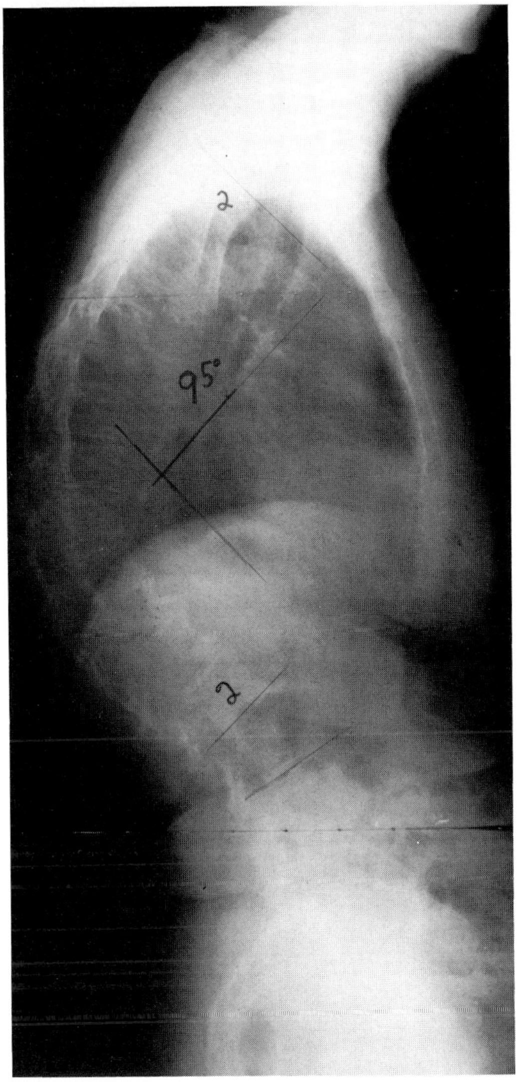

Figure 41 □ Woman, 37 years old. Preoperative kyphosis measures 95 degrees at T2–L2.

used for 6 months. The early success of this technique is attributed to the fusion mass being under compression. The anterior instrumentation prevents collapse of interbody grafts which occur without instrumentation, as has been pointed out by White and Panjabi,[35] Morscher,[23] and Malcolm and Bradford.[22]

Iliac crest grafts are preferred; these are bicortical in younger and tricortical in older osteopenic people. There are preferred to fibula grafts because iliac crest grafts revascularize quickly. Fibular grafts do not begin to revascularize often until 6 months postoperatively. Anterior instrumentation is necessary, however, if iliac crest grafts are to be used, because as White and Panjabi[35] have pointed out, these grafts alone are unable to stand the loads in the erect position, particularly in the thoracolumbar and lumbar spine.

MORBIDITY AND MORTALITY

The treatment of spinal deformities in the adult is not without risk. The incidence of

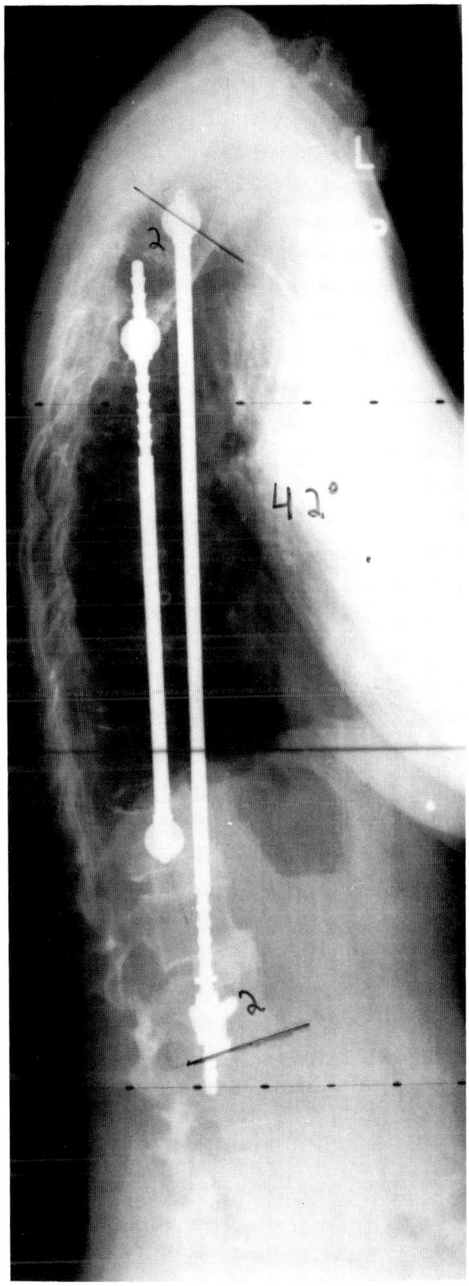

Figure 42 □ Postoperative kyphosis at 2 years. Curve has been corrected and maintained at 42 degrees with relief of pain.

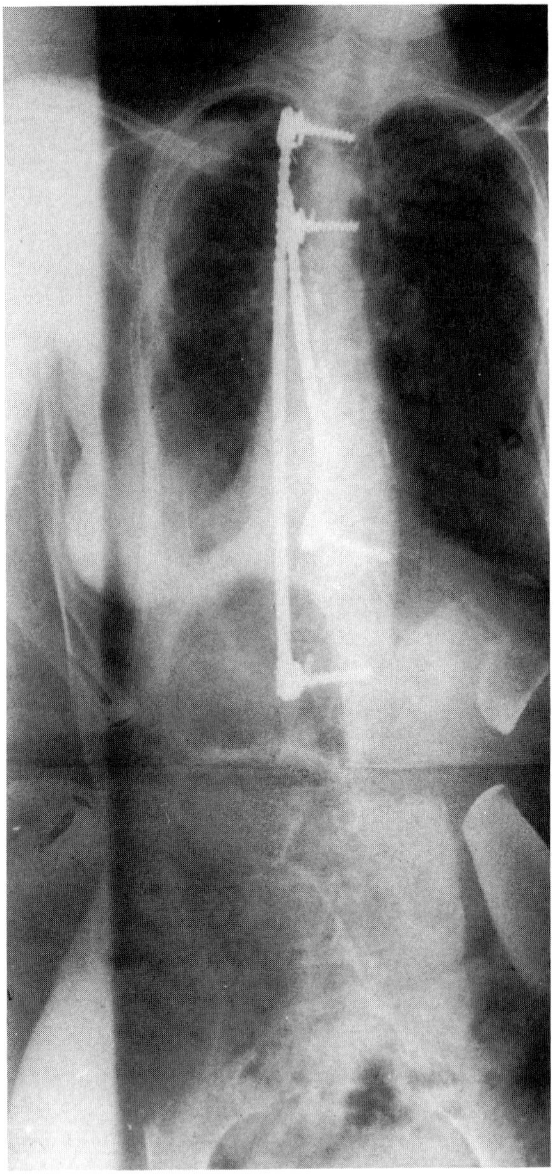

Figure 43 □ AP radiograph demonstrates full screw penetration of the vertebral bodies. In this case, T2–T4–T12 and L2 have been used.

neurologic complications in the adolescent has been repeatedly reported as being approximately 1%. Morbidity reports indicate that the incidence of neurologic complications in the adult lies between 2% and 3%. In the author's review of the first 1,000 patients, there is an incidence of paraparesis of 0.7% (seven patients). Only two patients remained unable to walk at follow-up. The incidence of nerve root irritation of single root motor weakness occurred in 3%. The vast majority of these recovered. The second most frequent complication is that of pulmonary embolus. Two deaths have occurred as a result of this dreaded complication, but none have occurred in the last 5 years, since the advent of prophylaxis consisting of an intravenous minidose of heparin, 2,500 units daily, and intravenous dipyridamole (Persantine), 150 mg daily, run as a continuous drip; it is started preoperatively and maintained for an average of 10 days postoperatively. The deep infection rate has been 1%, with no major sequelae. Prophylactic antibiotics are used for 48 hours.

There has been a 0.8% mortality rate. Two

instances of this have resulted from pulmonary embolus, three from adult respiratory distress syndrome, one from a disseminated intervascular coagulopathy, and two from vascular problems.

Other complications, such as instrumentation failure rates, pseudarthroses, and loss of lumbar lordosis, have been discussed under sections.

References

1. Cochran, T., Irstram, L., and Nachemson, A.: Long-term anatomic and functional changes in patients with adolescent idiopathic scoliosis treated by Harrington rod fusion. Spine 8:576–584, 1983.
2. Collis, D. K., and Ponseti, I. V.: Long-term follow-up of patients with idiopathic scoliosis not treated surgically. J. Bone Joint Surg. 51A:425–445, 1969.
3. Dewar, F. P.: Incidence of scoliosis in an adult population using miniature chest radiographs. Unpublished data. Toronto General Hospital, 1947.
4. Drummond, D., Guadagni, J., Keene, J. S., et al.: Interspinous process segmental spinal instrumentation. J. Pediatr. Orthop. 4:397–404, 1984.
5. Dubousset, J.: Proceedings of the International Congress on Cotrel-Dubousset Instrumentation, Sauramps Medical. Montpellier, France, June, 1986.
6. Dwyer, A. F.: Experience of anterior correction of scoliosis. Clin. Orthop. 93:191, 1973.
7. Edgar, M. A., and Mehta, M. H.: A long-term review of adults with fused and unfused idiopathic scoliosis. Orthop. Trans. 6:462–463, 1982.
8. Simmons, E. H., Jackson, R. P., and Stripinus, D.: Incidence and severity of back pain in adult idiopathic scoliosis. Spine 8:749–756, 1983.
9. Kostuik, J. P., and Bentivoglio, J.: The incidence of low back pain in adult scoliosis. Spine 6:268–273, 1981.
10. Kostuik, J. P.: Recent advances in the treatment of painful adult scoliosis. Clin. Orthop. 147:238–252, 1980.
11. Kostuik, J. P., Israel, J., and Hall, J. E.: Scoliosis surgery in adults. Clin. Orthop. 93:225–234, 1973.
12. Kostuik, J. P., and Hall, B. B.: Spinal fusions to the sacrum in adults with scoliosis. Spine 8:489–500, 1983.
13. Kostuik, J. P., Gleason, T. F., Errico, T. J., and Errico, C. C.: The surgical correction of flat back syndrome (iatrogenic lumbar kyphosis). Orthop. Trans. 9:131, 1985.
14. Kostuik, J. P., Maurais, G. R., Richardson, W. J., and Okajima, Y.: Combined single stage anterior and posterior osteotomy for correction of iatrogenic lumbar kyphosis. Spine 13:257–266, 1988.
15. Kostuik, J. P., and Lorenz, M.: Long-Term Results of Posterior Instrumentation for the Treatment of Scheuermann's Kyphosis in Adults. Presented at the Scoliosis Research Society Meeting, Montreal, 1981.
16. Kostuik, J. P.: Anterior fixation for burst fractures of the thoracic and lumbar spine with or without neurological involvement. Spine 13:286–293, 1988.
17. Kostuik, J. P., and Matsusaki, H.: Anterior stabilization, instrumentation and decompression for post-traumatic kyphosis. Spine, 14:379–386, 1989.
18. Kostuik, J. P.: Anterior Kostuik-Harrington distraction systems. Orthopedics (Special Issue-Spinal Techniques) 11:1371–1379, 1988.
19. Lagrone, M. O., Bradford, D. S., Moe, J. H., et al: Treatment of symptomatic flatback after spinal fusion. J. Bone Joint Surg. 70-A:569–580, 1988.
20. Luque, E. R.: Segmental Spinal Instrumentation. Thorofare, NJ, Slack Publishers, 1984.
21. Macnab, I.: Backache. Baltimore, Williams & Wilkins, 1977.
22. Malcolm, B. W., and Bradford, D.: Post traumatic kyphosis. A review of forty-eight surgically treated patients. J. Bone Joint Surg. 63:891–899, 1981.
23. Morscher, E.: Unpublished data. Department of Orthopedics, Basel, Switzerland.
24. Nachemson, A.: A long-term follow-up study of non-treated scoliosis. Acta Orthop. Scand. 39:466–476, 1968.
25. Nachemson, A.: A long-term follow-up study of non-treated scoliosis. J. Bone Joint Surg. 50A:203, 1969.
26. Nilsonne, U., and Lundgren, K. D.: Long-term prognosis in idiopathic scoliosis. Acta Orthop. Scand. 39:455–465, 1968.
27. Ponseti IV: The Pathogenesis of Adult Scoliosis. *In* Zorab, P. A. (ed.): Proceedings of Second Symposium on Scoliosis Causation. Edinburgh, E. & S. Livingstone, 1968.
28. Simmons, E. H., and Jackson, R. P.: The management of nerve root entrapment syndromes associated with the collapsing scoliosis of idiopathic lumbar and thoracolumbar curves. Spine 4:533–541, 1979.
29. Smith-Peterson, M. N., Larson, C. B., and Aufranc, O. E.: Osteotomy of the spine for correction of flexion deformity in rheumatoid arthritis. J. Bone Joint Surg. 27:1–11, 1945.
30. Stagnara, P.: Scoliosis in adults. Surgical treatment of severe forms. Excerpta Medical Foundation International Congress Series No. 192, Paris, 1969.
31. Stagnara, P., Gonon, G. P., and Faucher, P.: Surgical Treatment of Idiopathic Rigid Lumbar Scoliosis in the Adult in Management of Spinal Deformities (Orthopaedics 2) London, Butterworths, 1984, pp. 303–321.
32. Stagnara, P.: Utilization of Harrington's device in the treatment of adult kyphoscoliosis above 100 degrees. *In* Fourth International Symposium, 1971. Nijmegen, Stuttgart, George Thieme Verlag, 1973.
33. Stagnara, P., Fleury, D., Pauchet, R., et al.: Scolioses majeures de l'adultes superieures a 100–183 cas traites chirurgicalement. Rev. Chir. Orthop. 61:101–122, 1975.
34. Vanderpool, D. W., James, J. I. P., and Wynne-Davies, R.: Scoliosis in the elderly. J. Bone Joint Surg. 51A:446–455, 1969.
35. White, A. A., and Panjabi, M. M.: Clinical Biomechanics of the Spine. Philadelphia, J. B. Lippincott, 1978.
36. Weinstein, S. L., and Ponseti, I. V.: Curve progression in idiopathic scoliosis. J. Bone Joint Surg. [Am.] 65:447–455, 1983.
37. Zielke, K., and Pellin, B.: Ergebnisse operativer Skoliosen-und kyphoskoliosen-behandlung beim adoleszenten uber 18 jahre und beim erwachsenen. Z. Orthop. 113:157, 1975.

21 □ Spinal Instrumentation

Martin H. Krag
Bruce E. Fredrickson
Hansen A. Yuan

■ BIOMECHANICS OF TRANSPEDICLE SPINAL FIXATION

Martin H. Krag

Extensive interest has recently developed in spinal instrumentation that uses transpedicle screws as the method of vertebral attachment. This interest has been stimulated by certain major advantages of this approach, although much remains to be learned about its limitations and the best methods for avoiding potential complications. Many of these issues are biomechanical ones. Here is presented a history of the development of these devices as well as a review of the topic, which is organized by biomechanical subject and which includes our current understanding as well as certain remaining questions.

DEVELOPMENT OF TRANSPEDICLE IMPLANTS

Attachment sites other than the pedicles were used for a number of decades for spinal implants. The spinous processes were the attachment sites for the upper and lower ends of pairs of tin-plated steel rods implanted by Lange[96, 97] in 1910 for treating "spondylitis." Plates that are bolted together on each side of four or five spinous processes for stabilization of traumatic injury or lumbosacral degeneration were first described by Wilson in 1943 (Wilson and Straub[174]), and then by Williams in 1956 (Williams[173]). A similar approach was used by Reimers[131] and Sicard and Menegaux.[147] A wire loop passed around adjacent spinous processes for thoracolumbar fracture/dislocations was described by Stanger.[150]

At about this same time, the facet joints were used as attachment sites for metal screws, which were placed across the joints for partial immobilization of the lower lumbar and lumbosacral spine. In the 1940s, apparently independently, both Toumey[160] and King[76, 77] described the same method almost simultaneously, which was then also used by others (Baker and Hoyt,[14] Pennal and coworkers,[126] Thompson and Ralston[159]). A fairly high pseudarthrosis rate with this method led Boucher[21] to redirect the screws more medially so that they still went across the facet joint but continued into the pedicle, rather than exiting the lateral cortex of the superior articular process. Others (Pennal,[126] and Andrew and coworkers[4]) have reported their experience with this method. Yet another method (described by Magerl[112, 113] and also used by Jacobs and coworkers[70]) was to increase the angulation of the screw in the opposite direction so that it was oriented more laterally: the screw enters at the base of the spinous process on the contralateral side, passes through the ipsilateral lamina, crosses the facet joint, and exits the lateral cortex of the superior articular process. This probably provides for a stronger grip on the inferior articular process, which appears to be the "weak link" in the other facet screw methods. Casey and Jacobs[25] showed that this method provides stiffness in the lumbosacral region comparable to that provided by Luque rods (see below).

A quite different line of development was based upon attachment of implants to the laminae. Harrington distraction rods were described in 1962,[62] and the choice of hook attachment site was based upon strength testing of various possible attachment sites. This implant was designed for realignment of scoliosis but was also used for spondylolisthesis[63, 64] and for trauma and other causes of instability.[61] The history of this device has been described elsewhere.[60, 63]

As experience with Harrington rods grew, problems with their use were identified.[55] The range of their usefulness was explored, and clinical problems that posed greater biomechanical demands were treated. A number of refinements and modifications resulted: (1) the hook shape was modified,[46, 51] (2) two or more upper hooks on each rod were used,[20, 120] (3) an enclosed two-part hook was developed,[69, 72] (4) the ratchets on the rod were replaced by threads[69, 72, 161] or eliminated altogether,[163] (5) the lower rod end was made square to prevent rod rotation after the rod was bent into lordosis,[31, 118] (6) a plastic spacer between the lamina and the central portion of the rod was used to allow increased lordosis without rod bending,[44, 45] (7) wires passed through the bases of the spinous processes spanned by the rods were used to increase the number of attachment sites of the implant,[38, 39, 154] and (8) increased length of rods (to the third vertebra above and third vertebra below) either with no graft[40] or a short graft,[26, 71, 72] which has caused some concern regarding the spanned but ungrafted facet joints.[73, 74] In conjunction with the Harrington distraction rods, compression rods were also developed.[62] These too have been subsequently modified[75] and mechanically tested (e.g., by Laborde and coworkers[95]). These rods were initially intended to be used in combination with distraction rods for realignment of scoliotic spines, but they have also been used in combination for stabilization of traumatized spines.[143]

Other devices have been attached to the laminae by means of hooks. Knodt and Larrick,[82] beginning in 1961, used a threaded rod to produce distraction between a pair of hooks. Attenborough and Reynolds[13] stretched a spring between a pair of hooks to achieve compression and extension. Weiss,[170] apparently independent of Attenborough, and extending the work of Gruca,[57] devised a similar system.

Another method of attachment to the laminae was described by Luque;[108, 109] wires were passed around the laminae and tied to a longitudinal smooth L-shaped rod, dorsal to the laminae. The major feature of this method was that it allowed (1) multiple vertebrae to be attached to the implant (previously described by Resina and Alves,[132] based upon his experience with a similar system since 1963), and (2) long-segment deformities such as scoliosis or kyphosis to be gradually corrected by transverse rather than longitudinal forces.

One variation of this method is to join the 2 L rods into a solid rectangle.[22, 37] Another variation is to replace the wires with Mersilene tapes, which are much more flexible and thus safer to pass around the laminae.[56] Yet another approach has been to use the circumlaminar wires with Harrington distraction rods instead of L rods.[3, 24, 36, 52, 135] Various wire closure techniques have been described and mechanically tested.[167] Comparison between wires placed around the lamina and those placed through the spinous processes has also been made.[168, 171] The risk that wire passage around or removal from the lamina may cause neural damage is not insignificant,[36] particularly when the wires are used with Harrington distraction rods[36] or compression rods,[135] although others have not emphasized this.[3, 24] Mersilene tapes may be significantly safer in this regard.[56]

Use of the pedicle specifically as an attachment site for spinal implants to the vertebra has a history of more than 20 years. In 1969 Harrington and Tullos[64] described two cases of L5 spondylolisthesis, operated upon in 1967, in which "lag screws" were placed one each through the pedicles and into the body of L5 and were wired to Harrington distraction rods to produce and maintain a partial reduction (Fig. 1). Because these authors believed that this method was not particularly helpful for the problem,[63] they stopped using it. On the contrary, Roy-Camille and coworkers,[137, 138] under the initial

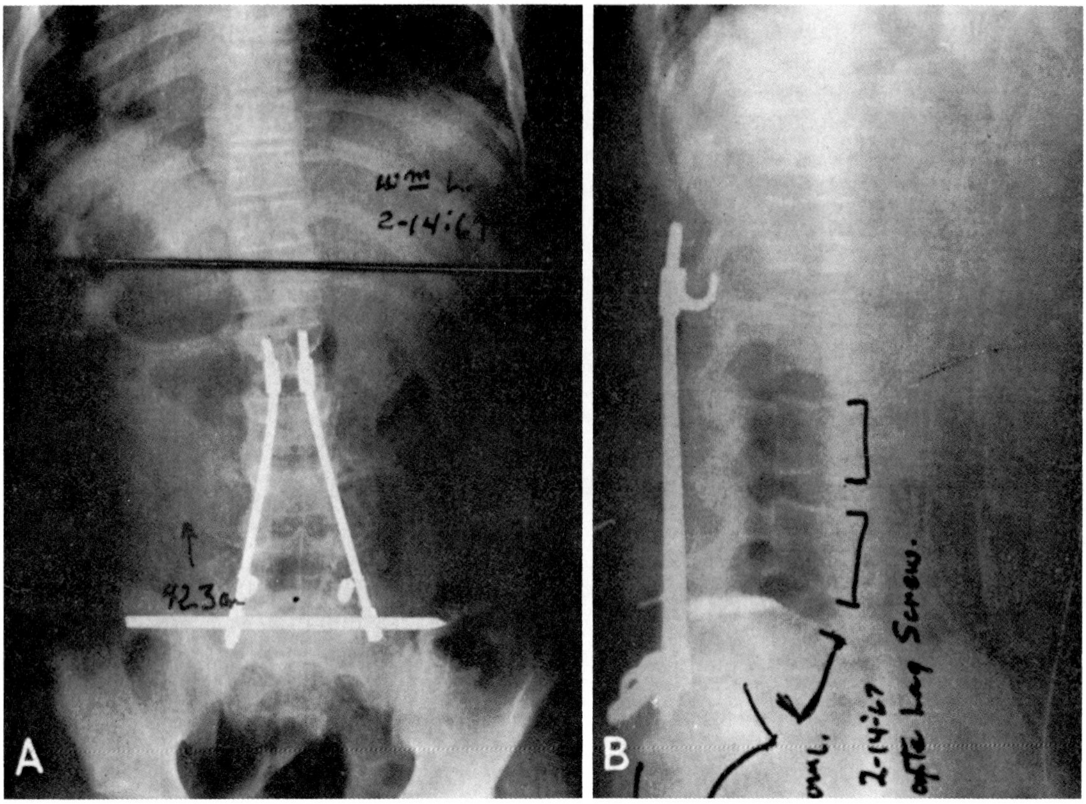

Figure 1 □ Earliest reported case (February, 1967) of transpedicle screws used for attachment to a vertebra. *A,* Anteroposterior x-ray film shows transpedicular screws in L5 medial to the rods. *B,* Lateral x-ray film shows screws inserted into L5 vertebrae, attached by wires to Harrington distraction rods from L1 to a sacral bar below. (From Harrington, P.R., and Tullos, H. S.: Reduction of severe spondylolisthesis in children. Reprinted by permission from the Southern Medical Journal 62:1–7, 1969.)

guidance of Judet,[104] have reported since 1970 an extensive positive experience using transpedicle screws (which apparently they began in 1963) to attach specially designed posterior plates for spinal stabilization of various conditions. Other authors also have described their experience with this implant system.[19, 29, 66, 78] The extensive and pioneering work by Roy-Camille appears to have been directly or indirectly the origin of most of the current transpedicle fixation systems.

Plates and screws were thus the first really successful transpedicle screw-based spinal implants, and a family of such implants has developed. Louis, drawing upon his experience with the Roy-Camille system, modified the design.[104–106] Since at least 1979, the use of tibial AO *dynamic compression plates* (AO-DCP) has been described[119, 157] for posterior spinal fixation; the use of a somewhat different AO plate *(notched plate)* has also been described.[19, 33] More recently, Steffee has also made modifications of *standard AO neutralization plates,*[151–153] so that the screw could be adjusted along the plate and could be clamped perpendicularly to it by means of nuts both anterior to and posterior to the plate. Other authors have reported their experience with this method.[67, 68, 172] The longitudinal adjustability of the screw along the plate introduced by Steffee has been further increased by Luque.[110]

Another large family of transpedicle screw-based implants uses rods as the longitudinal element. It may be useful to consider these in two subgroups: (1) those in which the screws provide supplemental fixation sites for rods, which are also attached by either hooks or circumlaminar wires, and (2) those in which the screws alone are used for rod attachment. In the first subgroup, a number of systems were devised specifically for obtaining and maintaining reduction of spondylolisthesis. Harrington and Tullos,[64]

Sijbrandij,[148] Vercauteren and DeGroote,[163] and Zielke and Strempel[177] attached the transpedicle screw to a Harrington distraction rod between the upper and lower hooks. In contrast, placement of the screw above the two attachment points to the sacrum was the approach used by Schöllner,[144] Edwards,[41] and Matthiass and Heine.[115] Vidal and coworkers[164] described yet a different use for transpedicle screws: as an attachment point for the lower hook of a Harrington distraction rod to the sacrum. Other devices in this subgroup were not specifically designed for management of spondylolisthesis. Kostuik[84, 85] used a screw, its attachment to a Harrington distraction rod being identical to standard Harrington hooks. Although he used this for anterior stabilization, apparently it was originally intended for posterior stabilization in the presence of myelomeningocele, in which no lamina was available for a hook attachment. Luque[107] describes screws that are wired to Luque L-shaped rods, in a manner somewhat analogous to the early work of Harrington and Tullos.[64] Similarly, Mehdian and coworkers[116] wired Dwyer screws to a Luque rectangular frame. Edwards and Weigel[47] used compression rods to join a proximal hook to a sacral screw bilaterally, for low lumbar nonunions. More recently Cotrel and coworkers[20] have described a system in which various screws or hooks can be attached along a knurled rod. Others (such as Birch and coworkers[18]) have also reported their experience with this system.

The second of the two subgroups of implants described above used screws alone for rod attachment. Because these systems are typically used with at least three screws on each side, in general either the rods must be bent to contact the screws,[59, 125, 128, 129, 145, 149] or care must be taken to align the posterior ends of the screws colinearly.[145] Apparently since the early 1980s (inferring from publication date and length of patient follow-up), two such systems, both of which use threaded rods, have been implanted: the Zielke system[129, 149] and the Balgrist system,[145] the latter inspired by experience with Roy-Camille and Louis plates. Since 1985, the Wiltse system has been implanted and a fairly extensive experience acquired.[59, 125, 158] Even more recently, Puno and colleagues[128] have presented mechanical testing of a new system.

The third family of transpedicle screw-based implants is that of the fixators, the two major characteristics of which are (1) three-dimensional positional adjustability between screw and longitudinal linking component without bending of either one, and (2) three-dimensional positional control of each screw (and thus of each vertebra). Two subgroups of this family have developed—external fixators and internal fixators. For the former, Magerl[112, 113] certainly was the pioneer. He apparently combined the idea of transpedicle screw attachment popularized by Roy-Camille and the idea of external fixation for limb fractures, the use of which had been evolving for decades. Substantial experience with this spinal external fixator was acquired in Western Europe.[29, 81, 112, 113] Arnold[7, 8] in Leipzig developed one modification of this device, and Ölerud and coworkers[123] in Uppsala adapted a Hoffman fixation frame for temporary lumbosacral fixation as a diagnostic test for degenerative "instability." The following features have inhibited widespread use of this device: use of these devices requires a special mattress to accommodate the posteriorly protruding device; pin track infections can develop as with any external fixator; and accidental penetration of the pins through the anterior vertebral cortex is possible.

Internal spinal fixator development began almost simultaneously along two separate lines that have proceeded independently and that were both directly influenced by Magerl. According to Dick,[32, 33] Magerl suggested such an internal fixator, which was subsequently designed in late 1982 by Dick and coworkers and first implanted in December, 1983. Its use was first reported in 1984,[33] and in English in 1985.[34] More extensive clinical experience has since been reported by Dick[32] as well as by others.[1, 2, 29, 49, 156] Experience with this device was the basis for its modification by Kluger and Gerner[81] from West Germany in 1985, whose design has also been used by others.[19] Similarly, Ölerud from Uppsala has described his modification, apparently in use since late 1985.[122]

The other separate line of internal fixator development was stimulated not only by Magerl but also by Roy-Camille. In 1981, the author was able to meet with Roy-Camille concerning his internal plate and screw system, and with Magerl and Schläpfer regarding their work on the external fixator. These visits helped solidify our own ideas concerning how best to internalize an external fixator. It was only after our own early publications on this topic in 1985[90] that we were able to learn, through published reports, of the efforts of others (see above) who pursued the same basic goal. Because in 1981 even the basic morphometric issues needed further research, at that time we began a program of implant design development, extensive biomechanical testing,[89–91] and anatomic studies,[94] which eventually led to the initial clinical implantation in July, 1986, of the Vermont Spinal Fixator (VSF).

It seems clear that further testing and design development in the area of transpedicle screw-based spinal implants will continue. Improved understanding of the various benefits, complications, and risks associated with such devices is needed, which in turn will help guide future design improvements. Because biomechanical issues play a central role in this development, some of these topics are reviewed below.

MORPHOMETRY

The factor limiting the diameter of a transpedicular screw is the mediolateral width of the pedicle. Saillant[139] has reported certain important cadaver data; however, these have certain limitations. First, only average values were given and not the ranges or standard deviations. Second, the length of the screw that could be implanted was reported for only a purely sagittal placement: other screw placement angles may be preferable,[80, 81, 86, 87, 89–91, 112, 113] and their use would usually alter this length. Third, only the pedicle diameter perpendicular to the pedicle axis was reported: screws not oriented along the pedicle axis may encounter an effectively smaller diameter. Finally, no clinically usable radiographic confirmation to the caliper measurements from cadaveric specimens was provided.

For these reasons, a study was undertaken by the author to provide the desired data,[89, 94] some of which are shown in Figure 2 and Table 1. Subsequently, additional morphometric data have confirmed or extended this work. Zindrick and coworkers[178] measured not only T9 to L5, but also T1 to T8, and included sagittal height and angulation of the pedicle. Berry and colleagues[17] studied T2, T7, T12 and L1–L5. They included a number of other measurements relative to the vertebral body, spinous process, and

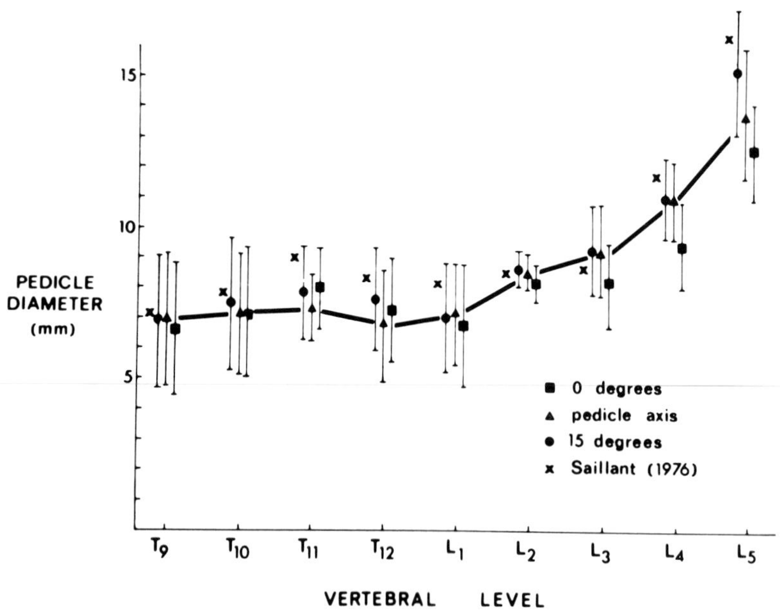

Figure 2 □ Pedicle diameter means ± 15 degrees for each vertebral level, measured from computed tomographic (CT) transverse plane images. Effective diameter was measured parallel to the frontal plane (0 degrees), perpendicular to the pedicle axis or in a plane 15 degrees anterolateral from the frontal plane (15 degrees). The data means given by Saillant[139] are provided for comparison. (From Krag, M. H., Beynnon, B. D., Pope, M. H., et al.: An internal fixator for posterior application to short segments of the thoracic, lumbar, or lumbosacral spine: Design and testing. Clin. Orthop. Rel. Res. 203:75–98, 1986.)

Table 1 □ Pedicle Diameter and Distribution by Size

LEVEL	MEAN	SD	NUMBER	3–3.9 mm (%)	4–4.9 mm (%)	5–5.9 mm (%)	6–6.9 mm (%)	7–7.9 mm (%)	8–19.4 mm (%)
T9	6.88	2.23	14	14	7	14	21	7	35
T10	7.47	2.24	18	11		11	39		39
T11	7.83	1.56	22			14	18	14	55
T12	7.63	1.79	24			21	21	12	46
L1	7.01	1.84	22	9		18	18	14	41
L2	8.67	0.64	14					7	92
L3	9.30	1.51	24				8	12	79
L4	11.03	1.36	24						100
L5	15.15	1.97	20						100

spinal canal. Banta and coworkers[15] compared pedicle dimensions of cadaveric vertebrae obtained by anteroposterior (AP) and lateral x-ray studies, as well as by direct measurement with calipers. Although they conclude that the lateral x-ray film is not very helpful (pedicle height-to-width ratios are not constant), they unfortunately do not report the correlation between width measurements from AP x-rays and those from calipers. Misenheimer and coworkers[117] confirmed the accuracy of computed tomography (CT), showed that sequential insertion into the pedicle of probes of increasing diameter did not give an accurate assessment of pedicle endosteal diameter, and demonstrated that pedicle cortical disruption did not occur if screw diameter was less than the endosteal diameter or less than 80% of the cortical diameter. Finally, Asher and Strippgen[11] studied the sacrum and described the path lengths of six different screw sites in both female and male cadaveric sacra.

TRANSPEDICLE SCREW DESIGN

Even though there is a fairly extensive literature characterizing the strength of various screws implanted into limb bones, only one study in this area has been done that independently varies the different screw design features of tooth profile, pitch, and minor diameter (DeCoster and coworkers[30]). Bechtol[16] did compare pull-out strength of screws from dog limb bones with one each of eight different tooth profiles, but the minor diameters were unspecified and the use of different pitches was done in a way that did not allow isolation of the effect of this variable. Koranyi and coworkers[83] reported equal pull-out strengths for both V-toothed Sherman screws and buttress-toothed AO screws, using dog or cattle femora. However, neither major nor minor diameters were specified, although tooth heights were the same. Diehl and coworkers[35] concluded that the pull-out strengths of AO cortical and cancellous screws were approximately the same when these were inserted into epiphyseal or metaphyseal sites (i.e., those that were predominantly cancellous bone). Lyon and colleagues,[111] Nunamaker and Perren,[121] and Schatzker and coworkers[140] each studied various groups of different commercially available screws, but their study designs did not assess the individual effects of pitch, major diameter, and minor diameter to be segregated.

Martin and coworkers[114] focused attention upon a feature of screw design other than just axial or pull-out loads, namely, flexural rigidity (i.e., bending stiffness). In the case of screws used to hold plates against tubular long bones, sufficient friction must be present to shield screws from such flexural loads. However, when loosening occurs (e.g., screw back-out, or resorption of bone under plate) such shielding may break down, leading to failure of screws that were not designed to tolerate such loads.[27, 124, 127, 176] Shielding of screws from flexural loads may be especially difficult to maintain under plates applied to the spine posteriorly, since the surface is fairly irregular, even if the facet joints are partially removed. Herrman[66] emphasized the relation between facet trimming and plate contact area. Failure to design screws to tolerate flexural loads may be the explanation for the high screw breakage or bending rate encountered with use of various implant systems.[68, 137, 138, 152, 172]

Studies specifically directed at transpedicle screws are few. Only one such study, by the author and coworkers,[89, 91] has systematically varied pitch, minor diameter, and tooth profile. For screw pull-out strength testing it showed that (1) the V and buttress tooth profiles were the same, (2) 2-mm pitch screws were only somewhat (21%) stronger than 3-mm pitch screws in only one of three subgroups tested, and (3) smaller minor diameter screws (3.8 mm) were only somewhat stronger (19% to 26% depending upon subgroup) than larger minor diameter screws (5 mm), but that this was offset by a reduction to less than half ($[3.8/5]^3 = 44\%$) of the flexural rigidity of the 5-mm minor diameter screws.

Other issues concerning transpedicle screw design have also been studied. Liu and coworkers[103] showed experimentally that the above-described and predictable sensitivity of flexural rigidity to minor diameter was in fact present: increasing the minor diameter of Steffee screws from 3 to 3.8 mm doubled the static and fatigue strength ($[93.8/3]^3 = 2.04$). We determined[88] the fatigue response of VSF screws and showed that the limiting factor for fatigue life was not the clamps that joined screw to rod, but rather the first thread root. Liu and colleagues[102] showed that nitrogen-ion implantation into the metal of 7-mm Steffee screws could improve fatigue life by 98% (significant, $p < .05$) at lower bending loads (3.96 N•m or 35 inch-pounds), although only 20% (insignificant, $p < .01$) at higher bending loads (5.09 N•m or 45 inch-pounds). Most recently, Geiger and coworkers[53] measured four-point bending fatigue strengths of a number of screw types subjected to various cyclic loads (haversine pattern, 2.9–10.8 N•m, lever arm of 28 mm, requency of 4 Hz). The screws studied were Cotrel-Dubousset 5 mm, Ölerud 5mm, Steffee 5.5 mm, AO modified 6.5 mm, Luque 6.5 mm, and Steffee 7 mm with and without integral nut. The authors noted the importance of avoiding stress risers in screw design and the lack of correlation between major diameter and fatigue life. Unfortunately, the minor diameters of the screws tested are not specified; this measure may correlate fairly well with fatigue life. It has also been emphasized[68] that bending the screws may cause a significant decrease in screw fatigue life, and thus should clearly be avoided during either reduction maneuvers or during attachment between screw and longitudinal linking device (plate or rod). It seems clear that further work in the area of transpedicle screw design remains to be done.

TRANSPEDICLE SCREW PLACEMENT

The basic principles involved in optimal screw placement include (1) strength of the resulting bone–metal interface, (2) avoidance of damage to neurologic structures by screw penetration through pedicle cortex or vertebral body cortex, (3) avoidance of damage to the adjacent facet joint, and (4) ease and convenience of implantation procedure. Various aspects of screw implantation will be considered with these four principles in mind.

Entry Site and Orientation

Because the desired orientation affects the entry site, these will be considered together. Two different approaches have been advocated. Roy-Camille[137, 138] has adopted the motto of "straight ahead," based on his recommendation (followed by others[101, 104, 122, 151, 152]) that transpedicle screws be placed parallel to the sagittal plane, as well as to the vertebral end plates. The resulting entry point (Fig. 3*A*) is at the intersection between a transverse line bisecting the transverse process, and a longitudinal line bisecting the facet joint. In contrast, Magerl,[112, 113] and later others,[1, 2, 32–34, 89, 94, 169] used an "inward" or anteromedial approach. For this, the longitudinal guide line for the entry site (Fig. 3*B*) is along the lateral aspect of the superior articular process rather than through the facet joint. Through this entry site the screw is oriented along the pedicle axis, obliquely to the sagittal plane, but parallel to the end plate.

An even further departure from the straight-ahead approach that the author has found to be useful may be described as "up and in" (Fig. 3*C*). The entry site is as far lateral as in the Magerl approach but is also somewhat lower, along a transverse line between the upper two thirds and lower one third of the transverse process. The orientation is still medially angulated along the pedicle axis but is also inclined somewhat cephalad, although not so far as to intersect the superior end plate. This up-and-in approach allows the dorsally protruding screw

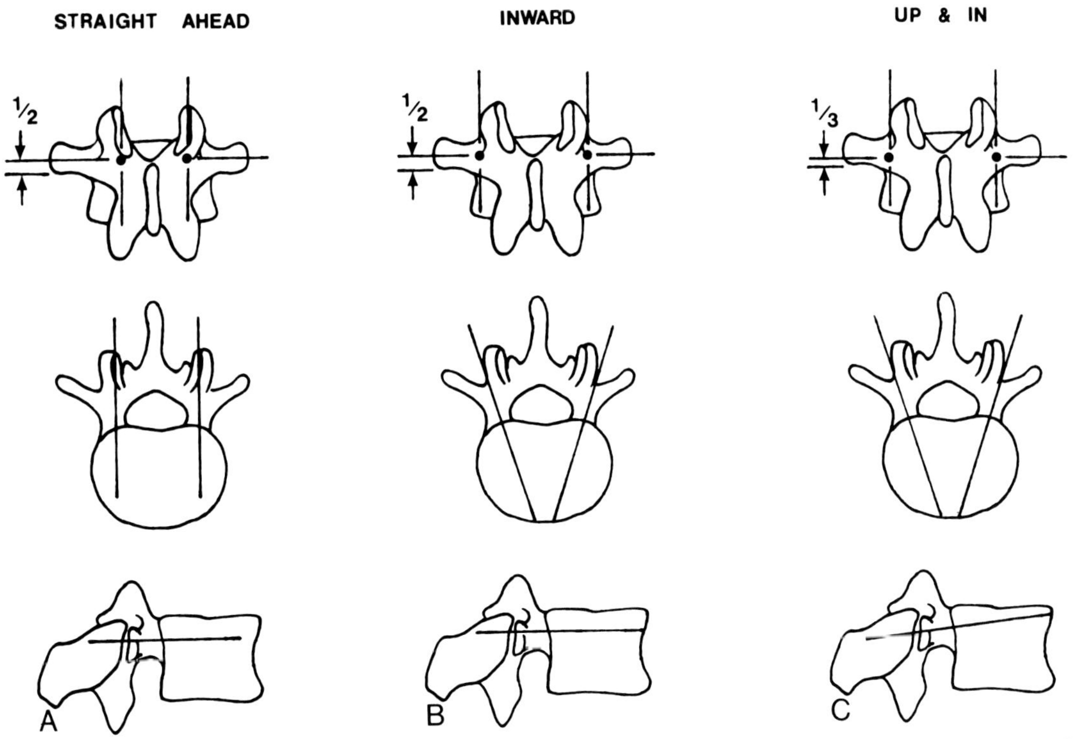

Figure 3 □ Entry point and orientation alternatives for transpedicle screws. *A*, "Straight ahead." The entry point is the intersection of a line that bisects the transverse process and a line that bisects the facet joint. Orientation is parallel to the sagittal plane and parallel to the end plates. *B*, "Inward." The entry point is more lateral, and the orientation is anteromedial along the pedicle. The longitudinal line is along the lateral aspect of the facet joint (superior articular process). *C*, "Up and in." The entry point is both more lateral and lower (more caudad). The transvere line divides the upper and lower thirds of the transverse process. The orientation is still anteromedial but also anterocephalad (up and in), although not enough to intersect the superior end plate.

head to remain "down and out," relative to the superjacent facet joint (also mentioned by Levine and associates[101]). This in turn has at least three implications. First, there is less interference with the superjacent facet joint,[86] which may be a more important factor than implant stiffness in causing the accelerated degeneration of the superjacent motion segment that has been reported.[67] Second, a screw along the oblique path may be longer than one along the straight-ahead path,[94, 178] without anterior cortex penetration, thereby increasing the bone–metal interface strength.[87, 98] Third, the "toenailing" effect produced by the interaction between obliquely oriented instrumentation on the right and on the left sides of the vertebral column (Fig. 4), will resist lateral translation of the upper vertebra relative to the lower, even without any cross-bridging.

Placement of screws into the sacrum poses a particular problem because of the unique anatomy in this region, and the somewhat greater difficulty of intraoperative visualization of structures, even radiographically. Perhaps for these reasons, a wide variety of recommendations have been given for screw entry site and orientation (Table 2).

Not only do these clinically based recommendations vary, but also there are no strength measurements available that allow well-controlled comparisons among different proposed insertion sites. Asher and Strippgen[11] measured the path lengths of various screw placements in the sacrum. The lengths anteromedially to the sacral promontory in females and males were 47 and 50 mm, respectively, while the lengths anterolaterally into the S1 ala were 37 and 39 mm. Using these length data as a basis, the authors conjecture that the stronger screw would be the one directed anteromedially into the promontory. However, no measurements of strength were made to confirm this. Zindrick and coworkers[180] did perform strength measurements, using 6.5-mm

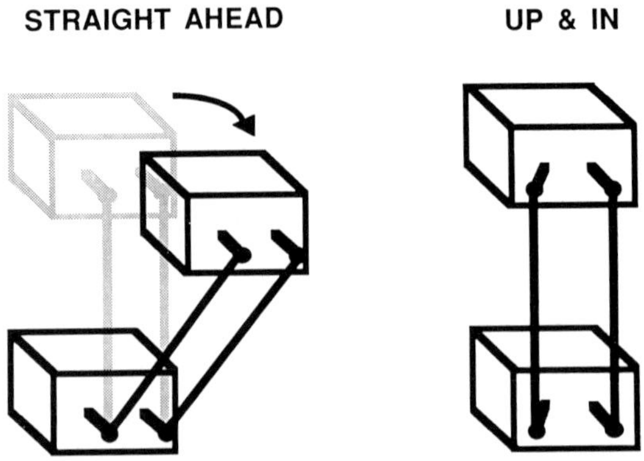

Figure 4 □ Straight-ahead orientation of the screws causes them to be parallel, and thus lateral shifting meets with little resistance (friction between screw and bone). Up-and-in orientation causes an interlocking or toenailing effect, which resists this lateral shifting.

screws placed into various sites in the sacrum. Unfortunately, they noted a very high interspecimen variation and yet did not perform right-to-left comparisons of different screw sites within the same specimen. Thus, it is not clear whether the mean differences observed between screw sites were significant. Also, the type of load used was a pull-out of the screw along its own axis; yet clinically this does not appear to be an important failure mode. Although limited, these are the only strength data available, and they show no conclusive difference between the anteromedial and the anterolateral placements.

We are presently completing a study that compares the strength of an anteromedially directed screw in one S1 pedicle to the strength of an anterolaterally directed screw in the opposite S1 pedicle of the same specimen. This design controls for the known large interspecimen variation. The study also uses flexion loads rather than pull-out along the screw axis, because we believe this to be more clinically relevant. In addition, to address the issue of safety in screw placement we are measuring the location of important neurovascular structures relative to sacral bony landmarks.

A final issue concerning screw entry and orientation is that of monitoring the process in order to ensure safe and accurate placement of screws through the pedicles. The most direct approach is to completely remove the posterior elements, down to the pedicles, so that the process of screw placement into the pedicle is continuously visi-

Table 2 □ Methods for Sacral Screw Placement

AUTHOR	LEVEL	ENTRY SITE	TRANSVERSE PLANE ANGLE	SAGITTAL PLANE ANGLE	DEPTH
Cotrel et al[28]	S1	Midpoint between L5–S1 facet and S1 foramen	30 deg lateral	?	?
Edwards et al[46]	S1	Base of L5–S1 facet	From inferodorsal corner of L5 spinous process to entry site		Through anterior cortex
Guyer et al[59]	S1	Caudal and just lateral to S1 superior articular process	25 deg medial	?	To anterior cortex
Krag[86]	S1	Center of S1 pedicle seen by x-ray oriented along S1 pedicular axis	Toward midline (from preop CT)	Toward promontory	To anterior cortex
Louis[104]	S1	Lateral to L5–S1 facet and S1 foramen	35–45 deg lat	35–45 deg caud	?
Magerl[112]	S1	Intersection of lines along lateral and inferior edges of S1 superior articular process	15–20 deg med	Toward promontory	To anterior cortex
Roy-Camille et al[138]	S1	?	30 deg lat	?	?
Steffee et al[151]	S1	Just below S1 superior articular process	0 deg	0 deg	To anterior cortex
Guyer et al[59]	S2	Midway between 1st and 2nd dorsal foramina	40–50 deg lat	10–15 deg ceph	?
Steffee et al[151]	S2	?	45 deg lat	?	?

Note: lat = anterolateral; med = anteromedial orientation; ceph = anterocephalad; caud = anterocaudal orientation.

ble.[68, 107, 152] A smaller amount of resection will allow direct palpation with a curved probe of the borders of the pedicle, which allows semidirect visualization; various guides for assisting this process have been described.[68] Yet another approach is to use anatomic landmarks to guide an initial insertion of drill bit, awl, or guide wire and then afterward to obtain an x-ray to identify proper (or improper) placement. Even in quite experienced hands, however, this method has been reported to yield pedicle "miss" rates (screw out of pedicle) that are disturbingly high. Saillant[139] in 1976 reported a 10% miss rate, and Roy-Camille[136] in 1987 reported a 13.5% rate; elsewhere, Roy-Camille[138] described the rate in their more recent experience with trauma as "near to nil." Robbins and Gertzbein[133] described use of image intensification to guide screw replacement, although which x-ray views were used is not described, and they report a miss rate of 28.8%. Even though a miss may not cause neurologic deficit, it probably does affect the screw–vertebra interface strength.

An alternative to using surface landmarks alone is to use x-ray to properly locate and orient the drill bit (or guide wire), even before insertion is accomplished. For this, however, the choice of x-ray technique may be quite important. Using AP and lateral views alone, Weinstein and coworkers[169] showed an initial miss rate of approximately 21% for screws implanted into cadaveric spine specimens. However, other x-ray views are also possible, as described by the author.[86] If the central x-ray beam is positioned obliquely to pass along the axis of the pedicle (the orientation of which is readily available either accurately from a preoperative CT scan or approximately from morphometric data[17, 89, 94, 139, 178]), the pedicle cortex can be quite clearly seen as an oval. The drill bit tip can then be positioned in the middle of this oval. Next, the drill bit shaft (with no driver attached) is rotated up to an orientation parallel to the x-ray central beam: the drill bit will then appear as a spot in the center of the pedicle ("bull's eye" or "pedicle-coaxial" x-ray view), as shown in Figure 5. The image intensifier can then be rotated aside and the driver (power or manual) attached to the drill bit, which is then advanced to proper depth. The author has used this method since 1986, and routinely probes all four quadrants of the drill hole before screw placement, to establish cortical intactness. In 54 patients (216 screws) there have been two pedicles with cortical disruption. Although these results have obviously not been confirmed by transecting the pedicles (as done in a cadaver study), postoperative CT scans have been obtained for many of these patients. The probe and CT results have established that the miss rate can be very low when this specific x-ray view is used instead of the more traditional AP and lateral views.

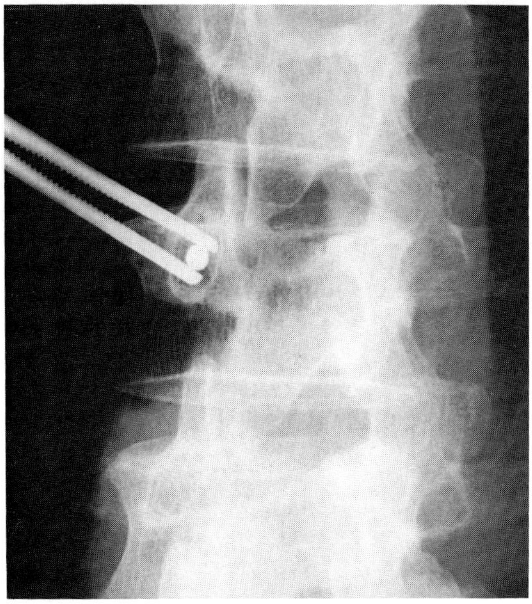

Figure 5 □ Coaxial, or "bull's eye," x-ray view. Oblique view of L3 vertebra is shown, with central beam along left pedicle axis. Drill bit is seen end-on as a black spot, centered within the oval cortex of the pedicle, adjacent to the left L2-L3 facet joint. The drill bit is held from below by the jaws of a Kocher clamp. (From Krag, M. H., Van Hal, M. E., and Beynnon, B. D.: Placement of transpedicular vertebral screws close to anterior cortex: Description of methods [in press, Spine, 1989].)

Depth of Penetration

The optimal depth of screw penetration through the pedicle and into the vertebral body is not yet well established. A variety of clinically based opinions have been reported. Roy-Camille,[138] for example, describes it as "dangerous and pointless" to insert the screw so deeply that it contacts the anterior cortex of the vertebral body. In contrast, Magerl[112, 113] and Dick[32] recommend placement of the screw tip close to the anterior cortex.

Although the relationship between strength and screw penetration depth has been well established for tubular bones,[5, 16, 83, 162] few studies have been done for transpedicle screws. Lavaste[98, 99] measured pull-out strength of various commercially available screws and concluded that depth was not an important determinant of strength. However, his analysis failed to take advantage of the right-to-left comparisons that were possible with his data, and thus his conclusions were heavily influenced by interspecimen variability, which he emphasized was large. A reanalysis of Lavaste's data performed by the author,[87] based upon the 10 of his specimens that allow right-to-left comparison, leads to a conclusion that is the opposite of the one he drew: a significant ($p < .05$) increase in pull-out strength is in fact produced by a depth increase of only 5 mm.

Zindrick and colleagues[180] conducted both pull-out and cyclic transverse displacement testing. In pull-out, the through-anterior-cortex group had a mean strength of 220% for the 4.5-mm cortical screw and 130% for the 6.5-mm cancellous screw, compared with the to-anterior-cortex group. In contrast, there was no significant difference between the mean strengths of the to-anterior-cortex group and the 50% depth group. Whether younger specimens (mean age was 74.5 years in that study) or a different analysis (e.g., matched-pairs *t*-test) would have altered the results is not clear. For the cyclic transverse displacements, both the through-cortex versus to-cortex and to-cortex versus 50% depth comparisons showed the deeper screw to be significantly stronger. However, the clinical significance of this test mode is not clear, as is discussed in more detail elsewhere.[87]

We compared the peak strength of screws at 50% versus 80% depth of penetration and 80% versus 100% depth of penetration, using a right-to-left comparison within each vertebral specimen.[87] Each pair of screws was exposed to a load mimicking vertebral flexion or axial rotation. Matched-pairs *t*-testing was used, and showed that strength varied approximately linearly with penetration depth (Fig. 6), for both load types. The strength of screws at 50% depth was 75% to 77% (depending on load type) of that at 80% depth. Strength for screws at 100% (to-cortex) depth was 124% to 154% of that at 80% depth.

Thus, on the basis of at least the reanalysis[87] of Lavaste's data[99] and our work, it can be concluded that deeper screw insertion provides increased screw–vertebra interface strength. Of course this also increases the risk of anterior vertebral cortex penetration. The optimal balancing between these two features must take into account surgeon skill and experience, the availability of an adequate x-ray visualization source, anticipated postoperative loading, as well as other factors.

Particularly with the deeper screw penetration, monitoring of the depth by one or more methods is desirable in order to avoid breaking through the anterior cortex. One method is based upon the increased resistance to further drill bit or screw advancement that can sometimes be felt when the cortex is reached. Another method (mallet method[93]) is to insert the drill bit or probe almost to the anterior cortex, and then to tap it lightly with a mallet: a distinct change in sound (rise in pitch) and increased vibration

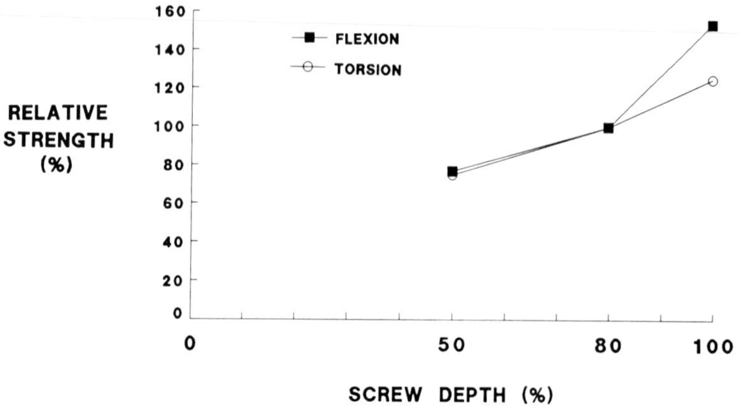

Figure 6 □ Mean strength of the 100% and 50% depth screws relative to the mean strength of the 80% depth screws. Each vertebra had implanted either an 80% or a 50% depth screw, or an 80% and a 100% depth screw. Relative strength is plotted against percentage of depth penetration, both for flexion and for torsion loads. (From Krag, M. H., Beynnon, B. D., DeCoster, T. A., and Pope, M. H.: Depth of insertion of transpedicular vertebral screws into human vertebrae: Effect upon screw-vertebra interface strength. J. Spinal Dis. 1:287–294, 1988.)

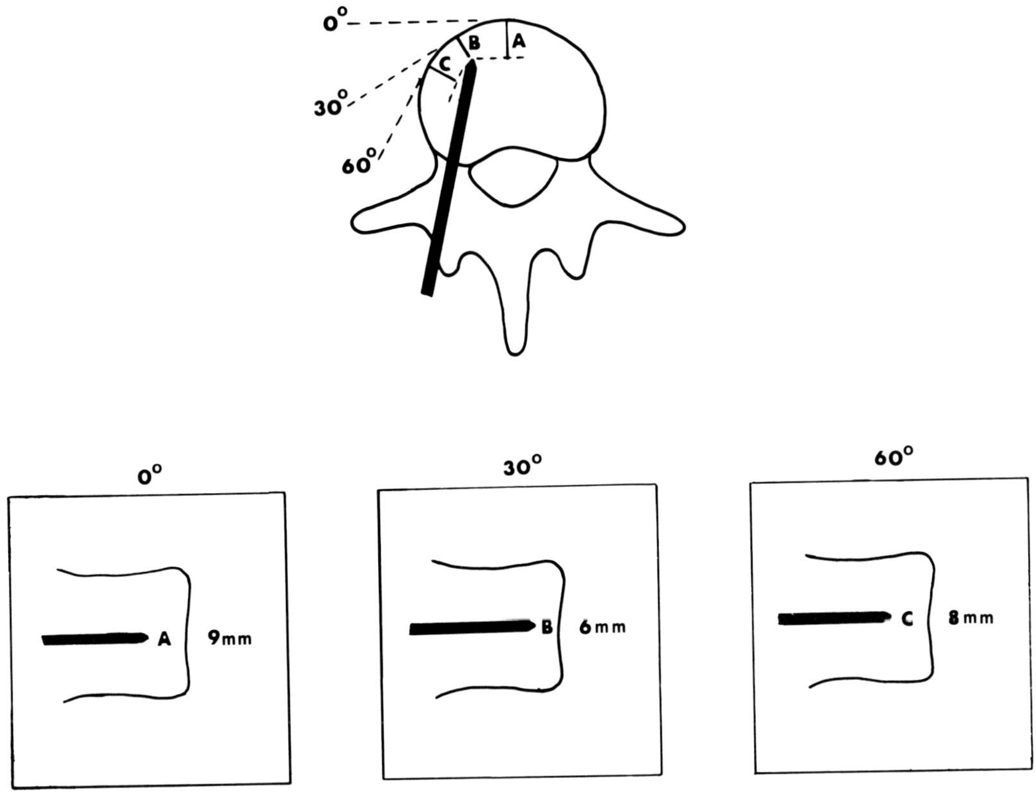

Figure 7 □ Apparent distance from drill bit tip to anterior cortex varies with the angle of view (SPTL—1954.1-001). *A,* On lateral view, the apparent distance A = 9 mm. *B,* on oblique view 30 degrees from lateral, the apparent distance, B = 6 mm, is also the true distance. This is the near-approach view. *C,* On oblique view at 60 degrees from lateral, the apparent distance, C = 8 mm, is larger than the value seen at the near-approach view. (From Krag, M. H., Van Hal, M. E., and Beynnon, B. D.: Placement of transpedicular vertebral screws close to anterior vertebral cortex: Description of methods [in press, Spine, 1989]).

in the instrument shaft may be detected when the tip of the instrument contacts the anterior cortex. In osteopenic bone, however, caution must be used; the anterior cortical thinning may prevent either change from being detected.

A third method is to use x-rays to provide a direct assessment of the distance between screw tip and anterior cortex; however, the choice of x-ray view may be important to avoid a misleading appearance. This same problem can occur during internal fixation of the hip[23, 100, 134, 146, 165, 166] and knee[48] and has been described by the author and coworkers in more detail elsewhere[93] for transpedicular screw placement. The lateral view has been suggested to be the most accurate,[101, 112, 122] but this may not be true. If the screw tip is close to penetrating the anterior cortex at a location away from the midline, the lateral view will promote a false sense of security as shown in Figure 7. The apparent distance from screw tip to cortex will be greater than the actual distance, since the screw tip is "over the horizon." When the beam is tangential to the point on the anterior cortex at which the screw would penetrate, the distance from screw tip to cortex is at a minimum (near-approach view). Final screw advancement using this orientation will generally provide a more direct view of the relationship between screw tip and cortex than will a true lateral x-ray.

Hole Preparation Method

It may be useful to consider four phases of hole preparation. The first phase is to break through the posterior cortex overlying the pedicle. Tools recommended for accomplishing this vary, from drill bit to rongeur to air-driven dental bur. The second phase is to deepen the hole past the narrow waist, or midportion, of the pedicle. This can be done by drill bit,[86, 87, 112, 113, 137, 138] curet,[42, 98] curved probe,[59, 151] or straight probe or guide wire.[122] The third phase is to complete the hole to the maximum desired depth. Here, the options are drill, curved probe, or straight probe. The fourth phase is to use a tap for cutting threads in bone, if desired.

Various methods for accomplishing these four phases of hole preparation have been recommended and are summarized in Table 3. Although the assessment of each method could include safety, ease or speed of insertion, or effect on screw–vertebra interface strength, very few of these parameters have actually been studied. Concerning the issue of tapping, no data from vertebral testing appear to be available; although Zindrick and coworkers[179] mention that they studied this matter, little overall difference was seen—no benefit in osteopenic bone and a decrease in strength in some specimens. For sites other than the spine, Nunamaker and Perren[121] showed in bovine cancellous limb bone that tapping added no strength, and Koranyi and coworkers[83] and Vangsness and colleagues[162] showed similar results for screws placed across the femoral diaphysis. Thus, there appear to be no data in support of tapping to increase screw strength, and some data against it.

Table 3 □ Pilot Hole Preparation Techniques for Transpedicle Screws

AUTHOR	METHOD
Dick[32]	K wire (2-mm) into body (approximately 3 cm deep) Drill (3.5-mm) 5–10 mm deep Screw under x-ray control
Edwards[42]	Hole developed with 3–0 curet Replacement with guide wire; x-ray Screw
Guyer et al[59]	Awl Pedicle probe through pedicle Blunt K wire driven in under x-ray control K wire removed; threads tapped to 2 cm
Krag[86]	Bur to enter cortex, centered over pedicle by x-ray "coaxial view" Drill along pedicle axis to anterior cortex; monitor by x-ray "near-approach view" Screw; orientation with nearby guide wire; depth by x-ray "near-approach view"
Louis[104]	2.8-mm drill (depth?) Screw
Luque and Rapp[110]	Enter pedicle (use drill?) Curet through pedicle Drill in blunt K wire to anterior cortex Cannulated tap over K wire Cannulated screw over K wire
Magerl[113]	Drill 3.5-mm approximately 4 cm deep Replacement with K wire; x-ray Screw to anterior cortex; monitor with x-ray
Ölerud et al[122]	K wire and x-ray to define entry site Drill through cortex Screw to anterior cortex; monitoring with lateral view
Roy-Camille et al[138]	Awl to locate entry Drill (3.2 mm) Screw
Steffee et al[151]	Awl or probe through pedicle Tap through pedicle Screw

On the subject of probe versus drill bit, we have shown on a small number of specimens that use of a drill bit versus a straight 2-mm cylindric probe (with blunt conical tip) produces no significant difference for transpedicle screw pull-out.[54] In choosing between the two methods, one should consider not only the laboratory results, but also the important issues of safety, dependability, ease, and speed. Regarding pilot hole depth, no specific data are available for vertebrae, although the work of Lyon and coworkers[111] suggests (on the basis of very limited data) that this may be an important issue for screw strength in human femora. For pilot hole diameter as well, there is no specific testing on vertebrae. Banta and coworkers[15] raise the concern that use of too small a hole may lead to pedicle blow-out during screw insertion. This may bear upon the choice made between probe and drill to form the pilot hole; the former compacts bone, whereas the latter removes it. Whether this significantly affects the blow-out tendency remains to be established.

Insertion of the screw after completion of hole preparation requires proper orientation of the screw relative to the central axis of the hole. Because the cortical bone is quite thin, because the cancellous bone does not provide substantial resistance to screw malalignment, and because the deep end of the hole is not visible for use as a guide, the screw will not necessarily "follow" the hole. A useful technique is to insert a short Kirschner wire into an adjacent bony prominence (e.g., spinous process, or posterior ilium), approximately parallel to the drill bit or probe. This will provide a visual guide to the correct screw orientation, even after drill bit or probe removal.

Polymethylmethacrylate Augmentation

Should the screw–vertebra interface be prophylactically strengthened by insertion of polymethylmethacrylate (PMMA) into the pilot hole before screw insertion into osteopenic bone? If a screw becomes loose intraoperatively, should PMMA be inserted, or should the screw be redirected or moved to another site? Few data relevant to these questions have been reported. Kleeman and coworkers[79] tested human calcanei and tibiae into which screws were (1) inserted in the usual fashion, (2) pulled out using an Instron materials testing machine, (3) reinserted after the holes had been manually filled with PMMA, and (4) again pulled out after setting of the PMMA. The reinforced-screw pull-out force was 226% of the initial pull-out force. Zindrick and coworkers[180] performed similar testing on human cadaveric vertebrae with transpedicle screws and also tested the effect of PMMA pressurization before screw reinsertion. They showed that PMMA placement without pressurization provides a screw strength approximately equal to normal (contralateral pedicle used as a control), whereas PMMA placed under pressure provides a strength of approximately twice the normal. The authors caution, however, against the possibility of nerve root or cord damage from PMMA extrusion through any cortical defects that may be present, especially when pressurization is used.

The difficulty of such PMMA removal (e.g., for débridement of infection) is a sobering counterbalance to the relatively easy gain in strength achieved by the technique. Perhaps placement of the screws all the way to, or even slightly through, the anterior cortex would be a better option. The answer is not yet available.

LONGITUDINAL LINKAGE BETWEEN SCREWS

Transpedicle screw-based fixation devices are still under active development and will likely undergo further changes. Other than the screw itself, the linkage between screw and longitudinal component (rod or plate) is the most varied design feature in current devices, and it will probably continue to be a focus of future improvement. Thus, certain general aspects of this linkage may be worth considering.

Positional Adjustability

Although there is a certain range of adjustability (prior to screw insertion) between vertebra and screw, it is limited by the anatomic constraints. Further adjustability must come between the screw and the plate or rod. Current devices exhibit a wide spectrum of such adjustability. For plates with individual, separate, circular holes,[19, 104–106, 119, 137, 138, 157] mediolateral angulation and cephalocaudal angulation are continuously adjustable, but longitudinal translation is adjustable stepwise in fairly coarse intervals. For example, the holes in Roy-Camille plates are 13 mm apart.[138] Mediolateral translation is only adjustable by bending of the plate in the coronal plane, if there is a screw above and below the site in question already fixing the plate in position. Finer stepwise adjustability of longitudinal translation (a few millimeters) is provided by the Steffee[151] and Luque[110] plates and by the Edwards rods.[43] These plates use longitudinal slots instead of circular holes, and they have scalloped edges (or "screw nests") to provide some mechanical interlocking between screw head and plate. The Edwards rods are ratcheted for stepwise adjustment. In the Steffee system, the continuous adjustability of angulation between screw and plate is restricted by the use of a nut on each side of the plate to lock together the two components. If the screw is not positioned in the vertebra so as to be perpendicular to the adjacent segment of the plate, tightening of the lock nut tends to bend the screw shaft (thereby weakening it) or to loosen the screw in the vertebra.[68] A newly available 5-degree wedge-shaped washer provides an alternative angular position for the screw.

The Balgrist,[145] Cotrel-Dubousset,[28] Edwards,[43] Puno,[128] Wiltse[59] and Zielke[129] systems all require a perpendicular orientation between screw and longitudinal linking component; however, because these systems use a rod instead of a plate, the following two adjustability restrictions are lessened: (1) bending of the rod is significantly easier than bending of the plate within the coronal plane (mediolateral direction), and (2) a wider range of difference in mediolateral angulation between adjacent screws is allowed, since the range of this angulation for the screw about the rod is greater than that for the screw within the plate hole (mediolateral "toggle").

Fully three-dimensional adjustability between screw and rod is allowed by the internal fixators (Dick,[32] Kluger,[81] Vermont,[89] and Ölerud[122]). These devices combine the cephalocaudal angular adjustment of some of the plate systems with the continuous adjustability of longitudinal translation in the previously described rod systems, and they maintain the mediolateral angular adjustability. Cephalocaudal angulation is adjustable in 6-degree increments (maximum mismatch is ±3 degrees) for all of these internal fixators except for the Ölerud, which allows continuous adjustability. Mediolateral angulation is continuously adjustable in all of these fixators, except for the Dick, which is adjustable in 6-degree increments.

Positional Control

Control between vertebra and screw is determined by the screw design and bone strength, as discussed before. Positional control between screw and longitudinal component has a range across devices that is as great as that for positional adjustability.

For most of the plate and screw systems[19, 104–106, 110, 119, 137, 138, 157] the screw is free to toggle within the plate and is prevented from doing so only by the ligamentous interconnections between adjacent vertebrae, the friction between plate and subjacent bone, and the friction between plate and screw head. The first of these control elements is subject to soft tissue elongation or stretching, which is one of the problems associated with Harrington distraction rods. The second control element, plate-bone friction, is subject to bone resorption, especially if the bone surface is irregular. Bone graft placed underneath the plate may also add to this problem. The final control element, friction between screw head and plate, is quite small. Because of the above, toggling of screw in the plate may be predicted to be a fairly likely occurrence. This will allow the screws to be subjected to bending loads, which in turn can cause screw breakage, especially if the screws have not been specifically designed to tolerate such loads. In addition, such motion may contribute to nonunion of the bone graft. It probably is relevant to this topic that (1) 25% of trauma patients (21 of 84) had distal screws break with Roy-Camille instrumentation,[138] (2) 24% of trauma patients (5 of 21) had 10% to 12% of loss of reduction at follow-up with this same implant system,[78] and (3) a solid union rate of 53% in primary operations, an 11% screw loosening rate (5 of 46 patients), and a 6.5% rate of screw breakage and nonunion (3 of 46 patients) were seen with DCP plates.[157] Blauth and coworkers[19] refer to screw toggle as "a major disadvantage."

Substantial but incomplete positional control of the screw or the rod is provided by the Edwards[43] and the Puno[128] implants. Edwards[40] conjectures that the partial motion allowed between screw and rod may protect the system from peak loads. Puno[128] describes micromotion present between screw and rod and speculates that this may lessen the degree of stress shielding of the bone graft by the implant. Whether such motion actually occurs in vivo, and if so whether it produces either of these effects, remains to be established.

Complete positional control between the screw and longitudinal linking component is provided by the Balgrist,[145] Cotrel-Dubousset,[28] Dick,[32] Kluger,[81] Ölerud,[122] Steffee,[151] Vermont,[89] and Wiltse[59] devices. These devices allow only motion that occurs by elastic deflection or (if the loads are high enough) plastic deformation of bone, screw, or longitudinal linking component. Future research will have to determine the amount of positional control that provides the optimal balance among all the biologic factors affected by it.

Stiffness

The stiffness of the assembled implants varies considerably. Based upon dimensions, the stiffest is probably the Steffee and the least stiff is the Wiltse single-rod construct, although complete data have not been published. Geiger and coworkers[53] have tested some of the longitudinal components in four-point bending: the stiffness of the Steffee plate is 11.6 kN/mm, and that of the C-D rod is 7 kN/mm, or 60% of the Steffee. The stiffness level that is optimal remains to be established in terms of (1) preventing dangerous intervertebral deflections before healing, (2) facilitating development of bony union during healing, and (3) preventing excessive stress shielding after healing. Whether or not implant stiffness, in addition, affects the rate of degeneration at adjacent motion segments (as conjectured by Hsu and coworkers[67, 68]) remains to be established. Bony fusion alone produces a segmental stiffness so much greater than that of a normal disc that the incremental stiffness from addition of hardware may in fact be relatively small.

Fatigue Strength

Typically, the fatigue strength of a structure is determined by applying a specific load amount to it over and over again, until either it fails or a sufficiently high number of load cycles is reached. This is then repeated using each of a number of different load amounts to characterize the fatigue strength of that structure. Such testing for plates and rods has not been published; however, limited testing at a single load amount (24.1 N•m at a frequency of 4 Hz) has been performed by Geiger and coworkers,[53] who showed a wide range of cycles to failure for different devices. Differences among the Cotrel-Dubousset rod (65,000 cycles), Ölerud rod (80,000 cycles), and Luque plate (100,000 cycles) were not significant. The Steffee plate (210,000 cycles) and Harrington 1/4-inch rod (220,000 cycles) were also not significantly different from each other, but both were stronger than the former group.

Performance of Reduction

If a fusion in situ is to be performed, no alteration in the relative position of one vertebra with respect to another (reduction or realignment) needs to be accomplished. If realignment is needed, it must be accomplished either before or after the transpedicle screws are inserted into the vertebra and attached to the longitudinal link (rod or plate). For systems in which the longitudinal link must be positioned before screw insertion,[104, 110, 138] reduction must be accomplished either by traction upon or positioning of the patient (described in further detail elsewhere[104, 138]), or by means of another temporarily implanted device, such as Harrington distraction rods (although these may require additional dissection). If the longitudinal link can be applied after screw insertion, then it becomes possible to use the screw as a "handle" for controlling vertebral position and performing the reduction. In some patients this may allow the performance of a successful reduction, which otherwise might be attempted only by a separate anterior approach.[104]

Various instruments that attach to individual screws have been mentioned,[68, 81, 110] and the dorsally protruding shaft of a Schanz pin can be used in this fashion before it is cut off.[32, 113] Positioning such screw extensions to produce realignment can be accomplished either manually or by means of an instrument. Whatever method is used, caution must be exercised to prevent placing excessive force on any one screw; otherwise screw-vertebra loosening or screw bending can occur. To decrease the chance of this complication, we have developed a reduction frame that rigidly links together the right and left screws at each vertebral level, thereby producing balanced load-sharing between the screws. The biomechanical relevance of this is indicated by the cadaveric testing performed by Kling and coworkers,[80] who showed that such cross-linked screws are more than twice as strong as a single screw alone ($p<.05$).

The use of this reduction frame (1) provides an accurate control of position, (2) allows slower, more gradual reductions with less chance of excessive transient loads than might be feasible during manually driven reductions in difficult cases, (3) may be used to provide bridging between right and left screws for load equalization, (4) frees surgical hands for other tasks, and (5) allows the implanted device to remain simple; the "tool" used for the reduction is not implanted in the patient but is returned to the "toolbox."

One special consideration exists for reduction of spondylolisthesis, since this is a situation in which an unusually large amount of anteroposterior positional adjustment may be needed. If the two screws into the spondylolisthetic vertebra are oriented obliquely (which seems to provide a stronger attachment than nonoblique screws), the distance between the screws will decrease anteriorly. If the reduction mechanism used does not have sufficient adjustability, the two screws will tend to be forced apart as the reduction is accomplished, causing either screw-bone loosening or screw bending.

Other Characteristics

The design used for connection between screws and longitudinal link is one of the major determinants of the bulk of the implant, the simplicity of the device, and the ease of assembly. Although these aspects are not as readily quantified as mechanical characteristics (e.g., positional adjustability, stiffness, and fatigue strength), they may be quite important. Bulky devices may encroach on adjacent facet joints, displace muscle tissue away from normal position, produce more dead space (possibly increasing infection), cause tenderness from adjacent tissue irritation, and occupy space otherwise available to the bone graft. Devices that are not simple and easy to assemble may be associated with longer operative times, increased risk of holes in sterile gloves, greater chance of incorrect implantation, and an overall greater "fiddle factor."

TRANSVERSE CONNECTION BETWEEN RIGHT AND LEFT IMPLANTS

Transverse connectors were initially used to improve deformity correction for scoliosis. The history for this has been reviewed by Asher and coworkers.[10] More recently, attention has been focused on using such connectors to improve overall implant stiffness, although testing apparently has not yet been done upon transpedicle screw-based implants. Asher and coworkers[10] measured the improved stiffness from cross-bridging between Harrington distraction rods without and with circumlaminar wires; Ashman and colleagues[12] studied Luque and Cotrel-Dubousset rods attached by such wires. The effect of the cross-bridging was to increase stiffness in response to certain load types, but not to others. The relationship of these results to transpedicle screw-based devices is not clear: the interface between screw and vertebral pedicle and/or body is highly different from that between hook and lamina.

For transverse connectors attached to transpedicle screw-based devices, Gurr and coworkers[58] describe biomechanical testing of whole implants attached to fresh calf lumbar spines that had the laminae excised and that were exposed to torsional and flexural loads. Cotrel-Dubousset implants spanning three or five vertebra were tested without and with transverse connectors. No significant stiffening effect was produced by these connectors. Thus, clinical experience–based statements that such connectors are important[28] do not yet have an experimentally validated basis.

Another type of connector involves the use of diagonal wires in an X pattern attached to the dorsal ends of the screws. This has been described by Dick[32] and Ölerud and associates[122] and is intended to increase implant resistance to lateral shifting of the upper vertebra relative to the lower. The same kind of resistance provided by the wires may instead be accomplished by orienting the screws "up and in" (see Fig. 4), which also provides certain other benefits (see Entry Site and Orientation, above). If the screws are oriented parallel to each other (e.g., when the pedicles are oriented sagittally and have a narrow mediolateral diameter), only friction between screw and bone resists the lateral shifting. Under this circumstance, especially in the case of a highly unstable fracture, the diagonal wiring may be quite helpful. The combination of transverse connectors & diagonal wiring may provide even more stiffening than either one alone, since the force distribution between screw and bone produced by a laterally directed load is different for each method.

BIOMECHANICAL TESTING OF WHOLE IMPLANTS

The testing of individual components such as screws, rods, and plates does not yield information concerning either the connecting device between the screw and longitudinal component or the interface between screw and vertebra. Such information can be obtained by testing the entire assembled device, implanted into some appropriate model. Human cadaveric spines can be used, but interspecimen variation can be a problem. It is possible to obtain animal spines that are more consistent in their properties, but their relevance to the human situation is an important issue. Nonbiologic specimens, such as plastic blocks, are highly repeatable but differ even more from the human specimens. Not only does each model have its own special drawback, but all have in common the absence of muscular and ligamentous forces, which may be the major feature of these models that makes difficult their application to the in vivo situation.

As an example of how such forces may be important, an axial compressive load along the central axis of the vertebral bodies would tend to produce substantial bending loads in the implanted screws, even if the "middle column" or posterior portion of the vertebral bodies and discs were intact to function as a fulcrum. When posterior muscle forces are present, however, the bending loads are "converted" into shear loads, to which the screws are much more resistant. Our knowledge of such loads in the human is quite limited,[92] as is our understanding of the relationship between human and nonhuman spinal loads; thus, simulating such loads is difficult. Even less is known of the load distribution in various injury states[141] or of the relationship between experimental models of such injuries and the in vivo reality. These model limitations should not preclude such testing but should be kept clearly in mind during the interpretation of results and application of conclusions.

Table 4 summarizes certain major features

Table 4 □ Static Tests of Whole Implants in Vitro

AUTHOR	DEVICE	SPECIMEN	INJURY MODEL	LOADS: Type	LOADS: Amount	OUTCOME MEASURE
Asazuma et al[9]	Steffee Vermont Zielke	Pig (L5, L6, L7, S1)	Intact	Flexion Extension Lateral bend Torsion	<11.2 N•m <11.2 N•m <11.2 N•m <11.2 N•m	3 rotations and 3 translations for each
Ashman et al[12] Herring and Ashman[65]	Steffee	Calf (L5, L6, S1, S2)	Spondylolisthesis (Cut pars and disc)	Compression Flexion Torsion	? ? ?	Major motion for each
Falahee et al[50]	Dick	Human (T10–L3)	Trauma (L1 burst, cut multiple ligaments)	Flexion Extension Lateral bend Torsion	10 N•m 10 N•m 10 N•m 10 N•m	3 rotations and 3 translations for each
Gurr et al[58]	Cotrel-Dubousset Steffee	Calf (L1, S1)	Laminectomy (L4 and L5, partial L4–L5 and L5–S1 facetectomy, L4–L5 discectomy)	Compression Flexion Torsion	100, 200 N (5 cm) 5 Nm	Major motion for each
Jacobs et al[71]	Roy-Camille	Human (T9–L3)	Trauma (flex to failure)	Flexion	25 N•m	Flexion
Puno et al[128]	Steffee Screw-rod fixator	Human (L4–S2)	Intact	Compression Flexion Extension Lateral bend Torsion	450 N 31.2 N•m 31.2 N•m 31.2 N•m 11.2 N•m	Energy absorption to failure for each
Schläpfer et al[142]	Magerl	Human (T11–L5)	Trauma (Wedge osteotomy and cut posterior ligaments; also cut anterior ligaments)	Flexion	≤40 N•m	Flexion
Tencer et al[155]	Roy-Camille Vermont	Human (T10–L2)	Trauma (Remove anterior ⅔ body and cut posterior ligaments; remove rest of body)	Flexion Extension Lateral bend Torsion	<310 N <310 N <310 N <18 N•m	Rotation; AP and lateral translation for each

of reports on static testing in vitro of various transpedicle screw-based implants. In most cases other devices were also tested (not shown in Table 4) to provide a comparison. Some work using fatigue testing has also been done. Tencer and coworkers,[155] in addition to the static loads indicated in Table 4, also exposed each construct to 4,320 cycles at 0.5 Hz (over 6 hours) of a combined compression, flexion, and lateral bending load. Although full details are not provided in the abstract, the transpedicle screw-based devices appear to have fared substantially better than the hook and/or wire-based devices. We performed[88] fatigue testing on assembled implants attached to plastic blocks (simulating vertebrae) used to model a highly unstable injury (no interconnections). Up to 1,000,000 cycles of various magnitudes of a combined flexion-compression load were applied. In no case did clamp loosening occur, although at high loads screw failure could eventually be obtained at the root of the first thread.

As can be seen, these reports of both static and fatigue tests involve a wide variety of devices, applications (spine specimen and injury model), and methods (loads and outcome measures). From this diversity, the following major conclusions may be drawn:

1. Transpedicle screw-based devices definitely convey better overall positional control than do other devices.
2. One component of this improved positional control is the improved security of the screw–pedicle/body interface compared with the hook–lamina or wire–lamina interface.
3. Devices that have secure screw–plate or screw–rod interface control can return normal stiffness to an injury model even if only one vertebra above and below the injury site is instrumented (rather than two or three above and below as with other devices).
4. When screw–vertebra interface failure occurs, it does not appear to threaten neural elements (i.e., the spinal canal and foramina remain intact).
5. The significance of different mechanical characteristics for the clinical situation needs to be kept in mind. Ultimate strength is an important measure, since it may describe screw-bone failure, but stiffness is also important because the amount of deflection may affect bone or disc fragment motion.
6. Overall response of an implant to a variety of load types should be assessed because device response may be quite load-type dependent, and in vivo loads are reasonably likely to be quite varied.
7. Much remains to be learned concerning the in vivo load reality and the applicability of various experimental injury models to clinical situations.

POSTOPERATIVE MANAGEMENT

The major issues that are generally considered to be important are length of time spent on bed rest, type and duration of external support (if any), and restrictions on activities. Major reports that address these topics are summarized in Table 5. The extent to which mechanical loads are affected by such intervention is by no means clear. Clinical studies available to the present are sufficiently varied that generalizations concerning these issues cannot yet be made. The spectrum of bracing recommended (from none to total contact trunk orthosis with a thigh cuff for 3 months) is sufficiently wide that some conclusions should be forthcoming. Little information has been given in available reports concerning activity restrictions. Although patient compliance with recommended restrictions may be difficult to assess, nontheless some description of this in future clinical reports would probably be useful.

IMPLANT REMOVAL

Should these implants be routinely removed, or only if specific clinical conditions so require? A consensus has by no means been reached. Most authors have made no mention of the topic, although concern has been raised about a number of issues that retained implants present, such as (1) impaired assessment of fusion solidity,[19, 104] (2) impaired visualization by diagnostic radiographic techniques, (3) accelerated degeneration or altered function at adjacent motion segments,[67, 68] (4) prolonged stress shielding of the fusion mass, (5) irritation to overlying tissue, (6) possibility of its being a site for hematogenous spread of infection, (7) altered local damage in the event of future regional trauma, and (8) long-term metal

Table 5 □ Postoperative Management

ORTHOSIS Type	Weeks	RESTRICTIONS	DEVICE	DIAGNOSIS	SITE*	REPORT
None	—	?	Ölerud	Trauma	T/L	Ölerud et al[122]
None		?	Steffee	Various	L, L/S	Steffee et al[151]
Corset	12	Walking ≤1 mile Minimal sitting	Steffee	Degeneration	L, L/S	Hsu et al[68]
Chairback	≤12	Cautious exercise	AO plates	Degeneration	L, L/S	Thalgott et al[157]
Jewett	8	?	Kluger	Trauma	T, L	Blauth et al[19]
Jewett	8	?	Dick	Various	T, L	Dick[32]
Lumbar brace	8	?	Dick	Trauma	T, L	Aebi et al[2]
Lumbar brace	≤12	?	Roy-Camille	Trauma	T, L	Kinnard et al[78]
Lumbar brace	25	Progressive over 3 months	Vermont	Various	L/S	Krag[86]
Lumbar brace	25	No sitting (? number weeks)	Louis	Various	L/S	Louis[104]
Lumbar brace	≤16	?	Roy-Camille	Various	T/L, L	Roy-Camille et al[138]
Brace and thigh	12	?	Edwards	Trauma	Low L	Levine and Edwards[101]
Thigh out	12					
Bed rest,	12	?	Roy-Camille	Spondylolisthesis	L/S	Roy-Camille et al[138]
then brace	12					

*T = thoracic, T/L = thoracolumbar, L = lumbar, L/S = lumbosacral.

toxicity. Ölerud[20] does not remove his device before at least 1 year has passed. Dick[32] and Kinnard[78] recommend routine removal if discs are spanned that have not also been grafted. The author recommends its routine removal, as for most other metallic hardware. Only the long-term results will establish which approach provides the best balance between the risks and costs of an additional surgical procedure for device removal, and the functional benefits thereby achieved.

CONCLUSION

A very high level of interest has grown over the past few years in the area of transpedicle screw fixation. Clearly such fixation can be used in a way that is effective and safe, as demonstrated by a growing number of patients who have had extremely satisfactory outcomes but who have not been condemned to a lifetime of dealing with a relatively long fused spinal segment. Equally clearly, this fixation brings with it certain demands and risks. The challenge is to find ways to meet the demands and simultaneously to reduce the risks.

Accomplishing this will require further research not only in the area of biomechanics (e.g., implant design, materials, testing methods, manufacturing standards), but also in the area of clinical practice (surgical indications, implantation techniques, outcome studies). As in any relatively new field, the number of good questions far exceeds that of good answers, but at least there is a substantial beginning. Part of that beginning is the biomechanical research already completed—that which has been reviewed here.

References

1. Aebi, M., Etter, C., Kehl, T., and Thalgott, J.: The internal skeletal fixation system: A new treatment of thoracolumbar fractures and other spinal disorders. Clin. Orthop. Rel. Res. 227:30–43, 1988.
2. Aebi, M., Etter, C., Kehl, T., and Thalgott, J.: Stabilization of the lower thoracic and lumbar spine with the internal spinal skeletal fixation system: Indications, techniques, and first results of treatment. Spine 12:544–551, 1987.
3. Akbarnia, B. A., Fogarty, J. P., and Tayob, A. A.: Contoured Harrington instrumentation in the treatment of unstable spinal fractures: The effect of supplementary sublaminar wires. Clin. Orthop. Rel. Res. 189:186–194, 1984.
4. Andrew, T. A., Brooks, S., and Piggott, H.: Long-term followup evaluation of screw-and-graft fusion of the lumbar spine. Clin. Orthop. Rel. Res. 203:113–119, 1986.
5. Ansell, R. H., and Scales, J. T.: A study of some factors which affect the strength of screws and their holding power in bone. J. Biomech. 1:279–302, 1968.
6. Armstrong, G. W. D.: Harrington instrumentation for spinal fractures. Proceedings of the Scoliosis Research Society Annual Meeting, 1976.
7. Arnold, W.: Early surgical treatment using an external fixation device in traumatic paraplegia. Beitrag Orthop. Traumatol. 32:6–14, 1985.
8. Arnold, W.: Early surgical treatment of traumatic paraplegia with an external fixation device and

diagonal vertebroplasty. Der Unfallchir. 88:293–298, 1985.
9. Asazuma, T., Stokes, I. A. F., Moreland, M. S., and Suzuki, N.: An intersegmental spinal flexibility with lumbo-sacral instrumentation: In vitro biomechanical investigation. Proceedings of the I.S.S.L.S. Kyoto, Japan, 1989.
10. Asher, M, Carson, W., and Heinig, C.: A modular spinal rod linkage system to provide rotational stability. Spine 13:272–277, 1988.
11. Asher, M. A., and Strippgen, W. E.: Anthropometric studies of the human sacrum relating to dorsal transsacral implant designs. Clin. Orthop. Rel. Res. 203:58–62, 1986.
12. Ashman, R. B., Birch, J. G., Bone, L. B., et al.: Mechanical testing of spinal instrumentation. Clin. Orthop. Rel. Res. 227:113–125, 1988.
13. Attenborough, C. G., and Reynolds, M. T.: Lumbosacral fusion with spring fixation. J. Bone Joint Surg. 57:283–288, 1975.
14. Baker, L. D., and Hoyt, W. A.: The use of interfacet vitalium screws in the Hibbs fusion. South. Med. J. 41:419–426, 1948.
15. Banta, C. J., King, A. G., Dabezies, E. J., and D'Ambrosia, R.: Direct measurement of effective pedicle diameter. Proceedings of the North American Spine Society Annual Meeting. Banff, Canada, 1987.
16. Bechtol, C. O.: Internal fixation with plates and screws. *In* Bechtol, C. O., Ferguson, A. B., Jr., and Laing, P. B. (eds.): Metals and Engineering in Bone and Joint Surgery. Baltimore, Williams & Wilkins, 1959, pp. 152–171.
17. Berry, J. L, Moran, J. M., Berg, W. S., and Steffee, A. D.: A morphometric study of human lumbar and selected thoracic vertebrae. Spine 12:362–367, 1987.
18. Birch, J. G., Herring, J. A., Roach, J. W., and Johnston, C. E.: Cotrel-Dubousset instrumentation in idiopathic scoliosis. Clin. Orthop. Rel. Res. 227:24–29, 1988.
19. Blauth, M., Tscherne, H., and Haas, N.: Therapeutic concept and results of operative treatment in acute trauma of the thoracic and lumbar spine: The Hannover experience. J. Orthop. Trauma 1:240–252, 1987.
20. Bobechko, W. P.: The instant Harrington. Proceedings of the Scoliosis Research Society Annual Meeting, 1981.
21. Boucher, H. H.: A Method of Spinal Fusion. J. Bone Joint Surg. 41:248–259, 1959.
22. Bridwell, K. H.: The treatment of flexion/distraction spinal fractures with SSI and Luque rectangles. Proceedings of the Scoliosis Research Society Annual Meeting, 1984.
23. Brodsky, J. W., Barnes, D. A., and Tullos, H. S.: Unrecognized pin penetration of the hip joint. Contemp. Orthop. 9:13–20, 1984.
24. Bryant, C. E., and Sullivan, J. A.: Management of thoracic and lumbar spine fractures with Harrington distraction rods supplemented with segmental wiring. Spine 8:532–537, 1983.
25. Casey, M. P., and Jacobs, R. R.: Internal fixation of the lumbosacral spine: A biomechanical evaluation. Proceedings of the I.S.S.L.S. Annual Meeting, Montreal, 1984.
26. Casey, M., Jacobs, R. R., and Asher, M.: The rod long-fuse short technique in the treatment of thoraco-lumbar and lumbar spine fractures. Proceedings of the Scoliosis Research Society Annual Meeting, 1984.
27. Cordey, J., and Perren, S. M.: Limits of plate on bone friction in internal fixation of fractures. Proceedings of the Orthopaedic Research Society Annual Meeting, Las Vegas, 1985, p. 186.
28. Cotrel, Y., Dubousset, J., and Guillaumat, M.: New universal instrumentation in spinal surgery. Clin. Orthop. Rel. Res. 227:10–23, 1988.
29. Daniaux, H.: Transpedikuläre Reposition und Spongioplastik bei Wirbel-Körperbruchen den unteren Brust- und Lendenwirbelsäule. Unfallchirurgie 89:197–213, 1986.
30. DeCoster, T., Jones, W., and Heetderks, D.: Bone Screw Pullout Strength as a Function of Thread Design. Proceedings of the Orthopaedic Trauma Association Annual Meeting, Dallas, 1988, p. 89.
31. Denis, F., Ruiz, H., and Searls, K.: Comparison between square-ended distraction rods and standard round-ended distraction rods in the treatment of thoracolumbar spinal injuries: A statistical analysis. Clin. Orthop. Rel. Res. 189:162–167, 1984.
32. Dick, W.: The "fixateur interne" as a versatile implant for spine surgery. Spine 12:882–900, 1987.
33. Dick, W.: Innere fixation von Brust—und Lendenwirbelfrakturen. Bern, Hans Huber, 1984.
34. Dick, W., Kluger, P., Magerl, F., et al.: A new device for internal fixation of thoracolumbar and lumbar spine fractures: The "fixateur interne". Paraplegia 23:225–232, 1985.
35. Diehl, K., Hanser, U., Hort, W., and Mittelmeier, H.: Biomechanische Untersuchungen über die maximalen Vorspannkräfte der Knochenschrauben in verschiedenen Knochenabschnitten. Acta Orthop. Unfallchir. 80:89, 1974.
36. Dove, J.: Segmental wiring for spinal deformity. A morbidity report. Spine 14:229–231, 1989.
37. Dove, J.: Internal fixation of the lumbar spine: The Hartshill rectangle. Clin. Orthop. Rel. Res. 203:135–140, 1986.
38. Drummond, D. W., Guadagni, J., Keene, J. S., et al.: Interspinous process segmental spinal instrumentation. J. Pediatr. Orthop. 4:397–404, 1984.
39. Drummond, D., Narechania, R., Wenger, D., et al.: Wisconsin segmental spinal instrumentation. Proceedings of the Scoliosis Research Society Annual Meeting, 1981.
40. Edwards, C. C.: New method for direct sacral fixation: Rationale and clinical results. Proceedings of the I.S.S.L.S. Annual Meeting, 1986.
41. Edwards, C. C.: Reduction of spondylolisthesis: Biomechanics and fixation. Proceedings of the I.S.S.L.S. Annual Meeting, 1986.
42. Edwards, C. E.: Spinal screw fixation of the lumbar and sacral spine: Early results treating the first 50 cases. Proceedings of the Scoliosis Research Society Annual Meeting, 1986.
43. Edwards, C. C.: Sacral fixation device: Design and preliminary results: Proceedings of the Scoliosis Research Society Annual Meeting, 1984.
44. Edwards, C. C., Griffith, P., Levine, A. M., and DeSilva, J. B.: Early clinical results using the spinal rod sleeve method for treating thoracic and lumbar injuries. Proceedings of the American Academy of Orthopaedic Surgeons Annual Meeting, 1982.
45. Edwards, C. C., and Levine, A. M.: Early rod-

sleeve stabilization of the injured thoracic and lumbar spine. Orthop. Clin. North Am. 17:121–145, 1986.

46. Edwards, C. C., Levine, A. M., York, J. J., and Holt, E. S.: A new spinal hook: Rationale and clinical trials. Proceedings of the Scoliosis Research Society Annual Meeting, 1984.
47. Edwards, C. C., and Weigel, M. C.: A prospective study of 51 low lumbar non-unions. Proceedings of the I.S.S.L.S. Annual Meeting, 1988.
48. El-Khoury, G. Y., and McWilliams, F. E.: A simple radiological aid in the diagnosis of small avulsion fractures of the knee. J. Trauma 18:275–277, 1978.
49. Esses, S. I.: The AO spinal internal fixator. Proceedings of the North American Spine Society Annual Meeting, Colorado Springs, 1988.
50. Falahee, M., Mann, K., Yuan, H., et al.: Biomechanical evaluation of augmented anterior and posterior short segment internal fixation for thoracolumbar burst fractures. Proceedings of the I.S.S.L.S. Annual Meeting, 1988, pp. 65–66.
51. Freedman, L. S., Houghton, G. R., and Evans, M.: Cadaveric study comparing the stability of upper distraction hooks used in Harrington instrumentation. Spine 11:579–582, 1986.
52. Gaines, R. W., Breedlove, R. F., and Munson, G.: Stabilization of thoracic and thoracolumbar fracture—dislocations with Harrington rods and sublaminar wires. Clin. Orthop. Rel. Res. 189:195–203, 1984.
53. Geiger, J. M., Udovic, N. A., and Berry, J. L.: Bending and fatigue of spine plates and rods and fatigue of pedicle screws. Proceedings of the American Academy of Orthopaedic Surgeons Annual Meeting, 1989.
54. George, D. C., Krag, M. H., Johnson, C. C., et al.: Hole preparation techniques (drill versus probe) for transpedicular screws: Effect upon pullout strength from human cadaveric vertebrae (submitted to Spine, 1989).
55. Gertzbein, S. D., MacMichael, D., and Tile, M.: Harrington instrumentation as a method of fixation in fractures of the spine: A cortical analysis of deficiencies. J. Bone Joint Surg. 64:526–529, 1982.
56. Grobler, L. J., Kempff, P. G., and Gaines, R. W., Jr.: Comparing Mersilene tape (M. T.) and stainless steel wire (S.S.W.) during segmental spinal instrumentation—evaluation of the macroscopical and microscopical tissue response in the baboon (*Papio urinus*). Proceedings of the Scoliosis Research Society Annual Meeting, Vancouver, 1987.
57. Gruca, A.: Pathogenesis and treatment of idiopathic scoliosis: A preliminary report. J. Bone Joint Surg. 40:570–584, 1958.
58. Gurr, K. R., McAfee, P. C., and Shih, C. M.: Biomechanical analysis of posterior instrumentation systems following decompressive laminectomy: An unstable calf model. J. Bone Joint Surg. 70:680–691, 1988.
59. Guyer, D. W., Wiltse, L. L., and Peek, R. D.: The Wiltse pedicle screw fixation system. Orthopaedics 11:1455–1460, 1988.
60. Harrington, P. R.: The history and development of Harrington instrumentation. Clin. Orthop. Rel. Res. 93:110–112, 1973.
61. Harrington, P. R.: Instrumentation in spine instability other than scoliosis. South Afr. J. Surg. 5:7–12, 1967.
62. Harrington, P. R.: Treatment of scoliosis. Correction and internal fixation by spine instrumentation. J. Bone Joint Surg. 44:591–610, 1962.
63. Harrington, P. R., and Dickson, J. H.: Spinal instrumentation in the treatment of severe progressive spondylolisthesis. Clin. Orthop. Rel. Res. 117:157–163, 1976.
64. Harrington, P. R., and Tullos, H. S.: Reduction of severe spondylolisthesis in children. South. Med. J. 62:1–7, 1969.
65. Herring, J. A., and Ashman, R. B.: Biomechanical testing of instruments for the fixation of spondylolisthesis. Proceedings of the Scoliosis Research Society Annual Meeting, 1986.
66. Herrman, H. D.: Transarticular (transpedicular) metal plate fixation for stabilization of the lumbar and thoracic spine. Acta Neurochir. (Wien) 48:101–110, 1979.
67. Hsu, K. Y., Zucherman, J., White A., et al.: Deterioration of motion segments adjacent to lumbar spine fusions. Proceedings of the North American Spine Society Annual Meeting, Colorado Springs, 1988.
68. Hsu, K., Zucherman, J. F., White, A. H., and Wynne, G.: Internal fixation with pedicle screws. *In* White, A. H., Rothman, R. H., and Ray, C. D. (eds.): Lumbar Spine Surgery: Techniques and Complications. St. Louis, C. V. Mosby, 1987.
69. Jacobs, R. R., Dahners, L. E., Gertzbein, S. D., et al.: A locking hook-spinal rod: Current status of development. Paraplegia 21:197–200, 1983.
70. Jacobs, R. R., Montesano, P. X., and Jackson, R. P.: Enhancement of lumbar spine fusion by use of translaminar facet joint screws. Spine 14:12–15, 1989.
71. Jacobs, R. R., Nordwall, A., and Nachemson, A.: Stability and strength provided by internal fixation systems for dorso-lumbar spinal injuries. Clin. Orthop. Rel. Res. 171:300–308, 1982.
72. Jacobs, R. R., Schlaepfer, F., Mathys, R., Jr., et al.: A locking hook spinal rod system for stabilization of fracture–dislocations and correction of deformities of the dorsolumbar spine: A biomechanic evaluation. Clin. Orthop. Rel. Res. 189:168–177, 1984.
73. Kahanovitz, N., Arnoczky, S. P., Levine, D. B., and Otis, J. P.: The effects of internal fixation on the articular cartilage of unfused canine facet joint cartilage. Spine 9:268–272, 1984.
74. Kahanovitz, N., Bullough, P., and Jacobs, R. R.: The effect of internal fixation without arthrodesis on human facet joint cartilage. Clin. Orthop. Rel. Res. 189:204–208, 1984.
75. Keene, J. S., Drummond, D. S., and Narechania, R. G.: Mechanical performance of the Wisconsin compression system. Proceedings of the Orthopaedic Research Society Annual Meeting, Atlanta, 1980.
76. King, D.: Internal fixation for lumbosacral spine fusions. J. Bone Joint Surg. 30:560–565, 1948.
77. King, D.: Internal fixation for lumbosacral fusion. Am. J. Surg. 66:357–361, 1944.
78. Kinnard P., Ghibely, A., Gordon, D., et al.: Roy-Camille plates in unstable spinal conditions: A preliminary report. Spine 11:131–135, 1986.
79. Kleeman, B. C., Gerhart, T. N., and Hayes, W. C.: Augmenting screw fixation in osteopenic trabecular bone. Proceedings of the Society of Biomaterials Annual Meeting, 1987.

80. Kling, T. F., Jr., Vanderby, R., Jr., Belloli, D. M., and Thomsen, E. L.: Cross-linked pedicle screw fixation in the same vertebral body: A biomechanical study. Proceedings of the Scoliosis Research Society Annual Meeting, 1986.
81. Kluger, P., and Gerner, H. J.: Das Mechanische Prinzip des Fixateur Externe zur Dorsalen Stabilisierung der Brust–und Lendenwirbelsäule. Unfallchirurgie 12:68–79, 1986.
82. Knodt, H., and Larrick, R. B.: Distraction fusion of the spine. Ohio State Med. J. 60:1140–1142, 1964.
83. Koranyi, E., Bowman, C. E., Knecht, C. D., and Janssen, M.: Holding power of orthopaedic screws in bone. Clin. Orthop. Rel. Res. 72:783–786, 1970.
84. Kostuik, J. P.: Anterior Kostuik-Harrington distraction systems. Orthopaedics 11:1379–1391, 1988.
85. Kostuik, J. P.: Anterior fixation for fractures of the thoracic and lumbar spine with or without neurologic involvement. Clin. Orthop. Rel. Res. 189:103–115, 1984.
86. Krag, M. H.: Lumbosacral fixation with the Vermont spinal fixator. *In* Lin, P. M., and Gill, K. (eds.): Lumbar Interbody Fusion: Principles and Techniques of Spine Surgery. Rockville, Maryland, Aspen Publishers, 1988.
87. Krag, M. H., Beynnon, B. D., DeCoster, T. A., and Pope, M. H.: Depth of insertion of transpedicular vertebral screws into human vertebrae: Effect upon screw-vertebra interface strength. J. Spinal Dis. 1:287–294, 1988.
88. Krag, M. H., Beynnon, B. D., Frymoyer, J. W., and Haugh, L. D.: Fatigue testing of an internal fixator for posterior spinal stabilization. Proceedings of the American Academy of Orthopaedic Surgeons 54th Annual Meeting, San Francisco, 1987.
89. Krag, M. H., Beynnon, B. D., Pope, M. H., et al.: An internal fixator for posterior application to short segments of the thoracic, lumbar, or lumbosacral spine: Design and testing. Clin. Orthop. Rel. Res. 203:75–98, 1986.
90. Krag, M. H., Beynnon, B. D., Pope, M. H., and Frymoyer, J. W.: Vermont spinal fixator for posterior thoracic, lumbar, or lumbosacral spinal stabilization; initial mechanical testing and implantation. Proceedings of the I.S.S.L.S. Annual Meeting, Sydney, Australia, 1985.
91. Krag, M. H., Frymoyer, J. W., Beynnon, B. D., and Pope, M. H.: An internal fixator for posterior application to short segments of the thoracic, lumbar, or lumbosacral spine: Design and testing. *In* White, A. H., Rothman, R. H., and Ray, C. D. (eds.): Lumbar Spine Surgery: Techniques and Complications. St. Louis, C. V. Mosby, 1987, pp. 339–367.
92. Krag, M. H., Pope, M. H., and Wilder, D. G.: Mechanisms of spine trauma and features of spinal fixation methods. Part I: Mechanisms of injury. *In* Ghista, D. (ed.): Spinal Cord Medical Engineering. Springfield, Charles C Thomas, 1986, pp. 133–157.
93. Krag, M. H., Van Hal, M. E., and Beynnon, B. D.: Placement of transpedicular vertebral screws close to anterior vertebral cortex: Description of methods (in press, Spine, 1989).
94. Krag, M. H., Weaver, D. L., Beynnon, B. D., and Haugh, L. D.: Morphometry of the thoracic and lumbar spine related to transpedicular screw placement for surgical spinal fixation. Spine 13:27–32, 1988.
95. Laborde, J. M., Bahniuk, E., Bohlman, H. H., and Samson, B.: Comparison of fixation of spinal fractures. Clin. Orthop. Rel. Res. 152:303–310, 1980.
96. Lange, F.: Support for the spondylitic spine by means of buried steel bars attached to the vertebrae. (Reprinted from the original.) Clin. Orthop. Rel. Res. 203:3–6, 1986.
97. Lange, F.: Support for the spondylitic spine by means of buried steel bars attached to the vertebrae. Am. J. Orthop. Surg. 8:344–361, 1910.
98. Lavaste, F.: Biomechanique du rachis dorso-lombaire. Deux. J. Orthop. Pitie pp. 19–23, 1980.
99. Lavaste, F.: Étude des Implants Rachidiens: Mémoire de Biomechanique. Thesis Ingeneur, École Nationale Supériore des Arts et Metiers á Paris, 1977.
100. Lehman, W. B., Grant, A., Rose D., et al.: A method of evaluating possible pin penetration in slipped capital femoral epiphysis using a cannulated internal fixation device. Clin. Orthop. Rel. Res. 186:65–70, 1984.
101. Levine, A. M., and Edwards, C. C.: Low lumbar burst fractures. Orthopaedics 11:1427–1432, 1988.
102. Liu, Y. K., Njus, G. O., Bahr, P. A., and Geng, P.: Fatigue life improvement of nitrogen-ion implanted pedicle screws. Proceedings of the I.S.S.L.S. Annual Meeting Miami, 1988.
103. Liu, Y. K., Njus, G. O., and Singerman, R.: Improvement in the mechanical properties of pedicle screws used in spinal internal fixation. Proceedings of the I.S.S.L.S. Annual Meeting, Dallas, 1986.
104. Louis, R.: Fusion of the lumbar and sacral spine by internal fixation with screw plates. Clin. Orthop. Rel. Res. 203:18–33, 1986.
105. Louis, R., and Maresca, C.: Stabilisation Chirurgical avec Réduction des Spondylolyses et des Spondylolisthésis. Int. Orthop. (S.I.C.O.T.). 1:215–225, 1977.
106. Louis, R., and Maresca, C.: Les arthrodèses stables de la charnière lombo-sacrée (70 cas). Rev. Chir. Orthop. 62(Suppl. II):70–79, 1976.
107. Luque, E. R.: Interpeduncular segmental fixation. Clin. Orthop. Rel. Res. 203:54–57, 1986.
108. Luque, E. R.: Anatomic basis and development of segmental spinal instrumentation. Spine 7:256–259, 1982.
109. Luque, E. R., Cassis, N., and Ramirez-Wiella, G.: Segmental spinal instrumentation in the treatment of fractures of the thoracolumbar spine. Spine 7:312–317, 1982.
110. Luque, E. R., and Rapp, G. F.: A new semirigid method for interpedicular fixation of the spine. Orthopaedics 11:1445–1450, 1988.
111. Lyon, W. F., Cochran, J. R., and Smith, L.: Actual holding power of various screws in bone. Ann. Surg. 114:376–384, 1941.
112. Magerl, F.: External spinal skeletal fixation. *In* Weber, B. G., and Magerl, F. (eds.): The External Fixator. New York, Springer-Verlag, 1985.
113. Magerl, F. P.: Stabilization of the lower thoracic and lumbar spine with external skeletal fixation. Clin. Orthop. Rel. Res. 189:125–141, 1984.
114. Martin, D., Cordey, J., Rahn, B. A., and Perren, S. M.: Bone screw displacement under lateral loading. Proceedings of the 2nd Meeting of the European Society of Biomechanics, Strasbourg, 1979.
115. Matthiass, H. H., and Heine, J.: Surgical reduction

of spondylolisthesis. Clin. Orthop. Rel. Res. 203:34–44, 1986.

116. Mehdian, H., Jaffray, D., and Eisenstein, S. M.: Dwyer/Hartshill transpedicular segmental fixation. Proceedings of the I.S.S.L.S. Annual Meeting, Miami, 1988.

117. Misenheimer, G. R., Peek, R. D., Wiltse, L. L., et al.: Anatomic analysis of pedicle cortical and cancellous diameter as related to screw site. Proceedings of the I.S.S.L.S. Annual Meeting, Dallas, 1988.

118. Moe, J. H., and Denis, F.: The iatrogenic loss of lumbar lordosis. Proceedings of the Scoliosis Research Society Annual Meeting, 1976.

119. Müller, M. E., Allgöwer, M., Schneider, R., and Willenegger, H.: Techniques recommended by the AO Group: Manual of internal fixation (2nd revised edition), Berlin, Springer-Verlag, 1979.

120. Nasca, R. J., and Johnson, L. P.: Harrington-Bobechko instrumentation in the treatment of scoliosis: A preliminary report. Spine 13:246–249, 1988.

121. Nunamaker, D. M., and Perren, S. M.: Force measurements in screw fixation. J. Biomech. 9:669–675, 1976.

122. Ölerud, S., Karlström, G., and Sjöstrom, L.: Transpedicular fixation of thoracolumbar vertebral fractures. Clin. Orthop. Rel. Res. 227:44–51, 1988.

123. Ölerud, S., Sjöström, L., Karlström, G., and Hamberg, M.: Spontaneous effect of increased stability of the lower lumbar spine in cases of severe chronic back pain: The answer of an external transpeduncular fixation test. Clin. Orthop. Rel. Res. 203:67–74, 1986.

124. Pawluk, R. J., Musso, E., Tzitzikalakis, G. I., and Dick, H. M.: Effects of internal fixaltion techniques on altering plate screw strain distribution. Proceedings of the Orthopaedic Research Society Annual Meeting, Las Vegas, 1985.

125. Peek, R. D., Thomas, J. C., Weinstein, J., et al.: Lumbar spine fusion with pedicle screw and rods. Proceedings of the I.S.S.L.S. Annual Meeting, Dallas, 1988.

126. Pennal, G. F., McDonald, G. A., and Dale, G. G.: Method of spinal fusion using internal fixation. Clin. Orthop. Rel. Res. 35:86–94, 1964.

127. Perren, S. M., Cordey, J., Enzler, M., et al.: Mechanics of bone screw with internal fixation plates. Unfallheilkunde 81:211–218, 1978.

128. Puno, R. M., Bechtol, J. E., Byrd, J. E., et al.: Biomechanical analysis of five techniques of fixation for the lumbosacral junction. Proceedings of the Orthopaedic Research Society Annual Meeting, San Francisco, 1987.

129. Puschel, J., and Zielke, K.: Transpedicular vertebral instrumentation using VDS instruments in ankylosing spondylitis. Proceedings of the Scoliosis Research Society 19th Annual Meeting, 1984.

130. Reed, S., and Wagner, T.: Preliminary report on lumbo-sacral fusion with pedicle screws and Steffee plates. Proceedings of the Scoliosis Research Society 21st Annual Meeting, 1986.

131. Reimers, C.: Die Dorsale Spannverstrebung von Wirbelsäulenabschnitten mittels innerer Schienung. Chirurgie 17:10, 1956.

132. Resina, J., and Alves, A. F.: Technique of correction and internal fixation for scoliosis. J. Bone Joint Surg. 59(B):159–165, 1977.

133. Robbins, S., and Gertzbein, S.: Accuracy of pedicle screw placement in vivo. Proceedings of the Orthopaedic Trauma Association Annual Meeting, Dallas, 1988.

134. Rooks, M. D., Schmitt, E. W., and Drvaric, D. M.: Unrecognized pin penetration in slipped capital femoral epiphysis. Clin. Orthop. Rel. Res. 234:82–89, 1988.

135. Rossier, A. B., Cochran, T. P.: The treatment of spinal fractures with Harrington compression rods and segmental sublaminar wiring: A dangerous combination. Spine 9:796–799, 1984.

136. Roy-Camille, R.: Experience With Roy-Camille Fixation for the Thorocolumbar and Lumbar Spine. Acute Spinal Injuries: Current Management Techniques. University of Massachusetts Continuing Medical Education Course, Sturbridge, Massachusetts, October, 1987.

137. Roy-Camille, R., and Demeulenaere, C.: Ostéosynthèse du rachis dorsal, lombaire et lombosacrée par plaque métalliques vissées dans les pédicules vertébraux et les apophyses articulaires. Presse Médicale 78:1447–1448, 1970.

138. Roy-Camille, R., Saillant, G., and Mazel, C.: Internal fixation of the lumbar spine with pedicle screw plating. Clin. Orthop. Rel. Res. 203:7–17, 1986.

139. Saillant, G.: Étude anatomique des pédicules vertébraux: Application chirurgicale. Rev. Chir. Orthop. 62:151–160, 1976.

140. Schatzker, J., Sanderson, R., and Murnaghan, P. J.: The holding power of orthopaedic screws *in vivo*. Clin. Orthop. Rel. Res. 108:115–126, 1975.

141. Schläpfer, F., Magerl, F., Jacobs, R., et al.: In vivo measurements of loads on an external fixation device for human lumbar spine fractures. Institute of Mechanical Engineers. C131/80:59–64, 1980.

142. Schläpfer, F., Wörsdörfer, O., Magerl, F., and Perren, S. M.: Stabilization of the lower thoracic and lumbar spine: Comparative in vitro investigation of an external skeletal and various internal fixation devices. *In* Uhthoff, H. K., and Stahl, E. (eds.): Current Concepts of External Fixation of Fractures. New York, Springer-Verlag, 1982.

143. Schlicke, L., and Schulak, J.: The simultaneous use of Harrington compression and distraction rods in a thoracolumbar fracture-dislocation. J. Trauma. 20:177–179, 1980.

144. Schöllner, O.: Ein neues Verfahren zur Reposition und Fixation bei Spondylolisthesis. Orthop. Praxis 4:270, 1975.

145. Schreiber, A., Suezawa, Y., and Jacob, H. A. C.: Preliminary report of 40 patients. Dorsal spinal fusion with a transpedicular distraction and compression system. Orthop. Rev. 15:93–96, 1986.

146. Shaw, J. A.: Preventing unrecognized pin penetration into hip joint. Orthop. Rev. 13:142–152, 1984.

147. Sicard, A., and Menegaux, J.: L'abord anterieur de l'articulation sacroiliaque. J. Chir. 77:29, 1959.

148. Sijbrandij, S.: A new technique for the reduction and stabilization of severe spondylolisthesis. J. Bone Joint Surg. 63:266–271, 1981.

149. Simmons, E. H., and Capicotto, W. N.: Posterior Zielke instrumentation of the lumbar spine with transpedicular fixation. Proceedings of the Scoliosis Research Society Annual Meeting, 1986.

150. Stanger, J. K.: Fracture-dislocation of the thoracolumbar spine. With special reference to reduction by open and closed operations. J. Bone Joint Surg. 29:107–118, 1947.

151. Steffee, A. D., Biscup, R. S., and Sitkowski, D. J.: Segmental spine plates with pedicle screw fixation: A new internal fixation device for disorders of lumbar and thoracolumbar spine. Clin. Orthop. Rel. Res. 203:45–53, 1986.
152. Steffee, A. D., and Sitkowski, D. J.: Posterior lumbar interbody fusion and plates. Clin. Orthop. Rel. Res. 227:99–102, 1988.
153. Steffee, A. D., and Sitkowski, D. J.: Reduction and stabilization of grade IV spondylolisthesis. Clin. Orthop. Rel. Research. 227:82–89, 1988.
154. Tello, C. A.: Early results with a variation of spinal instrumentation. Proceedings of the Scoliosis Research Society Annual Meeting, 1984.
155. Tencer, A. F., Ferguson, R. L., Woodard, P. L., and Allen, B. L., Jr.: Biomechanical evaluation of posterior fixation of spine fractures. Proceedings of the Orthopaedic Research Society 33rd Annual Meeting, San Francisco, 1987.
156. Thalgott, J. S., Aebi, M., and LaRocca, H.: Internal spinal skeletal fixation system. Orthopaedics 11:1465–1468, 1988.
157. Thalgott, J. S., LaRocca, H., Aebi, M., et al.: Reconstruction of the lumbar spine using AO DCP plate internal fixation. Spine 14:91–95, 1989.
158. Thomas, J. C., Jr., Haye, W., Wiltse, L. L., et al.: Review of deep wound infection complicating pedicle screw fixation of the lumbar spine. Proceedings of the I.S.S.L.S. Annual Meeting, Miami, Florida, 1988.
159. Thompson, W. A. L., and Ralston, E. L.: Pseudarthrosis following spine fusion. J. Bone Joint Surg. 31:400–405, 1949.
160. Toumey, J. W.: Internal fixation in fusion of the lumbo-sacral joints. Lahey Clin. Bull. 3:188–191, 1943.
161. Trias, A., Bourassa, P., and Massoud, M.: Dynamic loads experienced in correction of idiopathic scoliosis using two types of Harrington rods. Spine 4:228–235, 1979.
162. Vangsness, C. T., Carter, D. R., and Frankel, V. H.: In vitro evaluation of the loosening characteristics of self-tapped and non-self-tapped cortical bone screws. Clin. Orthop. Rel. Res. 157:279–286, 1981.
163. Vercauteren, M., and DeGroote, W.: Reduction of spondylolisthesis with severe slipping. Acta Orthop. Belgica 47:502–511, 1981.
164. Vidal, J., Fassio, B., Buscayret, C., and Allieu, Y.: Surgical reduction of spondylolisthesis using a posterior approach. Clin. Orthop. Rel. Res. 154:156–165, 1981.
165. Volz, R. G., and Martin, M. D.: Illusory biplane radiographic images. Radiology 122:695–697, 1977.
166. Walters, R., and Simon, S. R.: Joint destruction: A sequel of unrecognized pin penetration in patients with slipped capital femoral epiphysis. Proceedings of the Eighth Open Scientific Meeting of the Hip Society. St. Louis, C. V. Mosby, 1980.
167. Wang, G. J., Reger, S. I., Jennings, R. L., et al.: Variable strengths of wire fixation. Orthopaedics 5:435–436, 1981.
168. Ward, J. J., Nasca, R. J., and Lemons, J. E.: Biomechanical evaluation of the neural arch. Proceedings of the Scoliosis Research Society Annual Meeting, 1984.
169. Weinstein, J. N., Spratt, K. F., Spengler, D., and Brick, C.: Spinal pedicle fixation: Reliability and validity of roentgenogram-based assessment and surgical factors on successful screw placement. Spine 13:1012–1018, 1988.
170. Weiss, M.: Dynamic spine alloplasty (spring-loading corrective devices) after fracture and spinal cord injury. Clin. Orthop. Rel. Res. 112:150–158, 1975.
171. Wenger, D., Miller, S., and Wilkerson, J.: Evaluation of fixation sites for segmental instrumentation of the human vertebra. Proceedings of the Scoliosis Research Society Annual Meeting, 1981.
172. Whitecloud, T. S., Butler, J. C., Cohen, J. L., and Candelora, P. D.: Complications with the variable spinal plating system. (in press, Spine, 1989).
173. Williams, E. W. M.: Traumatic paraplegia. *In* Matthews, D. N. (ed.): Recent Advances in Surgery of Trauma. London, Churchill, 1963, pp. 171–186.
174. Wilson, P. D., and Straub, L. R.: Lumbosacral fusion with metallic-plate fixation. Am. Acad. Orthop. Surg. Instruct. Course Lect. 9:53–57, 1952.
175. Yamagata, M.: Biomechanical study of posterior spinal instrumentation for scoliosis. J. Jpn. Orthop. Assoc. 58:523–534, 1984.
176. Zand, M. S., Goldstein, S. A., and Matthews, L. S.: Fatigue failure of cortical bone screws. J. Biomech. 16:305–312, 1983.
177. Zielke, K., and Stremple, A. V.: Posterior lateral distraction spondylodesis using the twofold sacral bar. Clin. Orthop. Rel. Res. 203:151–158, 1986.
178. Zindrick, M. R., Wiltse, L. L., Doornik, A., et al.: Analysis of the morphometric characteristics of the thoracic and lumbar pedicles. Spine 12:160–166, 1987.
179. Zindrick, M. R., Wiltse, L. L., Holland, W. R., et al.: Biomechanical study of intrapedicular screw fixation in the lumbosacral spine. Proceedings of the I.S.S.L.S. Annual Meeting, Sydney, Australia, 1985.
180. Zindrick, M. R., Wiltse, L. L., Widell, E. H., et al.: Biomechanical study of interpeduncular screw fixation in the lumbosacral spine. Clin. Orthop. Rel. Res. 203:99–111, 1986.

INTERNAL FIXATION

Bruce E. Fredrickson
Hansen A. Yuan

Instrumentation of the lumbar spine and lumbar sacral junction has become more commonly accepted since the late 1970s. Instrumentation systems are available today that can be implanted either anteriorly or posteriorly or in various combinations. These systems can be classified in a number of ways. The first classification system is based on rigidity. Rigid implants do not rely on the ligaments or articulations of the spine for their support. Semirigid implants derive some of their stability from the normal articulations and ligamentous attachments of the individual motion segments. Flexible implants usually apply only one corrective force, and the stability of the spine is basically dependent on its normal articulations and ligamentous attachments. The second major classification system is segmental versus nonsegmental. Implants that are segmental allow for attachment of the device to each individual vertebra.

Indications for the use of a device to internally fix the spine are varied. In degenerative disease of the lumbar spine, devices have been used to increase the fusion rate and to distract the intervertebral foramen. In specific diagnoses, such as spondylolisthesis, they have been used not only to enhance the rate of fusion but also, at times, to afford some reduction of the deformity. In scoliosis, devices have commonly been used for correction of the deformity and maintenance of position while a fusion is consolidating. In the case of trauma to the lumbar spine, devices have been used to reduce and to hold the reduction while a fusion is taking place. Specific problems, such as osteomyelitis, Pott's disease, and metastatic disease of the spine, have required various anterior internal fixation devices or combinations of anterior and posterior devices to afford stability while the lesions themselves are being treated.

The first use of internal fixation in the spine was by Hadra[23] in 1891. He used a wire to fix a cervical fracture/dislocation posteriorly. The history of internal fixation of the spine is then intimately associated with the history of spinal fusion from the time of Hibbs and Albe in the early 1900s. Attempts at fixation of the spine were carried out by various surgeons in the early 1900s. Lange[44] was the first to implant a metal rod in an attempt to increase spinal stability. Jenkins[31] of New Zealand in 1936 used a peg of tibia to anteriorly fix L5 to S1 in a patient with spondylolisthesis. Mercer[58] in 1936 and Speed[75] in 1938 described similar procedures involving the use of a bone peg as a form of internal fixation at the L5–S1 junction for spondylolisthesis.

The first extensive use of internal fixation, posteriorly, with the exception of wire, was by King[37] in 1948. He used screws placed across the facet joints to increase the fusion rate for lumbosacral fusions. Boucher[8] in 1959 and Andrew[4] in 1986 described a similar procedure. Wilson and Straub[81] in 1952 described the use of a metal plate held to the spinous processes by a series of bolts. He listed four specific objectives in his use of internal fixation: (1) to provide absolute immobilization of the operative area while fusion was occurring; (2) to shorten the period of postoperative recovery; (3) to reduce postoperative discomfort; and (4) to reduce the number of failed fusions.

Anterior fixation techniques continued to rely on the use of rigid bony implants through the 1950s. The work of Wiltburger[82] and Harmon[25] illustrates the two approaches taken. Harmon advocated the anterior approach to the intervertebral disc space, whereas Wiltburger recommended the posterior interbody technique. Both techniques relied on fixation by the graft itself.

The report of Harrington[27] in 1962 was the beginning of the current techniques used in internal fixation of the lumbar spine. His device was applied posteriorly and relied on hooks placed around the lamina for purchase on the spine. Fixation was not segmental, and the construct is classified as semirigid. Roy-Camille[10] developed a system utilizing screws placed into the pedicle. This system was segmental and rigid. Its further development was carried out in Europe during the 1960s by both Roy-Camille and Louis.[47] The report of Harrington and Dickson in 1976 reviewed their experience with pedicle screws. They were used in the attempted reduction of spondylolistheses but were discarded when it was believed that they were not needed.

Modifications of the Harrington device have been made by several authors. A distraction rod was specifically developed for the lumbar spine by Knodt and reported on by Beattie.[7] It was designed for use over one or two segments and provided a semirigid construct. Jacobs and coworkers[30] reported on a stronger threaded device with a locking proximal hook to try and decrease the incidence of hook dislodgment.

White and colleagues,[80] Selby,[74] and Lee and deBari,[45] reported on their results using the Knodt device. Kaneda and associates[34] reported on a similar device supplemented with compression hooks to help further with stability. Edwards[18] increased the torsional stability of the basic Harrington rods by the addition of rod sleeves.

Segmental posterior systems were introduced to North American orthopedists by Luque[49] and subsequently refined with better fixation techniques to the pelvis by Allen and Ferguson.[2] Fixation was by sublaminar wires twisted to solid contoured rods. The technique is segmental but only semirigid.

Segmental techniques involving purchase by transpedicular screws were initially developed in Europe by Roy-Camille[10] and later popularized by Louis.[47] External peduncular fixation was introduced by Magerl.[54] Modification of his concept by Dick[13] was reported by Aebi and coworkers.[1] The peduncular systems are all segmental and provide rigid immobilization, except for that of Edwards, which is semirigid. Systems utilizing the transpedicular technique in North America include those developed by Steffee,[77] Edwards,[17] Wiltse,[83] and Krag.[42]

The development of anterior fixation devices generally has lagged behind that of posterior instrumentation. Dwyer[15] developed the first commonly used device for anterior fixation. This was a flexible device and generally used only for correction of spinal deformity, secondary to scoliosis. Hall[24] reviewed its current status in spinal surgery in 1981. Zielke[88] modified the Dwyer approach to include a rod rather than a flexible cable. The device then became semirigid and had greater applicability to severe spinal deformities and injuries. Moe and colleagues[59] and Kaneda and associates[36] have reported on its use.

Anterior devices have been developed by other surgeons for specific problems. Humphries and colleagues[29] reported on the use of an anterior plate for either one- or two-level anterior spinal fusions. They considered the device to be rigid and allowed early ambulation. Werlinich[79] reported on the use of an anterior staple for single-level fusions. He considered the fixation to be rigid. Kostuik[39] reported on the development of an anterior device utilizing Harrington distraction rods and modified Dwyer screws. Advantages sighted were a decreased nonunion rate and an increased ability to correct kyphotic deformities. He cautioned that the device did not provide good control of rotation and lateral bending, and therefore the use of a supplementary system, such as a solid Hall rod and an external orthosis, was needed. Dunn[14] described the evolution of an anterior fixation system from a semirigid to rigid classification. This device has subsequently been removed from the market because of several reported incidences of aortic erosion resulting from its use. Kaneda and coworkers[33] described an anterior device similar to that of Dunn with two solid, threaded rods placed laterally over the vertebra. This device[85] has been further modified to have a cross-linking member to provide enhanced torsional stability. To date, there have been no reported instances of aortic erosion with this device. It is currently available on a limited basis in the United States.

At present, many systems for both anterior and posterior use are being developed and tried on a clinical basis. They generally rely on segmental fixation and are either rigid or semirigid.

GOALS AND DEFINITIONS

The goals for all fixation devices used in the spine are the same. First a device should allow correction of a deformity, if one is present, and should prevent deformity during the postoperative period. Second, the fusion rate should be at least equal to that without the device in place, and preferably it should be improved. Third, early mobilization of the patient should be possible, with the use of less external immobilization.

In order to meet these goals, the implant must have certain characteristics. No single implant will be able to be used for every problem; however, the overall characteristics of the implants should be the same. First, the implant itself should be compatible with the body. Currently used materials include stainless steel and titanium. The use of materials that would allow ingrowth of bone have been used on an experimental basis.[48] The use of porous ingrowth devices is advantageous if the device is not to be removed. However, if the device has to be removed in the future, large quantities of bone may have to be removed, resulting in a significant defect in the spinal column and requiring extensive reconstructive surgery. Second, the device must allow instrumentation of a minimum number of segments. Third, the device should be at least semirigid and preferably rigid so that it can be used either with or without intact ligamentous and bony structures. Further development in the area of disc replacement would change this characteristic, making a flexible implant advantageous for some applications. Fourth, adequate room must be left for the application of an adequate bone graft for solid fusion, if needed. Only in specific instances, such as in the case of metastatic disease, can one expect the device to remain stable throughout a patient's life. Fifth, safe and easy implantation of the device must be possible. Instrumentation systems that require a great deal of specialized instrumentation and manual dexterity tend not to be implanted appropriately and greatly prolong the surgical time. Sixth, the device must be adaptable to various situations and allow correction of deformity, if one is present.

BIOMECHANICS

The actual loads that a spinal implant are expected to support in the spine are not known. Attempts to assess these loads have been carried out by various techniques. Nachemson[63] measured the in vitro hydrostatic properties of the nucleus pulposus in various positions of the body. He determined that the pressures within the normal disc were 1.3 to 1.6 times the vertical load applied per unit area and that there was a linear increase in pressure for external loads of up to 2,000 N. The load on the L3 disc varied from 20 to 270 kg, in various body positions without lifting, in a 70-kg individual. Nachemson and coworkers reported the load distribution between the anterior disc and the posterior elements to be 85% to 90% anterior and only 10% to 15% posterior in the erect position.[61]

Harrington rods instrumented with strain gauges have been implanted in patients with idiopathic scoliosis. Monitoring of the forces seen by the rods has been carried out both at the time of the procedure with the patients under general anesthesia and also postoperatively in the sitting and upright positions.[78] Forces of 196 to 294 N were generally sufficient to produce correction of 60% to 75% in flexible curves.[28] Forces increased up to 669 N during such activities as coughing and vomiting. The highest values seen during sitting and standing were only about 196 N. Nachemson and Elfstrom[64] carried out similar experimentation using telemetry. They recorded a maximum force during distraction of 412 N, but generally the maximum distraction force was in the range of 196 to 245 N. They noted a rapid decrease of 25% to 40% in this force during the first hour postoperatively. Forces of 98 to 245 N were noted during supine bed rest and log rolling. Forces similar to those reported by Hirsch up to 226 N were reported during standing and walking. These forces could be reduced by approximately 49 N with the addition of a Milwaukee brace.

Schläpfer and coworkers[71] reported on the in vitro measurements of loads on an external fixation device. Nagel and colleagues[65] instrumented Harrington distraction rods, which were implanted in sheep; their data, however, are difficult to convert to the human model.

Loads in the lumbar spine have also been computed by numerous authors using various mathematical models. Schultz and colleagues[72] predicted moments on the lumbar spine of as much as 2,400 N•m during standing and holding an 8-kg weight. Their model showed that these large net reaction moments were not attributable to the external forces so much as to the large trunk muscle contraction forces. Anderson and coworkers[3] and Morris and associates[60] have also constructed various biomechanical models to explain these large forces.

Krag and coworkers[42] have suggested that the answer to the question of how strong an implant and the implant bone junction needs to be could be answered by looking at the available implants and their relative strengths. They reasoned that an implant in current use and associated with both a low breakage rate and a high fusion rate must be meeting the biologic demands of the spine. They extrapolated that 3.5- to 4.5-mm screws are strong enough when used in pedicle systems, because screw breakage has not been reported to be a problem in devices utilizing a screw of this size. They further reasoned that the bending loads applied to a pedicle plate must be less than 11.3 N•m based on mechanical testing of Roy-Camille plates and the clinical experience with this device.

It appears, based on the work of Nachemson and Hirsch, that a posteriorly applied spinal implant must be able to support forces, on the average, of up to 245 N in compressive loading if there are intact bony and ligamentous structures. In addition, based on the assumptions of Krag, 4.5-mm screws applied through the pedicles are large enough to resist physiologic forces in an intact spine. Care should be taken in interpreting all of these in vivo data when applying them to assess the needed strength and stability of implants in spines that are not intact. This is because they were gathered from basically intact spines and not with a major disruption of either the osseous or ligamentous structures. Recent research has produced information on the destabilized spine to help with this problem. Peek and associates[70] and McGowan and coworkers[52] reported on biomechanical investigations in which the spine was destabilized by serial sectioning of ligaments and bone, and instrumented with various implants.

Testing techniques in the laboratory setting have varied among investigators trying to assess the actual strength of implants and the implant-bone complex. The earliest techniques used were simple tests to failure. More recent techniques have included the following: relative stiffness of implanted devices, stress measurements of implanted devices loaded to physiologic forces with secondary mathematical modeling of failure modes, and cyclic testing of implanted devices loaded to physiologic stresses.

Harrington,[27] in the development of his system, evaluated the various posterior purchase sights for hooks on the thoracic and lumbar spine by loading to failure. Dwyer and colleagues[15] evaluated the mechanical properties of his cable and screw system by testing to failure the cable and cable screw junctions. They did not perform any in-vitro testing of the screw-bone complex, but in-vivo measurements suggested that the screw-staple complex could withstand forces in excess of 445 N.

Investigators such as Guyer and coworkers[22] and Mann and colleagues[55, 56] have tested devices in vitro, using loads that were known to not result in permanent deformities of the intact spine. The stiffness of various implants in the same spine was established. Johnston and colleagues[32] have recorded the strain in a fixation device implanted in vitro and subjected to known loads. The mode of failure and number of repetitions to failure of a specific device were then calculated.

Nasca and coworkers[66, 67] have applied cyclic physiologic loads to both noninstrumented and instrumented spines. Information has been obtained regarding failure of the implant and the implant-bone junction.

IN VITRO BIOMECHANICAL EVALUATIONS OF SPECIFIC DEVICES

Relative stiffness and modes of failures of various devices have been studied by numerous authors.[6, 14, 19, 20, 22, 30, 38, 52, 55, 56, 68, 70]

Posterior Devices

Jacobs and coworkers[30] reported on the development of the modified Harrington system and spinal stability when using a long-rod versus short-rod method for fracture fixation. The bending strength of their modified rod was approximately 1.5 times that of a Harrington rod. The yield point of the threaded portion was only 1.5 times less than that of the solid portion, compared with the 2.5 times weakening effect of the notches on the standard Harrington rod. Edwards[16] has also studied the strength of the Harrington rod and has modified it by increasing the inner diameter of the notches and by doubling the number of notches per inch. This has led to an increase in strength similar to that of the rod developed by Jacobs.

The strength of the standard upper Harrington hook-bone complex was tested by Jacobs and found to fail at 794 N, as compared with 1275 N for his locking hook. The force reported by Jacobs that was required to cause failure at the upper hook site for the standard Harrington hook was significantly above that reported by Waugh[78] and is less than that reported by Harrington.[27] This reflects the problems in trying to assess and compare data from different studies on tests carried out to failure.

Jacobs and coworkers[30] evaluated four systems of lumbar sacral fixation that are applied posteriorly. Flexion bending moments were applied to each device until failure occurred. The four systems were the Roy-Camille plates, Harrington distraction rods attached to a sacral bar (the bending moment being resisted by contact of the rod with the sacral ala), Harrington distraction rods attached to a sacral bar reinforced with a four-holed plate over the iliac spine, and Allen's modification of the Luque system known as the Galveston technique. The strongest system was the Luque-Allen and the weakest was the plate system of Roy-Camille.

Schläpfer and coworkers[71] measured the stiffness of a lumbar spine fixed with four different systems. They evaluated the External Fixator, conventional Harrington rod system, Jacobs modified Harrington rod system, and a plate pedicle screw system. The stiffest system was found to be the plate pedicle screw system. The Jacobs modified Harrington system was almost as stiff, and it was followed by the External Fixator supplemented with facet screws. The External Fixator was stiffer than the standard Harrington rod.

Guyer and colleagues[22] observed the stiffness and modes of failure of seven internal fixation devices implanted at the lumbar sacral junction when it was subjected to flexion bending moments and extension distraction forces (Fig. 1). The seven devices included the standard Harrington rod, Harrington rods with sublaminar wires, Knodt rods, the Luque rectangular ring, the Kaneda device, the Synthes pelvic fixator, and interfacet screws. All systems were significantly stiffer than the intact spine in extension. The Luque, Kaneda, Synthes, and Knodt systems were approximately equal in their stiffness values. The Harrington rod and Harrington rods with sublaminar wires and facet screws were not as stiff as the other four. In flexion, the Synthes, interfacet screws, and the Kaneda system had approximately similar stiffnesses, and all were much stiffer than the normal spine. The other systems were of decreasing stiffness; the Harrington and Harrington with sublaminar wires approached the stiffness of the normal intact spine. The Kaneda and Synthes systems were found to provide the stiffest fixation in both flexion and extension. Failure of the first sacral lamina was seen in implants requiring attachment to the first sacral lamina within the range of physiologic forces used. Devices relying on fixation to this area were therefore considered to be potentially unstable.

Studies by Peek and associates[70] on the effect of decompressive laminectomy on the stiffness of an instrumented spine suggest that pedicle screw systems are preferred. Evaluation of pedicle screw designs and placement has been carried out by numerous authors, including Steffee and coworkers,[77] Zindrick and colleagues,[89] Asher and Strippgen,[5] Roy-Camille and associates,[10] and Krag and colleagues.[42] Various characteristics of the screw have been evaluated, including inner and outer core diameters, profile, and pitch. The effect of these variables both on pull-out strength and on toggle secondary to shear forces has been evaluated.

Anterior Devices

Evaluation of anterior devices has been carried out in a manner similar to that for posterior devices. Dunn,[14] in the development of his three anterior devices, evaluated the pull-out strength of the Dwyer screw. Subsequently, in a fracture model, he compared each of his designs with standard posterior instrumentation with two Harrington rods. His Type II and Type III devices were stiffer and stronger. Mann and colleagues[55, 56] tested five different devices in a fracture model under a compressive load of 400 N and a maximum bending moment of 10 to 14 N•m. The model consisted of excision of the posterior two thirds of the body of L1 and both adjacent discs. A wood block was used to simulate a solid cortical strut graft. The constructs tested included the graft alone and subsequently the grafted model plus the Kostuik, Kaneda, I-plate, or revised I-plate. Stiffness data were compared with the intact spine prior to removal of the vertebral body. Testing consisted of application of the load during flexion, extension, and right and left lateral bend. All instru-

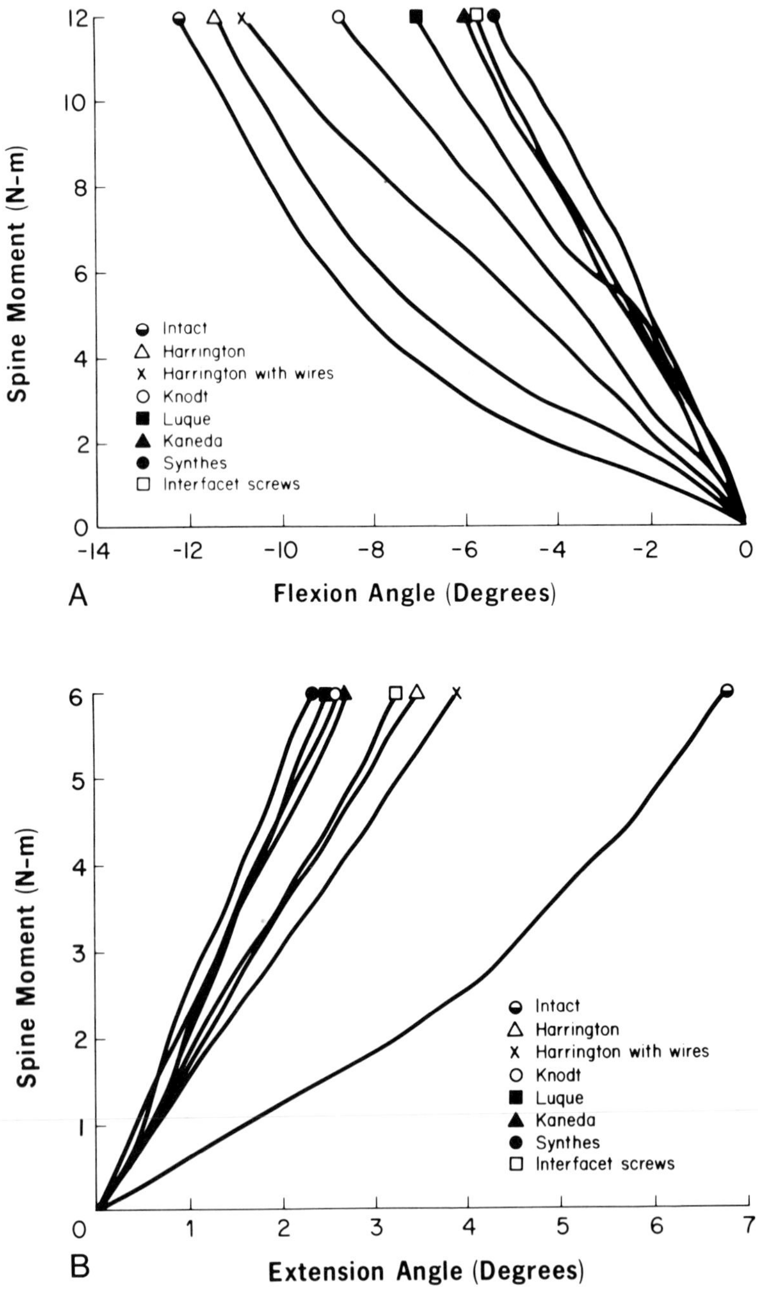

Figure 1 □ *A, B,* Deformation of instrumented spines in both flexion and extension is shown in terms of degrees per applied moment. Testing of this nature allows comparison between various instrumentation systems in regard to stiffness. The forces applied were not of sufficient magnitude to cause failure of the device or the bone.

mented constructs, with the exception of the Kostuik, in flexion had stiffness equal to or greater than the normal spine. The revised I-plate and Kaneda device provided the greatest stiffness in all planes. McGowan and colleagues[52] reported on a similar study with serial destabilization of the spine by sectioning and removing the posterior ligaments and facets. He recommended that a posterior implant be combined with any anterior device if the posterior elements were severely destroyed.

Nasca and colleagues[66, 67] reported on the cyclic loading of spinal implants in a calf spine model. The maximum number of times that any one construct was cycled was 10,000. They have not reported any definite conclusions regarding the advantages of specific implants.

CURRENTLY AVAILABLE IMPLANTS: ADVANTAGES AND DISADVANTAGES

Each device that can be used for fixation of the lumbar spine, be it anterior or posterior, has its obvious advantages and disadvantages. Some devices have had highly significant complications relating to either their implantation or secondary deformities. Falling into this category are the Knodt rods and standard Harrington rods. Both produce unacceptable kyphosis of the lumbar spine and are contraindicated. Modifications of the standard Harrington system, such as the Moe square-ended rods and Jacobs ratcheted rods, do allow for control of the lumbar lordosis and therefore have some use in the lumbar spine. In regard to the anterior approach, the Type III Dunn device has been removed from the market because of complications associated with vascular erosion.

Most surgeons today think that the fewest possible segments in the lumbar spine should be instrumented for any particular problem. Instrumentation extending down from the thoracolumbar junction should stop at L3, if possible, in order to reduce the incidence of late degenerative changes in the lumbar spine.[21] In fusions of the lumbosacral junction, the previous practice of long distraction fusions carried out with Harrington hooks from the sacral ala up to L1 and L2 should be abandoned. This not only avoids the major complication of loss of the normal lumbar lordosis but also leaves as many segments mobile as possible. The devices currently favored by most surgeons today, therefore, involve some form of segmental instrumentation, either sublaminar wires as advocated by Luque, pedicle screws as advocated by numerous authors, or the Cotrel-Dubousset system, which allows segmental fixation by means of hooks (Fig. 2).[19]

Anterior fixation systems are generally segmental in nature. The Dwyer system is a flexible implant and has been associated with high nonunion rates. It generally has been superseded by the VDS system of Zielke. This has resulted in higher fusion rates and fewer problems with iatrogenic lumbar kyphosis, which was also highly associated with the previously used Dwyer system. Kostuik has developed a semirigid system using modified Dwyer screws and

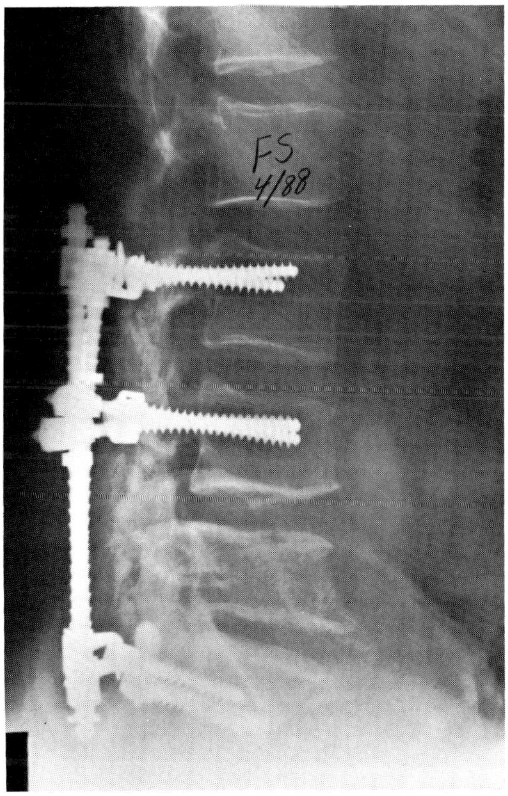

Figure 2 □ Pedicle screw fixation allows segmental instrumentation of the lumbar sacral junction. Significant lordotic forces can be generated by some of the pedicle screw devices. Bowing of the distraction rods can be seen, indicating the presence of a large antilordotic force. The inherent stiffness of the spine in this case, however, cannot be overcome by a purely posterior approach.

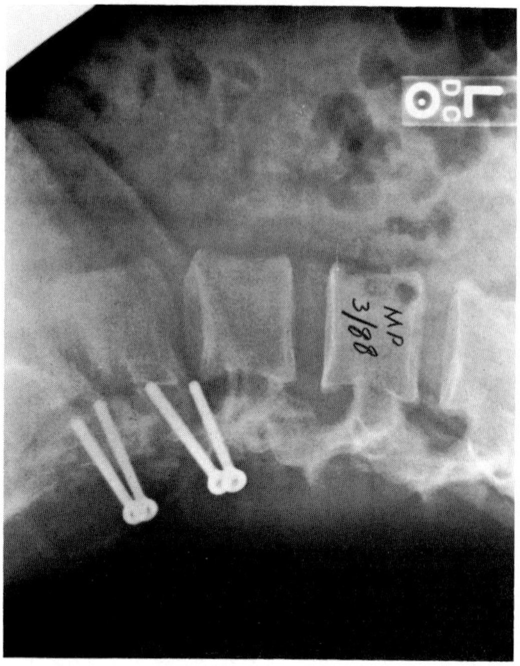

Figure 3 □ The relative stiffness of various constructs used with the anterior approach are illustrated. Laboratory data help the operating surgeon arrive at a better choice of the particular device required in a specific patient.

standard Harrington rods. This allows for correction of kyphosis and some stability when combined with a Hall rod. The more rigid anterior systems either in development or in currently limited use include the Kaneda[33] and the I-plate of Yuan (Fig. 3).[85, 86]

RESULTS OF TREATMENT

The use of posterior segmental instrumentation via pedicle screws, sublaminar wires, or the Cotrel-Dubousset system has resulted in universally higher rates of fusion, compared with the rates for noninstrumented spines. DePalma and Rothman[12] reported a pseudarthrosis rate of 5% for lumbosacral fusions. Fusions extending from L4 to S1 are reported to have a pseudarthrosis rate of 20%. Fusions of more than two motion segments are reported to show increasingly higher rates of pseudarthrosis. Steffee and colleagues[77] report only a 5% nonunion rate with multiple-level lumbar fusions utilizing pedicle screws and plates. Kostuik and associates[41] reported a 15% pseudarthrosis rate in 20 patients fused using Luque rods from either L2 or L3 to the sacrum. They caution against the use of sublaminar wires around the S1 lamina because of a high incidence of neurologic damage to the sacral roots. Kostuik's subsequent evaluation of the problem has identified the female patient as being particularly prone to the disorder. Louis[47] reported a 5% nonunion rate with pedicle screws and plates. Kornblatt and coworkers[38] reported a fusion rate of 84% with internal fixation versus 76% without it. A similar rate of 96% with internal fixation was reported by Kaneda.[35]

The results of anterior fixation with rigid or semirigid devices have also led to an improvement in fusion rate. Humphries and coworkers[29] reported on a series of patients fused anteriorly from either L4 or L5 to S1 with an anterior plate. They reported no evidence of plate or screw breakage in 23 patients with a follow-up of more than 1 year. They reported solid fusions in 18 of the 23, questionable fusions in 3, and definite nonunions in 2. This would be a nonunion rate of approximately 10%. Kostuik[39, 40] has reported on results of anterior stabilizations and fusion for various problems, including congenital kyphosis, infection, and fracture. Anterior fixation consisted of a modified Harrington system usually combined with a solid Hall rod. He reported that primary bone union occurred in 40 of 42 patients.

The results of treatment with the current segmental devices, be they anterior or posterior, show an improved rate of fusion. Other advantages cited by the various authors include a decreased use of external immobilization, a faster rate of mobilization, and better correction of deformity, if present at the time of surgery. These results would justify the continued use of these devices, as they meet the original goals.

THE AUTHORS' CURRENT APPROACH TO LUMBAR FIXATION

The use of a specific internal fixation device in the lumbar spine is dependent upon the goals of a particular surgical procedure and the limitations of the device. The most important factors in the decision-making process are as follows: (1) the specific segment or segments of the spine that are involved, (2) the specific diagnosis, and (3) the knowledge and expertise of the operating surgeon. Our current indications for use of a particular device are also changing as our knowledge of its capabilities and limitations become better known.

Degenerative disease of the lumbosacral junction is the most common underlying pathologic process currently being treated. Primary fusion of one or two segments, regardless of whether it is combined with a limited decompression, can be accomplished without the use of internal fixation with an acceptable anticipated rate of nonunion. Internal fixation of some kind is definitely indicated in secondary procedures, in extensive decompressions, and in all cases involving more than two disc levels. Facet screws are the preferred method of fixation if the lamina is still intact (Fig. 4). The technique used is that popularized by Magerl.[53] Pedicle fixation is indicated for patients in whom the posterior elements have been removed (Fig. 5). The choice of a specific device is dependent upon the needs of a particular patient for rigid versus semirigid immobilization, and the ease of insertion at a particular level. Current devices being used include the AO internal fixator, the Edwards pedicle screw system, and the Wiltse pedicle screw system. The AO internal fixator allows for insertion of two pairs of pedicle screws, but it is difficult to afford fixation at additional levels. Furthermore, the use of the fixator at the lumbosacral junction is difficult because of the proximity of the ilium. We currently favor it for fractures of the thoracolumbar junction and lumbar spine. The Edwards pedicle screw system is semirigid and allows placement of screws either laterally or medially at the S1 level. The lumbar lordosis can be increased or decreased in the Edwards systems by the addition of pedicle connectors (Fig. 6). Fusion rates have been acceptable with this device, even though it is semirigid. The Long Beach pedicle screw system as developed by Wiltse[83] is rigid. It allows for multisegmental fixation. Distraction and correction of some limited rotational deformities are possible but not as easily accomplished as in the Edwards system. However, it is less bulky than the Edwards system and is therefore preferable, particularly in thin individuals. Plates systems such as those developed by Steffee[77] and Luque have some use in limited lumbar fusions but do not have the flexibility to be used in more difficult spinal deformities and are therefore not generally recommended for primary use. In addition, the use of plates removes a large area of potential fusion.

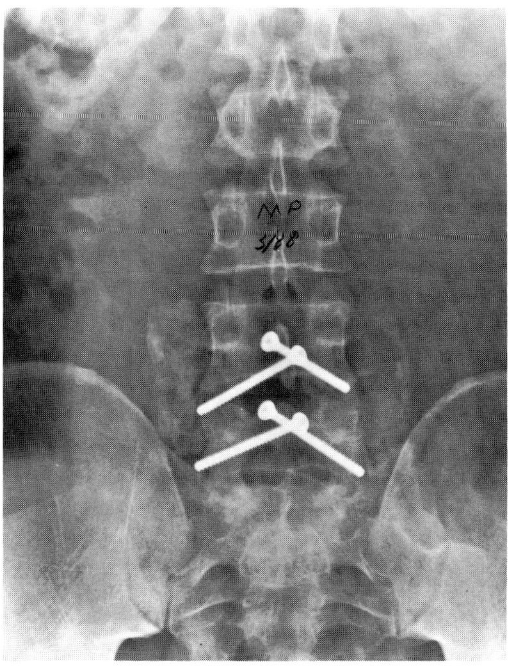

Figure 4 □ Facet screws allow secure fixation of the facet joints but require an intact spinous process and lamina.

Stabilization of the lumbosacral junction is difficult even with pedicle systems. For patients in whom it is not possible to fix to the sacrum, the only method of attachment is that developed by Jacobs (Fig. 7).[30] This technique, as mentioned previously, is the same as that of Allen but allows for the use of either a modified Harrington hook or a pedicle screw system proximally, in addition to segmental wire. The device crosses the sacroiliac joint, and there have been reported incidences of late pain secondary to this placement. In addition, placement of the rod involves extensive dissection of both iliac wings; this can be avoided with the more commonly used pedicle screws. Nevertheless, it is a valuable technique if fixation to the sacrum is impossible.

Anterior fixation techniques in degenerative disease of the lumbar spine are currently used only above the L5–S1 level. They are predominantly used either in failed posterior fusions or in isolated cases of one- or two-level instability with secondary collapse of the disc space, in which distraction of the space is preferred. The I-plate is preferred with fibula struts. Isolated anterior fusions of the L5–S1 junction have been carried out

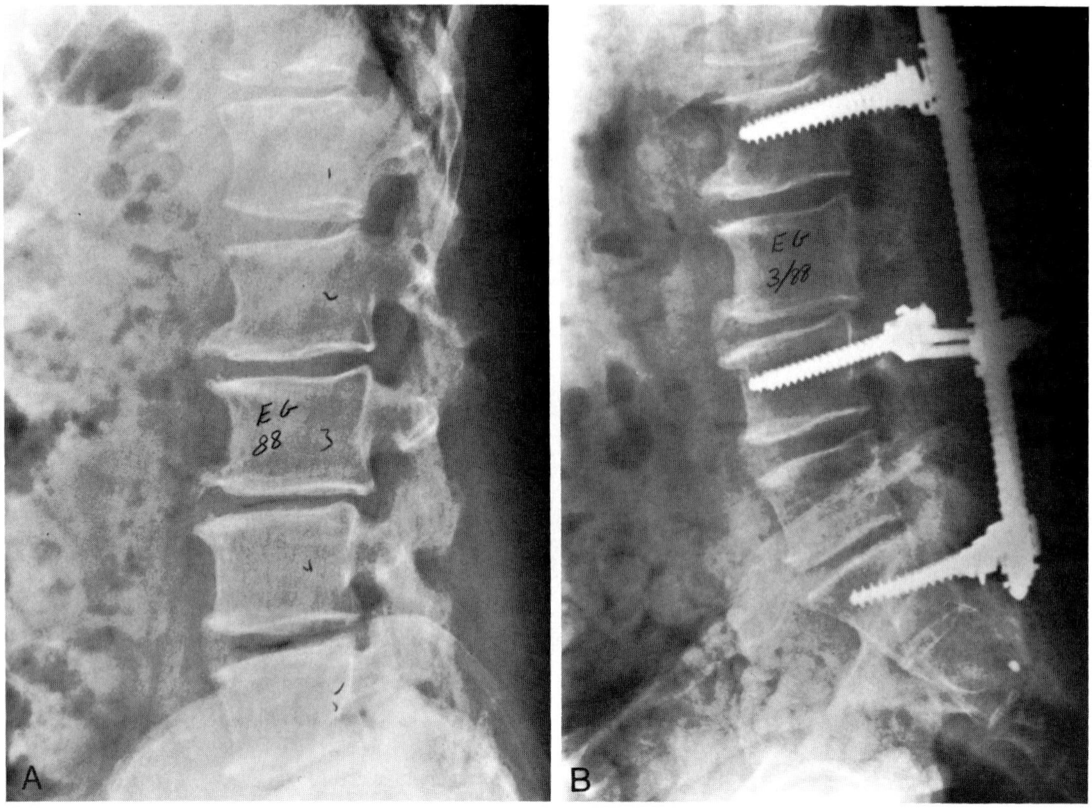

Figure 5 □ *A, B,* Pedicle fixation has allowed distraction of the vertebral bodies, opening of the intervertebral foramen, and a return to normal lumbar lordosis.

by Selby,[74] using the bone graft as a form of internal fixation and distraction. He reports a very high rate of fusion in addition to good clinical results. Currently, we are not using this technique, relying instead on posterior pedicle fixation and fusion. We have not been using anterior instrumentation, with the exception of the I-plate, below L4 because of the fear of vascular erosion. All anterior implants are placed far laterally to avoid undue pressure against the vascular structures.

Spondylolisthesis of L5 is generally treated with an isolated in situ posterior fusion. Postural reduction is used for patients with a large slip angle. In those with a high-grade slip or with an unacceptable slip angle, consideration is given to the possibility of reduction. The current technique used is that advocated by Edwards, involving his pedicle screw system. He has reported an acceptable level of reduction with few neurologic complications to date. We do not believe that this technique currently should be used in patients over the age of 20 years. Edwards[16] himself has reported its use in people in their thirties with good results. The use of anterior reduction techniques with either bone pegs or screw fixation is not indicated, in our opinion, because of the better results obtained by the posterior approach.

Internal fixation devices are definitely indicated in the treatment of lumbar scoliosis, regardless of whether it is primary or due to degenerative changes. Treatment of the adolescent with a primary lumbar curve is best carried out with an anterior device such as the VDS. This limits the length of the fusion and can save an important one or two levels that would have to be fused with more conventional techniques. The recent development of the Cotrel-Dubousset system does allow for posterior instrumentation in the adolescent and may prove to be as effective as the VDS device in the future. Maintenance of normal lumbar lordosis can be obtained by either technique. The adult with either

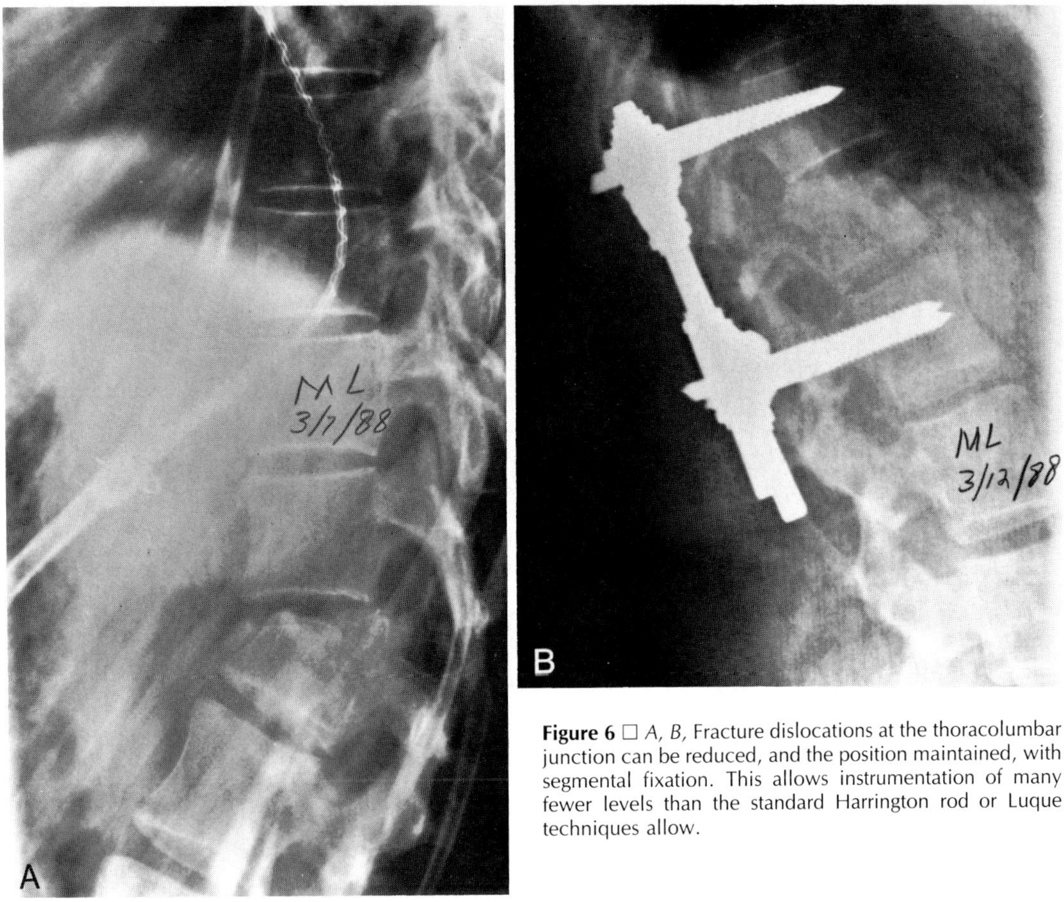

Figure 6 □ *A, B,* Fracture dislocations at the thoracolumbar junction can be reduced, and the position maintained, with segmental fixation. This allows instrumentation of many fewer levels than the standard Harrington rod or Luque techniques allow.

primary lumbar scoliosis or degenerative lumbar scoliosis is best managed by a two-stage procedure. We currently perform an anterior discectomy combined with a second posterior pedicle screw system. The posterior system used is either the Edwards device or the Cotrel Dubousset. This allows for a circumferential fusion and better correction of the overall deformity than attempting to treat the problem by either an isolated anterior or a posterior approach. Maintenance or creation of a lumbar lordosis is extremely important in treatment of this problem. In cases of degenerative scoliosis, distraction of the spine is also extremely important in order to resolve coexisting radiculopathies secondary to foraminal encroachment.

Fractures of the lumbar spine are treated surgically if (1) neurologic deficits are present, (2) the kyphosis is more than 20 degrees, or (3) the degree of canal compromise is greater than 50%.[43] We believe that a posterior approach can be carried out in patients treated within the first 24 to 48 hours with the use of the AO internal fixator. In a small percentage of patients this will not afford reduction of the intracanal fragment, and an anterior approach will have to be carried out. A primary anterior approach is used in patients who have a canal compromise greater than 75% or for those in whom there are associated fractures of the vertebrae above or below, a condition that would preclude the use of pedicle screws. In the unusual injuries involving L4 or L5, either the AO internal fixator or the Edwards device is used, depending on the physical characteristics of the sacrum. Posterolateral fusions are always carried out in conjunction with the use of either the AO internal fixator or the Edwards device. The Jacobs pelvic rods are used in the rare instances of associated sacral fractures that preclude the use of sacral screws.

Metastatic disease requires an individual-

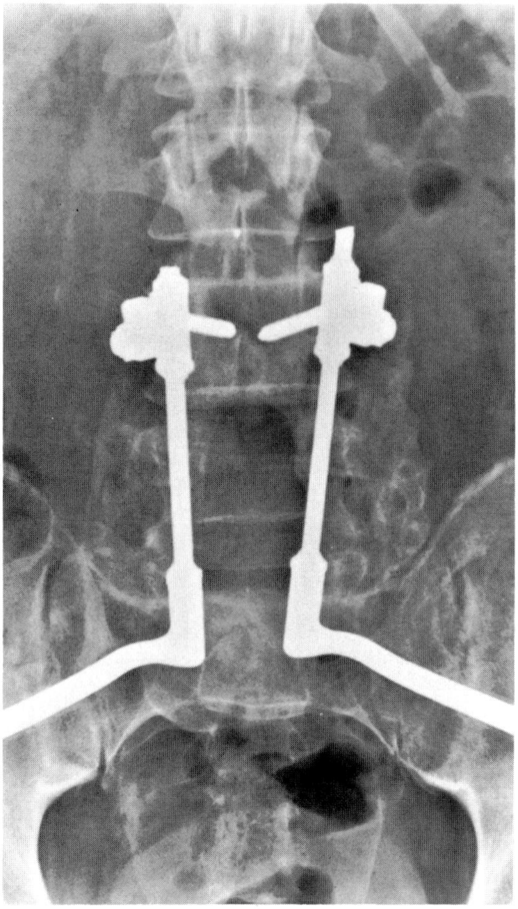

Figure 7 □ The Jacobs pelvic fixator allows secure fixation within the alla of the ilium and also allows use of pedicle screws or hooks above.

ized approach to each problem. In patients with impending pathologic fractures or actual fractures, some form of internal fixation is definitely indicated. A patient's projected life span is an important consideration in determining the type of fixation to be used and whether or not it is combined with bone grafting or supplemental methyl methacrylate. The anterior approach is preferred for isolated cases of metastasis. Fixation is obtained with the I-plate in conjunction with either bone graft or methyl methacrylate, as indicated above (Fig. 8). In cases involving multiple-level disease, posterior fixation is generally preferable. Some form of segmental fixation should be obtained, by the use of Harrington rods with multiple segmental wires, the Cotrel-Dubousset system, or pedicle screws. Some form of external support is required in most patients to prevent failure of the fixation device or the bone metal junction.

FUTURE AREAS OF DEVELOPMENT

The pedicle screw systems currently used will be modified to allow multiple sites of attachment in the systems that currently do not allow this to be done. In addition, either distraction or compressibility of the systems will be enhanced, allowing easier correction of spinal deformities and relief of foraminal entrapment syndromes. In conjunction with the ability to distract and compress, the correction of pre-existing lordotic or kyphotic deformities needs to be an inherent function of these systems. One of the major problems with these systems is their size and prominence; this has to be addressed in the future. Plate systems limit the available area for grafting and are difficult to apply to multiplanar deformities. For these reasons, rod systems will most likely be preferred for most patients.

Changing the currently available materials to allow bony ingrowth would solve some of the problems of implant loosening. This may be carried out by some form of sintering or perhaps by using hollow titanium screws, as are currently being developed by the AO School for their anterior cervical plating system. The thrust will unquestionably continue to focus on the pedicle, as no other area affords the strength and accessibility to the vertebrae. Lamina hooks will continue to be used on a limited basis, as will various forms of segmental wiring.

The currently available anterior devices will most likely be radically changed. The most important device to be developed will be a replacement for the vertebral discs. Spengler and coworkers[76] have recently reported experimental results in this area. Lee[46] is developing a composite material that could be used to replace the disc in its early stages of degeneration. This is probably the most important goal in implant surgery today.

Replacement of the intervertebral disc with some form of metal implant with the capability of biologic ingrowth also has some limited applicability. Lubicky and coworkers[48] have proved that implants in monkeys do become incorporated. The use of such an implant in the human would allow for distraction of the disc space and,

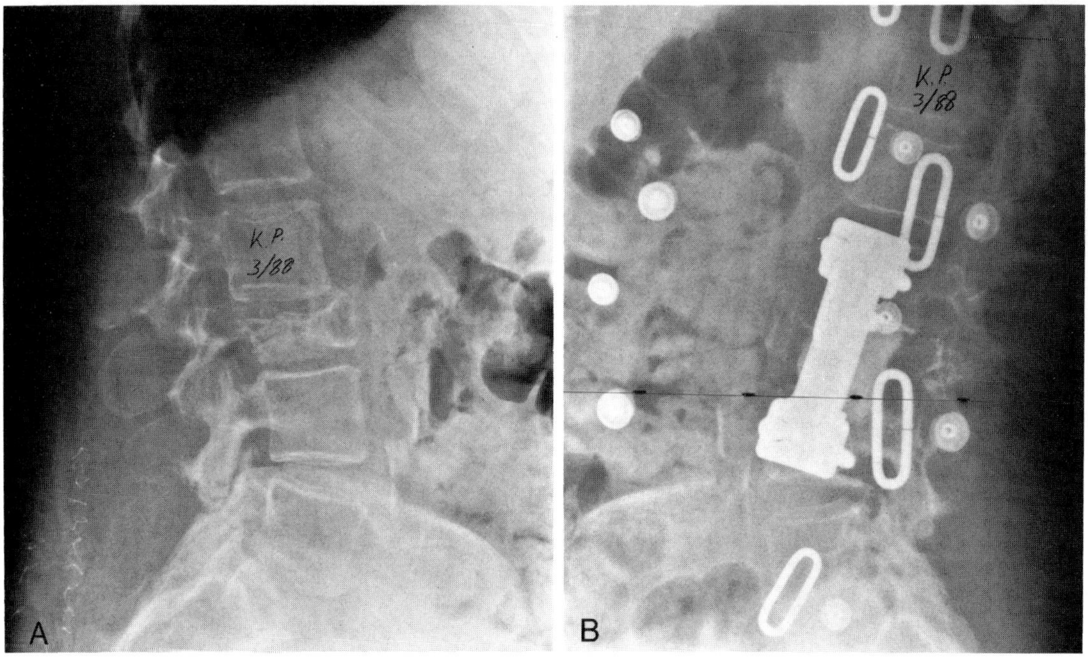

Figure 8 □ *A, B,* Metastatic disease of L3 with resulting collapse and early cauda equina syndrome can be stabilized by a combination of methylmethacrylate and a I-plate.

if combined with bone graft, would allow for solid fusion, reducing the possibility of late collapse that currently occurs in some patients in whom bone graft only was used.

An implant that could replace one or two vertebral segments is definitely needed in the treatment of metastatic disease. This implant needs to be self-contained within the vertebrae to avoid the problems seen with devices applied externally to the spine. The device must allow the use of either bone graft or other material to be added for further stabilization. For this use, the other anterior devices involving screws, cables, and rods will most likely be superseded by such a device.

Devices for use in the lumbar spine will definitely be developed in the future. Factors limiting their distribution to the treating orthopedists, however, will continue to be a problem. Their use will become more technically demanding, and their release to those involved in care of the lumbar spine will likely be very limited.

References

1. Aebi, M., Etter, C., Kehl, T., and Thalgott, J.: Stabilization of the lower thoracic and lumbar spine with the internal spinal skeletal fixation system. Spine 12:544–551, 1987.
2. Allen, B. L., and Ferguson, R. L.: The Galveston technique of pelvic fixation with L-rod instrumentation of the spine. Spine 9:388–394, 1984.
3. Anderson, C. K., Chaffin, D. B., Herrin, G. D., and Matthews, L. S.: Biomechanical model of the lumbosacral joint during lifting activities. J. Biomech. 18:571–584, 1985.
4. Andrew, T.A., Brooks, S., and Piggott, H.: Long-term follow-up evaluation of screw-and-graft fusion of the lumbar spine. Clin. Orthop. Rel. Res. 203:113–119, 1986.
5. Asher, M.A., and Strippgen, W.E.: Anthropometric studies of the human sacrum relating to dorsal transsacral implant designs. Clin. Orthop. Rel. Res. 203:58–62, 1986.
6. August, A.C., Tencer, A.F., and Mooney, V.: A Biomechanical Comparison of Methods of Posterior Fixation in Lumbosacral Spine Fusion. Presented at the 31st Annual Orthopedic Research Society, Las Vegas, Nevada, Jan. 21–24, 1985.
7. Beattie, F.C.: Distraction rod fusion. Clin. Orthop. Rel. Res. 62:218–222, 1969.
8. Boucher, H.H.: A method of spinal fusion. J. Bone Joint Surg. 41B:248–259, 1959.
9. Boxall, D., Bradford, D.S., Winter, R.B., and Moe, J.H.: Management of severe spondylolisthesis in children and adolescents. J. Bone Joint Surg. 61A:479–495, 1979.
10. Camille, R.-R., Saillant, G., and Mazel, C.: Internal fixation of the lumbar spine with pedicle screw plating. Clin. Orthop. Rel. Res. 203:7–17, 1986.
11. Cotrel, Y., and Dubousset, J.: Nouvelle technique d'osteosynthese rachidienne segmentarie par voie posterieure. Rev. Chir. Orthop. 70:489–494, 1984.
12. DePalma, A.F., and Rothman, R.H.: The nature of pseudarthrosis. Clin. Orthop. Rel. Res. 59:113–118, 1968.

13. Dick, W.: Spinal system: The "fixateur interne" (F.I.). AO/ASIF Dialogue Vol. 1, 1987.
14. Dunn, H.K.: Anterior stabilization of thoracolumbar injuries. Clin. Orthop. Rel. Res. 189:116–124, 1984.
15. Dwyer, A.F., Newton, N.C., and Sherwood, A.A.: An anterior approach to scoliosis. Clin. Orthop. Rel. Res. 62:192–202, 1969.
16. Edwards, C.C.: Scoliosis Research Society Meeting. Vancouver, Canada, Sept., 1987.
17. Edwards, C.C.: A New Method for Direct Sacral Fixation: Rationale and Clinical Results. I.S.S.L.S., Dallas, 1986.
18. Edwards, C.C., and Levine, A.M.: Early rod-sleeve stabilization of the injured thoracic and lumbar spine. Orthop. Clin. North Am. 17:121–145, 1986.
19. Farcy, J.-P., Weidenbaum, M., Michelson, C., et al.: A comparative biomechanical study of spinal fixation using Cotrel-Duboussett instrumentation. Spine 12:877–881, 1987.
20. Fidler, M.W.: Posterior instrumentation of the spine: An experimental comparison of various possible techniques. Spine 11:367–372, 1986.
21. Goldstein, L.: Personal communication.
22. Guyer, D.W., Yuan, H.A., Werner, F.W., et al.: Biomechanical comparison of seven internal fixation devices for the lumbosacral junction. Spine 12:569–573, 1987.
23. Hadra, B.E.: Wiring of the vertebrae as a means of immobilization in fracture and Potts disease. Med. Times Reg. 22:423, 1901.
24. Hall, J.E.: Current concepts review Dwyer instrumentation in anterior fusion of the spine. J. Bone Joint Surg. 63A:1188–1190, 1981.
25. Harmon, P.H.: Anterior excision and vertebral body fusion operation for intervertebral disk syndromes of the lower lumbar spine: Three to five year results in 244 cases. Clin. Orthop. 26:107–127, 1963.
26. Harrington, P.R., and Dickson, J.H.: Spinal instrumentation in the treatment of severe progressive spondylolisthesis. Clin. Orthop. Rel. Res. 117:157–163, 1976.
27. Harrington, P.R.: Treatment of scoliosis. J. Bone Joint Surg. 44A:591–634, 1962.
28. Hirsch, C. and Waugh, T.: The introduction of force measurements guiding instrumental correction of scoliosis. Acta Orthop. Scand. 39:136–144, 1968.
29. Humphries, A.W., Hawk, W.A., and Berndt, A.L.: Anterior interbody fusion of lumbar vertebrae: A surgical technique. Surg. Clin. North Am. 41:1685–1700, 1971.
30. Jacobs, R.R., Schlaepfer, F., Mathys, R., Jr., et al.: A locking hook spinal rod system for stabilization of fracture-dislocations and correction of deformities of the dorsolumbar spine. Clin. Orthop. Rel. Res. 189:168–177, 1984.
31. Jenkins, J.A.: Spondylolisthesis. Br. J. Surg. 24:80–85, 1936.
32. Johnston, C.E., II, Ashman, R.B., Sherman, M.C., et al.: Mechanical consequences of rod contouring and residual scoliosis in sublaminar segmental instrumentation. J. Orthop. Res. 5:206–216, 1987.
33. Kaneda, K., Abumi, K, and Fujiya, M.: Burst fractures with neurologic deficits of the thoracolumbar-lumbar spine. Results of anterior decompression and stabilization with anterior instrumentation. Spine 9:788–793, 1984.
34. Kaneda, K., Satoh, S., Nohara, Y., and Oguma, T.: Distraction rod instrumentation with posterolateral fusion in isthmic spondylolisthesis, 53 cases followed for 18–89 months. Spine 10:383–389, 1985.
35. Kaneda, K., Kazama, H., Staoh, S., and Fujiya, M.: Follow-up study of medial facetectomies and posterolateral fusion with instrumentation in unstable degenerative spondylolisthesis. Clin. Orthop. Rel. Res. 203:159–167, 1986.
36. Kaneda, K., Fujiya, N., and Satoh, S.: Results with Zielke instrumentation for idiopathic thoracolumbar and lumbar scoliosis. Clin. Orthop. Rel. Res. 203, 1986.
37. King D.: Internal fixation for lumbosacral fusion. J. Bone Joint Surg. 39A:560–565, 1948.
38. Kornblatt, M.D., Casey, M.P., and Jacobs, R.R.: Internal fixation in lumbosacral spine fusion: A biomechanical and clinical study. Clin. Orthop. Rel. Res. 203:141–150, 1986.
39. Kostuik, J.P.: Anterior fixation for fractures of the thoracic and lumbar spine with or without neurologic involvement. Clin. Orthop. Rel. Res. 189:103–115, 1984.
40. Kostuik, J.P.: Anterior spinal cord decompression for lesions of the thoracic and lumbar spine; techniques, new methods of internal fixation results. Spine 8:512–531, 1983.
41. Kostuik, J.P., Errico, T.J., and Gleason, T.F.: Techniques of internal fixation for degenerative conditions of the lumbar spine. Clin. Orthop. Rel. Res. 203:219–231, 1986.
42. Krag, M.H., Beynnon, B.D., Pope, M.H., et al.: An internal fixator for posterior application to short segments of the thoracic, lumbar, or lumbosacral spine. Clin. Orthop. Rel. Res. 203:75–98, 1986.
43. Krompinger, J., Fredrickson, B.E., Mino, D.E., et al.: Conservative treatment of fractures of the thoracic and lumbar spine. Orthop. Clin. North Am. 17:161–170, 1986.
44. Lange, F.: The classic: Support for the spondylitic spine by means of buried steel bars, attached to the vertebrae. Clin. Orthop. Rel. Res. 203:3–6, 1986.
45. Lee, C.K., and deBari, A.: Lumbosacral spinal fusion with Knodt distraction rods. Spine 11:373–375, 1986.
46. Lee, C.K.: Personal communication.
47. Louis, R.: Fusion of the lumbar and sacral spine by internal fixation with screw plates. Clin. Orthop. Rel. Res. 203:18–33, 1986.
48. Lubicky, J.P., Fredrickson, B.E., Yuan, H.A., and Froehling, A.: Sintered Fibermetal Spinal Implants; An Experimental Evaluation. Presented at The Scoliosis Research Society Meeting, Orlando, FL, 1984.
49. Luque, E.R.: Segmental spinal instrumentation: A method of rigid internal fixation of the spine to induce arthrodesis. Orthop. Trans. 4:391, 1980.
50. Luque, E.R.: Interpeduncular segmental fixation. Clin. Orthop. Rel. Res. 203:54–57, 1986.
51. Luque, E.R.: Segmental spinal instrumentation of the lumbar spine. Clin. Orthop. Rel. Res. 203:126–134, 1986.
52. McGowan, D.P., Mann, K.A., Yuan, H.A., et al.: A Biomechanical Study of Anterior Spinal Fixation for Thoracolumbar Burst Fractures with Varying Degrees of Posterior Disruption. Presented at The International Society for the Study of the Lumbar Spine. Rome, 1987.
53. Magerl, F.P.: A.O. Spine Course. Davos, Switzerland, 1986.
54. Magerl, F.P.: Stabilization of the lower thoracic and lumbar spine with external skeletal fixation. Clin. Orthop. Rel. Res. 189:125–141, 1984.
55. Mann, K.A., Found, E.M., Yuan, H.A., et al.: Biomechanical Evaluation of the Effectiveness of An-

terior Spinal Fixation Systems. 33rd Annual Meeting, Orthopaedic Research Society, Jan. 19–22, 1987, San Francisco, California.

56. Mann, K.A., Yuan, H.A., Found, E.M., et al.: A biomechanical study of the stability of thoracolumbar anterior decompression surgery and anterior spinal fixation. (Submitted for publication.)
57. Matthiass, H.H., and Heine, J.: The surgical reduction of spondylolisthesis. Clin. Orthop. Rel. Res. 203:34–44, 1986.
58. Mercer, W.: Spondylolisthesis: With a description of a new method of operative treatment and notes of ten cases. Edinburgh Med. J. 43:545–572, 1936.
59. Moe, J.H., Purcell, G.A., and Bradford, D.S.: Zielke instrumentation (VSS) for the correction of spinal curvature. Analysis of results in 66 patients. Clin. Orthop. Rel. Res. 180:133–153, 1983.
60. Morris, J.M., Lucas, D.B., and Bresler, B.: Role of the trunk in stability of the spine. J. Bone Joint Surg. 43A:327–351, 1961.
61. Nachemson, A.L., Schultz, A.B., and Berkson, M.H.: Mechanical properties of human lumbar spine motion segments. Influences of age, sex, disc level, and degeneration. Spine 4:1–8, 1979.
62. Nachemson, A.: The load on lumbar discs in different positions of the body. Clin. Orthop. 45:107–122, 1965.
63. Nachemson, A.L.: Disc pressure measurements. Spine 6:93–97, 1981.
64. Nachemson, A., and Elfstrom, G.: Intravital wireless telemetry of axial forces in Harrington distraction rods in patients with idiopathic scoliosis. J. Bone Joint Surg. 53A:445–465, 1971.
65. Nagel, D.A., Cordey, J., Schneider, E., et al.: In Vivo Measurement of Load on Harrington Distraction Rods In Sheep Spines With and Without Fusion. Presented at the 30th Annual Orthopedic Research Society. Atlanta, Feb. 7–9, 1984.
66. Nasca, R.J., Lemons, J.E.: Biomechanical Testing of Spinal Implants. Presented at the North American Spine Association in Canada, 1987.
67. Nasca, R.J., Hollis, M., Lemons, J.E., and Cool, T.A.: Cyclic axial loading of spinal implants. Spine 10:792–798, 1985.
68. Ogilvie, J.W., and Schendel, M.: Comparison of lumbosacral fixation devices. Clin. Orthop. Rel. Res. 203:120–125, 1986.
69. Olerud, S., Sjostrom, L., Karlstrom, G. and Hamberg, M.: Spontaneous effect of increased stability of the lower lumbar spine in cases of severe chronic back pain: The answer of an external transpeduncular fixation test. Clin. Orthop. Rel. Res. 203:67–74, 1986.
70. Peek, R.D., Wiltse, L.L., Widell, E.H., et al.: Biomechanical Effects of Decompressive Laminectomy on Internal Fixation of the Lumbosacral Spine. Presented at The North American Spine Society. June, 1987.
71. Schläpfer, F., Worsdorfer, O., Magerl, F., and Perren, S.M.: Stabilization of the lower thoracic and lumbar spine: Comparative in vitro investigation of an external skeletal and various internal fixation devices. Curr. Concepts Extern. Fix. Fract. 1982, pp. 367–380.
72. Schultz, A., Anderson, G., Ortengren, R., et al.: J. Bone Joint Surg. 64A:713–720, 1982.
73. Selby, D.: Internal fixation with Knodt's rods. Clin. Orthop. Rel. Res. 203:179–184, 1986.
74. Selby, D.: The Role of Anterior Lumbar Fusion for Internal Disc Disruption. I.S.S.L.S., Dallas, 1986.
75. Speed, K.: Spondylolisthesis: Treatment by anterior bone graft. Arch. Surg. 37:175–189, 1938.
76. Spengler, D.M., Keller, T.S., and Main, J.A.: Dynamic vertebral body replacement: A proposed prosthetic device. 1987 Advances in Bioengineering, B.E.D. 3:DE 12:75–76, 1987.
77. Stefee, A.D., Biscup, R.S., and Sitkowski, D.J.: Segmental spine plates with pedicle screw fixation: A new internal fixation device for disorders of the lumbar and thoracolumbar spine. Clin. Orthop. Rel. Res. 203:45–53, 1986.
78. Waugh, T.R.: Intravital measurement during instrumentated corrections of idiopathic scoliosis. Acta Orthop. Scand. 93(Suppl.):58–87, 1966.
79. Werlinich, M.: Anterior interbody fusion and stabilization with metal fixation. Int. Surg. 59:269–273, 1974.
80. White, A., Wynne, G., and Taylor, L.W.: Knodt rod distraction lumbar fusion. Spine 8:434–437, 1983.
81. Wilson, P.D., Straub, L., Ramsay, M.D.: Lumbosacral fusion with metallic plate fixation. Instructural course lecture. Am. Acad. Orthop. Surg. 9:53–65, 1952.
82. Wiltburger, B.R.: Intervebral body fusion by the use of posterior bone dowel. J. Bone Joint Surg. 39A:284, 1957.
83. Wiltsie, L.L.: A.O. Spine Course. Davos, Switzerland, 1986.
84. Yamamoto, I.: Personal communication.
85. Yuan, H. A., Mann, K. A., Fredrickson, B. E., and Lubicky, J.P.: Anterior Decompression of Furst Fractures with Spinal I-Plate Fixation: A Clinical and Experimental Study. Presented at the American Spinal Injury Association, 1986.
86. Yuan, H.A., Found, E.M., Mann, K.A., and Fredrickson, B.E.: Clinical and Biomechanical Evaluation of an I-Plate System for Anterior Spinal Surgery. Presented at the North American Spine Society, June, 1987.
87. Zielke, K., and Stremple, A.V. Posterior lateral distraction spondylodesis using the twofold sacral bar. Clin. Orthop. Rel. Res. 203:151–158, 1986.
88. Zielke, K., and Stunkat, R.: Derotation and fusion: Anterior spinal instrumentation (abstr.) Orthop. Trans. 2:270, 1978.
89. Zindrick, M.R., Wiltse, L.L., Widell, E.H., et al.: A biomechanical study of intrapeduncular screw fixation in the lumbosacral spine. Clin. Orthop. Rel. Res. 203:99–112, 1986.

22 □ Surgical Approaches

John Getty
Kiyoshi Kaneda
Noboru Nakano
Tohru Nakano

LAMINECTOMIES

John Getty

The term *laminectomy* is often used to describe any spinal procedure involving decompression of the spinal cord and/or nerve roots in the back. As a result of current advances, the term is to some extent a misnomer. It is now realized that in degenerative disorders of the lumbar spine, the symptom most effectively relieved by surgical intervention is radicular leg pain. In the preoperative assessment, every attempt is made to establish that the leg pain is of root origin and then to identify the affected root, so that the operative procedure is carefully planned and surgical trauma is minimized. This change has led to the development of more limited surgical approaches, the aim being to adequately decompress the affected neural tissue but with a minimum of trauma. In cases of spinal cord compression, it is also often possible to identify a specific level as being responsible for symptoms and accordingly to decompress that level alone instead of performing the more classical extensive decompression of the past.

The concept of a carefully planned spinal procedure is partly derived from the introduction of advanced technology, such as computed tomography (CT) and magnetic resonance imaging (MRI); more importantly, it is derived from an increased appreciation of certain clinical and etiologic factors that play a part in degenerative disorders of the lumbar spine, in which there is a compromise of neurologic function. Therefore, a true laminectomy, as such, is now much less commonly employed than it was formerly. As more attention is directed toward the root and as the importance of identifying a specific organic lesion before offering surgical intervention is increasingly appreciated, the term laminectomy should possibly be discarded, because it is misleading.

Patient selection for surgical intervention has thus become more stringent in the light of these developments.

DEFINITION

Many terms are used by lumbar spine surgeons to describe the various operative procedures, and it is useful to consider what some of these terms actually mean.

Laminectomy is often used to describe any operative procedure in the lumbar spine that is undertaken from behind. The term implies the removal of a whole lamina, whereas *hemilaminectomy* implies the removal of half of the lamina.

The term *fenestration* indicates the removal of the ligamentum flavum in an interlaminar space, whereas *laminotomy fenestration* implies removal of ligamentum and a small amount of lamina in a cephalic and/or caudal direction.

The term *discectomy* is also a misnomer in that one does not remove the entire disc when this procedure is undertaken. Spengler has indicated that limited disc excision in selected patients is as effective as the more classical radical clearance.[47] Other techniques of discectomy include the use of the percutaneous nucleotome, and some have even attempted to use lasers.

Chemical laminectomy or discectomy implies the use of enzymes such as chymopapain or collagenase.

The dominance of the concept of the disc as the prime source of nerve root irritation in the lumbar spine has been usurped by the realization that bony entrapment, usually due to osteoarthrosis of the facetal joint complex, is the most common cause of sciatica in the older patient. This has resulted in the development of alternative operative procedures designed to decompress the nerve roots in such circumstances. Complete facetectomies have been used, but they are virtually unnecessary because of the development of the technique of partial undercutting facetectomy, which in essence preserves stability and the depth of the spinal canal.[15]

Although it is not be discussed in detail in this subchapter, some surgeons undertake a simultaneous spinal arthrodesis at the time of spinal decompression; sometimes, this is done as an alternative to spinal decompression as a means of treating acute disc prolapses.

In summary, therefore, the tendency has been to move away from the more extensive to more limited surgical procedures and to concentrate on a specific lesion, as identified by the preoperative assessment.

DIAGNOSTIC CRITERIA AND TECHNIQUES

Clinical Assessment

Accepting current surgical philosophy regarding treatment demands careful delineation of the site and type of lesions, it is clear that prior to undertaking an operation, stringent diagnostic criteria must be employed. The usual indication for operative therapy is evidence of the need to decompress a nerve root that is in some way compromised.

Irrespective of whether the underlying etiology is a herniated disc, facetal arthritis, or spinal stenosis, the first essential step is to determine whether the pain results from neural compromise. The distinction between referred and radicular leg pain must be made. The attempted distinction between these two types of pain constitutes the basis of clinical assessment of patients with suspected lumbar nerve root entrapment. As a result of electric stimulation of lumbar nerve roots, McCulloch and Waddell showed that referred pain rarely radiates beyond the upper calf, tends to be dull and poorly localized, and has rarely been described as a paresthesia.[31] Radicular pain due to L5 or S1 irritation, on the other hand, nearly always radiates to the ankle or below it and is sharp, well localized, and often associated with paresthesia (Table 1). The presence of paresthesia and the extent of the radiation of leg pain are valuable in the clinical assessment in distinguishing radicular from referred pain.

The actual distribution is less reliable. McCulloch and Waddell showed that pain patterns of L5 and S1 are often difficult to distinguish.[31] Below the ankle, they tend to follow the recognized dermatomal distribution, whereas above the ankle, the patterns overlap. Kortelainen and coworkers, analyzing the symptoms and signs of sciatica in relation to the level of lumbar disc protrusion, noted that pain projection into the L5 dermatome was important in establishing the clinical findings of L5 root irritation; however, pain projection into the S1 dermatome was less reliable, particularly if two roots were involved.[27] In patients with two roots compromised, pain projection into the L5 dermatome was usually referred to an L4–L5 disc. In order to establish a clinical diagnosis of S1 root involvement, multiple signs were necessary for a diagnosis of the correct level of a lumbosacral prolapse.

A further important feature of clinical assessment is the recognition of spinal or so-called neurogenic claudication. This may be

Table 1 □ Clinical Features Useful in Differentiating Radicular from Referred Pain

RADICULAR PAIN
Commonly radiates beyond upper calf
Often associated with paresthesiae
REFERRED PAIN
Seldom beyond upper calf
Rarely described as paresthesiae

present in patients with spinal stenosis, bony entrapment, or cauda equina compression and occasionally in those with lateral disc herniations. It is a condition that is often overdiagnosed.[43] The distinction between neurogenic and vascular claudication is important. In some patients, the two conditions coexist, in which case Doppler testing may be of value.[24]

Patient examination also affords useful diagnostic information. When allied to the patient's symptoms, this information provides a basis upon which a diagnosis can often be achieved without resorting to extensive sophisticated investigations.

Nerve root tension is a sign that is often misdiagnosed. It is essential to note the important features of the two commonly used diagnostic tests, the femoral stretch and the straight-leg raising tests, as described by Macnab, before reaching a diagnosis of root tension.[33] The femoral stretch test is carried out with the patient prone and is only significant if pain is reproduced down the front of the thigh. Straight-leg raising involves five components, as shown in Figure 1. In the author's opinion, all five components should be carried out in a straight-leg raising test. Macnab has indicated that reproduction of back and/or leg pain is irrefutable evidence of root compression when the bowstring test is applied.[33]

A careful neurologic examination is essential to the assessment of any patient with a suspected lumbar spinal disorder. However, it should be noted that the absence of neurologic signs in itself does not exclude a diagnosis of nerve root pain.

The three components of neurologic assessment are the assessment of motor function, sensory function, and reflex activity. Identification of the compromised nerve root depends on the segmental innervation of the lower limb muscles, which is still a subject of controversy. In a detailed study of perioperative lumbar nerve root stimulation, Young and coworkers confirmed that the accepted patterns are essentially reliable.[61] It was also shown that a dual innervation is present for most muscles, with one root being dominant, as shown in Table 2.

An important feature of this study is the demonstration that in the presence of bony segmentation anomalies, variations in innervation patterns may be present, especially if there is sacralization of the L5 vertebra. Thus, the interpretation of neurologic signs must be allied to an analysis of plain lumbar spine radiographs and, in particular, to the determination of the number of mobile lumbar vertebrae. The surgeon should be aware that Young and coworkers recommended that in the presence of segmental anomalies, the L5 and S1 roots should be explored at operation.[61] An L5 sensory deficit is strong evidence of an L4–L5 prolapse, whereas S1 sensory changes should be analyzed with care.[27]

Table 2 □ Segmental Innervation of Seven Muscles in the Lower Limb

MUSCLE	SEGMENT
Tibialis anterior	L5
Extensor hallucis longus	L5
Extensor digitorum brevis	L5 (80%) S1 (20%)
Lateral gastrocnemius	L5 (75%) S1 (25%)
Soleus	S1
Medial gastrocnemius	S1
Abductor hallucis (mainly)	S1

The roots given are the dominant supply.
From Young, A., Getty, J., Kirwan, E.O'G., et al.: Variations in the pattern of muscle innervation by the L5 and S1 nerve roots. Spine 8:616–624, 1983.

An analysis of the reflex pattern of the lower limbs also should be interpreted with care. The absence of ankle jerks is not unusual in the elderly or in individuals in whom there has been a previous episode of S1 embarrassment that may well have been subclinical. The ankle reflex is of multiple root origin, and the absence of an ankle jerk alone is of limited diagnostic value. Kortelainen and colleagues have demonstrated that alteration in the status of the knee reflex is of no value in diagnosing the level of low lumbar lesions, nor indeed is its alteration typical for high prolapses.[27]

The importance of clinical assessment in determining the place for "laminectomy" cannot be emphasized sufficiently. The appreciation of the symptoms and signs should dominate a decision to intervene surgically, not the results of the various diagnostic tests (discussed below). Thus, the clinical assessment is the cornerstone of all diagnostic criteria that are employed to determine the need for surgical intervention.

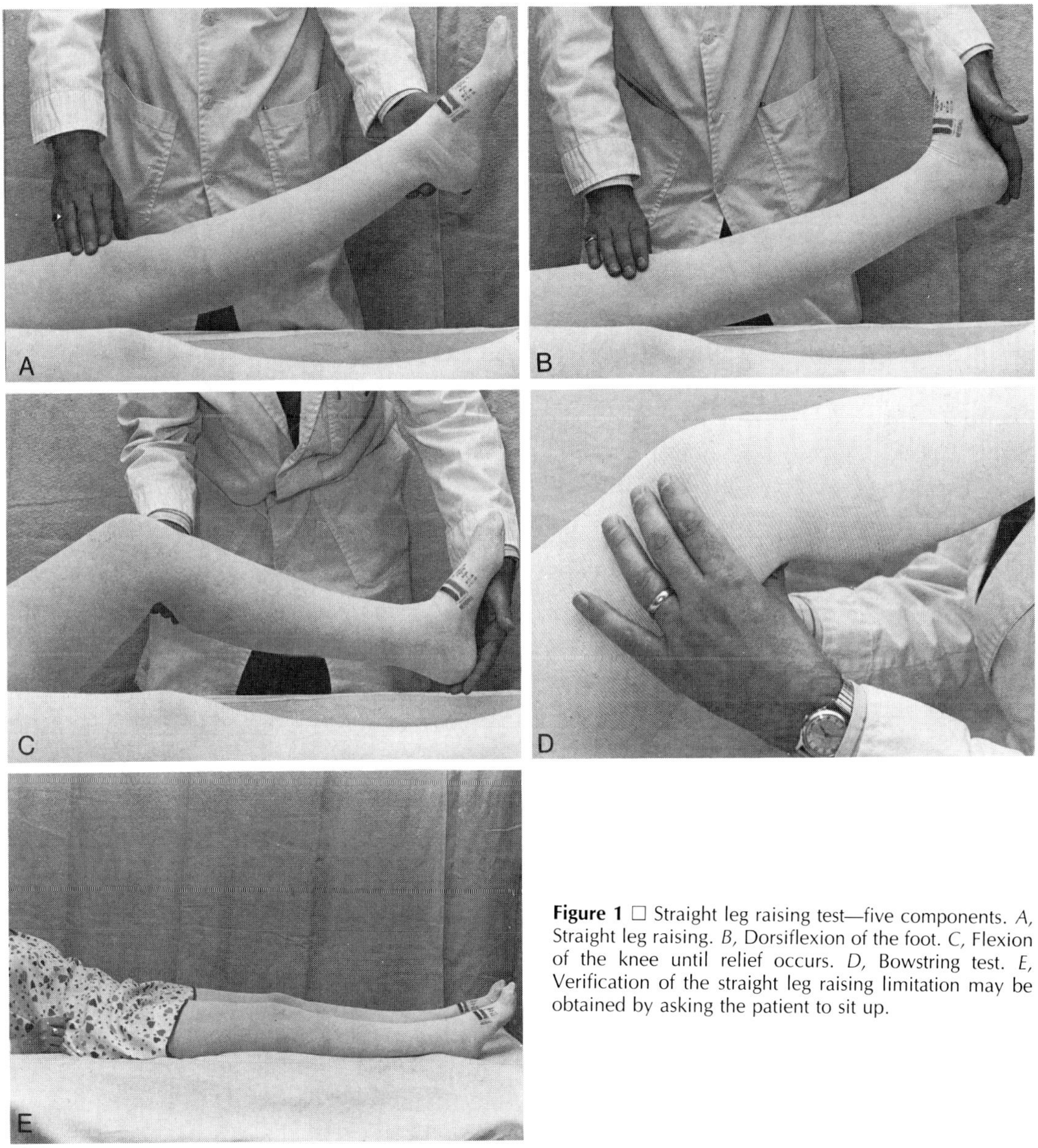

Figure 1 □ Straight leg raising test—five components. *A*, Straight leg raising. *B*, Dorsiflexion of the foot. *C*, Flexion of the knee until relief occurs. *D*, Bowstring test. *E*, Verification of the straight leg raising limitation may be obtained by asking the patient to sit up.

Clinical Syndromes of Nerve Root–Spinal Cord Compromise

The three most common causes of lumbar root compromise are disc prolapse, bony entrapment, and spinal stenosis.

The clinical presentation of the prolapsed disc is well established. It is now appreciated in older patients that the most common cause of sciatica, which is leg pain of root origin, is degenerative change in the posterior joint complexes. The clinical presentation is somewhat different from that of a disc prolapse and has previously been described by Macnab and by Getty and colleagues.[15, 33]

Patients with bony entrapment tend to be 40 years of age or older, often with a long history of backache and subsequently developing root pain in the leg. Spinal claudication may be present. Examination of most patients indicates no limitation of straight-leg raising, and spinal movements are relatively free.

The clinical features of spinal stenosis have previously been well documented.[14, 54] This condition is better thought of as a clinical spectrum, rather than as a clinical syndrome. The presentation may be variable.

A useful summary of the clinical symptoms and signs of root entrapment due to these three different causes is presented in Table 3. In all three conditions, the most common presenting symptoms are low back and/or leg pain. Rydevik and colleagues have indicated that the difference in the clinical picture may possibly result from the different types of neural deformation produced in the various conditions.[46]

The most important recent advance in patient assessment has been the appreciation of the importance of the functional contribution to disability. The most common cause of a failed laminectomy is an incorrect diagnosis associated with an inappropriate operation. One cannot assess patients on the basis of purely physical signs alone, or on sophisticated technologic investigations, without appreciating the functional contribution to their disability. The identification of the so-called nonorganic physical signs (Table 4) in low back pain as described by Waddell and coworkers allows the clinician to recognize the presence of a significant functional contribution.[55] This in turn helps identify patients who require further psychosocial assessment.

The importance of the identification of such a functional contribution to the patient's disability is that it enables the surgeon to avoid unnecessary investigation and therapy and to plan an appropriate management campaign, which may involve a multidisciplinary approach to managing the patient's disorder.

If a significant organic lesion is established in a well-balanced individual, then further investigation may be indicated to confirm the diagnosis and establish which treatment option should be offered. It is essential that each patient be treated on the basis of the characteristics of his or her individual disorder.

Investigations

Most patients with low back pain receive a plain radiograph of the lumbar spine. Nachemson has indicated that clinically unsuspected positive findings are unusual in patients between the ages of 20 and 50 years.[37] In the present context of assessing patients

Table 3 □ Clinical Presentation of Disc, Bone, and Spinal Stenosis

	DISC	BONE	SPINAL STENOSIS
Age: Range	16–58 yr	23–75 yr	18–75 yr
Mean	77% < 40 yr	44.8 yr	52 yr
Mean duration of symptoms	77% < 5 yr	10.6 yr	5.8 yr
Paresthesiae	70%	58%	26%
Claudication	?	17%	39%
Reduction in spinal mobility	100%	71%	39%
↓ SLR	99%	29%	23%
Motor deficit	96%	49%	52%
Sensory deficit	80.6%	38%	58%
Reflex deficit	78%	42%	71%

Modified from O'Connell, 1951 (Ref. 41); Getty et al, 1981 (Ref. 15); and Getty, 1980 (Ref. 14).

Table 4 □ Nonorganic Physical Signs in Low Back Pain

Detection of tenderness—superficial/nonanatomic
Simulation testing causing low back pain
Axial loading on the skull
Rotation of shoulders/pelvic as one unit
Inappropriate straight-leg raising
Regional weakness and/or sensory deficit
Over-reaction
To be clinically significant three or more of the five signs should be present.

for surgical therapy, the most important value of a plain radiograph is the determination of the number of mobile lumbar vertebrae. The possibility of anomalous root innervation in the presence of bony segmental anomalies has already been mentioned. Plain radiographs in patients who have had previous operative therapy will often provide information as to the level of the previous procedure and give some indication of its nature.

The introduction of CT and MRI has revolutionized investigation of the lumbar spine. However, as with radiculography, these techniques should probably be used only in patients being seriously considered for surgical treatment on the basis of their clinical assessment. In addition, it is also well established that interpreting images involves a degree of observer bias. Despite popular claims, no single imaging technique has exclusive superiority over the other. One should consider that the information provided is often complementary, rather than alternative.

Formerly, radiculography was the imaging technique of choice. The technique involves the introduction of a contrast medium into the subarachnoid space, the aim being to identify and confirm the level of neural compromise and to exclude the occasional neoplasm. Although the role of this investigation in the diagnosis of disc prolapse is well established, its place in identifying root canal stenosis is less clear.[30]

Euinton and coworkers found that in patients with bony entrapment, for only half did the radiculogram and operative findings exactly correlate.[12] They suggested that the reason for failure was that the contrast-filled root sheath did not extend far enough distally to allow the contrast medium to outline the site of entrapment (Fig. 2).

In patients under consideration for revision laminectomy, radiculography has a limited role, largely because of the common existence of postoperative extradural fibrosis.[21] Radiculography may also identify root anomalies, knowledge of the existence of which is important in planning surgical decompression.[25]

CT provides a noninvasive method of visualizing the vertebral canal and its contents. Care is required in the interpretation of CT scans. The incidence of false-positive scans is less well appreciated than that of false-positive radiculograms.

In the diagnosis of bony entrapment, comparing CT and radiculography, Stockley and coworkers noted that although radiculography correctly identified root entrapment in 54% of patients undergoing primary or revision laminectomy, the accuracy with CT was higher, specifically 75%.[50] Although they considered CT the investigation of choice in degenerative disease of the lumbar spine, they stressed that CT and radiculography were complementary, not alternative, investigations.

For patients who have had previous surgery, CT also provides valuable information outlining the extent of previous surgery and allowing the surgeon to plan the subsequent surgical intervention. The differentiation of scar tissue from disc material can be difficult. Contrast-enhanced CT has been developed to aid in this situation.[51]

CT scanning is currently regarded as the first line of investigation in degenerative disorders of the lumbar spine, particularly in patients with suspected disc prolapse and bony entrapment. Radiculography, in this author's opinion, remains the investigation of choice in patients with suspected spinal stenosis. One disadvantage of CT is that only a limited area of the spine is scanned, and therefore, there is a potential risk of missing unsuspected neoplastic lesions.

MRI is the newest of the imaging modalities for assessing disorders of the lumbar spine. Although it is available in only a limited number of institutions, clearly the technique is one of great potential. Its definitive role in this context remains to be defined, not least because of its continuing and rapid technologic development. Burton has indicated that the information provided relates more to the quality and nature of a tissue than to its structural delineation.[3] If we confine our attention to its role in the

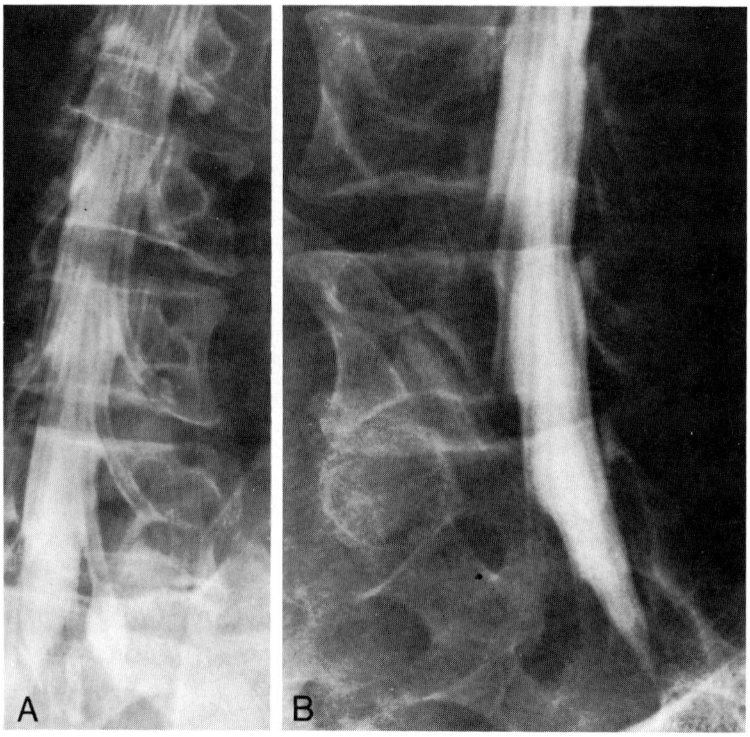

Figure 2 □ *A,* Root sleeves in this patient are long, thus bony entrapment is more likely to be demonstrable. *B,* Short root sleeves are present, thus bony entrapment is unlikely to be demonstrated.

identification of the level of nerve root involvement, it is of interest that Boumphrey and colleagues found MRI to be more accurate in assessing disc degeneration, whereas they found CT to be more accurate in root canal compression.[2] MRI also seems to have a further role in assessing spinal canal dimensions and in turn in diagnosing spinal stenosis.[17] The great advantage of MRI is that it is noninvasive and involves no exposure to ionizing radiation.

A number of other diagnostic techniques are also available in the preoperative assessment of patients.

Nerve root injection studies have had a limited application, despite Macnab's contention that the abolition of leg pain after root sheath infiltration is powerful evidence of the level of the lesion.[33] The technique has the advantage of identifying the level involved but does not indicate (1) the underlying etiology or (2) whether that etiology is reversible. The technique is time consuming, and personal experience has indicated that its effectiveness depends on regular application. The advantage of nerve root injection would seem to lie in the fact that in the majority of patients with spondylosis, as Kikuchi and coworkers have demonstrated, abolition of root pain and/or intermittent claudication can be achieved by a single root infiltration.[26] This is obviously a great advantage in establishing the level of operative intervention and in turn minimizing the surgical trauma. The experience in the Sheffield Problem Back Unit tends to confirm this.[49] In addition, it is a valuable test for determining whether the leg pain is referred or radicular. Stanley and coworkers identified 56% of their patients as having leg pain that was not predominantly of root origin.[49] In patients undergoing operative treatment, the findings correlated closely in 72%, bony entrapment being the main etiologic agent in the group studied. It is of interest that there was one false-positive result. Although this test is time consuming and can be uncomfortable for the patient, the author has used it increasingly in the older patient with spondylosis and suspected root involvement for which the level is uncertain.

Controlled electromyogram (EMG) studies, particularly in patients with bony entrapment, have not supported earlier claims of success at the levels reported for this technique.[28] Jarratt and coworkers, in a preliminary report and subsequently on further analysis, have indicated that the EMG has value in determining the presence of root compression but that it is of limited value in identifying the level involved.[23] The EMG is also valuable in patients with diabetes presenting with a lumbar radiculopathy by helping distinguish radiculopathy from diabetic neuropathy. Dermatomal sensory evoked potentials have also been found useful in patients with disc prolapses, with approximately an 86% accuracy in determining the level.[9] Their role in bony entrapment has yet to be defined.

Liquid crystal thermography has been recommended by several authors as a valuable technique in diagnosing spinal root syndromes.[42] However, although it is attractive as a noninvasive technique, a controlled study in patients with suspected bony entrapment has demonstrated that the technique is of no significant value in this context.[35]

In summarizing this section on diagnostic criteria and techniques, one can state that although the aim is to establish the presence and the level of root involvement or the symptomatic stenotic levels, undoubtedly the over-riding component is the clinical assessment of the patient. Plain x-ray studies and routine blood tests are commonly employed for most patients. CT probably remains the radiologic investigation of choice, but the information provided by radiculography should be regarded as complementary, not as alternative. MRI will undoubtedly play a major role, but it has yet to be carefully defined. EMGs provide a useful method of screening, particularly in the older patient, for the presence of radicular pain; nerve root injection studies can provide valuable information, not only regarding the presence or absence of root pain but also in identifying the level involved.

METHODS OF TREATMENT VERSUS NATURAL HISTORY

The success of treatment of disorders of the lumbar spine is difficult to evaluate because most patients improve spontaneously. Thus, the natural history of nerve root compromise becomes extremely important. There are three main conditions associated with nerve root compromise in degenerative disorders of the lumbar spine: (1) herniated nucleus pulposus, (2) bony entrapment of nerve roots, and (3) stenosis of the lumbar spine. The diagnostic features of these conditions have already been considered above.

O'Connell and Weber have written two classic papers on the subject of the herniated nucleus pulposus.[41, 57] O'Connell thought that a history of a definite and remembered injury was important in understanding the etiology of a lumbar disc herniation.[41] He noted that the greatest problem was not establishing the diagnosis but rather deciding upon the correct treatment regimen, because of the tendency toward spontaneous recovery. He advised rest during the acute phase, followed later by exercises for the lumbar muscles and joints. Surgery was to be considered only when such a regimen failed. He emphasized that in his personal series of 500 discs that were operated on, these represented only a small proportion of the patients seen in his outpatient department in whom the clinical diagnosis of lumbar disc herniation had been made. He believed it difficult to determine exactly what proportion of patients with disc protrusions required surgery, but his estimate was that only one fifth of the patients referred to the outpatient clinic underwent surgical intervention, this being a preselected population. Weber carried out a controlled prospective study of lumbar disc herniation over a 10-year period.[57] For most patients, initially conservative therapy is preferred; surgical intervention is considered only if recovery is delayed. However, the indications for operative intervention vary among doctors, so Weber thought it important to compare the results of operative and nonoperative treatment in two randomized groups with disc herniation. Others have reported no significant difference between the final outcome of surgical or conservative therapy after periods varying from 7 to 20 years of follow-up.[19, 39] Weber studied 126 patients, with ages ranging from 25 to 55 years, who after 14 days of rest still had radicular pain with indications of increased dural tension. The choice of further treatment in these patients was debatable. To this extent, Weber thought it reasonable to randomize them into two groups, one for operative treatment and one for conservative treatment.

Subsequent analysis of the results indicated several important factors that have a major influence on the decision of whether to undertake surgery. No profession showed striking preponderance regarding the onset of low back pain and the onset of sciatica. Psychosocial problems were noted in nearly a third of the individuals, which is the same as the proportion found in the normal Scandinavian population.

Weber assessed his patients on the basis of their ability to work, the presence or absence of neurologic deficit, pain, and the mobility of the spine. The overall assessment at follow-up examination indicated that after 1 year, the results were significantly better in the surgically treated group. Comparison after 4 years did not show a statistically significant difference, although there was still a tendency for the surgically treated group to have a more favorable outcome. At 10 years there was hardly any difference in the results between the two treatment groups. The mean duration of recurrences in the two groups was the same. The rehabilitation period after leaving the hospital was shorter in the conservatively treated group. Restoration of muscle strength was found to be unrelated to the treatment modality and continued over several years. Sensory function followed a similar pattern. No difference was noted in either group with reference to pain or to spinal mobility.

After 10 years of observation, only age was found to correlate with unsatisfactory results; older patients had poor results as compared with younger patients. All other variables were noted to be without prognostic importance.

This carefully controlled study is important because it demonstrates the natural history of the disorder and the influence of conservative treatment and surgical intervention. In summary, in a group of patients who have disc herniation and debatable operative indications, the results of surgical treatment compared with conservative treatment are significantly better after 1 year, but during the course of the following 9 years the difference becomes less pronounced. Moreover, as Weber also noted, the natural course of radiculopathies in disc disease is more encouraging than one might anticipate.

Natural History of Bony Entrapment

The importance of bony entrapment has been appreciated over the past 10 years. Porter and colleagues have described the natural history of root entrapment syndrome.[44] They noted that the clinical findings for the syndrome are distinct from those due to an acute disc lesion. The condition was diagnosed in approximately one tenth of patients attending Porter's Back Pain Clinic, which was an incidence higher than that of patients with a disc lesion. Although root symptoms were severe, signs were less common. Spinal movement was freer than in patients with an acute disc prolapse.

Table 5 □ Etiology of Root Compromise in Different Age Groups

0–40 yr	Herniated nucleus pulposus (HNP)
40–50 yr	HNP/bony entrapment
50 yr or older	Bone

No specific therapy was offered in nearly 80% of the patients because of the fact that they were either improving or were prepared to wait, having had the diagnosis explained. Approximately 10% were treated operatively. Assessment of the operated patients 1 year after surgery indicated that the pain was completely relieved in 3 patients, less severe in 15, but no better in 6.

The progress of the patients who were not operated on and seen 1 to 4 years previously was assessed by a postal questionnaire. Most had root pain, but the vast majority of all the conservatively treated patients were sufficiently satisfied, in spite of discomfort, not to have sought treatment elsewhere.

Thus, bony encroachment on a lumbar nerve root does not, in most patients, require specific intervention. Porter believes that once root symptoms were sufficiently severe to require hospital assessment, the condition was likely to become chronic and only one in four would be asymptomatic 12 months later. However, the majority of the remainder found their pain to be manageable. This is certainly the author's impression. It is of interest that Getty and colleagues reported a mean time of 10.5 years from onset of symptoms to operation in this group of patients; the corresponding time for disc prolapses is much shorter.[15]

The cause of nerve root compromise in the different age groups is shown in Table 5.

Natural History of Spinal Stenosis

The natural history of spinal stenosis is less clear. The most common cause is degenerative spinal stenosis (Fig. 3). Wiltse and co-

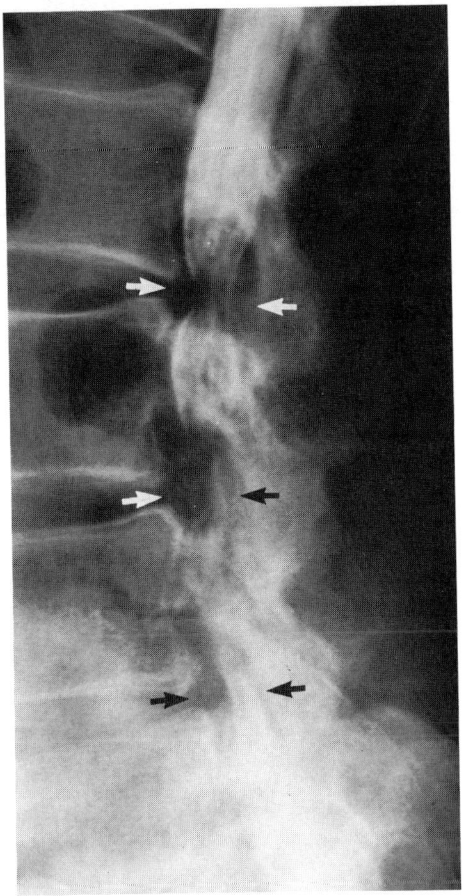

Figure 3 □ Myelogram of degenerative lumbar spinal stenosis.

workers believed some degree of spinal stenosis was very common in humans.[60] Symptoms do not usually develop until the seventh decade of life.[48] An insidious onset of slowly progressive symptoms is characteristic. Once severe symptoms are established in this condition, the patient is unlikely to improve with time, as, for example, does the younger patient with a disc herniation. Surgical intervention is often the only effective therapy. Undoubtedly, for many patients spinal stenosis goes undetected, and they are diagnosed as having mechanical back pain, sometimes with referral to the legs.

The natural history of spinal stenosis has been studied by Wardlaw and Macnab, particularly in patients with spinal claudication treated conservatively.[56] The regimen consists of rest, a nonsteroidal agent, an epidural injection, and a rigid lumbar brace. Patients who responded had backache of less than a 5-year duration and leg pain of less than 6 months, whereas those with backache lasting longer than 1 year and a tendency for bilateral symptoms remained the same or deteriorated. All the patients in this study had radicular leg pain. On the basis of this assessment it was therefore believed that in spinal stenotics, a history of backache of less than 5 years and leg pain of less than 6 months was associated with a reasonable rate of success for conservative treatment. However, once symptoms and signs are established in this condition, operative intervention is often indicated.

Conservative Treatment of Sciatica

The evaluation of conservative treatment of sciatica is fraught with difficulty, owing to the spontaneous recovery of most patients. This will be apparent from the foregoing analysis of the natural history of the main causes. For most patients, once a diagnosis of sciatica has been established, conservative treatment will initially be offered.

It is not proposed to describe all the methods available. The regimen advocated by Bell and Rothman utilizes the two methods that, on the evidence available, seem to provide the most effective means of relieving root pain.[1] This regimen consists of a period of bed rest, which may be 2 weeks, although many recommend 3 weeks. The patient is provided with an anti-inflammatory agent. Bed rest is followed by 7 to 10 days of mobilization, at which stage a program of back care and exercise is encouraged. In the absence of a definite indication for surgical intervention, up to 3 months of conservative treatment are thought to be reasonable before one considers operative intervention.

In the absence of deteriorating neurologic or sphincter function, the author advises 3 weeks of rest. Patients are allowed to get up to use the bathroom, if they so wish. The majority of patients can be treated at home; many find this more relaxing than being confined to a hospital environment. Sphincter function must be checked at the initial assessment, the patient must be fully advised, and the general practitioner must be agreeable to visiting during the period of conservative treatment.

A nonsteroidal anti-inflammatory agent is used together, if necessary, with a muscle relaxant, over the 3-week period. The nonsteroidal agent is continued during the initial mobilization period. Occasionally it may be necessary to provide a strong analgesic for the first 24 to 48 hours of the treatment regimen. Additionally, a laxative is provided until the patient is mobile.

In the presence of neurogenic claudication, the regimen of Wardlaw and Macnab is utilized.[56] Calcitonin has proved unreliable in this situation and is no longer used by the author.[43]

In patients with chronic sciatica, it is essential to define the exact disability, including an assessment of the patient's psychologic profile, if so indicated. If the disability is significant, a period of ambulant treatment with a nonsteroidal agent, often with attention to spinal hygiene, exercise, and possibly a course of physiotherapy, may afford relief to the extent that the patient does not require additional treatment. In the event of failure, further investigation may be indicated.

Surgical Treatment of Sciatica

It is important to define the indications for ceasing conservative therapy and undertaking a different treatment. The indications are summarized in Table 6. Although up to 3 months of conservative treatment have been advocated, the time scale depends on the prevailing circumstances. In degenerative disorders of the lumbar spine, operative intervention undoubtedly produces the best results when undertaken for root entrapment syndromes.

An analysis of the outcome of any therapy for disorders of the lumbar spine will be predetermined first by the surgeon's selection criteria and, secondly, by appreciation of the therapeutic methods prejudiced by one's own practice. Within the International Society for the Study of the Lumbar Spine, a constant goal is to achieve an objective assessment of the patient and his or her sciatica and thereby to provide a rationale for the treatment program offered. However, every surgeon has his or her own proven method for excising a disc, for decompressing a nerve root due to bony entrapment, or for decompressing a spinal stenosis.

Table 6 □ Indications for Surgical Decompression of Lumbosacral Nerve Roots

Progressive neurologic deficit
Radicular pain interfering with function—failure to respond to conservative treatment
Impending cauda equina syndrome

The decision to operate on a patient is based on an overall assessment of the patient. There is a tendency for us to rely too heavily on investigations and not to appreciate that the main factor in deciding whether to operate rests with the clinical assessment of the patient. Morris and coworkers, in a prospective study of 185 patients undergoing primary lumbar spine surgery, compared how accurately the clinical criteria and radiculography predicted the operative findings.[36] They stated that although surgeons agree in principle that diagnosis and decisions to operate should be based on an overall assessment of the patient and that investigations should be used to complement and not replace clinical judgment, to their knowledge this study was the first that actually showed that clinical diagnosis supplemented by radiology was still better than an overdependence on radiology alone.

The advent of new technologic advances in imaging may well lead us incorrectly to decisions to operate. This has undoubtedly occurred in the earlier days of our use of CT. It is an easy trap into which to fall and one that is essential for the surgeon to appreciate when interpreting the results of treatment.

Treatment of Disc Prolapse

As a "halfway house" between conservative treatment and surgical intervention, chemonucleolysis gained great popularity. A number of different agents were used, the most popular of which was chymopapain. McCulloch and Macnab have described in detail the pathophysiology and the pros and cons of using this agent.[32] These have all been previously well discussed. However, it is useful to assess the results reported by McCulloch and Macnab, who indicated that the procedure was effective in relieving sciatic pain in 70% of properly selected patients.[32] The results, however, have been blighted by the occurrence of neurologic complications well documented in the literature to the extent that many lumbar spine surgeons have abandoned the use of this technique. In most cases, it is probably true that needle misplacement has been the responsible factor, but in a number of cases the complications remain inexplicable. This is obviously a worrisome phenomenon.

Postacchini and colleagues conducted a prospective study comparing the results of chemonucleolysis and surgery in 156 patients with lumbar disc herniation considered suitable for chemonucleolysis. They found the success of chymopapain in patients with large herniations to be significantly less than that of surgery.[45] It appeared that chemonucleolysis was the treatment of choice in most patients with small disc herniations. Thus, chymopapain was recommended as an effective alternative to surgery in most patients with medium-sized herniations when the preoperative clinical pattern indicated slight or moderate root compression. However, surgery was preferable in patients with large, small, or medium-sized herniations, who had severe nerve root impingement.

Percutaneous nuclectomy offers an alternative method of decompressing the disc prolapse. This method has been recommended for the treatment of uncomplicated "contained" herniated discs.[8] No significant complications have been reported to date, although obvious risks include nerve root damage, dural tears, and possible damage to retroperitoneal structures.

Should the technique prove effective, its advantage, like that of chemonucleolysis, is that the spinal canal is not breached. It is claimed that subsequent surgical intervention, if indicated, is no different from a primary procedure, and the results are as effective. An overall success rate of 74% has been claimed for its use. The technique is still under evaluation.

The least invasive of the classic surgical techniques is microlumbar discectomy. This technique was developed specifically for patients with surgically undisturbed lumbar anatomy, who had a soft disc herniation without any degree of lumbar spinal stenosis.[59] The aim was to decompress only that part of the disc producing nerve root pressure in a minimum amount of time with minimal blood loss and tissue morbidity. In Williams' hands, the operating time averaged approximately half an hour with a postoperative stay of 3 days.[59] Fourteen percent of his series required reoperation, the most common cause being a true recurrent disc. In only 0.3% was the cause a missed disc, whereas 17 of the 903 patients in his series had recurrent sciatica due to adhesions. Williams claimed a 99.1% surgical cure in his series at 12 years. He noted that most of the disc reherniations occurred within 9 months of the initial procedure. Further investigations led him to conclude that rigorous restrictions should be placed on the "lumbar" activities of microlumbar discectomized patients for a period of 1 year after the operation in an attempt to prevent new lumbar injury. The aim of decompressing a nerve root is to decompress with a minimum of trauma. Surgeons using microdiscectomy techniques emphasize a better operating field, faster procedure, and smaller incision with more rapid rehabilitation. However, the limited access may produce difficulties of identifying the level involved, of increasing the risk of leaving herniated disc material outside the operative field, and of failing to adequately decompress stenotic canals.[20] CT and MRI may allow more accurate patient selection. In comparing chemonucleolysis and microsurgical discectomy, it has been noted that results for the chemonucleolysis group were less successful than results for those treated with the microsurgical lumbar discectomy.[62] There was a lower incidence of treatment success and a higher incidence of patients suffering morbidity in the chemonucleolysis group.

There is considerable variation among surgeons in the extent to which they excise disc material from within the disc space. Some favor an extensive exploration with thorough curettage, and others remove only the disc prolapse. Spengler reported the results of a study of 54 patients who underwent a limited discectomy.[47] If the disc was sequestered, the free fragment was removed and the annulus was not entered. In extruded disc herniations, the extruded fragment was excised, and loose fragments near the annular defect were removed with a small rongeur. In the case of a protruded disc, the annulus was incised and all loose disc material removed. The neural foramen was treated, as appropriate, in each case after disc excision. The results indicate that the technique was reliable, safe, and effective in selected patients with disc herniation. The prior concern that the incidence of recurrent disc herniation would increase with limited disc excision was not borne out.

The classic technique of lumbar disc excision was described by O'Connell.[41] In his series, 92% of the patients were completely symptom-free or were significantly improved postoperatively. He claimed an incidence of 2% for postoperative recurrent symptoms requiring re-operation.

The role of simultaneous fusion is controversial. In a prospective study, White and colleagues compared two groups receiving bilateral lumbar laminectomy and disc excision; one group had an intratransverse fusion with internal fixation.[58] Both groups were studied approximately 3 years after operation, at which stage it was found that although the general success rate of both groups was 87%, the best results were in the nonfusion group. Thus simultaneous fusion would appear unnecessary in patients with a simple herniated lumbar disc.

Although we are concerned with the posterior approach, disc prolapses may be excised anteriorly with interbody fusion.

On occasion, the herniated nucleus pulposus is located in the foramen or is extraforaminal. In the past, some have considered it reasonable to excise the facets to gain access, thereby creating potentially symptomatic instability. However, it has been clearly shown that this is not necessary.[22] Adequate exposure is invariably gained by a partial facetectomy and foraminotomy. If it is not, then a lateral exposure through the intratransverse ligament should be considered, while keeping the facetal complex intact.

Posterior lumbar interbody fusion is used by some in the treatment of disc herniation. Cloward quoted a success rate of 85% "long-term cures."[4] The exact long-term success rate in other surgeons' hands remains to be clearly defined. Cloward recommended posterior lumbar interbody fusion for patients with low back pain, with or without sciatica, due to lumbar disc disease as the ultimate answer to the treatment of disease of the lumbar spine.[5] He has stated that simple discectomy, decompression laminectomy, and chemonucleolysis should be eliminated. This remains to be proven.

The current treatment of choice in patients with simple lumbar disc protrusion would appear, after appropriate investigation and trial of conservative treatment, to be surgical decompression by microdiscectomy, limited lumbar discectomy, or a classic lumbar discectomy with curettage of the disc space through a laminotomy fenestration. Chemonucleolysis has fallen into some disrepute but may well, with better understanding of the biochemistry and pathophysiology, be restored to an appropriate place. The initial results with percutaneous nuclectomy seem promising. Simultaneous fusion does not appear to play a role in the treatment of this group of patients.

The author does not subscribe to the concept of a routine bilateral procedure, which is based on the idea that the patient may develop problems on the opposite side in the future. The operative therapy should be directed specifically toward the demonstrated site of pathology in the vast majority of patients. This is in keeping with the concept of minimal surgical trauma to achieve relief of the compromised root. Less radical decompressions currently available are associated with a reduced likelihood of instability and thus potential problems, immediately or long-term, on the opposite side.

A bilateral laminectomy may be indicated in the case of a central disc prolapse. Newer imaging techniques such as CT and MRI, however, now allow more careful preoperative planning, and so they do help reduce the extent of surgical exposure. The final decision is, of course, always dictated by the surgeon's judgment at operation.

Treatment of Bony Entrapment

The findings at operation in patients with this condition are often more subtle than those in patients with a true disc prolapse.

As previously mentioned, although in the older patient facetal arthritis is the most common cause of root compromise, in patients in the 40- to 50-year-old age range root compromise is frequently caused by a mixture of disc and bone. It may be impossible, particularly in this older group, to define the etiologic lesion until the time of operation. The decision to carry out a partial undercutting facetectomy, with or without disc excision, is often made at that stage. Likewise, in this group the appearance of the nerve root is extremely variable; often it is invisible until the partial undercutting facetectomy has been carried out. Microsurgery does not appear to yield acceptable results in patients with lateral recess stenosis.[13]

The results of operation in patients with

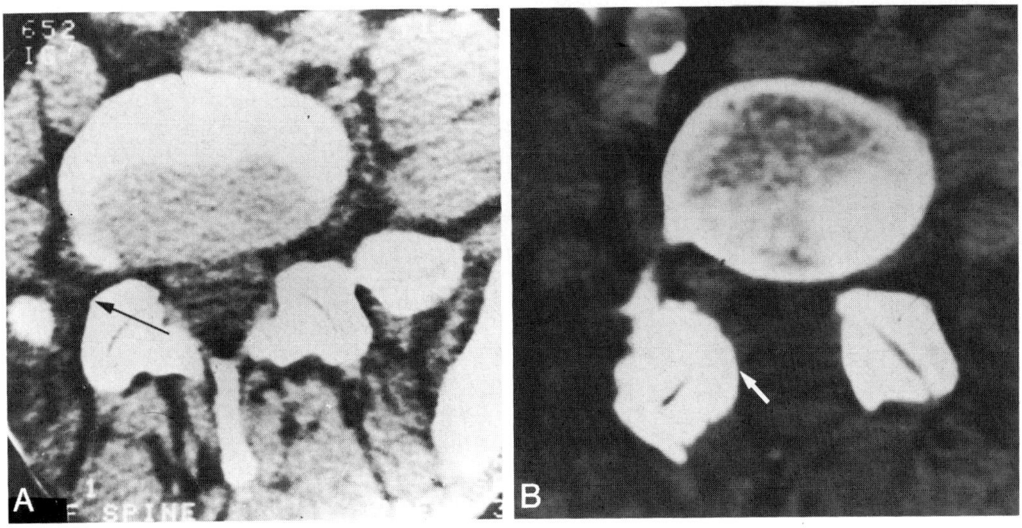

Figure 4 □ *A,* The *arrow* indicates the direction of the osteotomy cut in a partial undercutting facetectomy. *B,* CT appearance after a partial undercutting facetectomy.

bony entrapment have previously been reported.[15] The mean age at operation in this group of 78 patients was 45 years old, with leg pain being the predominant symptom. In half of the patients there was evidence of motor involvement. The decompression is carried out by means of a partial undercutting facetectomy, which in essence preserves stability and helps maintain the tent of the spinal canal (Fig. 4). Eighty-five percent of the patients in this group were satisfied with the outcome.

In this series, the cause of nerve root compromise was degenerative change in the posterior joint complex. Although in one third of the patients the disc was removed simultaneously, subsequent experience has been associated with a much lower incidence of disc excision. Because there is degenerative change in the spine, patients with bony entrapment are advised that the aim of the procedure is to ease leg pain. Interestingly, however, a substantial proportion gain relief from their back pain. Surgery should be directed toward the symptomatic root. Prophylactic bilateral decompression is not indicated. There is little evidence to support its routine use, especially if a partial facetectomy is used.

Treatment of Spinal Stenosis

The third group of conditions causing sciatica is spinal stenosis, the clinical spectrum of which has already been considered. It may be congenital, developmental, or acquired. Here we will concentrate on acquired stenosis. Conservative therapy has already been outlined. Once symptoms are firmly established and cause disability, operative therapy is usually indicated. In the past, unnecessarily wide and extensive decompressions have been performed, often with a poor outcome. Such procedures are now seldom indicated, because it is understood that one level alone is often responsible for symptoms, despite the presence of extensive stenosis. Additionally, the introduction of newer surgical techniques, such as partial facetectomy, has obviated the need of most patients for wide destructive laminectomies often associated with postoperative symptomatic instability. This concept also applies in patients with degenerative spondylolisthesis. Similarly, there is no statistically significant evidence to indicate that prophylactic decompression of the opposite side in patients with unilateral symptoms is routinely warranted, especially when these newer operative techniques are used. Further perioperative refinements, such as monitoring with sensory evoked potentials, remain controversial as a means of determining the required extent of operative treatment.

Spengler reported that after posterior decompression, he did not have to carry out a stabilization procedure in any patient with acquired degenerative spinal stenosis.[45] This author's experience is similar. Although postoperative slipping in degenerative spondylolisthesis may occur, it does not appear to influence the outcome of surgery.

The results of surgical treatment of idiopathic developmental lumbar spinal stenosis have been reported in a classic paper by Verbiest.[54]

Getty reported a series of 31 patients treated for spinal stenosis.[14] In 28 of the patients (90%), degenerative change was the principal etiologic factor. Following therapy, the condition of over 50% of the patients was classified as good, and that of 84% was satisfactory. Partial undercutting facetectomies were used for the lateral decompression, and spinal fusion was not carried out either simultaneously or subsequently in the patients studied in the series. A relatively long decompression was commonly done in this group over several levels.

Nasca reported a heterogeneous group of patients who had spinal stenosis, with 71% of the patients obtaining good results from their surgical treatment. The role of fusion was not clearly defined in the various groups.[38] Natelson noted that in patients who had osteoporosis and a small compression fracture, with spinal stenosis decompression intensified the stenosis and the compression fractures increased.[40] He considered simultaneous bilateral fixation and fusion to be beneficial to this group.

Tile, in a discussion of how wide and how long a spinal decompression should be, indicated that the nerve should be fully decompressed.[52] In most patients this did not necessitate a complete facetectomy. He further noted that long laminectomies were no longer indicated, because the symptoms of spinal stenosis are segmental. Although a limited approach was favored in this context, he believed that surgical judgment was required.

However, the use of nerve root infiltration allows one to be more precise. Macnab and associates reported that most patients with spinal stenosis present with clinical evidence of a single unilateral root compression, which can be confirmed by nerve root injection.[34] In their series, over 90% of patients had a satisfactory outcome after decompression of the offending root, and the results were maintained over time. He found the existence of stenosis at other levels did not influence the results of a single root decompression and rarely caused subsequent symptoms.

Thus, current concepts in the treatment of spinal stenosis are moving toward the identification of the symptomatic segmental level followed by a limited decompression. Extensive laminectomies have become less common, and their efficacy is already seriously doubted.

In summarizing this section on treatments, it is noted that several techniques of treatment have changed. Surgical exposure has been limited in an attempt to minimize scarring and the problems it creates in the spine. It is not so much the introduction of advanced technology that has led to these changes, but rather the appreciation of certain clinical and etiologic factors. The decision to operate is ultimately based on clinical findings.

THE AUTHOR'S APPROACH

When a surgeon is asked to describe his or her current approach to the treatment of a specific problem, naturally the account is likely to be somewhat eclectic. This is understandable in that we each believe our philosophy to be correct; otherwise, how could we justify our practices?[6]

In order to understand a surgeon's approach to a specific disorder, one has to understand something of his or her conception of the problem. Surgeons are concerned with relieving nerve root compromise, whether it is by conservative treatment, by injection treatment, or by surgical intervention. The symptom they are best equipped to treat is radicular leg pain. (I do not discuss fusion at length here, as this topic is outside the present context.)

In Table 7, the factors contributing to this author's philosophy in the treatment of this problem are outlined.

We have already referred to diagnostic criteria, to techniques, to current treatment options, to their results, and to the natural history of the conditions encountered.

The clinical assessment mentioned above is followed closely by this author. If nerve root involvement is suspected, then initial investigations consist of a full blood count, erythrocyte sedimentation rate, and plain x-ray films of the lumbar spine. The value of plain x-ray films is twofold. First and most

Table 7 □ Concepts in the Treatment of Lumbosacral Nerve Root Dysfunction

Patients have back complaints, not problem backs.
"Think root."
Clinical assessment dominates decision-making.
Leg pain is the symptom most effectively treated.
Extensive investigations are unwarranted, unless the presence of root dysfunction is established and further treatment is indicated.
In using most imaging techniques the radiologist should be blinded as to the suspected lesion until after reporting the results, in order to obviate risks of subjective interpretation.
Treat the symptomatic lesion.
Prophylactic decompressions are seldom indicated.

importantly, they identify the segmental pattern in the lumbar spine. Second, the presence of an unsuspected spondylolisthesis or a degree of degenerative change not previously suspected may be detected. Rarely will one find a lesion more sinister than already anticipated.

The importance of bony segmental anomalies, which has already been considered,[61] lies in the fact that sometimes one finds during clinical assessment, an apparent overlap of the clinical symptoms and signs, suggesting multiple root involvement. This may be explained on the basis of bony segmental anomalies, and simple plain x-rays films may solve what initially seemed to be a rather confusing pattern. In this context, the furcal nerve also requires consideration.[26]

Irrespective of etiology, the conservative treatment of root entrapment is as already outlined: a period of bed rest and the use of a nonsteroidal anti-inflammatory drug, followed by a period of mobilization. For most patients this regimen is adequate. Further investigation is undertaken if it is not and their disability is sufficient to warrant it.

Currently, the investigation of choice for the lumbar spine is CT. MRI provides complementary information; whether it will supplant CT will remain unclear until the technique becomes more widely available. However, radiculography also has a significant role to play. It has been shown that the information obtained from CT and myelography is complementary, and the investigations are not to be regarded as alternatives to each other.[50]

Usually, the information gained from these imaging modalities is sufficient to complement the clinical assessment and to allow the surgeon to plan the operation, if one is indicated. For patients with apparent multilevel disease (e.g., those with bony entrapment or spinal stenosis) nerve root infiltration studies are used to identify the symptomatic level. This author, as a result of his experience in these groups regards nerve root infiltration studies as a front-line investigative tool. Discometric analysis and facetal studies are rarely used in the current context. Currently, liquid crystal thermography has also been abandoned in the investigation of these patients. Similarly, EMG studies are seldom used. They may be employed before proceeding to imaging, if there is difficulty distinguishing radicular from referred pain. They are useful in assessing diabetic patients with lumbar spine problems and in helping differentiate radiculopathy from diabetic neuropathy.

In the cases of an acute disc and a bony entrapment, the preparations for operation (if indicated) are similar, once the patient's lesion has accurately been identified. A general medical assessment is carried out. The orthopedic surgeon determines whether the patient is fit for the knee–chest position (Fig. 5). Contraindications to this position include significant cervical spondylosis, obesity, and peripheral vascular disease. The author uses this position routinely, if it is considered safe for the patient. It has been shown that this position permits the best interlaminar exposure. It ensures free respiration and a low intra-abdominal pressure, and it prevents venous congestion in the extradural space.[10] Serious complications with the position are rare and largely avoidable.

Positioning the patient is important and requires an adequate number of experienced staff members. The patient is anesthetized on the bed, rolled into the prone position onto the operating table, and then lifted into the knee–chest position. The abdomen must lie free. The position of the head is controlled at all times by the anesthetist, and the neck must not be twisted, as there is a potential risk of vertebral artery thrombosis.

Preoperative Planning

In preoperative planning the surgeon must be aware of the number of mobile vertebral bodies, the level of the lesion, and the symptomatic side. It is this author's practice to

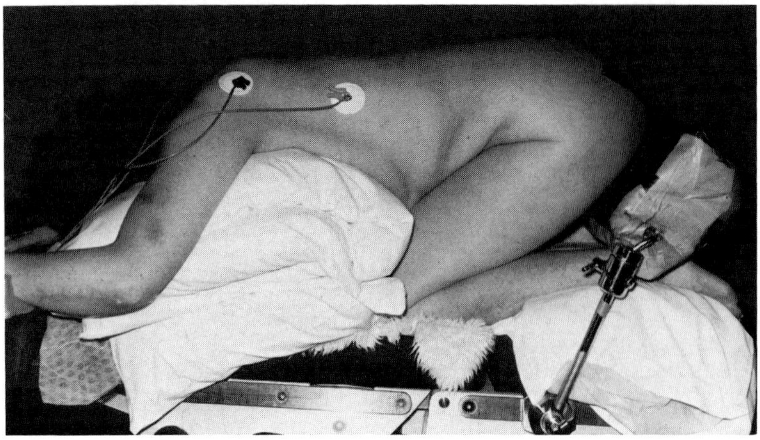

Figure 5 □ Patient in the knee/elbow position.

mark the symptomatic leg from behind. It is all too easy to forget that sides change when the patient is turned to the prone position. This is a small but significant cause of failed back surgery.

Technique of Surgical Decompression

With induction, a broad-spectrum antibiotic is given, usually a cephalosporin, which routinely is administered 8 and 16 hours after operation. It is not this author's practice to infiltrate the skin with lidocaine and adrenalin. Diathermy is used with blending to divide the muscle from the spinous processes, staying close to the spinous processes and thereby ensuring a bloodless plane. The muscle is swept out to expose the appropriate operative field. The level is confirmed radiologically or by identification of the sacrum. It is this author's practice to identify the pars interarticularis, as this defines the extent of the dissection. The spinal canal is then entered.

Discectomy

For discectomy, a laminotomy fenestration is usually adequate. The principle of nerve root decompression is to mobilize the neural tissue, retract it and disturb it as little as possible, and at the same time achieve decompression. The use of loupes and a head lamp facilitate the decompression, but they are not essential. Once exposure is adequate, the nerve is identified and mobilized, and the disc excised. It is this author's practice to excise the disc on the basis of a limited discectomy.[47] This technique has been used in the past 50 patients, and no recurrent disc has occurred to date. Vigorous curettage of the disc space is usually unrewarding and potentially dangerous. Once the nerve root is adequately decompressed, it is essential to search carefully in all directions for free fragments.

It is this author's practice to have the anesthetist forcibly hand-ventilate the patient to determine whether there are any undetected dural leaks. A fat graft is then placed over the laminotomy fenestration site.

Currently, fat grafting would appear to be the most effective means of minimizing scar formation.[53] Meticulous hemastasis is essential throughout the procedure. Hypotensive anesthesia is essential.

In the presence of anomalous roots, which are often detectable by the preoperative imaging, it is essential that damage is not done to them. In this author's experience, it has never been necessary to cause any iatrogenic trauma to such roots in order to mobilize and remove the disc or, in the presence of bony entrapment, in order to decompress the root. It may be necessary to extend a laminotomy fenestration to a wider exposure in order to allow access to the disc prolapse. In this context, adequate exposure is essential.

Closure of the muscles is done in layers. It is not usual to drain the laminectomy wound.

Postoperative mobilization is largely determined by the patient's progress. Straight-leg raising is encouraged at once, and the patient is allowed to mobilize as soon as control of the back is achieved. Sitting is allowed after several days for as long as the patient feels comfortable. Instructions in back hygiene are supplied. Excessive physical activity is to be avoided for at least a 3-month period.

If a catheter is necessary, it is usually covered with an appropriate antibiotic until 24 hours after the successful removal of the catheter.

Treatment of Bony Entrapment

The technique of partial undercutting facetectomy may be used in patients with isolated bony entrapment.[15] Osteotomes ranging from 1 to 10 mm in width are used. The direction of the cut is always in the longitudinal axis of the nerve. It is important that no instruments, such as punches, are forced beneath the facets, as the nerve may become crushed and damaged. Once the partial facetectomy has begun, however, one can use fine punches to complete the decompression.[11] At the conclusion of decompression, the nerve must lie free throughout the root canal, from its origin at the dural sac to its passage through the intervertebral foramen. Occasionally, it is necessary to shave the pedicle with an osteotome to achieve this. In true bony entrapment, it is usually unnecessary to violate the disc. However, in cases of mixed bone and disc disorders, the disc is removed; the ultimate decision is made perioperatively.

The same principles of closure and mobilization are used. A nonsteroidal anti-inflammatory agent is used during the postoperative period for 2 to 3 weeks.

To date, bony regrowth has not proved to be a problem. Undoubtedly, preoperative identification of the level involved will serve to minimize surgical trauma and, one hopes, to improve the results.[26, 49]

Treatment of Spinal Stenosis

The identification of the symptomatic root or segmental level has revolutionized the surgical treatment of this condition. Now there is seldom an indication for extensive laminectomy. Central decompression should aim to leave a ridge of lamina, whereas lateral decompression may be accomplished by a partial undercutting facetectomy. Fat grafts are used, and the postoperative regimen is essentially the same as for bony entrapment.

In patients with degenerative spondylolisthesis, a similar technique is used. It has not been this author's practice to simultaneously perform fusion in such patients, although this topic is still a matter of debate.[7, 29]

THE FUTURE

Much progress has been made in recent years, with the increasing emphasis on the root and the development of newer investigative modalities to delineate the site and cause of nerve root compromise. Refinements in surgical techniques and in techniques such as chemonucleolysis and percutaneous nuclectomy will undoubtedly continue.

However, future research should also be directed toward the pathophysiology of nerve root compromise. An attractive long-term proposition concerns the possibility of using sophisticated medication to counteract this problem.

The role of fusion in treating the entire range of patients with degenerative lumbar spine disease is still a matter of debate, largely because of ignorance about pathophysiology and recognition of symptomatic lumbar instability. The situation may be summarized simply: patient selection is important, not implant selection. Undoubtedly research into this area must continue.

Another major area of research must be the development of techniques to determine adequacy of nerve root decompression perioperatively. Currently this determination is largely subjective, and a reliable objective method remains to be developed.

It is perhaps worth reiterating a basic concept: in patients presenting with lumbar spine disorders, a precise anatomic diagnosis is seldom achieved. As a result, the term *problem back* has evolved, which is unfortunate because patients should be treated on the basis of their specific disorders. Some of the confusion surrounding this group of patients could be readily dismissed.

In any case, one should not talk of a "problem back" but of a patient with a back complaint.[16]

References

1. Bell, G.R., and Rothman, R.: The conservative treatment of sciatica. Spine 9:54–56, 1984.

2. Boumphrey, F.R.S., Modic, M., and Bell, G.: Nuclear Magnetic Resonance of the Lumbar Spine. A Comparative Study. Read at the meeting of the I.S.S.L.S. Montreal, 1984.
3. Burton, C.V.: High-resolution CT scanning: Present and future. Orthop. Clin. North Am. 14:539–551, 1983.
4. Cloward, R.B.: Posterior lumbar interbody fusion. Treatment of ruptured lumbar intervertebral disc by vertebral body fusion. Indications, operative technique, after care. Clin. Orthop. Rel. Res. 193:5–15, 1985.
5. Cloward, R.B.: Posterior lumbar interbody fusion, updated. Clin. Orthop. Rel. Res. 193:16–19, 1985.
6. Colton, C.L.: Slipped upper femoral epiphysis *In* Catterall, A. (ed.): Recent Advances in Orthopaedics. Edinburgh, Churchill Livingstone, 1987, pp. 61–77.
7. Dall, B.E., and Wroe, D.E.: Degenerative spondylolisthesis, its surgical management. Spine 10:668–672, 1985.
8. Davis, G.W.: Personal communication, 1988.
9. Dvonch, V., Scarff, T., Bunch, W.H., et al.: Dermatomal somatosensory evoked potentials: Their use in lumbar radiculopathy. Spine 9:291–293, 1984.
10. Eie, N., Solgaard, T., and Kleppe, H.: The knee/elbow position in lumbar disc surgery: A review of complications. Spine 8:897–900, 1983.
11. Epstein, J.: Personal communication, 1981.
12. Euinton, H.A., Locke, T.J., Barrington, N.A., et al.: Is water soluble radioculography accurate in predicting the level of bony entrapment of lumbosacral nerve roots? J. Bone Joint Surg. (Br.) 67B:499, 1985.
13. Feldman, R.J., and McCulloch, J.A.: Microsurgical Experience in the Treatment of Degenerative Lumbar Spine Disorders. Read at the meeting of the I.S.S.L.S. Rome, 1987.
14. Getty, C.J.M.: Lumbar spinal stenosis. J. Bone Joint Surg. (Br.) 62B:481–485, 1980.
15. Getty, C.J.M., Johnson, J.R., Kirwan, E. O'G., and Sullivan, M.F.: Partial undercutting facetectomy for bony entrapment of the lumbar nerve root. J. Bone Joint Surg. (Br.) 63B:330–335, 1981.
16. Getty, C.J.M.: Management of the problem back. *In* Catterall, A.: Recent Advances in Orthopaedics. Edinburgh, Churchill Livingstone, 1987, pp. 79–100.
17. Gibson, M.J., Szypryt, E.P., Buckley, J.H., et al.: Magnetic resonance imaging of adolescent disc herniation. J. Bone Joint Surg. (Br.) 69B:699–703, 1987.
18. Gill, G.G., Scheck, M., Kelley, E.T., and Rodrigo, J.J.: Pedicle fat grafts for the prevention of scar in low back surgery. Spine 10:662–667, 1985.
19. Hakelius, A.: Prognosis in sciatica. A clinical follow-up of surgical and non-surgical treatment. Acta Orthop. Scand. (Suppl.):129, 1970.
20. Hudgins, W.R.: The role of microdiscectomy. Orthop. Clin. North Am. 14:589–603, 1983.
21. Irstam, L.: Differential diagnosis of recurrent lumbar disc herniation and post operative deformation by myelography. Spine 9:759–763, 1984.
22. Jackson, R.P., and Glah, J.J.: Foraminal and extra foraminal disc herniation: Diagnosis and treatment. Spine 12:577–585, 1982.
23. Jarratt, J.A., Getty, C.J.M., Stockley, I., et al.: Electromyography and bony sciatica. J. Bone Joint Surg. (Br.) 67B:499, 1985.
24. Johansson, J.E., Barrington, T.W., and Ameli, M.: Combined vascular and neurogenic claudication. Spine 7:150–158, 1982.
25. Kadish, L.J., and Simmons, E.H.: Anomalies of the lumbar sacral nerve roots. J. Bone Joint Surg. (Br.) 66B:411–416, 1984.
26. Kikuchi, S., Hasue, M., Nishiyama, K., and Tsukasa, I.: Anatomic and clinical studies of radicular symptoms. Spine 9:23–30, 1984.
27. Kortelainen, P., Puranen, J., Koivisto, E., and Lahde, S.: Symptoms and signs of sciatica and their relation to the localisation of the lumbar disc herniation. Spine 10:88–92, 1985.
28. Leyshon, A., Kirwan, E. O'G., and Wynn Parry, C.B.: Electrical studies in the diagnosis of compression of the lumbar root. J. Bone Joint Surg. (Br.) 63B:71–75, 1981.
29. Lombardi, J.S., Wiltse, L.L., Reynolds, J., et al.: Treatment of degenerative spondylolisthesis. Spine 10:821–827, 1985.
30. Love, B.R., Davies, A.A., Kirwan, E. O'G., and Sullivan, M.F.: The normal radiculogram: The relation between operative findings and clinical and electrical investigations. J. Bone Joint Surg. (Br.) 64B:135, 1982.
31. McCulloch, J.A., and Waddell, G.: Variations of the lumbo-sacral myotomes with bony segmental anomalies. J. Bone Joint Surg. (Br.) 62B:475–480, 1980.
32. McCulloch, J.A., Macnab, I.: Sciatica and chymopapain. Baltimore, Williams & Wilkins, 1983.
33. Macnab, I.: Backache. Baltimore, Williams & Wilkins, 1977.
34. Macnab, I., McBroom, R.J., Wardlaw, D., and Parrott, T.: Unilateral Root Decompression in Lumbar Spinal Stenosis. Read at the meeting of the I.S.S.L.S. Rome, 1987.
35. Mills, G.H., Davies, G.K., Getty, C.J.M., and Conway, J.: The evaluation of liquid crystal thermography in the investigation of nerve root compression due to lumbo sacral lateral spinal stenosis. Spine 11:427–432, 1986.
36. Morris, E.W., Di Paola, M., Vallance, R., and Waddell, G.: Diagnosis and decision making in lumbar disc prolapse and nerve entrapment. Spine 11:436–439, 1986.
37. Nachemson, A.L.: The lumbar spine: An orthopaedic challenge. Spine 1:59–61, 1976.
38. Nasca, R.J.: Surgical management of lumbar spinal stenosis. Spine 12:809–816, 1987.
39. Nashold, B.S., and Hrubec, Z.: Lumbar Disc Disease: A 20-Year Clinical Follow-up Study. St. Louis, C.V. Mosby, 1971.
40. Natelson, S.E.: The injudicious laminectomy. Spine 11:966–969, 1986.
41. O'Connell, J.E.A.: Protrusions of lumbar intervertebral disc. J. Bone Joint Surg. (Br.) 33B:8–30, 1951.
42. Pochaczevsky, R., Wexler, C.E., Meyers, E.N., et al.: Liquid crystal thermography of the spine and extremity: Its value in the diagnosis of spinal root syndromes. J. Neurosurg. 56:386–395, 1982.
43. Porter, R.W., and Hibbert, G.: Calcitonin treatment for neurogenic claudication. Spine 8:585–592, 1983.
44. Porter, R.W., Hibbert, C., and Evans, C.: Natural history of root entrapment syndrome. Spine 9:418–421, 1984.
45. Postacchini, F., Lami, R., and Massobrio, M.: Chemonucleolysis versus surgery in lumbar disc her-

niation: Correlation of the results to pre-operative clinical pattern and size of the herniation. Spine 12:87–96, 1987.
46. Rydevik, B., Brown, M.D., and Lundborg, G.: Pathoanatomy and pathophysiology of nerve root compression. Spine 9:7–15, 1984.
47. Spengler, D.M.: Lumbar discectomy, results with limited disc excision and selective foraminotomy. Spine 7:604–607, 1982.
48. Spengler, D.M.: Degenerative stenosis of the lumbar spine. J. Bone Joint Surg. (Am.) 69A:305–308, 1987.
49. Stanley, D.S., Euinton, H.A., Getty, C.J.M., and McLaren, M.: The Diagnostic Value of Nerve Root Injection (in press, Spine, 1989).
50. Stockley, I., Getty, C.J.M., Dixon, A.K., et al.: Lumbar lateral canal entrapment: Clinical, radiculographic and computer tomography findings (in press, Radiology, 1988).
51. Teplick, J.G., and Haskin, M.E.: Intravenous contrast/enhanced CT of the post operative lumbar spine. A.J.R. 143:845–855, 1984.
52. Tile, M.: The role of surgery in nerve root compression. Spine 9:57–64, 1984.
53. Van Akkerveekan, P.F., Van De Kraan, W., and Muller, J.W.T.H.: The fate of the free fat graft. Spine 11:501–504, 1986.
54. Verbiest, H.: Results of surgical treatment of idiopathic developmental stenosis of the lumbar vertebral canal. J. Bone Joint Surg. (Br.) 59B:181–188, 1977.
55. Waddell, G., McCulloch, J.A., Kummel, E., and Venner, R.M.: Non-organic physical signs in low back pain. Spine 5:117–125, 1980.
56. Wardlaw, D., and Macnab, I.: The Natural History of Spinal Stenosis. Read at the meeting of the I.S.S.L.S. Cambridge, 1983.
57. Weber, H.: Lumbar disc herniation: A controlled prospective study with ten years of observation. Spine 8:131–140, 1983.
58. Whight, A.H., Von Rogov, P., Zucherman, J., and Heiden, D.: Lumbar laminectomy for herniated disc: A prospective controlled comparison with internal fixation fusion. Spine 12:305–307, 1987.
59. Williams, R.W.: Micro lumbar discectomy: A twelve year statistical review. Spine 11:851–852, 1986.
60. Wiltse, L.L., Kirkaldy-Willis, W.H., and McIvor, G.W.D.: The treatment of spinal stenosis. Clin. Orthop. Rel. Res. 115:83–91, 1976.
61. Young, A., Getty, J., Kirwan, E. O'G., et al.: Variations in the pattern of muscle innervation by the L5 and S1 nerve roots. Spine 8:616–624, 1983.
62. Zeiger, H.E.: Comparison of chemonucleolysis and microsurgery discectomy for the treatment of herniated lumbar discs. Spine 12:796–799, 1987.

■ ANTERIOR SURGICAL APPROACH TO THE THORACOLUMBAR, LUMBAR, AND LUMBOSACRAL SPINE

Kiyoshi Kaneda

For most patients, the choice of approach to the thoracolumbar to lumbar spine should be made based on the site of the primary pathologic condition. Diseases or deformities that primarily involve the vertebral bodies may be approached directly through the transpleural-retroperitoneal, the retroperitoneal, or the transperitoneal route. The anterolateral approach to the lumbar vertebral bodies through a long and oblique flank incision (Fig. 1A–C) affords direct access to all the upper lumbar vertebral bodies and to the anterior lumbosacral junction. It may be indicated for extensive resection, débridement, or bone grafting in the treatment of tumors or infections at multiple levels, spinal deformities (e.g., scoliosis, kyphosis), vertebral body fractures, and other disorders.

THORACOLUMBAR JUNCTION AND LUMBAR SPINE

The vertebral bodies in this area (T12, L1) are exposed by the transpleural-retroperitoneal approach or the extrapleural-retroperitoneal approach.

Extrapleural-Retroperitoneal Approach

In this approach, the procedure of detaching the pleura from the chest wall should be performed with care, because the pleura is easily ruptured, resulting in a thoracotomy. The extrapleural-retroperitoneal approach is recommended in patients with infectious diseases of the vertebral body or of the intervertebral disc.

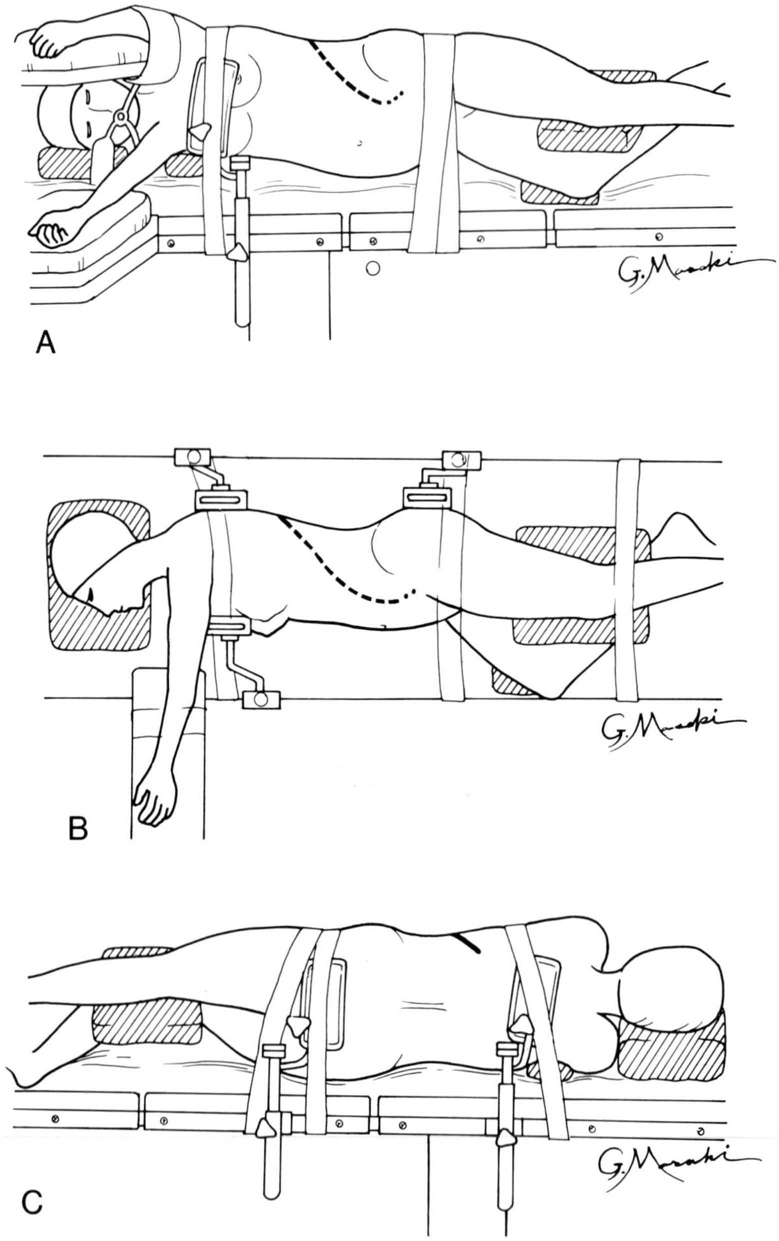

Figure 1 □ *A,* Positioning and skin incision: anterolateral approach to thoracolumbar and lumbar spine (from front). *B,* Positioning and skin incision to thoracolumbar and lumbar spine (from top). *C,* Positioning (from back).

Transpleural-Retroperitoneal Approach

In this approach, vertebral bodies from T9 to L5 can be exposed. In general, this can be accomplished by a left-sided or a right-sided approach, depending on the location of the pathologic condition. Usually, the left-sided approach is preferable for the following anatomic reasons: the liver on the right side is large and difficult to retract; the vena cava, also on the right, is easily torn, and bleeding from it may be difficult to control. The spleen, on the left, is fragile but smaller than the liver and is more easily retractable. The aorta, owing to its pulsation, is easier to locate than the vena cava, even among infectious or scarring tissues; furthermore, it is less susceptible to damage, and bleeding from it is much easier to control.

Positioning

The patient is placed on the operating table with the side to be operated upon facing superiorly (thus, the patient most frequently lies on the right side, for a left-sided approach) (see Fig. 1*A–C*). An axillary pad is used for prevention of circulatory disturbance of the right upper extremity (see Fig. 1*A*). Pressure on the peroneal nerve of the right side should be eliminated, to avoid nerve palsy. The skull is kept on a pillow, with the cervical spine straight. The chest cage is supported on the sternum and the back by pads and adhesive tape. The pelvis is fixed by a gluteal pad and adhesive tape on the greater trochanter. After placement of the patient with the trunk supported in this way, the position remains stable, even when the table is tilted during surgery. By tilting the operating table, the patient can be placed at the angle required by any surgical procedure. This position tends to shift the abdominal and retroperitoneal contents toward the nonoperated side and also facilitates retraction.

Skin Incision and Thoracoabdominal Exposure

To best gain access to the vertebral bodies of T12 and L1, resection of the tenth rib is made, allowing exposure between T10 and L2. A curvilinear skin incision is made, following the tenth rib, with the ability to extend either the cephalic or caudal end. If necessary, the incision may be extended obliquely downward and anteriorly to the lateral margin of the rectus sheath at the level of the anterosuperior iliac spine. When performing the extrapleural-retroperitoneal approach, the skin incision is made on the eleventh or twelfth rib, and it may be extended obliquely downward, as described above (see Fig. 1*A–C*). After cutting the skin (Fig. 2), the incision of the muscles (latissimus dorsi, external oblique muscle of the abdomen) is continued along the course of the tenth rib with the diathermy knife; complete hemostasis has to be ensured during the operation (Fig. 3). The periosteum of the tenth rib is transected with a cutting diathermy knife along its entire length, and the rib is stripped subperiosteally. The rib is then dissected with a knife at the costochondral junction, is elevated dorsally, and is transected with a rib cutter at the exposed proximal end. After removing the rib, the thoracic cavity is opened by a longitudinal

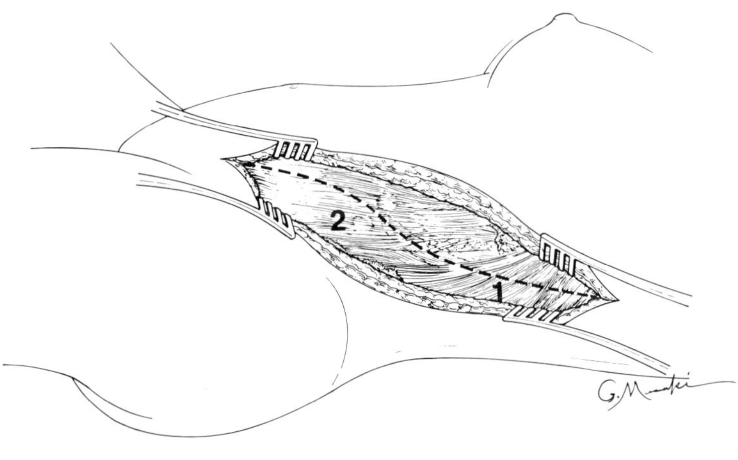

Figure 2 □ Exposure of the operative area after transection of skin and subcutaneous tissue: *1,* lattissimus dorsi muscle; *2,* external abdominal oblique muscle.

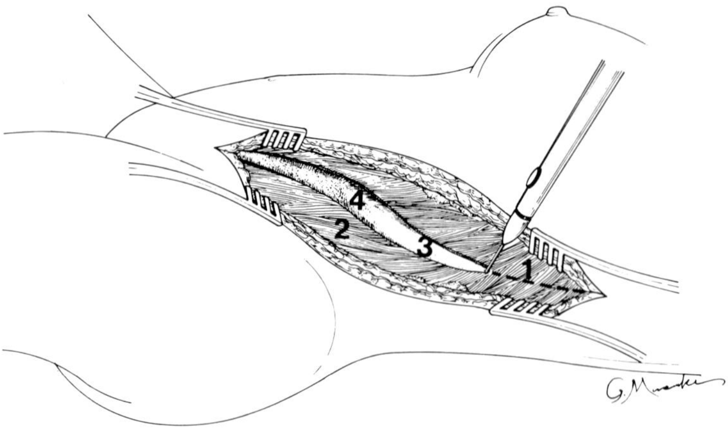

Figure 3 □ Exposure of the tenth rib after transection of external abdominal oblique muscle and lattisimus dorsi muscle: *1,* lattisimus dorsi muscle; *2,* external oblique abdominal muscle; *3,* tenth rib; *4,* cartilage of tenth rib.

incision of the parietal pleura along the bed of the resected rib (Fig. 4).

The abdominal muscle layers (external and internal oblique muscles of abdomen, transverse muscle of abdomen) are transected along the skin incision line. The peritoneum is forced apart bluntly from the abdominal wall using a sponge, and retracted medially. Further dissection of the abdominal wall is conducted, following the course of the vessels and nerves. Then the costal cartilage is divided with a knife; this divided cartilage is useful as a landmark for resuturing (Fig. 4).

After the peritoneum under the diaphragm is forced apart bluntly, a diathermy knife is used to transect the diaphragm circumferentially at a point about 2 cm away from the rib attachment, and the incision is extended dorsally to the vertebral body (Fig. 5). It is beneficial to apply marking sutures in the dissected edges of the diaphragm. These facilitate more accurate resuturing. (Fig. 6).

By means of these procedures, the chest cavity and the retroperitoneal space are connected. Using manual retraction, the lung is displaced cranially, and the peritoneal contents medially (see Fig. 6). The left diaphragmatic crus is dissected about 2 cm above the lateral and medial arcuate ligaments (Fig. 7). Then, the left psoas major and the thoracolumbar vertebrae are exposed. The kidney and the ureter are retracted medially with the peritoneum (see Fig. 6). The psoas major is retracted posteriorly at L1, L2, and other relevant vertebral bodies. A longitudinal scissor incision is made on the parietal pleura along the axis of the lower thoracic vertebral column. This exposes segmental vessels, which run transversely over the vertebral bodies. They are then ligated and transected to the extent needed (see Fig. 7).

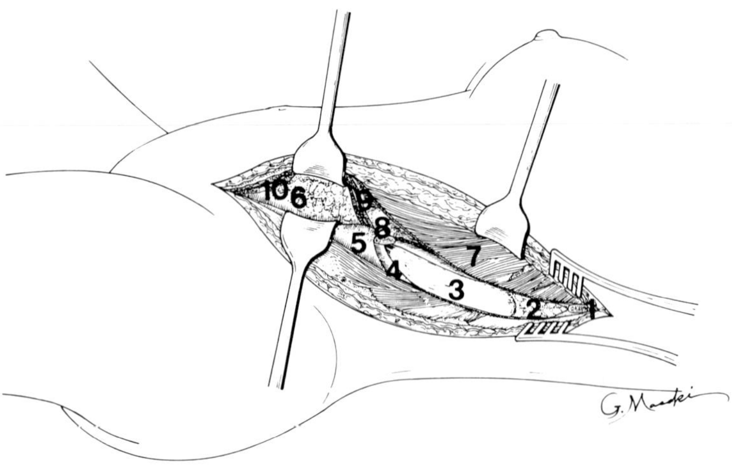

Figure 4 □ Resection of the tenth rib and opening of thoracic cavity: *1,* stump of tenth rib; *2,* lung; *3,* diaphragm; *4,* periosteum of tenth rib; *5, 9,* internal abdominal oblique muscle; *6,* peritoneum; *7,* external abdominal oblique muscle; *8,* cartilage of tenth rib; *10,* transverse abdominal muscle.

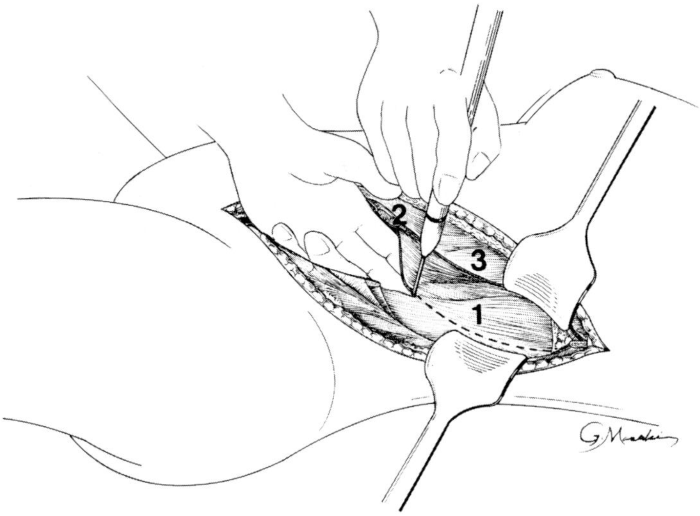

Figure 5 □ Transection of thoracic diaphragm: *1,* thoracic diaphragm; *2,* divided costal cartilage; *3,* external abdominal oblique muscle.

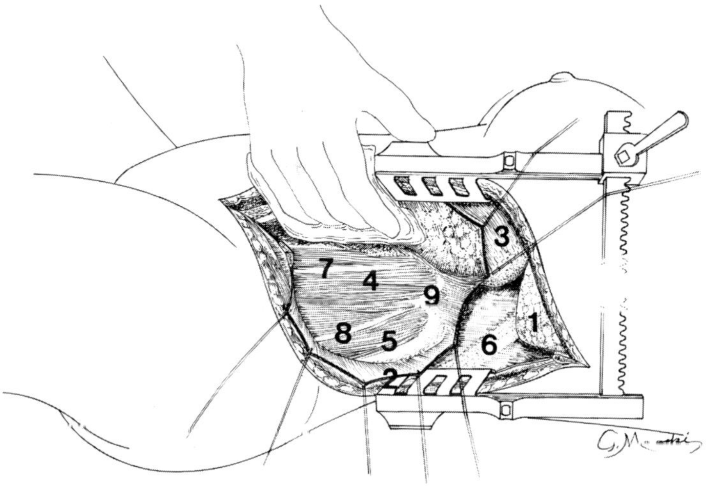

Figure 6 □ Transection of diaphragm and exposure of retroperitoneal space: *1,* lung; *2, 3,* diaphragm; *4,* psoas major muscle; *5,* quadratus lumborum muscle; *6,* eleventh rib; *7,* ilioinguinal nerve; *8,* iliohypogastric nerve; *9,* medial arcuate ligament.

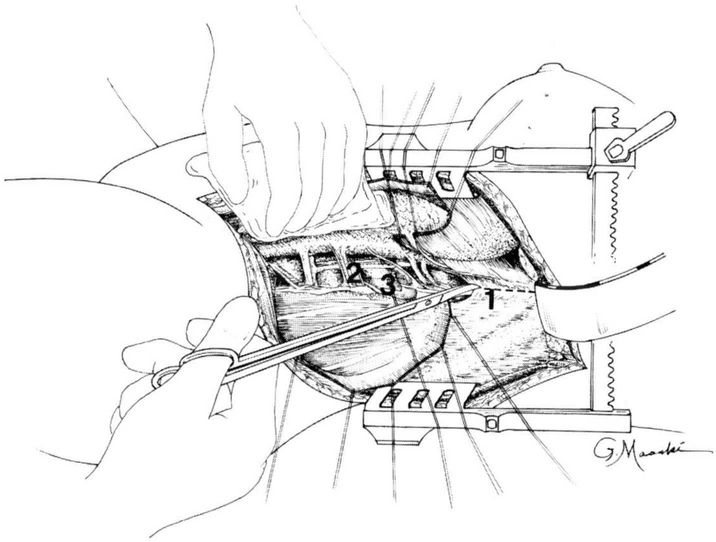

Figure 7 □ Exposure of vertebrae by splitting parietal pleura and retroperitoneal tissues: *1,* parietal pleura, *2,* lumbar segmental vessels; *3,* left medial crus.

Exposure of the Vertebrae

When one is exposing the vertebral bodies, dissection should be started over the intervertebral discs, which are the prominent areas; no vessels are present there. Tissues over the intervertebral discs and the vertebral bodies, including the psoas major, are retracted until the base of the transverse processes is touched. This procedure is performed using a sponge applicator, scissors and Cobb elevators. The sympathetic trunk is retracted laterally. The psoas origins are detached from the intervertebral discs (Fig. 8). Bleeding from the vertebral cortex resulting from damage of nutrient vessels is controlled with bone wax.

Making a sufficiently long incision, this transpleural-retroperitoneal approach affords exposure of the vertebral bodies from the thoracolumbar region to the upper portion (the promontory) of the sacrum. With this approach, all kinds of surgical procedures involving the thoracolumbar-lumbar vertebral bodies can be performed.

Wound Closure

After the required anterior procedures are completed, wound closure is begun. The psoas major is replaced into the original area without any suture. Anatomic reattachment of the diaphragm is important. The parietal pleura over the vertebral column is then closed by a continuous suture. The diaphragm is closed in a posteromedial to anteromedial direction using an interrupted suture (Fig. 9). The costal cartilage of the tenth rib, which was divided as a landmark, is sutured. A chest tube for drainage is inserted through the chest wall. A retroperitoneal drain is inserted, if necessary. The parietal pleura over the resected rib bed is sutured. The thoracic wall muscles (intercostal muscle, latissimus dorsi, anterior serratus), as well as the abdominal wall (transverse muscle, internal oblique muscle, external oblique muscle) are sutured in layers (Fig. 10).

If the lung is compressed for a long time during surgery, its inflation will sometimes be indicated.

LUMBOSACRAL JUNCTION AND LUMBAR SPINE: RETROPERITONEAL APPROACH TO LUMBAR SPINE (L2–L5) AND SACRUM (S1)

The anterolateral approach to the lumbar spine and the lumbosacral junction has been used by general surgeons for lumbar sympathectomy. A long incision from the twelfth rib posteriorly to the lower abdomen anteriorly provides broad access to all the lumbar vertebral bodies and the upper sacrum, in

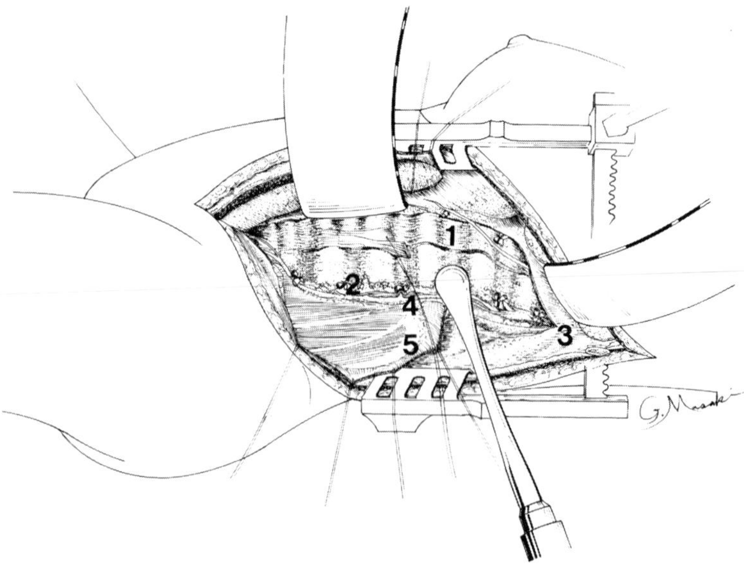

Figure 8 □ Exposure of vertebral bodies by transection of segmental vessels and retraction of psoas major muscle: *1*, anterior longitudinal ligament; *2*, lumbar segmental vessels (ligated and dissected); *3*, parietal pleura; *4*, medial arcuate ligament; *5*, lateral arcuate ligament.

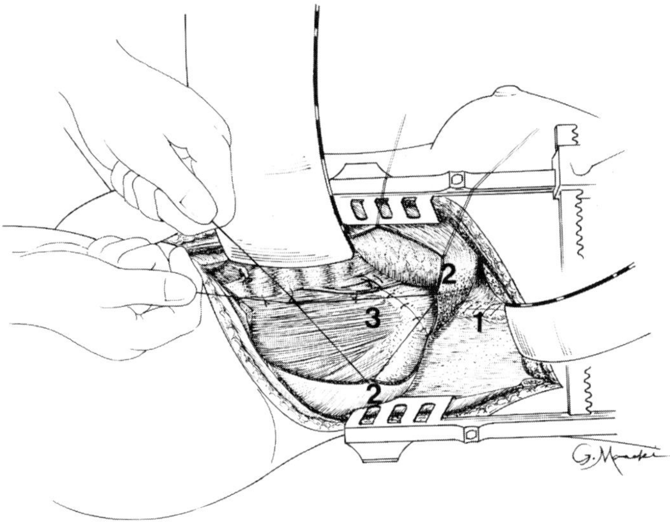

Figure 9 □ Closure of medial and lateral arcuate ligament, parietal pleura and diaphragm: *1,* parietal pleura; *2,* thoracic diaphragm; *3,* psoas major muscle.

continuity. The transectional route from the skin incision to the vertebra at the first lumbar vertebral level is shown (Fig. 11).

Positioning

Positioning of the patient is the same as that in the transpleural-retroperitoeal approach to the thoracolumbar junction (see Fig. 1*A*–*C*). In exposing the lower lumbar area, the patient is placed on the operating table with the side to be operated upon tilted upward at an angle of 45 to 60 degrees. This approach can be made from the left as well as from the right. The left-sided approach is generally used, if there are no special reasons for which the vertebrae have to be exposed on the right side, such as tumor or infection, or a scoliotic component in kyphoscoliosis.

Skin Incision; Exposure

The skin incision is started over the lateral half of the twelfth rib and extended obliquely downward and anteriorly to the lateral margin of the rectal fascia at the level of the anterosuperior iliac spine. The lower distal incision is then curved to direct the anterosuperior iliac spine (see Fig. 1*A*, *B*). This makes the working space broader, especially in exposure of the lumbosacral junction, owing to the extensive posterior retraction of the abdominal muscles. In the exposure of the upper lumbar spine, the latissimus dorsi is dissected on the twelfth rib. The external oblique muscle is divided parallel to the direction of the muscle fibers. Then, the inferior posterior serratus, which lies in the posterior portion, is transected. The internal oblique and transverse muscles

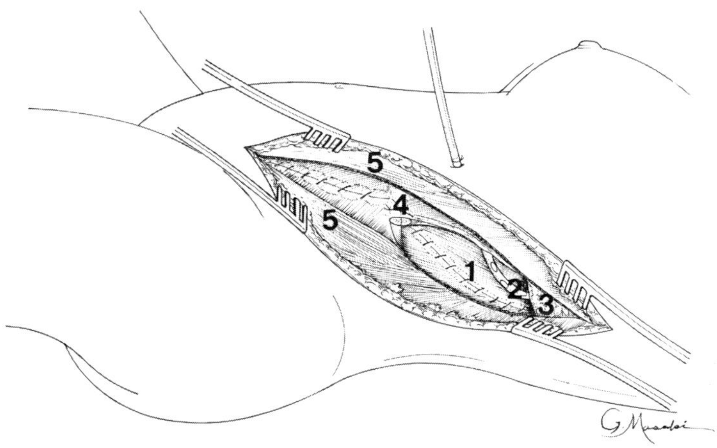

Figure 10 □ Closure of thoracic and abdominal walls: *1,* sutured thoracic diaphragm; *2,* chest tube (drain); *3,* lung; *4,* sutured costal cartilage; *5,* external abdominal oblique muscle.

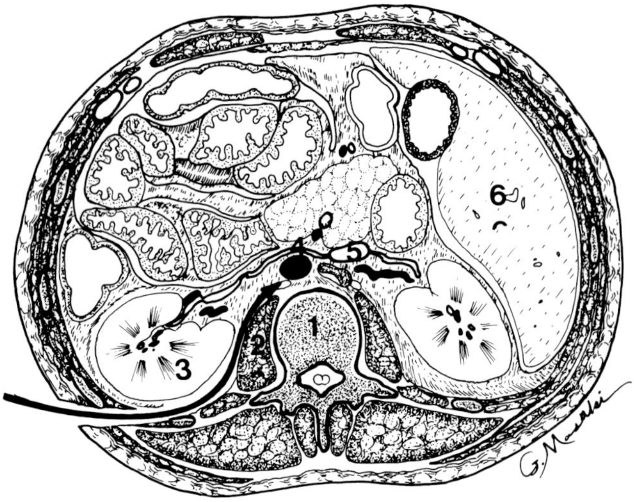

Figure 11 □ Cross section at L2–vertebra: *1,* L2–vertebral body; *2,* left psoas major; *3,* left kidney; *4,* abdominal aorta; *5,* inferior vena cava; *6,* right liver.

of the abdomen are transected, in line with the skin incision. The peritoneum is separated from the abdominal wall at the anterior and lateral portions, and under the twelfth rib (Figs. 12 to 14). Following this, the twelfth rib is resected. (In the exposure of the lower lumbar region and the lumbosacral junction, the rib resection is not necessary.) Then, the quadratus lumborum and the psoas major are exposed. The kidney and the ureter are retracted medially with the peritoneum (Fig. 15). The renal fascia is continuous with the peritoneum and extends posteriorly behind the kidney, surrounding the kidney, ureters, and the adrenals. The peritoneal fat is loosely adhered to the quadratus lumborum and psoas major muscles. Dissection of the peritoneal fat, along with that of the peritoneum and the renal fascia, is carried out by sponge and the fingers. The segmental lumbar vessels tether the abdominal aorta and the inferior vena cava. Therefore, in order to expose the anterior portion of the lumbar vertebral bodies, these should be ligated and cut to the extent needed (Fig. 15). The sympathetic trunk is retracted laterally. Vertebral bodies and intervertebral discs from L2 to L4 (5) can be exposed by this approach (Fig. 16).

Wound Closure

After completion of the necessary anterior procedures, wound closure is carried out. The rib bed is sutured if the twelfth rib is resected. Other closing procedures are almost the same as those in the transpleural-retroperitoneal approach.

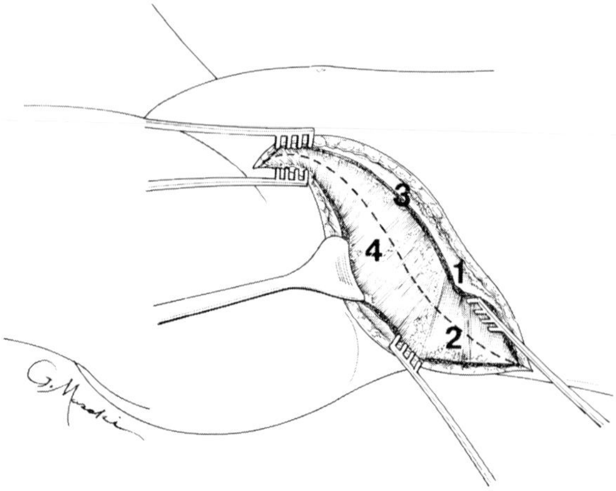

Figure 12 □ Exposure for retroperitoneal approach: transection of lattisimus dorsi and external abdominal oblique muscles: *1,* lattisimus dorsi muscle; *2,* posterior inferior serratus muscle; *3,* external abdominal oblique muscle; *4,* internal abdominal oblique muscle.

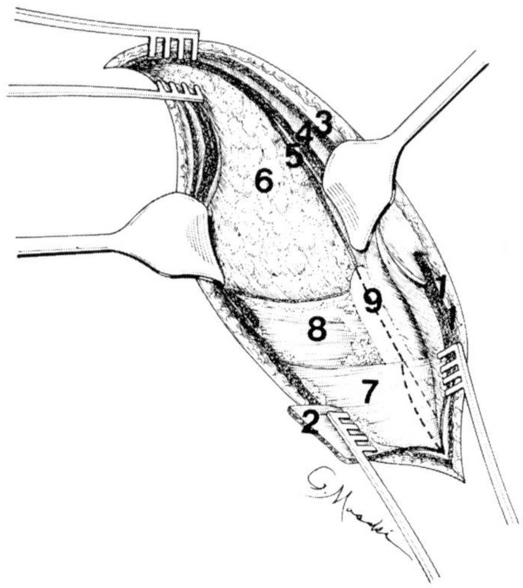

Figure 13 □ Exposure of peritoneum and twelfth rib: *1,* lattisimus dorsi muscle; *2,* posterior inferior serratus muscle; *3,* external abdominal oblique muscle; *4,* internal abdominal oblique muscle; *5,* transverse abdominal muscle; *6,* peritoneum; *7,* iliocostal muscle; *8,* quadratus lumborum muscle.

LUMBOSACRAL JUNCTION: TRANSPERITONEAL APPROACH TO L4–S1

This approach is useful for the anterior procedures in patients with lumbosacral spondylolisthesis and tumors of the lower lumbar spine and sacrum.

Positioning

The patient is positioned on the back. The lumbosacral junction is placed on the angled

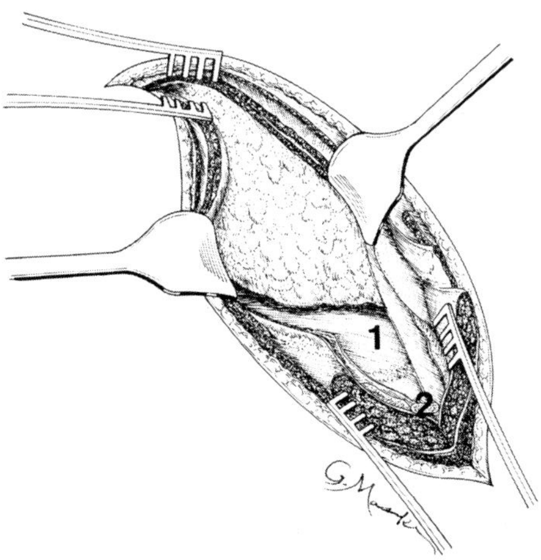

Figure 14 □ Resection of twelfth rib: *1,* quadratus lumborum muscle; *2,* stump of twelfth rib.

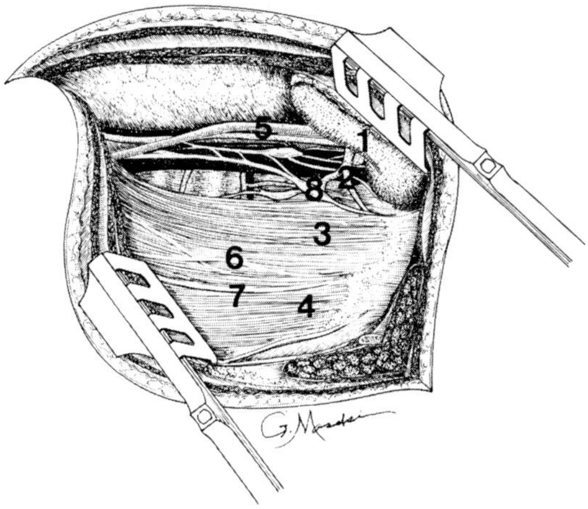

Figure 15 □ Retroperitoneal tissues after retraction of peritoneal contents: *1,* kidney; *2,* renal vein; *3,* psoas major muscle; *4,* quadratus lumborum muscle; *5,* ureter; *6,* ilioinguinal nerve; *7,* iliohypogastric nerve; *8,* sympathetic trunk.

portion at the center of the operating table in a position of lumbar hyperlordosis. This posture permits an easy approach to the sacral promontory.

Skin Incision; Exposure

A skin incision is made—a median laparotomy curving around the navel on the left (Fig. 17). When exposing the lumbosacral junction only, an incision from just under the navel to just above the symphysis pubis

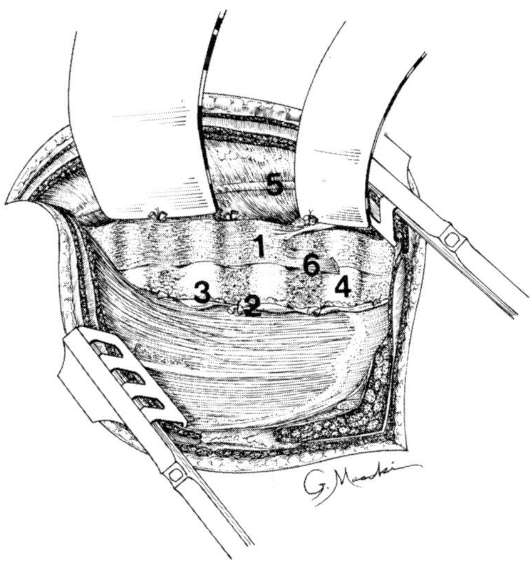

Figure 16 □ Exposure of lumbar vertebral bodies: *1,* anterior longitudinal ligament; *2,* ligated and dissected segmental vessels; *3, 4,* intervertebral disc; *5,* ureter.

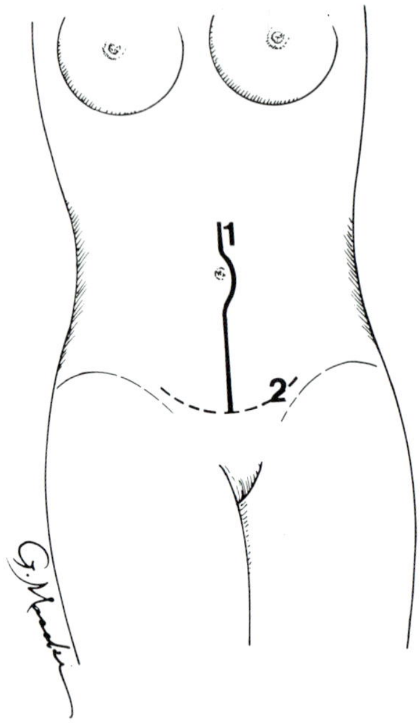

Figure 17 □ Transperitoneal approach for exposure of lumbosacral junction: *1*, midline incision; *2*, transverse incision.

is usually sufficient. The abdominal wall is divided at the linea alba. The peritoneum is cut longitudinally, in line with the skin incision, while the bowel beneath is protected from injury. The wound is distracted with large laparotomy retractors. The intra-abdominal contents are packed upward with a large towel compress, to expose the posterior peritoneal layer at the lumbosacral junction. The bilateral mesocolons are also retracted with a wet towel. The sigmoid colon is retracted to the left and downward by a wide flexible spatula. The parietal peritoneal layer is then incised, from 2 to 3 cm proximal and to the left of the bifurcation of the aorta to 2 to 3 cm distal to the sacral promontory (Fig. 18). In this incision, great care should be taken not to damage the underlying adjacent superior hypogastric plexus, which provides the sympathetic innervation of the urogenital system. Saline infiltration under the posterior peritoneal layer may facilitate the differentiation of the superior hypogastric plexus from the peritoneal layer (Fig. 19). Duncan and Jonk[3] recommended an eccentric approach to this area through the right side to avoid most of these hypogastric nerve fibers. Following the posterior peritoneal incision, the fatty connective tissue, which covers the superior hypogastric plexus and the retroperitoneal vessels, must be bluntly opened just to the right of the midline and over the right common iliac artery, and retracted to the left with the aid of cotton applicators. At this point, the right ureter, which crosses the external iliac artery, must be identified. In these procedures, the left side of the peritoneum and all the tissues subadjacent to it (including the prevertebral tissues, vessels, and the hypogastric plexus) may be moved as a unit to the left of the vertebrae, without dissecting them separately. This technique reduces the risk of injuring the hypogastric nerve fibers. The middle sacral artery in front of the L5–S1 intervertebral disc is ligated and sectioned, if encountered. This approach provides a broad view of the lumbosacral junction (Fig. 20). The fourth lumbar vertebral body can be exposed from the left side (Fig. 21).

Wound Closure

After completion of the required procedures, wound closure is begun. The posterior parietal peritoneal layer is sutured with absorbable thread. The wet compressive towels are removed, and the bowel contents and

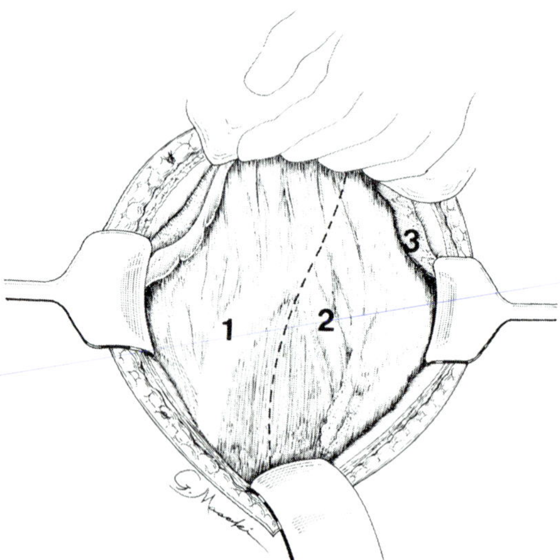

Figure 18 □ Transperitoneal exposure of posterior peritoneal layer: *1*, right common iliac artery and posterior parietal peritoneum; *2*, left common iliac artery; *3*, sigmoid colon. Dotted line shows incision of posterior parietal peritoneum.

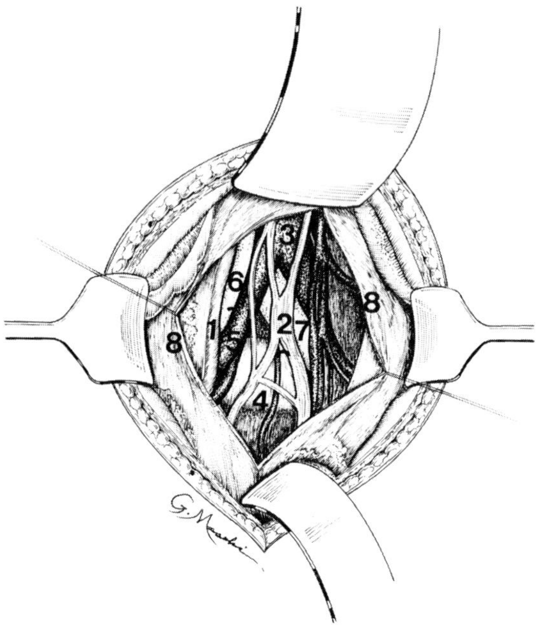

Figure 19 □ Anatomic relationship of vessels, hypogastric nerves, and ureter behind posterior parietal pleura around lumbosacral junction: *1*, ureter; *2*, superior hypogastric nerve; *3*, bifurcation of abdominal aorta; *4*, promontory; *5*, right external iliac artery; *6*, right common iliac vein; *7*, left common iliac artery; *8*, posterior parietal peritoneum.

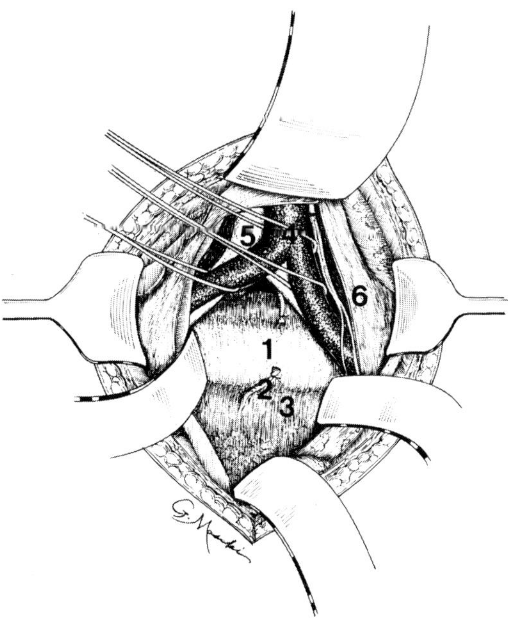

Figure 20 □ Exposure of lumbosacral junction: *1*, L5–S1 intervertebral disc; *2*, ligated and dissected median sacral artery; *3*, promontory; *4*, bifurcation of abdominal aorta; *5*, inferior vena cava.

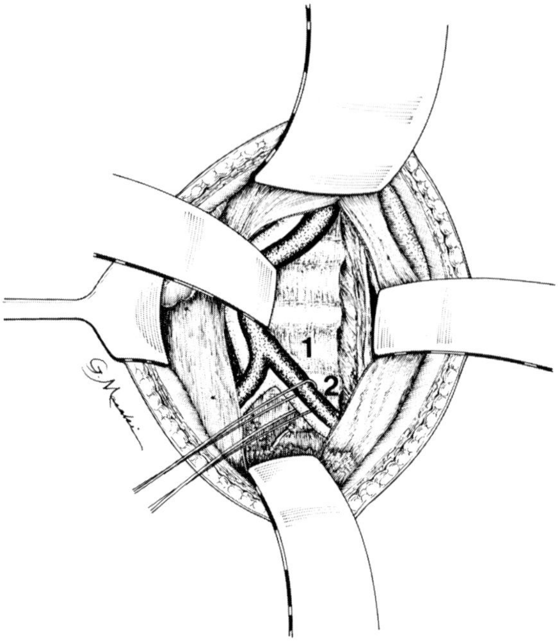

Figure 21 □ Exposure of L4 and L5 vertebral bodies: *1,* L5–vertebral body; *2,* L5–S1 intervertebral disc.

the greater omentum are re-placed into their normal positions. Closure of the abdominal wall is the same as in an ordinary laparotomy.

Complications

In the transperitoneal approach to the lumbosacral junction, the superior hypogastric plexus may be injured, which in males results in sexual disturbances, including retrograde ejaculation. There is a possibility of damage to the ureters, the common iliac vein, or the inferior vena cava, which are sometimes difficult to repair.

References

1. Bauer, R., Kerschbaumer, F., and Poisel, S.: Spine, Anterior Approaches to Thoracolumbar Junction, Lumbar and Lumbosacral Spine: Operative Approaches in Orthopedic Surgery and Traumatology. New York, Georg Thieme Verlag, 1987, pp. 37–66.
2. Burrington, J.O., Brown, C., Wayne, E.R., and Odom, J.: Anterior approach to the thoracolumbar spine—technical considerations. Arch. Surg. 3:456–463, 1976.
3. Duncan, H.J.M., and Jonck, L.M.: The presacral plexus in anterior fusion of the lumbar spine. S. Afrik. Tydskrif Chirurg. 3:93–96, 1965.
4. Goldner, J.L., McCollum, D.E., and Urbaniak, J.R.: Anterior disc excision and interbody spine fusion for chronic low back pain. *In* American Academy of Orthopaedic Surgeons, Committee On Publications: Symposium on the Spine. St. Louis, C.V. Mosby, 1969, pp. 111–131.
5. Harmon, P.H.: Anterior excision and vertebral body fusion operation for intervertebral disc syndromes of the lower lumbar spine: Three- to five-year results in 244 cases. Clin. Orthop. 26:107–127, 1963.
6. Hodgson, M.B., and Wong, S.K.: A description of a technic and evaluation of results in anterior spinal fusion for deranged intervertebral disc and spondylolisthesis. Clin. Orthop. 56:133–162, 1968.
7. Johnson, R.M., and Southwick, W.O.: Surgical approaches to the lumbosacral spine. *In* Rothman, R.H., and Simeone, F.A. (eds.): The Spine. Philadelphia, W.B. Saunders, 1982, pp. 171–187.
8. Louis, R.: Surgery of the Spine, Surgical Anatomy and Operative Approaches. New York, Springer-Verlag, 1983, 232–261; 292–313.
9. Sacks, S.: Anterior interbody fusion of the lumbar spine. Indications and results in 200 cases. Clin. Orthop. 44:163–170, 1966.
10. Stauffer, R.N., and Coventry, M.B.: Anterior interbody lumbar spine fusion, Analysis of Mayo Clinic series. J. Bone Joint Surg. 54A:756–768, 1972.

ANTERIOR EXTRAPERITONEAL LUMBAR DISCECTOMY WITHOUT FUSION

Noboru Nakano
Tohru Nakano

For the surgical treatment of lumbar disc lesions, the posterior approach is customarily used. Some surgeons try to restrict the exposure; problems with hemostasis and nerve root relations in persons with facet arthrosis make the surgical exposure difficult. Wide exposure for laminectomy invites irritation of the dura, arachnoid adhesions produce other problems. It is not always easy to achieve good results. Recently microsurgery has been recommended to improve the results. Once a correct diagnosis is made by means of myelography or other methods, it is more logical to remove the disc by approaching it from the front, without disturbing the spinal canal. On the basis of this idea, anterior extraperitoneal lumbar discectomy and fusion have been performed.

Because excellent results were obtained by simply removing the disc without fusion in one young patient (anterior lumbar interbody fusion could not be done because of severe adhesion of the iliac vessels), this procedure was tried with other young patients, then used with even older patients.

Surgeons have performed anterior discectomy without fusion in at least 304 patients suffering from low back pain and/or sciatica and have been impressed by the absence of complications following anterior surgical exposure. Follow-up studies have been done on 159 patients after more than 5 years, with an average interval of 7 years.

Narrowing of the intervertebral disc space was found to occur but could not be equated with poor clinical results, as satisfactory results have been obtained in most patients (excellent grade without any residuals in 90.6%). Retrograde ejaculation with or without poor erection was not seen in this series. With correct clinical diagnosis refined by myelography, computed tomography (CT), and magnetic resonance imaging (MRI), the surgeon gains confidence in removing the disc from the front. Thereby, the large posterior muscles are not disturbed, and the spinal canal is not entered. The surgical technique and long-term follow-up procedures are presented herein.

SURGICAL TECHNIQUE

The patient is placed in the supine position under general anesthesia after muscle relaxants have been used to secure abdominal muscle relaxation. A left paramedian extraperitoneal approach is used. A 7-cm slightly oblique left abdominal incision is made. The anterior layer of the sheath of the rectus abdominis is incised, and the rectus abdominis is retracted laterally (Fig. 1). Then the posterior sheath of the rectus abdominis is incised after it is separated from the anterior surface of the peritoneum with a small stick-sponge (Fig. 2). The peritoneum and its contents are pulled to the right side. As the peritoneum is mobilized, it is easily lifted from the anterior surface of the psoas (Fig. 3). The exposure of the L4 disc is made from the left anterolateral aspect. The sympathetic chain and the fourth lumbar ganglion lie in the lateral gutter and are not disturbed, but the branches communicating with the hypogastric plexus are pushed out of the way. It is usually unnecessary to ligate the lumbar vessels, because wide exposure does not require removing the disc. The peripheral disc ligament annulus is opened, and a small hole of 5 to 7 mm in diameter is created. Residual nucleus and fragments of degenerated annulus are carefully removed with special attention, especially from the posterior area of the disc (Fig. 4). In the case of the L5 disc, sometimes the large vein is in the way, but it is easy to push it upward after ligation of small terminal sacral vessels. The hypogastric sympathetic plexus is carefully displaced.

CLINICAL MATERIAL

This operation has been performed on 304 patients including 215 males and 89 females

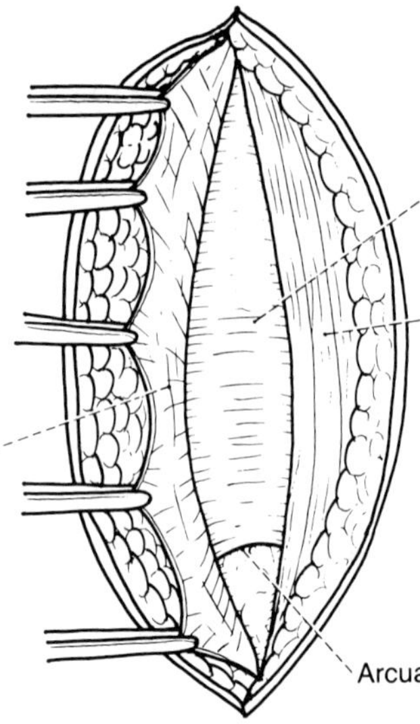

Figure 1 □ The anterior layer of the sheath of the rectus abdominis is incised and the rectus abdominis is retracted laterally.

at Nakano Orthopaedic Hospital between February, 1967, and March, 1988.

The age distribution was from 9 to 80 years, averaging 36.1 years (Table 1).

Illustrative Cases

A 46-year-old man had been treated by pelvic traction elsewhere, but he became unable to walk because of severe low back pain and sciatica with 20-degree straight-leg raising (Fig. 5). Metrizamide myelograms revealed a complete defect at the level of the L4 disc (Fig. 6). Extraperitoneal anterior lumbar discectomy was done, and one large disc fragment with a degenerative disc, weighing 5.6 g, was removed from a posterior protruded pocket on the right side (Figs. 7 to 9). Straight-leg raising was improved to up to 85 degrees on both sides 1 week following operation (Fig. 10).

Postoperative myelography was performed 2 months after operation and showed some improvement, but a filling defect was still recognized. Clinical symptoms, however, disappeared completely (Fig. 11). The patient has since worked without difficulty on a fishing boat for 7 years.

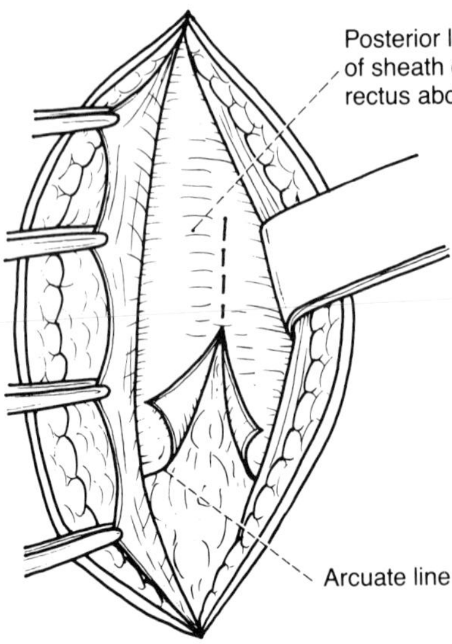

Figure 2 □ The posterior sheath of the rectus abdominis is incised as laterally as possible.

Results

Operating time was 30 to 305 minutes, averaging 57.9 minutes. Blood loss was 7 to 337 ml, averaging 76.6 ml.

The weight of the removed nucleus and degenerated annulus ranged from 0.5 to 10

Text continued on page 993

Table 1 □ Number of Patients

AGE RANGE	NUMBER OF MALES	NUMBER OF FEMALES	TOTAL NUMBER (PERCENTAGE)
9–19	14	14	28 (9.2%)
20–29	77	11	88 (29.0%)
30–39	55	12	67 (22.0%)
40–49	39	26	65 (21.4%)
50–59	21	21	42 (13.8%)
60–80	9	5	14 (4.6%)
Total	215 (70.7%)	89 (29.3%)	304 (100%)

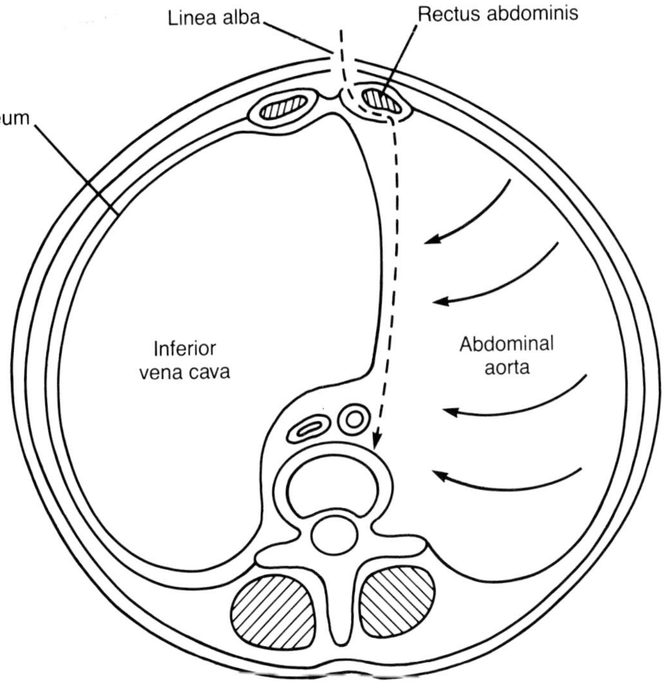

Figure 3 □ The peritoneum and its contents are pulled to the right side.

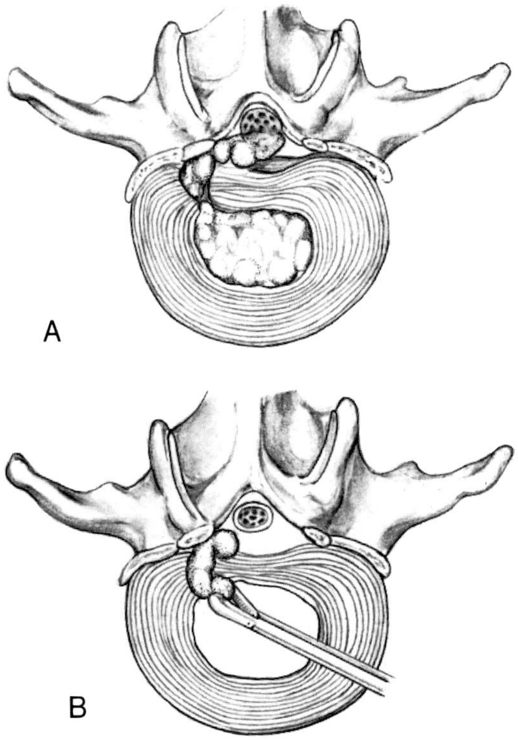

Figure 4 □ Portion of the sequestered nucleus fragments are retrieved through a naturally occurring defect in the posterior annulus (*A*). This results in a large protruded fragment moving forward into the disc space after removing the anterior part of the disc. This fragment can then be removed easily (*B*).

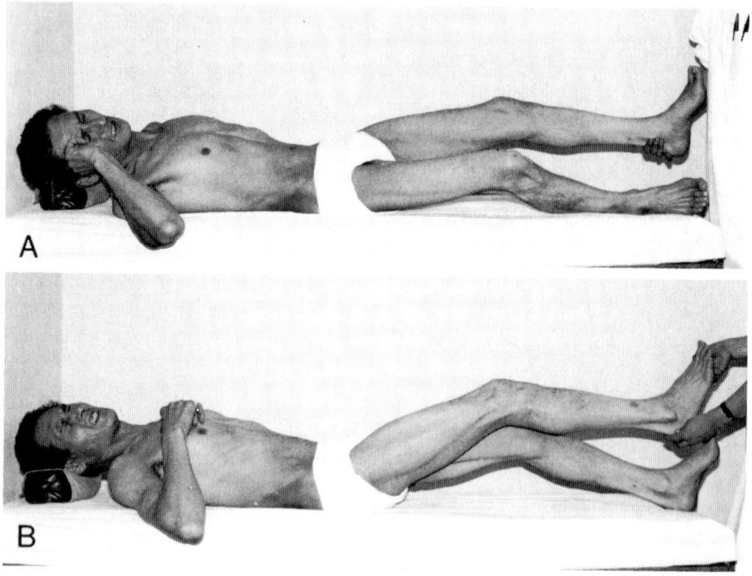

Figure 5 □ *A, B,* A 46-year-old man complained of severe low back pain and sciatica.

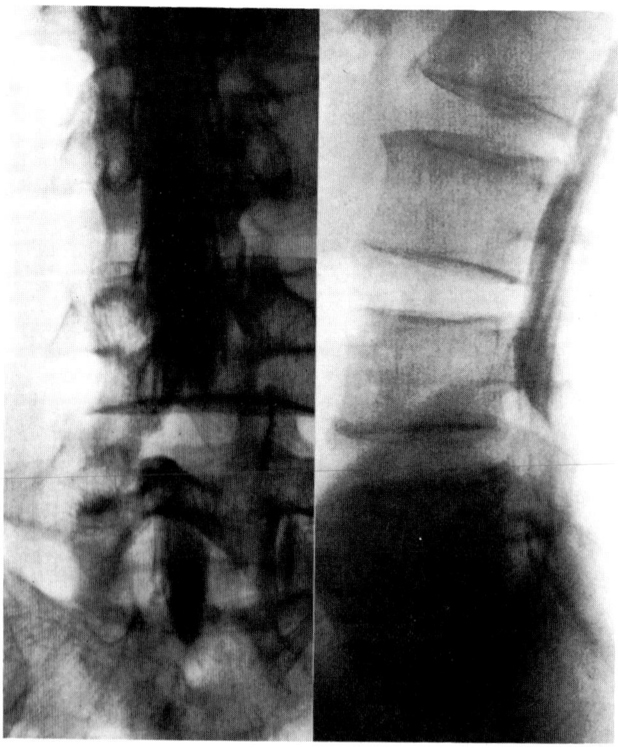

Figure 6 □ Metrizamide myelograms revealed complete defect at the level of the L4 disc.

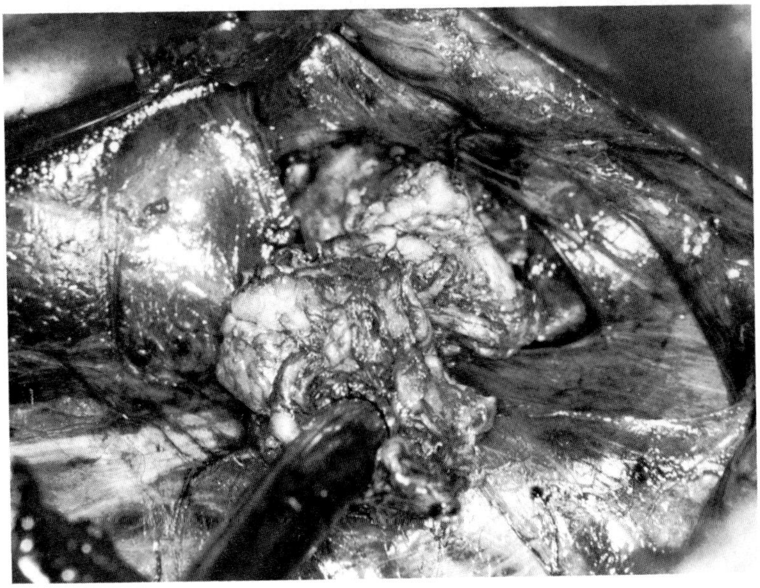

Figure 7 □ The peripheral disc ligament-annulus is opened, creating a small hole, 5 mm to 7 mm in diameter. Fragments of degenerated annulus are removed easily.

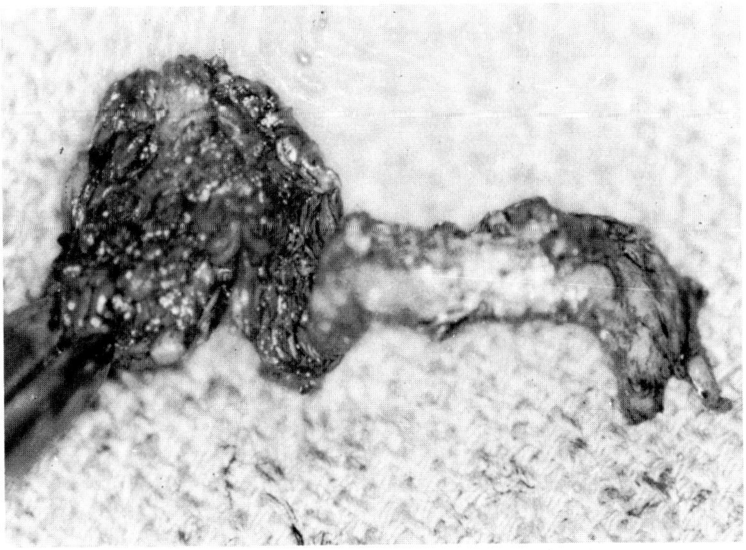

Figure 8 □ This large disc fragment was removed last.

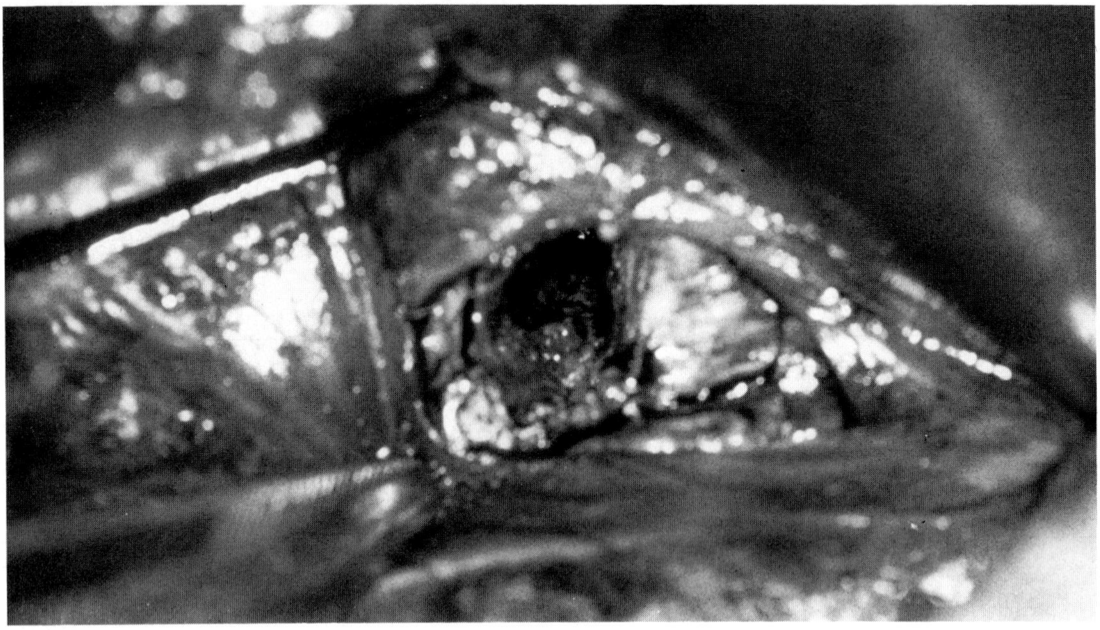

Figure 9 □ Normal part of disc was not removed.

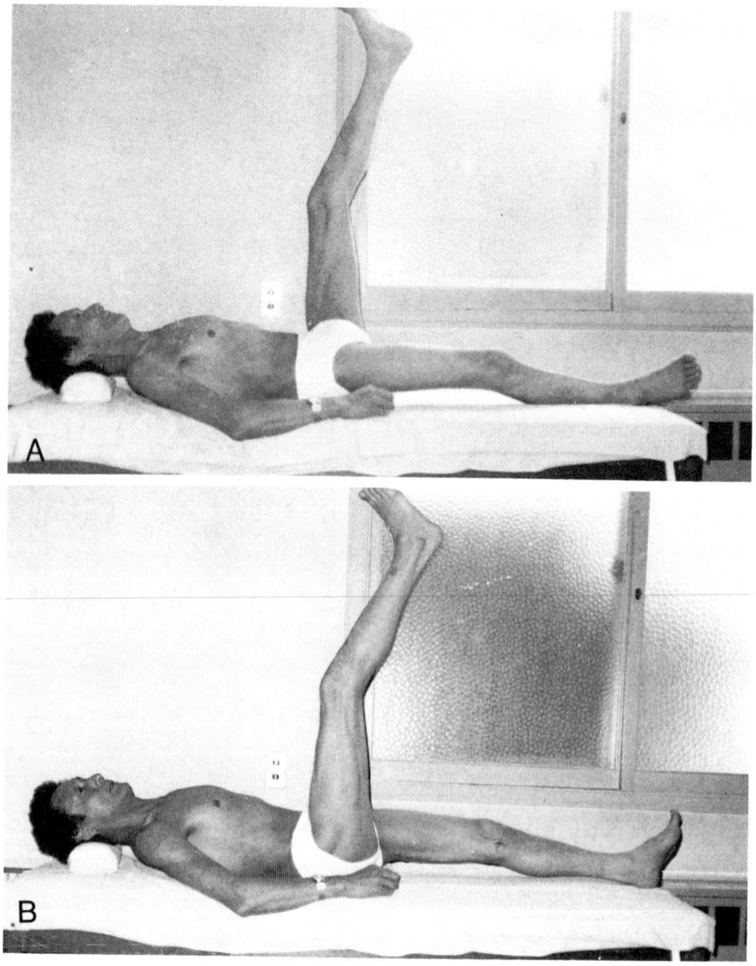

Figure 10 □ *A, B,* Straight-leg raising was improved up to 85 degrees on both sides 1 week after the operation.

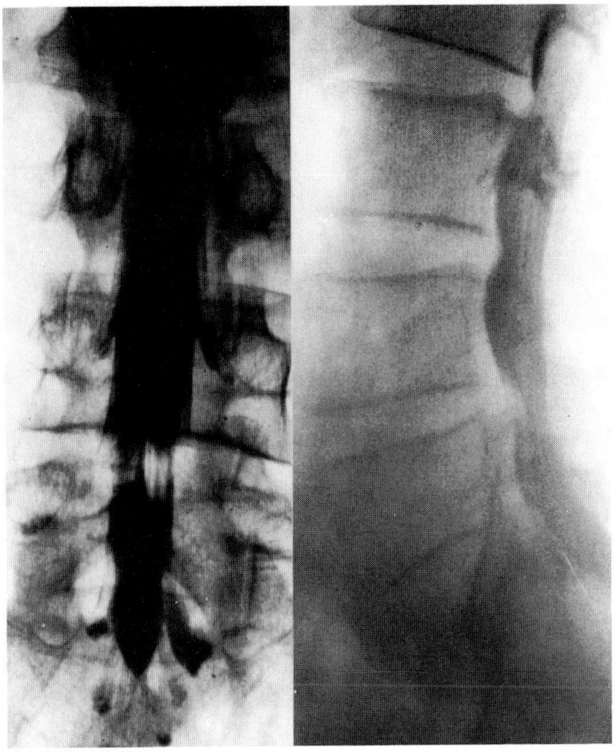

Figure 11 □ Postoperative myelography was done 2 months after operation, but filling defect was still recognized. Clinical symptoms, however, had disappeared completely.

g, averaging 2.9 g, at L4–L5 and from 0.4 to 5.0 g, averaging 2.3 g at L5–S1. There was no relation between age and weight of removed disc.

Narrowing of the disc had progressed as far as it was going to, in most patients by 6 months after the operation. This narrowing averaged 28.6% at the L4 disc space and 26.3% at the L5 disc space after 7 years (Fig. 12).

After anterior discectomy, slight instability was seen in three patients (1.9%), but no further operation has been required in any patients. Figure 13 is a postoperative radio-

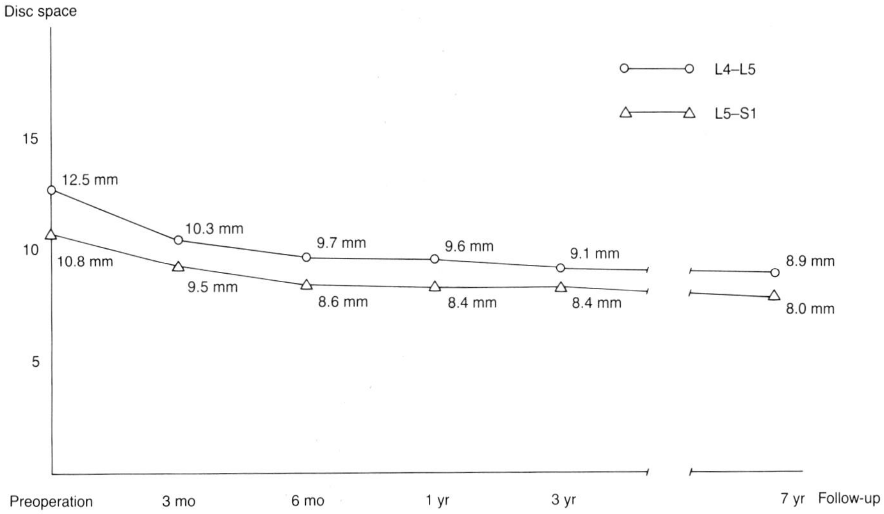

Figure 12 □ Narrowing of the disc had progressed by 6 months after the operation, but it had not increased markedly. This narrowing averaged 28.6% at L4/5 and 26.3% at L5/S1 after 7 years.

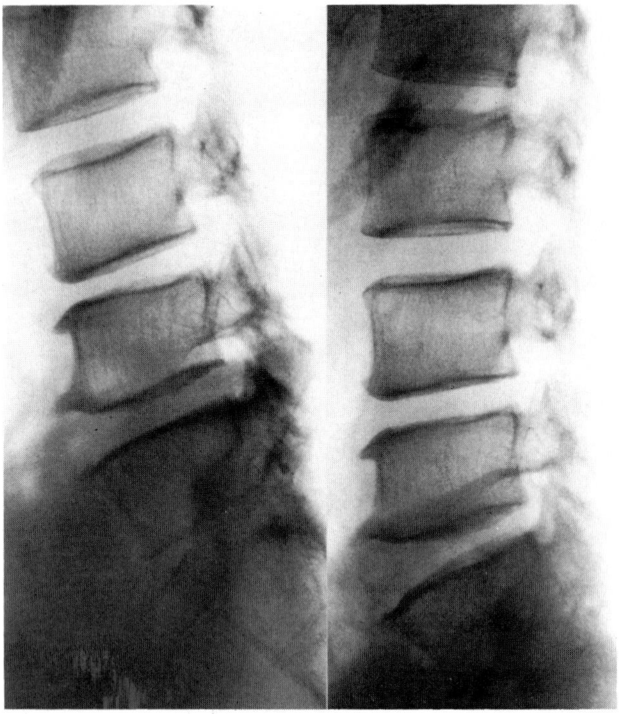

Figure 13 □ Slight instability was seen by flexion at L4/5 5 years after operation, but the patient has worked as a heavy laborer without symptoms.

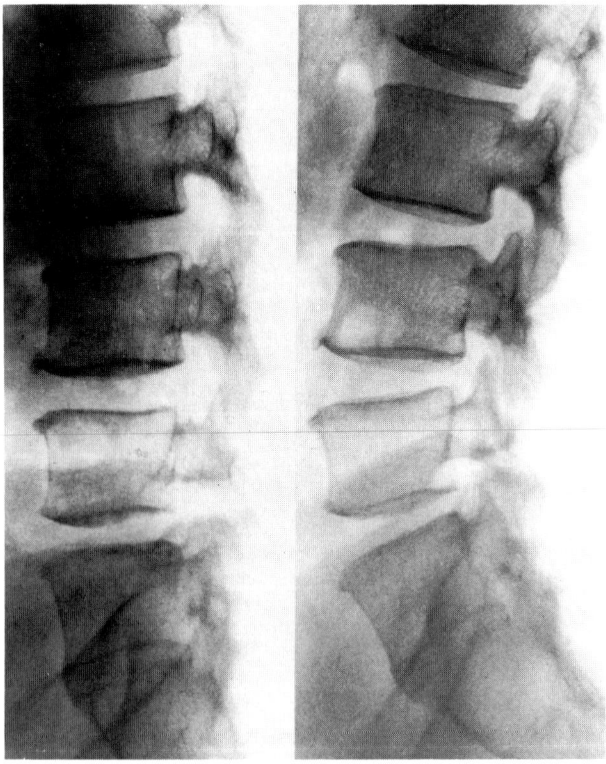

Figure 14 □ A 17-year-old male was going to have anterior interbody fusion at L5/S1 but adhesion of big vessels was severe, so only anterior discectomy was done. This is an 18 years postoperative flexion-extension film, which shows no instability.

graph of a patient who was operated on at the L3 and L4 disc spaces. Slight instability was seen by flexion at the L4 space in a radiograph 5 years after the operation. He has worked as a heavy laborer without symptoms. Figure 14 is a 7 years' postoperative flexion–extension film, which shows no instability; the patient has been working as a carpenter without any difficulty.

Complications

Two superficial infections and one deep one were recognized, but in the case of deep infection, anterior discectomy was performed. Secondly, infection might have occurred in the first operation, which was done at another hospital. Retrograde ejaculation was not seen in this series.

Four patients underwent reoperation posteriorly. Three of them were operated on at the same level; but the fourth, whose symptoms had not completely improved, was operated on at another hospital. One patient was operated on within 1 year, and one patient after 10 years. Recurrence in one patient was at a different level. One was unsatisfied, owing to misdiagnosis.

Clinical Results

Anterior extraperitoneal lumbar discectomy without fusion was performed on 304 patients, and a follow-up study was done on 159 cases after more than 5 years, with an average interval of 7 years. The criteria used for the postoperative clinical evaluation are shown in Table 2. Overall results were as follows: excellent, 144 (90.6%); good, 9 (5.7%); fair, 5 (3.1%); and poor, 1 (0.6%) (Table 3).

The relationship between results and age is shown in Tables 4 and 5. Among all age groups, women in their forties received the lowest proportion of "excellent" ratings—69%. All but two patients went back to their original occupations, including heavy labor.

Table 2 □ Criteria for Clinical Results of Low Back Pain

Excellent	All symptoms disappear, and patients can work without difficulty.
Good	Occasional low back pain exists, not sufficient to disturb daily life.
Fair	Symptoms are the same as they were before surgery or have slightly improved.
Poor	Symptoms have worsened.

Table 3 □ Results According to Sex

RESULT	NUMBER OF MALES	NUMBER OF FEMALES	TOTAL
Excellent	108 (94.7%)	36 (80.0%)	144 (90.6%)
Good	2 (1.8%)	7 (15.6%)	9 (5.7%)
Fair	3 (2.6%)	2 (4.4%)	5 (3.1%)
Poor	1 (0.9%)	0 (0.0%)	1 (0.6%)
Total	114 (100%)	45 (100%)	159 (100%)

Discussion

Hult[2] reported anterior discectomy with lumbar sympathetic ganglionectomy performed on 30 patients who had chronic low back pain with sciatica and negative myelography (degenerated disc without protrusion or extrusion). He thought that the addition of sympathectomy produced better results. Unfortunately, there has been much disagreement about the combining of an anterior operation and this surgery; there have been no reports on this method.

Excellent results were obtained by just removing the disc in a young patient for whom anterior lumbar interbody fusion had been planned but failed because adhesion of the iliac vessels was severe. As a result, this procedure was tried in patients with sciatica and low back pain and has produced satisfactory results.

The anterior extraperitoneal lumbar discectomy has been performed, following failure of conservative treatments, on patients with positive myelograms and more than two of the following symptoms: low back pain, pain or numbness at the lower extremity, a positive straight-leg raising test, muscle weakness of the lower extremity, and disturbance of urinary bladder function. These are, similarly, indications for posterior discectomy without fusion.

Some surgeons pointed out that extruded fragments might be impossible to remove anteriorly. Occasionally, portions of the sequestered nucleus fragments are retrieved through a naturally occurring defect in the posterior annulus. This sometimes results in a large protruded fragment moving forward into the disc space because of reduced pressure in the disc space after the anterior area of the disc has been removed. This fragment can then be removed easily. Therefore, re-

Table 4 □ Results According to Age (Males)

AGE RANGE	NUMBER EXCELLENT	NUMBER GOOD	NUMBER FAIR	NUMBER POOR	TOTAL
9–19	7	0	0	0	7
20–29	42 (95.6%)	1 (2.2%)	1 (2.2%)	0	44 (100%)
30–39	25 (89.3%)	0	2 (7.1%)	1 (3.6%)	28 (100%)
40–49	16 (94.1%)	1 (5.9%)	0	0	17 (100%)
50–59	13	0	0	0	13
60–80	5	0	0	0	5
Total	108 (94.7%)	2 (1.8%)	3 (2.6%)	1 (0.9%)	114 (100%)

moval of disc materials from the spinal canal should not be attempted (Fig. 15).[5–8] Extensive laminectomy and certainly rough handling of the dura produced some poor results.[4] Anterior discectomy with interbody fusion became an accepted operation,[3] but some cases of male sterility were reported. Flynn and Hogue[1] have put this complication into proper focus, finding that surgeons who have performed a large number of anterior discectomies and fusion operations do not experience this complication. It is now believed that most poor results and/or complications from an anterior operation are due to unfamiliarity with retroperitoneal anatomy and to poor exposure. Retrograde ejaculation with or without poor erection has not been seen in this series.

The anterior approach is more appropriate than the posterior one because portions of a disc can be removed, without disturbing the spinal canal, for decompression of the posterior disc area. Low back pain and sciatica are caused by a combination of posterior disc protrusion or high intradiscal pressure, produced by degeneration, nucleus absorption, or a segmented disc annulus pressing against the posterior longitudinal ligament.

The disc space had narrowed in most of the patients (about 90%) by 6 months after the operation, but not markedly thereafter. This narrowing averaged 28.6% at L4–L5 and 26.3% at L5–S1 after 7 years (see Fig. 12). There was no statistical correlation between narrowing of the space and clinical results, because it is the decompression of the posterior longitudinal ligament that relieves the symptoms. After anterior discectomy, flexion–extension films were taken for every patient to reveal any instability. Slight instability was recognized in three patients, but no further operation was required.

An excellent result among women of the fifth decade occurred less frequently than for other groups (see Tables 4 and 5.) This might be related to menopause and an incorrect indication for surgery.

This method does not disturb the muscle at all. Therefore, it is a good procedure for athletes suffering from low back pain and sciatica. Postoperative details, however, are very important for these patients, as they are in all lumbar spinal surgery. These details include light postural exercise, muscle strengthening of both anterior and posterior muscle groups, and care in lifting, stooping, and twisting. There should be both a limitation on riding in motor vehicles and a minimum rest period of 4 weeks before normal activities are resumed.

Table 5 □ Results According to Age (Females)

AGE RANGE	NUMBER EXCELLENT	NUMBER GOOD	NUMBER FAIR	NUMBER POOR	TOTAL
9–19	7	0	0	0	7
20–29	6	0	0	0	6
30–39	6 (85.7%)	1 (14.3%)	0	0	7 (100%)
40–49	9 (69.2%)	3 (23.1%)	1 (10.7%)	0	13 (100%)
50–59	8 (80.0%)	2 (20.0%)	0	0	10 (100%)
60–80	0	1 (50.0%)	1 (50.0%)	0	2 (100%)
Total	36 (80.0%)	7 (15.6%)	2 (4.4%)	0	45 (100%)

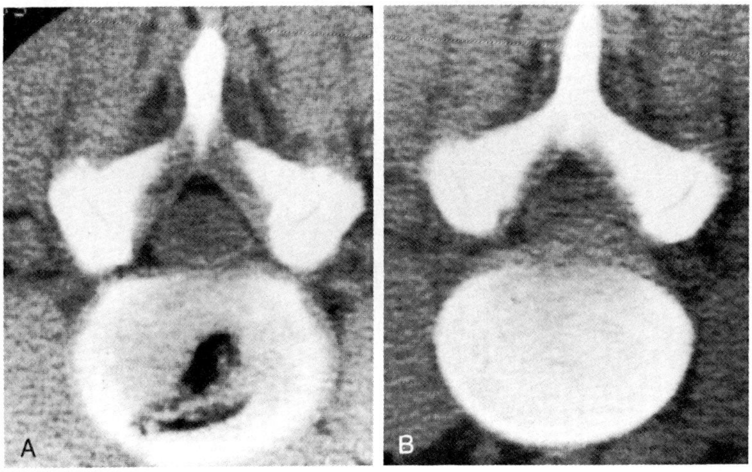

Figure 15 □ These are CT after (*A*) and before (*B*) and anterior discectomy. It is seen that disc was removed anteriorly.

References

1. Flynn, J.C., and Hogue, M.A.: Anterior fusion of lumbar spine: End result study with long-term follow-up. J. Bone Joint Surg. 61A:1143–1150, 1979.
2. Hult, L.: Retroperitoneal disc fenstration in low back pain sciatica. A preliminary report. Acta Orthop. Scand. 20:342–348, 1950.
3. Harmon, P.H.: Anterior extraperitoneal lumbar disc excision and vertebral body fusion: A study of long-term results. Clin. Orthop. 18:169–185, 1961.
4. Nakano, N.: Multiple back operations. J. West. Pacific Orthop. Assoc. 14:67–74, 1977.
5. Nakano, N.: Anterior extraperitoneal discectomy in lumbar disc herniation. J. Jpn. Orthop. Assoc. 52:1530–1531, 1978.
6. Nakano, N., and Tomita, T.: Results of surgical treatment of low back pain: A comparative study of the anterior and posterior approach. Int. Orthop. 4:101–106, 1980.
7. Nakano, N.: Lower lumbar anterior discectomy without fusion: A several year follow-up indicating usefulness of this technique in surgery of the lower lumbar spine—a report of 110 cases. J. Jpn. Orthop. Assoc. 57:321–328, 1983.
8. Nakano, N., and Nakano, T.: Surgical technique of anterior extraperitoneal lumbar discectomy to the lumbar disc herniation. Operation 41:1–6, 1987.

23 □ Fusion: Where It's Been and Where It's Going

Charles V. Burton

Fusion is a term that appears to have a different meaning for almost every professional involved in spinal therapy or surgery today, despite general agreement that it relates to rigid fixation by bone and/or other materials with or without associated internal fixation devices. In regard to the subject of fusion, it is particularly important to review the past so that we can explore how, in the future, the word and the associated concept of fusion may come to be perceived.

According to Wiltse,[1] the history of modern spinal fusion began with Albee[2] and Hibbs[3] in New York City in 1911, based on the efforts of earlier surgeons to correct unstable spines by dorsal bone placement. Lateral placement of bone to the transverse processes was described by Campbell in 1927,[4] but surprisingly, it took about 35 years before this technique became common practice.

Wiltse credits Burns[5] with the first anterior lumbar interbody fusion (ALIF) in 1933. The genesis of the posterior lumbar interbody fusion (PLIF) occurred in the 1940s, led by Briggs and Milligan,[6] Cloward,[7] and Jaslow.[8] By the 1930s, metallic implants were being tried, but it was not until Venable and Stuck[9] solved the problem of dissimilar metals producing electromotive force (EMF) currents (with alloyed chrome-cobalt) that internal fixation became truly feasible. Credit is due to Harrington and coworkers[10, 11] for the next quantum step forward. Since their contribution, there has been a progression of innovation in metallic internal fixation devices by Knodt and Larrick,[12] Luque,[13, 14] Judet,[15] Roy-Camille,[16] Louis,[17] Magerl,[18] Kraag and colleagues,[19] Zielke and Strempel,[20] Cotrel and Dubousset,[21] and Steffee.[22] The ultimate goal of these systems has been to obtain rigid fixation. In clinical use it soon became evident that the "stand-alone" rigid devices progressively loosened with the passage of time. For this reason, these systems have typically required associated bone fusions, usually of the dorsolateral variety.

POSTERIOR FUSION

It has been interesting to observe the modern evolution of metallic fixation devices utilizing pedicle screws as their basic support. As these systems have become more technically efficient in achieving rigid fixation, they have also been associated with certain increased clinical problems and failures. The study of these data has made it possible to develop a greater appreciation of the biomechanical forces normally present in lumbar motion and has begun to open new vistas of investigation for the future.

It has been pointed out by Liu and coworkers[23] that "pedicle screws are to posterior spinal instrumentation as pilings are to a building." It has now become evident that as the rigidity of pedicle screw systems has increased, the price paid for this has been greater system failure resulting from shearing and other adverse phenomena related to the focusing of stress and loading on these "pilings."

The general response to these observations has been to increase the size and strength of the pilings. The diameter of a pedicle screw is, however, inherently limited by the size and geometry of the vertebral pedicle itself. For this reason, strength optimization has been directed toward improving alloys and increasing the mean fatigue life of the metal by means of special techniques, such as nitrogen ion implantation, to create metal strength greater than the forces of segmental stress and loading. In this situation, metal strength is potentiated by means of nitrogen ion bombardment under conditions of varying intensity, temperature, and age.

An important consideration is the fact that the mechanical strength of some modern pedicle screw systems now appears to be substantially greater than "normal" local spine stress. This means that loading and stress are not being dissipated locally and have now been transferred to the adjacent motion segments and other surrounding structures.

Since the advent of modern spinal computed tomography (CT) and magnetic resonance imaging (MRI), it has become possible, by noninvasive and sophisticated means, to appreciate the changes induced by the continued stress of and insult to multilevel rigid fusions to adjacent motion segments. These disc and facet joint stress-related degenerative changes are now being routinely identified and have become referred to as the *transitional syndrome*. This syndrome typically reflects local or referred pain but can also produce neurologic problems, such as central spinal stenosis with cauda equina compression. A recent review by Hsu and coworkers[24] has observed, once again, that the deterioration of adjacent vertebral motion segments in the transitional syndrome directly relates to the degree of rigid fixation produced by the fusion.

These data and observations now suggest and support what has previously been considered to be unthinkable. We have been working to improve rigid fixation when we might have better focused our attention on *flexible stabilization*. Burton[25] more recently reviewed the liabilities of rigid fixation and noted:

> The requirement for both instrumentation and bony fusion represents a long and costly surgical procedure for the patient, often involving significant blood loss and replacement, with lengthy hospitalization. Another disadvantage of metallic fusion devices is subsequent reduction in the quality of postoperative imaging techniques. These liabilities represent a persuasive argument for reexamination of the concept of fusion as a treatment modality.

As the practice of spinal therapy and surgery becomes progressively more dependent upon modern imaging, it is certain that a point will be reached at which the routine destruction of imaging efficiency by all implanted metal will no longer be acceptable.

Wiltse has recently introduced an advanced metallic pedicle screw internal fixation device in which the support bars contain a degree of flexibility.[26] Despite the liabilities of its metal construction, this fixator appears to be one of the first devices to recognize the logic inherent in moving away from the principle of rigid fixation.

For quite some time, many spinal surgeons (including this author) have been progressively more concerned with the problems associated with rigid fixation. Consequently,

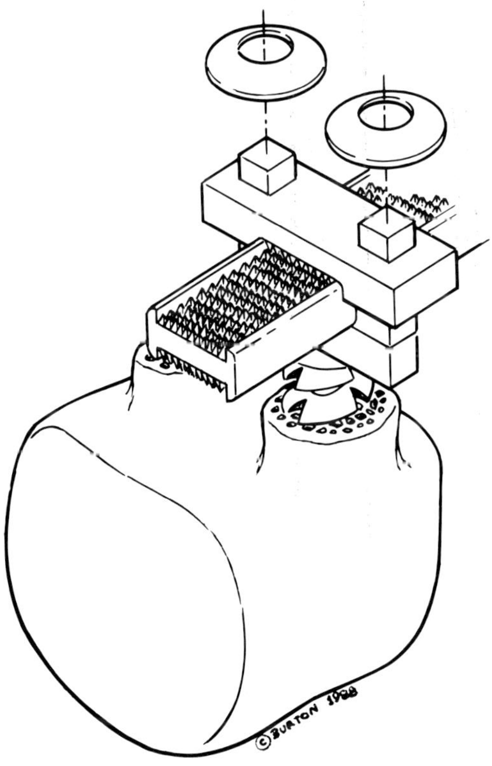

Figure 1 □ The basic components of a new polymeric nonmetallic flexible stabilization (NFS) system, designed by the author but not yet clinically employed, is shown. An advanced pedicle screw design with cross bars is used to support a flexible rod. (Courtesy of Charles V. Burton, M.D.)

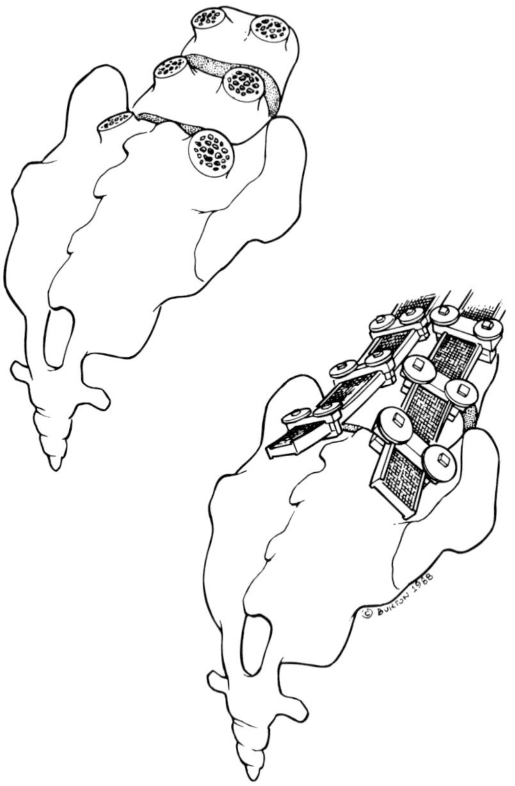

Figure 2 □ The ideal application of this device would be in the case of a lumbar claudication syndrome characterized by multilevel central and lateral spinal stenosis, requiring removal of the posterior elements. Because the system is flexible and conforms to the pedicle screws, the spine influences the device (rather than the converse). Note that the flexible rod is bending in three planes. For the sake of graphic simplicity, spacers between the pedicle and the device are not shown. (Courtesy of Charles V. Burton, M.D.)

this author has, during the past 8 years, been working on the development of nonmetallic flexible stabilization (NFS) systems as a means of avoiding some of the problems previously reviewed. Figures 1 and 2 represent one example of a new *flexible* pedicle screw stabilization device constructed of nonmetallic polymeric materials. This example is intended to function as a "stand-alone" device for which associated bone fusion is unnecessary. Aside from the potential physiologic and biomechanical advantages of NFS systems, these devices introduce the likelihood of significantly decreasing operating time, the extent of operative exposure, the associated blood loss, the length of hospital stay, and the overall cost.

Although this author believes that the future belongs to NFS systems, the following cautions exist:

1. We do not presently accurately understand the "normal" biomechanical functioning of an in vivo neuromotion segment.
2. The determination of "optimal" device flexibility for a given patient may be a challenge.
3. The risks inherent in the placement of pedicle screws remain.
4. Potential fatigue failure of an NFS system is ultimately determined in clinical practice only.
5. The long-term response of the body to implanted polymers is only now becoming known.

POSTERIOR INTERBODY FUSION

As with posterior fusion, the efforts in PLIF have also focused on achieving rigid fixation, usually with an osseous allograft or homograft. The major advantages of PLIF have been in decreasing operative time and blood loss, as well as in placing a fusion closer to the central axis of spinal support. Its major disadvantage is proximity to neural structures and the lack of immediate mechanical stabilization. For patients with patent intervertebral foramina, Simmons[27] has popularized the *chip PLIF,* in which bone harvested from the primary incisional area is used to create a fibro-osseous intervertebral union. At this time, the data for PLIF do not allow us to biomechanically compare it with flexible stabilization systems. This is certain to be an important area of study in the future.

Through the insight provided by spinal MRI we have been given pathophysiologic information that seems likely to increase the importance of PLIF as a procedure in the future. The ability of MRI to detect quality of tissue as well as topographic anatomy has led to a better understanding of end-plate dynamics and the fate of degenerated and dehydrated intervertebral discs. In Figure 3, the "normal" process of disc degeneration and progressive absorption across the end plate, which ultimately results in self-stabilization, is reviewed.

Owing to influences that are not yet well

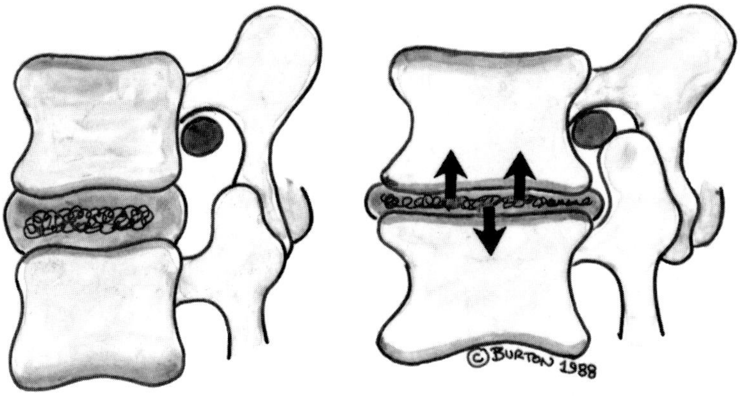

Figure 3 □ As disc degeneration and dehydration progress, disc volume appears to be progressively decreased by absorption across the end plate (*arrows*). At the same time segmental dysfunction promotes subperiosteal bone deposition (osteophytes) and hypertrophy of the zygoapophyseal joints. At the end of the healing process the segment has stabilized, and, although the foraminal opening has decreased in size, clinically symptomatic spinal nerve compression has not occurred. (Courtesy of Charles V. Burton, M.D.)

understood but may involve an autoimmune response to injured cartilage or reparative collagen, the end plate may undergo sclerosis and thickening. When this occurs, the degenerated disc material appears not to be absorbed. This phenomenon appears to be accompanied by early adjacent bone marrow changes of an inflammatory nature (increased water content demonstrated by MRI) and more chronic changes that appear to represent avascular necrosis (red marrow changing to white marrow with high fat content shown by MRI). These changes produce a situation that is conducive not only to recurrent disc herniation but also to the potential development of a degenerative spondylolisthesis at that level (Fig. 4). Another consideration of significance is the relationship of these pathophysiologic changes to the production of the *discogenic pain syndrome.*

Kenneth Heithoff, at the Center for Diagnostic Imaging in Minneapolis, and Michael Modic, at Case Western Reserve University in Cleveland, have contributed a great deal to identifying and explaining the MRI changes described above. For patients in whom vertebral end-plate sclerosis and adjacent marrow change have been diagnosed, the operative findings of "ivory-like" densely sclerotic end plates and degenerated disc (often mucinous in consistency) material serving as a "lubricant" tending to encourage segmental hypermobility, correlate well with the MRI findings and the subsequent clinical course.

When these changes are appreciated in individuals who have experienced recurrent

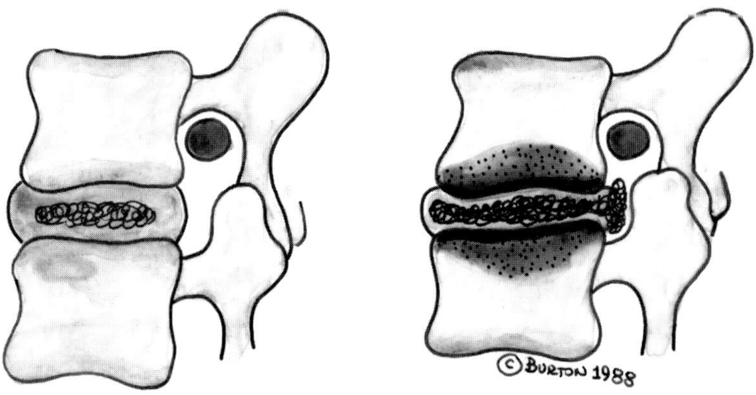

Figure 4 □ Because of progressive sclerosis of the end plates and pathologic changes in the adjacent bone marrow, degenerated disc material has not been absorbed but has acted as a lubricant to further enhance segmental dynamic dysfunction, in some cases leading to degenerative spondylolisthesis. The nonabsorption of disc material also enhances the likelihood of recurrent disc herniations. (Courtesy of Charles V. Burton, M.D.)

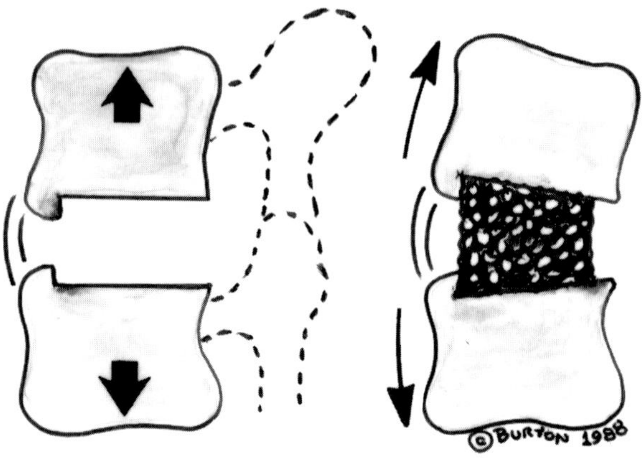

Figure 5 □ To remove the degenerated or herniated disc and the pathologic end plates, a posterior lumbar interbody fusion (PLIF) is being performed with a microporous cancellous block implant of chromium cobalt (S + G Implants, Lubeck, West Germany). The implant is placed under vertebral distraction so that mechanical impaction will allow early stability to be further enhanced by bone ingrowth. Note that the implant's configuration enhances preservation of the lordotic curve (*arrows*). (Courtesy of Charles V. Burton, M.D.)

disc herniations at the same level, PLIF becomes an operative procedure worthy of consideration. At this time, essentially all PLIF is carried out with bone. The disadvantages of this are lack of immediate mechanical stabilization, the possibility of absorption or collapse of the graft, and a number of other considerations, including the potential transmission of slow viruses from allograft material.

By studying hip endoprosthesis systems incorporating cancellous metals, Waisbrod[28] has introduced microporous cancellous block implants (CBI) for PLIF and ALIF. The Institute for Low Back Care in Minneapolis has been serving as the North American test site for these implants as applied to degenerative spinal disease (Fig. 5). On the basis of approximately 50 cases performed since the end of 1987, preliminary observations suggest that CBI may offer significant insights into the future development of PLIF devices.

If the concept of flexible stabilization rather than rigid fixation remains sound, the future for PLIF may well become the era of the "functional artificial disc." Various combinations of metals and polymers are being devised to attach to adjacent vertebrae but to allow some degree of flexibility between these surfaces. This concept is presently being explored at a number of institutions in North America.

SUMMARY

A review of the past and a look to the future suggest that the best devices for spine stabilization have yet to be developed. The theoretical basis upon which they will be prescribed is only now in the process of being defined. The author believes that NFS systems will represent a key element in the exploration of this most challenging frontier.

Acknowledgments

The author would like to express his appreciation to the pioneers of neurosurgery and orthopedics who established the foundation upon which the clinicians of today can build, to my associates Richard Salib and William Akins for their review and support, and to Robert Watkins for his review and suggestions.

References

1. Wiltse, L.L.: History of lumbar spine surgery. *In* White, A.H., Rothman, R.H., and Ray, C.D. (eds.): Lumbar Spine Surgery. St. Louis, C. V. Mosby, 1987.
2. Albee, F.H.: Transplantation of a portion of the tibia into the spine for Pott's disease. J.A.M.A. 57:885, 1911.
3. Hibbs, R.H.: An operation for progressive spinal deformities. New York J. Med. 93:1013, 1911.
4. Campbell, W.C.: An operation for extra articular arthrodesis of the sacroiliac joint. Surg. Gynecol. Obstet. 45:218, 1927.
5. Burns, B.B.: An operation for spondylolisthesis. Lancet 1:1233, 1933.
6. Briggs, B., and Milligan, P.: Chip fusion of the low back following exploration of the spinal canal. J. Bone Joint Surg. 24:125, 1944.
7. Cloward, R.B.: New treatment of ruptured intervertebral discs. Paper read at the Annual Meeting of the Hawaii Territorial Medical Association, May, 1945.
8. Jaslow, I.: Intercorporal bone graft in spinal fusion after disc removal. Surg. Gynecol. Obstet. 82:215, 1946.

9. Venable, C.S., and Stuck, W.G.: Electrolysis controlling factor in the use of metals in treating fractures. J.A.M.A. 3:349, 1939.
10. Harrington, P.R., and Tullos, H.S.: Spondylolisthesis in children. Clin. Orthop. 79:75, 1971.
11. Harrington, P.R., and Dickson, J.H.: Spinal instrumentation in treatment of severe spondylolisthesis. Clin. Orthop. 117:157, 1976.
12. Knodt, T.H., and Larrick, R.: Distraction fusion of the lumbar spine. Ohio State Med. J. 12:140, 1964.
13. Luque, E.: The anatomic basis and development of segmental spinal instrumentation. Spine 7:270–275, 1982.
14. Luque, E.: Interpeduncular segmental screw fixation. Clin. Orthop. 203:20, 1986.
15. Judet, R., et al.: Osteosynthese: Material, techniques, complications. Actualities. Chirurg. Orthop. Hosp. Raymond Pain Care (Paris) 7:196, 1970.
16. Roy-Camille, R.: Internal fixation of the lumbar spine (submitted for publication, 1986).
17. Louis, R.: Fusion of the lumbar and sacral spines by internal fixation with screw plates. Clin. Orthop. 203:18, 1986.
18. Magerl, F.: External skeletal fixation of the lower thoracic and lumbar spine. *In* Current Concepts of External Fixation of Fractures. Berlin, Springer-Verlag, 1982.
19. Kraag, M.H., et al.: An internal fixator for posterior application to short segments of the thoracic, lumbar, or lumbosacral spine: Design and testing. Clin. Orthop. 203:75–98, 1986.
20. Zielke, K., and Strempel, A.V.: Posterior lateral distraction spondylodesis using the twofold sacral bar. Clin. Orthop. 203:151–158, 1986.
21. Cotrel, Y., and Dubousset, J.: The use of pedicle screws and universal instrumentation for spinal fixation. Paper presented to the AO Trauma Course, Davos, Switzerland, Dec., 1985.
22. Steffee, A.: Segmental spine plates with pedicle screw fixation. Clin. Orthop. 203:45, 1986.
23. Liu, Y.K., et al.: Fatigue life improvement of nitrogen-ion implanted pedicle screws.
24. Hsu, K.Y., et al.: Deterioration of motion segments adjacent to lumbar spine fusions. Presented at the annual meeting of the I.S.S.L.S., Miami, April, 1988.
25. Burton, C.V.: The liabilities of fusion. *In* Cauthen, J.C. (ed.): Lumbar Spine Surgery. Baltimore, Williams & Wilkins, 1987, p. 336.
26. Wiltse, L.L.: Personal communication, 1987 to 1988.
27. Simmons, J.W.: Posterior lumbar interbody fusion with posterior elements as chip grafts. Clin. Orthop. Rel. Res. 76:85, 1985.
28. Waisbrod, H.: Personal communication, 1986 to 1988.

Index

Note: Page numbers in *italics* refer to illustrations; page numbers followed by (t) refer to tables.

Abdominal muscles, exercise of, dynamic stretching, for spondylolisthesis, 504, *505–507*
for low back pain, 8
isometric, for spondylolisthesis, 501
Abdominal wall, anatomy of, 409, *409*, *410*
closure of, in transpleural-retroperitoneal approach, 980, *981*
transection of, in anterior extraperitoneal discectomy, 987, *989–990*
in retroperitoneal approach, 982, *982–983*
in transperitoneal approach, 984, *984*
in transpleural-retroperitoneal approach, 978, *978*
Abscess(es), epidural, 717
surgery for, 720–721
treatment of, conservative, 718
paravertebral, in spinal tuberculosis, 702
Absorptiometry, of osteoporosis, 766
Acetylsalicylic acid, for disc herniation, 386–387
Achondroplasia, developmental spinal stenosis in, 558–559, 596(t), 597, *599*
Acromegaly, developmental idiopathic spinal stenosis with, 577
osteoporosis and, 764
Actinobacillus actinomycetemcomitans, vertebral infection from, 721
Acupuncture, for disc herniation, 387
Acute back syndrome, symptomatology of, 385
Adhesions, postoperative, nonsurgical treatment of, 21
Adrenocorticotrophic hormone, for disc herniation, 12
Aging, and bone loss, 763. See also *Osteoporosis*.
and low back pain, 91, 882
disc degeneration from, 246, 369, 375
biochemical changes in, 9, 11, 371–372
composition changes in, 241
facet joint deterioration from, 424–425, *425*
pathoanatomic disc changes in, 371
scoliosis from, 882
Aircraft, vibrations of, low back disorders from, 181–182
Albers-Schönberg disease, pathologic spondylolisthesis from, 484, *485*
Alexithymia, and chronic low back pain, 814
Amniotic sac, development of, 71–72, *72*
Amyloidosis, in ankylosing spondylitis, 641–642
Analgesics, for chronic low back pain, 818–819
Aneurysmal syndrome, in spinal tuberculosis, 701, *703*
Annulus fibrosus, anatomy of, 79, 246, *246*
biomechanics of, 6–8
collagen structure of, 9–10
deterioration of, and postural deformity, 799
in disc degeneration, 261–262
fragmentation of, removal of, in anterior extraperitoneal discectomy, 988, *991*, 995–996, *997*
herniation of, level of, and nerve root canal stenosis, 602
imaging anatomy of, 267, *268*, *272*
innervation of, 13
MRI of, 321, *321*
in degenerative disc disease, *327*
syndesmophytosis of, in ankylosing spondylitis, 639
tangential stressing of, and lumbar loading, 245, *245*
vascular supply of, and low back pain, 10
Anterolisthesis, in degenerative spondylolisthesis, *84*
Antibiotics, for discitis, 736, 738
Antidepressants, tricyclic, for chronic low back pain, 818–819
Anti-inflammatory agents, nonsteroidal, for sciatica, 965–966
for scoliosis, 885
Anus, sphincter of, electrostimulation of, in spinal cord lesion diagnosis, 154, *155*
AO internal fixator, for burst fractures, 680, *684*
Aorta, anatomy of, 409, *410*
incompetence of, in ankylosing spondylitis, 641
Apophyseal joint, and ankylosing spondylitis, 639
asymmetry of, in isthmic spondylolisthesis, 592, *593*
damage to, during spinal surgery, 873(t), 874
dysfunction of, low back pain from, 90
history of, 422
hypoplasia of, with congenital spinal stenosis, 558
Apophysis, fracture of, anterior discectomy for, interbody fusion with, 407, *408–413*, 409–414
Aprotonin, intradiscal, for lumbar disc disease, 20
Arachnoiditis, after laminectomy, fibrinolytic defects in, 660

Arachnoiditis *(Continued)*
classification of, 650
fibrinolytic defects in, 656–658, *657*, *659*
fibrinolytic enhancement therapy for, 658
inflammation and scarring in, 650–651, 651(t), *651–652*
MRI of, 329
pathologic studies of, 651, 653, *653–655*, 655, 655(t)
postoperative, nonsurgical treatment of, 21
Arthritis, peripheral, inflammatory bowel disease in, 646
psoriatic. See also *Spondyloarthropathy, psoriatic.*
classification of, 644(t)
reactive, 642(t), 642–644
bacteria in, 642, 642(t)
clinical presentation of, 642–643
diagnosis of, 642(t), 643–644
evolution of, 643
extra-articular symptoms in, 643
treatment of, 644
rheumatoid, low back pain with, and pregnancy, 842, *842*, 843
Arthrodesis. See *Fusion.*
Arthrography, of facet joints, 112–113, *113–120*, 115, 118, 120
diagnostic value of, 115
history of, 112
indications for, *114*, 115, *116–120*, 118, 120
technique of, 113, *113*, 115
Arthrogryposis, pathologic spondylolisthesis from, 484
Articular cartilage, MRI of, 323, *323*
physical model of, 231–232, *232*
Articular nerve, denervation of, 433–434
Articular process(es), anatomy of, 77, *78*
compression fracture of, degenerative spondylolisthesis from, 483
degeneration of, spinal stenosis from, 285, *286*
dysplastic, congenital spondylolisthesis from, *472*, 473, 476
hypertrophy of, degenerative spondylolisthesis from, 540
developmental idiopathic spinal stenosis from, 562, *563*
vertebral canal narrowing from, 549
inferior, radiographic anatomy of, in developmental spinal stenosis, 560, *561*
stress fracture of, after laminectomy, spondylolisthesis from, 484
malorientation of, in congenital spondylolisthesis, *478*, 479
osteoarthritic changes in, combined spinal stenosis from, *602*
nerve root canal stenosis from, 601–602
superior, enlargement of, spinal stenosis from, 287
erosion of, in degenerative spondylolisthesis, 300, *301*
hypertrophy of, *555*
hypoplasia of, spondylolisthesis from, 480–481
Athletics, contact sports in, stabilization training for, 779, *783–786*
lumbar disc disease from, 173–174
risk factors of, 176–177
Athletics *(Continued)*
stress fractures from, of pars interarticularis, 482
treatment of, 495, *495*, 497
Atrioventricular block, in ankylosing spondylitis, 641
Automanipulation, 807, *807*
Autonomic nervous system, anatomy and physiology of, 450
Axons, anatomy and physiology of, 132, *133*

Back Pain Classification Scale, of chronic low back pain, 817
Back school. See also *Exercise.*
disease-training match in, 787–788
during pregnancy, 844–845
education in, 770–771, 783, 786, 788
exercise in, 771–772
goal acheivement in, 783, 786(t), 786–787
in hospital, 779, 782–883
public education in, 788–789
stabilization training in, 772, *773–778*, 776, 779, *780–786*
Backache, managment strategy for, 50–51, 51(t)
Basivertebral vein, MRI of, 322
Bayonet deformity, in spinal tuberculosis, 701, *704*
Becs de perroquet, in spinal tuberculosis, 701
Bed rest, for disc herniation, 386
Behavioral therapy, operant, for chronic low back pain, 820–821
Bending, biomechanics of, 214, *215*
Benzodiazepines, in chronic low back pain therapy, 818
Biofeedback, for chronic low back pain, 821–822
Biopsy, needle, in pyogenic spondylitis, 711
in septic intervertebral discitis, 718
of vertebral body, in osteoporosis diagnosis, 767
percutaneous, of spinal tumors, 742, *743*
open, after discography, results of, 733(t)
Bladder, dysfunction of, cauda equina injury and, 452–454
clinical neurophysiologic diagnosis of, *154–156*, 156–157
disc herniation and, 385
electrodiagnosis of, 153, *153*
nucleus pulposus herniation and, 399
sacral nerve injury and, 452
functional recovery of, after cauda equina syndrome treatment, 454–455
Bone, cancellous, bone grafting with, in posterior fusion, 463, *467*
replacement of, by granulation tissue, 725, *727*
stressing of, in instrumentation, 204–205, *205*, 205(t)
cortical, bone grafting with, in posterior fusion, 463, *467*
stressing of, in instrumentation, 204–205, *205*, 205(t)
formation of, in pyogenic spondylitis, 711, *714*
metaplastic, in developmental idiopathic spinal stenosis, 577
haversian system of, 762

Bone *(Continued)*
loss of. See *Osteoporosis.*
maturation of, 763
metabolism of, 762
mineral content of, and exercise, 176–177
loss of, measurement of, 766–767
radiography of, 340
physiology of, 761–762
resorption of, causes of, metabolic studies of, in posterior fusion, 457–458
in psoriatic spondyloarthropathy, 645
sclerosis of, in pyogenic spondylitis, 711, *714*
subchondral, sclerosis of, in septic discitis, 716, *716*
types of, 761
Bone grafts, autogenous, in posterior fusion, 463, *466–468*, 469
for pyogenic spondylitis, 718, *719*, 720
interbody, Steffe plates with, biomechanical evaluations of, 204–207, *205*, 205(t)–206(t)
with decompression, in burst fracture treatment, 680, *685*
Bone marrow, disease of, MRI of, 331
Bone scanning. See *Radionuclide imaging.*
Braces. See *Orthosis(es).*
Breast, metastatic carcinoma of, MRI of, 331, *334*
Broom's model, of extracellular matrix, 231–232, *232*
Brown-Séquard syndrome, chymopapain injection and, 441
Brucellosis, vertebral, 721
Bulbocavernosus reflex response testing, of spinal cord lesions, 153–154, *154–155*
Burst fracture. See *Fracture(s), burst.*

Calcitonin, and calcium metabolism, 762
for neurogenic claudication, 19
for spinal stenosis, 603
Calcium, metabolism of, 762
supplementation of, for osteoporosis, 767
Capillaries, constriction of, and intervertebral disc nutrition, 257, *257*, 258
Carcinoma. See also *Tumor(s).*
endometrial, estrogen and, 767
of breast, estrogen and, 707
metastases from, MRI of, 331, *334*
of spine, metastatic, internal fixation of, 951–952, *953*
Cardiovascular disease, in ankylosing spondylitis, 641
Cardiovascular fitness, and industrial back pain, 852–853, *853*
compromise of, smoking and, 257, *257*
Carisoprodol, for muscle spasm, 362
Cauda equina, anatomy of, 132, *133*
avulsion of, treatment of, *688*
compression of, in osteoporosis, 765
in spondylolisthesis, 482
nerve root deterioration from, 137
spinal stenosis from, surgery for, 604
treatment of, 361
imaging anatomy of, 267, *269*, *271–272*, 277, 280, *281*
ischemia of, intermittent neurogenic claudication from, 572
lesions of, electrodiagnosis of, 153, *153*

Cauda equina *(Continued)*
MRI of, 323, *323*
nerve roots of, 134, *134*
compression of, 141–142, *142*
imaging anatomy of, 277, *277*
size of, and vertebral canal size, 591–592
Cauda equina syndrome, 452–454
acute, 453
chronic, 453–454
congenital spondylolisthesis and, 476
in ankylosing spondylitis, 641
physical findings in, 454
prognosis of, 454–455
radiography of, 454
treatment of, 454
Caudal nerve root, compression of, in spinal stenosis, 557
absolute, 572–575, 573(t)–574(t)
secondary, 597, *600*
intermittent neurogenic claudication from, 572–574
injury to, iatrogenic spinal stenosis from, 579
types of, in developmental idiopathic spinal stenosis, 573
vulnerability of, in developmental idiopathic spinal stenosis, 574
Caudography, of developmental idiopathic spinal stenosis, 560, 562, *562–563*
Central nervous system, development of, deficiencies of, malnutrition and, 593
Centrum, development of, 72–73, *75–76*
Cephazolin, in discography, 736
iatrogenic discitis from, 724–725
Cerebrospinal fluid, perfusion of, in cauda equina, 134, *134*
in nerve root sheath, 14–15
Chance fracture, automobile accidents and, 668, *669*, 670
Chemonucleolysis, 441–449
alternative enzymes in, 447
anaphylactic reactions from, 443–445
complications of, prevention of, 446–447
discitis from, 723
failure of, surgical confirmation of, 442–443
for disc herniation, 388
vs other treatments, 443
for disc prolapse, results of, 966–967
for low back pain, 366
for sciatica, with disc herniation, 144–145
history of, 441–442
MRI after, 329
neurologic reactions to, 445–446
patient selection in, 443, 446, 447
results of, 447
technique of, precautions in, 446–447
Chemotherapy, bone marrow replacement in, MRI of, 333
for spinal tuberculosis, 702, 706
Chiropractic. See also *Manipulation; Physiotherapy.*
manipulation in, 793
Chlamydia trachomatis, in reactive arthritis, 642, 642(t)
Chlorpromazine, for chronic low back pain, 819
Chondrification, of vertebrae, 73
Chondrocytes, synthetic activity of, anti-inflammatory drugs in, 12

Chondroitinase ABC, in chemonucleolysis, clinical trials of, 447
Chondroma, in later spinal stenosis, *288–289*
Chondromalacia, of facet joint, 425–426
Chondrosarcoma, of spine, 746, 750, 750(t)
Chordoma, of spine, 746, 750, 750(t)
  surgery for, 753, *754–755*
Chymopapain, anaphylactic reactions to, 443–445
  clinical trials of, history of, 441–442
  for disc herniation, results of, 389–390
  in chemonucleolysis, 366. See also *Chemonucleolysis.*
  intradiscal, for lumbar disc disease, 19–20
  neurologic reactions to, 445–446
Claudication, differential diagnosis of, in low back pain, 88–89
  neurogenic, assessment of, in surgical planning, 957–958
    definition of, 120
    diagnosis of, lumbar nerve root sheath infiltration in, 120–121, 125–126, *126–127*
    in disc herniation, 383
    intermittent, and spinal stenosis treatment, 584–585, 584(t)–585(t)
      in spinal stenosis, 559
        developmental idiopathic, causes of, 572–575
          diagnosis of, 573–574
      radiculopathy in, 573–574, 573(t)–574(t)
    sciatica with, treatment of, 966
    vascular deficiencies in, spinal stenosis with, 18–19, 88–89
  prevalence of, in low back pain, 33
Clear cell sarcoma, surgery for, 753, *756*
Collagen, deposition of, in arachnoiditis, 650, *651*
  laxity of, pregnancy and, low back pain from, 843
  molecular structure of, 232–233, *233*
  MRI appearance of, 267
  network of, 234
    and lumbar loading, 248
  organization of, *246*, 248
  synthesis of, 242
    in disc degeneration, 10–11
  types of, 233(t), 233–234, 247–248
    degenerative changes in, 262–263
Collagenase, clinical trials of, 442
  in chemonucleolysis, 366. See also *Chemonucleolysis.*
  intradiscal injection of, for lumbar disc disease, 20
Compression fracture. See *Fracture(s), compression.*
Computed tomography, 3–D reconstruction in, of pinhole stenosis, *304*
    of spinal stenosis, 287, *289*
      developmental idiopathic, 563, 565, *565–567*
  discography with, in chemonucleolysis, 443
    of recurrent disc herniation, vs postoperative scarring, 352, *354*
    risks of, 356
  lamincetomy planning with, operative results from, 313–317, *316*
Computed tomography *(Continued)*
  myelography with, of foraminal disc herniation, accuracy of, 352–353, *353*
  of disc herniation, with nerve root compression, 308–310, 309(t), *309–310*
  of low back pain, history of, 21
    origin of, reliability of, 341–342
  of lumbar spine anatomy, in axial plane, 267, *268–276*, 277
    in coronal plane, 280, *281–282*, 282
    in sagittal plane, 277–278, *277–281*
    in surgical planning, 961
  of lumbar spine disorders, 283–319. See also specific disorder; e.g., *Spinal stenosis.*
    principles of, 283–285, *284*
  of nucleus pulposus herniation, 347–348
  of osteoporosis, 766
  of pyogenic spondylitis, 711, 715
  of scoliosis, 885
  of spinal fractures, 674, *676*, 677
  of spinal stenosis, developmental idiopathic, 562–563, 565–568, *565–568*, *570*
      midsagittal diameter measurement in, 565–568, *568–570*
    lateral, types of, 286–287, *288*
  of spinal tumors, 742–743
  of vertebral canal, 18
  preoperative, of nucleus pulposus herniation, 400, 401(t)
  vs myelography, of disc herniation and spinal stenosis, 310–317, 312(t)–313(t), *316*
    of lumbar disc disease, 346
    with discography, of nucleus pulposus herniation, 346–353, 349(t)–351(t), *353–355*, 356
      accuracy of, 349–353, 351(t)
      radiographic diagnoses in, 348–349, 349(t)–350(t)
Congenital abnormalities, and low back pain, employment screening for, 846
Construction machinery, vibrations of, low back disorders from, 182
Conus medullaris, anatomy and physiology of, 450
  compression of, spinal stenosis from, surgery for, 604
  imaging anatomy of, 277, *277*, *281*
  injury to, urologic dysfunction from, 452
  ultrasonography of, *679*
Conus medullaris syndrome, 452
Corsets. See *Orthosis(es).*
Corticosteroids, epidural injection of, for sciatica, 365–366
    results of, 388
  facet joint injection of, for inflammation, results of, 434–435
  for disc herniation, 387
  osteoporosis and, 764, *764*
Costal process(es), formation of, 73, *76*
Cotrel-Dubousset instrumentation, for kyphoscoliosis, *890–891*, *896–898*
  for metastatic disease, 952, *953*
  for scoliosis, 889–890, 950–951
    paralytic, 902
  for thoracolumbar spinal deformities, in elderly patients, 903–904

Cotrel-Dubousset instrumentation *(Continued)*
in rib hump excision, 901–902
posterior, results of, 948
sacral fusion with, 898
segmental instrumentation with, advantages of, 947
Crohn's disease, peripheral arthritis in, 646
Cryptococcus, vertebral infection from, 721
Cushing's syndrome, bone resorption from, in posterior fusion, 457
osteoporosis and, 764
Cyst(s), aneurysmal bone, of spine, 743, *748*
synovial, in later spinal stenosis, *288–289*
Cysteine-EDTA, for disc herniation, clinical trials of, 442
Cystometrography, of bladder dysfunction, 156, *156*
Cystometry, of spinal cord lesions, 153–154, *154–155*

Débridement, anterior, for pyogenic spondylitis, 718, *719*, 720
Decompression, for degenerative spondylolisthesis, *496*, 497
segmental instability after, 632–633
for spinal stabilization, biomechanical evaluations of, 197–198, *198*
for spinal stenosis, 605–606
extent of, 606
levels of, 605
segmental instability after, *632*, 633
types of, 606
unilateral vs bilateral procedure in, 605–606
foraminal, for spinal stenosis, 581, *582–583*, 584
fusion with, for disc prolapse, 968
indications for, 966, 966(t)
of disc prolapse, results of, 966–968
of lumbar spine, nerve root sheath infiltration after, 121
pain after, facet arthrography of, 118, *119–210*, 120
orthoses after, 229
posterior, in scoliosis treatment, contraindications to, 903
posterolateral, for burst fractures, 689, *692–695*
repetition of, results of, 875–878, 876(t)–877(t)
undercutting facetectomies in, 957
with bone grafting, in burst fracture treatment, 680, *685*
Defecation, impairment of, in cauda equina syndrome, 453
neural reflexes of, 451, 451(t)
Depression, and chronic low back pain, psychosocial factors in, 811–813
Dermatome(s), definition of, *111*, 111–112
distribution of, in low back pain, 90
in radicular pain, *107*
skin stimulation of, in radiculopathy detection, 150, *150*
Dermomyotome, development of, 72, *73–74*
Desimipramine, for chronic low back pain, 819
Diabetes, anterior thigh pain in, 367
bone resorption from, in posterior fusion, 457
Diabetes *(Continued)*
osteoporosis and, 764
translational segmental instability in, 630
Diaphragm, transection of, in transpleural-retroperitoneal approach, 978, *979*
Diazepam, for disc herniation, 387
for low back pain, 362
addiction in, 365
chronic, 818
Disc space, infection of, after laminectomy, 724
in microsurgery, 406
nomenclature of, 739
narrowing of, after anterior extraperitoneal discectomy, 993, *993*, 996
degenerative, lytic spondylolisthesis with, 295
discitis and, 734, 736, *736*
in pyogenic spondylitis, 711, *713*
in septic discitis, 716, *716*
lateral spinal stenosis from, 290–291, *292*
sciatica resolution from, 144–145
Discectomy. See also *Intervertebral disc(s), excision of.*
anterior, interbody fusion with, advantages of, 407, *408*
extraperitoneal approach to, 412–413, *413*
indications for, 407, *408*
postoperative care in, 413–414
surgical anatomy in, 409, *409–410*
technqiue of, 409–413, *411–413*
transperitoneal approach to, 409–412, *411–412*
lumbar sympathetic ganglionectomy with, results of, 995
vs posterior, 995–996, *997*
definition of, 957
extraperitoneal, anterior, without fusion, 987–988, 988(t), *988–994*, 995–996, 995(t)–996(t), *997*
complications of, 995
disc fragments in, removal of, 995–996, *997*
for low back pain and sciatica, 988, *990–993*
operative findings in, 988, 993, *993–994*, 995
patient age in, 987–988, 988(t)
results of, 995–996, 995(t)–996(t), *997*
technique of, 987, *989–990*
for disc prolapse, results of, 967–968
for low back pain, history of, 4–5
for nerve root canal stenosis, 610–611
for nerve root compression, 972–973
percutaneous, 414, *415*, 420
posterior, vs anterior, 995–996, *997*
Discitis, chemonucleolysis and, 446
developmental stages of, intradiscal procedures and, 728, *730*
diagnosis of, age in, 91
discography and, 353
anterior disc clearance and fusion for, 732, 734, *734–735*, 736, *738*
open biopsy for, 733(t)
iatrogenic, 723–725, *725*, 726(t), *727–730*, 728, 731–732, *732*, 733(t), 734, *734–738*, 736, 738–740
clinical presentation of, 728, 731
etiology of, 724–725

Discitis *(Continued)*
intradiscal procedures and, 723–724
laboratory studies of, 731
nomenclature of, 739
pathology of, 725, *725*, 726(t), *727–730*, 728
radiography of, 731–732, *732*
treatment of, 736, 738–739
intervertebral, septic, 715–717, *716*
MRI of, 716–717
radiography of, 715–716, *716*
treatment of, conservative, 718
surgical, 720
Discogenic pain syndrome, pathophysiology of, 1001
Discography, chemonucleolysis with, neurologic complications from, 445–446
contrast material extravasation in, 352
CT scanning with, of recurrent disc herniation, vs postoperative scarring, 352, *354*
discitis after, 723–724. See also *Discitis, iatrogenic.*
developmental stages of, 728, *730*
histopathology of, 725, 726(t)
prevention of, 736, 738–739
treatment of, 732, 734, *734–735*
of disc degeneration, pain correlation with, 374
of disc herniation, accuracy of, 353, *353*, *355*
of low back pain, history of, 22
in scoliosis, 883, 889
reliability of, 342
of nuclear pulposus degeneration, 734, *735*
of nucleus pulposus herniation, 347
injection pain in, 349, 350–351
of pain origin, reliability of, 342
side effects of, 348, 351, 353
vs CT scanning, of lumbar disc disease, 346
vs myelography, with CT scanning, of nucleus pulposus herniation, 346–353, 349(t)–351(t), *353–355*, 356
accuracy of, 349–353, 351(t)
radiographic diagnoses in, 348–349, 349(t)–350(t)
Distraction, techniques of, for chronic low back pain, 821
Diving, lumbar disc disease from, 173–174
Dorsal root ganglion, anatomy of, and spinal stenosis, 556
compression of, radicular pain from, 138
imaging anatomy of, 267, *272–274*, 277, *279*, *281*
MRI of, 321, 322, *322*
vascular supply of, 134–135
Dorsiflexion, assessment of, 96–97
weakness of, disc herniation and, 384, *384*
Drug(s), anti-inflammatory, and synovial cellular response, 12
for spinal stenosis, 603
nonsteroidal, for ankylosing spondylitis, 641–642
for scoliosis, 885
antimicrobial, for discitis, 736, 738
antituberculous, for spinal tuberculosis, 702, 706
bone resorption from, in posterior fusion, 457
for disc herniation, 386–387
for low back pain, 362
Drug(s) *(Continued)*
chronic, 818–819, 837
in pregnancy, 844
Dura mater, injury to, during microsurgery, 406
Dural sac, compression of, spinal stenosis from, 595
Dwarfism, developmental spinal stenosis in, 558–560, 596(t), 597, *599*
Dwyer instrumentation, anterior, biomechanical evaluation of, 945
for thoracolumbar spinal deformities, in elderly patients, 903–904
segmental instrumentation with, advantages of, 947–948
vs Zielke instrumentation, 892
Dysentery, reactive arthritis from, 642(t), 642–643
Dysostosis, cheirolumbar, 577

Ectoderm, development of, 72
Edward's sleeves, for burst fracture, *692–693*
Ejaculation, neural reflexes of, 451(t), 451–452
Electrodiagnostic testing. See also *Neurophysiology, clinical.*
of low back pain, 146(t)–147(t), 146–154, *148–150*, *153–156*, 156–159
Electromyography. See also *Electrodiagnostic testing; Neurophysiology, clinical.*
neurologic deficit detection with, 146, 146(t), 148, *148*
of lumbar spine, in surgical planning, 962–963
of spinal musculature, 191
Electrophysiology, advances in, in low back pain diagnosis, 21–23
Electrotherapy, for disc herniation, 387
Embryo, development of, 71–72, *72*
End plate, anatomy of, 246, *246*
burst fracture of, 664, 666
destruction of, discitis and, 731, 732, *732*, *734*, 736, *737–738*
nucleus pulposus herniation and, discitis and, 725, *727–728*
granular invasion of, discitis and, 725, *725*, *729*
imaging anatomy of, 267, *274*, *280*
irregularity of, in septic discitis, 716, *716*
osteophytic spurring of, nerve root entrapment from, 295, *297*
postoperative changes of, in disc degeneration, MRI of, 327, *329*
sclerosis of, and disc degeneration, 1000–1001, *1001*
imaging anatomy of, *281*, *282*
posterior interbody fusion for, 1002, *1002*
Endoderm, development of, 72, *72*
Endorphins, CSF diffusion of, in nerve root compression, 14–15
production of, by exercise, 65
Enterobacteria, reactive arthritis from, 642(t), 642–643
Enthesis, inflammation of, in ankylosing spondylitis, 639–640
Enthesopathy, in ankylosing spondylitis, 639–640
Enzymes, disc degeneration from, 241
Epidural fat, in later spinal stenosis, *288–289*

Epidural fat *(Continued)*
MRI of, 321, 322, *322*
Epidural vein, MRI of, 322
Erector muscle, imaging anatomy of, *270, 275–276*
Ergonomics, of work environment, postural considerations in, 217–218
Erythrocyte sedimentation rate, elevation of, in discitis, 731
in epidural abscesses, 717
in pyogenic spondylitis, 708
Estrogen therapy, for osteoporosis, 767–768
Ewing's sarcoma, of spine, 746, 750, 750(t)
Exercise. See also *Back school; Rehabilitation.*
and disc nutrition, 10, 253–255, *254*, 258
during pregnancy, 844–845
dynamic, of abdominal muscles, for spondylolisthesis, 504, *505–507*
for disc herniation, 387
for low back pain, abdominal strengthening in, 8
principles of, 771–772
for lumbar spine disorders, 802–803
for osteoporosis, 767
for postural correction, in spondylolisthesis, 504, 507–508, *507–509*
in hospital, 779, 782–883
isometric, of abdominal muscles, for spondylolisthesis, 501, 502, *503*
stabilization training in, 772, *773–778*, 776, 779, *780–786*
stretching, of spinal muscles, for spondylolisthesis, 502, *503–504*
Exostosis(es), in developmental idiopathic spinal stenosis, with degenerative spondylolisthesis, *565–567*
multiple, in developmental spinal stenosis, 560
Extension injury, treatment of, 689

F response testing, of neurologic deficits, 148–149, *149*
Facet joint(s), aging of, 424–425, *425*
anatomy of, *77, 78*, 424–429, *425–429*
and axial rotational segmental instability, 630, *630*
ankylosis of, 639
arthritis of, 373
nerve root irritation from, history of, 422–423
arthrography of, 112–113, *113–120*, 115, 118, 120. See also *Arthrography, of facet joints.*
arthropathy of, inflammation from, corticosteroid injections for, results of, 434–435
pathogenesis of, 439
asymmetry of, low back pain from, history of, 422
biomechanics of, 8, 427
capsular entrapment of, manipulation for, 807–808, *808*
cartilage-bone interface of, *114–115*
chondromalacia of, 425–426
decortication of, in posterior fusion, 463, *466*
degeneration of, in degenerative spondylolisthesis, 118, *119–210*, 120, *286, 301*
Facet joint(s) *(Continued)*
nerve root entrapment from, 969
radiography of, in degenerative spondylolisthesis, 540
denervation of, results of, 432–434
enlargement of, spinal stenosis from, *84–85*
failure of, cyclic loading and, 613
fixation of, for lumbosacral disc degenerative disease, 949, *949*
history of, 916–917
functions of, 423–424, *425*
hypertrophy of, front-back spinal stenosis from, 302, *303*
lateral spinal stenosis from, 290
MRI of, in disc degeneration, 325, 327, *328*
hypoplasia of, spondylolisthesis from, 481–482
imaging anatomy of, *281*
injection of, pain correlation with, 429–432
injury to, spinal instability from, 189, *189*
innervation of, 423–424, 428–429, *428–429*
instability of, pain from, 427
loading of, 426–427
absorbing capacity of, 666
meniscus of, 425, *426*
neural blockage of, in pain assessment, 14
in scoliosis, 889
orientation of, in congenital spondylolisthesis, *478*
osteoarthrosis of, nerve root entrapment from, 957
posterior fusion of, 456
referred pain from, 423
sclerosis of, in scoliosis, 883
stress to, transpedicle fixation and, 999–1000, *999–1000*
synovial reaction of, in disc degeneration, 370–371
tropism of, in degenerative spondylolisthesis, 483
Facet syndrome, 422–441, *425–429, 437–438*
anatomy of, 424–429, *425–429*
corticosteroid injections for, patient selection in, 435–436
results of, 434–435
technique of, 435–436, *437–438*, 438–439
definition of, 14
degenerative arthritis in, nerve root compression from, *427*, 427–428
denervation for, history of, 423–424
results of, 432–434
diagnosis of, 59
criteria for, 429–432
history of, 90, 422–424
innervation in, 428–429, *428–429*
nerve root entrapment in, history of, 551
pain localization in, and treatment, 438–439
symptoms of, 431
treatment of, 435–436, *437–438*, 438–439
options in, 432
results of, 432–435
Facetectomy, undercutting, for nerve root compression, 968–969, *969*, 973
Femoral nerve, irritation of, vs sciatic nerve irritation, 99
Femoral stretch test, 99
Fenestration, definition of, 956
Fetus, development of, stages in, 71

Fibrin, deposition of, chronic tissue damage from, 655–656
Fibrinolytic enhancement therapy, for low back pain, 658, *660*
Fibrinolytic system, 656, *656*
Fibromyalgia syndrome, in low back pain, 57–58
Fibrositis, in low back pain, 57
Flexion-distraction injury, 666, 668, *668–669*, 670, *676–677*
  burst type, 670–671, *674–675*
  treatment of, 680, *686–688*, 689
Flexion-rotational injury, 670, *671*
Fluoride, supplementation of, for osteoporosis, 768
Fluorosis, spinal stenosis in, classification of, 579
Football, spondylolisthesis from, 174–175
Foraminal fat, MRI of, 321, *322*
Foraminal recess, nerve root entrapment in, history of, 551
Fracture(s), axial loading, of lumbar spine, 662
  burst, 664, 666, *667*
    biomechanics of, 662–663, *663*
    decompression for, 689, *692–693*
    failure patterns in, 664, 664(t)
    flexion-distraction injuries with, 668
    Kostuik-Harrington instrumentation for, 909, *911*
    treatment of, 680, *682–685*
  Chance, trauma and, 668, *669*, 670
  classification of, 664, 664(t)
  compression, 664, *665–666*
    failure patterns in, 664, 664(t)
    flexion-distraction injuries with, 668
    osteoporosis and, 763–765, *764–765*
      MRI of, 331, *332*
    scoliosis from, 882
    treatment of, 680, *681*
  evaluation of, 671, 674
  extension, 670, *670*
    treatment of, 689
  failure patterns of, 664, 664(t)
  fatigue, repetitive lumbar loading and, 172, 177–178, *178*
  flexion-distraction, 666, 668, *668–669*, 670
    classification of, 668, *668*
    failure patterns in, 664, 664(t)
  of lumbar spine, internal fixation of, 951
  of posterior arch, 671, *675*
  of spine, secondary spinal stenosis from, 597
  orthoses for, 691, 696
  osteoporosis and, 763
  radiography of, 674, *676–679*, 677
  secondary spinal stenosis from, 597
  segmental instability from, 629(t)
  stress, of pars interarticularis, 473, *473*
    vs fatigue, 172
  treatment of, algorithm for, 696
    goals of, 678–680
    nonoperative vs operative, 678–680
Fracture(s)-dislocation(s), 670–671, *670–674*
  failure patterns in, 664, 664(t)
  flexion-distraction injury in, *676–677*
    burst type, 670–671, *675*
    treatment of, 680, *686–688*, 689
  flexion-rotational injury in, 670, *671*
Fracture(s)-dislocation(s) *(Continued)*
  segmental instability from, 629(t)
  shear injuries in, 670, *672–674*
  treatment of, 689, *690*
Fusion, acquired spondylolisthesis after, 634
  and disc nutrition, 255, *255–256*
  anterior, for pyogenic spondylitis, 718, *719*, *720*
    for spondylolisthesis, in children and adolescents, 519
    radical resection with, for spinal tuberculosis, 707–708, *709–712*
  definition of, 998
  discectomy with, for low back pain, 17
    pseudarthrosis after, 634
    results of, 195–196
  extension of, in scoliosis treatment, 899–900, *899–902*
  for kyphosis, complications of, 908
  for low back pain, rationale of, 195–196
    results of, 375
      vs nonoperative treatment, 373
  for lumbar disc disease, rationale of, 195–196
  for nerve root canal stenosis, 611
  for progressive degenerative scoliosis, 631
  for segmental instability, in low back pain, 363–364
    retrolisthetic, 631
  for spondylolisthesis, congenital, 491, *491*
    degenerative, *496*, 497
    in children and adolescents, 517, 519
    isthmic, 488, *488–490*, 491
  history of, 998
  indications for, in spinal stenosis, 607
  interbody, anterior, discectomy with, advantages of, 407, *408*
        extraperitoneal approach to, 412–413, *413*
        indications for, 407, *408*
        postoperative care in, 413–414
        surgical anatomy in, 409, *409–410*
        technique of, 409–413, *411–413*
        transperitoneal approach to, 409–412, *411–412*
      discitis after, 734, 736, *736–737*
      for discitis, 738–739
    for disc herniation, disadvantages of, 1002
    microporous cancellous block implants in, 1002, *1002*
    posterior, for disc herniation, results of, 968
      future trends in, 1000–1002, *1001–1002*
  MRI after, 327, 329, *330*
  pedicle screw fixation in. See also *Transpedicle fixation.*
    for spondylolisthesis, 491, *492–493*
  posterior, 456–460, *460–468*, 463, 466, 469–470
    anesthesia in, 459
    bone grafts in, 463, 466, *466–468*
    bone resorption in, metabolic studies of, 457–458
    clinical presentation in, 457
    future trends in, 998–1000, *999–1000*
    history of, 456–457
    indications for, 457
    internal fixation in, 459
    pain control after, 469
    patient positioning in, 459

Fusion *(Continued)*
postoperative care in, 466, 469
preoperative care in, 457–459
smoking cessation before, 457
technique of, 456, 460, *461–466*, 463
vascular anatomy in, 459–460, *460*
posterolateral, for spondylolisthesis, degenerative, in spinal stenosis, 610
in children and adolescents, *525*, 525–526
postoperative pain in, facet arthrography of, 118, *119–210*, 120
repetition of, results of, 875–878, 876(t)–877(t)
rerotational, of facet joint, 630
sacral, Cotrel-Dubousset instrumentation in, 898
in scoliosis treatment, 897–899
Zielke instrumentation in, 892, 898
segmental instability after, *633*, 633–634
spinal stenosis after, classification of, 597, 601
iatrogenic, 579
with decompression, for disc prolapse, 968
for spondylolisthesis, in adults, 540, 542–543

Gallium, imaging with, of pyogenic spondylitis, 715
Gastrointestinal tract, assessment of, in scoliosis, 884
dysfunction of, bone resorption from, in posterior fusion, 457
clinical neurophysiologic diagnosis of, *154–156*, 156–157
electrodiagnosis of, 153, *153*
nucleus pulposus herniation and, 399
Genitalia, dysfunction of, electrodiagnosis of, 153, *153*
Genitourinary tract, assessment of, in scoliosis, 884
functional recovery of, after cauda equina syndrome, 454–455
neural elements of, 450
Gluteal artery, superior, anatomy of, in posterior fusion, 460, *460*
Gluteal muscles, assessment of, in low back pain, 99
weakness of, disc herniation and, *384*, 384–385
Glycosaminoglycans, in articular cartilage, 234–236, *235*
in intervertebral disc, associated disease with, 9
in low back pain, 6
polysulfated, biochemical studies of, in disc degeneration, 13
synthesis of, in disc degeneration, 10–11
Granuloma, eosinophilic, of spine, 743, *749*
Guillain-Barré syndrome, chemonucleolysis and, 446
Gymnastics, spondylolisthesis from, 174–175

H reflex testing, of neurologic deficits, 148–149, *149*
Hall-Fairbank-Pynsent classification, of low back pain, 100–103, 101(t)–102(t)
Haloperidol, for chronic low back pain, 819
Hamstring(s), reflex of, in low back pain, 99–100
tightening of, in spondylolisthesis, fusion for, 493, *494–495*
Harrington rods, complications of, 947
for burst fractures, *692–693*
for fracture-dislocation injuries, 680, *686–688*, 689
for kyphotic deformities, complications of, 909
for metastatic disease, 952, *953*
for thoracolumbar spinal deformities, in elderly patients, 903–904
history of, 917, 919
lumbar lordosis loss from, 904, *906*
posterior, evaluation of, 944–945
for scoliosis, 889–890
sacral fusion with, lumbar lordosis loss from, 897
Hemangioma, of spine, 743, *745*, 746
Hematoma, postoperative, in recurrent disc herniation, *317*
Hemilaminectomy, definition of, 956
Hemivertebra, vs spinal tuberculosis, 701, *704*
Hemorrhage, cerebral, chemonucleolysis and, 446
Hensen's node, development of, 71, *72*
Hepatic insufficiency, bone resorption from, in posterior fusion, 457
Hernia, anterior thigh pain in, 367
Hip joint, assessment of, 96, 97, 99
degeneration of, diagnosis of, nerve root sheath infiltration in, 126, 128, *129–130*
pain in, 94
from anterior thigh, 367
vs low back pain, 97
Hockey, spondylolisthesis from, 174–175
Homocystinuria, osteoporosis and, 764
Hormones, in sexual response, 451–452
Hydroxypyridinium, in disc degeneration, 263
Hyperparathyroidism, bone resorption from, in posterior fusion, 457
Hyperthyroidism, osteoporosis and, 764
Hypnosis, for chronic low back pain, 822–823
Hypochondriasis, and chronic low back pain, 813–814
Hypochondroplasia, developmental spinal stenosis in, 559
Hypogastric plexus, superior, anatomy of, 409, *410*
Hypothyroidism, bone resorption from, in posterior fusion, 457
Hysteria, and chronic low back pain, 813–814

Iliac crest, bone grafts from, in burst fracture treatment, 680, *685*
in kyphosis treatment, *912*, 913
in posterior fusion, 463, *466–468*, 469
in sacral fusion, 898–899
Iliac vein, anatomy of, 409, *410*
Ilium, imaging anatomy of, *275–276*
Illness, biopsychosocial concept of, in low back pain, 44–45, *45*
disease model of, in low back pain, 43–44

Illness *(Continued)*
in low back disorders, 46–48, *47*, 47(t)
Imagery techniques, for chronic low back pain, 821
Imaging. See also *Computed tomography; Magnetic resonance imaging (MRI).*
3–D, of lateral spinal stenosis, 284–285
of lumbar spine anatomy, 266–267, *268–282*, 277–278, 280, 282
in axial plane, 267, *268–276*, 277
in coronal plane, 280, *281–282*, 282
in sagittal plane, 277–278, *277–281*
Immobilization, after spondylolisthesis repair, 521
Immune system, dysfunction of, malnutrition and, 593
Impotence, clinical neurophysiologic diagnosis of, 156–157
Incontinence, in spinal fracture, *692–693*
sacral nerve injury and, 452
Infection(s), bacterial, in discitis, 724–725
of bone, pathologic spondylolisthesis from, 484
of disc space, in microsurgery, 406
pyogenic, of spine, 708, 711, *713–715*, 715–718, *716*, *719*, 720–721
classification of, 708
secondary spinal stenosis from, 597
tuberculous, of spine. See *Tuberculosis, of spine.*
Inflammatory bowel disease, with inflammatory spondyloarthropathies, 646
Instrumentation, anterior, biomechanical evaluation of, 945, 947
for degenerative disc disease, 949–950
segmental fixation with, advantages of, 947–948, *948*
results of, 948
AO internal fixator in, for burst fractures, 680, *684*
biomechanical evaluations of, 196–201, *198–200*, 200(t)
technique of, 201–204, *202–204*
Cotrel-Dubousset. See *Cotrel-Dubousset instrumentation.*
dual locking hook spinal rods in, for burst fractures, 680, *682–683*
for compression fractures, 680, *681*
for fracture-dislocations, *690*
Dwyer. See *Dwyer instrumentation.*
future development of, 952–953
Harrington. See *Harrington rods.*
implants in, advantages and disadvantages of, *947*, 947–948
desired characteristics of, 942–943
internal fixation in, 941–945, *946–953*, 947–955
extent of, 947
goals of, 942–943
history of, 941–942
indications for, 941
techniques of, 948–953, *949–953*
loading of, biomechanics of, 943–944
Luque. See *Luque instrumentation.*
nonmetallic flexible stabilization in, 999–1000, *999–1000*
posterior, biomechanical evaluations of, 944–945, *946*
for burst fractures, 680, *682–685*

Instrumentation *(Continued)*
segmental fixation with, advantages of, 947
results of, 948
rigid fixation in, complications of, 999
segmental fixation with, techniques of, 948–953, *949–953*
theories of, 999
transitional syndrome from, 999
transpedicle fixation in. See *Transpedicle fixation.*
Zielke. See *Zielke instrumentation.*
International Society for the Study of the Lumbar Spine (ISSLS), lumbar spine disease studies of, 5
Interspinous ligament, imaging anatomy of, 277
Intervertebral disc(s), aging of, 369
vs degeneration, 261–264
anatomy of, 77, *78*, 79
biochemistry of, 9–13, 231–239, *232–233*, 233(t), *235*, *237*, *239–240*, 240(t), 241–242
biomechanics of, history of, 5–9
blood supply of, and low back pain, 10
chemical structure of, and fluid content, 9–10
collagen network of, 6–7, 234, 247–248
collagen/proteoglycan matrix of, 246, *247*
composition of, 239, 240(t), 241, *245–247*, 245–248
and hydration, loading in, 239, *240*
cellular, 248, *249*
degeneration of, biochemistry of, 262–264
physicochemical function and, 248–250, *250*
cyclic loading of, experimental models of, 614, *614–616*, 616
degeneration of, 81, *82*, 83. See also *Lumbar disc disease.*
abnormal motion in, radiography of, 623, *625*
aging and, 246, 375, 623(t)
radiography of, 374
autoimmune activity in, 11–12
biochemistry of, 9
and pain syndromes, 371
animal models of, 263–264
causes of, 58
CT scanning of, with discography, radial fissures in, 352, *353*
definitions of, 369
disc volume reduction in, 1000–1001, *1001*
disease model of, 369, 372
enzyme regulation in, 11
genetic factors in, 12
histologic, 261–262
internal fixation for, 949–950, *949–952*
low back pain from, 191
etiology of, 369–370
macroscopic, 261
motion segment instability from, 374–375
pathoanatomic analysis of, 372–373
MRI of, 324–325, *324–328*, 327
nerve root compression and, criteria of, 394
pain correlation with, 369, 370, 374
pathoanatomy of, 370–371
radicular leg pain in, discography of, 355

Intervertebral disc(s) *(Continued)*
radiography of, pain correlation with, 373–374
reliability of, 340–341
sex distribution in, 623(t)
spinal stenosis from, 285
venous congestion in, 278, 280, *280*
vs aging, 261–264
embryology of, 73, *74*
notochordal tissue in, *76*
excision of. See also *Discectomy.*
failure of, prevention of, 874–875
rates of, 872
reasons for, 873(t)–874(t), 873–875, 878
initial, results of, 872–873, 873(t)
repetition of, results of, 875–878, 876(t)–877(t)
segmental instability after, 632
technical considerations in, 875
extracellular matrix of, 248
fat pads of, imaging anatomy of, 267, *269*
fluid transport in, 249–250, *250*
granulation tissue in, discitis and, 736, *738*
herniation of, abnormal lateral bending in, radiography of, 342
after fusion, *633*, 633–634
biochemistry of, 9
biomechanics of, 6–8
bladder dysfunction from, 385
cauda equina syndrome from, 453
chemonucleolysis for, 19–21, 388, 441–449. See also *Chemonucleolysis.*
contained, 394, *394*
CT scanning of, vs myelography and discography, 346–353, 349(t)–351(t), *353–355*, 356. See also specific imaging technique.
definition of, 382
developmental idiopathic spinal stenosis from, *562–563*
diagnosis of, 382–385, *384*
CSF examination in, 385
patient history in, 382–383
physical examination in, 383
sensory disturbance in, 385
sensory-evoked potentials in, 385
straight-leg raising in, 383–384
discectomy for, 14, 23
anterior, interbody fusion with, 407, *408–413*, 409–414
fusion with, 17
history of, 4–5
percutaneous, 414, *415*
discitis and, 736, *738*
discography of, accuracy of, 353, *353*, *355*
vs CT scanning and myelography, 346–353, 349(t)–351(t), *353–355*, 356. See also specific technique.
epidemiology of, 7
fusion for, interbody, posterior, 1002, *1002*
history of, 2–5, 381
hypermobility in, radiography of, 342–343
in degenerative spondylolisthesis, *286*
in developmental idiopathic spinal stenosis, MRI of, *564*
in pregnancy, 840
lateral, and lytic spondylolisthesis, 296, *298–299*, 300

Intervertebral disc(s) *(Continued)*
MRI of, *308*
manipulation for, 810
motor deficits in, *384*, 384–385
MRI of, 324–325, *324–328*, 327
accuracy of, 356
multiple, in developmental idiopathic spinal stenosis, 559, 577
myelography of, vs CT scanning and discography, 346–353, 349(t)–351(t), *353–355*, 356. See also specific technique.
natural history of, conservative vs operative treatment in, 963–964
nerve root compression from, 135–136, *136*
biomechanics of, 141–145, *142–144*
CT scanning of, 308–310, 309(t), *309–310*
functional changes in, 138–139, *139*
noncontained, *394*, 394–395
pain differeniation in, 13–14
pain mechanisms in, 137–138
radiography of, 385
recurrent, and surgery failure, 873(t), 873–874
imaging of, *317*
pathophysiology of, 1001, *1001*
vs postoperative scarring, 352, *354*
reflex changes from, 385
sciatica in, patient age in, *143–144*, 143–145
segmental motion in, radiography of, 342–343
spinal stenosis with, CT scanning of, vs myelography, 310–317, 312(t)–313(t), *316*
staging of, 382, 395, *396–399*, 397
stenotic compression from, 557
surgery for, 366–367, 388. See also *Discectomy; Intervertebral disc(s), excision of.*
anatomy in, 395, *396–397*
contraindications to, 400, 400(t)
history of, 393(t)
repetition of, results of, 875–876, 876(t)
techniques of, 401–414, *402–403*, 402(t)–404(t), *405–413*, 407(t). See also *Nucleus pulposus, herniation of, surgery for.*
treatment of, back school in, 386
bed rest in, 386
conservative, 386–387
vs surgery, 963–964
drug therapy in, 386
options in, 386
physiotherapy in, 387
protocol for, 390
results of, 388–390
vs aging, biochemical changes in, 371–372
vs stenosis, 594–595
hydration of, 248
and aging, 372
and proteoglycans, 238–239, *239*
imaging anatomy of, 267, *268*, 277, *277*
infections of, surgery for, extrapleural-retroperitoneal approach to, 975
inflammation of. See also *Discitis.*
pathology of, 728, *728*
injury to, lumbar torsion and, 178–179

Longitudinal ligament *(Continued)*
posterior, hypertrophy of, spinal stenosis from, 579–580
Lordosis, lumbar, caudal nerve root compression in, intermittent neurogenic claudication from, 572, 574–575
loss of, consequences of, 904, *905*
etiology of, 904–905
in degenerative spondylolisthesis, 540
pregnancy and, 843
prevention of, in scoliosis, 886–887, *886–887*
radiographic measurement of, 338
restoration of, 904–907, *905–909*
Cotrel-Dubousset instrumentation for, *890–891*, 895–897, *896–898*
in kyphoscoliosis, instrumentation for, 889, *890–891*
Low back pain, acute, as potential chronic problem, 815–816
treatment of, conservative, results of, 16
aging and, 882
vs disc degeneration, 261–264
assessment of, in spinal surgery failure, 879
biomechanics of, history of, 5–9
biopsychosocial concept of, 44–45, *45*
cauda equina syndrome in, 361, 453
chronic, alexithymia in, 814
behavioral therapy for, 837
operant, 820–821
depression with, psychosocial factors in, 811–813
disability from, 854
fitness and, 836–837
functional recovery from, 827–839
barriers to, 835–836
program of, 836–838, 837(t)
interpersonal stressors in, 815
organic vs psychogenic basis of, 816–817
personality in, 814–815
psychiatric evaluation of, 817–818
psychodynamic psychotherapy for, 823
psychophysiologic model of, 814–815
psychosocial factors in, 813–814, 836
and disability, 854
reconditioning for, 837
somatosensory model of, 811
treatment of, bed rest in, disability from, 49–50, 50(t)
biofeedback in, 821–822
cognitive approaches in, 822
distraction in, 821
follow-up in, 837–838
group therapy in, 823
hypnosis in, 822–823
imagery techniques in, 821
psychologic approaches to, 811–827
relaxation in, 821
respondent techniques in, 821–822
results of, 16–17
vs acute, 42–43, 43(t)
classification of, 100–103, 101(t)–102(t)
claudication in, 88–89. See also *Claudication.*
prevalence of, 33
congenital abnormalities and, employment screening for, 846
CT scanning of, principles of, 283–285, *284*
derangement syndrome in, 798–800, 803–804
Low back pain *(Continued)*
description of, 94
diagnosis of, 59, 360
categories of, 59, 60(t)
clinical neurophysiology in. See *Neurophysiology, clinical.*
facet arthrography in. See *Arthrography, of facet joints.*
historical aspects of, 89–91
laboratory studies in, 364
lumbar nerve root sheath infiltration in. See *Lumbar nerve, root sheath infiltration of.*
mechanical, 794–796
medical evaluation in, 364
musculoskeletal assessment in, 95–100
neurologic assessment in, 13–16, 96–100
limitations of, 829–830
patient history in, 91–95, 360
physical examination in, 95–100, 361
vs clinical neurophysiologic testing, 147
physical vs psychologic factors in, 41(t), 46–48, *47*, 47(t)
disability from, 34–35, 38, 39(t), *40–41*, 41–43, 41(t)–43(t)
assessment of, 94–95
economic factors of, 828
disc degeneration with. See also *Intervertebral disc(s), degeneration of.*
pain correlation with, 373–374
disc herniation with. See also *Intervertebral disc(s), herniation of.*
pain mechanisms in, 137–138
discectomy for. See *Discectomy.*
discogenic, assessment of, 99
discography of. See *Discography.*
disease model of, 43–44
dysfunction syndrome in, 798, 803
economic consequences of, 35(t), 35–37, *36*, 36(t)
epidemiology of, 7
etiology of, asymptomatic vs symptomatic, 107
mechanical fatigue failure in, 176–177, 213, *213*
multifactorial aspects of, 589–590
muscular dysfunction in, 57–58, 433
overexertion in, 212–214, *213*
pathoanatomic changes in, 371
fibrinolytic defect in, hypothesis of, *660*, 660–661
fibrinolytic enhancement therapy for, 658, *660*
fibrinolytic studies of, 656–658, *657*, 657(t), *659*
fibrosis and, 649–650
fusion for. See *Fusion.*
glycosaminoglycans in. See *Glycosaminoglycans.*
history of, 1–31
idiopathic, industrial occupations and, 869
impairment from, 34–35
in ankylosing spondylitis, 638, 638(t)
in degenerative spondylolisthesis, 540
in discitis, 731
in pregnancy, 840–845, *841–842*. See also *Pregnancy, low back pain in.*
in scoliosis, 882–883, 889
treatment of. See *Scoliosis, surgery for.*

Low back pain *(Continued)*
inflammation and, 649–650
leg pain with. See also *Leg pain.*
facet arthropathy and, 430
management of, results of, 16
magnitude of, *32*, 32–38, 33(t)–36(t), *36*
manipulation for. See *Manipulation.*
mechanisms of, 90–91
motion segment in. See *Motion segment.*
myofascial, 432
natural history of, 38, *39*, *41*, 41–43, 42(t)–43(t)
occupational factors in. See *Occupations, industrial, low back pain from.*
origin of, CT scanning of, reliability of, 341–342
facet joint injection of, 429–432
myelography of, reliability of, 341–342
radiography of, reliability of, 341–342
structural vs neural, 13–14
orthoses for, 224–229. See also *Orthosis(es).*
pathogenesis of, 793–794
factors in, 649–650
patterns of, 92–94
physician visits for, 33, 33(t)
physiotherapy for. See *Physiotherapy.*
postoperative, facet arthrography of, 118, *119–120*, 120
postpartum, 844
postural syndrome in, 796, 798, 803
posture for, 508
recumbent, 218
predisposing factors of, 381–382
prevention of, cardiovascular fitness in, 64
exercise in, 64
public education in, 788–789
prognosis of, 388–389
psychologic factors in, 15–16, 56–57, 61, 64, 94
radicular pain in, 367–368, 375
radiography of, 59, 363–364. See also specific techniques and disorders; e.g., *Computed tomography; Spinal stenosis.*
and pain symptoms, 342–343
in surgical planning, 960–963, *962*
interpretation of, 338
referred pain in, 367
repetitive lumbar loading and, 172–177
research on, treatment advances from, 16 23
sacroiliac joint defects and, 3–5
sciatica with. See *Sciatica.*
segmental instability and. See *Segmental instability.*
signs and symptoms of, neurogenic vs vascular, 93
nonorganic, in surgical planning, 960, 961(t)
onset of, 92
parameters in, 244–245, *245*
smoking and, 658
spa treatment for, 508–509
spinal instability and. See *Spinal instability.*
spondylolysis and, 363
surgery for, 358, 360
failure of, 46, 61
indications for, 366–367
prevalence of, 34, *34*
results of, 43, 43(t)

Low back pain *(Continued)*
systemic disease in, 94
thigh pain with, *367*, 367–368
treatment of, algorithm of, 358, *359*, 360–368
back school in, 364–365. See also *Back school.*
bed rest in, 48(t), 48–50, 50(t)
chemonucleolysis in, 19–21
indications for, 366
clinical models of, 38, 39(t), *39–41*, 41(t)–43(t), 41–51, *45*, *47*, 47(t)–48(t), 50(t)–51(t)
conservative, 361. See also *Back school; Exercise; Physiotherapy.*
diagnostic basis of, 61, 62(t)–63(t)
drug therapy in, 362
economic costs of, 360
exercise in, 15, 61, 64–66, 363, 502, *502–508*, 504, 507, 771–772. See also *Back school; Exercise.*
goals of, 358, 360
history of, 2
management strategy in, 50–51, 51(t)
orthoses in, 362–363. See also *Orthosis(es).*
persistent pain in, 365
physical activity in, 49–50, 50(t)
physical vs psychologic factors in, 42(t), 43(t), 48
psychologic assessment in, 15–16, 365
research in, 16–23
rest in, 361–362
results of, *40–41*, 45–48, *47*, 47(t)
stabilization training in, 772, *773–778*, 776, 779, *780–786*
success of, 42
surgery in, results of, 17
vs nontreatment, 42, 42(t)
types of, 102(t), 102–103
vascular changes and, 649–650
vertebral canal size in, 17–18, 589, *590*
vibration and, 180–184
vs hip joint pain, 97
vs sciatica, 363–366
without radiculopathy, sources of, 432
Lumbar artery, arteriosclerosis of, leg weakness from, 18
Lumbar disc disease. See also entries under *Intervertebral disc(s); Low back pain.*
among industrial workers, 173
and scoliosis, low back pain with, 882–883
anterior extraperitoneal discectomy for, 987–988, 988(t), *988–994*, 995–996, 995(t)–996(t), *997*. See also *Discectomy, extraperitoneal, anterior.*
CT scanning of, 308–310, 309(t), *309–310*
principles of, 283–285, *284*
definitions of, 369
diagnosis of, evoked responses in, 148–150, *148–150*
disc composition changes from, 241
fusion for, rationale of, 195–196
natural history of, 397, 397(t)
neurologic deficit in, imaging of, 147–151, *148–150*
pain in, pathology and, 799
posterior microdiscectomy for, results of, 403–404, 403(t)–404(t)

Lumbar disc disease *(Continued)*
radiography of, vs facet arthrography, *114–118*, 115, 118
spinal instability in, nucleus pulposus herniation with, 414
spinal stenosis in, 17–18
surgery for, anterior approach in, 407, *408–413*, 409–414
complications of, nonsurgical approaches for, 21
treatment of, surgical vs nonsurgical, 23
Lumbar nerve, anatomy and physiology of, 450
imaging anatomy of, *274*, 277, *281*, 282
root sheath infiltration of, 120–121, *121–124*, 123–126, *126–127*, 128, *129–130*, 130–131
diagnostic value of, 124–125
in surgical planning, 962
indications for, 125–126, *126–127*, 128, *129–130*
technique of, 121, *121–124*, 123–124
therapeutic value of, *130*, 130–131
roots of, compression of. See *Nerve root(s), compression of.*
Lumbar spine, anatomy of, 77, *78*, 79, 662–663, *663*
backrests for, biomechanics of, *216*, 216–217
biomechanics of, facet joint in, 427
occupational factors in, 212–214, *213*, *215–223*, 216–219, 221–223
blood supply of, imaging of, 280, *281*
curvature of. See also *Scoliosis.*
surgery for, indications for, *886–888*, 886–889
Zielke instrumentation in, 890. See also *Zielke instrumentation.*
deformities of, in elderly patients, treatment of, 902–904
degeneration of, classification of, 190
imaging anatomy of, *280–281*
instability from, 190–191, *191*
phases of, 85–87, *86*
types of, 81, *82–85*, 83, 85
dysfunction of, cardiovascular evaluation in, 834
deconditioning syndrome in, 829–830
measurement of, design of, 829–830
principles of, 828–829
fixation of. See *Instrumentation.*
flexibility of, and industrial back pain, 852
fractures of, 662–698. See also *Fracture(s); Fracture(s)-dislocation(s).*
hyperextension of, athletics and, 174–175
imaging of, computer reconstruction in, 266
CT scanning vs MRI in, 266
in coronal plane, 280, *281–282*, 282
segmental image interpretation in, 266
infections of, 699–740. See also *Discitis; Infection(s), pyogenic; Tuberculosis.*
instability of. See *Segmental instability; Spinal instability.*
ligamentous attachments of, biomechanics of, 8–9
loading of, athletics and, risk factors in, 176–177
biomechanics of, and backrest inclination, 216–218, *216–218*
and spinal implants, 943–944

Lumbar spine *(Continued)*
experimental models of, 160–162, *161*, 161(t), 163(t), 164–166, *167*, 167(t), 168, 169(t), 170
disc degeneration in, biomechanics of, 190–191, *191*
injury mechanisms of, 212–214, *213*
lifting capacity in, 834–835
lifting strength in, and industrial back pain, 852
manual labor and, 218–219, *219–223*, 221–223
muscle contraction force calculations of, 161–162, 163(t)
comprehensive model in, 166, *167*, 167(t), 168, 169(t), 170
validity of models in, 162, 163(t), 164–166
musculoskeletal reaction to, 160–161, *161*, 161(t)
repetitive, athletics and, 174–175
biomechanical terms about, 172
disorders from, 172–177
load cycle of, 175–176
mechanical effects of, 177–180, *178*
voluntary, vs vibration, 171–172
vibration in, biomechanical terms about, 172
MRI of, 321–323, *321–323*
musculature of, anatomy of, 80
and spinal instability, 191
neural elements of, injury to, 449
range of motion of, and spinal instability, 192–193
biomechanical evaluations of, 198–201, *199–200*, 200(t)
after stabilization, 201–204, *202–204*
functional evaluation of, 830–832, *832*
in flexion-extension, and low back pain, 191–192
stabilization of, biomechanics of, 195–212, *198–200*, *202–205*, 205(t)–206(t), *208*
instrumentation in, biomechanical evaluations of, 196–201, *198–200*, 200(t)
orthoses in, 224–229
stenosis of, history of, 3
structures of, and low back pain, 370
surgery of, extrapleural-retroperitoneal approach to, 975
retroperitoneal approach to, 980–982, *982–983*
exposure in, *976*, 981–982, *982–983*
patient positioning in, *976*, 981
wound closure in, 982
transpleural-retroperitoneal approach to, *976–981*, 977–978, 980
patient positioning in, *976*, 977
thoracoabdominal exposure in, 977–978, *977–979*
vertebral exposure in, *979–980*, 980
wound closure in, 980, *981–982*
torsion of, 178–179
trunk muscles of, strength of, evaluation of, 832–834, *833–834*
measurement of, 859–861, 860(t), 862(t), 863–864, 864(t), *865–866*, 867. See also *Trunk muscles.*
tuberculosis of, 699–708, *700*, *702–705*, 707(t), *709–712*. See also *Tuberculosis, of spine.*

Lumbar spine *(Continued)*
tumors of, surgery for, transperitoneal approach to, 983–984, *984–986*, 986
vibration of, resonant frequency of, 182–184
Lumbosacral muscles, activity of, backrests and, *216*, 216–217
straining of, low back pain from, 213–214
orthoses for, 228
vibration of, response to, 183
Lumbosacral nerve, compression of, in cauda equina syndrome, 454
Lumbosacral plexus, anatomy and physiology of, 450
Lumbosacral space, lateral spinal stenosis of, 290
Lumbosacral spine, anatomy of, and orthosis use, 225
variations of, history of, and back pain, 3
degenerative disc disease of, internal fixation for, 949–950, *949–952*
extent of, 947
imaging of, anatomic differences in, 267, *274*
in axial plane, 267, *268–276*, 277
in sagittal plane, 277–278, *277–281*, 280
immobilization of, orthoses in, 691, 696
stabilization of, internal fixation for, 949, *952*
surgery of, indications for, 966, 966(t)
retroperitoneal approach to, 980–982, *982–983*
exposure in, *976*, 981–982, *982–983*
patient positioning in, *976*, 981
wound closure in, 982
transperitoneal approach to, 983–984, *984–986*, 986
complications of, 986
exposure in, 983–984, *984–986*
patient positioning in, 983
wound closure in, 984, 986
tuberculosis of, 708, *712*
Luque instrumentation, for scoliosis, 889–890
paralytic, 902
for spinal stabilization, biomechanical evaluations of, 197–201, *198–200*
for thoracolumbar spinal deformities, in elderly patients, 903–904
history of, 917, 919
posterior, biomechanical evaluation of, 945
sacral fusion with, lumbar lordosis loss from, 897
segmental fixation with, advantages of, 947
Lymphoma, of spine, 746, 750, 750(t)

Magnetic resonance imaging (MRI), advantages of, 320
in later spinal stenosis, 306
after fusion, 327, 329, *329–331*
axial myelographic contrast in, 322–323, *323*
clinical evaluation with, 323–324
of developmental idiopathic spinal stenosis, 562–563, *564*
of disc degeneration, 310
and clincial course, 1001
of disc herniation, accuracy of, 356
lateral, 296, *299*, 300
of fractures, 331, *332*, 677, *677*
Magnetic resonance imaging (MRI) *(Continued)*
of infection, 331, *333*
of low back pain, history of, 21–22
of lumbar disc disease, 324–325, *324–328*, 327
of lumbar spine anatomy, 321–323, *321–323*
in axial plane, 267, *268–276*, 277, 322–323, *323*
in coronal plane, 280, *281–282*, 282
in sagittal plane, 277–278, *277–281*, 321, *321–322*
in surgical planning, 961–962
of lumbar spine disorders, 320–325, *321–335*, 327, 329, 331, 333, 335–336. See also under specific disorder; e.g., *Intervertebral disc(s), herniation of.*
of metastatic tumors, 331, 333, *334–335*
of muscular rupture, 57
of septic discitis, 716–717
of soft tissue abnormalities, 318
of spinal stenosis, lateral, 307–308, *308*
preoperative, of nucleus pulposus herniation, 400, 401(t)
protocols in, 320–321
vs contrast-enhanced CT scanning, in postoperative evaluation, 316, *317*
Malnutrition, and vertebral canal development, 591
osteoporosis from, 763–764
Manipulation, for disc herniation, 387
of lumbar spine, automanipulation in, 807, *807*
benefits of, 800–802
contraindications to, 809
definition of, 806
history of, 792–793, 807
indications for, 808–809, *808–809*
limitations of, 809–810, *810*
mechanical basis of, 805–806
mechanical diagnoses in, 795–796
pain site in, 432
practitioners of, 793
purpose of, 807–808, *807–808*
techniques of, 806(t), 806–807
Massage, for disc herniation, 387
for lumbar spine disorders, 802
McGill Pain Questionnaire, on chronic low back pain, 817
Median nerve, compression of, experimental models of, 137
neuropathy from, 573
Menopause, bone loss after, 763. See also *Osteoporosis.*
Mensana Clinic Back Pain Test, of chronic low back pain, 817
Mesoderm, development of, 72, *72*
Methocarbamol, for muscle spasm, 362
Methylmethacrylate cement, for spinal stabilization, 753, *757*
Microdiscectomy, posterior, for lumbar disc disease, results of, 403–404, 403(t)–404(t)
Microsurgery, disc space identification in, 404, *405–406*
for nucleus pulposus herniation, complications of, 404–406, *405–407*, 407(t)
Micturition, neural reflexes of, 451, 451(t)
Minnesota Multiphasic Personality Inventory, in chronic low back pain management, 813–814, 817

Minnesota Multiphasic Personality Inventory *(Continued)*
in failed spinal surgery evaluation, 879
in industrial back pain prediction, 853–854
in low back pain management, 15–16
in surgical decision making, 876
Mithramycin, for spinal stenosis, 603
Morphine, continuous epidural perfusion of, for chronic pain control, 15
Morquio's disease, developmental spinal stenosis in, 559–560
Motion segment, as model of spinal dynamics, 80–81
biomechanics of, and orthoses, 225–227
degeneration of, 81, *82–85*, 83, 85
discal involvement in, 374–375
fusion for, vs nonoperative treatment, 373
imaging anatomy of, 278
low back pain from, pathoanatomic analysis of, 372–373
nerve root compression from, 280, *281*
fracture of, repetitive lumbar loading and, 177–178, *178*
immobility of, age and sex in, 623(t)
injury/stabilization of, biomechanical evaluations of, 198–201, *199–200*, 200(t)
analysis of, 204–207, *205*, 205(t)–206(t)
3–D finite element model of, 207–211, *208*
technique of, 201–204, *202–204*
instability of. See *Segmental instability; Spinal instability.*
lesions of, nonradicular pain from, 108, *108*
loading of, repetitive, in extension, 179
response to, 614, *616*
loss of stiffness of. See *Segmental instability; Spinal instability.*
mechanics of, in low back pain, 58–59
movement of. See also *Intervertebral motion.*
radiography of, and lumbar spinal disorders, 342–343
neuroanatomic definition of, 428–429, *428–429*
stress to, transpedicle fixation and, 998–1000, *999–1000*
torsion of, repetitive, disc injury from, 178–179
transitional syndrome in, 999
Motor vehicles, vibrations of, low back disorders from, 181
Myelitis, acute transverse, chemonucleolysis and, 445–446
Myelography, arachnoiditis from, 650
contrast material extravasation in, 352
intraoperative, in decompression, 689
iophendylate in, arachnoditis from, 316
of cauda equina syndrome, 454
of developmental idiopathic spinal stenosis, 560, 562, *562–563*
of disc herniation, in anterior extraperitoneal discectomy, *990*
of low back pain, history of, 21
of nucleus pulposus herniation, 347
of pain origin, reliability of, 341–342
of sciatica, indications for, 366
of scoliosis, 888–889
of vertebral canal, 18
preoperative, of nucleus pulposus herniation, 400
Myelography *(Continued)*
side effects of, 348, 351, 353
vs CT scanning, of disc herniation and spinal stenosis, 310–317, 312(t)–313(t), *316*
of lumbar disc disease, 346
with discography, of nucleus pulposus herniation, 346–353, 349(t)–351(t), *353–355*, 356
accuracy of, 349–353, 351(t)
radiographic diagnoses in, 348–349, 349(t)–350(t)
with CT scanning, of foraminal disc herniation, accuracy of, 352–353, *353*
Myofascial pain syndromes, patterns of, 93–94

Narcotics, in chronic low back pain therapy, 818
National Institute of Occupational Safety and Health (NIOSH), lifting guidelines of, 222–223, *223*
Neisseria gonorrhoeae, in reactive arthritis, 642, 642(t)
Nerve conduction, deficits of, evoked response testing of, 146(t), 148–150, *148–150*
studies of, during posterior reduction, 533, *536*
for peripheral entrapment neuropathy, 152
Nerve fibers, anatomy and physiology of, 132–134, *133–134*
Nerve root(s), anatomy and physiology of, 132–135, *133–134*
bony entrapment of, clinical presentation of, in surgical planning, 960, 960(t)
natural history of, conservative vs operative treatment in, 964, 964(t)
treatment of, 968–969, *969*
undercutting facetectomy for, 973
compression of, anatomy in, 141–142, *142*
and disc prolapse, 655(t)
and pain syndromes, 90
assessment of, 96
biomechanics of, 135–137, *136*
bony segmental anomalies in, 971
COMPRESSION mechanism in, *142–144*, 142–145
CSF perfusion after, 14–15
decompression for, 972
disc degeneration from, criteria of, 394
disc herniation and, 135–136, *136*
biomechanics of, 141–145, *142–144*
CT scanning of, 308–310, 309(t), *309–310*
discectomy for, 972–973
edema in, and spinal stenosis, 306–307, *307*
etiology of, 960, 960(t), 964(t)
functional changes from, 138–139, *139*
hemangioma and, 746
manipulation for, 810, *810*
nonradicular pain from, 109, *110*
nucleus pulposus herniation and, osteophytic spurring in, *394*, 395
osteophytic spurring and, 287, *288–290*
of uncinate process, *292*
pain mechanisms in, 137–138
posterior fusion for, 457

Nerve root(s) *(Continued)*
radicular pain from, disc herniation and, 382–383
radiography of, 971
spinal stenosis and, 595
surgery for, 973
surgery for, concepts of, 970, 971(t)
decompression technique in, 972
indications for, 366–367
patient positioning in, 971, *972*
preoperative planning in, 971–972
TENSION mechanism in, *142–144*, 142–145
treatment of, conservative, 971
conduction of, mechanical stimulation of, in pain control, 15
decompression of. See also *Decompression.*
in posterior reduction, 533, *535–536*
indications for, 966, 966(t)
displacement of, in disc herniation surgery, 402, *402*
dysfunction of, in axial rotational segmental instability, 630
entrapment of, diagnosis of, root sheath infiltration in. See *Lumbar nerve, root sheath infiltration of.*
in lumbar disc disease, 4
in root sheath infiltration, 124, *124*
in scoliosis, 883
in spinal stenosis, 285–286, *286*
history of, 551
pathogenesis of, 285–286, *286*
postoperative imaging of, *317*
fibrosis of, disc prolaspe and, 653, *654*
identification of, in root sheath infiltration, *123*, 123–124
imaging anatomy of, *271*, 278, *279–281*, 280, *281*
inflammation of, pathophysiology of, 138–139, *139*
injury to, disc prolapse and, pain response in, 649–650
during spinal surgery, 873–874, 873(t)–874(t)
irritation of, assessment of, 98, 99
causes of, 957
radicular pain from, *107*, 107–108
spinal deformity treatment and, 914
ischemia of, in spinal stenosis, 18
mechanical properties of, 135
motion of, and injury, 135
MRI of, 322
surgical anatomy of, 395, *396*
tension of, diagnosis of, in surgical planning, 958, *959*
vascular supply of, 134–135
Nerve root canal, anatomy of, 132, *133*
and nerve root compression, 141–145, *142–144*
compression of, osteophytic spurring in, *288–289*
of uncinate process, 293, *294–296*
identification of, 291, *292*
spinal stenosis from, far-out type, 304, *305*, 306
lateral, 290–291, *291–292*, *294*
definition of, 554–555, *555*
stenosis of, classification of, 596, 596(t), 601–602
3–D imaging of, 287, *289*
Nerve root canal *(Continued)*
definition of, 595–596
surgery for, *610*, 610–611
Nerve root ganglion, compression of, in dynamic spinal stenosis, 306, *307*
in lateral spinal stenosis, with lytic spondylolisthesis, 295–296, *298–299*, 300
osteophytic spurring in, of uncinate process, 293, *294–296*
edema of, in degenerative spondylolisthesis, *301*
Neural arch, development of, 73
repetitive loading of, 179–180
Neural plate, development of, 72, *72*
Neural tube, development of, 72, *73*
Neurogenic bowel disturbance, clinical neurophysiologic diagnosis of, 157
Neuropathy, entrapment type, electrodiagnosis of, 152
peripheral, anterior thigh pain and, 367
electrodiagnosis of, 152
vs radiculopathy, 152
Neurophysiology, clinical, of low back pain, 146(t)–147(t), 146–154, *148–150*, *153–156*, 156–159
of neurologic deficit, documentation of, 147–150, *148–150*
localization of, 151–154, *153–155*
severity of, 151
patient questions in, 146–147, 147(t)
tests in, 146, 146(t)
Neurosurgery, history of, 1
Nocardia, vertebral infection from, 721
Nociceptors, activation of, biomechanics of, 195
Nonmetallic flexible stabilization, in posterior fusion, 999–1000, *999–1000*
Notochord, development of, 71–72, *72*
intervertebral disc formation from, *76*
remnants of, malignant chordoma from, 73
Nuclectomy, percutaneous, for disc prolapse, results of, 967
MRI after, 329
Nucleus pulposus, anatomy of, 79, 246, *246*
biomechanical studies of, in low back pain, 5–6
circulation of, in low back pain, 10
collagen structure of, 9–10, 248
deterioration of, in disc degeneration, 261–262
granular invasion of, in discitis, *729*
herniation of. See also *Intervertebral disc(s), herniation of.*
acute radicular syndrome from, diagnosis of, 420, 420(t)
anatomic level of, 420, 420(t)
and postural deformity, 799
artifactual changes in, 397, *399*
characteristics of, 393–394
CT scanning of, vs myelography and discography, 346–353, 349(t)–351(t), *353–355*, 356
discography of, vs CT scanning and myelography, 346–353, 349(t)–351(t), *353–355*, 356
foraminal, 414, *416–417*
in adolescents, 414
in discitis, 725, *727–728*
in spinal stenosis, 414
instability with, 414

Nucleus pulposus *(Continued)*
microsurgery for, complications of, 404–406, 407(t)
posterior discectomy in, results of, 403–404, 403(t)–404(t)
myelography of, 346
vs CT scanning and discography, 346–353, 349(t)–351(t), *353–355*, 356
natural history of, conservative vs operative treatment in, 963–964
recurrent, 419, *419*
sciatica in, recurrent, surgery for, 399–400, 400(t)
signs and symptoms of, nonorganic causes in, 420, 420(t)
spondylolisthesis with, 414, *418–419*
staging of, 395, 397, *398–399*
surgery for, contraindications to, 400, 400(t)
indications for, 399–400, 400(t)
kneeling position in, 401, *402*, 402(t)
nerve root displacement in, 402, *402*
options in, 401
posterior approach to, 401–406, *402–403*, 402(t)–404(t), *405–407*, 407(t)
preoperative imaging in, 400–401, *401*, 401(t)
scar formation in, 402–403, *403*
techniques of, 401–414, *402–403*, 402(t)–404(t), *405–413*, 407(t)
treatment of, conservative, failure of, 399
results of, 397, 397(t)
imaging anatomy of, 267, *268*, *272*
MRI of, 321, *321*
oxygen tension gradients of, and fusion, *256*

Occupations, industrial, disc disease from, 173
low back pain from, disability from, 854
etiology of, 847
injury mechanisms in, 212–214, *213*
management of, 869–870
perceptions of, and claim-filing process, 847–849
prevention of, 855
risk factors of, 846–850, 849(t), 851(t), 852–859, *853*
prospective studies of, 850, 851(t), *853*, 853–854
retrospective studies of, 849(t), 849–850
screening for, 846–847
treatment of, 869–870
vs back injury claims, 847
work factors in, 859
repetitive lumbar loading in, load cycle of, 175–176
low back pain from, 91–92
biomechanics of, 212–214, *213*, *215–223*, 216–219, 221–223
frequency of, 160
manual material handling in, biomechanics of, 218–219, *219–223*, 221–223
preference for, among scoliotic patients, 882
repetitive lumbar loading in, 170–171
Ocular lesions, in reactive arthritis, 643
Oophorectomy, bone loss after, 763
Orgasm, neural reflexes of, 451(t), 451–452
Orthopedics, history of, 1
Orthosis(es), for disc herniation, 387
for low back pain, in pregnancy, 844
for scoliosis, 886
for spinal fractures, 691, 696
for spinal stenosis, 603–604
lumbosacral, 224–229
biomechanical effects of, 225–227
clinical applications of, 227–229
history of, 225
negative effects of, 229
Ossification, of vertebrae, 75, *76*
Osteoarthritis, of vertebral arch, in developmental idiopathic spinal stenosis, 570
Osteoblastoma, of spine, 743, *745*
Osteoblasts, in bone formation, 761
Osteochondroma, of spine, 743, *747*
Osteoma, osteoid, of spine, 743, *745*, 746
scoliosis with, treatment of, 746, *749*
Osteomalacia, scoliosis from, 882
Osteomyelitis, vertebral, 721
MRI of, 331, *333*
nomenclature of, 739
Osteopenia, vs osteoporosis, 760
Osteopetrosis, pathologic spondylolisthesis from, 484, *485*
Osteophytosis, in facet joint, 425
in segmental instability, 618, *619*
in spinal stenosis, 287, *288–290*
developmental, 559
lateral, 290–291, *294*
Osteoporosis, 760–769, *764–765*
compression fractures in, 763–765, *764–765*
definition of, 760–761
idiopathic, definition of, 761
in Zielke instrumentation, 890–892
involutional, bone resorption from, in posterior fusion, 457
definition of, 761
natural history of, 760
physiology of, 763
postmenopausal, and scoliosis progression, 886
fractures from, 763
radiography of, 766–767
scoliosis from, 882
senile, definition of, 761
systemic disease and, 763–764
treatment of, 767–768
Osteosarcoma, of spine, 746, 750, 750(t)
Osteotomy, in lumbar lordosis restoration, 904–907, *905–909*
Oswestry Disability Questionnaire, 91
Oxycodone hydrochloride, addiction to, and low back pain, 365
Oxygen, concentrations of, in intervertebral disc, 251–252, *252*
after fusion, 255, *255*

Paget's disease, bone resorption from, in posterior fusion, 457
calcitonin for, 603
spinal stenosis in, classification of, 579
Pain. See also *Low back pain.*
chronic, management of, neurologic studies in, 15
placebos in, 15

Pain *(Continued)*
clinical neurophysiologic diagnosis of, 157
conceptual models of, 44–45, *45*
control of, exercise in, 65
neurologic studies of, 13–16
cross-over, 98
description of, physical and psychologic aspects in, 46–48, *47*, 47(t)
discogenic, orthoses for, 228
types of, 102, 102(t)
gate control theory of, 45
and chronic low back pain, 811
and spinal manipulation, 806
mechanisms of, 90
neurologic studies of, 13–16
neurologic modulation of, 56, *57*
nonradicular, definition of, 108, *108*
diagnosis of, facet arthrography for, *114*, 115, *116–118*, 118
synonyms for, 108(t)
vs radicular, 108–109, *110*, 111
origin of, in disc herniation, 383
radiography of, reliability of, 341–342
patterns of, low back pain syndromes and, 93–94
radicular, definition of, *107*, 107–108
disc herniation and, 382–383
nerve root inflammation in, 138
synonyms for, 108(t)
vs nonradicular, 108–109, *110*, 111
referred, 93
and sclerotomes, 112, *112*
assessment of, 97–98
from facet joint, 423
from spinal structures, vs nerve root pain, 13–14
vs nerve root pain, in disc herniation, 383
Pain Drawing Test, of chronic low back pain, 817
Para-aminosalicylic acid, for spinal tuberculosis, 706
Paracetamol, for disc herniation, 386–387
Paralysis, in scoliosis, treatment of, 902
Paraparesis, polyostotic metastatic breast cancer and, surgery for, 753, *757*
Paraplegia, chemonucleolysis and, 445–446
in pyogenic spondylitis, 718
septic discitis and, 716
spinal tuberculosis and, 700–701
Paraspinal muscles, imaging anatomy of, *268*
Parasympathetic nervous system, anatomy and physiology of, 450
Parathyroid hormone, and calcium metabolism, 762
Paresis, chemonucleolysis and, 445
Pars interarticularis, anatomy of, in posterior fusion, 459, *460*
cleaning of, in posterior fusion, 460, *462*
elongation of, in congenital spondylolisthesis, 476
in isthmic spondylolisthesis, 472, *473–475*, 480, *481*, 592
fracture of, in congenital spondylolisthesis, *477*
in isthmic spondylolisthesis, *479*, 479–482, *481*
natural history of, 487
repetitive lumbar loading and, 174–175
stress, athletics and, 482
treatment of, 495, *495*, 497
Pars interarticularis *(Continued)*
fusion of, in spondylolisthesis, 497
sclerosis of, in spondylolisthesis, *517*
Pedicle(s), defects of, in axial rotational segmental instability, 630, *630*
fixation of, in spinal instrumentation. See *Transpedicle fixation.*
mediolateral width of, in spinal fixation, *920*, 920–921, 921(t)
Pelvic-visceral function, anatomy and physiology of, 450
impairment of, cauda equina syndrome and, 454. See also *Cauda equina syndrome.*
Penile tumescence, measurement of, 156–157
Pericarditis, in ankylosing spondylitis, 641
Perineurium, innervation of, 133–134, *134*
Peripheral joint disease, in ankylosing spondylitis, 639
Peripheral nerve, anatomy of, 132, *133*
compression of, experimental models of, 137
neural fibers of, 133–134, *134*
Personality, and chronic low back pain, 814–815
Phenobarbital, for low back pain, 362
Phenothiazines, for chronic low back pain, 818–819
Phenylbutazone, for ankylosing spondylitis, 641–642
Physiotherapy, end-range motion in, and pain patterns, 795–796, *797*
exercise in, 802–803. See also *Back school; Exercise.*
for derangement syndrome, 798–800, 803–804
for disc herniation, 387
for dysfunction syndrome, 798, 803
for postural syndrome, 796, 798, 803
for scoliosis, 885–886
for spinal stenosis, 603
manipulation in, 793, 800–802
massage in, 802
mechanical diagnoses in, 794–796
traction in, 802
Plantar flexion, assessment of, 96
Plasmacytoma, of spine, 746, 750, 750(t)
Polymethylmethacrylate, in transpedicle fixation, 929
Posterior arch, fracture of, 671, *675*
Posterior joint, degeneration of, 81, *82*
Posterior joint syndrome, 83
Posture, correction of, kinesitherapy in, for spondylolisthesis, 504, 507–508, *507–509*
orthoses in, 227
deformity of, in spondyloptosis, *518*
during lifting, biomechanics of, 219, *219–221*, 221
during pushing and pulling, biomechanics of, 223
low back pain from, 796, 798–800
occupational, biomechanics of, 214, *215–218*, 216–218
recumbent, biomechanics of, 218
sitting, biomechanics of, 214, 216–218, *216–218*
standing, biomechanics of, 214, *215*
Pott's disease. See *Tuberculosis, of spine.*
Pregnancy, low back pain in, 840–845, *841–842*

Pregnancy *(Continued)*
clinical presentation of, *841*, 841–842
epidemiology of, 840
pathogenesis of, 842–843
physical examination for, 843
prevention of, 844–845
treatment of, 843–844
Prostaglandins, in chronic pain, 15
Prostate, metastatic carcinoma of, MRI of, 331, *334*
Proteoglycans, cartilaginous structure of, 234–235, *235*
concentration of, and disc loading, disc hydration from, 239, *240*
and pore size distribution, 236–238, *237*
degenerative changes in, animal models of, 263–264
disc hydration by, 235–236, 238–239, *239*
in disc loading, 248–249
molecular system of, 246–247, *247*
osmotic pressure of, 236, *237*
reduction of, aging and, 371
synthesis of, 241–242
and exercise, 254–255
Pseudarthrosis, lumbar lordosis loss with, 905
repair of, in spondylolisthesis, 520–521
results of, 877, 877(t)
Pseudomeningocele, MRI of, 329, *330*
Pseudospondylolisthesis, age and sex in, 623(t)
in segmental instability, 618
Pseudostenosis, definition of, 596
Psoas muscle, imaging anatomy of, *270*
Psychiatric evaluation, of chronic low back pain, 817–818
Psychodynamic factors, and chronic low back pain, 813–814
and repeat spinal surgery failure, 875–878, 876(t)–877(t)
Psychologic assessment, of low back pain, 15–16, 365
chronic, psychogenic vs organic basis of, 816–817
of spinal surgery failure, 879
Psychotherapy, psychodynamic, for chronic low back pain, 823
Pudendal nerve, lesions of, electrodiagnosis of, 153, *153*
Pulling, low back pain from, 223
Pulmonary disease, in ankylosing spondylitis, 641
Pulmonary embolism, spinal deformity treatment and, 914–915
Pushing, low back pain from, 223
Pyrazinamide, for spinal tuberculosis, 702, 706

Quadriplegia, chemonucleolysis and, 446

Radiation therapy, marrow replacement in, MRI of, 333
of spinal tumors, 750(t), 750–751
Radicular vein, MRI of, *322*
Radiculitis, classification of, 650
Radiculography, of lumbar spine, in surgical planning, 961, *962*
Radiculopathy, clinical neurophysiologic diagnosis of, 148–150, *148–150*
documentation of, clinical neurophysiology in, 147
electrodiagnosis of, 151–152
in developmental idiopathic spinal stenosis, intermittent neurogenic claudication with, 572–575, 573(t)–574(t)
vs peripheral neuropathies, 152
Radiography, advances in, in low back pain diagnosis, 21–23
clinical uses of, 338
diagnostic capability of, 343
dynamic, difficulties of, 343
of bone mineral loss, 340
of disc degeneration, reliability of, 340–341
of failed spinal surgery, 879
of lumbar spine disorders, reliability of, 337–345, *339*
of pain origin, reliability of, 341–342
of spinal motion, and pain symptoms, 342–343
in spinal instability diagnosis, 191–192
reliability of, 338–339, *339*
of vertebral shape, reliability of, 338
reliability of, definitions in, 337
technique of, 337–338
Radionuclide imaging, of osteoporosis, 766
of pyogenic spondylitis, 715
of spinal tumors, 742
Range of motion, evaluation of, 830–832, *832*
Rectum, examination of, in low back pain, 100
Reduction, of spondylolisthesis, in adults, 531–534, *532–539*, 536–537, 539
in children and adolescents, *524*, 524–525, *526*
with spondyloptosis, in children and adolescents, 520
Reflex(es), diminished, disc herniation and, 385
Reflex sympathetic dystrophy, thermography of, 157
Rehabilitation, back school in, 770–792. See also *Back school.*
education in, 770–771
exercise in. See also *Exercise.*
principles of, 771–772
stabilization training in, 772, *773–778*, 776, 779, *780–786*
Reiter's syndrome, ankylosing spondylosis with, 646–647
reactive arthritis in, 642(t), 642–643
Relaxation, techniques of, for chronic low back pain, 821
Renal function, impairment of, bone resorption from, in posterior fusion, 457
in ankylosing spondylitis, 642
Respiratory function, assessment of, in scoliosis, 884
Retrolisthesis, in degenerative spondylolisthesis, *84*
Retrovertebral plexus, MRI of, 322
Rhizotomy, denervation by, 433
repetition of, results of, 875–878, 876(t)–877(t)
Rib, embryology of, 73, *76*

Rib hump, assessment of, 884
excision of, 901–902
Rifampicin, for spinal tuberculosis, 702, 706

Sacral artery, anatomy of, in posterior fusion, 459–460, *460*
Sacral nerve, anatomy and physiology of, 450
compression of, bladder dysfunction from, 453
entrapment of, electrodiagnosis of, 153, *153*
imaging anatomy of, *275–276*
injury to, urologic dysfunction from, 452
sensory conduction testing of, for spinal cord lesions, 153, *154*
Sacroiliac joint, assessment of, 97–98
dysfunction of, 793–794
exercise and, 174
low back pain from, 89
imaging anatomy of, *275–276*
mechanical defects of, low back and leg pain from, 3–5
pain in, pregnancy and, 841, *842*
radiography of, in ankylosing spondylitis, 638–639, 639(t)
Sacroiliitis, Crohn's disease in, 646
in ankylosing spondylitis, 638–639, 638(t)–639(t)
in psoriatic spondyloarthropathy, 644
Sacrum, fixation of, screw placement in, 923, 924(t)
fusion of, for scoliosis, 897–899
imaging anatomy of, *275–276*, 277, 282, *282*
opening of, in congenital spondylolisthesis, 476, *477*
tumors of, surgery for, transperitoneal approach to, 983–984, *984–986*, 986
Sarcoma, clear cell, surgery for, 753, *756*
Ewing's, of spine, 746, 750, 750(t)
Scheuermann's kyphosis, Kostuik-Harrington instrumentation for, 908–909, 911, *912*
Sciatic nerve, irritation of, assessment of, 98
lesions of, clinical neurophysiologic diagnosis of, *149*
Sciatica, "burned-out" spinal stenosis with, 302
cauda equina syndrome in, 453
diagnosis of, 59, 60(t)
differential diagnosis of, 400(t)
disc herniation and, 370
nerve root compression mechanisms in, 141–145, *142–144*
pain in, 382–383
patient age in, *143–144*, 143–145
treatment of, results of, 397
discectomy for, results of, 872–873, 873(t)
epidural injections for, history of, 14
etiology of, 132–140, *133–134*, *136*, *139*
history of, 393, 393(t)
facet joint osteoarthrosis and, 957
history of, 1–2
low back pain with, anterior extraperitoneal discectomy for, 988, *990–993*
disability from, 854
treatment of, 365–366
lytic spondylolisthesis with, lateral spinal stenosis in, 296, *299*, 300
Sciatica *(Continued)*
nucleus pulposus herniation and, radicular syndrome in, 395, 395(t)
pain location in, *395*
prevalence of, in low back pain, *32*, 32–33
recurrent, in nucleus pulposus herniation, surgery for, 399–400, 400(t)
spontaneous resolution of, biomechanical mechanisms of, 144–145
surgery for, indications for, 966, 966(t)
treatment of, chemonucleolysis in, 19–21
conservative, 965–966
diagnostic basis of, 61, 62(t)–63(t)
Scintigraphy, with technetium, of sacroiliac joint disease, 4
Sclerotome(s), definition of, *111–112*, 112
development of, 72–73, *73–76*
Scoliosis, compensatory curve with, surgery for, 887–888, *888*
curvature progression in, assessment of, 884
definition of, 882
deformities from, treatment of, 900–909, *905–914*, 911, 913
cosmesis in, 900–902
in elderly patients, 902–904
degenerative, progressive, segmental instability in, 631
disc composition changes from, 241
epidemiology of, 882–883
evaluation of, 883–885
in osteoporosis, 765
in spinal tuberculosis, 701, *704*
internal fixation for, 950–951
osteoid osteoma in, treatment of, 746, *749*
pain in, assessment of, 889
curvature correlation with, 882–883
paralytic, treatment of, 902
radiography of, 885
rophlectoric, stretching exercises for, 502, *503*
spondylolisthesis with, treatment of, 521
surgery for, fusion extensions after, 899–900, *899–902*
indications for, *886–888*, 886–889
instrumentation in, degenerative changes after, 887
morbidity and mortality of, 913–915
techniques of, 889–900, *890–902*
Zielke instrumentation in, *888*, 889–895, *892–896*. See also *Zielke instrumentation.*
treatment of, age in, 883
conservative, 885–886
prognosis of, curvature degree and, 883
Seatbelt injury, 668, *669*, 670–671, *674*, *676–677*
treatment of, 680, *686–688*, 689
Segmental artery, development of, 73, *75*
imaging anatomy of, 267
Segmental instability. See also *Spinal instability.*
abnormal motion in, radiography of, 620, 623, *624–627*, 625, 626(t), 627
biomechanical analysis of, 625, *626*, 626(t)
center of movement in, 623, *625*
in flexion and extension, 623, *624*
acquired spondylolisthesis in, after fusion, 634
after decompression, *632*, 632–633

Segmental instability *(Continued)*
after discectomy, 629(t), 632
after fusion, 629(t), *633*, 633–634
and spinal tumors, 751–752
animal models of, 616–617, *617*
axial rotational, 629(t), 629–630, *630*
biomechanics of, 612–614, *613–617*, 616–617
classification of, 629(t), 629–634, *630–633*
cyclic loading in, experimental models of, 613–614, *614–615*
definitions of, 617–618
conceptual models of, 612–613, *613*
diagnosis of, clinical approach to, 628–629
immobilization in, 627
pain responses to, *627*, 627–628
spinal loading in, 627
disc disruption in, 629(t), 631
disc space narrowing and, 618
in low back pain, radiography of, 342–343, 363–364
surgery for, 364
pathology of, 612
primary, 629(t), 629–632, *630–631*
pseudarthrosis in, after fusion, 629(t), 634
radiography of, 342–343, 618–620, *619–622*, 623, 623(t), *624–627*, 625, 626(t), 627
biplanar motion, 625, 627, *627*
retrolisthetic, 629(t), 631
scoliosis in, progressive degenerative, 629(t), 631
secondary, 629(t), *632–633*, 632–634
spinal malalignment in, 618–619, *620–622*, 623(t)
static loading in, 613
theory of, 628
traction spurs in, 618, *619*
translational, 629(t), 630–631, *631*
vertebral body position in, 619–620, *624*
Segmental nerve, development of, 73, *76*
Seizures, chemonucleolysis and, 446
Selspot II system, for spinal stabilization evaluation, 201–204, *202–204*
Sensory nerves, stimulation of, in radiculopathy detection, 150, *150*
Serotonin, depletion of, and chronic low back pain, 819
Sexual function, and sympathectomy, 452
impairment of, clinical neurophysiologic diagnosis of, *154–156*, 156–157
neural reflexes of, 451(t), 451–452
Sexually transmitted diseases, reactive arthritis from, 642(t), 642–643
Shear injury, 670, *672–674*
Shigella flexneri, in reactive arthritis, 642, 642(t)
Sinuvertebral nerve, anatomy of, 79–80
Smoking, and disc nutrition, 256–258, *257*
and low back pain, 256, 658
in industry, 853, *853*
cessation of, before posterior fusion, 457
Soft tissue, abnormalities of, in degenerative spondylolisthesis, 300, 302
MRI of, 318
Somatoform disorders, chronic low back pain with, 813–814
Somatosensory evoked response testing, during spinal surgery, 154, 156
of neurologic deficits, *149*, 149–150
Somatosensory evoked response testing *(Continued)*
of spinal cord lesions, 153–154, *154–155*
Somites, development of, 72, *73*
Spina bifida, spondylolisthesis with, *592*, 592–593
congenital, 480
natural history of, 487
Spina bifida occulta, congenital spondylolisthesis with, 473, 476–477, *476–477*
Spinal canal. See *Vertebral canal.*
Spinal column, anatomy of, 75, 77, *78*, 79
formation of, *75–76*
imaging anatomy of, 277, *278*
instability of. See *Segmental instability*; *Spinal instability.*
Spinal cord, compression of, in ankylosing spondylitis, 641
in osteoporosis, 765
polyostotic metastatic breast cancer and, surgery for, 753, *757*
stenotic, 557
with dorsolumbar stenosis, 559
lesions of, electrodiagnosis of, 153–154, *154–155*
ultrasonography of, *679*
Spinal dysraphism, with congenital spinal stenosis, 558
Spinal instability. See also *Segmental instability.*
after anterior extraperitoneal discectomy, 993, *994*, 995
and spinal tumors, 751–752
bilateral laminectomy and, 607, *608*
biomechanics of, 8–9
causes of, 188–191, *189–191*
definition of, 188
degenerative spondylolisthesis from, 482–484, *483*
diagnosis of, 191–193
fractures and, orthoses for, 691, 696
kyphosis with, treatment of, 905–906, *906–907*
low back pain with, 58–59, 188–193, *189–191*, 383
radiography of, 191–192
posterior fusion for, 457
three-column model of, *663*, 663–664, 664(t)
trauma and, *663*, 663–664, 664(t)
treatment of, 193
Spinal ligament, injury to, spinal instability from, 189, *189*
Spinal muscles, stretching exercises for, dynamic, for spondylolisthesis, 504, *506–507*
for spondylolisthesis, 502, *503–504*
Spinal nerve, anatomy of, 79, 132, *133*
compression of, in spinal stenosis, 285
distribution of, 13
irritation of, sciatica from, 5
lesions of, radicular pain from, *107*, 107–108
response of, to mechanical stress, 14–15
swelling of, in spinal stenosis, CT scanning of, 306–307, *307*
vascular supply of, 134–135
Spinal stenosis. See also entries under *Stenosis*; *Vertebral canal.*
absolute, significance of, *561*, 570–572, *571*
vs relative, taxonomy of, 580
acquired, classification of, 577–579, 581

Spinal stenosis *(Continued)*
treatment of, results of, 969–970
after fusion, *633*, 633–634
classification of, 597, 601
"burned-out" type, CT scanning of, 302
cauda equina syndrome from, 453
caudal nerve root size in, and degree of stenosis, 572–575
central, 285–286, *286*
CT scanning of, vs myelography, 312, 312(t)–313(t)
degenerative spondylolisthesis and, 300, *301*
classification of, 287, 547, 596(t), 596–597, *598–602*, 601–603
principles of, limits to, 551–552
types of, 557–558
combined, classification of, 578–579, 596(t), 601, *601–602*
congenital, classification of, 581, 596(t), 597, *598*
pathomorphology of, 558
decompression for. See also *Decompression*.
foraminal, 581, *582–583*, 584
operative planning of, 605–606
segmental instability after, *632*, 633
spondylolisthesis after, 484
technique of, 973
definition of, 594–596
etymology in, 552–554
problems in, 554–556, *555*
degenerative, classification of, 601
developmental, classification of, 596(t), 597, *599*
of bony lumbar vertebral canal (DSBLVC), 557
classification of, 558
idiopathic, 560
areas of, 575–576, *576*
caudal nerve root vulnerability and, 574
classification of, 596(t), 597
compressive agents in, 576
3-D CT scanning of, 563, 565, *565–567*
etiology of, 576–577
ligamentum flavum hypertrophy in, 579–580
midsagittal diameter in, and disease extent, 575–576, *576*
measurement of, 565–568, *568–570*
MRI of, 562–563, *564*
posterior longitudinal ligament hypertrophy in, 579–580
radiculopathy in, 572–575, 573(t)–574(t)
radiodiagnostic features of, 560, *561–570*, 562–563, 565–568
skeletal growth errors and, 558–560
taxonomy of, 581
diagnosis of, 59
disc herniation with, 595
CT scanning of, vs myelography, 310–317, 312(t)–313(t), *316*
patient age in, 143, *144*
dynamic, CT scanning of, 306, *307*
fibrinolytic activity defects in, 656–658, *657*, *659*
fusion for, indications for, 607
historical review of, 547–551, *550*

Spinal stenosis *(Continued)*
iatrogenic, classification of, 579
in fluorosis, classification of, 579
in Paget's disease, classification of, 579
intermittent neurogenic claudication in, 572–575, 573(t)–574(t)
lumbar lordosis and, 572, 574–575
lateral, causes of, 287, 290
CT scanning of, 285–287, *286*, *288–290*, 290
vs myelography, 312–313, 312(t)–313(t)
3-D imaging of, 284–285
far-out type, classification of, 578
CT scanning of, 304, *305*, 306
front-back type, causes of, *288–289*
pinhole stenosis with, CT scanning of, 302, *303–304*
Kirkaldy-Willis type, *291*
segmental instability with, retrolisthetic, 629(t), 631
spondylolisthesis and, degenerative, 300, *301*
lytic, CT scanning of, 295–296, *298–299*, 300
structures affected by, 287, 290
"tram-track" spurring in, vs uncinate spurring, *297*
up-down type, causes of, *288–289*
CT scanning of, *288–289*, 290–291, *291–292*, 293, *294–295*, 295
uncinate spurring in, 290–291, *291–292*, 293, *294–295*, 295
low back and leg pain from, 17–18
mixed, classification of, 596(t), 601
narrow lateral gutter in, definition of, 557
narrow lateral recess in, definition of, 557
natural history of, conservative vs operative treatment in, 964–965, *965*
nerve root compression from, clinical presentation of, in surgical planning, 960, 960(t)
neural swelling in, CT scanning of, 306–307, *307*
neurovascular dysfunction with, 18–19
nomenclature of, history of, 548–549
nucleus pulposus herniation with, 414
orthoses for, 227, 228–229
pain types in, 102, 102(t)
pathogenesis of, 285–287
pathomorphology of, definitions in, 546–547
spatial nature of, 546
post-traumatic, classification of, 579
primary, classification of, 596, 596(t), *598–599*
pseudostenosis in, definition of, 596
radicular syndrome in, 573–574, 573(t)–574(t)
surgical indications for, 604
relative, significance of, 568–570, 574(t)
vs absolute, taxonomy of, 580
risk factors of, vertebral shape in, 338
secondary, classification of, 597, *600*, 601
degenerative spondylolisthesis in, 597, *600*
spondylolisthesis in, classification of, 579
degenerative, surgery for, 607, *609*, 610
surgery for, 604–607, *608–610*, 610–611
contraindications to, 604
indications for, 367, 604

Spinal stenosis *(Continued)*
taxonomy of, 580–581
nomenclature in, 580
three-joint complex degeneration and, 83, *83–85*
treatment of, conservative, 603–604
drug therapy in, 603
orthoses in, 603–604
physiotherapy in, 603
results of, 581, *582–583*, 584–585, 584(t)–585(t)
types of, postoperative disturbances in, 584–585, 585(t)
preoperative disturbances in, 584, 584(t)
vertebral canal size in, measurement of, history of, 548–549, *550*
midsagittal diameter in, and degree of stenosis, 572–573
and relative stenosis, 568–570, 574(t)
vs disc herniation, 594–596
Spinal surgery. See also specific procedure or organ; e.g., *Fusion*; *Intervertebral disc(s), herniation of, surgery for.*
activity after, 783
anterior approaches in, 975–997
diagnostic criteria for, 957–958, 957(t)–958(t), *959*, 960(t)–961(t), 960–963, *962*
electrodiagnositic monitoring during, 154, *156*, 156–157
failure of, 21, 46
causes of, 877
lateral spinal stenosis and, 307
lumbar nerve root sheath infiltration after, 121, 128
management of, 879–880
patient approach in, 878–879
prevention of, imaging in, 318
rates of, 872
initial, results of, 872–873, 873(t)
limited approaches in, 956
psychologic factors in, 876
repetition of, criteria for, 877
patient selection in, 878–879
procedure selection in, 877, 877(t), 878
results of, 875–878, 876(t)–877(t)
success factors in, 878
results of, 17, 43, 43(t)
retained debris after, arachnoiditis from, 650–651, 651(t)
scar tissue after, reduced spinal mobility from, 798
spondylolisthesis after, 484
unnecessary, 358, 360
Spine, anatomic arrangement of, vs spondylolisthetic condition, *534*
assessment of, in low back pain, 95–96, 97
curvature of. See also *Scoliosis.*
and intervertebral disc variations, 9
and pain, 882
radiographic measurement of, 338
vertebral canal narrowing from, 548
deformities of, in elderly patients, treatment of, 902–904
treatment of, morbidity and mortality in, 913–915
fractures of. See *Fracture(s).*
ligamentous attachments of, 79
loading of, kyphosis from, 907–908, *910*
malalignment of, in segmental instability, 618–619, *620–622*, 623(t)
Spine *(Continued)*
tuberculosis and, 701, *704–705*
mechanics of, intervertebral disc in, 246, *246*
motion of, measurement of, radiographic, reliability of, 338–339, *339–340*
surface techniques in, 339–340
radiography of, and pain symptoms, 342–343
studies of, results of, 343
motion segment of. See *Motion segment.*
three-joint complex of. See *Three-joint complex.*
tumors of. See entries under *Tumor(s).*
vascular supply of, imaging anatomy of, *272*
Spinous process(es), fixation of, history of, 916–917
flexion-distraction injuries of, 668, *669*
imaging anatomy of, *278*
synostosis of, with congenital spinal stenosis, 558
Spondylitis, ankylosing, 637–642, 638(t)–639(t)
diagnostic criteria for, 638, 638(t)
enthesopathies in, 639–640
epidemiology of, 641
etiology of, 641
morning stiffness from, 93
pathology of, 637–638
peripheral joint disease in, 639
prevalence of, 641
prognosis of, 641
radiography of, 638–639, 639(t)
sex distribution of, 641
systemic disease in, 640–641
treatment of, 641–642
ulcerative colitis in, 646
Crohn's disease in, 646
in psoriatic spondyloarthropathy, 644–645
pyogenic, 708, 711, *713–714*, 715
laboratory studies of, 708, 711
radiography of, 711, *713–714*, 715
surgery for, 718, *719*, 720
treatment of, conservative, 717–718
Whipple's disease in, 646
Spondyloarthropathy, inflammatory, 637–649, 638(t)–639(t), 642(t), 644(t)
definition of, 637
etiology of, 646–647
genetic factors in, 647
history of, 637
inflammatory bowel disease in, 646
pathogenesis of, 647
psoriatic, 644(t), 644–646
bone resorption in, 645
clinical presentation of, 644, 644(t)
extra-articular involvement in, 645
laboratory findings in, 645
sacroilitis in, 644
spondylitis in, 644–645
treatment of, 645–646
Spondylolisthesis, acquired, after fusion, 634
and spina bifida, *592*, 592–593
athletics and, 174–175
body contour in, 493, 495
classification of, *472–475*, 473
controversy in, 493, *494–496*, 495, 497–498
retrodisplacement in, 497

Spondylolisthesis *(Continued)*
congenital, *472*, 473, 476–477, *476–478*, 479
etiology of, 480–482
inheritance factors in, 480(t), 482
natural history of, 484, 486–487
clinical studies of, 486–487
surgery for, 491, *491*
treatment of, conservative, 487
vs isthmic, 493, 497
definitions of, 471, 472
degenerative, 473, 482–484, *483*
CT scanning of, *286*, 300, *301*, 302
decompression for, segmental instability after, 629(t), 632–633
facet joint degeneration in, 118, *119–210*, 120
fusion for, *496*, 497
in adults, biomechanics of, 540
clinical presentation of, 540
decompression for, fusion with, 540, 542–543
history of, 539–540
radiography of, 540
treatment of, 540, *541*, 542–543
conservative, 540
natural history of, 488
pathophysiology of, 1001, *1001*
segmental instability from, 619, *620–622*, 623(t)
translational, 629(t), 630–631, *631*
spinal stenosis with, classification of, *576*, 578
developmental idiopathic, 3–D CT scanning of, *565–567*
secondary, 597, *600*
surgery for, 607, *609*, 610
three-joint complex degeneration and, 83, *84*
treatment of, conservative, results of, 513, *514*, 515
vertebral body position in, 619–620, *624*
diagnosis of, spinal loading in, 627
discectomy for, anterior, interbody fusion with, 407, *408–413*, 409–414
dysplastic, treatment of, conservative, results of, 512–513, *513*
hamstring tightness in, fusion for, 493, *494–495*
in adults, decompression for, 530–531
fusion for, 530–531
lumbosacral kyphosis in, 529, *529*
pars interarticularis repair in, 531
reduction of, cast technique of, 532–533, *532–534*
rationale for, 531–532
surgical, anterior approach in, 534
combined approaches in, 534, 536–538, *537–539*
indications for, 537, 539, *539*
neurologic complications from, 537
posterior approaches in, 533, *535–536*
sagittal plane alignment in, 529, *529*
surgery for, clinical presentation in, 529, *529*
considerations in, 529–530
indications for, 530
in children and adolescents, after prior fusion, 521
fusion for, 517, 519

Spondylolisthesis *(Continued)*
anterior, 519–520
decompression with, 524
failure of, repair of, 520–521
guidelines for, 522(t), 522–523, *523*
posterior, 520
posterolateral, *525*, 525–526
iatrogenic, 521–522
kyphotic deformity reduction in, 523
reduction of, 520
pedicle screw fixation in, *524*, 524–526
risk factors of, 516
surgery for, 515–517, *517–518*, 519–527, 522(t), *523–525*
guidelines for, 522, 522(t)
indications for, 516–517, *517–518*
isthmic defect repair in, 519–520
options in, 515–517, 519–521
postoperative care in, 521
procedure selection in, 522(t), 522–525, *523–524*
instrumentation for, 495
history of, 916–920, *918*
internal fixation for, 950
isthmic, 473, *473–475*, *479*, 479–480, 480(t)
etiology of, 480–482
inheritance factors in, 480, 480(t), 482
natural history of, 484, 486–487
pseudostenosis in, 596
surgery for, 488, *488–490*, 491
treatment of, conservative, 487
results of, 510, 512, *512*
vertebral displacement in, 592–593, *592–593*
vs congenital, 493, 497
controversy in, 493, *494–496*, 495, 497
lumbosacral, surgery for, transperitoneal approach to, 983–984, *984–986*, 986
lytic, and lateral spinal stenosis, CT scanning of, 295–296, *298–299*, 300
nucleus pulposus herniation with, 401, *401*, 414, *418–419*
orthoses for, 227, 228
pain types in, 102, 102(t)
pars interarticularis fusion in, 497
pathologic, 473, 484
postsurgical, 473, 484
post-traumatic, 473, *475*, 484
reversed, in spinal tuberculosis, 701, *704*
scoliosis with, treatment of, 521
signs and symptoms of, 500
slippage calculation in, Meschanes method of, 510, *510*
spa treatment for, 508–509
spinal stenosis in, classification of, 579
surgery for, decompression in, 493
pedicle screw fixation in, 491, *492–493*
treatment of, autotraction in, 502, *502*, 504
bed rest in, 501, *501*
conservative, 500–502, *501–510*, 504, 507–510, 509(t), 511(t)–512(t), 512–513, *512–514*, 515
goals of, 500
results of, 509(t), 509–510, *510*, 511(t)–512(t), 512–513, *512–514*, 515
exercise in, 501–502, *503–504*, 504, *506–507*
kinesitherapy in, 504, 507–508, *507–509*
pelvic traction in, 501–502, *502*, 504, *504*

Spondylolisthesis *(Continued)*
physical therapy in, 501
types of, 473, 476–477, *476–479*, 479–484, 480(t), *481*, *483*
Spondylolysis, anterior discectomy for, interbody fusion with, 407, *408–413*, 409–414
athletics and, 177
in adults, surgery for, 531
inheritance factors in, 480, 480(t)
orthoses for, 227–228
repetitive lumbar loading and, 172–175
Spondyloptosis, in children and adolescents, fusion for, 523–524
reduction of, 520
Spondylosis, ankylosing, etiology of, 646–647
degenerative, spinal stenosis in, 286, *286*
fibrinolytic activity defects in, 656–658, *657*, 657(t), *659*
pathogenesis of, 285–287
pathologic studies of, 651, 653, *653–655*, 655, 655(t)
St. Thomas' Questionnaire, 91
Stabilization training, for low back pain, 772, *773–778*, 776, 779, *780–786*
Steffee plates, for spinal stabilization, biomechanical evaluations of, 198, *198*, 200–201
interbody bone grafts with, biomechanical evaluations of, 204–207, *205*, 205(t)–206(t)
Stenosimetry, vertebral canal diameter measurements with, 549, *550*
Stenosis. See also entries under *Spinal stenosis*; *Vertebral canal.*
combined, of vertebral canal, classification of, 601, *601–602*
compressive, definition of, 556–557
developmental, 548
fibrous, pseudostenosis in, 596
idiopathic, 549
mixed, of vertebral canal, classification of, 601
of intervertebral foramen, classification of, 596(t), 603
of vertebral canal, classification of, 596(t), 596–597, *598–602*, 601
pin-hole type, CT scanning of, *304*
primary, of vertebral canal, classification of, 596, 596(t), *598–599*
secondary, of vertebral canal, classification of, 597, *600*, 601
transport, definition of, 556
Stereophotogrammetry, of spinal stabilization, 201
Straight-leg raising, after anterior extraperitoneal discectomy, 988, *992*
in disc herniation diagnosis, 383–384
in surgical planning, 958, *959*
Streptomycin, for spinal tuberculosis, 702, *706*
Stress, interpersonal, and chronic low back pain, 815
Stromer's law, 71
Subarachnoid space, imaging anatomy of, *278*
Subarticular recess, stenosis of, 285, *286*, *291*
CT scanning of, 309, *310*
vs myelography, 312, 312(t)–313(t)
degenerative spondylolisthesis and, 300, *301*
Subluxation, dorsolumbar, in spinal tuberculosis, 701, *704*
with kyphosis, in pyogenic spondylitis, 711, *715*
Supraspinous ligament, imaging anatomy of, 277
Sympathectomy, lumbar, and sexual function, 452
Sympathetic nervous system, anatomy and physiology of, 450
Symphysiolysis, in pregnancy, 843
Syndesmophyte, in ankylosing spondylitis, 638, 638(t)
Synovial cells, synthetic activity of, anti-inflammatory drugs in, 12
Synthes instrumentation, posterior, biomechanical evaluation of, 945
Syphilis, pathologic spondylolisthesis from, 484

Technetium, imaging with, of pyogenic spondylitis, 715
Thecal sac, constriction of, in degenerative spondylolisthesis, 300, *301*
degenerative changes in, imaging of, 267
imaging anatomy of, 267, *269*, *272*, *278*
MRI of, 322
in degenerative disc disease, 325, 327, *328*
Thermography, of lumbar spine, in surgical planning, 963
of spinal pain, 157
Thermotherapy, for disc herniation, 387
Thigh pain, anterior, diagnosis of, 367
posterior, diagnosis of, 367–368
Thoracic cavity, closure of, in transpleural-retroperitoneal approach, 980, *981*
transection of, in retroperitoneal approach, 982, *982–983*
in transperitoneal approach, 984, *985*
in transpleural-retroperitoneal approach, 978, *978–979*
Thoracic spine, curvature of, and low back pain, 882–883
deformities of, in elderly patients, treatment of, 902–904
scoliotic, 900
treatment of, cosmesis in, 900–902
Thoracolumbar spine, curvature of, surgery for, indications for, *886–888*, 886–889
Zielke instrumentation in, 890. See also *Zielke instrumentation.*
deformities of, in elderly patients, treatment of, 902–904
fractures of, transpedicle fixation of, 949, *951*
scoliotic deformities of, 900
surgery of, extrapleural-retroperitoneal approach to, 975
transpleural-retroperitoneal approach to, *976–981*, 977–978, 980
patient positioning in, *976*, 977
thoracoabdominal exposure in, 977–978, *977–979*
vertebral exposure in, *979–980*, 980
wound closure in, 980, *981–982*

Three-joint complex, definition of, 81
degenerative changes in, 81, *82–85*, 83, 85
dysfunction phase of, 85–86, *86*
instability phase of, 86, *86*
pain from, 86–87
stabilization phase of, *86*, 86–87
treatment of, 87
pathoanatomic changes in, 370–371
Traction, for disc herniation, 387
for lumbar spine disorders, 802
Trampoline, lumbar disc disease from, 174
Transpedicle fixation, AO internal fixators in, for burst fractures, 680, *684*
history of, 918
biomechanical testing of, 932–934, 933(t)
development of, 916–920, *918*
fatigue strength of, 931
for burst fractures, 680, *682–685*
for lumbosacral disc degeneration, 949, *950*
for thoracolumbar spine fractures, 949, *951*
future trends in, 952, 998–1000, *999–1000*
implant removal in, 934–935
internal/external fixators in, history of, 919–920
morphometry in, *920*, 920–921, 921(t)
positional adjustability in, 929–930
positional control in, 930
posterior, results of, 948
postoperative management in, 934, 935(t)
reduction with, 931–932
screw design in, 921–922
screw implants in, history of, 918–919
screw placement in, 922–929, *923–927*, 924(t), 928(t)
depth of, 925–927, *926–927*
entry site and orientation of, 922–929, *923–925*, 924(t)
hole preparation for, 927–929, 928(t)
longitudinal linkage between, 929–932
polymethylmethacrylate in, 929
screw strength in, screw depth and, 926–927, *926–927*
segmental instrumentation with, advantages of, 947, *947*
stiffness in, 930–931
transverse connectors in, 932
Transverse foramen, formation of, 73
Transverse process, anatomy of, 77, *78*
cleaning of, in posterior fusion, 463, *464–465*
formation of, 73
fusion of, 456. See also *Fusion, posterior.*
technique of, 459–460, *460–468*, 463, 466
identification of, in posterior fusion, 460, *462–463*
imaging anatomy of, *270*
length of, and segmental instability, 619, *624*
vascular supply of, anatomy of, in posterior fusion, 459, *460*
Trauma, burst fractures from, 664, 666
Chance fracture from, 668, *669*, 670
spondylolisthesis from, 473, *475*, 484
to vertebral body, MRI of, 331, *332*
Trunk muscles, endurance of, measurement of, 861, 862(t), 863, *865–866*
measurement of, definitions in, 860, 860(t)
strength of, correlation of, with endurance, 864, 864(t), 867
Trunk muscles *(Continued)*
measurement of, 861, 862(t), 863
Tuberculosis, of spine, 699–708, *700*, *702–705*, 707(t), *709–712*
abscesses in, 702
chemotherapy for, 702, 706
clinical presentation of, 699–700
distribution of, 699, *700*
paraplegia in, 700–701
radiography of, 701–702, *703–705*
spinal malalignments in, 701, *704–705*
surgery for, 706–708, 707(t), *709–712*
vs hemivertebra, 701, *704*
Tumor(s), conus, myelography of, vs CT scanning, 315
giant cell, 743, *748*
of bone, pathologic spondylolisthesis from, 484
of lumbosacral spine, surgery for, transperitoneal approach to, 983–984, *984–986*, 986
of spine, anatomic staging of, and surgical planning, *752*, 752–753
and spinal instability, 751–752
benign, 743, *745–749*, 746, 746(t)
diagnostic approach to, *742*
incidence of, 741
laminectomy for, spondylolisthesis after, 521–522
malignant, 746, 746(t), 750, 750(t)
metastatic, 750–751
MRI of, 331, 333, *334–335*
primary, clinical presentation of, 741–742, 741(t)–742(t), *742–743*
location of, 743, *744*
radiography of, 742–743
surgery for, anatomic extent in, 753, 753(t), *754–757*
symptoms of, diurnal pain in, 93
of vertebral canal, pseudostenosis in, 596
retroperitoneal, anterior thigh pain and, 367
segmental instability from, 629(t)

Ulcerative colitis, ankylosing spondylitis in, 646
peripheral arthritis in, 646
Ultrasonography, intraoperative, in burst fracture treatment, 680
in decompression, 689, *694–695*
of spinal fractures, 677, *678–679*
burst, *692*
Uncinate process, osteophytic spurring of, lateral spinal stenosis from, 290–291, *291–292*, *294*
location of, *291–292*, *294–296*, 295
Ureaplasma urealyticum, in reactive arthritis, 642, 642(t)
Urethra, proximal, electrostimulation of, in spinal cord lesion diagnosis, 154, *155*
Urethritis, reactive arthritis from, 643
Urinary retention, in cauda equina syndrome, 453
Urination, neural reflexes of, 451, 451(t)
Urodynamic studies, of cauda equina syndrome, 454
Urologic function, assessment of, in spinal fracture, 674
Uveitis, in ankylosing spondylitis, 641

Venous plexus, compression of, disc prolapse and, 653, *653–654*
imaging anatomy of, 267, *269–272*, *274*, *278*
Vermont Spinal Fixateur, for translational segmental instability, 631, *631*
Vertebra(e), anatomy of, 75, 77, *78*, 79
embryology of, 71–73, *72–76*, 75
fractures of, mechanical stress and, 176
loading of, burst fractures from, 664, 666
failure from, 662
repetitive, 179–180
fatigue fractures from, 177–178, *178*
lumbar, formation of, 73, *76*
shape of, radiographic measurement of, reliability of, 338
symmetric destruction of, in pyogenic spondylitis, 711, *713*
Vertebral arch(es), anatomy of, 77, *78*
growth disturbance of, spinal stenosis from, 548
developmental, 558
pathology of, and midsagittal diameter, 570
Vertebral body(ies), aging of, and lateral spinal stenosis, 293, 295
anatomy of, 77, *78*, 246, *246*, 662–663
biopsy of, in osteoporosis diagnosis, 767
bone mineral content of, in disc degeneration, 8
development of, 72–73, *75–76*
disc herniation into, in discitis, 724, 728, *728*
enlargement of, spinal stenosis from, *85*
erosion of, discitis and, 734, 736, *736*
failure of, cyclic loading and, 613
fractures of, orthoses for, 228
imaging anatomy of, *268–270*, *274*, 277, *277–278*, *280*
infections of, surgery for, extrapleural-retroperitoneal approach to, 975
metastatic carcinoma to, 750
osteophytosis of, nerve root canal stenosis from, 602
position of, and segmental instability, 619–620, *624*
surgery of, retroperitoneal approach to, 980–982, *982–983*
transperitoneal approach to, 983–984, *984–986*, 986
transpleural-retroperitoneal approach to, *976–981*, 977–978, 980
surgical anatomy of, 395, *396–397*
trauma to, MRI of, 331, *332*
tuberculosis of, radiography of, 701, *703*
ultrasonography of, *679*
uncinate spurring of, *292*
Vertebral canal, achondroplastic stenosis of, 548–549
bony intrusion of, burst fractures and, 666, *667*
cervical, stenosis of, in developmental idiopathic spinal stenosis, 577
components of, and low back disorders, 590
compressive stenosis of, 556
3–D CT scanning of, 563, 565, *565–567*
development of, 590–591
imaging anatomy of, *269*, *271–272*, 277, *277–278*, *280*
loss of volume of, and cauda equina syndrome, 454
Vertebral canal *(Continued)*
maldevelopment of, malnutrition and, CNS and immune deficiencies from, 593
maturity of, 590, *591*
measurement of, imaging techniques for, 18
midsagittal diameter of, and bony maturity, 590
measurement of, and relative stenosis, 568–570, 574(t)
and spinal stenosis, 595
CT scanning in, 565–568, *568–570*
disease extent and, in developmental idiopathic spinal stenosis, 575–576, *576*
history of, 549, *550*
in combined spinal stenosis, 601, *601–602*
narrowing of. See also *Spinal stenosis.*
congenital, 17
history of, 547–548
neurovascular anatomy of, dysfunction of, in spinal stenosis, 18–19
pressure measurements of, in spinal stenosis, 19
residual bone in, after fracture, *692–693*
size of, and contents volume, 591–592
and low back disorders, 589, *590*
and neural compression, 595
in low back pain, 17–18
stenosis of. See also *Spinal stenosis.*
classification of, 596(t), 596–597, *598–602*, 601
MRI of, 325, 327, *328*
surgical anatomy of, 395, *397*
trefoil shape of, and low back pain, 589, *590*
in developmental idiopathic spinal stenosis, 570–572, *571*
Vibration, and disc nutrition, 258
biomechanical studies of, human response in, 182–184
low back disorders from, 180–184
Video display terminals, and postural disorders, 218
Visceral efferent nerve, anatomy and physiology of, 450
Vitamin D, and calcium metabolism, 762
supplementation of, for osteoporosis, 768
Vitamin deficiencies, spina bifida occulta from, 592

Walking, neurovascular compromise from, and intermittent neurogenic claudication, 572–573
in spinal stenosis, 18, 88–89
Weight lifting, lumbar disc disease from, 173
Whipple's disease, peripheral arthritis in, 646

Yersinia, in reactive arthritis, 642, 642(t)
Yolk sac, development of, 71, *72*

Zielke instrumentation, for scoliosis, *888*, 889–895, *892–896*
age limits in, 892, *892–893*

Zielke instrumentation *(Continued)*
compensatory curves in, results of, *888*, 894–895
disc degeneration with, complications of, 894
fusion extension in, 899–900, *899–902*
lordosis maintanence in, 886–887, *886–887*
osteoporosis in, 890–892
results of, 893, *895–896*
sacral fusion with, 892
for thoracolumbar spinal deformities, in elderly patients, 903–904
sacral fusion with, 898
segmental instrumentation with, advantages of, 947
Zygapophyseal joint, asymmetry of, degenerative spondylosis from, 285
degeneration of, degenerative spondylolisthesis from, *301*
spinal stenosis from, 285–286